SEVENTH EDITION

CARDIAC NURSING

The Red Reference Book for Cardiac Nurses

SEVENTH EDITION

CARDIAC NURSING

The Red Reference Book for Cardiac Nurses

Elizabeth M. Perpetua, DNP, ACNP-BC, ANP-BC, AACC

Founder, Empath Health Services LLC
Adjunct Professor, Seattle Pacific University
Seattle, Washington

Patricia A. Keegan, DNP, NP-C, AACC

Director, Strategic and Programmatic Initiatives, Emory Heart and Vascular
Lead Nurse Practitioner, Structural Heart and Valve Center
Emory Healthcare
Atlanta, Georgia

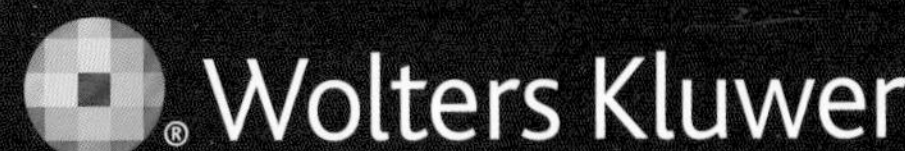

Philadelphia • Baltimore • New York • London
Buenos Aires • Hong Kong • Sydney • Tokyo

Acquisitions Editors: Nicole Dernoski and Michael Kerns
Development Editor: Maria M. McAvey
Editorial Coordinator: Ashley Pfeiffer
Production Project Manager: Barton Dudlick
Design Coordinator: Elaine Kasmer
Manufacturing Coordinator: Kathleen Brown
Marketing Manager: Linda Wetmore
Prepress Vendor: Aptara, Inc.

7th edition

9 8 7 6 5 4 3 2 1

Printed in China

978-1-9751-0632-4
Library of Congress Cataloging-in-Publication Data
available upon request

Library of Congress Control Number: 2020914253

DISCLAIMER

Care has been taken to confirm the accuracy of the information present and to describe generally accepted practices. **Case studies and case based learning examples are fictitious, including names, and are provided for teaching purposes only.** The authors, editors, and publisher are not responsible for errors or omissions or for any consequences from application of the information in this book and make no warranty, expressed or implied, with respect to the currency, completeness, or accuracy of the contents of the publication. Application of this information in a particular situation remains the professional responsibility of the practitioner; the clinical treatments described and recommended may not be considered absolute and universal recommendations.

The authors, editors, and publisher have exerted every effort to ensure that drug selection and dosage set forth in this text are in accordance with the current recommendations and practice at the time of publication. However, in view of ongoing research, changes in government regulations, and the constant flow of information relating to drug therapy and drug reactions, the reader is urged to check the package insert for each drug for any change in indications and dosage and for added warnings and precautions. This is particularly important when the recommended agent is a new or infrequently employed drug.

Some drugs and medical devices presented in this publication have Food and Drug Administration (FDA) clearance for limited use in restricted research settings. It is the responsibility of the health care provider to ascertain the FDA status of each drug or device planned for use in their clinical practice.

shop.lww.com

CCS1020

DEDICATION

To my parents, Gabriel and Josie; my sons, Carlos (Mucho) and Mateo, and their Papa Carlos; my grandparents; and everyone who has taught and uplifts my grateful heart

—Liz

To my loves, Gary, Kathryn, and Andrew; My parents, sister, nieces and nephews; and to the best tribe that inspires me on a daily basis

—Tricia

This book is dedicated to all of the nurses who will use this text on and off-the-job, as we did, to care for their patients

—EMP and TK

ACKNOWLEDGMENTS

"The true alchemists do not change lead into gold; they change the world into words."

—William H. Gass

We would like to acknowledge the community that has given voice to Cardiac Nursing and inspired the 7th edition.

The founding editors of *Cardiac Nursing*, Dr. Susan L. Woods, Dr. Erika S. Sivrajan Froelicher, Dr. Sandra L. Underhill Motzer, Dr. C. Jean Halpenny, and Dr. Elizabeth J. Bridges for advancing the knowledge and skills of generations of cardiac nurses.

Our contributors for devoting their time and expertise to continue this legacy—this edition is possible because of all of you.

Nicole Dernoski, Acquisitions Editor; Michael Kerns, Acquisitions Editor; and the Acquisitions Team at Wolters Kluwer for your belief and commitment to the Red Book and its impact on nurses.

Ashley Pfeiffer, Editorial Coordinator; Maria McAvey, Development Editor; Barton Dudlick, Production Project Manager, Indu Jawwad and the Wolters Kluwer Development Team for your tireless dedication and collaboration—all the way to the finish line.

Cardiac Nurses for making our patients' lives and the world better, everyday.

All nurses and healthcare workers who choose to lift each other up—let us rise the tide, together.

ABOUT THE EDITORS

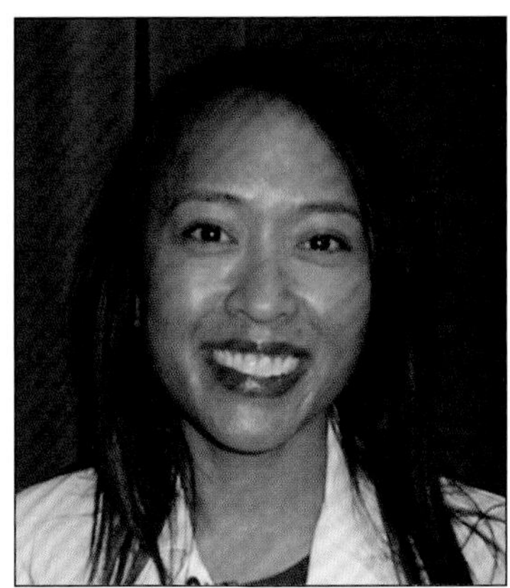

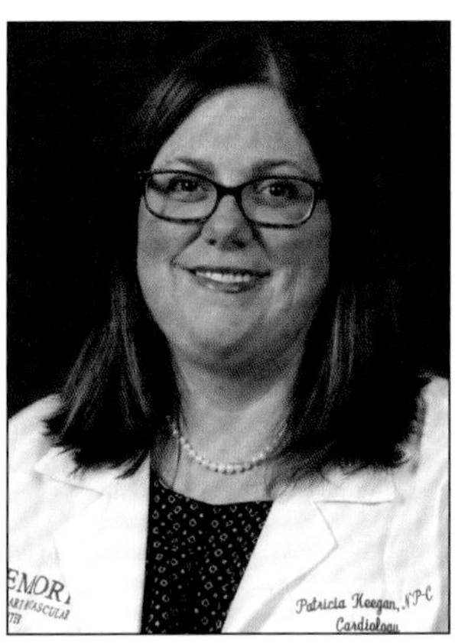

Elizabeth M. Perpetua, DNP, ACNP-BC, ANP-BC, AACC

Liz is a first-generation Filipina-American and second-generation Registered Nurse, inspired to come into the profession by her mother, Josephine, and her aunt, Lourdes. Liz has been a cardiac nurse since 2002. Liz received the Master of Nursing degree in 2008 and Doctor of Nursing Practice degree in 2009 from the University of Washington. She is a board certified adult and acute care nurse practitioner.

Her passions are education, innovation, and advancement in the profession of nursing. Her career focus has been the patient journey, multidisciplinary team care, and systems of care for structural and valvular heart disease. Liz has been an investigator for multiple cardiology clinical trials and has served in faculty and leadership roles in hospitals and academic medical centers. As faculty for Seattle Pacific University Doctor of Nursing Practice program, she teaches professional role identity and leadership, population health, and practice inquiry. Liz is an Associate Editor on the Editorial Board for *Structural Heart: The Journal of the Heart Team,* the peer-reviewed journal of her specialty. She is an Associate of the American College of Cardiology (ACC) and a founding member of the ACC Cardiovascular Team Section's Structural Heart Team Workgroup. Liz also founded Empath Health Services LLC, which provides consulting and cloud-based software solutions to heart and vascular programs.

Liz loves being with her two sons, Carlos and Mateo, and spending time with family and friends. She enjoys traveling, singing, reading, writing, playing games, nature walking, and mushroom foraging.

Patricia A. Keegan, DNP, NP-C, AACC

Tricia is a second career nurse, proving it is never too late to find your passion. As a child, her love of nursing was fostered by her desire to be Dixie McCall on *Emergency*. Her command of the situation, knowledge, and team work was an inspiration to become involved in nursing. Tricia has been a cardiac nurse for 15 years. She received her Masters in Nursing in 2010 from the University of Alabama, Birmingham, and Doctor of Nursing Practice in 2016 from University of South Alabama.

Her journey in cardiology began as a telemetry nurse at Emory Healthcare in Atlanta, GA. She worked on a unit staffed by nurses who loved to share their gifts of compassion and knowledge. This fostered her desire to continue learning and improving care of patients with cardiac disease. She became involved with the Structural Heart Center and worked with the team to implement practice improvements for this patient population. She participated in clinical trials as well as writing publications. Her work included implementation of Nurse Led Sedation and the minimalist pathway. She is very involved in the American College of Cardiology (ACC), including the Cardiovascular Team Section and the Society of Thoracic Surgeons/ACC Transcatheter Valve Therapies Research and Publications Committee. Her passion is working to improve education and outreach related to cardiac disease.

Tricia is married to Gary, and has two children, Kathryn and Andrew. She enjoys traveling to Disney, relaxing at the lake, and spending time with friends and family. She also notes that she loves her home state of New Jersey.

PREFACE TO THE 7TH EDITION

Thanks to the leadership of our predecessors, *Cardiac Nursing* is the reference book for nurses caring for patients who have or are at risk for developing cardiac disease. We aim to provide comprehensive, evidence-based content relevant to the cardiac nurse at all practice levels ranging from novice to expert. We believe that this edition highlights cardiac nurses' knowledge and skills in our many roles and practice settings, and that all stand to benefit from the content in this edition.

ABOUT THIS EDITION

Major changes in cardiac nursing and cardiology have occurred since the 6th edition of *Cardiac Nursing* was published. Revising this iconic book was therefore an exhilarating albeit formidable undertaking. We were inspired by the wisdom of the previous editors and contributors, and the current collective of authors recognized by our peers as experts in the field, actively practicing and shaping their specialties. As with prior editions, we anchor this work with the Scope and Standards for Cardiovascular Nursing, classic and landmark research, and the most recent evidence and guidelines.

A new chapter structure was created to cultivate the cardiac nurse's mental model of the content and its application. Each chapter is framed by objectives and critical questions to focus the reading. Full-color images, guideline-directed protocols, and easy-to-reference tables are incorporated to emphasize important concepts. Authors curated their best practice key resources, which are displayed prior to each chapter's respective reference list. To facilitate the development of critical thinking and decision-making skills, the clinician authorship synthesized personal experience with current evidence and guidelines to write case studies and case-based learning examples rich with real-world questions and practice challenges. This scaffolding aims to enhance the cardiac nurse's application of textbook knowledge to clinical practice.

Content was added, updated, and organized to incorporate over a decade of practice change. We begin the text with a chapter on evidence-based practice, which provides the language necessary to understand and implement this book and the science of our discipline. The subsequent parts are (1) fundamentals of cardiac nursing, (2) evaluation of the heart and heart disease, (3) risk assessment and prevention of heart disease, (4) pathophysiology and management of heart disease, and (5) expanded roles for the cardiac nurse. Of note, there are new chapters in each part, including women and heart disease; palliative care in cardiology; quality, economics, and policy in cardiovascular care; and advanced practice cardiac nursing. The text concludes with a chapter on leadership and team-based care, reflecting the philosophy that all cardiac nurses must be prepared as leaders and collaborators with the knowledge and skills necessary to provide and guide care across the lifespan.

Change is inevitable, challenging, and exciting. We hope you find that the 7th edition lives up to the standard of excellence of the past six editions, and that it becomes your primary reference source for cardiac nursing.

Elizabeth M. Perpetua, DNP, ACNP-BC, ANP-BC, AACC
Patricia A. Keegan, DNP, NP-C, AACC

STANDARDS OF PRACTICE[1]

STANDARD 1. ASSESSMENT

The cardiovascular registered nurse collects comprehensive data pertinent to the patient's health or the situation.

STANDARD 2. DIAGNOSIS

The cardiovascular registered nurse analyzes the assessment data to determine the nursing diagnoses or the issues.

STANDARD 3. OUTCOMES IDENTIFICATION

The cardiovascular registered nurse identifies expected outcomes for a plan individualized to the patient or the situation.

STANDARD 4. PLANNING

The cardiovascular registered nurse develops a plan that prescribes strategies and alternatives to attain expected outcomes.

STANDARD 5. IMPLEMENTATION

The cardiovascular registered nurse implements the identified plan.

STANDARD 5A: COORDINATION OF CARE

The cardiovascular registered nurse coordinates care delivery.

STANDARD 5B: HEALTH TEACHING AND HEALTH PROMOTION

The cardiovascular registered nurse employs strategies to promote health and a safe environment.

STANDARD 5C: CONSULTATION

The advanced practice registered nurse (APRN) provides consultation to influence the identified plan, enhance the abilities of others, and effect change.

STANDARD 5D: PRESCRIPTIVE AUTHORITY AND TREATMENT

The advanced practice registered nurse uses prescriptive authority, procedures, referrals, treatments, and therapies based on education, certification, credentialing, and APRN scope of practice in accordance with state and federal laws and regulations.

STANDARD 6. EVALUATION

The cardiovascular registered nurse evaluates progress toward attainment of outcomes.

STANDARD 7. ETHICS

The cardiovascular registered nurse practices ethically.

STANDARD 8. EDUCATION

The cardiovascular registered nurse attains knowledge and competence that reflects current nursing practice.

STANDARD 9. EVIDENCE-BASED PRACTICE AND RESEARCH

The cardiovascular registered nurse integrates evidence and research findings into practice.

STANDARD 10. QUALITY OF PRACTICE

The cardiovascular registered nurse contributes to quality nursing practice.

STANDARD 11. COMMUNICATION

The cardiovascular registered nurse communicates effectively in a variety of formats in all areas of practice.

STANDARD 12. LEADERSHIP

The cardiovascular registered nurse demonstrates leadership in the practice setting and the profession.

STANDARD 13. COLLABORATION

The cardiovascular registered nurse collaborates with patient, family, and others in the conduct of nursing practice.

STANDARD 14. PROFESSIONAL PRACTICE EVALUATION

The cardiovascular registered nurse evaluates her or his own nursing practice in relation to professional practice standards and guidelines, relevant statutes, rules and regulations.

STANDARD 15. RESOURCE UTILIZATION

The cardiovascular registered nurse utilizes appropriate resources to plan and provide nursing services that are safe, effective, and financially responsible.

STANDARD 16. ENVIRONMENTAL HEALTH

The cardiovascular registered nurse practices in an environmentally safe and healthy manner.

REFERENCE

1. American Nurses Association. *Cardiovascular nursing: Scope and standards of practice* (2nd ed). 2015, American Nurses Association: Silver Spring, MD.

PREVIOUS EDITION CONTRIBUTORS

Sushama D. Acharya, MS
Gaylene Altman, PhD, RN
Bradley E. Aouizerat, PhD, MAS
Kathleen A. Berra, MSN, ANP, FAHA, FPCNA, FAAN
Susan Blancher, MN, ARNP
Jean Marie Blue Verrier, MN, ARNP
Eleanor F. Bond, PhD, RN, FAAN
Lora E. Burke, PhD, MPH, FAHA, FAAN
Robert L. Burr, MSEE, PhD
Mary M. Canobbio, MN, RN, FAAN
Peter J. Cawley, MD
Michael A. Chen, MD, PhD
Susanna G. Cunningham, BScN, MA, PhD
Michaelene Hargrove Deelstra, MSN, ARNP
Cheryl R. Dennison, PhD, ANP
Sandra B. Dunbar, DSN, RN, FAAN, FAHA
Joan M. Fair, PhD, ANP
Linda Felver, PhD, RN
Polly E. Gardner, MN, ACNP, ARNP, FAHA
Rebecca A. Gary, PhD, RN
Donna Gerity, MN, RN
Mark Hawk, MSN, ACNP
Nancy Houston Miller, BSN, RN
Jon S. Huseby, MD
Carol Jacobson, MN, RN
M. Kaye Kramer, DrPH, MPH, BSN, CCRC
Shannon M. Latta, MN, RN
Denise LeDoux, MN, ARNP
Barbara S. Levine, PhD, CRNP, CS
Helen Luikart, MS, RN
Simone K. Madan, PhD
Kirsten Martin, BSN, MS, RN
Diana E. McMillan, PhD, RN
Margaret M. McNeill, PhD, RN, CCRN, CCNS, NE-BC
Philip Moons, PhD, RN
Nancy Munro, MN, CCRN, ACNP
Jonathan Myers, PhD
Katherine M. Newton, PhD, RN
Kathy P. Parker, PhD, RN, FAAN
Susan L. Reed, MN, CCRN, ARNP
Joseph O. Schmelz, PhD, RN, CIP, FAAN
Kawkab Shishani, PhD
Min Sohn, PhD, ACNP
Laurie A. Soine, PhD, ARNP, ACNP
Beverly Dyck Thomassian, MPH, RN, BC-ADM, CDE
Patricia K. Tuite, MSN, RN, CCRN
Melanie Warziski Turk, PhD, RN
Kyeongra Yang, PhD, MPH, RN

CONTRIBUTORS

Kelley M. Anderson, PhD, FNP, CHFN-K
Associate Professor
Georgetown University
School of Nursing and Health Studies
Department of Professional Nursing Practice
Washington, DC

Reiko Asano, PhD, RN
Postdoctoral Fellow
Georgetown University
School of Nursing and Health Studies
Washington, DC

Kathy Lee Bishop, PT, DPT, CCS, FNAP
Board-Certified Cardiovascular and Pulmonary Clinical Specialist
Program Manager, Emory St. Joseph's Cardiac Rehabilitation Program
Program Director, Emory Acute Care Residency Program
Assistant Professor, Emory University School of Medicine
Interim Assistant Director of Clinical Education, Doctor of Physical Therapy Program
Atlanta, Georgia

Russell Brandwein, MS, PA-C, AACC
Director, Outpatient Services, Structural Heart and Valve Center
Chief Physician Assistant
New York Presbyterian/Columbia University Medical Center
New York, New York

Kyle Briggs, PA-C
Adjunct Professor
Master of Physician Assistant Studies
Rocky Mountain College
Billings, MT
Physician Assistant
Emory University Hospital
Atlanta, GA

Julie Bumgardner, MSN, NP-C
Nurse Practitioner
Department of Vascular Surgery
Emory Healthcare
Atlanta, Georgia

Sarah E. Clarke, DNP, ACNP-BC
Nurse Practitioner
La Jolla, California

Sarah R. Coffey, MS, ARNP
Nurse Practitioner
Mayo Clinic
Rochester, Minnesota

Yvonne Commodore-Mensah, PhD, MHS, RN, FAHA, FPCNA
Assistant Professor
School of Nursing
Johns Hopkins University
Baltimore, Maryland

Beth Davidson, DNP, ACNP-BC, CCRN, CHFN
President, American Association of Heart Failure Nurses
Director, Heart Failure Disease Management Program
HCA TriStar Centennial Heart and Vascular
Nashville, Tennessee

Anna Dean, MSN, APRN, ACNS-BC
Nurse Practitioner
Emory Healthcare
Atlanta, Georgia

Nicole Dellise, DNP, FNP-BC, CHFN
Advanced Heart Failure Nurse Practitioner
Vanderbilt Heart and Vascular Institute
Instructor of Nursing
Vanderbilt University School of Nursing
Nashville, Tennessee

Adam M. Diesi, BSN, RN, CCRN
MSN/DNP Candidate, AGACNP Program
University of Colorado Anschutz Medical Campus
Aurora, Colorado

Laurie Beth DiMaggio, MSN, RN, APRN-C
Nurse Practitioner
Northside Hospital, HCA
Structural Heart and Valve Clinic
St. Petersburg, Florida

Sandra B. Dunbar, RN, PhD, FAAN, FAHA, FPCNA
Charles Howard Candler Professor
Senior Associate Dean for Academic Advancement
Nell Hodgson Woodruff School of Nursing
Emory University
Atlanta, Georgia

Joelle T. Fathi, DNP, RN, ARNP, ANP-BC, CTTS, NCTTP
Clinical Assistant Professor
Department of Biobehavioral Nursing and Health Informatics
School of Nursing
University of Washington
Seattle, Washington

Kimberly A. Guibone, DNP(c), MSN, ACNP-BC, AACC
Structural Heart Lead Nurse Practitioner
Beth Israel Deaconess Medical Center
Boston, Massachusetts

Divya Gupta, MD
Medical Director of Advanced Heart Failure and Transplantation
Associate Professor of Medicine
Division of Cardiology
Emory University School of Medicine
Atlanta, Georgia

Marian Hawkey, RN
Project Lead
Heart and Vascular Hospital
Hackensack University Medical Center
Hackensack, New Jersey

Cheryl Dennison Himmelfarb, PhD, MSN, RN, ANP, FAAN, FAHA, FPCNA
Vice Dean for Research, Sarah E. Allison Endowed Professor
School of Nursing
Johns Hopkins University
Baltimore, Maryland

Jeremy L. Iman, CNMT
Department of Radiology
University of Washington
Seattle, Washington

Katie N. Jaschke, MSN, RN, AGACNP-BC
Nurse Practitioner
Department of Cardiology
Saint Luke's Mid America Heart Institute
Kansas City, Missouri

Stacy Jaskwhich, BSN, MSN, FNP-C
Lead Nurse Practitioner
Preventive and General Cardiology and Women's Heart Center, The Emory Clinic
Adjunct Faculty, Emory Nell Hodgson Woodruff School of Nursing
Atlanta, Georgia

Maureen B. Julien, MSN, CRNP, AACC
Nurse Practitioner
Clinical Faculty
Penn Medicine
Interventional Cardiology
University of Pennsylvania
Philadelphia, Pennsylvania

Jasmina Katinic, MSN, RN, APRN-C, CCRN-K, AACC
Structural Heart Program Director
HCA West Florida Division
Palm Harbor, Florida

Josip Katinic, MSN, RN, APRN-C, AACC
Electrophysiology and Pacing Nurse Practitioner
The Heart Institute HCA
St. Petersburg, Florida

Patricia A. Keegan, DNP, NP-C, AACC
Director, Strategic and Programmatic Initiatives, Emory Heart and Vascular
Lead Nurse Practitioner, Structural Heart and Valve Center
Emory Healthcare
Atlanta, Georgia

Amanda M. Kirby, DNP, ACNP-BC
Nurse Practitioner
Milwaukee, Wisconsin

Monica Knapp, MSN, ARNP, FHRS
Electrophysiology Nurse Practitioner
Electrophysiology Lab
Virginia Mason Medical Center
Seattle, Washington

Binu Koirala, PhD, MGS, RN
Research Associate
School of Nursing
Johns Hopkins University
Baltimore, Maryland

Kristan N.D. Langdon, DNP, NP-C
Adjunct Faculty
School of Nursing
Nell Hodgson Woodruff School of Nursing
Atlanta, Georgia

Sandra Lauck, PhD, RN
Clinical Associate Professor
St. Paul's Hospital and Heart & Stroke Foundation Professorship in Cardiovascular Nursing at University of British Columbia
Clinician Scientist
St. Paul's Hospital
Vancouver, British Columbia
Canada

Dmitry B. Levin, BS
Associate Director, Center for Cardiovascular Innovation
Research Scientist and Engineer, Department of Cardiology
University of Washington School of Medicine
Seattle, Washington

Jane A. Linderbaum, MS, ARNP, AACC
Nurse Practitioner
Mayo Clinic
Rochester, Minnesota

Melissa Long, MSN, FNP-BC
Nurse Practitioner
Vanderbilt Heart and Vascular Institute
Nashville, Tennessee

Moses Mathur, MD, FACC
Interventional Cardiologist
Structural Heart Interventionalist
Penn State Hershey Medical Center
Hershey, Pennsylvania

Jan L. McAlister, DNP, APRN, CLS, AACC, FNLA, FPCNA
Nurse Practitioner
Piedmont Heart Institute
Atlanta, Georgia

Puja K. Mehta, MD, FACC, FAHA
Director, Women's Translational Cardiovascular Research
Emory Women's Heart Center
Associate Professor of Medicine (Cardiology)
Emory University School of Medicine
Atlanta, Georgia

William R. Miranda, MD, FACC
Assistant Professor of Medicine, College of Medicine and Science
Senior Associate Consultant in the Division of Structural Heart Disease
Department of Cardiovascular Medicine
Mayo Clinic
Rochester, Minnesota

Megan L. Morrison, PhD, RN, ARNP, FNP-BC, ACHPN
Assistant Professor
Advanced Certified Hospice and Palliative Care Nurse
Johns Hopkins University School of Nursing
Baltimore, Maryland

Dorothy L. Murphy, DNP, FNP-BC, AACC
Professor
Director, Family Nurse Practitioner-Doctor of Nursing Practice Program
Liberty University School of Nursing
Lynchburg, Virginia

Gabe Najarro, PA-C, MMSc
Intensivist Physician Assistant
Emory Healthcare
Atlanta, Georgia

Sunny M. Ohman, MSN, MN, RN, CRNA, ARNP, ANP-BC
Clinical Instructor
Department of Biobehavioral Nursing and Health Informatics
School of Nursing
University of Washington
Seattle, Washington

Melissa I. Owen, PhD, RN, CNE
Assistant Clinical Professor
Nell Hodgson Woodruff School of Nursing
Emory University
Atlanta, Georgia

Christina R. Paganelli, BSN, MPH
Public Health Analyst
Center for Applied Public Health Research
RTI International
Seattle, Washington

Victoria M. Pak, PhD, RN, MS, MTR
Assistant Professor
Nell Hodgson Woodruff School of Nursing
Emory University
Atlanta, Georgia

Angela D. Pal, PhD, RN, ACNP-BC
Assistant Professor
Specialty Director, Adult Gerontology Acute Care Nurse Practitioner Program
College of Nursing
University of Colorado
Aurora, Colorado

Roseanne Palmer, MSN, RN
Manager
Structural Heart Program
Dartmouth-Hitchcock Medical Center
Lebanon, New Hampshire

Pamela L. Patel, FNP-BC
Nurse Practitioner
Wellstar Health System
Comprehensive Care Clinic
Atlanta, Georgia

Elizabeth M. Perpetua, DNP, ACNP-BC, ANP-BC, AACC
Founder, Empath Health Services LLC
Adjunct Professor, Seattle Pacific University
Seattle, Washington

Christine Peverini, DNP, APRN, ANP-BC
Nurse Practitioner
Emory Adult Congenital Heart Center
Atlanta, Georgia

Marilyn A. Prasun, APRN, PhD, CCNS, CHFN, FAHA
Advocate BroMenn Endowed Professor
Mennonite College of Nursing
Illinois State University
Normal, Illinois

Laurie Quinn, PhD, RN, FAAN, FAHA, CDCES, APN-CS
Clinical Professor
Department of Biobehavioral Nursing Science
College of Nursing at University of Illinois at Chicago
Chicago, Illinois

Mario Ramos, RTR (CT)
Administration Officer, Diagnostic Imaging Services/ Radiolology
Veterans Administration Puget Sound Healthcare System
Seattle, Washington

Patricia Rantos, MSN, ARNP, AACC
Cardiology Nurse Practitioner
Heart Institute
Virginia Mason Medical Center
Seattle, Washington

Kumhee Ro, DNP, FNP-BC
Professor, Seattle University
Nurse Practitioner, University of Washington
Seattle, Washington

Ann E. Rogers, PhD, RN, FAAN, FAASM
Professor
Nell Hodgson Woodruff School of Nursing
Emory University
Atlanta, Georgia

Rajasree Roy, MD
Hospitalist, Assistant Professor of Medicine
Division of Hospital Medicine
Emory University
Atlanta, Georgia

Carrie L. Sanvick, RN, BSN
Registered Nurse
Mayo Clinic
Rochester, Minnesota

Meghan Sirochman, MSN, RN
Registered Nurse
Seattle, Washington

Martina K. Speight, MSN, FNP-BC
Nurse Practitioner
Stanford Health Care
Stanford, California

Nina Stefanie, MSN, ACNP-C
Registered Nurse
Coronary Care Unit
Emory Healthcare
Atlanta, Georgia

Courtney S. Swenson, MS, ARNP
Nurse Practitioner
Mayo Clinic
Rochester, Minnesota

Brandy Thomas, MSN, APRN, AGCNS-BC, AGPCNP-BC
Nurse Practitioner
Emory Healthcare
Atlanta, Georgia

Karen M. Vuckovic, PhD, APRN, ACNS-BC, FAHA
Clinical Associate Professor
Adjunct Faculty Division of Cardiology
University of Illinois
Champaign, Illinois

Kevin Widner
Department of Radiology
University of Washington
Seattle, Washington

Janet Fredal Wyman, DNP, APRN, ACNS-BC, AACC
Director Clinical Services, Structural Heart Disease
Henry Ford Health System
Detroit, Michigan

Alison Yam, MSN, APRN, AGCNS-BC, AGPCNP-BC
Clinical Nurse Specialist
Emory Healthcare
Atlanta, Georgia

Tao Zheng, MN, RN, CCRN-CSC-CMC, CHFN, PCCN
PhD Student/Fellow
Omics and Symptom Science Training Program
School of Nursing, University of Washington
Seattle, Washington

CONTENTS

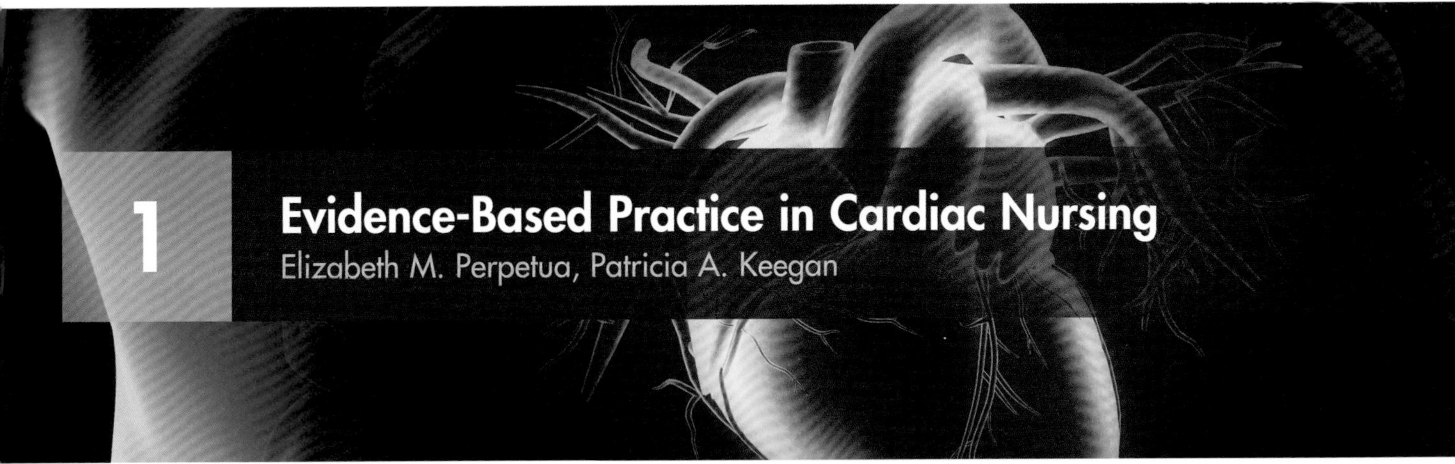

1 Evidence-Based Practice in Cardiac Nursing

Elizabeth M. Perpetua, Patricia A. Keegan

OBJECTIVES

1. Define evidence-based practice (EBP).
2. Describe the importance of evidence-based cardiac nursing.
3. Review the application of evidence and guidelines into cardiovascular nursing practice.
4. Discuss the use of EBP models in nursing practice.

KEY QUESTIONS

1. How does EBP influence practice?
2. What defines best practice?
3. How does qualitative research differ from quantitative research?

BACKGROUND

Cardiac nursing is a specialty dedicated to the care of patients with or at risk for heart and vascular disease, the most prevalent and deadly group of conditions worldwide. Heart disease is the leading cause of death for both men and women.[1] According to the World Health Organization, an estimated 17.9 million people died from cardiovascular disease (CVD), representing 31% of all global mortalities.[2] Heart attack and stroke comprise 85% of these deaths.[2] In the United States, approximately 50% of Americans have at least one of the risk factors for CVD: hypertension (HTN), high LDL cholesterol, and a history of smoking.[1] Most if not all nurses will care for a patient with CVD given its magnitude.

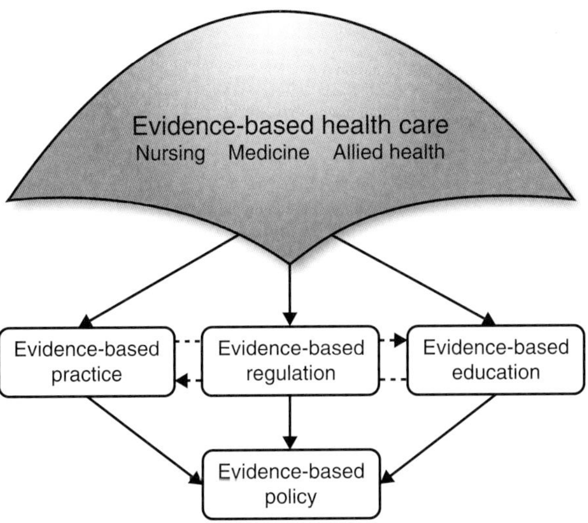

Figure 1-1. Evidence-based health care. (Used with permission from Spector N. Evidence-based nursing regulation: a challenge for regulators. *J Nurs Reg.* 2010;1(1):30–36.

The rapid advancements in technology and accelerated translation from bench to bedside means that caring for patients with CVD necessitates a spirit of inquiry with an appetite for evidence-based practice (EBP), such that the cardiac nurse is empowered to ask, "Why? What is the evidence and guideline? Is this best practice?" This chapter will review foundational terminology and resources for EBP literacy, and outline evidence-based models for asking clinical questions. The purpose of this chapter is to serve as a pragmatic overview for understanding research, guidelines, EBP, and the processes applied in the cardiovascular cllnical setting. For further instruction, the cardiac nurse is encouraged to seek rich and rigorous resources, as well as mentorship, on the critical appraisal of research and EBP.

PRIMER FOR EVIDENCE-BASED PRACTICE

Definition and Rationale

EBP is defined as the integration of the highest-quality evidence in research, practice, education, and regulations with clinical expertise and patient values (Fig. 1-1).[3,4] From novice to expert, cardiac nurses across many subspecialties and settings (Table 1-1) must be prepared to access, appraise, and implement EBP to improve patient care and outcomes.[5] To do so, cardiac nurses partner and serve with EBP champions to review the evidence from practice (e.g., data from the electronic health record, quality registries, staff/workflow observation, cost accounting, payer datasets) and research (e.g., guidelines and studies). Table 1-2 lists curated resources germane to the cardiac nurse, specified by professional society, publications, and nursing certification.

Case in point: The cardiac nurse provides patient education on HTN. The nurse must know how to access the most current multisocietal guidelines on the selection of pharmacologic therapy in HTN.[6] The nurse must understand the class of recommendation (COR), the level of evidence (LOE) supporting the guideline, and the decision pathways provided for patient and/or disease-specific

Table 1-1 • CARDIAC NURSING SUBSPECIALTIES

Subspecialty	Description	Common Disease States and Conditions
General and Preventative Cardiology	Prevention and management of heart and vascular disease. Practice settings include ambulatory/outpatient clinic, lipid clinic, diagnostic laboratories, and acute care.	• Coronary artery disease • Dyslipidemia • Heart failure • Valvular and structural heart disease • Cardiac arrhythmias • Vascular disease
Cardiac Imaging	Evaluation of heart and vascular disease. Practice settings include diagnostic imaging in cardiology (e.g., echocardiography laboratory) and radiology (e.g., CT, MRI, nuclear medicine, PET).	• Coronary artery disease • Dyslipidemia • Heart failure • Valvular and structural heart disease • Cardiac arrhythmias • Vascular disease
Interventional Cardiology	Evaluation and management of heart and vascular disease, including invasive, catheter-based techniques and device implantation. Practice settings include ambulatory/outpatient clinic, cardiac catheterization laboratory, and acute care.	• Coronary artery disease • Myocardial infarction • Valvular and structural heart disease • Heart failure
Valvular and Structural Cardiology	Evaluation and management of valvular and structural heart disease, including invasive, catheter-based techniques and device implantation. Practice settings include ambulatory/outpatient clinic, cardiac catheterization laboratory, and acute care.	• Aortic valve disease • Mitral valve disease • Tricuspid valve disease • Pulmonary valve disease • Atrial fibrillation • Septal defects
Congenital Heart Disease	Evaluation and management of congenital heart disease, including invasive, catheter-based techniques and device implantation. Practice settings include ambulatory/outpatient clinic, cardiac catheterization laboratory, and acute care.	• Septal defects • Tetralogy of Fallot • Single-ventricle defects • Pulmonary valve stenosis
Electrophysiology	Evaluation and management of cardiac arrhythmias, including invasive catheter-based techniques and device implantation. Practice settings include ambulatory/outpatient clinic, diagnostic laboratory, electrophysiology laboratory, and acute care.	• Atrial fibrillation/flutter • Supraventricular tachycardia • Ventricular arrhythmias • Syncope • Heart block • Heart failure
Heart Failure and Cardiac Transplant	Evaluation and management of heart failure, including medical therapy, cardiac rhythm/device management, mechanical circulatory support, and cardiac transplant. Practice settings include ambulatory/outpatient clinic, diagnostic laboratories, interventional and electrophysiology laboratories, and acute care.	• Systolic and/or diastolic heart failure with preserved or reduced ejection fraction • Cardiogenic shock • Heart transplant
Cardio-Oncology	Evaluation and management of cancer-related heart disease, particularly in patients prescribed high-risk chemotherapy and radiation therapy. Practice settings include ambulatory/outpatient clinic, diagnostic laboratories, and acute care.	• Cardiac arrhythmias • Drug-induced cardiomyopathy • Radiation heart disease • Heart failure
Vascular Medicine and Surgery	Evaluation and management of peripheral vascular disease, including medical therapy, catheter-based intervention, and open surgery. Practice settings include ambulatory/outpatient clinic (e.g., aortic clinic, vein clinic), diagnostic laboratories, and acute care.	• Aortic disease • Peripheral vascular disease • Claudication
Cardiac and Thoracic Surgery	Surgical management of cardiovascular disease, including catheter-based, open, and robotic surgical approaches. Practice settings include ambulatory/outpatient clinic, diagnostic laboratories, and acute care (e.g., cardiothoracic and transplant).	• Coronary artery disease • Myocardial infarction • Valvular and structural heart disease • Endocarditis • Heart failure

CT, computed tomography; MRI, magnetic resonance imaging; PET, positron emission tomography.

considerations. The nurse is then equipped with the knowledge that first-line therapy for HTN will vary according to the patient's risk factors and medical history (e.g., ethnicity, diabetes, and chronic kidney disease (CKD)).[7] As the nurse develops a deeper understanding of the medical management and therapeutic goals of this condition, care and education may now be individualized to the patient's particular needs, values, and preferences.

The role of the cardiac nurse in EBP and processes may be described at the patient-level, group- team- or unit-level, and the organizational-level. Consider the following examples.

Example 1—The cardiac nurse is caring for a 45 year old Black female, newly diagnosed with HTN. The medical history is notable for diabetes and renal disease. Knowledgeable of the evidence, guidelines, and therapy for HTN, the nurse understands that the recommended first-line agent for this patient is not a thiazide diuretic, but an angiotensin-converting enzyme inhibitor (ACE-I).[8] The cardiac nurse also anticipates that laboratory studies to evaluate renal function will be obtained.

Example 2—Cardiac nurses in the outpatient setting use this knowledge to (1) promote medication adherence and lifestyle changes for a goal blood pressure of less than 130/80 mm Hg instead of 140/90 mm Hg, and (2) educate on the surveillance of side effects and renal function via appropriate laboratory studies.

Table 1-2 • PROFESSIONAL ORGANIZATION PUBLICATIONS AND CERTIFICATIONS

Organization	Publications	Cardiac Nursing Certifications
Nursing		
American Association of Critical Care Nurses (AACN)	*American Journal of Critical Care* *Critical Care Nurse*	Critical Care Registered Nurse—Cardiac Surgery Certified (CCRN-CSC) Critical Care Registered Nurse—Cardiac Medicine Certified (CCRN-CMC) Progressive Critical Care Nurse (PCCN)
American Association of Heart Failure Nurses (AAHFN)	*Heart and Lung: Journal of Acute and Critical Care*	Certified Heart Failure Nurse (CHFN) Certified Heart Failure Nurse, Knowledge (CHFN-K [nonclinical])
American Nurses Association	*American Journal of Nursing*	Cardiac-Vascular Nurse Certification, Board Certified (RN-BC)
European Society of Cardiology	*European Journal of Cardiovascular Nursing*	Certified EAPCI NAP in Interventional Cardiology Nursing core curriculum available
Association of Cardiovascular Nursing and Allied Professions (ACNAP)		
European Association of Percutaneous Cardiovascular Interventions (EAPCI)		
Nurses and Allied Professional group (NAPs)		
Preventative Cardiovascular Nursing Association (PCNA)	*Journal of Cardiovascular Nursing*	Registered Nurse, Board Certified (RN-BC)
Medicine or Surgery		
American Association of Thoracic Surgeons (AATS)	*Journal of Thoracic and Cardiovascular Surgery*	
American College of Cardiology (ACC)	*Journal of the American College of Cardiology* and related publications	Cardiovascular Care Coordinator Certification Advanced Practice Provider (nurse practitioner and physician assistant) competencies published
American Heart Association (AHA)	*Circulation* and related publications	
European Society of Cardiology (ESC)	*European Heart Journal* and related publications	
Heart Rhythm Society (HRS)	*Heart Rhythm Journal*	
National Academies of Sciences, Engineering and Medicine—Health and Medicine Division (HMD) (formerly known as the Institute of Medicine [IOM])	Multiple publications and reports	
Society for Thoracic Surgeons (STS)	*Annals of Thoracic Surgery*	

Example 3—Nurses in the cardiothoracic (CT) intensive care unit (ICU) apply this knowledge to anticipate possible complications after emergency coronary artery bypass surgery (CABG), aware that (1) preoperative ACE-I therapy has historically been associated with increased mortality and morbidity, especially shock and atrial fibrillation,[9] and (2) a hypertensive patient with diabetes and CKD was likely on ACE-I therapy with no opportunity to discontinue prior to an emergent operation.

- The bedside nurse who recovers this patient post-CABG understands that there is an increased risk for postoperative hemodynamic instability, and determines whether the appropriate protocols are initiated in the postoperative orders.
- The charge nurse assimilates this patient's profile among those of the current and expected patients during the shift, and makes staffing assignments based on acuity, nursing skill mix, and the flow of postoperative patients per the operating room (OR) schedule.
- The CTICU nurse practitioner admitting the patient is equipped with comfort and concrete evidence when the family asks, "How can it be that a medication that's supposed to help him is now making him sicker? How long does its effect last? When is he 'out of the woods'?"

Example 4—For the home health nurse, this knowledge prompts him or her to question why the patient is not prescribed an ACE-I upon discharge status post-CABG, and to scrutinize the discharge summary for rationale and trends in blood pressure and renal function laboratory studies. The home health nurse coordinates with the primary care physician to obtain laboratory studies and determine the plan for reinitiating ACE-I if and when appropriate.

Example 5—At the organizational and system level, nurses use this knowledge to apply and assess/evaluate evidence-based best practices.

- In the inpatient setting, the ICU practice council revises protocols for CABG based on (1) hospital-specific outcomes reported by the quality assurance nurse responsible for the Society of Thoracic Surgeons (STS) Adult Cardiac Surgery database and (2) emerging evidence reviewed by practice council members including the clinical nurse specialist.[10]
- In the clinic, a performance initiative for multiple comorbid conditions such as HTN, coronary artery disease (CAD), diabetes, and CKD designates the cardiac nurse as a change agent in the implementation of a new care coordination model.
- Health system leadership in the ambulatory and acute care settings, including the Chief Nursing Officer evaluate practice change and impacts on quality, outcomes, and cost-effectiveness.

Terminology and Resources

Best practice is the synthesis of (1) highest-quality evidence; (2) top-of-license, skill–task-aligned clinical work; and (3) national, local, and site-specific policy, which is then implemented, evaluated, and iterated on an ongoing basis. To engage in this EBP cycle, a fundamental understanding of EBP terminology and resources is needed.[11]

Research Databases

Research databases are organized bibliographical collections of references (articles). Standard and advanced or comprehensive searches may be performed using key subject terms. A standard search will map initial search terms to corresponding fields and National Library of Medicine Medical Subject Heading (MeSH) terms, synonyms, and Boolean operators. To elaborate, the cardiac nurse performing a standard search of PubMed for "antihypertensive medications in diabetes and kidney disease" will match to MeSH terms "pharmaceutical preparations"; "diabetes insipidus"; "kidney diseases"; "diabetes mellitus"; "antihypertensive agents" and yield over 700 results. The nurse may use the advanced search in PubMed to further refine the results, combining specific fields including publication date(s), journal, and author with Boolean terms *and, or,* and *not.* Table 1-2 lists commonly used nursing and medical research databases.

Reference Types

To implement EBP, the cardiac nurse must understand the types and quality of references. A database search may produce many types of articles: abstracts, review articles, research studies, or practice guidelines. The nurse may search for a specific article or journal if known. Conversely, the nurse investigating a broader clinical question may search PubMed using particular terms (e.g., "antihypertensive medications in diabetes and kidney disease") and must be able to differentiate multiple results, which can also be filtered by the type of article.

Examples of article types are defined.

- *Abstract:* An overview (200 to 300 words) of a scientific paper (research, thesis, review, conference proceedings), deconstructed into four sections: background or introduction, methods, results or findings, conclusion.
- *Literature Review:* A manuscript summarizing the current state of a topic, including the primary clinical experts, major advances and discoveries, gaps in research, debates, and future areas of study. A high-quality review article can provide a thorough understanding of a topic and its key evidence and is often a good place for the cardiac nurse to begin inquiry on an area of interest. Note that a review article is not the same as a quantitative or qualitative research review (i.e., systematic review or meta analysis).
- *Research Study*: A scientific study that includes people and processes involved in health and disease and aims to answer a specific question. Most databases allow the user to search various types of research studies (e.g., randomized controlled trials [RCTs], multicenter trials).
- *Practice Guideline:* A statement that includes recommendations intended to optimize care, informed by expert stakeholders' opinions (usually affiliated with professional societies) review of evidence and the related benefit, risk, and harm of diagnosis and management.

Of great importance is to understand which types of articles constitute a primary source. The primary source, also known as an original source, is the first-hand account or documentation by the authors directly involved. A research study report written by the investigators is a primary source. A textbook or review article will name primary sources but both are in fact secondary sources. Whenever possible, the primary source is preferred.

Key information is derived from a cursory overview of the search results. First, note the *number and type of results.* Consider whether a new or advanced search using specific article types (e.g., clinical trial, review, practice guideline) or additional keywords would produce more relevant content. Next, identify the *publication title and year.* Does the title accurately describe the article and its content? What is the year of publication? Publications from the last 2 to 5 years are generally considered current and most desirable, excepting seminal works (i.e., landmark or pivotal trials or articles that define or influence a field).

Next, consider whether the journal is reputable, which may be readily evaluated via an affiliation with a professional society of nursing or medicine, or publishing organizations such as the International Association of Scientific, Technical and Medical (STM) Publishers. Further, is the journal peer reviewed? Information about the journal may be found on the journal's website. Note the journal's impact factor if reported. The impact factor is the measure of frequency with which an average article in a journal has been cited in a particular year (i.e., the more frequent the citations, the greater the impact of the article and thus the journal). High-impact journals are considered the most influential in their respective fields.[12] For example, *New England Journal of Medicine* carries the highest-impact factor (79.258 in 2017) of all general medical journals.[13] With the rise in "predatory journals" that charge for publication, lack a peer-review process, or do not adhere to publishing standards, understanding the credibility of information sources is paramount.

Types of Research

Quantitative Research. Quantitative research is based on the traditional scientific method and generates numerical data by examining the relationship among variables. Statistical analysis is used to test the strength and significance of these relationships. Study design determines the quality of evidence, depicted as a pyramid (Fig. 1-2). Evidence quality and study availability are inversely related; there are generally fewer studies of high quality and more studies of lower quality. To answer a clinical question, the nurse moves up the pyramid for study design that is more rigorous and reduces bias or systematic error. However, if there are few high-quality studies, the nurse may need to move down the pyramid for available evidence. Quantitative research study types are defined.

Case Series/Case Reports. These are collections of reports on the treatment of individual patients or a report on a single

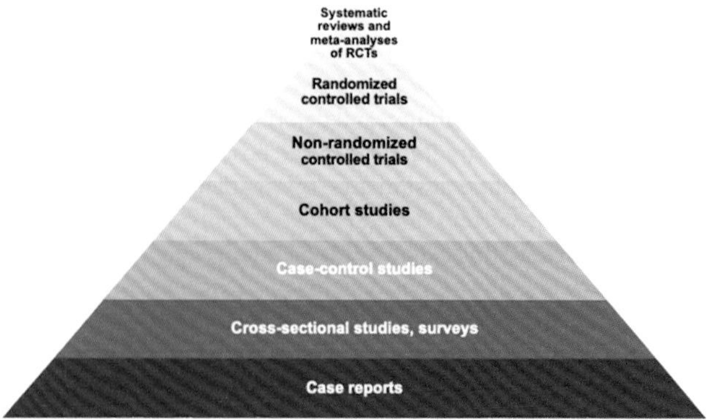

Figure 1-2. Evidence quality pyramid.

patient. No control group is used to compare outcomes. These are descriptive, not analytical, and carry little statistical validity.

Observational Studies. These studies observe the effects of risk factors, diagnostic test, treatment, or other intervention without manipulation or intervention. Data collection relies on medical records and patient recall. As the two groups studied may differ in ways other than the variables under study, a statistical relationship between variables is not necessarily causal.

Case Control Study. This is a study in which patients with a specific condition are compared with patients who do not have the condition to identify possible associated factors.

Cohort Study. This study investigates patients already exposed to a particular treatment or intervention, followed prospectively for specific outcomes, and compared with a similar patient group that has not been exposed by the treatment or intervention studied.

Randomized Controlled Trial. Known as an RCT, this is a study in which patients are allocated randomly and blindly to receive clinical interventions. One clinical intervention is a standard of comparison, or control, which may be a standard practice, a placebo, or no intervention. Careful planning reduces the potential for bias and allows for comparison between intervention and control groups to evaluate cause and effect. The randomized clinical trial has long been the "gold standard" of evidence.

Systematic Review. This is a study focused on a clinical topic to answer a specific question via an extensive literature search. Studies are reviewed, assessed for quality, and results are summarized.

Meta-Analysis. Considered the highest LOE, a meta-analysis examines valid studies on a topic and mathematically combines the results using an accepted statistical methodology to report the results as if it were one large study. A meta-analysis is predicated on the tenet that there is common (pooled) truth behind conceptually similar scientific studies.

Qualitative Research. Qualitative research aims to provide an understanding of experience, motivations, perceptions, and behaviors based on description and observation of subjects and the contextual setting. Examples of qualitative research study types are outlined.

Case Study. This is a single case example of an individual person, group, or institution, which aims to shed light on a phenomenon.

Grounded Theory. This design involves reading a textual database (field notes) and discovering and/or labeling variables (categories, concepts, and properties) and examining their relationships. It aims to understand the social and psychological processes characterizing a situation.

Historical Cohort. Similar to a cohort study, this study type uses information collected in the past and kept in files or databases. Patients begin with the presence or absence of an exposure or risk factor and are prospectively followed until the outcome of interest is observed.

Practice Guidelines. Professional society guidelines underpin cardiac nursing practice. Guidelines for clinical practice are ranked according to the COR and LOE (Fig. 1-3).[14,15] A Class IA recommendation, for example, is the strongest recommendation (I) with the highest-quality LOE (RCTs). Other recommendations in the form of scientific statements, expert consensus documents, appropriate use criteria, and treatment decision pathways may also guide patient care.

Clinical practice incorporates many types of recommendations. To elaborate, consider the documents informing the care of the patient with congestive heart failure (CHF) due to mitral regurgitation (MR).

- Guidelines for disease management (valvular heart disease,[16,17] heart failure,[18] ischemic heart disease[19]) detail various recommendations
- Appropriate use criteria (AUC) for clinically indicated, high-quality, cost-effective tests and procedures (diagnostic imaging,[20] coronary revascularization[21])
- Institutional and system-level recommendations specify the infrastructure and qualifications for the clinicians, hospitals, and health systems providing care (transcatheter mitral valve repair and replacement[22]; systems of care for valvular heart disease[23])

Searching the Literature vs Reviewing the Literature. The cardiac nurse must have working knowledge of these basic terms in order to search and read literature. General questions that may arise in an informal search of a topic include:

- What question is being asked? Does this question need to be refined?
- How do I search for the answers? What is the credibility of the source?
- What types of research studies best answer this question?
- Are there professional society guideline recommendations that answer this question?

When the problem is broad and the question is not yet clear it can be very helpful to peruse a highly credible quality resource such as UpToDate. UpToDate is a point-of-care software system recognized as the most comprehensive and current clinical resource available. The authors are widely recognized as international experts in their fields, and the peer-review process is rigorous. This ubiquitous clinical decision support tool covers 25 medical specialties and over 10,000 topics categorized by clinical questions.

Reading literature is not the same as a formal literature review. According to Hart, "a literature review is an account of what has been published on a topic by accredited scholars and researchers. It is an objective, thorough summary of the relevant available research and nonresearch literature on the topic being studied."[24] A more specific, systematic approach to literature review requires explicit definition of the problem or question at hand and foundational knowledge of the quality of evidence. These distinctions are further discussed in the context of EBP models.

EVIDENCE-BASED PRACTICE MODELS

EBP models use a process for framing a question, and locating and evaluating evidence in the literature. There are multiple EBP models to translate research into practice. Models help to organize the process to ensure the basic tenets are followed. The nomenclature may vary; however, these tenets are found in all models: **5 As: Ask, Attain, Appraise, Apply, and Assess**.

CLASS (STRENGTH) OF RECOMMENDATION	
CLASS I (STRONG)	**Benefit >>> Risk**
Suggested phrases for writing recommendations: ■ Is recommended ■ Is indicated/useful/effective/beneficial ■ Should be performed/administered/other ■ Comparative-Effectiveness Phrases†: ○ Treatment/strategy A is recommended/indicated in preference to treatment B ○ Treatment A should be chosen over treatment B	
CLASS IIa (MODERATE)	**Benefit >> Risk**
Suggested phrases for writing recommendations: ■ Is reasonable ■ Can be useful/effective/beneficial ■ Comparative-Effectiveness Phrases†: ○ Treatment/strategy A is probably recommended/indicated in preference to treatment B ○ It is reasonable to choose treatment A over treatment B	
CLASS IIb (WEAK)	**Benefit ≥ Risk**
Suggested phrases for writing recommendations: ■ May/might be reasonable ■ May/might be considered ■ Usefulness/effectiveness is unknown/unclear/uncertain or not well established	
CLASS III: No Benefit (MODERATE) *(Generally, LOE A or B use only)*	**Benefit = Risk**
Suggested phrases for writing recommendations: ■ Is not recommended ■ Is not indicated/useful/effective/beneficial ■ Should not be performed/administered/other	
CLASS III: Harm (STRONG)	**Risk > Benefit**
Suggested phrases for writing recommendations: ■ Potentially harmful ■ Causes harm ■ Associated with excess morbidity/mortality ■ Should not be performed/administered/other	

LEVEL (QUALITY) OF EVIDENCE‡	
LEVEL A	
■ High-quality evidence‡ from more than 1 RCT ■ Meta-analyses of high-quality RCTs ■ One or more RCTs corroborated by high-quality registry studies	
LEVEL B-R	**(Randomized)**
■ Moderate-quality evidence‡ from 1 or more RCTs ■ Meta-analyses of moderate-quality RCTs	
LEVEL B-NR	**(Nonrandomized)**
■ Moderate-quality evidence‡ from 1 or more well-designed, well-executed nonrandomized studies, observational studies, or registry studies ■ Meta-analyses of such studies	
LEVEL C-LD	**(Limited Data)**
■ Randomized or nonrandomized observational or registry studies with limitations of design or execution ■ Meta-analyses of such studies ■ Physiologic or mechanistic studies in human subjects	
LEVEL C-EO	**(Expert Opinion)**
Consensus of expert opinion based on clinical experience	

COR and LOE are determined independently (any COR may be paired with any LOE).

A recommendation with LOE C does not imply that the recommendation is weak. Many important clinical questions addressed in guidelines do not lend themselves to clinical trials. Although RCTs are unavailable, there may be a very clear clinical consensus that a particular test or therapy is useful or effective.

* The outcome or result of the intervention should be specified (an improved clinical outcome or increased diagnostic accuracy or incremental prognostic information).

† For comparative-effectiveness recommendations (COR I and IIa; LOE A and B only), studies that support the use of comparator verbs should involve direct comparisons of the treatments or strategies being evaluated.

‡ The method of assessing quality is evolving, including the application of standardized, widely used, and preferably validated evidence grading tools; and for systematic reviews, the incorporation of an Evidence Review Committee.

COR indicates Class of Recommendation; EO, expert opinion; LD, limited data; LOE, Level of Evidence; NR, nonrandomized; R, randomized; and RCT, randomized controlled trial.

Figure 1-3. Example of the American Heart Association/American College of Cardiology Guideline Recommendation Classification System. Note that the specific details for each class of recommendation and level of evidence may vary across guidelines statements.

Ask the Question (Define the Problem)

Perhaps a quote, commonly attributed to Einstein, best conveys the importance of defining the problem: "If given an hour to solve a problem, one should spend 55 minutes thinking about what problem is actually being solved and 5 minutes finding solutions."[26]

Perhaps a clinical situation prompts several key elements or questions. Clinical questions are generally categorized as background or foreground questions. Background questions ask who, what, where, when, how, or why, and obtain general knowledge about an illness, condition, or disease. Foreground questions are more complex inquiries that deal with a specific patient or population and ask for specific knowledge to inform clinical decisions.

Table 1-3 • EXAMPLES OF MAJOR NURSING AND MEDICINE RESEARCH DATABASES

Database	Organization	Description (+ Full-Text Database)
CINAHL (Cumulative Index of Nursing and Allied Health Literature) Database	EBSCOhost	Database of nursing and allied health literature. More than 6 million records. Full text for more than 1200 journals, dating back to 1937. Indexing for nearly 5500 journals. • CINAHL Complete (full text)
Cochrane Library	Cochrane Group	Databases of high-quality, independently reviewed research to guide healthcare decision making. • Cochrane Database of Systematic Reviews • CENTRAL (Cochrane Central Register of Controlled Trials) • Cochrane Clinical Answers
MedLine via PubMed	National Library of Medicine	Databases covering medicine, nursing, dentistry, veterinary medicine, healthcare system, and preclinical sciences. Over 12 million citations dating back to the mid-1950s. Contains bibliographic citations for more than 4,600 biomedical journals published in the United States and 70 other countries. • PubMed Central (full text)
PsycInfo	American Psychological Association	Databases covering psychology and the psychological aspects of related disciplines, including medicine, psychiatry, nursing, sociology, education, pharmacology, physiology, business, and law. More than 3 million citations dating back to the 1800s. • PsycArticles (full text) • PsycBooks (full text) • PsycTest (Psychological tests and measures)

Foreground questions are further classified into four types: therapy, diagnosis, prognosis, and etiology/harm. These questions are best answered by evidence from particular types of studies (Table 1-3). Formulating a question that can be answered is the foundation of a quality search for evidence.

Construct the PICO Question

Identify PICO Elements. In EBP the elements of this question form the acronym PICO(T). A PICO question is synonymous with a clinical question.

Population (Patient): Who are the relevant patients and what are their characteristics (age, sex, disease state, geographic location)?

Intervention (Indicator): What is the management strategy (diagnostic or screening test, or exposure) of interest?

Comparison: What is the control or alternate management strategy to compare to the intervention or indicator?

Outcome: What is the desired result or patient-relevant consequences of the intervention? What is being affected, measured, or improved (mortality, morbidity, accuracy, timeliness)?

Time Interval (optional): What is the time required to demonstrate an outcome? Or what is the time period during which patients are observed?

Formulate the Question. Next, craft the question. The form will be shaped by whether the clinical inquiry pertains to intervention, diagnosis, etiology, prevention, prediction/prognosis, or quality of life. To elaborate, the PICO question may have a template according to the type of clinical scenarios.

Intervention: These questions address the treatment of a condition or disease state.

- In [Population], how does [Intervention] compared to [Comparison] affect [Outcome] within [Time interval]?
- In [Population], what is the effect of [Intervention] on [Outcome] compared to [Comparison] within [Time interval or Type of study]?
- Example: In patients with nonvalvular atrial fibrillation, how does a rhythm control strategy compared to a rate control strategy affect morbidity, mortality, and quality of life?

Diagnosis: These questions address the evaluation used to identify or determine the nature and cause of a condition or disease state.

- Is [Intervention] more accurate in diagnosing [Population] compared with [Comparison] for [Outcome]?
- In [Population] is [Intervention] compared with [Comparison] more accurate in diagnosing [Outcome]?
- Example: Is a cardiac CT angiography more accurate than MR angiography in diagnosing patients with flow-limiting CAD?

Etiology: These questions address the causes of disease or the predisposing factors for a condition or disease state.

- Are [Population] who have [Intervention] at (increased/decreased) risk for/of [Outcome] compared with [Patients] with/without [Comparison] over [Time]?
- Are [Population] who have [Intervention] compared with those without [Comparison] at (increased/decreased) risk of/for [Outcome] over [Time]?
- Example: Are patients with nonischemic dilated cardiomyopathy at increased risk for sudden cardiac death as compared to patients with ischemic dilated cardiomyopathy?

Prevention: These questions address how to decrease the prevalence and progression of disease by early screening, and in identifying and modifying risk factors.

- For [Population], does the use of [Intervention] reduce the future risk of [Outcome] compared with [Comparison]?
- Example: For women at risk for CAD, does adherence to daily mindfulness practice delay onset and overall future risks?

Prognosis/Prediction: These questions address the prediction of the course of a disease.

- Does [Intervention] influence [Outcome] in [Population] over [Time]?
- In [Population], how does [Intervention] compared to [Comparison] influence [Outcome] over [Time]?

- Example: In Asian Americans aged 40 to 65 with pre-HTN, how does exercise compared to smoking cessation influence blood pressure control?

Quality of Life: These questions address patient-reported perceptions and experiences.

- How do [Patients] who receive [Intervention] perceive [Outcome] during [Time]?
- Example: How do patients with severe aortic stenosis who undergo aortic valve replacement perceive their quality of life before the procedure, and at 30 days and 1 year after the procedure?

As demonstrated, there is no "correct" question to construct from the PICO elements. Asking an answerable question relies upon identifying PICO elements relevant to the clinical scenario. Furthermore, a clinical situation may have more than one PICO question. The clinical question(s) should be specific enough to guide the search, without making it too limiting to find evidence.

Attain and Appraise the Evidence

Plan and Execute the Search Strategy

Select Key Terms. Translate the natural language PICO elements of the question into subjects, MeSH terms (see the previous section), or descriptors. An initial search may start with key terms for the **P**opulation/**P**atient and **I**ntervention/**I**ndicator. Take the previous example of an Intervention-based PICO question: In patients with nonvalvular atrial fibrillation, how does a rhythm control strategy compared to a rate control strategy affect morbidity, mortality, and quality of life?

- Population:
  - Natural language: Patients with nonvalvular atrial fibrillation
  - MeSH: atrial fibrillation
- Intervention:
  - Natural language: Rhythm control and rate control
  - MeSH: antiarrhythmic agents; antiarrhythmic drugs; heart rate control

For a scoping search of the literature, synonyms for all key PICO terms should be considered. These alternative terms may be used as needed in various combinations.

Select Databases. An initial scoping search for most clinical questions frequently starts with MedLine/PubMed and CINAHL. If there is a psychological component (e.g., behavioral interventions, quality of life) or the research design is qualitative, PsycInfo should be used. If the question has been answered via systematic reviews, the Cochrane Database should be included.

Apply Limits. The PICO question may specify certain limits such as age, publication year, and type of study. As seen in Table 1-4, the clinical question determines the research design(s) used, which are ranked according to the LOE generated. These limits may be applied to the initial search and modified for subsequent searches.

A systematic approach to EBP is made easier with tools. A worksheet for the PICO question and search strategy is provided (Fig. 1-4).

Appraise the Evidence

Review/Modify Search Results. Note the number of results and the first impression of whether the publication titles appear to answer the clinical question. Depending upon the terms and limits used, these results may be quite broad or narrow. After viewing the initial results, the search may be expanded using terms for the Comparison, Outcome, or Time elements of the PICO question in various combinations of "and" or "or." Various database filters may also be applied.

Table 1-4 • IDEAL TYPE OF STUDY BASED ON QUESTION TYPE

Type of Question	Ideal Type of Study
Therapy	Randomized controlled trial (RCT)
Prevention	RCT > cohort study > case control
Diagnosis	Prospective, blind controlled trial comparison to gold standard
Etiology/Harm	RCT > cohort study > case control
Cost Analysis	Economic analysis, cost-effectiveness analysis

Evaluate the Quality of the Evidence and Guidelines. Clinical decisions made from research and guidelines are only as good as the quality of the research and guidelines themselves. Quality of the study and appraisal of the validity, reliability, and applicability of results is determined by what the authors report in the manuscript.

For those interested in deepening their understanding of evidence appraisal, four tools are widely used to evaluate how studies and guidelines are reported. While further instruction on these tools is outside of the scope of this chapter, it is worthwhile to review their criteria and to know how to reference them if needed.

- CONSORT (Consolidated Standards of Reporting Trials) checklist, initially for randomized trials[26] and expanded to other trial designs.[27,28] The CONSORT flow diagram is provided to depict the criteria for quality report of randomized trials (Fig. 1-5).
- PRISMA-P (Preferred Reporting Items for Systematic Reviews and Meta-Analysis for Protocols) checklist for systematic review and meta-analyses.[29]
- AGREE-II (Appraisal of Guidelines for Research and Evaluation; 2nd version) instrument for practice guidelines.[30]

An initial, general however imperfect indicator of evidence quality is the source itself. Look for reputable peer-reviewed journals and authors affiliated with recognized professional societies. Review the results for practice guidelines and scientific statements that systematically rate the LOE of the primary sources.

Apply the Evidence and Assess the Process

Multiple models have been created to (1) apply the evidence and (2) assess the effectiveness, efficiency, and the ability to improve how to ask, acquire, appraise, and apply. While most begin with a clinical practice question that generally follows the PICO(T) format, the steps for applying evidence and assessing the process are distinctive to the model. The model chosen is specific to the institution and the clinician interested in implementing change. Models commonly used in nursing are described.

Iowa Model for Evidence-Based Practice to Promote Quality Care. The Iowa Model (Fig. 1-6) is an application-based model used to implement EBP. The model is heuristic; it is comprised of rule-of-thumb strategies to transform knowledge into

PICO Worksheet and Search Strategy

1. Define the question using **PICO**.

Population	
Intervention	
Comparison	
Outcome	

2. Write the question.

____

____

____

3. List the question's main topics and terms to use for the search.

	Natural language terms	**Database terms**	**Synonyms/other terms**
Population			
Intervention			
Comparison			
Outcome			

4. Check any limit that may pertain to your search.

_ Age
_ Language
_ Year of publication

5. Identify the type of study/publication you want to include in your search.

_ Systematic review or meta-analysis
_ Clinical practice guidelines
_ Critically appraised research studies
_ Qualitative research studies
_ Individual research studies
_ Electronic textbooks

6. Check the databases and sources you searched.

_ Cochrane library
_ PubMed
_ CINAHL
_ Joanna briggs institute
_ AHRQ evidence reports
_ Guidelines clearinghouse
_ Up to date
_ American Heart Association
_ American College of Cardiology
_ European Society of Cardiology
_ American Association of Heart Failure Nurses
_ Preventive Cardiology Nurses Association

Figure 1-4. Example of PICO question and search strategy worksheet.

action. Steps include: identify the problem- or knowledge-focused trigger, determine priority of trigger for organization, department, or unit, and lastly the formation of a team to work on research and implementation.[31]

Advancing Research and Clinical Practice Through Close Collaboration Model. This people-oriented model is used to amass resources and educate of clinicians in their role of implementing EBP at the point of care as well as throughout the organization. The model has seven steps: cultivating a spirit of inquiry; asking a PICOT-formatted clinical question; collecting, critically appraising, and integrating the best evidence with clinical expertise and patient preferences; and evaluating and disseminating practice change outcomes.[32]

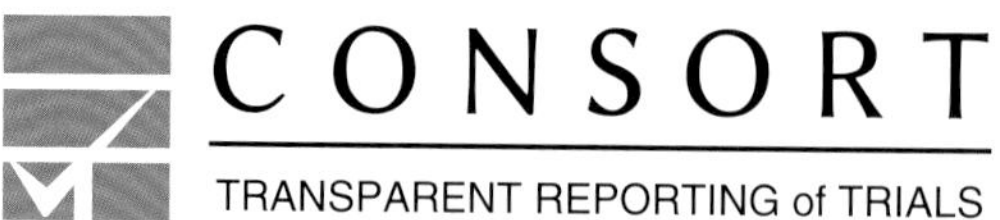

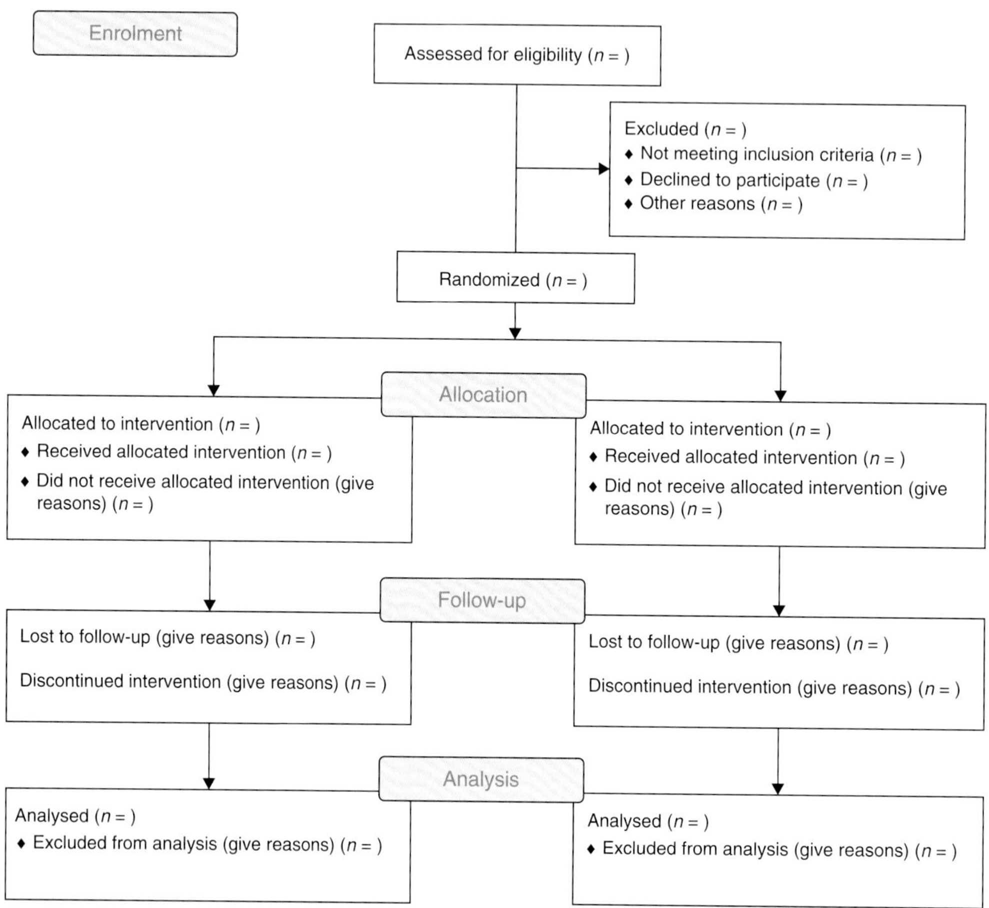

Figure 1-5. CONSORT flow diagram.

Johns Hopkins Nursing Evidence-Based Practice Model. This model (Fig. 1-7) is clinician-focused, allowing for rapid evaluation and utilization of best practices. It has three overall steps: practice question, evidence, and translation.[33]

Promoting Action on Research Implementation in Health Services (PARiHS) Framework. The PARiHS model (Fig. 1-8) asserts that the successful implementation is dependent upon the evidence available, care setting, and how facilitation occurs. This model stresses the strength and weakness of evidence and the context for change, and the clinical team's readiness to embrace and sustain change.[34]

Stevens Star Model of Knowledge Transformation. Formerly known as the Academic Center for Evidence-Based Practice (ACE) Star Model, the Stevens Star Model (Fig. 1-9) is composed of five major stages: knowledge discovery, evidence summary, translation into practice recommendations, integration into practice, and evaluation. This model utilizes the nurses' knowledge base within EBP and mainstreams nursing innovations into an EBP model.[35]

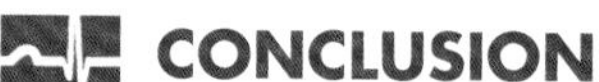

CONCLUSION

Engaging nurses in the EBP process encourages ownership of practice and empowers them to positively impact patient care and the profession. Every day, a clinical scenario arises that should prompt the cardiac nurse to attain new knowledge, to investigate, and to evaluate practice. This primer provides the EBP literacy needed to critically read this text, rich with high-quality evidence, guidelines, best practice examples, and considerations for the cardiac nurse. The next frontier for you, the reader, is to reflect on the problems you've already solved, the recurrent challenges that still need solving, and the ample opportunities that exist right now for you to engage in the EBP process in your current practice setting. The question is not *do* but *how* do you want to improve healthcare quality, outcomes, costs, and patient and clinician experience? Envision your unique contribution to nurse-driven, patient-centered practice change. The cardiac nurse is a champion and change agent of EBP.

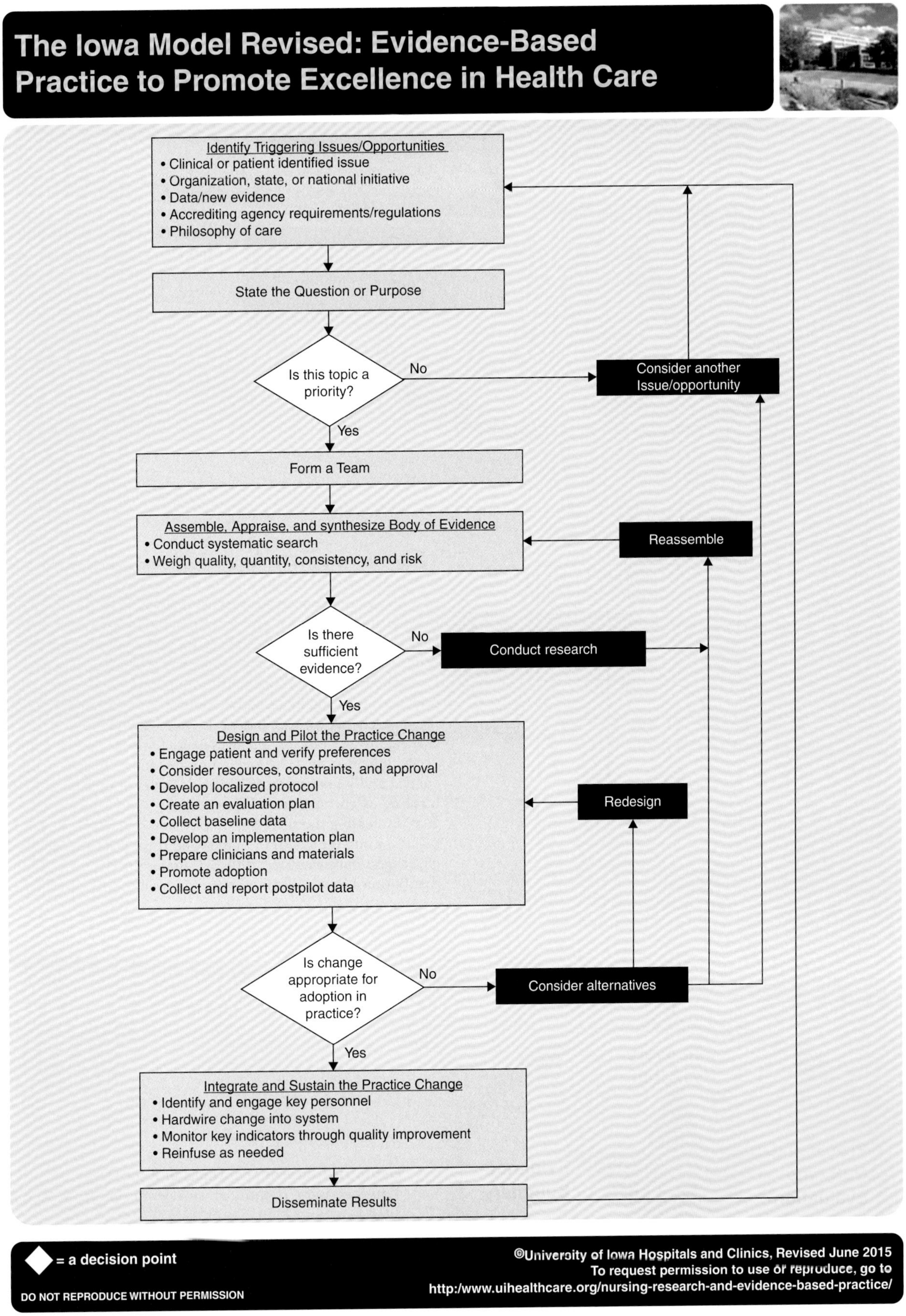

Figure 1-6. Iowa model for evidence-based practice to promote quality care. (Used/reprinted with permission from the University of Iowa Hospitals and Clinics, copyright 2015; Iowa Model Collaborative, Buckwalter KC, Cullen L, et al. Iowa model of evidence-based practice: revisions and validation. *Worldviews Evid-Based Nurs.* 2017;14[3]:175–182.)

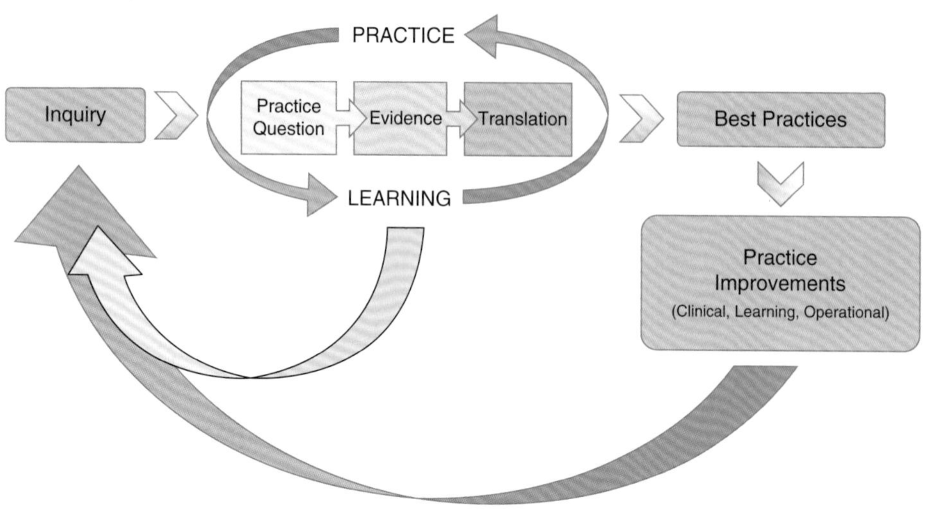

Figure 1-7. The Johns Hopkins nursing evidence-based practice model. (Reprinted with permission from Dang D, Dearholt SL, eds. *Johns Hopkins Nursing Evidence Based Practice: Model and Guidelines.* 3rd ed. Indianapolis, IN: Sigma Theta Tau International; 2017.)

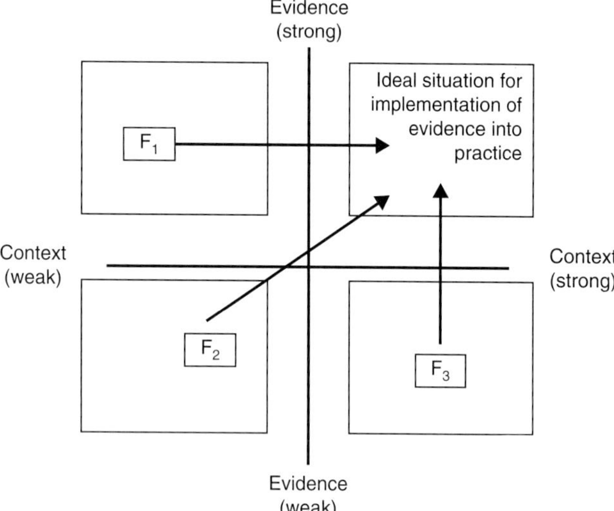

Figure 1-8. PARiHS framework diagnostic and evaluative grid. Diagnosis refers to the position of the team in terms of the strength of evidence and context for practice change. Evaluation describes the preparedness of the team to embrace and sustain practice change. Facilitation(s) (F) is/are active intervention(s) to promote team readiness to embrace new practice, evidence, or innovation. F_1: facilitation method for transforming weak context and strong evidence into a highly receptive context. F_2: facilitation method to manage weak context and weak evidence situation—most challenging and possibly involves issues of safety, basic competence needs to be managed. F_3: facilitation method to manage strong context and weak evidence situation—issues of routine and power involved. (Reprinted from Kitson AL, Rycroft-Malone J, Harvey G, et al. Evaluating the successful implementation of evidence into practice using the PARiHS framework: theoretical and practical challenges. *Implement Sci.* 2008;3:1; under the Creative Commons Attribution License [http://creativecommons.org/licenses/by/2.0].)

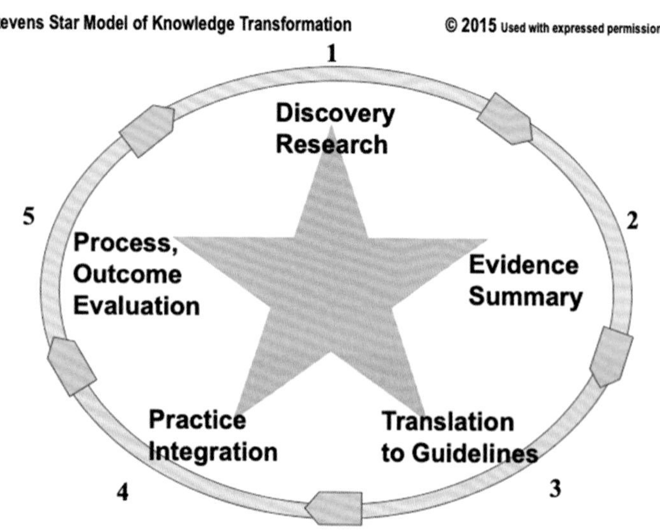

Figure 1-9. Stevens Star Model of Knowledge Transformation. (Reprinted with permission c/o K Stevens, 2015.)

CASE-BASED LEARNING

Patient Profile

The nurses in telemetry collectively note an increase in patient admissions due to rapid atrial fibrillation and hypotension after elective noncardiac surgery. This observation is communicated to the charge nurse team and clinical practice council. It is known that atrial fibrillation is the most common postoperative arrhythmia, seen in up to 20% to 40% of patients undergoing cardiac surgery and 10% to 20% of patients undergoing noncardiac surgery, and ranges from 5% after total joint replacements to up to 20% following abdominal surgery.[36] However, a more intensive utilization review reveals a recent "spike" in these admissions to telemetry while admissions to the ICUs, surgical volumes, and case mix index (patient acuity) remain stable. The nurses suspect that perioperative management of these patients may be playing a role and endeavor to define the problem. The clinical practice council begins the process of practice inquiry.

1. Ask the question.

	Natural Language	**Database (MeSH) Terms**
Population	• Surgical patients • Noncardiac surgery patients	• Surgery • (Non)cardiac surgery • (Non)cardiothoracic surgery
Intervention/ Indicators	• Perioperative medications • Perioperative management • Risk factors	• Medications • Risk factors • Preoperative • Perioperative care
Comparison	• No perioperative medications or perioperative medications • Perioperative management or no perioperative management • Risk factors or no risk factors	• Medications • Risk factors • Preoperative care • Perioperative care
Outcome	• Postoperative atrial fibrillation (POAF) • Prevention of POAF	• Atrial fibrillation • Atrial arrhythmia
Time	• Perioperative	• Perioperative period • Postoperative period

The nurses realize that many broad search terms are listed and subsequently peruse UpToDate on the general topic of POAF and its clinical question categories. They soon realize that the search terms considered pertain to both background and foreground clinical questions.

The background PICO(T) question: In patients undergoing noncardiac surgery, what are the modifiable risk factors for POAF?

The foreground PICO(T) question: In patients undergoing noncardiac surgery, what risk factors for POAF can be effectively modified during the perioperative period to decrease the incidence of POAF?

2. Attain and appraise evidence.

The clinical practice council searched Medline, the Cochrane database, and PubMed from 2010 through 2014 for research or review articles using combinations of MeSH terms: "postoperative atrial fibrillation" and "risk factors postoperative atrial fibrillation," "postoperative atrial fibrillation noncardiothoracic surgery," "postoperative atrial fibrillation noncardiac surgery," "postoperative arrhythmias" and "management postoperative atrial fibrillation," and "postoperative atrial fibrillation and prevention." They reviewed the references/bibliographies of the selected studies and medical texts for additional references. A total of 39 high-quality articles were focused on POAF/postoperative arrhythmias including 17 which focused on noncardiac surgery. Additionally, the U.S. multisocietal clinical practice guideline for perioperative management of patients undergoing noncardiac surgery was reviewed.[37]

A cursory chart review of the patients admitted for postoperative rapid atrial fibrillation during the last quarter revealed that nearly all of these patients had a history of coronary artery disease and hypertension but may not have had a history of atrial fibrillation. It appeared that these patients did not take their long-term beta-blockers or calcium-channel blockers preprocedure. This practice was found to be inconsistent with the clinical practice guideline, and with the hospital's preoperative instructions for medications.

3. Apply evidence.

While other root causes and risk factors were being evaluated, a common thread was revealed. Pre-operative documentation indicated these patients discontinued their long-term beta blockers and/or calcium channel blockers, which is notable in the literature as one of the most frequent, and readily modifiable, precipitating factors for PAOF. Applying the evidence, the clinical practice council sought to review and if needed revise the preoperative instructions for these medications, and the clinician workflow for providing and documenting this critical information to patients. It was found that recent changes to functionality of the electronic health record eliminated the historical facilitators (established order sets, smart texts, printer access) and created many new barriers to disseminating (printing) and documenting these patient instructions. A performance improvement group led by nurses and information technology specialists formed to propose, implement, and assess a solution to this problem, continuing the EBP cycle. This group has adopted the Stevens Star Model of Knowledge Transformation as the EBP framework.

KEY READINGS

Gawlinski A & Rutledge D. Selecting a Model for Evidence Based Practice Changes: A Practical Approach. *AACN Adv Crit Care.* 2008;19(3): 291–300. doi: https://doi.org/10.4037/15597768-2008-3007

Polit DF & Beck CT. Nursing research: Generating and assessing evidence for nursing practice (10th ed.). 2016. Wolters Kluwer: Philadelphia, PA.

Rycroft-Malone J & Bucknall T. Models and frameworks for implementing evidence-based practice: Linking evidence to action. 2015. Wiley-Blackwell: Hoboken, NJ.

REFERENCES

1. Centers for Disease Control and Prevention. Heart Disease Fact Sheet. 2018; Available at https://www.cdc.gov/dhdsp/data_statistics/fact_sheets/fs_heart_disease.htm. Accessed March 23, 2018.
2. World Health Organization. Cardiovascular Disease Fact Sheet. 2017; Available at https://www.who.int/en/news-room/fact-sheets/detail/cardiovascular-diseases-(cvds). Accessed March 23, 2018.
3. Sackett DL SS, Richardson WS, Rosenberg W, et al. *Evidence Based Medicine: How to Practice and Teach EBM.* London: Churchill Livingstone; 2001.
4. Spector N. Evidence-based nursing regulation: a challenge for regulators. *J Nurs Reg.* 2010;1(1):30–36.
5. Benner P. *From Novice to Expert: Excellence and Power in Clinical Nursing Practice.* Upper Saddle River, NJ: Prentice Hall; 1984.
6. Whelton PK, Carey RM, Aronow WS, et al. 2017 ACC/AHA/AAPA/ABC/ACPM/AGS/APhA/ASH/ASPC/NMA/PCNA guideline for the prevention, detection, evaluation, and management of high blood pressure in adults: a report of the American College of Cardiology/American Heart Association Task Force on clinical practice guidelines. *Hypertension.* 2018;71(6):e13–e115.
7. Whelton PK, Carey RM, Aronow WS, et al. 2017 ACC/AHA/AAPA/ABC/ACPM/AGS/APhA/ASH/ASPC/NMA/PCNA guideline for the prevention, detection, evaluation, and management of high blood pressure in adults: a Report of the American College of Cardiology/American Heart Association Task Force on clinical practice guidelines. *J Am Coll Cardiol.* 2018;71(19):e127–e248.
8. James PA, Oparil S, Carter BL, et al. 2014 evidence-based guideline for the management of high blood pressure in adults: report from the panel members appointed to the Eighth Joint National Committee (JNC 8). *JAMA.* 2014;311(5):507–520.
9. Miceli A, Capoun R, Fino C, et al. Effects of angiotensin-converting enzyme inhibitor therapy on clinical outcome in patients undergoing coronary artery bypass grafting. *J Am Coll Cardiol.* 2009;54(19):1778–1784.
10. Diepen SV, Norris CM, Zheng Y, et al. Comparison of angiotensin-converting enzyme inhibitor and angiotensin receptor blocker management strategies before cardiac surgery: a pilot randomized controlled registry trial. *J Am Heart Assoc.* 2018;7(20):e009917.
11. Straus SE, Glasziou P, Richardson WS, et al., eds. *Evidence-Based Medicine: How to Practice and Teach It.* 4th ed. Edinburg: Churchill Livingstone/Elsevier; 2011.
12. Garfield E. Citation indexing for studying science. *Nature.* 1970; 227(5259):669–671.
13. Web of Science Group. 2018 Journal Citation Reports. 2019; as cited by New England Journal of Medicine in About NEJM. Available at https://www.nejm.org/about-nejm/about-nejm. Accessed March 11, 2019.
14. Halperin Jonathan L, Levine Glenn N, Al-Khatib Sana M, et al. Further evolution of the ACC/AHA clinical practice guideline recommendation classification system. *Circulation.* 2016;133(14):1426–1428.
15. European Society of Cardiology. Governing Policies and Procedures for the Writing of ESC Clinical Practice Guidelines. 2010; Available at https://www.escardio.org/static_file/Escardio/Guidelines/ESC Guidelines for Guidelines Update 2010.pdf. Accessed March 23, 2019.
16. Nishimura RA, Otto CM, Bonow RO, et al. 2014 AHA/ACC guideline for the management of patients with valvular heart disease: a Report of the American College of Cardiology/American Heart Association Task Force on practice guidelines. *J Am Coll Cardiol.* 2014;63(22):e57–e185.
17. Nishimura RA, Otto CM, Bonow RO, et al. 2014 AHA/ACC Guideline for the management of patients with valvular heart disease: a Report of the American College of Cardiology/American Heart Association Task Force on Practice Guidelines. *J Am Coll Cardiol.* 2014;63(22):e57–e185.
18. Yancy CW, Jessup M, Bozkurt B, et al. 2017 ACC/AHA/HFSA focused update of the 2013 ACCF/AHA guideline for the management of heart failure: a Report of the American College of Cardiology/American Heart Association Task Force on Clinical Practice Guidelines and the Heart Failure Society of America. *Circulation.* 2017;136(6):e137–e161.
19. Wolk MJ, Bailey SR, Doherty JU, et al. ACCF/AHA/ASE/ASNC/HFSA/HRS/SCAI/SCCT/SCMR/STS 2013 multimodality appropriate use criteria for the detection and risk assessment of stable ischemic heart disease: a Report of the American College of Cardiology Foundation Appropriate Use Criteria Task Force, American Heart Association, American Society of Echocardiography, American Society of Nuclear Cardiology, Heart Failure Society of America, Heart Rhythm Society, Society for Cardiovascular Angiography and Interventions, Society of Cardiovascular Computed Tomography, Society for Cardiovascular Magnetic Resonance, and Society of Thoracic Surgeons. *J Am Coll Cardiol.* 2014;63(4):380–406.
20. Doherty JU, Kort S, Mehran R, et al. ACC/AATS/AHA/ASE/ASNC/HRS/SCAI/SCCT/SCMR/STS 2017 appropriate use criteria for multimodality imaging in valvular heart disease: a Report of the American College of Cardiology Appropriate Use Criteria Task Force, American Association for Thoracic Surgery, American Heart Association, American Society of Echocardiography, American Society of Nuclear Cardiology, Heart Rhythm Society, Society for Cardiovascular Angiography and Interventions, Society of Cardiovascular Computed Tomography, Society for Cardiovascular Magnetic Resonance, and Society of Thoracic Surgeons. *J Nucl Cardiol.* 2017;24(6):2043–2063.
21. Patel MR, Calhoon JH, Dehmer GJ, et al. ACC/AATS/AHA/ASE/ASNC/SCAI/SCCT/STS 2017 appropriate use criteria for coronary revascularization in patients with stable ischemic heart disease. A Report of the American College of Cardiology Appropriate Use Criteria Task Force, American Association for Thoracic Surgery, American Heart Association, American Society of Echocardiography, American Society of Nuclear Cardiology, Society for Cardiovascular Angiography and Interventions, Society of Cardiovascular Computed Tomography, and Society of Thoracic Surgeons. *J Am Coll Cardiol.* 2017;69(17):2212–2241.
22. Bonow RO, O'Gara PT, Adams DH, et al. 2019 AATS/ACC/SCAI/STS expert consensus systems of care document: operator and institutional recommendations and requirements for transcatheter mitral valve intervention. A Joint Report of the American Association for Thoracic Surgery, the American College of Cardiology, the Society for Cardiovascular Angiography and Interventions, and the Society of Thoracic Surgeons. *J Am Coll Cardiol.* 2020;76(1):96–117.
23. Nishimura RA, O'Gara PT, Bavaria JE, et al. 2019 AATS/ACC/ASE/SCAI/STS expert consensus systems of care document: a proposal to optimize care for patients with valvular heart disease. A Joint Report of the American Association for Thoracic Surgery, American College of Cardiology, American Society of Echocardiography, Society for Cardiovascular Angiography and Interventions, and Society of Thoracic Surgeons. *J Am Coll Cardiol.* 2019;73(20):2609–2635.
24. Hart C. *Doing a Literature Review: A Comprehensive Guide for the Social Sciences.* London: Sage; 2012.
25. Spradlin, D. Are you solving the right problem? *IEEE Eng Manag Rev.* 2016:44(4):47–54. doi: 10.1109/EMR.2016.7792409
26. Schulz KF, Altman DG, Moher D. CONSORT 2010 Statement: Updated Guidelines for reporting parallel group randomised trials. *BMJ.* 2010;340:c332.
27. Eldridge SM, Chan CL, Campbell MJ, et al. CONSORT 2010 statement: extension to randomised pilot and feasibility trials. *BMJ.* 2016;355:i5239.
28. Dwan K, Li T, Altman DG, et al. CONSORT 2010 statement: extension to randomised crossover trials. *BMJ.* 2019;366:l4378.
29. Moher D, Shamseer L, Clarke M, et al. Preferred reporting items for systematic review and meta-analysis protocols (PRISMA-P) 2015 statement. *Syst Rev.* 2015;4(1):1.
30. Brouwers MC, Kho ME, Browman GP, et al; AGREE Next Steps Consortium. AGREE II: advancing guideline development, reporting and evaluation in healthcare. *CMAJ.* 2010;182(18):E839–E842.
31. Iowa Model Collaborative, Buckwalter KC, Cullen L, et al. Iowa model of evidence-based practice: revisions and validation. *Worldviews Evid-Based Nurs.* 2017;14(3):175–182.
32. Melnyk BM, Fineout-Overholt E. *Evidence-Based Practice in Nursing & Healthcare: A Guide to Best Practice.* Philadelphia, PA: Lippincott Williams & Wilkins; 2005.
33. Dang D, Dearholt SL, eds. *Johns Hopkins Nursing Evidence Based Practice: Model and Guidelines.* 3rd ed. Indianapolis, IN: Sigma Theta Tau International; 2017.
34. Kitson AL, Rycroft-Malone J, Harvey G, et al. Evaluating the successful implementation of evidence into practice using the PARiHS framework: theoretical and practical challenges. *Implement Sci.* 2008;3:1.
35. Stevens KR. *ACE Star Model of EBP: Knowledge Transformation.* Academic Center for Evidence-based Practice, The University of Texas Health Science Center at San Antonio; 2004.
36. Dobrev D, Aguilar M, Heijman J, et al. Postoperative atrial fibrillation: mechanisms, manifestations and management. *Nat Rev Cardiol.* 2019;16(7):417–436.
37. Fleisher LA, Fleischmann KE, Auerbach AD, et al. 2014 ACC/AHA guideline on perioperative cardiovascular evaluation and management of patients undergoing noncardiac surgery. *J Am Coll Cardiol.* 2014;64(22):e77.

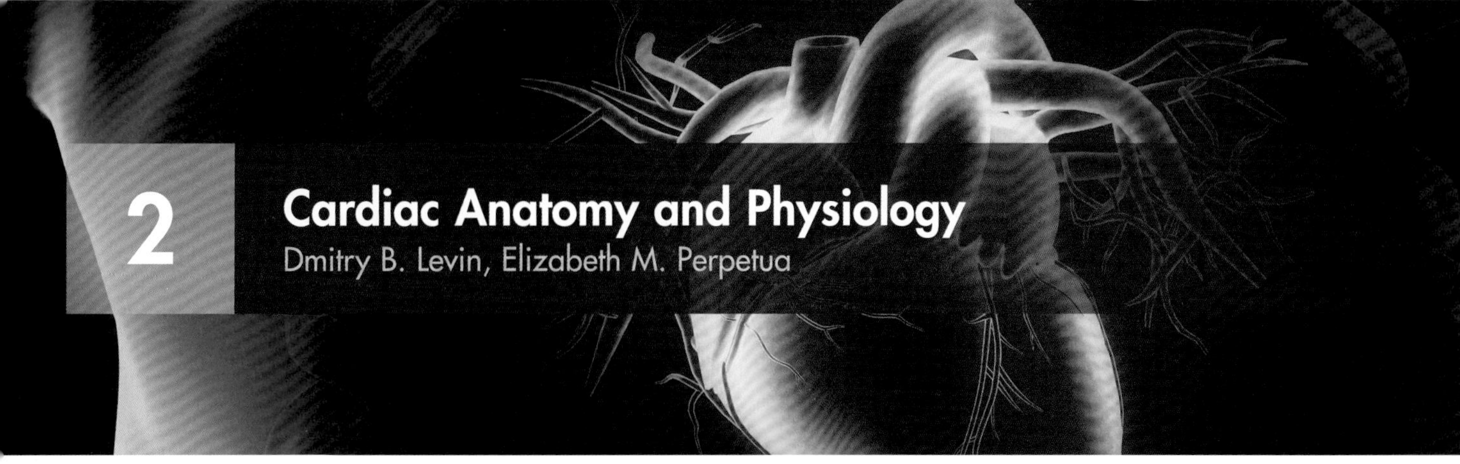

2 Cardiac Anatomy and Physiology

Dmitry B. Levin, Elizabeth M. Perpetua

OBJECTIVES

1. Acquire a foundational understanding of cardiac anatomy.
2. Apply the knowledge of cardiac anatomy in order to understand cardiac physiology.
3. Describe the cardiac cycle.
4. Understand the coronary circulation and the supply and demand of cardiac tissue.
5. Discuss the electrical, mechanical, and metabolic activities underlie cardiac performance.

KEY QUESTIONS

1. What are the correct terms and orientations of the heart's structures?
2. How does structure (anatomy) affect the function (physiology) of the heart?
3. What are the electrical, mechanical, and metabolic events of the cardiac cycle?
4. What physiologic processes impact cardiac performance?

BACKGROUND

Structure determines and supports function: this is the key tenet of anatomy and physiology. The cardiac nurse with strong foundational knowledge of cardiac anatomy will therefore have a deeper, richer understanding of cardiac physiology. Further, the cardiac nurse must understand normal anatomy and physiology to grasp the pathoanatomic and pathophysiologic changes of diseases and their functional consequences. This chapter describes normal human adult cardiac anatomy, cellular structure, and ultrastructure. The chapter also discusses electrical, mechanical, and metabolic activities that underlie cardiac pump performance. The coronary circulation is described in the context of its linkage to changing demands of cardiac tissue for nutrient delivery and waste removal. Finally, cardiac performance is discussed.

GENERAL ANATOMIC DESCRIPTION

Location and Dimensions

The heart is a hollow muscular organ encased and cushioned in its own serous membrane, the pericardium. It lies in the middle mediastinal compartment of the thorax between the two pleural cavities (Fig. 2-1). Two thirds of the heart extends to the left of the body's midline (Fig. 2-2).

The average adult heart is approximately 12 cm long from its base at the beginning of the root of the aorta to the left ventricular apex. It is 8 to 9 cm transversely at its greatest width, and 6 cm thick anteroposteriorly. Tables have been derived to indicate normal ranges of heart size for various body weights and heights.[1]

The adult male heart comprises approximately 0.43% of body weight, typically 280 to 350 g, with an average weight of 300 g. The adult female heart comprises approximately 0.40% of body weight, 230 to 300 g, with an average weight of 250 g.[2,3] Age, body build, frequency of physical exercise, and heart disease influence heart size and weight.

Anatomical Orientation

Understanding cardiac anatomy requires amassing a lexicon of terminology, which may in fact be confusing descriptions of the heart's structures and their orientation. Take, for example, the incorrect terms of the major coronary arteries: the left anterior descending artery actually lies on the *superior* surface of the heart, and the posterior descending artery actually lies on the *inferior* surface.[4] The nomenclature in early anatomy literature was based upon examination of the heart outside of the body and standing on its apex in the valentine position (Figs. 2-3 and 2-4).[5] Advancements in cardiology such as cardiac imaging, minimally invasive surgery, and percutaneous therapy have brought to bear the challenges of using these historical, incorrect terms and gave rise to *attitudinally correct cardiac anatomy*: the description of cardiac structures and their orientation with the body in the standard anatomical position.

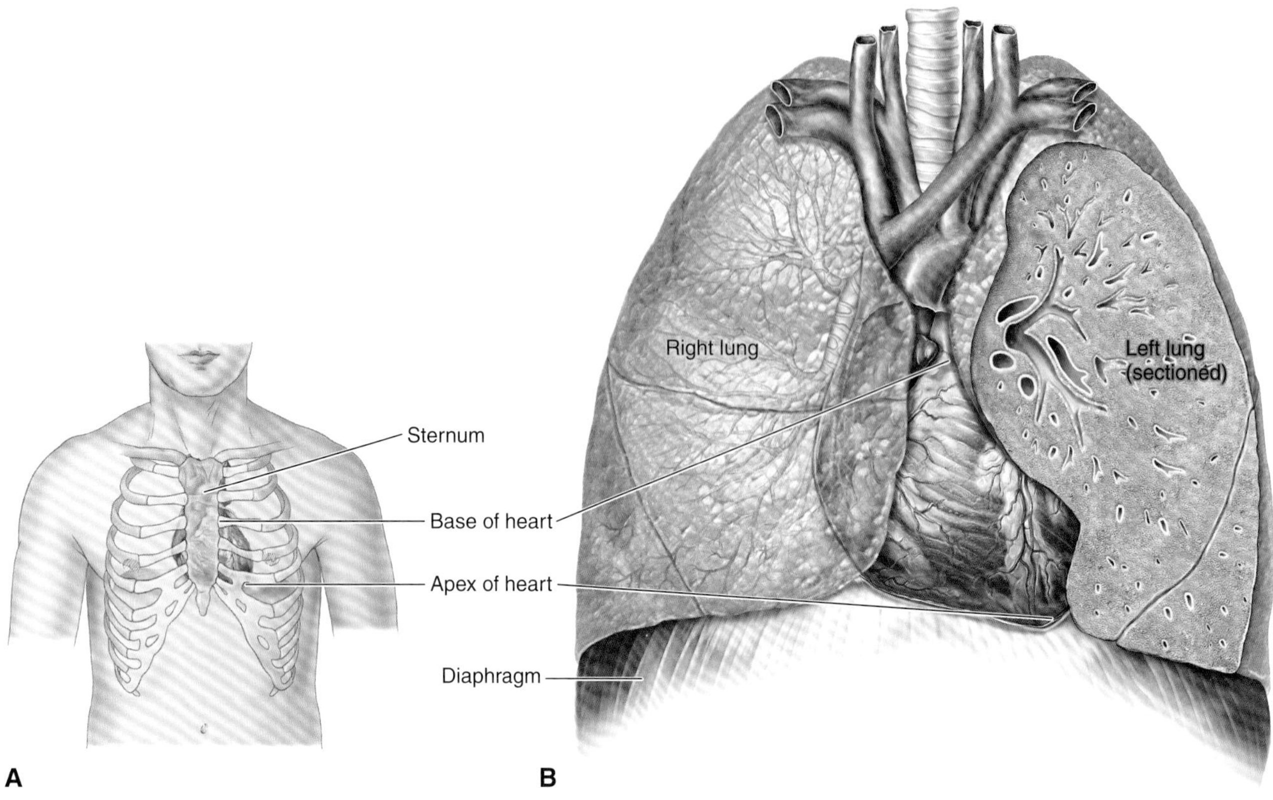

Figure 2-1. Location of the heart. **A:** Anterior view of the chest. The heart is partially visible behind the sternum. **B:** Anterior view of the thoracic cavity. The left lung is sectioned and the pericardium has been removed.

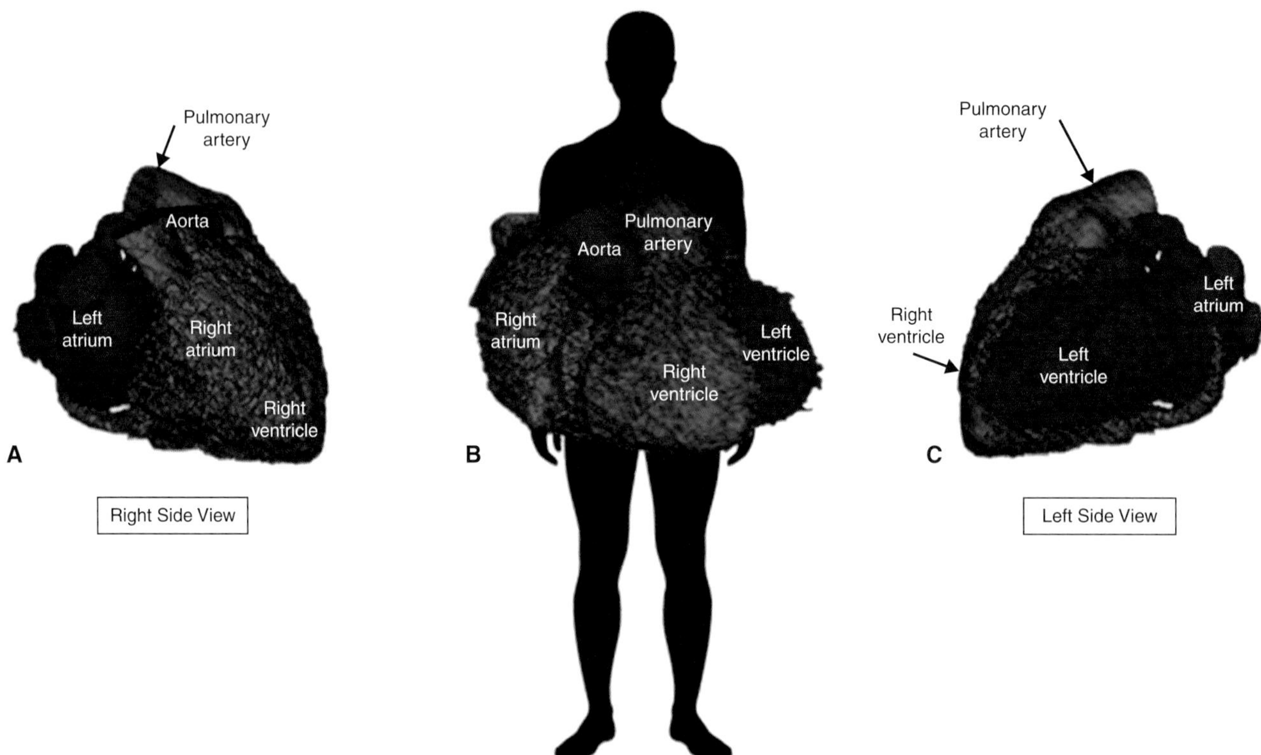

Figure 2-2. Anatomical perspective of the heart from three major angles. **A:** View of the heart from right side of the body. **B:** Anterior view of the heart. **C:** View of the heart from left side of the body.

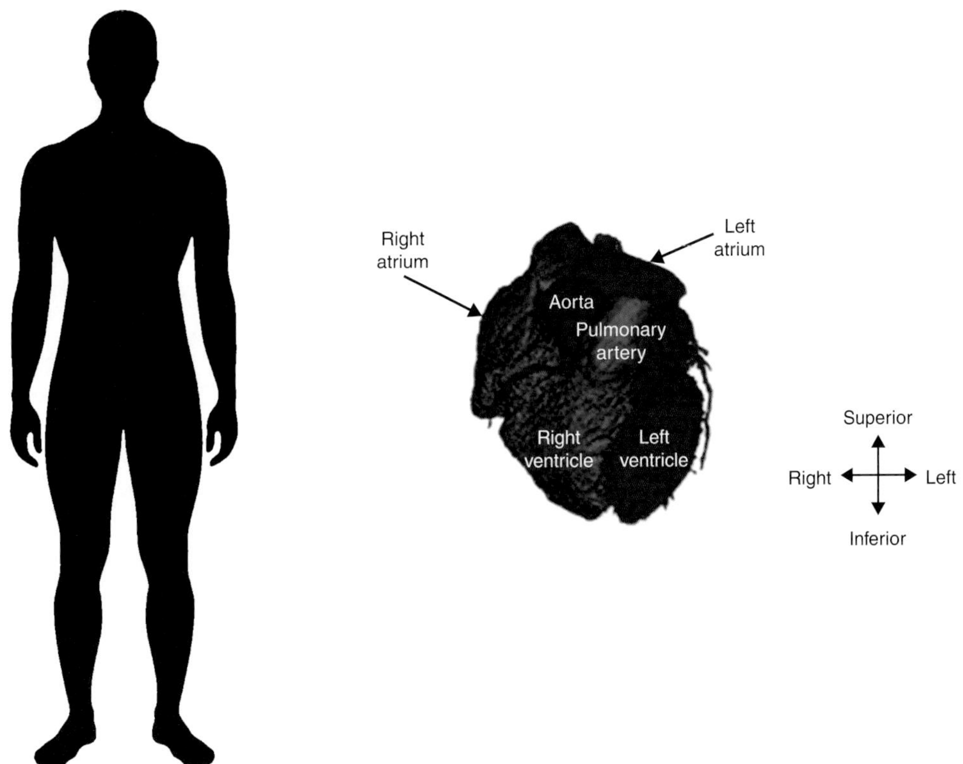

Figure 2-3. The "Valentine" heart orientation. Early anatomists examined and described the heart in the valentine position, as opposed to how it is actually oriented in the body, which resulted in confusing, or even incorrect, nomenclature.

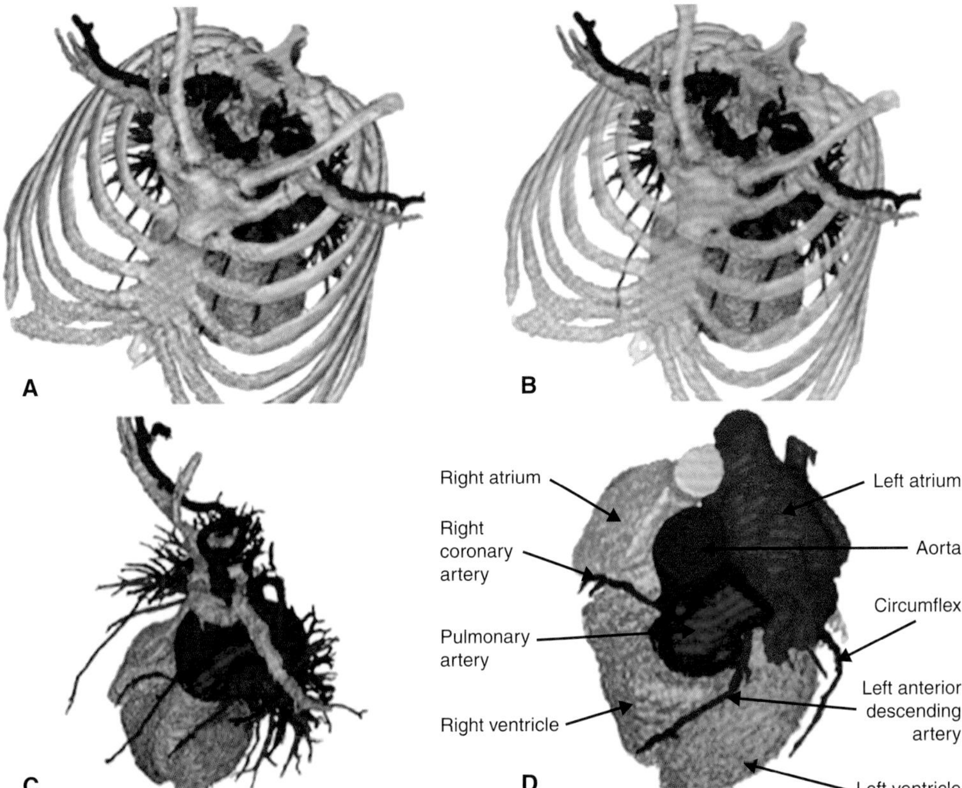

Figure 2-4. Body position (looking over the left shoulder) when the heart is in the valentine position. Note that the body is not in the standard anatomical position. **A:** Full anatomical perspective of the heart with vessels and rib cage intact. **B:** Transparent rib cage with heart and vessels present. **C:** Heart with major vessels coming of it from perspective over the left shoulder. **D:** Heart with four chambers in addition to pulmonic trunk and aorta with coronary vessels.

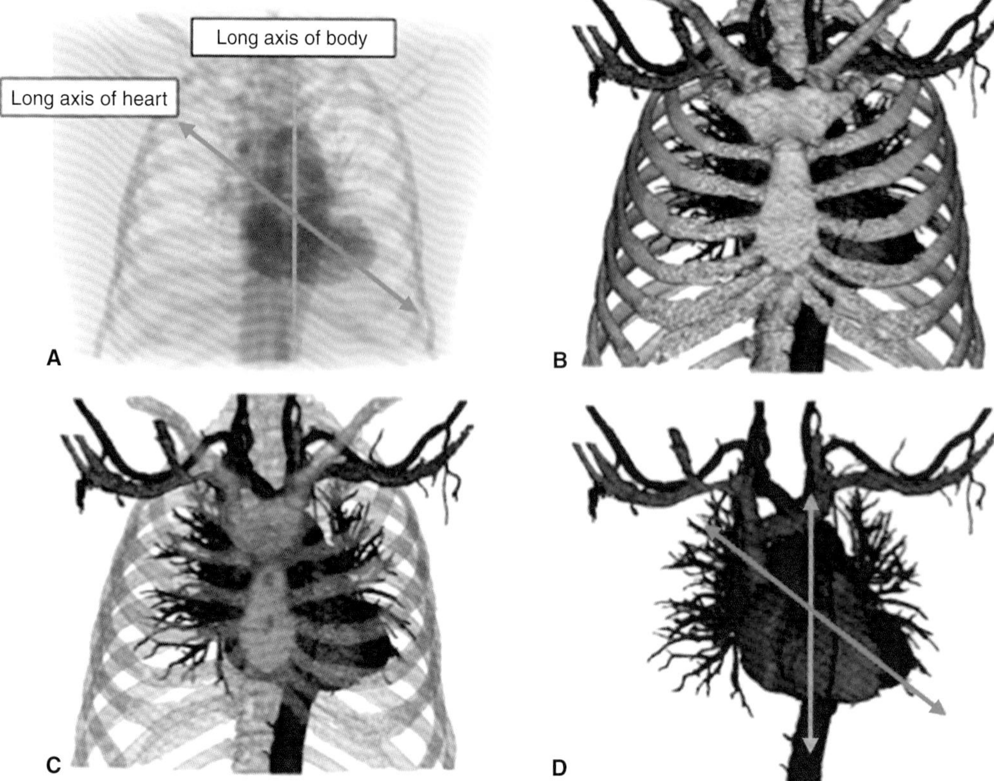

Figure 2-5. Attitudinally correct cardiac anatomy. Note that the body is in the standard anatomical position. The left side of the heart represented in *red* color, while the right side is in *blue*. **A:** Fluoroscopic reconstruction of an AP x-ray view of the chest. **B:** Full reconstruction of the heart with major vessels and rib cage. **C:** Transparent view of the chest. **D:** Anatomical reconstruction with representative heart and boxy axis noted. (Courtesy of Center for CardioVascular Innovation, University of Washington.)

The long axis of the heart is directed obliquely, leftward, downward, and forward (Fig. 2-5). Any factor that changes the shape of the thorax changes the position of the heart and modifies its directional axis. Respiratory alterations in the diaphragm and the rib cage constantly cause small changes in the cardiac axis. With a deep inspiration, the heart descends and becomes more vertical. Factors that may cause long-term axis variations in healthy people include age, weight, pregnancy, body shape, and thorax shape. A tall, thin person usually has a more vertical heart, whereas a short, obese person usually has a more horizontal heart. Pathologic conditions of the heart, lungs, abdominal organs, and other structures influence the cardiac axis.

The base of the heart, located at the level of the 3rd costal cartilage, is the superior surface to which the great veins (superior and inferior vena cava) and the great arteries (aorta and pulmonary trunk) are attached. The apex is the inferior tip of the heart and lies just to the left of the sternum between the 4th and 5th ribs near their articulation with the costal cartilages. The right side of the heart is deflected anteriorly and the left side is deflected posteriorly.

EXTERNAL SURFACE OF THE HEART

Pericardial Membranes

The layers of the heart wall are comprised of three layers (Fig. 2-6): pericardium, myocardium, and endocardium. Described later in the chapter are myocardium, the muscular layer, and endocardium, the innermost layer of the heart wall. This section describes the pericardium and its sublayers, which cover the surface of the heart.

Pericardium

The *pericardium* is the membrane that directly surrounds the heart and the roots of the great vessels (Figs. 2-7 and 2-8). The pericardium consists of two distinct sublayers, the outer *fibrous pericardium* and the inner *serous pericardium*. The fibrous pericardium is tough, dense connective tissue that protects the heart and maintains its position in the thorax. The serous pericardium consists of two layers: the *parietal pericardium*, which is fused to the fibrous pericardium, and the inner *visceral pericardium*, or *epicardium*, which is fused to the heart and is part of the heart wall. The pericardial membrane extends beyond the serous pericardium and is attached by ligaments and loose connections to the sternum, diaphragm, and structures in the posterior mediastinum.

The pericardium helps to retard ventricular dilation, helps to hold the heart in position, and forms a barrier to the spread of infections and neoplasia. Pathophysiologic conditions such as cardiac bleeding or an exudate-producing pericarditis may lead to a sudden or large accumulation of fluid within the pericardial sac. This may impede ventricular filling. From 50 to 300 mL of pericardial fluid may accumulate without serious ventricular impairment. When greater volumes accumulate, ventricular filling is impaired; this condition is known as cardiac tamponade. If the fluid accumulation builds slowly, the ventricles may be able to

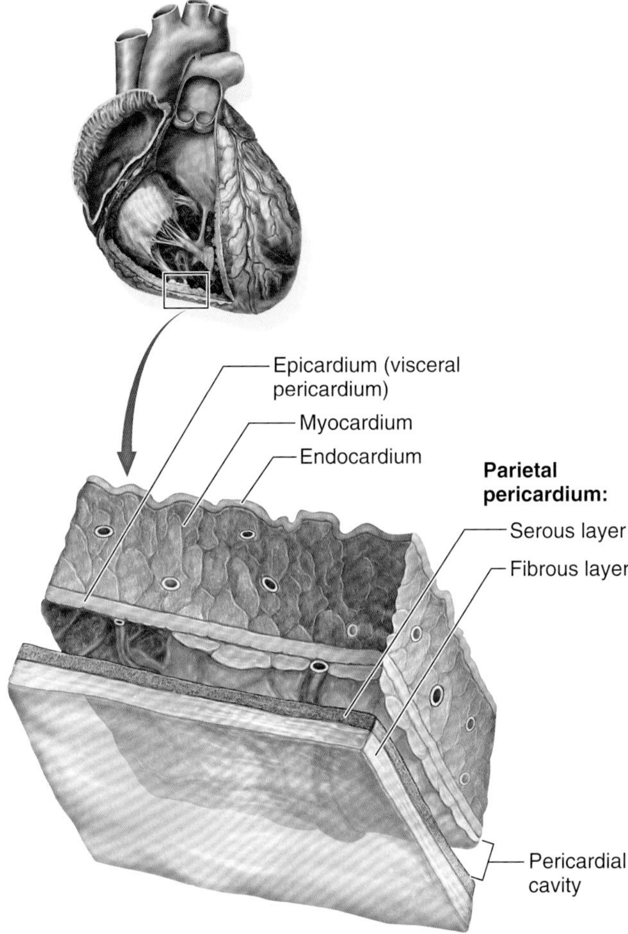

Figure 2-6. Heart membranes and heart wall. The **upper** diagram is a sectioned heart, provided to show the location of the heart membranes and wall. The **lower** diagram illustrates the pericardium and the layers of the heart wall: from exterior to interior, the parietal pericardium, visceral pericardium or epicardium, myocardium, and endocardium.

maintain an adequate cardiac output (CO) by contracting more vigorously. The pericardium is histologically similar to pleural and peritoneal serous membranes, so inflammation of all three membranes may occur with certain systemic conditions such as rheumatoid arthritis.

Epicardium

The epicardium completely encloses the external surface of the heart and extends several centimeters along each great vessel, encircling the aorta and pulmonary artery together. It merges with the tunica adventitia of the great vessels, at which point it doubles back on itself as the parietal pericardium. This continuous membrane thus forms the *pericardial sac* and encloses a potential space, the pericardial cavity. The *pericardial cavity*, which lies between the pericardium and the epicardium, usually contains 10 to 30 mL of thin, clear serous fluid.

Visceral serous membranes that surround other organs of the body are microscopic; however, the epicardium is not a microscopic but macroscopic layer that consists of a simple squamous epithelium called *mesothelium*, which is reinforced with loose areolar connective tissue that attaches to the pericardium. This mesothelium secretes the lubricating serous fluid that fills the pericardial cavity and protects the moving surfaces of the heart, reducing friction as the heart contracts. Branches of the coronary blood and lymph vessels, nerves, and fat are enclosed in the epicardium and the superficial layers of the myocardium.

Surfaces of the Heart

The surfaces of the heart (Figs. 2-9 and 2-10) are used to reference its position in relation to other structures and to describe the location of damage, as in a myocardial infarction.

The right ventricle and parts of the right atrium and the left ventricle form the sternocostal or *anterior cardiac surface* (see Fig. 2-9A,B). The right atrium and ventricle lie anteriorly and to the right of the left atrium and ventricle in the frontal plane. Thus, when viewed from the front of the body, the heart appears to be lying sideways, directed forward and leftward, with the right heart foremost. The small portion of the lower left ventricle that extends anteriorly forms a blunt tip composed of the apical part of the interventricular septum and the left ventricular free wall. Because of the forward tilt of the heart, movement of this apex portion of the left ventricle during cardiac contraction usually forms the *point of maximal impulse*, which can be observed in healthy people in the 5th intercostal space at the left midclavicular line, 7 to 9 cm from midline. The sternum, costal cartilages of the 3rd to 6th ribs, part of the lungs, and, in children, the thymus, overlie the anterior cardiac surface.

The left atrium and a small section of the right atrium and ventricle comprise the base of the heart, which is directed backward and forms the *posterior cardiac surface* (see Fig. 2-9C,D). The thoracic aorta, esophagus, and vertebrae are posterior to the heart. The inferior or diaphragmatic surface of the heart, composed chiefly of the left ventricle, lies almost horizontally on the upper surface of the diaphragm (see Fig. 2-9C,D). The right ventricle forms a portion of the *inferior cardiac surface.*

The right atrium forms the lateral *right heart border* (see Fig. 2-9A,B); therefore, the right atrium and right lung lie close together. The entire right margin of the heart extends laterally from the superior vena cava along the right atrium and then toward the diaphragm to the cardiac apex. The lateral wall of the left ventricle and a small part of the left atrium form most of the *left heart border* (see Fig. 2-9A,B). This portion of the left ventricle is next to the left lung and sometimes is referred to as the *pulmonary surface.*

Sulci

Prominent on the superior surface of the heart is a series of fat-filled grooves, each of which is referred to as a *sulcus.* Major coronary blood vessels are located in these sulci. The deep *coronary sulcus*, also called the *atrioventricular (AV) sulcus*, is the external landmark denoting the separation of the atria from the ventricles (see Fig. 2-9B–D). The AV sulcus encircles the heart obliquely and contains coronary blood vessels, cardiac nerves, and epicardial fat. The aorta and pulmonary artery interrupt the AV sulcus anteriorly. Two additional sulci lie more shallowly than the coronary sulcus and are located between the left and right ventricles: *anterior and posterior interventricular sulci* separate the right and left ventricles on the external heart surface. The *crux* of the heart is the point on the external posterior heart surface where the posterior interventricular sulcus intersects the coronary (AV) sulcus externally and where the interatrial septum joins the interventricular septum internally.

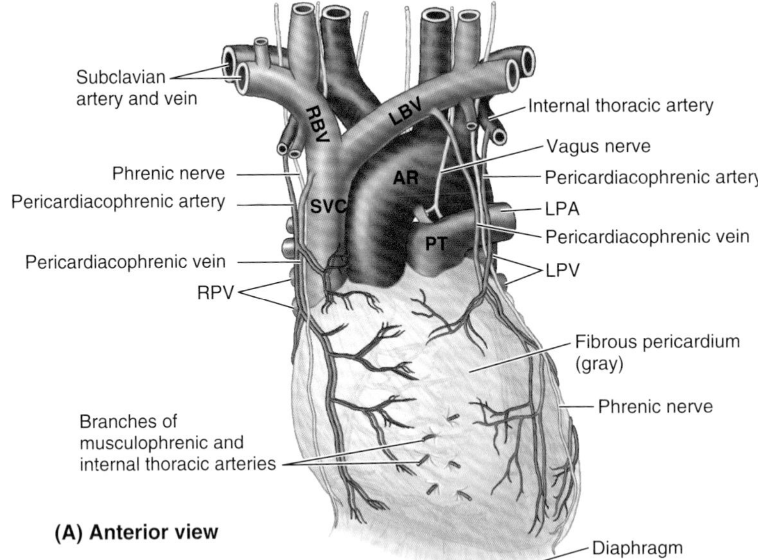

Figure 2-7. Pericardium. **A:** Arterial supply and venous drainage. **B:** Interior of pericardial sac, after removal of the heart. A, aorta; AR, arch of aorta; IVC, inferior vena cava; LBV, left brachiocephalic vein; LPA, left pulmonary artery; LPV, left pulmonary vein; PT, pulmonary trunk; RBV, right brachiocephalic vein; RPV, right pulmonary vein; SVC, superior vena cava. (Used with permission from Moore KL, Dalley II AF, Agur AMR. *Clinically Oriented Anatomy*. 8th ed. Philadelphia PA: Wolters Kluwer; 2017.)

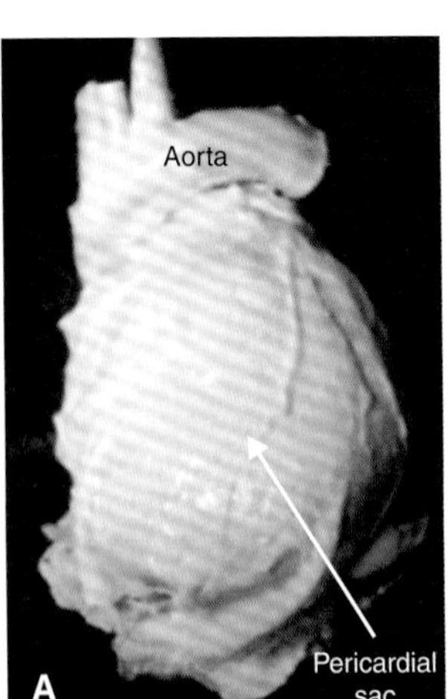

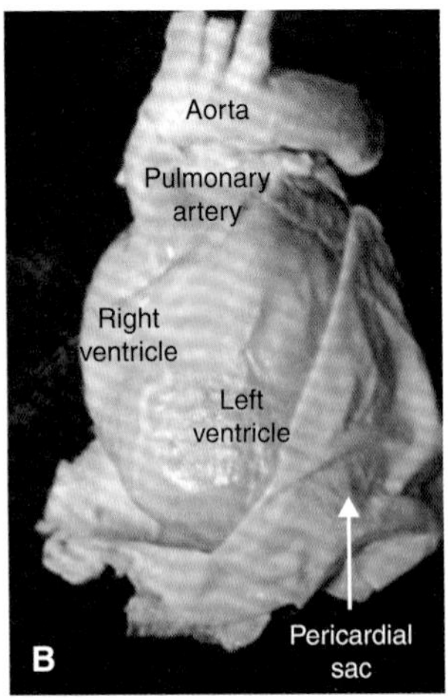

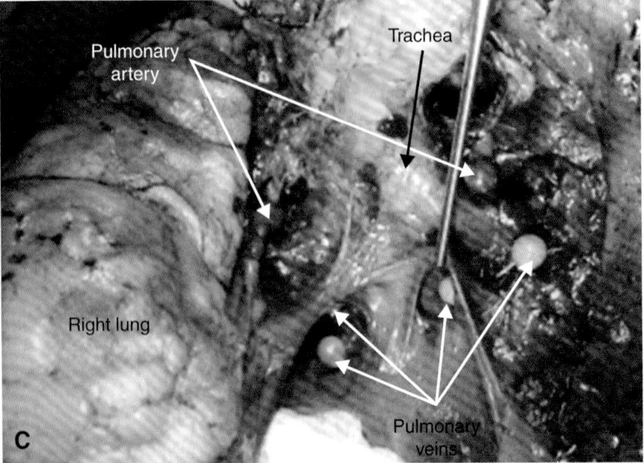

Figure 2-8. Anterior view of the heart and chest cavity behind the heart. **A:** Heart with pericardial sac intact. **B:** Heart with pericardial sac removed with view of the anterior surface of the heart. **C:** Posterior chest cavity with heart removed. Openings to pulmonary veins (*red dots*) and pulmonary artery (*blue dots*). (Courtesy of Center for CardioVascular Innovation, University of Washington.)

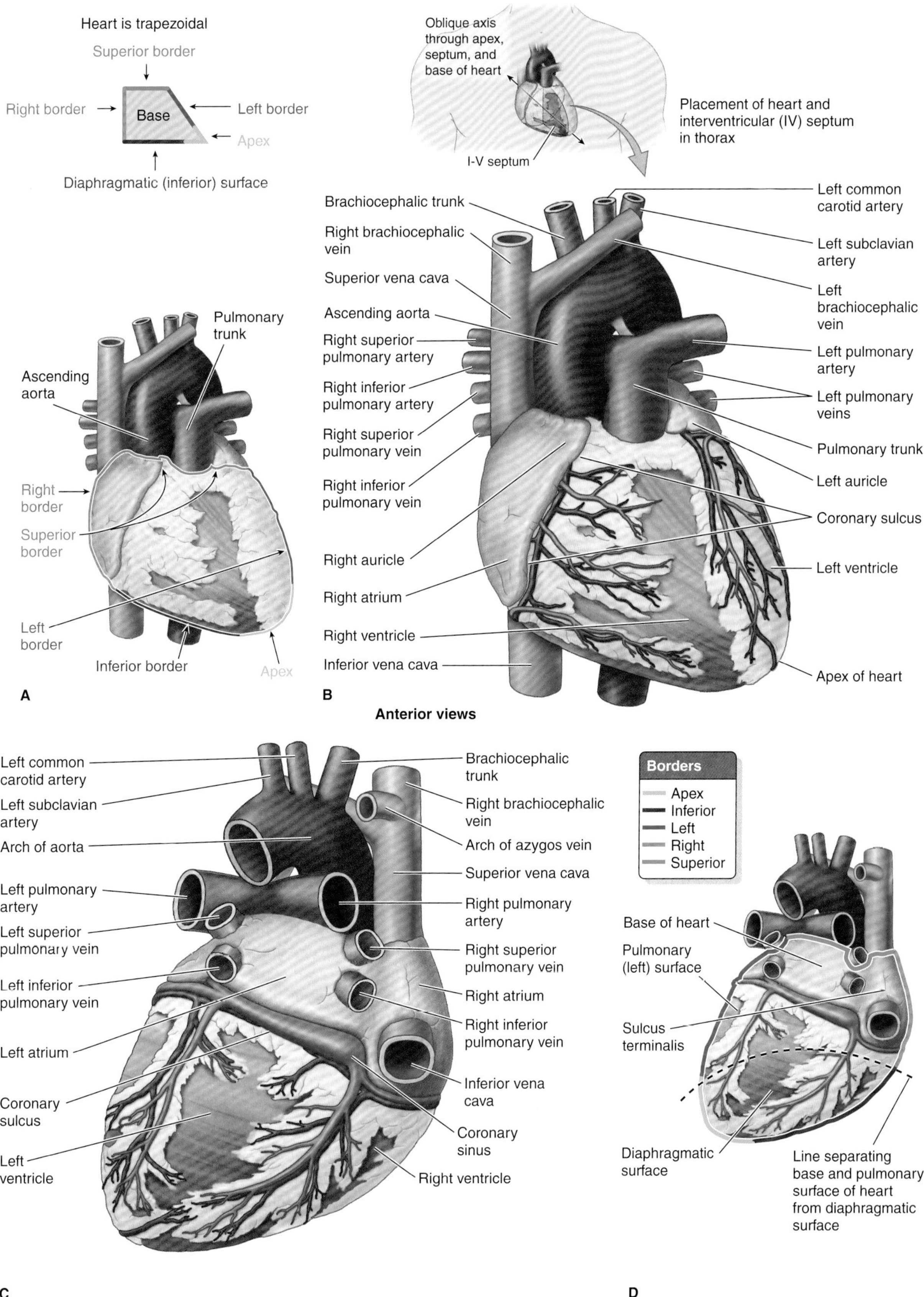

Figure 2-9. Shape, orientation, surfaces, and borders of heart. **A, B:** The sternocostal surface of the heart and the relationship of the great vessels are shown. The ventricles dominate this surface (two thirds right ventricle, one third left ventricle). **C, D:** The pulmonary (**left**) and diaphragmatic (inferior) surfaces and the base of the heart are shown as well as the relationship of the great vessels.

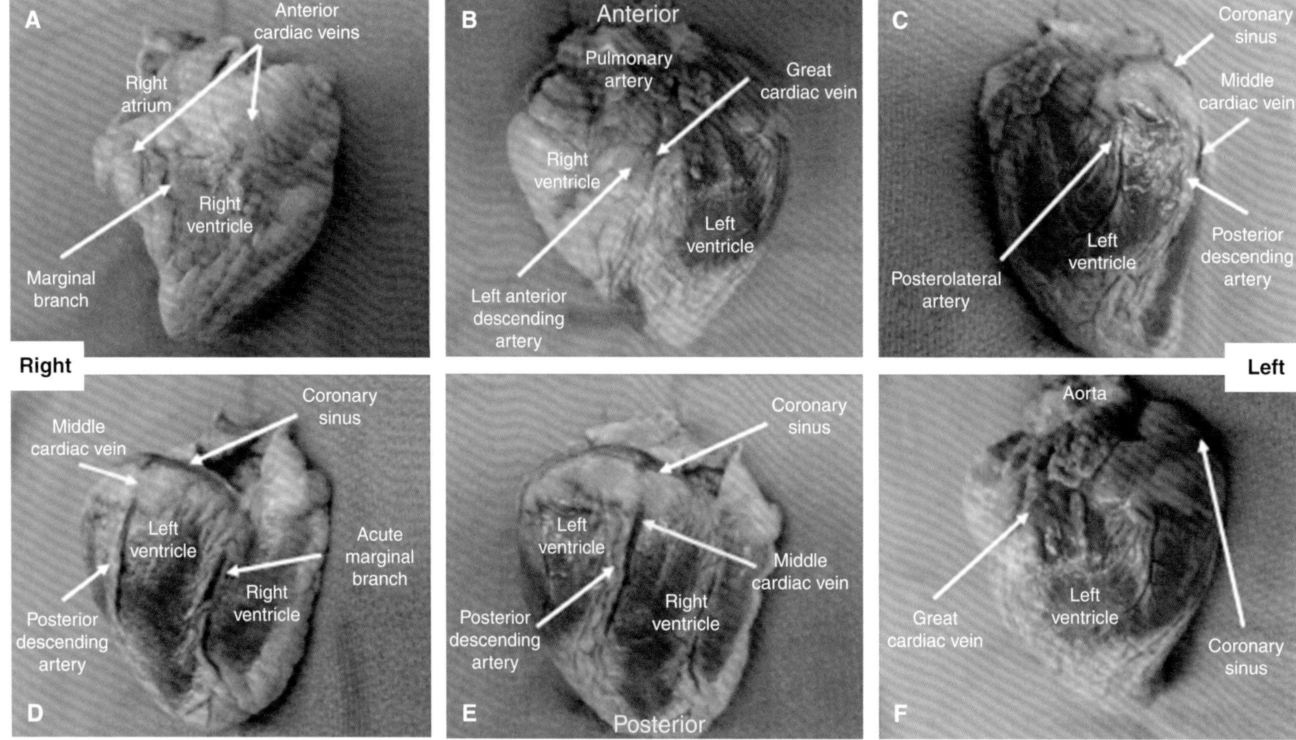

Figure 2-10. Shape, orientation, surfaces of the heart. Representative views of the heart from anterior and posterior, in addition to left to right perspective of the heart. **A:** Anterior and right-side view of the heart. **B:** Anterior view of the heart. **C:** Anterior and left-side view of the heart. **D:** Posterior and right-side view of the heart. **E:** Posterior view of the heart. **F:** Posterior and left-side view of the heart. (Courtesy of Center for CardioVascular Innovation, University of Washington.)

INTERNAL STRUCTURES OF THE HEART

Septa

Septum, derived from the Latin for "something that encloses," refers to a partition or wall that divides the heart into chambers. The septa are extensions of the myocardium, lined with endocardium. The heart has three septa.

The *interatrial septum* is located between right and left atria and extends obliquely forward from right to left. The lower portion of the interatrial septum is comprised of the lower medial right atrial wall on one side and the aortic outflow tract of the left ventricular wall on the other side. In the normal adult heart, the interatrial septum an oval-shaped depression called the *fossa ovalis*, a remnant of an opening in the fetal heart known as the *foramen ovale*. In the fetal heart, the foramen ovale allows blood to pass directly from the right to the left atrium thereby allowing some blood to bypass the pulmonary circuit. The *septum primum*, a flap of tissue that previously acted as a valve, closes the foramen ovale within seconds after birth, and establishes the typical cardiac circulation pattern. Autopsy studies have found that the prevalence of patent foramen ovale in adults is up to 30%; with aging, prevalence decreases and size increases.[6] This is clinically significant, providing a potential conduit for a shunt from the right atrium to the left atrium and accounting for increased risk of stroke[7] and migraine headache.[8]

The *interventricular septum* lies between the two ventricles. This septum is normally intact after its formation during fetal development. As the ventricles generate greater pressure than the atria during contraction, the interventricular septum is substantially thicker than the interatrial septum. The lower muscular portion of the interventricular septum extends downward from the upper membranous part of the interventricular septum.

The *AV septum* lies between the atria and ventricles. This septum is marked by the presence of four openings that allow blood to move from the atria into the ventricles and from the ventricles into the pulmonary trunk and the aorta. Located in each of these openings between the atria and ventricles is a valve that ensures the one-way flow of blood. Because these openings structurally weaken the AV septum, tissue is reinforced with dense connective tissue known as the cardiac fibrous skeleton.

Fibrous Skeleton

The *fibrous skeleton* (Fig. 2-11) is the internal support structure of the heart, formed of connective tissue and oriented obliquely within the mediastinum. The fibrous skeleton divides the atria from the ventricles, frames the membranous portions of the cardiac septa, encircles the four valves, and provides the attachment site for some of the atrial and ventricular cardiac muscle fibers.

Four rings of dense connective tissue (*annuli fibrosi*) surround the cardiac valves: two rings encircle the AV valves; two "coronets" encircle the semilunar valves and extend to the origins of the aorta and the pulmonary trunk. Occupying the central position of the fibrous skeleton is the aortic valve; the other valve annuli are attached to it. The triangular formation between the aortic

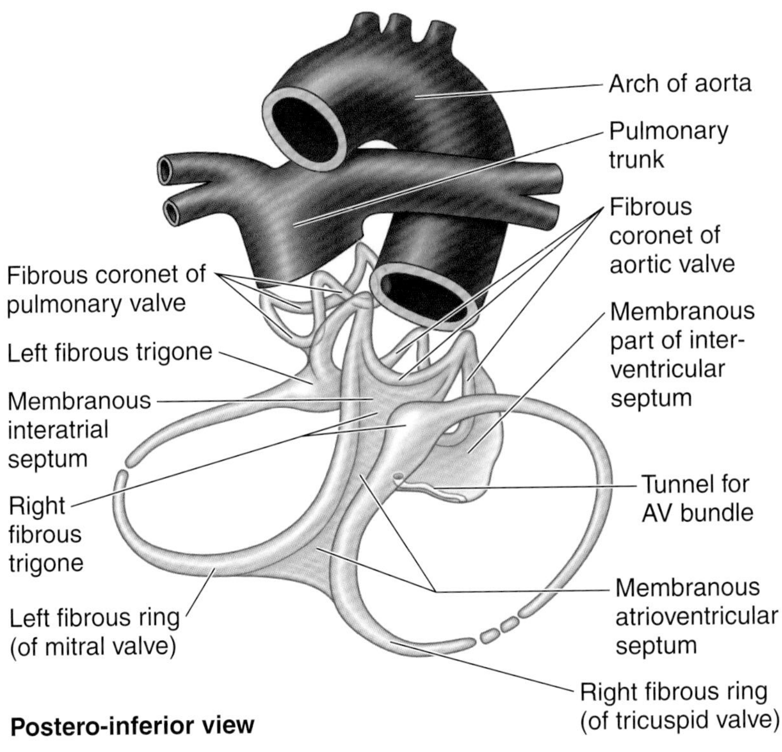

Figure 2-11. Fibrous skeleton of heart. (Used with permission from Moore KL, Dalley II AF, Agur AMR. *Clinically Oriented Anatomy*. 8th ed. Philadelphia, PA: Wolters Kluwer; 2017.)

valve and the medial parts of the tricuspid and mitral valve is the *right fibrous trigone*, which is the area of largest thickening and strongest portion of the cardiac skeleton. The right fibrous trigone links the aortic, mitral, and tricuspid valves and the membranous septi. Together the right fibrous trigone and membranous septum form the *central fibrous body*. The membranous interventricular septum is an inferior extension of the central fibrous body that attaches to the muscular interventricular septum. The membranous septum is crossed on its right aspect by the attachment of the tricuspid valve, dividing the septum into AV and interventricular components. The *left fibrous trigone* is a collagenous thickening of the most inferior aspect of the fibrous skeleton, attached to the noncoronary leaflet (posterior) of the aortic valve and the anterior leaflet of the mitral valve. The *intervalvular fibrous body,* also known as the *aortomitral curtain* or the aortomitral continuity, is a fibrous sheet between the noncoronary and left coronary leaflets of the aortic valve and the anterior leaflet of the mitral valve.[9] The intervalvular fibrous body is attached by the right and left fibrous trigones to the left ventricular myocardium.[10] These key fibrous structures are seen in Figure 2-12. A tendinous band, known as the *tendon of the conus arteriosus,* extends superiorly from the right AV fibrous ring, and connects the posterior surface of the conus arteriosus of the right ventricle to the aorta.

Chambers

The wall thickness of each of the four cardiac chambers reflects the amount of force generated by that chamber. The two thin-walled atria serve functionally as reservoirs and conduits for blood that is being funneled into the ventricles; they add a small amount of force to the moving blood. The left ventricle, which adds the greatest amount of energy to the flowing blood, is two to three times as thick as the right ventricle. The approximate normal wall thicknesses of the chambers are as follows: right atrium, 2 mm; right ventricle, 3 to 5 mm; left atrium, 3 mm; and left ventricle, 13 to 15 mm.

Cardiac circulation is comprised of two circuits: the pulmonary circulation including the right side of the heart and the arterial circulation including the left side of the heart (Fig. 2-13). It is useful to remember that the internal surfaces of the cardiac chambers affect blood flow and turbulence, that is, blood flows more smoothly and with less turbulence across walls that are smooth rather than ridged. Blood pools in atrial appendages (auricles) or other areas out of the direct path of blood flow.

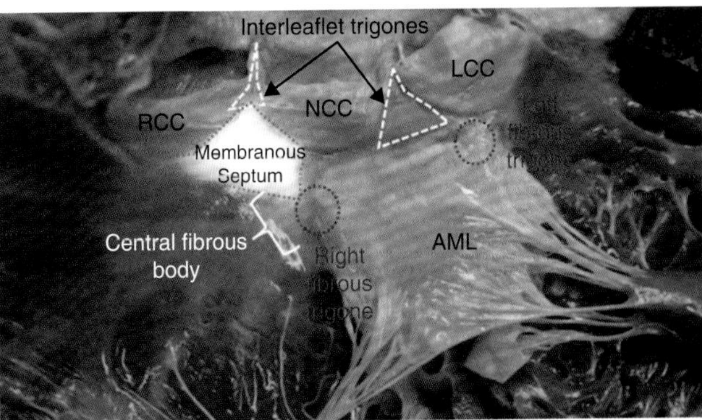

Figure 2-12. Fibrous continuities. This image of the aortic root opened from the left ventricle shows the fibrous continuities between the interleaflet triangles, the fibrous trigones, and the membranous septum. Note how the ends of the area of fibrous continuity between the aortic leaflet of the mitral valve and the noncoronary (NCC) and left coronary (LCC) leaflets of the aortic valve anchor the aortic-mitral curtain in the roof of the left ventricle. The ends of the area of fibrous continuity are the left and right fibrous trigones. As can be seen, the right fibrous trigone is itself continuous with the membranous septum, the conjoined are being known as the central fibrous body. RCC, right coronary cusp; AML, anterior mitral leaflet. (Courtesy of Center for CardioVascular Innovation, University of Washington.)

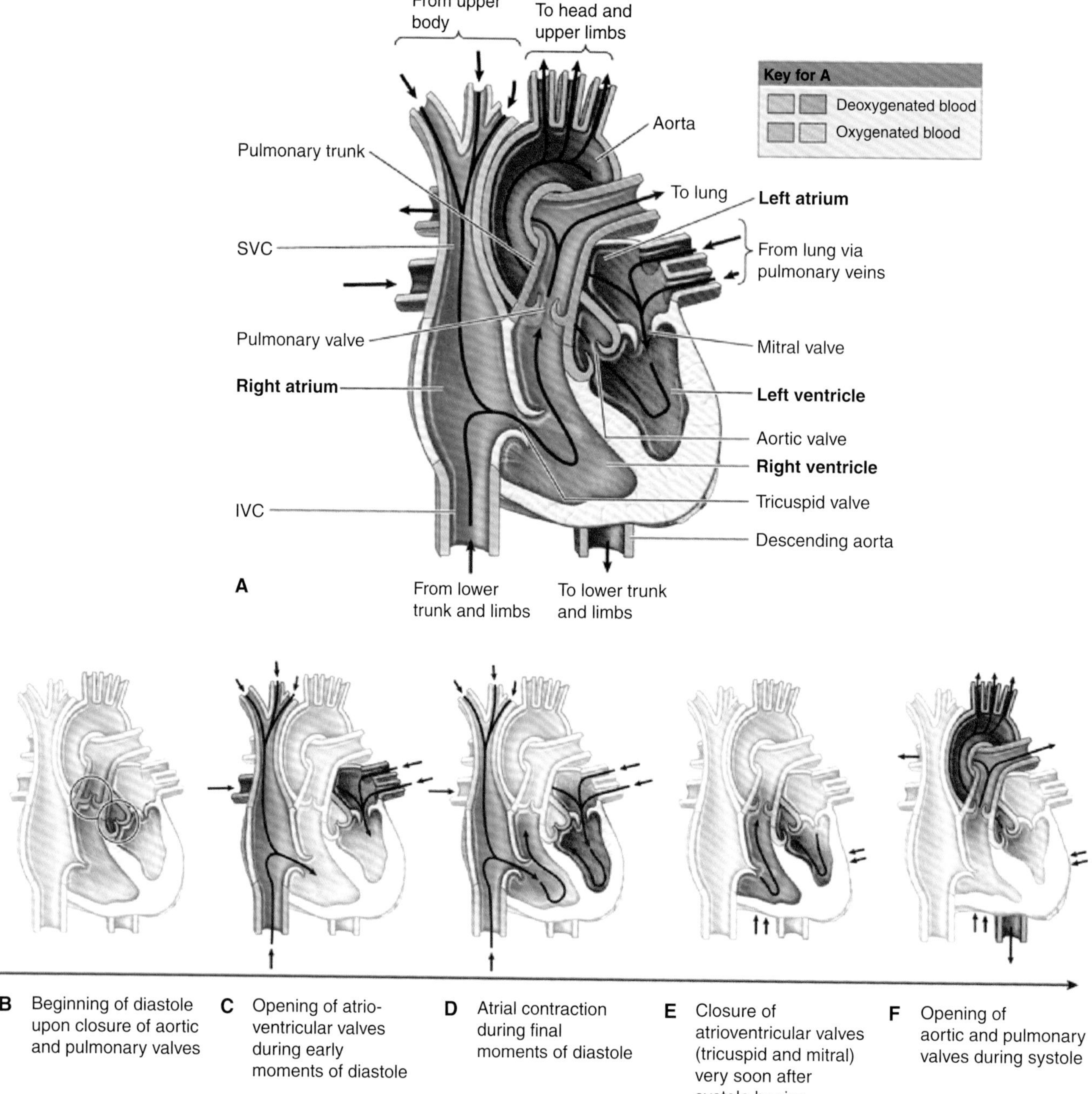

Figure 2-13. Blood flow through cardiac chambers and valves. **A:** Circulation of blood through the heart. The right heart (*blue side*) is the pump for the pulmonary circuit; the left heart (*red side*) is the pump for the systemic circuit. **B–F:** Stages of cardiac cycle. The cardiac cycle describes the complete movement of the heart or heartbeat and includes the period from the beginning of one heartbeat to the beginning of the next one. The cycle consists of diastole (ventricular relaxation and filling) and systole (ventricular contraction and emptying). (Used with permission from Moore KL, Dalley II AF, Agur AMR. *Clinically Oriented Anatomy*. 8th ed. Philadelphia, PA: Wolters Kluwer; 2017.)

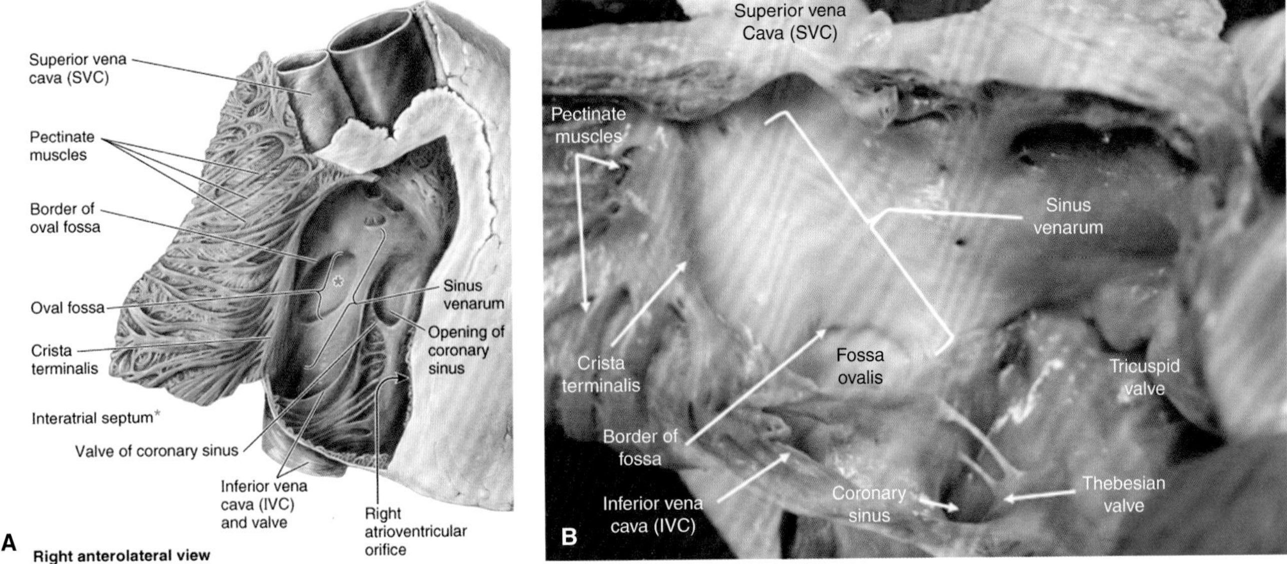

Figure 2-14. Interior of the right atrium. **A:** Schematic of the right atrium. (Used with permission from Moore KL, Dalley II AF, Agur AMR. *Clinically Oriented Anatomy*. 8th ed. Philadelphia, PA: Wolters Kluwer; 2017.) **B:** Right atrium has been dissected open along the atrioventricular groove. (Courtesy of Center for CardioVascular Innovation, University of Washington.)

Right Heart

The right atrium (Fig. 2-14) is smaller than the left atrium, and shaped like an irregular ellipsoid except for the right atrial appendage (auricle), which arises anteriorly. It is smooth at the posterior and septal walls, whereas the lateral wall and the right atrial appendage have parallel muscular ridges, termed *pectinate muscles.* The right auricle extends over the aortic root externally. The tricuspid valve forms the inferior wall of the right atrium and part of the superior wall of the right ventricle.

The right ventricle (Fig. 2-15) is lined anteriorly and inferiorly with *trabeculae carneae*; these muscle bundles form a rough-walled inflow tract for blood. One muscle group, the *septomarginal trabecula* or *moderator band,* extends from the lower interventricular septum to the anterior right ventricular papillary muscle. Another thick muscle bundle, the *crista supraventricularis,* extends from the septal wall to the anterolateral wall of the right ventricle. The crista supraventricularis helps to divide the right ventricle into an inflow and outflow tract. The smooth-walled outflow tract, called the *conus arteriosus* or *infundibulum,* extends to the pulmonary artery.

The concave free wall of the right ventricle is attached to the slightly convex septal wall. The internal right ventricular cavity is crescent or triangle shaped. The right ventricle also forms a crescent laterally around the left ventricle. Right ventricular contraction causes the right ventricular free wall to move toward the interventricular septum. This bellows-like action is effective in ejecting large and variable volumes into a low-pressure system.

Venous blood enters the right atrium from the upper and the lower posterior parts of the atrium through the superior and inferior venae cavae. Most of the venous drainage from the heart enters the right atrium through the *coronary sinus,* which is located between the entrance of the inferior vena cava into the right atrium and the orifice of the tricuspid valve. Blood flows medially and anteriorly from the right atrium through the tricuspid orifice into the right ventricle. Blood enters the right ventricle in an almost horizontal but slightly leftward, anterior, and inferior direction. The right ventricular outflow tract (RVOT) is tubular and extends from the *crista terminalis* to the pulmonary valve, which is usually referred to as part of the RVOT. Blood is ejected superiorly and posteriorly through the pulmonary valve.

Left Heart

The left atrium (Fig. 2-16) is a cuboid structure that lies between the aortic root and the esophagus. The left atrial appendage (auricle) extends along the border of the pulmonary artery. The walls of the left atrium are smooth except for pectinate muscle bundles in the highly trabeculated left atrial appendage.

The left ventricle (Figs. 2-16 and 2-17) has a cone-like or oval shape, bordered by the generally concave left ventricular free wall and interventricular septum. The mitral valve and its attachments form the left ventricular inflow tract. The outflow tract is formed by the anterior surface of the anterior mitral valve cusp, the septum, and the aortic vestibule. The lower muscular interventricular septum and free walls of the left ventricle are deeply ridged with trabeculae carneae muscle bundles, so most of the interior surface of the ventricle is rough. The upper membranous septum and aortic vestibule region have smooth walls. The interventricular septum is functionally and anatomically a more integral part of the left ventricle than the right ventricle. The septum is triangular, with its base at the aortic area. The upper septum separates the right atrium from the left ventricle and is often called the *AV septum.*

Blood is ejected from the left ventricle mainly by circumferential contraction of the muscular wall, that is, by decreasing the diameter of the cylinder. There is some longitudinal shortening. The ventricular cavity has a small surface area in relation to the volume contained, but high pressure can be developed because of

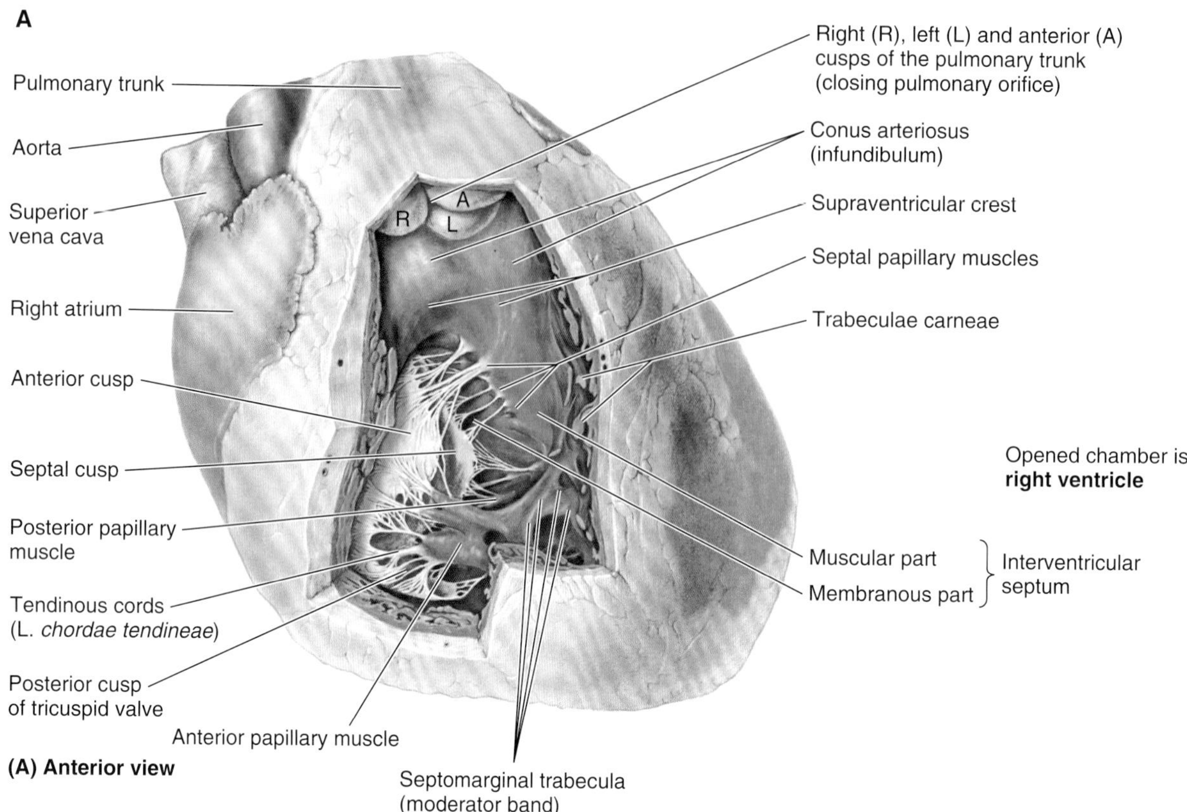

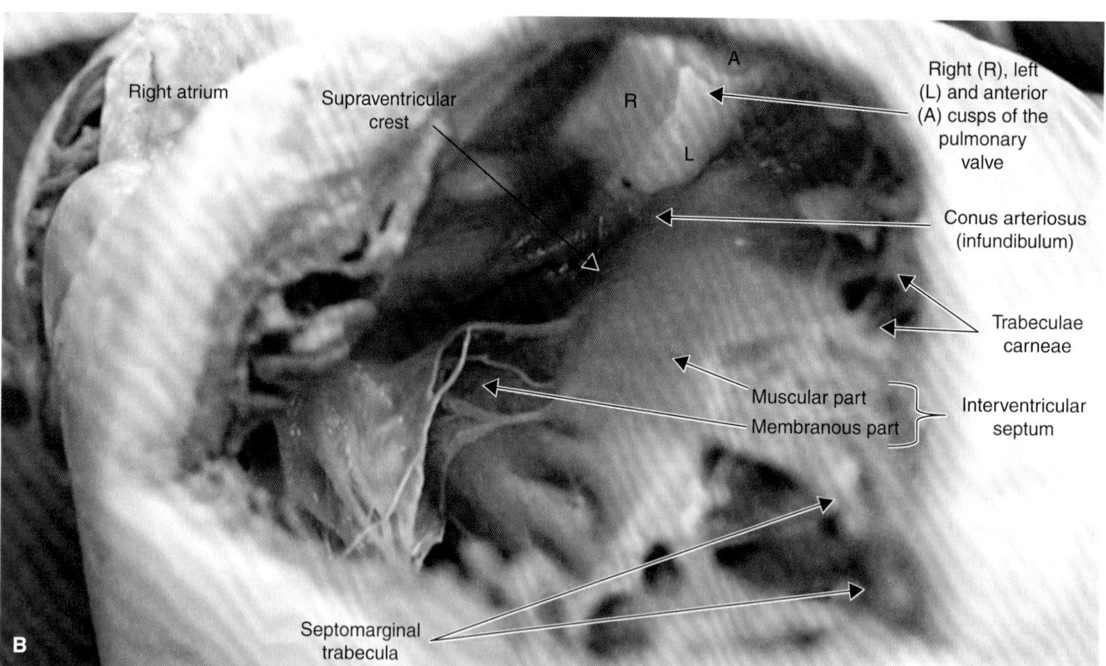

Figure 2-15. Interior of right ventricle. **A:** Schematic of the right ventricle. The *tricuspid valve* at the entrance to the ventricle (right atrioventricular [AV] orifice) is open and the pulmonic valve at the exit to the pulmonary trunk is closed, as they would be during ventricular filling (diastole). The smooth funnel-shaped *conus arteriosus is* the outflow tract of the chamber. L, Latin. (Used with permission from Moore KL, Dalley II AF, Agur AMR. *Clinically Oriented Anatomy*. 8th ed. Philadelphia, PA: Wolters Kluwer; 2017.) **B:** The sternocostal wall of the right ventricle has been excised. R, right pulmonary cusp; L, left pulmonary cusp; A, anterior pulmonary cusp. (Courtesy of Center for CardioVascular Innovation, University of Washington.)

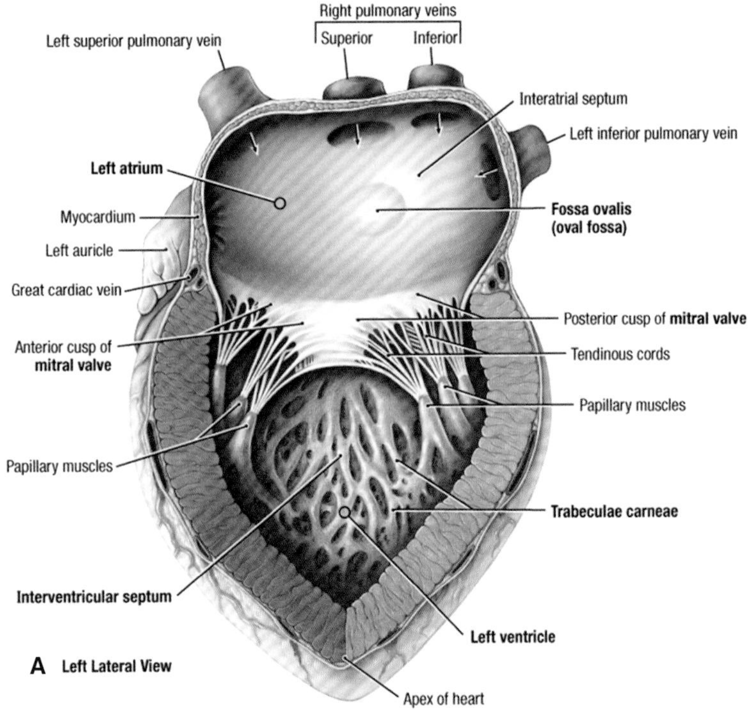

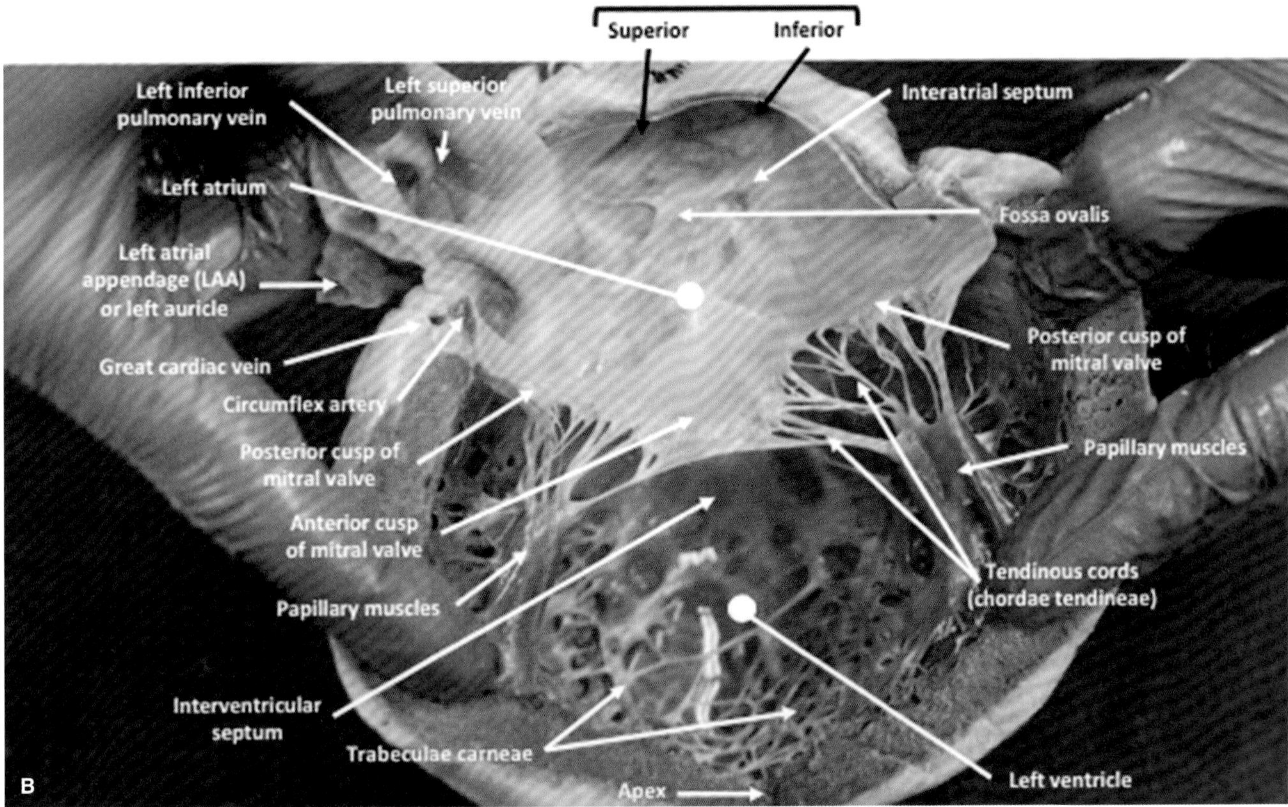

Figure 2-16. Interior of left atrium and ventricle. **A:** Schematic of the interior of left heart. (Used with permission from Moore KL, Dalley II AF, Agur AMR. *Clinically Oriented Anatomy*. 8th ed. Philadelphia, PA: Wolters Kluwer; 2017.) **B:** A diagonal cut was made from the base of the heart to the apex, passing between the left and right pulmonary veins and through the posterior cusp of the mitral valve, followed by retraction (spreading) of the left heart wall on each side of the incision. The entrances (pulmonary veins) to the left atrium are posterior, and the exit (left atrioventricular or mitral orifice) is anterior. The left side of the fossa ovalis is also seen on the left side of the interatrial septum, although the left side is not usually as distinct as the right side is within the right atrium. Except for that of the left atrial appendage (auricle), the atrial wall is smooth. (Courtesy of Center for CardioVascular Innovation, University of Washington.)

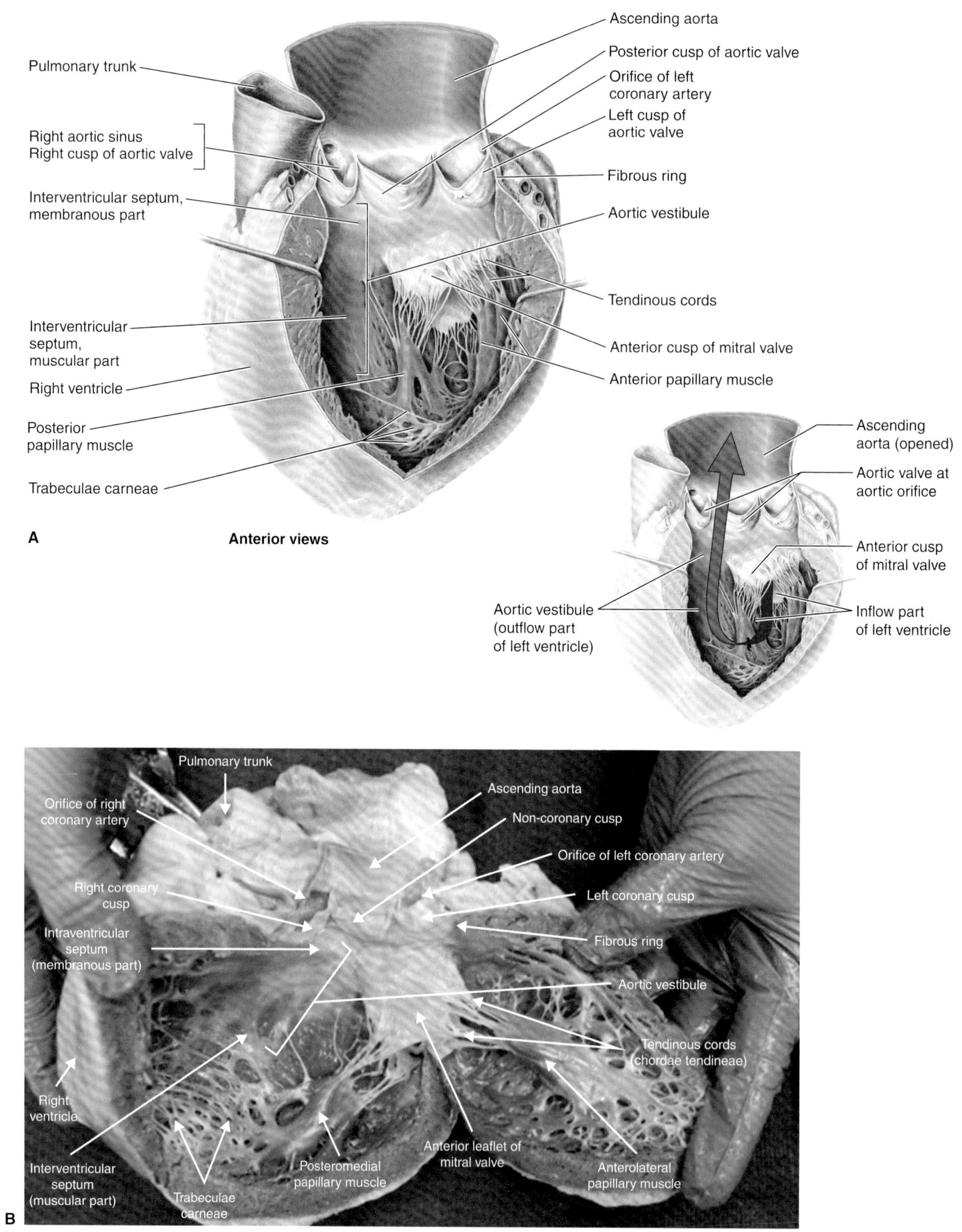

Ascending aorta
Pulmonary trunk
Posterior cusp of aortic valve
Orifice of left coronary artery
Left cusp of aortic valve
Right aortic sinus
Right cusp of aortic valve
Fibrous ring
Interventricular septum, membranous part
Aortic vestibule
Tendinous cords
Interventricular septum, muscular part
Anterior cusp of mitral valve
Right ventricle
Anterior papillary muscle
Posterior papillary muscle
Trabeculae carneae

A **Anterior views**

Ascending aorta (opened)
Aortic valve at aortic orifice
Anterior cusp of mitral valve
Aortic vestibule (outflow part of left ventricle)
Inflow part of left ventricle

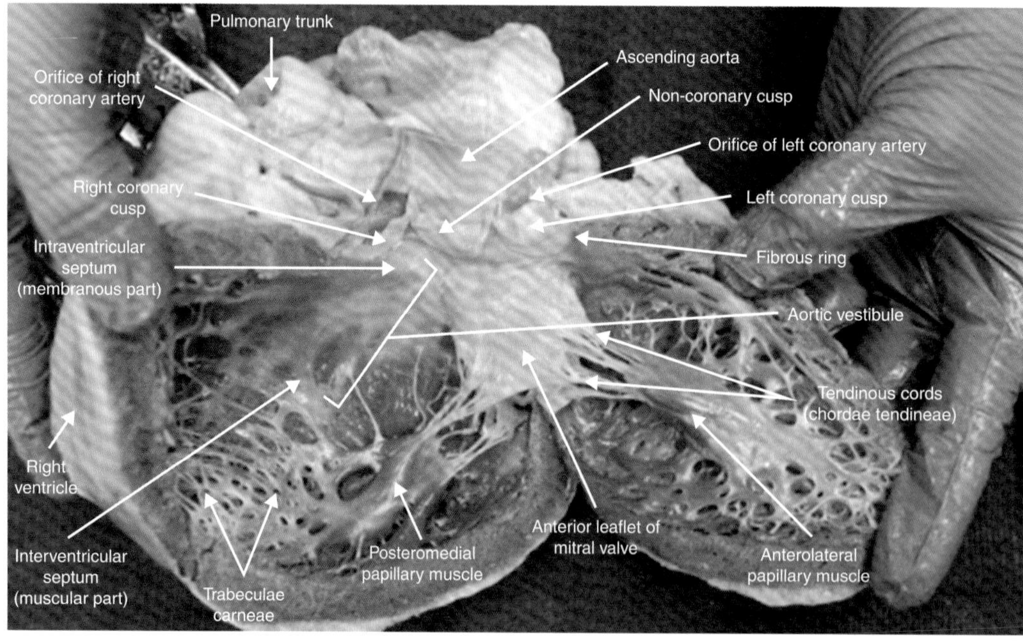

Figure 2-17. Interior and outflow tract of left ventricle of heart. **A:** Schematic of the interior of the left ventricle and outflow tract. Note that noncoronary cusp of the aortic valve is referred to as the posterior cusp. (Used with permission from Moore KL, Dalley II AF, Agur AMR. *Clinically Oriented Anatomy*. 8th ed. Philadelphia, PA: Wolters Kluwer; 2017.) **B:** The anterior surface of the left ventricle has been incised parallel to the interventricular groove, with the right margin of the incision retracted to the right, revealing an anterior view of the chamber. The left atrioventricular orifice and mitral valve are located posteriorly, and the aortic vestibule leads superiorly and to the right to the aortic valve. (Courtesy of Center for CardioVascular Innovation, University of Washington.)

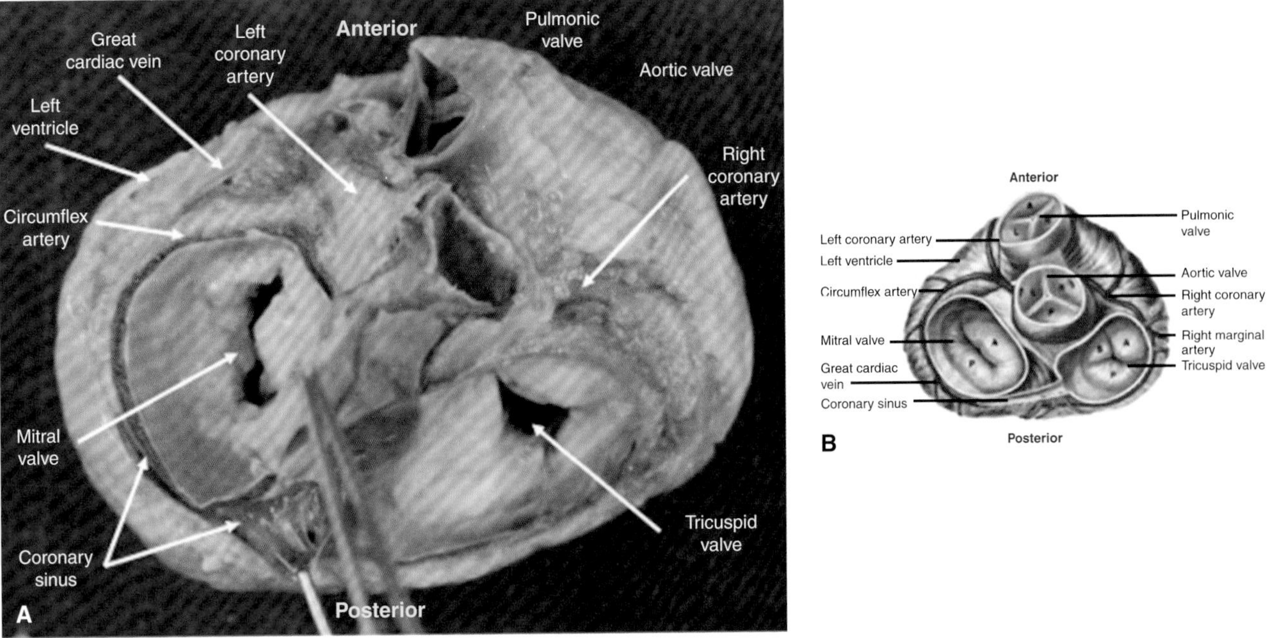

Figure 2-18. Cardiac valves. Seen in the same plane through a transverse section with the atria removed. **A:** Superior or "teapot" view of the heart. **B:** Schematic representation of the heart valves from superior view. Note that in **panel B** the noncoronary cusp of the aortic valve is referred to as (*P*), posterior. A, anterior; P, posterior; S, septal; L, lateral. (Courtesy of Center for CardioVascular Innovation, University of Washington.)

the amount of ventricular muscle, the shape of the cavity, and the way the muscles contract.

Four pulmonary veins return blood from the lungs to openings in the posterolateral wall of the left atrium. Blood is directed obliquely forward out of the left atrium and enters the left ventricle in an anterior, leftward, and inferior direction. The *left ventricular outflow tract* (LVOT) is ovoid in shape. Blood flows out of the ventricle from the apex through the LVOT and toward the aorta in a superior and rightward direction. Thus, blood flows from posterior orifices into both ventricles in a leftward direction and is ejected superiorly toward the center of the heart.

Valves

The four valves of the heart (Fig. 2-18) ensure the unidirectional flow of blood through the heart. During diastole, the AV valves open passively when pressure in the atria exceeds that in the ventricles. The papillary muscles are relaxed. The valve cusps part and project into the ventricle, forming a funnel and thus promoting blood flow into the ventricles. Each cusp of the semilunar valves bears a nodule in the midpoint of its free edge, flanked by a thin connective tissue area called the lunule. Toward the end of diastole, the deceleration of blood flowing into the ventricles, movement of blood and increasing pressures in the ventricle compared with lessening pressures in the atria causes the nodules and lunulae to meet centrally, closing the valve. Filling of the coronary arteries occurs during diastole (when ventricular walls are relaxed). During systole, the free edges of the valve cusps are prevented from being everted into the atria by contraction of the papillary muscles and tension in the chordae tendineae. Thus, in the normal heart, blood is prevented from flowing backward into the atria despite the high systolic ventricular pressures.

Atrioventricular Valves. The AV tricuspid and bicuspid (mitral) valve complexes (see Fig. 2-18) are composed of six components that function as a unit: the atria, the valve rings or annuli fibrosi of the fibrous skeleton, the valve cusps or leaflets, the chordae tendineae, the papillary muscles, and the ventricular walls. The mitral and tricuspid valve cusps are composed of fibrous connective tissue covered by endothelium. They attach to the fibrous skeleton valve rings. Fibrous cords called *chordae tendineae* connect the free valve margins and ventricular surfaces of the valve cusps to papillary muscles and ventricular walls. Each papillary muscle or muscle group controls the adjacent sides of two cusps, resisting valve prolapse during systole. The papillary muscles are bundles of trabeculae carneae oriented parallel to the ventricular walls, extending from the walls to the chordae tendineae. The chordae tendineae provide many cross-connections from one papillary muscle to the valve cusps or from trabeculae carneae in the ventricular wall directly to valves.

Tricuspid Valve. The tricuspid valve (Figs. 2-19 to 2-21) is named for its three cusps or leaflets. In the adult, the tricuspid orifice is larger (approximately 11 cm in circumference, or capable of admitting three fingers). The tricuspid valve annulus is a nonplanar shape. The combined surface area of the AV valve cusps, which resemble curtain-like, billowing flaps, is larger than the surface area of the valvular orifice.

Most commonly, there are three tricuspid valve cusps: the large *anterior*, the *septal*, and the *posterior* (inferior) *tricuspid valve leaflets*. There are usually two principal right ventricular papillary muscles, the anterior and the posterior (inferior), and a smaller set of septal (accessory) papillary muscles attached to the ventricular septum.

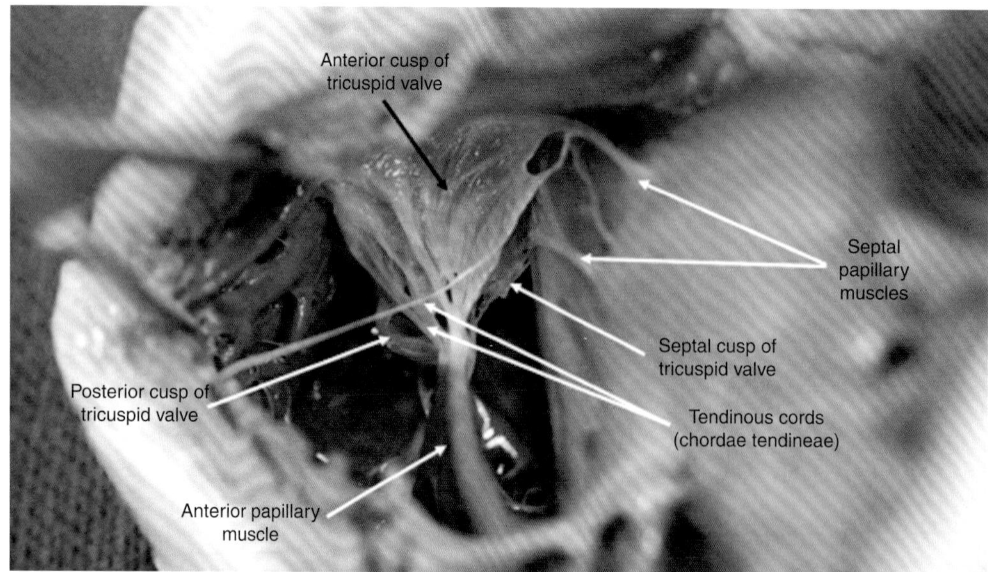

Figure 2-19. Tricuspid valve. View of the tricuspid valve from right ventricle with anterior portion of right ventricular wall removed. (Courtesy of Center for CardioVascular Innovation, University of Washington.)

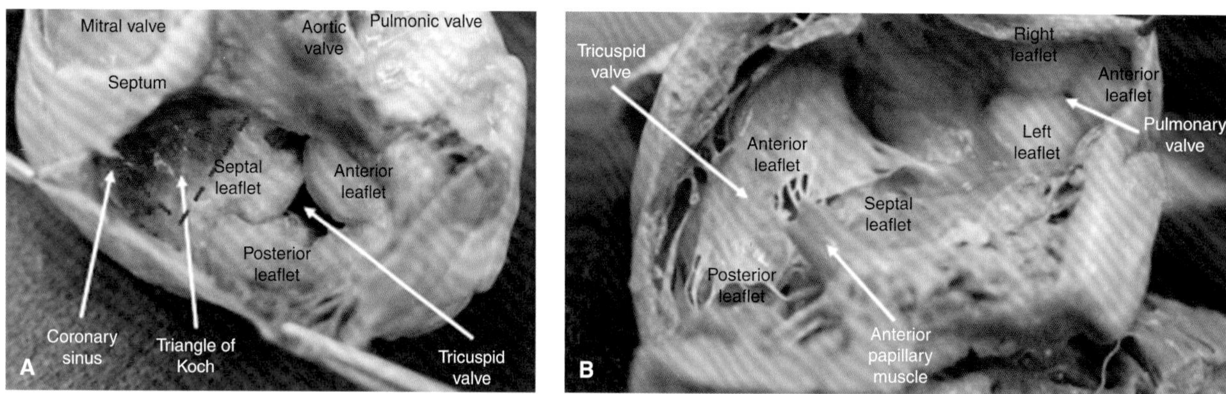

Figure 2-20. Tricuspid valve. **A:** View of tricuspid valve from right atrium. **B:** Ventricular view of the tricuspid valve. (Courtesy of Center for CardioVascular Innovation, University of Washington.)

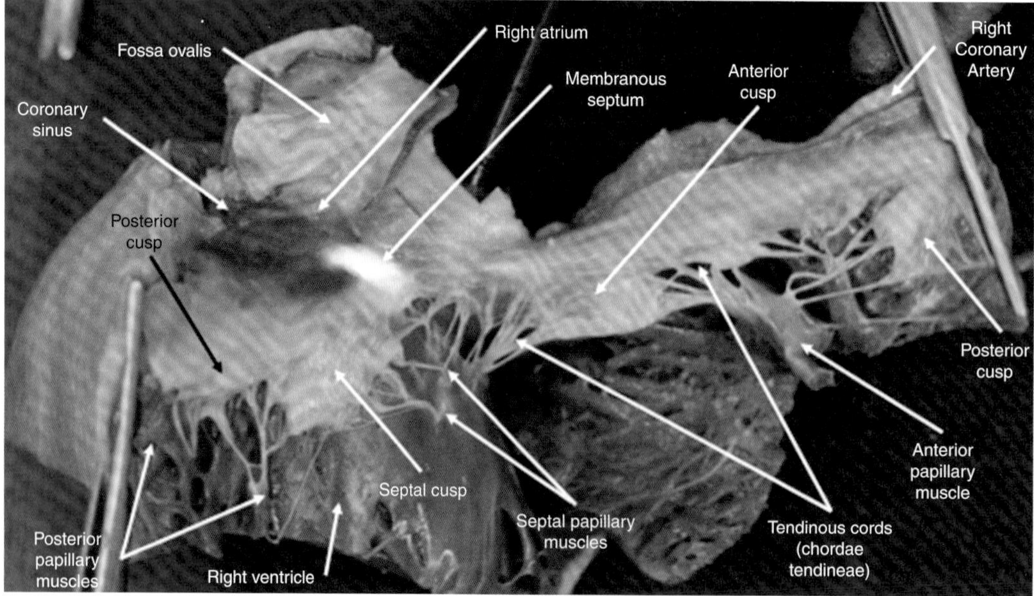

Figure 2-21. Tricuspid valve. Left atrium and ventricle have been dissected open. (Courtesy of Center for CardioVascular Innovation, University of Washington.)

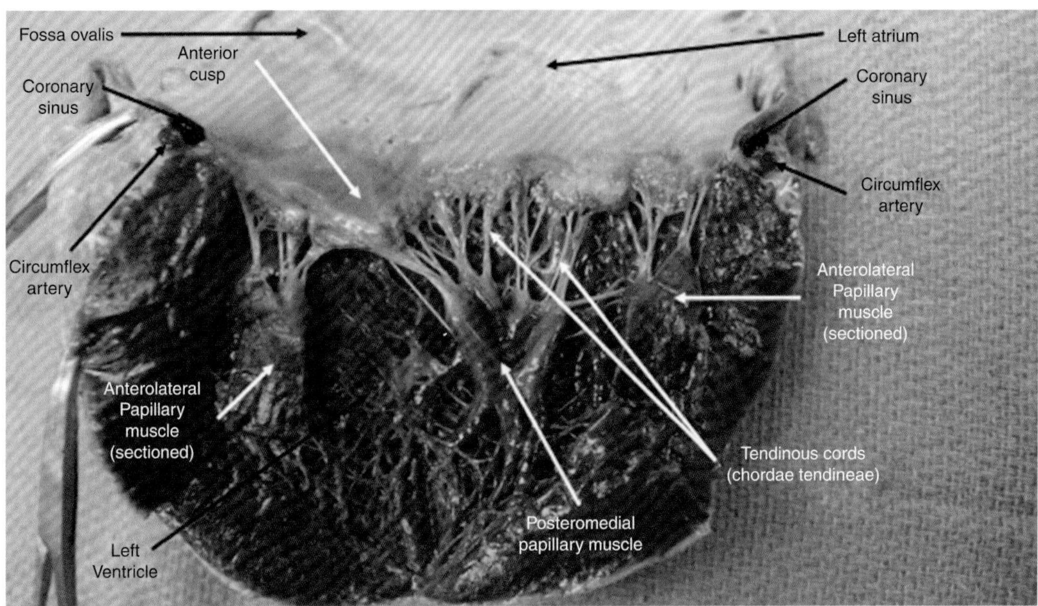

Figure 2-22. Mitral valve. Left atrium and ventricle have been dissected open. Coronary sinus (*blue*) and circumflex artery (*red*) have been injected with silicone to demonstrate their proximity to mitral valve annulus. (Courtesy of Center for CardioVascular Innovation, University of Washington.)

Mitral Valve. The bicuspid valve (Figs. 2-22 to 2-24) is named for a bishop's hat, or miter; hence the structure is called the "mitral" valve. The mitral orifice is approximately 9 cm in circumference, or capable of admitting two fingers. The mitral valve annulus is a nonplanar saddle shape, which decreases the strain on the posterior leaflet during systolic valve closure. From the atrial view when the valve is closed, the line where the leaflets meet looks like a smile. The areas where the two leaflets (commissures) insert into the annulus are named the *anterolateral commissure* and *posteromedial commissure*. The smaller, less mobile posterior cusp is situated

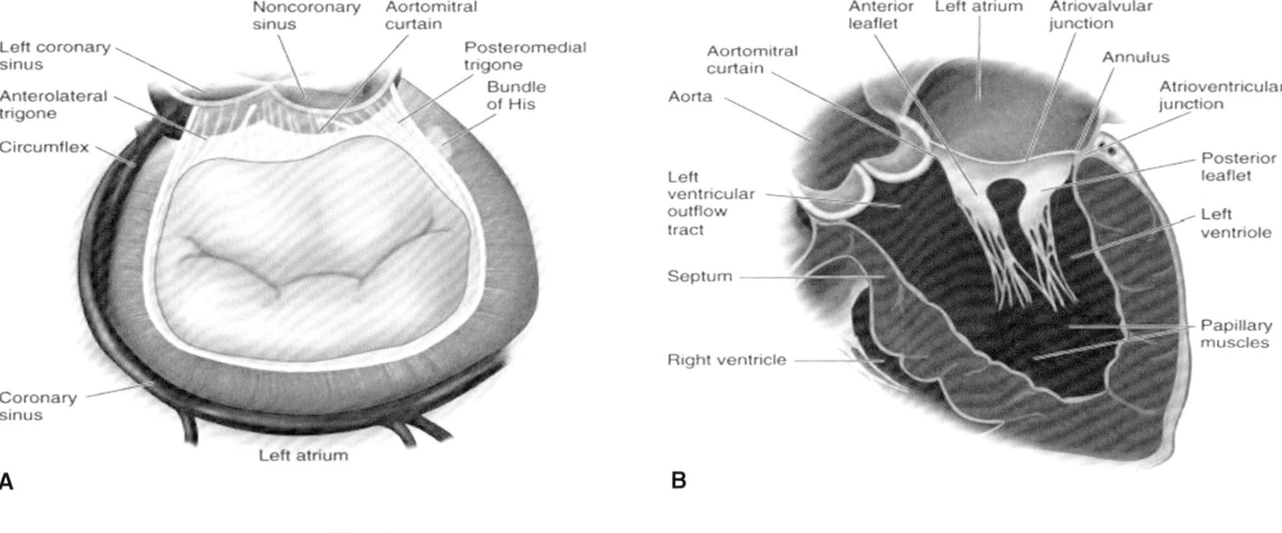

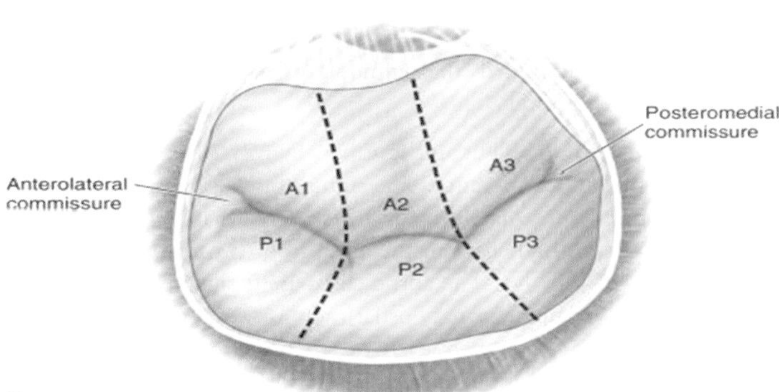

Figure 2-23. Schematic representation of the mitral valve. **A:** En face or surgeon's view of the mitral valve from the left atrium. **B:** Left ventricular outflow tract (LVOT) view including the left atrium, left ventricle, and the LVOT. **C:** En face or surgeon's view of the mitral valve; leaflet segments are labeled using Carpentier classification.

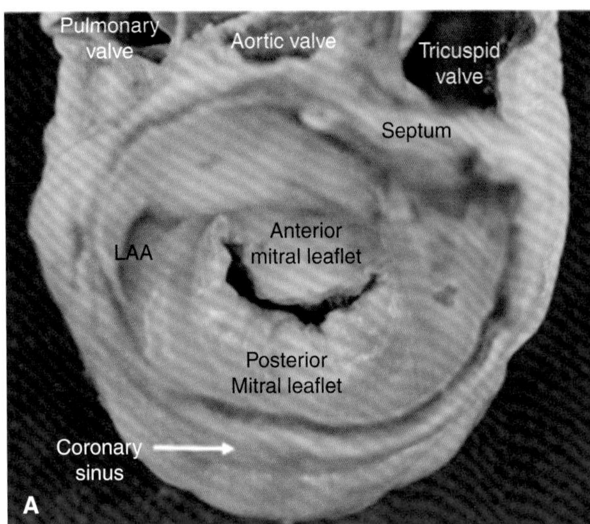

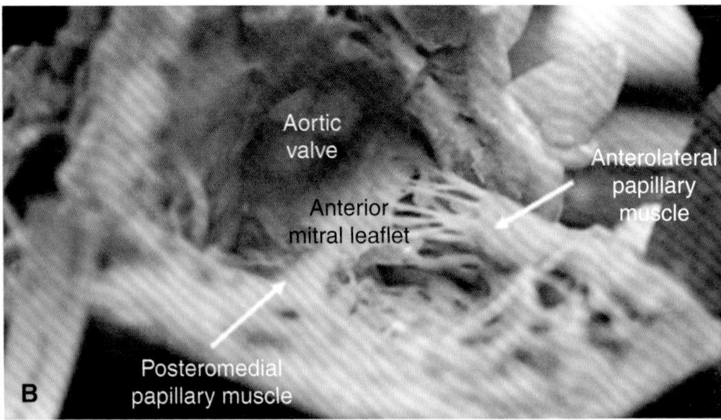

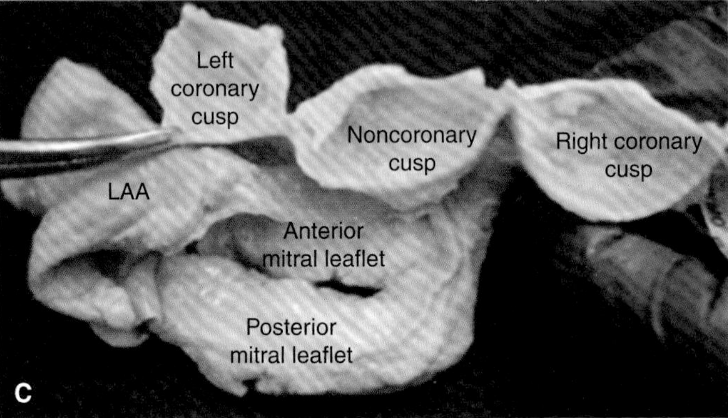

Figure 2-24. Mitral valve, multiple views. **A:** En face or surgeon's view of the mitral valve from the left atrium. **B:** Left ventricular outflow tract (LVOT) view including the left ventricle and the LVOT. **C:** En face or surgeon's view of the mitral valve with reference of the split aortic valve. LAA, left atrial appendage. (Courtesy of Center for CardioVascular Innovation, University of Washington.)

posterolaterally, behind, and to the left of the aortic opening. The *posterior mitral leaflet* has three indentations or scallops, which are thusly named in succession from the lateral to the medial commissure using Carpentier classification (see Fig. 2-23)[11]: P1 (adjacent to the anterolateral commissure), P2 (central scallop), and P3 (adjacent to the posteromedial commissure). The larger, tongue-shaped, highly mobile *anterior mitral leaflet* extends from the anterolateral papillary muscle to the interventricular septum. The anterior leaflet does not have indentations however its segments are named A1, A2 and A3 for the corresponding areas of the posterior leaflet.

The left ventricle most commonly has two major papillary muscles: the posteromedial papillary muscle attached to the diaphragmatic ventricular wall and the anterolateral papillary muscle attached to the sternocostal ventricular wall (see Fig. 2-24). Chordae tendineae from each papillary muscle go to both mitral cusps. The *rough zone* of each leaflet is thick and has chordae tendinae insertions at the ventricular surface; this zone is the region of *coaptation,* where the valve leaflets meet in systole.

Semilunar Valves. The semilunar pulmonary (or pulmonic) and aortic valves are each composed of three cup-shaped cusps of approximately equal size that attach at their base to the fibrous skeleton. The valve cusps are convex from below, with thickened nodules at the center of the free margins. The cusps are composed of fibrous connective tissue lined with endothelium. The endothelial lining on the nonventricular side of the valves closely resembles and merges with that of the intima of the arteries beyond the valves. The semilunar valve cusps are thicker than the AV valve cusps.

The aortic and pulmonic semilunar valves are approximately at right angles to each other in the closed position. The pulmonic valve is anterior and superior to the other three cardiac valves. When closed, the semilunar valve cusps contact each other at the nodules and along the crescent arcs (*lunulae*), below the free margins. During systole, the cusps are thrust upward as blood flows from an area of greater pressure in the ventricle to an area of lesser pressure in the aorta or the pulmonary artery. The effect of the deceleration of blood in the aorta during late systole on small circular currents of blood in the sinuses of Valsalva helps passively to close the semilunar valve cusps. Backflow into the ventricles during diastole is prevented because of the cusps' fibrous strength, their close approximation, and their shape.

Pulmonary Valve. The pulmonary valve (Fig. 2-25) is approximately 8.5 cm in circumference. The pulmonic valve cusps are termed *right anterior* (right), *left anterior* (anterior), and *posterior* (left). As mentioned, the pulmonic valve is typically considered part of the RVOT.

Aortic Valve. The aortic valve (Fig. 2-26) is approximately 7.5 cm in circumference. The sinuses of Valsalva are pouch-like structures immediately behind each semilunar cusp. The coronary arteries branch from the aorta from two of the pouches or sinuses of Valsalva. The aortic cusps are designated by the name of the associated coronary ostia: *right coronary* (right or anterior) aortic cusp, *left coronary* (left or left posterior) aortic cusp, and *noncoronary* (posterior or right posterior) aortic cusp. The aortic cusps are thicker than the pulmonic cusps.

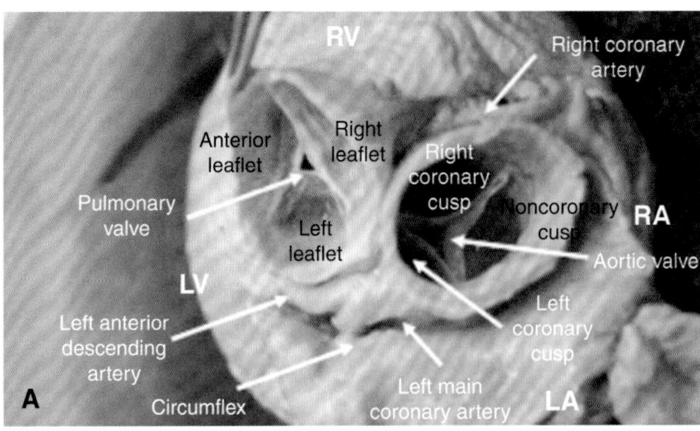

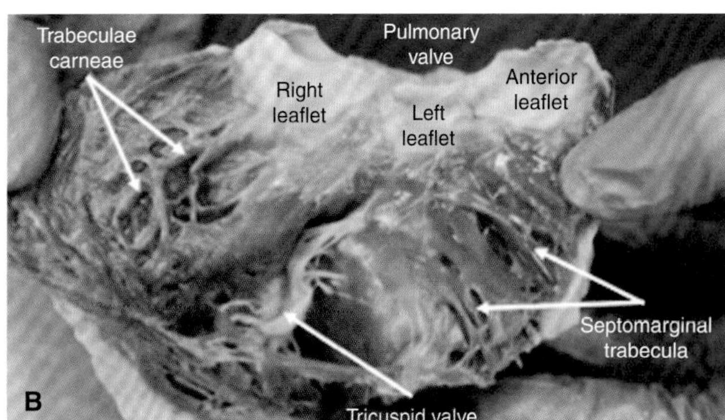

Figure 2-25. Pulmonary valve. **A:** Superior view of the pulmonary and aortic valves. **B:** Split view of the pulmonary valve. Right ventricular has been dissected open and pulmonary valve cut between right and anterior leaflets. LV, left ventricle; RV, right ventricle; RA, right atrium; LA, left atrium. (Courtesy of Center for CardioVascular Innovation, University of Washington.)

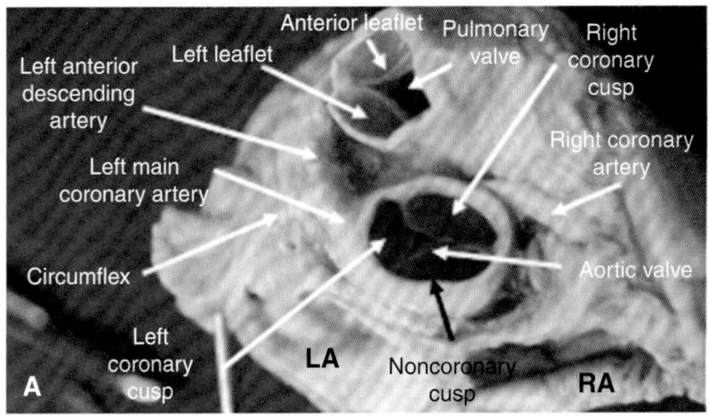

Figure 2-26. Aortic valve. **A:** Superior view of the aortic valve. **B:** Split view of the aortic valve. **C:** View of the aortic valve and left ventricular outflow tract (LVOT). LA, left atrium; RA, right atrium. (Courtesy of Center for CardioVascular Innovation, University of Washington.)

CORONARY CIRCULATION

The heart is continuously active. Like all tissues, it must receive oxygen and metabolic substrates; carbon dioxide and other wastes must be removed to maintain aerobic metabolism and contractile activity. However, unlike other tissues, it must generate the force to power its own perfusion. The heart requires continuous perfusion.

Coronary Arteries

The major coronary arteries (Fig. 2-27) in humans are the right coronary artery and the left coronary artery, sometimes called the *left main coronary artery.* These arteries branch from the aorta in the respective sinus of Valsalva and extend over the epicardial surface of the heart and branch several times. The branches usually emerge at right angles from the parent artery.[12] The arteries plunge inward through the myocardial wall and undergo further branching. The epicardial branches exit first. The more distal branches supply the endocardial (internal) myocardium. The arteries continue branching and eventually become arterioles, then capillaries. Partially because the blood supply originates more distally, the endocardium is more vulnerable to compromised blood supply than is the epicardial surface.

There is much individual variation in the pattern of coronary artery branching. In general, the right coronary artery supplies the right atrium and ventricle. The left coronary artery supplies much of the left atrium and ventricle. The following discussion describes the most common arterial pattern, depicted in Figures 2-28 and 2-29. Table 2-1 lists the major cardiac structures, their usual arterial supply, and some common variations (e.g., either the right or the left coronary artery may supply the AV node).

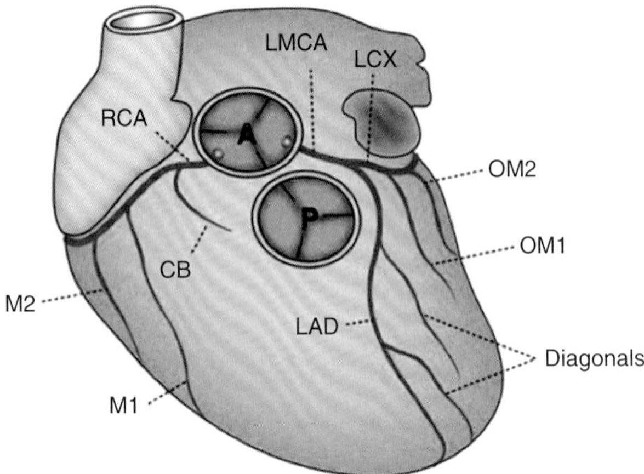

Figure 2-27. Schematic of normal coronary anatomy. A, aortic valve; CB, conus branch of the right coronary artery; diagonals, first and second diagonal branches of the left anterior descending coronary artery; LAD, anterior descending branch of left coronary artery; LCX, circumflex branch of the left coronary artery; LMCA, left main coronary artery; M1/2, first and second marginal branches of the right coronary artery; OM1/2, first and second obtuse marginal branches of the left coronary artery; P, pulmonic valve; RCA, right coronary artery.

Individual anatomic variation should be considered in analyzing patient data. For example, angiographic visualization of the left circumflex artery might show severe stenosis. Although it is not likely that AV node and His bundle perfusion would be affected (because the right coronary artery typically perfuses these structures), in approximately 10% of cases the structures would be at risk. Thus, angiographic information is validated with clinical data. Also, apparently attenuated or narrowed vessels may be normal anatomic variants.

Vessel Dominance

Dominance (or *preponderance*), a term commonly used in describing coronary vasculature, refers to the distribution of the terminal portion of the arteries. The artery that reaches and crosses the *crux* (where the right and left AV grooves cross the posterior interatrial and interventricular grooves) is said to be *dominant.* For most coronary anatomies, the dominant coronary artery is that which gives rise to the posterior descending artery. In approximately 85% of cases, the right coronary artery crosses the crux and this is "dominant." The term can be confusing because in most human hearts, the left coronary artery is of wider caliber and perfuses the largest proportion of myocardium. Thus, the dominant artery usually does not perfuse the largest percentage of myocardial mass. The dominant artery supplies the posterior diaphragmatic interventricular septum and diaphragmatic surface of the left ventricle.

Right Coronary Artery

The right coronary artery supplies the right atrium, right ventricle, and a portion of the posterior and inferior surfaces of the left ventricle. It supplies the AV node and bundle of His in 90% of hearts, and the sinus node in 55% of hearts.[12] It originates behind the right aortic cusp and passes behind the pulmonary artery, coursing in the right AV groove laterally to the right

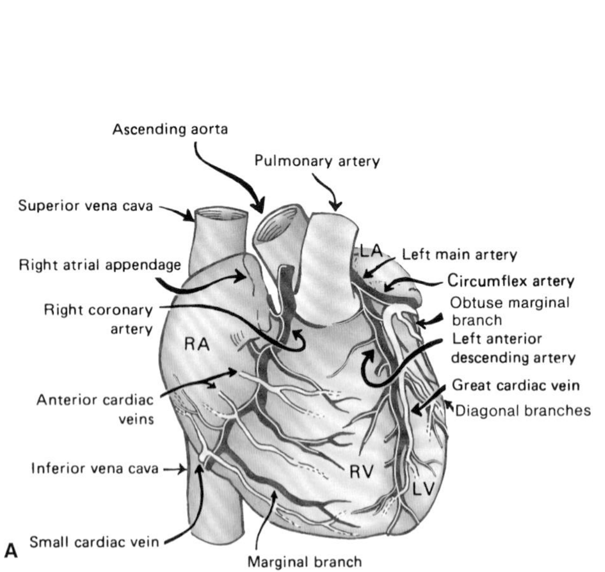

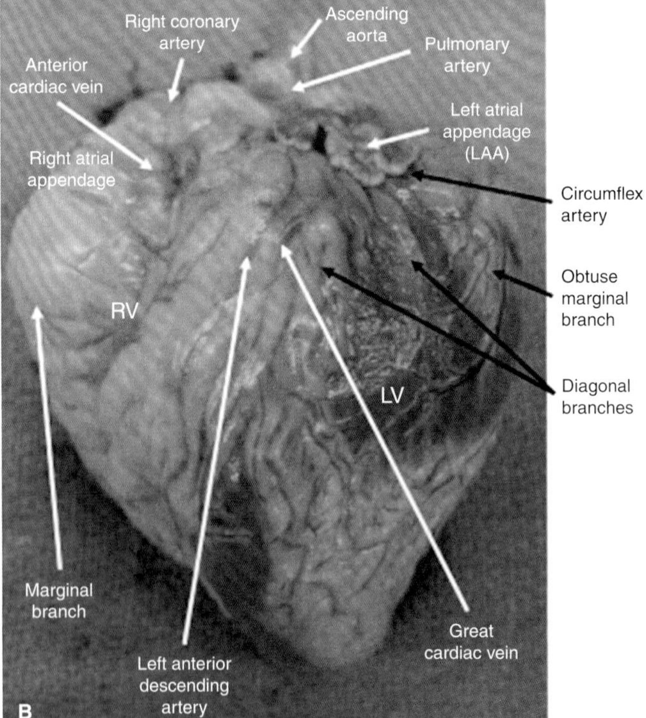

Figure 2-28. Principal arteries and veins on the anterior surfaces of the heart. Note that the left coronary artery arises from the left coronary aortic sinus behind the pulmonary trunk. **A:** Schematic representation of the surface coronary and venous circulation of the heart from anterior right-side view. (Adapted from Wamsley R, Watson H. *Clinical Anatomy of the Heart.* New York: Churchill Livingston; 1978:203.) **B:** Anterior view of the heart with silicone injections of coronary arteries (*red*) and veins (*blue*). RV, right ventricle; LV, left ventricle. (Courtesy of Center for CardioVascular Innovation, University of Washington.)

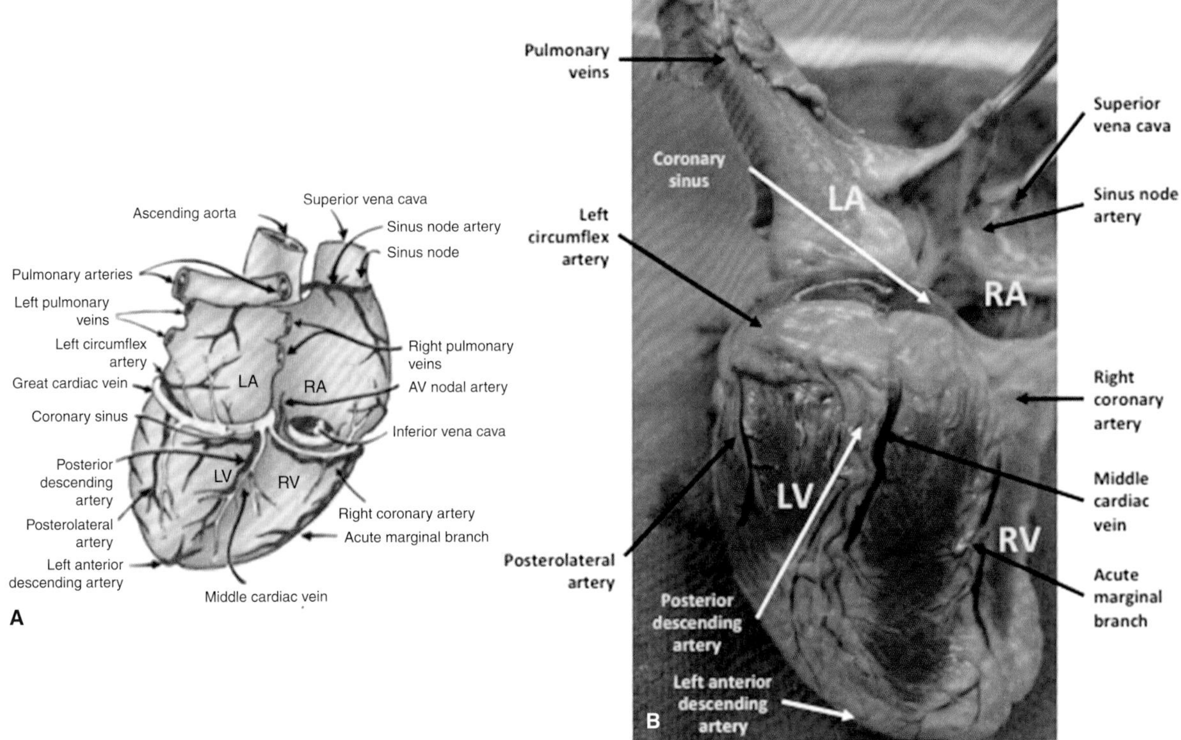

Figure 2-29. Principal arteries and veins on the posterior surfaces of the heart. **A:** Schematic representation of the surface coronary and venous circulation of the heart from the posterior view. (Adapted from Wamsley R, Watson H. *Clinical Anatomy of the Heart*. New York: Churchill Livingston; 1978:203.) **B:** Anterior view of the heart with silicone injections of coronary arteries (red) and veins (blue). RV, right ventricle; LV, left ventricle. (Courtesy of Center for CardioVascular Innovation, University of Washington.)

Table 2-1 • CORONARY ARTERIAL SUPPLY OF CARDIAC STRUCTURES[a]

Structure	Usual Arterial Supply	Common Variants
Right atrium	Sinus node artery, branch of RCA (55%)	Sinus node artery, branch of L circumflex (45%)
Left atrium	Major L circumflex[b]	Sinus node artery, branch of L circumflex (45%)
Right ventricle		
Anterior	Major RCA Minor LAD	
Posterior	Major RCA; posterior descending branch of RCA Minor LAD (ascending portion)	Posterior descending may branch from L circumflex (10%) LAD terminates at apex (40%)
Left ventricle		
Posterior (diaphragmatic)	Major L circumflex, posterior descending branch of RCA Minor LAD (ascending portion)	Posterior descending may branch from L circumflex (10%) LAD terminates at apex (40%)
Anterior	L coronary artery; L circumflex and LAD	
Apex	Major LAD	
Intraventricular septum	Major septal branches of LAD Minor posterior descending branch of RCA and AV nodal branch of RCA	Minor posterior descending may branch from L circumflex, AV nodal may branch from L circumflex
Left ventricular papillary muscles		
Anterolateral	Diagonal branch of LAD; other branches of LAD, other branches of L circumflex	Diagonal may branch from circumflex
Posteromedial	RCA and L circumflex	RCA and LAD
Sinus node	Nodal artery from RCA (55%)	Nodal artery from L circumflex (45%)
AV node	RCA (90%)	L circumflex (10%)
Bundle of His	RCA (90%)	L circumflex (10%)
Right bundle	Major LAD septal branches Minor AV nodal artery	
Left anterior bundle	Major LAD septal branches Minor AV nodal artery	
Left posterior bundle	LAD septal branches and AV nodal artery	

[a]Percentages in parentheses denote frequency of occurrence in autopsy studies.
[b]Major and minor refer to degree of predominance of an artery in perfusing a structure.
RCA, right coronary artery; LAD, left anterior descending artery; L, left; LV, left ventricle; AV, atrioventricular.
Data from James TN. *Anatomy of the Coronary Arteries*. New York: Paul B. Hoeber; 1961 and James TN. 1978.

margin of the heart and then posteriorly. The major branches of the right coronary artery, in order of origin, are as follows:

1. Conus branch
2. Sinus node artery
3. Right ventricular branches
4. Right atrial branch
5. Acute marginal branch
6. AV nodal branch
7. Posterior descending branch
8. Left ventricular branch
9. Left atrial branch

The *conus branch* is small; in 60% of cases it exits within the first 2 cm of the right coronary artery. It sometimes originates as a separate vessel with an ostium within a millimeter of the right coronary artery.[13] The branch proceeds centrally to the left of the pulmonic valve. It supplies the upper part of the right ventricle, near the outflow tract at the level of the pulmonic valve. When the conus branch anastomoses with a right ventricular branch of the left anterior descending artery, the resulting structure is called the *circle of Vieussens*, an important collateral link between left and right coronary arteries.

The sinus node artery arises from the right coronary artery in 55% of cases.[13] It proceeds in the opposite direction from the conus branch, coursing cranially and to the right, encircling the superior vena cava. It usually has two branches: one supplies the sinus node and parts of the right atrium and the other branches to the left atrium.

The right coronary artery courses along the AV groove, giving rise next to one or more *right ventricular branches* that vary in length and distribute to the right ventricular wall. The *right atrial branch* proceeds cranially toward the right heart border and it perfuses the right atrium.

The *acute marginal branch* is a fairly large branch of the right coronary artery. It originates at the acute margin of the heart near the right atrial artery and courses in the opposite direction, toward the apex. It perfuses the inferior and diaphragmatic surfaces of the right ventricle and occasionally the posterior apical portion of the interventricular septum.

The *AV nodal branch* is slender and straight. It originates at the crux and is directed inward toward the center of the heart. It perfuses the AV node and the lower portion of the interatrial septum.

The *posterior descending branch* is an important branch of the right coronary artery. It supplies the posterosuperior portion of the interventricular septum. It exits at the crux and courses in the posterior interventricular sulcus.

The *left ventricular branch* originates just beyond the crux. It runs centrally in the angle formed by the left posterior AV groove and the posterior interventricular sulcus. It perfuses the diaphragmatic aspect of the left ventricle.

A *left atrial branch* may course in the posterior left AV groove, perfusing the left atrium.

Left Coronary Artery

The left main coronary artery arises from the aorta in the ostium behind the left cusp of the aortic valve. This artery passes between the left atrial appendage and the pulmonary artery. Typically, it then divides into two major branches: the *left anterior descending artery* and *left circumflex artery*.

Left Anterior Descending Artery. The left anterior descending artery supplies portions of the left and right ventricular myocardium and much of the interventricular septum. The left anterior descending artery appears to be a continuation of the left main coronary artery. It passes to the left of the pulmonic valve region, courses in the anterior interventricular sulcus to the apex, and then courses around the apex to terminate in the inferior portion of the posterior interventricular sulcus. Occasionally, the posterior descending branch of the right coronary artery extends around the apex from the posterior surface and the left anterior descending artery ends short of the apex. The major branches of the left anterior descending artery, in the order in which they branch, are the following:

1. First diagonal branch
2. First septal branch
3. Right ventricular branch
4. Minor septal branches
5. Second diagonal branch
6. Apical branches

The *first diagonal branch* is usually a large artery. It originates close to the bifurcation of the left main coronary artery and passes diagonally over the free wall of the left ventricle. It perfuses the high lateral portion of the left ventricular free wall. Several smaller diagonal branches may exit from the left side of the left anterior descending artery and run parallel to the first diagonal branch. The one referred to as the *second diagonal branch* takes its origin approximately two thirds of the way from the origin to the termination of the left anterior descending artery. This second diagonal branch perfuses the lower lateral portion of the free wall to the apex.

The number of septal branches varies. The *first septal branch* is the first to exit the left anterior descending artery. The others are referred to as *minor septal branches.* The septal branches exit at a 90-degree angle. They then course into the septum from front to the back and caudally. Together, the septal branches perfuse two thirds of the upper portion of the septum and most of the inferior portion of the septum. The remaining superoposterior section of the septum is supplied by branches from the posterior descending artery, which usually derives from the right coronary artery.

There can be one or more *right ventricular branches.* One branch runs toward the conus branch of the right coronary artery; it can anastomose into the circle of Vieussens.

The final branches are the *apical branches.* These branches perfuse the anterior and diaphragmatic aspects of the left ventricular free wall and apex.

Circumflex Artery. The *circumflex artery* supplies blood to parts of the left atrium and left ventricle. In 45% of cases, the circumflex artery supplies the major perfusion of the sinus node; in 10% of cases, it supplies the AV node.[13] The circumflex artery exits from the left main coronary artery at a near-right angle and courses posteriorly in the AV groove toward, but usually not reaching, the crux. If the circumflex reaches the crux, it gives rise to the posterior descending artery. In the 15% of cases in which this occurs, the left coronary artery supplies the entire septum and possibly the AV node.[13] The branches of the circumflex artery, in order of origin, are as follows:

1. Atrial circumflex branch
2. Sinus node artery
3. Obtuse marginal branches
4. Posterolateral branches

The *atrial circumflex branch* is usually small in caliber but sometimes is as wide as the remaining portion of the circumflex. It runs along the left AV groove, perfusing the left atrial wall.

In 45% of cases, the *sinus node artery* originates from the initial portion of the circumflex; it runs cranially and dorsally, to the base of the superior vena cava in the region of the sinus node.[13] This artery perfuses portions of the left and right atria as well as the sinus node.

There are between one and four *obtuse marginal branches*. These branches vary greatly in size. They run along the ventricular wall laterally and posteriorly, toward the apex, along the obtuse margin of the heart. The marginal branches supply the obtuse margin of the heart and the adjacent posterior wall of the left ventricle above the diaphragmatic surface.

The *posterolateral branches* arise from the circumflex artery in 80% of cases.[13] These branches originate in the terminal portion of the circumflex artery and course caudally and to the left on the posterior left ventricular wall, supplying the posterior and diaphragmatic wall of the left ventricle.

The *posterior descending* and AV nodal arteries occasionally arise from the circumflex. When this is the case, branches of the left coronary artery supply the entire septum.

Coronary Capillaries

Blood passes from arteries into arterioles, then into capillaries (Fig. 2-30) where exchange of oxygen, carbon dioxide, metabolic compounds, and waste materials takes place. The heart has a dense capillary network with approximately 3,300 capillaries per mm^2 or approximately one capillary per muscle fiber.[14] Blood flow through coronary capillaries is regulated according to myocardial metabolic needs.

When myocardial cells hypertrophy, the cell radius increases. The capillary network, however, does not appear to proliferate.[15] The same capillaries must perfuse a larger tissue mass. The diffusion distance is increased. Thus, with hypertrophy, the mass of tissue to be perfused is increased but the efficiency of exchange is diminished.

Coronary Veins

Most of the venous drainage of the heart is through epicardial veins. The large veins course close to the coronary arteries. Two veins sometimes accompany an artery.[12] The major veins feed into the great cardiac vein, which runs alongside the circumflex artery, becomes the coronary sinus, and then empties into the right atrium (see Figs. 2-28 and 2-29). An incompetent (incompletely shut) semilunar valve, called the *valve of Vieussens*, marks the junction between the great cardiac vein and the coronary

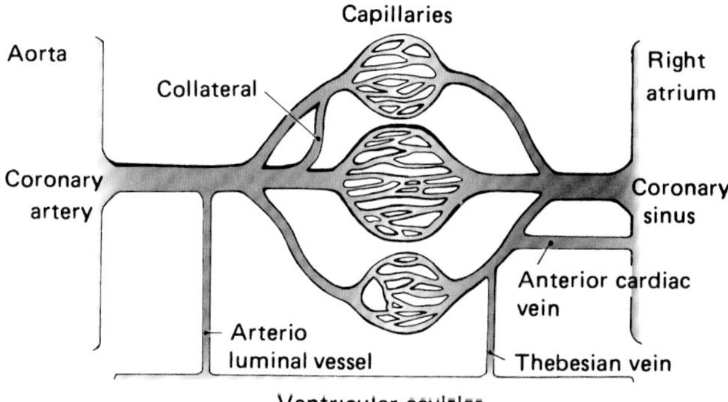

Figure 2-30. Schematic model of coronary circulation. As in other circulatory beds, the coronary circulation includes arteries, capillaries, and veins. Some veins drain directly into the ventricles. Collateral channels may link arterial vessels. Art, arterial. (Adapted from Ruch TC, Patton HD. *Physiology and Biophysics*. 20th ed. *Vol 2*. Philadelphia, PA: WB Saunders; 1974:249.)

sinus. A similar structure, the *Thebesian valve*, is also incompetent and is found at the entry of the coronary sinus into the right atrium. Venous blood from the right ventricular muscle is drained primarily by two to four anterior cardiac veins that empty directly into the right atrium, bypassing the coronary sinus.

The *Thebesian veins* empty directly into the ventricles. These are more common on the right side of the heart, where the pressure gradient is favorable for such flow. Only a small amount of venous blood is returned directly to the left ventricle. When blood is returned to the left ventricle, this flow is a component of physiologic shunt, or unoxygenated blood entering the systemic circulation. Many collateral channels are found in the venous drainage system.

Lymph Drainage

Cardiac contraction promotes lymphatic drainage in the myocardium through an abundant system of lymphatic vessels, most of which eventually converge into the principal left anterior lymphatic vessel. Lymph from this vessel empties into the pretracheal lymph node and then proceeds by way of two channels to the cardiac lymph node, the right lymphatic duct, and then into the superior vena cava.[16]

The importance of a normally functioning lymphatic system in maintaining an appropriate environment for cardiac cell function is frequently overlooked. Although complete cardiac lymph obstruction is rarely observed, experimental acute and chronic lymphatic impairment causes myocardial and endocardial cellular changes, particularly when occurring in conjunction with venous congestion.[16] Experimentally induced myocardial infarction in animals with chronically impaired lymphatic drainage causes more extensive cellular necrosis, an increased and prolonged inflammatory response, and a greater amount of fibrosis than infarction in animals without lymphatic obstruction.[16]

CARDIAC INNERVATION

Sensory nerve fibers from ventricular walls, the pericardium, coronary blood vessels, and other tissues transmit impulses by way of the cardiac nerves to the central nervous system. Motor nerve fibers to the heart are autonomic. Sympathetic stimulation accelerates firing of the sinus node, enhances conduction through the AV node, and increases the force of cardiac contraction. Parasympathetic stimulation slows the heart rate (HR), slows conduction through the AV node, and may decrease ventricular contractile force.

Sympathetic preganglionic cardiac nerves arise from the first four or five thoracic spinal cord segments. The nerves synapse with long postganglionic fibers in the superior, middle, and cervicothoracic or stellate ganglia adjacent to the spinal cord. Most postganglionic sympathetic nerves to the heart travel through the superior, middle, and inferior cardiac nerves. However, several cardiac nerves with variable origins have been identified.[15] Parasympathetic preganglionic cardiac nerves arise from the right and left vagus nerves and synapse with postganglionic nerves close to their target cardiac cells.

Both vagal and sympathetic cardiac nerves converge in the cardiac plexus. The cardiac plexus is situated superior to the bifurcation of the pulmonary artery, behind the aortic arch, and anterior to the trachea at the level of tracheal bifurcation. From the cardiac plexus, the cardiac nerves course in two coronary plexuses along with the right and left coronary blood vessels.

Sympathetic fibers are richly distributed throughout the heart. Right sympathetic ganglia fibers most commonly innervate the sinus node, the right atrium, the anterior ventricular walls, and to some extent the AV node. Most commonly, left sympathetic ganglia fibers extensively innervate the AV junctional area and the posterior and inferior left ventricle.[17]

A dense supply of vagal fibers innervates the sinus node, AV node, and ventricular conducting system. Consequently, many parasympathetic ganglia are found in the region of the sinus and AV nodes. Vagal fibers also innervate both atria and, to a lesser extent, both ventricles.[17] Right vagal fibers have more effect on the sinus node; left vagal fibers have more effect on the AV node and ventricular conduction system. However, there is overlap. The clinical importance of vagal stimulation for ventricular function continues to be debated. Although neurotransmitters from cardiac nerves are important modulators of cardiac activity, the success of cardiac transplantation illustrates the capacity of the heart to function without nervous innervation.

CARDIAC TISSUE

Recall that the heart wall is composed of three layers, the pericardium, myocardium, and endocardium. Of these, the predominant layer is the muscular layer, the myocardium. The endocardium covers the internal surface. The myocardium and endocardium are also further discussed in subsequent sections on myocardial contraction and electrical conduction.

Myocardium

The myocardial layer is composed of cardiac muscle cells interspersed with connective tissue and small blood vessels. Some atrial and ventricular myocardial fibers are anchored to the fibrous skeleton. The thin-walled atria are composed of two major muscle systems: one that surrounds both of the atria and another that is arranged at right angles to the first and that is separate for each atrium.

Each ventricle is a single muscle mass of nested figure eights of individual muscle fiber path spirals anchored to the fibrous skeleton. Ventricular muscle fibers spiral downward on the epicardial ventricular wall, pass through the wall, spiral up on the endocardial surface, cross the upper part of the ventricle, and go back down through the wall (Fig. 2-31). This vortex arrangement allows for the circumferential generation of tension throughout the ventricular wall; it is functionally efficient for ventricular contraction. Some fiber paths spiral around both ventricles. The fibers form a fan-like arrangement of interconnecting muscle fibers when dissected horizontally through the ventricular wall. The orientation of these fibers gradually rotates through the thickness of the wall (Fig. 2-31).

The myocardial tissue consists of several functionally specialized cell types. In areas of contact between diverse cell types, there is usually an area of gradual transition in which the cells are intermediate in appearance. These cell types are identified here and further discussed in subsequent sections on conduction tissues and myocardial cells.

Nodal cells are specialized for pacemaker function. They are found in clusters in the sinus node and AV node. These cells contain few contractile filaments, little sarcoplasmic reticulum (SR), and no transverse tubules. They are the smallest myocardial cells.

Purkinje cells are specialized for rapid electrical impulse conduction, especially through the thick ventricular wall. The large size, elongated shape, and sparse contractile protein composition reflect this specialization. These cells are found in the common His bundle and in the left and right bundle branches as well as in a diffuse network throughout the ventricles. Purkinje cell cytoplasm is rich in glycogen granules; thus, making these cells more resistant to damage during anoxia. A secondary function of

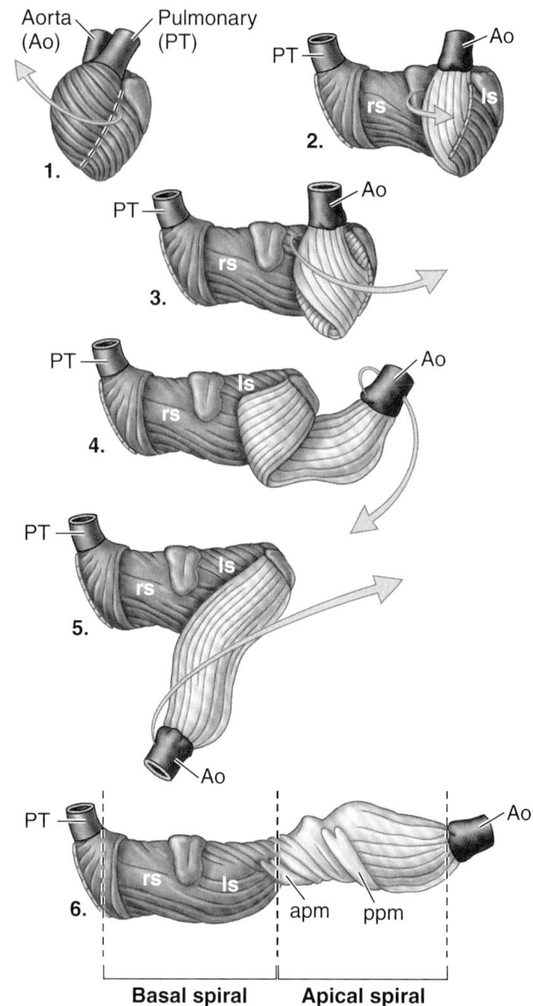

Figure 2-31. Arrangement of the myocardium and the fibrous skeleton of heart. The helical (double spiral) arrangement of the myocardium (modified from Torrent-Guasp et al., 2001). When the superficial myocardium is incised along the anterior interventricular groove (*dashed line* in 1) and peeled back starting at its origin from the fibrous ring of the pulmonary trunk (PT–2), the thick double spirals of the ventricular myocardial band are revealed (3). The ventricular myocardial band is progressively unwrapped (3–6). A band of nearly horizontal fibers forms an outer basal spiral (dark muscle–6) that constitutes the outer wall of the right ventricle (right segment, rs) and external layer of the outer wall of the left ventricle (left segment, ls). The deeper apical spiral (light muscle) constitutes the internal layer of the outer wall of the left ventricle. Its crisscrossing fibers make up the interventricular septum. Thus, the septum, like the outer wall of the left ventricle, is also double layered. The sequential contraction of the myocardial band enables the ventricles to function as parallel, sucking and propelling pumps; on contraction, the ventricles do not merely collapse inward but rather wring themselves out (apm, anterior papillary muscles; ppm, posterior papillary muscles). (Adapted with permission from Torrent-Guasp F, Buckberg GD, Clemente C, et al. The structure and function of the helical heart and its buttress wrapping. The normal macroscopic structure of the heart. *Semin Thorac Cardiovasc Surg*. 2001;13:30.)

the Purkinje cells is to serve as a potential pacemaker locus. In the absence of an overriding impulse from the sinus node, Purkinje cells initiate electrical impulses.

Working myocardial cells generate the contractile force of the heart. These cells have a markedly striated appearance caused by the orderly arrays of the abundant contractile protein filaments. Working myocardial cells comprise the bulk of the walls of both atrial and both ventricular chambers.

Endocardium

The endocardium is composed of a layer of endothelial cells and a few layers of collagen and elastic fibers. The endocardium is continuous with the tunica intima of the blood vessels.

Conduction Tissues

Conduction tissues (Fig. 2-32) are comprised of specialized nodal myocardial cells that, in the normal sequence of events, depolarize spontaneously and generate electrical impulses that are conducted to the larger mass of working myocardial cells. The sequential contraction of the atria and ventricles as coordinated units depends on the anatomic arrangement of the specialized cardiac conducting tissue. Small cardiac nerves, arteries, and veins lie close to the specialized conducting cells, providing neurohumoral modulation of cardiac impulse generation and conduction.

Keith and Flack first described the sinus node in 1907.[18] The sinus node lies close to the epicardial surface of the heart, above the tricuspid valve, near the anterior entrance of the superior vena cava into the right atrium. The sinus node is also referred to as the *sinoatrial node.* It is approximately 10 to 15 mm long, 3 to 5 mm wide, and 1 mm thick. Small nodal cells are surrounded by and interspersed with connective tissue. They merge with the larger working atrial muscle cells.

Bachmann[19] originally described an interatrial myocardial bundle conducting impulses from the right atrium to the left atrium. Later, James[20] presented evidence for three *internodal conduction pathways* from the sinus node to the AV node. It is unclear whether the pathways have functional significance. It is generally believed that the cardiac impulse spreads from the sinus node to the AV node via cell-to-cell conduction through the atrial working myocardial cells.

Tarawa[21] initially described the AV node in 1906. It is located subendocardially on the right atrial side of the central fibrous body, in the lower interatrial septal wall. The AV node is close to the septal leaflet of the tricuspid valve and anterior to the coronary sinus. A group of fibers connects the AV node to working myocardial cells in the left atrium. The AV node is approximately 7 mm long, 3 mm wide, and 1 mm thick.[22] Nodal fibers are interspersed with normal working myocardial fibers; it is difficult to precisely identify the AV node boundaries. There are several zones of specialized conducting tissue in the AV junction area: the compact AV node, a transition zone containing small nodal and larger working atrial myocardial cells, the penetrating AV bundle, and the branching AV bundle.[23,24]

Fibers from the AV node converge into a shaft termed the *bundle of His* (also called the *penetrating AV bundle* or *common bundle*). It is approximately 10 mm long and 2 mm in diameter.[22] The bundle of His passes from the lower right atrial wall anteriorly and laterally through the central fibrous body, which is part of the fibrous skeleton.

As first noted in 1893 by His,[25] the His bundle provides the only cellular connection between the atria and ventricles and is of pivotal functional importance. Cardiac impulse transmission is slowed at this site, providing time for atrial contraction to dispel blood from the atria into the ventricles. This slowing boosts ventricular volume and increases the CO during subsequent ventricular contraction. At the membranous septal region of the heart, the right atrium and left ventricle are opposite each other across the septum, with the right ventricle in close proximity. Three of the four cardiac valves are nearby. Thus, pathology of the fibrous skeleton, tricuspid, mitral, or aortic valves can affect functioning of one or more of the other valves or may affect cardiac impulse conduction. Dysfunction of the AV conducting tissue may affect the coordinated functioning of the atria and ventricles.

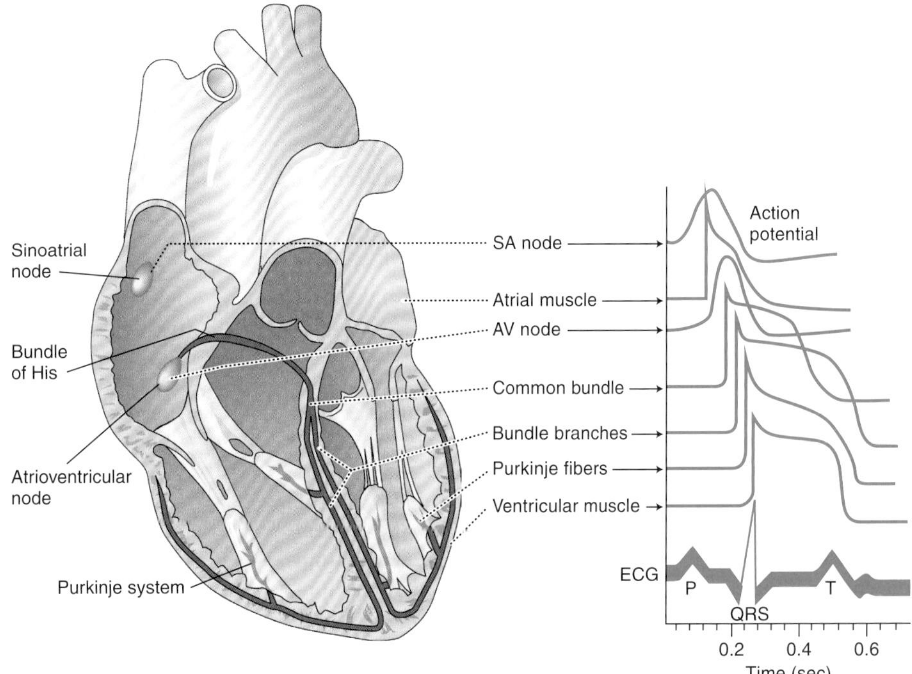

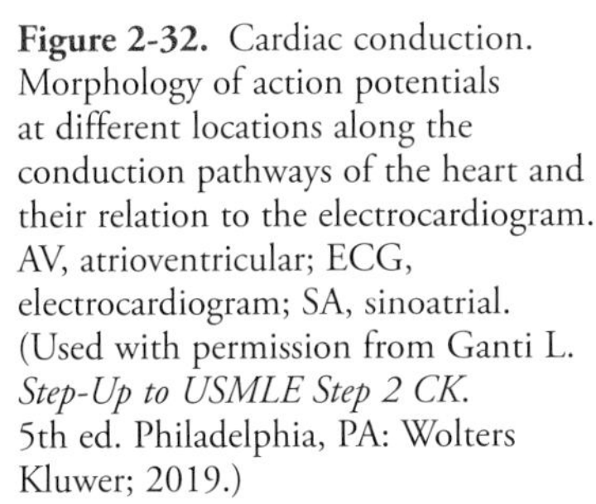
Figure 2-32. Cardiac conduction. Morphology of action potentials at different locations along the conduction pathways of the heart and their relation to the electrocardiogram. AV, atrioventricular; ECG, electrocardiogram; SA, sinoatrial. (Used with permission from Ganti L. *Step-Up to USMLE Step 2 CK.* 5th ed. Philadelphia, PA: Wolters Kluwer; 2019.)

Abnormal accessory pathways, termed *Kent bundles*, occasionally join the atria and ventricles through connections outside the main AV node and His bundle. Tracts from the His bundle to upper interventricular septum (termed *paraspecific fibers of Mahaim*) sometimes occur and are also abnormal.[26] AV conduction is accelerated when impulses bypass the delay-producing AV junction and travel instead through these abnormal connections. When accelerated AV conduction occurs, CO often decreases because there is inadequate time for atrial contraction to boost ventricular filling.[27]

The His bundle begins branching in the region of the crest of the muscular septum. The right bundle branch typically continues as a direct extension of the His bundle. The right bundle branch is a well-defined, single, slender group of fibers approximately 45 to 50 mm long and 1 mm thick. It initially courses downward along the right side of the interventricular septum, continues through the moderator band of muscular tissue near the right ventricular apex, and then continues to the base of the anterior papillary muscle. If a small segment of the bundle is damaged, the entire distal distribution is affected because of the right bundle's thinness, length, and relative lack of arborization.

The left bundle branch arises almost perpendicularly from the His bundle as the common left bundle branch. This common left bundle, approximately 10 mm long and 4 to 10 mm wide, then divides into two discrete divisions, the left anterior bundle branch and the left posterior bundle branch. The left anterior bundle branch, or left anterior fascicle, is approximately 25 mm long and 3 mm thick. It usually arises directly from the common left bundle after the origin of the posterior fascicle and close to the origin of the right bundle. It branches to the anterior septum and courses over the left ventricular anterior (superior) wall to the anterior papillary muscle, crossing the aortic outflow tract. Anterior and septal myocardial infarctions and aortic valve dysfunction often affect the left anterior bundle branch.

The large, thick, left posterior bundle branch, or left posterior fascicle, arises either from the first portion of the common left bundle or from the His bundle directly. The left posterior fascicle goes inferiorly and posteriorly across the left ventricular inflow tract to the base of the posterior papillary muscle; it then spreads diffusely through the posterior inferior left ventricular free wall. It is approximately 20 mm long and 6 mm thick. This fascicle is often the least vulnerable segment of the ventricular conducting system because of its diffuseness, its location in a relatively protected nonturbulent portion of the ventricle, and its dual blood supply (Table 2-1).

Three, rather than two, major divisions of the left bundle branch are sometimes found, with a group of fibers ramifying from the left posterior fascicle and terminating in the lower septum and apical ventricular wall.[24] This trifascicular configuration of the bundles explains some conduction defects involving partial bundle-branch block. Sometimes instead of three discrete bundles the common left bundle fans out diffusely along the septum and the free ventricular wall.[28]

Purkinje fibers, first described in 1845, form a complex network of conducting tissue ramifications that provide a continuation of the bundle branches in each ventricle.[29] The Purkinje fibers course down toward the ventricular apex and then up toward the fibrous rings at the ventricular bases. Purkinje fibers then spread over the subendocardial ventricular surfaces and then spread from the endocardium through the myocardium; thus, spreading from inside outward, providing extensive contacts with working myocardial cells, and coupling myocardial excitation with muscular contraction.

MYOCARDIAL CELLS

Myocardial Cell Structure

Myocardial cells are long, narrow, and often branched. A limiting membrane, the sarcolemma, surrounds each cell. Specialized surface membrane structures include the intercalated disc, nexus, and transverse tubules (T-tubules). Major intracellular components are contractile protein filaments (called myofibrils), mitochondria, SR, and nucleus. There is a small amount of cytoplasm, called *sarcoplasm* (Fig. 2-33).

The cell membrane or *sarcolemma* separates the intracellular and extracellular spaces. The sarcolemma is a thin phospholipid bilayer studded with proteins. Across the barrier of the sarcolemma are marked differences in ionic composition and electrical charge. The embedded proteins serve multiple functions.

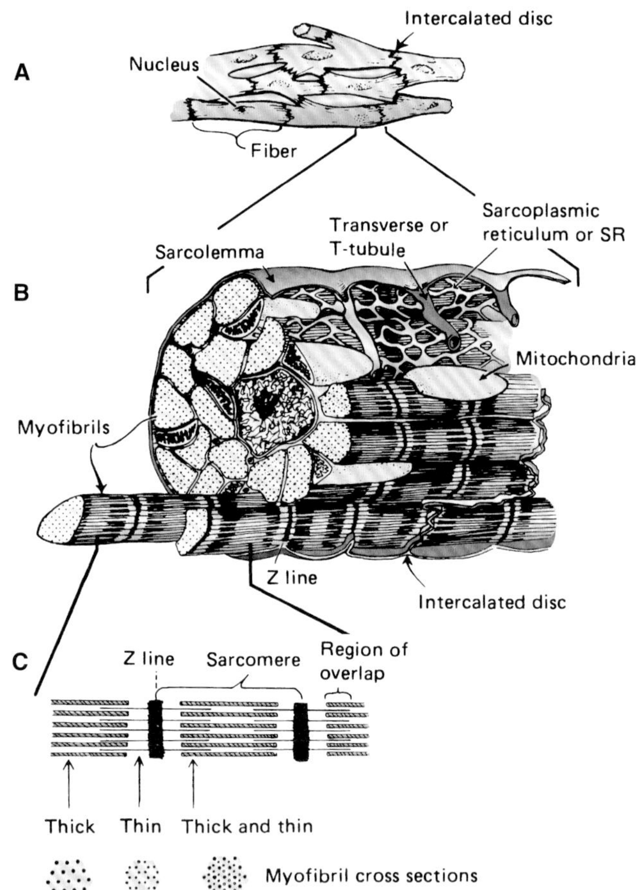

Figure 2-33. The microscopic structure of working myocardial cells. **A:** Working myocardial cells as seen under the light microscope. Note the branching network of fibers and intercalated discs. **B:** Schematic illustration of the internal structure of the working myocardial cell. Note the striated appearance of the myofibrils, the intimate association of the sarcoplasmic reticulum (SR) with the myofibrils, the presence of T-tubules, and the large number of mitochondria. **C:** Structure of the sarcomere, illustrating alignment of thick and thin filaments. Cross-sections taken at three different positions along the sarcomere illustrate a region with only thick filaments, a region with only thin filaments, and a region of overlap where the thick and the thin filaments interdigitate. (Adapted from Braunwald E, Ross J, Sonneblick E. *Mechanisms of Contraction of the Normal and Failing Heart.* 2nd ed. Boston, MA: Little, Brown; 1976:3.)

Embedded receptors bind extracellular substances; this binding in turn activates or inhibits cell electrical, contractile, metabolic, or other functions. Embedded ion channels regulate membrane ion permeability and electrical function. Various carrier proteins facilitate uptake of metabolic substrates such as glucose. Some sarcolemma proteins add structural stability, anchoring the cell's internal and external structural elements.

Structurally, each myocardial cell is distinct. An *intercalated disc* forms a junction between adjacent cells. A specialized type of cell-to-cell connection, the *nexus* (sometimes called the *gap junction*), is present in the intercalated disc. The nexus is the site of direct exchange of small molecules. The nexus also provides a low-resistance electrical path between cells, thus facilitating rapid impulse conduction. Physiologic conditions alter the permeability of the nexus. For example, two substances that vary with physiologic state are adenosine triphosphate (ATP)-dependent and cyclic adenosine monophosphate (cAMP)-dependent protein kinases. Both alter nexus permeability.[30,31] Because of these junctions, the heart functions as a syncytium of electrically coordinated cells, although anatomically the cells are discrete.

Another specialized membrane structure, the *T-tubule system*, is an extensive network of membrane-lined tubes systematically tunneling inward through each cell. T-tubules are formed by sarcolemma invaginations and are continuous with the surface membrane. The T-tubule lumen contains extracellular fluid. The T-tubular network carries electrical excitation to the central portions of myocardial cells, allowing near-simultaneous activation of deep and superficial parts of cells.

Myofibrils are long, rod-like structures that extend the length of the cell. They contain the contractile proteins, which convert the chemical energy of ATP into mechanical energy and heat. Muscle contraction involves generation of force, shortening, or both. The orderly alignment of contractile proteins into myofilaments gives the myocardial cell its striated (striped) appearance.

Mitochondria are small, rod-shaped membranous structures located within the cell. Substrate breakdown and high-energy compound synthesis occurs within the mitochondria. The relative abundance of mitochondria in cardiac muscle cells reflects the high level of biochemical activity required to support the heart's continuous contractile activity.

The SR is an extensive, self-contained internal membrane system. The T-tubules and SR link membrane depolarization to the mechanical activity of the contractile protein filaments. This functional coordination is called excitation–contraction coupling. The SR is the major storage depot for calcium ion, which releases then takes up calcium ions with each contraction of the heart.

The *nucleus* contains the genetic material of the cell. The nucleus is the site where new proteins are synthesized.

Myocardial Cell Electrical Characteristics

There is an electrical potential difference across the sarcolemma; it is measured in millivolts (mV). During the interim between excitations, the intracellular space is negative compared with the extracellular space. This potential difference is called the *membrane resting potential.* During excitation, the potential difference changes: the inside of the cell becomes less negative or slightly positive compared with the extracellular space. This type of potential difference change is called *depolarization*. After depolarization, the cell membrane *repolarizes*, or returns to the resting potential value. The normal depolarization–repolarization cycle is known as the *action potential.* The action potential is the signal-evoking contraction. Until the cell repolarizes sufficiently, there can be no action potential. If the potential difference becomes more negative than the usual resting potential, the membrane is said to be *hyperpolarized.* The more hyperpolarized the membrane, the more current is required to evoke an action potential.

Some myocardial cells have *automaticity*, that is, an intrinsic ability to depolarize spontaneously and initiate an action potential. The action potential generated in such a cell is then propagated throughout cardiac tissue. Depolarization of one cardiac cell initiates depolarization of adjacent cells and evokes contraction.

There are approximately 19 billion cells in the adult heart; these cells must depolarize in an orderly sequence if the heart is to undergo a coordinated contraction that is able to add force to moving blood. Impulses generated in ectopic sites in the heart are less likely to depolarize in an orderly sequence and less likely to contract in an orderly fashion that effectively pumps blood.

Basis for Myocardial Excitation: Characteristics of Biologic Membranes

Intracellular and extracellular spaces are separated by a thin insulating membrane, the sarcolemma. These spaces have very different ionic compositions. The intracellular space contains high concentrations of potassium ion (positively charged) and protein (negatively charged) and has low concentration of sodium ion (positively charged). The extracellular space consists of high concentrations of sodium ion and chloride ion (negatively charged); extracellular potassium ion concentration is low.

For each ion, concentration differences across the sarcolemma are determined by the sarcolemma's permeability to that ion and the balance of forces moving the ion from one to the other side of the membrane. Electrical and concentration differences are maintained by a number of active and passive processes. Typical concentration differences are outlined in Table 2-2.

The sarcolemma is composed of phospholipid molecules. Each molecule consists of a charged hydrophilic (water-attracting) globular head and a noncharged hydrophobic (water-repelling) tail. The molecules organize into thin sheets, with the heads oriented in a consistent direction. Two sheets are aligned tail to tail to form a double layer (bilayer). The tails form the core of the sheet, and the heads are directed outward in both directions. The result is a 7- to 9-nm, high-resistance, insulated barrier to ionic movement.

Proteins embedded within the phospholipid bilayer may compose more than half the mass of the membrane. Proteins function as receptors, channels, pumps, or structural stabilizers. The proteins may be inserted into the intracellular or extracellular side of the bilayer or span its full thickness. Some of the proteins contain a water-filled pore that spans the membrane, connecting the intracellular and extracellular spaces and forming a channel through which ions can pass. Membrane channels open and close in response to a stimulus (electrical, mechanical, or chemical), allowing passage of specific ions when open. The opening and closing properties of a channel are called its *gating* characteristics. The ability of a channel to selectively allow passage of certain ions while restricting other ions is called its *selectivity* property. Many ion channels are named after the ion for which they have selectivity. Some common types are sodium channels, potassium channels, and calcium channels (Fig. 2-34).

Table 2-2 • APPROXIMATE INTRACELLULAR AND EXTRACELLULAR ION CONCENTRATIONS AND ACTIVITIES IN CARDIAC MUSCLE[a]

Ion[b]	Extracellular Concentration[c] (mM)	Intracellular Concentration[d]	Ratio of Extracellular to Intracellular Concentration	E_I[e] (mV)	Intracellular Activity[f] (mM)
Na^+	145	15 mM	9.7	+60	7.0
K^+	4	150 mM	0.027	−94	125
Cl^-	120	5 mM	24	−83	15
Ca^{2+}	2	10^{-4} M	2×10^4	+129	8×10^{-6}

[a]Values given are approximations and vary according to the cardiac tissue, species, and method used for measurement.
[b]Na^+, sodium; K^+, potassium; Cl^-, chloride; Ca^{2+}, calcium.
[c]mM, millimolar.
[d]Most of the intracellular calcium is bound to proteins or sequestered in intracellular organelles; thus, total intracellular calcium content approximates 1 to 2 mm. During contraction, measurable intracellular calcium concentration approximates 10^{-5} mm.
[e]E_I, equilibrium potential; mV, millivolt
[f]Median values from summarized data; these values should be considered as subject to revision. Concentrations and equilibrium potentials from Sperelakis N. Origin of the cardiac resting potential. In: Berne RM, ed. *Handbook of Physiology, Section 2: The Cardiovascular System, Vol 1, the Heart*. Bethesda, MD: American Physiological Society; 1979:193. Activities are approximations from Lee CO. Ionic activities in cardiac muscle cells and application of ion-sensitive microelectrodes. *Am J Physiol.* 1981;241:H459–H478 and Fozzard HA, Wasserstrom JA. Voltage dependence of intracellular sodium and control of contraction. In: Zipes PP, Jalife J. *Cardiac Electrophysiology and Arrhythmias*. Orlando, FL: Grune & Tratton; 1985:52.

Mechanisms of Ion Distribution Across the Myocardial Membrane

Ions are distributed across the sarcolemma according to the membrane permeability to the ion and the electrical and diffusion forces on the ion. For each ion that can penetrate the membrane, there is a continual movement toward equilibrium. When equilibrium is reached, forces driving ion movement are balanced, and there is no additional net change in the ion distribution. The Nernst equation, discussed later, is useful in understanding the relationship between electrical and diffusional forces driving ion movement. It is useful to remember that the permeability properties of the living membrane change continually.

Diffusional Force. Particles in solution move, or diffuse, from an area of higher concentration to an area of lower concentration. In the case of uncharged, soluble molecules, diffusion proceeds until there is a uniform distribution of the molecules within the solution. The solution is then said to be in equilibrium. At equilibrium, there is still particle movement within the solution, but no net change in overall particle distribution. Charged particles also diffuse. The diffusion of charged particles is influenced not only by the concentration gradient but also by the electrical field.

Electrical Force and Current. Like charges repel, and opposite charges attract. Positively charged particles flow toward negatively charged particles and regions; similarly, negatively charged particles are attracted to positive ions and regions. The electrical (or electromotive) force difference between regions is called the *potential difference* and is expressed in volts (1 mV = 0.001 V). The net flow of charges is called *current* (measured in amperes). *Resistance* is the opposition to the flow of current, measured in ohms. Ohm law (electromotive force = current × resistance) describes the relation among current, voltage, and resistance.

When charged particles have different concentrations in the solutions separated by a cell membrane, and some of the particles are able to permeate the membrane and others are not, an electrical force is established. This force influences the distribution of all other charged particles. The potential difference across biologic membranes is described by comparing the interior of the cell with the external solution. In the typical quiescent or resting myocardial cell, the potential difference is −70 to −90 mV; that is, the cell interior is negative with respect to the exterior. When positively charged ions move from the extracellular fluid to the intracellular fluid, the current is said to be *inward*. With inward current, the

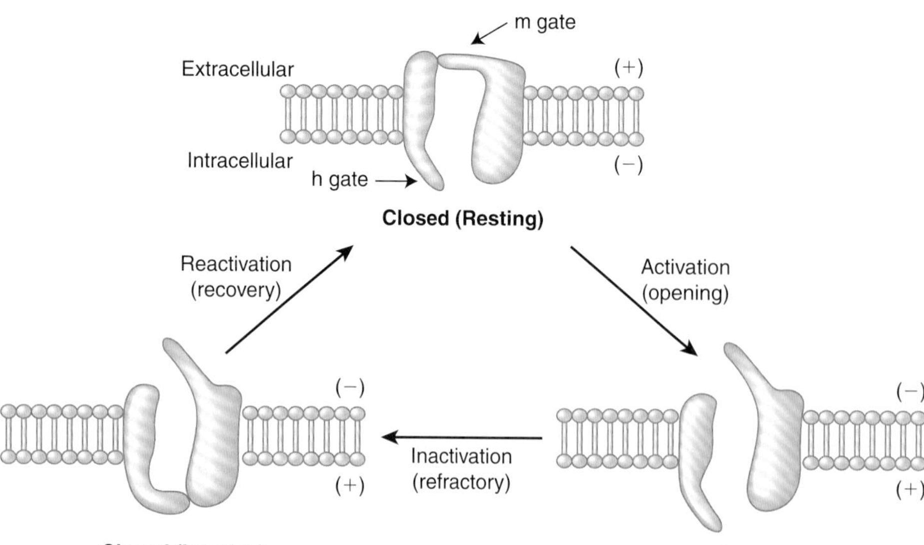

Figure 2-34. Three states of a voltage-gated ion channel. Depicted are the two closed and one open state. Transition between these states (*arrows*) open the channel (activation), close the channel in a refractory state where it cannot be reopened (inactivation), and reactivate the channel by ending this refractory state (recovery). (Used with permission from Katz A. *Physiology of the Heart*. 5th ed. Philadelphia, PA: Lippincott Williams & Wilkins; 2010.)

cell interior becomes less negative, that is, it depolarizes. When positively charged ions flow into the extracellular space from the interior of the cell, the current is said to be *outward*; the cell repolarizes or hyperpolarizes. Movement of negatively charged ions in one direction is electrically equivalent to an opposite-directed movement of positively charged ions. Thus, the inward movement of an anion such as chloride is called an outward current. This, too, causes repolarization or hyperpolarization.

Nernst Equation Calculation of Equilibrium Potential for Specific Ions. The Nernst equation is used to calculate the *equilibrium potential* for a particular ion. If the potential difference across the membrane is the same as that calculated by the Nernst equation for a particular ion, then the electrical force would counterbalance the concentration difference of that specific ion. If the membrane were permeable to the ion, there would be no net ion movement. An understanding of the equilibrium potential is basic to an understanding of the electrical characteristics of biologic membranes.

Potassium ion distribution across the sarcolemma provides a useful example in discussing the Nernst equation. Potassium ions (positively charged) are more concentrated in the sarcoplasm than in the extracellular space. To balance the force of the concentration difference, the inside of the myocardial cell would need to be approximately −94 mV compared with outside of the membrane. That charge, −94 mV, is known as the potassium ion equilibrium potential or the Nernst potential for potassium ion. The resting myocardial membrane is permeable to potassium ions. The large concentration gradient is maintained because the actual voltage across the membrane between activation cycles, approximately −90 mV (inside negative), is close to the Nernst potential for potassium ions in the myocardial cell, and thus nearly sufficient to retain potassium ions within the cell. The slow outward trickle of potassium ions is corrected by a membrane pump that moves potassium ions back into the cell (and moves sodium ions out of the cell). If the resting potential were −94 mV, there would be no net potassium ion movement.

The following illustrates the Nernst equation calculation of the equilibrium potential for potassium ion:

$$E_K = \frac{RT}{FZ_K} \ln \frac{[K^+]_o}{[K^+]_i}$$

where E_K = equilibrium potential for K^+
R = gas constant
T = absolute temperature
F = the Faraday (number of coulombs per mole of charge)
Z_K = the valence of K^+ (+1)
$[K^+]_o$ = K^+ concentration outside the cell (e.g., 4 mM)
$[K^+]_i$ = K^+ concentration inside the cell (e.g., 155 mM)

Converting from the natural log to the base 10 log and replacing the constants measured at 37°C with numeric values, the equation becomes approximately as follows:

$$E_K = 61 \log_{10} \frac{[K^+]_o}{[K^+]_i}$$

$$E_K = 61 \log_{10} \frac{4}{155} = -97 \text{ mV}$$

According to the Nernst equation, the higher the potassium ion concentration in the external solution, the more depolarized is the *potassium equilibrium potential*. If the resting membrane were highly permeable to potassium ion, then the higher the external potassium ion concentration, the more depolarized would be the *resting potential*. If one were to perform such an experiment, placing an intact muscle cell in a dish bathed in solutions with varying potassium ion concentrations as the potassium ion concentration in the external solution is raised, the membrane becomes more depolarized. When the concentration of potassium ion in the extracellular fluid becomes equal to the concentration in the intracellular fluid, the membrane potential is 0 mV.

In cardiac surgery, when it is important to have a heart without electrical and mechanical activity, the organ is sometimes perfused with cool cardioplegic solution. The perfusate typically contains 15 to 35 mM potassium. As would be predicted from the Nernst equation, the cell membranes depolarize. The depolarized cells no longer experience an action potential, resulting in a motionless surgical field.

Each ion has a different equilibrium potential that depends on the relative concentrations of that ion on the two sides of the membrane (see Table 2-2). In each case, the equilibrium potential can be calculated using the Nernst equation. For example, given typical sodium ion concentrations as in Table 2-2, the equilibrium potential for sodium ion is approximately +60 mV. This means that if the membrane were permeable to sodium ion, then the membrane potential would have to be +60 mV to halt net inward sodium current. At typical resting potentials of −90 mV, a large electromotive force favors inward sodium current. The sodium concentration is markedly higher in the extracellular space than it is in the intracellular space. Thus, diffusion forces also favor inward sodium current. At rest, however, there is minimal net movement of sodium ion because the sodium channels are closed. When the channels open during activation, the diffusional and electrical forces combine to produce a large, but transient, inward current carried by sodium ion. The result is rapid depolarization.

The chloride ion concentration is higher in the extracellular space than in the intracellular space. Thus, diffusional force favors inward movement of chloride ion. However, the resting membrane potential is at approximately the chloride ion equilibrium potential. Thus, the negative potential opposes the net inward movement of chloride ion. The resting muscle membrane is permeant to chloride ion, but there is scant net chloride ion movement.

The sarcoplasmic calcium ion concentration is extremely low. Calcium ions are actively removed from the sarcoplasm. Calcium ions are taken up into the SR and pumped outward to the extracellular space. The extracellular calcium ion concentration is in the millimolar range, approximately 10,000 times higher than the intracellular concentration. Thus, a powerful concentration gradient would move calcium ions inward if a path were available. A powerful electrical force also favors inward movement. The calcium ion equilibrium potential calculated from the Nernst equation is more positive than +100 mV. However, the resting membrane is not permeant to calcium ion. As with the sodium ion, the opening of a calcium ion channel evokes a large inward current. This inward current happens during activation. An increase in intracellular calcium ion signals metabolic and contractile changes.

Calculating Membrane Resting Potential. At high extracellular potassium ion concentrations, the Nernst equation for potassium ion predicts resting membrane potential with good accuracy. In and below the physiologic range of external potassium ion concentrations, the membrane potential is slightly less negative than would be predicted based on potassium ion concentrations. This state occurs because at very low external potassium ion concentrations, the membrane is slightly permeable to sodium ion. Because concentration and electrical gradients for sodium ion both favor inward sodium ion movement, an increase in sodium ion permeability allows an inward trickling of sodium ions (an inward current). The membrane depolarizes, becoming several millivolts more positive than the potassium ion equilibrium potential. The ratio of potassium and sodium permeabilities determines the extent to which the resting membrane potential deviates from the potassium ion equilibrium potential. Equations have been developed to predict resting membrane potential based on the relative permeabilities and concentrations of various ions. These computations assume that the membrane is in a steady state and that there are no active ion pumps producing current.

Typically, cardiac muscle cell resting membrane potential is approximately −90 mV. Excitation and propagation of excitation depend on the resting membrane potential. The more negative the resting membrane potential, the more current is required to initiate excitation, but the speed and amplitude of the subsequent depolarizing excitation are greater. The less negative is the resting membrane potential, the less is the current required to initiate excitation but the speed and amplitude of depolarization are reduced. If the resting potential is substantially depolarized, the cell can be impossible to activate.

The resting membrane potential is altered by changes in the ionic milieu on either side of the membrane and by hormones or drugs that alter the relative permeabilities of potassium or sodium ion. Factors that alter the action of the sodium–potassium pump alter the resting membrane potential. These include insulin and epinephrine (hyperpolarizing influences) and digoxin-like drugs (depolarizing influence).

Ionic Activity. Although electrochemical gradients are most frequently explained in terms of chemical concentration gradients, it is actually each ion's chemical activity that affects most cellular functions. Ionic activity reflects interactions between ions as well as the ion concentration. An ion's activity is equal to its concentration times its activity coefficient. It is possible to make reasonably accurate measurements of ionic activities within cells. However, most descriptions of ion movements are based on ion concentration.

Ion Movement Across the Myocardial Cell Membrane.

Passive Ion Movement. Ions traverse the sarcolemma passively through membrane-bound, water-filled pores called *channels.* When a channel is open, any ions that are able to pass through the channel move according to the concentration and electrical gradient, as constrained by the channel dimensions. When the channel is closed, ions do not penetrate. The opening and closing properties of an ion channel are referred to as its *gating* characteristics. The signal to open may be a change in the electrical field (voltage-gated channel) or a change in the chemical milieu (receptor-gated channel). Changes in the internal or external milieu may modify channel gating. Also, there can be time-dependent effects. For example, a small depolarization opens the sodium channel; it closes after a few milliseconds.

An important channel characteristic is its ability to allow passage of some ions while excluding others. This is called *selective permeability.* A theoretical model of an ionic channel is given in Figure 2-35.

The sodium channel is common in excitable cells and has been well characterized. In Nobel prize–winning work, Hodgkin and Huxley[32] described the sodium current of the squid giant axon. According to them, at rest, the membrane potential is negative, perhaps −90 mV, extracellular sodium ion concentration is high, and intracellular concentration low. Electrical and diffusion gradients favor inward sodium ion movement. Because the sodium channel is closed, there is no path for the ions to travel. With a small depolarization the sodium channel opens. This opening of the sodium channel in response to a small depolarizing current is sometimes described as opening the *activation (or m) gate.* When the activation gate opens, the sodium channel is then open; an inward depolarizing of sodium ion flows. Because both the electrical and concentration gradients are significant and favor inward movement, this inward current is intense. After a few milliseconds, however, another gate (sometimes called the *inactivation* or *h gate*) closes, halting the current. The h gate remains closed until the membrane is restored to a sufficiently negative voltage. At that time, the inactivation gate opens but no current flows because the activation gate has closed. With the closing of either gate, current is halted. To summarize, the sodium channel is conceptualized as having two gates. At resting membrane potential, the channel is closed because the activation gate is closed. Depolarization opens that gate but, after a brief lag, the inactivation gate closes, again closing the channel. Repolarization opens the inactivation gate but closes the activation gate.

Scores of channels have been described, each with characteristic gating and selectivity profiles. The mixing of channel types in

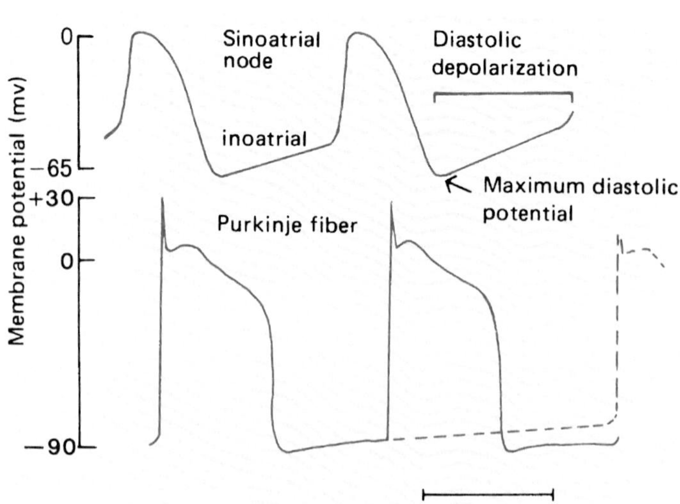

Figure 2-35. Action potentials of sinus node cells and Purkinje cells. Purkinje cells are not discharged by impulses from the sinus node or elsewhere, the Purkinje diastolic depolarization progresses enough to attain threshold. (Adapted from Vassale M. *Cardiac Physiology for the Clinician.* New York: Academic Press; 1976:35.)

various membranes can produce a rich repertoire of biologic operating characteristics. The membrane of vertebrate cardiac muscle is especially complex, with a diverse mix of channels. The result is a dynamic, responsive membrane that can be finely tuned to varying operating conditions. Some of the other major channels of the vertebrate heart are described later in this chapter.

Active Ion Transport. Any movement of ion against its electrochemical gradient is said to be *active movement* or *active transport.* To move any ion against its electrochemical gradient requires energy. The energy may be stored in ATP. In some cases, the energy stored in one ion's electrochemical gradient can be expended to power the movement of another ion against its electrochemical gradient. The former ion is said to be moving "downhill" or in the direction of a lower energy state. The ion that is moved against the gradient is said to be transported "uphill."

Sodium–Potassium–Adenosine Triphosphatase Pump. At resting potential, there is a slight inward trickle of sodium ions. During activation, there is transient inward sodium current. Sodium–potassium pumps on the cardiac muscle membrane (as well as on many other types of membranes) moves sodium ion back out of the cell in exchange for an inward movement of potassium ions. Both ions are moving against a concentration gradient. The pump is powered by the energy stored in ATP; hence, the pump is known as the *sodium–potassium pump* or *sodium–potassium–ATPase.* This pump helps to reestablish the resting concentrations of intracellular sodium and potassium after cardiac depolarization. The ratio of sodium ions pumped out to potassium ions pumped in is usually 3:2. This ratio of 3:2 results in a net outward charge movement, hyperpolarizing the membrane. A primary regulator of this pump is the intracellular sodium ion concentration. Other factors influencing pump activity include extracellular sodium concentration and intracellular and extracellular potassium concentration. Digoxin-like drugs block the sodium–potassium pump.[33] Epinephrine and insulin both stimulate the sodium–potassium pump, causing uptake of potassium into cells. Clinicians capitalize on this feature when they administer insulin and glucose to the hyperkalemic patient. Epinephrine and insulin can be associated with hypokalemia.

Sodium–Calcium Exchange. Another important cardiac membrane pump is the sodium–calcium pump. Calcium ion moves across the sarcolemma into the cell to activate contraction. It must be removed. Although there is some harvesting of calcium ion into the intracellular sequestering sites such as SR, the inward movement and storage cannot go on unopposed. Calcium ion is moved back into the extracellular space by means of an exchange pump. The energy stored in the sodium gradient powers the movement of calcium ion. In other words, sodium ion is moved downhill to pump calcium ion uphill.[34] Usually, this exchange mechanism transports three sodium ions into the cell for one calcium ion transported out of the cell. In this situation, the pump is electrogenic, but the direction or ratios of transmembrane ion exchanges may be reversed or changed. When the concentration of intracellular sodium ion is increased (e.g., when the use of digoxin-like drugs has partially blocked the sodium–potassium–ATPase pump), there is less energy stored in the sodium gradient. This exchange mechanism does not promote as great a sodium influx and calcium efflux. There is then more calcium ion stored in the SR and more calcium ion released during activation, with net positive inotropic effects.

Calcium ATPase Pumps. The cardiac SR actively pumps calcium ion uphill into its core in a process that hydrolyzes ATP as an energy source. An active calcium pump in the cardiac sarcolemma also extrudes calcium ion from the cell. The latter may be more important in vascular tissue than in cardiac muscle.

CARDIAC ACTION POTENTIAL

Each structural cardiac cell type (e.g., working myocardial, nodal, Purkinje cells) has characteristic action potential features. Electrically, there are two general types of cardiac cells: *fast-* and *slow-response* cells. Fast-response cells (e.g., Purkinje and working myocardial cells) have a fairly constant resting membrane potential, a rapid depolarization, and then a period of sustained depolarization (called *plateau phase*) before repolarizing to resting potential. Impulse conduction to adjacent cells is rapid. Slow-response cells (e.g., sinus and AV nodal cells) slowly and spontaneously depolarize during the interim prior to the action potential, and have a shorter, nonprominent plateau phase that merges into a slow repolarization period. These cells conduct more slowly (Fig. 2-36). Ionic current differences account for varying action potential shape.

In the following sections, the cardiac action potential is described. Table 2-3 summarizes the electrophysiologic properties of the various tissue types.

Fast-Type Myocardial Action Potentials

The fast response–type cell has a five-phase action potential (Fig. 2-37). Phase 0 is the initial period of rapid depolarization, the action potential upstroke. Membrane potential changes from resting potential (approximately −90 mV) to a value positive to 0 mV (e.g., +30 mV). After this brief (less than 1- to 2-millisecond) phase, the cell repolarizes slightly (phase 1) and then there is a period of sustained depolarization called the *plateau phase* (phase 2). In phase 3, repolarization becomes rapid, returning the membrane

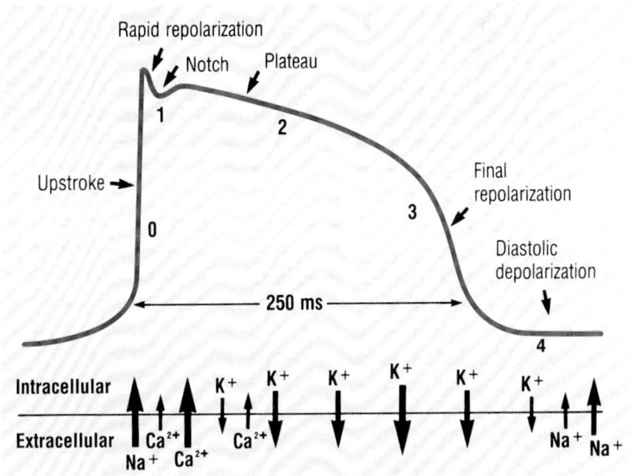

Figure 2-36. Schematic illustration of major ionic movements during a Purkinje cell action potential, with the cell depicted as exhibiting spontaneous depolarization. *Arrows* indicate approximate times when the indicated ion movement influences membrane potential. Pumps, exchanges, and leaks are not illustrated. Under normal physiologic conditions, Purkinje cells do not exhibit spontaneous depolarization. (Adapted from Ten Eick RE, Baumgarten CM, Sunger DH. Ventricular dysrhythmia: membrane basis of currents, channels, gates and cables. *Prog Cardiovasc Dis.* 1981;24:159 and Fozzard HA, Gibbons WR. Action potential and contraction of heart muscle. *Am J Cardiol.* 1973;31:183.)

Table 2-3 • CARDIAC ACTION POTENTIAL PROPERTIES[a]

	Fast-Conducting Tissue			Slow-Conducting Tissue	
	Purkinje	**Atrial Muscle**	**Ventricular Muscle**	**Sinus Node**	**Atrioventricular Node**
Resting Potential	−90 to −95 mV	−80 to −90 mV	−80 to −90 mV	−50 to −60 mV	−60 to −70 mV
Activation Threshold	−70 to −60 mV			−40 to −30 mV	
Action Potential					
Rate of Phase 0 (V_{max}) (V/s)	500–800	100–200	100–200	1–10	5–15
Amplitude (mV)	120	110–120	110–120	60–70	70–80
Overshoot (mV)	30	30	30	0–10	5–15
Duration (ms)	300–500	100–300	200–300	100–300	100–300
Diastolic Depolarization (Major Ion)		Not prominent		Prominent	
Depolarizing Current		Na^+		Ca^{2+}	
Channel Blocked by	Tetrodotoxin, type I antiarrhythmics, or sustained depolarization at −40 mV			Mn^{2+}, La^{3+}, verapamil, nifedipine, other inorganic substances, type IV antiarrhythmics	
Effect of Adrenergic Stimulation	Not pronounced			Pronounced	

[a]Values are approximations and vary with methods and specific tissue used.
Adapted from Bigger JT. Electrophysiology for the clinician. *Eur Heart J.* 1984;5(Suppl B):1–9; Opie L. *The Heart.* Orlando: Grune & Stratton; 1984:44; Sperelakis N. Origin of the cardiac resting potential. In: Berne RE, ed. *Handbook of Physiology, Section 2: The Cardiovascular System (Vol 1, the Heart).* Bethesda, MD: American Physiological Society; 1979:190; Zipes DP. Genesis of cardiac arrhythmias. In: Braunwald E, ed. *Heart Disease.* 2nd ed. Philadelphia, PA: WB Saunders; 1984:615.

to resting potential. Phase 4 is the interval between action potentials; the resting potential is fairly constant. The cardiac action potential may take hundreds of milliseconds. Duration and amplitude of each phase depends on the opening and closing of various ion channels, which in turn, depends on the ionic and neurohormonal milieu. Conduction to adjacent cells is rapid.

Phase 0: Action Potential Upstroke

The working myocardial cell action potential is initiated by an inward current flowing primarily by way of the low-resistance nexus. This small current depolarizes the cell to threshold (approximately −70 mV; Fig. 2-38). Once threshold voltage is reached, the sodium channel activation gate opens, thus, opening the sodium channel followed by a large inward current carried by sodium ions. The depolarizing current opens more sodium channels, producing the propagating, regenerating, swift depolarization of the action potential upstroke. Peak voltages attained are

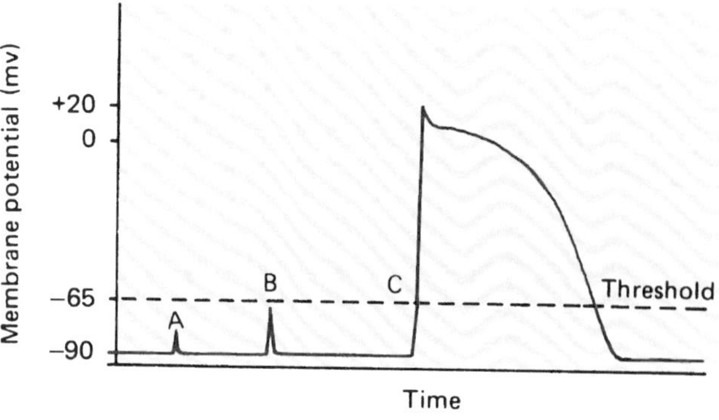

Figure 2-37. Schematic illustration of the initiation of an action potential when the membrane potential is depolarized to threshold. Small depolarizing stimuli (**A** and **B**) that fail to reach threshold (*dashed line*) are unable to initiate an action potential. When depolarization reaches threshold (**C**), a regenerative action potential is produced. Once the latter begins, further depolarization becomes independent of the initial stimulus. (Used with permission from Katz A. *Physiology of the Heart.* 5th ed. Philadelphia, PA: Lippincott Williams & Wilkins; 2010.)

+30 to +40 mV, approaching but not attaining the sodium equilibrium potential (approximately +65 mV). Depolarization closes the inactivation gate. The channel closes, halting the current and stopping depolarization.

The maximal velocity of phase 0 depolarization is sometimes called V_{max} (to be distinguished from the contractile variable, maximal shortening velocity, also called V_{max}). The speed of impulse conduction through the myocardium depends on V_{max} for the individual cells. V_{max} reflects sodium channel activity. Factors that alter the resting potential or the sodium gradient alter V_{max}. Such factors include ionic milieu and certain drugs, including many antiarrhythmic drugs. Class I antiarrhythmic agents (lidocaine, quinidine, procainamide, etc.) block the fast sodium channel, slowing the rate of phase 0 depolarization.

Generally, the more negative is the resting membrane potential, the faster is V_{max}, and the greater is the amplitude of depolarization. Hyperpolarization opens the inactivation gate. When depolarization opens the activation gate, the sodium channel is open, and the current is intense. Conversely, if the membrane potential preceding threshold depolarization is less negative, inactivation may be incompletely removed; V_{max} is slower. Hyperkalemia causes such depolarization; this condition is associated with arrhythmias.

Phase 1: Early Repolarization

The rapid upstroke ceases when sodium channels close spontaneously after a few milliseconds (caused by inactivation). Another transient current is activated, the transient outward current. This outward current is carried primarily by potassium ion (moving outward) but also by chloride ion (moving inward) and results in the slight repolarization of the cell to approximately +10 mV. When the voltage is positive, both the concentration gradient and the electrical force (inside positive) favor outflow of the positively charged potassium ion from the cell, an outward current. Similarly, with chloride ion, when the membrane potential is positive, the electrical gradient amplifies the concentration gradient, both favoring inward movement of the negatively charged chloride ion. Inward movement of negative ions is electrically indistinguishable from an outward movement of positive ions; both are called *outward currents.*

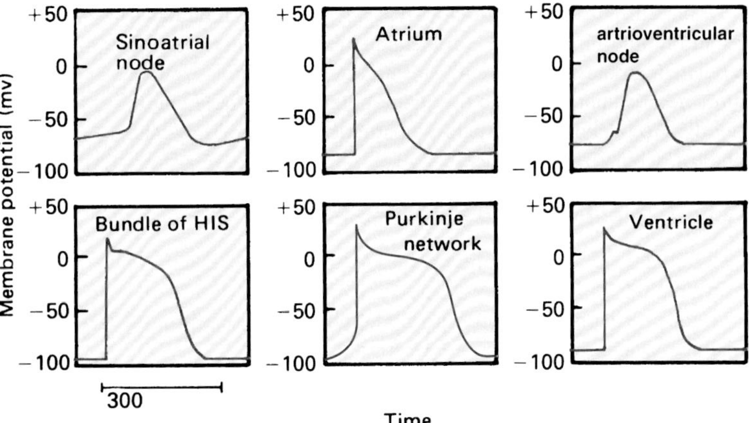

Figure 2-38. Characteristic action potentials in different regions of the heart. See text for description. (Used with permission from Katz A. *Physiology of the Heart*. 5th ed. Philadelphia, PA: Lippincott Williams & Wilkins; 2010.)

Phase 1 ends with the closure of the current-bearing channels. A "notch" appears on the action potential profile. The voltage of the notch region has important effects on subsequent gating of other channels and can affect the shape of the remainder of the action potential.

Phase 2: Action Potential Plateau

During the plateau, little net current flows. Inward (depolarizing) and outward (repolarizing) currents are nearly balanced; there is little change in membrane voltage. Inward currents are carried by sodium and calcium ions. Calcium ion in turn evokes additional calcium ion release from internal stores; contraction ensues. Outward currents are carried by potassium ion. Over time, calcium channels inactivate, repolarizing outward potassium currents predominate and the membrane repolarizes. This phase ends when the calcium channels close.

During the plateau, sodium currents travel through fast sodium channels that failed to inactivate and through at least two types of calcium channels. Both types of calcium channels open with depolarization, and then close spontaneously after a period of time. β-Adrenergic agonists potentiate calcium currents, increasing plateau amplitude and duration. Ultimately, the result is increased sarcoplasmic calcium ion concentration, which in turn has a positive inotropic effect on contraction. Calcium channel blockers, acidosis, and ATP depletion are negative inotropes, diminishing calcium currents, reducing plateau amplitude and duration, and diminishing the force generated during contraction.

The counterbalancing outward current is carried by potassium ion through multiple channel types. One type of potassium channel that is important in disease is the ATP-sensitive potassium current. This potassium channel is activated or opened when the ATP concentration falls, such as during ischemia, which in turn greatly shortens the duration of the plateau and hastens the onset of the rapid repolarization phase. Shortened depolarization decreases the calcium current and thus the contractile force (a negative inotropic influence).

The plateau phase distinguishes working myocardial cells from skeletal muscle cells and neuronal tissue. The plateau provides for greater inward calcium currents in cardiac muscle. Because the cell is refractory to stimulation for the duration of phase 2 and much of phase 3, cardiac muscle cannot experience tetany.

Phase 3: Late Rapid Repolarization

The calcium currents that sustained the plateau eventually stop when the calcium channels close and repolarization proceeds unopposed, caused by outward potassium ion movement. As membrane voltage becomes increasingly negative, sodium channel inactivation is removed. The sodium channel can once again be activated (as soon as a small depolarization opens the activation gate).

Phase 4: Interim Between Action Potentials

During rapid repolarization (phase 3), the membrane potential is restored to the resting potential. Phase 4 is the period between the end of rapid repolarization and the start of the next action potential. During phase 4, the membrane is permeable to potassium ion. The membrane voltage is close to the potassium equilibrium potential. The type of potassium channel open during this phase is called the *inward rectifier* (so called because it allows inward current more readily than outward current). Because the membrane potential is slightly more positive than the potassium equilibrium potential, potassium trickles outward.

Slow-Type Myocardial Action Potentials

Slow-response cells, such as cells of the sinus and AV nodes, spontaneously depolarize between action potentials. The action potential upstroke of depolarization is slower; the plateau phase is shorter and nonprominent; repolarization is slower; the maximum repolarization potential achieved is less negative than that in fast-response cells.

Phase 0 depolarization is slower in the slow-response cells; it is primarily carried by calcium ion rather than sodium ion. The transition between the depolarization rate before and after reaching threshold is less abrupt in the in slow-response cells. Phase 1 is absent: there is no large transient outward potassium current and no notch in the action potential. Phase 2 is present, but abbreviated. Slow repolarization begins after the maximal positive voltage. As in other cells, potassium efflux evokes repolarization in slow myocytes. Phase 3 repolarization is similar to that in fast myocytes, although the rate of repolarization is slower and the maximal diastolic potential attained is less negative than in fast-response cells. During phase 4, the slow-response cells continually depolarize toward threshold. Maximal negative voltage at the start of phase 4 is approximately −60 mV, termed the *maximal diastolic potential* (see Fig. 2-37). Phase 4 spontaneous depolarization is caused by the following sequence of currents: a nonselective channel opens, allowing inward sodium current; outward potassium current declines after some depolarization; transient (T)-type calcium channels open, allowing inward calcium current; long-lasting (L)-type calcium channels open, again allowing inward calcium current and evoking the action potential upstroke, phase 0.

Ionic currents flowing in slow-type myocytes are modulated by autonomic innervation. Adrenergic stimulation increases the repolarizing potassium current, causing the cell to repolarize to a more negative potential, and the action potential to proceed more swiftly. Acetylcholine, the parasympathetic mediator, slows the phase 4 depolarizing currents.

Action Potential of the Sinus Node Cells

Cells in the sinus node spontaneously depolarize to threshold more rapidly than do other automatic cardiac cells. Thus, the slope of phase 4 is steeper in sinus node cells and these cells normally set the pace for cardiac contraction.

Action Potential of Purkinje-Type Cells

The Purkinje cell action potential is similar to that of the working myocardial cell, although the plateau duration is somewhat prolonged. Hypoxia and acidosis in ischemic Purkinje cells may produce conditions in which the fast sodium channel is not opened. Phase 0 depolarization is then due to slow channel activation, carried primarily by calcium ion.

Action Potential of Atrial Cells

Atrial working myocardial cells undergo rapid depolarization. These cells have essentially no plateau period, but repolarization is slower than in Purkinje cells (Fig. 2-39). The total action potential duration of atrial cells is shorter than that of Purkinje cells. Atrial muscle cells do not spontaneously depolarize under physiologic conditions. Spontaneous depolarization can occur under nonphysiologic conditions.

Cells in the AV Node

In general, spontaneously depolarizing cells of the AV node are similar to sinus node cells in the rate of phase 0 depolarization and of maximal repolarization voltage. The AV node has several types of cells with different electrophysiologic characteristics; these are termed *atrionodal*, *nodal*, and *nodal-His*. These are located in the upper, middle, and lower junctional areas, respectively.[35]

Cells in the Bundle of His

The electrophysiologic characteristics of His bundle cells closely resemble those of Purkinje cells in the distal conducting system. The duration of the His bundle action potential, however, is slightly less than that of cells in the Purkinje network. The most rapid period of depolarization and the longest period of repolarization occur in Purkinje cells at the distal end of the conducting system.

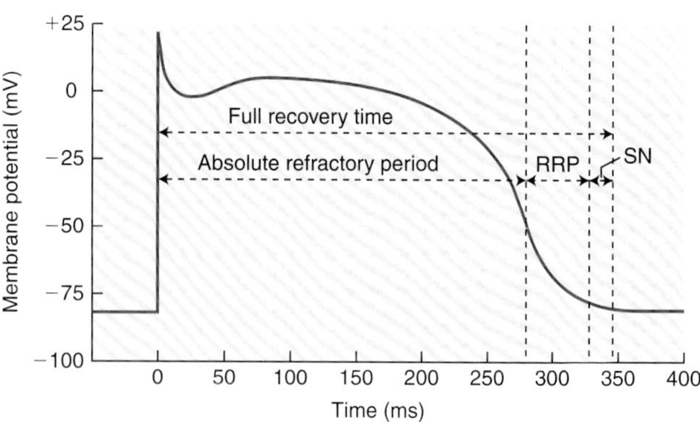

Figure 2-39. Refractory periods. Closing of the h gates immediately after membrane depolarization causes the absolute refractory period, during which no stimulus regardless of its strength is able to initiate a propagated action potential. This is followed by a relative refractory period (RRP) during which only stimuli that exceed the normal threshold can cause a propagated action potential. The functional refractory period, which includes the absolute and relative refractory periods, is followed by a supernormal (SN) period, during which subthreshold stimuli slightly less than those that reach the normal threshold can generate a propagated action potential. Action potentials generated during the relative refractory and supernormal periods are small and slowly rising because of incomplete recovery of the sodium channels. The full recovery time begins with depolarization and ends after the supernormal period, when normal stimuli produce normally propagated action potentials. (Used with permission from Katz A. *Physiology of the Heart*. 5th ed. Philadelphia, PA: Lippincott Williams & Wilkins; 2010.)

Refractory Periods

The period after depolarization, during which it is difficult or impossible to reexcite the cell, is termed the *refractory period* (Fig. 2-40). Refractoriness reflects the effects on depolarization of time and voltage requirements for the activation, inactivation, and recovery of ion channels.

During the *effective refractory period*, no action potential can be initiated by an external electrical stimulus. The duration of this period depends on the time it takes to remove inactivation from the sodium and calcium channels. The effective refractory period extends from phase 0 through the middle of phase 3.

During the *relative refractory period*, only a stimulus greater than normal can initiate an action potential. The relative

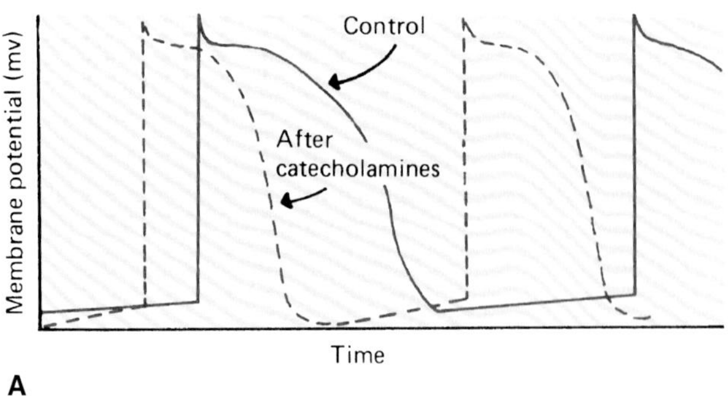

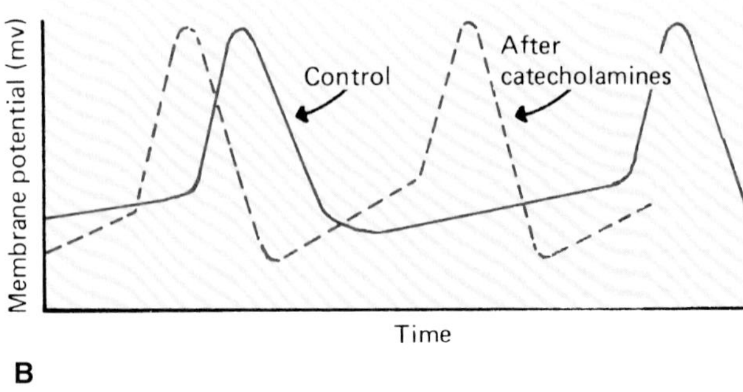

Figure 2-40. Schematic illustration of the general electrophysiological effects of catecholamines on **(A)** Purkinje cells and **(B)** sinus node cells. (Used with permission from Katz A. *Physiology of the Heart*. 4th ed. Philadelphia, PA: Lippincott Williams & Wilkins; 2006:449.)

refractory period occurs during the latter part of repolarization (late phase 3). Under certain conditions, a stimulus can initiate an action potential during the last part of phase 3 and the beginning of phase 4. Cardiac arrhythmias may occur during when this happens, especially when pathophysiologic situations, such as ischemia, promote abnormal refractory periods.

The entire period between depolarization and complete repolarization is termed the *full recovery time*. Under normal conditions, cardiac cells are not depolarized until they have had time to recover fully from the previous depolarization. Usually, cells with long refractory periods have long action potential durations. The upper limits of normal HR responses and the time allowed for ventricular filling depend on normal cardiac electrical refractoriness.

SARCOLEMMAL IONIC CURRENTS

The currents that combine to orchestrate the action potential can be studied independently. Neurohormonal and ionic milieu, pharmacologic agents, and pathologic processes variably influence each current. Techniques such as the patch clamp and molecular biology have extended our understanding of channels types and hold the promise of increasing our understanding of important issues such as the generation of arrhythmias in disease states. New treatments are being developed. Some of the major channels are discussed individually (Table 2-4).

Inward Currents

The inward currents are carried by sodium or calcium ions moving into the cell. For each ion, there are several different types of channels, each with its own gating characteristics.

Fast Inward Current I_{NA}

The fast sodium current is activated to cause rapid depolarization in phase 0 of fast-response cells. It was discussed in some detail previously. Briefly, the sodium channel opens with depolarization to threshold (−70 to −60 mV), but quickly closes because of inactivation. Repolarization is necessary to remove the inactivation.[32] The fast sodium current is blocked by the puffer fish poison tetrodotoxin. Many antiarrhythmic agents, particularly class I agents, alter this current.

Calcium Currents

The two major types of calcium channels are termed L (long-lasting) and T (transient). The L current activates with depolarizations beyond −40 mV and then slowly inactivates. The T current activates at −70 mV and rapidly diminishes. Both channels probably contribute to maintaining the plateau phase of the cardiac action potential. The T channels contribute to spontaneous depolarization in pacemaker cells and the L channels contribute to the action potential upstroke in these cells. These currents may be potentiated by β-adrenergic (catecholamine) stimulation and diminished by acetylcholine and acidosis.[30] The current is blocked by inorganic compounds such as lanthanum, cobalt, nickel, and manganese. Organic charged tertiary amines, such as verapamil, block the slow channel. The block depends on membrane potential and rate of stimulation. Organic dihydropyridines, such as nifedipine, also block this channel.

Pacemaker Current

Pacemaking results from the combination of at least four currents. There is a time-dependent inactivation of the potassium current, and thus a loss of outward current (which would tend to

Table 2-4 • CARDIAC IONIC CURRENTS

Current[a]	Charge Carrier	Activation Mechanism	Function
Inward Currents			
I_{Na}	Na^+	Voltage	AP upstroke
I_{Ca} (I_{Si}, I_{Caf}, I_{Cas})	Ca^{2+}	Voltage	AP plateau E–C coupling AP upstroke Sinus pacemaker
I_f (I_h)	Na^+ and K^+	Voltage	Spontaneous depolarization
I_{ti} ($I_{t'}$, $I_{Na,K}$)	Na^+ and K^+	?[(Ca^{2+}]$_i$	After-depolarization
Outward Currents			
I_K (I_x, I_{x1}, I_{x2})	K^+ (Na^+)	Voltage	Repolarization
I_{to}	K^+	Voltage, ?[Ca^{2+}]	Early repolarization
I_{K1}	K^+	Voltage	Resting potential Repolarization ?Plateau potential
I_{KCa}	K^+	[Ca^{2+}]$_i$	Repolarization
I_{KAch}	K^+	ACh, ? voltage	Inhibition
Pump/Exchange Currents			
I_p	Na^+, K^+	[K^+], [Na^+]	Na^+–K^+–ATPase pump
$I_{Na,Ca}$	Na^+, Ca^{2+}	[Ca^{2+}], [Na^+]	Na^+–Ca^{2+} exchange
Background Currents			
I_{bNa}	Na^+	?	Inward leakage
I_{bCa}	Ca^{2+}	?	? Inward leakage
? I_{bCl}	Cl^-	?	?

[a]Currents identified in multicellular preparations are labeled I and currents identified in single-cell preparations are labeled i. Some of these currents are speculative (see text).

Ach, acetylcholine; AP, action potential; E–C, excitation–contraction; [], concentration of ion indicated.

Adapted from Brown HF. Electrophysiology of the sinoatrial node. *Physiol Rev.* 1982;62(2):505–530; Nobel D. The surprising heart. *J Physiol.* 1981;353:43; Opie L. *The Heart.* Orlando, FL: Grune & Stratton; 1984:47; and Reuter H. Ion channels in cardiac cell membranes. *Ann Rev Physiol.* 1984;46:474.

hyperpolarize). This inactivation alone does not produce depolarization; channels that carry ions with an equilibrium potential positive to the membrane potential also must open. The currents involved are I_h, I_{Ca}, and background sodium current. I_h channels open at negative (hyperpolarized) potentials (hence the designation "h"), close at positive potentials, and allow passage of both sodium (hence a depolarizing influence) and potassium. Gating is slow. Similarly, a sodium leak current occurs and is a depolarizing influence. Calcium channels are activated with depolarization. With increasing depolarization, the calcium T channels open, carrying inward depolarizing calcium current (I_{Ca}).[36]

Transient Diastolic Inward Current I_{ti}

The transient diastolic inward current is a nonselective current that carries both sodium and potassium and may be activated by intracellular calcium. It is not normally active but may be involved in initiating delayed depolarizations and triggering arrhythmias in Purkinje and ventricular muscle cells, particularly when extracellular potassium concentration is low. Other inward currents have been identified. Sodium and calcium "leak" currents and the sodium–calcium exchange mechanisms can generate small inward currents.

Outward Currents

A cell can experience outward current in two primary ways: (1) potassium can flow out of the cell or (2) chloride can flow inward. Both ways tend to repolarize the membrane that had been depolarized and to stabilize the resting membrane potential. There are many types of potassium currents in cardiac muscle.

Outward Rectifying Current I_K

The outward rectifying current causes repolarization after an action potential. It opens slowly after depolarization, so it is also called the *delayed rectifying current.* It carries potassium, and it closes with repolarization. It also may be labeled I_x, and has been subdivided into I_{x1} early rapid component and I_{x2} late slower component.

Background Outward Current I_{K1}

This potassium current flows through channels that close with depolarization and open with repolarization. Thus, when the cell is depolarized during the plateau phase, the channel is closed. Were the channel open, potassium would flow outward, resulting in a repolarization. This repolarization would abort the plateau and halt the calcium current, which activates contraction. Hence, it is efficient that this channel is closed during depolarization. It is open with repolarization and serves to stabilize the membrane potential close to the potassium equilibrium potential. It is sometimes called the *inward rectifier* because it is highly permeant to inward potassium currents but less permeant to outward currents. When the membrane is depolarized and potassium can flow outward, the channel closes. It is sensitive to the extracellular potassium concentration.

Transient Outward Current I_{to}

This potassium current is linked with early (phase 1) rapid repolarization. It opens when a cell is depolarized after a period of hyperpolarization, and it closes quickly.

Other Potassium Currents

A nonvoltage-dependent potassium current, which is activated by an increase in the intracellular calcium concentration (I_{Kca}), may participate in the maintenance of the plateau and in repolarization. This current may be the same as or similar to the transient outward current (I_{to}).

Of potential importance in the diseased heart is the ATP-dependent potassium channel. This channel opens when the ATP concentration falls to 10% to 20% of normal.[35] The action potential becomes abbreviated during ischemia. This channel may account for such a phenomenon. It opens when the ATP level drops, shortens the action potential duration, and results in less contraction when the substrate needed for contraction is unavailable.[37]

Acetylcholine activates potassium channels whose outward currents decrease during depolarization. Although this phenomenon may be related to potentiation of the background outward potassium current (I_{K1}), there is evidence for a separate voltage-responsive potassium current (I_{KACh}), whose channels are regulated by muscarinic cholinergic receptors.

Other outward currents have been identified. The sodium–potassium–ATPase pump usually generates a small outward current (I_p).

FACTORS MODIFYING ELECTROPHYSIOLOGIC FUNCTION

Factors that alter cardiac cell depolarization and repolarization do so by affecting the rates of voltage changes, the magnitudes of voltage changes, or the timing of the phases of the cardiac action potential. Such changes affect cardiac impulse generation, impulse conduction, or both, and reflect the effects of environmental alterations on transcellular ionic fluxes.

Impulse generation, or *automaticity*, is influenced by a cardiac cell's maximal diastolic repolarization, threshold level, and rate of spontaneous depolarization to threshold (slope of phase 4). If maximal diastolic repolarization becomes more negative, threshold becomes less negative, or the slope of phase 4 becomes less steep, the rate at which the entire cell is spontaneously depolarized can become slower; opposite effects can lead to a more rapid rate of spontaneous depolarization.

Cardiac impulse conduction velocity is influenced by the rate of depolarization (slope of phase 0), the magnitude of depolarization (amplitude of phase 0), the distance from resting potential to threshold level, the action potential and refractory period durations, and the resistance to current flow. If the rate or amplitude of phase 0 is decreased, the difference between resting potential and threshold is increased, the action potential or refractory periods are lengthened, or the resistance to current flow is increased, the rate of conduction can slow. For example, Purkinje cells have faster conduction velocities than nodal cells because the Purkinje cells have rapid sodium channels that create fast and large depolarization.

The responsiveness of cardiac cells is described by the relation between the membrane potential before rapid depolarization and the maximal velocity of conduction during rapid depolarization. Cardiac cell excitability is described by the current required to alter the membrane potential from resting to threshold.[38] Although once threshold is reached, the cell rapidly depolarizes, the amplitude of the action potential can be decreased if the distance between the resting potential and the threshold potential is less than usual. Stimuli that are insufficient to depolarize a cell to threshold are not effective in initiating action potentials, but such stimuli can have an effect on ionic movements; in pathophysiologic situations, these stimuli may influence cardiac arrhythmia generation and conduction.

Cardiac impulse generation, conduction, or both can be altered by the effects on cardiac cells of changes in the ratio of extracellular to intracellular ionic concentrations, acid–base changes, sympathetic and parasympathetic stimulation, myocardial stretch, cooling, ischemia, and HR changes. These factors often affect different cardiac cells in different ways; the following section discusses general selected examples of some of these alterations. (The effects of alterations in extracellular ionic concentrations on cardiac electrical and mechanical functions are discussed in a subsequent chapter.)

Adrenergic and Cholinergic Effects

Catecholamines

This broad class of biologically active compounds includes many endogenous hormones and neurotransmitters (epinephrine, norepinephrine, and dopamine) as well as pharmacologic agents. These compounds have metabolic, endocrine, central nervous system, and other actions. In the heart they are generally excitatory, increasing the strength and/or the frequency of contraction. In the blood vessels, these substances can evoke constriction or dilation. There are several receptor subtypes producing complex and sometimes conflicting effects on cardiac cell action potentials. Generally, catecholamines increase the magnitude and rate of diastolic depolarization in both Purkinje and sinus nodal cells. Repolarization becomes faster, and the action potential duration is shortened. The increased rate of sinus node spontaneous depolarization (slope of phase 4) appears to be the most important mechanism by which adrenergic stimulation increases HR (Fig. 2-41). Catecholamines increase the amplitude and rate of rise of phase 0 in junctional cells, which increases conduction velocity through the AV node. Catecholamines also increase myocardial contractility. Most of catecholamine effects on the cardiac action potential are caused by stimulation of β-adrenergic receptors.

Acetylcholine

The cholinergic effects of parasympathetic (vagal) nerve stimulation are more pronounced on the sinus node, AV node, and atrial muscle than on ventricular muscle. Acetylcholine slows the rate of diastolic depolarization (slope of phase 4) in sinus node cells. The HR is slowed (Fig. 2-42). The sinus node action potential duration and refractory period are both shortened. There is a decreased rate of rise and amplitude of phase 0 in AV nodal cells in response to acetylcholine, leading to slowed AV conduction. The AV refractory period may also be prolonged. Atrial contractile strength is decreased. Cholinergic cardiac receptor stimulation inhibits cardiac catecholamine effects by inhibiting the β-adrenergic effects of cAMP and inhibiting prejunctional norepinephrine release.

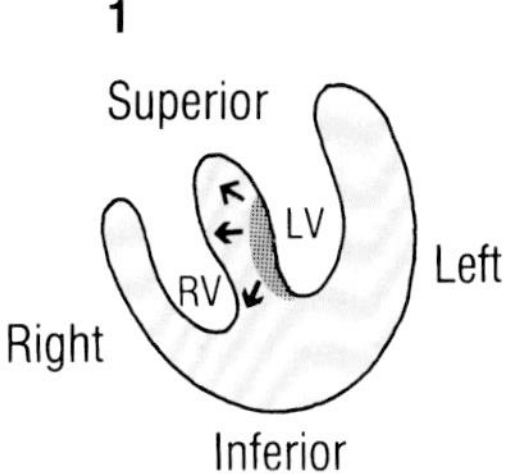

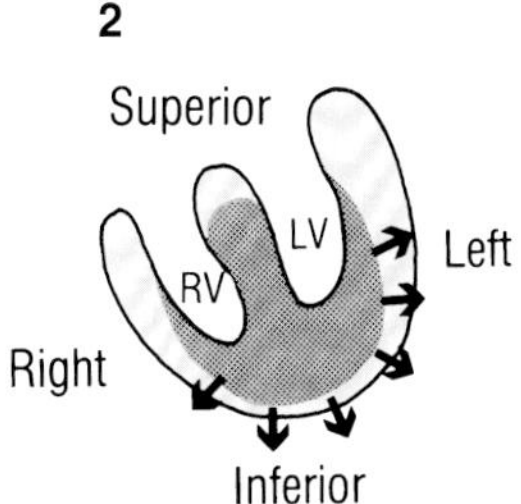

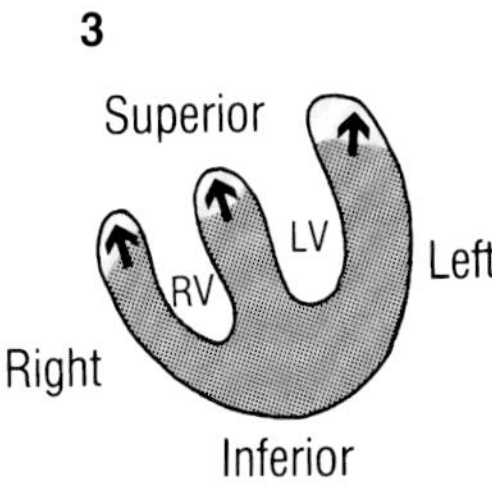

Figure 2-42. Schematic illustration of the sequence of ventricular depolarization. RV, right ventricle; LV, left ventricle. (Used with permission from Katz A. *Physiology of the Heart.* 4th ed. Philadelphia, PA: Lippincott Williams & Wilkins; 2006:447–448.)

Effects of Acidosis and Alkalosis

Acidosis slows repolarization and prolongs the action potential duration in Purkinje fibers. Cardiac calcium channels are blocked by acidosis, resulting in a cardiac action potential with a slower rate of rise, amplitude, and duration.[5] Acidosis decreases contractility by decreasing calcium ion influx and decreasing the sensitivity of the myofibrils to calcium ion.[39] Alkalosis can shorten the action potential duration. Purkinje automaticity is increased owing to an increased rate of diastolic depolarization.[38]

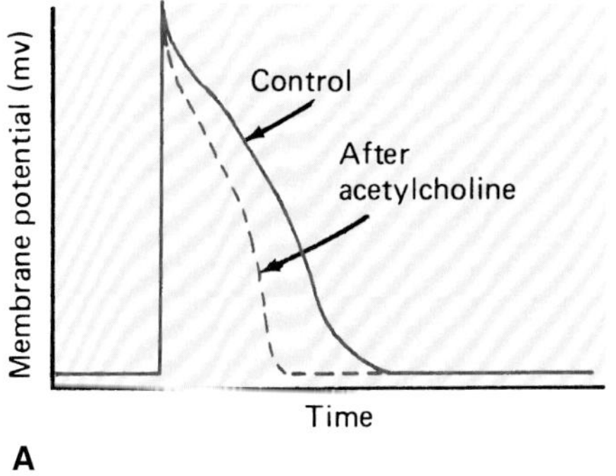

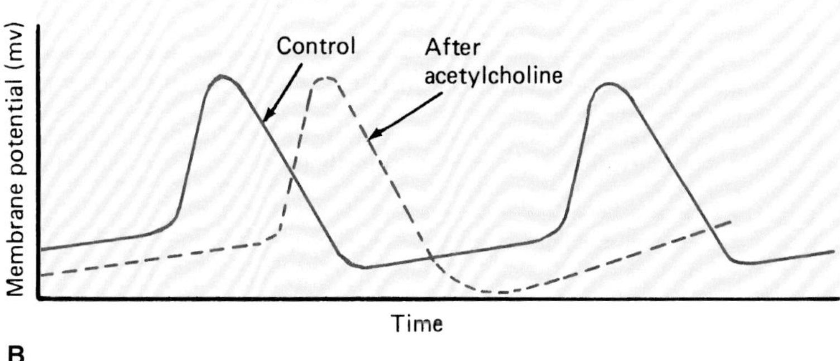

Figure 2-41. Schematic illustration of the general electrophysiologic effects of acetylcholine (vagal stimulation) on **(A)** atrial muscle cells and **(B)** sinus node cells. (Used with permission from Katz AM. *Physiology of the Heart.* 4th ed. New York: Raven Press; 1977:362, 363.)

Other Effects

The action potential duration is related to the length of the preceding diastolic interval. When HR increases (thus the interval between successive cardiac impulses decreases), then repolarization is usually also faster. The action potential is shorter in duration. At slower HRs, the action potential duration lengthens.

In experimental situations, the effects of *warming the heart* are somewhat similar to adrenergic effects (e.g., diastolic depolarization is increased in automatic fibers). *Cooling the heart* depresses spontaneous depolarization in automatic cells. Repolarization is delayed, and conduction is decreased. Arrhythmias may occur during cooling, which is clinically relevant for the cardiac surgical patient who has been subjected to hypothermia and for the patient experiencing hypothermia caused by exposure.

Stretching cardiac fibers increases the rate of diastolic depolarization and makes the maximal diastolic potential less negative in automatic fibers. Myocardial fiber stretch may cause arrhythmias during heart failure.

PROPAGATION OF THE CARDIAC IMPULSE

The spread of the cardiac impulse through the heart depends upon several factors, including (1) anatomic characteristics of the conducting system, (2) structural characteristics of cells (e.g., cardiac cell type and diameter, arrangement of low-resistance intercalated discs, and contiguity to other cells capable of conducting current), and (3) electrophysiologic state of the cell membrane (i.e., resting and threshold potentials, ionic concentrations and conductances, rate and magnitude of depolarization and repolarization, duration of the action potential and the refractory period). As in a battery, there is energy stored across the cell membrane. When one segment of the membrane depolarizes, positive charge enters the cell, and an electrical circuit is established along the cell.[5]

In general, current flows more easily inside the cell and to adjacent cells across the intercalated discs at tight junctions than laterally across adjacent, highly resistant areas of cell membranes. If the current is sufficient to depolarize adjacent cells, a wave of depolarization is propagated and spreads rapidly from cell to cell. Thus, the cardiac tissue behaves essentially as a syncytium, although propagation may be somewhat discontinuous.[40]

As the impulse spreads through the heart, it depolarizes tissue that has recovered and is excitable, but it cannot depolarize tissue that is still refractory. Because the cardiac impulse spreads rapidly through the atria, slowly through the AV junction, and then rapidly through the ventricles, both atria contract almost synchronously, the ventricles have time to receive blood from the contracting atria, and then both ventricles contract almost synchronously.

Atrial Conduction

Sinus node cells normally have the fastest rate of spontaneous depolarization and thus set the pace of cardiac excitation. The sinus node normally initiates the electrical impulse that is then conducted to other areas of the myocardium, depolarizing other cells of the conducting system before those cells have time to spontaneously depolarize to threshold. The electrical impulse appears to spread outward in relatively concentric circles from the sinus node through the atria, moving in approximately 0.1 second from the upper right atrium to the posterior left atrium. Conduction velocity (speed with which the impulse spreads) through the atria is approximately 0.8 to 1 m/s (Table 2-5). Conduction velocities are not equal through the atria; conduction is more rapid by way of the Bachmann bundle into the left atrium than in other areas of the interatrial septum. There are specialized conduction pathways in the atrium as in the ventricle, but the functional significance of the atrial fibers is less clear. Generally, the impulse travels radially within the atria. Atrial repolarization spreads in the same direction as depolarization.

Junctional Conduction

The cardiac impulse is not conducted through the connective tissue of the cardiac skeleton, so cardiac muscle tissue in the AV junction provides the only pathway for electrical conduction from the atria to the ventricles. Conduction velocity through the AV node is approximately 0.05 m/s, although in some areas it has been found to be as slow as 0.02 m/s.

The rate of impulse conduction through the AV junction is influenced by the atrial site at which the impulse enters the junctional area.[41] An initial normal slowing of conduction through the AV junction with a later increase in the speed of conduction is correlated with electrophysiologic differences in atrionodal, nodal, and nodal-His cells.[42] Other mechanisms have been postulated for the slowing of conduction through the junction, including the small size of the junctional conducting cells and the amounts of connective tissue interspersed among conducting cells.

The term *decremental conduction* describes the condition when a propagating impulse becoming successively weaker. The extent that decremental conduction normally occurs in the AV junction is debatable. Decremental conduction can lead to AV blocks. Slowing of the cardiac impulse at the AV junction prevents the atria and ventricles from contracting simultaneously and protects the ventricles from the abnormally fast HRs that can be generated

Table 2-5 • NORMAL CARDIAC ACTIVATION SEQUENCE

Normal Sequence of Activation	Conduction Velocity (m/s)	Time for Impulse to Traverse Structure (s)	Rate of Automatic Discharge (per min)
Sinoatrial node	—	~0.15	60–100
Atrial myocardium	0.8–1		None
AV node	0.02–0.05	~0.08	See text
AV bundle	1.2–2		40–55
Bundle branches	1.5–2		
Purkinje network	2–4	~0.08	25–40
Ventricular myocardium	0.3–1		None

AV, atrioventricular; m, meters; s, second; ~, approximately.
Adapted from Katz AM. *Physiology of the Heart*. New York: Raven Press; 1977:259.

in the atria under abnormal situations. Pre-excitation syndromes are evoked when there are accessory junctional pathways.[26]

Ventricular Conduction

The excitation impulse travels quickly through the His-Purkinje system. The His-Purkinje cells have the most rapid conduction velocities in the heart, approximately 1.5 to 2 m/s in the His bundle and 2 to 4 m/s in the Purkinje system.[38] The cardiac impulse next spreads rapidly (approximately 0.08 seconds), in a sequential manner from the common His bundle through the bundle branches, then through the extensive ramifications of the Purkinje fiber system, and finally through ventricular muscle. Ventricular activation occurs in three general phases: septal depolarization, apex depolarization, and basal depolarization (Fig. 2-43). The depolarization wave moves through the interventricular septum from left to right. The middle left septal area and the anterior and posterior left paraseptal areas are depolarized within the first 0 to 10 milliseconds.[43]

Most of the left and right ventricular muscle is depolarized within 20 to 40 milliseconds.[43] Activation spreads from the endocardium toward the epicardium. Although the impulse travels more rapidly through left ventricular tissue, the right ventricular wall is thinner. Thus, the full thickness of the right ventricle generally depolarizes prior to the left. The first epicardial depolarization usually occurs in the lower right ventricular wall.

Purkinje fibers are sparsely distributed in the basal (upper) sections of the ventricles and septum, particularly in the right ventricle and the septum. The basal and posterior portions of both ventricles and the basal interventricular septum are the last areas to be activated, at approximately 80 milliseconds.[43]

Although Purkinje fibers conduct the cardiac impulse more rapidly than other cardiac cells, Purkinje cells in the distal terminations of the conducting system have longer action potential durations and refractory periods than do ventricular muscle fibers (see previous). Because conduction is slower in cells with longer

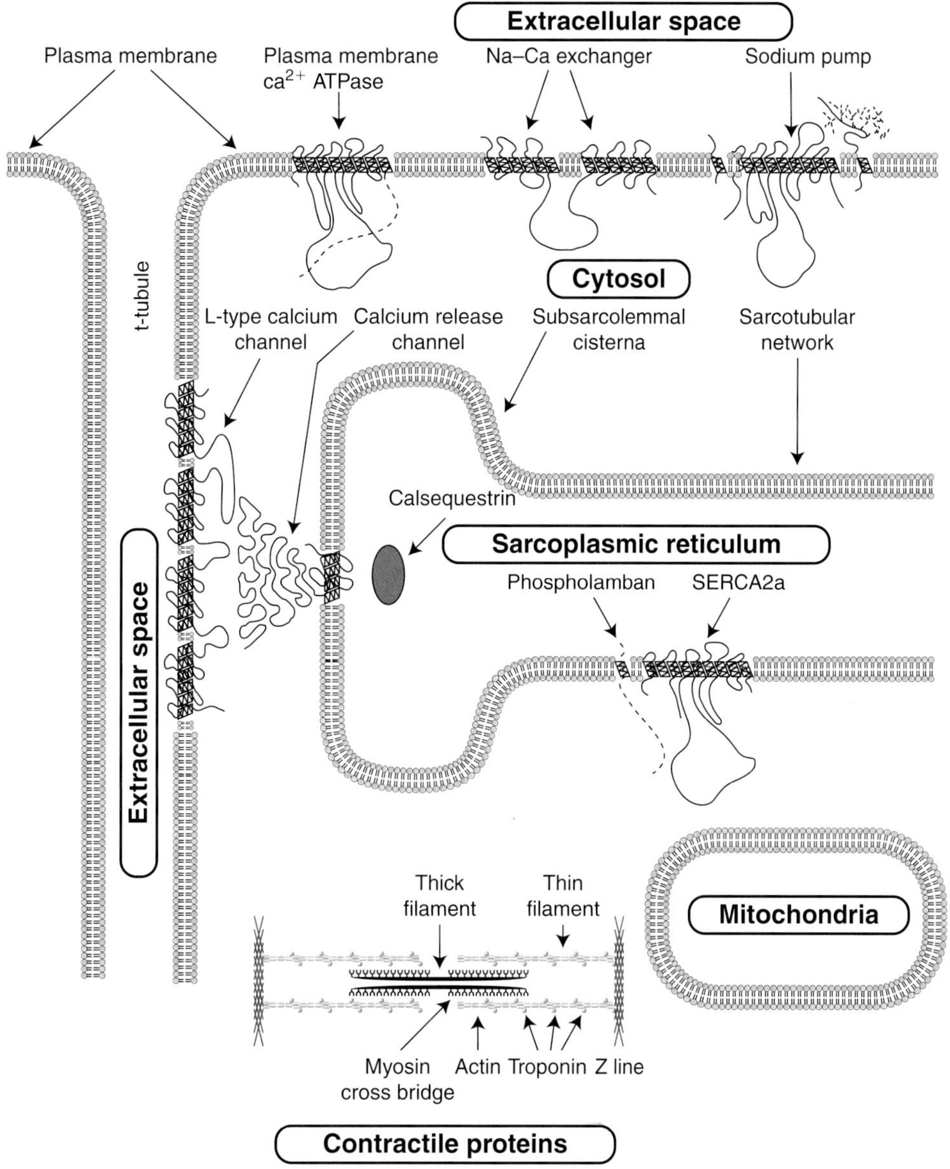

Figure 2-43. Schematic diagram showing extracellular and intracellular calcium cycles that control cardiac excitation–contraction coupling and relaxation. (Used with permission from Katz A. *Physiology of the heart.* 5th ed. Philadelphia, PA: Lippincott Williams & Wilkins; 2010.)

action potential durations and refractory periods, the conduction velocity of the cardiac impulse is slowed at the point where Purkinje fibers connect with ventricular muscle cells. In theory, the distal Purkinje fibers then function like a gate, the length of the refractory period in distal Purkinje fibers normally controlling the rate at which ventricular muscle fibers depolarize.[44] Excitation–contraction coupling and the rate of cardiac contraction may be controlled by this gating mechanism. The clinical importance of this gating mechanism is not clear.

Ventricular repolarization proceeds in general from the epicardium to the endocardium and spreads from the ventricular bases to the apices.[45] Thus, ventricular repolarization proceeds in a direction that is opposite to the direction of depolarization; thus, the QRS and T waves are generally oriented in the same direction under normal circumstances. All portions of the ventricle recover at approximately the same time. However, ventricular repolarization is not homogeneous; under pathophysiologic conditions, this may help create situations that promote ventricular arrhythmias.

Excitation–Contraction Coupling

Electrical excitation (i.e., depolarization of the myocardial cell membrane during the action potential) causes cardiac muscle contraction. Linking of electrical and mechanical activity is called *excitation–contraction coupling.* As identified by Ringer more than 100 years ago, an increase in cytosolic calcium concentration is necessary to trigger this process.[46] An increase in intracellular calcium ion concentration occurs with electrical excitation. Intracellular calcium ion in turn is the key that initiates contractile protein interaction during contraction. Calcium ion removal turns off the process and results in relaxation of the contractile apparatus. Thus, calcium ion is the link between electrical excitation and mechanical contraction. Calcium ion flows inward across the cell membrane during the action potential. Intracellular calcium ion stimulates release of calcium ion from internal stores such as the SR. Removal of calcium ion from the myoplasm evokes relaxation. The mechanisms by which ionic fluxes across the sarcolemma evoke contraction and relaxation are illustrated in Figure 2-44.

Calcium influx across the sarcolemma in response to cardiac membrane depolarization triggers calcium release by the SR.[15] The terminal cisternae of the SR press closely on the T-tubule. Bridges or "feet" spanning the distance between the two membrane systems are visible with electron microscopy.[47] These structures, called *ryanodine receptors* (because of binding properties), communicate the signal for SR calcium ion release.

The primary cardiac contractile proteins are actin, myosin, troponin, and tropomyosin. In cardiac cells, tropomyosin inhibits actin–myosin interaction. When calcium ion binds with troponin following electrical excitation, this alters tropomyosin in such a way that the resting inhibition by tropomyosin ceases. Myosin interacts with actin, binding and forming cross-bridges.

Calcium exerts some effects by combining with the intracellular protein *calmodulin.* In cardiac myocardial cells, the calcium–calmodulin complex promotes calcium ion binding to troponin and thus promotes contraction. Calcium–calmodulin also may stimulate calcium ion pumps on the SR and sarcolemma and may stimulate sodium–calcium exchange; these actions help remove calcium ion from the cytosol. Calcium–calmodulin influences the synthesis and breakdown of cAMP and may promote sarcolemmal calcium influx. Calcium may exert several other effects, either directly or by combining with other intracellular proteins, and thus may modulate myocardial cell contraction and relaxation through several different mechanisms.

Stimulation of β-adrenergic receptors on the cardiac cell membrane influences transmembrane calcium fluxes and cardiac contraction through the intracellular production of cAMP from ATP. cAMP in turn initiates several reactions involving intracellular protein phosphorylation (transfer of high-energy phosphates) by protein kinases. Phosphorylation of a sarcolemmal calcium channel membrane protein by cAMP creates a conformation or pore diameter change that places the calcium channel in a functional state available for voltage activation.[48] cAMP may also facilitate the SR release of calcium. Both actions promote an increased cytosolic calcium concentration and thus promote muscle contraction.

Phospholamban is an SR membrane protein that activates the SR calcium pump. Phosphorylation of phospholamban by cAMP and by calmodulin at a different site stimulates the calcium pump, increases SR calcium uptake, and promotes relaxation. cAMP phosphorylation of troponin influences the interaction between troponin and calcium, and promotes relaxation.

Although calcium ion uptake into the SR promotes relaxation, mechanisms increasing the amount of calcium ion in the SR cause increased calcium ion availability for tension generation during subsequent contractions. Thus, the increased rate and strength of contraction produced by β-adrenergic stimulation and other combined chronotropic–inotropic mechanisms appear to be matched by mechanisms that enhance the rate of cardiac relaxation.[48]

Calcium ion, the initiator and regulator of contraction, is the major link between excitation and contraction. The intracellular calcium concentration is directly and indirectly influenced by the amount of calcium transported in and out of the cell across

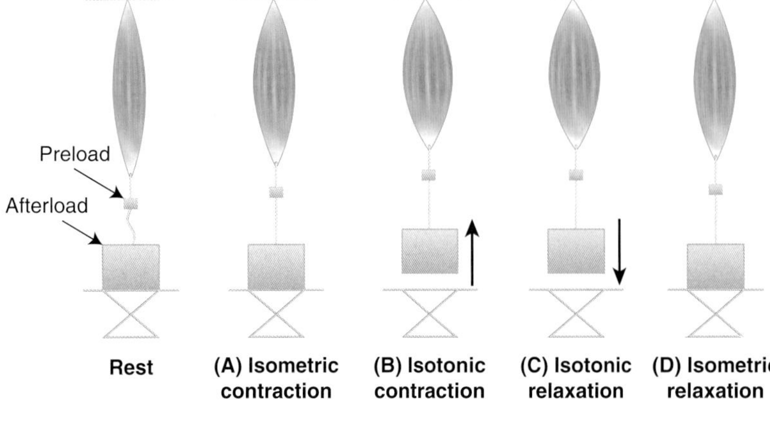

Figure 2-44. Cycle of contraction and relaxation in an afterloaded skeletal muscle. A small preload stretches the resting muscle, while the heavier afterload rests on a support until after the muscle has started to contract. The first phase in the cycle is isometric contraction **(A)**, during which tension developed by the muscle increases until it equals the afterload. In the second phase, isotonic contraction **(B)**, the muscle shortens while lifting the afterload. Relaxation is initially isotonic when the afterload is lowered to the support **(C)**. Isometric relaxation **(D)** begins when the afterload reaches the support and continues until muscle tension returns to zero. (Used with permission from Katz A. *Physiology of the Heart.* 5th ed. Philadelphia, PA: Lippincott Williams & Wilkins; 2010.)

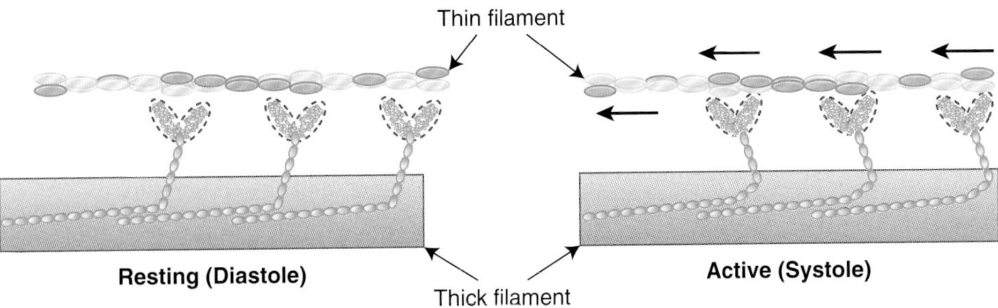

Figure 2-45. In resting muscle (**right**), the crossbridges project almost at right angles to the longitudinal axis of the thick filament. In active muscle (**left**), the crossbridges interact with the thin filaments, which are drawn toward the center of the sarcomere. (Used with permission from Katz A. *Physiology of the Heart.* 5th ed. Philadelphia, PA: Lippincott Williams & Wilkins; 2010.)

the sarcolemma.[48] Calcium sarcolemmal fluxes are affected by the membrane potential and by sodium and potassium ion concentrations and transcellular fluxes. Conversely, potassium flux through the calcium-regulated potassium channel and sodium flux during sodium–calcium exchange are affected by the intracellular concentration of calcium ion.

MECHANICAL CHARACTERISTICS OF CARDIAC CELLS

Overview of Contraction

As seen in Figure 2-45, the myofibril is composed of a series of repeating units, called *sarcomeres.* Sarcomeres are the basic functional and structural units of the myofibril. Dark-staining Z lines mark the ends of the sarcomere. Attached to the Z line are the thin filaments. The center of the sarcomere is composed of the dark-appearing thick filaments. Interdigitating thin and thick filaments overlap to a variable extent. Shortening alters the amount of thick and thin filament overlap: filament proteins interact causing the filaments slide past one another.

The individual thick and thin filaments do not themselves change in length; the sarcomere (and the muscle as a whole) shortens. If shortening of the sarcomere (or the muscle cell) is prevented, the interaction of thick and thin filaments is manifested as tension or force generation. Such a contraction is termed *isometric.* When a stimulated muscle is allowed to shorten, tension is not increased, and the contraction is said to be *isotonic* (Fig. 2-46). In the heart, early systolic contraction is primarily isometric, that is, tension increases and muscle length remains fairly constant. Later in systole, the contraction is primarily isotonic, that is, the heart muscle shortens and the blood is expelled into the aorta, whereas little additional tension is developed.

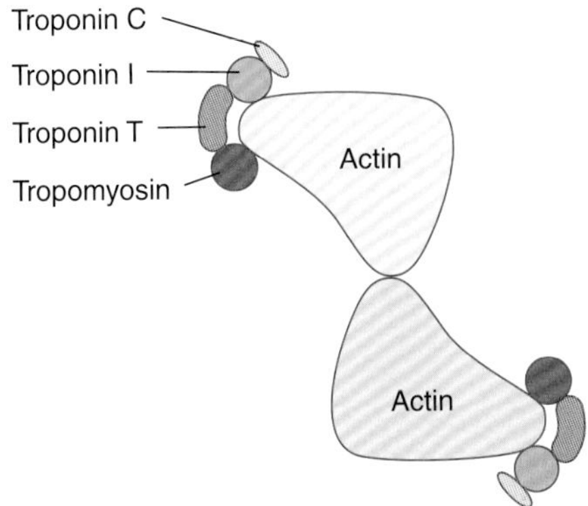

Figure 2-46. Cross-section of the thin filament in resting muscle at the level of a troponin complex showing relationship between actin, tropomyosin, and the three components of the troponin complex. (Used with permission from Katz A. *Physiology of the Heart.* 5th ed. Philadelphia, PA: Lippincott Williams & Wilkins; 2010.)

Molecular Basis for Contraction

The *thick filaments* are composed primarily of the protein myosin. Myosin is large, consisting of six subunits: two heavy chains and four light chains per molecule. The two heavy chain subunits are coiled to form a long, rod-like tail at one end. At the opposite end of the long myosin heavy chain, a head protrudes from each subunit. Groups of myosin tails are arranged to form the rigid backbone of the thick filament. The heads are the site of ATP breakdown and interaction with the thin filaments. Heads project outward in a spiral along the length of the thick filament. At the center of the filament, the molecules reverse direction, leaving a bare region from which no heads protrude. The small light chains are nestled in the angle between head and tail, two per heavy chain. Both heavy and light chains are members of multigene families and exist in several forms, called *isoforms.* Variation in isoform composition may modify the rate or intensity of myosin chemical activity, which may modify the contractile properties of the tissue. Age, mechanical loading, or metabolic or hormonal state may modify isoform composition.

The *thin filaments* are composed of bead-shaped molecules of the protein actin arranged in an intercoiled, double-stranded chain. Two other proteins, troponin and tropomyosin, are located on the thin filaments at periodic intervals (Fig. 2-47). Actin interacts with the thick-filament protein, myosin, resulting in the transduction of the chemical energy of ATP into mechanical energy. Troponin and tropomyosin are called *regulatory proteins* because they modify the interaction of actin and myosin (Fig. 2-48).

Myosin is an enzyme that breaks down the high-energy ATP molecule. During the resting state, the products of ATP breakdown remain bound to the myosin head. When myosin interacts with actin, the rate of ATP turnover is greatly increased. The chemical energy released from ATP is converted to the mechanical energy of contraction and heat.

According to the *cross-bridge theory,* a bond or crossbridge forms during muscle contraction, linking thick and thin filaments. The protuberant myosin head contains an actin-binding site and forms the crossbridge. This crossbridge is capable of binding, flexing, releasing, and binding again, thus pulling the thin filament toward the center of the sarcomere in an isotonic contraction. If the muscle is held at a fixed length and is unable to shorten (an isometric contraction), tension is generated by the pulling of the crossbridge.

When the muscle is relaxed during diastole, actin–myosin interaction is inhibited by tropomyosin and troponin. Depolarization initiates inward calcium ion currents across the sarcolemma and

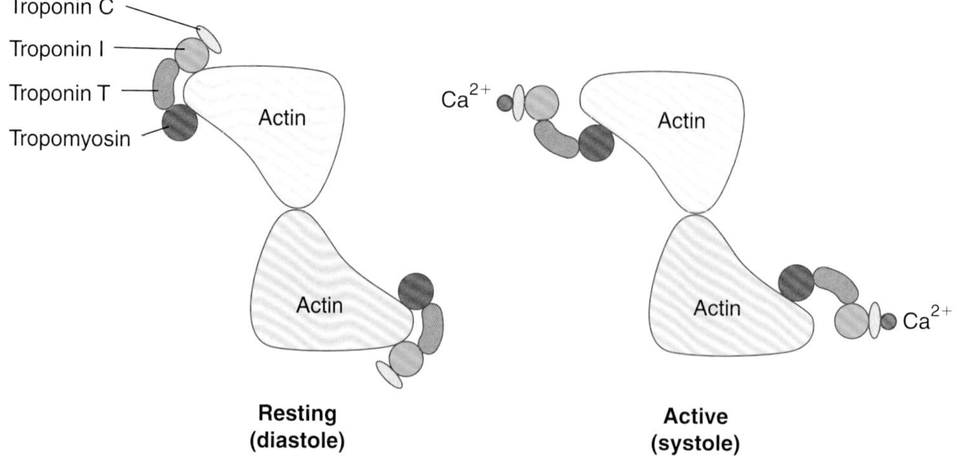

Figure 2-47. Cross-section of a thin filament at a region containing the troponin complex in resting (**left**) and active (**right**) muscle. At rest, the troponin complex holds the tropomyosin molecules toward the periphery of the groove between adjacent actin strands, which prevents actin from interacting with the myosin crossbridges. In active muscle, calcium binding to troponin C weakens the bond linking troponin I to actin. Loosening of this bond rearranges the regulatory proteins so as to shift tropomyosin deeper into the groove between the strands of actin, thereby exposing active sites on actin for interaction with the myosin crossbridges. (Used with permission from Katz A. *Physiology of the Heart.* 5th ed. Philadelphia, PA: Lippincott Williams & Wilkins; 2010.)

T-tubule membranes; calcium ion is then released from within the SR. The increased sarcoplasmic calcium ion concentration is in turn a trigger for contraction. Calcium ion binds troponin; tropomyosin rotates in a manner such that resting inhibition to cross-bridge formation is removed, and crossbridges form.

At relaxation, sarcoplasmic calcium ion concentration is very low. When calcium ion concentration rises, contraction occurs. The sarcoplasmic calcium ion concentration determines the forcefulness of contraction. Figure 2-49 illustrates the relationship; the higher the sarcoplasmic calcium ion concentration the greater the tension the heart muscle can generate until a saturating concentration is attained.

Molecular Basis for Relaxation

Contraction ceases when calcium ion is removed from the sarcoplasm. Troponin releases its bound calcium ion; tropomyosin returns to the position in which actin and myosin interaction was blocked. The cell relaxes.

Removal of calcium ion is essential in relaxation. Two mechanisms are important in this process. The SR pumps calcium ion into its core. This is an active process and requires chemical energy from ATP breakdown. Also, calcium ion is pumped outward across the sarcolemma. This removal process is also an active process because calcium ions must be moved against electrical and concentration gradients. Rather than using ATP directly, this process uses the energy stored in the sodium ion gradient. In conjunction with sodium ion moving inward down its concentration gradient, calcium ion is forced outward. The sodium ion gradient, in turn, is maintained by the sodium–potassium pump, which is powered by ATP.

The ATP required for the calcium ion removal from the sarcoplasm and for the cycling of crossbridges may be depleted,

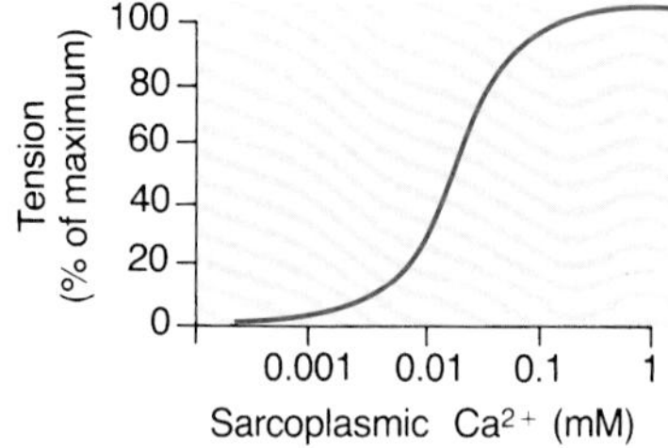

Figure 2-48. The calcium ion (Ca^{2+}) concentration versus tension relation. The higher the sarcoplasmic Ca^{2+} concentration, the more tension the heart muscle is able to generate until a maximum level is attained. Note the range of intracellular Ca^{2+} is significantly lower than the 1- to 2-mM concentration in the extracellular space.

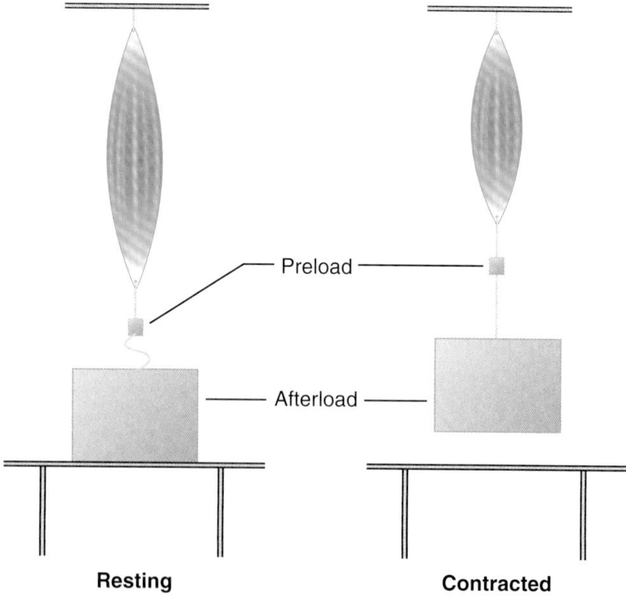

Figure 2-49. Preload and afterload. A preload is supported by a resting muscle before it begins to contract (**left**). An afterload, such as a weight resting on a support, is not encountered by the muscle until developed tension exceeds its weight (**right**). (Used with permission from Katz A. *Physiology of the Heart.* 5th ed. Philadelphia, PA: Lippincott Williams & Wilkins; 2010.)

for example, in myocardial ischemia. When this happens, cross-bridges form and are not broken and the muscle becomes stiff.

Modulation of Sarcoplasmic Calcium Ion Concentration

Interventions that alter sarcoplasmic calcium ion concentration alter the force generated during contraction. For example, β-adrenergic drugs, such as epinephrine, may increase inward calcium current through calcium channels opened during the action potential, increasing sarcoplasmic calcium ion concentration and thus the force of contraction. Certain antiarrhythmic drugs such as procainamide are associated with decreased calcium ion release from the SR and, thus, decreased systolic tension generation and blood pressure.[49]

Digitalis-like drugs increase the force of contraction. This is possibly caused by increased sarcoplasmic calcium ion concentration. Digitalis-like drugs partially block the sodium–potassium pump. As the transmembrane sodium ion gradient decreases, less calcium ion is pumped out across the sarcolemma. The intracellular calcium ion stores and calcium ion level during contraction increase. The end result is augmented contractile strength.

MECHANICAL PROPERTIES OF THE MYOCARDIUM

The heart is a pump. It functions to add energy to the flowing blood, thus propelling the blood through the systemic and pulmonary circulations. The performance of the heart as a pump can be described in terms of the *CO*. CO is the volume of blood pumped by one ventricle in 1 minute. CO is equal to the stroke volume (*SV*), or volume of blood pumped with each beat times the number of cardiac contractions (*HR*) in 1 minute (CO = SV × HR). Typical normal values in a 70-kg man at rest (HR: 68 beats/min; SV: 80 mL) produce a CO of 5,440 mL/min or 5.4 L/min.

SV is determined by the degree of ventricular filling during diastole (preload), the force against which the ventricle must pump (afterload), the contractile state of the myocardium, and HR. In the remainder of this section, these factors are discussed in more detail, and the manner in which they interact to influence the mechanical function of the heart is described.

Preload and Afterload

Preload is the distending force that stretches the ventricular muscle immediately before electrical excitation and contraction. Figure 2-50 further defines preload and illustrates the role of preload in the contraction of a simple muscle preparation. Left ventricular end-diastolic pressure is the left ventricular preload. In the absence of pathologic mitral valve changes, left atrial pressure is an indicator of left ventricular preload. In order to make clinical judgments about left ventricular preload, clinicians measure the pulmonary artery pressures and the pulmonary artery occlusion pressure. If there is no pulmonary hypertension as well as no mitral valve pathology, then these pressures are useful indices of left ventricular preload. Central venous pressure, in the absence of tricuspid valve disease, is an index of right ventricular preload.

A related term describing cardiac mechanical function is *afterload.* Afterload is the force that opposes ventricular ejection (i.e., the forces that the muscle must overcome to move the blood during contraction). Left ventricular afterload is determined by the *volume and mass of blood* ejected by the ventricle, the *resistance to blood flow*

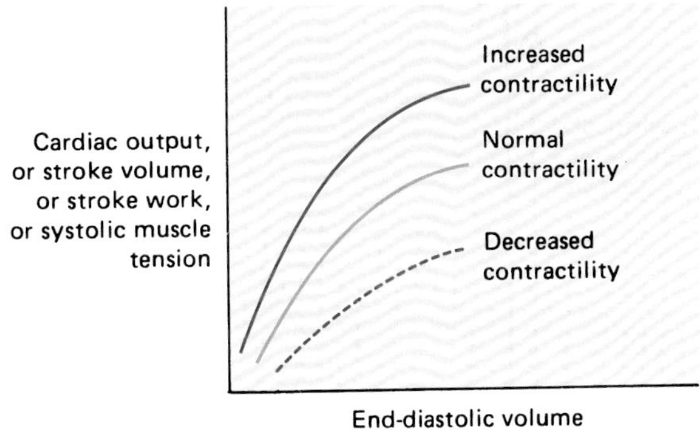

Figure 2-50. The length–tension relation of the heart. End-diastolic volume determines the end-diastolic length of the ventricular muscle fibers and is proportional to the tension generated during systole as well as to cardiac output, stroke volume, and stroke work. A change in cardiac contractility causes the heart to perform on a different length–tension curve.

(determined mainly by the cross-sectional area of the small arterioles, known as resistance vessels), *aortic impedance* (amount of pressure change for a given volume of blood ejected into the aorta; this depends on the elasticity of the aorta and branching arteries), and intrathoracic pressures. The arterial systolic pressure is a useful clinical indicator of the left ventricular afterload; pulmonary systolic pressure suggests right ventricular afterload. Total systemic vascular resistance and total pulmonary vascular resistance are also used to suggest left and right ventricular afterload, respectively.

Preload Role: Length–Tension Relationship

Early in the 20th century, Starling observed that within limits, an increase in left ventricular volume at the end of diastole resulted in the generation of increased active pressure and increased volume pumped during the ensuing contraction. Beyond a certain volume, this mechanism is no longer operational; increased end-diastolic volume results instead in decreased pressure developing and a decreased volume of blood being ejected.[50] This property is known as *Starling law of the heart* or the *length–tension relation of cardiac muscle* (or sometimes, the *Frank-Starling law of the heart*). This property is commonly illustrated in a graph (Fig. 2-51). Although the left ventricular *volume* at the end of diastole is a factor that determines the subsequent force of contraction, clinicians measure pressure increments, not volume. However, the volume and the pressure are related, as discussed later (see "Compliance" section).

The length–tension mechanism is useful; it likely contributes to overall matching of the left and right ventricular outputs. For instance, if a person reclines after being in a standing position (or elevates the legs when in a reclining position), the volume of blood returning to the heart transiently increases. The right ventricle is stretched and increases its force of contraction, pumping a larger SV into the pulmonary circulation. Pulmonary vascular pressures increase. This increased right ventricular output increases left ventricular filling volume and preload. The left ventricle pumps a larger SV and arterial vascular pressures increase. This intrinsic ability of the heart to match increased cardiac return with increased volume pumped is useful in case of the cardiac transplant patient, providing a mechanism to increase CO, particularly early in exercise.

Some treatment approaches take advantage of the length–tension characteristics of the heart. Examples of this are leg raising and intravascular volume expansion in the patient with shock. These therapies increase central blood volume

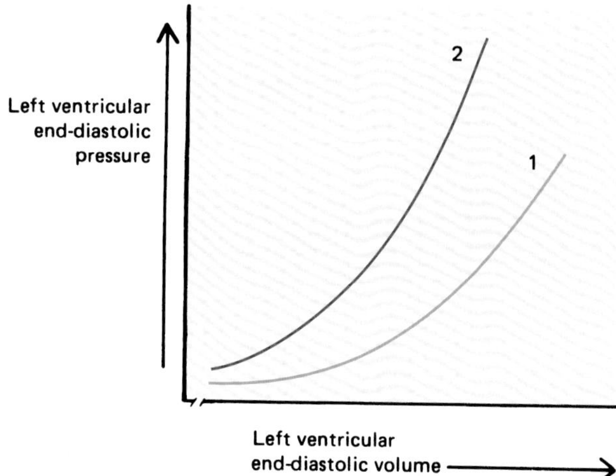

Figure 2-51. The stiffness of the left ventricle. Stiffness is the slope of the pressure–volume relation. Curve 1 represents normal stiffness; curve 2 represents an increase in stiffness such as that which might occur after a myocardial infarction. In both cases, increases in volume result in increased pressure and an increased increment in pressure for a given increment in volume. Compliance is the inverse of stiffness. (Adapted from Forrester JS, Diamone GA. Clinical application of left ventricular pressures. In: Corday E, Swan HJC, eds. *Myocardial infarction: New Perspectives in Diagnosis and Management.* Baltimore, MA: Williams & Wilkins; 1973:143–148.)

and improve cardiac contractile force; they are easily and rapidly accessible. They are, however, associated with an increase in myocardial oxygen consumption (MVO_2) and should be used carefully in the patient at risk for myocardial ischemia. These patients should be monitored for ECG signs of myocardial ischemia and for symptoms such as chest pain when interventions increase the preload.

It is often clinically useful to monitor an indicator of cardiac volume (such as jugular venous distension, pulmonary artery or central venous pressures, location of the point of maximum impulse) and a concurrently measured indicator of the tension generated (such as CO). The length–tension relationship characterizes the mechanical functioning of the heart and can be helpful in judging the efficacy of therapies. Positive inotropic factors, that is, factors that increase the contractility of the heart, such as sympathetic stimulation, alter the length–tension relation, so that a higher tension is generated at the same left ventricular end-diastolic volume. In the failing heart, the same stretch generates much less tension and CO does not substantially increase with volume. The heart is said to be refractory to inotropic stimulation; it could be said that the Starling curve is reduced.

The cross-bridge theory of muscle contraction partly accounts for the cardiac muscle length–tension relationship. Tension generated by muscle is proportional to the number of crossbridges formed. At short lengths, thin filaments overlap one another and interfere with cross-bridge formation. Maximal tension development occurs in the range of muscle lengths at which the myosin crossbridge regions maximally overlap the thin filaments without the thin filaments overlapping one another. If the muscle is stretched still further, then the region of cross-bridge overlap is diminished and less tension is developed.[51]

Other factors also contribute to the shape of the Starling curve. For example, when the heart is stretched, more cells may be brought into parallel with the axis of shortening and may be able to contribute more effectively to the total development of force within the ventricle. Calcium ion, which grades the force of contraction, may enter the sarcoplasm in larger quantities for longer periods of time. Contractile filaments may be more sensitive to calcium ion at longer sarcomere lengths.

Compliance. Starling law of the heart relates end-diastolic length, rather than end-diastolic pressure, to the strength of contraction. However, end-diastolic length and pressure are related. *Compliance* is the term used to describe that relation. Compliance (C) is the change in volume (ΔV) that results for a given change in pressure (ΔP):

$$C = \frac{\Delta V}{\Delta P}$$

Stiffness (S) is the inverse of compliance ($S = \Delta P/\Delta V$). Increased stiffness is the same as decreased compliance.

Cardiac compliance is determined by inherent properties of the cardiac muscle tissue, cardiac chamber geometry, and the state of the pericardium. Myocardial tissue is stiffer with hypoxia, ischemia, and scarring, such as after a myocardial infarction (curve 2 in Fig. 2-52).[52] Infiltrative myocardial diseases such as amyloidosis increase muscle stiffness. Geometry changes that result in increased stiffness include hypertrophy. When operating at a more distended volume, the heart is invariably stiffer: it requires larger increments in filling pressure to achieve a given increment in volume (see Fig. 2-53). Pericardial conditions that increase cardiac stiffness include pericarditis and tamponade. The ability of the cardiac muscle to relax, expand, and stretch in response to increased volume is called "lusitropy."

Implications for Patient Care. It is important to consider left ventricular compliance in patient care. In monitoring preload, the nurse commonly measures indices of ventricular filling *pressures*. Yet, therapeutic goals are related to achieving *volume* changes that will take advantage of the length–tension relation of the heart to maintain or increase CO. The pressure change is important, too, because elevated ventricular filling pressures may result in pulmonary congestion and edema. For example, immediately following a myocardial infarction, myocardial stiffness may be increased.[53] The same end-diastolic volume may be accompanied by such a markedly increased end-diastolic pressure that signs of left ventricular failure, such as crackles, appear. In this case, inotropic

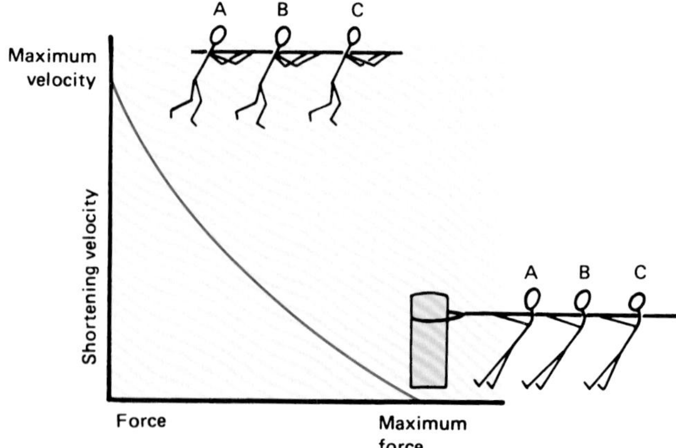

Figure 2-52. Approximation of the force–velocity of shortening relation of cardiac muscle. Velocity of shortening is maximal with extremely light afterload. Shortening is impossible with large afterload. (Adapted from Katz AM. *Physiology of the Heart.* 4th ed. New York: Raven Press; 1977:87, 126.)

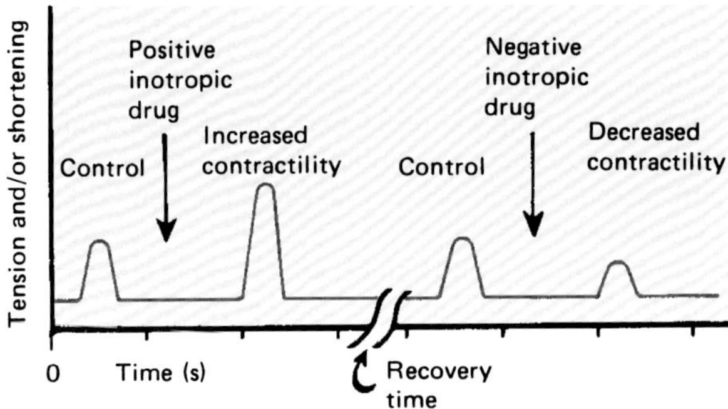

Figure 2-53. Positive and negative inotropic effects on tension development or myocardial shortening. An increase in myocardial contractility enhances the amount of tension developed, the rate of shortening, or both, without an increase in initial cardiac muscle length. A decrease in myocardial contractility reduces the amount of tension developed, the rate of shortening, or both, without a decrease in initial cardiac muscle length. (Used with permission from Katz A. *Physiology of the Heart*. 4th ed. Philadelphia, PA: Lippincott Williams & Wilkins; 2006:285–286.)

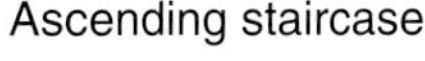

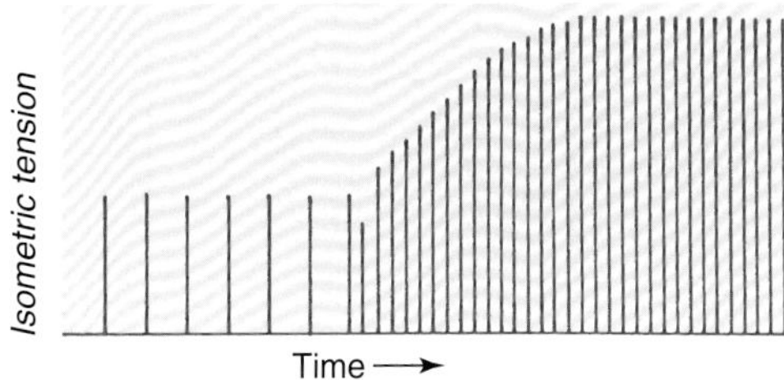

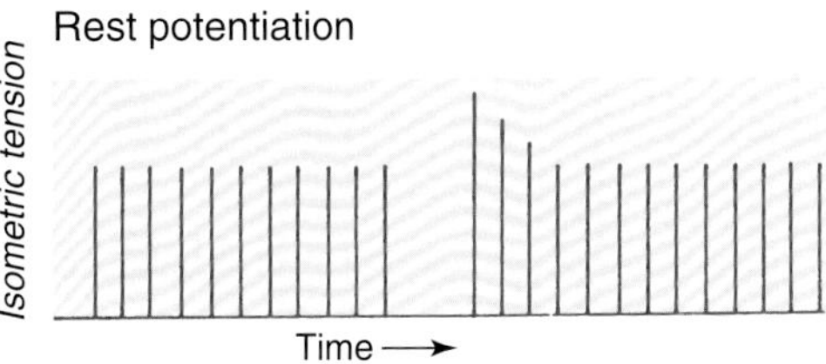

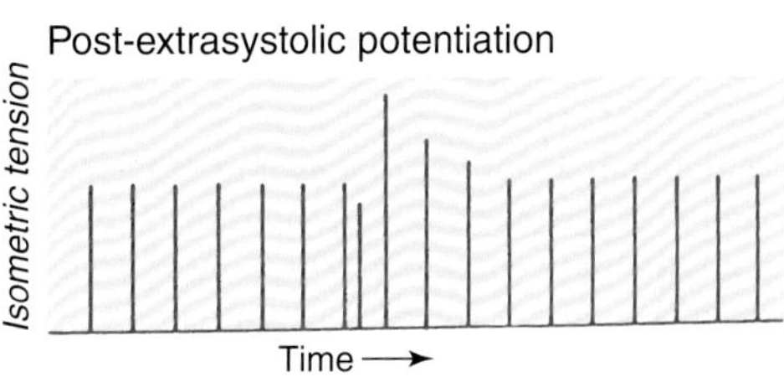

Figure 2-54. Changes in isometric force generated in cardiac muscle when the stimulation frequency is altered. (Used with permission from Feigl EO. *Physiology and Biophysics*. 20th ed. *Vol 2*. Philadelphia, PA: WB Saunders; 1974:37.)

agents, which increase the force of contraction, would be of little or no benefit. Unloading therapies, which may decrease the end-diastolic volume, can eliminate the damaging increase in end-diastolic pressures. Furthermore, decreased ventricular pressures throughout diastole may improve coronary artery filling. Better coronary perfusion can improve tissue oxygenation and further diminish stiffness.

Afterload Role: Force–Velocity Relationship

The heart's ability to shorten is influenced by the amount of pressure above preload it must actively generate. With a smaller afterload, the heart is able to contract more rapidly. Contraction is much slower against very large afterload. This interaction is referred to as the *force–velocity of shortening relation*, or simply the *force–velocity relation* (Fig. 2-54). Changes in the initial muscle length or changes in contractility can alter the force–velocity relation.

At the molecular level, the rate of cycling of crossbridges may be equated to the speed of shortening. Generation of tension may be equated to attachment and pulling by the crossbridges. The amount of tension the muscle can generate is determined by the number of crossbridges the muscle is able to form. The cross-bridge formation is determined in part by the preload, or the amount of diastolic stretch placed on the muscle. Once a critical amount of force equivalent to the afterload, or force opposing ejection, is generated, the muscle shortens. The speed of that shortening may be equated with the speed of cycling of crossbridges and is determined in part by the afterload.

Effect of Afterload on the Volume Ejected by the Ventricle. In addition to influencing the speed of shortening, afterload is related to extent of shortening. Increases in systemic vascular resistance, at a constant end-diastolic pressure, result in decreased volume pumped by the left ventricle. When pumping against decreased aortic pressure, the left ventricle pumps a larger SV. Note that this effect primarily occurs in individuals with impaired cardiac contractile function.

Implications for Patient Care. It is important to consider the force–velocity relation in myocardial performance. Vasopressors that increase vascular resistance increase the afterload. Because of the inverse nature of the force–velocity relation, development of greater force is accompanied by a slower velocity of shortening. There may be a concomitant decrease in SV and CO. Further, there is an increase in the oxygen requirements of the cardiac tissue when afterload is increased.

Conversely, therapies that decrease afterload are associated with faster, more extensive shortening and a larger SV. The CO increases. Increases in CO achieved in this manner have the unique advantage of decreasing MVO_2. Reduced afterload, however, may be associated with decreased coronary perfusion pressure.

Contractility of Cardiac Muscle

Contractility describes the heart's ability to contract; it describes the ability of the heart muscle to shorten, develop tension, or both. Altered contractility is a change in the ability of the heart to contract independent of variations induced by altering either preload or afterload (see Fig. 2-55).

Contractility is a property intrinsic to the muscle. Its physiologic basis is not well understood. Although contractility is difficult to define or measure, it is a property of critical importance because abnormalities in contractility are a major problem in the failing heart. Many therapies are designed to enhance contractility.

Contractility is not equivalent to cardiac performance, which can be influenced by valvular function and circulating blood volume as well as by myocardial contractility. *Inotropic agents* affect the contractility of the heart. Positive inotropic agents, which increase contractility, include sympathetic stimulation, excess thyroid hormone, exogenous epinephrine, norepinephrine,

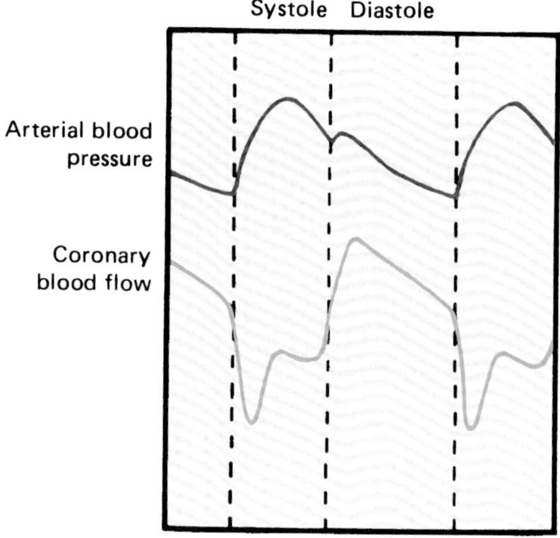

Figure 2-55. Effect of systolic compression on coronary blood flow. Note the decrease in flow during systole and the increase during diastole. (From Folkow B, Neil E. *Circulation*. Oxford: Oxford University Press; 1971:421.)

dopamine, dobutamine or isoproterenol infusions, and calcium salt infusion. Digitalis-like drugs have positive inotropic action. Increased contractility increases MVO_2. Agents such as catecholamines increase both contractility and afterload and result in substantial increase in MVO_2. Negative inotropic agents decrease contractility; these include myocardial hypoxia, ischemia, acidosis, barbiturates, alcohol, propranolol, and possibly lidocaine.

Treppe

HR is the fourth major determinant of the force of contraction. Alteration in the force of contraction with HR is called the *Treppe* or the *staircase phenomenon*. In an experimental preparation with the preload held constant, the faster the rate of stimulation, the stronger is the force of contraction. Conversely, in the same preparation, slower rates of stimulation result in less forceful contraction. In the intact organism, as HR increases, there is decreased time for filling. The Treppe phenomenon provides some compensation for the decrement (Fig. 2-54). Treppe is an intrinsic property of the heart muscle, independent of hormones or innervation. It is present in the transplanted heart. The physiologic basis for Treppe may be rate-driven variations in sarcoplasmic calcium ion concentration.

Two other types of rate-related alterations occur in force of contraction. A pause augments the force of the ensuing beat. This is called *rest potentiation*. After an extra beat, the force of the ensuing contraction is increased. This effect is called *postextrasystolic potentiation*. The manner in which variations in cardiac rate or rhythm induce changes in CO in the intact heart is complex. Rate-related variations in force of contraction and filling interact; the SV depends on that complex interaction.

Cardiac Reserve

The interaction of the mechanical properties of the heart can be illustrated by considering the reserve capacity of the heart. *Cardiac reserve* refers to the ability of the heart to increase its output. In the healthy person, the reserve capacity is used to meet demands for increased blood flow, such as during exercise. Normal CO is 5.5 L/min in a healthy, 70-kg man. This can be increased with activity to about 18 L/min. Heart disease often limits the total possible output and the patient may have to rely on reserve capacity simply to maintain a normal CO at rest. The two components of cardiac reserve are increase in HR and SV.

HR increases often increase the CO. However, as the heart beats more rapidly, there is less time for filling. The rate-related increase in force of contraction partially compensates for the lower end-diastolic filling. At rates exceeding about 180 beats/min, diastole is shortened and the diastolic filling is decreased. SV is then decreased, as predicted by the Starling relation. Furthermore, the coronary arteries are perfused during diastole, and a fast HR decreases coronary blood flow, which may result in ischemia, and in turn decrease myocardial compliance and contractility. The stiff ventricle requires greater filling pressures to expand it to the same diastolic volume and may operate at a smaller volume, further decreasing SV, as defined by the Starling relation.

During diastole, the heart can fill to a larger volume than usual, thereby increasing its SV. This is sometimes called the *diastolic cardiac reserve*. Increases in diastolic volume are accompanied by increases in end-diastolic pressure. Left ventricular end-diastolic pressures beyond approximately 20 to 25 mm Hg typically result in pulmonary congestion. The more dilated the ventricle, the more oxygen it requires; this may be a limiting problem in the patient with coronary artery disease.

The heart also has *systolic reserve*, an ability to eject a larger percentage of the end-diastolic volume. Increased contractility and decreased afterload increase SV and CO. Increases in velocity of contraction or contractility make extra demands on the heart in terms of oxygen requirements and pose risk for the patient with coronary artery disease.

Factors involved in mechanical performance interact continuously. For example, an increase in afterload decreases the SV. This in turn results in a larger volume of blood in the heart at the end of systole. The addition of an unchanged amount of blood during the subsequent diastole increases the end-diastolic volume. The ensuing contraction is more forceful, and SV is increased owing to the Starling effect.

In hemorrhage, the filling pressure may diminish; the SV decreases as predicted by the Starling relationship. However, the afterload (ventricular wall tension) may also decrease. This tends to raise the SV. Adrenergic outflow also contributes to increased SV. The CO may increase despite decreased filling pressures.

Assessment of the Pump Performance

Assessment of the patient includes the evaluation of numerous indices of overall pump performance as follows:

- urine output, mental status, skin color, and temperature are indices of the adequacy of CO to various organs and tissues;
- CO may be measured directly;
- left ventricular preload is estimated from the pulmonary artery occlusion pressure;
- systemic vascular resistance (index of left ventricular afterload) is calculated; and
- mean arterial blood pressure is the product of CO and vascular resistance.

These observations measure end products of many interacting variables that together compose the reserve capacity of the cardiovascular system. In making these assessments, the nurse not only should ask whether blood flow and pressure are adequate but also should probe more deeply.

- How much of the patient's reserve capacity must be used to maintain the current level of functioning?
- Is the patient already tachycardic, with a dilated left ventricle?
- Is the patient's heart already receiving a high level of endogenous catecholaminergic stimuli?
- How much of the patient's reserve capacity is left? Of the reserve capacity left, how much can be used in planning the patient's care?
- What is the cost of the patient's current functional state in terms of $M\dot{V}O_2$?

MYOCARDIAL METABOLISM

The chemical energy of ATP powers myocardial contraction, ion pumping, and many other activities. ATP is broken down (hydrolyzed) into adenosine diphosphate and inorganic phosphate. With hydrolysis, chemical energy is transformed into mechanical energy and heat. Because the heart is continuously active, ATP must be continuously available. The usual intramyocardial cellular concentrations of ATP (estimated at 5 mM) are sufficient to power contraction mechanical activity for only a few beats.

Creatine phosphate is a backup source of high-energy phosphate to replenish the ATP supply. However, energy stores in ATP and creatine phosphate together supply enough energy only for several minutes of activity. Thus, the heart depends on ongoing ATP synthesis. This occurs in a series of efficient, but complex, enzyme-dependent reactions. The bulk of myocardial ATP is synthesized in an aerobic environment. Myocardial cells have large amounts of mitochondria, the sites of aerobic synthesis of ATP.

Free fatty acids are the preferred myocardial fuel, particularly when the patient is in the fasting state. *Glucose* or its storage form, glycogen, can serve as an additional substrate for energy metabolism. Whereas glucose contributes only 15% to myocardial ATP synthesis in the fasting patient, its role increases to nearly 50% in the postprandial state. *Amino acids* play a minor role in energy metabolism of the heart. In starvation, however, amino acid intermediates are metabolized to maintain energy stores.

PHYSIOLOGY OF THE CORONARY CIRCULATION

Under normal conditions at rest, the heart extracts a large amount of oxygen from the blood perfusing the heart: the difference in oxygen content between coronary arterial and coronary sinus blood is approximately 11.4 mL O_2/100 mL blood.[54] The total oxygen content of arterial blood is normally approximately 20 mL O_2/100 mL blood, so this represents extraction of more than 50% of the arterial oxygen content. It is difficult to extract much more oxygen than this, yet the oxygen requirement of the heart may increase many fold. This additional oxygen can be supplied only by increasing coronary blood flow. Coronary blood flow is proportionate to myocardial metabolism and oxygen consumption.

Determinants of $M\dot{V}O_2$

Several factors contribute to the oxygen needs of the heart. A small and relatively constant volume is used in the "housekeeping" activities of heart cells. "Housekeeping" activities are independent of contraction and include repair or replacement of intracellular proteins and maintenance of the ionic environment. Each cardiac contraction involves ionic movement across cell membranes. The oxygen required for electrical depolarization and repolarization is small,[55] accounted for by the cycling of pumps that maintain sodium, potassium, and other ionic distributions.

In addition to these two fairly constant and low requirements for oxygen, factors related to activity and the state of the heart that determine how much oxygen the heart needs. These factors, which include intramyocardial tension, HR, shortening, and contractile state, constitute the major determinants of $M\dot{V}O_2$.

Intramyocardial Tension

The *law of Laplace* is used to calculate intramyocardial tension. This law states that intramyocardial tension is proportional to the internal pressure within the ventricular cavity times the ventricular cavity radius; it is inversely proportional to the ventricular wall thickness. An increase in left ventricular afterload causes the left ventricle to develop more pressure during the systolic period, thereby increasing intramyocardial tension and oxygen consumption. An increase in the preload or filling pressures of the left ventricle increases tension because both internal pressure and the radius of the ventricular cavity are increased and the thickness is decreased. Again, $M\dot{V}O_2$ is increased.

Heart Rate

Increased HR (at the same preload and afterload) increases $M\dot{V}O_2$. Each beat represents the generation of tension by the myocardium.

Shortening

In an *isotonic twitch*, there is a component of the oxygen consumption that is proportional to the amount of shortening by a muscle. That is, there is a metabolic cost that is related to shortening. This is sometimes called the *Fenn effect* and is a characteristic of cardiac as well as of skeletal muscle. In cardiac muscle, a contraction with a large amount of shortening is one that expels a large SV. Increased myocardial shortening increases $M\dot{V}O_2$.

Contractile State

Contractility correlates with the amount of oxygen consumed by the heart. Positive inotropic factors increase $M\dot{V}O_2$ and negative inotropic agents decrease $M\dot{V}O_2$.

Pressure versus Volume Work

Work done by the heart is proportional to the pressure generated times the volume pumped (stroke work = [mean arterial pressure–left atrial pressure] × SV). Pressure generated is a component of intramyocardial tension as described by the Laplace relationship, and contributes to overall $M\dot{V}O_2$. The size of the SV is related to the amount of myocardial shortening, and thus it too contributes to $M\dot{V}O_2$. Although equal amounts of work can be obtained by altering pressure or volume, the cost in terms of $M\dot{V}O_2$ is much greater for high-pressure work than for high-volume work. Thus, cardiac work is not well correlated with $M\dot{V}O_2$.

Indices of $M\dot{V}O_2$

There is no single accurate indicator of myocardial oxygen requirements. Ideally, such an indicator would take into account all major $M\dot{V}O_2$ determinants. The pressure–rate product and tension–time index are often used to estimate $M\dot{V}O_2$. The pressure–rate product is calculated by multiplying the HR by the systolic or mean arterial pressure and dividing by 100. The tension–time index (more appropriately should be called the pressure–time index) is calculated by multiplying the area under the left ventricular pressure curve by HR. Both pressure–rate product and tension–time index take HR (a major $M\dot{V}O_2$ determinant) into account. Because pressure, not tension, is included in these indicators, the other factors in the Laplace equation (i.e., ventricular cavity radius, ventricular wall thickness) must be constant if these indices are to accurately predict $M\dot{V}O_2$.

Myocardial Oxygen Supply

Control of Coronary Blood Flow

Flow of blood in the coronary circulation is, as in all vascular beds, proportional to the perfusion pressure and inversely proportional to the resistance of the bed. Resistance in the coronary bed is altered by compression on it during systole and by metabolic, neural, and hormonal factors. Coronary artery disease can impose significant resistance.

The pressure difference that drives cardiac perfusion is the gradient between aortic pressure and right atrial pressure because most of the coronary perfusion returns to the right atrium. Because the heart develops its own perfusion pressure, a fall in aortic pressure can reduce coronary perfusion, which in turn may further decrease cardiac function and pressure development. A cycle of deterioration may result. The coronary circulation, however, is autoregulated. This means that changes in the perfusion pressure over a range of pressures (approximately 60 to 180 mm Hg) make little difference in the amount of blood flowing to the heart if the other factors influencing perfusion are held constant.

During systole, myocardial wall tension is high. This compresses the coronary arteries, preventing perfusion. Thus, the heart has the unique property of receiving most of its blood flow during diastole. Rapid HRs decrease the time spent in diastole and may impinge on coronary perfusion.

Intramyocardial tension tends to be highest in the subendocardial regions of the left ventricle. Thus, $M\dot{V}O_2$ is probably highest in this region; yet systolic compression is also greatest here, which in part explains why this area has an increased incidence of infarction. In transmural infarctions (i.e., ones that involve the full thickness of the left ventricular wall), the area of involvement is typically greater on the subendocardial surface than on the subepicardial surface. Another factor contributing to this infarction pattern is the coronary artery distribution. Because arteries enter the myocardium on the epicardial surface and plunge inward through the wall, the most easily compromised distal segments of the coronary arteries perfuse the endocardium.

The coronary arteries are innervated by α-sympathetic and parasympathetic fibers. The direct effects of neural outflow are the same in the coronary bed as in other systemic beds; α-adrenergic stimulation (or norepinephrine) constricts arteries and parasympathetic (vagal) stimulation dilates them. Pharmacologic doses of the β-adrenergic drug isoproterenol dilate the coronary artery bed. Often, however, the direct effect of neural outflow on the coronary bed is masked because the autonomic nervous system also affects myocardial metabolism and contractility, and the effect of these latter factors predominates.

Local metabolic conditions are the predominant determinants of coronary perfusion. Increased metabolism or hypoxia leads to vasodilation and increased myocardial blood flow. The mechanism that mediates this effect is unknown.

With atherosclerosis, significant resistance can develop in the coronary arteries. Lesions that occupy more than two thirds of the vessel's cross-sectional area may impinge on flow at rest. Such lesions can prevent the increases in flow necessary when myocardial oxygen demand increases.

Collateral Circulation

Collateral arteries are interarterial vessels that can connect two branches of a single coronary artery or connect branches of the right coronary artery with branches of the left. In the human heart, collaterals are found through the full thickness of the myocardium, with the highest density near the endocardial surface. Although they are present at birth, collaterals do not become functionally significant unless the myocardium experiences hypoxic or ischemic insult. Before transformation, the collateral arteries are very narrow. They are devoid of smooth muscle and therefore are unable to respond to pharmacologic or metabolic vasoactive substances. After being stimulated to develop, the collateral tracts increase in diameter and develop a smooth muscle layer until, ultimately, the vessels are histologically similar to arterioles. When fully developed, these vessels are able to vasodilate when nitrates are administered and may autoregulate.[45] The time course from ischemic insult until significant enlargement is seen may be as short as 9 days.[56]

Three conditions are correlated with collateral development: coronary artery disease, chronic myocardial hypoxia, and myocardial hypertrophy. In coronary artery disease, the collateral diameter increases in proportion to the severity of coronary artery narrowing. Functionally significant increases in collateral structure are seen with a 75% or greater reduction in the luminal diameter of a major vessel. Chronic hypoxic myocardium is seen in patients with anemia, cyanotic heart disease, and chronic obstructive pulmonary disease.[57] There is also an increase in collateral diameter in hypertrophied hearts.[58] Attempts to stimulate development of collaterals with exercise programs have not been successful.[45] Collaterals frequently disappear after successful aortocoronary bypass grafting.[59]

Blood flow through collateral vessels may contribute significantly to myocardial perfusion. Patients with similar coronary occlusions have smaller areas of infarction when collateral development has occurred. Patients with abundant and well-developed collaterals sometime have a totally occluded coronary artery but no evidence of infarction. Blood flow through collateral vessels may be insufficient to meet increased demand, such as during exercise, and is insufficient to prevent necrosis in most cases.

Clinical Implications

It is important to analyze the effect of altered clinical states on the myocardial oxygen need. It is useful to consider the Laplace relation when evaluating oxygen demand in clinical states. For example, *hypertrophy of ventricular muscle* results in an increase in the thickness of the ventricular wall. This is advantageous in that wall tension is lower for the same left ventricular cavity size (same end-diastolic volume); hence, oxygen consumption is decreased. However, development of hypertrophy is a double-edged sword. At the same time that wall tension is decreased, the mass of tissue requiring oxygen is increased; the net result may well be a greater oxygen demand by the heart. Furthermore, because hypertrophy tends to increase the size of the muscle cells without increasing the tissue capillarity, diffusional distances are increased. The supply of oxygen to the interior of the fiber may be significantly impaired.

With *cardiac dilation*, left ventricular radius is increased. A larger end-diastolic volume is associated with higher end-diastolic pressure and increased pressure generation during systole. The Laplace relationship predicts that both factors lead to increased intramyocardial wall tension. Stretching of the heart wall is associated with decreased wall thickness, further increasing intramyocardial wall tension.

THE CARDIAC CYCLE

Every ventricular contraction that propels blood to the body or the lungs is the result of the sequential activation of the cardiac chambers through the coordinated functioning of electrical and mechanical factors. This section describes the changing cardiac pressures and volumes that coincide with the time sequence of cardiac events. An understanding of normal or abnormal cardiac functioning depends on familiarity with the cardiac cycle, which is represented graphically in Figure 2-56.

For the sake of simplicity, this description of events occurring during the cardiac cycle begins with events in the left heart. Figure 2-56 should be referred to frequently to obtain an understanding of what is occurring concurrently with respect to electrical activity; atrial, ventricular, and aortic pressures; atrial and ventricular volumes; valvular activity; and heart sounds.

Some general points about pressure and timing are useful to remember. Blood flows from the chamber with greater pressure to the chamber with lower pressure. When valves are open between two chambers, pressures in both chambers change until they are approximately equal. When valves between two chambers are closed, the pressures in the chambers change relatively independently of each other.

Ventricular systole and diastole divide the cardiac cycle into two major phases. The cardiac cycle can be further subdivided into several separate periods during systole and diastole. Because the cardiac cycle is continuous, the description of these periods can begin at any point.

Left Ventricular Cardiac Events

Ventricular Systole

Isovolumic Ventricular Contraction (Period a, Fig. 2-56). Ventricular contraction follows ventricular depolarization (reflected by the ECG QRS wave). Ventricular pressure increases rapidly. At the onset of this phase, pressures in the atrium and ventricle are approximately equal, but atrial pressure decreases with atrial muscle relaxation. Closure of the mitral valve buffers the atria from the high ventricular pressures.

The mitral valve closes when the ventricle contracts. Pressure in the ventricle becomes higher than in the atrium. The aortic valve remains closed until left ventricular pressure exceeds aortic pressure. Bulging of the cardiac valves due to abrupt ventricular pressure increases may cause slight increases in atrial and aortic pressures recorded during this period.

During the brief time when both mitral and aortic valves are closed, there are no actual changes in ventricular volume because no blood is flowing into or out of the ventricle. The ventricle changes shape during this period. The apparent increase in ventricular volume recorded on the ventricular volume curve in Figure 2-56 occurs when ventricular volume is calculated based on ventricular circumference.

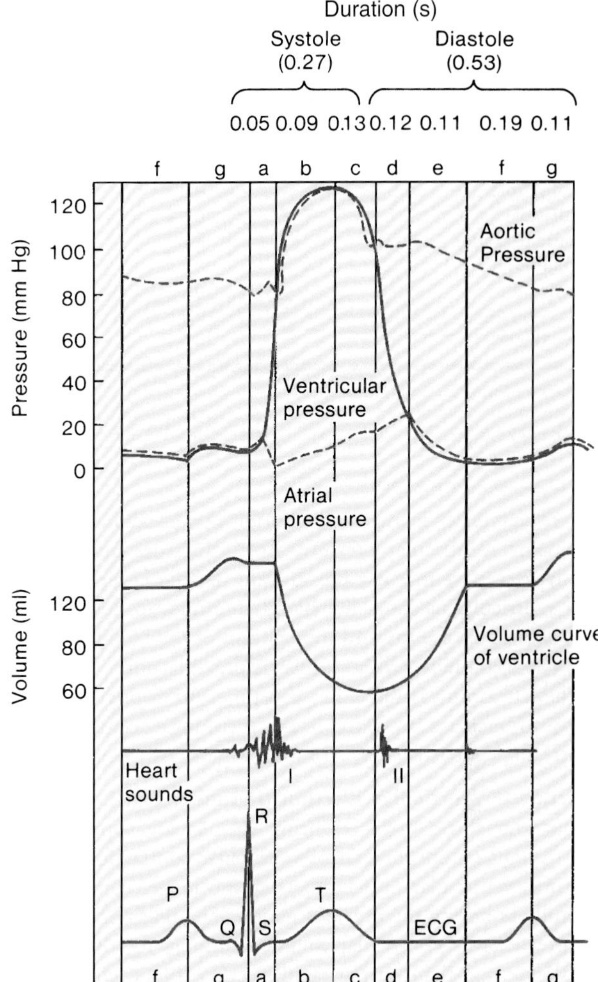

Figure 2-56. The cardiac cycle, illustrating the changes in aortic, left ventricular, and left atrial pressures, and in left ventricular volume in relation to phonocardiogram and the ECG. The duration of each phase at a heart rate of approximately 75 beats/min is indicated at the top of the figure. a, isovolumetric ventricular contraction; b, rapid ventricular ejection; c, slow ventricular ejection; d, protodiastole and isovolumetric relaxation; e, rapid ventricular filling; f, diastasis; g, atrial contraction; I, first heart sound; II, second heart sound. (Adapted from Wiggers CJ. *Circulatory Dynamics*. New York: Grune and Stratton; 1952:57.)

The *isovolumic* or *isovolumetric period* is also termed the *isometric phase* of ventricular contraction because tension is increasing rapidly, but the muscle fibers do not shorten much until they overcome the afterload of aortic pressure. Muscle contraction is not completely isometric, however, because the ventricles change dimensions.

Rapid Ventricular Ejection (Period b, Fig. 2-56). Ventricular muscle contraction continues, and the aortic valve remains open as long as left ventricular pressure exceeds aortic pressure. The aorta and left ventricle are essentially a common cavity at this time. Ventricular pressure continues to increase rapidly during the initial part of this period, and then rises less rapidly to approximately the systolic pressure (120 mm Hg in the figure) later during this period.

Ventricular volume decreases rapidly during ventricular ejection; two thirds or more of the SV is ejected during this approximately 0.09-second period (Table 2-6). Aortic flow reaches

Table 2-6 • DURATION OF CARDIAC CYCLE PERIODS[a]

Cycle Phase	Duration (s)
Isometric contraction	0.05
Maximal ejection	0.09
Reduced ejection	0.13
Total systole	0.27
Protodiastole	0.04
Isometric relaxation	0.08
Rapid inflow	0.11
Diastasis	0.19
Atrial systole	0.11
Total diastole	0.53

[a]Numbers shown are for heart rate of approximately 75 beats/min.
From Scher AM. Mechanical events of the cardiac cycle. In: Ruch TC, Patton HD, eds. *Physiology and Biophysics*. 20th ed. Vol. II. Philadelphia, PA: WB Saunders; 1974:102–116.

peak velocity early in the rapid ejection period before the point of maximal ventricular pressure. Aortic pressure may actually slightly exceed ventricular pressure during the latter period of rapid ventricular ejection, but blood continues to flow into the aorta because of the forward momentum of the blood. Much of the SV is accommodated in the elastic proximal aorta.

The left atrium is relaxed at this time. Atrial pressure slowly begins to increase as blood from the lungs accumulates in the atrium. Ventricular repolarization begins.

Reduced Ventricular Ejection (Period c, Fig. 2-56). Ventricular and aortic pressures begin to decrease approximately 0.13 seconds before the end of ventricular contraction. During this time, ventricular muscle fibers are no longer contracting as forcefully as during the previous period. The fibers have reached a shorter length. Ventricular volume continues to fall, although at a slower rate than during rapid ejection. Blood continues to flow into the aorta. This period of reduced ventricular ejection comprises approximately the latter two thirds of the total ejection period (see Table 2-6). Atrial pressure and volume continue to increase. Ventricular repolarization is usually complete by this time, as indicated by the end of the T wave.

Ventricular Diastole

Protodiastole (Initial Part of Period d, Fig. 2-56). As ventricular muscle relaxation begins, there is a brief period before ventricular pressure becomes lower than aortic pressure when no blood is being ejected from the ventricle. Blood flow momentarily reverses. This backflow at a time when ventricular pressure is becoming less than aortic pressure facilitates the closure of the aortic valve. The second heart sound occurs. During this time, a slight transient decrease in atrial pressure may occur, reflecting the effect of ventricular relaxation.

Isovolumic Ventricular Relaxation (Latter Part of Period d, Fig. 2-56). Ventricular pressure decreases rapidly as the ventricle relaxes. There is no change in ventricular volume during this period when all the cardiac valves are closed. After closure of the aortic valve, aortic pressure increases by a few millimeters of mercury, and the incisura or dicrotic notch is noted on the aortic pressure tracing. Atrial pressure continues to increase as the atrium continues to receive pulmonary venous blood.

Rapid Ventricular Filling (Period e, Fig. 2-56). The AV (mitral) valve opens when atrial pressure exceeds ventricular pressure. The ventricle fills rapidly with blood that has been accumulating in the atrium, but ventricular pressure continues to decrease during this period because ventricular relaxation continues. Most of the blood that was sequestered in the atrium during systole is emptied into the ventricle by the time the ventricle reaches maximal diastolic size. Atrial pressure decreases as the atria empty but remains slightly greater than ventricular pressure throughout this period.

Late Diastole (Diastasis; Period f, Fig. 2-56). The mitral valve remains open, and pressures in the atrium and ventricle equilibrate in the time after rapid ventricular filling and before the beginning of atrial contraction. Blood from the lungs continues to enter the left ventricle passively, so ventricular volume and pressure slowly increase. Coronary artery blood flow usually is maximal during late diastole. The beginning of atrial depolarization is indicated by the upstroke of the ECG P wave.

Atrial Contraction (Period g, Fig. 2-56). Atrial muscle contraction follows atrial depolarization and results in an increase in left atrial pressure. Ventricular volume and pressure are increased slightly as the atrium forces much of its remaining blood into the ventricles. Between 15% and 25% of the end-diastolic ventricular volume consists of blood that has been ejected from the atrium during atrial contraction. The contribution of atrial contraction to total ventricular volume depends on venous return and HR; it is greater at faster heart rates. This atrial contribution to ventricular volume may be lost when the atria and ventricles are electrically and mechanically dissociated, such as during atrial fibrillation or complete heart block. Aortic pressure continues to decrease as blood in the aorta flows into the periphery. Toward the end of this period, the ventricles begin to depolarize. Diastole ends with the onset of ventricular contraction. The cardiac cycle is repeated.

Right Ventricular Cardiac Cycle

The sequence of events in the right ventricle during the cardiac cycle is exactly the same as in the left ventricle, but the timing of events in the two ventricles is slightly different. Right ventricular and pulmonary artery pressures are much lower than left ventricular and aortic pressures and right atrial pressures are usually slightly less than left atrial pressures.

Several factors lead to differences in the timing of events between the right and left heart. Contraction of the left ventricle begins before contraction of the right ventricle. Left ventricular isovolumetric contraction and relaxation last longer than right ventricular isovolumetric contraction and relaxation, presumably because the left ventricle must develop more contractile force to overcome higher systemic pressures. Right ventricular ejection begins before, lasts longer than, and ends after left ventricular ejection. Thus, right ventricular filling and ejection periods are longer than left ventricular periods, but the durations of left and right ventricular electromechanical systole are almost equal.

Cardiac Valvular Events and Normal Heart Sounds

Valvular Events

The differences in timing of right and left ventricular events lead to differences in timing of right and left valvular events. The AV valves close at the onset of ventricular systole. The mitral valve normally closes before the tricuspid valve because left ventricular contraction begins before right ventricular contraction.

The aortic and pulmonic valves open when ventricular pressures exceed arterial pressures. The pulmonic valve opens before the aortic valve. Right ventricular isovolumetric contraction is shorter than left ventricular isovolumetric contraction.

The aortic and pulmonic valves close when ventricular pressures fall below arterial pressures. The aortic valve closes before the pulmonic valve. The right ventricular ejection period is longer than the left.

The AV valves open during diastole when ventricular pressures are lower than atrial pressures. The tricuspid valve opens before the mitral valve because of the more rapid isovolumetric right ventricular relaxation.

Normal Heart Sounds

The specific mechanisms responsible for heart sounds are disputed. Sudden accelerations and decelerations of blood, turbulent blood flow, and the movements of valves, heart walls, and blood vessels may all produce vibrations and sounds audible at the body surface.

First Heart Sound. Mitral valve closure and oscillations in the movement of blood in the ventricles are associated with vibrations of the entire valvular apparatus and of atrial and ventricular walls. This creates the early components of the first heart sound. Later components of the first heart sound may be due to the acceleration of blood ejected into the aorta.

Second Heart Sound. The second heart sound actually begins before semilunar valve closure. The mechanisms responsible for the second heart sound include arterial blood flow decelerations caused by ventricular relaxation, blood vessel wall vibrations, and semilunar valvular vibrations.

Pulmonic valve closure follows aortic valve closure and leads to a two-component sound, which is accentuated during inspiration. During inspiration, the time between closure of the aortic and pulmonic valves is increased, probably because a decrease in pulmonary vascular impedance leads to a longer right ventricular ejection time.

Clinical Applications of Cardiac Events

Systolic Events

The SV is the volume ejected by the ventricle in a single contraction. SV multiplied by the number of cardiac cycles per minute (heart rate) equals the CO. A typical volume ejected by the ventricle is 60 to 130 mL/m^2 body surface area/s, illustrated by the ventricular volume downstroke of Fig. 2-56. The SV, which is the difference between the ventricular end-diastolic and end-systolic volume, is approximately 24 to 36 mL/beat/m^2 of body surface area.

The *ejection fraction* is the percentage of total ventricular volume ejected during each contraction (i.e., SV divided by end-diastolic volume). The ejection fraction is a frequently used index of ventricular function; normally, it is greater than 55% and usually is approximately 65%.

The maximal rate of left ventricular force development and rise of left ventricular pressure over time (peak d*P*/d*t*) occurs during isovolumic ventricular contraction. Peak d*P*/d*t* is sometimes used as a clinical measure of ventricular contractility.

Diastolic Events

Diastole comprises a greater portion of the cardiac cycle (approximately 65%) than does systole (approximately 35%) at normal heart rates (see Table 2-6). At faster heart rates, both systole and diastole are shortened, diastole proportionally more so than systole. For example, at a heart rate of 180 beats/min, diastole comprises approximately 40% and systole approximately 60% of the cardiac cycle. At fast heart rates, diastolic filling is increasingly important in terms of the decreased amount of time available for ventricular and coronary artery filling, which may lead to impaired myocardial functioning.

The jugular venous and the carotid arterial pulses normally reflect right and left heart events, respectively. All cardiovascular assessment and treatment plans intimately depend on an appreciation of the cardiac cycle.

CONCLUSION

The cardiac nurse who deepens his or her knowledge of cardiac anatomy will have a more thorough understanding of cardiac physiology. While many cardiac nurse competencies and responsibilities focus on pathoanatomic and pathophysiologic changes of diseases and their functional consequences, the cardiac nurse must first understand normal anatomy and physiology to comprehend what and why cardiac structures and functions are abnormal. The synthesis of the anatomic and physiologic (electrical, mechanical, and metabolic) processes that underpin cardiac performance is applied to the individual patient and his or her preferences and values. In both individuals and populations, the cardiac nurse plays an important role in the preventing the onset and/or progression of cardiovascular disease and its complications.

KEY READINGS

Anderson R, Spicer D, Hlavacek A, et al. *Wilcox's Surgical Anatomy of the Heart.* Cambridge: Cambridge University Press; 2013.

Fuster V, Harrington RA, Narula J, et al. *Hurst's the Heart.* 14th ed. New York: McGraw-Hill; 2017.

University of Minnesota. The Atlas of Human Cardiac Anatomy: University of Minnesota's Visible Heart Laboratory's free-access educational website highlighting both functional and static human cardiac anatomy. Available at http://www.vhlab.umn.edu/atlas/

REFERENCES

1. Ungerleider H, Clark C. Study of the transverse diameter of the heart silhouette with prediction table based on the teleroentgenogram. *Am Heart J.* 1939;17:92–102.
2. Reiner L, Mazzoleni A, Rodriguez F, et al. The weight of the human heart. I. Normal cases. *AMA Arch Pathol.* 1959;68:58–73.
3. Smith H. The relation of the weight of the heart to the weight of the body and of the weight of the heart to age. *Am Heart J.* 1928;4:79–93.
4. Hill AJ. Attitudinally correct cardiac anatomy. In: Iaizzo PA, ed. *Handbook of Cardiac Anatomy, Physiology, and Devices.* Totowa, NJ: Humana Press; 2009:15–21.
5. Anderson RH, Spicer DE, Hlavacek AJ, et al. Describing the cardiac components—attitudinally appropriate nomenclature. *J Cardiovasc Transl Res.* 2013;6(2):118–123.
6. Hagen PT, Scholz DG, Edwards WD. Incidence and size of patent foramen ovale during the first 10 decades of life: an autopsy study of 965 normal hearts. *Mayo Clin Proc.* 1984;59(1):17–20.
7. Lamy C, Giannesini C, Zuber M, et al. Clinical and imaging findings in cryptogenic stroke patients with and without patent foramen ovale. *Stroke.* 2002;33(3):706–711.
8. Dowson A, Mullen Michael J, Peatfield R, et al. Migraine Intervention With STARFlex Technology (MIST) trial. *Circulation.* 2008;117(11):1397–1404.
9. Piazza N, de Jaegere P, Schultz C, et al. Anatomy of the aortic valvar complex and its implications for transcatheter implantation of the aortic valve. *Circ Cardiovasc Interv.* 2008;1(1):74–81.

10. Van Mieghem NM, Piazza N, Anderson RH, et al. Anatomy of the mitral valvular complex and its implications for transcatheter interventions for mitral regurgitation. *J Am Coll Cardiol.* 2010;56(8): 617–626.
11. Carpentier A. Cardiac valve surgery—the "French correction." *J Thorac Cardiovasc Surg.* 1983;86:323–337.
12. James T. *Anatomy of the Coronary Arteries.* New York: Paul B. Hober; 1961.
13. Kelly AE, Gensini GG. Coronary angiography and left heart studies. *Heart Lung.* 1975;4:85–98.
14. Weam J. Morphological and functional alterations of the coronary circulation. *Bull N Y Acad Med.* 1940;17:754–777.
15. Armour J, Hopkins D. Anatomy of the efferent autonomic nerves and ganglia innervating the heart. In: Randall W, ed. *Nervous Control of Cardiovascular Function.* New York: Oxford University Press; 1984: 20–45.
16. Miller A. *Lymphatics of the Heart.* New York: Raven Press; 1982.
17. Randall W. Selective autonomic innervation of the heart. In: Randall W, ed. *Nervous Control of Cardiovascular Function.* New York: Oxford University Press; 1984:44–67.
18. Keith A, Flack M. The form and nature of the muscular connections between the primary divisions of the vertebrate heart. *J Anat Physiol.* 1907;41:172–189.
19. Bachmann G. The inter-auricular time interval. *Am J Physiol.* 1916;41:309–320.
20. James TN. The connecting pathways between the sinus node and A-V node and between the right and the left atrium in the human heart. *Am Heart J.* 1963;66:498–508.
21. Tarawa S. *Das Reisleitungs system des Saugetierherzens [The conduction system of the mammalian heart].* Jena, Germany: Gustav Fischer; 1906.
22. Titus JL, Daugherty GW, Edwards JE. Anatomy of the normal human atrioventricular conduction system. *Am J Anat.* 1963;113:407–415.
23. Anderson RH, Becker AE, Brechenmacher C, et al. The human atrioventricular junctional area. A morphological study of the A-V node and bundle. *Eur J Cardiol.* 1975;3:11–25.
24. Hecht HH, Kossmann CE, Childers RW, et al. Atrioventricular and intraventricular conduction. Revised nomenclature and concepts. *Am J Cardiol.* 1873;31:232–244.
25. His W. Die Thätigkeit des embryonalen Herzens und deren Bedeutung für die Lehre von der Herzbewegung beim Erwachsenen. [The function of the embryonic heart and its significance in the interpretation of the heart action in the adult]. *Arbeit aus der Medizin Klinik zu Leipzig.* 1893;14–50. Translation from: Willius FA, Keys TE, His W, Jr. *Classics of Cardiology.* New York, NY: Dover Publications; 1941;2:695.
26. Kent A. The right lateral auriculo-ventricular junction of the heart. *J Physiol.* 1914;48:22–24.
27. Anderson RH, Becker AE, Brechenmacher C, et al. Ventricular pre-excitation: a proposed nomenclature for its substrates. *Eur J Cardiol.* 1975;3:27–36.
28. Massing GK, James T. Anatomical configuration of the His bundle and bundle branches in the human heart. *Circulation.* 1976;53: 609–621.
29. Purkinje J. Mikroskopisch-neurologische beobachtungen. *Arch Anat Physiol Wiss Med.* 1845;12:281–295.
30. Sperelakis N. Hormonal and neurotransmitter regulation of Ca^{++} influx through voltage-dependent slow channels in cardiac muscle membrane. *Membr Biochem.* 1984;5:131–166.
31. De Mello W. Effect of isoproterenol and 3-isobutyl-1-methylxanthine on junctional conductance in heart cell pairs. *Biochim Biophys Acta.* 1989;1012:291–298.
32. Hodgkin AL, Huxley AF. Currents carried by sodium and potassium ions through the membrane of the giant axon of Loligo. *J Physiol.* 1952;116:449–472.
33. Glynn IM. Annual review prize lecture. 'All hands to the sodium pump'. *J Physiol.* 1993;462:1–30.
34. Langer GA. Sodium-calcium exchange in the heart. *Annu Rev Physiol.* 1982;44:435–449.
35. Noma A, Shibasaki T. Membrane current through adenosine-triphosphate-regulated potassium channels in guinea-pig ventricular cells. *J Physiol.* 1985;363:463–480.
36. DiFrancesco D. A new interpretation of the pace-maker current in calf Purkinje fibres. *J Physiol.* 1981;314:359–376.
37. Nichols CG, Ripoll C, Lederer WJ. ATP-sensitive potassium channel modulation of the guinea pig ventricular action potential and contraction. *Circ Res.* 1991;68:280–287.
38. Singer DH, Baumgarten CM, Ten Eick RE. Cellular electrophysiology of ventricular and other dysrhythmias: studies on diseased and ischemic heart. *Prog Cardiovasc Dis.* 1981;24:97–156.
39. Donaldson SK, Goldberg ND, Walseth TF, et al. Inositol trisphosphate stimulates calcium release from peeled skeletal muscle fibers. *Biochim Biophys Acta.* 1987;927:92–99.
40. Spach MS, Kootsey JM. The nature of electrical propagation in cardiac muscle. *Am J Physiol.* 1983;244:H3–H22.
41. Maylie J, Morad M. Ionic currents responsible for the generation of pacemaker current in the rabbit sino-atrial node. *J Physiol.* 1984;355:215–235.
42. de Carvalho A, de Almeida D. Spread of activity through the atrioventricular node. *Circ Res.* 1960;8:801–809.
43. Durrer D, van Dam RT, Freud GE, et al. Total excitation of the isolated human heart. *Circulation.* 1970;41:899–912.
44. Weidmann S. Cardiac cellular physiology and its contribution to electrocardiography. *Jpn Heart J.* 1982;23(Suppl):12–16.
45. Cohen M. *Coronary Collaterals: Clinical and Experimental Observations.* Mt Kisco, New York: Futura; 1985.
46. Ringer S. A further contribution regarding the influence of the different constituents of the blood on the contraction of the heart. *J Physiol.* 1883;4:29–42.
47. Franzini-Armstrong C. Studies of the triad. IV. Structure of the junction in frog slow fibers. *J Cell Biol.* 1973;56:120–128.
48. Sperelakis N. Propagation mechanisms in heart. *Annu Rev Physiol.* 1979;41:441–457.
49. Hunter DR, Haworth RA, Berkoff HA. Cellular calcium turnover in the perfused rat heart: modulation by caffeine and procaine. *Circ Res.* 1982;51:363–370.
50. Patterson SW, Starling EH. On the mechanical factors which determine the output of the ventricles. *J Physiol.* 1914;48:357–379.
51. Gordon AM, Huxley AF, Julian FJ. The variation in isometric tension with sarcomere length in vertebrate muscle fibres. *J Physiol.* 1966;184:170–192.
52. Lewis BS, Gotsman MS. Current concepts of left ventricular relaxation and compliance. *Am Heart J.* 1980;99:101–112.
53. Hood WB Jr, Bianco JA, Kumar R, et al. Experimental myocardial infarction. IV. Reduction of left ventricular compliance in the healing phase. *J Clin Invest.* 1970;49:1316–1323.
54. Regan TJ, Frank MJ, Lehan PH, et al. Myocardial blood flow and oxygen uptake during acute red cell volume increments. *Circ Res.* 1963;13:172–181.
55. Klocke FJ, Braunwald E, Ross J Jr. Oxygen cost of electrical activation of the heart. *Circ Res.* 1966;18:357–365.
56. Siepser SL, Kaltman AJ, Mills N, et al. Coronary collateral flow after traumatic fistula between right coronary artery and right atrium. *N Engl J Med.* 1972;287:754–756.
57. Zimmerman HA. The coronary circulation in patients with severe emphysema, cor pulmonale, cyanotic congenital heart disease, and severe anemia. *Dis Chest.* 1952;22:269–273.
58. Barmeyer J. Postmortem measurement of intercoronary anastomotic flow in normal and diseased hearts: a quantitative study. *Vasc Surg.* 1971;5:239–248.
59. Levin DC, Beckmann CF, Sos TA, et al. The effect of coronary artery bypass on collateral circulation. *Radiology.* 1981;141:317–322.

3 Systemic and Pulmonary Circulation and Oxygen Delivery

Sunny M. Ohman, Joelle T. Fathi

OBJECTIVES

1. Describe blood flow, characteristics, and regulation through the vasculature and lymphatic system.
2. Explain the components and effects on distribution of blood flow that neural and local metabolic factors have.
3. Describe the physiologic factors that affect the oxyhemoglobin dissociation curve, the resulting shifts on the curve, and the effects these changes have on hemoglobin's affinity for oxygen.
4. Describe the mechanisms that alter pulmonary vascular resistance.
5. Discuss the transport and distribution of oxygen between the lungs and organs.

KEY QUESTIONS

1. What physiologic factors influence the function of vascular endothelium as a metabolically active barrier?
2. What are the local factors that affect vascular resistance and what are the mechanisms involved?
3. What are the components involved in the physiologic process of respiration?
4. How do ventilation/perfusion problems and diffusion defect problems arise and what are their effects?

BACKGROUND

The structural and functional characteristics of the systemic circulation determine the continuous adjustments in flow, pressure, and resistance that occur in each vascular bed and that are vital determinants of tissue function. Blood flow and nutrient exchange in various vascular beds are affected by the structural and metabolic characteristics of the vascular bed, the physical factors that affect flow and the exchange of materials across the blood vessel wall, the local factors originating from the metabolically active cells and vascular endothelium that regulate flow to individual vascular beds, and local and systemic neuroendocrine regulation. The combined regulation of cardiac output, blood pressure, and systemic vascular resistance determines tissue blood flow and, ultimately, the survival of each organ system and the body as a whole (Display 3-1). This chapter describes the basic anatomy and physiology of the systemic and pulmonary circulation; Chapter 4 describes the overall regulation of cardiac output and blood pressure.

STRUCTURAL CHARACTERISTICS OF THE VASCULATURE AND LYMPHATICS

Blood vessels are usually classified in the following manner: aorta, large arteries; main arterial branch, small arteries, arterioles; terminal arterioles, capillaries, postcapillary venules; venules, small veins, main venule branch, large veins, and the vena cava.[1–3] These classifications are based on structural characteristics such as diameter, wall thickness, and the presence of muscle. Although blood vessel diameter is often used to characterize different vessels, it is not an appropriate criterion to use for classification, because differences in vessel size reflect the state of vessel contraction as well as differences between organ systems and species (Fig. 3-1).[3,4]

With the exception of the capillaries, the systemic vasculature is composed of three layers: the tunica intima or internal layer, which consists of the endothelium and the basal membrane; the tunica media, which consists of smooth muscle and a matrix of collagen, elastin, and glycoproteins; and the tunica adventitia, which consists of connective tissue (Fig. 3-2).[5] The muscularis in the artery is a concentric ring, which allows for vasoconstriction. In contrast, the venous musculature is organized into small bundles at right angles.[6] In the larger arteries and veins, the tunica adventitia also contains blood vessels that supply the vessel wall

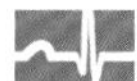

DISPLAY 3-1

Vascular System

The vascular system serves two primary functions, distribution and exchange.

Blood is distributed to and from the organs. Nutrients, gases, and cell excreta are exchanged.

Vessels can be organized by their primary function: distribution/resistance (aorta, large and small distributing arteries), exchange (capillaries, small venules, and capacitance [large venules, veins, and vena cava]).

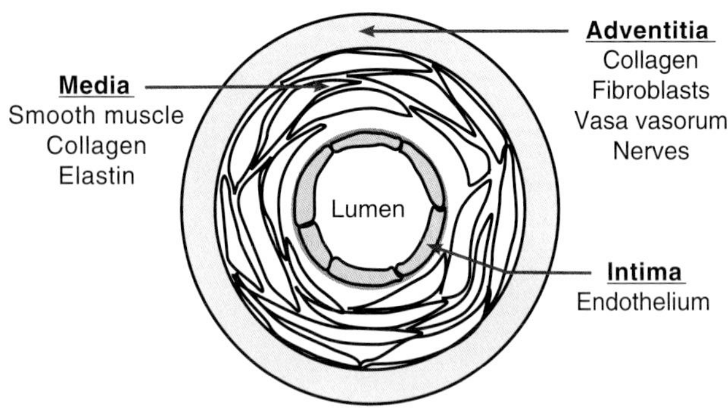

Figure 3-1. Blood vessel components. (Reprinted with permission from Klabunde RE. *Cardiovascular Physiology Concepts.* 2nd ed. Philadelphia, PA: Wolters Kluwer/Lippincott Williams & Wilkins; 2012:50.)

(vasa vasorum).[3] The vascular endothelium, which is a metabolically active barrier, is a primary mediator of vascular function and is discussed in detail.

Arteries

Arteries in which the media contains smooth muscle and elastin are called *elastic arteries.*[3] Because of the considerable amount of elastin, these large conducting arteries are able to distend to twice their unloaded length. The ability of the capacitive arteries to distend is important in cushioning pulsatile flow, such that the blood flow to the organs/tissue is almost a constant flow (Display 3-2). During systole, the aorta and proximal large vessels store approximately 50% to 60% of the stroke volume. During diastole, the distended vessels recoil and move the remaining blood to the periphery. This phenomenon is referred to as a "Windkessel function," which is the transformation of pulsatile flow in the central arteries to constant flow in the periphery.[7] As the arteries approach the periphery, they become smaller in diameter, and there is a relative decrease in elastin and a relative increase in smooth muscle in the tunica media.[8,9] These peripheral arteries are referred to as *muscular arteries.*

DISPLAY 3-2

Arterial System

Large arteries, such as the carotid, branch off the aorta to distribute blood flow to various regions of the body and specific organs. Once this large distributing artery reaches its target organ or region, it in turn branches into small arteries that distribute the blood flow within that organ or region. These smaller arteries, continue to branch into smaller and smaller vessels, the smallest termed arterioles.

The small arteries (prearteriolar vessels with a diameter less than 500 mm) receive nervous stimulation primarily from noradrenergic stimuli, with the nerve terminals located in the adventitia. Unlike the larger arteries, in which sympathetic neural constriction is activated by α_1 and postsynaptic α_2 receptors, the small arteries are noradrenergically constricted mainly by the postsynaptic α_2 receptors.[9,10] The small arteries are also sensitive to endothelium-derived relaxing and contracting factors. Of clinical importance, abnormal small artery wall structure is an independent

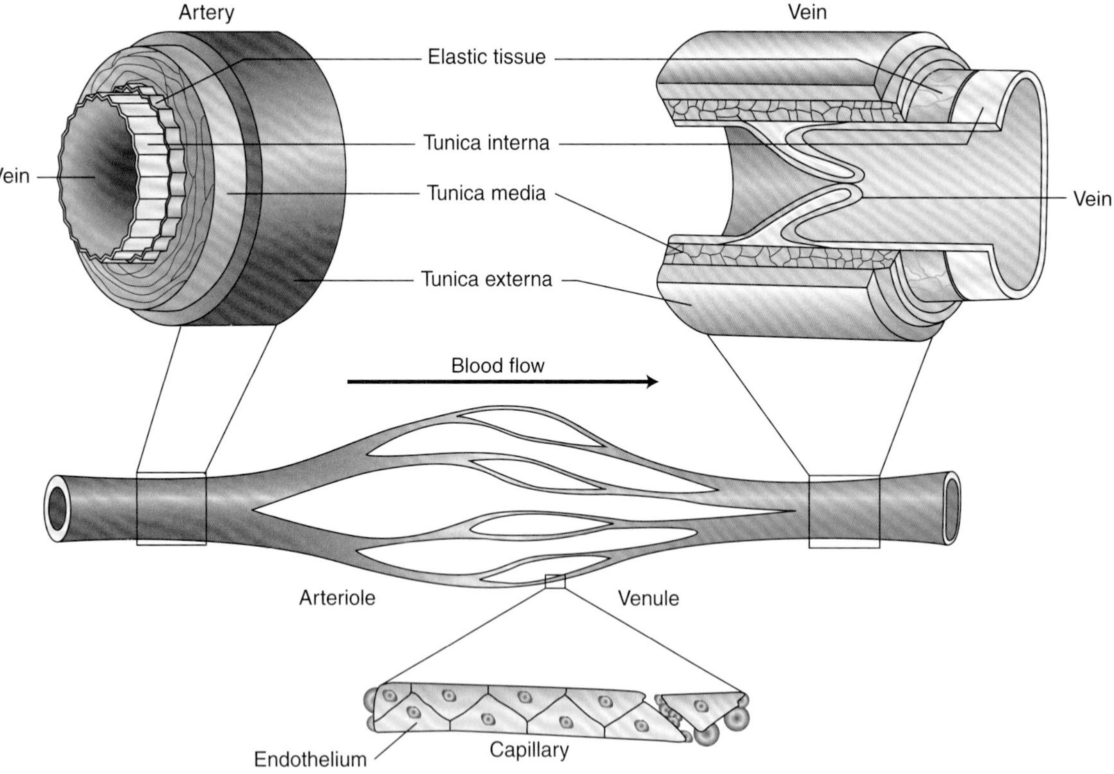

Figure 3-2. Schematic drawing of the major structural characteristics of the principal segments of blood vessels. The relative amounts of elastic tissue and fibrous tissues are largest in the aorta and least in small branches of the arterial tree. Small vessels have more prominent smooth muscle in the media. Capillaries consist only of endothelial cells. The walls of the veins are much like the arterial walls, but are thinner in relation to their caliber. (From iDAMS 3746-08-17.)

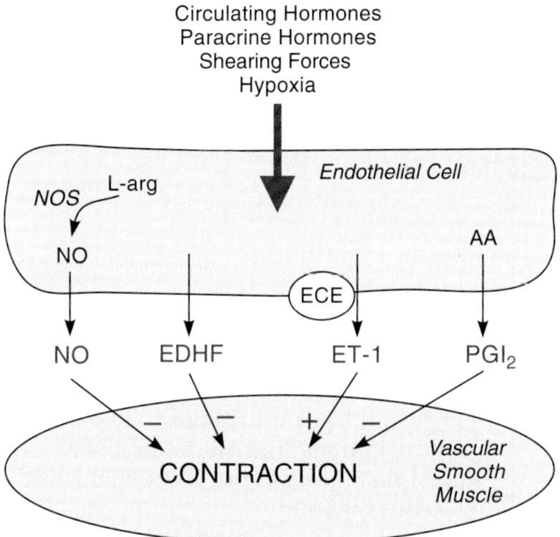

Figure 3-3. Endothelial-derived vasoactive factors. (Reprinted with permission from Klabunde RE. *Cardiovascular Physiology Concepts.* 2nd ed. Philadelphia, PA: Wolters Kluwer/Lippincott Williams & Wilkins; 2012:152.)

predictor of cardiovascular events (e.g., stroke, myocardial infarction, death).[11,12] However, it may be possible to reverse these changes with vasodilator therapy (Fig. 3-3).[13]

Microvascular Bed

The term *microcirculation* denotes the vascular and lymphatic microcirculation. The vascular microcirculation consists of (1) large and small arterioles (*precapillary resistance vessels*); (2) terminal arterioles, which in many tissues serve as the so-called precapillary sphincters; and (3) other precapillary structures such as capillaries; and (4) nonmuscular venules, known collectively as the exchange vessels, and muscular venules (postcapillary resistance vessels). The term lymphatic microvasculature refers specifically to the terminal lymphatic vessels.

Arterioles

As the vessel diameter decreases from the small arteries to the arterioles, the number of smooth muscle layers decreases from approximately six layers in the 300-μm vessels to a single layer of irregularly dispersed smooth muscle in the 30- to 50-μm vessels.[8] At this point, the vessels are referred to as *arterioles*. The smallest arteriolar branches (8 to 20 μm in diameter) are called the *terminal arterioles*.[14] In some cases, smooth muscle extends beyond the intersection of the terminal arterioles with the nonmuscular capillaries into structures known as *precapillary sphincters*.[15] The terminal arterioles and precapillary sphincters control the distribution of blood supply to the exchange vessels.[16]

Capillaries

Capillaries branch from terminal arteriolar segments. The capillary wall consists of endothelial cells and basal lamina; there is no tunica media or adventitia (Display 3-3). Capillary diameter is 4 to 8 mm, which is just large enough to allow the deformable red blood cells to pass through.[15,17] Not all exchange vessels in an area are simultaneously open. During periods of increased metabolism, capillary recruitment increases the number of open and perfused exchange vessels, thereby decreasing the distances for diffusion between exchange blood vessels and cells, as well as increasing the total surface area for exchange between the capillaries and cells.[14]

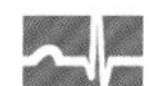 DISPLAY 3-3

Capillaries and the Microcirculation

Capillary walls are extremely thin single layer of highly permeable endothelial cells and basal lamina. This arrangement allows for the exchange of cell excreta, water, and nutrients to be efficiently exchanged between the tissue and circulating blood.

In the microcirculation metabolic waste, fluid, gases, substances such as nutrients, and hormones, as well as thermal energy is exchanged between the tissue and blood.

In microvascular beds located in the ears, fingers, and toes in humans and many other mammals, there are arteriovenous vascular channels that bypass the exchange vessels and allow blood to flow directly from arterioles to venules.[14] These arteriovenous anastomoses, which are richly innervated by the sympathetic nervous system, are important in local temperature control in these areas and even of the whole body in some conditions.[18]

Exchange Vessel Endothelium

The endothelium of exchange vessels in various organs contains at least four different structures that determine the rate of filtration and bulk transport of water and solutes and the exchange of larger molecules (Fig. 3-4). The structure of the membrane (continuous, fenestrated, discontinuous, and tight junction) varies depending on the location of the vascular bed.[19] All four types of endothelium have a continuous basement membrane, with the exception of the discontinuous endothelium.

Continuous endothelium is found in skin; skeletal, smooth, and cardiac muscle; and the lungs. There are several mechanisms by which substances pass through continuous endothelium. Water and solutes pass through intercellular junctions (40 to 1 Å) driven predominantly by a pressure gradient (ΔP) driving fluid out of the vessels. This outward flow is partly counterbalanced by forces drawing water back into the vessels. Lipid-soluble substances (CO_2, O_2) pass directly through the cell by diffusion; cytoplasmic vesicles transport solutes and water back and forth through the endothelium; and vesicles intermittently fuse to create channels in the cell. The junctions between the cells are responsible for the high permeability of the membrane to "ultrafiltrate," or protein-free fluid, and for the rapid diffusion of small ions. The continuous endothelium is relatively impermeable to plasma proteins and large molecules.

Fenestrated vascular endothelium is located in the gastrointestinal mucosa, glands, renal glomerular capillaries, and peritubular capillaries. The endothelium has openings (fenestrae) that expose the basement membrane (renal glomerular capillaries) or are covered by a thin diaphragm (gastrointestinal mucosa, renal peritubular capillaries). The fenestrated endothelium has a higher permeability to water and small solute molecules than continuous endothelium, whereas its permeability to plasma proteins is low, similar to continuous endothelium.[14]

Discontinuous endothelium is located in the hepatic cells, bone marrow, and splenic sinusoids. Discontinuous endothelium contains gaps in the endothelium and basement membrane and is permeable to proteins and other large molecules.

Tight-junction endothelium is located in the central nervous system and retina. It is the least permeable. The endothelial cells are connected by tight junctions that effectively restrict passage

Phenotype		Organ (function)
Continuous	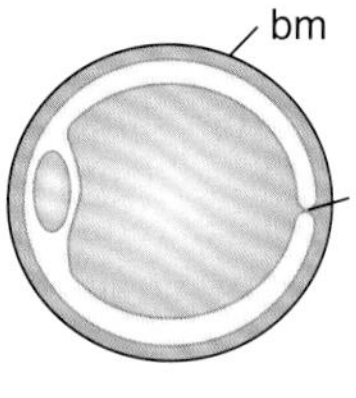 bm tj	CNS (blood—brain barrier) Lymph node (lymphocyte homing) Muscle (metabolic exchange)
Fenestrated	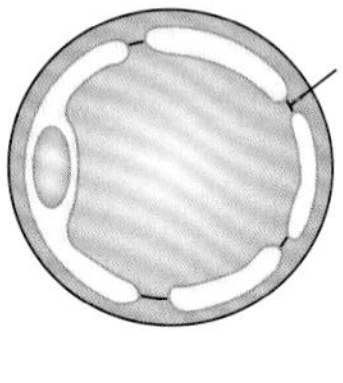 f	Endocrine glands (secretion) GI tract (absorption) Choroid plexus (secretion) Kidney glomeruli (filtration)
Discontinuous	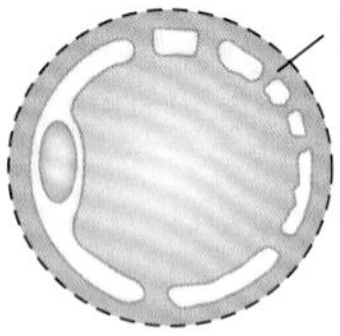 p	Liver (particle exchange) Bone marrow (hematopoiesis) Spleen (blood cell filter)

Figure 3-4. Different types of endothelial cells, their distribution to different organs and specific functional roles (bm, basal membrane; tj, tight junction; f, fenestrae; p, pores). (Reprinted with permission from Pries AR, Kuebler WM. Normal endothelium. *Handb Exp Pharmacol.* 2006; [176 Pt 1]:1–40.)

of all substances. Water- and lipid-soluble molecules pass directly through the endothelium, whereas ions and lipid-insoluble substances, such as glucose and amino acids, are transported by membrane carriers.[20]

Venules

Venous capillaries extend to the postcapillary venules (nonmuscular, 7 to 50 μm) and collecting venules. Along with the capillaries, the nonmuscular venules act as exchange vessels. Smooth muscle reappears in venules that are approximately 30 to 50 μm in diameter. These venules, which receive adrenergic innervation, are referred to as the muscular venules, postcapillary resistance vessels, or capacitance vessels.[2,14,17] As discussed later in the section on microcirculation, postcapillary resistance tends to be far less than precapillary resistance and has almost no effect on overall systemic vascular resistance (SVR). The veins contain approximately 70% of total blood volume, with approximately 25% of this volume in the venules.[2]

Veins

In general, veins have a larger diameter and thinner, more compliant walls than arteries at equivalent branches of the vascular tree.[2] However, the thickness of the venous walls is variable. For example, the veins in the legs and feet, which withstand the high hydrostatic pressure associated with standing, are thick-walled, whereas the veins near or above the level of the heart are thin-walled. The veins contain all three vascular layers found in the arteries; however, these layers are often indistinct.[3] Superficial veins form a rich anastomosis with deeper veins via vessels that perforate the muscles. These perforating veins allow venous return from cold skin to be diverted to warm muscle, providing a thermal short circuit, and they are particularly important for function of the muscle pump, which is described in Chapter 4.

Venous Valves

With the exception of the intrathoracic and intracerebral veins, the medium-sized veins contain valves that are oriented in the direction of blood flow, thus preventing retrograde blood flow into the muscle.[2] The presence of competent valves, in conjunction with the muscle pump in the lower extremities, is crucial to the ability to stand erect and in maintaining a reasonably low capillary pressure, because the valves interrupt the hydrostatic column that extends from the right atrium to the feet after each leg muscle contraction.[21] After humans with normal valvular function stand up, the valves in dependent veins initially interrupt the hydrostatic column. However, over a period of approximately 2 to 3 minutes, as the veins fill with blood, the valves can no longer interrupt the hydrostatic column as volume continues to accumulate. At this time, there is a displacement of approximately 600 mL of blood from the central circulation into the legs and pelvic organs.[22] In conditions in which blood flow is high, the hydrostatic effects associated with the loss of valvular function occur within 2 to 3 seconds. If the hydrostatic effects are not overcome by the muscle pump in the lower extremities, arterial hypotension, and syncope result. This phenomenon is readily seen in the soldier who faints while standing motionless at attention. There is also some evidence that there are microscopic venous valves located in the small veins and also in the postcapillary venules.[23] These microscopic valves may play a protective role against venous hypertension when there is valvular insufficiency in larger veins.

Venoconstriction

In contrast to the arteries, not all veins constrict when exposed to norepinephrine. For example, the postcapillary venules ranging from 0.007 to 2 mm in diameter do not have smooth muscle and therefore cannot constrict.[24] Most of the larger venules and small veins (including veins in the skeletal muscle) contain some smooth

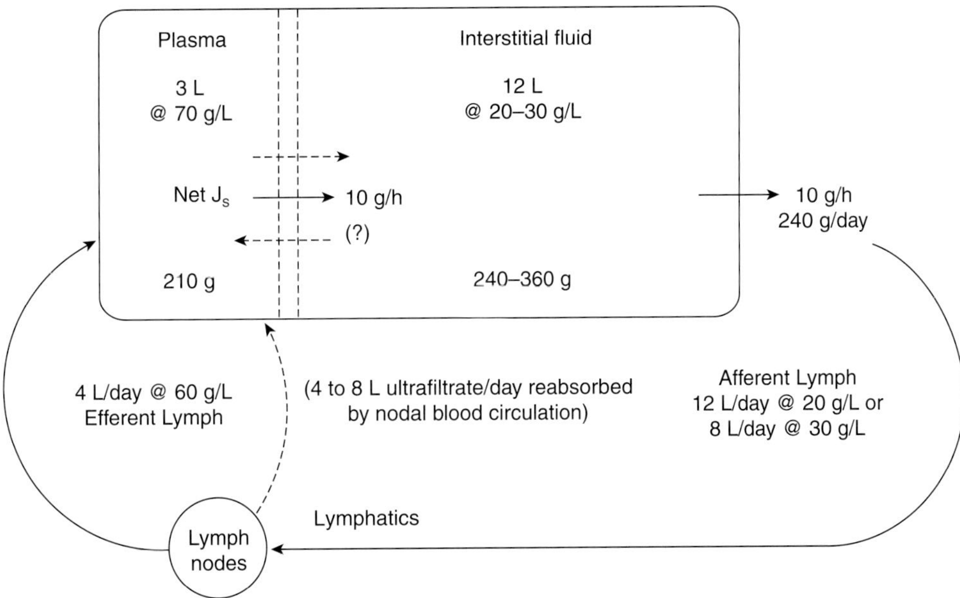

Figure 3-5. Steady-state distribution and circulation of fluid (ultrafiltrate) and plasma proteins in a normal human (weight, 65 kg). The *double-dashed line* between plasma and interstitial fluid represents exchange vessel endothelium. The weights at the bottoms of the boxes represent the total content of each. (Reprinted with permission from Renkin EM. Some consequences of capillary permeability to macromolecules: Starling's hypothesis reconsidered. *Am J Physiol.* 1986;250[5 Pt 2]:H706–H710.)

muscle,[2] but they are sparsely innervated and are not considered sites of vasoconstriction. The lack of venoconstriction in the skeletal muscle is important because the leg veins do not constrict in orthostasis. The splanchnic organs (liver, gastrointestinal tract, pancreas, and spleen) are the exception because they are richly innervated by sympathetic noradrenergic fibers and are capable of venoconstriction. In addition, the veins in the skin respond to thermoregulatory reflexes. In humans, significant venoconstriction occurs only in the splanchnic circulation; in response to thermoregulatory reflexes, the veins in the skin constrict and dilate.[18,25,26]

Lymphatics

The lymphatics are a system of thin-walled vessels that collect and conduct lymph through active contraction of the lymphatic microvasculature to the central circulation.[27–29] Lymph consists primarily of ultrafiltrate and proteins that have been filtered from exchange vessels. The initial lymphatic vessels (also known as terminal lymphatics or lymph capillaries), which consist of endothelialized tubes, originate in large, blind-terminal bulbs located in the connective tissue of most organ systems.[30] The lymphatic capillaries empty into collecting lymphatics, which in turn empty into transporting lymphatic vessels (Fig. 3-5). The central lymphatic vessels empty into the left and right lymphatic ducts, which empty into the subclavian veins.

A very small and transient pressure gradient between the interstitium and the terminal lymphatics promotes fluid movement into the lymphatics. Beginning at the level of the collecting capillaries, there are bicuspid valves, and the larger lymphatics contain smooth muscle that spontaneously contracts in a rhythmic manner.[31] The primary mechanism underlying the peristaltic like lymphatic flow is the intrinsic contraction of the lymphangions, which are the functional unit of lymphatic vessels, consisting of the valve and portion of the vessel surrounding the valve. The intrinsic contraction remains active during rest, anesthesia, and immobilization.[32] Lymphatic flow is also facilitated by lymph formation, skeletal muscle contractions (e.g., walking, foot flexing), respiration, fluctuations of central venous pressure, gastrointestinal peristalsis, and arterial pulsations.[33]

Vascular Smooth Muscle

Vascular smooth muscle contains the contractile filaments, actin and myosin; however, unlike striated smooth muscle (cardiac), the filaments are not organized in any fashion.[34] Although the sarcoplasmic reticulum is not as prominent in vascular smooth muscle as in cardiac muscle, it serves as the primary intracellular source of calcium.[35] Additionally, the amount of myosin in smooth muscle is approximately one-fifth that found in striated muscle. Despite this lower amount of myosin, smooth muscle develops higher force per cross-sectional area than striated muscle. Vascular smooth muscle also usually contracts more slowly than striated muscle, and it maintains tonic contractions with lower-energy (adenosine triphosphate [ATP]) expenditure.

Smooth muscle is characterized as "phasic" and "tonic." Phasic vascular smooth muscle, which is capable of high shortening velocities, is located in the portal veins. Tonic vascular smooth muscle is located in most of the small arteries and arterioles and has a slower shortening velocity, but it is capable of maintaining sustained vascular tone.[36] As in cardiac and skeletal muscle, contraction of vascular smooth muscle is related to the formation and release of crossbridges by the cyclic attachment and detachment of the heads of the contractile protein myosin with actin (see Chapter 1). Tonic contractions allow for the maintenance of a basal vascular tone, which is crucial for the maintenance of arterial blood pressure. These tonic contractions are the result of a "latch bridge," which is a slowing in the cross-bridge cycling rate. Other possible mechanisms for the tonic contraction include increased calcium sensitivity and inhibition by agonists of proteins

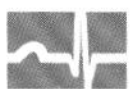

DISPLAY 3-4

Local regulation of tissue determines the diameter of the arterioles which in turn control the blood flow to each tissue. As a result, each tissue maintains control over its blood flow requirements in proportion to its metabolic needs.

The resistance vessels are innervated by autonomic nerves (sympathetic adrenergic) and dilate and contract in response to stimuli.

Resistance vessels are impregnated with receptors that bind circulating hormones such as catecholamines, angiotensin II and other substances such as adenosine, potassium ion, and nitric oxide that alter the vessel diameter.

Synthesized by the endothelium, endothelin-1, causes the contraction/constriction of vascular smooth muscle. Vascular endothelium also synthesizes nitric oxide and prostacyclin, which in turn, cause the relaxation/dilation of vascular smooth muscle.

Under normal physiologic conditions, nitric oxide appears to be the most important endothelial factor in regard to regulation of blood flow.

(e.g., caldesmon) that bind actin and interfere with the inhibitory effects of calcium–calmodulin.[37]

LOCAL REGULATION

In addition to the systemic factors that affect vascular resistance, there are local factors that control resistance. These factors include autacoids, endothelium-derived vasoactive substances, local metabolic factors that match blood flow (oxygen transport) to metabolism, autoregulation and local heating and cooling (Display 3-4).

Autacoids

The autacoids (vasoactive substances) include histamine, serotonin, prostaglandin, and bradykinin. These factors most often compete with adrenergic (vasoconstrictive) effects and exert a local vasodilatory effect, which can improve tissue perfusion. The autacoids are not involved in systemic regulation of blood pressure or total peripheral resistance; however, they initiate or modify the vascular response to other stimuli.

Endothelium-Derived Vasoactive Substances

The vascular endothelium, which is a single layer of squamous cells in the tunica intima that lines the entire vascular tree, modulates vascular tone by secreting dilator and constrictor substances. In addition, the endothelium affects platelet adhesion and aggregation and under basal conditions substances secreted by the endothelium affect the clotting cascade.[38] The endothelium is also involved in the regulation of vascular smooth muscle proliferation.[38] The proposed functions of the vascular endothelium (Table 3-1) require an intact endothelium.[39] The control of vascular tone involves cross talk between the vasodilators nitric oxide (NO), prostaglandins, and endothelial-derived hyperpolarizing factor (EDHF) and the vasoconstrictors endothelin-1 and prostacyclin (Fig. 3-6). A discussion of each of these factors related to vascular control follows. A summary of the stimuli that cause the release of each of the factors is presented in Table 3-2.

Table 3-1 • FUNCTIONS OF THE VASCULAR ENDOTHELIUM RELATED TO VASOMOTOR FUNCTION

Action	Factors Responsible
Release of vasodilatory agents	Nitric oxide Prostacyclin Endothelium-derived hyperpolarizing factor
Release of vasoconstrictor agents	Endothelin-1 Angiotensin/angiotensin II Prostaglandin H2 Thromboxane A_2 Superoxide anions
Antiaggregatory effects	Nitric oxide Prostacyclin Thromboresistant endothelium

Endothelium-Derived Relaxing Factors

The seminal observation that endothelium is a key mediator of vascular reactivity was made in 1980.[39] The ability of the artery to relax was attributed to the elusive substance, EDRF, which was later identified as NO.[40,41] Although NO is the major EDRF, other relaxing factors such as prostacyclin (prostaglandin I_2 [PGI_2]) EDHF are also produced (Fig. 3-7).

Nitric Oxide

NO is a gas with an extremely short half-life (seconds) that diffuses into vascular smooth muscle cells and causes vasodilation.[41–43] NO production is stimulated by the enzyme nitric oxide synthase (NOS). There are two constitutive forms of NOS: endothelial NOS (eNOS) and neurologic NOS (nNOS). Inducible NOS (iNOS), which is present only under pathologic conditions, generates 100- to 1000-fold more NO than the constitutive forms.

Shear stress and vasoactive substances are the primary factors involved in the release of NO for control of vasomotor tone (Fig. 3-8). The activation of eNOS is different for these two mechanisms. Shear stress through G proteins (Gs) leads to eNOS activation, which via the inositol triphosphate (IP_3) pathway causes

Table 3-2 • ENDOTHELIUM-DERIVED VASODILATING AND VASOCONSTRICTING FACTORS

Factors	Stimuli
Vasodilating Factors	
Nitric oxide Endothelium-derived relaxing factor Prostacyclin Endothelium-derived hyperpolarizing factor	Acetylcholine, histamine, arginine vasopressin, epinephrine, norepinephrine, bradykinin, adenosine diphosphate, serotonin (from aggregating platelets), thrombin (from coagulation cascade)
Vasoconstricting Factors	
Endothelium-derived contracting factor	Physical stimuli (mechanical stretch), arachidonic acid (endothelial injury and platelet aggregation), serotonin, adenosine platelet diphosphate
Endothelin-1	Thrombin, interleukin-1, epinephrine, angiotensin II, arginine vasopressin
Prostanoids	Endothelin-1, endothelial membrane damage
Superoxide anions	Physical stress (e.g., shear stress, postischemic reperfusion), chemical endothelial stimulants (bradykinin, cytokines)

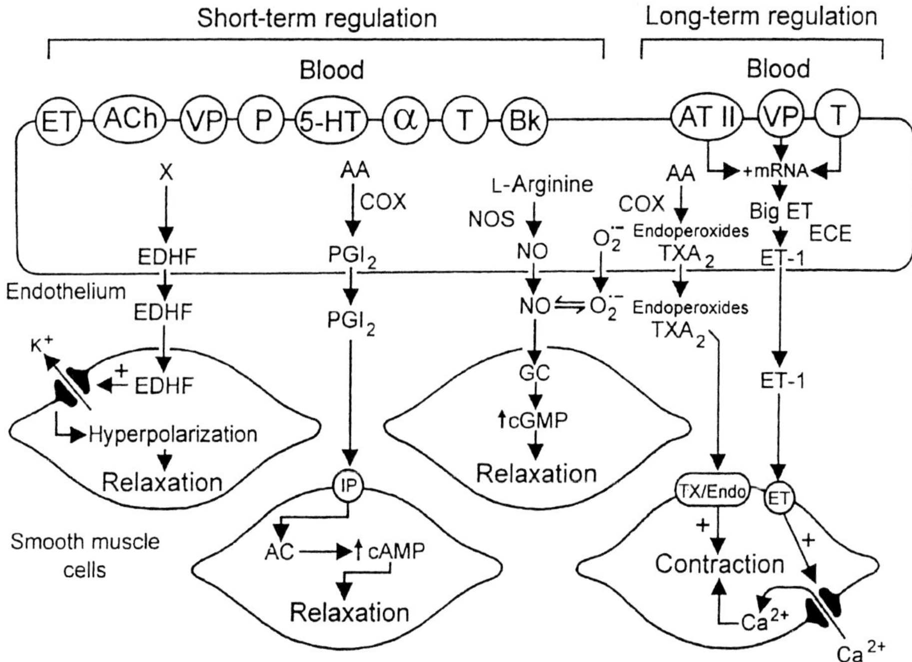

Figure 3-6. Activation of endothelial receptors can stimulate NO synthase (NOS, with the production of nitric oxide [NO]) and cyclooxygenase (COX), which produces prostacyclin (PGI_2) from arachidonic acid (AA) and can lead to the release of EDHF. NO causes relaxation by activating the formation of cyclic GMP (cGMP) from guanosine triphosphate (GTP) by soluble guanylate cyclase (GC). PGI_2 causes relaxation by activating adenylate cyclase (AC) leading to the formation of cyclic AMP (cAMP). EDHF causes hyperpolarization and relaxation by opening K^+ channels. Any increase in cytosolic calcium (including that induced by calcium ionophore A23187) causes the release of relaxing factors. In certain blood vessels, contracting substances can be released from the endothelial cells, which include superoxide anions (O_2^-), thromboxane A_2 (TXA_2), endoperoxides, and possibly ET_1. Thromboxane A_2 and endoperoxides activate specific receptors (TX/Endo) on the vascular smooth muscle, as does ET_1. Such activation causes an increase in intracellular Ca^{2+} leading to contraction. The production of ET_1 (catalyzed by endothelin-converting enzyme [ECE]) can be augmented by angiotensin II (ATII), vasopressin (VP), or thrombin (T). The neurohumoral mediators that cause the release of endothelium-derived relaxing factors (and sometimes contracting factors) through activation of specific endothelial receptors (*circles*) include acetylcholine (ACh), adenosine diphosphate (P), bradykinin (BK), endothelin (ET), adrenaline (α), serotonin (5-HT), T, and VP. (Reprinted with permission from Vanhoutte PM. How to assess endothelial function in human blood vessels. *J Hypertens.* 1999;17:1047–1058.)

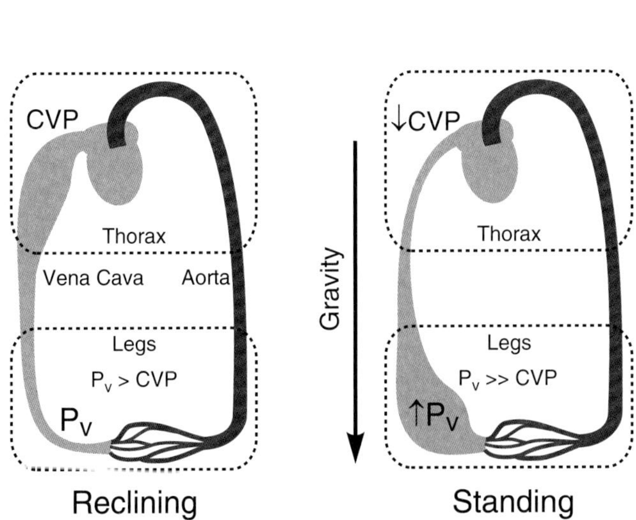

Figure 3-7. Effects of gravity on central venous pressure and venous pressure in the lower leg. (Reprinted with permission from Klabunde RE. *Cardiovascular Physiology Concepts.* 2nd ed. Philadelphia, PA: Wolters Kluwer/ Lippincott Williams & Wilkins; 2012:109.)

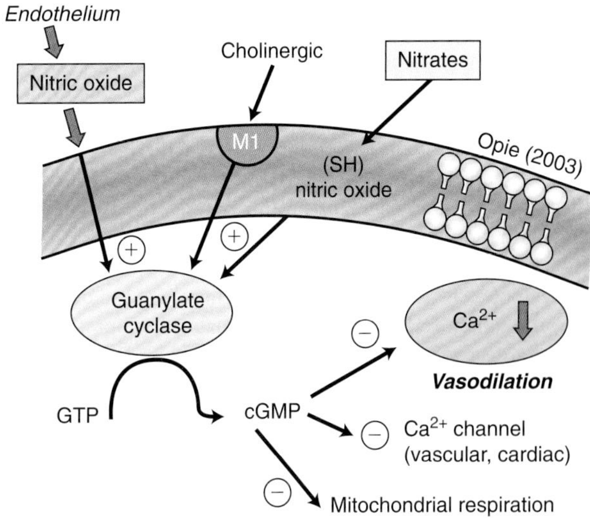

Figure 3-8. Nitric oxide messenger system. Proposed role in stimulating soluble guanylate cyclase and cyclic guanosine 3,5′-monophosphate to cause vasodilation and possibly a negative inotropic effect. Antianginal nitrates cause coronary vasodilation by this mechanism. M1, muscarinic receptor, subtype 1. (Reprinted with permission from Opie LH. *Heart Physiology: From Cell to Circulation.* Philadelphia, PA: Lippincott; 2004.)

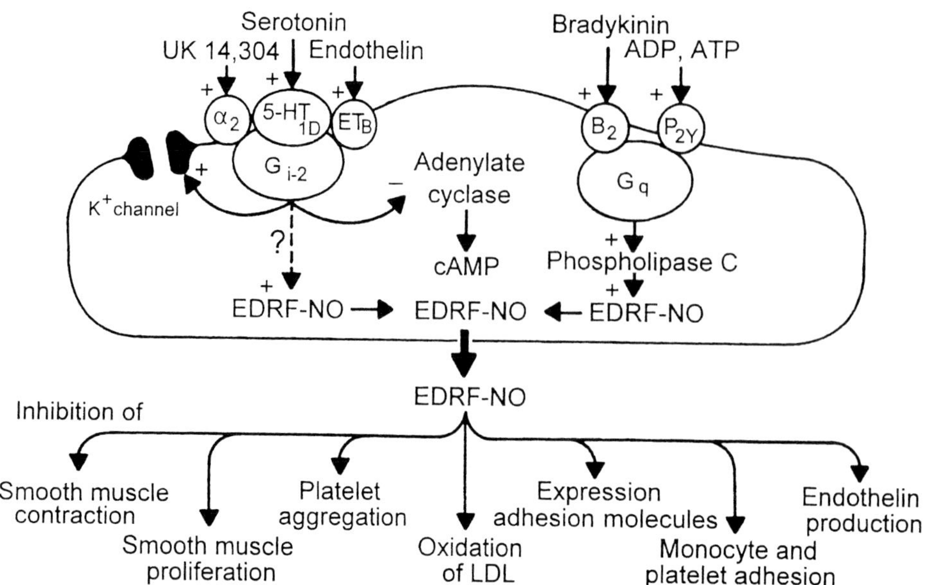

Figure 3-9. Postulated signal transduction processes in a normal endothelial cell. Activation of the cell causes the release of NO, which has important protective effects in the vascular wall. α, alpha-adrenergic; 5-HT, serotonin receptor; EDRF, endothelium-derived relaxing factor; ET, endothelin receptors; B, bradykinin receptor; P, purinoreceptor; G, coupling proteins; cAMP, cyclic adenosine monophosphate; NO, nitric oxide; LDL, low-density lipoproteins; +, activation; –, inhibition. (Reprinted with permission from Vanhoutte PM. Endothelial dysfunction and vascular disease. In: Panza JA, Cannon RO, eds. *Endothelium, Nitric Oxide and Atherosclerosis.* New York: Futura Publishing; 1999.)

hyperpolarization of the endothelial cells, which allows calcium to flow into the cell.[44,45] The increased intracellular calcium binds to calmodulin, which releases eNOS from the inhibitory protein calveolin. The eNOS catalyzes the conversion of L-arginine to NO. After NO is formed in the endothelial cells, it diffuses out of the endothelial cell to the vascular smooth muscle and as described below causes vasodilation. Nitric oxide also has secondary vasodilatory effects through the inhibition of the release of the vasoconstrictor endothelin-1 (ET_1), although this beneficial effect decreases with age.[46,47]

Autocoids and hormones cause the release of NO from the endothelium (Fig. 3-9).[48] These substances (Table 3-3) cause the release of IP_3, which leads to an increase in intracellular calcium and subsequently stimulates the release of NO. Additionally, NO decreases sympathetic vasoconstriction by inhibiting the release of norepinephrine at the supraspinal, spinal, and synaptic levels.[49] Clinically, nitrovasodilators (e.g., nitroglycerin and sodium nitroprusside) cause vasodilation by the donation of NO or NO-like compound.[50,51] Of note, nitroglycerin-induced coronary artery vasodilation does not require the presence of an intact endothelium. In addition, angiotensin-converting enzyme inhibitors (ACE-Is), calcium channel blockers, statins, and phosphodiesterase inhibitors indirectly stimulate NO release or enhance its bioavailability.[52]

Nitric oxide also inhibits platelet activation, aggregation, and adhesion (i.e., anticoagulant/profibrinolytic phenotype), leukocyte adhesion,[53] vascular smooth muscle proliferation, and it inhibits endothelial cell apoptosis but stimulates vascular smooth muscle apoptosis (Fig. 3-9).[38,54] With aging there is a decrease in NO production and increased endothelial cell apoptosis, which leads to a decrease in the protective effect of NO against platelet aggregation and vasoconstriction decreases. There is also diminished NO production with disease processes (e.g., hypertension, diabetes, postmyocardial infarction reperfusion injuries) and altered defense mechanisms.[45,55] The loss of the protective endothelium, decreased NO production, and increased NO degradation may foster increased platelet aggregation and vascular proliferation, which are keys to the development of atherosclerosis,[56] intimal hyperplasia that causes restenosis after a vascular intervention such as bypass surgery or angioplasty,[54] and the procoagulant state seen in septic shock.[38] The cytokine-induced increase in NO synthesis by iNOS may be responsible for the decreased vascular tone, vascular hyporeactivity, and hypotension observed in septic shock.[57] Nitric oxide also inhibits cytochrome c oxidase, which may be one factor associated with cytopathic hypoxia in sepsis.[58,59]

Prostacyclin

Prostacyclin (PGI_2) is a cyclooxygenase (COX)-dependent vasodilator prostaglandin, which is released transiently by stimulation

Table 3-3 • ABBREVIATIONS

V_T	Tidal Volume
V_E	Expired volume
V_D	Dead space volume
V_A	Alveolar volume
P_A	Alveolar pressure
P_a	Arterial pressure
P_v	Venous pressure
PA_{O2}	Alveolar partial pressure of oxygen
PA_{CO2}	Alveolar partial pressure of carbon dioxide
PA_{O2}	Arterial partial pressure of oxygen
Pa_{CO2}	Arterial partial pressure of carbon dioxide
$P\bar{v}O_2$	Mixed venous partial pressure of oxygen
P_{CO_2}	Partial pressure of carbon dioxide
PO_2	Partial pressure of oxygen
F_{IO2}	Fraction of inspired oxygen
P_{IO2}	Pressure of inspired oxygen
P_{50}	Partial pressure of oxygen at which Hgb is 50% saturated
Sa_{O2}	Arterial blood saturation
Ca_{O2}	Oxygen content of arterial blood
Cv_{O2}	Oxygen content of mixed venous blood
$C(a–v)_{O2}$	Difference between arterial and venous oxygen content
$S\bar{v}O_2$	Mixed venous oxygen saturation
O_2ER	Oxygen extraction ratio
Sp_{O2}	Pulse oximetry oxygen saturation
$\dot{V}/\dot{Q}$	Ventilation–perfusion ratio
$\dot{V}O_2$	Oxygen consumption
$\dot{D}O_2$	Oxygen delivery
$\dot{Q}O_2$	Oxygen transport
WOB	Work of breathing
Hgb	Hemoglobin

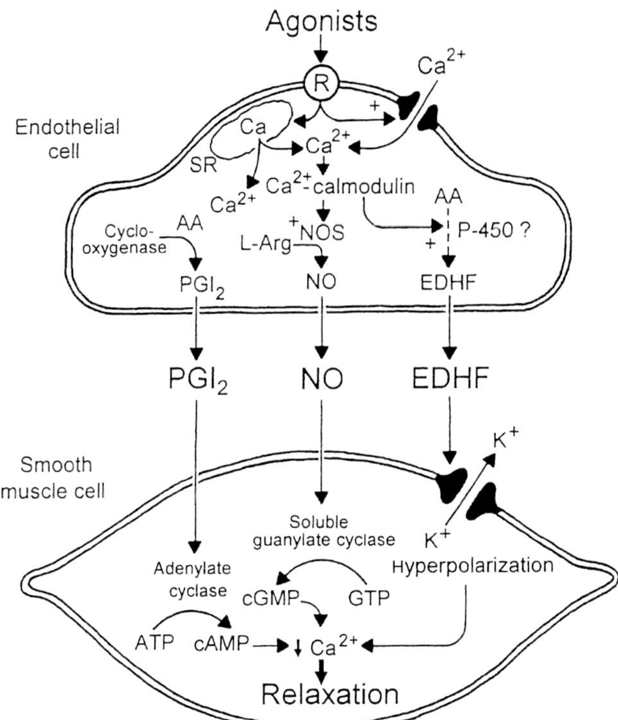

Figure 3-10. Schematic summarizing the release of relaxing factors from endothelial cells and their effect on vascular smooth muscle cells. (Reprinted with permission from Mombouli JV. Vanhoutte PM. Endothelial dysfunction: from physiology to therapy. *J Mol Cell Cardiol.* 1999;31:61–74.)

of endothelial-specific receptors. Prostacyclin receptor stimulation causes an increase in intracellular calcium, which activates phospholipase A_2 and subsequently releases arachidonic acid. Under basal conditions the arachidonic acid is then metabolized by COX-1, which results in the production of prostaglandin H2 (PGH_2) and subsequently PGI_2.[60] Prostacyclin binds to receptors on vascular smooth muscle and platelets and through G-protein–mediated activation of adenylate cyclase increases cyclic adenosine monophosphate (cAMP) (Fig. 3-10). Increased cAMP stimulates potassium-induced cellular hyperpolarization and the phosphorylation of protein kinase A (PKA), which increases calcium extrusion from the cell and causes vasodilation and also inhibits platelet activation.[61] Prostacyclin also act through peroxisome proliferator-activated receptor (PPAR)β/Δ, which causes a decrease in intracellular calcium and subsequent vasodilation and platelet inhibition through mechanisms that are still being studied. There is cross talk between PGI_2 and NO and they have synergistic vasodilatory and antithrombotic actions. Prostacyclin increases NO release and, concomitantly, NO prolongs the effect of prostacyclin by inhibiting its breakdown.[60,61]

Endothelium-Derived Hyperpolarizing Factors

Vasodilation of arterioles is also mediated by non NO/nonprostanoid EDHFs.[62,63] EDHF may be the predominant mechanism for vasodilation in smaller diameter vessels (i.e., resistance arteries less than 300 μm) in contrast to larger vessels where NO is the dominant vasodilator.[64] There are four putative EDHFs: the enzyme cytochrome p450 monooxygenase (cytochrome P-450), potassium, hydrogen peroxide, and C-type natriuretic peptide.[63] EDHFs, which may be considered a mechanism as much as a factor,[64] are synthesized in response to wall shear stress or the binding of bradykinin and acetylcholine or substance P to endothelial cell receptors. EDHF diffuses from the endothelium to the vascular smooth muscle where it causes endothelium-dependent hyperpolarization, which in turn decreases cytosolic calcium and causes vasorelaxation through the various mediator-specific pathways (Fig. 3-11).[62]

In hypertension or hypercholesterolemia, when NO-mediated vasodilation is decreased, there may be a compensatory upregulation of EDHF-mediated vasorelaxation.[65] Of note, there may be gender-specific EDHF compensatory response, with increased

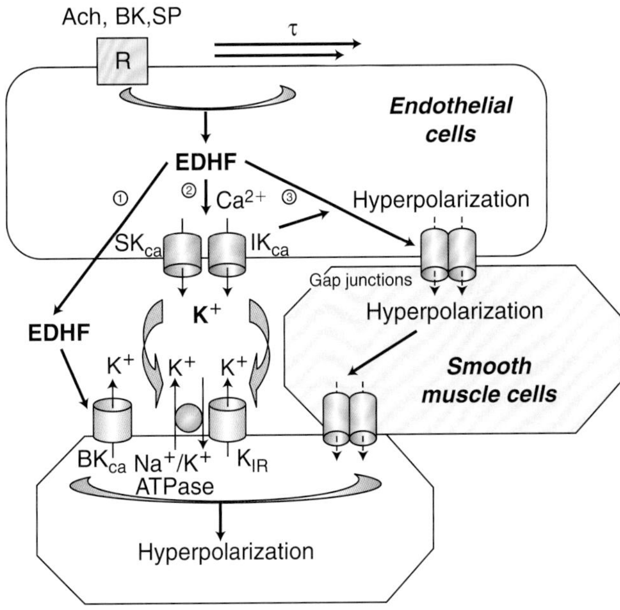

Figure 3-11. Schematic description of the main hyperpolarizing mechanisms mediated by endothelium-derived hyperpolarizing factor (EDHF). The binding of acetylcholine (Ach), bradykinin (BK), and substance P (SP) to their endothelial receptors and the increase in wall shear stress (τ) promote the synthesis of EDHF. EDHF can then hyperpolarize the smooth muscle cells by three principal pathways. EDHF can passively diffuse from the endothelium to activate calcium-activated potassium (K_{Ca}) channels of large conductance (BK_{Ca}) located on the smooth muscle cells thereby promoting the release of K^+ and membrane hyperpolarization. EDHF can act in an autocrine manner to facilitate the activation of the endothelial K_{Ca} channels of small (SK_{Ca}) and intermediate (IK_{Ca}) conductance directly mediated by Ca^{2+} inducing the release of K^+ and the hyperpolarization of the endothelial cells. Then, the hyperpolarization is transmitted electronically through the myoendothelial gap junctions into the smooth muscle cell layer and/or the K^+ released from the endothelial SK_{Ca} and IK_{Ca} channels into the myoendothelial space activates the Na^+/K^+ ATPase and the inward rectifying potassium channels (K_{IR}) located on the smooth muscle cells promoting the release of K^+ and subsequent hyperpolarization of these cells. EDHF can enhance gap junctional communication. Finally, the smooth muscle cells hyperpolarization decreases the open-state of voltage-gate Ca^{2+} channels lowering cytosolic Ca^{2+} and thereby provoking vasorelaxation. (Reprinted with permission from Bellien J, Thuillez C, Joannides R. Contribution of endothelium-derived hyperpolarizing factors to the regulation of vascular tone in humans. *Fundam Clin Pharmacol.* 2008;22[4]:363–377.)

EDHF activity in females but not in males.[63] However, oxidative stress associated with atherosclerosis, hyperhomocysteinemia, and possibly poorly controlled diabetes can decrease this compensatory response.[65–67]

Endothelium-Derived Contracting Factors

The endothelium-derived contracting factors include ET_1, the vasoconstrictor prostanoids, PGH_2, the precursor of thromboxane A_2 (TXA_2); superoxide anions (O_2^-); and components of the renin–angiotensin–aldosterone system. These substances are released in response to vasoconstrictive stimuli (Fig. 3-6). Vasoconstriction also occurs as a result of a decrease in endothelial production of NO.

Endothelin-1

In humans there are three isoforms of endothelin.[68] ET_1, which is the primary isoform in the cardiovascular system, is thought to be the most potent vasoconstrictor known. ET_1 is an amino acid peptide that binds to vascular smooth muscle membrane receptors ET_A (located on vascular smooth muscle) and ET_B (located on vascular smooth muscle and endothelial surfaces). Binding of ET_1 to the ET_A and ET_B receptors on the vascular smooth muscle activates the phospholipase C (PLC)-IP_3 pathway, which increases intracellular calcium and the phosphorylation of myosin kinase and causes prolonged muscle contraction. In contrast, under normal resting conditions, the circulating plasma level of ET_1 is very low and it acts locally, in a paracrine fashion, to cause vasodilation through the endothelial synthesis of NO and PGI_2.[69,70] The production of ET_1 can be augmented by shear stress, angiotensin II (AII), vasopressin, oxygen free radicals, thrombin, and platelet-derived transforming growth factor and inhibited by NO, atrial natriuretic polypeptide, B-type natriuretic peptide, and prostacyclin[71] (Fig. 3-12).

The effects of ET_1 are important clinically. In pathologic conditions such as heart failure, increased ET_1 levels are associated with increased morbidity and mortality[72] and may play an important role in the disease pathogenesis.[65] For example, ET_1 stimulates the renin–angiotensin–aldosterone system, which enhances the conversion of angiotensin I to AII, causing a synergistic augmentation of vasoconstriction and sodium retention.[71] In addition, in heart failure, ET_1 has a negative inotropic effect.[69] ET_1 may play a role in salt-sensitive hypertension although the mechanism remains unclear.[69,73] Unfortunately antagonism of ET_1 receptors has not been found to improve outcomes for patients with heart failure or hypertension.[74–76] ET_1 levels are

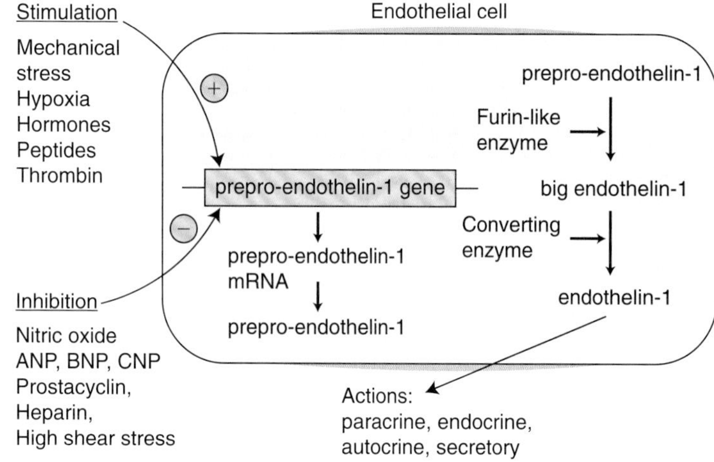

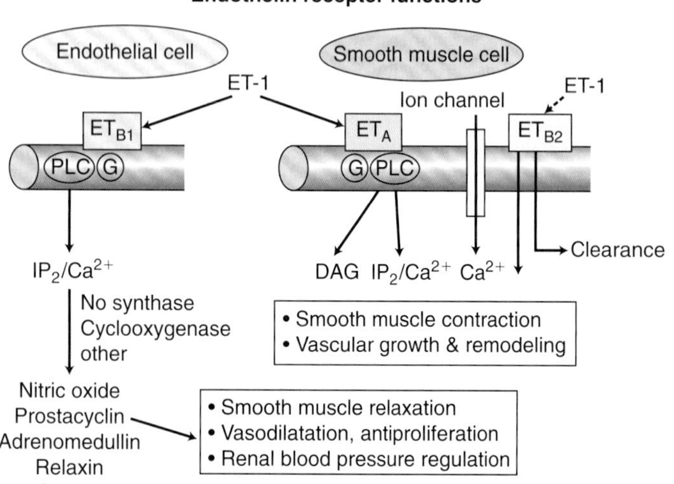

Figure 3-12. **A:** Synthesis of endothelin receptors (ET) and its regulation. The release of active ET_1 is controlled via regulation of gene transcription and/or endothelin-converting enzyme activity. ET_1 synthesis is stimulated by several factors, of which hypoxia seems to be the most important. ET_1 formation is downregulated by activators of the NO/cGMP pathway and other factors. **B:** Vascular actions of ET. In healthy blood vessels, the main action of ET_1 is indirect vasodilation mediated by ET_B receptors located on endothelial cells. Their activation generates a Ca^{2+} signal via PLC that turns on the generation of nitric oxide (NO), prostacyclin, adrenomedullin, and other mediators that are powerful relaxants of smooth muscle. On the other hand, binding of ET_1 to ET_A receptors located on smooth muscle cells will lead to vascular contraction (physiologic effect) and/or wall thickening, inflammation, and tissue remodeling (pathologic effects). These latter effects may be mediated by vascular ET_{B2} receptors in certain disease states. Smooth muscle cell signaling involves DAG formation, PKC activation, and extracellular calcium recruited via different cation channels. (Reprinted with permission from Brunner F, Bras-Silva C, Cerdeira AS, et al. Cardiovascular endothelins: essential regulators of cardiovascular homeostasis. *Pharmacol Ther.* 2006;111[2]:508–531.)

increased with hypercholesterolemia and increased ET_1 levels may be a marker for endothelial dysfunction. Possible pathologic mechanisms for ET_1 in atherosclerosis and restenosis after angioplasty include increased fibrous tissue formation, inhibition of eNOS formation, stimulation of platelet aggregation, vascular smooth muscle proliferation, and inflammation of the vessel wall.[70,77,78] There is also a link between ET_1 and idiopathic pulmonary arterial hypertension and inhibition of ET_1 has been shown to improve outcomes for these patients.[79,80]

Prostanoids

Two prostanoids that have vasoconstrictive actions are PGH_2 and TXA_2. Similar to prostacyclin, arachidonic acid is converted by COX-1 to PGH_2. PGH_2 is then converted to TXA_2 by thromboxane synthase or as discussed above, to prostacyclin.[81] TXA_2, which acts in a paracrine fashion, causes platelet activation, vasoconstriction, and smooth muscle proliferation, and it is thought to play an important role in the pathogenesis of myocardial infarction. The rationale for the administration of COX-1 antagonists (e.g., nonsteroidal anti-inflammatory drugs [NSAIDs], aspirin) in cardiovascular disease is to inhibit platelet production of TXA_2, which reduces cardiovascular morbidity and mortality[82,83]; however, in patients where there is incomplete TXA_2 inhibition, there is still a risk for cardiovascular events.[84] A negative side effect of the COX-1 antagonists is that they are toxic to the gastric mucosa.

Because of the negative side effects of COX-1 antagonists, the use of selective PGH2 or COX-2 inhibitors (coxibs), which are not toxic to the gastrointestinal tract, were evaluated. However, several studies of coxibs found an increased incidence of adverse serious cardiovascular events, including myocardial infarction and stroke.[85,86] This increased risk resulted in the Food and Drug Administration requiring labeling of all selective and nonselective NSAIDs to reflect the possibility of an increased risk for myocardial infarction and stroke with their use.[87] It is important to note that the increased risk varies depending on the medication[88–90] and a prospective clinical trial is ongoing to determine the cardiovascular risk of selective and nonselective NSAIDs. The probable mechanism of these adverse effects is that while COX-2 inhibitors do not inhibit thromboxane they do inhibit vascular prostacyclin causing increased systolic blood pressure and platelet activation, which increases the likelihood of thrombus formation.[91–93]

Reactive Oxygen Species

In response to physical stresses, such as oscillatory shear stress, postischemic reperfusion, and chemical endothelial stimulants (bradykinin, cytokines, AII), the endothelium and vascular smooth muscle produce reactive oxygen species (ROS), which are metabolites of oxygen. Example of ROS include superoxide (O_2^-), hydrogen peroxide, and peroxynitrite ($ONOO^-$), which is the product of NO and O_2^-.[94] These ROS inhibit NO, EDHF, and prostacyclin pathways and guanylyl cyclase (Fig. 3-13), increase calcium mobilization and the production of the vasoconstrictors PGH_2 and TXA_2, decrease NO-mediated vasorelaxation, and play a role in endothelial dysfunction.[65,94] Pathologic effects of ROS that contribute to the development of atherosclerosis include stimulation of vascular smooth muscle proliferation and migration, endothelial apoptosis, altered vasomotor reactivity, oxidation of low-density lipoprotein, which causes cholesterol accumulation in macrophages, the upregulation of adhesion molecules and the creation of a proinflammatory state.[95,96] In contrast antioxidant

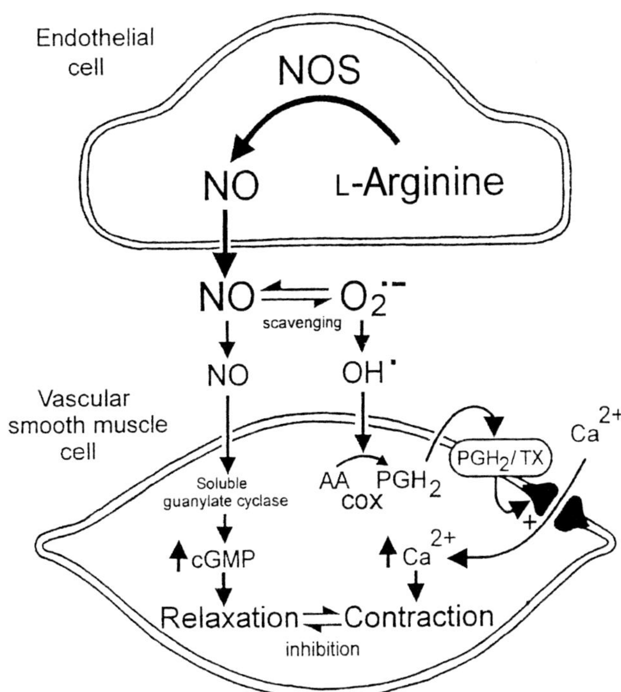

Figure 3-13. Interactions between nitric oxide (NO) and superoxide anions (O_2^-). Superoxide anions cause contraction of vascular smooth muscle by scavenging endothelium-derived NO and by activating the production of vasoconstrictor prostaglandins in the vascular smooth muscle cells, presumably after transformation of hydroxyl radicals (OH^-). AA, arachidonic acid; COX, cyclooxygenase; cGMP, cyclic guanosine monophosphate; NOS, nitric oxide synthase; PGH_2, endoperoxides; TX, thromboxane. (Reprinted with permission from Vanhoutte PM. Endothelial dysfunction and vascular disease. In: Panza JA, Cannon RO, eds. *Endothelium, Nitric Oxide and Atherosclerosis.* New York: Futura Publishing; 1999.)

systems, such superoxide dismutase (SOD) and glutathione peroxidase, scavenge, and inactivate ROS. SOD is an enzyme that breaks down the free radicals into nontoxic substances and inhibits the breakdown of NO by superoxide anions, inhibits pathologic ET_1 production, and augments endothelial relaxation.[96] Clinically, ACE-Is, which prevent angiotensin II from inducing oxidative stress, may improve NO availability,[97,98] and statins, which inhibit ROS formation have been found to improve cardiovascular outcomes.[99] However, studies and meta-analyses failed to find any beneficial effects from supplemental antioxidants (vitamin C and vitamin E) in the reduction of cardiovascular mortality or death.[100–102]

Local Metabolic Control of Blood Flow

Local metabolic factors that control arteriolar resistance play a role in matching blood flow (oxygen transport) to metabolism. These factors may accumulate in low-flow conditions and cause vasodilation by inhibition of basal tone. The increased flow that occurs as a result of the vasodilation is referred to as *reactive hyperemia.* Metabolic factors that have been shown to interact and contribute to reactive hyperemia include adenosine and ATP, NO, prostaglandins, and potassium.[103–105] An increase in flow-dependent shear stress on the endothelium has also been shown to cause vasodilation in skeletal muscle and venules. This vasodilation is mediated in part by the release of NO and prostaglandin.[106]

DISPLAY 3-5

Neurohormonal Stimulation

Sympathetic stimulation results in catecholamine release, primarily epinephrine. Epinephrine results in cardiac stimulation via β_1-adrenoceptors. Based upon plasma concentration, epinephrine also decreases or increases systemic vascular resistance via β_2 vascular receptors or β_1- and β_2 adrenoceptors.

Vasopressin, synthesized in the thalamus and released by the posterior pituitary, increases blood volume and venous pressure. This in turn affects preload and cardiac output through the Frank-Starling relationship. Increased blood volume increases cardiac output and arterial pressure.

NEUROHUMORAL STIMULATION

In addition to stimulation by endothelium-derived vasodilating and vasoconstricting factors, neurohumoral factors bind with receptors on vascular smooth muscle. The effects of this stimulation vary throughout the vascular system (Display 3-5).

Adrenergic Stimulation

α-Adrenergic Stimulation

The α-adrenergic receptors, which are a series of G_q-protein–coupled receptors that bind epinephrine and norepinephrine, are generally categorized as α_1 and α_2 receptors.[107] Molecular cloning techniques have led to a further division of the α-receptor subtypes. The α_1-adrenergic receptors, which are now characterized as subtypes α_{1A}, α_{1B}, and α_{1D}, are located in arteries, arterioles, and cutaneous and visceral veins. The α_{1A} receptors are responsible for vessel contraction. The α_{1B} receptors are thought to contribute to the maintenance of basal vascular tone and arterial blood pressure in conscious animals and are sensitive to exogenous agonists. Finally, the α_{1D} receptors also play a role in vascular contraction, although they have a lesser effect than the α_{1B} receptors.[108]

The α_2 receptors, which have presynaptic and postsynaptic functions, are characterized as $\alpha_{2A/D}$, α_{2B}, and α_{2C}. The $\alpha_{2A/D}$ and α_{2B} receptors are present in large arteries but are located with greater density on the terminal arterioles, which act as precapillary sphincters to control the number of open capillaries and total capillary blood flow. The $\alpha_{2A/D}$ receptors play the primary role in vasoconstriction.[109,110] The α_{2B} receptors also play a role in vasoconstriction and may contribute to the onset of hypertension. The α_{2C} receptors are responsible for venoconstriction.[108,111]

Whereas stimulation of the presynaptic α_2 receptors inhibits norepinephrine, stimulation of the postsynaptic α_2 receptors located on the vascular smooth muscle causes norepinephrine release and subsequent vasoconstriction. However, the α_2-mediated vasoconstriction is attenuated by the α_2 presynaptic inhibition of norepinephrine release. In addition, in contrast to α_1 receptor stimulation, the effect of norepinephrine on α_2 in terminal arterioles is inhibited by metabolites, thus fostering metabolic vasodilation even when vasoconstrictor tone to blood vessels in the skeletal muscle is high.

β-Adrenergic Stimulation

In the heart, β_1 receptors predominate (80%), although there are also a smaller number of β_2 receptors (20%), with the β_2 receptors playing a role in coronary vasodilation.[112] Of note, the β_2 vasodilation is impaired in severely atherosclerotic coronary vessels.[113] There is also a small number (less than 1%) of β_3-adrenergic receptors in cardiomyocytes.[114] The β_3 receptors, which mediate negative inotropy via an NO-dependent pathway,[115] become important during heart failure when they are upregulated and while protective may contribute to functional degradation of the failing heart.[114,116]

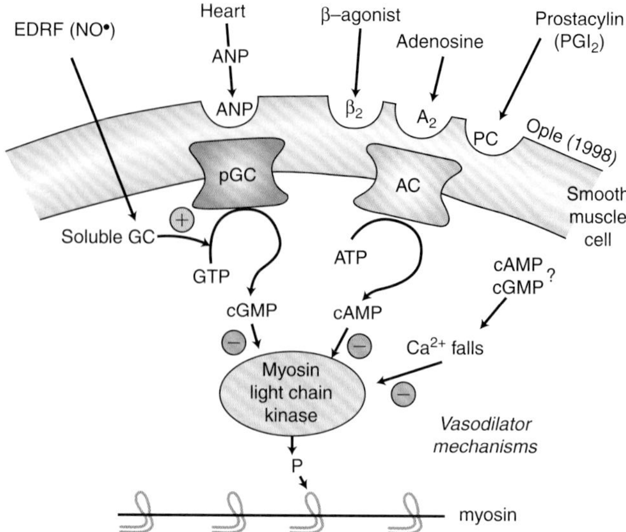

Figure 3-14. Vasodilatory mechanisms. Most act by formation of cyclic nucleotides, cyclic guanosine monophosphate (cGMP), and cyclic adenosine monophosphate (cAMP), both of which are vasodilatory, possibly through inhibition of myosin light-chain kinase. GMP is the messenger for guanylate cyclase (GC), which in turn is stimulated by atrial natriuretic polypeptide (ANP) or by EDRF (i.e., nitric oxide). Vasodilatory cAMP is formed by stimulation of adenylate cyclase (AC) in response to β_2-stimulation or by adenosine (A) stimulation through A_2-receptors, or by prostacyclin (PO; PGI_2) receptor. ATP, adenosine triphosphate; pGC, prostacyclin C (G kinase). (Reprinted with permission from Opie LH. *The Heart: Physiology From Cell to Circulation.* 3rd ed. Philadelphia, PA: Lippincott-Raven; 1998:240.)

In vascular smooth muscle, the β-adrenergic receptors are predominantly of the β_2-subtype. Stimulation of these receptors causes vasorelaxation[117] via activation of Gs protein, which binds to adenylate cyclase and catalyzes the conversion of ATP to cAMP. cAMP in turn activates PKA, which then phosphorylates myosin light-chain kinase (MLCK) (Fig. 3-14). Phosphorylation decreases MLCK's affinity for calmodulin, which decreases the promotion of the myosin kinase–calmodulin–calcium complex. Failure to form the calmodulin–calcium complex inhibits cross-bridge formation with subsequent vascular relaxation.[118] β_2-Adrenergic stimulation also decreases intracellular calcium by hyperpolarization of the vascular smooth muscle, which decreases the influx of calcium into the cell, increases cAMP-mediated extrusion of calcium from the cell, and promotes calcium uptake by the sarcoplasmic reticulum.[119] There is also a β_2-mediated release of NO, which is thought to involve the cAMP/PKA pathway.[118] The β_3 receptors in the vascular smooth muscle may mediate vasodilation, with the effects vary depending on the vascular bed.[115,120]

Vasopressin

Vasopressin, which is synthesized in the hypothalamus, is released in response to increased plasma osmolality and decreased blood pressure and cardiac output and exogenous vasopressin is used to

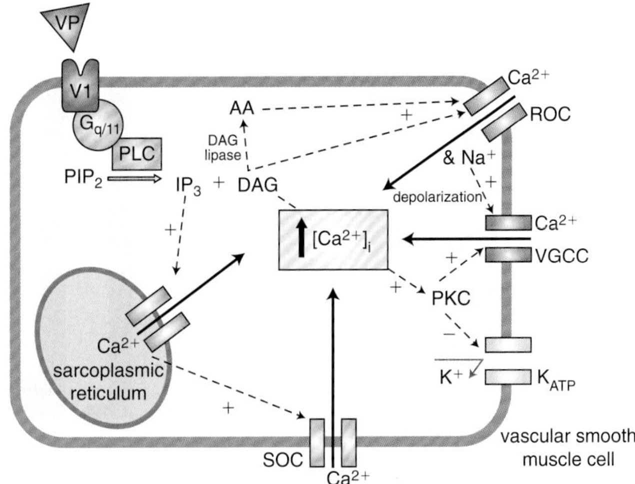

Figure 3-15. A schematic showing the pathways of intracellular calcium (Ca^{2+}) elevation following the binding of vasopressin (VP) to the V1 receptor (*V1R*) on a vascular smooth muscle cell. The weighting of the *black solid arrows* demonstrates the relative importance of the different pathways. V1Rs are coupled through Gq/11 to phospholipase C (PLC), which hydrolyzes phosphatidyl inositol bisphosphonate (PIP2) to produce inositol triphosphate (IP_3) and diacylglycerol (DAG). The latter, in turn, stimulates the activity of protein kinase C (PKC). A transient increase in intracellular Ca^{2+} is produced by the action of IP_3 on the sarcoplasmic reticulum, whereas a sustained increase is triggered by influx of extracellular Ca^{2+}. Store-operated channels (*SOCs*), activated by intracellular store depletion, appear to play a minor role in comparison to voltage-gated calcium channels (VGCCs) and receptor-operated channels (ROCs). VGCCs are opened by cell membrane depolarization, secondary to cation influx via ROCs and the PKC-mediated closure of adenosine triphosphate-sensitive potassium (KATP) channels. PKC can also open VGCCs directly. The opening of ROCs is G protein-dependent via PLC, with a downstream mechanism involving DAG and arachidonic acid (AA). They have significant permeability to Ca^{2+}, which is likely to contribute directly to contraction. (From Barrett LK, Singer M, Clapp LH. Vasopressin: mechanisms of action on the vasculature in health and in septic shock. *Crit Care Med.* 2007;35[1]:33–40.)

treat refractory hypotension.[121] There are three types of vasopressin receptors, with V1 receptors located on vascular smooth muscle. V1 receptor stimulation causes the activation of PLC, which catalyzes the conversion of IP_3, and subsequently causes calcium release from the sarcoplasmic reticulum.[122] The increased intracellular calcium causes vasoconstriction (Fig. 3-15). If the sympathetic and renin–angiotensin systems are in intact, vasopressin has minimal effect on vascular control. However, if these systems are impaired, vasopressin plays a larger role in acute blood pressure control. Exogenous vasopressin may be beneficial in refractory vasodilatory shock when there is a relative vasopressin deficiency (e.g., septic shock, intraoperative hypotension).[123] During cardiopulmonary resuscitation, vasopressin increases coronary and cerebral blood flow, and is part of the protocol for resuscitation of ventricular fibrillation.[124–126]

Intracellular Signals for Vasodilation and Vasoconstriction

The two major messengers for vasodilation are the intracellular nucleotides cAMP and cyclic guanosine monophosphate (cGMP). The primary messenger for vasoconstriction is IP_3.

Cyclic Guanosine Monophosphate

Nitric oxide, atrial natriuretic peptides, and nitrovasodilators (e.g., nitroglycerin and nitroprusside) activate membrane bound or soluble guanylate cyclase, which generates cGMP from guanosine triphosphate. The cGMP then activates phosphokinase G, which is thought to decrease intracellular calcium and subsequently cause vasorelaxation by (1) increasing the uptake or extrusion of calcium by the cytoplasm, (2) inhibiting calcium release from the sarcoplasmic reticulum, (3) regulating the levels of IP_3, (4) inhibiting calcium-activated potassium channels, and (5) decreasing contractile protein sensitivity to calcium.[127–129] Phosphokinase G also directly inhibits MLCK, thus inhibiting contraction. Additionally, cGMP hyperpolarizes the cell, which further decreases intracellular calcium.[43] Nitric oxide also, independent of cGMP, increases the uptake of cytosolic calcium into the sarcoplasmic reticulum.[129]

Inositol Triphosphate

In response to vasoconstrictor stimuli (e.g., norepinephrine, AII, and endothelin), the enzyme PLC located in the cell wall splits phosphatidyl inositol into IP_3 and diacylglycerol (Fig. 3-16). IP_3 is the primary messenger for vasoconstriction and acts on a special calcium-receptor channel on the sarcoplasmic reticulum to release calcium, which as described below leads to contraction. Conversely, cGMP inhibits the accumulation of IP_3, which leads to a decrease in cytosolic calcium levels and vasorelaxation.[130]

CALCIUM

The major endpoint of extrinsic neurohormonal factors and local regulation of vascular tone involves a cascade of messengers that influence calcium movement in and out of the cell or sarcoplasmic reticulum, thus influencing the contractile process.[131] Knowledge of the role of calcium is important because the modulation

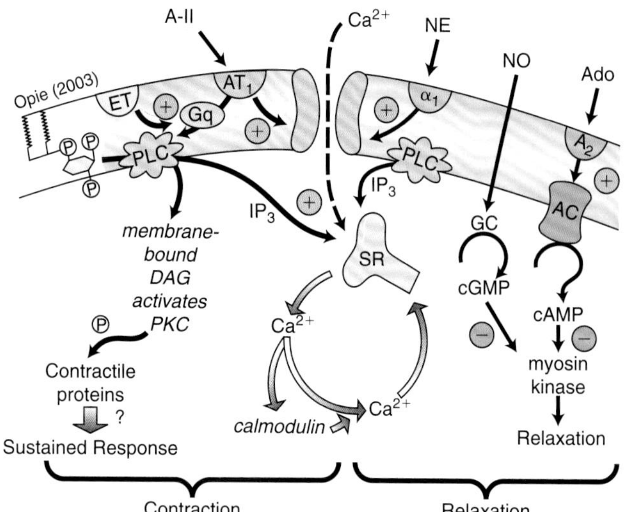

Figure 3-16. Protein kinase C (PKC)-linked receptors in vascular smooth muscle. For example, the α1-agonist signaling system is coupled via a G protein to phospholipase C (PLC), which breaks down phosphatidylinositol 4,5-biphosphate (PIP2) to 1,2-diacylglycerol (DAG) and inositol 1,4,5-triphosphate (IP_3). DAG is thought to translocate protein kinase C from cytosol to the sarcolemma, thereby activating protein kinase C. Signals beyond protein kinase C are not clear. IP_3 releases calcium from the sarcoplasmic reticulum to initiate contraction in vascular smooth muscle. Other vasoconstrictors such as angiotensin II and endothelin act by the same signal system. (From Opie LH. *The Heart: Physiology From Cell to Circulation.* 3rd ed. Philadelphia, PA: Lippincott-Raven; 1998:240.)

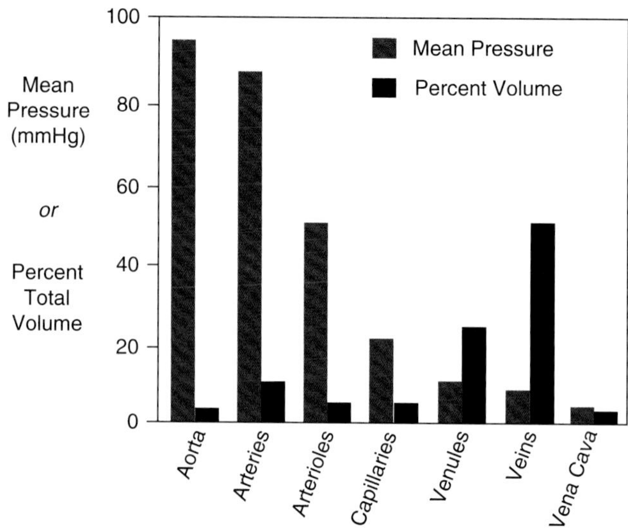

Figure 3-17. Distribution of pressure and volumes in the systemic circulation. (From Klabunde RE. *Cardiovascular Physiology Concepts.* 2nd ed. Philadelphia, PA: Wolters Kluwer Health; 2012:96.)

of calcium flux is the focus of pharmacologic control of vascular resistance.

As with cardiac and skeletal muscle, the changes in intracellular calcium are responsible for vascular smooth muscle contraction and relaxation. However, unlike skeletal and cardiac muscle in which calcium reverses the inhibitory effect of troponin on the actin–myosin interaction, vascular smooth muscle cross-bridge formation and muscle contraction result from the indirect activation of myosin by calcium.[36,132]

Sources of Calcium

The increased intracellular calcium comes from an influx of ***calcium across the sarcolemma and from the sarcoplasmic reticulum.***[132] The calcium influx across the sarcolemma is through voltage-gated ion channels, which are altered by the activation of the IP_3-regulated channels or ryanodine receptors. These receptors display calcium-induced calcium release.[133,134]

Calcium Signaling

The increased intracellular calcium binds with calmodulin, a small protein found in the cytosol of vascular smooth muscle. The calcium–calmodulin complex activates the enzyme MLCK, which in turn phosphorylates the light protein chains of the myosin head. The phosphorylation activates the myosin (increases the ATPase activity) such that the myosin can interact with actin. The process of phosphorylation is considered the primary mechanism of smooth muscle contraction. Conversely, a decrease in the cytoplasmic calcium concentration inactivates the MLCK and permits dephosphorylation of myosin by the enzyme myosin light-chain phosphatase. The dephosphorylation facilitates the detachment of myosin from actin, resulting in relaxation.[132]

The cytoplasmic calcium concentration is decreased through uptake of calcium into the sarcoplasmic reticulum and transport out of the cell across the plasma membrane by Ca^{2+}-ATPase exchanger or a probable Na^+/Ca^{2+} exchanger.[35] Additionally, calcium is decreased by closure of the membrane calcium channels through hyperpolarization[134] or pharmacologically with calcium channel blockers.

VOLUME AND FLOW DISTRIBUTION

Resistance

The pressure decrease from the aorta to the small arteries is relatively small, approximately 25 mm Hg (Fig. 3-17).[135] As much as 50% of the peripheral resistance appears to occur proximal to vessels with diameters of 100 mm. This finding indicates the primary sites for peripheral vascular resistance are the small arteries and the arterioles, although the exact location of the resistance vessels remains equivocal (Display 3-6).[136]

Alterations in the diameter of the terminal arterioles or precapillary blood vessels control capillary and venous pressures,

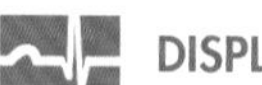

DISPLAY 3-6

Arterial Pressure and Flow

The aorta has the highest mean blood pressure, as blood flows further away from the heart the pressure exerted progressively decreases. A drop in pressure (βP) is related to the flow (F) and the resistance to flow (Q). βP = F • R

Arterial pressure regulation is primarily via the arteries and arterioles, the small resistance vessels.

Mean arterial pressure = (CO • SVR) + CVP

Vascular resistance is directly related to vessel length and blood viscosity, and inversely related to the radius of the vessel to the fourth power. The radius is the most important factor for regulating resistance.

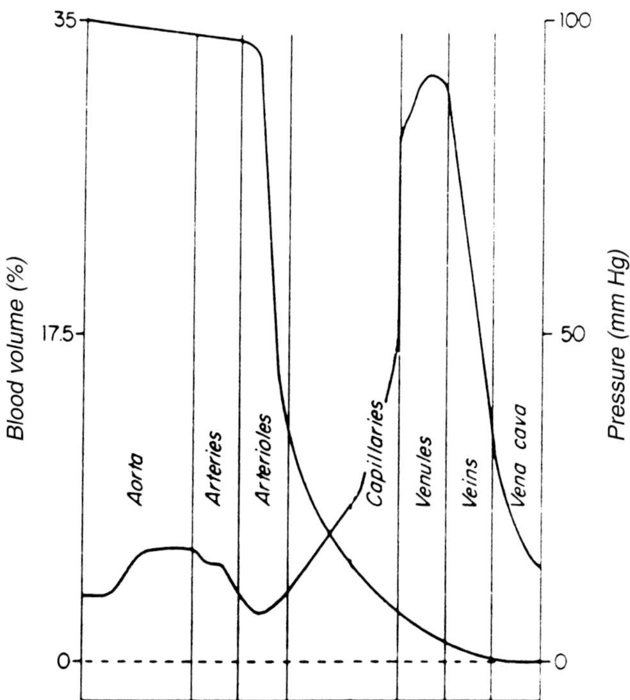

Figure 3-18. Changes in estimated blood volume (%) and blood pressure (mm Hg) in consecutive segments of the systemic blood vessels. Note that the volume is predominantly in the venules. The pressure is high in the aorta and arteries, falls rapidly in the arterioles, and then falls more slowly from the capillaries to the vena cava. (Reprinted with permission from Scher AM. The veins and venous return. In: Patton HD, Fuchs A, Hille B, et al., eds. *Textbook of Physiology.* Vol 2. 21st ed. Philadelphia, PA: WB Saunders; 1989:880.)

microvascular blood flow and exchange, and postcapillary venous volume.[137,138] Although the radius of the capillaries is considerably smaller than the radius of the arterioles, the resistance is lower because of the increase in cross-sectional area.

Volume Distribution

At rest, the systemic veins contain as much as 60% to 80% of the total blood volume, with 25% to 50% of this volume in the small veins (less than 1 mm in diameter). One-fourth of the total blood volume is in the capacious splanchnic circulation. Although the cross-sectional area is largest at the end of the capillaries, the largest volume of blood, as demonstrated in Figure 3-18, is in the venules because of the combination of cross-sectional area and the length of the venules.[139] The remainder of the blood is distributed in the aorta and systemic arteries (10%), the capillaries (5%), and the pulmonary bed and heart (15% to 25%).[2]

BLOOD FLOW

Definition of Flow

Blood flow ($\dot{Q}$) is expressed in terms of volume of blood per unit of time (volume/time). For example, the cardiac output, which is defined as the liters of blood pumped out of the left ventricle into the systemic circulation each minute, is usually expressed as liters per minute.

Determinants of Flow

Nonturbulent flow ($\dot{Q}$) in a segment of an isogravitational blood vessel (i.e., a blood vessel on the same horizontal level) is determined by the pressure difference (ΔP) between the inflow and outflow ends of that segment divided by the resistance (R) to flow provided by that segment. The relationship that demonstrates that flow will change as the result of a change in pressure or the change in resistance across a vascular bed is expressed in the following equation:

$$\dot{Q} = \frac{\Delta P}{R}$$

Substituting physiologic values into this equation gives:

$$\text{CO} = \frac{\text{MAP} - \text{RAP}}{\text{SVR}}$$

where MAP − RAP is the difference between the mean arterial pressure (MAP; as an indicator of aortic or upstream pressure) and right atrial pressure (RAP; downstream pressure) divided by the SVR.

Pressure

Blood pressure is the force exerted by the blood in a blood vessel. Clinically, pressure is expressed as millimeters of mercury, torr, or centimeters of H_2O. The relationship between these various measures is:

$$1 \text{ mm Hg} = 1 \text{ torr} = 1.36 \text{ cm } H_2O$$

Pressure in blood vessels has three components: (1) static pressure, which is related to the fullness of the vascular system at zero flow; (2) hydrostatic pressure, which is equal to the height of the column of liquid (h) multiplied by the density of the liquid (p) multiplied by the gravitational force (g), hydrostatic pressure = pgh; and (3) dynamic pressure, which is the pressure generated by the heart and is equal to flow multiplied by resistance (pressure = flow × resistance). The static pressure and the hydrostatic pressure are added to the dynamic pressure to give blood pressure. The hydrostatic pressure, and particularly the effect of the height of the fluid column, is especially important in the upright position, because the fluid column between the heart and the feet may add an additional 100 mm Hg of hydrostatic pressure to the dynamic pressure (100 mm Hg). In the systemic circulation, blood flows from the aorta, where the MAP is 100 mm Hg, to the right atrium (mean pressure = 0 to 6 mm Hg). Blood pressure control is discussed in Chapter 4.

Resistance

Based on an analogy to Ohm's law, resistance (R) is equal to a pressure gradient (ΔP) divided by blood flow ($\dot{Q}$):

$$R = \frac{\Delta P}{\dot{Q}}$$

According to Poiseuille's law for laminar nonpulsatile flow of a substance with uniform viscosity, vascular resistance is proportional to a constant ($8/\pi$), the viscosity of the blood (η), and the length of the vessel (L). It is inversely proportional to the fourth power of the radius (r^4):

$$R = \frac{8L\eta}{\pi r^4}$$

Thus, the resistance to flow depends on only the dimension length (L) and radius (r) of the vessel and the viscosity (η) of the fluid. The radius of the blood vessel is the primary factor determining resistance in the vascular system. For example, if all other factors are held constant, decreasing the vessel radius by 50% increases resistance 16-fold, because resistance is inversely proportional to the fourth power of the radius. An increase in the hematocrit (e.g., polycythemia caused by high altitude) can increase blood viscosity, causing resistance to increase.[140] A limitation of Poiseuille's law is that it is based on rigid tubes and predicts a linear relationship between pressure and flow. However, because of the elastic properties of blood vessels, the relationship between pressure and flow is nonlinear. Depending on the starting pressure and the vasoconstrictive state of the vessel, an initial increase in pressure may distend the vessel but have limited effect on flow. See the hemodynamics chapter for a discussion of the calculation and interpretation of the systemic and pulmonary vascular resistance.

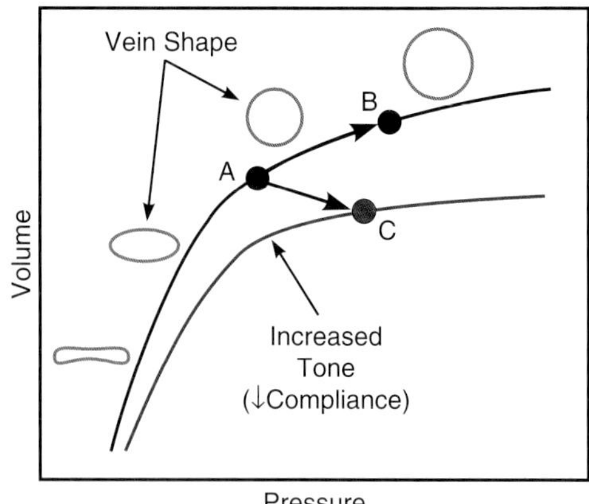

Figure 3-19. Compliance curves for a vein. (Reprinted with permission from Klabunde RE. *Cardiovascular Physiology Concepts*. 2nd ed. Philadelphia, PA: Wolters Kluwer Health; 2012:108.)

THE VENOUS SYSTEM

The venous system transports blood back to the heart from the microcirculation of each organ system and plays a crucial role in the maintenance of thoracic intravascular volume. The veins also serve as a low-pressure reservoir with the capacity to contain a large and variable volume of blood (similar to a giant capacitor sitting next to the right ventricle). The veins are innervated by α-adrenergic fibers but not β-adrenergic fibers. Only the splanchnic and cutaneous veins receive extensive innervation. The veins constrict in response to α-adrenergic stimuli and dilate as the result of withdrawal of the α-adrenergic stimuli or in response to increased transmural pressure (i.e., passive vasodilation). There are no active vasodilatory mechanisms in the veins.[24]

Venous Pressure and Resistance

In the supine position, the pressure generated by the heart in the large arteries is approximately 100 mm Hg. However, as demonstrated in Figure 3-17, the pressure decreases across the arterioles and capillaries, with a resultant pressure in the small veins of only 15 to 20 mm Hg. The right atrial pressure is approximately 0 to 5 mm Hg (depending on position, the state of hydration, and cardiac output). Thus, the pressure driving blood flow from the left side of the heart to the capillaries is approximately 80 mm Hg, whereas the driving pressure from the postcapillary vessels to the right atrium is only 15 to 20 mm Hg (difference between the postcapillary vessels and the right atrium). Interestingly, in the upright position this gradient is unchanged, despite the addition of hydrostatic pressure (determined by the height of a continuous column of blood between any given point and the heart).

Skeletal muscle contractions in the extremities (the muscle pump) and respiration (respiratory pump) play an essential role in propelling venous blood from the veins to the right atrium (see Chapter 4). In addition, the venous valves prevent backward flow into the muscle. Valvular function is particularly important during standing and exercise and the pathogenesis of venous insufficiency. The valves also promote the one-way flow of blood through perforating veins that lie between the superficial and deep veins (Fig. 3-7).

Venous Compliance

When empty, the thin walls of the veins are flattened and the vessels are elliptical. As the veins fill with blood, they passively change to a circular shape. Because of this passive accommodation to an increase in volume, the veins are capable of receiving large volumes of fluid with only small increases in transmural pressure; that is, they are compliant. Because of their ability to serve as a volume reservoir, the veins are referred to as capacitance vessels. At increased pressures, the veins become distended and less compliant; thus, any given pressure change is associated with a smaller change in volume (Fig. 3-19). Because of the compliant nature of the veins, the venous system plays an important role in altering thoracic intravascular volume.[25]

MICROCIRCULATORY EXCHANGE

Flow Through the Microvascular Circulation

Blood flow ($\dot{Q}$) through the microcirculation (or any organ) is directly related to the difference in pressure between the arterial end of the vascular segment (P_A) and venous pressure (P_v) and is inversely related to vascular resistance (R_T).[14,15]

$$\text{Flow} = \frac{P_A - P_V}{R_T}$$

In the absence of changes in arterial pressure (P_A), changes in local vascular resistance and intravascular pressure are caused by vasodilation and vasoconstriction of the arterioles. Any alteration in the tone of the muscular venules contributes little to the change in resistance (Display 3-7).

Microvascular Transport Mechanisms

Solutes and water passively move across the endothelium as the result of two processes, diffusion and ultrafiltration. Diffusion is the result of the random kinetic motion of ions and molecules. Diffusion results in the net transport of substances along a concentration gradient from high to low concentration. Ultrafiltration is the combined movement of fluid and solutes in a unilateral direction through a membrane, except that the movement of the solutes is restricted by the membrane. The driving force for ultrafiltration is the difference between hydrostatic pressure and oncotic pressure across the membrane. Ultrafiltration is the primary mechanism for controlling plasma and interstitial fluid volume.[14]

DISPLAY 3-7

Mechanisms of Exchange Across Capillary Endothelium

Capillary walls are extremely thin single layer of highly permeable endothelial cells and basal lamina. This arrangement allows for the exchange of cell excreta, water, and nutrients to be efficiently exchanged between the tissue and circulating blood.

Diffusion is the result of molecule movement from areas of high concentration to low concentration. The diffusion constant is the ease with which a molecule can move across the capillary wall.

The rate of diffusion is directly proportional to the concentration difference of molecules across the capillary wall, the diffusion constant, and the area of diffusion. It is inversely proportional to the distance of diffusion.

Diffusion, bulk flow, vesicular transport and active transport are methods fluids, electrolytes, gases and other substances transverse the capillary endothelium and are ruled by the same factors effecting blood flow in vessels.

Hydrostatic pressure is the driving force determining fluid movement across the capillary wall. Capillary wall pressure is determined by arterial and venous pressure, and the resistance in the pre- and postcapillary vessels.

Diffusion

Concentration gradients, created by the production or consumption of specific substances, are the primary driving forces for diffusion (with the exception of the tight-junction capillaries, which are affected by electrical gradients). Because diffusion in or out of a blood vessel creates a concentration gradient along the vessel, diffusion exchange is strongly influenced by blood flow, particularly for those substances that rapidly diffuse through the membrane wall.[15,141] The rate of diffusion of a solute across the capillary wall (J_s) is proportional to the concentration gradient, that is, the difference between the concentration in the plasma (C_p) and interstitial concentration (C_i), the permeability (P_s) of the endothelium to the solute, and the surface area (A) available for exchange.

$$J_s = P_s A(C_p - C_i)$$

For substances that diffuse rapidly through the capillary endothelium (e.g., O_2, CO_2), the transport of the solute depends on the concentration gradient and blood flow (through the delivery or removal of the substance). The rate of diffusion (J_s) is described as *flow-limited.*

$$J_s = (C_a - C_i)\dot{Q}$$

where C_a is the concentration of the substance in the arterial blood, C_i is the concentration of the substance in the interstitium, and $\dot{Q}$ is the rate of blood flow. Flow-limited diffusion has potentially important implications for oxygen delivery in the setting of decreased oxygen delivery (e.g., cardiogenic shock or during severe exercise when flow rates are so high that diffusion is limited). However, most substances have intermediate endothelial permeability, and the rate of diffusion depends on endothelial permeability and flow.[14]

Most solutes, including small lipophilic and hydrophilic molecules and macromolecules, move through membranes of exchange vessels by diffusion. The route of diffusion depends on the type of membrane (continuous, fenestrated, discontinuous, and tight-junction) and the characteristics of the substance (e.g., lipid soluble, ionic, large macromolecule) (Fig. 3-20). Water

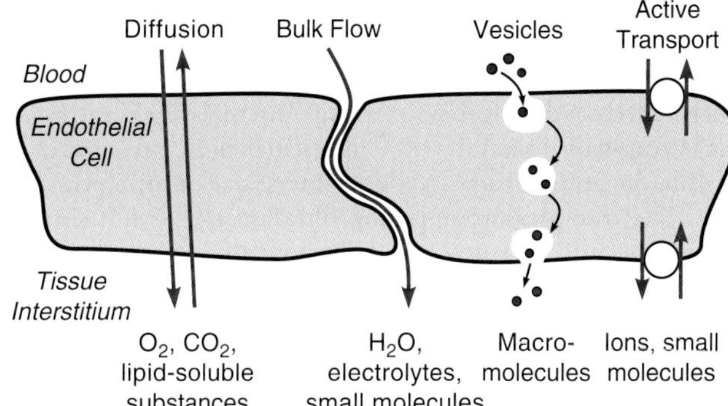

Figure 3-20. Mechanisms of exchange across the capillary endothelium. (Reprinted with permission from Klabunde RE. *Cardiovascular Physiology Concepts.* 2nd ed. Philadelphia, PA: Wolters Kluwer Health; 2012:181.)

diffuses through the endothelium primarily through intercellular clefts.[142,143] Lipid-soluble substances, such as O_2, CO_2, and anesthetic gases, which pass easily through the lipid bilayer of the microvascular wall, diffuse relatively rapidly through the endothelium. Small hydrophilic solutes, such as ions and simple sugars, pass primarily through fenestrae, junctions between cells, or intracellular clefts. The primary mode of macromolecular transport is through vesicles or possibly large pores.[143] The transport or movement of the macromolecules into the interstitium contributes to interstitial oncotic pressure.

Ultrafiltration

Starling's hypothesis of microvascular fluid exchange is described by the following equation[144–147]:

$$\frac{J_v}{A} = L_p\,([P_c - P_i]) - \sigma\,[\pi_c - \pi_i])$$

J_v/A = fluid filtration across the capillary wall per unit area
L_p = hydraulic permeability of the capillary wall
P_c = global value for capillary pressure
P_i = global value for interstitial pressure
σ = osmotic reflection coefficient
π_c = global value for capillary oncotic pressure
π_i = global value for interstitial oncotic pressure

In Starling's initial conceptualization of ultrafiltration, it was thought that at the arterial end of the capillary, the net forces favored the movement of fluid out of the vessel (filtration). Somewhere in the middle of the vessel, an equilibrium point was reached at which there was neither a gain nor a loss of fluid. Finally, on the venous end of the exchange vessel, the net forces favored reabsorption. Although the validity of Starling's equation has been repeatedly confirmed, the conceptualization of upstream filtration and downstream reabsorption has been questioned.[147] In general, the forces opposing filtration do not exceed capillary pressure, and filtration occurs along the entire length of the exchange vessel.[148] The net filtration is necessary to wash out the proteins that are continuously diffusing out of the vessels into the interstitium.[148,149] The ultrafiltrate and proteins that cross the vessel wall into the interstitial fluid are subsequently removed by the lymphatic system.

The primary direction of ultrafiltration is out of the vessel (filtration versus reabsorption), with the rate of fluid movement across a short segment of exchange vessel (J_v/A) having a curvilinear relationship to the net pressure difference (i.e., limited fluid movement at low P_c) across the vessel wall.[147] In Starling's initial conceptualization, the net pressure difference reflected the algebraic sum of four pressures: intravascular (capillary) pressure (P_c), interstitial fluid pressure (P_i), plasma oncotic pressure (π_c), and interstitial oncotic pressure (π_i). The true pressure opposing filtration (P_o) is not simply plasma oncotic pressure, but rather oncotic plasma pressure minus interstitial oncotic pressure plus interstitial hydrostatic pressure and the reflection coefficient:

$$P_o = \sigma(\pi_p - \pi_i) + P_i$$

However, the effective oncotic force that opposes fluid filtration across the microvessel wall is the local oncotic pressure difference across the endothelial surface glycocalyx (the structure that covers the entire capillary endothelium and is the primary filter for proteins) and not the global difference between the oncotic pressure in the plasma and tissue.[150] Models of this new conceptualization suggest that the oncotic pressure opposing filtration is greater than estimated from blood–tissue protein concentration differences, and transcapillary fluid flux is smaller than predicted from the original Starling equation. Therefore, in the Starling equation, the pressures P_i and π_i are the local hydrostatic pressure behind the glycocalyx and oncotic pressure on the tissue side of the matrix layer, respectively, and not the values from the tissue space.[150,151]

Capillary pressure (P_c) is the primary force behind filtration. Mean capillary pressure (P_c) is determined by the arterial and venous pressures and the ratio of postcapillary resistance (R_v) to precapillary resistance (R_a), as described by the following equation[152]:

$$P_c = (P_v + P_a) \times \frac{R_v}{R_a}$$

where P_v is venous pressure, P_a is arterial pressure, R_v is postcapillary midpoint resistance, and R_a is precapillary midpoint resistance (where $R_v + R_a = R_{Total}$). An increase in either P_a or P_v results in an increase in P_c, unless counteracted by a decrease in the R_v/R_a ratio. The lower the R_v/R_a ratio (i.e., increased precapillary resistance or decreased postcapillary resistance) the lower the capillary pressure. It is the adjustment in R_v/R_a ratio, primarily through regulation of precapillary resistance (R_a) in the skeletal muscle and skin, that constitutes the primary effector mechanism for the central nervous system–mediated control of plasma volume.[153,154] However, the centrally mediated decrease in mean capillary pressure occurs only to the extent allowed by local autoregulatory adjustments.

In response to hypovolemic hypotension, compensatory precapillary vasoconstriction (increased R_a) decreases the mean P_c, and the net pressure in the downstream (venous) segment of the exchange vessel favors transient reabsorption. This autotransfusion is the result of a change in the ratio of the postcapillary to precapillary resistance on mean capillary pressure.[155] Of note, this response is decreased in older individuals, which may impair their response to orthostasis or hemorrhage.[156]

In addition to the hydrostatic and oncotic forces, two other factors affect fluid movement across the exchange vessel: the hydraulic conductivity of the wall (L_p) and the reflection coefficient (σ). Hydraulic conductivity is a measure of the permeability of the exchange vessel to fluid, with the highest L_p values for fenestrated endothelia and lowest for tight-junction endothelia.[14] Hydraulic conductivity is difficult to measure and is estimated by the capillary filtration coefficient. The capillary filtration coefficient, which is equal to the product of hydraulic conductivity and the available area (L_pA), is expressed as milliliters of net filtrate formed in 100 g of tissue per minute for each milliliter increase in mean capillary filtration pressure (mL $\times$ min^{-1} mm Hg^{-1} $\times$ 100 g^{-1}). The capillary filtration coefficient is a useful indicator of capillary permeability.[149] A decrease in the capillary filtration coefficient, for example, by a decrease in the area available for exchange, reduces the rate of net capillary filtration for any given net filtration pressure. The second factor, the reflection coefficient (σ), represents the osmotic pressure exerted by a difference in the concentration gradient of a substance across a membrane (oncotic effect of the concentration gradient) and the greater the ratio of the solute size to pore size, the greater the ratio.[157]

The reflection coefficient is close to 1 for tight-junction endothelium, which is completely impermeable to protein. In normal systemic exchange vessels in the skin and skeletal muscle, with continuous or fenestrated endothelium, the reflection coefficient ranges from 0.8 to 0.95 for albumin and total protein,[148,149] which indicates that these vessels are not completely impermeable to proteins. In the lungs, the reflection coefficients are, in general, lower for albumin (0.5 to 0.6) and protein (0.5 to 0.7).[149] In cases of injury to the endothelium, the reflection coefficient is markedly reduced, allowing increased movement of large molecules (e.g., protein) out of the exchange vessels.

The Lymphatic System

Removal of fluid and plasma proteins from the interstitium by the terminal lymphatics is essential in the maintenance of equilibrium in microvascular-interstitial exchange.[157] Depending on the protein concentration in the lymph, 8 to 12 L/day of lymph, which reflects net filtration caused by movement of fluid out of the vascular bed, is removed from the interstitium by the lymphatic system[146,157] (Fig. 3-3). Approximately 4 to 8 L of the ultrafiltrate is directly reabsorbed from the lymphatic vessels back into the blood vessels, and the remaining 4 L of efferent lymph, which includes all of the filtered protein, is delivered back to the central circulation.[146,149] This high level of lymphatic flow supports the idea that filtration (return of lymph to the systemic vasculature) occurs along the entire length of lymphatic bed and not just in the central circulation (Fig. 3-21).

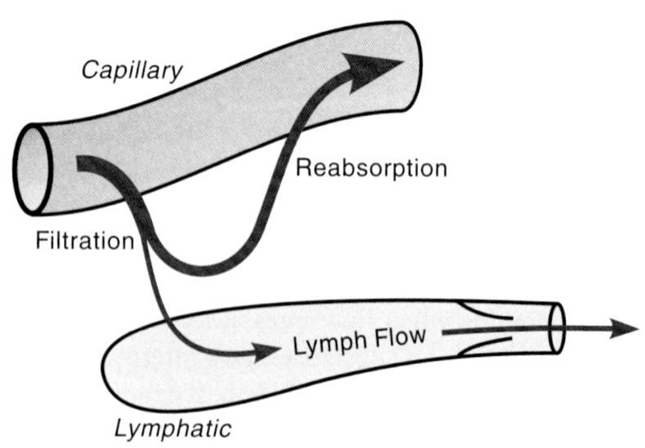

Figure 3-21. Capillary filtration, reabsorption, and lymph flow. (Reprinted with permission from Klabunde RE. *Cardiovascular Physiology Concepts.* 2nd ed. Philadelphia, PA: Wolters Kluwer Health; 2012:187.)

DISPLAY 3-8

Pressures and Gas Exchange in the Pulmonary and Systemic Circulation

Pressures and resistance in the pulmonary circulation are much lower than in the systemic circulation.

Cardiac output of the right ventricle is equal to pulmonary blood flow.

When supine, blood flow is almost equal throughout the lung. When standing, blood flow is unevenly distributed due to the effect of gravity. It is lowest in the apex (zone 1) and highest in the base (zone 3).

Lung Zones: Uneven blood flow in the lungs is due to hydrostatic pressure differences within the blood vessels. West describes the differences by dividing the lungs into three zones

- Zone 1 PA > P_a > P_v Lowest blood flow
- Zone 2 Pa > P_A > P_v Medium blood flow
- Zone 3 Pa > P_v > P_A Highest blood flow

In the lungs hypoxia results in vasoconstriction, the opposite of all other organs.

Four Causes of Hypoxemia

1. Hypoventilation
2. Diffusion limitations such as fibrosis
3. Shunt
4. Ventilation–perfusion mismatch

Oxygen is transported in the blood either dissolved in the blood or bonded to hemoglobin. Bonded to hemoglobin, the carrying capacity of blood for oxygen is approximately 70-fold.

Carbon dioxide exists in three forms: 1 to 6% dissolved state; 20 to 25% combined with hemoglobin; 3 to 70% combine with hydrogen to form bicarbonate.

Oxygen delivery to the tissues is determined by the arterial blood flow and the arterial oxygen content.

PULMONARY CIRCULATION

Gross Anatomy

The primary function of the pulmonary circulation is to expose the blood to alveolar air so that oxygen can be taken up by the blood and carbon dioxide can be excreted. The pulmonary circulation is in series with the systemic circulation and receives the same cardiac output, approximately 5 to 6 L/min at rest for an adult weighing 70 kg. The pulmonary circulation has only 10% the capacity of the systemic circulation, yet it must accommodate the same ejected volume (Display 3-8).

Although pulmonary blood flow is equal to that of the systemic system, its vascular resistance is seven to eight times lower than systemic resistance. The pulmonary vascular bed is regulated by passive factors, such as lung volume, and active factors, such as alveolar gas. These mechanisms alter pulmonary vascular resistance (Fig. 3-22)

Pulmonary blood volume decreases or is diverted to the systemic circulation in conditions such as generalized systemic vasodilation, the standing position, positive end-expiratory pressure, or circulatory shock. Conditions that increase pulmonary blood volume include generalized systemic vasoconstriction, the supine position, mitral stenosis, and left heart failure.[188]

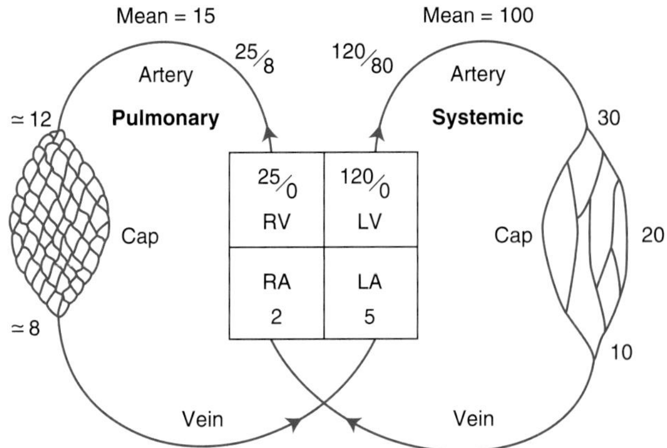

Figure 3-22. Comparison of pressures in the pulmonary and systemic circulations. (Reprinted with permission from West JB, Luks AM. *West's Respiratory Physiology: The Essentials.* 10th ed. Philadelphia, PA: Wolters Kluwer Health; 2016:42.)

The pulmonary circulation originates from the base of the right ventricle, extends 5 cm, and divides into the right and left pulmonary arteries. As the pulmonary artery rises, the right pulmonary artery is positioned posterior to the aorta and superior vena cava and anterior to the right mainstem bronchus. The left pulmonary artery extends over the left main bronchus and divides into lobar branches. The pulmonary arteries and segmental and lobar branches are composed of elastic arteries to maintain low vascular resistance. These arteries contain smooth muscle with the capability of vasoconstriction and vasodilation. The muscular arteries have internal and external elastic laminae with a layer of smooth muscle cells. The intra-acinar and supernumerary arteries (precapillary arteries) are muscular. Increases in pulmonary vascular resistance come from the precapillary arteries. Arterioles are vessels with a thin intima and a single elastic lamina. These vessels make up the accessory branches of the respiratory tree and end at the alveolar capillary network (see Table 4-3).

Cellular and Hormonal Effects

The pulmonary vascular bed is lined with endothelium. In the pulmonary vasculature, the primary endothelium-relaxing factors released by the endothelial cells are NO and prostacyclin (PGI_2). Nitric oxide plays an important role in baseline pulmonary vasodilation where it is most likely the common pathway for producing pulmonary vasodilation.[188] Nitric oxide–mediated vasodilation maintains low basal pulmonary vascular resistance, and it can cause further vasodilation in response to receptor-mediated stimulation.[189] Additionally, NO counteracts hypoxic pulmonary vasoconstriction (HPV), but its release is decreased with chronic hypoxia and primary pulmonary hypertension.[190] There is no evidence that EDHF exists in the pulmonary circulation.

Circulating factors that cause pulmonary vasoconstriction include endothelin, superoxide anion (O_2^-), TXA_2, serotonin, PGH_2, and angiotensin. Factors that cause vasodilation include histamine, bradykinin, and substance P. In addition, circulating catecholamines induce vasoconstriction via α_1 receptors (mediated by norepinephrine and epinephrine), whereas α_2 and β_2 receptors stimulation causes vasodilation (mediated by epinephrine). Vasoconstriction predominates in response to sympathetic stimulation.

The pulmonary vascular endothelium also plays a role in activation of vasoactive substances. For example, 80% of angiotensin I is converted to AII during one pass through the pulmonary

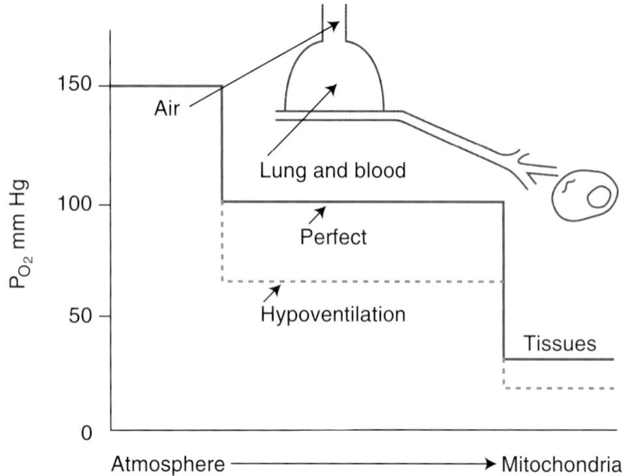

Figure 3-23. Scheme of the O_2 partial pressure from the air to tissues. (From West JB, Luks AM. *West's Respiratory Physiology: The Essentials.* 10th ed. Philadelphia, PA: Wolters Kluwer Health; 2016:64.)

circulation. This conversion is caused by the presence of ACE, which is located on the endothelial surface.[191] ACE-Is cover this enzyme and thus interfere with it action. Pulmonary vascular ACE also deactivates the peptide bradykinin. Other factors that may be altered as they pass through the pulmonary circulation include atrial natriuretic peptide and the endothelins.[188]

Physiology

Respiration is a process consisting of four major events: (1) pulmonary ventilation, which is the bulk movement of air between the atmosphere and the alveoli in the lungs; (2) diffusion of gases (O_2 and carbon dioxide) across the respiratory membrane between the alveoli and blood; (3) transport of gases to and from the cells of the body; and (4) other non–gas exchange functions (e.g., hormonal activity).

Maintenance of adequate tissue oxygenation depends on complex mechanisms, including transport of oxygen, microvascular control (systemic and local), and intact metabolic cellular function (Fig. 3-23).[192] Which illustrates the processes by which oxygen is transported from the atmosphere to the mitochondria, demonstrates the pressure gradient from 150 mm Hg in the atmosphere to 1 mm Hg at the mitochondria.

Ventilation

Ventilation is the process of the exchange of air between the atmosphere (external environment) and alveoli. It involves the distribution of air into the pulmonary structures of the tracheobronchial tree to the alveoli of the lung. Air flow in the conducting airways (first 17 airway generations) is along a pressure gradient. Air moves from higher outside pressure (atmospheric) to lower airway pressure (sub-atmospheric). As air enters the alveolar region of the lung, the movement of gases becomes less dependent on the pressure gradient and diffusion becomes increasingly important.[188]

Diffusion is the process of movement of gases from an area of high partial pressure to an area of low partial pressure. Toward the end of the airways, at the alveoli, diffusion is the driving force behind the movement of oxygen and carbon dioxide across the alveolar membrane into the pulmonary capillaries.

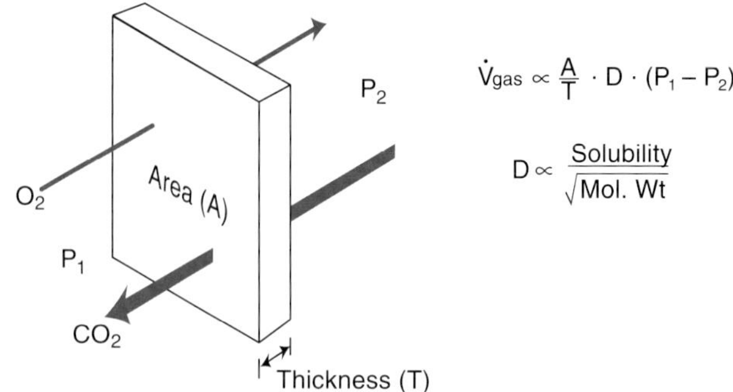

Figure 3-24. Gas diffusion and transport in the circuitry of the cardiovascular system. (From West JB, Luks AM. *West's Respiratory Physiology: The Essentials.* 10th ed. Philadelphia, PA: Wolters Kluwer Health; 2016:29.)

Perfusion is the process of transporting gases to and from the cells of the body (Fig. 3-24). This event includes mixed venous blood flow to the pulmonary capillaries where gases are exchanged between the alveoli and blood, and blood flow to the systemic capillaries where gases are exchanged between the blood and the surrounding body fluids.

Other lung functions that affect respiration but do not involve gas exchange include hormonal activity and the work of breathing. Work of breathing is the metabolic demand of breathing. It includes the energy needed to move the lung and chest wall and results in a demand for oxygen.

Dead Space

Ventilation must keep pace with the constant demand to replenish oxygen and eliminate carbon dioxide exchanged in the alveoli. Dead space is the volume of inspired air that does not participate in gas exchange. The volume of gas in a normal breath is measured as the tidal volume (V_T). This volume is multiplied by the number of breaths per minute to calculate minute volume (V_E). Minute volume represents the total volume of air moved through the airways to and from the alveoli. A portion of this volume will reach the alveoli where gas exchange can occur (alveolar volume), while the remainder will stay in the conducting airways and will not contribute to gas exchange (anatomic dead space) ($V_T = V_A + V_A$). In disease states, some lung regions may continue to receive ventilation but will not get normal blood flow. The result is wasted ventilation, adding to dead space volume (physiologic dead space).[193]

Lung Zones

Because the alveolar air spaces surround collapsible capillaries, intrapleural and alveolar pressures affect pulmonary capillary pressures. Pulmonary blood flow reflects this influence during respiration in the upright and lateral recumbent positions. Inspiration and expiration induce fluctuating intrathoracic pressures that influence the pulmonary vessels. Pulmonary capillaries are also affected by alveolar pressure to a certain degree. However, the capillary–alveolar membrane is thin and compliant enough to approximate pulmonary capillary pressure to alveolar pressure. With a change from supine to standing position, a hydrostatic pressure difference of 20 cm H_2O is created between the apex and base of the lung.

West[194] described the hydrostatic effect of body position on pulmonary capillary flow by dividing the lung into three regions

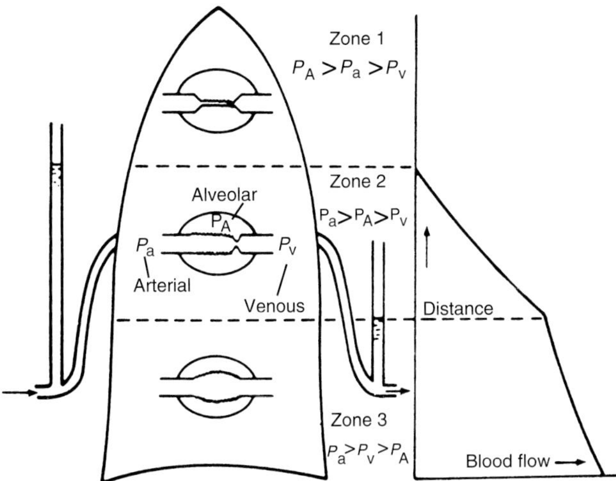

Figure 3-25. Model to explain the zones of the lungs. P_A, alveolar pressure; P_a, pulmonary arterial pressure; P_v, pulmonary venous pressure. (Reprinted with permission from West JB. *Respiratory Physiology: The Essentials.* 2nd ed. Baltimore, MD: Williams & Wilkins; 1979:43.)

(Fig. 3-25). Zone 1 is represented above the heart in an upright body position, where pulmonary alveolar pressure (P_A) may exceed pulmonary arterial pressure (P_a) and pulmonary venous pressure (P_v) ($P_A > P_a > P_v$). In a normal physiologic state, pulmonary arterial pressure is sufficient to maintain blood flow to the top of the lung. Thus, zone 1 does not usually develop. However, in conditions that decrease arterial pressure (e.g., hemorrhage) or increase alveolar pressure (e.g., positive end-expiratory pressure), a zone 1 region may be created. In this state, the apex of the lung is ventilated yet unperfused, which creates alveolar dead space that is ineffective for gas exchange.

The region of zone 2 is represented at the level of the left atrium of the heart, where pulmonary arterial pressure increases because of the hydrostatic effect. At this point, P_a exceeds P_A, which continues to exceed venous pressures ($P_a > P_A > P_v$). Although P_a exceeds P_A, alveolar pressure is still higher than the pressure of the left atrium.

The region of zone 3, below the left atrium, is where both P_a and left atrial pressures exceed P_A ($P_a > P_v > P_A$). Blood flow, which is determined by the difference between arterial and venous pressures, is increased markedly in this region of the lung because of capillary distention. The zone 3 region creates a continuous column of fluid between the pulmonary artery and the left atrium. Reliable pulmonary artery pressure measurements can be obtained when the tip of the pulmonary artery catheter is located in zone 3.

This general model of blood flow distribution is adequate for understanding the range of ventilation and perfusion relationships throughout the lung as a whole. However, high-resolution imaging technology has found that within a given isogravitational plane, there is greater heterogeneity than explained by the West zones most likely related to the asymmetrical branching of the bronchial and pulmonary vascular anatomy, and that gravity plays less of a role in the distribution of blood flow than previously thought.[195–198]

Diffusion

Each gas in a mixture of gases behaves as if it alone occupies the total volume and exerts a partial pressure independent of the other gases present. Diffusion is the process of movement of molecules. In conditions in which a gas has an area of high concentration and an area of low concentration, the net diffusion of gas will be from the area of high to low. In addition to the difference in pressure, the solubility of the gas in the body fluid (primarily water), the cross-sectional area of the exchange surface (alveolar–pulmonary capillary interface), and the distance the gas must travel are among the factors that affect the net diffusion in fluids. Carbon dioxide is approximately 20 times more soluble in water than in oxygen. Some pathologic conditions (e.g., pulmonary edema) can affect cross-sectional area and distance.

Ventilation–Perfusion Matching

Pulmonary precapillary vasomotor and bronchiolar responses serve to match pulmonary capillary perfusion to alveolar ventilation. Unlike in the systemic circulation where hypoxemia, decreased pH, or increased amounts of carbon dioxide cause local vasodilation, any of these conditions in the pulmonary circulation may cause arteriolar vasoconstriction. In well-ventilated regions, there is little vasoconstriction in response to deoxygenated blood. In poorly ventilated areas where the amount of alveolar oxygen is less than normal, such as when a bronchus is obstructed, vasoconstriction occurs and blood is shunted to other lung areas.

Distribution of pulmonary blood flow in normal adults is normally controlled to a greater extent by the hydrostatic pressure gradient discussed earlier. Active control of pulmonary circulation, for example, hypoxic vasoconstriction, serves a useful role in diverting blood flow to areas of the lung with more abundant oxygen, thus improving gas exchange. In contrast to peripheral vasculature, which vasodilates in response to hypoxia, pulmonary vessels constrict (e.g., HPV) to shunt blood away from poorly ventilated areas to match perfusion and ventilation.[199] HPV occurs within seconds in response to alveolar hypoxia and decreased mixed venous (pulmonary arterial) PO_2, with alveolar PO_2 exerting a greater effect.[188] The exact mechanism of HPV is unknown; however, the most likely cause is hypoxia-induced vascular smooth muscle hyperpolarization, which leads to increased intracellular calcium and subsequent vasoconstriction.[200–202] Other factors that are endothelium dependent, and may modulate hypoxic vasoconstriction and cause vascular remodeling, include inhibition of NO production, decreased effect of prostacyclin and increased endothelin.[188,203] Of clinical importance, while inhaled NO has been used to acutely treat pulmonary hypertension, its effectiveness is equivocal,[204] and a recent meta-analysis recommended that NO not be used for the treatment of acute respiratory distress syndrome.[205] In contrast, phosphodiesterase inhibitors, which enhance NO-mediated vasodilation have been found to improve outcomes and are traditional therapies, recently endothelin receptor antagonists have been proposed as alternative treatments.[206] In addition, endothelin receptor antagonists have become first-line therapy for pulmonary arterial hypertension,[207] selective phosphodiesterase-5 inhibitors have also been shown to be effective[208] and intravenous prostacyclin is reserved for severely ill patients.[209,210]

When blood flow to a region of the lung is decreased, there is also a decrease in alveolar CO_2. The bronchial smooth muscle responds to the decreased alveolar CO_2 levels by constricting; thus, shifting ventilation away from a poorly perfused area. This response occurs in conditions such as prolonged high altitude or in patients with chronic obstructive pulmonary disease or prolonged pulmonary hypertension.[211]

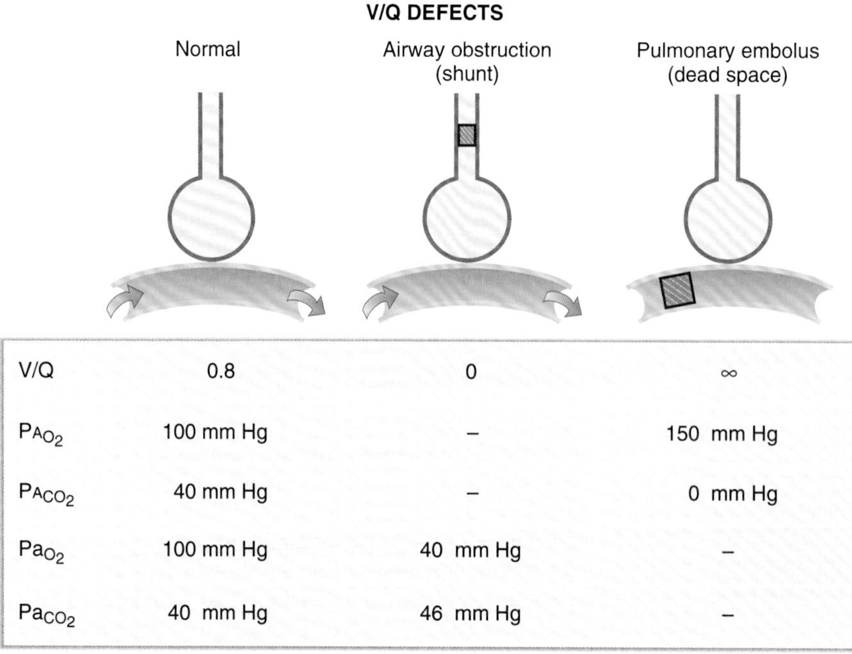

Figure 3-26. Effect of ventilation/perfusion (V/Q) defects on gas exchange. With airway obstruction, the composition of systemic arterial blood approaches that of mixed venous blood. With pulmonary embolus, the composition of alveolar gas approaches that of inspired air. PA$_{O2}$ = alveolar Po$_2$; PA$_{CO2}$, alveolar Pco$_2$; Pa$_{O2}$, arterial Po$_2$; Pa$_{CO2}$, arterial Pco$_2$. (From Costanzo LS. *Physiology.* 6th ed. Philadelphia, PA: Wolters Kluwer Health; 2015:135.)

Ventilation and perfusion must occur in equal proportion in the various regions of the lung to achieve adequate gas exchange. Gas exchange determines the levels of alveolar oxygen partial pressure (PA$_{O2}$) and carbon dioxide partial pressure (PA$_{CO2}$). An adequate alveolar Po$_2$ depends on a balance of two factors: the rate of removal of oxygen by the pulmonary arterial blood and the rate of replenishment of oxygen by alveolar ventilation. An adequate PA$_{CO2}$ depends on the rate of removal of carbon dioxide by alveolar ventilation. A key concept used to understand pulmonary gas exchange is the ventilation–perfusion ratio ($\dot{V}/\dot{Q}$). The concentration of gases (i.e., oxygen, carbon dioxide, nitrogen) in the various regions of the lung is determined by the ratio of the rate of ventilation to the rate of perfusion (blood flow). Obstruction to ventilation or perfusion leads to alteration in this ratio and, consequently, the composition of gases as noted in Figure 3-26.

Inequality in ventilation–perfusion hinders the lungs' ability to replenish oxygen and remove carbon dioxide. Impairment of gas exchange can result in a decrease in Pa$_{O2}$ and an increase in tissue Pco$_2$. Clinically, these conditions can result in hypoxemia.

Causes of Arterial Hypoxemia

There are six sources of arterial hypoxemia:

- Decreased partial pressure of inspired oxygen
- Decreased percentage of inspired oxygen (decreased fraction of inspired oxygen, Fi$_{O2}$)
- Diffusion limitation
- Hypoventilation
- $\dot{V}/\dot{Q}$ mismatch
- Shunt

Decreases in the atmospheric pressure related to higher altitude result in a proportional decrease in the partial pressure of inspired oxygen (Pi$_{O2}$). These conditions are common to high-altitude locations and air travel; however, they are rarely encountered in the clinical setting. Decreased percentage of inspired oxygen (Fi$_{O2}$) occurs in situations in which other gases may displace oxygen and lower the overall percentage of oxygen below 21% (e.g., diagnostic testing, fire). Diffusion limitation can potentially cause abnormal diffusion of oxygen across the alveolar–capillary membrane. Diffusion limitation can be caused by increases in the thickness of the diffusion pathway and/or decreased transit time through the pulmonary circulation. Hypoventilation can result in a decrease in alveolar Po$_2$ caused by insufficient gas exchange between the external environment and the alveoli. Hypoventilation can result from trauma to the chest wall, paralysis of the respiratory muscles, and medications such as morphine sulfate and barbiturates, which depress the respiratory center.[212]

Matching ventilation of the alveoli with perfusion of the pulmonary capillary bed is a delicate balance. $\dot{V}/\dot{Q}$ matching is a dynamic process with different distributions occurring simultaneously within the regions of the lungs. In disease, there are a myriad of $\dot{V}/\dot{Q}$ relationships exemplified by regions receiving excessive ventilation (dead space), normal ventilation and perfusion (ideal), and excessive perfusion (shunt).

Shunt refers to the condition when blood passes into the systemic circulation without passing through a ventilated region of the lung. Under normal conditions, there exists a small physiologic shunt because of the difference in Po$_2$ between alveolar gas and end-capillary blood. Physiologically, mixed venous blood from the pulmonary arterial bed mixes with capillary blood from pulmonary venous beds, thereby lowering the end-capillary Po$_2$. This difference can become larger in conditions such as ventricular septal defect, in which greater amounts of venous blood are added to arterial blood across the defect, resulting in a lower Pa$_{O2}$.

An important clinical characteristic of a shunt is that the hypoxemia cannot be completely resolved by placing the patient on an inspired oxygen fraction (Fi$_{O2}$) of 100% (Display 3-9). Because the shunt blood bypasses the ventilated regions of the lung, it is not exposed to the higher alveolar Po$_2$. In patients with shunt, the arterial Pco$_2$ may be low, normal, or high, depending on the capacity to increase respiratory drive in response to hypoxemia (Table 3-4).

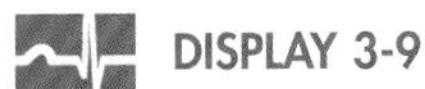
DISPLAY 3-9

Alveolar to Arterial Oxygen Gradient

The A-a gradient is used to compare causes of hypoxemia and is described by the following equation.

Normal A-a gradient (0–10 mm Hg)
A-a gradient = $PA_{O2} - Pa_{O2}$

In this equation A-a gradient equals the difference between alveolar PO_2 and arterial PO_2.

Alveolar PO_2 is derived from the alveolar gas equation:

PA_{O2} (alveolar PO_2) = **PI_{O2}** (inspired PO_2) – **PA_{CO2}/R**
PA_{CO2} = alveolar PCO_2 = arterial PCO_2 (via arterial blood sample)
R = respiratory exchange ration or respiratory quotient (CO_2 production/O_2 consumption)

GAS TRANSPORT

Gas Exchange

In the lungs, oxygen and carbon dioxide equilibrate across the alveolar–capillary membranes by simple passive diffusion, moving from an area of greater partial pressure to a region of lesser partial pressure. The partial pressure of oxygen in pulmonary arterial blood (venous blood from the body) is approximately 40 mm Hg, whereas pulmonary alveolar partial pressure of oxygen is approximately 100 mm Hg; thus, oxygen diffuses into the blood. The partial pressure of systemic arterial oxygen is slightly less than 100 mm Hg because of the admixture of oxygenated and deoxygenated blood. Blood from pulmonary veins is mixed with some deoxygenated blood from bronchial veins, and in the left heart it is mixed with deoxygenated blood from thebesian veins draining cardiac muscle tissue (physiologic shunt).

Carbon dioxide is removed in the pulmonary capillaries. The partial pressure of carbon dioxide in pulmonary arterial blood (systemic venous blood) is 46 mm Hg and that of blood leaving the lung (which becomes systemic arterial blood) is 40 mm Hg. The release of carbon dioxide is aided by the conversion of hemoglobin (Hgb) to oxyhemoglobin.

Oxygen reaching the tissues must dissociate from Hgb and pass out of the red blood cells and move to the mitochondria. Just as in the lungs, once the oxygen molecule leaves the cell, ***passive diffusion becomes the driving force in the movement of oxygen.*** Unlike the relatively short distances encountered in the lung, the oxygen diffusion from the blood to the mitochondria in the target cell is much greater. The partial pressure of oxygen at the arterial end of the capillary, approximately 90 mm Hg, quickly drops to approximately 30 mm Hg in the tissues and to approximately 1 to 3 mm Hg in the mitochondria.[188] Factors other than diffusion that influence oxygen delivery include the rate of oxygen delivery, the position of the P_{50} (right or left shift), and the rate of cellular oxygen consumption.[213]

Table 3-4 • CAUSES OF HYPOXEMIA

Cause	Pa_{O2}	A–a Gradient
High altitude (↓ PB)	Decreased	Normal
Hypoventilation (↓ PA_{O2})	Decreased	Normal
Diffusion defect (e.g., fibrosis)	Decreased	Increased
V/Q defect	Decreased	Increased
Right-to-left shunt	Decreased	Increased

A–a gradient, difference in PO_2 between alveolar gas and arterial blood; PB, barometric pressure; PA_{O2}, alveolar PO_2; Pa_{O2}, arterial PO_2; V/Q, ventilation/perfusion ratio.
From Costanzo LS. *Physiology*. 6th ed. Philadelphia, PA: Wolters Kluwer Health; 2015:130.

Transport of carbon dioxide in the blood begins with the diffusion of carbon dioxide out of the tissue cells. The PCO_2 of the tissues (50 mm Hg) is greater than the Pa_{CO2} in systemic capillaries (46 mm Hg). Thus, carbon dioxide diffuses from the tissues into the blood. The PCO_2 in the tissues is proportional to the amount of energy expended. Once carbon dioxide has diffused into the capillaries, a series of chemical reactions can occur. Carbon dioxide is carried in the blood by three mechanisms. Approximately 6% of carbon dioxide is carried in the dissolved state, 20% to 25% combines with Hgb, and the remainder (approximately 70%) of it combines with hydrogen to form bicarbonate. In the normal physiologic state, an average of 4 mL of carbon dioxide is transported from the tissues to the lungs in each 100 mL of blood. The amount of carbon dioxide carried in the blood can greatly alter the acid–base balance and must be carefully monitored in the critically ill patient. The diffusion of carbon dioxide into the blood is determined by two factors, the PCO_2 of the tissues and the oxygen content of the blood; both factors are in turn determined by the environment of the tissues. Thus, the physiochemical state that results from this exchange of gases is controlled by the metabolic demands of the tissues.

Oxygen Cascade

The oxygen cascade describes the partial pressure gradient for oxygen as it moves from air (PI_{O2} = 149 mm Hg at 37°C at sea level) through the respiratory tract where it is humidified to the alveolus (PA_{O2} = 100 mm Hg), across the alveolar–capillary membrane to arterial blood (PA_{O2} = 90 to 100 mm Hg) and the capillaries (P_{O2} = 30 to 40 mm Hg) and then into the tissues and finally to the cytoplasm and the mitochondria. The oxygen concentration at the tissue level varies based on the organ, by regional variations in perfusion, oxygen consumption, and the distance from the capillary. Mitochondrial function is generally not impaired until cellular oxygen drops below 1 to 2 mm Hg.[214]

Oxygen diffuses from the capillary to the mitochondria along a concentration gradient. In 1919, Krogh[215] defined a model of oxygen delivery that is characterized by a tissue cylinder surrounding each capillary. The Krogh model was based on the idea that oxygen consumption takes place along the capillary, with a progressive decrease in oxygen from the artery to the vein. This longitudinal oxygen gradient suggests that cells receiving oxygen from the venous end of the capillary would be at increased risk for decreased oxygen delivery under conditions of decreased flow or arterial oxygen. Current research indicates that while there is a longitudinal delivery gradient there is less heterogeneity than originally conceived.[216] In addition, oxygen delivery occurs not only along the capillaries, but also from the arterioles. The current models also suggest that oxygen consumption occurs not only within the tissue, but also in the arteriolar endothelium.[217,218] The implication of these findings is the need to redefine the radial gradient for oxygen delivery to include endothelial oxygen consumption and account for the relatively homogeneous delivery gradients.[217,218]

Mitochondrial Respiration

Ninety percent of the body's oxygen consumption occurs in the mitochondria. Inside the mitochondria the hydrogen ions produced during glycolysis are passed to the electron transport chain and through the step-wise process of oxidative phosphorylation they combine with molecular oxygen (dioxygen) to form water. The final step in the process is the reduction of oxygen by cytochrome a_3. Under aerobic conditions, the electron transport chain produces three ATP molecules during this process. Of clinical importance, mitochondrial respiration may be disrupted in sepsis by NO, which inhibits cytochrome a,a_3 and pyruvate dehydrogenase, which is responsible for the conversion of pyruvate.[58,219,220]

OXYGEN DELIVERY, CONSUMPTION, EXTRACTION

Oxygen Delivery

The delivery of adequate oxygen for normal cellular function depends not only on the total amount of oxygen in the arterial blood (arterial oxygen content) but also on the ability of the heart to provide adequate blood flow (cardiac output). Oxygen delivery ($\dot{D}o$) is defined as the transport of oxygen to the tissues per minute. Oxygen delivery is determined by the combined processes of ventilation and diffusion (pulmonary function), Hgb-binding capacity, convective movement of blood (cardiac function), microvascular distribution, and delivery of oxygen to the mitochondria (passive diffusion).

Cardiac Output

Cardiac output is a main determinant of oxygen delivery. Decrease in blood flow decreases the supply of oxygen to the cells, thereby initiating a series of compensatory mechanisms to increase oxygen transport and extraction. Careful monitoring of the determinants of cardiac output (preload, afterload, and contractility) and heart rate are necessary to optimize oxygen delivery. Arterial oxygen content and cardiac output are combined in the oxygen delivery ($\dot{D}o_2$) equation to measure the amount of oxygen delivered to the tissues in a given unit of time. Further discussion of the clinical implications of the oxygen consumption–delivery relationship is presented in Chapter 21.

Hemoglobin

In the red blood cell, the Hgb molecule acts as an oxygen-binding site responsible for carrying 97% of the oxygen in the blood. Hgb is a protein of four subunits of porphyrin and iron. The molecule is composed of two α and two β polypeptide chains, each with an iron-containing heme molecule capable of binding oxygen. Theoretically, 1 g of Hgb is capable of transporting 1.39 mL of oxygen. However, some of the heme sites are in an alternate form (methemoglobin) that is not capable of combining with oxygen. The maximum amount of oxygen that can be transported is approximately 1.34 to 1.36 mL/g of Hgb (some authors suggest this number may be lower, approximately 1.31 mL/g).[188,221] Hgb has a unique chemical structure that accounts for the differences in the speed at which oxygen binds with Hgb (affinity). Oxygen affinity increases as more Hgb is saturated with oxygen, so that the affinity of the last heme unit is greater than the first unit. This relationship explains the nonlinear curve represented in the oxyhemoglobin dissociation (or equilibrium) curve.[140]

Partial Pressure of Oxygen

Alveolar oxygen diffuses into the pulmonary capillaries. The amount of oxygen transferred depends on the mechanics of the ventilation–perfusion relationship of the lungs and the amount of inspired oxygen. The majority (97%) of the oxygen transported by the blood is bound to Hgb. The remaining 3% of the oxygen transported by the blood (0.3 mL/dL) comprises oxygen dissolved in plasma. The Pa_{O2}, a measurement of oxygen tension, is simply a reflection of the patient's plasma oxygenation. The Pa_{O2} is an indication of the patient's capacity for bonding oxygen to Hgb and the ability of oxygen to be released into the interstitial tissues. The body's plasma may carry a small percentage of the arterial oxygen, but measurement of its oxygen tension is an indirect method for determining the patient's oxygen–Hgb affinity.

Arterial Oxygen Saturation

As the partial pressure of oxygen in the pulmonary capillaries increases, oxygen binds with Hgb to form oxyhemoglobin. After leaving the pulmonary circulation, arterial blood can be sampled to measure the partial pressure of oxygen Pa_{O2}. Because oxygen binds with Hgb in a predictable manner, the saturation of Hgb in the arterial blood (Sa_{O2}) can be calculated (or measured directly by co-oximetry). The quantity of oxyhemoglobin, reflecting the amount of Hgb bound to oxygen, is measured as oxygen saturation. Saturation can be expressed as a percentage when multiplied by 100.

Oxyhemoglobin Dissociation Curve

The essential relationship between Pa_{O2} and Sa_{O2} is graphically illustrated by the oxyhemoglobin dissociation curve (Fig. 3-27).

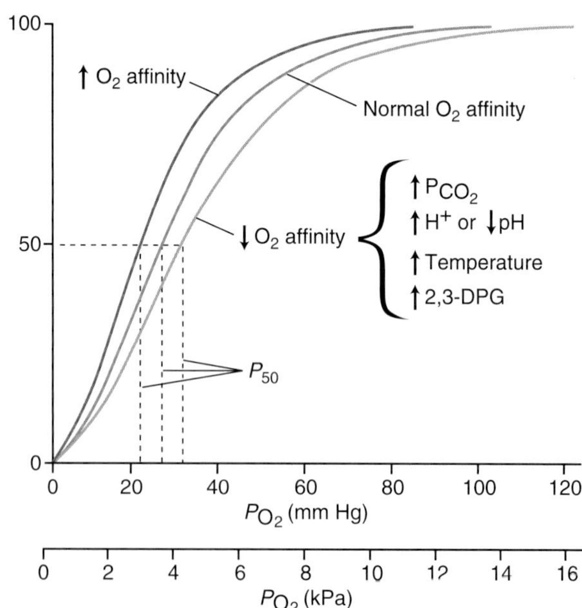

Figure 3-27. Changes in O_2 affinity of the O_2 saturation curve. Three curves are shown with progressively decreasing O_2 affinity indicated by increasing P_{50}. (From Hlastala MP, Berger AJ. *Physiology of Respiration.* 2nd ed. New York: Oxford University Press; 2001:99.)

The sigmoid, or S, shape of this curve reflects the optimal conditions that facilitate oxygen loading in the lungs and oxygen release to the tissues. To describe these processes in relation to the curve, the curve is often divided into two segments: the association segment and the dissociation segment.

The upper portion of the curve, or the association segment, represents oxygen uptake, where large decreases in Pa_{O2} elicit only small decreases in Sa_{O2}. For example, in the association segment of the curve, a 40% decrease in the Pa_{O2} (mm Hg) from 100 to 60 results only in a 7% decrease in oxygen saturation. The association segment also represents the body's protective mechanism to ensure that, even with a substantial decrease in Pa_{O2}, adequate arterial oxygen content is available for transport to the cells. The lower portion of the curve, or the dissociation segment, reflects the release of oxygen to the tissues. Here, small changes in Pa_{O2} result in large changes in Sa_{O2}, protecting the tissues by releasing large amounts of oxygen with minimal changes in oxygen tension. Unlike in the association segment, a 40% decrease in the Pa_{O2} causes a 20% decrease in oxygen saturation.

Changes in oxyhemoglobin affinity affect the oxyhemoglobin dissociation curve and need to be considered in tissue oxygen assessment. Increased affinity, caused by hypothermia, alkalosis, or decreased levels of 2,3-diphosphoglycerate (also referred to as biphosphoglycerate), decreases oxyhemoglobin affinity, shifting the curve to the right and thus allowing more oxygen to be released. In this way, tissue oxygenation is enhanced in the presence of decreased saturation and increased demand.

Change in the Pa_{CO2} and pH also cause shifts in the Hgb dissociation curve; this is termed the *Bohr effect.*[188,222] As blood perfuses through the lungs, carbon dioxide diffuses from the blood to the alveoli. As a result of this movement of carbon dioxide, the Pa_{CO2} is reduced, and there is a subsequent increase in pH. The Hgb dissociation curve shifts to the left, thus increasing the binding of Hgb to oxygen and allowing greater oxygen transport to the tissues. At the tissue level, however, carbon dioxide displaces oxygen from the hemoglobin. The Hgb dissociation curve shifts to the right at the tissue level, facilitating higher oxygen delivery to the tissues (opposite to what occurs in the lungs). Shifts in the oxygen–Hgb dissociation curve have greater effects on events in the tissues than in the lungs because the relationships in the lungs are described in the flat upper position of the curve.

The P_{50}, which is an index of right and left shifts of the dissociation curve, describes the Pa_{O2} at which Hgb is 50% saturated. A higher than normal P_{50} value indicates a lower than normal affinity for oxygen. Under normal conditions (37°C, pH 7.40, PCO_2 40 mm Hg, and normal Hgb), the P_{50} is 27 mm Hg.

Blood Oxygen Content

Blood oxygen content reflects the amount of oxygen dissolved in plasma ($0.0031 \times PO_2$) and the amount bound to Hgb ($1.36 \times \text{Hgb} \times Sa_{O2}$), where 1.36 is the maximum amount of oxygen carried by 1 gram of Hgb. This expression is depicted in the following equation:

$$\underbrace{\left(\text{Hgb} \times 1.36 \times Sa_{O2}\right)}_{97\%} + \underbrace{\left(0.0031 \times Pa_{O2}\right)}_{3\%}$$

Assuming a normal Hgb of 15 g, arterial Pa_{O2} equal to 100 mm Hg, and 98% saturation, the arterial oxygen content (Ca_{O2}) is 20 mL/dL. The equation can also be used to determine venous oxygen content (Cv_{O2}). Assuming no change in the Hgb and a venous Pa_{O2} of 40 mm Hg and 75% saturation, the venous oxygen content is 15 mL/dL.

Measurement of Oxygen Delivery

Measurement of oxygen delivery ($\dot{D}_{O2}$) or transport ($\dot{Q}_{O2}$) is calculated by multiplying total arterial oxygen content by cardiac output (CO):

$$\begin{aligned} \dot{D}_{O2} &= CO \times Ca_{O2} \times 10 \\ \text{where } Ca_{O2} &= (\text{Hgb} \times 1.36 \times Sa_{O2}) + (0.0031 \times Pa_{O2}) \\ &= CO \times \text{Hgb} \times Sa_{O2} \times 13.6 \end{aligned}$$

In patients with cardiac output of 5 L/min and a Ca_{O2} of 20 mL/dL, arterial oxygen delivery ($\dot{D}_{O2}$) is 1,000 mL of oxygen/min or on average 500 to 650 mL/min/m^2. Critical oxygen delivery, which reflects the point where oxygen delivery fails to satisfy metabolic needs for oxygen has not been definitively identified. Critical $\dot{D}_{O2}$ has been estimated to be less than 7 mL/kg/min in awake, healthy young adults and 330 mL/min/m^2 in anesthetized older adults.[223–225]

Delivery of oxygen to support aerobic metabolism can be limited anywhere along the route from the environment through the alveolar–pulmonary interface, the systemic circulation, and the capillary–tissue junction to the mitochondria. Hypoxia is the shortage of oxygen at the tissue level. Hypoxia can be classified as (1) hypoxic hypoxia, caused by a decreased PO_2; (2) anemic hypoxia, caused by decreased Hgb; (3) ischemic (stagnant) hypoxia, caused by a lack of blood flow to the tissue; and (4) histotoxic (cytopathic) hypoxia, normal oxygen delivery; however, the cell is unable to process the oxygen and produce ATP.

Oxygen Consumption

Oxygen consumption ($\dot{V}O_2$) is the body's demand for oxygen and is defined as the amount of oxygen consumed at the tissue level per minute. Oxygen consumption can be calculated by determining the difference between the quantity of oxygen carried by the arterial system to the tissues (Ca_{O2}) and the quantity remaining in the blood returning in the venous system to the lungs (Cv_{O2})[180]:

$$\begin{aligned} \dot{V}O_2 &= (CO \times Ca_{O2} \times 10) - (CO \times Cv_{O2} \times 10) \\ \dot{V}O_2 &= Ca_{O2} \times Cv_{O2} \end{aligned}$$

By combining the factors, the preceding can be simplified to the following equation:

$$\dot{V}O_2 = CO \times \text{Hgb} \times 13.6 \times (Sa_{O2} \times S\bar{v}_{O2})$$

This equation is a restatement of the Fick equation, placing $\dot{V}O_2$ on the left instead of cardiac output. This formula identifies all components of oxygen supply and demand. In a patient with normal values in a relatively steady state, normal $\dot{V}O_2$ is on average between 200 and 250 mL/min (or estimates of 3.5 mL/kg), as shown in the following equation:

$$\begin{aligned} \dot{V}O_2 &= 5 \text{ L/min} \times 15 \text{ g/dL} \times 13.6\ (0.98 - 0.75) \\ \dot{V}O_2 &= 234 \text{ mL/min} \end{aligned}$$

Oxygen consumption is affected by several factors. Blood flow depends on the cardiac output and on the degree of constriction of the vascular bed in the tissue (vasoregulatory mechanisms). Low Hgb decreases the amount of available oxygen to be delivered to the tissues. Reduced PaO_2 can affect the driving force needed to load the oxygen molecule on the Hgb. Decreased Sa_{O2} affects the affinity between oxygen and Hgb, enhancing the release of oxygen to the tissues. The metabolic rate of the tissues also affects the affinity of oxygen to be released.

Oxygen Extraction Ratio

The percentage of oxygen extracted by the tissues is a useful indicator of the balance between oxygen delivery and consumption. Oxygen extraction represents the difference between arterial and venous oxygen contents (normal 5 mL/dL or 25%) and is known as the $C(a\text{–}v)_{O_2}$ difference or oxygen extraction ratio (O_2ER). This ratio increases in pathologic conditions characterized by an imbalance between oxygen delivery and V_{O_2}. O_2ER is increased by factors such as decreased cardiac output, increased oxygen consumption (e.g., shivering), anemia, and decreased arterial oxygenation. O_2ER is decreased in conditions where V_{O_2} is relatively low in proportion to oxygen delivery, such as in sepsis, hypothermia, high-flow states, peripheral shunting, or cytopathic hypoxia.[213,220]

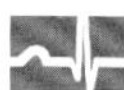

CONCLUSIONS

The systemic and pulmonary circulatory systems have evolved to provide the tissues of the body efficient oxygenation. Delivering exactly the amount of blood needed to meet each tissues requirement for oxygen and nutrients. This chapter has reviewed the network of the smallest vessels in the body and lymphatic vessels and delivery of oxygen.

CASE-BASED LEARNING 1

Sepsis and Microcirculation

Patient Profile

Mrs. Olsen is a 72-year-old female whom presents to the emergency room (ER) with complaints of intermittent nausea and vomiting, small volumes of emesis for 2 weeks, and 10/10 diffuse abdominal pain, getting worse instead of better. Her son became exceedingly concerned and brought her to the ER for further evaluation. She denies fever, chills, or night sweats. She reports anorexia but denies any weight loss. She denies syncope or near syncopal episodes. Denies chest pain, pressure, or palpitations, no dyspnea, cough, sputum, no hematemesis or hematochezia. Last bowel movement was loose, small volume, this morning. She denies dysuria, hematuria, urinary urgency or frequency.

Past Medical History

Gastroesophageal reflux
Hypertension
Abdominal aortic aneurysm
Cervical cancer in 2000

Past Surgical History

Appendectomy in 1988
Curative LEEP procedure 2000.

Family Medical History

Noncontributory

Social History

Former smoker, 45 pack-year history of smoking, quit 01/2012
Denies ETOH or other substance use
Retired librarian, married with 3 children, and 5 grandchildren

Medications

Lisinopril 10 mg daily
Pantoprazole 40 mg twice daily

Allergies

None

Patient Examination

Vital Signs

BP 221/126 mm Hg; PR 133 bmp; RR 26 rpm; Oxygen saturation on room air 94%; Wt. 56.2 kg; Temp 36.3°C

Physical Examination

General: Writhing in bed in obvious discomfort, complaining of severe pain and holding her abdomen. Accompanied by her son.

Neuro: Alert and oriented × 4, appropriately interacting with son and health care staff.

Skin: Warm, pale, poor turgor, and dry mucous membranes.

Cardiovascular: Normal S1, S2; tachycardic. RRR. No murmur, gallop, or rub.

Pulmonary: Clear to auscultation with diminished breath sounds in bilateral bases (unable to take a deep breath secondary to pain). Noted to be tachypneic.

Abdomen: Soft, nondistended with positive rebound tenderness, involuntary guarding, and hypoactive bowel sounds.

Extremities: Trace edema bilateral lower extremities.

Diagnostic Tests

Admission Labs

Complete Blood Count: White blood count of 33.3 K/uL, hemoglobin 15.9 gm/dL, hematocrit 49.7%, platelets 629 K/uL.

Chemistry Panel: Sodium 135 mmol/L, Potassium 3.1 mmol/L, Chloride 96 mmol/L, CO_2 23 mmol/L, Creatinine 2.5 mg/dL, BUN 30 mg/dL, Calcium 9.8 mg/dL, Magnesium of 1.8 mg/dL, Bilirubin Total 1.3 mg/dL, Alkaline phosphatase 228 U/L, AST 11 U/L, ALT 16 U/L, Lipase 107 U/L

Other Labs: Troponin I less than 0.02 ng/mL, Lactate 6.2 mmol/L

Coagulation Screen: aPTT 25 sec; PT 12 sec; INR 1.0; and Urine analysis negative.

ECG: Normal sinus rhythm, pulse rate: 116 bpm

Chest x-ray: Atelectasis bilateral bases. No acute cardiopulmonary findings

CT scan of abdomen/pelvis: Thoracic and infrarenal abdominal aneurysms, small bowel ischemia without pneumatosis, perforation or abscess.

Abdominal Angiogram: Occlusion of the superior mesenteric artery (SMA) and resulting bowel ischemia, trace pelvic free fluid, emphysema and probable small bilateral adrenal hemorrhages.

Assessment and Plan

1. Acute Superior Mesenteric Artery Occlusion and Mesenteric Ischemia. Emergent surgery planned for open thromboembolectomy of SMA.
2. Sepsis: As evidenced by lactic acid of 6.2 and leukocytosis with white blood cell count of 33 K/uL. Initiated on piperacillin/tazobactam 3.75 g.
3. Respiratory Distress: Monitor respiratory status closely.
4. Hypovolemia: Initiated on lactated ringers at 150 mL/h.
5. Hypertensive: Single dose of hydralazine 50 mg, intravenous, given in Emergency Room
6. Acute Kidney Injury: As evidenced by BUN 30 mg/dL and creatinine of 2.5 mg/dL. Underlying contributors may be hypoperfusion of kidneys due to hypovolemia and hemodynamic compromise.

CASE-BASED LEARNING 1 (*Continued*)

Sepsis and Microcirculation

Clinical Course

Intraoperative Assessment and Operation

Open laparotomy with thromboembolectomy of SMA and wound vacuum placement for an open abdomen secondary to diffuse soft tissue edema. Following surgery, perfusion to the bowels was noted to be improved.

Postoperative Course

Transferred to the intensive care unit (ICU) where she remained intubated, due to the following ABG values: pH 7.20; Pco_2 28; PO_2 104; HCO_3 20; Base Deficit 16; and her hypotensive state with blood pressure of 77/50 mm Hg that required blood pressure support with vasopressin and norepinephrine infusions. Hypoglycemia was also noted and felt to be secondary to septic shock.

While in the ICU she was started on famotidine 20 mg daily, continued on piperacillin-tazobactam 3.75 g, infusions of sodium bicarbonate 100 mEq and lactated Ringer's intravenous fluids for hydration, midazolam and fentanyl drips for sedation. Norepinephrine and vasopressin for blood pressure support continued, however, her blood pressure continued to decline, and epinephrine infusion was initiated.

Return to Operating Room

Approximately 12 hours after her first surgery, she returned to the operating room for a second look due to her worsening condition and open abdomen. At this time, she underwent small bowel resection, subtotal colectomy, and cholecystectomy secondary to gross abdominal organ ischemia.

Postoperative Day 1

In the ICU her condition continued to deteriorate despite supportive care. She remained intubated, with increasing ventilation and oxygenation requirements on 80% oxygen, developed worsening acidosis (pH 7.11; Pco_2 48; PO_2 88; HCO_3 11; Base Excess 14) on bicarbonate infusion. Mrs. Olsen continued in a hypotensive state (average blood pressures of 80/63 mm Hg) despite maximization of all vasoactive support medications. Her pulses were nonpalpable and absent by Doppler in the lower extremities but were appreciated by Doppler in the upper extremities, subsequently her skin became cold and mottled, with worsening turgor and dry, cracking mucous membranes. She developed acute renal failure (ARF) and anuria (BUN 43 mg/dL; creatinine 3.31 mg/dL) and was diagnosed with septic shock.

Diagnostic and Clinical Considerations

Incidence and Characteristics of Sepsis

Severe sepsis and septic shock are common and fatal complications for patients with chronic illness and acute organ dysfunction secondary to infection.[158] The incidence of severe sepsis and septic shock in adults ranges from 56 to 91 per 100,000 population per year.[159] Sepsis can be defined as a life-threatening organ dysfunction caused by a dysregulated host response to infection.[160] Septic shock, a subset of sepsis, where particularly profound circulatory, cellular, and metabolic abnormalities occur. Alterations related to septic shock include some degree of hypovolemia, a decrease in vascular tone, myocardial depression, and characterized by hemodynamic changes that are associated with a greater risk of mortality than with sepsis alone.[161]

Criteria for Septic Shock

Patients with septic shock are clinically identified by vasopressor requirements to maintain a mean arterial pressure of 65 mm Hg or greater and serum lactate level greater than 2 mmol/L (greater than 18 mg/dL) in the absence of hypovolemia.[160] Mrs. Olsen met this criteria for sepsis when she presented to the ER in a state of hypovolemia with a lactate level of 6.2 mmol/L despite intravenous hydration with 1 L of lactated ringers. Given that she had taken very little by mouth in the recent days and the underlying conditions of sepsis, she developed hypovolemia. Her clinical condition continued to decline, and she developed septic shock intraoperatively, as evidenced by the need for vasopressin, norepinephrine, and epinephrine drips to maintain her blood pressure with a mean arterial pressure greater than 65 mm Hg.

Pathogenesis and Pathophysiology of Septic Shock

The pathophysiology of sepsis involves a complex interaction of proinflammatory and anti-inflammatory mediators in response to pathogen invasion. This often involves a gram-positive bacteria[162] in concert with major modifications of the nonimmunologic pathways like the cardiovascular, neuronal, autonomic, hormonal, bioenergetic, metabolic, and coagulation pathways.[158,163,164] These significant contributors to this pathologic condition and physiologic interactions lead to endothelial damage, vascular permeability, microvascular dysfunction, coagulation pathway activation and impaired tissue oxygenation that result in sepsis. These pathophysiologic changes manifest as vasoplegic shock (distributive shock), myocardial depression, altered microvascular flow and diffuse injury to the endothelium.[165] The management of sepsis is primarily directed toward these changes.

Bacteria-Mediated Endothelium Dysfunction and Hypotension

An inflammatory stimulus, such as a bacteria toxin, triggers the production of proinflammatory mediators that launch a cascade of other mediators. The bacteria toxin or microbial agent causes microbial injury to the microcirculation through direct invasion of the endothelial cells or indirectly via attack by their byproducts leading to damage of the microvascular endothelium.[166] This damage results in endothelial dysfunction and sepsis with a decreased sensitivity to vasoconstricting and vasodilating agents.[167] This cascade of events triggered by bacteria toxin and the development of sepsis were evident in Mrs. Olsen's on postoperative day one. This was evidenced by her requirement for escalating doses of vasopressin, norepinephrine and addition of epinephrine to maintain support for hypotensive blood pressures ranging from 55/23 to 111/72 mm Hg, despite maximum support.

Compromised Microcirculation and Tissue Perfusion

The microcirculation, is comprised of the smallest blood vessels, precapillary arterioles, capillaries, and postcapillary venules. These small vessels are embedded in the body's organs and regulate their blood flow, tissue perfusion and oxygenation, blood pressure, and tissue temperature.[166] Damage to the endothelium of the microcirculation negatively impacts blood–tissue exchange and the regulation of blood flow, tissue perfusion, oxygenation, blood pressure and thermal regulation of tissues, all of which are witnessed in Mrs. Olsen's clinical course.[166,168,169]

Inflammatory Response Mediators

The inflammatory response of sepsis is exacerbated by inflammatory mediators (complement, cytokines, chemokines, adhesion molecules, inducible cyclooxygenase 2, and nitric oxide synthase metabolites) that the body manufactures. These inflammatory mediators inflict further damage to an already aggravated microvascular endothelium.[166] These changes

(*continued*)

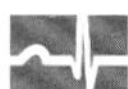

CASE-BASED LEARNING 1 (*Continued*)

Sepsis and Microcirculation

to the microcirculation culminate in a lethal insult upon the endothelial cells of the microvascular endothelium, through programmed cellular death (apoptosis) of the endothelial cells that have detached from the extracellular matrix.[166,170]

The physiologic changes, discussed thus far, may result in global tissue hypoxia, pan endothelial cell injury, activation of the coagulation cascade, and microcirculatory and mitochondrial distress syndrome.[171] Although it is the global hemodynamic profile of the macrovascular (heart, aorta, large arteries, main arterial branches, small arteries) bed that clinical management of septic shock is directed at, it is the microcirculation (arterioles; terminal arterioles, capillaries, postcapillary venules) that delivers blood from the macrocirculation to the tissue.[171] Alterations in this blood flow are attributed to altered local perfusion pressures in the microcirculation from distributive shock, endothelial cell dysfunction, increased leukocyte adhesion, microthrombi, rheologic abnormalities, and functional shunting.[172–175] The impairment in this flow has been shown to alter capillary oxygen extraction. These changes were notable when Mrs. Olsen returned from the operating room with cold mottled skin, loss of peripheral pulses, and increased ventilation and oxygen requirements.[176]

In the early stages of sepsis, the body's compensatory mechanisms may be stimulated and proinflammatory mediators are opposed by anti-inflammatory mediators, resulting in a negative feedback mechanism.[166] The initial response in this compensatory process causes arteries and arterioles to dilate which decreases the peripheral arterial resistance and cardiac output increases. On initial presentation Mrs. Olsen was likely experiencing an increased cardiac output as noted by the hypertension and rapid heart rate in the ER. Later, as sepsis progresses and cardiac output decreases, blood pressure falls. This phenomenon is noted during Mrs. Olsen's first surgery in her clinical appearance and onset of shock where her blood pressures were trending in the wrong direction (55/23 to 147/93 mm Hg) with pulse rate of 106 to 152 bpm and necessitated vasopressor medication support. Such hypotension, in the setting of sepsis, reflects the endothelial instability and dysfunction, manifested by the hyporesponsiveness to catecholamines.[177,178]

Profound hypotension, as experienced by Mrs. Olsen, leads to subsequent hypoprofusion and tissue dysfunction and organ failure in one or more organs. The prodrome of this organ dysfunction, due to hypoperfusion, can cause additional signs and symptoms specific to the organ involved such as gastric upset, nausea, vomiting, as seen in Mrs. Olsen. In this case, this perfusion compromise progressed and worsened, resulting in severe ischemia and clot formation in Mrs. Olsen's SMA and subsequent necrosis of other organs including her gallbladder, small bowel, and colon necessitating surgical excision of these organs in her second visit to the operating room.

Heterogeneity of Blood Flow in the Setting of Infection
The inflammatory response to infection also results in a complex hemodynamic situation known as the heterogeneity of blood flow, where vasodilation and vasoconstriction occur in tandem.[175] Compared to normal conditions in which there is a dense network of capillaries that are mostly perfused, sepsis causes a decrease in that capillary density. Sepsis is also accompanied by an increase in heterogeneity of perfusion. This heterogeneity reflects the presence of capillaries that are either intermittently perfused or have no perfusion and in close proximity to well perfused capillaries.[179] This dysregulated response effects the microcirculatory blood flow, and is one of the critical pathogenic events in sepsis and the major contributor to multiorgan failure,[179,180] as presented in Mrs. Olsen's case.

Experimental conditions have exhibited microvascular impairment that has been linked to signs of tissue hypoxia, localization of low PO_2, production of hypoxia inducible factor, and hypoperfused vessels.[181,182] The clinical presentation of such phenomena are absent peripheral pulses and mottled skin as seen in Mrs. Olsen's on postoperative day one, suggesting that the altered perfusion leads to altered tissue oxygenation.[181] Additionally, oxygen saturation at the capillary end of well-perfused capillaries is low, suggesting that the tissues are using the delivered oxygen.[167] Tissue perfusion is determined by vascular density and flow. In normal healthy conditions, the microcirculation is responsible for the fine tuning of perfusion to meet the local oxygen demands. This is achieved by mobilizing and demobilizing capillaries, shutting down and or limiting flow in capillaries that are perfusing areas with low oxygen requirements and increasing flow in areas with high oxygen requirements.[167] This normal function was eventually unable to compensate and resulted in the development of Mrs. Olsen's septic shock. Multiple organs and systems were compromised including her kidneys, lungs, and vessels.

An overwhelming infection that causes damage to the microcirculation can compromise of the function of multiple organs including the heart, lungs, liver, intestines, kidneys, and brain. This compromise leads to hypotension, myocardial dysfunction, microvascular leak, thrombocytopenia with or without disseminated intravascular coagulation, acute respiratory distress syndrome, acute kidney injury and/or acute brain injury. The common denominator for this multiorgan failure is hypothesized to be a perfusion-mediated phenomenon.[183–186]

Unfortunately, this condition contributed to Mrs. Olsen's suffering hypoperfusion of the myocardium, as evidenced by ECG changes consistent with ST elevation myocardial infarction (STEMI) that later deteriorated to asystole.

Conventional cardiovascular support measures, such as vasopressors, red blood cell transfusions, inotropic medications, and fluids, are aimed at achieving restoration of an acceptable arterial blood pressure in a septic shock patient, however, these interventions have a temporal limitation and often lead to persistent microcirculatory changes even after resuscitation.[187] Further decompensation occurs that may be irreversible. This was evidenced during the hours in between surgeries that Mrs. Olsen spent in the ICU and following the second surgery. She required large volumes of crystalloid fluid, multiple vasopressors to achieve minimally acceptable blood pressure with altered tissue perfusion. Nonetheless, fluids appear to improve the microcirculation in the early phase of sepsis as seen initially in the ER and operating room, although the magnitude of this effect varies largely from patient-to-patient. The ability to maintain sufficient perfusion pressure positively influences the microcirculation.[187]

Case Summary

The signs and symptoms of sepsis are highly variable and may be mistaken for manifestations of other disorders such as delirium, or pulmonary embolism. Typically, patients have fever, tachycardia, diaphoresis and tachypnea and blood pressure remains normal. Other signs of infection such as fever, chills, and extreme weakness, may be present.[166] In this

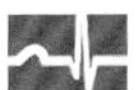

CASE-BASED LEARNING 1 *(Continued)*

Sepsis and Microcirculation

case, Mrs. Olsen presented with only tachycardia despite an otherwise critically ill appearance. A clinical diagnosis is often made before culture results are available, such as in this case presentation, relying on historical, clinical, and laboratory findings that are indicative of infection and/or organ dysfunction. As sepsis worsens or septic shock develops, blood pressure decreases (noted intraoperatively) resulting in the need for vasopressors. Initially, the skin may remain warm, later the extremities become cool and pale with peripheral cyanosis and mottling, noted during Mrs. Olsen's final hours.

As discussed, the impairments and severity of microvascular changes may directly impair tissue oxygenation and is associated with organ dysfunction and mortality in sepsis.[168] Less than 48 hours after her admission to the hospital Mrs. Olsen ultimately experienced severe hypotension that was unresponsive to vasoactive support. Additionally, she suffered myocardial dysfunction secondary to severe hypoperfusion of her tissues, including her myocardium, that resulted in an ST elevation myocardial infarction with further decompensation, and asystole unresponsive to resuscitation efforts.

The discussion in this chapter and case-based content illustrates that sepsis can lead to a constellation of changes to the microcirculation that if not reversed, may result in a significant cascade of consequences and deleterious outcomes.

LEEP, loop extrasurgical excision procedure; ETOH, alcohol; rpm, respirations per minute; RRR, regular rate and rhythm; BUN, blood urea nitrogen; AST, aspertate aminotransferase; ALT, alanine transaminase; aPTT, activated partial prothromboplastin time; PT, prothrombin time; INR, international normalized ratio; ICU, intensive care unit; ER, emergency room.

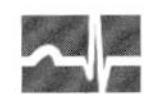

CASE-BASED LEARNING 2

Acute Respiratory Distress Syndrome and Impaired Gas Exchange

Patient Profile

History of Present Illness

Mr. Martinez is a 56-year-old Hispanic male with a 35 pack-year history of smoking and recent diagnosis of stage IIIB adenocarcinoma of the lung. He is admitted to the hospital for planned surgical resection of the left lower lobe following treatment with neoadjuvant chemotherapy and radiotherapy that were completed 1 month ago. On admit he states he is "feeling good and not as tired." He denies any residual complications from chemotherapy or radiation, no fever, chills, or night sweats. States his appetite has returned and he has re-gained 14 lb that he lost with chemotherapy. He denies syncope, chest pain, pressure, or palpitations. He states his shortness of breath is at baseline, he is usually able to walk 1 to 2 blocks before feeling fatigued, then needs to slow down or rest for 5 to 10 minutes before continuing. He endorses a productive cough, "the same stuff I usually cough up," a teaspoon size volume of slightly yellow-tinged mucus each morning with occasional streaks of bright red blood (felt to be related to lung cancer). He denies hematemesis or hematochezia. No bright red blood per rectum or changes in bowel function. He denies urinary urgency, frequency, hematuria, or dysuria.

Mr. Martinez underwent a surgical resection of the left lower lobe (lobectomy) for adenocarcinoma of the lung. Intraoperatively he was hypotensive and received 4 L of crystalloid fluids and 2 units of packed red blood cells with good response. He was breathing spontaneously, extubated and transferred to the post anesthesia care unit, followed by the surgical ward without incident in stable condition, with normal vital signs on 4-L nasal cannula.

Twenty-four hours following surgery he developed dyspnea and hypoxemia complaining of "not getting enough air" and demonstrated signs of air hunger that necessitated transfer to the intensive care unit (ICU).

Past Medical History

Adenocarcinoma of the lung, stage IIIb
Hypertension (HTN)
Hypercholesterolemia
Obstructive sleep apnea
Gout

Past Surgical History

Noncontributory

Family History

Mother: Alive, 77 years old with type 2 diabetes, obstructive sleep apnea, morbid obesity, HTN, hypercholesterolemia
Father: Deceased at 66 years old of acute coronary event, diabetes, hypercholesterolemia, former smoker
Brother: Alive, 54 years old with history of colon cancer, HTN, type 2 diabetes

Social History

35 pack-year history of smoking, current 1 pack per day
Consumes approximately 4 to 6 beers per day
Married to Alicia and father of 3 boys, works as a concrete laborer

Home Medication

Benazepril hydrochloride 20 mg daily
Furosemide 20 mg daily
Atorvastatin 40 mg daily

Allergies

None

Patient Examination

Preoperative Diagnostic Tests

Complete blood count: Within normal limits
Chemistry panel: Within normal limits
ECG: Normal sinus rhythm, pulse rate 77 bpm, occasional preventricular contractions (no evidence suggestive of coronary events)
Pulmonary Function Tests: Forced Expiratory Volume in 1 second (FEV1) was 1.69 L, 56% of the predicted value; calculated postoperative FEV1 was 46% of the predicted value

Physical Exam on Admission to ICU

Vital signs: BP 102/66; PR 133 bpm; RR 33/min; Oxygen saturation (SaO_2) of 86% on 100% nonrebreather; Wt. 112 kg; Temp 37.6°C

General: Sitting in bed, upright, in obvious distress, heaving chest rise and fall, speaking in one-word utterances.

Neuro: A&O X4, appropriate, nodding yes or no to questions

(continued)

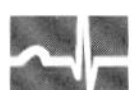

CASE-BASED LEARNING 2 (*Continued*)

Acute Respiratory Distress Syndrome and Impaired Gas Exchange

Skin: Warm, dry, moist mucous membranes.

Cardiovascular: Normal S1/S2, tachycardic, soft systolic mummer, no gallop or rub.

Respiratory: Shallow, decreased breath sounds over left lower lung field, diffuse inspiratory crackles throughout remaining fields, tachypneic with use of accessory muscles.

Abdomen: Soft, nondistended, nontender, bowel sounds present.

Extremities: Warm, dry, palpable pulses, 1 + pitting bilateral lower extremity edema.

ICU Labs and Diagnostic Tests

Complete blood count: Within normal limits

Chemistry panel: Within normal limits

Bronchoalveolar lavage and blood sent for microbiology analysis

Blood cultures: Results pending

Chest x-ray: Bilateral patchy infiltrates

Transthoracic echocardiography: Ejection fraction 60%, normal left ventricular systolic function. Mild right ventricular dilation.

Right Heart Data via Central Line: Cardiac output (CO): 7.74 L/min (normal 5–7 L/min)

Cardiac Index (CI): 4.8 L/min/m^2 (normal 3–5 L/min/m^2)

CVP: 8 mm Hg S (normal 3–8 mm Hg),

Pulmonary Artery Wedge Pressure: 11 mm Hg (normal 6–12 mm Hg)

Clinical Course

Postoperative Days Two and Three

His respiratory status continued to deteriorate, due to these ABG findings (pH 7.26; Pa_{O_2} 58 mm Hg; Pa_{CO_2} 52 mm Hg; and HCO_3 20 mmol/L) he was reintubated for continued monitoring and management and placed on volume control mechanical ventilation with settings of F_{IO_2} 0.06; V_T 450 mL; RR 18; PEEP 10 cm H_2O; V_E: 8 L/min.
Arterial Blood Gas Post Intubation: (F_{IO_2} 0.60) pH 7.28; Pa_{O_2} 60 mm Hg; Pa_{CO_2} 49 mm Hg; HCO_3 24 mmol/L; Pa_{O_2}/F_{IO_2} 117
Chest x-ray Post Intubation: Patchy infiltrates persist. ETT 1 cm below carina.
Additional supportive therapy included empiric broad-spectrum antibiotics and restrictive fluid management.

Postoperative Day Four

Due to further impairment of oxygenation saturations (Sa_{O2} less than 80%) that did not improve with an increase in positive end-expiratory pressure (PEEP) and increasing F_{IO2}, Mr. Martinez was placed on high-frequency oscillatory ventilation and diagnosed with acute respiratory distress syndrome (ARDS) based on radiographic findings, hypoxemia and acute onset of respiratory distress; all consistent with criteria for ARDS.

Clinical Considerations

Incidence of Acute Respiratory Distress Syndrome

Acute respiratory distress syndrome is a life-threatening form of respiratory failure that is the result of an acute alveolar injury. More than 3 million patients present with ARDS annually, representing 10% of ICU admissions.[226] Supportive care, including mechanical ventilation, aimed at reducing ventilator-induced lung injury remains the mainstay of therapy.[227]

The Berlin Definition

Acute respiratory distress syndrome is defined as an acute-onset, progressive, hypoxic condition characterized by bilateral lung infiltration on chest x-ray or computed tomography.[228] In 2011 a panel of experts developed the Berlin Definition. The Berlin Definition defines the clinical criteria for ARDS. Adult acute respiratory distress syndrome is represented by the following clinical findings[229]:

- Acute diffuse inflammatory lung injury
- Increased pulmonary vascular permeability
- Increased lung weight
- Loss of aerated lung tissue
- Hypoxemia
- Bilateral radiographic opacities
- Increased venous admixture (right-to-left shunt)
- Increased physiologic dead space
- Decreased lung compliance

Diagnosis of ARDS by the Berlin Definition also requires a minimum level of PEEP and mutually exclusive Pa_{O2}/F_{IO2} thresholds to differentiate between levels of severity based on degrees of hypoxemia[226,229]:

- Mild: 200 mm Hg < Pa_{O2}/F_{IO2} ≤300 mm Hg with PEEP or CPAP ≥5 cm H_2O
- Moderate: 100 mm Hg < Pa_{O2}/F_{IO2} ≤200 mm Hg with PEEP ≥5 cm H_2O
- Severe:
  - Pa_{O2}/F_{IO2} ≤100 mm Hg with PEEP ≥5 cm H_2O
  - Radiographic severity, respiratory system compliance (≤40 mL/cm H_2O)
  - PEEP (≥10 cm H_2O)
  - Corrected expired volume per minute (≥10 L/min)

Characteristics of Acute Respiratory Distress Syndrome

This life-threatening condition can be caused by a variety of pulmonary (pneumonia, aspiration, pulmonary contusion, pulmonary embolism, inhalational injury) or nonpulmonary (sepsis, pancreatitis, trauma, burns, multiple blood transfusions, shock) insults, leading to the development of nonhydrostatic pulmonary edema.[226,230,231] It appears that Mr. Martinez's respiratory difficulty developed as a result of the surgical trauma he encountered, although the possibility of pneumonia or festering sepsis cannot be ruled out and should remain high in the differential diagnosis. Alcohol abuse and smoking have also been implicated in the development of ARDS and may have contributed to his condition.[230]

Clinical Presentation of Acute Respiratory Distress Syndrome

The clinical presentation of ARDS is characterized by dyspnea, tachypnea, hypoxemia, and rapid progression to acute respiratory failure with poor lung compliance.[232] This is evidenced by Mr. Martinez's complaints that "I'm having difficulty taking in a breath, I feel like I'm being smothered," prior to his transfer to the ICU and reintubation. He exhibited tachypnea with a respiratory rate of 36/min, persistent hypoxemia (Sa_{O2} 86% on a nonrebreather) despite administration of high concentrations of inspired oxygen. Physiologically, this clinical scenario leads to an increase in shunt, decrease in pulmonary compliance and increase in the dead space ventilation; all contributing to his worsening overall clinical condition.[231]

In addition to his hypoxemia he demonstrated bilateral opacities on chest x-ray within 24 hours of his surgery,

CASE-BASED LEARNING 2 (*Continued*)

Acute Respiratory Distress Syndrome and Impaired Gas Exchange

necessitating his transfer to the ICU for increased ventilatory and oxygenation support via intubation with continued paralysis and sedation to reduce oxygen requirements. Mr. Martinez's presentation is classic for the development of the acute phase of ARDS. This likely occurred as a direct result of surgical insult to the lung cells and an indirect activation of local acute systemic inflammatory response.[233] These events resulted in the combination of pulmonary edema, hyaline membrane formation, loss of surfactant leading to hypoxemia, decreased lung compliance, poor air exchange, and pulmonary hypertension.[233–236] Given this scenario and clinical findings, Mr. Martinez met the Berlin Definition for diagnosis of ARDS.

Pathophysiology of Acute Respiratory Distress Syndrome
When Mr. Martinez sustained surgical trauma to his lung, a cascade of pathophysiologic events occurred that are consistent with compromised tissue perfusion and oxygenation leading to ARDS. This injury to the alveoli results in the release of proinflammatory cytokines, tumor necrosis factor, and interleukin (IL-1, IL-6, IL-8), which recruit neutrophils to the lungs where they become activated and release toxic mediators (reactive oxygen species and proteases) that damage the capillary endothelium and alveolar epithelium leading to alveolar edema.[234] This damage eventually leads to impairment of gas exchange, decreased lung compliance, and increased pulmonary arterial pressure.[237]

Mr. Martinez experienced these pathophysiologic changes which ultimately led to the accumulation of fluid in the epithelium and capillary endothelium of the alveoli, aka pulmonary edema, as evidenced on his chest x-ray.

Initially this exudative phase of ARDS, occurs within the first few days of the initial insult and is associated with diffuse alveolar damage.[232] The exudative/acute phase is followed by a proliferative stage within 72 hours of onset of symptoms, and can last for a week or more.[232] It is characterized by the proliferation of type II pneumocytes, fibroblasts, myofibroblasts, and repair of the epithelial and endothelial barriers.[235,238] If an improvement in pulmonary edema occurs it is likely due to repair of the epithelium in the setting of successful migration, proliferation, and differentiation of type II epithelial cells and their ability to repopulate the stripped basement membrane.[238] This may result in resolution of pulmonary edema and contribute to recovery in some cases. This process, if it occurs, is a gradual one, with resolution of hypoxemia, improved lung compliance and resolving radiographic abnormalities that occurs over many months.[234]

Clinical Course Interim Summary
Mr. Martinez continued to suffer respiratory complications requiring oscillatory ventilation for 2 weeks with minimal radiographic improvement. His recovery was slow but demonstrated steady resolution of hypoxemia with reduction in ventilatory requirements. With continued improvement over 3 weeks he passed spontaneous breathing trials and met criteria for extubation. He continued to improve over 2 additional weeks on the surgical ward and discharged to a skilled nursing facility.

Clinical Review

Consequences of Lung Injury and Development of Pulmonary Edema
During normal function, the endothelial and epithelial permeability is dynamically maintained via inter- and intracellular molecules, an interruption in this may result in increased vascular permeability to water.[239] Damage between the capillaries and alveoli is limited due to multiple barriers, such as the endothelial and epithelial cell layers—where water is actively regulated via the basement membrane, and the extracellular matrix.[239]

In normal and stable physiologic conditions, the lungs are protected from pulmonary edema by the pulmonary lymphatic system and epithelial water channels that are responsible for transporting water out of the extracellular space.[239] When vascular leakage overcomes the system, clinical pulmonary edema ensues. In the initial 12 to 24 hours postoperative, Mr. Martinez's pulmonary circulation and lymphatics were aggressively attempting to maintain this fluid balance. Ultimately, the lymphatics were unable to maintain balance, leading to the respiratory distress Mr. Martinez experienced.

Tissue injury and altered architecture result in damage to these layers leading to blood components leaking from the capillaries to the alveoli.[239] Edema is the accumulation of protein-rich fluid inside the alveoli and capillary endothelium; this causes the release of cytokines that result in wide spread alveolar damage.[240] The ability of the lung to perform gas exchange is made possible in part by the relationship between the alveolar epithelium and the endothelium of the pulmonary microvasculature.[231,241] When this normally existing barrier becomes compromised, in the setting of surgical trauma and Mr. Martinez's case, alveolar damage occurs and dysfunction between the endothelial–epithelial layers contributes to the development of ARDS.[231,237]

Increased pulmonary microvascular permeability is at the core of the pathophysiology of ARDS. Orbegozo et al. suggest that microvascular endothelial dysfunction is present in the earliest stages and is correlated with its severity.[242] It is characterized by an increased permeability of the pulmonary capillary and alveolar epithelial cells. Under normal physiologic conditions, the pressure in the microvasculature of the lung bases is higher than near the apex. This increase in hydrostatic pressure favors fluid filtration. An increase in the permeability of the microvascular bed ultimately leads to hypoxemia. In Mr. Martinez's case the hypoxemia was refractory to normal oxygen therapy, requiring escalating percentages of oxygen, up to a F_{IO_2} of 1.00 (100%) and PEEP of 15 mm Hg to maintain his saturations. This in part explains why Mr. Martinez rapidly decompensated following surgery.

Explaining Respiratory Compromise
Hypoxemia is a central component of ARDS and is mainly due to intrapulmonary shunt, where increased alveolar dead space determines the alteration of CO_2 clearance.[243] Gas exchange remains one of the main physiologic abnormalities in ARDS; understanding these factors will assist the clinician in the management of ARDS.

Traditionally, the increase in lung weight, that is, pulmonary edema and intrapleural pressure, raises the hydrostatic pressure transmitted throughout the lung, reducing the lung gas volume and promoting the development of nonaerated regions (consolidated or atelectatic regions).[244] These regions develop into areas without ventilation yet maintain intact perfusion, mostly affecting the more dependent lung regions, and is known as intrapulmonary shunt.[245] This right-to left shunt reduces

(*continued*)

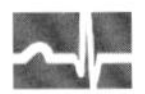

CASE-BASED LEARNING 2 *(Continued)*

Acute Respiratory Distress Syndrome and Impaired Gas Exchange

systemic arterial oxygen tension and concentrations due to the cardiac output being shunted, resulting in a ventilation-to-perfusion $\dot{V}/\dot{Q}$ ratio equal to zero. Post-operatively, due to inadequate pain control, Mr. Martinez remained largely recumbent, requiring large amounts of encouragement from staff to turn, sit up at the bedside, and use the incentive spirometer. These confounding factors all contributed to the atelectatic lung regions that were already insulted from surgical trauma and anesthesia.

Optimal and Impaired Gas Exchange

Optimal gas exchange between the alveoli and capillary depends on matching ventilation and perfusion. When a mismatch occurs, the microvasculature will constrict to minimize the ventilation-to-perfusion imbalance by diverting blood to areas with improved ventilation as an attempt to restore normal function. This is referred to as hypoxic vasoconstriction. The concept of alveolar $\dot{V}/\dot{Q}$ ratio implies that an optimal ratio exists and is necessary to obtain gas exchange under normal physiologic circumstances.[243] Ideally, the 4 L/min of alveolar ventilation is matched to 5 L/min of capillary blood flow in the lungs and this results in a normal alveolar $\dot{V}/\dot{Q}$ ratio. An imbalance in this ratio is one of the explanations of abnormal gas exchange seen in ARDS. Low $\dot{V}/\dot{Q}$ ratios are those areas where perfusion exceeds ventilation and leads to hypoxemia. This was experienced by Mr. Martinez on post-op day one, secondary to his limited physical activity and reduced respiratory effort, with oxygen saturation levels initially in the low 90s then deteriorating to the mid 80s. This deterioration necessitated an increased delivery of oxygen by increasing the flow of a nasal cannula, progressing to a nonrebreather face mask, and finally intubation to treat the hypoxemia. Consequently, a high $\dot{V}/\dot{Q}$ ratio, as in lung regions where ventilation exceeds perfusion, results in an increase in physiologic dead space in which the alveolar unit is ventilated but not perfused.[246,247]

Delivery of Oxygen

As noted in the core content of this chapter, under normal physiologic conditions, increases in oxygen utilization or consumption like during exercise, are met by an increase in cardiac output and oxygen extraction with increased ventilation and subsequent increase in oxygen uptake. This results in a widened gap between the arterial-mixed venous oxygen content. This relationship is represented by the Fick equation: cardiac output equals oxygen consumption $\dot{V}O_2$ divided by the arterial-mixed venous oxygen content difference [C (a – V)O_2] and can be measured with direct measurement of the $\dot{V}O_2$.[248] In the setting of fever, sepsis and acidosis, such as Mr. Martinez's case prior to intubation, this relationship can be considered via the Oxyhemoglobin Dissociation Curve. A left shift occurs in states of alkalosis, or hypothermia, oxygen has a higher affinity for hemoglobin. A patient's Sa_{O2} will increase at a given Pa_{O2}, but more of it will stay bound to hemoglobin and be transported back to the lungs unused. This may result in tissue hypoxia despite adequate oxygen in the blood. Conversely, states of acidosis and fever, result in a rightward shift of the curve. Oxygen is released more readily in the blood due to a lower affinity for hemoglobin. This results in more oxygen being released from to the cells, however, initially less oxygen is carried from the lungs.

Mr. Martinez's postintubation ABG reflected a pH 7.28; $Pa{O_2}$ 60 mm Hg; $Pa{CO_2}$ 49; HCO_3 24; and a $Pa{O_2}/Fi{O_2}$ 117; these values demonstrate hypoxemic respiratory failure likely due to a $\dot{V}/\dot{Q}$ mismatch, shunt, and or diffusion problem. In patients with ARDS, the pulmonary causes leading to impaired gas exchange are almost solely related to mismatched $\dot{V}/\dot{Q}$.[221,244,246,247] Hypoxemia is a result of increased physiologic shunt compared to total pulmonary blood flow originating from right-to-left shunt. Due to its simplicity, the ratio of Pa_{O2}/Fi_{O2} is used to characterize the severity of ARDS and is used as indices to characterize hypoxemia.[229] Based on the Berlin definition of ARDS, the Pa_{O2}/Fi_{O2} of 117 placed Mr. Martinez in the moderate to severe category that carried a significant risk of mortality. Fortunately, his condition was turned around and he recovered from the surgical insult and cascade of pathologic events that followed.

Case Summary

During times of normal physiologic functioning, the lungs regulate movement of fluid in the interstitium and alveoli via the microcirculation, as presented in the core content of the chapter. When the integrity of the tissue becomes compromised from insult, fluid accumulates in the interstitium and alveoli and gas exchange is disrupted. This impairs gas exchange and compliance and may result in acute respiratory distress syndrome.

KEY READINGS

Hawiger J, Veach RA, Zienkiewicz J. New paradigms in sepsis: from prevention to protection of failing microcirculation. *J Thromb Haemost.* 2015;13(10):1743–1756.

Trzeciak S, Cinel I, Phillip Dellinger R, et al. Resuscitating the microcirculation in sepsis: the central role of nitric oxide, emerging concepts for novel therapies, and challenges for clinical trials. *Acad Emerg Med.* 2008;15(5):399–413.

West JB, Luks AM. *West's Respiratory Physiology: The Essentials.* 10th ed. Philadelphia, PA: Wolters Kluwer Health; 2016:42.

REFERENCES

1. Wiedeman M. Dimensions of blood vessels from distributing artery to collecting vein. *Circ Res.* 1963;12:375–378.
2. Rothe C. Venous system: physiology of the capacitance vessels. In: Abbound JSF, ed. *Handbook of Physiology. The Cardiovascular System. Peripheral Circulation and Organ Blood Flow.* Bethesda, MD: American Physiological Society; 1983:397–452.
3. Rhodin J. Architecture of the vessel wall. In: Bohr DF, Somlyo AP, Sparks HV, eds. *Handbook of Physiology.* Bethesda, MD: American Physiological Society; 1980:1–31.
4. Rhodin J. Anatomy of the microcirculation. In: Effros RM, Schonbein-Schmid H, Ditzel J, eds. *Microcirculation.* New York: Academic Press; 1981:11–17.
5. Klabunde RE. *Cardiovascular Physiology Concepts.* 2nd ed. Philadelphia, PA: Wolters Kluwer/Lippincott Williams & Wilkins; 2012.
6. Dalton SR, Fillman EP, Ferringer T, et al. Smooth muscle pattern is more reliable than the presence or absence of an internal elastic lamina in distinguishing an artery from a vein. *J Cutan Pathol.* 2006;33(3):216–219.
7. O'Rourke MF. Arterial aging: pathophysiological principles. *Vasc Med.* 2007;12(4):329–341.
8. Mulvany MJ, Aalkjaer C. Structure and function of small arteries. *Physiol Rev.* 1990;70(4):921–961.

9. Mulvany MJ. The Seventh Heymans Memorial Lecture Ghent, February 18, 1995. Physiological aspects of small arteries. *Arch Int Pharmacodyn Ther*. 1996;331(1):1–31.
10. Faber JE. In situ analysis of alpha-adrenoceptors on arteriolar and venular smooth muscle in rat skeletal muscle microcirculation. *Circ Res*. 1988;62(1):37–50.
11. Rizzoni D, Porteri E, Boari GE, et al. Prognostic significance of small-artery structure in hypertension. *Circulation*. 2003;108(18):2230–2235.
12. De Ciuceis C, Porteri E, Rizzoni D, et al. Structural alterations of subcutaneous small-resistance arteries may predict major cardiovascular events in patients with hypertension. *Am J Hypertens*. 2007;20(8):846–852.
13. Mulvany MJ. Small artery structure: time to take note? *Am J Hypertens*. 2007;20(8):853–854.
14. Renkin E. Microcirculation and exchange. In: Patton H, Fuches A, Hille B, et al., eds. *Textbook of Physiology*. Philadelphia, PA: WB Saunders; 1989:860–878.
15. Renkin E. Control of microcirculation and blood-tissue exchange. In: Michel ERC, ed. *Handbook of Physiology*. Bethesda, MD: American Physiological Society; 1984:627–687.
16. Sarelius IH, Cohen KD, Murrant CL. Role for capillaries in coupling blood flow with metabolism. *Clin Exp Pharmacol Physiol*. 2000;27(10):826–829.
17. Simionescu M, Simionescu N. Ultrastructure of the microvascular wall: functional correlations. In: Renkin E, Michel C, eds. *Handbook of Physiology: Microcirculation*. Bethesda, MD: American Physiological Society; 1984:41–101.
18. Charkoudian N. Skin blood flow in adult human thermoregulation: how it works, when it does not, and why. *Mayo Clin Proc*. 2003;78(5): 603–612.
19. Pries AR, Kuebler WM. Normal endothelium. *Handb Exp Pharmacol*. 2006;(176 Pt 1):1–40.
20. Schneeberger EE, Lynch RD. The tight junction: a multifunctional complex. *Am J Physiol Cell Physiol*. 2004;286(6):C1213–C1228.
21. Raju S, Fredericks R, Lishman P, et al. Observations on the calf venous pump mechanism: determinants of postexercise pressure. *J Vasc Surg*. 1993;17(3):459–469.
22. Rowell L. *Human Cardiovascular Control*. New York: Oxford University Press; 1993.
23. Caggiati A, Phillips M, Lametschwandtner A, et al. Valves in small veins and venules. *Eur J Vasc Endovasc Surg*. 2006;32(4):447–452.
24. Rowell L. Human circulation: regulation during physical stress. In: *Human Circulation: Regulation during Physical Stress*. New York: Oxford University Press; 1986.
25. Hainsworth R. Vascular capacitance: its control and importance. *Rev Physiol Biochem Pharmacol*. 1986;105:101–173.
26. Rowell L, O'Leary D, Kellogg D. Integration of cardiovascular control systems in dynamic exercise. In: Rowell L, Sheperd J, eds. *Handbook of Physiology. Exercise: Regulation and Integration of Multiple Systems*. Bethesda, MD: Oxford University Press; 1996:770–838.
27. Aukland K. Arnold Heller and the lymph pump. *Acta Physiol Scand*. 2005;185(3):171–180.
28. Zawieja D. Lymphatic biology and the microcirculation: past, present and future. *Microcirculation*. 2005;12(1):141–150.
29. Muthuchamy M, Zawieja D. Molecular regulation of lymphatic contractility. *Ann N Y Acad Sci*. 2008;1131:89–99.
30. Schmid-Schonbein GW. Microlymphatics and lymph flow. *Physiol Rev*. 1990;70(4):987–1028.
31. Gashev AA. Lymphatic vessels: pressure- and flow-dependent regulatory reactions. *Ann N Y Acad Sci*. 2008;1131:100–109.
32. Olszewski WL. Contractility patterns of normal and pathologically changed human lymphatics. *Ann N Y Acad Sci*. 2002;979:52–63; discussion 76–79.
33. Gashev AA. Physiologic aspects of lymphatic contractile function: current perspectives. *Ann N Y Acad Sci*. 2002;979:178–187; discussion 188–196.
34. Small JV, Gimona M. The cytoskeleton of the vertebrate smooth muscle cell. *Acta Physiol Scand* 1998;164(4):341–348.
35. Somlyo AP, Somlyo AV. The sarcoplasmic reticulum: then and now. *Novartis Found Symp*. 2002;246:258–268; discussion 268–271, 272–276.
36. Horowitz A, Menice CB, Laporte R, et al. Mechanisms of smooth muscle contraction. *Physiol Rev*. 1996;76(4):967–1003.
37. Griendling KK, Harrison D, Alexander R. Biology of the vessel wall. In: Fuster V, Alexander RW, O'Rourke RA, eds. *Hurst's the Heart*. New York: McGraw-Hill; 2008.
38. Wiel E, Vallet B, ten Cate H. The endothelium in intensive care. *Crit Care Clin*. 2005;21(3):403–416.
39. Furchgott RF, Zawadzki JV. The obligatory role of endothelial cells in the relaxation of arterial smooth muscle by acetylcholine. *Nature*. 1980;288(5789):373–376.
40. Ignarro LJ, Buga GM, Wood KS, et al. Endothelium-derived relaxing factor produced and released from artery and vein is nitric oxide. *Proc Natl Acad Sci USA*. 1987;84:9265–9269.
41. Palmer RM, Ferrige AG, Moncada S. Nitric oxide release accounts for the biological activity of endothelium-derived relaxing factor. *Nature*. 1987;327(6122):524–526.
42. Luscher TF. Endothelium-derived nitric oxide: the endogenous nitrovasodilator in the human cardiovascular system. *Eur Heart J*. 1991;12(suppl E):2–11.
43. Moncada S, Palmer RM, Higgs EA. Nitric oxide: physiology, pathophysiology, and pharmacology. *Pharmacol Rev*. 1991;43(2):109–142.
44. Cohen RA. Role of nitric oxide in vasomotor regulation. In: Loscalzo J, Vita J, eds. *Contemporary cardiology: Nitric oxide and the cardiovascular system*. Totowa, NJ: Humana Press; 2000:105–122.
45. Moncada S, Higgs EA. Nitric oxide and the vascular endothelium. *Handb Exp Pharmacol*. 2006;(176 Pt 1):213–254.
46. Vanhoutte PM. Say NO to ET. *J Auton Nerv Syst*. 2000;81(1–3): 271–277.
47. Alonso D, Radomski MW. The nitric oxide-endothelin-1 connection. *Heart Fail Rev*. 2003;8(1):107–115.
48. Busse R, Fleming I. Vascular endothelium and blood flow. *Handb Exp Pharmacol*. 2006;(176 Pt 2):43–78.
49. Iida N. Nitric oxide mediates sympathetic vasoconstriction at supraspinal, spinal, and synaptic levels. *Am J Physiol*. 1999;276(3):H918–H925.
50. McHugh J, Cheek DJ. Nitric oxide and regulation of vascular tone: pharmacological and physiological considerations. *Am J Crit Care*. 1998;7(2):131–140; quiz 141–142.
51. Ignarro LJ. After 130 years, the molecular mechanism of action of nitroglycerin is revealed. *Proc Natl Acad Sci U S A*. 2002;99(12):7816–7817.
52. Ignarro LJ. Nitric oxide as a unique signaling molecule in the vascular system: a historical overview. *J Physiol Pharmacol*. 2002;53(4 Pt 1): 503–514.
53. Loscalzo J. Nitric oxide insufficiency, platelet activation, and arterial thrombosis. *Circ Res*. 2001;88(8):756–762.
54. Ahanchi SS, Tsihlis ND, Kibbe MR. The role of nitric oxide in the pathophysiology of intimal hyperplasia. *J Vasc Surg*. 2007;45(suppl A): A64–A73.
55. Friedewald VE, Giles TD, Pool JL, et al. The Editor's Roundtable: endothelial dysfunction in cardiovascular disease. *Am J Cardiol*. 2008; 102(4):418–423.
56. Behrendt D, Ganz P. Endothelial function. From vascular biology to clinical applications. *Am J Cardiol*. 2002;90(10C):40l–48l.
57. Fernandes D, Assreuy J. Nitric oxide and vascular reactivity in sepsis. *Shock*. 2008;30(suppl 1):10–13.
58. Galkin A, Higgs A, Moncada S. Nitric oxide and hypoxia. *Essays Biochem*. 2007;43:29–42.
59. Trzeciak S, Cinel I, Phillip Dellinger R, et al. Resuscitating the microcirculation in sepsis: the central role of nitric oxide, emerging concepts for novel therapies, and challenges for clinical trials. *Acad Emerg Med*. 2008;15(5):399–413.
60. Mitchell JA, Ali F, Bailey L, et al. Role of nitric oxide and prostacyclin as vasoactive hormones released by the endothelium. *Exp Physiol*. 2008;93(1):141–147.
61. Mollace V, Muscoli C, Masini E, et al. Modulation of prostaglandin biosynthesis by nitric oxide and nitric oxide donors. *Pharmacol Rev*. 2005;57(2):217–252.
62. Bellien J, Thuillez C, Joannides R. Contribution of endothelium-derived hyperpolarizing factors to the regulation of vascular tone in humans. *Fundam Clin Pharmacol*. 2008;22(4):363–377.
63. Lushka L, Agewall S, Kublickiene K. Endothelium-derived hyperpolarizing factor in vascular physiology and cardiovascular disease. *Atherosclerosis*. 2009;202(2):330–344.
64. Feletou M, Vanhoutte PM. Endothelium-derived hyperpolarizing factor: where are we now? *Arterioscler Thromb Vasc Biol*. 2006;26(6):1215–1225.
65. Feletou M, Vanhoutte PM. Endothelial dysfunction: a multifaceted disorder (The Wiggers Award Lecture). *Am J Physiol Heart Circ Physiol*. 2006;291(3):H985–H1002.
66. Feletou M, Vanhoutte PM. Endothelium-dependent hyperpolarizations: past beliefs and present facts. *Ann Med*. 2007;39(7):495–516.
67. Yang Q, Yim AP, He GW. The significance of endothelium-derived hyperpolarizing factor in the human circulation. *Curr Vasc Pharmacol*. 2007;5(1):85–92.

68. Yanagisawa M, Kurihara H, Kimura S, et al. A novel potent vasoconstrictor peptide produced by vascular endothelial cells. *Nature.* 1988; 332(6163):411–415.
69. Shah R. Endothelins in health and disease. *Eur J Intern Med.* 2007;18(4):272–282.
70. Stauffer BL, Westby CM, DeSouza CA. Endothelin-1, aging and hypertension. *Curr Opin Cardiol.* 2008;23(4):350–355.
71. Brunner F, Bras-Silva C, Cerdeira AS, et al. Cardiovascular endothelins: essential regulators of cardiovascular homeostasis. *Pharmacol Ther.* 2006;111(2):508–531.
72. Masson S, Latini R, Anand IS, et al. The prognostic value of big endothelin-1 in more than 2,300 patients with heart failure enrolled in the Valsartan Heart Failure Trial (Val-HeFT). *J Card Fail.* 2006;12(5):375–380.
73. Feldstein C, Romero C. Role of endothelins in hypertension. *Am J Ther.* 2007;14(2):147–153.
74. O'Connor CM, Gattis WA, Adams KF Jr, et al. Tezosentan in patients with acute heart failure and acute coronary syndromes: results of the Randomized Intravenous TeZosentan Study (RITZ-4). *J Am Coll Cardiol.* 2003;41(9):1452–1457.
75. Anand I, McMurray J, Cohn JN, et al. Long-term effects of darusentan on left-ventricular remodelling and clinical outcomes in the EndothelinA Receptor Antagonist Trial in Heart Failure (EARTH): randomised, double-blind, placebo-controlled trial. *Lancet.* 2004;364(9431):347–354.
76. Sica DA. Endothelin receptor antagonism: what does the future hold? *Hypertension.* 2008;52(3):460–461.
77. Van Guilder GP, Westby CM, Greiner JJ, et al. Endothelin-1 vasoconstrictor tone increases with age in healthy men but can be reduced by regular aerobic exercise. *Hypertension.* 2007;50(2):403–409.
78. Ivey ME, Osman N, Little PJ. Endothelin-1 signalling in vascular smooth muscle: pathways controlling cellular functions associated with atherosclerosis. *Atherosclerosis.* 2008;199(2):237–247.
79. Rubin LJ, Badesch DB, Barst RJ, et al. Bosentan therapy for pulmonary arterial hypertension. *N Engl J Med.* 2002;346(12):896–903.
80. Denton CP, Pope JE, Peter HH, et al. Long-term effects of bosentan on quality of life, survival, safety and tolerability in pulmonary arterial hypertension related to connective tissue diseases. *Ann Rheum Dis.* 2008;67(9):1222–1228.
81. Le Brocq M, Leslie SJ, Milliken P, et al. Endothelial dysfunction: from molecular mechanisms to measurement, clinical implications, and therapeutic opportunities. *Antioxid Redox Signal.* 2008;10(9):1631–1674.
82. Antithrombotic Trialists' Collaboration. Collaborative meta-analysis of randomised trials of antiplatelet therapy for prevention of death, myocardial infarction, and stroke in high risk patients. *BMJ.* 2002;324(7329):71–86.
83. Ridker PM, Cook NR, Lee IM, et al. A randomized trial of low-dose aspirin in the primary prevention of cardiovascular disease in women. *N Engl J Med.* 2005;352(13):1293–1304.
84. Eikelboom JW, Hankey GJ, Thom J, et al. Incomplete inhibition of thromboxane biosynthesis by acetylsalicylic acid: determinants and effect on cardiovascular risk. *Circulation.* 2008;118(17):1705–1712.
85. Bombardier C, Laine L, Reicin A, et al. Comparison of upper gastrointestinal toxicity of rofecoxib and naproxen in patients with rheumatoid arthritis. VIGOR Study Group. *N Engl J Med.* 2000;343(21):1520–1528.
86. Bresalier RS, Sandler RS, Quan H, et al. Cardiovascular events associated with rofecoxib in a colorectal adenoma chemoprevention trial. *N Engl J Med.* 2005;352(11):1092–1102.
87. U.S. Food and Drug Administration. *Alert for healthcare professionals: non-selective non-steroidal antiinflammatory drugs (NSAIDs).* U.S. Department of Health and Human Services. 2005.
88. McGettigan P, Henry D. Cardiovascular risk and inhibition of cyclooxygenase: a systematic review of the observational studies of selective and nonselective inhibitors of cyclooxygenase 2. *JAMA.* 2006;296(13): 1633–1644.
89. Warner JJ, Weideman RA, Kelly KC, et al. The risk of acute myocardial infarction with etodolac is not increased compared to naproxen: a historical cohort analysis of a generic COX-2 selective inhibitor. *J Cardiovasc Pharmacol Ther.* 2008;13(4):252–260.
90. Roumie CL, Mitchel EF Jr, Kaltenbach L, et al. Nonaspirin NSAIDs, cyclooxygenase 2 inhibitors, and the risk for stroke. *Stroke.* 2008;39(7):2037–2045.
91. Grosser T, Fries S, FitzGerald GA. Biological basis for the cardiovascular consequences of COX-2 inhibition: therapeutic challenges and opportunities. *J Clin Invest.* 2006;116(1):4–15.
92. Funk CD, FitzGerald GA. COX-2 inhibitors and cardiovascular risk. *J Cardiovasc Pharmacol.* 2007;50(5):470–479.
93. Friedewald VE Jr, Bennett JS, Packer M, et al. The editor's roundtable: nonsteroidal antiinflammatory drugs and cardiovascular risk. *Am J Cardiol.* 2008;102(8):1046–1055.
94. Harrison D, Griendling KK, Landmesser U, et al. Role of oxidative stress in atherosclerosis. *Am J Cardiol.* 2003;91(3A):7A–11A.
95. Forstermann U. Oxidative stress in vascular disease: causes, defense mechanisms and potential therapies. *Nat Clin Pract Cardiovasc Med.* 2008;5(6):338–349.
96. Bonomini F, Tengattini S, Fabiano A, et al. Atherosclerosis and oxidative stress. *Histol Histopathol.* 2008;23(3):381–390.
97. Hornig B, Landmesser U, Kohler C, et al. Comparative effect of ace inhibition and angiotensin II type 1 receptor antagonism on bioavailability of nitric oxide in patients with coronary artery disease: role of superoxide dismutase. *Circulation.* 2001;103(6):799–805.
98. McQueen MJ, Lonn E, Gerstein HC, et al. The HOPE (Heart Outcomes Prevention Evaluation) Study and its consequences. *Scand J Clin Lab Invest Suppl.* 2005;240:143–156.
99. Landmesser U, Bahlmann F, Mueller M, et al. Simvastatin versus ezetimibe: pleiotropic and lipid-lowering effects on endothelial function in humans. *Circulation.* 2005;111(18):2356–2363.
100. Lonn E, Bosch J, Yusuf S, et al. Effects of long-term vitamin E supplementation on cardiovascular events and cancer: a randomized controlled trial. *JAMA.* 2005;293(11):1338–1347.
101. Vivekananthan DP, Penn MS, Sapp SK, et al. Use of antioxidant vitamins for the prevention of cardiovascular disease: meta-analysis of randomised trials. *Lancet.* 2003;361(9374):2017–2023.
102. Bjelakovic G, Nikolova D, Simonetti RG, et al. Systematic review: primary and secondary prevention of gastrointestinal cancers with antioxidant supplements. *Aliment Pharmacol Ther.* 2008;28(6):689–703.
103. Marshall JM. Roles of adenosine in skeletal muscle during systemic hypoxia. *Clin Exp Pharmacol Physiol.* 2002;29(9):843–849.
104. Ralevic V. Hypoxic vasodilatation: is an adenosine-prostaglandins-NO signalling cascade involved? *J Physiol.* 2002;544(Pt 1), 2.
105. Ray CJ, Abbas MR, Coney AM, et al. Interactions of adenosine, prostaglandins and nitric oxide in hypoxia-induced vasodilatation: in vivo and in vitro studies. *J Physiol.* 2002;544(Pt 1):195–209.
106. Koller A, Bagi Z. On the role of mechanosensitive mechanisms eliciting reactive hyperemia. *Am J Physiol Heart Circ Physiol.* 2002;283(6):H2250–H2259.
107. Flavahan NA, Cooke JP, Shepherd JT, et al. Human postjunctional alpha-1 and alpha-2 adrenoceptors: differential distribution in arteries of the limbs. *J Pharmacol Exp Ther.* 1987;241(2):361–365.
108. Civantos Calzada B, Aleixandre de Artinano A. Alpha-adrenoceptor subtypes. *Pharmacol Res.* 2001;44(3):195–208.
109. Kable JW, Murrin LC, Bylund DB. In vivo gene modification elucidates subtype-specific functions of alpha(2)-adrenergic receptors. *J Pharmacol Exp Ther.* 2000;293(1):1–7.
110. Kanagy NL. Alpha(2)-adrenergic receptor signalling in hypertension. *Clin Sci.* 2005;109(5):431–437.
111. Leech CJ, Faber JE. Different alpha-adrenoceptor subtypes mediate constriction of arterioles and venules. *Am J Physiol.* 1996;270(2 Pt 2): H710–H722.
112. Feigl EO. Neural control of coronary blood flow. *J Vasc Res.* 1998;35(2): 85–92.
113. Barbato E, Piscione F, Bartunek J, et al. Role of beta2 adrenergic receptors in human atherosclerotic coronary arteries. *Circulation.* 2005;111(3):288–294.
114. Gauthier C, Seze-Goismier C, Rozec B. Beta 3-adrenoceptors in the cardiovascular system. *Clin Hemorheol Microcirc.* 2007;37(1–2): 193–204.
115. Gauthier C, Leblais V, Kobzik L, et al. The negative inotropic effect of beta3-adrenoceptor stimulation is mediated by activation of a nitric oxide synthase pathway in human ventricle. *J Clin Invest.* 1998;102(7): 1377–1384.
116. Moniotte S, Kobzik L, Feron O, et al. Upregulation of beta(3)-adrenoceptors and altered contractile response to inotropic amines in human failing myocardium. *Circulation.* 2001;103(12):1649–1655.
117. Lands AM, Arnold A, McAuliff JP, et al. Differentiation of receptor systems activated by sympathomimetic amines. *Nature.* 1967;214(5088):597–598.
118. Queen LR, Ferro A. Beta-adrenergic receptors and nitric oxide generation in the cardiovascular system. *Cell Mol Life Sci.* 2006;63(9):1070–1083.
119. Sperelakis N, Tohse N, Ohya Y, et al. Cyclic GMP regulation of calcium slow channels in cardiac muscle and vascular smooth muscle cells. *Adv Pharmacol.* 1994;26:217–252.

120. Rozec B, Gauthier C. Beta3-adrenoceptors in the cardiovascular system: putative roles in human pathologies. *Pharmacol Ther*. 2006;111(3): 652–673.
121. Treschan TA, Peters J. The vasopressin system: physiology and clinical strategies. *Anesthesiology*. 2006;105(3):599–612; quiz 639–640.
122. Barrett LK, Singer M, Clapp LH. Vasopressin: mechanisms of action on the vasculature in health and in septic shock. *Crit Care Med*. 2007; 35(1):33–40.
123. Dellinger RP, Levy MM, Carlet JM, et al. Surviving Sepsis Campaign: international guidelines for management of severe sepsis and septic shock: 2008. *Crit Care Med*. 2008;36(1):296–327.
124. Wenzel V, Lindner KH. Arginine vasopressin during cardiopulmonary resuscitation: laboratory evidence, clinical experience and recommendations, and a view to the future. *Crit Care Med*. 2002;30 (4 suppl):S157–S161.
125. ECC Committee, Subcommittees and Task Forces of the American Heart Association. 2005 American Heart Association guidelines for cardiopulmonary resuscitation and emergency cardiovascular care. *Circulation*. 2005;112(24 suppl):IV1–IV203.
126. Kleinman ME, Goldberger ZD, Rea T, et al. 2017 American Heart Association Focused Update on Adult Basic Life Support and Cardiopulmonary Resuscitation Quality: an update to the American Heart Association guidelines for cardiopulmonary resuscitation and emergency cardiovascular care. *Circulation*. 2018;137(1):e7–e13.
127. Loscalzo J, Vita J. *Contemporary Cardiology: Nitric Oxide and the Cardiovascular System*. Totowa, NJ: Humana Press; 2000.
128. Yao X, Huang Y. From nitric oxide to endothelial cytosolic Ca2+: a negative feedback control. *Trends Pharmacol Sci*. 2003;24(6):263–266.
129. Cohen RA, Adachi T. Nitric-oxide-induced vasodilation: regulation by physiologic s-gluthiolation and pathologic oxidation of the sarcoplasmic endoplasmic reticulum calcium ATPase. *Trends Cardiovasc Med*. 2006;16:109–114.
130. Komalavilas P, Lincoln T. Regulation of intracellular Ca+2 by cyclic GMP-dependent protein kinase in vascular smooth muscle. In: Kadowitz PJ, McNamara D, eds. *Nitric Oxide and the Regulation of Peripheral Circulation*. Boston: Birkhauser; 2000:15–32.
131. Berridge MJ. Smooth muscle cell calcium activation mechanisms. *J Physiol*. 2008;586(21):5047–5061.
132. Somlyo AP, Somlyo AV. Signal transduction and regulation in smooth muscle. *Nature*. 1994;372(6503):231–236.
133. Berridge MJ. The endoplasmic reticulum: a multifunctional signaling organelle. *Cell Calcium*. 2002;32(5–6):235–249.
134. Patterson AJ, Henrie-Olson J, Brenner R. Vasoregulation at the molecular level: a role for the beta1 subunit of the calcium-activated potassium (BK) channel. *Trends Cardiovasc Med*. 2002;12(2):78–82.
135. Sheperd J, Vanhoutte P. *The Human Cardiovascular System. Facts and Concepts*. New York: Raven Press; 1979.
136. Christensen KL, Mulvany MJ. Location of resistance arteries. *J Vasc Res*. 2001;38(1):1–12.
137. Duling B. *Coordination of Microcirculatory Function with Oxygen Demand in Skeletal Muscle*. Budapest: Akademiai Kaido; 1981.
138. Duling BR, Klitzman B. Local control of microvascular function: role in tissue oxygen supply. *Annu Rev Physiol*. 1980;42:373–382.
139. Scher A. The veins and venous return. In: Patton H, Fuchs A, Hille B, eds. *Textbook of Physiology*. Philadelphia, PA: WB Saunders; 1989:879–886.
140. Hlastala M, Berger A. *Physiology of Respiration*. New York: Oxford University Press; 2001.
141. Crone E, Levitt D. *Capillary Permeability to Small Solutes*. Bethesda, MD: American Physiological Society; 1984.
142. Curry R. *Mechanics and Thermodynamics of Transcapillary Exchange*. Bethesda, MD: American Physiological Society; 1984.
143. Michel CC. Transport of macromolecules through microvascular walls. *Cardiovasc Res*. 1996;32(4):644–653.
144. Starling EH. On the absorption of fluids from the connective tissue spaces. *J Physiol*. 1896;19(4):312–326.
145. Landis E. Micro-injection studies of capillary permeability II. *Am J Physiol*. 1927;82:217–238.
146. Renkin EM. Some consequences of capillary permeability to macromolecules: Starling's hypothesis reconsidered. *Am J Physiol*. 1986;250(5 Pt 2):H706–H710.
147. Michel CC. Starling: the formulation of his hypothesis of microvascular fluid exchange and its significance after 100 years. *Exp Physiol*. 1997;82(1):1–30.
148. Levick JR. Fluid exchange across endothelium. *Int J Microcirc Clin Exp*. 1997;17(5):241–247.
149. Aukland K, Reed RK. Interstitial-lymphatic mechanisms in the control of extracellular fluid volume. *Physiol Rev*. 1993;73(1):1–78.
150. Weinbaum S, Tarbell JM, Damiano ER. The structure and function of the endothelial glycocalyx layer. *Annu Rev Biomed Eng*. 2007;9:121–167.
151. Hu X, Weinbaum S. A new view of Starling's hypothesis at the microstructural level. *Microvasc Res*. 1999;58(3):281–304.
152. Pappenheimer J. *Contributions to Microvascular Research of Jean Leonard Marie Poiseuille*. Bethesda, MD: American Physiological Society; 1984.
153. Mellander S. On the control of capillary fluid transfer by precapillary and postcapillary vascular adjustments. A brief review with special emphasis on myogenic mechanisms. *Microvasc Res*. 1978;15(3):319–330.
154. Aukland K, Nicolaysen G. Interstitial fluid volume: local regulatory mechanisms. *Physiol Rev*. 1981;61(3):556–643.
155. Lanne T, Lundvall J. Mechanisms in man for rapid refill of the circulatory system in hypovolaemia. *Acta Physiol Scand*. 1992;146(3):299–306.
156. Olsen H, Vernersson E, Lanne T. Cardiovascular response to acute hypovolemia in relation to age. Implications for orthostasis and hemorrhage. *Am J Physiol Heart Circ Physiol*. 2000;278(1):H222–H232.
157. Levick JR. Capillary filtration-absorption balance reconsidered in light of dynamic extravascular factors. *Exp Physiol*. 1991;76(6):825–857.
158. Angus DC, Linde-Zwirble WT, Lidicker J, et al. Epidemiology of severe sepsis in the United States: analysis of incidence, outcome, and associated costs of care. *Crit Care Med*. 2001;29(7):1303–1310.
159. Jawad I, Luksic I, Rafnsson SB. Assessing available information on the burden of sepsis: global estimates of incidence, prevalence and mortality. *J Glob Health*. 2012;2(1):010404.
160. Singer M, Deutschman CS, Seymour CW, et al. The third international consensus definitions for sepsis and septic shock (Sepsis-3). *JAMA*. 2016; 315(8):801–810.
161. De Backer D, Donadello K, Sakr Y, et al. Microcirculatory alterations in patients with severe sepsis: impact of time of assessment and relationship with outcome. *Crit Care Med*. 2013;41(3):791–799.
162. Hotchkiss RS, Monneret G, Payen D. Sepsis-induced immunosuppression: from cellular dysfunctions to immunotherapy. *Nat Rev Immunol*. 2013;13(12):862–874.
163. Deutschman CS, Tracey KJ. Sepsis: current dogma and new perspectives. *Immunity*. 2014;40(4):463–475.
164. Singer M. The role of mitochondrial dysfunction in sepsis-induced multi-organ failure. *Virulence*. 2014;5(1):66–72.
165. Marik PE. Early management of severe sepsis: concepts and controversies. *Chest*. 2014;145(6):1407–1418.
166. Hawiger J, Veach RA, Zienkiewicz J. New paradigms in sepsis: from prevention to protection of failing microcirculation. *J Thromb Haemost*. 2015;13(10):1743–1756.
167. De Backer D, Donadello K, Taccone FS, et al. Microcirculatory alterations: potential mechanisms and implications for therapy. *Ann Intensive Care*. 2011;1(1):27.
168. Edul VS, Enrico C, Laviolle B, et al. Quantitative assessment of the microcirculation in healthy volunteers and in patients with septic shock. *Crit Care Med*. 2012;40(5):1443–1448.
169. Farquhar I, Martin CM, Lam C, et al. Decreased capillary density in vivo in bowel mucosa of rats with normotensive sepsis. *J Surg Res*. 1996;61(1):190–196.
170. Woywodt A, Blann AD, Kirsch T, et al. Isolation and enumeration of circulating endothelial cells by immunomagnetic isolation: proposal of a definition and a consensus protocol. *J Thromb Haemost*. 2006;4(3): 671–677.
171. Bateman RM, Sharpe MD, Ellis CG. Bench-to-bedside review: microvascular dysfunction in sepsis—hemodynamics, oxygen transport, and nitric oxide. *Crit Care*. 2003;7(5):359–373.
172. Aird WC. The role of the endothelium in severe sepsis and multiple organ dysfunction syndrome. *Blood*. 2003;101(10):3765–3777.
173. Dellinger RP, Levy MM, Rhodes A, et al. Surviving sepsis campaign: international guidelines for management of severe sepsis and septic shock: 2012. *Crit Care Med*. 2013;41(2):580–637.
174. De Backer D, Creteur J, Dubois MJ, et al. The effects of dobutamine on microcirculatory alterations in patients with septic shock are independent of its systemic effects. *Crit Care Med*. 2006;34(2):403–408.
175. Ince C, Sinaasappel M. Microcirculatory oxygenation and shunting in sepsis and shock. *Crit Care Med*. 1999;27(7):1369–1377.
176. Rivers EP, Yataco AC, Jaehne AK, et al. Oxygen extraction and perfusion markers in severe sepsis and septic shock: diagnostic, therapeutic and outcome implications. *Curr Opin Crit Care*. 2015;21(5). 381–387.
177. Sharawy N. Vasoplegia in septic shock: do we really fight the right enemy? *J Crit Care*. 2014;29(1):83–87.

178. Marshall JC. Why have clinical trials in sepsis failed? *Trends Mol Med.* 2014;20(4):195–203.
179. De Backer D, Orbegozo Cortes D, Donadello K, et al. Pathophysiology of microcirculatory dysfunction and the pathogenesis of septic shock. *Virulence.* 2014;5(1):73–79.
180. Trzeciak S, Dellinger RP, Parrillo JE, et al. Early microcirculatory perfusion derangements in patients with severe sepsis and septic shock: relationship to hemodynamics, oxygen transport, and survival. *Ann Emerg Med.* 2007;49(1):88–98, 98.e81–e82.
181. Bateman RM, Tokunaga C, Kareco T, et al. Myocardial hypoxia-inducible HIF-1alpha, VEGF, and GLUT1 gene expression is associated with microvascular and ICAM-1 heterogeneity during endotoxemia. *Am J Physiol Heart Circ Physiol.* 2007;293(1):H448–H456.
182. Kao R, Xenocostas A, Rui T, et al. Erythropoietin improves skeletal muscle microcirculation and tissue bioenergetics in a mouse sepsis model. *Crit Care.* 2007;11(3):R58.
183. Skibsted S, Jones AE, Puskarich MA, et al. Biomarkers of endothelial cell activation in early sepsis. *Shock.* 2013;39(5):427–432.
184. Ye X, Ding J, Zhou X, et al. Divergent roles of endothelial NF-kappaB in multiple organ injury and bacterial clearance in mouse models of sepsis. *J Exp Med.* 2008;205(6):1303–1315.
185. London NR, Zhu W, Bozza FA, et al. Targeting Robo4-dependent Slit signaling to survive the cytokine storm in sepsis and influenza. *Sci Transl Med.* 2010;2(23):23ra19.
186. Trzeciak S, McCoy JV, Phillip Dellinger R, et al. Early increases in microcirculatory perfusion during protocol-directed resuscitation are associated with reduced multi-organ failure at 24 h in patients with sepsis. *Intensive Care Med.* 2008;34(12):2210–2217.
187. De Backer D, Creteur J, Preiser JC, et al. Microvascular blood flow is altered in patients with sepsis. *Am J Respir Crit Care Med.* 2002;166(1):98–104.
188. Lumb A. *Nunn's Applied Respiratory Physiology*. Philadelphia, PA: Elsevier; 2005.
189. Cooper CJ, Landzberg MJ, Anderson TJ, et al. Role of nitric oxide in the local regulation of pulmonary vascular resistance in humans. *Circulation.* 1996;93(2):266–271.
190. Ricciardolo FL, Sterk PJ, Gaston B, et al. Nitric oxide in health and disease of the respiratory system. *Physiol Rev.* 2004;84(3):731–765.
191. Brew K. Structure of human ACE gives new insights into inhibitor binding and design. *Trends Pharmacol Sci.* 2003;24(8):391–394.
192. West JB. *West's Respiratory Physiology: The Essentials* 10th ed. Lippincott Williams & Wilkins; 2015.
193. Weinberger S, Cockrill B, Mandel J. *Principles of Pulmonary Medicine.* Philadelphia, PA: Saunders/Elsevier; 2008.
194. West JB. Distribution of gas and blood in the normal lungs. *Br Med Bull.* 1963;19:53–58.
195. Hlastala MP, Glenny RW. Vascular structure determines pulmonary blood flow distribution. *News Physiol Sci.* 1999;14:182–186.
196. Galvin I, Drummond GB, Nirmalan M. Distribution of blood flow and ventilation in the lung: gravity is not the only factor. *Br J Anaesth.* 2007;98(4):420–428.
197. Glenny R. Last word on Point:Counterpoint: gravity is/is not the major factor determining the distribution of blood flow in the human lung. *J Appl Physiol.* 2008;104(5):1540.
198. Hughes M, West JB. Last word on Point:Counterpoint: Gravity is/is not the major factor determining the distribution of blood flow in the human lung. *J Appl Physiol.* 2008;104(5):1539.
199. Michiels C. Physiological and pathological responses to hypoxia. *Am J Pathol.* 2004;164(6):1875–1882.
200. Mauban JR, Remillard CV, Yuan JX. Hypoxic pulmonary vasoconstriction: role of ion channels. *J Appl Physiol.* 2005;98(1):415–420.
201. Moudgil R, Michelakis ED, Archer SL. Hypoxic pulmonary vasoconstriction. *J Appl Physiol.* 2005;98(1):390–403.
202. Aaronson PI, Robertson TP, Knock GA, et al. Hypoxic pulmonary vasoconstriction: mechanisms and controversies. *J Physiol.* 2006;570(Pt 1):53–58.
203. Gurney AM. Multiple sites of oxygen sensing and their contributions to hypoxic pulmonary vasoconstriction. *Respir Physiol Neurobiol.* 2002;132(1):43–53.
204. Griffiths MJ, Evans TW. Inhaled nitric oxide therapy in adults. *N Engl J Med.* 2005;353(25):2683–2695.
205. Adhikari NK, Burns KE, Friedrich JO, et al. Effect of nitric oxide on oxygenation and mortality in acute lung injury: systematic review and meta-analysis. *BMJ.* 2007;334(7597):779.
206. Liu C, Chen J, Gao Y, et al. Endothelin receptor antagonists for pulmonary arterial hypertension. *Cochrane Database Syst Rev.* 2013;2:CD004434.
207. Price LC, Howard LS. Endothelin receptor antagonists for pulmonary arterial hypertension: rationale and place in therapy. *Am J Cardiovasc Drugs.* 2008;8(3):171–185.
208. Barnes H, Brown Z, Burns A, et al. Phosphodiesterase 5 inhibitors for pulmonary hypertension. *Cochrane Database System Rev.* 2019;(1):CD012621.
209. Liu C, Liu K, Ji Z, et al. Treatments for pulmonary arterial hypertension. *Respir Med.* 2006;100(5):765–774.
210. Paramothayan NS, Lasserson TJ, Wells AU, et al. Prostacyclin for pulmonary hypertension in adults. *Cochrane Database Syst Rev.* 2005;2:CD002994.
211. Levitzky M. *Pulmonary Physiology*. New York: McGraw-Hill; 2007.
212. Pinsky M. *Role of Cardiorespiratory System in Delivering Oxygen*. Berlin: Springer-Verlag; 2002.
213. Leach RM, Treacher DF. The pulmonary physician in critical care* 2: oxygen delivery and consumption in the critically ill. *Thorax.* 2002;57(2):170–177.
214. Wilson DF. Quantifying the role of oxygen pressure in tissue function. *Am J Physiol Heart Circ Physiol.* 2008;294(1):H11–H13.
215. Krogh A. The number and distribution of capillaries in muscles with calculations of the oxygen pressure head necessary for supplying the tissue. *J Physiol.* 1919;52(6):409–415.
216. Tsai AG, Johnson PC, Intaglietta M. Is the distribution of tissue pO(2) homogeneous? *Antioxid Redox Signal.* 2007;9(7):979–984.
217. Tsai AG, Johnson PC, Intaglietta M. Oxygen gradients in the microcirculation. *Physiol Rev.* 2003;83(3):933–963.
218. Tsai AG, Friesenecker B, Cabrales P, et al. The vascular wall as a regulator of tissue oxygenation. *Curr Opin Nephrol Hypertens.* 2006;15(1):67–71.
219. Erusalimsky JD, Moncada S. Nitric oxide and mitochondrial signaling: from physiology to pathophysiology. *Arterioscler Thromb Vasc Biol.* 2007;27(12):2524–2531.
220. Fink MP. Bench-to-bedside review: cytopathic hypoxia. *Crit Care.* 2002;6(6):491–499.
221. Dantzker DR, Brook CJ, Dehart P, et al. Ventilation-perfusion distributions in the adult respiratory distress syndrome. *Am Rev Respir Dis.* 1979;120(5):1039–1052.
222. Jensen FB. Red blood cell pH, the Bohr effect, and other oxygen-ation-linked phenomena in blood O_2 and CO_2 transport. *Acta Physiol Scand.* 2004;182(3):215–227.
223. Shibutani K, Komatsu T, Kubal K, et al. Critical level of oxygen delivery in anesthetized man. *Crit Care Med.* 1983;11(8):640–643.
224. Ronco JJ, Fenwick JC, Tweeddale MG, et al. Identification of the critical oxygen delivery for anaerobic metabolism in critically ill septic and nonseptic humans. *JAMA.* 1993;270(14):1724–1730.
225. Lieberman JA, Weiskopf RB, Kelley SD, et al. Critical oxygen delivery in conscious humans is less than 7.3 ml $O_2 \times$ kg(-1) $\times$ min(-1). *Anesthesiology.* 2000;92(2):407–413.
226. Fan E, Brodie D, Slutsky AS. Acute respiratory distress syndrome: advances in diagnosis and treatment. *JAMA.* 2018;319(7):698–710.
227. Fan E, Needham DM, Stewart TE. Ventilatory management of acute lung injury and acute respiratory distress syndrome. *JAMA.* 2005;294(22):2889–2896.
228. Koh Y. Update in acute respiratory distress syndrome. *J Intensive Care.* 2014;2(1):2.
229. ARDS Definition Task Force; Ranieri VM, Rubenfeld GD, Thompson BT, et al. Acute respiratory distress syndrome: the Berlin Definition. *JAMA.* 2012;307(23):2526–2533.
230. Moazed F, Calfee CS. Environmental risk factors for acute respiratory distress syndrome. *Clin Chest Med.* 2014;35(4):625–637.
231. Cross LJ, Matthay MA. Biomarkers in acute lung injury: insights into the pathogenesis of acute lung injury. *Crit Care Clin.* 2011;27(2):355–377.
232. Monahan LJ. Acute respiratory distress syndrome. *Curr Probl Pediatr Adolesc Health Care.* 2013;43(10):278–284.
233. Villar J. What is the acute respiratory distress syndrome? *Respir Care.* 2011;56(10):1539–1545.
234. Ware LB, Matthay MA. The acute respiratory distress syndrome. *N Engl J Med.* 2000;342(18):1334–1349.
235. Pierrakos C, Karanikolas M, Scolletta S, et al. Acute respiratory distress syndrome: pathophysiology and therapeutic options. *J Clin Med Res.* 2012;4(1):7–16.
236. Saguil A, Fargo M. Acute respiratory distress syndrome: diagnosis and management. *Am Fam Physician.* 2012;85(4):352–358.
237. Rawal G, Yadav S, Kumar R. Acute respiratory distress syndrome: an update and review. *J Transl Int Med.* 2018;6(2):74–77.

238. Matthay MA, Ware LB, Zimmerman GA. The acute respiratory distress syndrome. *J Clin Invest.* 2012;122(8):2731–2740.
239. Fujishima S. Pathophysiology and biomarkers of acute respiratory distress syndrome. *J Intensive Care.* 2014;2(1):32.
240. Martin TR. Lung cytokines and ARDS: Roger S. Mitchell Lecture. *Chest.* 1999;116(1 suppl):2S–8S.
241. Orfanos SE, Mavrommati I, Korovesi I, et al. Pulmonary endothelium in acute lung injury: from basic science to the critically ill. *Intensive Care Med.* 2004;30(9):1702–1714.
242. Orbegozo Cortes D, Rahmania L, Irazabal M, et al. Microvascular reactivity is altered early in patients with acute respiratory distress syndrome. *Respir Res.* 2016;17(1):59.
243. Radermacher P, Maggiore SM, Mercat A. Fifty years of research in ARDS. Gas exchange in acute respiratory distress syndrome. *Am J Respir Crit Care Med.* 2017;196(8):964–984.
244. West JB. Understanding pulmonary gas exchange: ventilation-perfusion relationships. *Am J Physiol Lung Cell Mol Physiol.* 2004;287(6): L1071–L1072.
245. Pelosi P, D'Andrea L, Vitale G, et al. Vertical gradient of regional lung inflation in adult respiratory distress syndrome. *Am J Respir Crit Care Med.* 1994;149(1):8–13.
246. Calzia E, Radermacher P. Alveolar ventilation and pulmonary blood flow: the V(A)/Q concept. *Intensive Care Med.* 2003;29(8): 1229–1232.
247. West JB. State of the art: ventilation-perfusion relationships. *Am Rev Respir Dis.* 1977;116(5):919–943.
248. Weg JG. Oxygen transport in adult respiratory distress syndrome and other acute circulatory problems: relationship of oxygen delivery and oxygen consumption. *Crit Care Med.* 1991;19(5): 650–657.

4 Regulation of Cardiac Output and Blood Pressure

Nina Stefanie

OBJECTIVES

1. Learn the impact of neurohumoral control on the cardiovascular system.
2. Identify models used in the effect of cardiac output.
3. Discuss baroreflex responses on blood pressure.

KEY QUESTIONS

1. What two types of input do baroreceptors respond to?
2. How is the Bezold–Jarisch Reflex manifested?
3. What factors affect cardiac output?

This chapter reviews the neurohumoral control of the cardiovascular system as it relates to the rapid and more long-term control of cardiac output and blood pressure and the local control of blood flow (autoregulatory, metabolic, autacoid). Several models of cardiac function are presented, including the relationship between cardiac output and central venous pressure, the Krogh model of the effect of distribution of blood volume on cardiac output, and the arterial baroreflex responses to decreased and increased blood pressure.

AFFERENT INPUT AND RECEPTOR

Arterial Baroreceptors

The arterial baroreceptors are responsible for the reflex control of blood pressure. These baroreceptors are undifferentiated nerve fibers located in the adventitia of the carotid sinus (at the bifurcation of the carotid artery) and the aortic arch (between the arch of the aorta and the bifurcation of the subclavian artery; Fig. 4-1). The receptors are mechanoreceptors that respond to distortion or a change in transmural pressure or stretch of the vascular bed in which they are located. For example, the carotid baroreceptors are sensitive to external compression or massage, both of which unload them (decrease transmural pressure). Although baroreceptors are often referred to as "pressoreceptors," they in fact do not sense pressure directly, but instead only indirectly through change in stretch.

The baroreceptors respond to two types of input: static input (i.e., mean arterial pressure [MAP]) and phasic input (i.e., pulsatile changes). Therefore, the baroreceptors are responsive to MAP, pulse pressure, and the number of pulses per minute (e.g., heart rate).[1] The static response has a threshold effect, that is, below a certain threshold of MAP (20 to 50 mm Hg), the receptor stops firing. Above this threshold there is an increase in rate of receptor firing in proportion to the increase in mean pressure, until a plateau of the output is reached at saturation. The phasic response increases when the rate of change of pressure rises (increasing pressure) and decreases when the rate of change in pressure decreases.

Cardiopulmonary Receptors

Cardiopulmonary or low-pressure baroreceptors are located in the atria, ventricles, and pulmonary arteries and veins, with the cardiac baroreceptors providing the primary afferent input for the vagal cardioreflex.[2,3] The properties of the cardiopulmonary baroreceptors are similar to those of the arterial baroreceptors, that is, a decrease in transmural pressure in the chamber or vessel results in a decrease in the firing rate of receptors, and vice versa.

Input to the central nervous system from the ventricular receptors, which are sensitive to mechanical and chemical stimuli, is through nonmyelinated vagal afferents (C fibers).[4] In response to an increase in ventricular pressure, the mechanoreceptors were previously thought to stimulate a depressor response (decreased heart rate/vasodilation). The depressor reflex causes a decrease in heart rate, and may play a role in the alteration in vascular tone[5]; although this response is less than the vascular response induced by increases in carotid or coronary arterial pressure. The ventricular mechanoreceptors appear to play a role only in protection from gross overdistention, possibly during myocardial ischemia.[6,7] Chronic activation of cardiac receptors in heart failure cause increased activation of hypothalamic paraventricular neurons, which may contribute to resetting of the baroreceptor reflex and a sustained increase in sympathetic activation.[8]

Bezold–Jarisch Reflex

The Bezold–Jarisch reflex, which is the most commonly used model to explain the triggering of vasovagal (neurocardiogenic) syncope, is manifested as a triad of symptoms (bradycardia, apnea, and hypotension).[9] Neurocardiogenic syncope is thought to occur

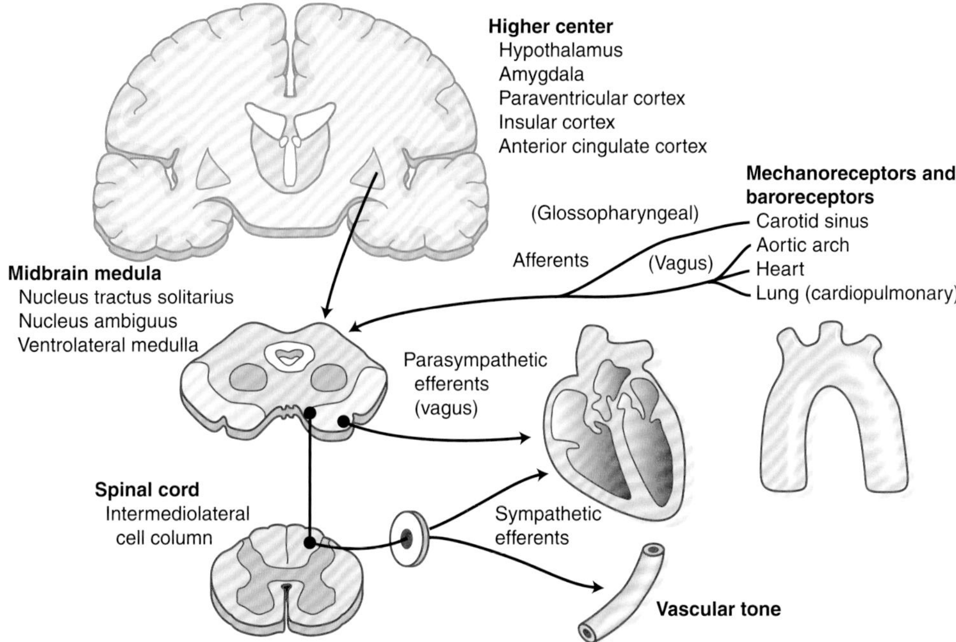

Figure 4-1. Autonomic nervous system regulation of cardiovascular hemodynamic responses. The baroreceptors (mechanoreceptors), which are located in the carotid sinus, in the aortic arch, and in the heart and lungs, send afferent impulses to the nucleus tractus solitarius. The vagal fibers to the heart arise from the vagal nucleus in the brainstem. This nucleus is governed by the nucleus tractus solitarius, which is the main receiving station for afferent information from the peripheral mechanoreceptors and chemoreceptors. The medullary centers also receive input from higher brain centers. The vagal nerve alters heart rate through its effect on the sinoatrial and atrioventricular nodes. Sympathetic fibers innervate the sinoatrial and atrioventricular nodes and the ventricular myocardium, and affect heart rate and contractility. In addition, the sympathetic fibers innervate the vasculature, and thus alter vascular tone. (From Fenton AM, Hammill SC, Rea RF, et al. Vasovagal syncope. *Ann Intern Med.* 2000;133:714–725.)

as a result of excessive venous pooling and a decrease in peripheral venous return. The decreased venous return leads to a hypercontractile state that stimulates the cardiac mechanoreceptors (particularly those in the inferoposterior wall of the left ventricle).[10] This hypercontractile state mimics hypertension and causes a paradoxical inhibitory or depressor reflex causing a vagally mediated decrease in heart rate and withdrawal of sympathetic stimulation to the peripheral vasculature with subsequent vasodilation.[11] Stimulation of this reflex may occur with pathologic conditions, such as myocardial infarction, administration of thrombolytic therapy, hemorrhage, aortic stenosis, or syncope. It is important to note that vasovagal syncope may also occur in patients with transplanted (denervated) hearts; thus, factors other than those traditionally attributed to the Bezold–Jarisch reflex must be considered.[9] Figure 4-2 characterizes the numerous putative causes of vasovagal syncope. During an acute inferoposterior myocardial infarction (particularly because of right coronary artery occlusion) and at the time of reperfusion of these infarctions, the transient bradycardia observed is thought to be a manifestation of the depressor effect of vagal receptors located in the inferoposterior wall of the left ventricle.[12] Research also suggests that this response occurs with more proximal lesions involving the right ventricle.[13] During ischemia, these receptors, which are mechanosensitive or chemosensitive, may be distorted by bulging of the ventricular wall during systole[14] or by the presence of reactive oxygen species, serotonin, bradykinin, thromboxane A_2, or adenosine.[15–17] During thrombolytic therapy, the occurrence of vagally mediated bradycardia may be an indicator of reperfusion and sustained vessel patency, particularly with an inferior myocardial infarction.[18] These receptors are also thought to mediate the reflex bradycardia and hypotension that occur during coronary angiography, particularly during injection of contrast material into the arteries that supply the inferoposterior surface of the left ventricle (e.g., circumflex, right coronary artery).[19] In severe aortic stenosis, some patients experience exertional syncope and even sudden death. The probable mechanism of the syncope is an exercise-induced increase in left ventricular pressure, which is extreme because of high aortic valve resistance, despite a decrease in aortic blood pressure. This high left ventricular pressure stimulates the ventricular baroreceptors and is manifested by a Bezold–Jarisch response.[20–23] Once these patients undergo surgical correction of the stenosis, however, the normal sympathetic vasoconstrictor response to exercise is restored. Similarly, in patients with hypertrophic cardiomyopathy, this abnormal response may be the cause of syncope, exercise-induced paradoxical peripheral vasodilation, or sudden cardiac arrest.[24–26] Finally, in cases of severe hemorrhage or during head-up tilt (particularly in patients receiving a concurrent infusion of isoproterenol), the ventricular depressor reflex is thought to be initiated by the acute distortion of the ventricular mechanoreceptors by a forceful ventricular contraction on a relatively empty ventricle or simply a forceful contraction.[27] Severe hypovolemia can lead to super ventricular tachycardia (SVT) and trigger the Bezold–Jarisch response.[28] This can be manifested by sudden bradycardia and even cardiac arrest due to triggering of the reflex. A trauma model, inhibition of Bezold–Jarisch-mediated bradycardia with β-adrenergic blockade may aid in resuscitation.[29]

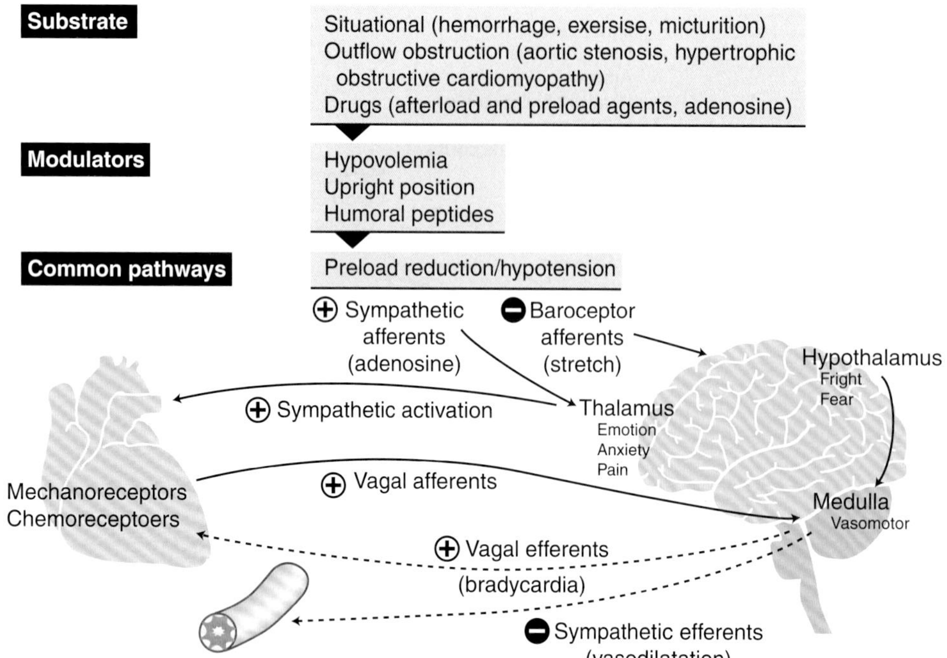

Figure 4-2. The Bezold–Jarisch reflex indicates that the neurocardiogenic reflex is initiated by cardiac mechanoreceptor activation. This information is transmitted by the vagal afferents to the cardiovascular respiratory center in the medulla. The negative feedback response is transmitted by an activation of the vagal efferents and an inhibition of the sympathetic efferents. Inputs to the medulla may originate from extracardiac locations as well as directly from the higher central nervous system. (From Fenton AM, Hammill SC, Rea RF, et al. Vasovagal syncope. *Ann Intern Med.* 2000;133:714–725.)

Chemoreceptors

Peripheral chemoreceptors located in the carotid and aortic bodies are sensitive to decreased arterial Pa_{O2} or an increase in Pa_{CO2} or [H^+], whereas central chemoreceptors, which are located in the medulla are sensitive to increased Pa_{CO2}.[30] Stimulation of these receptors leads to hyperventilation and sympathetic activation, which causes vasoconstriction in most vascular beds, except the brain and heart. While an increase in blood pressure is an outcome of the chemoreflex, an increase in baroreceptor stimulation (i.e., increased arterial blood pressure) inhibits the chemoreflex response. Conversely, the chemoreflexes potentiate the baroreflex-mediated vasoconstriction in response to decreased arterial blood pressure.[31] In hypertension and sleep apnea, the peripheral chemoreflex response to hypoxemia is enhanced, with a resultant increase in sympathetic activation. Of clinical importance, there is a strong relationship between hypertension and sleep apnea (i.e., individuals with sleep apnea have a high prevalence of hypertension).[32] In heart failure, both the peripheral and central chemoreflex responses may be enhanced, as manifested by increased sympathetic activation.[33] This enhanced response may contribute to genesis of sleep apnea in these patients, which is associated with a poorer prognosis.[34–36]

CENTRAL NERVOUS SYSTEM REGULATION

The *nucleus tractus solitarius* is an ovoid area located in the medulla that receives efferent input from cardiovascular, respiratory, and gastrointestinal sites. The *nucleus tractus solitarius* serves as the first relay station for reflexes (e.g., baroreceptor reflex, central and peripheral arterial chemoreceptors, and skeletal muscle receptors [ergoreceptors]) that control circulation and respiration.[37] From the *nucleus tractus solitarius*, there are multiple projections to areas such as: (1) the ventrolateral medulla, which is responsible for sympathetic efferent activity; (2) the *nucleus ambiguus* or "cardioinhibitory center" of the medulla, which is the location of the cell bodies of the vagal parasympathetic nerves; and (3) the median preoptic nuclei, which affect the release of vasopressin. The output from the medulla depends on the perturbation of the system (i.e., an increase or decrease in blood pressure). From the central nervous system, the efferent arm of the rapid control of blood pressure operates through the autonomic nervous system. From the carotid sinus, afferent input to the nucleus tractus solitarius in the medulla is through the carotid sinus nerve (nerve of Hering), which joins the ninth cranial nerve (glossopharyngeal). The sensory input from the aortic arch is through the 10th cranial nerve (vagus). Through synaptic connections to areas located in caudal and rostral ventrolateral medulla and *nucleus ambiguus*, sympathetic and parasympathetic output, respectively, is modified by afferent feedback from the baroreceptors. Output from the lateral ventrolateral medulla, which is directly projected to spinal sympathetic outflow via the bulbospinal (or medullospinal) tract, is responsible for maintaining tonic sympathetic activity, and thus resting arterial blood pressure.[38,39] In addition, baroreceptor signals are transmitted to the forebrain. Paraventricular nuclei in the forebrain play a role in the release of vasopressin in response to a sustained decrease in blood pressure and increased osmolarity (or hypernatremia) and influence the sympathoexcitatory vasomotor neurons in the medulla.[40,41] The excitation or inhibition of the sympathetic and parasympathetic systems depends on the direction of the change in arterial blood pressure. An example of the reflex response (increased parasympathetic activity in the heart and sympathetic activity in the heart and vasculature) to increased blood pressure is summarized in Figure 4-3.[42]

Of clinical importance, the baroreceptor reflex is reset at a higher point in hypertension, which is associated with adrenergic overdrive, decreased ability of cardiopulmonary receptors to control renin release, and altered control of blood pressure and blood volume.[43]

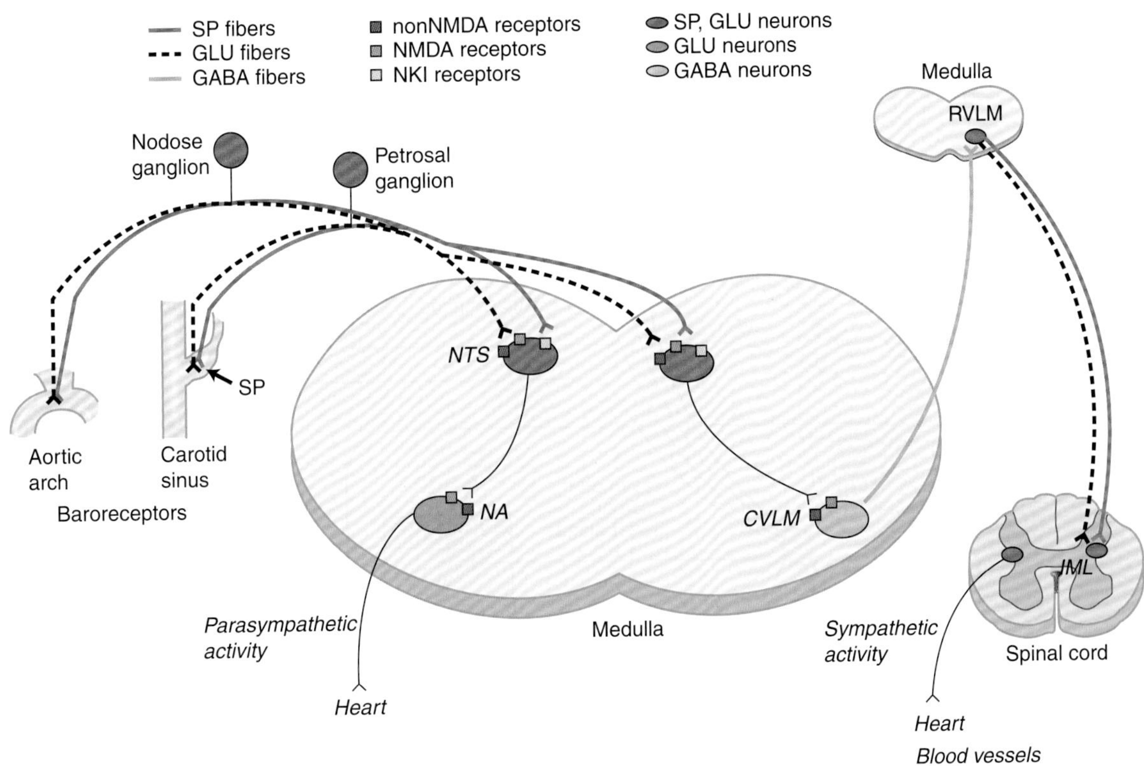

Figure 4-3. Schematic diagram indicating the baroreflex arc. Baroreceptor afferents, with cell bodies in the petrosal and nodose ganglia, are activated by high blood pressure (stretch) and excite neurons in the nucleus tractus solitarius (NTS). These neurons then activate neurons within the nucleus ambiguus (N. AMB) to increase parasympathetic activity to the heart or activate neurons in the caudal ventrolateral medulla (CVLM), which in turn inhibit presympathetic neurons in the rostral ventrolateral medulla (RVLM). This inhibition of RVLM neurons reduces activation of sympathetic preganglionic neurons in the intermediolateral cell column (IML) of the spinal cord, reducing sympathetic activity to the heart and vessels. Glutamate (GLU) has been identified as an excitatory neurotransmitter at many synapses in the reflex arc, while gamma-aminobutyric acid (GABA) has been identified as an inhibitory neurotransmitter at the RVLM. SP has been identified in presumptive baroreceptor fibers: in the carotid sinus and aortic arch, in fibers and neurons within the petrosal and nodose ganglia, in fibers and neurons in the NTS, within neurons in the RVLM, and in fibers in the IML. Release of SP within the NTS, RVLM, and IML has been found to excite neurons within the regions through activation of NK1 receptors. (From Helke CJ, Seagard JL. Subtance P in the baroreflex: 25 years. *Peptides*. 2004;25[3]:413–423.)

AUTONOMIC NERVOUS SYSTEM REGULATION

The autonomic nervous system, which is one branch of the peripheral nervous system, is responsible for coordination of body functions that ensure homeostasis. The autonomic nervous system is further divided into two major components: the sympathetic nervous system and the parasympathetic nervous system (Fig. 4-4).

Sympathetic Nervous System

Efferent projections from the hypothalamus and medulla terminate in the intermediolateral cells located in the gray matter of the thoracic and lumbar (thoracolumbar) sections of the spinal column (specifically, T-1 to L-2). Hence, the sympathetic nervous system is often referred to as the thoracolumbar division of the autonomic nervous system. The neuronal cell bodies, which are located in the spinal column, are generally the origin of short preganglionic efferent fibers that innervate postsynaptic sympathetic neurons located in three general groupings of ganglia (a group of nerve cell bodies). The paravertebral ganglia are located in a bilateral chain-like structure adjacent to the spinal column. This chain extends from the superior cervical ganglia, located at the level of the bifurcation of the carotid artery, to ganglia located in the sacral region. The prevertebral ganglia, which lie midline and anterior to the aorta and vertebral column, include the celiac, aorticorenal, and superior and inferior mesenteric ganglia. The third group of ganglia comprises the previsceral or terminal ganglia, which are located close to the target organs of the sympathetic nervous system. The previsceral ganglia have long preganglionic fibers and short postganglionic fibers. In contrast, the paravertebral and prevertebral ganglia give rise to long postganglionic fibers, which extend to the target organs of the sympathetic nervous system (e.g., heart, lungs, vascular smooth muscle, liver, kidneys, bladder, and reproductive organs). Of particular importance to the control of blood pressure are the sympathetic receptors located in the heart, vasculature, kidneys, and renal medulla.[44]

Adrenoreceptors

At the target organs, the postganglionic fibers terminate at the neuroeffector junction and are separated from the adrenergic

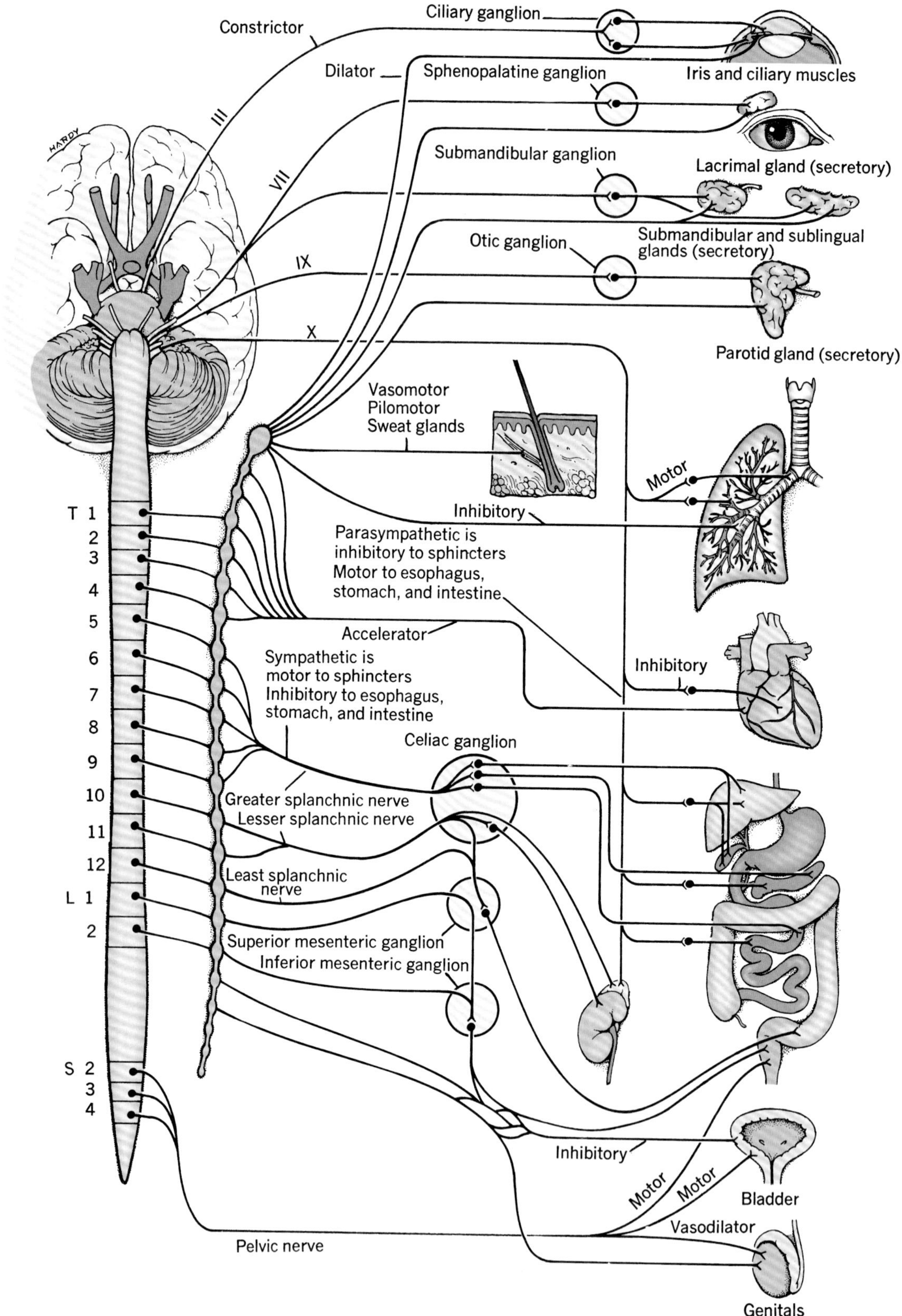

Figure 4-4. The autonomic nervous system. Parasympathetic (craniosacral) divisions send long preganglionic fibers that synapse with a second nerve in ganglia located close to or within the organs that are then innervated by short postganglionic fibers. The sympathetic (thoracolumbar) division sends relatively short preganglionic fibers to the chains of paravertebral ganglia and to certain outlying ganglia. The second cell then sends relatively long postganglionic fibers to the organs they innervate. (From Rodman MJ, Smith DW. *Pharmacology and Drug Therapy in Nursing*. 3rd ed. Philadelphia, PA: JB Lippincott; 1985:302.)

receptors (adrenoreceptors) by only a small junctional gap or cleft. The adrenoreceptors have been classified into two general groups: α-adrenergic receptors and β-adrenergic receptors. The receptor groups are further divided into general subtypes, β_1, β_2, and β_3 and α_1 and α_2 (Table 4-1).[45,46] Based on molecular cloning techniques, the α-receptors are further subdivided, with the α_1 subclassified as (α_{1A}, α_{1B}, α_{1D}).[47] The α_1-adrenergic receptors, which are now characterized as subtypes α_{1A}, α_{1B}, and α_{1D}, are located in arteries, arterioles, and cutaneous and visceral veins. The α_{1A} receptors are responsible for vessel contraction. The α_{1B} receptors are thought to contribute to the maintenance of basal vascular tone and arterial blood pressure in conscious animals and are sensitive to exogenous agonists. Finally, the α_{1D} receptors also play a role in vascular contraction, although they have a lesser effect than the α_{1B} receptors.[48] The α_2 receptor has also been subclassified (α_{2A}, α_{2B}, and α_{2C}). The α_2 receptors, which have presynaptic and postsynaptic functions, are characterized as $\alpha_{2A/D}$, α_{2B}, and α_{2C}. The $\alpha_{2A/D}$ and α_{2B} receptors are present in large arteries but are located with greater density on the terminal arterioles, which act as precapillary sphincters to control the number of open capillaries and total capillary blood flow. The $\alpha_{2A/D}$ receptors play the primary role in vasoconstriction.[49,50] The α_{2B} receptors also play a role in vasoconstriction and may contribute to the onset of hypertension. The α_{2C} receptors are responsible for venoconstriction.[51,52]

The effects of dopamine are mediated by two families of receptors (D_1 and D_2). The D_1-like receptors (D_1 and D_5 receptor subtypes) couple with G proteins to activate adenyl cyclase and the D_2-like receptors (D_2, D_3, and D_4 receptor subtypes) inhibit adenyl cyclase release and activate potassium channels.[53,54] Dopamine is a precursor of norepinephrine. In the heart, dopamine exerts its indirect inotropic and chronotropic effects through the release of norepinephrine. Stimulation of postjunctional D_1 receptors in the renal, mesenteric, and splenic arteries produces vasodilation and natriuresis. Defects in the D_1 and D_5 receptor may be associated with the development of hypertension.[53,55] Stimulation of prejunctional D_2 receptors in blood vessels inhibits norepinephrine release causing vasodilation. Additionally, in the kidneys stimulation of the D_2 receptor inhibits norepinephrine release and plays a synergistic role in modulating natriuresis via inhibition of aldosterone secretion.[54–57] Exogenous administration of low-dose dopamine (less than 4 μg/kg per minute) causes vasodilation of the renal and splanchnic vascular beds and increases sodium excretion. However, low-dose dopamine is not renoprotective.[58–60] Intermediate doses of exogenous dopamine (2 to 10 μg/kg per minute) stimulate β_1-adrenergic receptors in the heart and increases contractility. Higher doses (greater than 10 μg/kg per minute) stimulate α-adrenergic receptors in the peripheral vasculature and cause vasoconstriction.

Heart. In the heart, β_1 receptors predominate (80%), although there are also a smaller number of β_2 receptors (20%), with the β_2 receptors playing a role in coronary vasodilation.[61] Stimulation of the β_1 and β_2 receptors in the heart increases: (1) the rate of discharge of the sinoatrial node, (2) conduction across the atrioventricular node, and (3) speed of contraction in the atria and ventricles (chronotropic effect). In addition, β_1 stimulation increases cardiac contractility (inotropic effect). There is also a small number (less than 1%) of β_3 adrenergic receptors in cardiomyocytes.[62]

The β_3 receptors, which mediate negative inotropy via a nitric oxide–dependent pathway,[63] become important during heart failure when they are upregulated. While the receptors are protective, they may contribute to function degradation of the failing heart.[64–66]

There are small number (approximately 14%) of α_1 receptors located in the atria and ventricles.[67] Stimulation of the α_1 receptors creates a modest inotropic response.[68]

Vasculature. Sympathetic stimulation of the arterial tree extends to the level of the terminal arterioles and is also present on capacitance vessels, primarily in the splanchnic bed. The primary transmitter of the vascular smooth muscle sympathetic neuroeffector junction is norepinephrine. Binding of norepinephrine to the vascular smooth muscle α_1 receptor initiates vasoconstriction. The distribution of the α_1 subtypes varies depending on the vascular bed. For example, α_{1A} adrenoreceptors predominate in coronary, splanchnic, renal, and pulmonary vessels, whereas central arteries and veins express all three α_1 receptor subtypes.[69] Stimulation of presynaptic α_2 receptors inhibits norepinephrine release and decreases vasoconstriction, a process called *passive vasodilation.* Conversely, stimulation of the postsynaptic α_2 receptors, which are located on large arterioles and perhaps most importantly on the terminal arterioles, causes vasoconstriction.[51] This vasoconstriction determines the number of open capillaries, and thus capillary blood flow. The α_2-mediated vasoconstriction of the terminal arterioles can be inhibited by metabolic vasodilators (e.g., oxygen, potassium), particularly in the skeletal muscles. In vascular smooth muscle, the β-adrenergic receptors are predominantly of the β_2-subtype. Stimulation of these receptors causes vasorelaxation.[46]

Table 4-1 • CARDIOVASCULAR EFFECTS OF AUTONOMIC NERVOUS SYSTEM INNERVATION

		Effects	
Organ	**Site**	**Sympathetic Stimulation**	**Parasympathetic Stimulation**
Heart	Sinoatrial/atrioventricular nodes, His–Purkinje system	+ Chronotrope (β_1, β_2)	– Chronotrope
	Myocardium	– Inotrope (β_1, β_2, presynaptic α_1, presynaptic α_{2c})	– Inotrope (minor)
	Coronary arteries	Vasoconstriction (α_{1D}, α_2) Vasodilation (β_2)	Dilation
Systemic vasculature	Skeletal muscle	Vasodilation ($\beta_1 < \beta_2$, β_3, presynaptic α_2) Vasoconstriction (postsynaptic α_2)	—
	Splanchnic bed	Vasoconstriction (α, α_2)	—
	Renal	Vasoconstriction (α_1)	—
	Cutaneous veins	Vasoconstriction (postjunctional α_1, α_2)	Vasodilation

Cutaneous Vasculature

Control of the cutaneous circulation arises from both thermoregulatory and nonthermoregulatory reflexes. The cutaneous circulation has an extensive distribution of both α_1 and α_2 adrenoreceptors, but virtually no β adrenoreceptors.[70] The glabrous skin (e.g., palms/soles) is innervated only by vasoconstrictive nerves. In contrast, nonglabrous skin receives both vasoconstrictive and vasodilator innervations.[71] The sympathetic vasoconstrictor nerves release norepinephrine and may also release vasoconstrictive cotransmitters (neuropeptide Y [NPY] or adenosine triphosphate [ATP]), which augments vasoconstriction.[72,73]

In a thermoneutral environment, the cutaneous resistance vessels in the acral regions (e.g., ears) are tonically constricted, whereas the nonacral regions (limbs, head, and trunk) have minimal constriction.[74,75] Vasodilation in the acral regions is primarily caused by withdrawal of vasoconstrictive tone (passive vasodilation), whereas vasodilation in nonacral regions is the result of an active process, which is sympathetically (but not adrenergically) mediated. Within a "neutral zone," thermoregulation is controlled entirely by changes in cutaneous vasomotor tone.[76] An active increase in adrenergic tone causes vasoconstriction in response to hypothermia. Conversely, a decrease in adrenergic stimulation causes passive vasodilation and is responsible for 10% to 20% of vasodilation in response to hyperthermia.[71,72,77] Cholinergic nerves, which innervate the sweat glands, release a yet to be described cotransmitter that may be functionally linked to the large and important active cutaneous vasodilation seen in heat stress.[73,77,78] Additionally, under conditions of hyperthermia, nitric oxide is necessary for the vasodilatory response.[79] Endothelial nitric oxide (eNOS) is responsible for vasodilation in response to local cutaneous heating,[78] whereas neuronal nitric oxide (nNOS) is responsible for vasodilation in response to whole-body heating.[80] The cutaneous veins constrict in response to local cold and are reflexly constricted in response a decrease in skin or core body temperature.[81]

Nonthermoregulatory control of the cutaneous circulation via the arterial and cardiopulmonary baroreflexes plays a role in blood pressure control. For example, under normothermic conditions, "unloading" of the baroreflex causes cutaneous vasoconstriction. Because of the normally low cutaneous blood flow during normothermia, this vasoconstriction contributes little to blood pressure maintenance. However, under conditions of hyperthermia and during exercise, when there is significant blood flow to the cutaneous vasculature, baroreflex-mediated vasoconstrictive may offset thermoregulatory vasodilation and play an important role in maintenance of blood pressure.[82] Of note, the baroreflex sensitivity is not impaired by whole-body heating as previously thought; however, heat stress may decrease peripheral vasoconstrictor responsiveness, which contributes to an increased susceptibility to orthostatic intolerance.[83]

Neurotransmitters

The sympathetic postganglionic fibers that innervate the arterial tree are in general noradrenergic (i.e., release norepinephrine). The only exceptions are the postganglionic fibers that innervate the sweat glands (sudomotor neurons), which have acetylcholine as their neurotransmitter and the extrapyramidal system, which has dopamine as the primary neurotransmitter. Norepinephrine is synthesized from tyrosine and is stored in sympathetic nerve terminals. In response to neuronal stimulation, the "packets" or quanta of norepinephrine are extruded from the axon vesicles by exocytosis. The vesicular release of norepinephrine is enhanced by angiotensin II and cold, whereas the prejunctional effects of potassium, decreased P_{O_2}, heat, autacoids (adenosine, bradykinin, serotonin, and prostaglandins), nitric oxide, and acetylcholine inhibit its release (Fig. 4-5).[84] The neurotransmitters diffuse over varying small distances, depending on the width of the junctional cleft, to receptors located on effector organs. Norepinephrine is also considered a systemic hormone because of its spillover into the interstitial space.

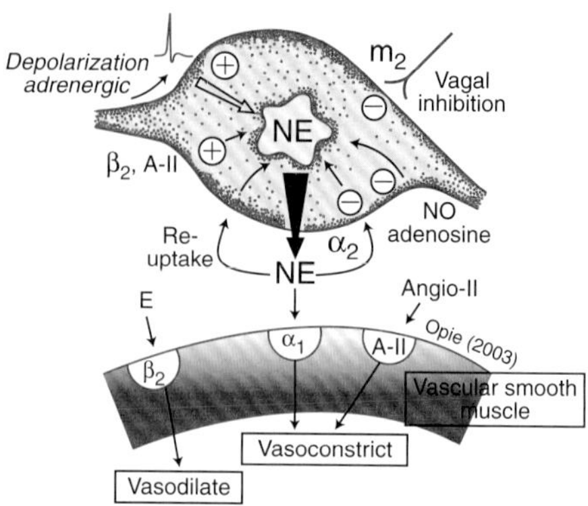

Figure 4-5. Role of neuromodulation in arteriolar constriction and dilation. Norepinephrine is released from the storage granules of the terminal neurons into the synaptic cleft that separates the terminals from the arterial wall. Norepinephrine has predominantly vasoconstrictive effects acting through postsynaptic α_1 receptors. In addition, norepinephrine stimulates presynaptic α_2 receptors to invoke feedback inhibition of its own release, to modulate excess release of NE. Parasympathetic cholinergic stimulation inhibits the release of norepinephrine and thereby indirectly causes vasodilation. Circulating epinephrine stimulates vascular vasodilatory β_2 receptors, but also presynaptic receptors on the nerve terminal that promotes release of norepinephrine. Angiotensin II, formed ultimately in response to renin released from the kidneys, is also powerfully vasoconstrictive, acting both by inhibition of norepinephrine release (presynaptic receptors, schematically shown to the left of the terminal neuron) and also directly on arteriolar receptors. E, epinephrine; NE, norepinephrine; A-II, angiotensin II; M2, muscarinic receptor, subtype 2. (From Opie LH. *Heart Physiology: From Cell to Circulation*. 4th ed. Philadelphia, PA: Lippincott Williams & Wilkins; 2003:25.)

Parasympathetic Nervous System

The second branch of the autonomic nervous system is the parasympathetic nervous system. The primary parasympathetic outflow is through four cranial nerves (III, VII, IX, and X). Of importance to blood pressure and cardiac output control, cardiac vagal (cranial nerve X) *motorneurons* are located in the nucleus ambiguus and dorsal vagal nucleus of the medulla. In addition, there are cell bodies located in the spinal cord gray matter at S-2 through S-4. Hence, the parasympathetic nervous system is referred to as the *craniosacral* branch of the autonomic nervous system. In contrast to the sympathetic nervous system, the preganglionic fibers of the parasympathetic nervous system are long fibers, synapsing on ganglia that are close to or directly attached to the effector organ. The postsynaptic fibers are relatively short, in contrast to the fibers of the sympathetic nervous system.

Receptors

In the parasympathetic nervous system, the nerve fibers are cholinergic, which means they liberate acetylcholine. Despite a common neurotransmitter (acetylcholine), stimulation of various receptors in the parasympathetic nervous system causes different effects. The reason for the variable response is that there are two general types of cholinergic receptors: nicotinic and muscarinic.

Preganglionic cholinergic receptors, which are found in the sympathetic and parasympathetic nervous systems, are nicotinic. The nicotinic receptors are located on autonomic ganglia and skeletal muscle end plates. Stimulation of the nicotinic receptors is excitatory and short term (milliseconds). These receptors are blocked by curare. In clinical practice, blockade of the nicotinic receptors with various neuromuscular-blocking agents (e.g., succinylcholine, pancuronium) causes musculoskeletal paralysis (blockade at the skeletal muscle end plate) and may potentially cause hypotension because of blockade at the autonomic ganglia.[85]

The primary postganglionic receptor in the heart, smooth muscle, and glandular tissue is muscarinic. These receptors are stimulated by muscarine and can be antagonized by atropine and scopolamine. There are subtypes of the muscarinic receptors that result in varied responses. The primary muscarinic receptors in the heart are the muscarinic subtype 2 (M_2), which are specifically associated with vagal nerve endings in the heart. The M_2 receptors have direct and indirect negative inotropic and chronotropic effects.[86] The direct effects are secondary to occupation of the β-adrenergic receptors and inhibition of norepinephrine release, and the indirect effects occur through inhibition of the adrenergic second messenger cAMP.[87,88] There are also M_1, M_3, and M_5 receptors in the heart, which may have pharmacologic implications.[89] Of clinical importance, the negative chronotropic and inotropic effects associated with the M_2 receptor are blocked by atropine.

Cotransmitters

At the preganglionic synapse, the primary neurotransmitter for the sympathetic and parasympathetic nervous systems is acetylcholine. At the neuroeffector junction in the sympathetic nervous system, the primary neurotransmitters are norepinephrine and its precursor, dopamine, whereas the primary neurotransmitter of the postganglionic fibers of the parasympathetic nervous system is acetylcholine. However, other neurotransmitters that augment or modify the effects of the primary neurotransmitter are coreleased, and are referred to as *cotransmitters* (Fig. 4-6).[90–92] The most prominent cotransmitters in the sympathetic nervous system ganglia are NPY and ATP.[91,93] Vasoactive intestinal peptide (VIP) is the prominent cotransmitter in the parasympathetic nervous system ganglia and nonadrenergic, noncholinergic nerves.[94]

Neuropeptide Y

NPY is an amino acid peptide released with norepinephrine from sympathetic nerve terminals. NPY has direct pressor effects and also exerts a prejunctional modulation of the release of other

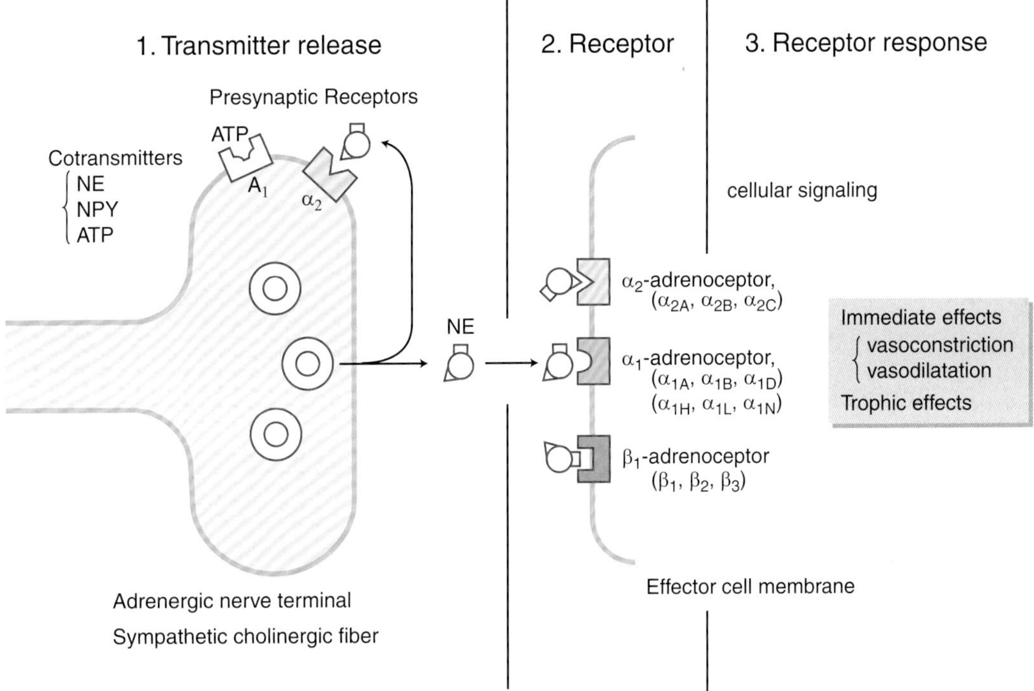

Figure 4-6. Diagram of the sympathetic nerve and adrenergic neuroeffector mechanism. (1) Transmitter release from the sympathetic terminal. Sympathetic nerve may contain three cotransmitters, that is, norepinephrine (NE), neuropeptide Y (NPY), and adenosine triphosphate (ATP). Release of main transmitter NE may be presynaptically modulated by α_2-adrenoreceptor, A_1 adenosine receptor, and so on. (2) Adrenoreceptors on the effector cell membrane. There are α- and β-adrenoreceptors and subtypes α_1 (α_{1A}, α_{1B}, and α_{1D}; α_{1H}, α_{1L}, and α_{1N}), α_2 (α_{2A}, α_{2B}, and α_{2C}), and β_1, β_2, and β_3. There may be regional differences in the population of adrenoreceptors. (3) Effector responses. Sympathetic nerves have both immediate effects—contraction and dilation, differing from vessel to vessel—as well as long-term trophic effect on blood vessels. (From Tsuru H, Tanimitsu N, Hirai T. Role of perivascular sympathetic nerves and regional differences in the features in sympathetic innervation of the vascular system. *Jpn J Pharmacol.* 2002;88[1]:9–13.)

neurotransmitters. For example, NPY inhibits the release of acetylcholine from vagal nerve endings, thus attenuating the effects of the parasympathetic system on heart rate, atrioventricular conduction, and atrial contractility.[95,96] In addition, NPY potentiates the postjunctional contractile effects of norepinephrine. In the mesentery, 30% of the sympathetic nervous system–induced vasoconstriction depends on NPY,[97,98] although the role of NPY varies depending on the vascular bed. NPY is also associated with vascular remodeling (Y_1 receptor) and angiogenesis (Y_2). Pharmacologic strategies that promote angiogenesis but inhibit the proatherosclerotic effects of NPY may be useful in preventing or treating pathologic vascular remodeling.[99,100]

Vasoactive Intestinal Peptide

VIP is present in the peripheral and central circulation, where it acts as a nonadrenergic, noncholinergic neurotransmitter, or neuromodulator. Endogenous VIP is a potent vasodilator, although its effects vary in different vascular beds. It is released in response to vagal stimulation in the heart, where it produces coronary vasodilation (effect greater on the arteries than the veins) as well as positive inotropic (particularly in the right atria and ventricle) and chronotropic effects.[101,102] VIP-induced peripheral vasodilation is caused by increased calcium extrusion or sequestration induced by VIP or natriuretic protein-C receptor stimulation. This peripheral vasodilation enhances the VIP-mediated inotropic effects.[103]

SYSTEMIC HORMONES

In addition to the rapid control of arterial pressure by the autonomic nervous system, hormones such as epinephrine and arginine vasopressin (AVP) directly and indirectly affect the baroreceptor reflex and play an important role in the rapid control of blood pressure. Three interrelated systems (natriuretic peptide system, renin–angiotensin–aldosterone system [RAAS], and the kallikrein–kinin system [KKS]) also contribute to the regulation of the arterial blood pressure and fluid volume (Fig. 4-7). Finally, a spillover of norepinephrine into the systemic circulation also affects blood pressure and cardiac output.

Epinephrine

In response to physical or emotional stressors (mental stress, exercise, hyperthermia, hypoglycemia), epinephrine is secreted into the plasma by the adrenal medulla, causing the plasma level of epinephrine to increase. Epinephrine stimulates β_1 receptors in the heart and has positive chronotropic and inotropic effects. The net effect of this cardiac stimulation is an increase in cardiac output. Epinephrine also acts on the vasculature and stimulates the β_2 receptors in the skeletal muscles and splanchnic arterioles, which cause vasodilation in these two large regions and potentially large decrements in the systemic vascular resistance. In the skin and kidneys, epinephrine stimulates the α-adrenergic receptors and causes vasoconstriction.[104]

Exogenously administered epinephrine has dose-specific effects. Low-dose epinephrine (0.1 mcg/kg per minute) stimulates the β_1 and β_2 adrenoreceptors and causes vasodilation and increased heart rate and contractility. Increased doses (greater than 0.2 mcg/kg per minute) stimulate the α-adrenoreceptors and increases vascular resistance and blood pressure.[105] Knowledge of these dose-specific effects is important, and although epinephrine is often administered for its vasoconstrictive effects, it may cause vasodilation with a smaller dose.

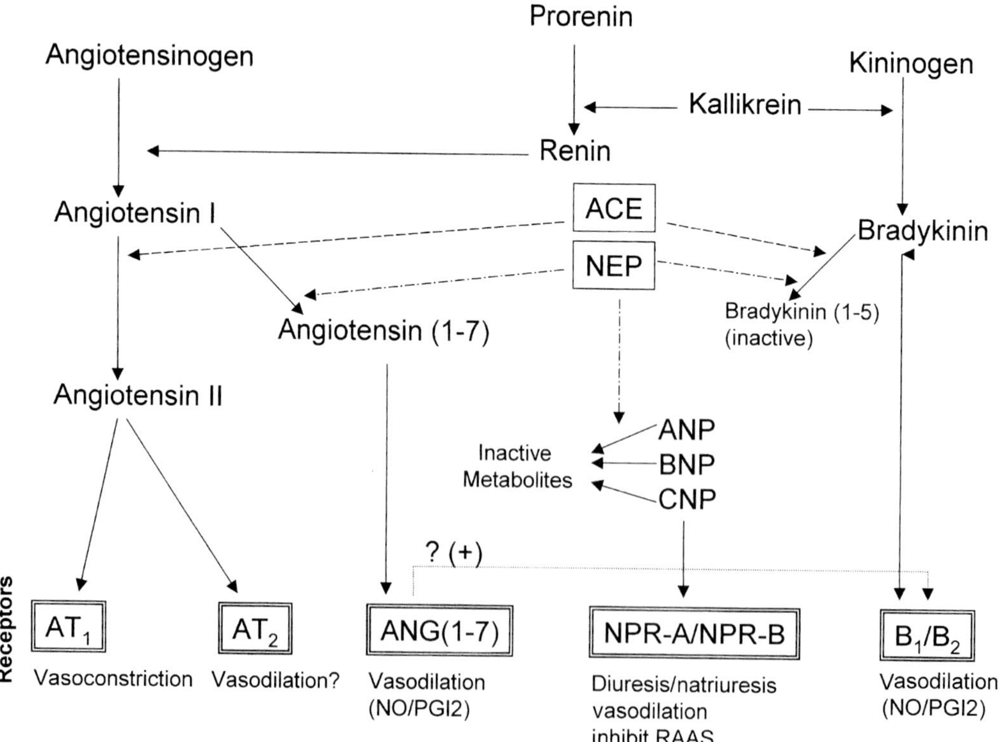

Figure 4-7. Interaction of the renin–angiotensin–aldosterone system (RAAS), kallikrein–kinin system (KKS), and natriuretic peptides.

Arginine Vasopressin

AVP, or antidiuretic hormone (ADH), is a neurotransmitter synthesized in the hypothalamus and released from the neurohypophysis of the pituitary gland (posterior pituitary gland). Vasopressin is primarily released in response to changes in plasma osmolality; however, AVP may also be released in response to a decrease in blood volume or blood pressure. As the osmolality increases, AVP secretion increases. In humans, the primary effect of AVP is its antidiuretic effect, which is caused by stimulation of water absorption at the distal and collecting tubules of the kidney.[106,107] The change in water absorption affects plasma osmolality. Vasopressin is exquisitely sensitive to changes in osmolality; for example, a 5- to 10-mOsm increase in osmolality causes an increase in plasma AVP.[108,109] The close relation between osmolality and AVP maintains plasma osmolality within 1% of normal under most conditions.[110,111]

The sensitivity of the baroreceptor system is less than that of the osmoreceptors, as demonstrated by the large (5% to 10%) iso-osmotic change in plasma volume required before vasopressin secretion is altered. However, during hemorrhage (plasma volume decreased by greater than 5% to 10%), plasma levels of vasopressin are increased, in some cases 100-fold (Fig. 4-8).[112] In this case, vasopressin acts in a manner similar to renin and norepinephrine, causing vasoconstriction and playing a supporting role to the sympathetic nervous system in the maintenance of blood pressure. The primary reflex controllers of the plasma volume–mediated release of vasopressin are the arterial baroreceptors and not the cardiac receptors.[74,113] In hemorrhage, the change in intrathoracic volume alters the arterial systolic blood pressure, which decreases arterial baroreceptor stimulation, and leads to increased vasopressin secretion.[114]

Natriuretic Peptides

There are three natriuretic peptides (A, B, and C) that contribute to the regulation of blood pressure and electrolyte and volume homeostasis.[115,116] Atrial natriuretic peptide (ANP)[117] and brain natriuretic peptide (B-type natriuretic peptide [BNP]) are released from granules in the atria and ventricles in response to increased stretch (increased preload and afterload) and hormonal stimuli (e.g., angiotensin II, glucocorticoids, endothelin I, catecholamines).[118,119] Of note, factors that stimulate BNP release may be different in a normal versus hypertrophied ventricle and after myocardial infarction, with hypoxia acting independent of ventricular dilation to stimulate BNP release.[118] The actions of BNP are similar to ANP. C-type natriuretic peptide is widely distributed in the brain, kidneys, lungs, heart, and endothelial cells, and is released in response to shear stress.

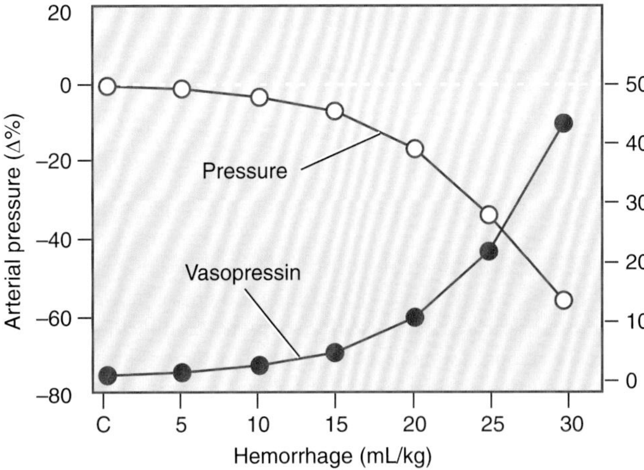

Figure 4-8. Mean percentage changes in arterial blood pressure and in plasma vasopressin concentration in response to blood loss (0.5 mL/kg/min) in a group of 12 dogs; the maximal volume of blood withdrawn was 30 mL/kg. (Redrawn from Shen YT, Cowley AWJ, Vatner SF. Relative roles of cardiac and arterial baroreceptors in vasopressin regulation during hemorrhage in conscious dogs. *Circ Res*. 2001;68:1422; from Koeppen BM, Stanton BA. *Berne and Levy Physiology*. 6th ed. Philadelphia, PA: Mosby Elsevier; 2008.)

The heart has endocrine functions[118] via the cardiac natriuretic peptides (ANP and BNP) that bind with natriuretic peptide receptors A and B (NPR-A and NPR-B) and cause diuresis and natriuresis. These actions subsequently decrease preload and blood pressure.[120] Preload reduction may occur because of shifting of fluid from the intravascular to the extravascular space (increased vascular endothelial permeability) and possibly increased capillary hydrostatic pressure along with natriuresis.[115,121] Additionally, ANP and BNP decrease sympathetic tone to the peripheral vasculature both centrally and peripherally, inhibit the RAAS by inhibiting angiotensin II-stimulated sodium and water transport in the proximal tubules, inhibit endothelin-1 production, improve ventricular relaxation, and lower the activation threshold for the vagal afferents, which suppresses the reflex tachycardia and vasoconstriction associated with the decrease in preload and cardiac output (Fig. 4-9).[122,123] In severe heart failure, increased levels of ANP may offset the detrimental effects of increased angiotensin–aldosterone and the sympathetic nervous system.[116,124]

In 2001, Natrecor, a synthetic BNP intravenous infusion was approved for use in acute decompensated heart failure. After randomized controlled studies (ROSE-AHF, ASCEND-HF) showed that it was no more effective than other less expensive heart failure medications, its usage diminished.[125] However, BNP blood levels are utilized to evaluate treatment effect and heart failure severity.[126]

C-type natriuretic peptide, which is stored in endothelial cells, acts in a paracrine fashion and binds to natriuretic peptide receptor C (NPR-C), which is located in vascular smooth muscle. Note that other texts refer to binding to NPR-A.[96] CNP couples to inhibitory G proteins (G_i) and causes inhibition of adenylate cyclase and activation of phospholipase-C leading to vasodilation. ANP also binds to NPR-C with similar inhibitory effects.[122] Recent research suggests that CNP may be an endothelium-dependent hyperpolarizing factor, with actions in the peripheral and coronary vasculature[122,127–129] The peripheral vascular effect of CNP decreases venous return and subsequently decreases cardiac filling pressures, cardiac output, and arterial blood pressure. Unlike ANP and BNP, CNP has minimal renal actions.[130] CNP is a potent coronary vasodilator and also has an antimitogenic effect on vascular smooth muscle, which may be protective against atheroma development and restenosis.[131] Additionally, in an experimental model of myocardial infarction, CNP administration decreased the size of the infarct and myocardial dysfunction and protected against ischemic reperfusion injury, with possible mechanisms including CNP/NPR-C related coronary vasodilation and decreased heart rate.[121]

Renin–Angiotensin–Aldosterone System

The RAAS plays an important role in the long-term control of arterial blood pressure, regional blood flow, and sodium balance.

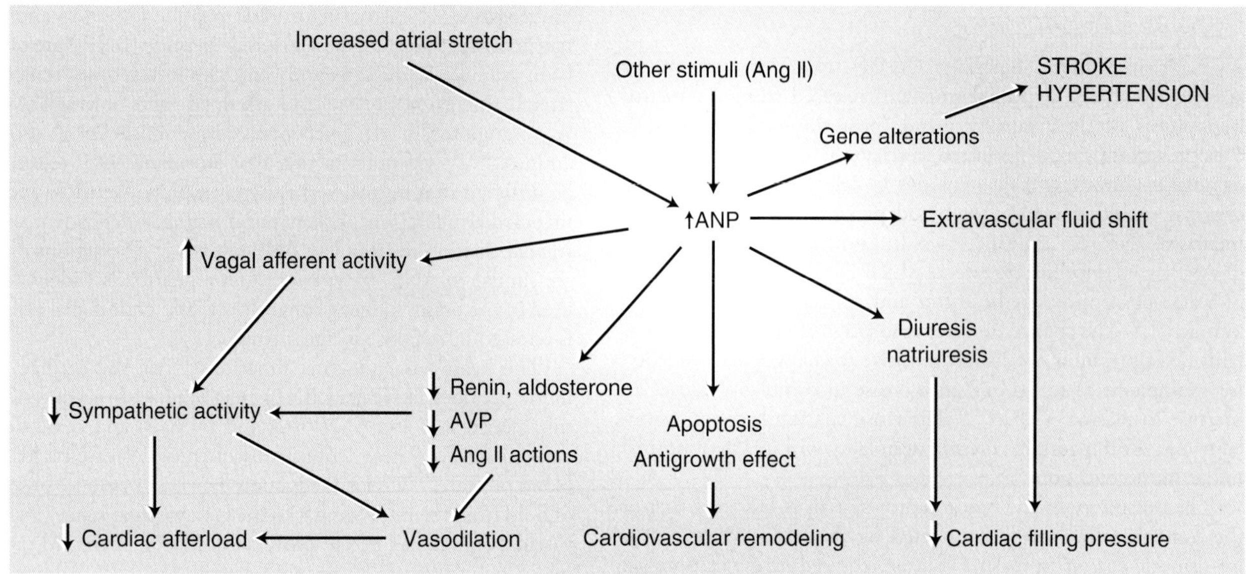

Figure 4-9. Schematic representation of the regulation and function of atrial natriuretic peptide (ANP). Along with the classical circulatory effects, the new emerging functional properties of the atrial natriuretic peptides are shown. AVP, vasopressin; ANG II, angiotensin II. (From Rubattu S, Volpe M. The atrial natriuretic peptide: a changing view. *J Hypertens.* 2001;19:1925.)

The RAAS acts in a cascade fashion, initiated by the stimulation of renin release from the kidney. Renin is stored in and released from the juxtaglomerular cells near the renal afferent arterioles. Renin release is stimulated by three mechanisms. First, renin release occurs in response to increased sympathetic nervous system stimulation of the afferent and efferent arterioles in the renal glomeruli. The β-adrenergic receptors in the cells of the juxtaglomerular apparatus are sensitive to neurally released and systemic catecholamines. This neurally mediated response can be blocked by β-adrenergic blockers (e.g., propranolol). Second, renin release is stimulated by decreased renal perfusion pressure, distending the afferent arterioles (intrarenal baroreceptor pathway). Below a MAP of 80 to 90 mm Hg, renin secretion is a steep and linear function of renal perfusion pressure. Finally, decreased sodium chloride concentration in the macula densa, which is located in the early distal tubule, stimulates the juxtaglomerular apparatus to secrete renin. Increased blood pressure decreases renin release by activating the baroreceptors causing a decrease in sympathetic tone, increasing pressure in the renal arterioles, and decreasing sodium chloride reabsorption in the proximal tubule, causing increased sodium chloride to reach the macula densa.

Angiotensin II is released through the proteolytic effects of renin on the plasma protein, angiotensinogen, which is synthesized and released into the plasma from the liver. Renin converts angiotensinogen to angiotensin I. Angiotensin I, which is inactive, is converted to angiotensin II by an angiotensin-converting enzyme (ACE) located in the plasma and vascular endothelium (primarily pulmonary).[132] Pharmacologically, ACE inhibitors exert their effect at this level of the RAAS.[133]

Angiotensin II has two receptors (AT_1 and AT_2). The classic actions of angiotensin II, which are primarily mediated through AT_1, include vasoconstriction and stimulation of aldosterone release. Angiotensin II causes vasoconstriction of the arterioles through a direct effect on the vascular smooth muscle and indirectly affects vascular tone by stimulating the formation of superoxide anions, which inhibit nitric oxide–mediated vasodilation, and by inducing endothelin-1 formation to cause further vasoconstriction.[134–136] Angiotensin receptor blockers work primarily on the AT_1 receptors.

The renal and splanchnic circulations are particularly sensitive to angiotensin II. Angiotensin II increases vascular resistance and stimulates the heart indirectly through its potentiating actions on the sympathetic nervous system. These effects include: (1) accelerating the synthesis and release of norepinephrine; (2) delaying neuronal reuptake of norepinephrine; (3) directly stimulating the sympathetic ganglia; and (4) facilitating the response to sympathetic activity and vasoconstrictor drugs.[74] Synthetic angiotensin II is reemerging as an adjuvant treatment for vasodilatory shock.[137] However, studies show that it worsens heart failure. It is not recommended for cardiogenic shock.[131]

Angiotensin II also has a long-term effect on blood pressure through stimulation of aldosterone synthesis and secretion, which increases blood volume. Aldosterone, a mineralocorticoid synthesized and secreted by the adrenal cortex, increases sodium reabsorption in the loop of Henle and decreases sodium excretion, which together lead to retention of water and expansion of blood volume. The change in blood volume is a slow process, which is important in the long-term control of blood pressure. Angiotensin II may also play a role in a sustained increase in sympathetic vasomotor or cardiac sympathetic activity by modification of sympathetic nervous system activity perhaps by action at the level of the paraventricular nucleus.[8,39] This latter mechanism may contribute to long-term control of sympathetic activity.

In 2000 ACE2 was discovered.[138,139] This enzyme hydrolyzes angiotensin (Ang) I to produce Ang-(1-9), which is subsequently catalyzed by neutral endopeptidase 24.11 (NEP) to produce Ang-(1-7). Angiotensin II can also be converted to Ang-(1-7). The receptor for Ang-(1-7) is Mas, which is located in the vascular wall and in myocardial cells. Ang-(1-7) has antiproliferative and vasodilator effects, which counterbalance the effects of the RAAS.[140] The role of Ang-(1-7) and the potential therapeutic benefit of Ang-(1-7) remains under investigation.

Kallikrein–Kinin System

The tissue KKS plays a role in blood pressure control and has protective cardiovascular effects. Kinins (e.g., bradykinin and kallidin or lys-BK), which are produced by the action of the enzyme hK1 (a kallikrein) on kininogens, bind with B_1 and B_2 receptors. Bradykinin is inactivated rapidly (less than 15 seconds) by ACE. Binding of kinins with the inducible B_1-receptor, which is upregulated during inflammation and tissue injury, causes the release of nitric oxide and prostacyclin (PGI_2) from endothelial cells and subsequent vasodilation. The constitutive B_2 receptors play a role in pathologic conditions such as pain, inflammation, and hypertension. Stimulation of the B_2 receptor causes the release of nitric oxide and PGI_2 and may be cardioprotective via vasodilation and anti-ischemic and antiproliferative effects.[141,142] Bradykinin plays a role in blood pressure regulation via antagonism of angiotensin-induced vasoconstriction and vasodilation (decreased vascular resistance), diuresis, and natriuresis.[141,143]

A deficient KKS (decreased levels of hK1 and kininogen deficiency and altered B_1 and B_2 genotypes) plays a role in the pathogenesis of hypertension through altered sodium excretion.[141,144] Bradykinin, which is released during ischemia, may also play a cardioprotective role in myocardial infarction and heart failure. After a myocardial infarction, ACE inhibition decreases cardiac dilation and failure by decreasing angiotensin II, but also by preventing the breakdown of kinins. Possible mechanisms for the KKS effect include increasing coronary blood flow and the promotion of angiogenesis and cardiac regeneration, which decrease the infarct size and inhibit ventricular remodeling.[141,144,145] The beneficial effects of the KKS suggest the possible role for pharmacologic treatment of hypertension, postmyocardial infarction, and heart failure.[141,146] However, kinins may contribute the adverse side effects (e.g., increased microvascular permeability, cough, and angioedema) associated with ACE inhibitors.[147]

Interaction Between the KKS, RAAS, and Natriuretic Hormones

The KKS, RAAS, and the natriuretic hormones interact via the actions of ACE and neuropeptidase (NEP) (see Fig. 4-7). ACE stimulates the conversion of angiotensin I to angiotensin II and degrades kinins. NEP is involved in the metabolism of ANP, BNP, CNP, bradykinin, endothelin-1, and angiotensin II and also stimulates the formation of angiotensin (1–7) from angiotensin I. Angiotensin (1–7) has vasodilatory and antiproliferative effects that inhibit ACE and also counteract the actions of angiotensin II.[148] Angiotensin (1–7) also enhances the effects of bradykinin. Kallikrein, which is the enzyme involved in the formation of bradykinin, may also stimulate the conversion of prorenin to renin.[149,150] Renin subsequently causes the conversion of angiotensinogen to angiotensin I. Exploitation of the physiologic interactions between these three systems may be useful in the treatment of heart failure and hypertension. For example, ACE inhibition exerts its antihypertensive effects by decreasing angiotensin II, increasing angiotensin (1–7) levels, and potentiating the effects of bradykinin by increasing its level and through direct effect on the B_2-receptor.[147,148] Triple vasopeptidase inhibitors, which inhibit NEP as well as ACE and endothelin-1–converting enzyme may offer a multimodal approach to the management of cardiovascular disease.[147] However, side effects may limit the utility of some of these medications. For example, omapatrilat (an ACE/NEP inhibitor), which decreased the risk of death and hospitalization in chronic heart failure compared to ACE inhibition alone,[151] was removed from development because of an increased incidence of angioedema,[152] possibly due to increased bradykinin or increased endothelin-1–induced nitric oxide production.[147]

Norepinephrine Spillover

Approximately 80% of the norepinephrine secreted at the neuroeffector junction is either taken up by sympathetic neurons (neuronal reuptake) or broken down by the enzymes monoamine oxidase or catechol-*O*-methyl transferase. The remaining 20% may spill into the systemic circulation. The spillover is usually proportional to the increase in sympathetic nervous system activation; thus, the plasma norepinephrine level can be used as an approximate indicator of sympathetic nervous system activity.[153] Factors such as the nerve firing rate, blood flow, neuronal uptake of norepinephrine, capillary permeability, and width of the junctional cleft can also affect the level of plasma norepinephrine. The width of the junctional cleft is particularly important in the pulmonary vasculature, where spillover is predominantly the result of the wide junctional clefts and not of a high rate of sympathetic nervous system activation or norepinephrine release.[154–156]

ARTERIAL BLOOD PRESSURE

Systolic and diastolic blood pressures describe the high and low values of pressure fluctuations around the mean of the arterial pressure wave. The mean arterial pressure (MAP) in the ascending aorta depends on the cardiac output and systemic vascular resistance (SVR):

$$\text{MAP} = \text{CO} \times \text{SVR}$$

whereas arterial distensibility and left ventricular stroke volume determine the amplitude and contour of the pressure wave.[157] The peak systolic pressure is determined by the volume and velocity of left ventricular ejection (i.e., the larger the stroke volume [SV], the larger the pulse pressure at any given distensibility), peripheral arterial resistance, the distensibility of the arterial wall, the viscosity of blood, and the end-diastolic volume in the arterial blood.[158] During diastole, arterial pressure decreases until the next ventricular contraction, so the minimal diastolic pressure is determined by factors that affect the magnitude and rate of the diastolic pressure drop including blood viscosity, arterial distensibility, peripheral resistance, and the length of the cardiac cycle. Central blood pressure measurements (aorta and carotid), which reflect both the antegrade pressure and the reflected pressure, may be different from peripheral blood pressure measurements.[159]

During systole, the elastic walls of the aorta and large arteries stretch as more blood enters than runs off into the periphery. Thus, a portion of the stroke volume is stored in the relatively distensible aorta during systole. During diastole, there is passive elastic recoil of the arterial walls, causing continued, but decreasing, ejection of blood out of the aorta and into the peripheral arteries. The elastic recoil transforms pulsatile flow into more continuous flow in the smaller vessels and explains why the blood pressure does not drop to zero during periods of no flow (e.g., diastole).

Pulse pressure is the difference between the systolic and diastolic pressures. The aortic pulse pressure is directly proportional to left ventricular stroke volume and inversely related to arterial compliance, with changes in stroke volume responsible for most acute changes.

$$\text{Pulse pressure} \cong \text{Stroke volume/arterial compliance}$$

A normal pulse pressure at the brachial artery is approximately 40 mm Hg. A higher pulse pressure may reflect where the pressure is measured in the body (increased pulse pressure in the periphery). Ejection velocity also affects the pulse pressure, whereas the SVR does not affect the pulse pressure as it affects both systolic and diastolic pressures.

HEART RATE

Control of Heart Rate

The intrinsic heart rate at rest, without any neurohumoral influence, is approximately 100 to 120 beats per minute. The heart rate in the intact, resting person reflects a balance between the tonically active sympathetic and parasympathetic nervous systems, with the parasympathetic nervous system predominating.[160–162] The predominance of the parasympathetic nervous system is manifested by a resting heart rate that is lower than the intrinsic rate. Parasympathetic predominance may also be demonstrated by abolishing the vagal influence with the administration of atropine.

Vagal stimulation of the sinoatrial and atrioventricular nodes leads to a rapid (within one to two beats) decrease in heart rate. When vagal stimulation is discontinued, the heart rate increases rapidly. The rapid response to vagal stimulation and the presence of a large amount of cholinesterase (the enzyme that degrades the acetylcholine that is released from the parasympathetic fibers) allows the vagus nerve to exert beat-to-beat control of heart rate. Conversely, the heart rate response to sympathetic stimulation is gradual in onset, and once the sympathetic stimulation is terminated, the heart rate slowly decreases.[161]

There is an inverse relation between heart rate and arterial blood pressure (Fig. 4-10).[163,164] The inverse changes in heart rate are in response to baroreceptor stimulation, with the response most pronounced over a MAP of 70 to 160 mm Hg. The alterations in heart rate are achieved by a reciprocal relationship between sympathetic and parasympathetic cardiac stimulations.

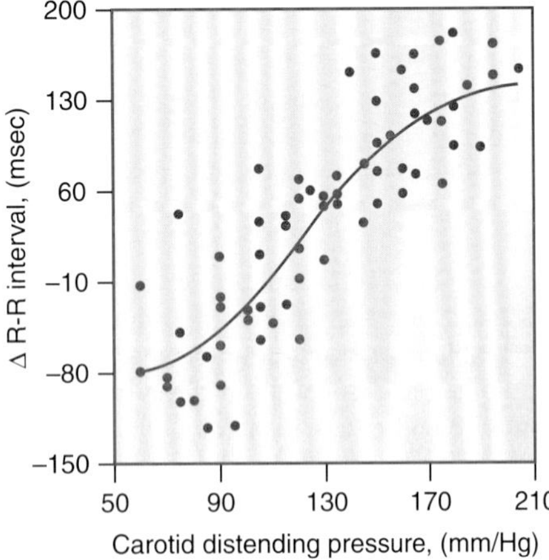

Figure 4-10. Stimulus–response curve for the cardiac arm of the baroreflex determined during application of positive and negative pressures over the anterior aspect of the neck in humans. Relations between carotid distending pressure and changes in *R-R* interval are presented. Data are the mean responses of 10 trials for each subject at each level of neck pressure and suction. The stimulus variable varies depending on the method used to assess baroreflex sensitivity. In this case, the stimulus is carotid sinus pressure (systolic pressure minus neck pressure). (From Rea RF, Eckberg DL. Carotid baroreceptor-muscle sympathetic response in humans. *Am J Physiol.* 1987;253[6, Pt. 2]:R929–R934.)

Changes in heart rate also occur as a result of chemosensor reflexes (Pa_{O_2} and Pa_{CO_2}) mediated by the carotid chemoreceptors. For example, a relatively slight excitation of the chemoreceptors leads to stimulation of the vagal center in the medulla and a decrease in heart rate. This response, which is seldom seen clinically, is considered the primary reflex effect of chemosensor stimulation. With increased levels of stimulation (e.g., a marked decrease in Pa_{O_2}), a secondary reflex is initiated that leads to depression of the primary chemoreceptor reflex and an increase in heart rate. This reflex is caused by pulmonary hyperventilation, which leads to hypocapnia and activation of pulmonary stretch receptors.[165] The chemosensor reflex plays only a minimal role in the control of heart rate because the primary and secondary reflexes tend to offset one another.[38] In heart failure, abnormal central and peripheral chemosensor responses may contribute to sympathetic overactivity and suppression of baroreceptor function.[166,167]

Respiratory Sinus Arrhythmia

There is a direct relation between heart rate and respiration. During inspiration the heart rate increases, then it decreases during expiration. This respiratory-induced cyclical variation in heart rate is referred to as a *respiratory sinus arrhythmia.* There is an ongoing debate whether this arrhythmia is due to a central mechanism, a baroreflex, or a combination of both.[168] The effector arm of this response is via vagal cardiac nerve activity. Respiratory activity phasically alters vagal motor neuron responsiveness, with decreased vagal output during inspiration compared to expiration.[169]

Heart Rate and Cardiac Output

The relationship between heart rate and cardiac output is defined by the equation: cardiac output = stroke volume × heart rate. The effect of heart rate on cardiac output can vary over a wide range because of changes in stroke volume. A small increase in heart rate causes an increase in cardiac output and a decrease in stroke volume. The decrease in stroke volume is due to the effect of increased cardiac output on the peripheral volume, and a subsequent decrease in central venous pressure.[170,171] In this case, the increase in heart rate is not the direct cause of the decrease in stroke volume. Only when the heart rate exceeds 150 beats per minute does the cardiac output decrease, due to inadequate diastolic filling time and decreased stroke volume.[172]

Conversely, below a heart rate of 50 beats per minute, the stroke volume is relatively fixed, and a further decrease in heart rate causes a decrease in cardiac output.[160,173–175]

INTRINSIC CARDIAC CONTROL

In addition to cardiac control through the autonomic nervous system and systemic hormones, cardiac output is modified by the intrinsic factors: preload, afterload, and contractility. The following discussion focuses on how these factors affect cardiac output.

Preload

At the level of the muscle fiber, preload is defined as the force acting to stretch the ventricular fibers at end-diastole. Preload is related to cardiac output by the Frank–Starling law of the heart (length–tension relationship), which states that an increase in myocardial muscle fiber length is associated with an increase in the force of contraction,[176,177] and the subsequent increase in stroke volume and cardiac output.[178,179] Preload-induced changes in cardiac output allow for beat-to-beat equalization of right and left ventricular stroke volume. In the case of preload-/afterload-dependent changes in contractile function, the mechanism of increased contractile force is known as length-dependent activation, whereby the myofilaments increase their sensitivity to cytosolic calcium as the sarcomere length increases to maximum.[180] This mechanism is contrary to traditional descriptions of Starling law of the heart, which had maximal cardiac function occurring at a sarcomere length where there was optimal overlap of actin and myosin.[181]

Afterload

In muscle fiber experiments, preload is the tension in the muscle before contraction and afterload is the additional tension that must develop in the muscle during contraction before shortening occurs.[176,182] At the level of the ventricle, afterload is defined as ventricular wall tension during the shortening phase of contraction and reflects the sum of the forces against which the ventricle must act to eject blood.[183] However, given the heterogeneous direction of myocardial fibers and the torsion or twisting of the ventricle during systole, a single measure of ventricular wall tension is inadequate to define afterload. In the intact system in vivo, afterload is defined as the pressure in the aorta during systole[184] thus, these values are interchangeable. The key factors that affect aortic blood pressure during ejection are arterial compliance, arterial resistance, and the reflection of pulse waves from the periphery.[185]

As described by the force–velocity relation, for any given preload there is an inverse relation between afterload and muscle shortening, and thus stroke volume.[186] Although this relationship is observed in the isolated muscle fiber, it is not clinically apparent in people with normal cardiac function.[170] However, in individuals with a chronically depressed inotropic state (e.g., heart failure, cardiomyopathy), a steady state with altered ventricular dimensions (hypertrophy, dilatation) and maximal use of the length–tension relation occurs. Therefore, in these people in the face of an increase in afterload, the reserve provided by the length–tension relationship is exhausted and stroke volume decreases acutely.[187,188] These findings help to explain the use of afterload-reducing agents in patients with heart failure.

In clinical practice, systemic vascular resistance, which is often considered *the* indicator of afterload, is used interchangeably with afterload. This conceptualization is incorrect because afterload can change independently of vascular resistance. For example, in a patient who has experienced a severe hemorrhage, despite the fact that the systemic vascular resistance is increased (often to extreme), afterload is actually decreased. Recalling the original definition of afterload as the additional tension that develops in the muscle during contraction before shortening occurs helps to clarify this area of confusion. The tension or stress that develops in the ventricular wall according to the Laplace relation is:

$$T = \frac{PR}{2h}$$

where T is average circumferential wall stress (force/cross-sectional area), P is intraventricular pressure, R is the radius of curvature of the wall, and h is wall thickness. In hemorrhage, the radius of the ventricle is decreased, and if the compensatory actions of increased heart rate and systemic vasoconstriction are inadequate to maintain pressure, the intraventricular pressure also decreases. Thus, despite an increase in systemic vascular resistance, ventricular afterload decreases.

Contractility

Contractility refers to the intrinsic properties of cardiac myocytes that reflect the activation, formation, and cycling of crossbridges between actin and myosin filaments. In the heart, a change in contractility is defined as an alteration in cardiac performance that is independent of preload and afterload. An increase in contractility results in greater magnitude and velocity of shortening and augmented stroke volume. Contractility, which reflects the availability of calcium to the myofilament and sensitivity of the myofilament to calcium, can be increased by an increase in circulating epinephrine and norepinephrine released from cardiac sympathetic nerves, and a decrease in the interval between beats, known as the Bowditch treppe (staircase) effect.[189,190] There is an also important relationship between heart rate and β-adrenergic stimulation and myocardial contractility, with the effects of β-adrenergic stimulation expressed only when there is a concomitant increase in heart rate (positive force–frequency relation).[191] The positive force–frequency relation is considered the fourth intrinsic factor influencing myocardial contractility, along with length-dependent activation, basal force frequency effect, and direct positive inotropic effect of myocardial β-adrenergic receptor stimulation.[186] Clinically, loss of the force–frequency relationship during heart block and downregulation of β-adrenergic stimulation during heart failure contributes to impaired cardiac function.[189,190] In patients with diastolic dysfunction, the positive force–frequency relation is maintained, whereas the positive force–relaxation relation is impaired, resulting in decreased stroke volume with increasing heart rate.[192]

EXTRINSIC CONTROL: PERICARDIAL LIMITATION

Under normal resting conditions, the pericardium has little or no effect on cardiac filling; however, during acute increases in cardiac volume, the pericardium affects ventricular interaction and plays a role in the compensatory increase or decrease in stroke volume between the two ventricles.[193] Additionally, in the face of increased filling pressures, the pericardium restricts cardiac filling, which is important in preventing excessive dilation during acute increases in cardiac volume.[194] Under conditions of acute failure, the pericardium augments ventricular interaction with decreased stroke volume.[195,196] In chronic cardiac dilation, however, there is growth of new pericardial tissue or slippage of the collagen fibers, and the pericardium actually enlarges in size and mass. As a result of this pericardial distortion or remodeling, there is limited increase in pericardial constraint in chronic cardiac dilation.[197,198]

After pericardiectomy there is an increase in the maximal cardiac output, O_2 consumption, and left ventricular end-diastolic segment length.[199] The increase in cardiac output is caused by an increase in stroke volume, which is caused by an increase in end-diastolic volume and myocardial fiber length, as described by the Frank–Starling law of the heart.[200]

However, the effects of pericardiectomy on stroke volume and cardiac output are apparent only during exercise.[199,201]

In cases in which the pericardium has been opened and reapproximated, pericardial constraint increases because of development of adhesions between the pericardium and the heart.[202] The increased constraint is manifested as an increase in intraventricular pressure for any given volume, which reflects an increase in juxtacardiac pressure.[203] Consideration of the increased juxtacardiac pressure is important in the interpretation of hemodynamic data (increased pressure for any given volume) in postcardiac surgery patients who have had pericardial reapproximation.

LONG-TERM CONTROL OF BLOOD PRESSURE

The mechanism for the long-term control of blood pressure has traditionally been considered to involve fluid volume regulation, with the mechanism being renal pressure diuresis–natriuresis.[204,205] There are alternative models which suggest that volume diuresis–natriuresis and central baroreceptors play a role in long-term blood pressure control. This section presents the pressure diuresis–natriuresis model, introduces the alternative models of long-term arterial blood pressure control, and discusses the importance of basal tone on the maintenance of blood pressure.

Pressure Diuresis–Natriuresis Model

The classic model of long-term blood pressure control is based on the principle that arterial pressure is maintained at a level required by the kidneys to excrete a volume of urine approximately equivalent to the daily fluid intake (minus extrarenal fluid losses).[204,206] The kidneys sense a change in blood volume through the arterial pressure.[204,207] According to this model, that arterial pressure and not fluid volume is sensed is demonstrated in disease processes associated with a combination of increased extracellular volume and decreased arterial pressure (e.g., heart failure or cirrhosis with ascites). In these cases, the kidneys retain fluid despite expanded fluid volume. Based on this hypothesis, an increase in renal perfusion pressure causes a decrease in sodium reabsorption and an increase in sodium and water excretion. This model may involve autoregulation of renal medullary blood flow, although the exact mechanism remains unknown.[205,208] According to this model, as long as sodium and water intake remained stable, the enhanced sodium excretion will decrease extracellular volume and blood volume, and arterial pressure will decrease. Additionally, an increase in systemic vascular resistance and subsequent increase in renal perfusion pressure would not cause a long-term increase in arterial pressure, unless renal function was impaired.[204]

Alternative Models of Long-Term Blood Pressure Control

An alternative model for long-term blood pressure control suggests that the pressure diuresis–natriuresis mechanism may play less of a role under normal circumstances than previously conceptualized; rather that volume diuresis–natriuresis may be the primary mechanism for long-term blood pressure role.[209] According to this model sodium excretion is based on extracellular volume, with the renin system playing a key role.

Another model suggests that while the sympathetic nervous system, through the sinoaortic baroreceptor reflex, plays the primary role in the rapid regulation of blood pressure it may also play a role in long-term blood pressure control.[210–212] The clinical importance of the involvement of the sympathetic nervous system in long-term blood pressure control may be in the development to hypertension. Resetting of the baroreflex at a higher pressure threshold may limit their ability to buffer changes in blood pressure and increased sympathetic nervous system activity at any given pressure.[213,214] Further research is needed to support this model.[210,215] Baroreflex independent control of the blood pressure via a central baroreceptor (rather than a pressor–sensor in the kidney) has been proposed, with the primary goal of maintaining cerebral blood flow.[216,217] The paraventricular nuclei in the hypothalamus may also play a role in modulating renal sympathetic nerve activity.[8]

Basal Tone

All arterioles exhibit a basal level of vasoconstriction or tone. Basal tone, which is the intrinsic level of vascular tone, is independent of neural or humoral influences and serves as the baseline around which neural or humorally mediated vasoconstriction or vasodilation occurs (Fig. 4-11). Basal tone varies among organs; it is lowest in the kidneys and highest in the skeletal muscles, heart, and brain.[218] The maintenance of arteriolar tone through tonic rhythmic vasoconstriction is essential for the maintenance of blood pressure. For example, it is estimated that if this basal myogenic tone were eliminated, a minimal cardiac output of 60 to 75 L/min would be required to maintain a normal blood pressure.[104,218] In contrast, if the sympathetic input associated with resting tone were withdrawn, the blood pressure would decrease only from 100 to 86 mm Hg. This small decrease in blood pressure occurs

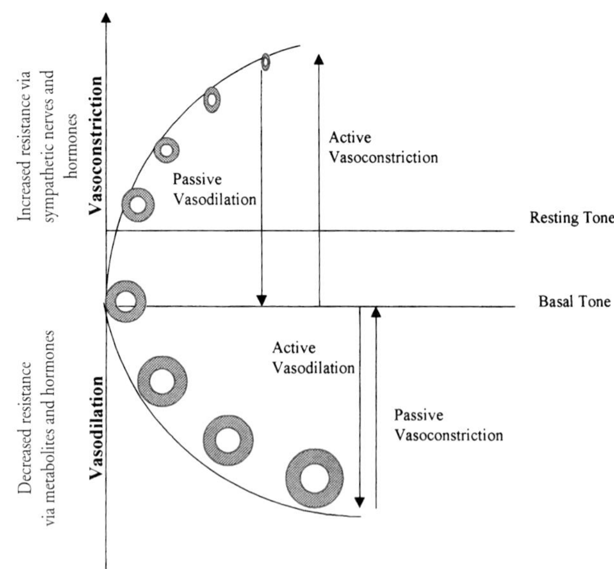

Figure 4-11. Schematic of active and passive changes in vascular resistance. The vascular bed is tonically constricted (basal tone) as a result of neurohumoral and local factors (autoregulation). In addition, some vascular beds have a higher level of tone (resting tone) indicating sympathetic nervous system stimulation. Passive vasodilation is the passive release of sympathetic nervous system stimulation, dilating the vessel toward basal tone. Passive vasoconstriction is the release of active vasodilatory stimuli. Active vasodilation is vascular dilation below basal tone and active vasoconstriction is constriction above basal tone. (Courtesy of Loring B. Rowell, University of Washington, Seattle, WA.)

because the vascular bed with the highest resting tone (skeletal muscle) normally receives only 15% of the cardiac output.

Nitric oxide (eNOS and nNOS) affects basal arteriolar and microvascular tone, with a greater effect in larger resistance vessels (greater than 200 μm) than in smaller resistance vessels (less than 200 μm).[219,220] Recent research suggests that nNOS generated nitric oxide is important for the regulation of basal vasomotor tone, which influences blood pressure, and eNOS generated nitric oxide affects the dynamic alterations in blood flow distribution.[219] Nitric oxide also affects large-artery distensibility.[221,222] The reduction or absence of tonic nitric oxide release causes increased mean arterial blood pressure and may be a cause of pathologic conditions characterized by increased blood pressure.[222,223]

As demonstrated in Figure 4-11, active and passive vasomotion occurs around the basal and resting tone of the vascular bed. Four terms define this vasomotion[104,224]:

1. *Active vasoconstriction*, which is mediated by sympathetic stimulation, is the increase in vascular resistance above the basal level.
2. *Passive vasodilation*, in contrast to active vasoconstriction, is the reduction in vascular resistance back to the basal level caused by the withdrawal of the sympathetic stimulation associated with active vasoconstriction. In some vascular beds, resistance may be increased above basal tone by tonic sympathetic stimulation. This increase in vascular tone is referred to as *resting tone.* Passive vasodilation is most easily seen in vascular beds with increased resting tone (e.g., acral regions).
3. If a vascular bed has high basal tone, *active vasodilation*, which is a decrease in vascular resistance below the level maintained by basal tone, may occur (i.e., vasodilation beyond that which exists after all neural and hormonal influences are removed). In this case, the vasodilation is not merely the result of withdrawal of sympathetic tone, because this action causes passive vasodilation.
4. *Passive vasoconstriction* is caused by withdrawal of the stimulation causing active vasodilation.

The skeletal muscle arterioles have a high basal tone and therefore are capable of a wide range of vasoconstriction and vasodilation, because there is an increased level of basal tone to be modulated. In contrast, the renal vasculature has a low basal and resting tone that can be markedly increased through sympathetic stimulation, but has little capability to undergo active vasodilation because there is so little basal tone to inhibit.

LOCAL REGULATION OF SYSTEMIC MICROVASCULAR BEDS

Arteriolar resistance vessels are partially constricted under normal circumstances by a tonic rhythmic myogenic tone, and this level of tone is modulated by neurogenic or other factors that cause active vasoconstriction or vasodilation. In the intact organism, blood flow and vascular hydrostatic pressure in the microvasculature of each organ system are controlled by complex interrelations among the effects of physical factors, locally released substances, circulating hormones, and above all by neurotransmitters secreted in response to central activation of the sympathetic nervous system. The relative predominance of local versus centrally mediated control of the microvascular bed varies among vascular beds, and it also varies among resistance, precapillary, and postcapillary blood vessels within a given vascular bed.

The large- and medium-sized arterioles, which are the predominant sites of vascular resistance, are primarily under the control of the sympathetic nervous system and centrally mediated neurohumoral factors (e.g., angiotensin II). These vascular segments are influential in the control of arterial blood pressure and, by virtue of their position; they control the total amount of blood entering a specific vascular area, and therefore, the distribution of blood flow between the different vascular beds. The terminal arterioles or precapillary vascular segments control the number of open capillaries and are under sympathetic nervous system and local control.[225] Local control mechanisms (autoregulation) that affect the terminal arterioles may have a substantial influence on exchange vessel pressures and flows and on the vascular tissue exchange of fluid and solutes.

Autoregulation

Autoregulation, which appears to occur in all organs except the lung, is the intrinsic tendency of an organ or vascular bed to maintain constant blood flow through alteration in its arteriolar tone, despite changes in arterial pressure. Autoregulation can occur in some organs over a range of perfusion pressure of 60 to 80 mm Hg to an upper limit of 150 mm Hg (Fig. 4-12), and is independent of neural and hormonal control. There are three hypotheses to explain autoregulation: the myogenic, metabolic, and tissue pressure hypotheses.[226,227] It appears that none of these mechanisms works in isolation and the tissue pressure hypothesis may apply only in pathologic conditions. A recent model suggests that myogenic and metabolic regulations overcome myogenic (shear-induced) effects.[228]

Myogenic Hypothesis

The myogenic hypothesis refers to the acute reaction of a blood vessel to a change in intraluminal pressure. For example, increasing intraluminal pressure between 20 and 120 mm Hg causes a pressure-induced stretch in vascular smooth muscle, which results

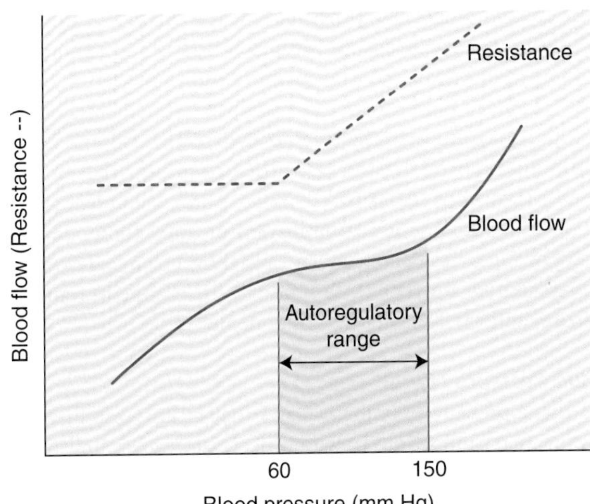

Figure 4-12. A schematic representation of autoregulation. The blood flow is relatively constant between an arterial pressure of 60 and 150 mm Hg because of an active increase in resistance. Below a mean pressure of 60 mm Hg and above 150 mm Hg, the flow is directly related to pressure.

in vasoconstriction and a decrease in the flow.[226,229] However, above an intraluminal pressure of 140 mm Hg the blood vessels dilate.[228] Shear stress, which is also associated with increased pressure, causes an increase in the release of eNOS and subsequent vasodilation. Conversely, when the intraluminal pressure is decreased, the stimulus for the myogenic response is decreased, the vessel dilates, and blood flow is returned toward control levels. Research suggests that, in isolation the myogenic response exerts only a small autoregulatory response.[228]

Metabolic Hypothesis

The metabolic hypothesis is based on the idea that the concentration of metabolites and metabolic substrates (e.g., ATP, potassium, hydrogen, O_2, CO_2, adenosine) in the interstitial space controls vascular tone. In this case, the vascular smooth muscle acts as a chemosensor. According to this hypothesis, a decrease in blood flow leads to an increase in the local concentration of a metabolite and causes vasodilation and increased blood flow.[227,230] For example, red blood cells release ATP in response to increased oxygen demand. Increased venular ATP may trigger an upstream response that causes arteriolar vasodilation.[228,231,232] The metabolic hypothesis has been suggested as a mechanism for autoregulation in organs or tissues where the primary function of blood supply is to support local metabolism. In this case, there is a close relation between blood flow and metabolic needs. However, in organ systems with high blood flow (e.g., kidney, skin), where blood flow occurs in excess of metabolic needs, there is a limited relationship between blood flow and metabolism,[104] and the metabolic hypothesis as a factor in the autoregulatory control of blood flow has not been supported. A combination of metabolic and myogenic responses generates autoregulatory flow changes despite the opposing effects of shear.[228]

An important point is that metabolic autoregulation is not the same as metabolically induced active and reactive hyperemia (increased blood flow), which occur in response to increased metabolic demand (e.g., intestinal vasculature during digestion or cardiac and skeletal muscle during activity) or interruption of blood flow to a vascular bed, respectively.[227] Active hyperemia is the adaptive increase in blood flow in response to changes in the local metabolic rate caused by variation in the functional activity of the surrounding cells. In response to this change in functional status, the vascular resistance decreases almost immediately. In addition, there is an increase in the number of perfused capillaries (capillary recruitment) in response to metabolic stimulation. The magnitude of the reactive hyperemia response depends on the duration of the vascular obstruction and the metabolic rate of the given vascular bed. Unlike "pure" metabolic autoregulation, this response is a combination of three components: (1) passive changes in vessel diameter caused by a change in transmural pressure; (2) a myogenic response to the change in transmural pressure; and (3) a metabolic component.[227,233,234]

Tissue Pressure Hypothesis

The tissue pressure hypothesis states that an increase in external pressure (e.g., interstitial pressure) decreases transmural pressure (pressure inside minus pressure outside the vessel), which passively decreased the vessel diameter and decreases flow.[227] The effect of external compression on blood flow normally occurs during ventricular systole, when the coronary arteries are compressed. Clinically, the effect of transmural compression is more likely to be observed in organs constrained in a rigid container (e.g., brain, where increased cerebrospinal fluid pressure may compress cerebral blood vessels) or a stiff capsule (e.g., kidney).[104,227] In the lung, vascular compression caused by increased external (alveolar) pressure, such as with the application of high levels of positive end-expiratory pressure (PEEP), may also affect blood flow.

Under physiologic conditions, tissue pressure probably does not play a major role in the control of blood flow, but it may be particularly important under pathologic conditions such as: edema, hemorrhage into the interstitial space, or cellular swelling caused by injury or hypoxemia (compartment syndrome).[227] In the latter cases, external compression my decrease blood flow below a physiologically safe level.

VENOUS SYSTEM

The primary functions of the venous system are to return blood from the capillaries to the heart and to serve as a reservoir that counterbalances the transient imbalance between cardiac output and venous return. However, because of its capacious nature, the venous system serves not only as a reservoir, storing approximately 70% of the total blood volume (approximately 33% of total blood volume is stored in the splanchnic bed—liver, stomach, spleen, and intestines), but also as a buffer against changes in cardiac output and blood pressure. The venous system plays both an active (venoconstriction) and, more importantly, a passive role in the maintenance of thoracic blood volume.

Neurohumoral Stimulation

The only neural control of veins is through the α-adrenergic fibers of the sympathetic nervous system.[235] Release of norepinephrine from α-adrenergic fibers causes constriction in the splanchnic and cutaneous veins, whereas withdrawal of sympathetic stimulation results in passive vasodilation. The cutaneous veins are densely innervated with α-adrenergic receptors, predominantly postsynaptic α_2-receptors.[72,236] There is limited β-adrenergic stimulation in the cutaneous veins and the veins of the skeletal muscle and the small venules have virtually no innervation. Epinephrine is the primary humoral factor that affects the veins, with actions on cutaneous vessels and, more importantly, splanchnic vessels. Given the preponderance of α-adrenergic receptors on the veins, epinephrine stimulation causes venoconstriction.

Passive versus Active Effects

Neurohumoral stimulation primarily affects the most capacious volume reservoirs (splanchnic and cutaneous venous bed). The question is whether translocation of blood from the venous system is primarily the consequence of active venoconstriction or of the passive effects that stem from the substantial changes in venous transmural pressure caused by arteriolar vasoconstriction or vasodilation.

Changes in upstream arteriolar tone alter downstream venous transmural pressure and the volume of blood that flows through the venous system. For example, arteriolar vasodilation increases blood flow into the highly capacious postcapillary venous beds, and the increase in their transmural venular pressure passively expands their volume. Given that total blood volume is constant, an increase in blood volume in the peripheral venous system means a decrease in the volume of the central veins that fill the heart. Conversely, vasoconstriction decreases flow into the postcapillary venous system, venous transmural pressure decreases,

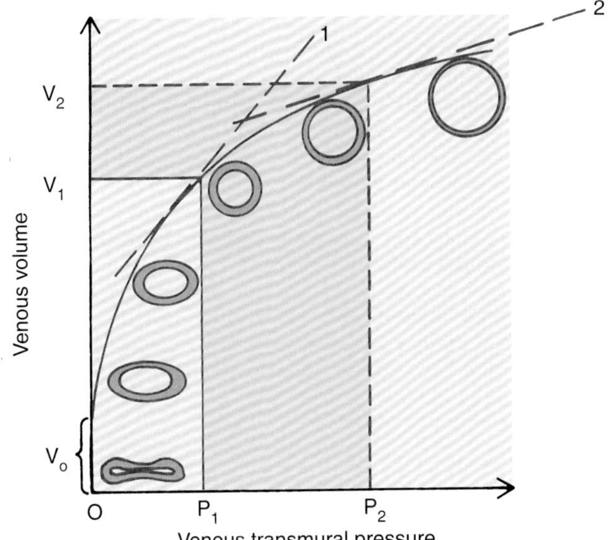

Figure 4-13. Typical volume–pressure curve of an isolated vein. *Dashed lines* (*1* and *2*) show the compliance ($\Delta V/\Delta P$) at two venous transmural pressures, P_1 and P_2. Note that compliance varies with pressure, being greatest at the lower pressures (*line 1*) and decreasing as the pressure increases (*line 2*). V_0 is the unstressed volume, which is the volume contained at 0 transmural pressure. The change in volume from V_2 to V_1 is the passive effect of changing pressures from P_2 to P_1. Note how changing cross-sectional geometry contributes to passive emptying. (From Rowell LB. *Human circulation: Regulation during physical stress*. New York: Oxford University Press; 1986:46.)

and the elastic recoil of the veins passively expels their volume toward the central thoracic veins.[235]

The magnitude of passive change in venous transmural pressure depends on where the changes occur along the venous volume–pressure curve. For example, as demonstrated in Figure 4-13, at a low venous transmural pressure, the pressure–volume curve is steep. A small change in distending pressure causes a large change in volume, that is, arteriolar vasodilation, which increases venous blood flow and venous transmural pressure, which causes a larger increase in venous volume expansion when the veins are not initially distended compared with the volume expansion that would occur if the veins were fully distended with decreased compliance. Conversely, passive vasoconstriction translocates a larger volume of blood to the central circulation when venular volume is normal or increased, in contrast to a situation such as hemorrhage, in which the volume is already diminished (e.g., no further volume to move into the central circulation). The passive effects of an alteration in blood flow on venous volume are exemplified in a study that evaluated the effect of a pacing-induced increase or decrease in cardiac output on central venous pressure.[171] A decrease in cardiac output, which resulted in a 17 mm Hg decrease in arterial pressure, was associated with a 3.9 mm Hg increase in central venous pressure. The increase in central venous pressure reflects the decrease in venous flow and transmural pressure associated with the decrease in cardiac output and the resultant passive recoil of the veins and the translocation of their blood centrally. The relation between venous volume and cardiac output is addressed further in the sections on the relation between cardiac output and central venous pressure, and the Krogh model.

The dominance of passive venous volume mobility can be altered in conditions such as hemorrhage, in which active venoconstriction of the richly innervated splanchnic veins can also play a role in the translocation of blood back to the central circulation.[104,237,238] In a study that examined the effects of a 27% decrease in cardiac output, with and without the presence of reflexes, active constriction of the splanchnic veins accounted for 21% of the translocated blood volume, whereas passive vasodilation accounted for the remaining 79%.[239] Thus, when active and passive effects are combined, the passive effects of decreased blood flow on venous volume mobility exceed the effect of simultaneous active venoconstriction.[74,239]

RELATION BETWEEN CARDIAC OUTPUT AND CENTRAL VENOUS PRESSURE—RETROGRADE VERSUS ANTEGRADE MODELS

In the 1950s, Guyton et al.[240–242] developed a model in which central venous pressure was presumed to affect cardiac output in a retrograde fashion. However, an opposing conceptualization is a model of the anterograde relationship between cardiac output and central venous pressure, that is, cardiac output affects central venous pressure.[74,243,244] A recent point–counterpoint discussion has failed to resolve these opposing models, with issues around the concept of mean circulatory pressure, the clarification of the components of the pressure gradient (mean circulatory pressure vs. right atrial pressure) and its effect on cardiac output, and the application of the models in static versus dynamic states.[245–249]

There are several implications of this discussion for clinical practice. For example, does increasing heart rate increase cardiac output? In experiments, an increase in cardiac output secondary to an increase in heart rate was limited by a decrease in central venous pressure.[175] Consideration of the resistive and capacitive properties of the arteries and veins within the context of an antegrade model may help to explain this effect.[104,170] In response to increased blood flow (increased cardiac output), transmural pressure in the veins rises, and thus their volume rises as well. The consequent shift in blood volume from the central to the peripheral veins lowers the central venous pressure.[77,170,171] If cardiac output continues to increase, the central venous pressure approaches 0 mm Hg, and eventually the central venous vasculature collapses, making it impossible to increase cardiac output further. This inverse relationship constitutes an autolimitation on our ability to increase cardiac output when there is no extra cardiac force available to match increased venous return with cardiac output. Factors that offset this autolimitation and allow us to stand and exercise are the muscle pump and the respiratory pump.

Muscle Pump

Initially when standing, there is an immediate translocation of 500 to 700 mL of blood to the periphery, which causes a decrease in central venous pressure and cardiac output and if allowed to continue could cause a person to faint. To offset this effect, contraction of the skeletal muscles in the legs causes compression of the veins and generates a gradient for flow between the venous beds and the right atrium, which can expel blood against the 100 mm Hg venous hydrostatic pressure that develops during quiet standing. The muscle pump, with a pumping capability *equal to that of the left ventricle*, is so important (particularly with exercise) that it is often referred to as the "second heart."[77,250,251] Clinically, encouraging the patient to actively contract their calf

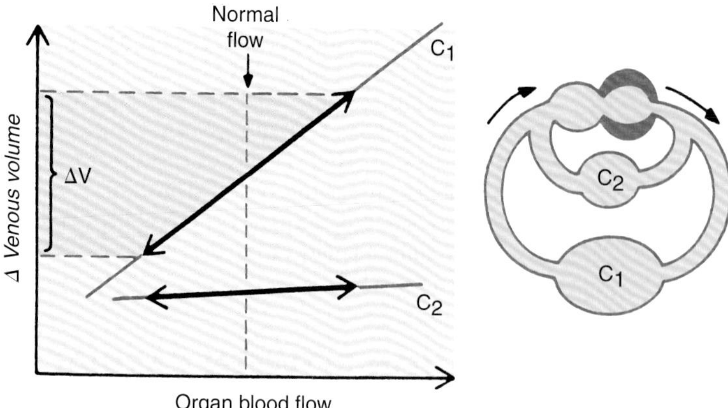

Figure 4-14. **Right**: The Krogh model divides the circulation between two circuits, one compliant (C_1) and the other noncompliant (C_2). **Left**: The relation between the change in organ venous volume and blood flow through a compliant organ (C_1) and a noncompliant organ (C_2). The volume of blood available to the heart is determined by the distribution of blood flow between such circuits. For example, in hyperthermia there is increased blood volume in the compliant vascular beds of the skin, and the amount of blood available to the heart is decreased. (From Rowell LB. *Human Circulation: Regulation during Physical Stress*. New York: Oxford University Press; 1986:60.)

muscles when arising from bed will augment the muscle pump and potentially decrease the risk for orthostasis.

Respiratory Pump

The respiratory pump augments the effect of the muscle pump on venous blood flow.[252,253] The pressure difference promoting flow from the venules to the right atrium is affected by changes in intrathoracic and intra-abdominal pressures. During inspiration, the diaphragm descends and intrathoracic pressure decreases and intra-abdominal pressure increases. These pressure changes create a gradient for blood flow from the point where the vena cava enters the thoracic cavity to the right atrium and thereby increases venous return to the heart. During expiration, the diaphragm relaxes and intrathoracic pressure increases, whereas intra-abdominal pressure decreases. The increased intrathoracic pressure impedes thoracic venous flow; however, there is an increase in blood flow from the lower extremities. During mechanical ventilation, the relation between the respiratory cycle and venous return is reversed.[254] These ventilatory-induced changes in preload have been exploited to aid in determining if a patient will respond to a fluid bolus with a clinically significant increase in stroke volume.

As described by the Krogh model (Fig. 4-14), the relative distribution of the cardiac output to compliant vascular beds (splanchnic—liver, gastrointestinal tract, pancreas, and the skin) and the remaining noncompliant vascular beds affects cardiac filling pressures.[74,235,255] For example, the administration of an α-adrenergic agent to a patient who is vasodilated will cause vasoconstriction of vessels leading into compliant vascular beds (e.g., splanchnic), which results in a passive collapse of the vascular bed with translocation of blood into the central circulation and a subsequent increase in blood return to the heart. However, a decrease in blood flow to the splanchnic region is not risk free as decreased gastrointestinal tract perfusion and ischemic bowel can occur if the vasoconstrictor-induced decrease in flow is too great. Conversely, the Krogh model is also useful for understanding the potentially negative consequences of recreational hyperthermia (i.e., hot tub or sauna) on coronary blood flow and cardiac output in a person with coronary artery disease. With hyperthermia, the highly compliant cutaneous vascular bed dilates, with up to 60% of the cardiac output directed to the skin to facilitate heat dissipation.[71,77] Generally, the redistribution of blood volume does not compromise oxygen delivery to vital organs. However, in individuals with compromised coronary circulation, there is a potential for a decrease in blood volume available to the heart and a subsequent decrease in cardiac output and coronary artery perfusion. The effects of environmental thermal stress plus exercise can also precipitate problems. In this case, the ability to increase cardiac output is limited by the decrease in central venous pressure and stroke volume, which is caused by vasodilation of the cutaneous vascular bed and the subsequent large increase in venous volume. This finding has important implications for exercise programs that are a part of cardiac rehabilitation and highlights the need for control of ambient temperature to maximize the benefits of exercise.[74,104]

VALSALVA MANEUVER

Extreme changes in intrathoracic pressure (Valsalva maneuver) also have potentially serious consequences for patients with cardiovascular disease. The Valsalva maneuver, which is a deep breath followed by straining to expire against a closed glottis, causes an abnormal increase in intrathoracic pressure. The hemodynamic response to the sudden increase in intrathoracic pressure associated with the Valsalva maneuver can be subdivided into four phases (Fig. 4-15).[256–258] During the initial phase (phase 1:

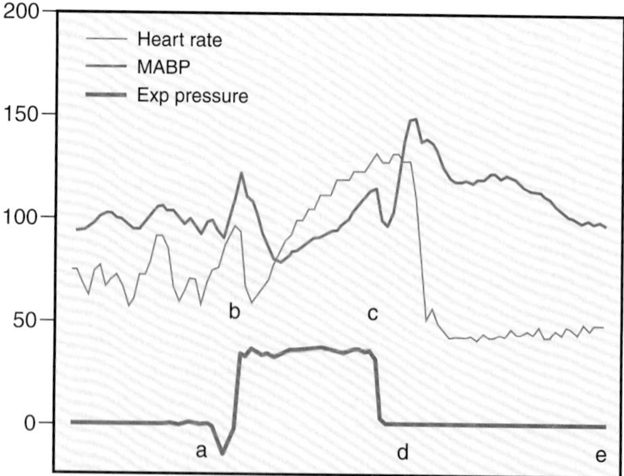

Figure 4-15. The normal hemodynamic response to a Valsalva maneuver. Phase 1: *a–b*, phase 2: *b–c*, phase 3: *c–d*, and phase 4: *d–e*. MABP, mean arterial blood pressure; Exp pressure, expiratory pressure. (From Freeman R. Noninvasive evaluation of heart rate variability. In: Low PA, ed. *Clinical Autonomic Disorders*. 2nd ed. Philadelphia, PA: Lippincott-Raven; 1997:302.)

strain phase), which is produced by forcefully exhaling against a closed glottis, there is a transient increase in arterial systolic and diastolic pressures due to aortic compression caused by increased intrathoracic pressure, and a marked decrease in venous return subsequent to compression of the vena cava and a decrease in pulse pressure and heart rate. During the remainder of the strain phase (phase 2), there is a progressive decrease in blood pressure and cardiac output due to a decrease in venous return and left ventricular filling and stroke volume subsequent to compression of the vena cava. The decrease in cardiac output and arterial pulse pressure, which increases baroreflex-mediated sympathetic activity, is manifested as a compensatory increase in heart rate and peripheral resistance. On release of the strain (phase 3), there is an abrupt decrease in arterial pressure (release of aortic compression) and a rapid rise in venous return (decreased caval compression with restoration of the inferior vena cava to right atrial pressure gradient) without a change in heart rate. Finally, during phase 4 (overshoot), when the increased venous return reaches the left ventricle, there is a progressive increase in left ventricular stroke volume, blood pressure, and pulse pressure above baseline caused by an increase in cardiac output, secondary to the increased venous return into the vasoconstricted systemic vasculature. The overshoot of blood pressure, pulse pressure, and cardiac output stimulates vagal activity, leading to reflex bradycardia.[259,260]

In the clinical setting, the effects of the Valsalva maneuver may be observed when a patient strains during defecation or vomiting.[261] It is the reflex bradycardia and the sequelae of the Valsalva maneuver (cardiac arrhythmias, sudden cardiac arrest, cerebral and subarachnoid hemorrhage, rupture of a dissecting aortic aneurysm) that are observed clinically.[262] Patients who may be at increased risk for an adverse response to the Valsalva maneuver include those with cardiac disease (e.g., heart failure) and older individuals.[258,263] Interventions to protect this high-risk group from the sequelae of the Valsalva maneuver (e.g., positioning, and avoiding straining during a bowel movement or vomiting) should be performed.

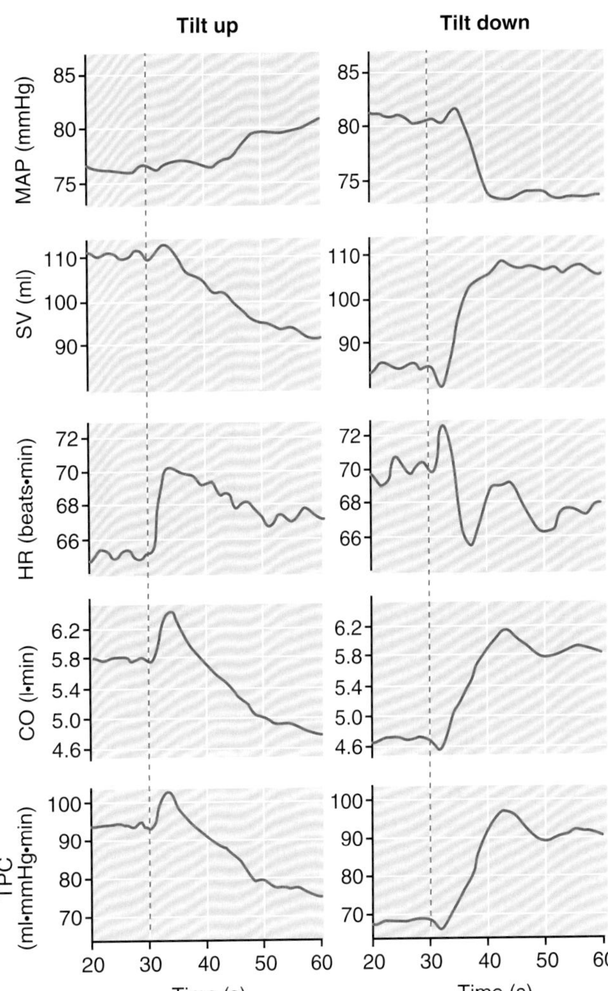

Figure 4-16. Average response to 30-degree head-up tilt and tilt back to supine position in seven subjects (41 experiments). (From Toska K, Walløe L. Dynamic time course of hemodynamic responses after passive head up tilt and tilt back to supine position. *J Appl Physiol.* 2002;92:1674.)

OVERALL CONTROL

Baroreflex Control of Blood Pressure

The arterial baroreflex is the primary mechanism of control for the short-term or rapid control of arterial blood pressure.[264–267] Neurohumoral factors (predominantly the control of sodium excretion) are primarily responsible for long-term or slower blood pressure control, although the sympathetic nervous system may also play a role in long-term control of blood pressure.

Arterial Baroreceptor Response to Decreased Arterial Pressure

A decrease in blood pressure may be the result of loss of blood (hemorrhage) or a shift in blood away from the heart (standing up) or standing up too quickly after bending over. In response to a decrease in arterial pressure, the baroreceptor-firing rate decreases, and the firing rate through the sinus node and vagal afferents is reduced. The clinical manifestations of this response are relatively slow in contrast to the almost instantaneous response to an increase in blood pressure (Fig. 4-16).[268] The response to a decrease in arterial pressure is described in the following section (Fig. 4-17).

Increased Sympathetic Nervous System Activity. The primary response to a decrease in arterial blood pressure is an increase in total vascular resistance.[269] This response is relatively slow (5 to 15 seconds). A small increase in stroke volume secondary to β_1 stimulation and increased contractility also occurs. The increase in vascular resistance is the primary mechanism for restoring blood pressure, because an increase in heart rate is relatively ineffective in raising cardiac output. As described previously, if the cardiac output increases without an increase in peripheral vascular tone, then the central venous pressure decreases. The sympathetic nervous system-mediated vasoconstriction decreases blood flow to the splanchnic region, thereby causing a passive release of 300 to 500 mL of blood from its capacious veins into the central circulation.[74,270] An individual who experiences dizziness or faints after bending over and then standing up to quickly is first exposed to increased blood pressure in the head followed by a rapid decrease. In this case, the dizziness is caused by an exaggerated rate of blood flow to the legs compared to an individual who moves from supine to upright.[270,271] The mechanism for this unique response to a "push–pull" maneuver has not been identified, but it may include myogenic vasodilation during the head-down phase or

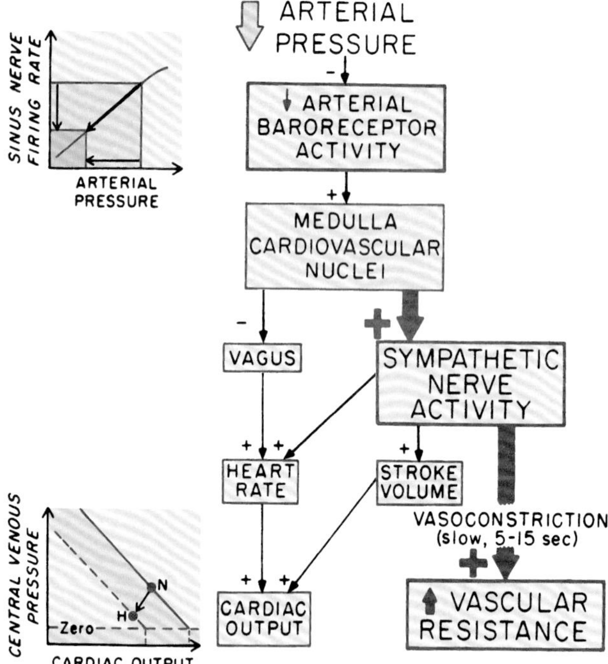

Figure 4-17. Summary of how the arterial baroreflex restores blood pressure back toward normal during arterial hypotension. Correction is by relatively slow (5 to 15 seconds) vasoconstriction. Increased heart rate has little or no effect if cardiac filling pressure is low and cardiac output cannot be increased, for reasons illustrated in the small graph next to "cardiac output" (central venous pressure vs. cardiac output). When normal (N) cardiac output increases, central venous pressure falls. When both cardiac output and central venous pressure are low during hemorrhage (H), cardiac output cannot rise much without collapsing central veins as central venous pressure goes to 0. (From Rowell LB. *Human Cardiovascular Control.* New York: Oxford University Press; 1993:57.)

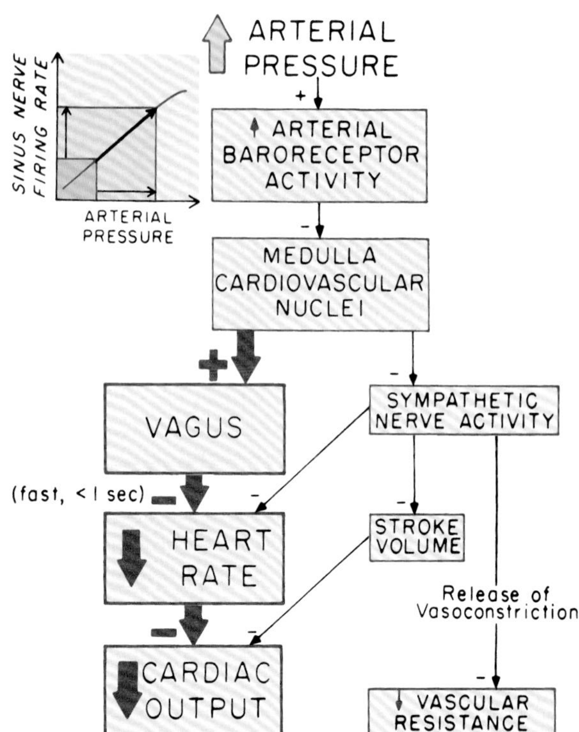

Figure 4-18. Summary of how the arterial baroreflex restores blood pressure back toward normal after sudden hypertension. Correction is rapid and achieved by immediate vagal activation and reduced heart rate and cardiac output. Release of tonic vasoconstriction is slow and has a minimal effect because only skeletal muscle has significant tonic vasoconstriction to be withdrawn in resting humans. (From Rowell LB. *Human Cardiovascular Control.* New York: Oxford University Press;1993:58.)

rapid refilling of the emptied veins. In this case, the relatively slow sympathetic response cannot offset these effects.

Decreased Vagal Activity Causing an Increase in Heart Rate. The cardiovagal arm of the baroreflex involves modulation of the heart rate. An increase in heart rate is not a primary compensatory response to a decrease in blood pressure,[269] although altered vagal function is associated with lower blood pressure.[272] As described by the cardiac output–central venous pressure relation, an increase in heart rate-induced central venous pressure is of limited efficacy in increasing the cardiac output and offsetting the decrease in blood pressure.

Arterial Baroreceptor Response to Increased Arterial Pressure

An acute increase in blood pressure results in increased stimulation of the sinoaortic baroreceptors. The increased baroreceptor-firing rate increases sinus and vagal afferent input into the nucleus tractus solitarius of the medulla (see Figs. 4-1 and 4-3). In response to the increased baroreceptor input, the following occur (Fig. 4-18):

1. A rapid (within one beat) decrease in heart rate, secondary to a sudden increase in vagal tone.
2. A secondary decrease in stroke volume due to the negative inotropic effects of the increased vagal tone (minor effect).
3. A sympathetic nervous system-mediated decrease in vascular tone (minor effect).

The net result or this response is a decrease in heart rate, with a subsequent decrease in cardiac output and blood pressure. The most important point is that the response, which occurs within one beat, is mediated by a vagally induced decrease in heart rate and cardiac output.[273] Passive vasodilation due to a decrease in sympathetic tone occurs only in the skeletal muscles, and thus does not contribute greatly to the sudden lowering of arterial blood pressure.[74]

The rapid baroreflex response is extremely important in the protection of the cerebral vessels.[274] An impaired baroreflex response can be observed in patients after a stroke, where over 70% of these individuals exhibit increased blood pressure.[275] There is also a decrease in baroreflex-mediated buffering with aging,[163] which may place older individuals at increased risk for the negative effects of blood pressure perturbations.

CONCLUSION

Cardiac output is the amount of blood the heart pumps in one minute. It is dependent on four factors: heart rate, contractility, preload, and afterload. The amount of blood the heart pumps is dependent on both cardiac and extracardiac factors. The interpretation of cardiac output, its four determinants and the extrinsic control can help to understand some of the complex pathophysiologic alterations in illness. This can also help to appreciate the effects of various interventions to augment cardiac output.

KEY READINGS

Corley A, Barnett A, Mullaney J, et al. Nurse-determined assessment of cardiac output. Comparing a non-invasive cardiac output device and pulmonary artery catheter: a prospective observational study. *Int J Nurs Stud.* 2009;46(10):1291–1297.

REFERENCES

1. Scher A. Cardiovascular control. In: Patton H, Fuchs A, Hille B, et al., eds. *Textbook of Physiology. Circulation, Respiration, Body Fluids, Metabolism, and Endocrinology.* Philadelphia, PA: WB Saunders; 1989:972–990.
2. McMahon NC, Drinkhill MJ, Myers DS, et al. Reflex responses from the main pulmonary artery and bifurcation in anaesthetised dogs. *Exp Physiol.* 2000;85:411–420.
3. Minisi AJ. Vagal cardiopulmonary reflexes after total cardiac deafferentation. *Circulation.* 1998;98:2615–2620.
4. Hainsworth R. Cardiovascular reflexes from ventricular and coronary receptors. *Adv Exp Med Biol.* 1995;381:157–174.
5. Kincaid K, Ward M, Nair U, et al. The coronary baroreflex in humans. *J Extra Corpor Technol.* 2005;37:306–310.
6. Wright C, Drinkhill MJ, Hainsworth R. Reflex effects of independent stimulation of coronary and left ventricular mechanoreceptors in anaesthetised dogs. *J Physiol.* 2000;528(Pt. 2):349–358.
7. Wright CI, Drinkhill MJ, Hainsworth R. Responses to stimulation of coronary and carotid baroreceptors and the coronary chemoreflex at different ventricular distending pressures in anaesthetised dogs. *Exp Physiol.* 2001;86:381–390.
8. Dampney RA, Horiuchi J, Killinger S, et al. Long-term regulation of arterial blood pressure by hypothalamic nuclei: some critical questions. *Clin Exp Pharmacol Physiol.* 2005;32:419–425.
9. Fenton AM, Hammill SC, Rea RF, et al. Vasovagal syncope. *Ann Intern Med.* 2000;133:714–725.
10. Aviado DM, Guevara Aviado D. The Bezold-Jarisch reflex. A historical perspective of cardiopulmonary reflexes. *Ann N Y Acad Sci.* 2001;940:48–58.
11. Grubb BP. Clinical practice. Neurocardiogenic syncope. *N Engl J Med.* 2005;352:1004–1010.
12. Serrano CV Jr., Bortolotto LA, Cesar LA, et al. Sinus bradycardia as a predictor of right coronary artery occlusion in patients with inferior myocardial infarction. *Int J Cardiol.* 1999;68:75–82.
13. Goldstein JA, Lee DT, Pica MC, et al. Patterns of coronary compromise leading to bradyarrhythmias and hypotension in inferior myocardial infarction. *Coron Artery Dis.* 2005;16:265–274.
14. Thoren P. Left ventricular receptors activated by severe asphyxia and by coronary artery occlusion. *Acta Physiol Scand.* 1972;85:455–463.
15. Fu LW, Guo ZL, Longhurst JC. Undiscovered role of endogenous thromboxane A2 in activation of cardiac sympathetic afferents during ischaemia. *J Physiol.* 2008;586:3287–3300.
16. Fu LW, Phan A, Longhurst JC. Myocardial ischemia-mediated excitatory reflexes: a new function for thromboxane A2? *Am J Physiol Heart Circ Physiol.* 2008;295(6):H2530–H2540.
17. Longhurst JC, Tjen ALSC, Fu LW. Cardiac sympathetic afferent activation provoked by myocardial ischemia and reperfusion. Mechanisms and reflexes. *Ann N Y Acad Sci.* 2001;940:74–95.
18. Chiladakis JA, Patsouras N, Manolis AS. The Bezold-Jarisch reflex in acute inferior myocardial infarction: clinical and sympathovagal spectral correlates. *Clin Cardiol.* 2003;26:323–328.
19. Perez-Gomez F, Garcia-Aguada A. Origin of ventricular reflexes caused by coronary arteriography. *Br Heart J.* 1977;39:967–973.
20. Mark AL, Kioschos JM, Abboud FM, et al. Abnormal vascular responses to exercise in patients with aortic stenosis. *J Clin Invest.* 1973;52:1138–1146.
21. Mark A, Abboud F, Schmid P, et al. Reflex vascular response to left ventricular outflow obstruction and activation of ventricular baroreceptors in dogs. *J Clin Invest.* 1973;52:1147–1153.
22. Mark A, Mancia G. Cardiopulmonary baroreflexes in humans. In: Sheperd J, Abboud F, eds. *Handbook of Physiology. Section 2. The Cardiovascular System.* Bethesda, MD: American Physiological Society; 1983:795–813.
23. Omran H, Fehske W, Rabahieh R, et al. Valvular aortic stenosis: risk of syncope. *J Heart Valve Dis.* 1996;5:31–34.
24. Prasad K, Williams L, Campbell R, et al. Episodic syncope in hypertrophic cardiomyopathy: evidence for inappropriate vasodilation. *Heart.* 2008;94:1312–1317.
25. Thaman R, Elliott PM, Shah JS, et al. Reversal of inappropriate peripheral vascular responses in hypertrophic cardiomyopathy. *J Am Coll Cardiol.* 2005;46:883–892.
26. Lim PO, Morris-Thurgood JA, Frenneaux MP. Vascular mechanisms of sudden death in hypertrophic cardiomyopathy, including blood pressure responses to exercise. *Cardiol Rev.* 2002;10:15–23.
27. Lee TM, Chen MF, Su SF, et al. Excessive myocardial contraction in vasovagal syncope demonstrated by echocardiography during head-up tilt test. *Clin Cardiol.* 1996;19:137–140.
28. Campagna JA, Carter C. Clinical relevance of the Bezold-Jarisch reflex. *Anesthesiology.* 2003;98(5):1250–1260.
29. Lim R, Kilgar J, Cayo S, et al. Complication after treatment for resistant supraventricular tachycardia: the Bezold-Jarisch reflex. *Am J Emerg Med.* 2013;31(9):1425.e3–e4.
30. Wisbach G, Tobias S, Woodman R, et al. Preserving cardiac output with beta-adrenergic receptor blockade and inhibiting the Bezold-Jarisch reflex during resuscitation from hemorrhage. *J Trauma.* 2007;63:26–32.
31. Hlastala M, Berger A. *Physiology of Respiration.* New York: Oxford University Press; 2001.
32. Kara T, Narkiewicz K, Somers VK. Chemoreflexes—physiology and clinical implications. *Acta Physiol Scand.* 2003;177:377–384.
33. Floras JS. Hypertension, sleep apnea, and atherosclerosis. *Hypertension.* 2008:53(1);1–3.
34. Narkiewicz K, Somers VK. Sympathetic nerve activity in obstructive sleep apnoea. *Acta Physiol Scand.* 2003;177:385–390.
35. Javaheri S. Central sleep apnea-hypopnea syndrome in heart failure: prevalence, impact, and treatment. *Sleep.* 1996;19:S229–S231.
36. Floras JS. Should sleep apnoea be a specific target of therapy in heart failure? *Heart.* 2009;95:1041–1046.
37. Somers VK, White DP, Amin R, et al. Sleep apnea and cardiovascular disease: An American Heart Association/American College Of Cardiology Foundation Scientific Statement from the American Heart Association Council for High Blood Pressure Research Professional Education Committee, Council on Clinical Cardiology, Stroke Council, and Council On Cardiovascular Nursing. In collaboration with the National Heart, Lung, and Blood Institute National Center on Sleep Disorders Research (National Institutes of Health). *Circulation.* 2008;118:1080–1111.
38. Schmidt H, Francis DP, Rauchhaus M, et al. Chemo- and ergoreflexes in health, disease and ageing. *Int J Cardiol.* 2005;98:369–378.
39. Dampney RA, Coleman MJ, Fontes MA, et al. Central mechanisms underlying short- and long-term regulation of the cardiovascular system. *Clin Exp Pharmacol Physiol.* 2002;29:261–268.
40. Pilowsky PM, Goodchild AK. Baroreceptor reflex pathways and neurotransmitters: 10 years on. *J Hypertens.* 2002;20:1675–1688.
41. Stocker SD, Osborn JL, Carmichael SP. Forebrain osmotic regulation of the sympathetic nervous system. *Clin Exp Pharmacol Physiol.* 2008;35:695–700.
42. Coote JH. Landmarks in understanding the central nervous control of the cardiovascular system. *Exp Physiol.* 2007;92:3–18.
43. Kougias P, Weakley SM, Yao Q, et al. Arterial baroreceptors in the management of systemic hypertension. *Med Sci Monit.* 2010;16(1):RA1–RA8.
44. Sata Y, Head GA, Denton K, et al. Role of the Sympathetic nervous system and its modulation in renal hypertension. *Front Med (Lausanne).* 2018;5:82.
45. Helke CJ, Seagard JL. Substance P in the baroreceptor reflex: 25 years. *Peptides.* 2004;25:413–423.
46. Grassi G, Trevano FQ, Seravalle G, et al. Baroreflex function in hypertension: consequences for antihypertensive therapy. *Prog Cardiovas Dis.* 2006;48:407–415.
47. Bylund DB, Eikenberg DC, Hieble JP, et al. International Union of Pharmacology nomenclature of adrenoceptors. *Pharmacol Rev.* 1994;46:121–136.
48. Lands AM, Arnold A, McAuliff JP, et al. Differentiation of receptor systems activated by sympathomimetic amines. *Nature.* 1967;214:597–598.
49. Guimaraes S, Moura D. Vascular adrenoceptors: an update. *Pharmacol Rev.* 2001;53:319–356.
50. Civantos Calzada B, Aleixandre de Artinano A. Alpha-adrenoceptor subtypes. *Pharmacol Res.* 2001;44:195–208.
51. Kable J, Murrin L, Bylund DB. In vivo gene modification elucidates subtype-specific functions of alpha (?)-adrenergic receptors. *J Pharmacol Exp Ther.* 2000;293:1–7.
52. Kanagy NL. Alpha(2)-adrenergic receptor signalling in hypertension. *Clin Sci (Lond).* 2005;109:431–437.

53. Leech CJ, Faber JE. Different alpha-adrenoceptor subtypes mediate constriction of arterioles and venules. *Am J Physiol.* 1996;270:H710–H722.
54. Banday AA, Lokhandwala MF. Dopamine receptors and hypertension. *Curr Hypertens Rep.* 2008;10:268–275.
55. Missale C, Nash SR, Robinson SW, et al. Dopamine receptors: from structure to function. *Physiol Rev.* 1998;78:189–225.
56. Zeng C, Armando I, Luo Y, et al. Dysregulation of dopamine-dependent mechanisms as a determinant of hypertension: studies in dopamine receptor knockout mice. *Am J Physiol Heart Circ Physiol.* 2008;294:H551–H569.
57. Jose PA, Eisner GM, Felder RA. Regulation of blood pressure by dopamine receptors. *Nephron Physiol.* 2003;95:19–27.
58. Jose PA, Eisner GM, Felder RA. Dopamine and the kidney: a role in hypertension? *Curr Opin Nephrol Hypertens.* 2003;12:189–194.
59. Zeng C, Eisner GM, Felder RA, et al. Dopamine receptor and hypertension. *Curr Med Chem Cardiovasc Hematol Agents.* 2005;3:69–77.
60. Kellum J, Decker J. Use of dopamine in acute renal failure: a meta-analysis. *Crit Care Med.* 2001;29:1526–1531.
61. Marik PE. Low-dose dopamine: a systematic review. *Intensive Care Med.* 2002;28:877–883.
62. Friedrich JO, Adhikari N, Herridge MS, et al. Meta-analysis: low-dose dopamine increases urine output but does not prevent renal dysfunction or death. *Ann Intern Med.* 2005;142:510–524.
63. Feigl EO. Neural control of coronary blood flow. *J Vasc Res.* 1998;35:85–92.
64. Gauthier C, Seze-Goismier C, Rozec B. Beta 3-adrenoceptors in the cardiovascular system. *Clin Hemorheol Microcirc.* 2007;37:193–204.
65. Gauthier C, Leblais V, Kobzik L, et al. The negative inotropic effect of B3-Adrenoreceptor stimulation is mediated by activation of nitric oxide synthase pathway in human ventricle. *J Clin Invest.* 1998;102:1377–1384.
66. Moniotte S, Kobzik L, Feron O, et al. Upregulation of beta(3)-adrenoreceptors and altered contractile response to inotropic amines in human failing myocardium. *Circulation.* 2001;103:1649–1655.
67. Bristow M, Monobe W, Pasmussen R, et al. Alpha-1 adrenergic receptors in the nonfailing and failing human heart. *J Pharmacol Exp Ther.* 1988;247:1039–1045.
68. Franchini K, Cowley AJ. Autonomic control of cardiac function. In: Robertson D, Low P, Polinsky R, eds. *Primer on the Autonomic Nervous System.* San Diego, CA: Academic Press; 1996:42–48.
69. Rudner XL, Berkowitz DE, Booth JV, et al. Subtype specific regulation of human vascular alpha(1)-adrenergic receptors by vessel bed and age. *Circulation.* 1999;100:2336–2343.
70. Borbujo J, Garcia-Villalon A, Valle J, et al. Postjunctional alpha-1 and alpha-2 adrenoreceptors in human skin arteries. An in vitro study. *J Pharmacol Exp Ther.* 1989;249:284–287.
71. Johnson J, Proppe D. Cardiovascular adjustments to heat stress. In: Fregly M, Blatteis C, eds. *Handbook of Physiology: Section 4. Environmental Physiology.* New York: Oxford University Press; 1996:215–243.
72. Charkoudian N. Skin blood flow in adult human thermoregulation: how it works, when it does not, and why. *Mayo Clinics Proceeding.* 2003;78:603–612.
73. Kellogg DL Jr. In vivo mechanisms of cutaneous vasodilation and vasoconstriction in humans during thermoregulatory challenges. *J Appl Physiol.* 2006;100:1709–1718.
74. Rowell L. *Human Cardiovascular Control.* New York: Oxford University Press; 1993.
75. Pergola PE, Kellogg DL Jr, Johnson JM, et al. Reflex control of active cutaneous vasodilation by skin temperature in humans. *Am J Physiol.* 1994;266:H1979–H1984.
76. Savage MV, Brengelmann GL. Control of skin blood flow in the neutral zone of human body temperature regulation. *J Appl Physiol.* 1996;80:1249–1257.
77. Rowell L, O'Leary D, Kellogg D. Integration of cardiovascular control systems in dynamic exercise. In: Rowell L, Sheperd J, eds. *Handbook of Physiology, Exercise: Regulation and Integration of Multiple Systems.* Bethesda, MD: Oxford University Press; 1996:770–838.
78. Kellogg DL Jr., Pergola PE, Piest KL, et al. Cutaneous active vasodilation in humans is mediated by cholinergic nerve cotransmission. *Circ Res.* 1995;77:1222–1228.
79. Kellogg DL Jr, Zhao JL, Wu Y. Endothelial nitric oxide synthase control mechanisms in the cutaneous vasculature of humans in vivo. *Am J Physiol Heart Circ Physiol.* 2008;295:H123–H129.
80. Kellogg DL Jr, Zhao JL, Wu Y. Neuronal nitric oxide synthase control mechanisms in the cutaneous vasculature of humans in vivo. *J Physiol.* 2008;586:847–857.
81. Joyner MJ, Dietz NM. Sympathetic vasodilation in human muscle. *Acta Physiol Scand.* 2003;177:329–336.
82. Crandall CG. Heat stress and baroreflex regulation of blood pressure. *Med Sci Sports Exerc.* 2008;40(12):2063–2070.
83. Crandall CG, Cui J, Wilson TE. Effects of heat stress on baroreflex function in humans. *Acta Physiol Scand.* 2003;177:321–328.
84. Vanhoutte P, Leusen I. *Vasodilatation.* New York: Raven Press; 1981.
85. Palmer T. Agents acting at the neuromuscular junction and autonomic ganglia. In: Brunton LL, Lazo JS, eds. *Goodman & Gilman's The Pharmacological Basis of Therapeutics.* New York: McGraw-Hill; 2008.
86. Myslivecek J, Trojan S. Regulation of adrenoceptors and muscarinic receptors in the heart. *Gen Physiol Biophys.* 2003;22:3–14.
87. Brodde OE, Michel MC. Adrenergic and muscarinic receptors in the human heart. *Pharmacol Rev.* 1999;51:651–690.
88. Brodde OE, Bruck H, Leineweber K, et al. Presence, distribution and physiological function of adrenergic and muscarinic receptor subtypes in the human heart. *Basic Res Cardiol.* 2001;96:528–538.
89. Myslivecek J, Novakova M, Klein M. Receptor subtype abundance as a tool for effective intracellular signalling. *Cardiovasc Hematol Disord Drug Targets.* 2008;8:66–79.
90. Burnstock G. Cotransmission. *Curr Opin Pharmacol.* 2004;4:47–52.
91. Burnstock G. Physiology and pathophysiology of purinergic neurotransmission. *Physiol Rev.* 2007;87:659–797.
92. Burnstock G. Non-synaptic transmission at autonomic neuroeffector junctions. *Neurochem Int.* 2008;52:14–25.
93. Tsuru H, Tanimitsu N, Hirai T. Role of perivascular sympathetic nerves and regional differences in the features of sympathetic innervation of the vascular system. *Jpn J Pharmacol.* 2002;88:9–13.
94. Burnstock G. Purines and cotransmitters in adrenergic and cholinergic neurones. *Prog Brain Res.* 1996;68:193–203.
95. Herring N, Lokale MN, Danson EJ, et al. Neuropeptide Y reduces acetylcholine release and vagal bradycardia via a Y2 receptor-mediated, protein kinase C-dependent pathway. *J Mol Cell Cardiol.* 2008;44:477–485.
96. Herring N, Paterson DJ. Neuromodulators of peripheral cardiac sympatho-vagal balance. *Exp Physiol.* 2009;94(1):46–53.
97. Han S, Yang CL, Chen X, et al. Direct evidence for the role of neuropeptide Y in sympathetic nerve stimulation-induced vasoconstriction. *Am J Physiol.* 1998;274:H290–H294.
98. Westfall TC, McCullough LA, Vickery L, et al. Effects of neuropeptide Y at sympathetic neuroeffector junctions. *Adv Pharmacol.* 1998;42:106–110.
99. Abe K, Tilan JU, Zukowska Z. NPY and NPY receptors in vascular remodeling. *Curr Top Med Chem.* 2007;7:1704–1709.
100. McDermott BJ, Bell D. NPY and cardiac diseases. *Curr Top Med Chem.* 2007;7:1692–1703.
101. Henning RJ, Sawmiller DR. Vasoactive intestinal peptide: cardiovascular effects. *Cardiovasc Res.* 2001;49:27–37.
102. Dvorakova MC. Cardioprotective role of the VIP signaling system. *Timely Top Med Cardiovasc Dis.* 2005;9:E33.
103. Lundberg JM. Pharmacology of cotransmission in the autonomic nervous system: integrative aspects on amines, neuropeptides, adenosine triphosphate, amino acids and nitric oxide. *Pharmacol Rev.* 1996;48:113–178.
104. Rowell L. *Human Circulation: Regulation During Physical Stress.* New York: Oxford University Press; 1996.
105. Westfall TC, Westfall DP. Adrenergic agonists and antagonists. In: Brunton L, Parker K, Murri N, et al., eds. *Goodman & Gilman's Pharmacology.* New York: McGraw-Hill; 2008.
106. Barrett L, Singer M, Clapp L. Vasopressin: mechanisms of action on the vasculature in health and septic shock. *Crit Care Med.* 2007;35:33–40.
107. Treschan T, Peters J. The vasopressin system: physiology and clinical strategies. *Anesthesiology.* 2006;105:599–612.
108. Bie P. Osmoreceptors, vasopressin, and control of renal water excretion. *Physiol Rev.* 1980;60:961–1048.
109. Ramsay DJ, Thrasher TN, Bie P. Endocrine components of body fluid homeostasis. *Comp Biochem Physiol.* 1988;90:777–780.
110. Voisin DL, Bourque CW. Integration of sodium and osmosensory signals in vasopressin neurons. *Trends Neurosci.* 2002;25:199–205.
111. Bourque CW. Central mechanisms of osmosensation and systemic osmoregulation. *Nat Rev Neurosci.* 2008;9:519–531.
112. Shen YT, Cowley AW Jr, Vatner SF. Relative roles of cardiac and arterial baroreceptors in vasopressin regulation during hemorrhage in conscious dogs. *Circ Res.* 1991;68:1422–1436.
113. Thrasher TN, Chen HG, Keil LC. Arterial baroreceptors control plasma vasopressin responses to graded hypotension in conscious dogs. *Am J Physiol.* 2000;278:R469–R475.

114. Thrasher TN, Keil LC. Systolic pressure predicts plasma vasopressin responses to hemorrhage and vena caval constriction in dogs. *Am J Physiol.* 2000;279:R1035–R1042.
115. Levin ER, Gardner DG, Samson WK. Natriuretic peptides. *N Engl J Med.* 1998;339:321–328.
116. Rubattu S, Sciarretta S, Valenti V, et al. Natriuretic peptides: an update on bioactivity, potential therapeutic use, and implication in cardiovascular diseases. *Am J Hypertens.* 2008;21:733–741.
117. de Bold AJ, Borenstein HB, Veress AT, et al. A rapid and potent natriuretic response to intravenous injection of atrial myocardial extract in rats. *Life Sci.* 1981;28:89–94.
118. Clerico A, Recchia FA, Passino C, et al. Cardiac endocrine function is an essential component of the homeostatic regulation network: physiological and clinical implications. *Am J Physiol Heart Circ Physiol.* 2006;290:H17–H29.
119. Ruskoaho H. Atrial natriuretic peptide: synthesis, release, and metabolism. *Pharmacol Rev.* 1992;44:479–602.
120. Dhingra H, Roongsritong C, Kurtzman NA. Brain natriuretic peptide: role in cardiovascular and volume homeostasis. *Semin Nephrol.* 2002;22:423–437.
121. Sabrane K, Kruse MN, Fabritz L, et al. Vascular endothelium is critically involved in the hypotensive and hypovolemic actions of atrial natriuretic peptide. *J Clin Invest.* 2005;115:1666–1674.
122. Rose RA, Giles WR. Natriuretic peptide C receptor signalling in the heart and vasculature. *J Physiol.* 2008;586:353–366.
123. Rubattu S, Volpe M. The atrial natriuretic peptide: a changing view. *J Hypertens.* 2001;19:1923–1931.
124. Nishikimi T, Maeda N, Matsuoka H. The role of natriuretic peptides in cardioprotection. *Cardiovasc Res.* 2006:69;318–328.
125. Wong YW, Mentz RJ, Felker GM, et al. Nesiritide in patients hospitalized for acute heart failure: does timing matter? Implication for future acute heart failure trials. *Eur J Heart Fail.* 2016;18(6):684–692.
126. Brunner-La Rocca HP, Eurlings L, Richards AM, et al. Which heart failure patients profit from natriuretic peptide guided therapy? A meta-analysis from individual patient data of randomized trials. *Eur J Heart Fail.* 2015;17(12):1252–1261.
127. Hobbs A, Foster P, Prescott C, et al. Natriuretic peptide receptor-C regulates coronary blood flow and prevents myocardial ischemia/reperfusion injury: novel cardioprotective role for endothelium-derived C-type natriuretic peptide. *Circulation.* 2004;110:1231–1235.
128. Sandow SL, Tare M. C-type natriuretic peptide: a new endothelium-derived hyperpolarizing factor? *Trends Pharmacol Sci.* 2007;28:61–67.
129. Villar IC, Panayiotou CM, Sheraz A, et al. Definitive role for natriuretic peptide receptor-C in mediating the vasorelaxant activity of C-type natriuretic peptide and endothelium-derived hyperpolarising factor. *Cardiovasc Res.* 2007;74:515–525.
130. Stingo AJ, Clavell AL, Aarhus LL, et al. Cardiovascular and renal actions of C-type natriuretic peptide. *Am J Physiol.* 1992;262:H308–H312.
131. Scotland RS, Ahluwalia A, Hobbs AJ. C-type natriuretic peptide in vascular physiology and disease. *Pharmacol Ther.* 2005;105:85–93.
132. Bader M, Ganten D. Update on tissue renin-angiotensin systems. *J Mol Med.* 2008;86:615–621.
133. Dzau VJ, Bernstein K, Celermajer D, et al. Pathophysiologic and therapeutic importance of tissue ACE: a consensus report. *Cardiovasc Drugs Ther.* 2002;16:149–160.
134. Griendling KK, Ushio-Fukai M. Reactive oxygen species as mediators of angiotensin II signaling. *Regul Pept.* 2000;91:21–27.
135. Harrison D, Griendling KK, Landmesser U, et al. Role of oxidative stress in atherosclerosis. *Am J Cardiol.* 2003;91:7A–11A.
136. Touyz RM. Reactive oxygen species as mediators of calcium signaling by angiotensin II: implications in vascular physiology and pathophysiology. *Antioxid Redox Signal.* 2005;7:1302–1314.
137. Bussard RL, Busse LW. Angiotensin II: a new therapeutic option for vasodilatory shock. *Ther Clin Risk Manag.* 2018;14:1287–1298.
138. Donoghue M, Hsieh F, Baronas E, et al. A novel angiotensin-converting enzyme-related carboxypeptidase (ACE2) converts angiotensin I to angiotensin 1–9. *Circ Res.* 2000;87:E1–E9.
139. Tipnis SR, Hooper NM, Hyde R, et al. A human homolog of angiotensin-converting enzyme. Cloning and functional expression as a captopril-insensitive carboxypeptidase. *J Biol Chem.* 2000;275:33238–33243.
140. Raizada MK, Ferreira AJ. ACE2: a new target for cardiovascular disease therapeutics. *J Cardiovasc Pharmacol.* 2007;50:112–119.
141. Madeddu P, Emanueli C, El-Dahr S. Mechanisms of disease: the tissue kallikrein-kinin system in hypertension and vascular remodeling. *Nat Clin Pract Nephrol.* 2007;3:208–221.
142. Sharma JN. Does the kinin system mediate in cardiovascular abnormalities? An overview. *J Clin Pharmacol.* 2003;43:1187–1195.
143. Granger JP, Hall JE. Acute and chronic actions of bradykinin on renal function and arterial pressure. *Am J Physiol.* 1985;248:F87–F92.
144. Sharma JN. The kallikrein-kinin system: from mediator of inflammation to modulator of cardioprotection. *Inflammopharmacology.* 2005;12:591–596.
145. Westermann D, Schultheiss HP, Tschope C. New perspective on the tissue kallikrein-kinin system in myocardial infarction: role of angiogenesis and cardiac regeneration. *Int Immunopharmacol.* 2008;8:148–154.
146. Sharma JN. Cardiovascular activities of the bradykinin system. *Scientific World Journal.* 2008;8:384–393.
147. Daull P, Jeng AY, Battistini B. Towards triple vasopeptidase inhibitors for the treatment of cardiovascular diseases. *J Cardiovasc Pharmacol.* 2007;50:247–256.
148. Tschope C, Schultheiss HP, Walther T. Multiple interactions between the renin-angiotensin and the kallikrein-kinin systems: role of ACE inhibition and AT1 receptor blockade. *J Cardiovasc Pharmacol.* 2002;39:478–487.
149. Schmaier AH. The kallikrein-kinin and the renin-angiotensin systems have a multilayered interaction. *Am J Physiol.* 2003;285:R1–R13.
150. Shen B, El-Dahr SS. Cross-talk of the renin-angiotensin and kallikrein-kinin systems. *Biol Chem.* 2006;387:145–150.
151. Packer M, Califf RM, Konstam MA, et al. Comparison of omapatrilat and enalapril in patients with chronic heart failure: The Omapatrilat Versus Enalapril Randomized Trial of Utility in Reducing Events (OVERTURE). *Circulation.* 2002;106:920–926.
152. Messerli FH, Nussberger J. Vasopeptidase inhibition and angio-oedema. *Lancet.* 2000;356:608–609.
153. Esler M. Clinical application of noradrenaline spillover methodology: delineation of regional human sympathetic nervous responses. *Pharmacol Toxicol.* 1993;73:243–253.
154. Bevan JA. Some functional consequences of variation in adrenergic synaptic cleft width and in nerve density and distribution. *Fed Proc.* 1977;36:2439–2443.
155. Bevan JA. Some bases of differences in vascular response to sympathetic activity. *Circ Res.* 1979;45:161–171.
156. Bevan JA, Su C. Variation of intra- and perisynaptic adrenergic transmitter concentrations with width of synaptic cleft in vascular tissue. *J Pharmacol Exp Ther.* 1974;190:30–38.
157. Gallagher D, O'Rourke M. What is the arterial pressure? In: O'Rourke M, Safar M, Dzau V, eds. *Arterial Vasodilation. Mechanisms and Therapy.* Philadelphia, PA: Lea & Febiger; 1993:134–148.
158. O'Rourke M. What is blood pressure? *Am J Hypertens.* 1990;3:803–810.
159. Agabiti-Rosei E, Mancia G, O'Rourke MF, et al. Central blood pressure measurements and antihypertensive therapy: a consensus document. *Hypertension.* 2007;50:154–160.
160. Hainsworth R. The control and physiological importance of heart rate. In: Malik M, Camms A, eds. *Heart Rate Variability.* Armonk, NY: Futura Publishing; 1995:3–19.
161. Levy MN. Neural control of cardiac function. *Baillieres Clin Neurol.* 1997;6:227–244.
162. Spyer M. Vagal preganglionic neurons innervating the heart. In: Page E, Fozzard H, Solaro R, eds. *Handbook of Physiology, Section 2: The Cardiovascular System, Vol I: The Heart.* Bethesda, MD: American Physiological Society; 2000:213–239.
163. Monahan KD. Effect of aging on baroreflex function in humans. *Am J Physiol Regul Integr Comp Physiol.* 2007;293:R3–R12.
164. Rea RF, Eckberg DL. Carotid baroreceptor-muscle sympathetic relation in humans. *Am J Physiol.* 1987;253:R929–R934.
165. Skow RJ, Day TA, Fuller JE, et al. The ins and outs of breath holding: simple demonstrations of complex respiratory physiology. *Adv Physiol Educ.* 2015:39(3);223–231.
166. Ponikowski P, Banasiak W. Chemosensitivity in chronic heart failure. *Heart Fail Monit.* 2001;1:126–131.
167. Ponikowski P, Chua TP, Anker SD, et al. Peripheral chemoreceptor hypersensitivity: an ominous sign in patients with chronic heart failure. *Circulation.* 2001;104:544–549.
168. Eckberg DL. Point: counterpoint: respiratory sinus arrhythmia is due to a central mechanism vs. respiratory sinus arrhythmia is due to the baroreflex mechanism. *J Appl Physiol (1985).* 2009;106(5):1740–1744.
169. Mazzone SB, Undem BJ. Vagal afferent innervation of the airways in health and disease. *Physiol Rev.* 2016;96(3):975–1024.
170. Janicki J, Sheriff D, Robotham J, et al. Cardiac output during exercise: contributions of the cardiac, circulatory, and respiratory systems. In:

Rowell L, Sheperd J, eds. *Handbook of Physiology. Exercise: Regulation and Integration of Multiple Systems*. Bethesda, MD: Oxford University Press; 1996:649–704.

171. Sheriff D, Zhou X, Scher A, et al. Dependence of cardiac filling pressure on cardiac output during rest and dynamic exercise in dogs. *Am J Physiol.* 1993;265:H316–H322.
172. Young DB. *Control of Cardiac Output.* San Rafael, CA: Morgan & Claypool Life Sciences; 2010. Chapter 3, Cardiac Function. Available at https://www.ncbi.nlm.nih.gov/books/NBK54477/
173. Miller D, Gleason W, Whalen R. Effect of ventricular rate in the cardiac output in the dog with chronic heart block. *Circ Res.* 1962;10:658–663.
174. Rushmer R. Constance of stroke volume in ventricular responses to exertion. *Am J Physiol.* 1959;196:745–750.
175. Bevegård S, Jonsson B, Karlof I, et al. Effect of changes in ventricular rate on cardiac output and central pressures at rest and during exercise in patients with artificial pacemakers. *Cardiovasc Res.* 1967;1:21–33.
176. Sonnenblick EH. Force-velocity relations in mammalian heart muscle. *Am J Physiol.* 1962;202:931–939.
177. Starling E. *The Linacre Lecture on the Law of the Heart, Given at Cambridge, 1915.* London: Longmans, Green; 1918.
178. Sarnoff SJ. Myocardial contractility as described by ventricular function curves; observations on Starling's Law of the Heart. *Physiol Rev.* 1955;35:107–122.
179. Weber K, Janicki J, Reeves R, et al. Determinants of stroke volume in the isolated canine heart. *J Appl Physiol.* 1974;37:742–747.
180. de Tombe PP, Mateja RD, Tachampa K, et al. Myofilament length dependent activation. *J Mol Cell Cardiol.* 2010;48(5):851–858.
181. Lakatta EG. Starling's law of the heart is explained by an intimate interaction of muscle length and myofilament calcium activation. *J Am Coll Cardiol.* 1987;10:1157–1164.
182. Brady A. Mechanical properties of isolated cardiac myocytes. *Physiol Rev.* 1991;71:413–428.
183. Delicce AV, Makaryus AN. Physiology, Frank Starling Law. [Updated 2020 Jan 19]. In: *StatPearls [Internet].* Treasure Island, FL: StatPearls Publishing; 2020. Available at https://www.ncbi.nlm.nih.gov/books/NBK470295/
184. Tedford RJ. Determinants of right ventricular afterload (2013 Grover Conference series). *Pulm Circ.* 2014;4(2):211–219.
185. Homan TD, Bordes S, Cichowski E. Physiology, Pulse Pressure. [Updated 2020 Jun 7]. In: *StatPearls [Internet].* Treasure Island, FL: StatPearls Publishing; 2020. Available at https://www.ncbi.nlm.nih.gov/books/NBK482408/
186. Covell J, Ross J. Systolic and diastolic function (mechanics) of the intact heart. In: Page E, Fozzard H, Solaro R, eds. *Handbook of Physiology: Section 2. The Cardiovascular System.* Bethesda, MD: American Physiological Society; 2002:741–784.
187. Ross J Jr. Afterload mismatch and preload reserve: a conceptual framework for the analysis of ventricular function. *Prog Cardiovasc Dis.* 1976;18:255–264.
188. Ross J Jr, Franklin D, Sasayama S. Preload, afterload, and the role of afterload mismatch in the descending limb of cardiac function. *Eur J Cardiol.* 1976;4(Suppl.):77–86.
189. Bombardini T. Myocardial contractility in the echo lab: Molecular, cellular and pathophysiological basis. *Cardiovasc Ultrasound.* 2005;3:27.
190. Endoh M. Force-frequency relationship in intact mammalian ventricular myocardium: physiological and pathophysiological relevance. *Eur J Pharmacol.* 2004;500:73–86.
191. Ross J Jr, Miura T, Kambayashi M, et al. Adrenergic control of the force-frequency relation. *Circulation.* 1995;92:2327–2332.
192. Yamanaka T, Onishi K, Tanabe M, et al. Force- and relaxation-frequency relations in patients with diastolic heart failure. *Am Heart J.* 2006;152:966.e1–966.e7.
193. Kroeker CA, Shrive NG, Belenkie I, et al. Pericardium modulates left and right ventricular stroke volumes to compensate for sudden changes in atrial volume. *Am J Physiol.* 2003;284:H2247–H2254.
194. Spodick D. *The Pericardium. A Comprehensive Textbook.* New York: Marcel Dekker, Inc; 1997.
195. Belenkie I, Sas R, Mitchell J, et al. Opening the pericardium during pulmonary artery constriction improves cardiac function. *J Appl Physiol.* 2004;96:917–922.
196. Belenkie I, Smith ER, Tyberg JV. Ventricular interaction: from bench to bedside. *Ann Med.* 2001;33:236–241.
197. Horne SG, Belenkie I, Tyberg JV, et al. Pericardial pressure in experimental chronic heart failure. *Can J Cardiol.* 2000;16:607–613.
198. Kardon DE, Borczuk AC, Factor SM. Mechanism of pericardial expansion with cardiac enlargement. *Cardiovasc Pathol.* 2000;9:9–15.
199. Hammond H, White F, Bhargava V, et al. Heart size and maximal cardiac output are limited by the pericardium. *Am J Physiol.* 1992;263:H1675–H1681.
200. De Hert SG, ten Broecke PW, Rodrigus IE, et al. The effects of the pericardium on length-dependent regulation of left ventricular function in coronary artery surgery patients. *J Cardiothorac Vasc Anesth.* 2001;15:300–305.
201. Stray-Gundersen J, Musch T, Haidet G, et al. The effect of pericardiectomy on maximal oxygen consumption and maximal cardiac output in untrained dogs. *Circ Res.* 1986;58:523–530.
202. Hunter S, Smith GH, Angelini GD. Adverse hemodynamic effects of pericardial closure soon after open heart operation. *Ann Thorac Surg.* 1992;53:425–429.
203. Rao V, Komeda M, Weisel RD, et al. Should the pericardium be closed routinely after heart operations? *Ann Thorac Surg.* 1999;67:484–488.
204. Cowley AJ. Long-term control of arterial blood pressure. *Physiol Rev.* 1992;72:231–300.
205. Granger JP, Alexander BT, Llinas M. Mechanisms of pressure natriuresis. *Curr Hypertens Rep.* 2002;4:152–159.
206. Guyton AC. Blood pressure control—special role of the kidneys and body fluids. *Science.* 1991;252:1813–1816.
207. Brooks V, Osborn J. Hormonal-sympathetic interactions in long-term regulation of arterial pressure: an hypothesis. *Am J Physiol.* 1995;268:R1343–R1358.
208. Evans RG, Majid DS, Eppel GA. Mechanisms mediating pressure natriuresis: What we know and what we need to find out. *Clin Exp Pharmacol Physiol.* 2005;32:400–409.
209. Bie P, Wamberg S, Kjolby M. Volume natriuresis vs. pressure natriuresis. *Acta Physiol Scand.* 2004;181:495–503.
210. Brooks VL, Sved AF. Pressure to change? Re-evaluating the role of baroreceptors in the long-term control of arterial pressure. *Am J Physiol Regul Integr Comp Physiol.* 2005;288:R815–R818.
211. Joyner MJ, Charkoudian N, Wallin BG. A sympathetic view of the sympathetic nervous system and human blood pressure regulation. *Exp Physiol.* 2008;93:715–724.
212. Lohmeier TE, Hildebrandt DA, Warren S, et al. Recent insights into the interactions between the baroreflex and the kidneys in hypertension. *Am J Physiol Regul Integr Comp Physiol.* 2005;288:R828–R836.
213. Thrasher TN. Baroreceptors, baroreceptor unloading, and the long-term control of blood pressure. *Am J Physiol Regul Integr Comp Physiol.* 2005;288:R819–R827.
214. Thrasher TN. Arterial baroreceptor input contributes to long-term control of blood pressure. *Curr Hypertens Rep.* 2006;8:249–254.
215. Barrett CJ, Malpas SC. Problems, possibilities, and pitfalls in studying the arterial baroreflexes' influence over long-term control of blood pressure. *Am J Physiol Regul Integr Comp Physiol.* 2005;288:R837–R845.
216. Osborn JW, Jacob F, Guzman P. A neural set point for the long-term control of arterial pressure: Beyond the arterial baroreceptor reflex. *Am J Physiol Regul Integr Comp Physiol.* 2005;288:R846–R855.
217. Osborn JW. Hypothesis: Set-points and long-term control of arterial pressure. A theoretical argument for a long-term arterial pressure control system in the brain rather than the kidney. *Clin Exp Pharmacol Physiol.* 2005;32:384–393.
218. Mellander S. Functional aspects of myogenic vascular control. *J Hypertens.* 1989;7(Suppl. 4):S21–S30.
219. Seddon MD, Chowienczyk PJ, Brett SE, et al. Neuronal nitric oxide synthase regulates basal microvascular tone in humans in vivo. *Circulation.* 2008;117:1991–1996.
220. Vallance P, Collier J, Moncada S. Effects of endothelium-derived nitric oxide on peripheral arteriolar tone in man. *Lancet.* 1989;189:997–1000.
221. Sugawara J, Komine H, Hayashi K, et al. Effect of systemic nitric oxide synthase inhibition on arterial stiffness in humans. *Hypertens Res.* 2007;30:411–415.
222. Wilkinson I, MacCallum H, Cockcroft J, et al. Inhibition of basal nitric oxide synthesis increases aortic augmentation index and pulse wave velocity in vivo. *Br J Clin Pharmacol.* 2002;53:189–192.
223. Sugawara J, Komine H, Hayashi K, et al. Relationship between augmentation index obtained from carotid and radial artery pressure waveforms. *J Hypertens.* 2007;25:375–381.
224. Celander O. The range of control exercised by sympathicoadrenal system. *Acta Physiologica Scandinavia.* 1954;32(Suppl. 116):1–132.
225. Johanson B. Myogenic responses of vascular smooth muscle. In: Stevens N, ed. *Smooth Muscle Contraction.* New York: Marcel Dekker; 1980:457–472.
226. Johnson P. Autoregulation of blood flow. *Circ Res.* 1986;59:483–495.
227. Renkin E. Control of microcirculation and blood-tissue exchange. In: Renkin E, Michel C, eds. *Handbook of Physiology.* Bethesda, MD: American Physiological Society; 1984:627–687.

228. Carlson BE, Arciero JC, Secomb TW. Theoretical model of blood flow autoregulation: roles of myogenic, shear-dependent, and metabolic responses. *Am J Physiol Heart Circ Physiol.* 2008;295:H1572–H1579.
229. Schubert R, Mulvany MJ. The myogenic response: established facts and attractive hypotheses. *Clin Sci.* 1999;96:313–326.
230. Feigl E. The arterial system. In: Patton H, Fuchs A, Hille B, et al., eds. *Textbook of Physiology.* Philadelphia, PA: WB Saunders; 1989:849–859.
231. Arciero JC, Carlson BE, Secomb TW. Theoretical model of metabolic blood flow regulation: roles of ATP release by red blood cells and conducted responses. *Am J Physiol Heart Circ Physiol.* 2008;295:H1562–H1571.
232. Hester RL, Hammer LW. Venular-arteriolar communication in the regulation of blood flow. *Am J Physiol.* 2002;282:R1280–R1285.
233. Johnson P. The myogenic response. In: Bohr D, Somlyo A, Sparks H, eds. *Handbook of Physiology, Section 2, Vol II, Vascular Smooth Muscle.* Bethesda, MD: American Physiological Society; 1980:409–442.
234. Lombard J, Duling B. Relative importance of tissue oxygenation and vascular smooth muscle hypoxia in determining arteriolar response to occlusion in the hamster cheek pouch. *Circ Res.* 1977;41:365–373.
235. Rothe C. Venous system: physiology of the capacitance vessels. In: Shepherd J, Abboud F, eds. *Handbook of Physiology. The Cardiovascular System. Peripheral Circulation and Organ Blood Flow.* Bethesda, MD: American Physiological Society; 1983:397–452.
236. Flavahan N, Linblad L, Verbeuren T, et al. Cooling and alpha-1 and alpha-2 adrenergic response in cutaneous veins: role of receptor reserve. *Am J Physiol.* 1985;249:H950–H955.
237. Hainsworth R. Vascular capacitance: its control and importance. *Rev Physiol Biochem Pharmacol.* 1986;105:101–173.
238. Rowell L. Regulation of splanchnic blood flow in man. *Physiologist.* 1973;16:127–142.
239. Rothe C, Gaddis M. Autoregulation of cardiac output by passive elastic characteristics of the vascular capacitance system. *Circulation.* 1990;81:360–368.
240. Guyton A. Determination of cardiac output by equating venous return curves with cardiac response curves. *Physiol Rev.* 1955;35:123–129.
241. Guyton A, Abernathy B, Langston J, et al. Relative importance of venous and arterial resistances in controlling venous return and cardiac output. *Am J Physiol.* 1959;196:1008–1014.
242. Guyton A, Lindsey A, Abernathy B, et al. Venous return at various right atrial pressures and the normal venous return curve. *Am J Physiol.* 1957;189:609–615.
243. Brengelmann GL. A critical analysis of the view that right atrial pressure determines venous return. *J Appl Physiol.* 2003;94:849–859.
244. Bridges E. Hemodynamic monitoring. In: Woods S, Sivarajan Froelicher E, Motzer S, et al., eds. *Cardiac Nursing.* Philadelphia, PA: Lippincott; 2005:81–108.
245. Brengelmann GL. Counterpoint: the classical Guyton view that mean systemic pressure, right atrial pressure, and venous resistance govern venous return is not correct. *J Appl Physiol.* 2006;101:1525–1526; discussion 1526–1527.
246. Brengelmann GL. Learning opportunities in the study of Curran-Everett's exploration of a classic paper on venous return. *Adv Physiol Educ.* 2008;32:242–243.
247. Magder S. Point: the classical Guyton view that mean systemic pressure, right atrial pressure, and venous resistance govern venous return is/is not correct. *J Appl Physiol.* 2006;101:1523–1525.
248. Rothe CF. Mean circulatory filling pressure: its meaning and measurement. *J Appl Physiol.* 1993;74:499–509.
249. Rothe C. The classical Guyton view that mean systemic pressure, right atrial pressure, and venous resistance govern venous return is/is not correct. *J Appl Physiol.* 2006;101:1529.
250. Casey DP, Hart EC. Cardiovascular function in humans during exercise: role of the muscle pump. *J Physiol.* 2008;586:5045–5046.
251. Rowland TW. The circulatory response to exercise: role of the peripheral pump. *Int J Sports Med.* 2001;22:558–565.
252. Osada T, Katsumura T, Hamaoka T, et al. Quantitative effects of respiration on venous return during single knee extension-flexion. *Int J Sports Med.* 2002;23:183–190.
253. Miller JD, Pegelow DF, Jacques AJ, et al. Skeletal muscle pump versus respiratory muscle pump: modulation of venous return from the locomotor limb in humans. *J Physiol.* 2005;563:925–943.
254. Michard F, Teboul JL. Using heart-lung interactions to assess fluid responsiveness during mechanical ventilation. *Critical Care.* 2000;4:282–289.
255. Krogh A. The regulation of the supply of blood to the right heart. *Skandinavisches Archiv fur Physiologie.* 1912;27:227–248.
256. Hamilton W, Woodbury R, Harper H. Physiologic relationships between intrathoracic, intraspinal, and arterial pressures. *JAMA.* 1936;107:853–856.
257. Hamilton W, Woodbury R, Harper H. Arterial, cerebrospinal and venous pressures in man during cough and strain. *Am J Physiol.* 1944;141:42–50.
258. Levin A. A simple test of cardiac function based upon the heart rate changes induced by the Valsalva Maneuver. *Am J Cardiol.* 1966;18:90–99.
259. Smith M, Beightol L, Fritsch-Yelle J, et al. Valsalva's maneuver revisited: a quantitative method yielding insights into human autonomic control. *Am J Physiol.* 1996;271:1240–1249.
260. Junqueira LF Jr. Teaching cardiac autonomic function dynamics employing the Valsalva (Valsalva-Weber) maneuver. *Adv Physiol Educ.* 2008;32:100–106.
261. McGuire J, Green RS, Courter S, et al. Bed pan deaths. *Trans Am Clin Climatol Assoc.* 1948;60:78–86.
262. Metzger B, Therrien B. Effect of position on cardiovascular response during the Valsalva Maneuver. *Nurs Res.* 1990;39:198–202.
263. Sharpey-Schafer E. Effects of Valsalva's manoeuvre on the normal and failing circulation. *BMJ.* 1955;1:693–695.
264. Eckberg DL, Sleight P. *Human Baroreflexes in Health and Disease.* Oxford, UK: Clarendon Press; 1992.
265. Mancia G, Mark A. Arterial baroreflexes in humans. In: Sheperd J, Abboud FM, eds. *Handbook of Physiology. The Cardiovascular System. Peripheral Circulation and Organ Blood Flow.* Bethesda, MD: American Physiologic Society; 1983:755–794.
266. Prakash ES, Madanmohan Pal GK. What is the ultimate goal in neural regulation of cardiovascular function? *Adv Physiol Educ.* 2004;28:100–101.
267. Sagawa K. Baroreflex control of systemic arterial pressure and vascular bed. In: Sheperd J, Abboud FM, eds. *Handbook of Physiology. The Cardiovascular System. Peripheral Circulation and Organ Blood Flow.* Bethesda, MD: American Physiologic Society; 1983:452–496.
268. Toska K, Walloe L. Dynamic time course of hemodynamic responses after passive head-up tilt and tilt back to supine position. *J Appl Physiol.* 2002;92:1671–1676.
269. Ogoh S, Yoshiga CC, Secher NH, et al. Carotid-cardiac baroreflex function does not influence blood pressure regulation during head-up tilt in humans. *J Physiol Sci.* 2006;56:227–233.
270. Rowell LB. Reflex control of the cutaneous vasculature. *J Invest Dermatol.* 1977;69:154–166.
271. Scott-Douglas NW, Robinson VJ, Smiseth OA, et al. Effects of acute volume loading and hemorrhage on intestinal vascular capacitance: a mechanism whereby capacitance modulates cardiac output. *Can J Cardiol.* 2002;18(5):515–522.
272. Wray DW, Formes KJ, Weiss MS, et al. Vagal cardiac function and arterial blood pressure stability. *Am J Physiol Heart Circ Physiol.* 2001;281(5):H1870–H1880.
273. Toska K, Eriksen M, Walloe L. Short-term cardiovascular responses to a step decrease in peripheral conductance in humans. *Am J Physiol.* 1994;266(1):H199–H211.
274. Heistad DKH. Cerebral circulation. In: Shepherd J, Aboutt F, Geiger S, eds. *Handbook of Physiology. The Cardiovascular System: Peripheral Circulation and Organ Blood Flow.* Bethesda, MD: American Physiological Society; 1983:137–182
275. Qureshi AI. Acute hypertensive response in patients with stroke: pathophysiology and management. *Circulation.* 2008;118(2):176–187.

5 Hematopoiesis, Coagulation, and Bleeding

Angela D. Pal

OBJECTIVES

By the end of the chapter, the learner should be able to:

1. Describe the types of blood cells.
2. Describe the physiologic roles of each of the blood cells.
3. Identify the major factors involved in coagulation.
4. Explain how the body maintains hemostasis.
5. Describe the pathophysiologic process of disseminated intravascular coagulation (DIC).
6. Describe the management and nursing care of a patient with DIC.
7. Describe the pathophysiologic process of venous thromboembolism (VTE), including deep vein thrombosis (DVT) and pulmonary embolus (PE).
8. Describe the management and nursing care of a patient with VTE.
9. Describe the pathophysiologic process of heparin-induced thrombocytopenia (HIT).
10. Describe the management and nursing care of a patient with HIT.

KEY QUESTIONS

1. How does the body maintain hemostasis?
2. What clinical manifestations might one see in a patient presenting with
   a. Disseminated intravascular coagulation?
   b. Venous thromboembolism, including deep vein thrombosis and pulmonary embolus?
   c. Heparin-induced thrombocytopenia?
3. What are the key nursing interventions for patients with
   a. Disseminated intravascular coagulation?
   b. Venous thromboembolism, including deep vein thrombosis and pulmonary embolus?
   c. Heparin-induced thrombocytopenia?

BACKGROUND

The hematologic system is a key organ system linked to the cardiovascular system and thus should be discussed in detail. This chapter will focus on the basic components of the hematologic system, as well as the main diseases or illnesses involving bleeding (disseminated intravascular coagulation [DIC]); clotting defects (venous thromboembolism [VTE], including deep vein thrombosis or DVT and pulmonary embolism or PE); and heparin-induced thrombocytopenia or HIT.

Current State and Context

The physiologic functions of blood include nutrition, oxygenation, respiration, and excretion. These various components of blood accomplish these functions. Approximately 55% of blood volume is composed of plasma, which is a transport medium for ions, proteins, hormones, and end products of cellular metabolism. The most important ions carried in the plasma are sodium, potassium, chloride, hydrogen, magnesium, and calcium. Examples of proteins transported in the plasma are immunoglobulins and the coagulation proteins. Formed elements or cells including red blood cells (RBCs; erythrocytes), white blood cells (WBCs; leukocytes), and platelets (thrombocytes) constitute the other 45% of blood volume. Erythrocytes transport oxygen to the tissues and carbon dioxide to the lungs for excretion. Leukocytes protect against infection and play a major role in the inflammatory process. Thrombocytes, along with coagulation proteins, protect against blood loss through the formation of blood clots.[1]

Because these functions are vital, a significant blood loss has devastating consequences for all body tissues. A complex series of events leading to hemostasis achieves protection against such blood losses and potential exsanguination from injuries. The endothelium of the vasculature plays a vital role in the coagulation process and is now considered an organ by the Margaux III Conference on Critical Illness: The Endothelium: An Underrecognized Organ in Critical Illness.[2] The endothelial cell participates by releasing mediators that effect coagulation and the role of the vessel's participation in hemostasis. The equally complex mechanism of fibrinolysis, which dissolves clots, balances this system. Normal blood flow through the vasculature depends partly on the balance of these two systems, hemostasis, and fibrinolysis. Knowledge of these normal processes is important as a basis for understanding the many alterations that may result from disease states or drug administration.

Hematopoietic Cells

Hematopoiesis, or the production of blood cells, occurs primarily in the bone marrow. The liver, spleen, lymph nodes, and thymus are involved in hematopoiesis during embryonic life, but after birth, extramedullary (outside the bone marrow) hematopoiesis occurs only during abnormal circumstances. If it occurs at all after birth, extramedullary hematopoiesis occurs mainly in the liver and spleen. The hematopoietic stem cell resides mainly in the bone marrow and in small numbers in the peripheral blood. The hematopoietic stem cell is the source of all the types of blood cells: RBCs, WBCs, and platelets.

The stem cell is an immature (undifferentiated) cell that has the capacity to reproduce itself and to mature (differentiate) into any of the different types of blood cells. As the stem cell divides and matures, it differentiates into one of two committed cell lines: lymphoid or myeloid progenitor cells. The committed lymphoid progenitor cell eventually matures into T and B lymphocytes and natural killer cells. The committed myeloid stem progenitor cell develops into (1) the megakaryocyte–erythrocyte precursors leading to the development of platelets and RBC and (2) the granulocyte–monocyte precursors leading to the development of the granulocyte and monocyte.[3] Maturation of these cell lines is influenced by multiple growth factors such as granulocyte colony-stimulating factor, erythropoietin, thrombopoietin, interleukins, interferon, and many others.[3] As the various types of blood cells mature, they are released into the peripheral circulation. Figure 5-1 shows a model for hematopoietic cell differentiation.

Red Blood Cells

The major role of the RBC is respiration, which is the exchange of gases. The mature RBC is a biconcave disc filled with hemoglobin, but it does not have a nucleus. The lack of a nucleus allows the RBC to change shape and facilitates movement through small capillary beds. Heme, the iron-containing pigment, is the actual oxygen-transporting portion of the hemoglobin molecule. Oxygen diffuses from the alveoli into the alveolar capillaries and binds to each of four to five sites on the heme portion of hemoglobin. One gram of hemoglobin can carry 1.34 to 1.36 mL of oxygen. The remarkable oxygen-binding capacity of the RBC is influenced by three factors that affect the oxyhemoglobin dissociation curve: pH, temperature, and the amount of 2,3-diphosphoglycerate. Tissue metabolism produces carbon dioxide as a waste product that is also transported from the tissues by the RBC. Carbon dioxide diffuses into the RBC and combines with water to form carbonic acid that further dissociates to the hydrogen and bicarbonate ions. The bicarbonate ion is inactivated when combined with hydrogen ions to again form water and carbon dioxide, which is eliminated at the alveoli.

The rate of bone marrow stem cell differentiation into erythrocytes is primarily controlled by erythropoietin. Most of this hormone is produced by the kidney. The creation of RBC is influenced by the oxygen content of the blood as sensed by the kidneys. Production also requires necessary substrates including vitamin B_{12}, vitamin B_6, folic acid, and iron. The vitamins and folic acid are obtained from dietary sources, as is iron. However, most iron is gained through the recycling of the RBC in the spleen. RBC production is increased at times of blood loss, at high altitude, and in pulmonary diseases which affect the transport of oxygen from the lungs to the blood. It takes approximately 3 to 5 days for a RBC to mature in the marrow and be released into the peripheral circulation. RBCs live approximately 120 days, at which time they are recycled by the spleen.

White Blood Cells

WBCs can be divided into two major categories: phagocytes and lymphocytes. The primary role of phagocytes is to locate and kill

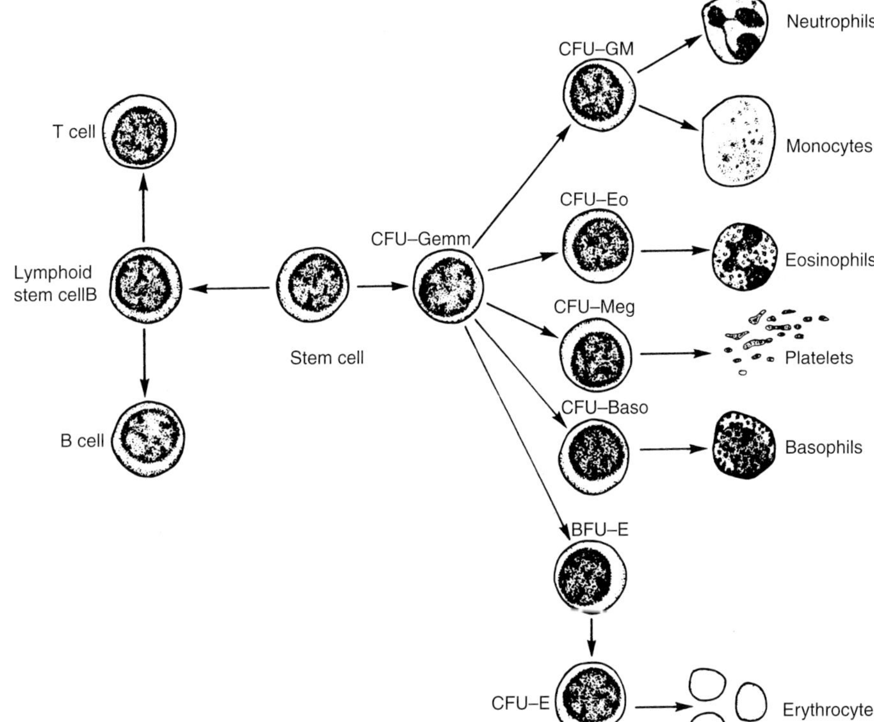

Figure 5-1. The hematopoietic hierarchy. As hematopoietic stem cells divide, they give rise to common lymphoid and common myeloid precursor cells that eventually generate all mature blood lineages of the body. LT-HSC, long-term hematopoietic stem cells; GMP, granulocyte–monocyte precursors; MEP, megakaryocyte–erythrocyte precursors; NK, natural killer; ST-HSC, short-term hematopoietic stem cells. (Reproduced with permission from Hoffman R, Benz E, Shattil S, et al. *Hematology: Basic Principles and Practice*. Philadelphia, PA: Elsevier/Churchill Livingstone; 2005.)

invading microorganisms or foreign antigens. The primary role of lymphocytes is to initiate and direct the immune response including the manufacture of antibodies. WBCs travel throughout the body and will migrate into different tissues depending on chemical mediators that signal the cells. Phagocytes perform their role primarily out in the tissues, where they travel toward the site of an inflammation (chemotaxis) and kill microbes by engulfing them (phagocytosis). Many substances, including complement fragments and bacterial products, stimulate this chemotactic migration. Phagocytosis is an active process that uses energy derived from anaerobic glycolysis. Phagocytic cells are divided into two subgroups: granulocytes (granular substances within the cell after staining) and monocytes. The granulocytes include neutrophils ("polys"), basophils, and eosinophils. Neutrophils compose 60% to 70% of all WBCs. Neutrophil maturation in the marrow takes 7 to 10 days. Their main function is to find and kill bacteria, especially resident microorganisms such as staphylococci and gram-negative enteric flora.[1] They also play an important role in acute inflammatory processes. Neutrophils are one of the first phagocytic cells to appear at the site of an acute inflammation. During severe inflammatory reactions, neutrophils can cause damage to surrounding tissues by releasing proteolytic enzymes and oxygen-free radicals. Once in the bloodstream, some of the neutrophils freely circulate while others linger along the blood vessel wall, which is called margination. Adhesion molecules emanating from an injury or from an organism make the blood vessel wall sticky so that the marginated neutrophils adhere to the vessel walls. The neutrophil releases substances allowing the endothelial cells to separate and permit the neutrophil to crawl into the connective tissue (diapedesis). The neutrophil migrates to the area of injury through chemotaxis. The migration of neutrophils to the tissues takes place rapidly, within 12 hours on entering the bloodstream. Once in the bloodstream, the neutrophil must be able to differentiate cells or substances that are foreign. Opsonization is a process in which molecules in the plasma coat the microorganism, making it more recognizable to the neutrophil.

Eosinophils and basophils are WBCs that have specific functions that are also important in the defense of the body. Eosinophils compose approximately 4% of a normal WBC count. Eosinophils have been postulated to play a defensive role against parasites and allergic reactions. Basophils account for only 0.5% to 1% of the total WBC count. Agranular leukocytes are WBCs without granular substances within the cells after staining. Monocytes and lymphocytes are agranular leukocytes. Monocytes constitute 4% to 8% of the total WBC count. Within 24 to 36 hours of entering the circulation, they migrate into the tissues where they undergo further maturation and are called macrophages. Hepatic Kupffer cells, alveolar macrophages, and peritoneal macrophages are examples of tissue macrophages.

Once lodged in their target organ, macrophages can live for up to 60 days. In the bloodstream, monocytes have similar functions to the neutrophil. However, in addition, monocytes and macrophages play a crucial role in recognizing foreign invaders and presenting foreign antigens to lymphocytes, thus stimulating the immune response. They are important in killing bacteria, protozoa, cells infected with viruses, and tumor cells. In addition to their phagocytic activity, macrophages secrete biologically active products, including cytokines that modulate the immune response.

Lymphocytes are essential components of the immune system. They recognize and are instrumental in the elimination of foreign proteins, pathogens, and tumor cells. Lymphocytes control the intensity and specificity of the immune response. There are two general types of lymphocytes, T lymphocytes (or T cells), which provide cell-mediated and B lymphocytes (B cells), which produce the antibodies of humoral immunity. Stem cell differentiation for the production of lymphocytes occurs in the bone marrow. It is in the thymus that T cells learn to differentiate self from nonself. There are four separate subsets of T cells: helper T cells, suppressor T cells, cytotoxic T cells, and memory T cells. Cell-mediated activities are of great importance in delayed hypersensitivity reactions; graft rejection; graft-versus-host disease; and in defense against fungal, protozoal, and most viral infections. Another important function of T cells is to regulate immune activities through the secretion of lymphokines.

B lymphocytes mature into cells that respond to stimulation from foreign proteins by differentiating into memory cells and plasma cells. The plasma cells produce specific antibodies that inactivate or destroy foreign proteins and pathogens. These antibodies are particularly effective against bacterial infections, especially encapsulated bacteria, such as pneumococci, streptococci, meningococci, and *Haemophilus influenzae,* as well as certain viruses. The helper cells of the T cells stimulate B cells to produce antibodies.

Natural killer cells, another subset of lymphocytes, kill tumor cells and cells infected by viruses. They play an important role in tumor surveillance. The activities of phagocytes and immune cells overlap in numerous mutually beneficial ways. For example, immune cells often participate in chronic inflammatory reactions. Conversely, engulfment of foreign protein by macrophages is a preparatory step leading to antibody production.

Table 5-1 summarizes the WBCs and their function.[4]

Because blood cells have a limited life span, they need to be replaced constantly. Usually, the number of cells produced is fairly constant, but depending on environmental stimuli such as bleeding, infection, or inflammation, various cells may be needed in larger than normal quantities at times. Thus, each of these cell lines is regulated by cytokines that influence the rate of growth and differentiation of the stem cells in the marrow. Cytokines are proteins that are made by cells of the immune system and regulate the immune response. Some examples of cytokines are granulocyte–macrophage colony-stimulating factor, which stimulates

Table 5-1 • WHITE BLOOD CELLS

Name	Function
WBC or leukocyte	Combat pathogens and other foreign substances that enter the body
Granular Leukocytes	
Neutrophils	Phagocytosis or the destruction of bacteria with lysozyme, defensins, and strong oxidants
Eosinophils	Combat the effects of histamine in allergic reactions, phagocytize antigen–antibody complexes
Basophils	Liberate heparin, histamine, and serotonin in allergic reactions that intensify the overall inflammatory response
Agranular Leukocytes	
Lymphocytes (T cells, B cells, natural killer cells)	Mediate immune responses including antigen–antibody reactions
Monocytes	Phagocytosis after transforming into macrophages

Adapted from Tortora G, Grabowski S. *Principles of Anatomy and Physiology.* New York: John Wiley & Sons, Inc.; 2003.

the growth of granulocytes and macrophages, and interleukin-3 (IL-3), which stimulates the stem cell. Cytokines also stimulate the function of mature immune cells.[4]

Platelets

Platelets are small cell fragments that are produced by the disintegration of megakaryocytes in the bone marrow, producing several thousand platelets that are released into the circulation. They are tiny, disc-shaped fragments that are capable of changing shape and have a high metabolic rate. It takes approximately 5 days for a stem cell to differentiate along the megakaryocyte line and produce platelets. Under normal circumstances, platelets circulate in the bloodstream for approximately 10 days. The production of platelets is regulated by thrombopoietin, which is a humoral hormonelike substance. Platelets are also called thrombocytes, which means *clot cell.* They play a major role in hemostasis by adhering to a damaged blood vessel wall and aggregating together to form a mechanical barrier to the flow of blood thereby preventing blood loss. Platelets will then release various mediators to attract other cells and components to the site so that fibrin formation can start. There are three storage granules in the platelets: alpha granules, dense bodies, and lysosomes. Alpha granules contain and release fibrinogen. Dense bodies release adenine nucleotides, serotonin, and platelet factor 4 (PF4). Lysosomes contain degradative acid hydrolases.[1] Platelets are sequestered in the spleen and are released as needed to combat bleeding. Their function is vital to the coagulation process, so much so that many cardiac interventions are now aimed at disabling platelet function.

Coagulation Factors

The major component of blood, plasma, contains many particles including proteins (clotting factors) that are involved in coagulation. To standardize the identification of these proteins, an international committee assigned a nomenclature for these proteins using Roman numerals listed in order of their discovery. However, the order does not refer to the sequence of reactions in the coagulation cascade. A lowercase "a" is also used to indicate the activated form of a clotting factor. Table 5-2 lists these clotting factors.[4] The liver plays a significant role in maintaining adequate amounts of these clotting factors, because it is the primary site of protein synthesis. Tissue thromboplastin, or tissue factor (III), is an exception that can be found in most body tissues, especially around vessels and organs.

Table 5-2 • BLOOD COAGULATION FACTORS

Factor Number	Name(s)
I	Fibrinogen
II	Prothrombin
V	Proaccelerin, labile factor, or accelerator globulin
VII	Proconvertin, serum prothrombin conversion accelerator (SPCA), or stable factor
VIII	Antihemophilic factor (AHF), antihemophilic factor A, or antihemophilic globulin (AHG)
IX	Christmas factor, plasma thromboplastin component (PTC), or antihemophilic factor B
X	Stuart-Prower factor, or thrombokinase
XI	Plasma thromboplastin antecedent (PTA) or antihemophilic factor C
XII	Hageman factor, glass factor, contact factor, or antihemophilic factor D
XIII	Fibrin-stabilizing factor

Adapted from Tortora G, Grabowski S. *Principles of Anatomy and Physiology*. New York: John Wiley & Sons, Inc.; 2003.

Antihemophilic factor (VIII) is a factor that is synthesized in the endothelial cells. It is also important to recognize that there are multiple enzymes and mediators that play key roles in the activation of these clotting factors. Synthesis of factors II, VII, IX, and X requires vitamin K to be present, and these are known as vitamin K–dependent factors. Calcium is also a coagulation factor whose role can be underestimated. To balance the coagulation process, there are also several proteins and systems that will inhibit coagulation including antithrombin III, proteins C and S, as well as components of the fibrinolytic cascade. The interaction of all these proteins in a chemical sequence will produce a clot to repair blood vessels and then dissolve the clot so that normal flow can be restored.

HEMOSTASIS

The normal hemostatic system is designed to protect against bleeding from injured blood vessels. Hemostasis is usually accomplished by a sequence of interrelated processes involving blood vessels and endothelial activity, platelets, and coagulation proteins. This complex system is highly regulated to ensure that clotting occurs only at a site of injury and only as long as the integrity of the vessel is compromised. The process of hemostasis consists of several components: (1) blood vessel spasm; (2) formation of a platelet plug; (3) contact between damaged blood vessel, blood platelet, and coagulation proteins; (4) development of a blood clot around the injury; and (5) fibrinolytic removal of excess hemostatic material to reestablish vascular integrity.[5] Coagulation proteins make up the coagulation cascade. The coagulation cascade consists of three components: the intrinsic pathway (vascular trauma), the extrinsic pathway (tissue trauma), and the common pathway leading to fibrin formation. The clotting processes are balanced by the complex mechanism of fibrinolysis, which breaks down clots and maintains or reestablishes blood flow once the vessel damage has healed. The balance between these two mechanisms and their activators and inhibitors is vital. An imbalance in one direction leads to excessive bleeding, whereas an imbalance in the other direction leads to excessive clotting. The following sections present the normal sequence of coagulation and fibrinolysis, as well as selected coagulation disorders most commonly associated with the patient experiencing cardiovascular disease.

Vascular Spasm

The sympathetic nervous system is automatically stimulated when a blood vessel is injured. Epinephrine and norepinephrine are released causing contraction of the vascular smooth muscle and vasoconstriction. Endothelin 1, which is a peptide produced by the endothelial cell, angiotensin II, and vasoconstrictor prostaglandins are additional agents that contribute to vasoconstriction.[5] The vasoconstriction of arterioles may be sufficient to decrease blood flow and close disrupted capillaries. Larger vessels may require longer periods of more intense vasoconstriction to assist with hemostasis but may ultimately require surgical intervention.

Role of the Endothelium in Hemostasis

The endothelial cell was once thought to be inert and have no specific role in maintaining vascular integrity. Research over the years has proven this hypothesis to be incorrect. The endothelial cell is a vital component of normal homeostasis. Under normal conditions, the endothelium surface is intact and there is minimal interaction with platelets or the coagulation proteins. The function of the endothelium is to promote blood flow. The endothelial cell inhibits blood coagulation by: (1) expressing thrombomodulin, a clotting enzyme that binds thrombin; (2) changing the specificity of thrombomodulin from fibrin to protein C, which blocks the ability to convert fibrinogen to fibrin; (3) using proteoglycans on their surfaces to bind and potentiate the coagulation inhibitors antithrombin III and tissue factor pathway inhibitor; (4) releasing small amounts of plasminogen activator tissue-type plasminogen activator (tPA); (5) inhibiting platelet aggregation by producing prostacyclin and nitric oxide, which vasodilate the microcirculation; and (6) inhibiting adherence of peripheral blood cells.[6] These interactions maintain the anticoagulant properties of the endothelium by keeping platelets inactive and inhibiting key coagulation proteins such as tissue factor and thrombin.

Once the endothelial surface is disrupted by various factors, including physical injury or circulating mediators, it will develop procoagulant properties. When the endothelium is stimulated by inflammatory cytokines such as IL-α, IL-β, or tumor necrosis factor-α, it is referred to as activated endothelium. Once the subendothelial connective tissue is exposed and activated, it will lose thrombomodulin and heparin sulfate and begin to synthesize tissue factor (factor III). Factor III interacts with factor VII to start the extrinsic pathway. Therefore, protein C is not activated, and the action of clotting inhibitor systems will be lost. This activation of the cascade will further incite the endothelial cell to produce more inflammatory mediators (cytokines and chemokines) that will start the expression of adhesion molecules. Leukocytes will adhere to the endothelial cell and become activated by the production of leukocyte agonists such as platelet-activating factor.[6] Platelets are now attracted to the site and augment the coagulation process.

Platelet Phase

The platelet phase refers to the formation of a soft mass of aggregated platelets that provides a temporary patch over the injured vessel. Almost immediately after vascular injury, platelets begin to adhere to the exposed subendothelial basement membrane and collagen fibers. Adherent platelets release adenosine diphosphate, which causes platelets to change from their normal disc shape into a spherical form with pseudopods that attach along the surface and allow platelets to clump together.[5] During activation, the platelets become sticky when bridges formed by fibrinogen in the presence of calcium cause platelets to adhere to each other, increasing the size of the platelet plug. Adenosine diphosphate and collagen also trigger formation of arachidonic acid from phospholipids in the platelet membrane. Arachidonic acid leads to the formation of thromboxane A_2, a substance that induces further platelet aggregation. Thromboxane A_2 causes conformational changes in glycoprotein IIb/IIIa, a receptor on the platelet surface, which exposes fibrinogen-binding sites. Fibrinogen builds bridges to adjacent platelets, a process called platelet adhesion, which advances platelet aggregation. When these aggregates are reinforced with fibrin, they are referred to as a thrombus.[5] Ultimately, aggregated platelets plug the injured vessel.

Coagulation Cascade

The final phase of hemostasis is the formation of a fibrin blood clot. The coagulation process is most commonly viewed as a series of enzymatic reactions in which clotting factors are sequentially activated. This process is known as the coagulation cascade. The clotting factors are all present in the circulating blood in their inactive form until a stimulus for clot formation occurs. Twelve different substances have been officially designated as clotting factors (see Table 5-2). As studied in the laboratory, the coagulation process can be initiated by two different pathways: the extrinsic pathway and the intrinsic pathway. Although differentiating between them is helpful for understanding pathologic mechanisms, medication actions, and coagulation tests, these two pathways are functionally inseparable in vivo. The extrinsic pathway, whose major mediators are rapidly inactivated, is the primary initiator of the clotting cascade. The intrinsic pathway, whose major mediators are more slowly degraded, is thought to be important for maintenance and amplification of the clotting cascade. Both extrinsic and intrinsic mechanisms eventually lead to the activation of factor X, with the remaining steps of the coagulation sequence being identical and referred to as the common pathway. The sequence of the coagulation process is shown in Figure 5-2.[4]

Extrinsic Pathway

The extrinsic pathway is initiated by the combination of tissue factor with factor VIIa and ionized calcium, which together convert factor X to its activated form, factor Xa. The function of the extrinsic pathway is tested in the laboratory by the prothrombin time (PT). Tissue factor, also called tissue thromboplastin (formerly factor III), is a membrane glycoprotein that is particularly prevalent in tissues, where it plays a vital role in the prevention of hemorrhage. Tissue factor is exposed to and binds to factor VII, which is activated to factor VIIa. Factor VIIa is a potent enzyme that activates factor X to Xa. The reactions from this step on are referred to as the common pathway. Calcium plays a significant role in each step leading to the formation of thrombin.[5]

Intrinsic Pathway

Because the intrinsic pathway is initiated by a separate set of factors that is not degraded by rapid-acting inhibitors, the process may proceed more slowly, and the results may last longer and be more pronounced than those initiated by the extrinsic pathway.

The function of the intrinsic pathway is commonly analyzed by the partial thromboplastin time (PTT). Intrinsic activation is initiated when blood is exposed to a negatively charged surface, such as the site of blood vessel injury. The negative charge, along with collagen and endotoxin, attracts factor XII, which binds to the surface and autoactivates to factor XIIa. Factor XIIa converts prekallikrein to kallikrein, which in turn converts circulating factor XII to its activated form, XIIa. Both the activated form of factor XII and kallikrein catalyze the activation of factor XI into XIa. Factor XIa, together with ionized calcium, cleaves factor IX at two sites to produce factor IXa. Factor IXa, together with factor VIII, phospholipid, and ionized calcium, converts factor X to its activated form, factor Xa. As discussed previously, factor X can also be activated through the extrinsic pathway. From here, the coagulation process proceeds along the common pathway, regardless of whether initiation was extrinsic or intrinsic.[5]

Common Pathway and Fibrin Formation

The final common sequence involves the combination of factors Xa and V, phospholipid, and ionized calcium into a complex that

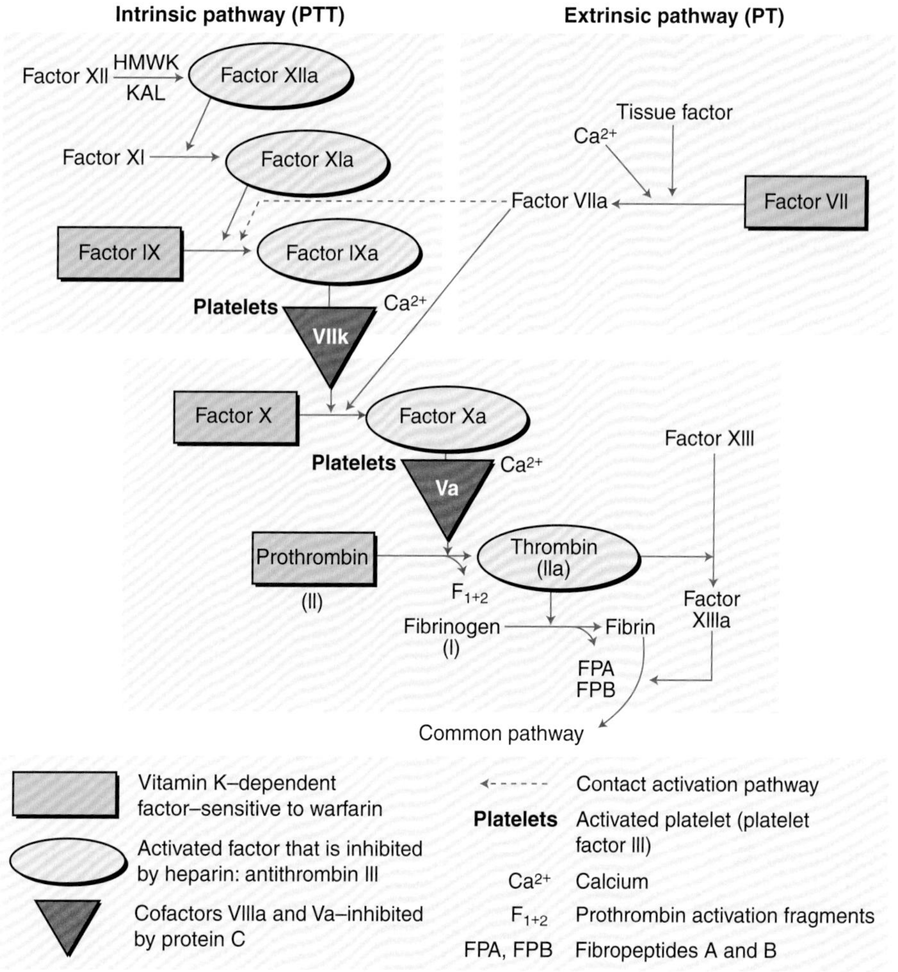

Figure 5-2. The intrinsic, extrinsic, and common coagulation pathways. Lower case "a" denotes an activated factor. The protime (PT) measures the function of the extrinsic and common pathways; the partial thromboplastin time (PTT or aPTT) measures the activity of the intrinsic and common pathways. HMWK, high–molecular-weight kininogen; KAL, kallikrein. (Reproduced with permission from Dipiro JT, Talbert RL, Yee GC, et al. *Pharmacotherapy: A Pathophysiologic Approach*. 6th ed. New York: McGraw-Hill; 2006.)

converts prothrombin to thrombin. The thrombin formed subsequently cleaves the long molecule fibrinogen to fibrin. The fibrin monomer is able to polymerize spontaneously to form a loose web of fibers that is capable of stopping the bleeding in small- and medium-sized arteries and veins. The fibrin clot is eventually stabilized and thickened by the action of factor XIII, which is activated by the presence of ionized calcium and thrombin. Fibrin forms a loose covering over the injured area and reinforces the platelet plug. After a short period of time, the clot begins to retract. This process is thought to be a reaction of the platelets, which send out cytoplasmic processes that attach to the fibrin and pull the fibers closer. Plasminogen and other components of the fibrinolytic mechanism are incorporated into the fibrin clot as it solidifies.

Fibrinolysis

The removal of clots when the site of vessel injury has healed is as important as the formation of the clot itself. Fibrinolysis is the physiologic process that removes insoluble fibrin deposits by enzymatic digestion of the stabilized fibrin polymers.[5] The process of fibrinolysis reestablishes blood flow. Plasmin dissolves clots by digesting fibrin and fibrinogen using hydrolysis. Plasminogen is a glycoprotein and an inactive form of plasmin, which is synthesized by the liver. It is activated to plasmin by the activity of proteolytic enzymes, the kinases that cleave a bond on the plasminogen molecule. Activators of plasminogen are found in various tissues, blood, and urine. The best-known endogenous activators are tPA and urokinase, which is a urinary activator of plasminogen. Some exogenous plasminogen activators are related to types of bacteria such as streptokinase and staphylokinase.[5] Drugs have been developed to mimic the activity of these kinases to dissolve clots. Fragments of the fibrin clot, known as fibrin degradation products (FDPs), are released into the circulation as the clot is broken down. FDPs are potent inhibitors of coagulation. They act by binding to thrombin, thus inhibiting its action, and by interfering with the binding of fibrin threads to form the fibrin clot. Except in some abnormal situations, FDPs are present in such small numbers that their anticoagulant effect is not clinically important. Plasminogen is then converted back to plasmin and neutralized by a number of antiplasmin and inhibitor systems. All these reactions that occur in the coagulation cascade and fibrinolytic system are time dependent and can be monitored using laboratory testing as listed in Table 5-3.[7–9]

Natural Anticoagulant Systems

Coagulation is regulated by three major mechanisms: the elimination of activated clotting factors, the protease inhibitors (inhibitors of coagulation), and the destruction of the fibrin clot. There must be a balance between coagulation and anticoagulation processes in the body to maintain homeostasis. The natural anticoagulant

Table 5-3 • COAGULATION LABORATORY TESTS

Test	Normal Value	Coagulation Correlation	Clinical Significance
Activated partial thromboplastin time (aPTT)	<35 seconds	Generation of thrombin and fibrin via intrinsic and common pathways	**Increased** with heparin or thrombin inhibitor therapy
Prothrombin time (PT)	10–13 seconds	Generation of thrombin and fibrin via extrinsic and common pathways	**Increased** with liver disease, extrinsic factor deficiencies, or oral anticoagulants
International normalized ratio (INR)	Therapy goal dependent	Standardized values used to correct for different thromboplastin reagents used in PT calculations	
Thrombin time (TT)	<20 seconds	Rate of thrombin-induced cleavage of fibrinogen to fibrin	**Increased** with low fibrinogen levels, DIC, liver disease, increased FDP
Anti-Xa assay	Therapy goal dependent	Indirectly measures the amount of heparin by measuring its inhibition of factor Xa activity;	**Increased** with unfractionated heparin, low–molecular-weight heparins May be useful in patients with heparin resistance
Fibrinogen	200–400 mg/dL	Deficiencies in fibrinogen and alterations in conversion of fibrinogen to fibrin	**Increased** with inflammatory response or tissue damage **Decreased** with liver disease or consumption of fibrinogen with intravascular clotting
Fibrin degradation products (FDPs)	8–10 μg/mL	Generation of fibrin fragments upon degeneration	**Increased** in fibrinolysis, DIC
Platelet count	150,000–400,000/mm^3	Amount of circulating platelets; does not reflect functional ability	**Increased** in myeloproliferative disorders, inflammation, postsplenectomy **Decreased** in consumptive states, DIC, drug reactions, platelet disorders
Bleeding time (BT)	2–9 minutes, depending on reagent	Determines platelet adhesion and aggregation	**Increased** with platelet abnormalities, aspirin, severe liver disease
Protein C	4–5 μg/mL	Determines activity of natural anticoagulation systems	**Increased** in inflammation **Decreased** in consumptive disorders
D-dimer assay	<400 ng/mL	Determines the level of endogenous thrombolysis; plasmin activity on fibrin	**Increased** with excessive endogenous thrombolysis
Activated clotting time (ACT)	46–70 seconds or 1.5–2.5 times control	Alternative test that can be performed at the bedside to determine heparin's anticoagulation level	**Increased** with heparin therapy **Decreased** with protamine administration
Functional platelet assessment Thromboelastography (TEG)[a]	Graph analysis; maximum amplitude (MA) normal 55–73 mm	Monitors the dynamic process of hemostasis; can determine the number and functional capacity of platelets	Maximum amplitude or width of graph estimates the number of platelets and their functioning capacity
Heparin-induced thrombocytopenia PF4 antibody		Detects and measures antibodies produced by some during or after heparin therapy	

[a]Sorensen E, Lorme T, Heath D. Thromboelastography: a means to transfusion reduction. *Nursing Management.* 2005;36:27–34.
Modified from Kinney M, Brooks-Brunn J, Molter N, et al. *AACN Clinical Reference for Critical Care Nursing.* St. Louis, MO: C.V. Mosby; 1998; Munro N. Hematopoiesis, coagulation, and bleeding. In: Wood SL, Sivarajan Froelicher ES, Motzer SU, et al., eds. *Cardiac Nursing.* 6th ed. Baltimore, MD: Wolters Kluwer Health/ Lippincott Williams & Wilkins; 2010; and Smythe MA, Priziola J, Dobesh PP, et al. Guidance for the practical management of the heparin anticoagulants in the treatment of venous thromboembolism. *J Thromb Thrombolysis.* 2016;41(1):165–186.

systems include antithrombin III, heparin cofactor II, and protein C and its cofactor, protein S.

Antithrombin III is an α2-globulin glycoprotein, which is considered the major inhibitor of coagulation. It slowly inactivates thrombin as well as factors Xa, IXa, XIa, and XIIa. In the presence of heparin, antithrombin III–thrombin binding is increased significantly. This is thought to be the main mechanism for heparin's anticoagulation ability and its interaction with antithrombin III and tissue factor pathway inhibitor.

Heparin cofactor II is a heparin-dependent thrombin inhibitor whose activity is also accelerated by the presence of heparin. This cofactor not only inhibits thrombin but also thrombin-induced platelet aggregation and release.[5]

Protein C and protein S are major natural anticoagulants in the body and have a powerful role in anticoagulation. Deficiency in either of these proteins can lead to the development of thrombus. Protein C is a vitamin K–dependent protein, which is synthesized in the liver and circulates as a zymogen, an inactive precursor form in the blood. Activation occurs faster when thrombin, in the presence of thrombomodulin, assists with proteolytic cleavage that converts protein C to its active enzymatic form, activated protein C (APC). Protein S must also be present to help APC proteolytically cleave factors Va and VIIIa, which will decrease the conversion of prothrombin to thrombin, and act as a regulatory feedback loop to balance coagulation. The dual role of thrombin in both coagulation and anticoagulation is exemplified here. Protein C also has a function in promoting fibrinolysis by neutralizing the inhibitors of tPA, which allows the conversion of plasminogen to plasmin. Inactivation of APC is a slower process with a plasma protease inhibitor that has a short half-life intimating the other unidentified direct cell mechanisms.[5] The properties of protein C have been applied clinically with the development of the medication, drotrecogin alfa.

Drotrecogin alfa was a recombinant human form of APC (rhAPC), which was used in severely ill patients with sepsis to decrease microemboli formation and inhibit immune function and was part of the Surviving Sepsis Guidelines in 2008.[10] APC has a major role as an agent that suppresses inflammation and prevents microvascular coagulation. Initial studies had shown the efficacy and safety of APC for severe sepsis.[10,11] However, the PROWESS SHOCK study investigators reported recombinant human APC (rhAPC) did not reduce mortality in patients with septic shock.[9] The medication was withdrawn from the market. Therefore, there was no recommendation about rhAPC in the Surviving Sepsis Guidelines in 2012 and more recently, 2016.[10,12]

COAGULATION-INFLAMMATION LINK

The role of the inflammatory process has become a major focus of study in many areas of medicine, especially inflammation's role in the atherosclerotic process. The study of the relationship between coagulation and inflammation is focused on the integrity of the endothelium and the recruitment of leukocytes.[13] Normally, the endothelium does not encourage the binding of WBCs to the wall.

However, with elevated levels of low-density lipoproteins, the excess low-density lipoprotein molecules will begin to infiltrate the endothelial wall and experience oxidation and glycation.[14] These chemical changes will cause the endothelial cell to express an adhesion molecule, vascular cell adhesion molecule I, which will bind various types of leukocytes, especially monocytes and T lymphocytes. This process occurs especially at arterial branch points where the endothelial cells are exposed to abnormal laminar flow. This abnormal laminar flow decreases the endothelial cell's protective ability to secrete nitric oxide and to limit the expression of vascular cell adhesion molecule I.[13]

Once the monocyte is attached to the endothelial wall, it releases monocyte chemoattractant protein-1, which will help the migration of the monocyte into the intima. With the assistance of macrophage colony-stimulating factor, the monocyte starts to ingest the excess lipids and transform itself into a macrophage foam cell. The macrophage foam cells are the trigger for activating the coagulation system. They release proteolytic enzymes that degrade the collagen fibers that compose the fibrous cap, so that it weakens and can rupture. The macrophage foam cell also produces tissue factor (factor III) and once the plaque cap ruptures and exposes the tissue factor to the circulating blood, coagulation will ensue.[13] The T cells also release cytokines such as tumor necrosis factor-β, which stimulates the macrophages, endothelial cells, and the smooth muscles. Peptide growth factors are released that promote the replication of smooth muscle cells into an extracellular matrix, which is characteristic of an atherosclerotic lesion.[13]

However, this link between coagulation and inflammation may not only be limited to the atherosclerosis process. Hypertension may also be linked to inflammation because angiotensin II not only may be a vasoconstrictor but also may cause intimal inflammation by stimulating the smooth muscle and endothelial cells to express proinflammatory cytokines such as IL-6 and monocyte chemoattractant protein-1.[13] Hyperglycemia associated with diabetes can lead to the formation of advance glycation end products that may augment the secretion of proinflammatory cytokines.[13] Even chronic extravascular infections such as gingivitis, prostatitis, bronchitis, etc., can augment extravascular production of inflammatory cytokines, which can accelerate the evolution of atherosclerotic lesions.[13] This new scientific insight into the role of inflammation in the development of atherosclerosis has led to using new markers to determine the degree of inflammation. Findings of a relationship between increased C-reactive protein levels and unfavorable cardiovascular outcomes have led to new therapeutic considerations for acute coronary syndrome.[13]

BLEEDING DISORDERS

Bleeding can occur when the intricate relationship between the various elements of the hemostatic system is disturbed. Bleeding defects in the hemostatic system can be categorized into three areas: vascular issues, platelet dysfunction, or coagulation dysfunction. Vascular issues generally cause endothelial damage by an autoimmune process (allergy-induced), endotoxins from infections, or abnormal vascular structure. Platelet dysfunction can present as thrombocytopenia (low platelet count) or thrombocytosis (high platelet count). Thrombocytopenia can result from decreased production, decreased distribution, or increased destruction of platelets. Thrombocytosis can result from either a primary or a secondary cause.

Coagulation dysfunction can be either congenital or acquired deficiencies in the coagulation factors (Display 5-1). In each case, bleeding is the primary manifestation. The bleeding may be minor, such as petechiae and easy bruising of the skin, or major, with massive hemorrhage.

The focus of cardiac interventions today emphasizes maintaining blood flow with percutaneous interventions (vascular injury) and anticoagulation to prevent thrombus formation. This intentional disruption of the coagulation system can potentially lead to bleeding disorders or even shock with excessive blood loss from percutaneous interventions and/or thrombolysis. Shock can lead to hypoperfusion and decreased oxygen delivery, which can trigger the intrinsic and extrinsic pathways simultaneously. DIC is a complication of shock. Although DIC is actually a disorder of coagulation, it is discussed as a bleeding disorder because its major manifestation is bleeding.

DISSEMINATED INTRAVASCULAR COAGULATION

DIC is a pathologic syndrome resulting in the indiscriminate formation of fibrin clots throughout all or most of the microvasculature. Paradoxically, diffuse bleeding occurs as a result of the consumption of clotting factors and is usually the hallmark sign of the syndrome. It is a disorder in which the coagulation cascade has been "pathologically activated" either by the extrinsic pathway releasing tissue factor or by the intrinsic pathway with endothelial injury.[1] It is considered a complication of many different diseases and is known as a consumptive coagulopathy or defibrination syndrome.[5] Successful treatment of DIC must include treatment of the primary cause of the disorder as well as the hematologic consequences (see Table 5-4 for clinical conditions associated with DIC).[15–17]

Etiology

Inappropriate coagulation results from the presence of thromboplastic substances in the bloodstream. These thromboplastic

DISPLAY 5-1

Conceptual Etiology of Bleeding Disorders

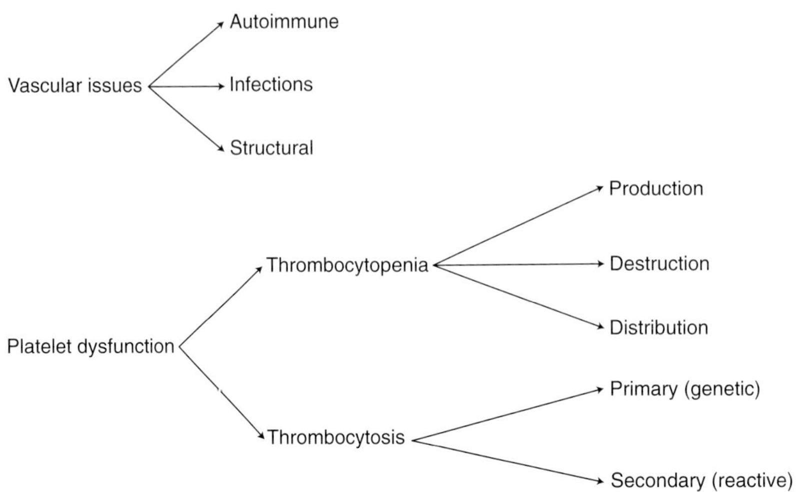

Table 5-4 • CONDITIONS ASSOCIATED WITH DISSEMINATED INTRAVASCULAR COAGULATION

Clinical Condition	Causes of DIC
Obstetrical	• Placental abruption • Placenta previa • Amniotic fluid embolism • Intrauterine death • Preeclampsia/eclampsia • HELLP syndrome
Malignancy	• Solid tumors • Hematologic malignancies (Leukemia)
Trauma	• Multitrauma • Head injury • Burns • Fat embolism • Surgery • Heat stroke of shock • Massive transfusion
Toxic and Immunologic Reactions	• Graft-versus-host disease • Transplant rejection • Severe transfusion reactions • Snake bites
Organ Destruction	• Pancreatitis, severe inflammation, tissue necrosis
Sepsis and Severe Infections	• Potentially any microorganism (gram-negative or gram-positive) • Viral infections • Malaria • Rickettsia infection
Vascular Abnormalities	• Aortic aneurysm (large) • Giant hemangiomas • Vasculitis • Other vascular malformations
Liver Disease	• Cirrhosis • Acute hepatic necrosis
Postcardiopulmonary resuscitation	

HELLP, hemolysis elevated liver enzyme levels and low platelet count; ARDS, acute respiratory distress syndrome.
Adapted from Levi M, Scully M. How I treat disseminated intravascular coagulation. *Blood.* 2018;131(8):845–854; Levi M, Toh CH, Thachil J, et al. Guidelines for the diagnosis and management of disseminated intravascular coagulation. British Committee for Standards in Haematology. *Br J Haematol.* 2009;145(1):24–33; and Papageorgiou C, Jourdi G, Adjambri E, et al. Disseminated intravascular coagulation: an update on pathogenesis, diagnosis, and therapeutic strategies. *Clin Appl Thromb Hemost.* 2018;8S–28S.

substances stimulate clotting despite the lack of actual bleeding. Tissue thromboplastin (tissue factor) is released into the circulation by damaged cells in massive burns, injuries, and systemic infections. DIC is a common complication of serious infections, especially gram-negative sepsis. The fetus, placenta, and amniotic fluid contain thromboplastic substances that are released into the maternal circulation during obstetric complications such as abruptio placentae and amniotic fluid embolism. Certain malignant tumors release small amounts of thromboplastic substances into the circulation. Chemotherapy or radiation treatment can cause tumor cells to die and release massive amounts of thromboplastin into the circulation.[18] In the patient with cardiovascular disease, DIC is most likely to develop as a result of cardiogenic, septic, or hemorrhagic shock; acidosis; or extracorporeal circulation, which can all lead to cellular death and thromboplastin release. Figure 5-3 provides a conceptual model of the cause of DIC.[8]

Pathophysiology

The two major consequences of DIC are bleeding and organ ischemia (Fig. 5-3). Endothelial damage and/or tissue damage initiate the pathways and activation of the coagulation factors that lead to the formation of thrombin. Thrombin influences the coagulation system by (1) cleaving fibrinogen to fibrin, (2) activating factor XIII, (3) stimulating platelets resulting in decreased circulating numbers, and activating protein C.[5] Widespread intravascular clotting resulting in the deposition of fibrin in the microcirculation leads to ischemia in organs such as the kidney, lungs, brain, skin, and gastrointestinal system. RBCs are damaged as they pass through the fibrin strands. These damaged RBC are called schistocytes. As the disseminated clotting continues, circulating platelets and clotting factors are consumed and bleeding ensues. Fibrinolysis is activated as a result of the widespread fibrin deposition, converting plasminogen to plasmin, which destroys fibrin and fibrinogen, yielding abnormally large amounts of circulating FDP.[5] In these large numbers, FDPs aggravate bleeding because they (1) inhibit platelet aggregation by coating receptor sites, (2) act as anticoagulants by competing with thrombin, and (3) impair fibrin polymerization.[5] Consumption of the factors is so rapid that repletion cannot be maintained.

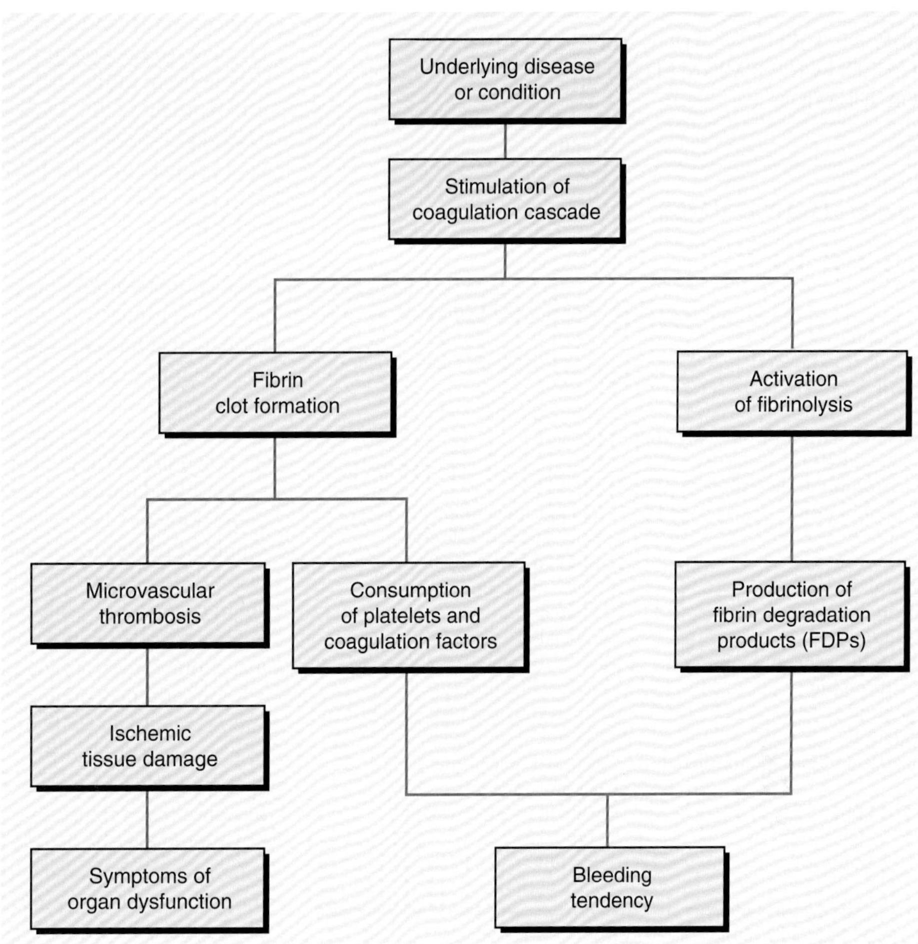

Figure 5-3. Pathophysiology of disseminated intravascular coagulation. (From Kinney M, Dunbar S, Brooks-Brun J, et al. *AACN's Clinical Reference for Critical Care Nursing.* St. Louis, MO: C.V. Mosby; 1998.)

Clinical Manifestations

DIC can occur in a chronic or acute form. The chronic form is subtler and easily goes unrecognized. The body may be exposed to smaller amounts of thrombin over a more extended period. The acute form tends to be more severe and sudden in onset. The astute clinician should have a high index of suspicion when patients experience any of the aforementioned conditions, observing for subtle signs of DIC. All organ systems are susceptible to the intravascular clotting that can occur.

Classically, skin disruptions such as petechiae, purpura, and ecchymosis are very common. Continual bleeding and/or oozing from any skin disruption such as venipunctures or vascular access sites are another familiar sign. Neurologic signs and symptoms can range from decreased level of consciousness and restlessness to seizures or coma. Respiratory dysfunction can be manifested by increased work of breathing with long expiratory times, use of accessory muscles, tachypnea, and adventitious breath sounds. Cardiac decompensation can encompass changes in rhythm and blood pressure as the sympathetic nervous system attempts compensation. The clinical presentation can range from hypertension to hypoperfusion. Hemodynamic indices may be decreased with hypovolemia or pulmonary artery pressures may be increased in the presence of a PE. Hypovolemic shock may result if blood loss is severe. Potential spaces for bleeding, especially the retroperitoneal space and thighs, need to be closely observed when femoral vascular access devices are in place or are removed. Acute abdominal signs such as distention, tenderness, pain, and decreased or absent bowel sounds may indicate major gastrointestinal dysfunction. Urine output may be decreased and signs of renal failure, such as an increase in creatinine, may occur. It is important to remember that the primary disorder that led to DIC must also be treated to correct DIC.

Medical Management

The diagnosis of DIC should be suspected whenever abnormal bleeding occurs in association with any of the primary disorders described previously. Multiple coagulation test abnormalities are found in DIC. These include prolonged PT, PTT, and thrombin time; decreased fibrinogen and platelet counts; and decreased levels of factors II, V, VIII, and X indicate the consumption of clotting factors. The elevation of FDP and the D-dimer levels confirm fibrinolysis. Table 5-5 includes an extensive list of coagulation tests and the expected results in DIC.[19] D-dimer levels indicate the level of activity of plasmin on fibrin, that is, thrombolysis. Schistocytes may also be present.[20] The presence of clotting and fibrinolysis with a suspicious clinical presentation can assist the practitioner in making the diagnosis of DIC. The prognosis of DIC varies markedly depending on the underlying cause and the amount of intravascular clotting. DIC may cease spontaneously, it may respond to prompt and aggressive treatment or it may lead to organ ischemia, bleeding, and potentially death. DIC always occurs as the result of some other underlying abnormality, and thus the treatment of DIC is directed toward improvement of the underlying disorder. For example, infection requires the use

Table 5-5 • COAGULATION-RELATED LABORATORY RESULTS IN DISSEMINATED INTRAVASCULAR COAGULATION[a]

Test	Results
Platelet count	Decreased—consumed
Activated partial thromboplastin time	Prolonged
Prothrombin time	Prolonged
Thrombin time	Prolonged—due to low fibrinogen and elevated D-dimer
Fibrinogen	Decreased—consumed
Coagulation factors	Decreased—consumed
Fibrin degradation products	Increased
Platelet count	Decreased (consumed)
Activated partial thromboplastin time (aPTT)	Prolonged
Prothrombin time (PT)	Prolonged
Thrombin time	Prolonged (due to low fibrinogen and elevated D-dimer)
Fibrinogen	Decreased (consumed)
Coagulation factors	Decreased (consumed)
Fibrin degradation products	Increased
D-dimer	Increased
Thrombin generation markers	Increased
Antithrombin	Decreased (consumed)
Protein C	Decreased (consumed)
Protein S	Decreased (consumed)
Thrombomodulin, endothelial	Decreased by neutrophil elastase + proinflammatory cytokines
tPA trauma	Early DIC—increased; late DIC—decreased
PAI-1 trauma	Early DIC—low levels; late DIC—elevated

[a]Typically, the only coagulation laboratory tests routinely performed to evaluate for DIC are platelet count, prothrombin time, activated partial thromboplastin time, fibrinogen, and D-dimer.
DIC, disseminated intravascular coagulation; PAI-1, plasminogen activator inhibitor 1; tPA, tissue plasminogen activator.
Adapted from Boral BM, Williams DJ, Boral LI. Disseminated intravascular coagulation. *Am J Clin Pathol.* 2016;146(6):670–680.

of antibiotics. General supportive measures such as fluid and blood replacement, mechanical ventilation, and vasoactive drugs to maintain tissue perfusion are essential.[21] Transfusions of platelets, fresh frozen plasma, RBC, and cryoprecipitate will be needed to attempt to replace consumed coagulation factors. The use of heparin, a potent anticoagulant that inactivates the intravascular clotting and thus inhibits consumption of the coagulation factors, is very controversial and probably inappropriate in the face of active bleeding.[21]

Nursing Interventions

Perceptive nursing skill can be the pivotal factor in the patient with DIC. Early recognition of the subtle signs could avert further decompensation. If the patient displays any sign of restlessness or agitation, physiologic factors such as hypoxemia should be the first consideration. Monitoring oxygenation using pulse oximetry will give some estimate of oxygenation that can be confirmed with an arterial blood gas (ABG). If gas exchange is adequate and restlessness and agitation persist, neurologic causes must be considered, and sedation should be avoided unless indicated. The patient's heart rate, rhythm, and blood pressure should be continually monitored for any changes. If manual or noninvasive blood pressure monitoring is being used, rotation of the cuff should be implemented because ecchymotic areas under the cuff can develop. Hemodynamic monitoring may be used and variations in indices may indicate cardiac failure, hypovolemia, or pulmonary complications such as PE. Monitoring urine output for at least 0.5 to 1 mL/kg/h should be routine practice. Removal of large catheters used for percutaneous interventions should always be performed with care. Achieving and maintaining hemostasis is dependent on technique. Manual pressure should be applied slightly above the insertion site of the vessel and minimal padding should be used to control bleeding. This technique will allow visualization of the site for continual monitoring and lessen the chance of hematoma formation. Once adequate hemostasis is achieved, other devices can be applied to assure adequate clot formation at the puncture site. Proper technique in hemostasis control is especially important for patients with a coagulopathy.

If hemorrhage is present, the priority should be volume resuscitation. Blood products should be replaced depending on estimated blood loss and laboratory values. Aggressive fluid resuscitation should be performed through short, large-bore venous access using pressure bags if the patient is hypotensive to assure fast intravascular volume repletion. While infusing blood products, the nurse should observe for allergic reactions (see Table 5-5). Continual bleeding may require massive blood product replacement, which can cause a "washout" effect of most of the functioning coagulation proteins, and paradoxically cause further coagulopathy. It is also important to keep accurate records as to the number of various blood products received. RBC loss needs to be replaced, but it is important to realize that a transfusion is not a benign intervention. Critically ill patients may be at risk for immunosuppressive and microcirculatory complications with red cell transfusions.[22] A restrictive transfusion strategy (transfuse for a hemoglobin less than 7.0 g/dL) has been shown to be as effective as a liberal strategy (transfuse for a hemoglobin less than 10 g/dL) with a decrease in mortality.[22] The only two groups of patients that may require the more liberal transfusion strategy are patients with an acute myocardial infarction or unstable angina.[22] In cases of massive bleeding that is not responsive to the usual interventions as described above, recombinant factor VIIa has been used as an additional intervention. Originally used for treatment of hemophilia, off-label use of factor VIIa has increased markedly over the last 10 years. Recombinant factor VIIa binds to the surface of activated platelets and promotes thrombin formation, thereby enhancing clot formation.[1] Dosing of this drug for off-label use varies greatly depending on the setting (surgery, trauma, hemorrhagic stroke, reversal of oral coagulation therapy, or impaired hepatic function).[23] Caution should be used when using factor VIIa due to the risk of thromboembolic adverse events.[23,24] Table 5-6 highlights pharmacologic therapy used to promote coagulation.[25] Observation for bleeding should include monitoring of all vascular accesses as well as the area around the site. Vigilant surveys by the nurse of the skin surface and digits are necessary to observe for petechiae, ecchymosis, and other skin disruptions that may provide early warning signs of impending DIC (see Table 5-3).

CLOTTING DISORDERS

Excessive or inappropriate coagulation is also of great clinical significance.

Venous thrombosis involves the interacting conditions of stasis, vascular damage, and hypercoagulability. The most common life-threatening complication, PE, is a major cause of mortality in

Table 5-6 • BLOOD PRODUCTS USED IN BLEEDING DISORDERS

Product	Standard Volume	Administration	Clinical Response	Factor Replaced
Platelets (from whole blood)	50–70/RD unit pool of 4–6 RD unit	Rapid administration increases possible allergic reaction	Increase platelet count 5,000–10,000/µL/RD unit	
Platelets (from apheresis)	200–400	Rapid administration possible allergic reaction	For pooled RD and SDAP: CCI ≥10× 10^9/L within 1 hour and ≥7.5 × 10^9 within 24 hours posttransfusion	
Packed red blood cells (PRBCs)	250–300	Rapid administration; blood type mismatch	Increase hemoglobin 10 g/L and hematocrit 3%	
Fresh frozen plasma (FFP)	200–250	Rapid administration increases possible allergic reaction	Increases coagulation factors about 2%	II, V, VII, IX, X, XI, XII
Cryoprecipitate	10–15/unit, pool of 4–5 units	Rapid administration increases possible allergic reaction	Increase plasma fibrinogen 5–10 mg/dL, increase factor VIII	I

RD, random donor; SDAP, single-donor apheresis platelets; CCI, corrected count increment.
Modified from Dzieczkowski JS, Tiberghien P, Anderson KC. Transfusion biology and therapy. In: Jameson J, Fauci AS, Kasper DL, et al., eds. *Harrison's Principles of Internal Medicine*. 20th ed. 2018. New York: McGraw-Hill; Sharma S, Sharma P, Tyler LN. Transfusion of blood and blood products: indications and complications. *Am Fam Physician*. 2011;83(6):719–724.

hospitalized patients. Recognition of patients likely to have any of these conditions is a nursing responsibility.

Clot Formation

A thrombus is a clot or solid mass formed by blood components. Thrombosis refers to the formation or presence of blood clots in a vessel. A thrombus that breaks loose and travels in the blood vessel is termed an embolus, hence the term thromboembolism. The potential outcome from either thrombosis or embolism is ischemia, leading to infarction with cellular and tissue necrosis. A thrombus develops when the normal process of hemostasis is inappropriately activated. Three factors (vessel injury, venous stasis, and hypercoagulability) can predispose a patient to thrombosis. These three factors are commonly known as Virchow triad (Fig. 5-4).[26,27]

First, the vessel involved must have suffered some type of injury, particularly damage to the endothelial layer. Vessel injury may be the result of sustained pressure on the vessel or surrounding tissue, as might occur from prolonged immobility of an extremity or pressure points caused by crossed legs, elastic-topped knee socks, or a bed where the knee gatch is raised too high. Vessel wall injury can also result from direct trauma by surgery or, more commonly, by intravenous (IV) or arterial catheters. Underlying vascular disease also creates vessel wall abnormalities. Chemical irritation may result from IV solutions and drugs. Anything that exposes collagen fibers in the vessel wall of arteries and veins may cause rapid platelet adhesion, aggregation, and thrombus formation. In addition, injury to vessels activates an inflammatory response that can be seen histologically and, in most cases, is seen most vividly in the lower extremities. When an extremity is immobile for any period of time, the pumping action is lost, resulting in venous stasis. For example, during the postoperative period, there is a decrease in total limb blood flow because of immobility. Stasis may also result from reduced cardiac output (CO) caused by heart failure or shock. Alteration in blood flow leading to arterial thrombosis may be caused by turbulent flow at points of arterial bifurcation or stenosis, or with aneurysms. Fortunately, the rapid blood flow in arteries tends to discourage thrombus formation. Reduced blood flow in the atria occurs with atrial fibrillation, leading to thrombus formation. When the patient's cardiac rhythm converts to a regular sinus rhythm, these thrombi can be expelled into the lungs or systemic circulation.[27]

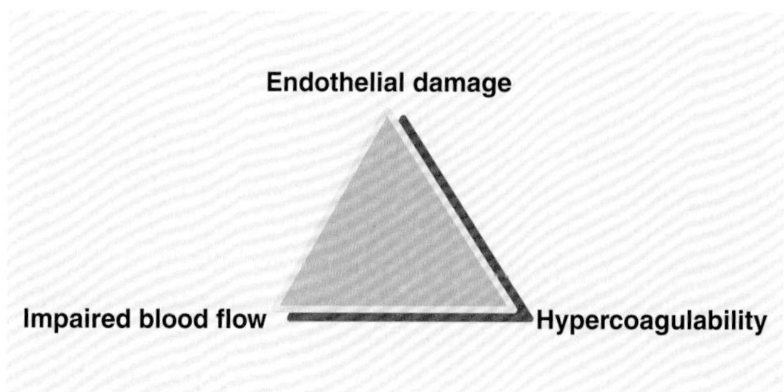

Figure 5-4. Virchow triad.

The final predisposing factor of Virchow triad is hypercoagulability of the blood. Changes in blood leading to hypercoagulability may occur during pregnancy or in women using oral contraceptive drugs, which can cause elevated levels of coagulation factors. Changes in blood constituents may also occur in polycythemia, in severe anemia, or with circulating endotoxins from systemic infections. Deficiencies in antithrombin III and decreased hepatic function may be thrombogenic in patients with liver disease and in premature infants. The type of thrombus formed usually differs between arteries and veins. Arterial thrombi usually begin at the site of endothelial injury or turbulence. A venous thrombus is almost always occlusive. In the slower-moving blood of the veins, the thrombus frequently creates a long cast in the lumen of the vessel. No matter what type of clot is present, embolic disorders are a clinical challenge in which tissue perfusion will be compromised and intervention needed.

Deep Vein Thrombosis

VTE affects approximately 300,000 to 600,000 individuals annually in the United States. VTE is now the appropriate term to include both DVT and pulmonary embolus (PE).

Patients can present with DVT and/or PE if diagnosed with VTE. Approximately two-thirds of patients diagnosed with VTE have DVTs and approximately one-third have a PE. However, these rates vary according to race, age, and gender. Higher rates have been reported in blacks, individuals over the age of 80 years, and males (with the exception of women and VTE in pregnancy).[28]

VTE causes great mortality and morbidity in the United States. Although diagnostic and therapeutic modalities have improved over the years, PE remains a challenging clinical entity.

VTE causes death in about 10% to 30% of patients with VTE within 30 days. Up to one-fourth of all PE patients have sudden death on presentation.[28] Furthermore, VTE causes complications such as recurrence of VTE, venous insufficiency, and pulmonary hypertension. Recurrence is as high as one-third of VTE patients, even in patients who are anticoagulated for the recommended duration of therapy. The risk of recurrence continues throughout their life.[28]

The clinical problems associated with VTE include DVT and PE. One of the most common and potentially life-threatening problems confronting health care professionals is the diagnosis, prophylaxis, and treatment of DVT and PE in both medical and surgical patients. The major risk associated with DVT is that it can lead to PE. Venous thrombosis in the lower extremity can involve superficial leg veins, the deep veins of the calf (calf vein thrombosis), and the more proximal veins, including the popliteal veins, the superficial femoral, common femoral, and iliac veins. In superficial vein thrombosis, sometimes called thrombophlebitis, the thrombosis is the result of inflammation in the venous wall of the superficial venous system and is benign and self-limiting.

Etiology

The risk factors associated with VTE can be divided into two categories: primary (or inherited) and secondary (or acquired) hypercoagulable states.

Virchow triad (see Fig. 5-4) theory can be applied to some of these risk factors (Table 5-7).[29–31]

Pathophysiology

Thrombi can form because the balance that is maintained in normal homeostasis has been disrupted. Coagulation is enhanced or fibrinolysis is impaired, which can lead to a hypercoagulable state. Primary inherited disorders that cause a hypercoagulable state are usually deficiencies in factors that inhibit coagulation, so there is less counterbalance to the coagulation process. The three main deficiencies are antithrombin III, protein C, and protein S.[5,31]

Table 5-7 • RISK FACTORS FOR VENOUS THROMBOEMBOLISM

Inherited (Primary) Hypercoagulable States
Activated Protein C resistance due to factor V Leiden mutation
Prothrombin gene mutation
Antithrombin III deficiency
Protein C deficiency
Protein S deficiency
Dysfibrinogenemias (rare)
Acquired (Secondary) Hypercoagulable States
Trauma
Pregnancy (especially postpartum period)
Immobilization (stroke or paralysis, extended bed rest, or sitting)
Advancing age
Postoperative state
Obesity
Prolonged air travel
Malignancy or treatment for malignancy
Estrogens (hormone replacement therapy, oral contraceptive therapy)
Lupus anticoagulant or antiphospholipid antibody syndrome
Previous venous thromboembolism
Presence of central venous lines
Chronic heart failure

Goldhaber SZ. Risk factors for venous thromboembolism. *J Am Coll Cardiol.* 2010;56(1):1–7; Kesieme E, Kesieme C, Jebbin N, et al. Deep vein thrombosis: a clinical review. *J Blood Med.* 2011;2:59–69.

Secondary hypercoagulable states may result from endothelial activation by cytokines that will lead to loss of normal vessel wall anticoagulant surface functions with conversion to proinflammatory thrombogenic functions.[32,33] Vascular endothelial damage can expose circulating blood components to subendothelial structures that initiate thrombosis. This process can also lead to vasoconstriction, which causes stasis and makes it easier for platelets to detach from flowing blood. The accumulation of platelets can furnish phospholipid for the intrinsic pathway, promoting thrombin formation by absorbing activated factor X to their surface.[33] Platelets can also undergo alterations in their surface area that can lead to spontaneous aggregation or increased adhesiveness.[33] Increased blood viscosity may also predispose thrombosis. Patients with increased levels of fibrinogen can induce erythrocyte aggregation, increasing viscosity and decreasing blood flow.

Clinical Manifestations

The classic signs and symptoms of pain, edema, warmth, erythema, and tenderness of the leg are common with DVT, but can also be caused by nonthrombotic events. However, some patients may be asymptomatic.[30,33] The size of the thrombus, the location of the affected vein, and the adequacy of collateral channels are some of the factors that cause the variability of the clinical presentation.[31,34] In the past, a positive Homans sign, which is pain occurring in the affected calf with forceful dorsiflexion of the foot, was thought to be diagnostic for a DVT. However, a positive Homans sign is not specific for thrombotic disease and could indicate minor muscle injury or other lower leg disorder.[34] Therefore, caution must be used when interpreting Homans sign because any inflammation near the calf muscles may also elicit similar pain. Asymmetry between two extremities may also be present, with the affected limb being slightly larger because of the congestion and edema associated with the inflammatory process. These signs and symptoms in combination with the presence of the associated risk factors should assist in the diagnostic process. The clinical manifestations of DVT are sometimes elusive and should always be confirmed by further evaluation with objective diagnostic tests.

Medical Management

Objective testing and a careful history and physical examination should be obtained if a DVT is suspected. The patient's history and physical examination are important components of the diagnostic process, because they may reveal an alternative cause of the patient's symptoms. Diagnostic studies for DVT include D-dimer assay, venography, and venous compression ultrasonography.

The D-dimer assay testing has a high sensitivity but has poor specificity and cannot always be used to rule out DVT. A negative D-dimer likely eliminates DVT and PE, but false-positive results have been reported in other conditions such as malignancy, inflammatory conditions, and infections.[30,33] Some form of ultrasound, either compression or color duplex, is usually the most common test used for diagnosing DVT because it is more specific and sensitive, especially for diagnosing DVTs in the femoral or popliteal veins. Compression ultrasound is less sensitive for calf vein DVT, but sensitivity can be enhanced with serial ultrasound.[33] Venography is used but is technically difficult to perform and requires experience to execute the test accurately. Venography can cause complications such as superficial phlebitis and DVT, if not performed correctly.[33] Once the diagnosis of DVT is confirmed, anticoagulation should be initiated immediately. Prevention is also an important priority to deter further decompensation of the patient's condition. Both these interventions will be discussed, along with more invasive interventions, such as venous filters for the treatment of PE.

Anticoagulation

The main goal of therapy for VTE, of any origin, is anticoagulation to prevent further formation of thrombi, prevent death from PE, and reduce morbidity.[33] Depending on the severity of the embolism, anticoagulation can be used conservatively or aggressively if thrombolytic therapy is needed to lyse a life-threatening clot. While some patients with VTE may be admitted and initiated on anticoagulation in the hospital setting, most patients can be treated in the outpatient setting because of newer treatment options, such as direct oral anticoagulants (DOACs), low–molecular-weight heparin (LMWH) and fondaparinux. Health care providers consider several factors when deciding whether a patient would best be treated in an acute care setting. Some of these factors may be, but are not limited to, hemodynamic instability, have contraindications to anticoagulation therapy, medical therapy noncompliance, and severe symptoms that may be difficult to manage.[33]

The most recent updates to the 9th Edition and 2016 Update of the Antithrombotic Guidelines published in *Chest* by the American College of Chest Physicians recommend these drugs to be used for anticoagulation with VTE: the heparins (unfractionated heparin [UFH] and LMWH), fondaparinux, oral anticoagulants, and thrombolytic agents.[35,36] The most common and one of the oldest medications used for anticoagulation is heparin. Heparin is a glycosaminoglycan that binds to and activates antithrombin III and reduces the formation of thrombin and fibrin.

UFH is used less commonly these days, but is still an option for specific hospitalized patients who might be at a higher risk of bleeding or have renal disease. However, UFH requires IV dosing, frequent lab testing (usually every 6 hours), and nursing care for dose adjustment based on aPTT lab results. UFH is typically administered with a bolus-loading dose intravenously, followed by a continuous IV infusion according to weight-based protocols, with dose adjustments to a therapeutic goal of the aPTT 1.5 to 2.5 times the normal aPTT. The anti-Xa activity can also measure therapy.[33]

Another group of drugs in the same class are the heparin derivatives, such as low–molecular-weight heparin and fondaparinux, which have a reduced ability to catalyze the inhibition of thrombin while retaining the ability to inhibit the activity of factor Xa. Preference of LMWH over UFH was reported in the 9th Edition Antithrombotic Therapy and Prevention of Thrombosis Guidelines.[36] The advantage to the LMWH is that they do not bind to most plasma proteins, which contribute to a more predictable anticoagulant dose, and there is no need for laboratory monitoring. Enoxaparin is the more common LMWH used currently and it can be administered either once or twice per day subcutaneously (SC). If prescribed once daily, the dose is 1.5 mg/kg and if prescribed twice daily (BID), the dose is 1.0 mg/kg. If needed, enoxaparin therapy can be monitored by using anti-factor Xa assay laboratory testing. Other LMWHs include dalteparin, tinzaparin, ardeparin, nadroparin, and reviparin, although the last three are not available in the United States. These agents differ and thus should not be used interchangeably.[37] Fondaparinux is another option for anticoagulation and involves administration once daily SC weight based. Fondaparinux also does not require frequent monitoring for therapeutic effect. Both LMWH and fondaparinux should be avoided in patients with creatinine clearances of less than 30 mL/min.[33] LMWH is the preferred treatment for patients' lower extremity DVT or PE with cancer over oral anticoagulants discussed below.[33,36]

The next drug category used for anticoagulation for VTE is oral anticoagulants which are used to prevent VTE progression or recurrence.[37] The two medication classes discussed here will include vitamin K antagonists (warfarin) and DOACs. Warfarin has been the primary oral anticoagulant drug used for many decades.[37] Originally, once a diagnosis of VTE was confirmed, a patient was started on heparin (to achieve a rapid therapeutic aPTT) and then given warfarin, with a typical starting dose of 2 to 5 mg orally. Warfarin dosing was then adjusted accordingly to the international normalized ratio (INR).

When administering warfarin, it is important to remember that the effect of the dose administered today will not be reflected in the PT/INR until approximately 3 days after that dose is administered. Typically, oral anticoagulant therapy overlaps with heparin therapy for at least 5 days until a therapeutic INR is obtained for 2 consecutive days.[37] Once the target for INR (typically 2 to 3) is reached and the level remains stable, the heparin can be discontinued, and the warfarin dose adjusted further until stable and then followed-up by intermittent INR sampling. Oral anticoagulation with warfarin is continued for at least 3 months and may be continued indefinitely, depending on the reason for the development of VTE.[36]

The newer class of oral anticoagulants is the direct oral anticoagulants or DOACs. Dabigatran targets thrombin. Other DOACs, such as rivaroxaban, apixaban, and edoxaban, inhibit factor Xa.[37] These oral anticoagulants were included on the updated recommendations of the 9th Edition Antithrombotic Therapy and Prevention of Thrombosis Guidelines as the preferred treatment for VTE of the leg or PE.[36] DOACs have less food and drug interactions (as compared to warfarin) and do not require routine monitoring for therapeutic dosing. However, some of the DOACs (dabigatran and edoxaban) require treatment with LMWH for at least 5 days prior to these medications.[33]

Length of therapy of oral anticoagulant therapy has been the topic of many studies and discussions. The 9th Edition Antithrombotic Therapy and Prevention of Thrombosis Guidelines recommend therapy for 3 months for patients with VTE provoked by a transient risk factor, such as surgery. However, in those patients with unprovoked VTE, therapy should be considered for a minimum of 3 months, and possibly extended therapy based on the risks and benefits of therapy. If therapy is extended indefinitely, then providers should reassess periodically for continued treatment.[33,36]

When a VTE dislodges and becomes a massive or life-threatening PE, thrombolytic agents can be used. Thrombolytic agents can be used in patients with hemodynamically unstable PE, and in those who are also at low risk for bleeding.[33,36] Streptokinase is the oldest plasminogen activator approved for use with VTEs and is administered intravenously with a loading. A limiting factor in the use of streptokinase is that patients can have an allergic reaction to the drug if they have had a recent streptococcal infection that can generate antibodies. Urokinase is another plasminogen activator that is administered intravenously with a loading dose followed by an infusion. Tissue plasminogen activator or tPA is also approved for use in the treatment of these patients. It is also administered intravenously and for VTE.[33] There is no laboratory test that correlates with clinical efficacy of fibrinolytic therapy.

Table 5-8 • MEDICATIONS USED TO PROMOTE ANTICOAGULATION

Medication Category	Mechanism of Action	Dose
Heparin (unfractionated heparin)	Binds to and activates antithrombin III and reduces the formation of thrombin and fibrin	Load: 5,000 u or 75 u/kg followed by initial infusion 18 units/kg/min; adjust according to weight-based protocol using aPTT (goal is usually 1.5–2.5 times the normal aPTT value)
Low–molecular-weight (LMWH), Enoxaparin	Similar to heparin but reduced ability to catalyze the inhibition of thrombin with retained ability to inhibit activity of factor Xa	1.5 mg/kg SC if dosed daily or 1.0 mg/kg if dosed q12h (treatment doses); if CrCl <30 mL/min, 1 mg/kg SC every 24 hours
Fondaparinux	Inhibits factor Xa but not thrombin	5–10 mg every 24 hours SC; avoid in patients with CrCl <30 mL/min; use caution for CrCl 30–50 mL/min
Warfarin (oral anticoagulant)	Antagonist of vitamin K	Dosed according to PT/INR (goal is related to reason for anticoagulation; usual INR goal is 2.0–3.0)
Dabigatran (DOAC)	Targets thrombin	150 mg orally twice daily after 5–10 days of initial parenteral anticoagulation; avoid if CrCl <30 mL/min and liver impairment
Rivaroxaban (DOAC)	Inhibits factor Xa	15 mg orally twice daily ×3 weeks, then 20 mg orally once daily; avoid if CrCl <30 mL/min and liver impairment
Apixaban (DOAC)	Inhibits factor Xa	10 mg orally twice daily ×7 days, then 5 mg orally twice daily; avoid if CrCl <25 mL/min, serum creatinine >2.5 mg/dL, or hepatic dysfunction
Edoxaban (DOAC)	Inhibits factor Xa	60 mg orally daily, or 30 mg once daily if CrCl 15–50 mL/min or body weight ≤60 kg; avoid in patients with CrCl <15 mL/min and liver impairment
Tissue Plasminogen activator, tPA	Induce a conformational change in plasminogen by proteolytically cleaving plasminogen to plasmin, enhancing fibrinolysis; has relative fibrin specificity	100 mg over 2 hours
Argatroban	Directly inhibits thrombin formation, enhancing fibrinolysis	No bolus; initial infusion rate 2 mcg/kg/min
Lepirudin	Directly inhibits thrombin formation, enhancing fibrinolysis	No bolus; initial IV infusion rate 0.05–0.10 mg/kg/h
Bivalirudin	Directly inhibits thrombin formation, enhancing fibrinolysis	No bolus; initial infusion rate 0.15–0.20 mg/kg/h

Warkentin T. Heparin-induced thrombocytopenia. *Hematol Oncol Clin North Am.* 2007;21(4):589–607.
SC, subcutaneous; CrCl, creatinine clearance.

Table 5-8 summarizes the anticoagulants used for treating DVT and VTE.[38–40]

Another intervention for DVT is catheter-directed thrombolysis (CDT) for select patients at low risk for bleeding. This intervention involves insertion of a catheter into the affected vein with the DVT and injection of a thrombolytic agent, with or without mechanical removal of the thrombus. However, there is an increased risk of bleeding with CDT. There has not been any evidence from clinical trials in which investigators showed an increase in quality of life with this therapy.[33] Thus recent guidelines suggest oral anticoagulation therapy over CDT for patients diagnosed with acute proximal leg DVT.[36]

The obvious side effect of any type of anticoagulation is bleeding. If the INR goal of 2.0 to 3.0 is attained, the risk of bleeding is minimal.[41] Careful consideration must be given to the patient's situation before starting anticoagulation, especially with the use of fibrinolytic therapy. Absolute contraindications for fibrinolytic therapy include prior intracranial hemorrhage, known structural cerebral vascular lesion, malignant intracranial neoplasm, ischemic stroke within 3 months, suspected aortic dissection, active bleeding or bleeding diathesis, or significant closed-head trauma or facial trauma within 3 months. Relative contraindications include uncontrolled hypertension (systolic blood pressure less than 180 mm Hg or diastolic blood pressure greater than 110 mm Hg), traumatic or prolonged cardiopulmonary resuscitation or major surgery within 3 weeks, recent internal bleeding (within 2 to 4 weeks), noncompressible vascular punctures, pregnancy, active peptic ulcer, current use of warfarin and INR greater than 1.7, and prior streptokinase exposure (greater than 5 days) or prior allergic reaction to streptokinase (if considering streptokinase).[37] The use of thrombolytic agents in the treatment of VTE should be individualized and careful consideration must be given to the risks and benefits of this type of intervention.[33,37]

Bleeding associated with anticoagulant therapy can be treated with various reversal agents such as protamine sulfate for heparin and vitamin K for Coumadin. While the DOACs have less associated bleeding events than other oral anticoagulants, there is still the possibility of bleeding or other situations, such as emergent surgery, requiring reversal of therapy. For reversal of dabigatran, idarucizumab is preferred in major bleeding or prior to urgent/emergent procedures.[31,42] For the direct Xa inhibitors, andexanet alfa has been approved for the reversal of apixaban and rivaroxaban.[42] Treatment is also directed at correction of coagulopathies, as indicated by abnormal coagulation studies (e.g., PT/PTT). Use of blood products such as fresh frozen plasma, cryoprecipitate, and platelets may be able to stop or decrease bleeding. Repletion of blood loss may also be necessary. Locating the major site of bleeding is very important but can be a challenging task, especially if the site is more occult in nature. Surgical intervention may be required, and this type of high-risk patient will need to be optimized before surgery.

Prophylaxis

Although treatment for VTE has become more delineated over the years, the key intervention with DVT and possible PE is prevention. The most common and oldest intervention is the use of low-dose unfractionated subcutaneous heparin of 5000 units every 8 to 12 hours. LMWH has also been shown to be effective in preventing VTE in medical and surgical patients and does not require anticoagulation monitoring.[31] Fondaparinux may also be used for prophylaxis for those at risk.[31] Oral anticoagulants are not used often because of the higher rate of bleeding. However, vitamin K antagonists can effectively prevent VTE in postoperative patients when given at the time of surgery or immediately postoperatively.[31] External intermittent pneumatic compression is a nonpharmacologic intervention that has proven valuable in many types of surgical patients including hip procedures. However, there have been few rigorous studies that support the effectiveness of lower extremity pneumatic compression.

Sequential compression devices have few side effects and are thus placed on patients in the operating room for prolonged surgical procedures.[31] The compression devices are attached to a machine that typically is placed on the footboard of the hospital bed and requires electrical connection for power. The tubing from the compression device contains cords that go from the lower extremities to the machine as well as the electrical outlet. There may be an increased risk of falls as patients begin mobilizing more and attempt to get out of bed.

Elastic stockings or graduated compression stockings are also used and found to be useful in the low- and moderate-risk surgical patient.[31]

Nursing Interventions

The primary approach to nursing management of the patient at risk for DVT includes identifying the risk category for a patient and implementing preventive strategies. Such strategies include active or passive leg exercises and early ambulation to increase muscle activity, thereby improving venous blood flow.

Frequent turning, coughing, and deep breathing help to improve venous return. Other measures to promote venous return are pneumatic compression stockings, graduated compression stockings, elevating the foot of the bed 6 to 8 in, and not raising the knee gatch to avoid excessive popliteal pressure. A thorough history of the patient's risk factors along with the vigilant physical assessment of extremities for any evidence of inflammation, such as redness, swelling, asymmetry, and tenderness, is critical. If any signs and symptoms are observed, objective diagnostic testing should be pursued. Bleeding is the most common complication of anticoagulant and fibrinolytic therapy. The patient must be observed for subtle signs of bleeding. Careful monitoring of all puncture sites is mandatory, especially femoral interventional sites, with special attention to the abdomen and flank areas where large amounts of blood can sequester before the patient becomes symptomatic. Gastrointestinal bleeding is also another mechanism for blood loss.

Assessing for symptoms of abdominal discomfort as well as guaiac testing of excretions of patients on anticoagulation should be routine nursing interventions.

Patient education regarding lab monitoring, anticoagulant medications and their side effects, and interactions with other drugs should be reviewed. Leg elevation while sitting should be emphasized and the importance of physical activity when discharged should be emphasized. Risk factors such as obesity, smoking, and estrogen therapy should be identified and interventions designed to assist the patient to modify them as appropriate.[34] Because embolization is always a threat, special attention to the assessment of cardiopulmonary indicators is paramount. PE may present with sudden onset of dyspnea, chest pain, and tachypnea, accompanied by other symptoms that will be discussed in the next section.

Pulmonary Embolism

PE may be the result of either arterial or venous thrombi. Common sources of PE include deep venous thrombi from the lower legs, right atrial thrombi, septic foci (often related to IV drug abuse or infected vascular access sites), and tumors. Other sources of emboli are amniotic fluid, fat, air, bone marrow, and other foreign bodies. These latter sources have a pathophysiology that is different from the usual venous source and occur less frequently. Many factors predispose patients to PE and are similar to those risk factors for development of DVT discussed earlier.

Pathophysiology

A PE is a mechanical complete or partial obstruction to blood flow from the right to left heart. The physiologic response of the patient is dependent on the degree of obstruction and the underlying cardiopulmonary function.[27] A patient with good cardiopulmonary function and a complete obstruction may have the same outcome as a patient with poor cardiopulmonary function and a partial obstruction. Cardiac failure with a massive PE is caused by increased wall stress and ischemia that comprises the right ventricular (RV) function quickly and eventually impacts left ventricular (LV) function.[27] Increased afterload develops due to obstruction of blood flow out of the right ventricle. Additional factors that increase afterload are neural reflexes, the release of humoral factors, mediators that are released by platelets (platelet-activating factor and serotonin), and systemic arterial hypoxemia.[27] The CO is initially maintained by increased catecholamine release resulting in an increased heart rate and contractility. The RV will attempt to contract against the resistance presented by the embolism but will eventually decompensate leading to an increase in RV volume. This increased RV preload leads to increased wall stress and compromised RV coronary blood flow and ischemia. Increased RV volume will also cause a septal shift that will decrease LV distensibility and decrease LV preload. This alteration in preload will lead to a decrease in CO and mean arterial pressure (MAP). RV coronary perfusion pressure is dependent on the gradient between the MAP and the RV subendocardial pressure.[27] The decrease in MAP will aggravate the compromised RV oxygen supply. Further RV ischemia will perpetuate decreased RV performance and the cycle will continue until complete decompensation occurs. This pathophysiologic cycle is summarized in Figure 5-5.

The emboli itself can lead to a local aggregation of platelets and the release of vasoactive substances, which increase vasoconstriction. Gas exchange abnormalities are related to the size and type of embolic material, the extent of the occlusion, and the underlying cardiopulmonary status and length of time since embolization.[27] With PE, there is initial adequate ventilation coupled with inadequate perfusion (i.e., alveolar dead space). The persistent obstruction and associated vasoconstriction can lead to bronchoconstriction, which produces shunting, another ventilation–perfusion (VQ) imbalance. Any sustained VQ mismatch results in arterial hypoxemia. The hemodynamic and gas exchange consequences of a massive PE can lead to a dramatic clinical presentation.

Clinical Manifestations

PE may occur with a sudden, abrupt onset, or have an insidious onset that mimics other cardiopulmonary disorders. Dyspnea is

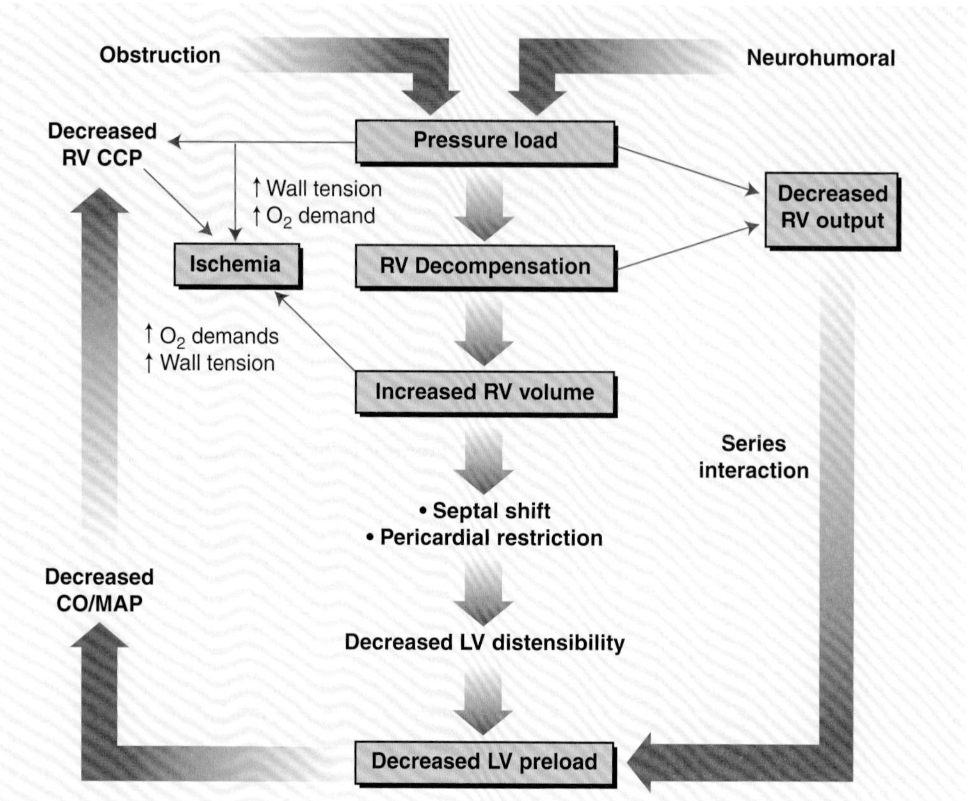

Figure 5-5. Pathophysiology of pulmonary embolism. (From Wood K. Major pulmonary embolism. Review of pathophysiologic approach to the golden hour of hemodynamically significant pulmonary embolism. *Chest.* 2002;121[3]:877–905.)

the most common symptom associated with PE. Other signs such as pleuritic pain, cough, or hemoptysis can be present.[31] The chest pain is typically sharp and sometimes related to respiratory excursions.[43] Classic cardiac signs such as tachycardia, low-grade fever, and neck vein distention can also be observed on presentation but may also be the function of age, the size of the PE, and the underlying cardiopulmonary status.[33] There may also be vague complaints of chest discomfort, which can also be associated with acute coronary ischemic syndromes.

The presentation of a patient with a massive PE can be very similar to the signs and symptoms mentioned above. The only difference is that the signs and symptoms are a more extreme and exaggerated response to the embolic event. The classic clinical presentation of a massive PE can include syncope, cyanosis, tachycardia (heart rate 120 beats/min), and tachypnea (respiratory rate greater than or equal to 30 breaths/min).[31] Because symptoms of a massive PE can be so vague, it is important to gather data about patients and continually consider what their risk factors are for having a PE.

Medical Management

The diagnosis of PE is challenging, because PE can mimic other cardiorespiratory or musculoskeletal disorders such as myocardial infarction, pneumonia, congestive heart failure, asthma, or costochondritis. The diagnosis of PE should always be confirmed by objective tests. However, there are few tests that are specific for PE. Because the protective mechanism of fibrinolysis is triggered with the formation of a clot, tests reflecting fibrinolysis have been helpful in making the diagnosis of PE. The quantitative plasma D-dimer enzyme-linked immunosorbent assay (ELISA) level is elevated (500 ng/mL) in more than 95% of patients with PE but is not specific and therefore not useful when considering hospitalized patients. Levels may also be elevated in other conditions previously mentioned.[44] ABG values are not valuable in the diagnosis of PE, which is contrary to classic teaching. The expected hypoxemia associated with PE was not found to be consistently present in patients with documented PE. The ECG may be abnormal with an S wave in lead I, a Q wave in lead III, and inverted T wave in lead III; however, these changes are usually seen in patients with a massive PE. A normal chest radiograph in a dyspneic patient could suggest a possible PE.[44]

A definitive diagnosis of PE is best made by pulmonary angiography because a well-performed pulmonary angiogram excludes the diagnosis of PE. Although the time and costs involved with the invasive pulmonary angiography preclude its routine use in the diagnosis of PE, it remains the most reliable clinical study available.[27] However, diagnosis can be made by means of a computed tomographic pulmonary angiography (CTPA) using spiral computed tomography (CT), which is now the preferred diagnostic testing with sensitivity (83%) and specificity (96%) with experienced personnel and validated protocols.[33]

Lung VQ scans are another diagnostic testing used for diagnosis of PE. In PE, a defect is evident in the perfusion portion of the scan in conjunction with a normal ventilation scan. An abnormal VQ scan suggests PE. If the VQ scan is normal, the likelihood of PE is low. This test needs to be carefully evaluated since preexisting cardiopulmonary disease can distort the interpretation and both the ventilation and perfusion portions of the test should be performed.

As CTPA has become more available, VQ scanning popularity has decreased, except for young patients and those with decreased renal function. CTPA requires significant contrast dye load. Thus, renal function should be considered when deciding which diagnostic test is safest for individual patients. Contrast-induced nephropathy may be caused by direct toxic effects on the tubular epithelial cells by the formation of reactive oxygen species or reduced antioxidant activity.[45] Decreased renal function from contrast dye load may also be caused by an alteration in renal hemodynamics resulting in renal vasoconstriction and erythrocyte aggregation.[45] The hallmark intervention for prevention of contrast-induced nephropathy is hydration, usually with normal saline.[45] While there have been studies in which hydration with sodium bicarbonate has been as effective[20] if not superior to hydration with normal saline, these results are inconclusive.[46] The most recent 2012 Kidney Disease: Improving Global Outcomes (KDIGO) Guidelines recommend use of either normal saline or sodium bicarbonate hydration prior to contrast-enhanced testing. Furthermore, it is not recommended to hydrate patients by oral solutions alone. The other option for prevention of contrast-induced nephropathy for increased-risk patients is using oral *N*-acetylcysteine with IV isotonic crystalloids. Fenoldopam, theophylline, and intermittent hemodialysis or hemofiltration are not recommended for prevention of contrast-induced nephropathy.[47]

Once PE is diagnosed, anticoagulation is the first intervention. The previous section on anticoagulation for DVT discusses the usual approach for treatment.

Systemic thrombolytic therapy is preferred over CDT for treatment of acute PE when deciding on thrombolytic therapy.[33] If the patient is severely compromised and experiencing cardiopulmonary failure due to a PE, thrombolytic therapy is indicated.[33] Inferior vena cava filter can also be used to prevent a PE in patients with a DVT who have contraindications to anticoagulation therapy.[33] This intervention helps prevent passage of emboli to the lung and is used in cases where anticoagulation may not be appropriate. IVC filters are not without risks,[33] so careful consideration of the risks and benefits should be considered in these patients.

Patients with a recent history of PE (previous 2 years) are at risk for chronic thromboembolic pulmonary hypertension (CTEPH). While CTEPH will not be discussed in detail here, thromboendarterectomy is a treatment option for CTEPH patients.[33] In rare and urgent instances, pulmonary embolectomy may be performed in conjunction with cardiopulmonary bypass. Mortality rates with this procedure can exceed 50% with high rates of complications and should be performed only in institutions that can quickly mobilize a cardiac surgery team.[27] With prompt identification and treatment, prognosis is good for patients with PE. Successful treatment results in little long-term morbidity. Sequelae such as pulmonary hypertension and cor pulmonale may be seen in patients with underlying cardiopulmonary disease or those with massive emboli.

Nursing Interventions

Because PE can be a life-threatening event, the emphasis of nursing management is on prevention. As discussed previously, prevention of thrombus formation and early detection of PE are essential. Fifty percent of those patients who die of PE do so within the first hour. Any patient experiencing a sudden onset of dyspnea, tachypnea, and possible chest pain must be evaluated for the possibility of PE. Assessing the character of the patient's chest pain is important because most patients describe their pain as pleuritic. A 12-lead ECG and an ABG also provide useful data. Explaining all procedures and tests helps reassure patients during a time of discomfort and anxiety about the sudden change of their condition. Once the diagnosis of PE has been established, continued nursing management of the patient's cardiopulmonary function is essential.

Because profound arterial hypoxemia can accompany PE, the primary goal is to normalize gas exchange. By normalizing the exchange of gases and minimizing the VQ mismatch, other systemic effects of impaired gas exchange can also be ameliorated.

Interventions to support respiratory function by patient positioning and the use of supplemental oxygen may help decrease the degree of hypoxemia accompanying PE. Supplemental oxygen may be administered by face mask or, if necessary, by endotracheal intubation and mechanical ventilation. Positioning the patient with the head of the bed elevated allows for better chest expansion with respiration. Coaching of the patient to promote the best respiratory pattern can be very important and maintaining a calm environment and approach to the patient can make the difference in the patient's course. The administration of prescribed analgesics and sedatives may help relieve the patient's discomfort and anxiety. By reducing discomfort and anxiety, respiratory rate may also decrease, thus reducing the additional vasoconstriction and bronchoconstriction caused by lower $PaCO_2$ levels. Anticoagulants and thrombolytic agents, as described earlier, are usually ordered by the physician. These agents help decrease the recurrence of emboli and may help lyse the embolus, thus restoring normal blood flow through the pulmonary vasculature.

Frequent assessment of cardiopulmonary function is also important. Vital signs, particularly respiratory rate, heart rate, and blood pressure should be assessed and documented hourly and as needed. Normal vital signs may indicate improved gas exchange. ABG analysis offers a quantitative assessment of gas exchange. Because of the prolonged duration of anticoagulant therapy, patients require extensive teaching about the administration and follow-up schedules of oral anticoagulants, a medication identification card or band, potential hazards associated with therapy, and the signs and symptoms of bleeding and recurrent VTE. Dietary restrictions and foods that contain large amounts of vitamin K should be reviewed for patients who are prescribed warfarin or vitamin K antagonist therapy. This is a disease with long-term implications that can be successfully managed with patient participation and education.

Heparin-Induced Thrombocytopenia

Anticoagulation is a key intervention in treating cardiovascular disease. The primary agent that has been used for years is heparin. However, heparin use is not without adverse effects. HIT is a challenging immunohematologic issue that was originally described in the early 1960s. Key elements of the syndrome were discovered in the mid 1970s, and the antigen target of the HIT antibody was identified in 1992.[48] With more patients exposed to heparin or related drugs, the occurrence of HIT has been increasing. HIT can have detrimental thromboembolic complications such as PE, myocardial infarction, stroke, and ischemic limb necrosis.[49] One issue with the disease is that it is difficult to diagnose and unpredictable in incidence but can have some devastating outcomes.

Unlike other clotting disorders, HIT is the result of an immunohematologic reaction.

Pathophysiology

The development of the pathogenic IgG is the key to this disorder. The heparin binds with PF4, which leads to the development of a highly reactive antigenic complex. Pathogenic IgG is formed and activates the platelets.[50] The major target antigen is a macromolecular complex comprising heparin or other high-sulfated oligosaccharides and PF4 which binds to the platelet surface.[50]

HIT is an immune-mediated adverse drug reaction that is caused by heparin-dependent, platelet-activating IgG antibodies that recognize complexes of PF4 bound to "heparin."[39] These antibodies are known as HIT antibodies because once they "see" heparin, the autoimmune response is triggered and they become anti-PF4/heparin, platelet-activating IgG antibodies. The activated platelets release procoagulant and PF4 neutralizes heparin that leads to increased thrombin generation.[39] With more thrombin available, a hypercoagulable state develops and can lead to the formation of thrombi (arterial and venous). The HIT antibodies are also thought to activate the endothelium and monocytes leading to the expression of tissue factor at cell surfaces, which can also lead to thrombin formation (see Fig. 5-6).[51] With this immunologic cascade of events, HIT is a potentially devastating thrombotic disorder.

Etiology

The cause of HIT is the exposure to heparin leading to the development of anti-PF4/heparin platelet-activating IgG antibodies, which leads to thrombocytopenia. Patients generally experience a 50% decrease in platelet count, but it is important to note that the postoperative patient's "baseline" platelet count is the highest postoperative count prior to the decrease suspected with HIT.[39]

An immune response requires time for the reaction to develop. Because of this aspect of the disease, HIT can have varying time onsets and is important in diagnosing HIT. The usual onset for 70% of patients is a decrease in platelet count 5 to 10 days after starting heparin (first day of heparin use equals day 0).[39] If patients have an exposure to heparin within the past few weeks or months leading to HIT antibody development, a "rapid-onset" HIT presentation can occur within 24 hours of subsequent heparin administration.[39] When the platelet count decreases after all heparin has been stopped, this is a "delayed presentation" HIT and thought to be due to high levels of circulating antibodies.[39] Although HIT can develop in any patient who has exposure to heparin; there are certain patient populations that seem to have a higher incidence (Table 5-9).[39,52]

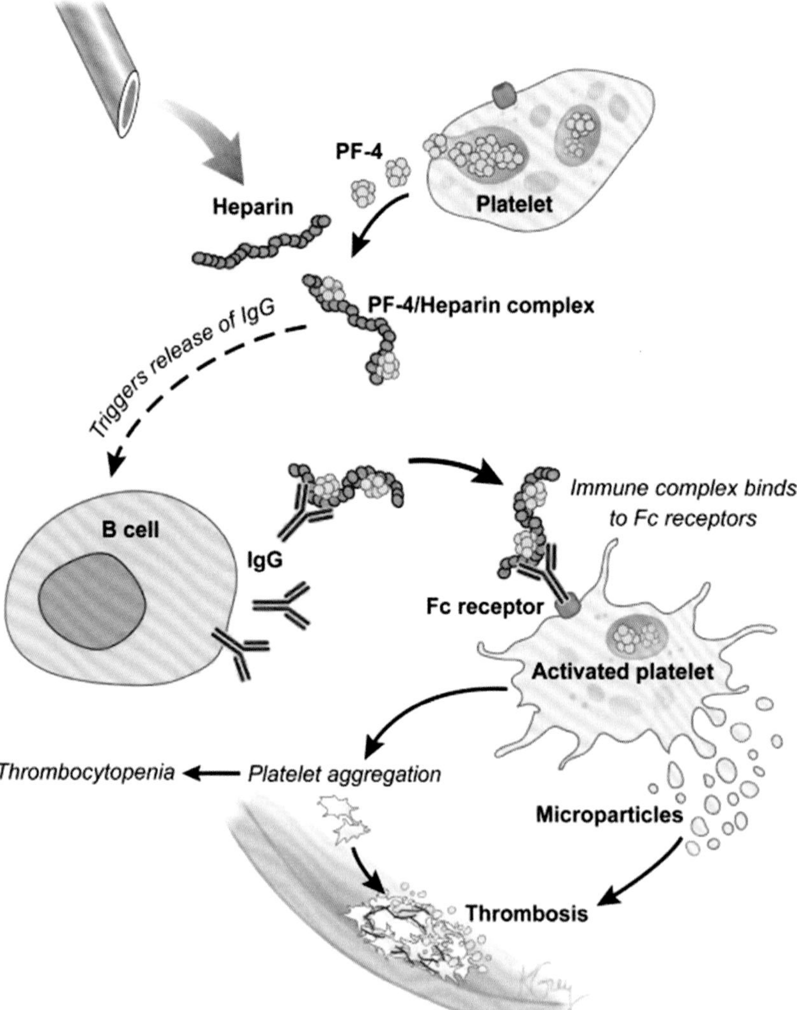

Figure 5-6. Pathogenesis of HIT. The PF4 protein released by platelets attaches to heparin, forming PF4/heparin complexes. This complex triggers the release of the IgG antibody from beta cells which attach to the PF4/heparin complex. This immune complex activates platelets and the release of platelet microparticles that initiate thrombotic activity. (Reproduced with permission from Roberts MK, Chaney S. Heparin-induced thrombocytopenia. *J Nurse Pract.* 2018;14[5]:402–408.e403.)

Table 5-9 • RISK FACTORS FOR HIT

Heparin type	Unfractionated > low–molecular-weight heparin > fondaparinux
Patient type	Postoperative (major > minor surgery) > medical > obstetric/pediatric
Dose	Prophylactic dose > therapeutic dose > flushes
Duration	11–14 days > 5–10 days > 4 days or fewer
Sex	Female > male

Adapted from Hoffman RS, Benz E, Silberstein LE, et al. *Hematology: Basic Principles and Practice*. 7th ed. Philadelphia, PA: Elsevier; 2018.

Clinical Presentation

The initial presentation of HIT in most patients is thrombocytopenia during or after heparin therapy leading to the development of thrombosis.[39,40] Venous thrombotic complications are most common including DVT (50%) and PE (25%).[51] Venous thrombosis of the adrenal vein occurs and can lead to adrenal hemorrhage.[39] Arterial thrombotic complications include limb artery thrombosis, thrombotic stroke, myocardial infarction, or other arterial thrombosis (mesentery or spinal).[39,51] Skin necrosis at heparin injection sites is another presentation that can range from painful erythematous papules to dermal necrosis. Warfarin necrosis with HIT is characterized by venous limb gangrene usually with DVT or classic necrosis in nonacral sites (breasts, abdominal wall, thigh, calf, or forearm). Overt DIC is another sequelae of HIT that occurs in 10% to 20% of patients. There has even been anaphylactic reaction to IV heparin 5 to 30 minutes after administration with symptoms ranging from cardiac arrest to an inflammatory presentation, that is, fever, chills, rigors, or flushing.[39]

Arterial thrombosis usually involves the distal portion of the aorta, and the symptoms can vary in degree depending on the thrombus size. Absent pulses indicate total arterial thrombosis occlusion, whereas pulses with distal extremity ischemia indicate microvascular occlusion.[39] The classic presentation for acute arterial thrombosis is known as the "6 Ps": pallor, pulselessness, pain, paresthesias, paralysis, and poikilothermy (coolness).[34] Either the arms or the legs can be involved. The pain and paralysis are the result of nerve and skeletal muscle ischemia that can occur as early as 4 to 6 hours after the occlusion. Beyond this time period, the situation can progress to potential compartment syndrome with severe pain, tense swelling, and muscle tenderness of the affected extremity.[34] In HIT, limb amputation is common.

Medical Management

Medical management is challenged with making the diagnosis of HIT. The diagnosis of HIT is based on the patient's exposure to heparin, which can extend to 100 days before the event.[53] The diagnostic process continues with the assessment of the platelet count. Thrombocytopenia after heparin exposure is the hallmark signal to indicate HIT, but other reasons for a decrease in platelets also need to be considered. Because of the complexity of diagnosing HIT, Warkentin[39] developed a "4Ts" scoring system (thrombocytopenia severity, timing of onset, thrombosis, and other causes of thrombocytopenia) to help estimate the pretest probability of HIT (Table 5-10).[40] Any source of heparin or LMWH must be discontinued. Even the smallest amounts of heparin such as heparin-coated catheters or heparin flush solutions must be eliminated.

The next step is to pursue laboratory detection of HIT antibodies. Platelet activation assays or functional testing tests patient serum against donor platelets "washed" in apyrase-containing buffer (potentiator of HIT antibody–induced platelet activation) and have high sensitivity.[39,40] PF4-dependent enzyme immunoassays (EIAs or ELISAs) were one of the original tests developed for HIT and a negative test essentially rules out the diagnosis of HIT.[40] However, the EIAs/ELISAs detect more clinically insignificant antibodies, which can lead to overdiagnosis of HIT.[39,40,54] A combination of the platelet activation assays and the EIAs/ELISAs should be used in the diagnosis of HIT. Varying laboratory practices in North America may impact the correct detection of the HIT diagnosis.[54] The presence of antibodies

Table 5-10 • 4Ts SCORING SYSTEM: ESTIMATING THE PRETEST PROBABILITY OF HEPARIN-INDUCED THROMBOCYTOPENIA

	Points (0, 1, or 2 for Each of Four Categories: Maximum Possible Score = 8)		
	2	**1**	**0**
Thrombocytopenia (acute)	Platelet fall >50% (nadir ≥20 × 10^9/L) and no surgery within preceding 3 days	Nadir, 10–19 × 10^9/L; or any 30–50% fall; or >50% fall within 3 days of surgery	Nadir, <10 × 10^9/L; or any <30% fall
Timing[a] of platelet count fall, thrombosis, or other sequelae	Clear onset between days 5–10; or ≤1 day (if prior heparin exposure in the past 5–30 days)	Consistent with day 5–10 fall, but not clear (e.g., missing platelet counts); or ≤1 day (heparin exposure within the past 31–100 days); or platelet fall after day 10	Platelet count fall begins in ≤4 days without recent heparin exposure
Thrombosis or other clinical sequelae	New proven thrombosis; skin necrosis[b]; anaphylactoid reaction after IV heparin bolus; adrenal hemorrhage	Progressive or recurrent thrombosis; erythematous skin lesions[b]; suspected thrombosis (awaiting confirmation with imaging)	None
OTher cause for thrombocytopenia not evident	No other explanation for platelet count fall is evident	Possible other cause is evident	Definite other cause is present

Pretest probability score: 6 to 8, HIGH; 4 to 5, INTERMEDIATE; 0 to 3, LOW.

The scoring system shown here has undergone minor modifications from previously published scoring systems.

[a]First day of immunizing heparin exposure considered day 0; immunizing heparin is usually that given during or soon after surgery (e.g., unfractionated heparin [UFH] during cardiac surgery is more immunogenic than UFH given during preceding acute coronary syndrome or with heart catheterization); the day the platelet count *begins* to fall is considered the day of onset of thrombocytopenia.

[b]Skin lesions occurring at heparin injection sites.

Reproduced with permission from Hoffman RS, Benz E, Silberstein LE, et al., eds. *Hematology: Basic Principles and Practice*. 7th ed. Philadelphia, PA: Elsevier; 2018.

may not always confirm the diagnosis of HIT. HIT antibodies develop and can be transient emphasizing the importance to test acute plasma or serum.[39] Clinical as well as laboratory data need to be compiled and interpreted to properly diagnose HIT. This is the reason why Warkentin has described HIT as a "clinicopathologic syndrome."[40]

The major clinical decision will be starting anticoagulation using one of the two types of nonheparin anticoagulants approved for the treatment of HIT: Direct thrombin inhibitor (DTI)—argatroban, recombinant hirudin (lepirudin) and bivalirudin; and long-acting indirect factor Xa inhibitors—danaparoid and fondaparinux. The indirect factor Xa inhibitors are not currently approved in the United States for the treatment of HIT.[40]

The DTIs are the primary medication to treat HIT. This class of medications inhibits thrombin produced by HIT, while not attaching to PF4. This class consists of argatroban, lepirudin, and bivalirudin. Lepirudin is no longer available from the manufacturer[40] and will not be discussed in further detail. Argatroban is FDA approved in the United States for the treatment of HIT, prevention of thrombosis, and for anticoagulation in patients with acute HIT and/or a history of HIT undergoing PCI.[39,40] Bivalirudin also inhibits thrombin directly, has a short half-life, is only partially renally eliminated, and is also approved for patients undergoing PCI with acute HIT and/or a history of HIT.[40] All of the DTIs can be administered intravenously. Dosing recommendations for the DTIs can be found in Table 5-7. A baseline aPTT should be obtained before the start of therapy. Infusion doses of these drugs are maintained to achieve an aPTT 1.5 to 2.5 times the normal value, similar to the goal of heparin therapy. The aPTT is usually sampled every 6 hours.

The long-acting indirect factor Xa inhibitors include danaparoid and fondaparinux. As mentioned, danaparoid is not FDA approved for the treatment of HIT in the United States and was discontinued in the early 2000s in the United States. However, fondaparinux has been used in the treatment of HIT for several reasons. It has a long half-life, does not require monitoring, and is cheaper. Because fondaparinux does not affect the aPTT, the only laboratory monitoring available is the anti-Xa activity, although rarely obtained in the United States.[40,51] Table 5-7 includes dosing recommendations for these medications.

Warkentin[39] summarized the principles of HIT to include suspected or confirmed HIT. It is important to (1) stop all heparin including LMWH and heparin administered as flushes and (2) start alternative nonheparin anticoagulation. Evidence supports the use of the nonheparin anticoagulants described previously. Warfarin is contraindicated in the acute phase of HIT due to the risk of warfarin-induced necrosis manifested by venous limb gangrene or classic skin necrosis.[40] Warfarin can also prolong the aPTT values, which could lead to underdosing of the DTIs.[40] Prophylactic platelet transfusions should not be given.[51] Diagnostic laboratory testing should include ELISA testing, which can rule in or out the HIT diagnosis in 80% to 90% of cases in the appropriate clinical context. Platelet activation assays should be used with the remaining percentage of patients.[39] Finally, duplex ultrasonography should be performed to investigate for lower limb DVT.[39] For patients with a history of HIT who have an important indication for heparin, it is recommended that sufficient time has elapsed since the episode (more than 2 to 3 months) to ensure that the antibodies are no longer present.[39]

Nursing Interventions

This "clinicopathologic syndrome"[40] requires the most astute observational and correlation skills of a nurse. A high index of suspicion is needed especially with postoperative surgical patients who are receiving prophylactic doses of UFH for at least 5 days.[53] A thorough history of the patient's possible exposure to heparin, including 100 days before the event, must be obtained. Platelet count should be measured promptly in high-risk patient populations and monitored closely at least every other day until day 14 or stopping heparin (whichever comes first).[40] Medical and postoperative patients receiving UFH and LMWH are considered moderate risk for HIT and platelet counts should be monitored at least two to three times weekly.[40,55]

A decreasing platelet count should cause suspicion and the search for possible thrombosis formation should begin. Vigilant physical assessment of extremities for any evidence of embolic events such as erythema, asymmetrical edema of the extremities, and/or tenderness is critical. The "6 Ps" should provide guidelines for monitoring limb perfusion.[34] Early observation of limb compromise may allow appropriate vascular intervention, which could avert amputation.

Further evaluation and observation of all body systems, especially neurologic, pulmonary, and cardiac, may reveal early signs and symptoms of embolic events. If the patient displays any sign of restlessness or agitation, physiologic factors such as hypoxemia should be the first consideration. Monitoring oxygenation using pulse oximetry will give some estimate of oxygenation that can be confirmed with an ABG. If gas exchange is adequate and restlessness and agitation persist, neurologic causes must be considered and sedation should be avoided unless indicated.

Respiratory distress with tachypnea, dyspnea on exertion (DOE), prolonged expiratory time as well as restlessness, and agitation could be indications of pulmonary emboli. The patient's heart rate, rhythm, and blood pressure should be continually monitored for any changes. Hemodynamic monitoring may be used and variations in indices may indicate cardiac failure, myocardial infarction, or pulmonary complications such as PE depending on the situation and the primary disorder. Gastrointestinal dysfunction can present with a wide range of signs and symptoms from nausea and vomiting to acute abdominal pain. Assessment of the abdomen, as well as monitoring trends in liver function test, should never be omitted and given special attention if HIT is suspected. Any abdominal discomfort should be carefully considered and monitored for any progression. Monitoring urine output for at least 0.5 to 1 mL/kg/h should be routine practice. The BUN and creatinine trends should also be closely reviewed. If these organ systems are severely compromised, multisystem organ dysfunction may be the end result, with poor outcomes. HIT can be a devastating syndrome.

Summary

Nurses play an integral part of the care of patients with hematologic conditions or illnesses. Understanding the pathophysiology, etiology, medical management, and nursing care of DIC, VTE, and HIT is essential to be able to care for these patients. Furthermore, as newer medications are recommended for these and many other conditions, nurses need to stay up-to-date on evidence-based practice in order to be knowledgeable and educate patients and families in the best manner.

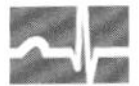

CASE STUDY 1

Patient Profile

Name/Age/Sex: **Marybeth Smith, 45-year-old female**

History of Present Illness
Marybeth presented to her local ED with complaints of left lower leg pain for 1½ days. She initially felt it was a pulled muscle in the groin region. However, the morning she presented to the ED, she noticed the considerable swelling and difference in her thighs. With her and her family history, she suspected a DVT.

Past Medical History
Protein S deficiency (no history of VTE), iron-deficiency anemia

Surgical History
Tonsillectomy as a child

Family History
Protein S deficiency (father, brother, and sister); Type I diabetes mellitus (father); Type II diabetes mellitus (mother); Hyperlipidemia (mother, paternal grandfather, maternal grandmother)

Social History
Nonsmoker, no marijuana or recreational drugs, occasional glass of wine. Recent travel to Asia for vacation; returned 12 days ago.

Medications
Aspirin 81 mg orally daily.

No known drug allergies.

Patient Examination

Vital Signs
BP 118/64; RR 16 bpm; Temp 37.3°C; HR 88 bpm; Ht. 164 cm; Wt. 78 kg

Physical Examination
General: Awake, alert, and oriented. No acute distress. Well developed, hydrated, and nourished. Appears stated age.

Skin: Warmness noted to left lower extremity. Skin intact.

Cardiac: The external chest is normal in appearance without lifts, heaves, or thrills. No murmurs, gallops, or rubs are auscultated. S1 and S2 are heard and are of normal intensity.

Respiratory: The chest wall is symmetric and without deformity. No signs of trauma. Chest wall is nontender. No signs of respiratory distress. Lung sounds are clear in all lobes bilaterally without rales, ronchi, or wheezes.

Abdominal: Abdomen is soft, symmetric, and nontender without distention. No masses, hepatomegaly, or splenomegaly are noted.

Psychiatric: Appropriate mood and affect. Good judgment and insight. No visual or auditory hallucinations. No suicidal or homicidal ideation.

Testing
Lower extremity US confirms diagnosis of left lower leg DVT

Considerations

Key Questions

- What is the appropriate medication to start for DVT?
- She was started on enoxaparin treatment dose of 1 mg/kg twice-daily dosing and was discharged home. She was changed to a DOAC (in this case, apixaban)
- What is the timeline for follow-up?
  - Within one week from discharge from the ED.
  - Given her family history of DVT as well as protein S deficiency it was recommended to follow up with a hematology provider.
  - Additionally, Marybeth's sister, who had a history of DVTs, had a warfarin-induced skin necrosis after her initial DVT. Therefore, Marybeth was concerned the same might happen to her if she chose warfarin. Marybeth and her hematologist had a good conversation about the pros and cons of the recommended anticoagulants for DVT.

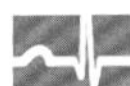

CASE STUDY 2

Patient Profile

Name/Age/Sex: **Nicole Thomas, 55-year-old female**

History of Present Illness
Nicole Thomas presented to her local emergency department (ED) with complaints of chest pain approximately 4 weeks ago. She described the pain as mid-chest discomfort, similar to a tightening of viselike gripping pain. She rated her pain as 10/10 on a scale of 0–10 with zero as no pain and 10 being the worst pain ever in her life. She reported she had never felt a pain like this before. She was diagnosed with acute inferior myocardial infarction and underwent cardiac catheterization. She was then diagnosed with multivessel CAD, started on aspirin therapy, β-blocker therapy, and her statin was increased to high-intensity therapy (atorvastatin 80 mg daily). Cardiac surgery was consulted and because she was chest pain free at the time, she was discharged to home until her coronary artery bypass (CABG) surgery could be performed.

She was admitted and underwent CABG surgery and progressed well immediately after surgery. However, on postoperative day 3, it was noted she had thrombocytopenia on her daily CBC.

Past Medical History
Hyperlipidemia, diagnosed age 53 years and type II diabetes

Surgical History
CABG

Family History
Father deceased age 72 years from cancer; mother deceased age 45 years from myocardial infarction secondary coronary artery disease (CAD); history of CAD in maternal grandparents and paternal grandmother.

Social History
Exercises 5–7 times/wk (walking with neighbor every evening); enjoys gardening and being a member of a local book club; denies use of tobacco, marijuana, or recreational drugs; drinks wine socially. Retired and lives with husband alone.

Medications
Atorvastatin 20 mg orally daily at bedtime.

Hospital (current) Medications
Aspirin 81 mg orally daily, atorvastatin 80 mg orally daily at bedtime, metoprolol tartrate 50 mg orally twice daily, amiodarone 400 mg orally three times daily, heparin

(continued)

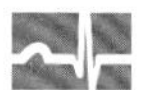

CASE STUDY 2 *(Continued)*

subcutaneous twice daily (DVT prophylaxis), docusate sodium 100 mg orally twice daily, and laxative of choice as needed, hydrocodone/acetaminophen 5 mg orally every 4–6 hours as needed for pain, acetaminophen 500 mg orally every 6 hours as needed for pain.

No known drug allergies.

Patient Examination

Vital Signs

BP 104/58; RR 16 breaths per minute; Temp 37.0°C; HR 75 beats per minute; Ht. 160 cm; Wt. 68 kg

Physical Examination

General: Awake, alert, and oriented. No distress noted.

Skin: Sternal incision intact. Well approximated. Drain sites with dressing intact. Bruising to abdomen at site of heparin injections.

Cardiac: No murmurs, gallops, or rubs are auscultated. S1 and S2 are heard and are of normal intensity.

Respiratory: Mild respiratory distress. Lung sounds are clear in all lobes bilaterally without rales, ronchi, or wheezes.

Abdominal: Abdomen is soft, symmetric, and nontender without distention. No masses, hepatomegaly, or splenomegaly are noted. Bruising to abdomen.

Psychiatric: Appropriate mood and affect. Good judgment and insight. No visual or auditory hallucinations. No suicidal or homicidal ideation.

Testing

HIT panel, CBC

Considerations

Key Questions

A CBC was obtained at postoperative day 3, which showed thrombocytopenia.

The nurse taking care of her on this day recalled that this patient was high risk for HIT and calculated her 4Ts score to estimate the pretest probability of Ms. Thomas having HIT. The following table highlights how her nurse calculated this probability.

4Ts	Ms. Thomas's Score
Thrombocytopenia	1
Timing	2
Thrombosis or other clinical sequelae	1
Other cause for thrombocytopenia not evident	2
Total Score	**6**

The nurse notified the provider of the recent lab results, her calculation of the 4Ts, and requested to obtain further laboratory testing, such as a repeat CBC (to confirm the thrombocytopenia), DIC testing, and testing for HIT antibodies, preferably the platelet activation test. The nurse and provider also discussed cessation of all heparin products, including heparin flushes and low–molecular-weight heparin. Additionally, the nurse and provider discussed treatment options for possible HIT and decided treatment should be initiated with an alternative anticoagulant if HIT was strongly suspected. The provider decided to start argatroban at the recommended dose until laboratory testing ruled out HIT.

KEY READINGS

Cuker A, Burnett A, Triller D, et al. Reversal of direct oral anticoagulants: guidance from the Anticoagulation Forum. *Am J Hematol.* 2019; 94(6):697–709.

Goldhaber SZ. Risk factors for venous thromboembolism. *J Am Coll Cardiol.* 2010;56(1):1–7.

Roberts MK, Chaney S. Heparin-induced thrombocytopenia. *J Nurse Pract.* 2018;14(5):402–408.e3.

Shaw JR, Siegal DM. Pharmacological reversal of the direct oral anticoagulants—a comprehensive review of the literature. *Res Pract Thromb Haemost.* 2018;2:251–265.

REFERENCES

1. Lichtman M, Beutler E, Kipps T. *Williams Hematology.* New York: McGraw-Hill; 2006.
2. Dhainault J, Abraham E, Opal S. Proceedings of the Third Margaux Conference on critical illness: the endothelium--an underrecognized organ in critical illness? Sedona, Arizona, USA. November 14–18, 2001. *Crit Care Med.* 2002;30(5 Suppl):S179–348.
3. Hoffman RS, Benz EJ, Shattil SJ, et al. *Hematology: Basic Physiology and Practice.* 4th ed. Philadelphia, PA: Churchill Livingstone; 2005.
4. Tortora G, Grabowski S. *Principles of Anatomy and Physiology.* New York: John Wiley & Sons; 2003.
5. Turgeon M. *Clinical Hematology: Theory and Procedures.* Philadelphia, PA: Williams & Wilkins; 2005.
6. Hack CE, Zeerleder S. The endothelium in sepsis: source of and a target for inflammation. *Crit Care Med.* 2001;29(7 Suppl):S21–S27.
7. Sorenson ER, Lorme TB, Heath D. Thromboelastography: a means to transfusion reduction. *Nurs Manag (Harrow).* 2005;36:27–34.
8. Kinney MR, Brooks-Brunn J, Molter N, et al. *AACN's Clinical Reference for Critical Care Nursing.* 4th ed. Maryland Heights, MO: Mosby; 1998.
9. Smythe MA, Priziola J, Dobesh PP, et al. Guidance for the practical management of heparin anticoagulants in the treatment of venous thromboembolism. *J Thromb Thrombolysis.* 2016;41(1):165–186.
10. Dellinger RP, Levy MM, Carlet JM, et al. Surviving Sepsis Campaign: international guidelines for management of severe sepsis and septic shock: 2008. *Crit Care Med.* 2008;36(1):296–327.
11. Bernard GR, Vincent JL, Laterre PF, et al. Efficacy and safety of recombinant human activated protein C for severe sepsis. *N Engl J Med.* 2001; 344(10):699–709.
12. Dellinger RP, Schorr CA, Levy MM. A user's guide to the 2016 surviving sepsis guidelines. *Crit Care Med.* 2017;45(3):381–385.
13. Libby P, Ridker PM, Maseri A. Inflammation and atherosclerosis. *Circulation.* 2002;105(9):1135–1143.
14. Libby P. Atherosclerosis: the new view. *Sci Am.* 2002;286(5):46–55.
15. Levi M, Scully M. How I treat disseminated intravascular coagulation. *Blood.* 2018;131(8):845–854.
16. Levi M, Toh CH, Thachil J, et al. Guidelines for the diagnosis and management of disseminated intravascular coagulation. British Committee for Standards in Haematology. *Br J Haematol.* 2009;145(1):24–33.
17. Papageorgiou C, Jourdi G, Adjambri E, et al. Disseminated intravascular coagulation: an update on pathogenesis, diagnosis, and therapeutic strategies. *Clin Appl Thromb Hemost.* 2018;1076029618806424.
18. Owen D, Webster J. *Hematology: Clinical Physiology AACN Clinical Reference for Critical Care Nursing.* St. Louis, MO: C.V. Mosby; 1998.
19. Boral BM, Williams DJ, Boral LI. Disseminated intravascular coagulation. *Am J Clin Pathol.* 2016;146(6):670–680.
20. Merten GJ, Burgess WP, Gray LV, et al. Prevention of contrast-induced nephropathy with sodium bicarbonate: a randomized controlled trial. *JAMA.* 2004;291(19):2328–2334.
21. Liebman H, Weltz I. Disseminated intravascular coagulation. In: Hoffman RS, Benz EJ, Shattil SJ, et al., eds. *Hematology: Basic Physiology and Practice.* 4th ed. Philadelphia, PA: Churchill Livingstone; 2005.
22. Hebert PC. Anemia and red cell transfusion in critical care. Transfusion requirements in Critical Care Investigators and the Canadian Critical Care Trials Group. *Minerva Anestesiol.* 1999;65(5):293–304.

23. Goodnough LT, Shander AS. Recombinant factor VIIa: safety and efficacy. *Curr Opin Hematol.* 2007;14(5):504–509.
24. O'Connell KA, Wood JJ, Wise RP, et al. Thromboembolic adverse events after use of recombinant human coagulation factor VIIa. *JAMA.* 2006;295(3):293–298.
25. Dzieczkowski JS, Tiberghien P, Anderson KC. Transfusion biology and therapy. In: Jameson J, Fauci AS, Kasper DL, et al., eds. *Harrison's Principles of Internal Medicine.* 20th ed. New York: McGraw-Hill; 2018.
26. Jimenez D, Yusen RD, Hull RD. Pulmonary embolism. In: Vincent JL, Abraham E, Moore FA, et al., eds. *Textbook of Critical Care.* 7th ed. Philadelphia, PA: Elsevier; 2017.
27. Wood KE. Major pulmonary embolism: review of a pathophysiologic approach to the golden hour of hemodynamically significant pulmonary embolism. *Chest.* 2002;121(3):877–905.
28. Beckman MG, Hooper WC, Critchley SE, et al. Venous thromboembolism: a public health concern. *Am J Prev Med.* 2010;38(4 Suppl):S495–S501.
29. Goldhaber SZ. Risk factors for venous thromboembolism. *J Am Coll Cardiol.* 2010;56(1):1–7.
30. Kesieme E, Kesieme C, Jebbin N, et al. Deep vein thrombosis: a clinical review. *J Blood Med.* 2011;2:59–69.
31. Shaw JR, Siegal DM. Pharmacological reversal of the direct oral anticoagulants—a comprehensive review of the literature. *Res Pract Thromb Haemost.* 2018;2:251–265.
32. Crowther M. Venous thromboembolism. In: Hoffman RS, Benz EJ, Shattil SJ, et al., eds. *Hematology: Basic Physiology and Practice.* 4th ed. Philadelphia, PA: Churchill Livingstone; 2005.
33. Siegal D, Lim W. Venous thromboembolism. In: Hoffman RS, Benz EJ, Silberstein LE, et al., eds. *Hematology: Basic Principles and Practice.* 7th ed. Philadelphia, PA: Elsevier; 2018.
34. Fahey V. *Vascular Nursing.* Philadelphia, PA: WB Saunders; 1999.
35. Kearon C, Akl EA, Comerota AJ, et al. Antithrombotic therapy for VTE disease: antithrombotic therapy and prevention of thrombosis, 9th ed: American College of Chest Physicians Evidence-Based Clinical Practice Guidelines. *Chest.* 2012;141(2 Suppl):e419S–e496S.
36. Kearon C, Akl EA, Ornelas J, et al. Antithrombotic therapy for VTE disease: CHEST guideline and expert panel report. *Chest.* 2016;149(2):315–352.
37. Blood coagulation and anticoagulant, fibrinolytic, and antiplatelet drugs. In: Hilal-Dandan R, Brunton LL, eds. *Goodman and Gilman's Manual of Pharmacology and Therapeutics.* 2nd ed. New York: McGraw-Hill.
38. Streiff MB, Agnelli G, Connors JM, et al. Guidance for the treatment of deep vein thrombosis and pulmonary embolism. *J Thromb Thrombolysis.* 2016;41(1):32–67.
39. Warkentin TE. Heparin-induced thrombocytopenia. *Hematol Oncol Clin North Am.* 2007;21(4):589–607, v.
40. Warkentin TE. Heparin-induced thrombocytopenia. In: Hoffman RS, Benz E, Silberstein LE, et al., eds. *Hematology: Basic Principles and Practice.* 7th ed. Philadelphia, PA: Elsevier; 2018.
41. Dalen JE. Pulmonary embolism: what have we learned since Virchow?: treatment and prevention. *Chest.* 2002;122(5):1801–1817.
42. Cuker A, Burnett A, Triller D, et al. Reversal of direct oral anticoagulants: guidance from the Anticoagulation Forum. *Am J Hematol.* 2019;94(6):697–709.
43. Bělohlávek J, Dytrych V, Linhart A. Pulmonary embolism, part I: epidemiology, risk factors and risk stratification, pathophysiology, clinical presentation, diagnosis and nonthrombotic pulmonary embolism. *Exp Clin Cardiol.* 2013;18(2):129–138.
44. Goldhaber SZ. Deep venous thrombosis and pulmonary thromboembolism. In: Jameson JL, Fauci AS, Kasper DL, et al., eds. *Harrison's Principles of Internal Medicine.* 20th ed. New York: McGraw-Hill Education; 2018.
45. Bartorelli AL, Marenzi G. Contrast-induced nephropathy. *J Interv Cardiol.* 2008;21(1):74–85.
46. Kidney International. KDIGO clinical practice guideline for acute kidney injury. *Kidney Int.* 2012;2. Available at https://kdigo.org/wp-content/uploads/2016/10/KDIGO-2012-AKI-Guideline-English.pdf
47. Lameire N, Kellum JA. Contrast-induced acute kidney injury and renal support for acute kidney injury: a KDIGO summary (part 2). *Crit Care.* 2013;17(1):205.
48. Warkentin TE. Heparin-induced thrombocytopenia: a clinicopathologic syndrome. *Thromb Haemost.* 1999;82(2):439–447.
49. Linkins LA, Dans AL, Moores LK, et al. Treatment and prevention of heparin-induced thrombocytopenia: antithrombotic therapy and prevention of thrombosis, 9th ed: American College of Chest Physicians Evidence-Based Clinical Practice Guidelines. *Chest.* 2012;141(2 Suppl):e495S–e530S.
50. Warkentin TE, Chong BH, Greinacher A. Heparin-induced thrombocytopenia: towards consensus. *Thromb Haemost.* 1998;79(1):1–7.
51. Roberts MK, Chaney S. Thrombocytopenia, C S. H-. *J Nurse Pract.* 2018;14(5):402–408.e3.
52. Hoffman RS, Benz E, Silberstein LE, et al. *Hematology: Basic Principles and Practice.* 7th ed. Philadelphia, PA: Elsevier; 2018.
53. Warkentin TE. Platelet count monitoring and laboratory testing for heparin-induced thrombocytopenia. *Arch Pathol Lab Med.* 2002;126(11):1415–1423.
54. Price EA, Hayward CP, Moffat KA, et al. Laboratory testing for heparin-induced thrombocytopenia is inconsistent in North America: a survey of North American specialized coagulation laboratories. *Thromb Haemost.* 2007;98(6):1357–1361.
55. Warkentin TE, Greinacher A. Heparin-induced thrombocytopenia: recognition, treatment, and prevention: the Seventh ACCP Conference on Antithrombotic and Thrombolytic Therapy. *Chest.* 2004;126(3 Suppl):311s–337s.

6 Fluid and Electrolyte and Acid–Base Balance and Imbalance

Gabriel Najarro, Kyle Briggs

OBJECTIVES

1. Describe the compartment model of fluid distribution within the body.
2. Understand the factors that lead to dysregulation of this fluid balance and the effects of abnormal fluid balance.
3. Detail the role of potassium, calcium, magnesium, and phosphate balance in normal physiology.
4. Explore the implications of elevated or decreased electrolyte concentrations on cardiac physiology.
5. Explore the principles of acid–base balance, including the primary drivers of imbalance and compensatory mechanisms.

KEY QUESTIONS

1. What are the primary mechanisms by which the body maintains fluid balance?
2. Why do abnormalities in electrolyte concentrations affect the heart and vasculature?
3. How does acidosis contribute to cardiovascular abnormalities?
4. How does alkalosis contribute to cardiovascular abnormalities?

PRINCIPLES OF FLUID BALANCE

The fluid in the body serves many vital functions. In addition to being the environment in which cellular chemistry occurs, it provides the transport medium for oxygen and other nutrients to reach the cells and for carbon dioxide and other metabolic waste products requiring removal from the body. Technically, *fluid* is water and the substances dissolved in it.

With aging, the amount of water in the body decreases. The body ranges from 70% water by weight (newborn infant) to 60% (young or middle-aged adult) to 45% (older adult woman). Women have less water by weight than men because a higher percentage of their weight is fat. Similarly, water is a lower percentage of body weight in obese patients. One liter of water weighs 1 kg (2.2 lb). Thus, a standard 70-kg (154-lb) middle-aged man (60% water) has 42 L of body water (70 kg × 0.60 = 42 kg; 42 kg = 42 L).[1]

Body Fluid Compartments

The fluid in the body lies in several compartments. The *extracellular fluid* consists of vascular and interstitial fluids. Some extracellular fluid is located in bone and dense connective tissue; this fluid is not considered accessible for dynamic exchange. *Intracellular fluid*, as the name indicates, lies within the cells. The *transcellular fluid* is fluid that is secreted by epithelial cells. Examples of transcellular fluid are cerebrospinal fluid (CSF), saliva, and intestinal secretions. Many of the transcellular fluids are reabsorbed by the body after they have been secreted.

More water is located inside the cells than outside of them. Clinically, approximately two thirds of body water in adults is considered intracellular and one third extracellular. Thus, the 70-kg man who has 42 L of body water can be regarded as to have approximately 28 L of water inside the cells and 14 L of extracellular water. This extracellular water is roughly one third vascular and two thirds interstitial. For clinical purposes, the 70-kg man can be considered to have approximately 4.5 L of water in the vascular compartment and about 9.5 L in the interstitial compartment.

Osmolality

The relative proportion of water to particles in body fluid is measured as osmolality. Osmolality can be considered to be the degree of concentration. Technically, osmolality is defined as the number of moles of particles per kilogram of water. The normal range of osmolality of the blood is 280 to 300 mOsm/kg.[2] Fluids that have osmolality within this normal range are called *isotonic*. Extracellular and intracellular fluids have the same osmolality. If the osmolality of the extracellular fluid is increased or decreased, then the osmolality of the intracellular fluid changes rapidly until intracellular and extracellular fluids again have the same osmolality. This process is discussed later in the "Fluid Distribution" section.

Although the osmolality of intracellular and extracellular fluids is the same, the ion composition of the two fluids differs. Thus, they have the same particle concentration, but the specific kinds of particles are different in the two fluids. The intracellular fluid has a higher concentration of protein and potassium, magnesium, and phosphate ions; the extracellular fluid has a higher concentration of sodium, calcium, chloride, and bicarbonate ions.[3] Transcellular fluids are usually hypotonic; their ion composition varies widely depending on their physiologic function.

Processes Involved in Fluid Balance

Fluid balance is the net result of fluid intake, fluid distribution, fluid excretion, and fluid loss by abnormal routes. Fluid balance is maintained when excretion and loss through any abnormal pathways are matched by fluid intake and when the fluid is distributed normally into its compartments.[3]

Fluid Intake

Habit is the primary determinant of fluid intake in a healthy adult. Thirst, another critical determinant of fluid intake, can be triggered by several physiologic mechanisms.[4] These include dryness of the oral mucous membranes, an increase in osmolality of the body fluids (osmoreceptor-mediated thirst), decrease in extracellular fluid volume (ECV) (baroreceptor-mediated thirst), and increased renin secretion (angiotensin-mediated thirst). Osmoreceptor-mediated thirst is the most common cause of thirst in healthy adults. This mechanism becomes less effective with aging. Thus, older adults often have a greater need for water before they become thirsty. Cultural factors have an important influence on fluid intake. For example, consumption of specific herbal teas may be considered necessary by some individuals when they become ill. Many patients refuse to drink cold water when they have certain illnesses due to their cultural beliefs. In clinical settings, health care professionals often regulate fluid intake. Routes of fluid intake include oral, rectal, intravenous, and intraosseous, as well as through tubes into body cavities. Oral fluid intake includes liquids and the water contained in food, as well as water made by cellular metabolism of ingested nutrients.

Fluid Distribution

Two types of fluid distribution operate in the body. First, fluid is distributed between the vascular and interstitial spaces, the two subcompartments of the extracellular compartment. Second, fluid is distributed between the extracellular and intracellular compartments. Different processes regulate these two types of fluid distribution.

Filtration is regulated by the fluid distribution between the vascular and interstitial spaces. Filtration is the net result of four opposing forces. Two of these forces tend to move fluid out of the capillaries, whereas the other two tend to move fluid into the capillaries. Which direction the fluid moves in any one location depends on which forces are stronger. The two primary forces that drive fluid out of capillaries are the blood hydrostatic pressure (outward force against the capillary walls) and the interstitial fluid osmotic pressure (inward pulling force caused by particles within interstitial fluid). The two forces that tend to move fluid into capillaries are the blood osmotic pressure (inward pulling force caused by particles in the blood) and the interstitial fluid hydrostatic pressure.

Usually, the blood hydrostatic pressure is highest at the arterial end of a capillary, and there is filtration from the capillary into the interstitial fluid (Fig. 6-1). This flow of fluid out of the capillaries is useful in carrying oxygen, glucose, amino acids, and other nutrients to the cells that are surrounded by interstitial fluid. Most

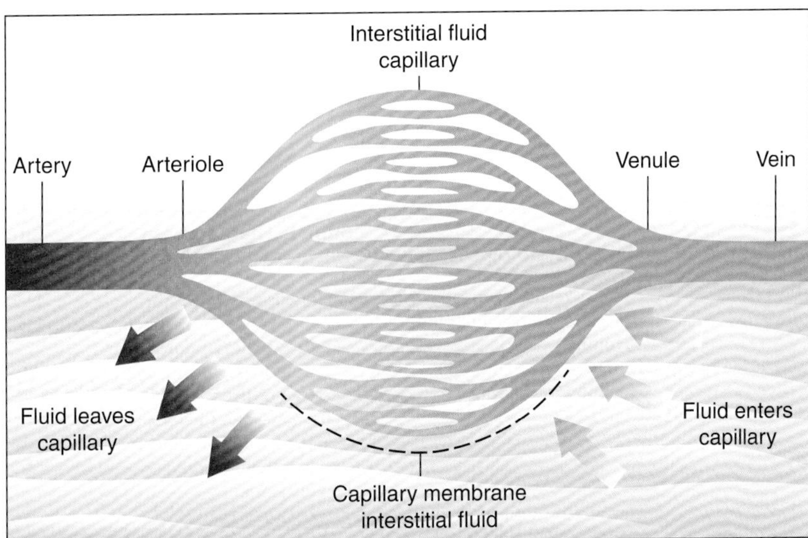

Figure 6-1. Understanding Fluid Balance. Normally, fluid moves freely between the interstitial and intravascular spaces to maintain homeostasis. Four basic types of pressure control fluid shifts across the capillary membrane that separates these spaces: capillary hydrostatic pressure (internal fluid pressure on the capillary membrane), interstitial fluid pressure (external fluid pressure on the capillary membrane), osmotic pressure (fluid-attracting pressure from protein concentration within the capillary), and interstitial osmotic pressure (fluid-attracting pressure from protein concentration outside the capillary). Here's how these pressures maintain homeostasis: Normally, capillary hydrostatic pressure is greater than plasma osmotic pressure at the capillary's arterial end, forcing fluid out of the capillary. At the capillary's venous end, the reverse is true: The plasma osmotic pressure is greater than the capillary hydrostatic pressure, drawing fluid into the capillary. Normally, the lymphatic system transports excess interstitial fluid back to the intravascular space. Edema results when this balance is upset by increased capillary permeability, lymphatic obstruction, persistently increased capillary hydrostatic pressure, decreased plasma osmotic or interstitial fluid pressure, or dilation of precapillary sphincters. (From Lippincott's Nursing Advisor, 2009.)

proteins are too large to cross into the interstitial fluid and remain in the capillary. At the venous end of a capillary, the blood's hydrostatic pressure is usually lower and the blood osmotic pressure higher because fluid has left the capillary, but the proteins have remained. These changes cause a net flow of fluid from the interstitial space back into the venous end of a capillary. The flow of fluid back into the capillaries is physiologically useful in carrying carbon dioxide, metabolic acids, and other waste products into the blood for further metabolism or excretion.

Changes in any of the four forces that determine the direction of filtration at the capillaries can cause abnormal distribution between the vascular and interstitial compartments. The most common abnormal distribution is edema, which is an expansion of the interstitial space. Edema can be caused by increased blood hydrostatic pressure (e.g., venous congestion), increased microvascular permeability that allows proteins to leak into interstitial fluid, increased interstitial fluid osmotic pressure (e.g., inflammation), decreased blood osmotic pressure (e.g., hypoalbuminemia), or blockage of the lymphatic system, which normally removes excess fluid from the interstitial space and returns it to the vascular compartment.

The second type of fluid distribution occurs between the extracellular and intracellular compartments. This process is regulated by osmosis. Cell membranes are freely permeable to water, but the passage of ions and other particles depends on membrane transport processes. Osmotic pressure is an inward-pulling force caused by particles in a fluid. Both the extracellular and intracellular fluids exert osmotic pressure. Because the osmolality of the two compartments is typically the same, the osmotic pressures are the same.

Therefore, the force pulling water into the cells balances the force pulling water into the interstitial space, maintaining the normal fluid distribution. If the osmolality of the extracellular fluid changes, however, then osmosis occurs, altering the fluid distribution until the osmolality in the extracellular and intracellular compartments again is the same. For example, if the extracellular fluid becomes more concentrated (increased osmolality), then the osmotic pressure of the extracellular fluid becomes higher than the osmotic pressure of the intracellular fluid. Water leaves the intracellular compartment until the intracellular fluid becomes as concentrated as the extracellular fluid. This process decreases the amount of water that is distributed into the intracellular compartment.

Similarly, if the extracellular fluid becomes more dilute (decreased osmolality), then the osmotic pressure of the extracellular fluid becomes lower than the osmotic pressure of the intracellular fluid. Water moves by osmosis into the intracellular compartment until the intracellular fluid becomes as dilute as the extracellular fluid. This process increases the amount of water that is distributed into the intracellular compartment.

In summary, fluid distribution between the vascular and interstitial compartments depends on filtration, the net result of four forces that act on fluid at the capillary level. The fluid distribution between the extracellular and intracellular compartments depends on osmosis, the movement of water across cell membranes to equilibrate particle concentrations.

Fluid Excretion

Normal routes of fluid excretion are respiratory tract, urine, feces, and skin. In a standard adult, approximately 400 mL of water is excreted daily through the respiratory tract, even if the person is fluid depleted. This amount increases during fever. The urine volume of a healthy adult averages 1500 mL/day and varies according to the fluid intake, the needs of the body, and the hormonal status. Major hormones that regulate urinary excretion of fluid are summarized in Table 6-1. Diuretics, ethanol, and high doses of caffeine increase urine volume.[5,6] Fecal excretion of water averages 200 mL/day in healthy adults who have a normal fluid balance

Table 6-1 • HORMONES THAT REGULATE RENAL FLUID EXCRETION

Hormone	Physiologic Source	Major Physiologic Actions	Stimuli That Increase Hormone Secretion	Stimuli That Decrease Hormone Secretion
Aldosterone	Adrenal cortex (zona glomerulosa)	Kidneys retain more saline (this expands extracellular fluid volume) Kidneys excrete more potassium and hydrogen ions	Angiotensin II (from the renin–angiotensin system; kidneys release more renin during hypovolemia and other causes of decreased blood flow through the renal artery and by stimulation of renal sympathetic nerves) Hypokalemia	Decreased angiotensin II Hyperkalemia
Natriuretic peptides	*A-type natriuretic peptide*: atrial myocardium *B-type natriuretic peptide*: ventricular myocardium *C-type natriuretic peptide*: endothelial cells	Natriuresis (kidneys excrete more saline, which reduces extracellular fluid volume) Vasodilation (suppresses endothelin; arterioles dilate, which reduces peripheral vascular resistance and lowers blood pressure) Suppression of renin–angiotensin system	*A-type natriuretic peptide*: atrial dilation (stretch) *B-type natriuretic peptide*: increased ventricular end-diastolic pressure and volume *C-type natriuretic peptide*: vascular shear stress	*A-type natriuretic peptide*: lack of atrial dilation (decreased stretch) *B-type natriuretic peptide*: normal or decreased ventricular end-diastolic pressure and volume *C-type natriuretic peptide*: reduced vascular shear stress
Antidiuretic hormone (ADH)	Synthesized in preoptic and paraventricular nuclei of hypothalamus Secreted from posterior pituitary gland	Kidneys retain more water (this dilutes body fluids, decreasing osmolality)	Increased osmolality of body fluids Hypovolemia Physiologic and psychological stressors, surgery/anesthesia, trauma, pain, nausea	Decreased osmolality of body fluids Hypervolemia Ethanol

and a fully functioning bowel. Diarrhea causes a dramatic increase in fecal excretion of water.

Fluid is excreted through the skin as either insensible or sensible perspiration. Insensible perspiration is fluid excretion through the skin that is not visible. It averages 500 mL/day in a healthy adult. Insensible perspiration occurs even if the person is fluid depleted. It increases during fever. Sensible perspiration or sweat is visible fluid excretion through the skin. The volume of sweat varies greatly depending primarily on thermoregulatory needs.

Fluid Loss by Abnormal Routes

Examples of abnormal routes of fluid loss are emesis, drains, suction, paracentesis, and hemorrhage. Third-spacing (e.g., ascites) can be considered abnormal fluid loss, even though the fluid remains in the body because the fluid is not freely available to the normal fluid compartments.

Summary of Fluid Balance

In summary, the processes of fluid intake, fluid distribution, fluid excretion, and fluid loss by abnormal routes act together to determine fluid balance or imbalances. A change in one of these processes must be matched by a change in another to maintain fluid balance. For example, if increased urine output and increased fluid intake are matched, then the fluid balance can be maintained. Fluid imbalance occurs when one or more of these processes are altered in isolation. Fluid imbalances are characterized by an altered volume of fluid (ECV imbalances), the altered concentration of fluid (osmolality imbalances), or a combination of both.

EXTRACELLULAR FLUID VOLUME BALANCE

The ECV is the net result of fluid intake, fluid distribution, fluid excretion, and fluid loss by abnormal routes. A normal ECV is maintained when fluid excretion and any fluid loss are balanced by fluid intake, and when the fluid distribution is normal. The body's responsiveness to the administration of a fluid load has a circadian rhythm (i.e., varies cyclically over 24 hours). The kidneys can excrete an excess fluid load more efficiently if it is administered during the time that the person is normally active than if it is administered during a person's customary sleeping time.

The blood volume is a key determinant of the work of the heart and provides the medium for oxygen delivery to tissues. Therefore, ECV imbalances can interfere with cardiac function and tissue oxygenation.

Extracellular Fluid Volume Deficit

ECV deficit is caused by the removal of sodium-containing fluid from the vascular and interstitial spaces. Usually, the fluid is removed from the body; however, in some cases, fluid is sequestered in the peritoneal cavity, the intestinal lumen, or some other "third space." ECV deficits occur when intake of sodium-containing fluid does not keep pace with increased fluid excretion or loss of fluid through abnormal routes. Clinical causes of ECV deficit are presented in Table 6-2. ECV deficit may develop in patients with cardiac disease who use diuretics if the dosage is excessive.

Clinical manifestations of ECV deficit include sudden weight loss (unless there is third-spacing), poor skin turgor, dryness of opposing mucous membranes, hard dry stools, longitudinal furrows in the tongue, absence of tears and sweat, and soft, sunken eyeballs. Although weight loss occurs immediately, most of these signs appear only after substantial fluid depletion. Cardiovascular manifestations are among the early signs; these are discussed next.

Table 6-2 • CAUSES OF EXTRACELLULAR FLUID VOLUME DEFICIT

Category	Clinical Examples
Excessive removal of gastrointestinal fluid	Diarrhea Emesis Gastrointestinal fistula drainage Nasogastric or intestinal tube suctioning or drainage
Excessive renal excretion of saline	Adrenal insufficiency Diuresis due to bed rest Excessive use of diuretics
Excessive removal of sodium-containing fluid by other routes	Hemorrhage Third-space accumulation Burns Excessive diaphoresis

Many of the clinical manifestations of ECV deficit are evident in the cardiovascular system. Decreased volume in the vascular compartment causes postural blood pressure drop with postural tachycardia, delayed capillary refill, prolonged small vein filling time, flat neck veins when supine (or neck veins that collapse during inspiration), and decreased central venous pressure.

A postural blood pressure drop is assessed by measuring blood pressure and heart rate with the individual supine and then standing or sitting with the legs dependent (not horizontal). If systemic blood pressure decreases substantially and heart rate increases significantly, then these postural changes are due to ECV deficit. The increased heart rate indicates that autonomic reflexes are functioning and rules out autonomic insufficiency, which may cause standing blood pressure to decrease when the ECV is normal. Postural blood pressure drop is not a reliable assessment for ECV deficit in individuals who have a transplanted heart due to surgical denervation. Thus, the heart rate may not increase in these individuals when their blood pressure drops from ECV deficit.[7]

The venous fluid load may be assessed by examining jugular vein distention. While the patient is sitting at 30 degrees, have the patient turn their head to the left. Identify jugular vein pulsations posterior to the sternocleidomastoid muscle. Measure the height of the wave above the clavicle and add 5. This value results in an estimate of right atrial pressure, generally between 8 and 12, and correlates with total ECV.[8]

The decreased preload of ECV deficit leads to decreased cardiac output, with resulting dizziness, syncope, and oliguria. If ECV deficit becomes severe, tachycardia, pallor caused by cutaneous vasoconstriction, and other manifestations of hypovolemic shock occur.

Extracellular Fluid Volume Excess

Excess ECV is an overload of fluid in the vascular and interstitial compartments. It is common in individuals with heart failure because their decreased cardiac output activates the renin–angiotensin–aldosterone system (RAAS).[9] Aldosterone causes renal retention of sodium and water, which expands the extracellular volume. Patients who have hypertension caused by elevated renin also develop ECV excess. Other causes of ECV excess are listed in Table 6-3. Clinical manifestations of ECV excess include sudden

Table 6-3 • CAUSES OF EXTRACELLULAR FLUID VOLUME EXCESS

Category	Clinical Examples
Excessive infusion of isotonic, sodium-containing solutions	Excessive normal saline (0.9% NaCl) Excessive Ringer's or lactated Ringer's
Renal retention of saline	Endocrine: Excessive aldosterone (CHF, cirrhosis, hyperaldosteronism); excessive glucocorticoids (Cushing syndrome, pharmacologic doses of glucocorticoids) Renal: Oliguric renal failure

CHF, congestive heart failure.

weight gain, peripheral edema, and the cardiovascular effects described next.

Increased vascular volume is manifested by bounding pulse, distended neck veins when upright, and elevated central venous pressure. The crackles, dyspnea, and orthopnea of pulmonary edema may be present. A sudden overload of isotonic fluid increases cardiac work and may cause heart failure, especially in an older adult or an infant.

OSMOLALITY BALANCE

The osmolality of body fluids is determined by the relative proportion of particles and water. The serum sodium concentration usually parallels the osmolality of the blood. When the serum sodium concentration is abnormally low, the osmolality is decreased; in other words, the blood is relatively too dilute (Fig. 6-2). Conversely, when the serum sodium concentration is elevated, the osmolality is increased; in that case, the blood is relatively too concentrated. Antidiuretic hormone (ADH), also called vasopressin (see Table 6-1), is the principal regulator of osmolality.

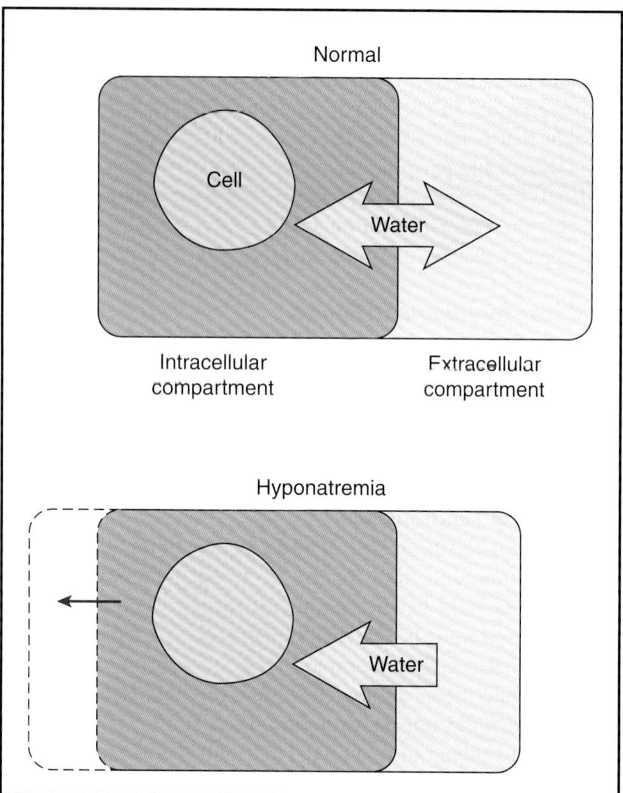

Figure 6-2. Osmolality in Hyponatremia. The hypo-osmolality of hyponatremia causes water to enter cells by osmosis. (From Lippincott's Professional Development Programs, February 2013 release.)

Hyponatremia

Hyponatremia is a relative excess of water that causes a decreased serum sodium concentration (Fig. 6-3). It is caused by a gain of water relative to salt or a loss of salt relative to water (Table 6-4). ADH increases the reabsorption of water by the distal renal tubules and collecting ducts, thus diluting body fluids. After cardiac surgery, hyponatremia may occur in the first few days after surgery from excess free water administration, the physiologic stress of surgery, anesthesia, pain, and nausea which all increase the secretion of ADH.[1] Hyponatremia is common in individuals with chronic heart failure as decreased cardiac output stimulates arterial baroreceptors, triggering nonosmotic release of ADH.[10] Diuretic therapy also contributes to hyponatremia, as discussed below. Hyponatremia in hospitalized heart failure patients is associated with prolonged hospitalization and increased in-hospital and postdischarge mortality.[11,12] Although clinical trials have shown that vaptans, aquaretic drugs that block vasopressin-2 receptors in the kidney, are capable of correcting hyponatremia in hyponatremic heart failure patients, any improvement in morbidity or mortality has yet to be demonstrated.[13] In patients with either ST-elevation myocardial infarction (MI) or suspected acute coronary syndrome, non–ST-elevation MI, hyponatremia is associated with adverse outcomes such as death or recurrent MI.

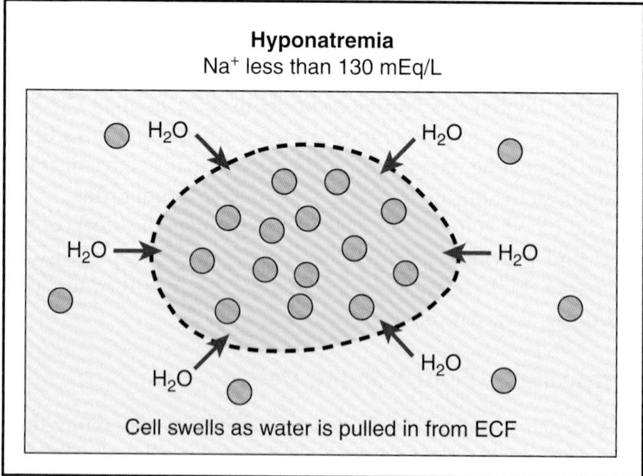

Figure 6-3. Hyponatremia. Hyponatremia may be due to excessive sodium loss or excessive water intake. Sodium can be lost through the kidneys, the GI tract, or the skin. Aggressive use of diuretics, especially if the patient is not ingesting sodium, can produce severe hyponatremia. Excess intake of water can cause dilutional hyponatremia. This may be due to compulsive water drinking, called psychogenic polydipsia, or it may be due to excessive parenteral administration of dextrose and water solutions. (From Lippincott's Professional Development Programs, February 2013 release.)

Table 6-4 • CAUSES OF HYPONATREMIA

Category	Clinical Examples
Gain of water relative to salt	Endocrine: Excessive ADH (ectopic production; stimulation by surgery/anesthesia, stressors, pain, nausea) Iatrogenic: Excessive infusion of D5W, tap water enemas, or water ingestion (after poisoning or before ultrasound examination); absorption of water from hypotonic irrigation solution Other: Near-drowning in fresh water; excessive ingestion of low-sodium fluid such as water (psychogenic polydipsia) or beer (beer potomania)
Loss of salt relative to water	Gastrointestinal: Replacement of water but not salt after emesis, diarrhea, or nasogastric suction; removal of sodium with hypotonic irrigation Renal: Diuretics, especially thiazides; salt-wasting renal diseases Other: Replacement of water but not salt after excessive diaphoresis

The most common medications used by patients with cardiovascular disease that may cause hyponatremia are diuretics, especially the thiazide diuretics and the thiazide-like diuretic indapamide.[14] Hyponatremia from thiazide diuretics occurs more frequently in women than men, especially in older women. However, this observation has been variable in more recent data.[13]

The hypo-osmolality of hyponatremia causes water to enter cells by osmosis. The clinical manifestations of hyponatremia are primarily nonspecific markers of cerebral dysfunction: malaise, confusion, lethargy, seizures, and coma. The extent of these manifestations depends on the speed with which hyponatremia develops as well as its severity. Hyponatremia rarely has significant clinical effects on cardiac electrophysiology and has been limited to case studies.[15]

Hypernatremia

Hypernatremia is a relative deficit of water that causes an increased serum sodium concentration (Fig. 6-4). It is caused by a loss of water relative to salt or a gain of salt relative to water (Table 6-5). The hyperosmolality of hypernatremia causes water to leave cells by osmosis. The clinical manifestations are similar to those of hyponatremia: malaise, confusion, lethargy, seizures, and coma.[3] Thirst (except in some older adults) and oliguria (except in hypernatremia caused by decreased ADH) may also occur. As with hyponatremia, the extent of these manifestations depends on the speed with which hypernatremia develops as well as its severity. Hypernatremia is much less common than hyponatremia in cardiac patients who do not have other pathophysiologies, although it is common in critically ill patients. Hypernatremia also does not have significant clinical effects on cardiac electrophysiology but has been shown to decrease left ventricular contractility.[16]

Mixed ECV and Osmolality Imbalances

ECV and osmolality imbalances may occur at the same time in the same person. For example, in a person who has severe gastroenteritis without proper fluid replacement, concurrent ECV deficit, and hypernatremia (clinical dehydration) will develop. Fluid lost from emesis and diarrhea, plus the usual daily fluid

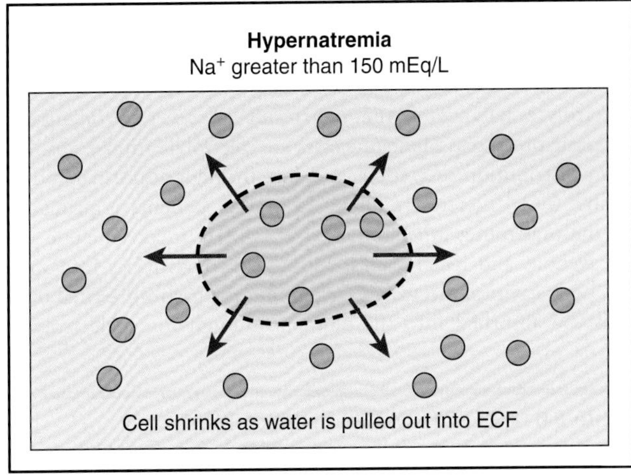

Figure 6-4. Hypernatremia. Hypernatremia may be due to an excessive intake of sodium, or from a loss of water. Sodium intake may be increased by rapid infusion of saline, especially hypertonic saline, and by rapid infusion of sodium bicarbonate. Near-drowning in salt water can also be responsible. Excessive water loss may be due to watery diarrhea, excessive sweating, hypertonic tube feedings, diabetes insipidus, and even through rapid breathing. Being deprived of water can also cause hypernatremia. It may be due to a physical inability to obtain or ingest water, such as when a fluid deprivation test is being done or an oral injury has occurred. It may also be due to injury of the thirst center in the brain. (From Lippincott's Professional Development Programs, February 2013 release.)

excretion (urine, feces, respiratory, insensible sweat), is hypotonic sodium-containing fluid (analogous to isotonic saline that has extra water added). Frequently, patients with chronic heart failure develop concurrent ECV excess and diuretic-induced hyponatremia, also known as hypervolemic hyponatremia.

The signs and symptoms of such mixed fluid imbalances are a combination of the clinical manifestations of the two separate imbalances. In the example of clinical dehydration, the individual has the sudden weight loss, indications of decreased vascular volume, and signs of decreased interstitial volume that result from ECV deficit plus the thirst and nonspecific signs of cerebral dysfunction that result from hypernatremia. In heart failure, the clinical manifestations include the weight gain, distended neck veins, and edema of ECV excess plus the nonspecific signs of cerebral dysfunction of hyponatremia.

Table 6-5 • CAUSES OF HYPERNATREMIA

Category	Clinical Examples
Loss of water relative to salt	Endocrine: Lack of ADH (diabetes insipidus) Renal: Osmotic diuresis; renal concentrating disorders Other: Inadequate water replacement after diarrhea or excessive diaphoresis
Gain of salt relative to water	Decreased intake of water: Inability to respond to thirst (coma, aphasia, paralysis, confusion); lack of access to water; difficulty swallowing fluids (advanced parkinsonism); prolonged nausea Increased intake of salt: Excessive hypertonic NaCl or $NaHCO_3$; near-drowning in salt water; tube feedings without adequate water intake

PRINCIPLES OF ELECTROLYTE BALANCE

Electrolyte balance is the net result of several concurrent dynamic processes. These processes are electrolyte intake, absorption, distribution, excretion, and loss through abnormal routes (Table 6-6).[3] Electrolyte intake in healthy patients is primarily by the oral route; other routes of electrolyte intake include the intravenous and rectal routes, and also through tubes into various body cavities. Electrolytes taken into the gastrointestinal tract must be absorbed into the blood. Although some electrolytes (e.g., potassium) are absorbed readily by mechanisms based on gradients, the absorption of other electrolytes (e.g., calcium and magnesium) is more complex and can be impaired by many factors.

Electrolytes are distributed into all body fluids, but their concentrations in the different body fluid compartments vary greatly. Substantial amounts of most electrolytes are located in pools outside the extracellular fluid. For example, the primary repository of potassium is inside cells; the primary repository of calcium is in the bones.

Electrolyte excretion occurs through the normal routes of urine, feces, and sweat. Any removal of electrolytes through other

Table 6-6 • ELECTROLYTE HOMEOSTASIS

Electrolyte	Sources of Intake	Absorption	Electrolyte Pool	Distribution	Excretion
Potassium (K^+)	*Foods:* Almonds Apricots Bananas Cantaloupe Coffee (instant) Dates Molasses Oranges Peaches Potatoes Prunes Raisins Strawberries *Intravenous:* Packed red blood cells or whole blood; penicillin G	Based on gradient between lumen and blood concentrations	Inside cells	*Cause shift into cells:* β-Adrenergic agonists Insulin Alkalosis *Cause shift out of cells:* Acidosis caused by mineral acids Lack of insulin Cell death	*Urinary:* Increased by increased flow in distal nephron, glucocorticoids Aldosterone causes K^+ excretion *Fecal:* Increased with diarrhea *Sweat*
Calcium (Ca^{2+})	*Foods:* Beet greens Broccoli Dairy products Farina Kale Milk chocolate Oranges Salmon (canned) Sardines Tofu	Most efficient in duodenum; increased by vitamin D Decreased by phosphates, phytates, oxalates, increased intestinal pH, undigested fat, diarrhea, glucocorticoids	Physiologically unavailable when bound in blood to proteins and small organic anions Bones	*Cause more binding in blood:* Alkalosis Citrate in blood products Protein plasma expanders Increased free fatty acids *Cause shift into bones:* Lack of parathyroid hormone *Cause shift from bones:* Parathyroid hormone High-protein diet Glucocorticoids Immobility	*Urinary:* Decreased by parathyroid hormone Increased by saline diuresis, high-protein diet *Fecal:* Increased with undigested fat *Sweat*
Magnesium (Mg^{2+})	*Foods:* Cocoa Chocolate Dried beans and peas Green leafy vegetables Hard water Nuts Peanut butter Sea salt Whole grains	Most efficient in terminal ileum Decreased by phosphates, phytate, undigested fat, alcohol, diarrhea Increased by lactose	Physiologically unavailable when bound in blood to proteins and small organic anions Bones Inside cells	*Cause more binding in blood:* Citrate in blood products Increased free fatty acids *Cause shift from bones:* Parathyroid hormone *Cause shift into cells:* Epinephrine Insulin	*Urinary:* Increased with extracellular fluid volume expansion, rising blood alcohol, high-protein diet, acidosis *Fecal:* Increased with undigested fat, increased aldosterone *Sweat*
Phosphate (P_i)	*Foods:* Eggs Meat Milk Processed foods Almost all foods have some phosphates	Decreased by aluminum and magnesium antacids, diarrhea	Inside cells	*Cause shift into cells:* Epinephrine Insulin Increased cellular metabolism *Cause shift out of cells:* Ketoacidosis Cell death *Cause shift out of bones:* Parathyroid hormone Immobility	*Urinary:* Increased by parathyroid hormone, phosphatonins, extracellular fluid volume expansion *Fecal* *Sweat*

From Felver L. Fluid and electrolyte balance and imbalances. In: Woods SL, Froelicher ES, Halpenny CJ, et al., eds. *Cardiac Nursing*. 3rd ed. Philadelphia, PA: JB Lippincott; 1995:126.

routes could be considered a loss of electrolytes through an abnormal route. Examples of these abnormal routes are emesis, nasogastric suction, fistula drainage, and hemorrhage.

To maintain the balance of any specific electrolyte, intake and absorption must equal to excretion and loss through abnormal routes, and the electrolyte must be distributed properly within the body. Alterations in any of these processes can cause an electrolyte imbalance.[3]

ELECTROLYTE IMBALANCES

Plasma electrolyte imbalances can have profound effects on cardiovascular function. Because cardiac function depends on ion currents across myocardial cell membranes, action potential generation, impulse conduction, and myocardial contraction are all vulnerable to alterations in electrolyte status. In addition to their effects on the myocardium itself, some electrolyte imbalances have vascular effects.

Potassium Balance

Potassium balance is the net result of potassium intake and absorption, distribution, excretion, and abnormal losses. These components are summarized in Table 6-6. Although the plasma potassium concentration describes the status of potassium in the extracellular fluid, it does not necessarily reflect the amount of potassium inside the cells. The plasma potassium concentration has a circadian rhythm, rising during the hours a person is usually active and reaching its trough when a person is typically asleep. A classic study demonstrated that the kidneys handle an intravenous potassium load much less efficiently during the hours a person is customarily sleeping, which has implications for potassium administration to ICU patients.[17]

The potassium concentration of the extracellular fluid has a major influence on the function of the myocardium. Specifically, the resting membrane potential of cardiac cells is proportional to the ratio of potassium concentrations in the intracellular and extracellular fluids. The potassium concentration within cardiac cells is approximately 140 mEq/L; the normal potassium concentration of the extracellular fluid is 3.5 to 5 mEq/L. A small change in the extracellular concentration of potassium has a significant effect on the intracellular to extracellular concentration ratio because the initial extracellular value is relatively small. A similar change in the intracellular potassium concentration has a lesser effect because the initial intracellular value is relatively large.

Hypokalemia

Hypokalemia, a decrease in the plasma potassium concentration, is caused by decreased potassium intake, the shift of potassium ions from the extracellular fluid into the cells, increased excretion of potassium, loss of potassium through an abnormal route, or any combination of these factors.[3] Some specific etiologic factors in these categories are listed in Table 6-7. Hypokalemia is common in patients with heart failure because of their increased activation of the RAAS and their diuretic therapy, and it is associated with increased mortality in ambulatory patients who have chronic heart failure.[18,19]

Catecholamine and β-agonist drugs cause potassium ions to shift into cells by a β_2-adrenergic mechanism. This effect can produce hypokalemia.[20] Plasma catecholamines increase rapidly during MI, and hypokalemia is common during acute coronary syndromes. This hypokalemic effect is not as strong in patients who have diabetic autonomic neuropathy.[21] Transient hypokalemia associated with catecholamine release during an MI may cause further impairment of an already compromised myocardium.

Table 6-7 • CAUSES OF HYPOKALEMIA

Category	Clinical Examples
Decreased potassium intake	NPO orders Anorexia Fad diets Fasting Prolonged IV therapy without K^+
Potassium shift into cells	Alkalosis Excessive β_2-adrenergic stimulation (epinephrine, β-agonists) Hypothermia (accidental or induced) Excessive insulin Rapid correction of acidosis during hemodialysis Familial periodic paralysis
Increased potassium excretion	Diarrhea (includes laxative overuse) Hyperaldosteronism (increases renal excretion of potassium) Chronic excessive ingestion of black licorice (contains aldosterone-like compounds) Excessive glucocorticoids (Cushing syndrome; glucocorticoid therapy) Hypomagnesemia (causes renal potassium wasting) Diuretic therapy with loop or thiazide diuretics or mannitol Polyuria High-dose penicillin therapy (nonreabsorbable anion effect in kidney)
Potassium loss by abnormal route	Emesis Nasogastric suction Drainage from gastrointestinal fistula Dialysis

IV, intravenous.

The increased potassium excretion caused by many types of diuretics is well known.[19,22] Hypokalemia caused by diuretic therapy occurs most frequently within 2 to 8 weeks, although it may arise after more than 1 year.[23] The necessity of monitoring the plasma potassium concentration in individuals using diuretics, especially hospitalized older adults, is clear.[24] Individuals with hypokalemia have significantly more ventricular arrhythmias after MI than do normokalemic individuals. The hypokalemic effect of catecholamines is stronger in patients who are using thiazide diuretics than it is in those who are not using diuretics.

Because of the cardiac effects of hypokalemia, the National Council on Potassium in Clinical Practice has established guidelines for potassium replacement.[25] For individuals with hypertension, the guideline is to maintain a serum potassium concentration of at least 4.0 mEq/L. Potassium replacement should be considered routinely in patients with congestive heart failure, even with a serum potassium level of 4.0 mEq/L. Potassium levels of at least 4.0 mEq/L are necessary for individuals who have cardiac arrhythmias. The guidelines also emphasize the necessity of routine monitoring of serum potassium in patients who have congestive heart failure or cardiac arrhythmias.

Clinical manifestations of hypokalemia include diminished bowel sounds, abdominal distention, constipation, polyuria, skeletal muscle weakness, flaccid paralysis, cardiac arrhythmias, and postural hypotension. Cardiac and vascular effects of hypokalemia are discussed next.

Cardiac Effects of Hypokalemia. The cardiac effects of hypokalemia center on the resulting changes to the membrane resting potential of the cardiac myocyte. When the extracellular potassium concentration decreases, the gradient between extracellular and intracellular potassium increases. This increased gradient causes a decrease in resting membrane potential. In this hyperpolarized state, the myocytes are less responsive to stimuli from neighboring myocytes and can make the initiation of depolarization more difficult. Additionally, hypokalemia will prolong the action potential duration and refractory periods as the cell works to reestablish the cellular membrane gradient.[26] The specific alteration of cardiac cell membrane resting potential thus depends on the degree of hypokalemia. Furthermore, as the action potential is different between myocytes in the sinoatrial node, atria, atrioventricular node, bundle branches, and myocardium, the combination of these effects can cause a wide variety of arrhythmias and conduction delays.

Hypokalemia-induced arrhythmias include supraventricular premature depolarizations and tachycardias, ventricular ectopic beats, ventricular tachycardia, torsade de pointes, and ventricular fibrillation.[27,28] Hypokalemia-induced arrhythmias are particularly prevalent in the setting of heart failure or acute MI.[29] Hypokalemia also potentiates digoxin toxicity, which in turn may produce various arrhythmias.[30]

As might be expected from the previous discussion, electrocardiographic (ECG) changes are seen in individuals with hypokalemia. While a characteristic change is the development of U waves, typically, T-wave flattening is the earliest ECG change.[31,32] Other ECG changes include the increased amplitude of P waves, prolonged PR interval, prolonged QT or QU interval, inverted T waves, and ST-segment depression.[33]

Long-standing hypokalemia is associated with selective myocardial cell necrosis. Selective myocardial cell necrosis is associated with sudden cardiac death.

Vascular Effects of Hypokalemia. In addition to the multiple cardiac effects discussed previously, hypokalemia has vascular effects. Postural hypotension often occurs in hypokalemia, most likely caused by impaired smooth muscle function.

Classic studies indicate that chronic potassium depletion in humans impairs vasodilation during strenuous exercise.[34] The resulting impaired muscle blood flow decreases oxygen delivery and contributes to the rhabdomyolysis that occurs with whole-body potassium depletion.[35]

Hyperkalemia

Hyperkalemia, an increased plasma potassium concentration, results from increased potassium intake, the shift of potassium ions from the cells to the extracellular fluid, decreased potassium excretion, or any combination of these factors. Examples of specific etiologic factors in each of these categories are listed in Table 6-8. Hyperkalemia may occur during hemorrhagic or hypovolemic shock and cardiopulmonary resuscitation.

Several medications commonly administered to individuals with cardiac disease may cause hyperkalemia. *Angiotensin-converting enzyme inhibitors* such as captopril and enalapril, *angiotensin II receptor blockers* such as losartan, *selective aldosterone blockers* such as eplerenone, and *direct renin inhibitors* such as aliskiren decrease the release of aldosterone. Aldosterone normally facilitates renal excretion of potassium. When these drugs decrease the availability of aldosterone, hyperkalemia may occur. The *potassium-sparing diuretics* spironolactone, triamterene, and amiloride may cause hyperkalemia, especially if given with potassium supplementation or angiotensin-converting enzyme inhibitors or used by patients who have any degree of renal impairment. *Nonselective β-adrenergic blockers* promote the development of hyperkalemia by blocking catecholamine action at β_2 receptors that normally stimulate potassium entry into cells.[36] The hyperkalemic effect of β-blockade is especially pronounced during exercise, which has relevance to treadmill stress testing and is enhanced in patients who take digitalis.[37,38] Administration of either unfractionated or low–molecular-weight *heparin*, even in low-dose therapy, decreases the synthesis of aldosterone; hyperkalemia is likely to occur in heparinized individuals who only have mild renal insufficiency.[38] A *digitalis overdose* causes hyperkalemia by impairing its movement back into cells and thus accumulating in the extracellular space.[36]

Table 6-8 • CAUSES OF HYPERKALEMIA

Category	Clinical Examples
Increased potassium intake	Excessive IV potassium
	Insufficiently mixed KCl in flexible plastic IV bag
	Massive transfusion of blood stored longer than 3 days (K^+ leaves red blood cells)
	Large doses of IV potassium penicillin G (contains 1.6 mEq K^+/million units)
	Large oral intake only if decreased renal excretion
Potassium shift out of cells	Acidosis due to mineral acids (not organic acids like ketoacids)
	Insulin deficiency
	Massive cell death (crushing injuries, burns, cytotoxic drugs)
	Large digitalis overdose
	Familial periodic paralysis
Decreased potassium excretion	Oliguria
	Extracellular fluid volume depletion
	Oliguric renal failure
	Decreased aldosterone from any cause (Addison disease, chronic heparin administration, lead poisoning, ACE-Is, angiotensin II receptor antagonists, selective aldosterone blockers, direct renin inhibitors)
	Potassium-sparing diuretics

IV, intravenous; ACE, angiotensin-converting enzyme.

Another cardiovascular-related source of hyperkalemia is a massive blood transfusion. While blood is stored, potassium ions leak from the erythrocytes into the plasma. The longer the storage time, the greater the potassium load contained in a unit of blood.[39] A classic study indicates that if the blood has been in storage for more than 3 days, rewarming the blood before administration causes only minimal return of potassium to the cells.[40] Individuals receiving more than 7 or 8 units of stored blood within a few hours are considered at high risk for severe hyperkalemia; however, fatal hyperkalemia has occurred with transfusion of fewer units, especially when they are administered rapidly.[41]

Hyperkalemia may be manifested clinically by intestinal cramping and diarrhea, skeletal muscle weakness, paresthesias, flaccid paralysis, cardiac arrhythmias, and cardiac arrest. The cardiac effects of hyperkalemia are potentially fatal; they are discussed in the next section.

Cardiac Effects of Hyperkalemia. Hyperkalemia alters myocardial cell function in several ways, including altered resting membrane potential, decreased action potential duration, and more rapid repolarization. When the extracellular potassium concentration increases, the gradient between extracellular and intracellular potassium decreases. This decreased gradient causes an increase in resting membrane potential. The degree of hyperkalemia may move the resting membrane potential toward the threshold potential, in mild hyperkalemia, or may prevent repolarization completely in severe hyperkalemia. In this hypopolarized state of mild hyperkalemia, myocyte excitability is increased; this can lead to ectopic beats and may trigger reentrant tachycardias. In severe hyperkalemia, successful depolarization and/or repolarization may not be possible. Cardiac cells vary in their sensitivity to the effects of hyperkalemia. Atrial cells are more sensitive than ventricular cells; the conduction system is the last to be affected.[38] Depending on the location of this myocyte malfunction, this can lead to nodal blockade, bundle branch blocks, ventricular fibrillation, or asystole.[32,42] In fact, the ability of hyperkalemia to cause asystolic cardiac arrest is exploited by using potassium as a cardioplegic agent during cardiac surgery.[43]

The characteristic ECG changes of hyperkalemia arise from the electrophysiologic changes previously described. The first ECG abnormality is the T waves becoming peaked (tented) with a narrow base and symmetric shape.[42] The QRS complex widens; ST depression may occur. Occasionally, ST elevation occurs, mimicking an MI.[44–46] Hyperkalemia also causes decreased amplitude and prolongation of P waves and PR prolongation.[47,48] As the plasma potassium concentration increases to high levels, the P waves disappear. A sine-wave pattern appears in severe, often terminal, hyperkalemia.[28,32,48]

The ECG changes of hyperkalemia are not well correlated with plasma potassium levels.[32,49–51] Although the ECG usually is abnormal with severe hyperkalemia (serum potassium greater than 8 mEq/L), minimal ECG changes have been observed in individuals with serum potassium concentrations greater than 9 mEq/L. The rate of increase of the plasma potassium concentration may contribute more to the ECG changes in hyperkalemia than does the absolute plasma potassium level. Hemodialysis patients may not exhibit the characteristic peaked T wave or other ECG signs when they are severely hyperkalemic.[52] The ECG changes of hyperkalemia also are blunted during hypothermia.[53]

ECG interpretation software may double or triple count the heart rate during severe hyperkalemia.[54,55] Individuals who have implantable defibrillators have received multiple inappropriate shocks in the setting of acute hyperkalemia.[56]

During myocardial ischemia, potassium concentration increases quickly in the extracellular spaces of the myocardium and promotes the development of lethal ventricular reentry arrhythmias.[57,58] During exercise, elevated catecholamines counteract the negative cardiac effects of hyperkalemia in normal hearts; this protective effect is diminished in ischemic hearts.

Hyperkalemia also has an indirect cardiac effect in that it stimulates aldosterone secretion. Through its saline-retaining action on the kidneys, aldosterone expands the ECV, which may have a detrimental effect on individuals in heart failure.

Vascular Effects of Hyperkalemia. Hyperkalemia reduces the smooth muscle relaxation normally mediated by endothelium-derived hyperpolarizing factor.[59] In very high concentrations, potassium ions cause cardioplegia and contraction of the smooth muscle of coronary arteries.[60]

Calcium Balance

Calcium balance is the net result of calcium intake and absorption, distribution, excretion, and abnormal losses. These components are summarized in Table 6-6. Calcium in the plasma exists in three forms: protein-bound, complexed, and ionized (free). The calcium that is bound to plasma proteins or complexed with small anions (e.g., citrate) is physiologically inactive. Only the ionized calcium is physiologically active. Two laboratory measures for extracellular calcium are available in many settings: total calcium concentration (includes bound, complexed, and ionized) and ionized calcium concentration.

Calcium ions play crucial roles in the automaticity of the sinus and atrioventricular nodes, in the plateau phase of the Purkinje and ventricular cell action potentials, in excitation–contraction coupling, and in cardiac and vascular muscle contraction. Not unexpectedly, one of the cardiac effects of an abnormal extracellular calcium concentration is an altered duration of the plateau phase. Extracellular fluid calcium imbalances are less likely to cause cardiac arrhythmias than are potassium imbalances, but arrhythmias associated with hypercalcemia have been fatal. In addition to their cardiac effects, acute calcium imbalances also affect the vasculature.

Hypocalcemia

Hypocalcemia may be defined as a decreased extracellular *total* calcium concentration or as a decreased extracellular *ionized* calcium concentration. The first definition refers to the commonly measured total calcium value. The second definition of hypocalcemia, however, is used in this chapter because decreases in ionized calcium concentration cause physiologic effects even if the total plasma concentration is within normal limits. Ionized hypocalcemia occurs frequently in intensive care units.[61]

Hypocalcemia results from decreased calcium intake or absorption, decreased physiologic availability of calcium, increased calcium excretion, loss of calcium by an abnormal route, or any combination of these factors.[3] Table 6-9 lists specific causative factors for hypocalcemia. Several of these specific factors may cause hypocalcemia in individuals with cardiac disease. Firstly, the preservative used in the storage of blood contains citrate, which complexes with calcium ions. Large or rapid transfusions of citrated blood cause hypocalcemia by decreasing the physiologic availability of calcium in the blood.[62] Similarly, rapid administration of proteinaceous plasma expanders such as albumin also reduces the physiologic availability of plasma calcium and may cause hypocalcemia.[63]

Hypocalcemia increases neuromuscular excitability. The clinical manifestations of hypocalcemia may include digital and perioral paresthesias, positive Chvostek sign, positive Trousseau sign, muscle twitching, and cramping, grimacing, hyperactive reflexes, tetany, carpopedal spasm, laryngospasm, seizures, cardiac arrhythmias, cardiac arrest, and hypotension (with acute hypocalcemia).

Cardiac Effects of Hypocalcemia. Hypocalcemia prolongs the plateau phase of cardiac myocyte action potentials. Hypocalcemia does cause characteristic alterations in the ECG. This manifests as QTc prolongation on an ECG tracing. It is important to note that this is primarily driven by the prolonged ST segment duration. Hypocalcemia prolongs the ST segment.[64] This finding is not unexpected because hypocalcemia prolongs the plateau phase of the action potential. The prolongation of the ST segment causes a prolonged QT interval.[28] The degree of prolongation of the QT interval is not a reliable indicator of the degree of

Table 6-9 • CAUSES OF HYPOCALCEMIA

Category	Clinical Examples
Decreased calcium intake or absorption	Diet deficient in calcium Diet deficient in vitamin D Malabsorption syndromes Chronic diarrhea (including laxative overuse) Steatorrhea Pancreatitis
Shift of calcium into physiologically unavailable form or into bones	Alkalosis Massive blood transfusion (citrate binds Ca^{2+}) Rapid infusion of albumin Pancreatitis Lack of PTH (hypoparathyroidism; surgical removal of parathyroid gland during thyroid surgery) Hypomagnesemia Hyperphosphatemia (overuse of phosphate-containing laxatives or enemas; excessive oral or IV phosphate intake; tumor lysis syndrome) Acute fluoride poisoning
Increased calcium excretion	*Gastrointestinal:* pancreatitis *Renal:* chronic renal insufficiency

PTH, parathyroid hormone; IV, intravenous.

hypocalcemia or the decrease in ionized calcium concentration, but it is influenced by the rate of decrease of the ionized calcium. Concurrent hypomagnesemia magnifies the effects of hypocalcemia.

These hypocalcemia-related changes in the myocardium usually are not great enough to give rise to significant cardiac arrhythmias in clinical settings. However, they may occasionally predispose to ventricular arrhythmias, including torsade de pointes.[65]

Hypocalcemia impairs myocardial contractility and thus may cause heart failure.[63,66–68] Patients who already have heart failure may decompensate if they become hypocalcemic. Hypocalcemia-associated heart failure may be unresponsive to digitalis until the hypocalcemia is corrected. The role of calcium ions in the regulation of myocardial contraction is clear. Although most of the calcium ions that initiate myocardial contraction come from the sarcoplasmic reticulum rather than directly from the extracellular fluid, entry of calcium from the extracellular fluid is necessary to trigger calcium release from the sarcoplasmic reticulum. In a normal heart, hypocalcemia reduces stroke work at any particular left ventricular end-diastolic pressure. This impairment is even greater in an ischemic heart. A classic study showed that patients who are administered albumin for resuscitation during hypovolemic shock also exhibit impaired myocardial contractility when the ionized calcium binds to the albumin and becomes physiologically unavailable.[63]

Vascular Effects of Hypocalcemia. Calcium ions play several important roles in the contraction of vascular smooth muscle. They are involved in the action potential, the regulation of cell membrane permeability, and in excitation–contraction coupling. In smooth muscle, as well as in cardiac muscle, contraction is initiated by an increase in cytoplasmic calcium. Most of the calcium ions that initiate the contraction come from the sarcoplasmic reticulum rather than from the extracellular fluid. Any short-term effects of hypocalcemia on the vasculature are more likely to arise from alterations in cell membrane permeability than from alteration in the contractile mechanisms. Acute (but not chronic) hypocalcemia causes hypotension. The mechanisms involved are not completely understood but likely include decreased peripheral vascular resistance and impaired cardiac function.

Table 6-10 • CAUSES OF HYPERCALCEMIA

Category	Clinical Examples
Increased calcium intake or absorption	Milk-alkali syndrome Excessive vitamin D
Shift of calcium out of bone	Hyperparathyroidism Prolonged immobility Bone tumors Multiple myeloma Cancers that produce parathyroid hormone–related peptide and other bone-resorbing factors
Decreased calcium excretion	Thiazide diuretics Familial hypocalciuric hypercalcemia

Hypercalcemia

Hypercalcemia results from increased intake or absorption of calcium, the shift of calcium from the bones into the extracellular fluid, decreased calcium excretion, or any combination of these factors. Specific causative factors are listed under these categories in Table 6-10. Note that thiazide diuretics, often administered to patients with cardiac disease, decrease the urinary excretion of calcium and thus may raise serum calcium levels.[69,70] Another type of diuretic should be substituted if hypercalcemia develops.

The clinical manifestations of hypercalcemia include anorexia, nausea, vomiting, constipation, abdominal pain, polyuria, renal calculi, skeletal muscle weakness, diminished reflexes, confusion, lethargy, possible personality change, frank psychosis, cardiac arrhythmias, and hypertension (with acute hypercalcemia).

Cardiac Effects of Hypercalcemia. Hypercalcemia shortens the plateau phase of the cardiac action potential, thereby decreasing the duration of the action potential. Also, it increases the rate of diastolic depolarization of sinus node cells and may increase the initial rate of increase and amplitude of the action potential. It may also delay atrioventricular conduction.[71]

Cardiac arrhythmias that have been reported to arise from hypercalcemia are rare but may include various types of heart block, paroxysmal atrial fibrillation, and severe bradycardia.[72,73] Hypercalcemia potentiates digitalis toxicity.[74] Patients using digitalis may acquire heart block if they become hypercalcemic. Sudden death has occurred in severe hypercalcemia, possibly caused by ventricular fibrillation.

The ECG in hypercalcemia reflects the short plateau phase in a shortened ST segment. The QT interval is decreased as a result.[28] The length of the QT interval is a clinically unreliable index of the extent of hypercalcemia. Hypercalcemia has been accompanied by lengthening of the QRS complex and diffuse flattening of T waves.[75]

Vascular Effects of Hypercalcemia. In patients who have intact parathyroid glands, acute hypercalcemia causes vasoconstriction and raises systolic blood pressure by impairing the vasodilatory function of the endothelium.[76,77] Increased intracellular calcium in vascular smooth muscle also causes increased vascular resistance. In many patients with essential hypertension, increased intracellular calcium occurs with normal plasma calcium levels. Parathyroid hormone and parathyroid hormone–related factors are implicated in transepithelial calcium transport and likely play a role in the hypertensive mechanism.

Magnesium Balance

Magnesium balance is the net result of magnesium intake and absorption, distribution, excretion, and abnormal losses. These components are summarized in Table 6-6. Similar to calcium, magnesium in the serum exists in three forms: protein bound, complexed with various anions, and ionized (free).[78] While the most physiologically active form is ionized magnesium, the only widely available clinical laboratory measure for magnesium is the total serum magnesium concentration (bound, complexed, and ionized).

Magnesium, like potassium, is primarily an intracellular ion with extracellular magnesium representing approximately 1% of total-body magnesium.[78] For this reason, plasma levels of magnesium do not necessarily reflect the intracellular magnesium content. Total-body magnesium depletion may be present even when the plasma magnesium is normal. Intracellular magnesium is a cofactor for many enzymes, including Na^+–K^+ adenosine triphosphatase (ATPase). Changes in magnesium balance, particularly hypomagnesemia, cause alterations in ion transport across membranes. Because the function of cardiac and smooth muscle depends on ion fluxes, magnesium imbalances have myocardial and vascular effects.

Hypomagnesemia and Total-Body Magnesium Depletion

Hypomagnesemia and total-body magnesium depletion are caused by decreased magnesium intake or absorption, decreased physiologic availability of magnesium, increased magnesium excretion, loss of magnesium by an abnormal route, or any combination of these factors. Specific causative factors for hypomagnesemia are listed in Table 6-11. Hypomagnesemia and total-body magnesium depletion are common in chronic alcoholism; therefore, patients who have alcoholic cardiomyopathy need assessment for hypomagnesemia.[79]

Diuretics (except for spironolactone, triamterene, and amiloride) cause increased renal excretion of magnesium and can lead to hypomagnesemia.[80] Individuals with heart failure are at high risk for hypomagnesemia or total-body magnesium depletion.[81] In addition to diuretic therapy, patients with heart failure often have congestion of the splanchnic vessels, which decreases magnesium absorption. Also, the secondary hyperaldosteronism and elevated catecholamines of heart failure increase urinary excretion of magnesium.[82] Among patients with heart failure, those who are hypomagnesemic have more arrhythmias than those with normal magnesium levels, and hypomagnesemia is associated with shorter survival.[83,84] Individuals with acute MI often have ionized hypomagnesemia.[84] Hypomagnesemia may be a causative factor for MI as well as a result of pathophysiologic changes immediately after MI.

Table 6-11 • CAUSES OF HYPOMAGNESEMIA

Category	Clinical Examples
Decreased magnesium intake or absorption	Prolonged IV therapy without Mg^{2+} Chronic malnutrition Chronic diarrhea Steatorrhea Pancreatitis Malabsorption syndromes Chronic alcoholism Ileal resection
Increased magnesium excretion	*Gastrointestinal:* Steatorrhea *Renal:* Diabetic ketoacidosis; diuretic therapy; increased aldosterone (CHF, cirrhosis, hyperaldosteronism); chronic alcoholism; renal damage from drugs (amphotericin B, aminoglycosides)
Magnesium loss by abnormal route	Emesis Nasogastric suctioning Drainage from GI fistula

IV, intravenous; GI, gastrointestinal.

Hypomagnesemia causes increased neuromuscular excitability. The signs and symptoms of hypomagnesemia include hyperreflexia (positive Chvostek or Trousseau sign), leg and foot cramps, muscle twitching, grimacing, tremors, dysphagia, nystagmus, ataxia, tetany, seizures, extreme confusion, cardiac arrhythmias, and hypertension.

Cardiac Effects of Hypomagnesemia and Total-Body Magnesium Depletion. Magnesium is a cofactor for Na^+–K^+ ATPase, the enzyme that plays a major role in the regulation of intracellular potassium concentration in the myocardium. When magnesium is deficient, the decreased intracellular magnesium leads to decreased activity of this enzyme. As a result, the intracellular potassium ion concentration decreases, and intracellular sodium concentration increases in myocardial cells. Decreased activity of Na^+–K^+ ATPase interferes with the reentry of potassium ions into depolarized cells and promotes diastolic leak of potassium from cells that are already depolarized. Also, hypomagnesemia causes increased membrane permeability to potassium, an effect that also tends to decrease intracellular potassium concentration in the myocardium.

In hypomagnesemia, the sinus node has an increased spontaneous firing rate, and there is a rate-dependent decrease in the duration of the cardiac action potential. The absolute refractory period is shortened, and the relative refractory period is lengthened. Hypomagnesemia thus predisposes to arrhythmias, especially tachyarrhythmias. The imbalance is associated with supraventricular tachycardia, supraventricular ectopy, ventricular ectopic beats, ventricular tachycardia, ventricular fibrillation, and torsade de pointes.[85–87] Whether these arrhythmias are caused directly by the hypomagnesemia itself or by hypomagnesemia-induced changes in potassium transport across myocardial membranes is uncertain. What is clear, however, is that both hypomagnesemia and total-body magnesium depletion lead to cardiac arrhythmias that can be corrected only by the administration of magnesium. Clinical studies demonstrate that correction of ionized hypomagnesemia during coronary artery bypass graft (CABG) surgery leads to fewer postoperative episodes of ventricular tachycardia.[87] Administration of magnesium reduces postoperative arrhythmias in CABG patients and also in children having surgery for congenital heart defects, regardless of whether they are initially hypomagnesemic.[88,89] In individuals with normal levels, magnesium has been used pharmacologically to treat arrhythmias, including atrial fibrillation, ventricular tachycardia, and torsade de pointes, and to reduce arrhythmias in acute MI and heart failure.[90,91]

A classic study demonstrated that heart muscle magnesium content decreases after acute MI.[92] This post-MI magnesium decrease may be caused by leakage of magnesium from necrotic cells and interference with ion transport in hypoxic cells. Another mechanism for myocardial magnesium decrease after MI may be the action of catecholamines. It is likely that the localized decrease of myocardial magnesium after acute MI is a predisposing factor for cardiac arrhythmias. Animal studies show decreased tolerance to ischemic stress with chronic magnesium deficiency.[93]

Hypomagnesemia potentiates digitalis toxicity. Hypomagnesemia-related digitalis toxicity arises in part from the intracellular potassium deficiency caused by the magnesium imbalance. Digitalis toxicity arrhythmias have been observed in individuals with therapeutic digitalis levels and either decreased serum magnesium levels or normal serum levels with total-body magnesium depletion.

The ECG changes in hypomagnesemia are not easily characterized; rather, they are somewhat nonspecific. Prolongation of the QT interval is frequently observed in hypomagnesemia.[94] This ECG change probably occurs because of altered potassium transport caused by hypomagnesemia. Other ECG changes that have been seen with hypomagnesemia, such as ST-segment depression, prolonged PR interval, wide QRS complex, and T-wave abnormalities, may be caused by multiple electrolyte imbalances that occur in conjunction with hypomagnesemia, or by the hypomagnesemia itself.[95]

Vascular Effects of Hypomagnesemia and Total-Body Magnesium Depletion. Hypomagnesemia has important effects on vascular smooth muscle. A decrease in the extracellular magnesium concentration causes arteriolar vasoconstriction, in part by increasing the intracellular calcium concentration in vascular smooth muscle and by reducing endothelial production of the vasodilators, nitric oxide and prostacyclin.[96] The resulting increased peripheral vascular resistance causes hypertension that often accompanies acute or chronic hypomagnesemia. Low levels of dietary magnesium and low serum magnesium are associated with an increased prevalence of hypertension.[97] Meta-analysis of clinical trials shows that magnesium supplementation has a small blood pressure–lowering effect in hypertension.[98]

Total-body magnesium depletion (with or without hypomagnesemia) appears to play an important role in the development of atherosclerosis and ischemic heart disease.[99] Low serum magnesium levels have been shown to increase the prevalence of peripheral arterial disease. Animal studies show hypertension, endothelial dysfunction, and vascular remodeling with chronic magnesium deficiency.[100] Animal studies also demonstrate plasma elevation of proinflammatory cytokines and neuropeptides that stimulate free radical formation.[101] Thus, magnesium deficiency can cause changes that are part of the atherosclerotic process.

In summary, the vascular effects of hypomagnesemia include increased peripheral resistance, hypertension, and impaired vasodilation. Current evidence relates total-body magnesium depletion, with or without hypomagnesemia, to congestive heart failure, ischemic heart disease, peripheral arterial disease, and essential hypertension.[96]

Hypermagnesemia

Hypermagnesemia is caused by increased magnesium intake or absorption, increased physiologic availability of magnesium, decreased magnesium excretion, or any combination of these factors.[3] Specific causative factors for hypermagnesemia are listed in Table 6-12. Overall, the risk of hypermagnesemia is rare; however, older adults who use magnesium-containing antacids and laxatives are at higher risk for the development of hypermagnesemia, in part because they may have unrecognized renal insufficiency.[102]

The cardiac effects (bradycardia, arrhythmias, cardiac arrest) and vascular effects (flushing, hypotension) of hypermagnesemia are discussed next. In addition to these effects, hypermagnesemia may cause a subjective sensation of warmth, diaphoresis, drowsiness, lethargy, coma, diminished deep tendon reflexes, flaccid skeletal muscle paralysis, and respiratory depression.

Table 6-12 • CAUSES OF HYPERMAGNESEMIA

Category	Clinical Examples
Increased magnesium intake or absorption	Excessive use of Mg^{2+}-containing laxatives, antacids, or urologic irrigation solutions
	Excessive IV infusion of Mg^{2+}
	Aspiration of sea water
Decreased magnesium excretion	Oliguric renal failure
	Adrenal insufficiency

IV, intravenous.

Cardiac Effects of Hypermagnesemia. A plasma excess of magnesium interferes with cardiac conduction throughout the heart. Atrioventricular block or complete heart block may occur at high plasma levels of magnesium.[103] Hypermagnesemia inhibits myocardial contraction and depresses membrane excitability, although intracellular contractile mechanisms remain intact.

Hypermagnesemia suppresses the sinoatrial node and causes sympathetic nervous system blockade.[102] Both of these factors contribute to clinically significant sinus bradycardia. Cardiac arrest in asystole may be fatal in severe hypermagnesemia. ECG changes associated with hypermagnesemia include prolonged PR interval and increased duration of the QRS complex.[78] These changes are somewhat variable and do not present a classic, easily recognizable picture.

Vascular Effects of Hypermagnesemia. Hypermagnesemia reduces peripheral vascular resistance by inhibiting calcium movement into vascular smooth muscle cells, inhibiting calcium release from intracellular storage, and depressing contractile responses to vasoactive substances such as epinephrine and angiotensin II. The peripheral vasodilation caused by these mechanisms leads to hypotension.[78] Vasodilation of cutaneous vessels in hypermagnesemia causes flushing.

Phosphate Balance

Phosphate balance is the net result of phosphate intake and absorption, distribution, excretion, and abnormal losses. These components are summarized in Table 6-6. Phosphate is necessary for many cell metabolic processes and is a component of ATP, the cellular energy source.

The normal range of serum phosphate concentration is 2.5 to 4.5 mg/dL. Mild or moderate hypophosphatemia (1.0 to 2.4 mg/dL) may be asymptomatic. Severe hypophosphatemia, with a serum phosphate less than 1 mg/dL, can cause clinical manifestations. Symptoms depend on the severity and chronicity of phosphate depletion.[104,105]

Severe Hypophosphatemia

Hypophosphatemia is caused by decreased intake or absorption of phosphate, the shift of phosphate into cells, or increased phosphate excretion.[1] Specific causative factors included in these categories are presented in Table 6-13.

Of importance to patients with cardiac disease is the decrease in plasma phosphate concentration that occurs with intravenous glucose administration. Glucose infusion by itself does not usually cause severe hypophosphatemia; however, if glucose infusion is combined with other factors, such as diuretics that increase phosphate excretion, severe hypophosphatemia may occur. Insulin, as well as glucose, promotes the movement of phosphate into cells. Catecholamines and β-adrenergic agonist drugs also shift phosphate into cells and predispose hypophosphatemia.[106]

Hypophosphatemia is common in chronic alcoholism.[107] Individuals with newly diagnosed alcoholic cardiomyopathy need to

Table 6-13 • CAUSES OF HYPOPHOSPHATEMIA

Category	Clinical Examples
Decreased phosphate intake or absorption	Prolonged or excessive antacid use Starvation Malabsorption syndrome Chronic diarrhea Chronic alcoholism
Shift of phosphate into cells	Total parenteral nutrition Rapid cell proliferation (refeeding after starvation or malnutrition; leukemic blast crisis) Respiratory alkalosis (hyperventilation) Insulin Epinephrine, β-adrenergic agonists Infusion of IV glucose, fructose, or lactate
Increased phosphate excretion	Diabetic ketoacidosis Alcohol withdrawal Diuretic phase after severe burns Infusion of IV bicarbonate Renal tubular acidosis Diuretic therapy Glucocorticoid therapy
Phosphate loss by abnormal route	Emesis Hemodialysis

IV, intravenous.

have their phosphate levels checked.[108] If they undergo alcohol withdrawal, then they will likely be hyperventilating, and respiratory alkalosis will develop, which also causes hypophosphatemia; therefore, their phosphate levels will need continued monitoring.

The signs and symptoms of severe hypophosphatemia include anorexia, nausea, malaise, diminished reflexes, paresthesias, muscle aching, muscle weakness, rhabdomyolysis, severe debility, acute respiratory failure, hemolysis (possible hemolytic anemia), confusion, stupor, seizures, coma, and impaired cardiac function. These effects of hypophosphatemia are caused primarily by decreased intracellular ATP and by decreased 2,3-bisphosphoglycerate (BPG) in the red blood cells. Decreased erythrocyte BPG causes tissue hypoxia by increasing hemoglobin–oxygen affinity, which reduces oxygen release. Administration of phosphate to hypophosphatemic individuals increases erythrocyte BPG, which decreases hemoglobin–oxygen affinity and allows greater tissue oxygenation.[107]

Cardiac Effects of Severe Hypophosphatemia. Severe hypophosphatemia impairs myocardial function by decreasing cardiac contractility. This cardiac impairment may progress to acute congestive failure or congestive cardiomyopathy.[107,109] The decreased cardiac performance of hypophosphatemia is reversed by the intravenous administration of phosphate.[110,111]

Cardiac arrest can occur from sudden severe hypophosphatemia caused by refeeding syndrome, a situation that arises when a malnourished person with low phosphate stores begins to receive oral or parenteral nutrition. The plasma phosphate concentration falls rapidly within a few days of beginning nutritional repletion because a sudden increase in cellular metabolism depletes the individual's phosphate stores.[109,112] The sudden phosphate depletion leads to a lack of ATP and cellular dysfunction.

The role of severe hypophosphatemia in cardiac arrhythmias is not well understood. Arrhythmias do occur in these individuals. However, many patients who have severe hypophosphatemia also have hypokalemia or hypocalcemia or multiple electrolyte imbalances, so it may be difficult to isolate the effect of the decreased phosphate.

Vascular Effects of Severe Hypophosphatemia. Increased vasoactive medication support in patients with severe hypophosphatemia has been identified. This effect may be caused by a vascular as well as a myocardial action; however, the cardiac effect is likely predominant.[113]

SUMMARY OF FLUID AND ELECTROLYTES

Fluid balance is determined by the interplay of fluid intake, distribution, excretion, and fluid loss through abnormal routes. The two types of fluid imbalances are ECV imbalances and osmolality imbalances. ECV imbalances are increases or decreases in the amount of fluid in the vascular and interstitial compartments. Osmolality imbalances are alterations in the concentration of body fluids and result in movement of water into or out of cells caused by osmosis. Extracellular volume and osmolality imbalances may occur concurrently or separately in patients with cardiac disease.

A normal plasma electrolyte concentration is necessary for optimal cardiovascular function. Because electrolytes play important roles in the generation of action potentials and the contraction of cardiac and smooth muscle, electrolyte imbalances exert cardiac and vascular effects. The effects of a specific electrolyte imbalance depend on the specific role of that electrolyte in normal cardiovascular function.

Patients who do not have cardiovascular disease may acquire an electrolyte imbalance that subsequently causes cardiovascular impairment. Also, patients who have pre-existing cardiovascular disease have specific risk factors for electrolyte imbalances. If imbalances develop in these individuals, then the cardiovascular effects of the electrolyte imbalances may cause severe disturbance to an already compromised cardiovascular system. Successful management of these individuals involves a careful assessment of risk factors, elimination of those risk factors when possible, surveillance for the manifestations of fluid and electrolyte imbalances, and interventions to protect and support function during the correction of fluid and electrolyte imbalances.

PRINCIPLES OF ACID–BASE BALANCE

The degree of acidity of bodily fluids plays an important role in physiology. It influences the structure and function of many enzymes and also modifies the affinity between oxygen and hemoglobin. Deviations of acid–base balance from normal can affect cellular function and tissue oxygenation. In the extreme, these imbalances can be fatal.

Terminology Review

An *acid* is a substance that donates hydrogen ions (H^+) in solution. A *base* is a substance that accepts hydrogen ions. The degree of acidity is proportional to the number of hydrogen ions present in a solution. The degree of acidity of body fluids is reported as the pH. The pH is the negative logarithm of the hydrogen ion concentration. It ranges from 1 (very acidic) to 14 (very alkaline). Human serum is normally slightly alkaline, with a normal pH range of 7.35 to 7.45. If the pH of the blood falls below the normal range (i.e., becomes more acidic), the patient is deemed to have *acidemia.* The process that leads to *acidemia* is referred to as *acidosis.*

Table 6-14 • THE MAJOR BUFFERS

Extracellular Fluid	Intracellular Fluid	Bone	Urine
Bicarbonate	Proteins	Carbonates	Inorganic phosphates
Inorganic phosphates	Organic and inorganic phosphates	Phosphates	
Plasma proteins	Hemoglobin (in erythrocytes)		

Similarly, if the pH of the blood rises above the normal range (i.e., becomes more alkaline), the patient is deemed to have *alkalemia.* The process that leads to the *alkalemia* is referred to as *alkalosis.*[3]

Processes Involved in Acid–Base Balance

Normal cellular metabolism continually produces acids, which can cause dangerous acidemia without the closely regulated processes by which the body maintains pH within the normal range. After acid production, the processes of acid buffering and acid excretion work to maintain or reestablish a normal pH.

Acid Production

Cellular metabolism produces two types of acids: carbonic acid and metabolic acids. Carbonic acid (H_2CO_3) is produced as carbon dioxide (CO_2); the enzyme carbonic anhydrase combines the CO_2 with water (H_2O) to produce carbonic acid. In a standard adult, approximately 15,000 mmol of CO_2 is generated per day from the metabolism of carbohydrates and fats.[3] Because carbonic acid is excreted as a gas, CO_2, it sometimes is called *volatile acid.*

Metabolic acids are produced primarily from the metabolism of phosphate-containing compounds and amino acids that contain sulfur. These metabolic acids include sulfuric and phosphoric acids. Metabolic acids are handled differently by the body than is carbonic acid. For this reason, they sometimes are called *noncarbonic, fixed,* or *nonvolatile acids.*

Cellular metabolism also produces small amounts of base (bicarbonate ions; HCO_3^-) as a result of oxidation of small organic anions such as citrate. Much more metabolic acid is produced than base. In a standard adult with a North American diet, approximately 1 mmol/kg/day of nonvolatile acids is produced.[3]

Acid Buffering

Buffers in the body act to minimize changes in pH because of the gain of acid or base. They neutralize acids by taking up excess hydrogen ions and neutralize bases by releasing hydrogen ions. Buffers are located in all body fluids; however, the most important buffers are those in the extracellular fluid, intracellular fluid, bone, and urine. Different body fluids contain different buffers, which meet specific needs (Table 6-14).

The major extracellular buffer is the carbonic acid–bicarbonate–carbon dioxide buffer system (commonly termed the *bicarbonate buffer system*). Carbonic acid is a weak acid, which means that it dissociates partially when in solution so that it is in equilibrium with bicarbonate and hydrogen ions. The carbonic acid concentration can be altered by variations in alveolar ventilation (variations in CO_2 excretion). The chemical equation for the bicarbonate buffer system is written as follows:

$$\underset{\text{carbon dioxide}}{CO_2} + \underset{\text{water}}{H_2O} \rightleftharpoons \underset{\text{carbonic acid}}{H_2CO_3} \rightleftharpoons \underset{\text{hydrogen ion}}{H^+} + \underset{\text{bicarbonate ion}}{HCO_3^-}$$

To maintain the pH of blood within a normal range, there must be 20 bicarbonate ions for every carbonic acid molecule. The Henderson–Hasselbalch equation, a mathematical description of the pH of a buffered solution, demonstrates how this 20:1 ratio is necessary:

$$pH = pKa + \log\frac{[A^-]}{[HA]} \quad \text{(general equation)}$$

$$pH = 6.1 + \log\frac{[HCO_3^-]}{[H_2CO_3]} \quad \text{(substituting values for bicarbonate buffer system)}$$

$$pH = 6.1 + \log\frac{20}{1}$$

$$pH = 6.1 + 1.3$$

$$pH = 7.4$$

A buffer system cannot buffer its own acid. Thus, the bicarbonate buffer system cannot buffer carbonic acid. The carbonic acid that is produced by cells (as CO_2 and H_2O) is buffered primarily by intracellular buffers. The bicarbonate buffer system is a major buffer for metabolic acids. Table 6-15 summarizes the role of buffers with respect to acid or base loads.

Acid Excretion

Even though the buffers minimize pH changes while acid is produced, they have a limited capacity. Therefore, mechanisms to excrete acid are necessary to maintain balance. The body has two acid excretion methods: the lungs excrete carbon dioxide, thus reducing carbonic acid, and the kidneys excrete metabolic acids and H^+.

Role of the Lungs. The lungs excrete carbon dioxide and water, thereby reducing the amount of carbonic acid in the body. They cannot excrete metabolic acids. When alveolar ventilation increases (a product of rate and volume of ventilation), more carbon dioxide is excreted. Conversely, when alveolar ventilation decreases, less carbon dioxide is excreted. By regulating the partial pressure of carbon dioxide ($PaCO_2$) within the serum, the body can control the contribution of carbonic acid to the body's acid–base balance.

If acidemia develops (via increased $PaCO_2$), chemoreceptors in the medulla and carotid and aortic bodies are stimulated by the increased $PaCO_2$ and decreased pH.[114] This stimulation results in increased alveolar ventilation and causes increased excretion of the excess carbon dioxide. Similarly, if too little acid is present

Table 6-15 • ROLE OF BUFFERS WITH RESPECT TO AN ACID OR BASE LOAD

Buffer	Role With Carbonic Acid Load	Role With Metabolic Acid Load	Role With Base (Bicarbonate) Load
Extracellular bicarbonate	Not effective	Major role (immediate action)	Not effective
Other extracellular buffers	Minor role (immediate action)	Minor role (immediate action)	Minor role (immediate action)
Intracellular buffers	Major role (10–30 minutes)	Important role (2–4 hours)	Important role (hours)
Bone buffers	Probably not important	Important role (2–4 hours)	Important role (hours)

(decreased $PaCO_2$), the chemoreceptors are less stimulated, and alveolar ventilation decreases to retain carbonic acid in the body. Hypoxia, sensed by the carotid chemoreceptors, stimulates alveolar ventilation and may override the suppression of ventilation from decreased $PaCO_2$. In a healthy person, alveolar ventilation changes rapidly in response to changes in $PaCO_2$, and thus carbonic acid is reduced at a rate effective in maintaining acid–base balance.

Role of the Kidneys. The kidneys excrete metabolic acids. They cannot excrete carbonic acid. The renal epithelial cells that line the proximal tubules secrete hydrogen ions into the renal tubular fluid and reabsorb bicarbonate ions in the process.[115] Bicarbonate is the primary extracellular buffer of metabolic acids. Therefore, the bicarbonate ion concentration indicates how much metabolic acid is present. A decreased serum bicarbonate concentration indicates increased amounts of metabolic acid. When the proximal tubular cells secrete hydrogen ions into the tubular fluid (urine), they reabsorb bicarbonate ions, replenishing the bicarbonate ions that were used in buffering. Hydrogen ions also are secreted into the renal tubular fluid by cells that line the distal tubules and collecting ducts, and these cells also can secrete bicarbonate into the tubular fluid or reabsorb it into the blood.[116]

If the urine were to become too acidic, it could damage the cells that line the urinary tract. Fortunately, the urine does not become dangerously acidic because the hydrogen ions in the renal tubules are buffered by the urine buffers or combine chemically with ammonia. Ammonia (NH_3) is produced by renal tubular cells and then diffuses into the tubular fluid.[117] Hydrogen ions combine with the ammonia in the tubular fluid to produce ammonium ions (NH_4^+). Because ammonium ions are charged particles, they cannot cross the cell membranes to enter the blood; thus, they are retained in the renal tubular fluid and excreted in the urine. An increase of acid in the body (decreased pH) causes the production of more ammonia, which facilitates renal excretion of acid. This process begins within 2 hours but takes several days to be maximally effective.[3]

Thus, the kidneys have several mechanisms that result in the compensation of acidosis arising from metabolic acids produced by cellular metabolism. These mechanisms can be adjusted to excrete more H^+ or less H^+, thereby maintaining the bicarbonate ion concentration within normal limits. Changes in renal function with normal aging cause older adults to excrete an acid load more slowly than younger adults.

SUMMARY OF ACID–BASE BALANCE

Cellular metabolism produces carbonic acid and metabolic acids. These acids must be excreted to maintain normal acid–base balance. Buffers in all body fluids act to minimize changes in pH due to an acid load or a bicarbonate (base) load. Carbon dioxide is excreted by the lungs, thereby reducing carbonic acid loads; increases or decreases in alveolar ventilation regulate the amount of carbonic acid. The $PaCO_2$ is the clinical indicator of carbonic acid. Metabolic acids are excreted by the kidneys, which can excrete more or less acid as needed. The plasma bicarbonate ion concentration (HCO_3^-) is the clinical indicator of the amount of metabolic acid. Table 6-16 summarizes the physiologic responses that maintain acid–base balance.

ACID–BASE IMBALANCES

Acid–base imbalances occur when the capacity of the buffers to modulate pH changes is exceeded. Two terms are important in understanding the physiologic responses to acid–base imbalances. *Correction* of the imbalance occurs when the original problem is fixed so that the pH, $PaCO_2$, and plasma bicarbonate ion concentration can return to normal.[3] *Compensation* for an acid–base imbalance restores the pH toward normal but does not correct the underlying problem causing the imbalance. In many cases, an acid–base imbalance persists long enough that compensatory physiologic processes occur. A *partially compensated* acid–base imbalance is characterized by abnormal pH, $PaCO_2$, and plasma bicarbonate ion concentration. However, the pH is not as abnormal as it was before the partial compensation. When an acid–base imbalance is *fully compensated*, the pH is in the normal range, but the $PaCO_2$ and plasma bicarbonate ion concentration are both abnormal. By moving the pH toward normal, compensation for an acid–base imbalance helps to protect cells from death.

Acidosis

An individual who has acidosis has processes that tend to decrease the pH of the blood below normal by creating a relative excess of acid. The resulting acidemia may persist or may be lessened by the body's compensatory response. A pH below 6.9 is usually fatal. Acidosis is classified as respiratory or metabolic, depending on what type of acid is primarily excessive.

Respiratory Acidosis

Respiratory acidosis occurs when too much carbonic acid accumulates in the blood. Clinically, the increase of carbonic acid is measured as an increase in $PaCO_2$. Carbon dioxide is normally excreted by the lungs through ventilation. Thus, any factor that decreases ventilation can cause respiratory acidosis (Table 6-17). Chronic respiratory acidosis can lead to chronic lung disease and pulmonary artery hypertension. This persistent elevation of afterload on the right ventricle can lead to cor pulmonale or right ventricular dysfunction.

Carbon dioxide diffuses readily through the blood–brain barrier. Thus, the pH of CSF decreases when respiratory acidosis

Table 6-16 • SUMMARY OF PHYSIOLOGIC RESPONSES THAT MAINTAIN ACID–BASE BALANCE

Physiologic Mechanism	Response to Decreased pH (Too Much Acid in Blood)	Response to Increased pH (Too Much Bicarbonate in Blood)
Buffers	Accept hydrogen ions	Release hydrogen ions
Respiratory system	Excretes carbonic acid by increasing rate and depth of respiration	Retains carbonic acid in the body by decreasing rate and depth of respiration
Kidneys	Excrete more metabolic acid by increasing secretion of H^+ into renal tubular fluid, increasing reabsorption of bicarbonate, and increasing production of NH_3	Excrete less metabolic acid by decreasing secretion of H^+ into renal tubular fluid, decreasing reabsorption of bicarbonate, and decreasing production of NH_3

Table 6-17 • CAUSES OF RESPIRATORY ACIDOSIS

Category	Clinical Examples
Decreased gaseous exchange (problem in the airways or alveoli of lungs)	Decreased alveolar ventilation for any reason
	Acute airway obstruction by foreign body
	Severe asthma
	Sleep apnea (obstructive type)
	Chronic obstructive pulmonary disease (COPD) type A (emphysema) in end stage
	Chronic obstructive pulmonary disease (COPD) type B (chronic bronchitis)
	Atelectasis
	Pneumonia
	Adult respiratory distress syndrome (ARDS)
	Pulmonary edema
	Hypoventilation with mechanical ventilation
Impaired neuromuscular function of chest (problem in the chest muscles or nerves)	Chest injury
	Surgical incision in chest or upper abdomen (pain limits chest expansion)
	Respiratory muscle fatigue
	Severe hypokalemia
	Poliomyelitis
	Guillain–Barré syndrome
	Myasthenia gravis
	Kyphoscoliosis
	Pickwickian syndrome (obesity limits chest expansion)
Suppression of respiratory neurons in brainstem (medulla) (problem in the brainstem)	Opioids
	Barbiturates
	Anesthetics
	Sleep apnea (central type)

occurs. As excess CO_2 enters brain cells, intracellular acidosis alters enzyme activity and central nervous system (CNS) depression results. Clinical manifestations of respiratory acidosis are CNS depression (disorientation, lethargy, somnolence), headache, blurred vision, tachycardia, and cardiac arrhythmias.

Respiratory acidosis can be corrected only by restoring lung function because the lungs are the only route of excretion of carbon dioxide. If the respiratory acidosis lasts long enough, the kidneys compensate by excreting more than the usual amount of metabolic acids, moving the pH back toward normal, even though the blood chemistry remains abnormal. Excretion of more metabolic acids raises the bicarbonate ion concentration because fewer bicarbonate ions committed to buffering. Thus, renal compensation for respiratory acidosis restores the 20:1 ratio of bicarbonate to carbonic acid, even though the absolute values of both are elevated. Restoring the 20:1 ratio normalizes the pH. Renal compensation for respiratory acidosis can take 3 to 5 days to be fully effective.[3] Compensated respiratory acidosis is characterized by elevated $PaCO_2$ (the sign of the primary problem), elevated bicarbonate ion concentration (the sign of the renal compensation), and pH that is decreased (partially compensated) or normal (fully compensated).

In respiratory acidosis, excess CO_2 diffuses into cardiac cells. Although intracellular buffering of carbonic acid may protect intracellular pH in cardiac cells more effectively than in many other types of cells, the intracellular pH in cardiac cells does decrease. Respiratory acidosis depresses cardiac contractility.[118] The adverse effects of decreased myocardial cell contractility in respiratory acidosis are offset partially by increased sympathetic neural discharge and increased catecholamine levels.[119] While cardiac arrhythmias in individuals who have respiratory acidosis may be caused by the increased circulating catecholamines, the intracellular acidosis also causes changes in the myocyte action potentials.[120]

Respiratory acidosis also affects vascular beds, altering both peripheral vascular resistance and the distribution of blood flow. Acidosis can cause vasodilation in large arteries and vasoconstriction in small arteries.[121] Specifically, acidosis can cause coronary vasodilation.[122] The peripheral vasculature becomes less sensitive to α- and β-adrenergic stimulation. Decreased peripheral vascular resistance and decreased cardiac contractility can cause hypotension, which may be diminished by constriction in splanchnic and peripheral venous beds (the venous capacitance beds). This response may increase central arterial blood volume.

The decreased pH in the CSF increases the synthesis of nitric oxide, which causes cerebral vasodilation, increasing cerebral blood flow.[122] This is the source of the headache that is experienced by many individuals with respiratory acidosis. Increased cerebral blood flow from cerebral vasodilation may also raise CSF pressure and cause papilledema. In contrast to its effect on other vascular beds, respiratory acidosis causes vasoconstriction in the pulmonary vasculature.[123] The resulting increase in pulmonary vascular resistance may worsen the clinical status of patients with pre-existing right heart failure.

In summary, the significant cardiovascular effects of respiratory acidosis are cardiac arrhythmias, decreased cardiac contractility, decreased peripheral vascular resistance, increased pulmonary vascular resistance, and shift of blood flow from the venous capacitance beds into the central and cerebral arterial beds.

Metabolic Acidosis

Metabolic acidosis is caused by relatively too much metabolic acid. It can be due to a gain of acid or a loss of base. Acid can be gained from the intake of acids or substances that are converted to acid in the body, from an increased rate of normal metabolism, from the production of unusual acids due to altered metabolic processes, or from factors that decrease renal excretion of acid. Bicarbonate ions (base) can be lost in the urine or through the gastrointestinal tract. Table 6-18 lists clinical conditions that cause metabolic acidosis by each of these mechanisms. Cardiogenic shock causes metabolic acidosis by the accumulation of lactic acid from anaerobic metabolism and through the failure of the decreased circulation to deliver metabolic acids to the kidneys for excretion. No matter what its cause, metabolic acidosis is characterized by a decreased plasma bicarbonate ion concentration. The bicarbonate either is depleted by being used to buffer excess metabolic acids or is lost directly from the body.

Some clinicians use the *anion gap* when evaluating metabolic acidosis.[124] The anion gap is the difference between the concentrations of the major positive and negative ions in plasma or serum:

$$\text{Anion gap} = (Na^+ + K^+) - (Cl^- + HCO_3^-)$$

Some patients omit the potassium concentration, a relatively small number, from the calculation to simplify it. The normal range of anion gap varies with the laboratory procedures used for electrolyte measurements, so that it may be reported as 6 to 16 mEq/L, 12 to 20 mEq/L, or another such range.[125,126] If unmeasured anions such as lactate or β-hydroxybutyrate accumulate in the body, the anion gap increases. Calculation of the anion gap is rapid and uses clinically available parameters, but it is less informative for individuals who have hypoalbuminemia unless a correction is used and may be misleading when two primary acid–base imbalances coexist.[127]

Table 6-18 • CAUSES OF METABOLIC ACIDOSIS

Category	Clinical Examples
Acid accumulation by ingestion or infusion of acid or acid precursors	Aspirin (acetylsalicylic acid) Boric acid Ammonium chloride (releases H^+) Methanol (converts to formic acid) Antifreeze (ethylene glycol converts to oxalic acid) Paraldehyde (converts to acetic and chloroacetic acids) Elemental sulfur (converts to sulfuric acid)
Acid accumulation by increased production of normal metabolic acids	Hyperthyroidism Hypermetabolic state after burns, trauma, or sepsis Lactic acidosis Shock
Acid accumulation by utilization of abnormal or incomplete metabolic pathways	Alcoholic ketoacidosis Diabetic ketoacidosis Starvation ketoacidosis
Acid accumulation by impaired acid excretion	Prolonged oliguria from any cause Oliguric renal failure Severe hypovolemia Shock Renal tubular acidosis (type 1) Hypoaldosteronism
Loss of base (bicarbonate ions)	Severe diarrhea Intestinal decompression Fistula drainage from pancreas or intestine Vomiting of intestinal contents Ureterosigmoidostomy Renal tubular acidosis (type 2)

Calculating the anion gap allows further differentiation of metabolic acidosis into two groups: *high serum anion gap metabolic acidosis* and *normal serum anion gap metabolic acidosis.*[3,125] The anion gap increases when an abnormal metabolic acid accumulates in the body, such as with lactic acidosis or ketoacidosis. Normal anion gap acidosis, also called *hyperchloremic acidosis,* typically occurs with diarrhea or loss of HCO_3^- from the kidneys, which retain NaCl in response, or with excessive administration of normal saline. Critically ill patients who have lactic acidosis, a type of anion gap acidosis, have been shown to have a higher mortality rate than those without acidosis.[127]

In research and some clinical settings, metabolic acid–base imbalances may be evaluated using a quantitative physical chemistry method, often called the *Stewart approach* or the *strong ion gap* (SIG).[128,129] The SIG is the apparent strong ion difference minus the charge on buffer base:

$$\text{Strong ion gap} = (Na^+ + K^+ + Ca^{2+} + Mg^{2+}) - (Cl^- \text{ lactate}) - (\text{charge on albumin } + \text{charge on phosphate} + HCO_3^-)$$

One advantage of the SIG over the traditional anion gap is that it enables quantification of the unmeasured anion, but disadvantages are that the calculation is time-consuming and includes clinical parameters such as serum magnesium and lactate concentrations that frequently are not readily available.[129] Whether or not the SIG is useful in predicting outcomes of metabolic acidosis is controversial.[128,129]

Metabolic acidosis can be corrected physiologically only by the kidneys, which are the sole excretory route for metabolic acids. Renal correction of metabolic acidosis may take several days. Meanwhile, respiratory compensation occurs within hours. The respiratory compensation for metabolic acidosis is hyperventilation. By increasing the excretion of carbonic acid, hyperventilation makes the blood less acidic. This makes the blood chemistry more abnormal (decreased $PaCO_2$), but tends to restore the 20:1 ratio of bicarbonate to carbonic acid and move the pH toward the normal range, thus helping to preserve cellular function. Compensated metabolic acidosis is characterized by a decreased $PaCO_2$ (the sign of the respiratory compensation), a decreased bicarbonate ion concentration (the sign of the primary problem), and a pH that is decreased (partially compensated) or normal (fully compensated).

The clinical manifestations of metabolic acidosis include headache, abdominal pain, cardiac arrhythmias, and CNS depression (confusion, drowsiness, lethargy, stupor, and coma). The CNS depression arises from decreased pH of the CSF and resultant intracellular acidosis of brain cells. The exact cause of abdominal pain is not clearly understood. Tachypnea reflects the compensatory hyperventilation.

Although intracellular pH in myocardial cells is regulated to some extent through the action of H^+ transporters in the sarcolemma, these mechanisms become overwhelmed in metabolic acidosis, and intracellular acidosis occurs.[130] Myocardial intracellular acidosis depresses cardiac contractility because it changes the charge on many different proteins. This alters intracellular signaling and delivery of calcium ions to the myofilaments and inhibits myofilament responsiveness to calcium.[131] Cardiac arrhythmias may be related to an increase in circulating catecholamine levels caused by metabolic acidosis or other concurrent pathophysiologic processes, including inhibiting the transient outward potassium ion current from myocytes. The catecholamine increase helps to preserve cardiac output during mild metabolic acidosis, but in more severe metabolic acidosis, the decreased myocardial contractility predominates. Coronary artery occlusion also causes myocardial acidosis, such that these cardiac effects occur in individuals who have acute MI without the systemic effects of metabolic acidosis.

The action of increased circulating catecholamines on the heart also helps to protect the arterial blood pressure from the peripheral vasodilation caused by acidosis. This peripheral vasodilation is caused by several factors, including increased release of nitric oxide by the vascular endothelium. Arterial vascular smooth muscles relax due to activation of ATP-sensitive potassium (K_{ATP}) channels that cause cell membrane hyperpolarization, with less entry of extracellular calcium through voltage-dependent calcium channels. These mechanisms contribute to peripheral, coronary, and cerebral vasodilation.[121] As acidosis progresses, the peripheral vasculature becomes hyporesponsive to adrenergic vasopressors. Contrary to other arterioles, pulmonary vessels respond to acidosis with vasoconstriction, in part due to suppression of nitric oxide synthesis.[123] Vascular effects of acid–base imbalances are summarized in Table 6-19.

Alkalosis

An individual who has alkalosis has processes that tend to increase the pH of the blood above normal by creating a relative excess of base (a relative deficit of acid). The resulting alkalemia may persist or may be modulated by a compensatory response. A pH above 7.8 usually is fatal. Alkalosis is classified as respiratory or metabolic, depending on what type of acid initially is relatively deficient.

Table 6-19 • VASCULAR EFFECTS OF ACID–BASE IMBALANCES

Vascular Bed	Respiratory Acidosis	Metabolic Acidosis	Respiratory Alkalosis	Metabolic Alkalosis
Peripheral	Vasodilation	Vasodilation	Vasoconstriction (debatable)	Vasoconstriction (likely)
Coronary	Vasodilation	Vasodilation	Vasoconstriction	Vasoconstriction
Cerebral	Vasodilation	Vasodilation	Vasoconstriction	Vasoconstriction
Pulmonary	Vasoconstriction	Vasoconstriction	Vasodilation	Vasodilation

Respiratory Alkalosis

Respiratory alkalosis occurs when there is too little carbonic acid in the blood. Clinically, the decreased carbonic acid is measured as a decreased $PaCO_2$. Any factor that causes hyperventilation can cause excretion of too much carbonic acid, leading to respiratory alkalosis (Table 6-20).

Note that hypoxia, as from pulmonary embolism or severe anemia, causes appropriate hyperventilation with resultant respiratory alkalosis. In such cases, the cause of the hypoxia should be the primary focus of treatment rather than the respiratory alkalosis.

Individuals who have respiratory alkalosis may evidence light-headedness, diaphoresis, paresthesias (digital and circumoral), muscle cramps, carpal and pedal spasms, tetany, syncope, and cardiac arrhythmias.[132] Most of these manifestations are the result of increased neuromuscular excitability and may also be associated with changes in the levels of calcium circulating in plasma.[133]

Respiratory alkalosis can be corrected only by the lungs. If any compensation occurs, it is performed by the kidneys, which decrease the reuptake of urinary bicarbonate ions to restore the 20:1 ratio of bicarbonate ion to carbonic acid. Renal compensation for a respiratory acid–base imbalance requires several days. Most cases of respiratory alkalosis have a short duration; therefore, the disorder is often uncompensated or partially compensated. Compensated respiratory alkalosis is characterized by a decreased $PaCO_2$ (the sign of the primary problem), a decreased bicarbonate ion concentration (the sign of the renal compensation), and a pH that is increased (partially compensated) or normal (fully compensated).

Respiratory alkalosis causes increased pH inside myocardial cells and increases cardiac contractility by increasing the calcium sensitivity of myofibrils.[134] The imbalance also increases sympathetic nervous system activity and circulating catecholamines that may cause cardiac arrhythmias. Although respiratory alkalosis may cause transient peripheral vasodilation, which decreases peripheral vascular resistance, it is most likely to cause peripheral vasoconstriction and increased peripheral vascular resistance.[135] Respiratory alkalosis also causes pulmonary artery vasodilation and cerebral vasoconstriction.[136] This latter effect reduces intracranial pressure and cerebral blood flow and may be the reason for the light-headedness and syncope experienced by some individuals with respiratory alkalosis. In contrast to its effect on other blood vessels, respiratory alkalosis causes pulmonary vasodilation.[137] This effect is decreased in conditions with chronically increased pulmonary blood flow, such as some congenital heart defects.[138]

Table 6-20 • CAUSES OF RESPIRATORY ALKALOSIS

Category	Clinical Examples
Hyperventilation due to hypoxemia	Pulmonary disease that causes decreased PaO_2 Pulmonary embolism High altitude
Hyperventilation due to situational factors	Anxiety or fear Pain Prolonged crying and gasping Hyperventilation with mechanical ventilation
Hyperventilation due to stimulation of respiratory neurons in brainstem (medulla)	High fever Encephalitis Meningitis Salicylate overdose Gram-negative sepsis

Metabolic Alkalosis

Metabolic alkalosis is caused by relatively too little metabolic acid. It can be due to a loss of acid or a gain of base. Acid can be lost through the gastrointestinal tract or in the urine. Acid may also be shifted into cells and thus "lost" from the blood. Base (bicarbonate ions) may be gained from the intake of bicarbonate or of substances that are converted to bicarbonate in the body. More commonly, base is gained through renal bicarbonate reabsorption. For example, loop and thiazide diuretic therapy often cause a mild "contraction alkalosis." This is a metabolic alkalosis generated by the loss of chloride and potassium ions. These ion losses lead to increased bicarbonate urinary losses. As is common in heart failure, excessive mineralocorticoid stimulation leads to further loss of H^+ secretion, thereby leading to maintained metabolic alkalosis.[3] In patients requiring large volumes of blood transfusions, metabolic alkalosis may develop due to the metabolism of citrate preservative into bicarbonate.[139] Additional causes of metabolic alkalosis are listed in Table 6-21.

Table 6-21 • CAUSES OF METABOLIC ALKALOSIS

Category	Clinical Examples
Decrease of acid	Emesis Gastric suction Hyperaldosteronism (increases renal excretion of acid) Chronic excessive ingestion of black licorice (contains aldosterone-like compounds) Glucocorticoid excess Loop or thiazide diuretics Hypokalemia (acid moves into cells)
Increase of base (bicarbonate ions)	Excess ingestion of baking soda or bicarbonate antacids Excess infusion of $NaHCO_3$ Excess administration of lactate or acetate (convert to bicarbonate) Massive blood transfusion (citrate converts to bicarbonate) Citrate anticoagulation during chronic renal replacement therapy (citrate converts to bicarbonate) Extracellular fluid volume deficit (contraction alkalosis)

The initial clinical manifestations of metabolic alkalosis are often milder than those of respiratory alkalosis because bicarbonate ions cross membranes (and thus alter CSF and intracellular pH) less rapidly than does carbon dioxide. These clinical manifestations may include light-headedness, paresthesias, muscle cramps, carpal and pedal spasms, and cardiac arrhythmias. An initial CNS excitation is followed by the CNS depression of severe metabolic alkalosis: confusion, lethargy, and coma.

Correction of metabolic alkalosis must be accomplished by the kidneys because they are the excretory organs for bicarbonate ions. Compensation for the disorder, therefore, is the role of the lungs. Because the bicarbonate ion concentration is increased in metabolic alkalosis, the 20:1 ratio of bicarbonate ion to carbonic acid that creates a normal pH can be restored by increasing the amount of carbonic acid in the blood. Thus, the respiratory compensation for metabolic alkalosis is decreased rate and depth of respiration.[140] This compensatory hypoventilation retains carbonic acid (carbon dioxide and water) in the body, which tends to normalize the pH. Compensatory hypoventilation, however, is limited by the body's need for oxygen, so full compensation for metabolic alkalosis is not common. Compensated metabolic alkalosis is characterized by an increased $PaCO_2$ (the sign of the respiratory compensation), an increased bicarbonate ion concentration (the sign of the primary problem), and a pH that is somewhat increased (partially compensated).

Metabolic alkalosis causes increased cardiac contractility by increasing calcium sensitivity, although intracellular pH does not increase in myocardial cells as it does in respiratory alkalosis.[134] Cardiovascular effects include vasoconstriction, pulmonary vasodilation, and cerebral vasoconstriction resulting in decreased cerebral blood flow and light-headedness.[3]

Principles of Interpreting Arterial Blood Gas Reports

Arterial blood gases are used to assess an individual's acid–base status. The material presented earlier in this chapter provides the basis for understanding and interpreting acid–base aspects of arterial blood gases. The principles are summarized in this section. PaO_2 is a measurement of oxygenation.

The first laboratory value to consider is the pH.[141] If the pH is below the normal range (i.e., less than 7.35 or the reported laboratory normal), then the individual has acidosis. If the pH is above the normal range (greater than 7.45 or the reported laboratory normal), then the individual has alkalosis. If the pH is within the normal range, there may be no acid–base imbalance or the individual may have a fully compensated imbalance. For purposes of interpretation, then, if the pH is less than 7.40, the individual is tentatively considered to have acidosis; if the pH is greater than 7.40, the individual is tentatively considered to have alkalosis.

The next value to consider is $PaCO_2$. If $PaCO_2$ is above the normal range, then the individual has respiratory acidosis. This respiratory acidosis may be the primary problem, or it may be compensatory. On the other hand, if the $PaCO_2$ is below the normal range, then the individual has respiratory alkalosis. This respiratory alkalosis may be the primary problem, or it may be compensatory. If the $PaCO_2$ is within the normal range, then the individual does not have a respiratory acid–base disorder.

A basic understanding of acid–base imbalances facilitates differentiating between primary and compensatory respiratory imbalances. If the individual has *primary respiratory acidosis*, then the pH would be expected to be below 7.40. A *compensatory respiratory acidosis* would occur in response to metabolic alkalosis, so the pH would be above 7.40.

The third laboratory value to consider is the bicarbonate ion concentration. If it is above the normal range, the individual has metabolic alkalosis, which may be the primary problem or may be compensatory. If the bicarbonate ion concentration is below the normal range, then the individual has primary or compensatory metabolic acidosis. A bicarbonate ion concentration within the normal range indicates no metabolic acid–base disorder. The differentiation between primary and compensatory imbalances is made by considering the pH. An individual who has a *primary metabolic acidosis* would be expected to have a pH below 7.40. A *compensatory metabolic acidosis* would be a response to a primary respiratory alkalosis, so the pH would be above 7.40. Following similar logic, with a *primary metabolic alkalosis*, the pH would be above 7.40; with a *compensatory metabolic alkalosis*, the pH would be below that value.

Once the three values have been examined, the final step in interpreting arterial blood gas values is to correlate the interpretation with the individual's history and condition. The principles of laboratory value interpretation presented in this section apply to patients who have only one primary acid–base imbalance. Mixed acid–base imbalances (more than one concurrent primary imbalance) are presented briefly in the next section.

Mixed Acid–Base Imbalances

Occasionally, an individual may have more than one primary acid–base imbalance at the same time. In this circumstance, coexisting primary acidosis and alkalosis may somewhat neutralize each other so that the pH is near normal while the $PaCO_2$ and bicarbonate ion concentration are grossly abnormal. Alternatively, two primary disorders that cause the same pH alteration (e.g., types of coexisting alkalosis) can create a pH that rapidly approaches the fatal limit. Examples of mixed acid–base imbalances are presented in Table 6-22.

Summary of Acid–Base

Cellular metabolism generates carbonic acid, which the lungs excrete via carbon dioxide, and metabolic acids, which the kidneys excrete. Respiratory acid–base imbalances are disorders of too much or too little carbonic acid (carbon dioxide and water). Their laboratory marker is an altered $PaCO_2$. The body compensates for an ongoing respiratory acid–base disorder by excreting more or fewer metabolic acids in the urine to normalize the pH. Metabolic acid–base imbalances are disorders of too many or too few metabolic acids. Their laboratory marker is an altered bicarbonate ion concentration. The body compensates for metabolic acid–base disorders by adjusting alveolar ventilation to excrete more or less carbonic acid to normalize the pH. In addition to their other effects, acid–base imbalances alter cardiac contractility and may cause cardiac arrhythmias. These disorders also influence the degree of vasomotor tone in various vascular beds. Thus, an understanding of acid–base balance and imbalance is essential in the care of patients who have heart failure and other cardiovascular pathophysiology.

Cardiac nurses apply knowledge of fluid, electrolyte, and acid–base balance and imbalance to patients with cardiovascular disease or consequences on the cardiovascular system due to noncardiovascular disease. To summarize the chapter content as a whole, Figure 6-5 conceptualizes fluid, electrolyte, and acid–base balance, and general nursing considerations are encompassed in Table 6-23.

Table 6-22 • MIXED ACID–BASE IMBALANCES

Concurrent Primary Acid–Base Imbalances	Effect on pH	Clinical Examples	Blood Gas Values
Respiratory acidosis plus metabolic alkalosis	Opposing effect on pH	Person with type B COPD (chronic bronchitis) develops repeated emesis	pH possibly near normal $PaCO_2$ increased HCO_3^- increased
Respiratory alkalosis plus metabolic acidosis	Opposing effect on pH	Person with encephalitis develops circulatory shock	pH possibly near normal $PaCO_2$ decreased HCO_3^- decreased
Metabolic acidosis plus metabolic alkalosis	Opposing effect on pH	Person with chronic renal failure develops repeated emesis	Vary, depending on severity and duration of imbalances
Respiratory acidosis and metabolic acidosis	Same effect on pH	Person with type B COPD (chronic bronchitis) develops prolonged diarrhea	pH greatly decreased $PaCO_2$ increased HCO_3^- decreased
Two different types of metabolic acidosis	Same effect on pH	Person with diabetic ketoacidosis becomes dehydrated and develops lactic acidosis from poor tissue perfusion	pH greatly decreased $PaCO_2$ likely decreased (compensation) HCO_3^- greatly decreased
Metabolic alkalosis and respiratory alkalosis	Same effect on pH	Person who received massive blood transfusion hyperventilates from pain and fear	pH greatly increased $PaCO_2$ decreased HCO_3^- increased

Table 6-23 • NURSING CONSIDERATIONS FOR FLUID, ELECTROLYTE, AND ACID–BASE BALANCE/IMBALANCE

Patient presentation	Do the patient's chief complaint, admitting or primary diagnosis, or overt signs and symptoms suggest a fluid, electrolyte, or acid–base imbalance? • Shock • Sepsis • Respiratory failure • Heart failure • Liver failure • Renal failure • Dehydration
Past medical and surgical history	Does the past medical history suggest a diagnosis consistent with a known or likely fluid, electrolyte, or acid–base imbalance? • Diabetes • Heart failure • Colon cancer s/p total colectomy • Renal failure
Physical examination	Are there overt signs that suggest a known or likely fluid, electrolyte, or acid–base imbalance? • Altered mental status • Abnormal heart sounds • Abnormal lung sounds • Increased or decreased respiratory rate • Ascites • Hepatojugular reflux • Jaundice • Decreased urine output • Peripheral edema • Poor skin turgor
Laboratory studies	Are there laboratory studies available or being obtained to assess fluid, electrolyte, or acid–base balance? • Complete blood count • Basic or comprehensive metabolic panel • BNP • Arterial blood gas
Medications	Does the patient require medications that are known to impact fluid, electrolyte, or acid–base balance? • Diuretics • Electrolyte supplementation • Nutritional supplementation • Insulin • Certain medications that may cause acidosis: biguanides, propofol, diazepam, salicylates, amphotericin B, nonsteroidal anti-inflammatory drugs • Certain medications that may cause alkalosis: diuretics, penicillin, aminoglycosides, laxatives, bicarbonate or citrate administration
Interventions/procedures	Are there planned interventions or procedures that will impact fluid, electrolyte, or acid–base balance? • Fluid administration/resuscitation • Enteral or parenteral nutrition • Invasive procedures • Surgery, especially if requires cardiopulmonary bypass pump

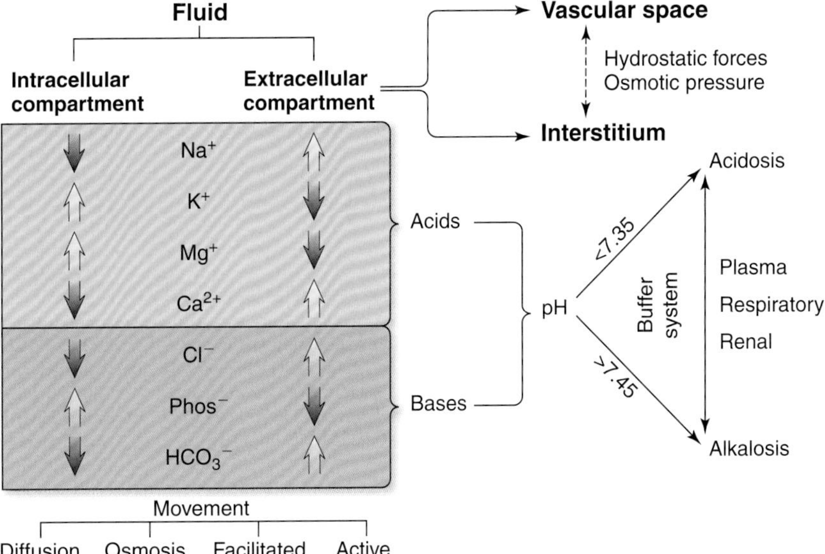

Figure 6-5. Concept Map of Fluid, Electrolyte, and Acid–Base Balance. (Used with permission from Braun C, Anderson C. *Applied Pathophysiology*. 3rd ed. Philadelphia, PA. Wolters Kluwer; 2016.)

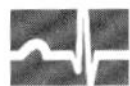

CASE STUDY 1

Patient Profile

You are caring for a 52-year-old female with a history of nonischemic cardiomyopathy, poorly controlled hypertension, and concerns for early kidney disease. Her antihypertensive regimen was recently changed to add spironolactone (aldosterone antagonist) and lisinopril (ACE-I, angiotensin converting enzyme inhibitor). She reports 1 week of progressive malaise and paresthesias (numbness) in her arms and legs. An ECG is obtained and demonstrates peaked T waves. What electrolyte abnormality might you expect, and what is the most likely etiology?

Her lab results demonstrate an increase in serum creatinine from a baseline of 1.1–1.8, and her potassium is now 5.5. The most likely cause of hyperkalemia is the addition of a potassium-sparing diuretic, such as spironolactone and ACE inhibition. This is exacerbated by an acute kidney injury causing an increase in her serum creatinine.

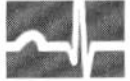

CASE STUDY 2

Patient Profile

You are caring for a 65-year-old male with a history of ischemic cardiomyopathy who has been hospitalized for the past 3 days for acute decompensated heart failure. As part of his therapy, he has been diuresed daily with high-dose loop diuretics. He has urinated a total of 6 L over the past 3 days for a net negative fluid balance of −4 L. A blood gas was obtained out of concern for persistent oxygen requirements of 4 L nasal cannula and an inability to obtain a reliable oxygen saturation with pulse oximetry. The blood gas results as pH 7.5; PCO_2 50 mm Hg; PO_2 110 mm Hg; HCO_3 37 mEq/L. Demonstrates adequate oxygenation. What other acid–base disorder is present, and what is the likely etiology?

His pH of 7.5 demonstrates alkalemia, which is the primary problem. His PCO_2 is well above normal (40 mm Hg), indicating respiratory acidosis; however, since the pH is alkalemic, this elevation in PCO_2 must be compensatory. His HCO_3 is also well above normal (24 mm Hg), indicating an excess of base, metabolic alkalosis. Thus, this patient has primary metabolic alkalosis with a partially compensated respiratory acidosis. In the setting of profound urine output from loop diuretics, this is an example of contraction alkalosis.

KEY READINGS

Cooper HA, Dries DL, Davis CE, et al. Diuretics and risk of arrhythmic death in patients with left ventricular dysfunction. *Circulation.* 1999;100(12):1311–1315.

Diercks DB, Shumaik GM, Harrigan RA, et al. Electrocardiographic manifestations: electrolyte abnormalities. *J Emerg Med.* 2004;27(2):153–160.

Evans KJ, Greenberg A. Hyperkalemia: a review. *J Intensive Care Med.* 2005;20(5):272–290.

Jahnen-Dechent W, Ketteler M. Magnesium basics. *Clin Kidney J.* 2012;5(Suppl 1):i3–i14.

Reddi AS. *Fluid, Electrolyte and Acid-Base Disorders: Clinical Evaluation and Management.* New York: Springer; 2013.

Verbalis JG, Goldsmith SR, Greenberg A, et al. Diagnosis, evaluation, and treatment of hyponatremia: expert panel recommendations. *Am J Med.* 2013;126(10 Suppl 1):S1–S42.

REFERENCES

1. Hall JE. *Guyton and Hall Textbook of Medical Physiology*. 13th ed. Philadelphia, PA: Elsevier; 2016.
2. Blackburn S. *Maternal, Fetal, & Neonatal Physiology*. Philadelphia, PA: WB Saunders; 2003.
3. Reddi AS. *Fluid, Electrolyte and Acid-Base Disorders: Clinical Evaluation and Management.* New York: Springer; 2013.

4. Johnson AK. The sensory psychobiology of thirst and salt appetite. *Med Sci Sports Exerc.* 2007;39(8):1388–1400.
5. Maughan RJ, Griffin J. Caffeine ingestion and fluid balance: a review. *J Hum Nutr Diet.* 2003;16(6):411–420.
6. De Marchi S, Cecchin E. Ethanol-induced water diuresis: one of a spectrum of renal defects resulting from ethanol toxicity. *Nephron.* 1986;43(1):79–80.
7. Awad M, Czer LS, Hou M, et al. Early denervation and later reinnervation of the heart following cardiac transplantation: a review. *J Am Heart Assoc.* 2016;5(11):e004070.
8. Chua Chiaco JM, Parikh NI, Fergusson DJ. The jugular venous pressure revisited. *Cleve Clin J Med.* 2013;80(10):638–644.
9. Selektor Y, Weber KT. The salt-avid state of congestive heart failure revisited. *Am J Med Sci.* 2008;335(3):209–218.
10. LeJemtel TH, Serrano C. Vasopressin dysregulation: hyponatremia, fluid retention and congestive heart failure. *Int J Cardiol.* 2007;120(1):1–9.
11. Gheorghiade M, Abraham WT, Albert NM. Relationship between admission serum sodium concentration and clinical outcomes in patients hospitalized for heart failure: an analysis from the OPTIMIZE-HF registry. *Eur Heart J.* 2007;28:980–988.
12. Rossi J, Bayram M, Udelson JE. Improvement in hyponatremia during hospitalization for worsening heart failure is associated with improved outcomes: insights from the Acute and Chronic Therapeutic Impact of a Vasopressin Antagonist in Chronic Heart Failure (ACTIV in CHF) trial. *Acute Card Care.* 2007;9:82–86.
13. Verbalis JG, Goldsmith SR, Greenberg A, et al. Diagnosis, evaluation, and treatment of hyponatremia: expert panel recommendations. *Am J Med.* 2013;126(10 Suppl 1):S1–S42.
14. Chapman M, Hanrahan R, McEwen J, et al. Hyponatraemia and hypokalaemia due to indapamide. *Med J Aust.* 2002;176:219–222.
15. Kottwitz J, Akdis D, Duru F, et al. Severe hyponatremia leading to complete atrioventricular block. *Am J Med.* 2016;129(10):e243–e244.
16. Lindner G, Funk GC. Hypernatremia in critically ill patients. *J Crit Care.* 2013;28(2):216.e11–216.e20.
17. Moore-Ede MC, Meguid MM, Fitzpatrick GF, et al. Circadian variation in response to potassium infusion. *Clin Pharmacol Ther.* 1978;23(2):218–227.
18. Ahmed A, Zannad F, Love TE, et al. A propensity-matched study of the association of low serum potassium levels and mortality in chronic heart failure. *Eur Heart J.* 2007;28(11):1334–1343.
19. Papadopoulos DP, Papademetriou V. Metabolic side effects and cardiovascular events of diuretics: should a diuretic remain the first choice therapy in hypertension treatment? The case of yes. *Clin Exp Hypertens.* 2007;29(8):503–516.
20. Hahn RG, Lofgren A. Epinephrine, potassium and the electrocardiogram during regional anaesthesia. *Eur J Anaesthesiol.* 2000;17(2):132–137.
21. Foo K, Sekhri N, Deaner A, et al. Effect of diabetes on serum potassium concentrations in acute coronary syndromes. *Heart.* 2003;89(1):31–35.
22. Ives H. Diuretic agents. In: Katzung B, ed. *Basics and Clinical Pharmacology.* New York: Lange Medical Books, McGraw-Hill; 2007:236–254.
23. Blanning A, Westfall JM, Shaughnessy AF. Clinical inquiries. How soon should serum potassium levels be monitored for patients started on diuretics? *J Fam Pract.* 2001;50:207–208.
24. Zuccala G, Pedone C, Cocchi A, et al. Older age and in-hospital development of hypokalemia from loop diuretics: results from a multicenter survey. GIFA Investigators. Multicenter Italian Pharmacoepidemiologic Study Group. *J Gerontol A Biol Sci Med Sci.* 2000;55(4):M232–M238.
25. Cohn JN, Kowey PR, Whelton PK, et al. New guidelines for potassium replacement in clinical practice: a contemporary review by the National Council on Potassium in Clinical Practice. *Arch Intern Med.* 2000;160(16):2429–2436.
26. Schaefer TJ, Wolford RW. Disorders of potassium. *Emerg Med Clin North Am.* 2005;23(3):723–747, viii–ix.
27. Maeder M, Rickli H, Sticherling C, et al. Hypokalaemia and sudden cardiac death—lessons from implantable cardioverter defibrillators. *Emerg Med J.* 2007;24(3):206–208.
28. Slovis C, Jenkins R. ABC of clinical electrocardiography: conditions not primarily affecting the heart. *BMJ.* 2002;324:1320–1323.
29. Skogestad J, Aronsen JM. Hypokalemia-induced arrhythmias and heart failure: new insights and implications for therapy. *Front Physiol.* 2018;9(1500):1500.
30. Steiness E, Olesen KH. Cardiac arrhythmias induced by hypokalaemia and potassium loss during maintenance digoxin therapy. *Br Heart J.* 1976;38(2):167–172.
31. Spodick DH. Hypokalemia. *Am J Geriatr Cardiol.* 2008;17(2):132.
32. Webster A, Brady W, Morris F. Recognising signs of danger: ECG changes resulting from an abnormal serum potassium concentration. *Emerg Med J.* 2002;19(1):74–77.
33. Humphreys M. Potassium disturbances and associated electrocardiogram changes. *Emerg Nurse.* 2007;15(5):28–34.
34. Knochel JP, Schlein EM. On the mechanism of rhabdomyolysis in potassium depletion. *J Clin Invest.* 1972;51(7):1750–1758.
35. Lane R, Phillips M. Rhabdomyolysis. *BMJ.* 2003;327(7407):115–116.
36. Raebel MA. Hyperkalemia associated with use of angiotensin-converting enzyme inhibitors and angiotensin receptor blockers. *Cardiovasc Ther.* 2012;30(3):e156–e166.
37. Sejersted OM, Sjogaard G. Dynamics and consequences of potassium shifts in skeletal muscle and heart during exercise. *Physiol Rev.* 2000;80(4):1411–1481.
38. Evans KJ, Greenberg A. Hyperkalemia: a review. *J Intensive Care Med.* 2005;20(5):272–290.
39. Smith HM, Farrow SJ, Ackerman JD, et al. Cardiac arrests associated with hyperkalemia during red blood cell transfusion: a case series. *Anesth Analg.* 2008;106(4):1062–1069.
40. Eurenius S, Smith RM. The effect of warming on the serum potassium content of stored blood. *Anesthesiology.* 1973;38(5):482–484.
41. Aboudara MC, Hurst FP, Abbott KC, et al. Hyperkalemia after packed red blood cell transfusion in trauma patients. *J Trauma.* 2008;64(2 Suppl):S86–S91; discussion S91.
42. Somers MP, Brady WJ, Perron AD, et al. The prominent T wave: electrocardiographic differential diagnosis. *Am J Emerg Med.* 2002;20:243–251.
43. Chambers DJ, Fallouh HB. Cardioplegia and cardiac surgery: pharmacological arrest and cardioprotection during global ischemia and reperfusion. *Pharmacol Ther.* 2010;127(1):41–52.
44. Cook LK. An acute myocardial infarction? *Am J Crit Care.* 2005;14(4):313–315.
45. Sims DB, Sperling LS. Images in cardiovascular medicine. ST-segment elevation resulting from hyperkalemia. *Circulation.* 2005;111(19):e295–e296.
46. Tatli E, Buyuklu M, Onal B. Electrocardiographic abnormality: hyperkalaemia mimicking isolated acute inferior myocardial infarction. *J Cardiovasc Med (Hagerstown).* 2008;9(2):210.
47. Petrov D, Petrov M. Widening of the QRS complex due to severe hyperkalemia as an acute complication of diabetic ketoacidosis. *J Emerg Med.* 2008;34:459–461.
48. Scarabeo V, Baccillieri MS, Di Marco A, et al. Sine-wave pattern on the electrocardiogram and hyperkalaemia. *J Cardiovasc Med (Hagerstown).* 2007;8(9):729–731.
49. Mitra JK, Pandia MP, Dash HH, et al. Moderate hyperkalaemia without ECG changes in the intraoperative period. *Acta Anaesthesiol Scand.* 2008;52:444–445.
50. Montague BT, Ouellette JR, Buller GK. Retrospective review of the frequency of ECG changes in hyperkalemia. *Clin J Am Soc Nephrol.* 2008;3(2):324–330.
51. Aslam S, Friedman EA, Ifudu O. Electrocardiography is unreliable in detecting potentially lethal hyperkalaemia in haemodialysis patients. *Nephrol Dial Transplant.* 2002;17:1639–1642.
52. Nemati E, Taheri S. Electrocardiographic manifestations of hyperkalemia in hemodialysis patients. *Saudi J Kidney Dis Transpl.* 2010;21(3):471–477.
53. Mattu A, Brady WJ, Perron AD. Electrocardiographic manifestations of hypothermia. *Am J Emerg Med.* 2002;20(4):314–326.
54. Littmann L, Brearley WD Jr, Taylor L 3rd, et al. Double counting of heart rate by interpretation software: a new electrocardiographic sign of severe hyperkalemia. *Am J Emerg Med.* 2007;25(5):584–586.
55. Oudit GY, Cameron D, Harris L. A case of appropriate inappropriate device therapy: hyperkalemia-induced ventricular oversensing. *Can J Cardiol.* 2008;24(3):e16–e18.
56. Khan E, Voudouris A, Shorofsky SR, et al. Inappropriate ICD discharges due to "triple counting" during normal sinus rhythm. *J Interv Card Electrophysiol.* 2006;17:153–155.
57. Terkildsen JR, Crampin EJ, Smith NP. The balance between inactivation and activation of the Na^+-K^+ pump underlies the triphasic accumulation of extracellular K+ during myocardial ischemia. *Am J Physiol Heart Circ Physiol.* 2007;293:H3036–H3045.
58. Long C, Li W, Lin DM, et al. Effect of potassium-channel openers on the release of endothelium-derived hyperpolarizing factor in porcine coronary arteries stored in cold hyperkalemic solution. *J Extra Corpor Technol.* 2002;34(2):125–129.

59. Krassoi I, Pataricza J, Papp JG. Thiorphan enhances bradykinin-induced vascular relaxation in hypoxic/hyperkalaemic porcine coronary artery. *J Pharm Pharmacol.* 2003;55(3):339–345.
60. Matsuda N, Morgan KG, Sellke FW. Preconditioning improves cardioplegia-related coronary microvascular smooth muscle hypercontractility: role of KATP channels. *J Thorac Cardiovasc Surg.* 1999;118(3):438–445.
61. Chernow B, Zaloga G, McFadden E, et al. Hypocalcemia in critically ill patients. *Crit Care Med.* 1982;10(12):848–851.
62. Giancarelli A, Birrer KL, Alban RF, et al. Hypocalcemia in trauma patients receiving massive transfusion. *J Surg Res.* 2016;202(1):182–187.
63. Kovalik SG, Ledgerwood AM, Lucas CE, et al. The cardiac effect of altered calcium homeostasis after albumin resuscitation. *J Trauma.* 1981;21(4):275–279.
64. Mishra A, Wong L, Jonklaas J. Prolonged, symptomatic hypocalcemia with pamidronate administration and subclinical hypoparathyroidism. *Endocrine.* 2001;14(2):159–164.
65. Keegan MT, Bondy LR, Blackshear JL, et al. Hypocalcemia-like electrocardiographic changes after administration of intravenous fosphenytoin. *Mayo Clin Proc.* 2002;77(6):584–586.
66. Iwazu Y, Muto S, Ikeuchi S, et al. Reversible hypocalcemic heart failure with T wave alternans and increased QTc dispersion in a patient with chronic renal failure after parathyroidectomy. *Clin Nephrol.* 2006;65(1):65–70.
67. Kazmi AS, Wall BM. Reversible congestive heart failure related to profound hypocalcemia secondary to hypoparathyroidism. *Am J Med Sci.* 2007;333(4):226–229.
68. Tsironi M, Korovesis K, Farmakis D, et al. Hypocalcemic heart failure in thalassemic patients. *Int J Hematol.* 2006;83(4):314–317.
69. Wermers RA, Kearns AE, Jenkins GD, et al. Incidence and clinical spectrum of thiazide-associated hypercalcemia. *Am J Med.* 2007;120(10):911.e9–e15.
70. Mannstadt M, Kronenberg HM. Parathyroid hormone gene: structure, evolution, and regulation. In: Bilezikian JP, ed. *The Parathyroids.* 3rd ed. Academic Press; 2015:37–44.
71. Vosnakidis A, Polymeropoulos K, Zarogoulidis P, et al. Atrioventricular nodal dysfunction secondary to hyperparathyroidism. *J Thorac Dis.* 2013;5(3):E90–E92.
72. Kiewiet RM, Ponssen HH, Janssens EN, et al. Ventricular fibrillation in hypercalcaemic crisis due to primary hyperparathyroidism. *Neth J Med.* 2004;62(3):94–96.
73. Diercks DB, Shumaik GM, Harrigan RA, et al. Electrocardiographic manifestations: electrolyte abnormalities. *J Emerg Med.* 2004;27(2):153–160.
74. Vella A, Gerber TC, Hayes DL, et al. Digoxin, hypercalcaemia, and cardiac conduction. *Postgrad Med J.* 1999;75(887):554–556.
75. Longo D, Fauci A, Kasper D, et al. *Harrison's Principles of Internal Medicine.* 18th ed. McGraw-Hill; 2011.
76. Nilsson IL, Rastad J, Johansson K, et al. Endothelial vasodilatory function and blood pressure response to local and systemic hypercalcemia. *Surgery.* 2001;130(6):986–990.
77. Kamycheva E, Jorde R, Haug E. Effects of acute hypercalcaemia on blood pressure in subjects with and without parathyroid hormone secretion. *Acta Physiol Scand.* 2005;184:113–119.
78. Jahnen-Dechent W, Ketteler M. Magnesium basics. *Clin Kidney J.* 2012;5(Suppl 1):i3–i14.
79. Leevy CM, Moroianu SA. Nutritional aspects of alcoholic liver disease. *Clin Liver Dis.* 2005;9(1):67–81.
80. Cohen N, Almoznino-Sarafian D, Zaidenstein R, et al. Serum magnesium aberrations in furosemide (frusemide) treated patients with congestive heart failure: pathophysiological correlates and prognostic evaluation. *Heart.* 2003;89(4):411–416.
81. Cooper HA, Dries DL, Davis CE, et al. Diuretics and risk of arrhythmic death in patients with left ventricular dysfunction. *Circulation.* 1999;100(12):1311–1315.
82. Oladapo OO, Falase AO. Congestive heart failure and ventricular arrhythmias in relation to serum magnesium. *Afr J Med Med Sci.* 2000;29(3–4):265–268.
83. Gao X, Peng L, Adhikari CM, et al. Spironolactone reduced arrhythmia and maintained magnesium homeostasis in patients with congestive heart failure. *J Card Fail.* 2007;13(3):170–177.
84. Elming H, Seibaek M, Ottesen MM, et al. Serum-ionised magnesium in patients with acute myocardial infarction. Relation to cardiac arrhythmias, left ventricular function and mortality. *Magnes Res.* 2000;13(4):285–292.
85. Klevay LM, Milne DB. Low dietary magnesium increases supraventricular ectopy. *Am J Clin Nutr.* 2002;75(3):550–554.
86. Mela T, Galvin JM, McGovern BA. Magnesium deficiency during lactation as a precipitant of ventricular tachyarrhythmias. *Pacing Clin Electrophysiol.* 2002;25:231–233.
87. Wilkes NJ, Mallett SV, Peachey T, et al. Correction of ionized plasma magnesium during cardiopulmonary bypass reduces the risk of postoperative cardiac arrhythmia. *Anesth Analg.* 2002;95(4):828–834.
88. Dorman BH, Sade RM, Burnette JS, et al. Magnesium supplementation in the prevention of arrhythmias in pediatric patients undergoing surgery for congenital heart defects. *Am Heart J.* 2000;139(3):522–528.
89. Speziale G, Ruvolo G, Fattouch K, et al. Arrhythmia prophylaxis after coronary artery bypass grafting: regimens of magnesium sulfate administration. *Thorac Cardiovasc Surg.* 2000;48(1):22–26.
90. Kaye P, O'Sullivan I. The role of magnesium in the emergency department. *Emerg Med J.* 2002;19(4):288–291.
91. Priori SG, Blomstrom-Lundqvist C, Mazzanti A, et al. 2015 ESC Guidelines for the management of patients with ventricular arrhythmias and the prevention of sudden cardiac death: The Task Force for the Management of Patients with Ventricular Arrhythmias and the Prevention of Sudden Cardiac Death of the European Society of Cardiology (ESC)Endorsed by: Association for European Paediatric and Congenital Cardiology (AEPC). *Europace.* 2015;17(11):1601–1687.
92. Speich M, Bousquet B, Nicolas G. Concentrations of magnesium, calcium, potassium, and sodium in human heart muscle after acute myocardial infarction. *Clin Chem.* 1980;26(12):1662–1665.
93. Kramer JH, Mak IT, Phillips TM, et al. Dietary magnesium intake influences circulating pro-inflammatory neuropeptide levels and loss of myocardial tolerance to postischemic stress. *Exp Biol Med (Maywood).* 2003;228(6):665–673.
94. Haigney MC, Berger R, Schulman S, et al. Tissue magnesium levels and the arrhythmic substrate in humans. *J Cardiovasc Electrophysiol.* 1997;8(9):980–986.
95. Baker WL. Treating arrhythmias with adjunctive magnesium: identifying future research directions. *Eur Heart J Cardiovasc Pharmacother.* 2017;3(2):108–117.
96. Kolte D, Vijayaraghavan K, Khera S, et al. Role of magnesium in cardiovascular diseases. *Cardiol Rev.* 2014;22(4):182–192.
97. de Baaij JHF, Hoenderop JGJ, Bindels RJM. Magnesium in man: implications for health and disease. *Physiol Rev.* 2015;95(1):1–46.
98. Dickinson HO, Nicolson DJ, Campbell F, et al. Magnesium supplementation for the management of essential hypertension in adults. *Cochrane Database Syst Rev.* 2006;3(3):CD004640.
99. Del Gobbo LC, Imamura F, Wu JHY, et al. Circulating and dietary magnesium and risk of cardiovascular disease: a systematic review and meta-analysis of prospective studies. *Am J Clin Nutr.* 2013;98(1):160–173.
100. Mazur A, Maier JA, Rock E, et al. Magnesium and the inflammatory response: potential physiopathological implications. *Arch Biochem Biophys.* 2007;458(1):48–56.
101. Mubagwa K, Gwanyanya A, Zakharov S, et al. Regulation of cation channels in cardiac and smooth muscle cells by intracellular magnesium. *Arch Biochem Biophys.* 2007;458(1):73–89.
102. Zaman F, Abreo K. Severe hypermagnesemia as a result of laxative use in renal insufficiency. *South Med J.* 2003;96:102–103.
103. Birrer RB, Shallash AJ, Totten V. Hypermagnesemia-induced fatality following epsom salt gargles. *J Emerg Med.* 2002;22(2):185–188.
104. Weisinger JR, Bellorin-Font E. Magnesium and phosphorus. *Lancet.* 1998;352(9125):391–396.
105. Knochel JP. The pathophysiology and clinical characteristics of severe hypophosphatemia. *Arch Intern Med.* 1977;137(2):203–220.
106. Liamis G, Milionis HJ, Elisaf M. Medication-induced hypophosphatemia: a review. *QJM.* 2010;103(7):449–459.
107. Shiber JR, Mattu A. Serum phosphate abnormalities in the emergency department. *J Emerg Med.* 2002;23(4):395–400.
108. Claudius I, Sachs C, Shamji T. Hypophosphatemia-induced heart failure. *Am J Emerg Med.* 2002;20(4):369–370.
109. Korbonits M, Blaine D, Elia M, et al. Metabolic and hormonal changes during the refeeding period of prolonged fasting. *Eur J Endocrinol.* 2007;157(2):157–166.
110. Miller DW, Slovis CM. Hypophosphatemia in the emergency department therapeutics. *Am J Emerg Med.* 2000;18(4):457–461.
111. Subramanian R, Khardori R. Severe hypophosphatemia. Pathophysiologic implications, clinical presentations, and treatment. *Medicine (Baltimore).* 2000;79(1):1–8.
112. Lin KK, Lee JJ, Chen HC. Severe refeeding hypophosphatemia in a CAPD patient: a case report. *Ren Fail.* 2006;28(6):515–517.

113. Heames RM, Cope RA. Hypophosphataemia causing profound cardiac failure after cardiac surgery. *Anaesthesia.* 2006;61(12):1211–1213.
114. Barrett KE, Barman SM, Brooks HL, et al., (eds.). Regulation of respiration. In: *Ganong's Review of Medical Physiology.* 26th ed. New York: McGraw-Hill Education; 2019.
115. Barrett KE, Barman SM, Brooks HL, et al., (eds.). Gas transport & pH. In: *Ganong's Review of Medical Physiology.* 26th ed. New York: McGraw-Hill Education; 2019.
116. Schoolwerth AC, Kaneko TM, Sedlacek M, et al. Acid-base disturbances in the intensive care unit: metabolic acidosis. *Semin Dial.* 2006;19(6):492–495.
117. Boron WF. Acid-base transport by the renal proximal tubule. *J Am Soc Nephrol.* 2006;17(9):2368–2382.
118. Mizukoshi Y, Shibata K, Yoshida M. Left ventricular contractility is reduced by hypercapnic acidosis and thoracolumbar epidural anesthesia in rabbits. *Can J Anaesth.* 2001;48:557–562.
119. Avidan MS, Ali SZ, Tymkew H, et al. Mild hypercapnia after uncomplicated heart surgery is not associated with hemodynamic compromise. *J Cardiothoracic Vasc Anesth.* 2007;21:371–374.
120. Crampin EJ, Smith NP, Langham AE, et al. Acidosis in models of cardiac ventricular myocytes. *Philos Trans A Math Phys Eng Sci.* 2006;364(1842):1171–1186.
121. Crimi E, Taccone FS, Infante T, et al. Effects of intracellular acidosis on endothelial function: an overview. *J Crit Care.* 2012;27(2):108–118.
122. Najarian T, Marrache AM, Dumont I, et al. Prolonged hypercapnia-evoked cerebral hyperemia via K(+) channel- and prostaglandin E(2)-dependent endothelial nitric oxide synthase induction. *Circ Res.* 2000;87(12):1149–1156.
123. Barnes PJ, Liu SF. Regulation of pulmonary vascular tone. *Pharmacol Rev.* 1995;47(1):87–131.
124. Kraut JA, Madias NE. Serum anion gap: its uses and limitations in clinical medicine. *Clin J Am Soc Nephrol.* 2007;2(1):162–174.
125. Chernecky C. *Laboratory Tests and Diagnostic Procedures.* St. Louis, MO: Elsevier Saunders; 2008.
126. Emmett M. Anion-gap interpretation: the old and the new. *Nat Clin Pract Nephrol.* 2006;2(1):4–5.
127. Gunnerson KJ, Saul M, He S, et al. Lactate versus non-lactate metabolic acidosis: a retrospective outcome evaluation of critically ill patients. *Critical Care.* 2006;10(1):R22.
128. Dubin A, Menises MM, Masevicius FD, et al. Comparison of three different methods of evaluation of metabolic acid-base disorders. *Crit Care Med.* 2007;35(5):1264–1270.
129. Gunnerson KJ. Clinical review: the meaning of acid-base abnormalities in the intensive care unit part I—epidemiology. *Crit Care.* 2005;9(5):508–516.
130. Orchard C. Downhill all the way: H(+) gradients within cardiac myocytes. *Biophys J.* 2007;92(2):371–372.
131. Du Z, Chaoqian X, Shan H, et al. Functional impairment of cardiac transient outward K+ current as a result of abnormally altered cellular environment. *Clin Exp Pharmacol Physiol.* 2007;34:148–152.
132. Han JN, Stegen K, Simkens K, et al. Unsteadiness of breathing in patients with hyperventilation syndrome and anxiety disorders. *Eur Respir J.* 1997;10(1):167–176.
133. Somjen GG, Allen BW, Balestrino M, et al. Pathophysiology of pH and Ca2+ in bloodstream and brain. *Can J Physiol Pharmacol.* 1987;65(5):1078–1085.
134. Hunjan S, Mason RP, Mehta VD. Simultaneous intracellular and extracellular pH measurement in the heart by 19F NMR of 6-fluoropyridoxol. *Magnetic Reson Med.* 1998;39(4):551–556.
135. Steinback CD, Poulin MJ. Cardiovascular and cerebrovascular responses to acute isocapnic and poikilocapnic hypoxia in humans. *J Appl Physiol (1985).* 2008;104(2):482–489.
136. Raichle ME, Plum F. Hyperventilation and cerebral blood flow. *Stroke.* 1972;3(5):566–575.
137. Jundi K, Barrington KJ, Henderson C, et al. The hemodynamic effects of prolonged respiratory alkalosis in anesthetized newborn piglets. *Intensive Care Med.* 2000;26(4):449–456.
138. Cornfield DN, Resnik ER, Herron JM, et al. Pulmonary vascular K+ channel expression and vasoreactivity in a model of congenital heart disease. *Am J Physiol Lung Cell Mol Physiol.* 2002;283(6):L1210–L1219.
139. Li K, Xu Y. Citrate metabolism in blood transfusions and its relationship due to metabolic alkalosis and respiratory acidosis. *Int J Clin Exp Med.* 2015;8(4):6578–6584.
140. Barrett KE, Barman SM, Brooks HL, et al., (eds.). Acidification of the urine & bicarbonate excretion. In: *Ganong's Review of Medical Physiology.* 26th ed. New York: McGraw-Hill Education; 2019.
141. Cowley NJ, Owen A, Bion JF. Rational testing: interpreting arterial blood gas results. *BMJ.* 2013;346(7895):36–38.

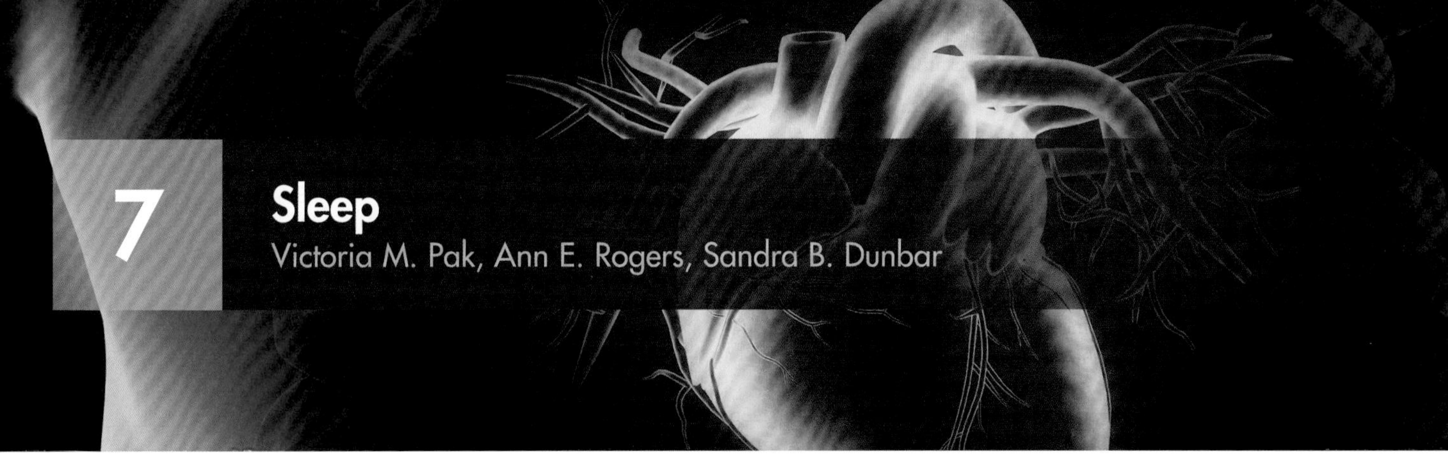

7 Sleep

Victoria M. Pak, Ann E. Rogers, Sandra B. Dunbar

OBJECTIVES

1. Describe normal sleep patterns in adults and identify behaviors and other factors that adversely affect normal sleep.
2. Describe sleep physiology and processes in terms of selected body systems.
3. Describe subjective, objective, and behavioral assessment of sleep including measures.

KEY QUESTIONS

1. Name symptoms and treatment approaches for selected sleep disorders.
2. Name interactions among sleep disorders, obstructive sleep apnea, and selected cardiovascular risk factors and conditions.
3. Name nursing care approaches for sleep disorders in CV patients incorporating pharmacologic and nonpharmacologic treatment.

INTRODUCTION

Physiologic changes that accompany normal sleep may have adverse effects on patients with cardiovascular disease (CVD). Cardiac patients as a group have a high prevalence of sleep abnormalities, and because sleep disorders have also been increasingly identified as a contributor to the development of or progression of CVD, attention to sleep in overall cardiovascular care has become essential.[1] Cardiovascular nurses are well positioned to assess sleep patterns and sleep-disordered breathing (SDB), identify poor sleep quality and quantity, intervene to prevent sleep loss, educate and counsel cardiovascular patients regarding sleep, refer patients for sleep consultation, and work with the interdisciplinary team to assure treatments for sleep and sleep-related problems. To assist nurses in helping patients with or at risk for CVD achieve adequate, restful, and restorative sleep, this chapter reviews normal sleep and sleepiness, changes in cardiopulmonary and other system functions during sleep, sleep problems commonly seen in patients with CVD, and appropriate management.

NORMAL SLEEP

Sleep and Sleepiness

The human need for sleep has been recognized throughout the centuries, and few physiologic phenomena have received as much attention from scholars, scientists, poets, and other literary figures. Before the 20th century, sleep was thought to be a simple, passive phenomenon—a state often described as existing between waking and death.[2] Although much remains to be fully understood about the topic, the modern study of sleep has revealed some of its secrets. Sleep is now understood as an active process regulated by a multiplicity of behavioral, neuroendocrine, and central nervous system factors.[3] Insufficient and/or poor quality nocturnal sleep and daytime sleepiness adversely affect important clinical outcomes.[4–7] Over 60 sleep disorders[8] have been recognized, and the field of sleep medicine is now a bona fide, empirically based subspecialty.[9]

The modern definition of sleep is "a reversible behavioral state of perceptual disengagement from and unresponsiveness to the environment."[3] Sleep is further defined according to behavioral and physiologic criteria. Behavioral criteria include quiescence, closed eyes, decreased response to external stimuli, recumbent position, and reversible unconsciousness. Physiologic criteria are based on recordings from a polysomnogram that includes electroencephalography (EEG), electro-oculography (EOG), and electromyography (EMG).[3]

Daytime sleepiness refers to the tendency or propensity to fall asleep during the day. In normal individuals, sleepiness typically has a biphasic circadian rhythm,[10] with an increased sleep tendency in the midafternoon and, as is well known to night-shift workers, in the early morning hours.[3,10] In fact, a continuum between being very alert and very sleepy (often referred to as *arousal state*) provides a background for all waking endeavors and is a far more important dimension of human function than commonly recognized. Many adults are chronically sleepy in the daytime because of insufficient or disrupted nighttime sleep. The problem may initially go unnoticed when masked by stimulating factors such as movement, excitement, high motivation, or hunger. However, daytime sleepiness can be unmasked by situational factors such as boredom, a warm dark room, or a prolonged dull task.[10] Although poor nocturnal sleep can cause sleepiness, abnormal daytime sleep can also adversely affect nocturnal sleep. Thus, a complete assessment must include an examination of nocturnal and daytime sleep/wake patterns.

Normal Sleep

Most adults have their major sleep period at night, organized into a rhythmic sequence of sleep stages. Sleep is usually divided into nonrapid eye movement (NREM) and rapid eye movement (REM) sleep. NREM sleep is further divided into four stages (1, 2, 3, and 4) reflecting increasing depth of sleep and a reduction in the arousal threshold. Dreaming occurs during REM sleep.

In a young healthy adult, who is obtaining adequate sleep, sleep begins with a short period, for example, 1 to 7 minutes of stage 1 sleep. During this stage the sleeper is easily aroused and may not be aware that they are sleeping. Within a few minutes, sleep deepens and the individual becomes more difficult to arouse, and if aroused, is aware that they have been sleeping. Stage 2 sleep usually lasts from 20 to 40 minutes during the first sleep cycle of the night. Stages 3 and 4, collectively termed, slow wave or deep sleep, differ only in the percentage of delta waves that are recorded during a sleep study. SWS typically lasts from 20 to 40 minutes at the beginning of the night and the individual is very difficult to arouse. After a period of deep sleep, the individual's sleep "lightens" and they may have 5 to 10 minutes of stage 2 sleep before entering REM sleep. The first dreaming period is typically short, for example, less than 10 minutes and typically occurs 80 to 90 minutes after sleep onset. NREM and REM sleep periods then alternate throughout the night, with more slow wave or deep sleep occurring during the first third of the night and more REM sleep occurring during the last third of the night. In healthy young adults, 2% to 5% of the night is spent in stage 1 sleep, 45% to 55% of the night consists of stage 2 sleep, 10% to 20% of the night is spent in SWS (stages 3 and 4), and 20% to 25% consists of REM sleep.[3]

The below Figure 7-1 represents typical sleep of a healthy young adult. Both the duration of sleep and the distribution of sleep stages across the night can be altered by a variety of factors including age, volitional determinants (e.g., staying up late, waking by an alarm, etc.), circadian rhythms, sleep environment, alcohol and drug ingestion, health, and sleep disorders.

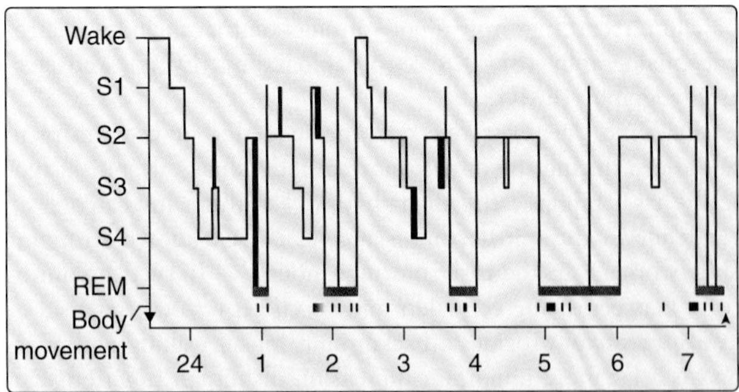

Figure 7-1. The progression of sleep stages across a single night in a normal young adult volunteer. The histogram was drawn on the basis of a continuous overnight recording of electroencephalogram, electro-oculogram, and electromylogram in a normal 19-year-old male. (Used with permission from Kryger M, Roth T, Dement WC. *Principles and Practice of Sleep Medicine.* 6th ed. Philadelphia, PA: Elsevier; 2017:21.)

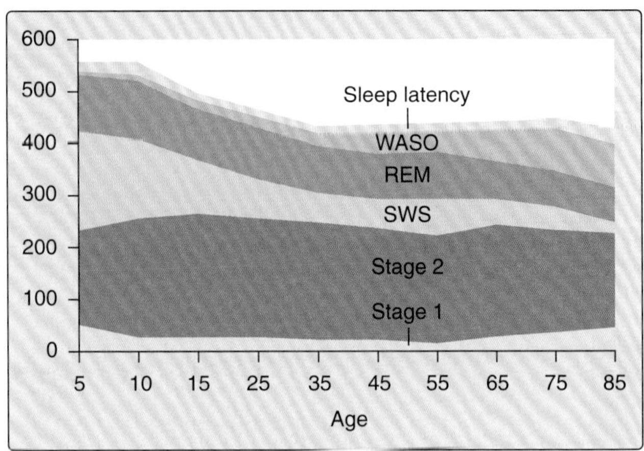

Figure 7-2. Time (in minutes) for sleep latency and wake time after sleep onset (WASO) and for REM sleep and NREM sleep stages 1,2, and slow wave sleep (SWS). Summary values are given for ages 5 to 85 years. (Used with permission from Kryger M, Roth T, Dement WC. *Principles and Practice of Sleep Medicine.* 6th ed. Philadelphia, PA: Elsevier; 2017:21.)

Age

Age is one of the major factors that affect sleep stages across the night. Unlike adults, infants enter REM (called active sleep in newborns) and then transition to NREM sleep, and their sleep is distributed throughout the 24-hour period. Sleep cycles are typically 60 minutes rather than 90 minutes in length. Within 6 months to 1 year, they develop the more mature pattern of entering NREM sleep before REM sleep, and sleep begins to be consolidated at night. Young children typically have longer periods of SWS and are particularly difficult to arouse during deep sleep. The first REM period may be skipped by children and young teens due to the quantity and quality of their SWS. By midadolescence, SWS decreases by approximately 40%[11] and their sleep pattern resembles that of a young adult (Fig. 7-2).

Older people may spend more time in bed but less time asleep (lower sleep efficiency) and are more easily awakened from sleep. Even healthy older people experience more arousals (short awakenings) after age, 60 and by age 55 to 60, SWS in men has declined to half of that of similarly aged women (8.2% compared to 17%).[12] REM sleep, as a percentage of sleep time, is relatively well maintained across the lifespan but may decline slightly with advanced age. Sleep latency (time required to fall asleep) shows little change with aging, however, bedtime and wake-up times come earlier (circadian phase advance), daytime sleep tendency may be increased, and daytime napping is more common.[13,14] Sleep disorders, such as obstructive sleep apnea (OSA) and periodic limb movements (PLMs) (involuntary repetitive leg jerks during sleep) are more common in older adults, and can contribute to sleep disruption.[14]

Although most adults require 7 to 8 hours sleep for optimal cognitive performance and maintenance of health,[15–17] studies have shown that approximately one third of all adults in the United States regularly obtain less than 7 hours sleep[14]; 23.0% of the 444,306 respondents to the Behavioral Risk Factor Surveillance System (BRFSS) reporting a sleep duration of 6 hours or less and 11.8% of the respondents reporting that they obtain

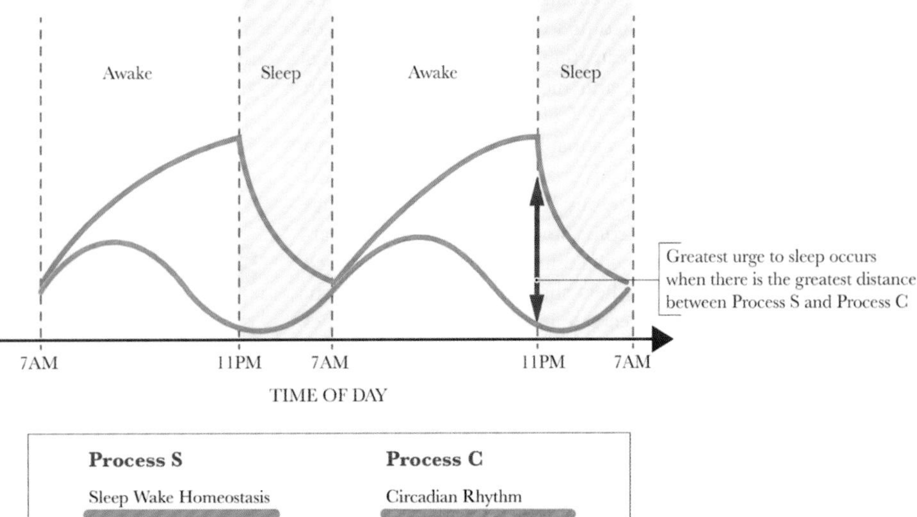

Figure 7-3. Two-process model of sleep regulation showing the interaction between Process S which rises during waking and declines during sleep and Process C which is not directly dependent on sleep and waking.

5 hours or less sleep/night. Mean sleep durations varied by (1) geographic region, for example, those in the southeastern United States and the Appalachian Mountains reporting less sleep; (2) age, with 73.7% of those over 65 reporting that they obtained at least 7 hours sleep/night; (3) marital status with those who were married obtaining more sleep than those who were divorced, widowed, or separated; (4) employment status; (5) educational attainment; and (6) ethnicity.[18]

Circadian Rhythms

The timing and duration of sleep is also highly influenced by the interaction of two different biologic mechanisms; homeostatic processes and circadian rhythms. The two-process model of sleep regulation describes how Process S (sleep/wake homeostasis) and Process C (circadian rhythm) interact. Process S refers to the sleep need which is dependent on the amount of previous amount of sleep and wakefulness. As seen in Figure 7-3, the physiologic need for sleep is low upon awakening, builds throughout the day, and dissipates throughout the night.[19] The circadian process (Process C), a sinusoidal rhythm of approximately 24 hours, is controlled by a biologic oscillator (suprachiasmatic nucleus). Perhaps one of the best known circadian rhythms is that of core body temperature; it is lowest around 4 AM, rises during the morning and early afternoon, then peaks in the late afternoon between 4 and 6 PM, and falls toward night time. Although night shift workers are often sleepy when they get off work in the morning, it can be very difficult to fall asleep due to the rising core body temperature. Likewise, when core body temperature is at its lowest during the early morning hours, it can be very difficult to remain awake.

The timing and duration of sleep are determined by the combined action of homeostatic and circadian processes.[20] Factors that either oppose or enhance these processes can have significant effects on the timing, duration, and structure of sleep as well as daytime alertness.

Although the shape of the sinusoidal circadian rhythm remains the same, the timing of peaks and troughs of daytime alertness and the timing of nocturnal sleep can be highly variable among healthy individuals.[21] Some individuals like to go to bed early and get up early (morning types), while others prefer to get up late and to sleep late (evening types). Studies among twin pairs, and population- and family-based cohorts have shown roughly 50% heritability for diurnal preference[22] and 22% to 25% for habitual bedtimes,[23,24] suggesting the contribution of additive, small effects of multiple genes in combination with the environment.[25]

Environment

The environment can play an important role in the quantity and quality of sleep. A thermoneutral environment (neither too hot nor too cold) is essential for normal thermoregulatory changes to optimize sleep.[26] Excessive noise disrupts subjective and objective sleep. Too much light, particularly associated with the use of electronic devices, alters melatonin production.[27,28] On a more macrolevel, living in disadvantaged neighborhoods is associated with more waking after sleep onset, shorter sleep durations, and daytime napping.[29–31]

Drug and Alcohol Exposure

Virtually all drugs with high abuse potential, including alcohol, cocaine, amphetamines, and opioids, have disruptive effects on sleep and daytime alertness.[32] Even more socially acceptable drugs, such as marijuana, nicotine, and caffeine, have adverse effects on sleep and wakefulness.

Approximately 30% of patients with insomnia report using alcohol to help them fall asleep, and 67% of these individuals report that alcohol was effective in inducing sleep.[33]

Although low doses of alcohol may initially reduce sleep latency, tolerance to its beneficial effect develops within three to five nights.[34] Higher doses of alcohol suppress REM during the first half of the night (before the alcohol has been completely metabolized), along with increased wakefulness and a REM rebound during the last half of the night after the alcohol has been metabolized. Patients with alcoholism frequently complain of difficulties falling asleep, daytime sleepiness, and parasomnias (sleep disruptions that occur due to arousals from NREM and REM sleep).[37] Sleep latencies and total sleep time are disturbed on both drinking and discontinuation nights.[35] These abnormal sleep patterns can persist up to 3 years in some patients with alcoholism, and may even predict the likelihood of relapse during abstinence.[32]

According to a recent Gallup poll,[36] approximately 45% of adults living in the United States have tried marijuana, and

12% to 13% report current use of marijuana. Although marijuana remains classified as a schedule I drug (no acceptable medical use) on the federal level, recreational use is legal in 9 states plus the District of Columbia, and medicinal use is allowed in another 30 states and the District of Columbia.[37,38] Most research on the effects of marijuana (or cannabis) on sleep date back to the 1970s, including a number of small studies which included objective measures (polysomnography [PSG]) of sleep.[32] Findings from that era were mixed with some studies suggesting that marijuana was associated with a decrease in sleep latency, decreased wake after sleep onset, while others showed no effects on sleep, or an increase in SWS and a decrease in REM sleep.[39–42] Studies also suggested that marijuana might have a short-term beneficial effect on sleep,[43] but that chronic use could be associated with habituation to the sleep-inducing and slow wave sleep–enhancing properties.[41,44,45] More recent systematic reviews have concluded that although there may be a decrease in SWS and a corresponding increase in stage 2 sleep, there is no consistent effect on sleep duration.[46,47] Subjective sleep quality, however, may be improved among individuals using medicinal marijuana to treat conditions such as pain, that are known to disrupt sleep.[46] Withdrawal symptoms, for example, difficulty sleeping, decreased total sleep time, decreased REM sleep, decreased sleep efficiency, and increased wake after sleep onset, tend to get worse during the first 14 days of abstinence, and persist for at least 45 days.[48,49]

Given the effects of nicotine on sleep, it is not surprising that many smokers complain of difficulties falling asleep and staying asleep.[50] Laboratory studies have demonstrated that the use of nicotine is associated with extended sleep latencies, decreased total sleep time, extended REM latency, and decreased SWS.[51] The effects of nicotine withdrawal, for example, decreased sleep quality, increased nocturnal awakenings, and altered mood, can last up to 20 days.[52]

Even though caffeine is not usually considered a drug of abuse, tolerance to its effects can develop with chronic use.[53] Caffeine typically prolongs sleep latency, reduces both total sleep time and sleep efficiency, and worsens perceived sleep quality.[50,54] Although there is significant individual variation in sensitivity to caffeine, SWS is usually reduced and stage 1 sleep, wakefulness, and arousals are increased. Withdrawal symptoms can include headaches, reduced vigor, and increased sleepiness, fatigue, and drowsiness.[32]

Health and Sleep Disorders

Sleep can also be shortened and/or disrupted by a variety of acute and chronic health conditions. For example, cancer patients often have symptoms of insomnia and disrupted sleep during treatment and even several years after treatment.[55–58] Other health conditions frequently associated with impaired sleep include asthma,[59,60] CVD,[61] fibromyalgia, chronic fatigue syndrome,[62] renal disease,[63] diabetes,[64] anxiety disorders,[65] depression,[65,66] and schizophrenia.[67]

The Function of Sleep

The function of sleep remains a topic surrounded by controversy. Some have postulated that it is important for mental and physical restoration,[68,69] and energy conservation.[70,71] Others propose that the primary function of sleep is the maintenance of synaptic and neuronal network function, information processing, and synaptic plasticity.[72–75] Sleep deprivation studies have shown that both total and partial sleep loss impair well-being and functioning, with mood being the most strongly affected, followed by cognitive and motor performance.[76–80] As a person ages, the effects of insufficient sleep on executive functioning, sustained attention, and long-term memory become more significant.[76] In summary, sleep fulfils a vital need, one that is essential to human health and well-being, even if the exact function of sleep remains to be discovered.[81]

SLEEP PHYSIOLOGY

Cardiovascular Function in Sleep

Cardiovascular control during sleep is primarily determined by variation in autonomic and sympathetic nervous system activity, which causes changes in blood pressure and heart rate, the major determinants of myocardial O_2 demand.[82–85] Increased parasympathetic tone and, to a lesser extent, decreased sympathetic tone, lead to a reduction in heart rate and cardiac output in NREM sleep.[86,87] REM sleep is associated with a simplification of cardiac mechanisms that could result in the cardiovascular system having an impaired ability to react to adverse cardiovascular events.[88] Vasodilation causes a reduction in systemic vascular resistance and a decrease in blood pressure which can impair blood flow through stenotic coronary blood vessels and trigger myocardial ischemia or infarction.[89] Baroreflex plays a significant role in the reduction and stability of blood pressure.[90] Brief surges in blood pressure and heart rate during sleep occur with K complexes, arousals, and large body movements.[87,91,92] Sympathetic and parasympathetic responses have shown significant decline in increasing age groups, possibly reflecting the decline in parasympathetic and sympathetic function that occurs with increasing age.[93] Sharp increases in heart rate and blood pressure occur with morning awakening and beginning the day's activities.[94,95] The morning hours after wakening are associated with a higher risk of adverse cardiovascular events, as sleep-to-wake transitions in the morning are associated with maximal shifts toward sympathetic autonomic activation as compared to those in the rest of the day.[96]

Respiratory Function in Sleep

Sleep alters breathing patterns, ventilation, and arterial blood gas values. Periodic breathing, a cyclic waxing and waning of tidal volume, sometimes with brief apnea, is common at sleep onset in association with fluctuations between wakefulness and light sleep.[97] Breathing is remarkably regular in SWS.[98] The breathing pattern becomes faster and more erratic during phasic REM sleep.[99]

Thermoregulation in Sleep

Sleep onset occurs after vasodilation of the hands and feet, increasing heat loss.[100] The normal temperature-regulating mechanisms are inhibited during REM sleep; during this stage of sleep, body temperature is influenced almost entirely by the environment instead of the hypothalamus.[101] Body temperature also has an independent circadian rhythm that typically peaks in the late afternoon and reaches a minimum in the early morning hours of sleep.[102]

In contrast, a sleep period that begins when temperature is high is relatively long because temperature drops and a subsequent rise in temperature does not occur for some time.[103] The body temperature rhythm shifts a little earlier (phase advance) with aging, which may partly explain why many older adults have an earlier wake-up time than younger adults.[104]

Cerebral Blood Flow in Sleep

Brain blood flow decreases in sleep in comparison to waking.[105] Brain imaging studies reveal that there is a small to moderate decrease in brain blood flow in NREM sleep in the brainstem and cortex.[106,107] Poor performance on tasks after sleep deprivation is associated with reduced metabolic activity in the bilateral intraparietal sulcus, bilateral insula, right prefrontal cortex, medial frontal cortex, and right parahippocampal gyrus, and an increase in metabolic activity in the bilateral thalamus compared to rested wakefulness.[108]

Renal Function in Sleep

Urine flow is reduced and more concentrated during sleep with a decreased excretion of sodium, chloride, potassium, and calcium.[109–111] The mechanisms involved in these changes are complex and include changes in renal blood flow, glomerular filtration, hormone secretion (vasopressin, aldosterone, prolactin, parathormone), and sympathetic neural stimulation.[112]

Endocrine Function in Sleep

Endocrine hormone secretion is influenced by sleep. For example, growth hormone secretion is highly sleep dependent and most secretion occurs during the first few hours after sleep onset during SWS. If sleep is advanced or delayed, growth hormone secretion shifts accordingly. In contrast, thyroid hormone and cortisol secretions have independent circadian rhythms. Thyroid hormone secretion increases in the late evening; cortisol concentration increases in the latter half of the night and peaks toward the end of the normal sleep period or soon after awakening.[113,114]

The hormone melatonin, secreted by the pineal gland, induces sleepiness and has a marked circadian rhythm that is closely linked to the light–dark cycle, temperature, and cortisol rhythms. A late evening surge in melatonin begins at darkness, approximately 2 hours before bedtime, and is considered a marker of the body's circadian timing system. Secretion peaks at approximately 3:00 AM but is suppressed by daylight to levels that are barely detectable. Bright light exposure suppresses melatonin secretion and can be used to help reset a person's circadian clock.[115,116]

CLINICAL EVALUATION, DIAGNOSIS, AND APPROACHES

There are three common ways that sleep and sleepiness are measured: subjectively, behaviorally, and objectively.

Subjective Measurement

Subjective measures of sleep can be particularly useful for screening, triage, and assessing the effects of treatment.[117,118] Types of information typically obtained include an individual's assessment of sleep latency (time from lights out to the onset of sleep), number of awakenings, depth and length of sleep, refreshing quality of sleep, satisfaction with sleep, and soundness of sleep. This information can be collected through the use of sleep questionnaires, such as the Pittsburgh Sleep Quality Index (PSQI),[119,120] St. Mary's Hospital Sleep Questionnaire,[121] sleep diaries, visual analogue scales, and interviews. Although obtaining subjective information about an individual's sleep is critical, it is important to note that information recorded in sleep diaries often overestimates sleep duration when compared to objective measures of sleep such as wrist actigraphy recordings.[122,123]

Daytime sleepiness can also be measured using subjective measures such as the Epworth Sleepiness Scale (ESS),[124–126] an instrument that has been widely used in the clinical and research settings. Test scores greater than 10 are frequently reported in patients with sleep disorders that cause excessive daytime sleepiness (EDS)[127]; the average score for control subjects is 6 (possible range of scores is 0 to 24; higher score = greater subjective sleepiness).[124,126] The ESS has been shown to be sensitive to and helpful in evaluating treatment for OSA and narcolepsy (another disorder of EDS).[127] Although gender and age do not affect scores on the ESS, studies have shown that African Americans have significantly higher scores than Caucasian Americans (Fig. 7-4).[128,129]

Behavioral Assessment

Assessment of behaviors related to sleep and sleepiness are an important part of a thorough assessment. Typically, individuals who are sleepy or sleep-deprived manifest characteristic behaviors including yawning, eye rubbing, head nodding, ptosis of the eyelids, irritability, and slowed movement. Other observable waking behaviors that may be noted include automatic behavior, unintentional sleep episodes, cataplexy (a stereotypical feature of narcolepsy in which there is a sudden decrease in muscle tone and loss of deep tendon reflexes leading to muscle weakness, paralysis, and/or postural collapse), and sleep drunkenness.[8]

Although lying quietly in a horizontal position is typical, movements and position changes can occur and are a normal part of sleep behavior. Abnormal sleep-related behaviors include bizarre postures, restless sleep, jerking of the extremities, seizure activity, and dream enactment. Video recordings of these behaviors during PSG are often made to assist in the assessment and diagnosis of sleep problems. Observations of patients' nocturnal behaviors by healthcare providers, bed partners, or parents often play an important role in the diagnosis and treatment of sleep disorders.

Objective Measurement

The structure and timing of sleep stages and cycles can be studied objectively using PSG, a procedure involving the simultaneous recording of the EEG, EMG, and EOG. At the usual recording speed of 1 cm/s, a standard 30-cm page represents a 30-second period, or *epoch*. Each epoch is assigned a single sleep-stage score based primarily on changes in EEG frequency (in cycles/s, or hertz [Hz]) and amplitude (in microvolts [μV]), with confirmation by the EOG and EMG patterns.[130] In addition to sleep-staging signals, PSG recordings include the measurement of other physiologic parameters, such as respiratory movements of the chest and abdomen, airflow at the nose and mouth, Sa_{O2}, electrocardiogram, and leg movements (anterior tibialis EMG). Additional EEG channels may be added if there are nocturnal seizures, and video recordings made if abnormal REM behaviors are suspected.

Unattended home sleep testing, using four-to-six channel recording systems, include measurements of oxygen saturation and pulse rate, oronasal airflow, and respiratory effort, and may include measurements of body position.[131] Home sleep testing is recommended only after an initial evaluation by a sleep specialist, is appropriate only for the diagnosis of a sleep-related breathing disorder (SRBD).[132,133] Home sleep tests should not be used for

Name: ______________________________

Today's date: ______________ Your age: ______________

Your sex (male = M; female = F): ______________

How likely are you to doze off or fall asleep in the following situations, in contrast to feeling just tired? This refers to your usual way of life in recent times. Even if you have not done some of these things recently, try to work out how they would have affected you. Use the following scale to choose the *most appropriate number* for each situation:

0 = would *never* doze

1 = *slight* chance of dozing

2 = *moderate* chance of dozing

3 = *high* chance of dozing

Situation	**Chance of Dozing**
Sitting and reading	
Watching TV	
Sitting, inactive in a public place (theater or meeting)	
As a passenger in a car for an hour without a break	
Lying down to rest in the afternoon when circumstances permit	
Sitting and talking to someone	
Sitting quietly after a lunch without alcohol	
In a care, while stopped for a few minutes in traffic	

Figure 7-4. Epworth Sleepiness Scale. (Used with permission from Johns MW. A new method for measuring daytime sleepiness: the Epworth sleepiness scale. *Sleep.* 1991;14[6]:540–545.)

the diagnosis of other sleep disorders or if there are any other comorbid pulmonary, cardiovascular, mental disorders, neurologic disorders, neuromuscular disorders, heart failure (HF), or if another sleep disorder is present.

Daytime sleepiness (daytime sleep propensity or tendency) can be quantified using the multiple sleep latency test (MSLT).[134] Beginning 2 hours at the end of a nocturnal polysomnographic recording, four to five 20-minute nap opportunities are typically given in 2-hour intervals. The sleep latency of any given nap opportunity is defined as the time from lights out to the first 30-second epoch scored as sleep. The average sleep latency across all naps is calculated and expressed as the mean sleep latency. Possible mean sleep latency scores on the MSLT range from 0 to 20 minutes, with low scores indicating greater sleepiness. Although traditionally sleep latencies of 5 minutes or less were considered indicative of pathologic sleepiness, current diagnostic standards consider a sleep latency of 8 minutes or less to be indicative of abnormal sleepiness.[8] Sleep latencies of 10 minutes or more are considered normal on the MSLT.

Actigraphy is an alternative method sometimes used to objectively measure sleep/wake patterns by monitoring periods of rest and activity.[135] Using a battery-operated-wristwatch-size microprocessor that senses movement with a piezoelectric beam, continuous motion data can be obtained for long periods. Computer algorithms allow for analysis of activity and nonactivity, as well as scoring of sleep and wakefulness. While sleep stages cannot be determined using actigraphy, information on total sleep time, percent of time spent awake, number of awakenings, time between awakenings, and sleep onset latency can be obtained. Estimates of sleep time from actigraphy vary according to the type of device being used, the setting, and the population being studied. Actigraphy data correlate well with PSG data, particularly when sleep is normal.[136,137] Correlations decrease when sleep is disturbed or activity is limited.[135,138]

Although there are numerous consumer smartphone apps, wearable devices (e.g., Fitbit and Jawbone) and other more elaborate devices (e.g., Beddit3, Smart Monitor, and Sense with Voice Sleep System) that purport to measure sleep duration, classify sleep into "light," "deep," and REM sleep, wake you during light sleep, and improve your sleep, these consumer sleep technologies are not reliable or accurate.[136,139–141] As long as patients and providers recognize the limitations of consumer sleep technologies, these applications and devices may promote greater awareness of sleep and greater patient engagement.[142]

IMPAIRED SLEEP, SLEEP DISORDERS, AND EXCESSIVE DAYTIME SLEEPINESS

Sleep disorders, specific diagnostic entities, include a wide array of problems characterized by insomnia (difficulty initiating or maintaining sleep or early morning awakening), EDS, and/or abnormal movements, behaviors, or sensations during sleep. There are eight groups of primary sleep disorders outlined in the International Classification of Sleep Disorders (see Table 7-1),[143] including the insomnias, SRBDs, hypersomnias of central origin, circadian rhythm disorders, parasomnias, sleep-related movement disorders, isolated symptoms and apparently normal sleep variants, and "other" (physiologic, nonphysiologic, and environmental sleep disorders).[143–145]

Sleep deprivation and sleep disruption result in sleep loss.[146] Sleep deprivation studies have shown that sleep loss has numerous adverse effects including fatigue, anxiety, increased illness, increased sensitivity to pain, decreased immune response, restlessness, cognitive impairment, decreased alertness/attention during the day, and decreased sense of well-being.[147–149] The consensus states that adults aged 18 to 60 years should sleep 7 or more hours per night on a regular basis to promote optimal health and well-being.[149–151]

EDS, the inability to maintain the alert awake state, is the most common consequence of sleep disorders and/or insufficient or

Table 7-1 • INTERNATIONAL CLASSIFICATION OF SLEEP DISORDERS

International Classification of Sleep Disorders—Third Edition[8]	
Insomnia	**Circadian Rhythm Sleep/Wake Disorders**
Chronic insomnia disorder	Delayed sleep/wake phase disorder
Short-term insomnia disorder	Advanced sleep/wake phase disorder
Other insomnia disorder	Irregular sleep/wake rhythm disorder
Sleep-Related Breathing Disorder	Non-24-hour sleep/wake rhythm disorder
OSA disorders	Shift work disorder
OSA, adult	Jet lag disorder
OSA, pediatric	Circadian sleep/wake disorder not otherwise specified
Central sleep apnea syndromes	**Parasomnias**
Central sleep apnea with Cheyne–Stokes breathing	***NREM-related parasomnias***
Central sleep apnea due to a medical disorder without Cheyne–Stokes breathing	Confusional arousals
Central sleep apnea due to high altitude periodic breathing	Sleepwalking
Central sleep apnea due to a medication or substance	Sleep terrors
Primary central sleep apnea	Sleep-related eating disorder
Primary central sleep apnea of infancy	***REM-related parasomnias***
Primary central sleep apnea of prematurity	REM sleep behavior disorder
Treatment-emergent central sleep apnea	Recurrent isolated sleep paralysis
Sleep-related hypoventilation disorders	Nightmare disorder
Obesity hypoventilation syndrome	***Other parasomnias***
Congenital central alveolar hypoventilation syndrome	Exploding head syndrome
Late-onset central hypoventilation with hypothalamic dysfunction	Sleep-related hallucinations
Idiopathic central alveolar hypoventilation	Sleep enuresis
Sleep-related hypoventilation due to a medication or substance	Parasomnia due to a medical disorder
Sleep-related hypoventilation due to a medical disorder	Parasomnia due to a medication or substance
Sleep-related hypoxemia disorder	Parasomnia, unspecified
Central Disorders of Hypersomnolence	**Sleep-Related Movement Disorders**
Narcolepsy type 1	Restless legs syndrome
Narcolepsy type 2	Periodic limb movement disorder
Idiopathic hypersomnia	Sleep-related leg cramps
Kleine–Levin syndrome	Sleep-related bruxism
Hypersomnia due to a medical disorder	Sleep-related rhythmic movement disorder
Hypersomnia due to a medication or substance	Benign sleep myoclonus of infancy
Hypersomnia associated with a psychiatric disorder	Propriospinal myoclonus at sleep onset
Insufficient sleep syndrome	Sleep-related movement disorder due to a medical disorder
	Sleep-related movement disorder due to a medication or substance
	Sleep-related movement disorder, unspecified

poor sleep and is the most prevalent symptom of patients seen in sleep disorders centers in the United States estimated to be as high as 18%.[152] EDS can be seen in otherwise healthy individuals who do not have an adequate opportunity or circumstances for sleep.[153] When severe, however, it can be debilitating, causing a broad range of neuropsychological deficits affecting daytime functioning and quality of life. EDS can be life-threatening due to associated alterations in alertness and reactivity.[152,154–157] Increased napping has also been associated with increased mortality in the elderly.[158–160]

Sleep-Related Disordered Breathing

Sleep-related changes in breathing and oxygenation have important cardiovascular consequences. This section focuses on the cardiovascular impact of OSA and central sleep apnea.

Obstructive Sleep Apnea

Patients with sleep apnea repeatedly stop breathing during sleep for periods of 10 seconds or longer. Apnea can be obstructive (a collapsed upper airway blocks airflow despite effort to breathe), central (no respiratory effort), or mixed (central, then obstructive component). A predominance of obstructive apnea is the most common pattern and can lead to repetitive episodes of hypoxemia that are terminated by brief arousals. Prevalence of OSA is approximately 22% in men and 17% in women.[161] Other risk factors include race (African Americans, Mexican Americans, Pacific Islanders, and East Asians),[162,163] obesity, menopause, age, fluid retention, smoking, and adenotonsillar hypertrophy.[164] Sleep apnea is likely to be worsened by sleep deprivation,[165] alcohol ingestion,[166] and sedative or hypnotic use.[167]

OSA has significant cardiovascular consequences and inflammatory processes have been heavily implicated as an important link between the two, although not conclusively established.[168] Sleep apnea is highly associated with and a risk factor for cardiac arrhythmias.[169,170] Apneas are often associated with a progressive sinus bradycardia, sometimes with a prolonged sinus pause, followed by an abrupt increase in heart rate when breathing resumes. A decrease and subsequent increase in cardiac output parallels the heart rate changes.[169–171]

To minimize possible complications, early diagnosis and treatment are critical. The treatment of choice for OSA is nasally applied continuous positive airway pressure (CPAP). A soft, firmly fitting nasal mask is held in place by straps and attached to a bedside blower that provides continuous pressure (usually 5 to 15 cm H_2O) to prevent collapse of the upper airway. In addressing long-term changes of CPAP usage on inflammatory markers in those who are CPAP adherent (greater than 4 hours/night) to those who are not compliant, CPAP adherence was shown to significantly reduced

ICAM-1 in a prospective observational study in patients with at least moderate OSA over 2 years.[172] These findings suggest that CPAP treatment reduces inflammatory biomarkers and prevents continued increases, which may decrease the rate of progression of CVD.[172]

While discontinuation of PAP for OSA is common, further research is needed on the drivers of nonadherence with diagnostic sleep testing and PAP treatment initiation.[173] A prior study showed that testing and treatment ordered by primary care providers, residence outside the Midwest region, and two or fewer office visits within 6 months of preauthorization in addition to an apnea–hypopnea index score less than 30 events/h were strong predictors of nonadherence.[173] Thus, healthcare providers should develop better strategies in order to engage this higher risk group for nonadherence.[173]

Conservative treatment strategies for OSA include weight loss, learning to sleep in a side-lying position (e.g., putting a ball in a pouch on the back), and avoidance of alcohol and sedatives.[174–177] Oral appliances, which move the lower mandible forward in order to increase the posterior airway space, are now also available and effective in improving OSA.[178,179]

Pharmacologic approaches with purported respiratory stimulants (e.g., acetazolamide, medroxyprogesterone, fluoxetine, and protriptyline) have had variable effectiveness.[180] Occasionally, surgery is performed to enlarge the airway through cranial reconstruction (maxillomandibular advancement),[181] improve nasal airflow (nasal surgery),[182] or use of tracheostomy for when respiratory failure occurs and standard CPAP or bilevel is not tolerated.[183]

Inspire is a remote-controlled device that is surgically implanted, consisting of a stimulation lead, pulse generator and breathing sensor to stimulate the upper airway for adults with OSA.[184] The Food and Drug Administration (FDA)–approved device is effective for patients intolerant to CPAP.[184] A Stimulation Treatment for Apnea Reduction[185] clinical trial published in the *New England Journal of Medicine* was a multicenter, prospective single-group, cohort design with surgically implanted upper-airway stimulation in 126 OSA patients.[186] The results of this study were that median apnea–hypopnea score at 12 months decreased 68%, from 29.3 events per hour to 9.0 events per hour ($P < 0.001$). The oxygen desaturation index (ODI) score decreased 70%, from 25.4 events per hour to 7.4 events per hour ($P < 0.001$). Overall, in the uncontrolled cohort study, upper-airway stimulation led to significant improvements in objective and subjective measurements of the severity of OSA.[186]

Central Sleep Apnea

Patients with severe congestive HF often have a pattern of periodic (Cheyne–Stokes) breathing during light sleep in which periods of central apnea alternate with hyperpnea.[187] This breathing pattern causes recurrent episodes of hypoxemia that can further impair the failing heart.[187,188] One mechanism for the abnormal breathing pattern is prolonged circulation time that delays the ventilatory responses to blood gas changes. The resulting hypoxemia sets up a vicious cycle whereby increased ventilation improves oxygenation but decreases carbon dioxide tension below the apneic threshold; the resulting apnea then leads to hypoxemia, which perpetuates the cycle. In addition, cardiac enlargement and pulmonary congestion decrease gas stores in the lungs, which allow wider swings in blood gas values with changes in ventilation.[188] Effective treatment of the HF and low-flow O_2 therapy during sleep help to correct the hypoxemia and stabilize the breathing pattern.[189] Use of adaptive servoventilation (ASV) has also been shown to decrease the severity of central apneas in patients with HF.[190]

Restless Legs Syndrome and Periodic Limb Movement

Restless legs syndrome (RLS) is a neurologic sensorimotor disorder characterized by disagreeable leg sensations that usually occur prior to sleep onset and accompanied by an almost irresistible urge to move the legs.[191] Vividly described by the English physician Willis in 1671,[192] the disorder was more completely characterized in 1945, when Ekbom described its classic clinical features and made recommendations for treatment.[191] Primary RLS usually develops in old age, whereas secondary RLS occurs at younger ages, may have a familial component, and is triggered by factors such as iron deficiency, pregnancy, renal failure, certain medications, and neuropathy.[193] Although, RLS has more recently received significant attention by the scientific and lay communities, it remains poorly understood and under diagnosed.

The five criteria necessary to make the clinical diagnosis of RLS include:

1. an urge to move the limbs usually associated with paresthesias or dysesthesias;
2. motor restlessness manifested by using different motor strategies to relieve the discomfort such as floor pacing, tossing and turning in bed, and rubbing the legs;
3. symptoms that become worse or are exclusively present at rest with at least partial and temporary relief by activity;
4. symptoms that are worse in the evening or night (typically between 6:00 PM and 4:00 AM); and
5. the above symptoms are not solely explained by any other medical or behavioral condition (e.g., positional discomfort, arthritis, myalgias, leg edema, peripheral neuropathy, radiculopathy, and habitual foot tapping).[194,195]

Other associated features commonly seen in patients with RLS—but that are not necessary for the diagnosis—are sleep disturbances, daytime fatigue/sleepiness, a family history of RLS, involuntary, repetitive, jerking limb movements during sleep, and an initial reduction in symptom severity when treated with dopaminergic medications.[195]

RLS is common and its prevalence is estimated to be between 5% and 15%.[196] The disorder can occur at any age, but there are bimodal peaks in age of onset. Early-onset or idiopathic RLS usually occurs around 20 years of age and is associated with more severe symptoms and a positive family history of RLS, whereas late-onset or secondary RLS tends to begin in the early 40s and is not associated with a family history of the disorder.[197] In adults, older than 40, RLS occurs approximately twice as often in women than men, but there are no gender differences for children and young adults.[195,198,199]

A related condition, PLMs was originally termed nocturnal myoclonus by Symonds in 1953.[200] The periodic nature of the movements and their common association with RLS were later described by Lugaresi et al.,[201] and Coleman et al.[202] PLMs usually involve the legs and consist of a sudden extension of the great toe (similar to the Babinski reflex) associated with flexion at the ankle, knee, and hip. Because the arms are sometimes included, many prefer the term PLMs rather than the previously used term, periodic leg movements. Similar to RLS, the expression of PLMs also appears to have a circadian component and is typically worse at night.

Both RLS and PLM occur in idiopathic and secondary forms. The idiopathic form, especially in the case of RLS, is often found in those who have afflicted first-degree relatives.[203] The exact mode of inheritance remains unclear, but the frequency with which offspring of affected individuals develop the condition suggests an autosomal-dominant genetic pattern.[195]

RLS and PLM may also develop in association with several medical, neurologic, and metabolic conditions and secondary to conditions characterized by iron deficiency such as anemia, pregnancy, and uremia.[195,204–206] Large epidemiologic studies have shown a significant association between RLS, CVD, and stroke.[207–209] RLS and PLM in children have also been associated with attention-deficit/hyperactivity disorder.[199,210,211]

The treatment of RLS and PLM is symptomatic. Patients with the mild forms of the disorders may respond favorably to nonpharmacologic interventions. Patients should be advised to refrain from drinking alcohol in the evening since it frequently exacerbates symptoms. Three reversible forms of RLS, including pregnancy, renal failure, and anemia, are each characterized by iron deficiency (as reflected in low ferritin levels; less than 50 ng/mL) and treatment with both oral and intravenous iron has been found to improve or resolve RLS symptoms. When symptoms occur two nights per week, are considered distressing, and interfere with functioning, pharmacologic therapy with dopaminergic agents, alpha-2-delta ligands (anticonvulsants acting on calcium channels), opioids, or benzodiazepines is indicated.[195]

Two types of dopaminergic medications are beneficial in the treatment of RLS and PLM. Both decrease symptoms and numbers of limb movements. Dopamine precursors, such as regular or sustained-release carbidopa/levodopa, increase the delivery of levodopa to the brain where it is converted to dopamine. The carbidopa is a dehydroxylase inhibitor, which decreases the peripheral breakdown of the levodopa so more can get to the brain. This medication is excellent for patients with sporadic, infrequent symptoms. However, with chronic use, there is frequent development of *rebound* (return of symptoms) or *augmentation*, the tendency for symptoms to develop earlier in the day, and/or to be more severe than prior to treatment. In these situations, it is often best to change to a dopamine agonist, in which case the symptoms of rebound and augmentation usually disappear in a few days or weeks. Although dopamine agonists have been traditionally used for Parkinson disease, several controlled clinical trials have also demonstrated the efficacy of pergolide,[212] pregabalin,[213] pramipexole,[213] and ropinirole[214] in the treatment of RLS and PLM. In fact, these agents are currently considered first-line drugs for most patients.[195] Side effects from these medications such as sleepiness, nausea, and hypotension occur infrequently, and can most often be avoided by slowly increasing the dose until symptoms abate. Symptoms may spontaneously remit for weeks or even months, allowing patients to use medications on an as needed basis when having symptoms.[195]

Initially, it is important to listen, support, and validate the experiences of both the patient and family, as they may have gone for years with their symptoms and concerns being dismissed by healthcare providers. Referral to support groups such as those offered through the Restless Legs Syndrome Foundation can help provide additional support and education. The Restless Legs Syndrome Foundation also has a web site with important and relevant patient and professional information (www.RLS.org). Patients should also be referred to a sleep disorders specialist for management, particularly if treatment involves dopaminergic agents or chronic opioid medications.

SLEEP IN PATIENTS WITH CARDIOVASCULAR DISEASE

Sleep in Coronary Heart Disease

An estimated 18.2 million Americans over the age of 20 years are estimated to have coronary heart disease (CHD),[215] and 720,000 Americans are expected to have a new coronary event of first hospitalized myocardial infarction (MI) or CHD death, with approximately 335,000 people expected to have a recurrent event each year. Several recent large studies, such as the Sleep Heart Health Study, and growing evidence have linked sleep symptoms and SDB with both risk factors and outcomes of CVD.[1] Assessing the independent contribution of sleep to cardiovascular outcomes is often complicated by confounding variations in age, sex, type and severity of cardiovascular impairment, and type and severity of the sleep disorder a well as other risk factors, and medications. For example, OSA was more contributory to stroke than CHD in elders over the age of 65 years.[216] The magnitude of the sleep disturbance may be the key in that mild, moderate, and severe OSA has been associated with all-cause mortality in a dose response fashion with only severe OSA associated with cardiovascular mortality. OSA may be associated with unstable coronary artery plaque characteristics.[217] Sleep duration may be a factor as well in that short sleep (less than 7 hours per night) is associated with total CVD and CHD but not stroke whereas long sleep duration was associated with total CVD, CHD, and stroke.[215] Growing evidence consistently links sleep disorders with increased cardiovascular risk and suggests that patients with CHD often have disturbed sleep.

While mechanisms linking sleep with adverse neurobehavioral and cardiovascular outcomes are currently being defined, sleep apnea and sleep-related disorders are known to contribute to increased CHD risk factors such as hypertension, obesity, inflammatory markers, and metabolic changes related to glucose and insulin.[218] Thus, during any assessment of cardiovascular risk, sleep patterns should be considered and evaluated for contribution to other risk factors. The threshold for sleep duration on risk factors appears to be a habitual sleep time around less than 5 to 6 hours per night, or over 8 to 9 hours per night.[219]

The relationship is reciprocal in that impaired cardiac function from multiple causes can produce symptoms such as chest pain and dyspnea which interfere with sleep. Even in patients with multiple comorbidities, cardiovascular symptoms are a major factor associated with symptoms of reduced total sleep and increased nighttime wakefulness. The psychological impact of heart disease also has a major impact on sleep. Acute MI, for example, not only affects physical health and comfort but also influences social relationships, living patterns, work options and income, and sense of personal vulnerability. Fear of death, reinfarction, anxiety, and depression, typically accompanied by poor sleep, are common after MI; many patients report troublesome insomnia that lasts for months and sometimes years. This may in fact be due to changes in perfusion and altered sleep architecture after acute MI due to the infarction itself and its associated physiologic and inflammatory changes.[1,220]

Sleep apnea may increase the risk of CHD via pathways mediated by hypertension and the metabolic consequences of increased oxidative stress, C-reactive protein, and insulin resistance. PSG-verified sleep disruptions and desaturations as well as insomnia are associated with adverse changes in neuroendocrine changes, coagulation proteins/factors, and increased prothrombotic state.[221] Patients with OSA may also be obese and have a greater prevalence of other underlying cardiovascular risk factors suggesting a bidirectional relationship. Poor sleep appears to be a precursor to MI as symptoms of insomnia, habitual short sleep, waking up exhausted, daytime sleepiness, and frequent napping are common in the preceding months.

Unusual fatigue and sleep disturbance are among prodromal symptoms reported as early as 1 month prior to an acute MI in men and women, and those younger (less than 55 years) in age, with women reporting more prodromal symptoms than men.[222–224] An underlying factor may be a period of depression, which is well linked to elevated inflammatory markers, as the possible explanation for these symptoms that may precede MI.[225] As OSA becomes more and more linked to subclinical CHD as measured by endothelial and vascular function, and in some studies to coronary artery calcification, attention to OSA as a modifiable cardiac risk factor is becoming increasingly important.[226,227]

Sleep in the Cardiovascular Intensive Care Unit and After Cardiac Surgery

Specialized units reduce in-hospital deaths after MI and cardiac surgery, but they are far from optimal environments for sleep. The setting is unfamiliar and frightening to patients, the schedule and bedtime routines differ from those at home, noise and lighting may never be completely suppressed, and interruptions for patient care procedures are frequent. Sedatives and analgesics are routinely used in cardiovascular patients, yet they have the potential for side effects, such as delirium and sleep architecture disruption. These medications are extremely important in providing patient comfort; however, the goals of care must focus on the right balance of sedative and analgesic administration while reducing unnecessary or overzealous use. Most staff believe that the intensive care unit environment does adversely affect sleep, as well as factors such as difficult emotions and anxiety also affect sleep.[228] True sleep versus the appearance of sleep due to sedating side effects of medications is important to assess in the cardiovascular intensive care unit (CICU).

In classic PSG studies, coronary care unit patients typically have a pattern of light, fragmented sleep with reduced slow wave and REM sleep, frequent stage changes, and considerable nighttime wakefulness.[229] Although total sleep time is not necessarily reduced, the normal circadian sleep/wake rhythm is disrupted, with sleep occurring off and on during the 24 hours. REM and slow wave (deep) sleep may be significantly decreased and disrupted. Sleep is more disturbed as illness severity increases. Sleep patterns may improve over time with improving health status, fewer interruptions for care, and increased adaptation to the CICU environment. In addition to noise in the CICU patient monitoring, pain, and treatments may contribute to sleep disruptions, and some studies or quality improvement projects to reduce environmental disruptions yielded increased patient and staff satisfaction, actual sleep for patients, and improved outcomes related to length of stay, nosocomial infections, and ventilator days. However, clustering of care to provide sleep and naps is not always feasible due to urgent care and complexity of coordinating the multiple departments involved in care.[230]

Sleep After Cardiac Surgery

Sleep disruption after surgery is related to the magnitude of procedure and associated postoperative care, asynchrony between patient needs and unit procedures, and temporary physiologic changes in brain stem and hypothalamus due to circulatory changes. Patients who undergo cardiac surgery experience dramatic sleep pattern disturbances (SPDs), which may extend for as long as 6 months after discharge from the hospital.[231] Severe sleep deprivation is common in the early postoperative period, with only a few hours of fragmented sleep each 24 hours and virtual absence of slow wave and REM sleep.[232] Asynchrony during partial ventilatory support (in which the ventilator applies pressure in proportion to the inspiratory effort) is associated with reduced quality of sleep,[233] although efforts to reduce postoperative ventilator time have helped to reduce this factor. Another factor is the type of circulatory assist used during the surgery. Off-pump CABG surgical procedures have been advocated to reduce the adverse effects of cardiopulmonary bypass on the brain. Sleep and mood disturbance comparing patients after on-pump and off-pump suggests that off-pump surgery was associated with better objective sleep continuity (decreased percentage of wake time after sleep onset and fewer awakenings) but no longer sleep duration after controlling for age and sex, and differences may not be retained at 6 months.[234]

As with the coronary care environment, cardiac surgical patients report sleep disturbances and distress at uninterrupted sleep because of nursing care. Contributing environmental and clinical factors to postoperative sleep problems include persistent interruptions and activity, high noise and lighting levels, anxiety, incisional pain, and medications. Additionally, cardiac surgery patients may be elderly with pre-existing sleep disorders. Sleep deprivation and insomnia are implicated as a risk factor for the postoperative delirium that develops in some cardiac surgical patients,[235] underscoring the need for attention to sleep-promoting interventions after cardiac surgery.

Although sleep patterns gradually improve after cardiac surgery, slow wave and REM sleep may be suppressed for several weeks after the patient returns home, with many patients reporting continuing sleep disturbances. The cause of sleeplessness after CABG surgery may be temporary deterioration of circulation in the centers of the brain stem and hypothalamus that control sleep and awakening. Improvement of the circulation in these centers occurs a few months after the operation helps to regain sleep control and reduce sleep disturbances over time. An initial contributing factor for some patients with heart valve replacements is noise generated by the mechanical valve prosthesis, including audible high-frequency closing clicks and low-frequency sounds conducted by body tissues that the patient becomes accustomed to over time.

Although very few interventions have been tested for their effects on promoting sleep after cardiac surgery, attention to reducing noxious environmental stimuli is an obvious approach. Examples are found in studies reporting positive effects of structured quiet time, guidelines to reduce noise, and providing patients with earplugs while in intensive care units, and use of white noise and music therapy; however the effectiveness of noise interventions in the ICU require sustained effort to retain behavior changes and mask effects for patients.[236] Because sleep disruptions after cardiac surgery are multifactorial and include environmental, treatment-related, and intrinsic factors, a comprehensive approach to management of these problems is essential.

Sleep and Heart Failure

Moderate to severe sleep apnea is found in about 50% to 75% of patients with HF including those with reduced or preserved ejection fraction and is considered the most common comorbidity.[61,237]

Patients with HF frequently have combinations of central and obstructive apneas with obstructive being the most common. The characteristic SRBDs of HF have been studied more widely in HF patients and have been referred to as Cheyne–Stokes respiration (CSR), or Hunter–Cheyne–Stokes respiration to acknowledge the original discoverer, and reflect the pathophysiology of HF leading to prolonged circulation time. However, insomnia (perceived difficulty initiating or maintaining sleep) is the most common sleep complaint occurring in 25% to 65% of persons with HF, and it significantly contributes to daytime symptoms, decreased functional performance, poor cognition, reduced quality of life, as well as inflammation and autonomic dysfunction and subsequent cardiac events.[238–242] Evidence suggests that up to 70% of patients with HF experience at least one sleep complaint, far exceeding the 10% to 15% reported in the general population. Factors that contribute to sleep disturbances in persons with HF include increased age, body mass index, comorbidities, fluid overload, medications, nocturia, low vitamin D intake, and psychological distress, particularly depression.[243–246]

SRBDs have been more widely studied in HF patients than SPDs. Estimates are that SRBD with apnea–hypopnea index of greater than 15 occurs in approximately 50% of HF patients compared to 13% of working adults age 30% to 70% in the general population.[61] Both obstructive apneas and CSR with central apneas or a mix of both are common in patients with HF. The hallmarks of CSR are higher NYHA class, atrial fibrillation (AF), frequent nocturnal ventricular arrhythmias, lower Pa_{CO2}, and a left ventricular ejection fraction of 20% or less. Patients with CSR and central apnea have interrupted sleep with frequent awakenings and poor sleep efficiency or light sleep. In addition, nocturnal O_2 desaturation and large negative changes in intrathoracic pressure are seen in CSR.

Heightened risk for cardiac arrhythmias, poor clinical outcomes including rehospitalization, and increased mortality are also associated with CSR and central apnea.[61] Similar to the general population, obstructive and central apneas in HF patients are more common in men than women although age and hormone status may be a factor in that women with HF over 60 years have six times the risk for CSA and OSA than younger women.[61] Women, however, have a greater risk of insomnia than men in the general adult population,[215] and this pattern has also been described in HF.[247]

Focused assessment of HF patient at risk for apnea and sleep disturbance should also include those with obesity, EDS, nocturnal angina, paroxysmal nocturnal dyspnea, restless sleep, RLS, PLM during sleep—all of which contribute to frequent arousals.[61,243] EDS is an important symptom to document and consider in care. The greater the degree to which adults perceive and report sleepiness symptoms, the greater the clinical relevance of their OSA, and the greater the risk for cardiovascular events; HF patients tend to report higher EDS.[248] Why some persons with OSA tend not to report EDS is unclear and is currently under study.[248,249] Importantly, EDS has been associated with reduced cognition in adults and those with HF,[241,250] accompanied by reductions in significant self-care behavior, primarily medication adherence.[251]

Interventions in HF

In patients with stable HF, interventions to improve sleep problems have included the standard use of CPAP for OSA and medications.[237] Observational and registry data suggest that CPAP in patients with HF is associated with reduced daytime heart rate and blood pressure, lower sympathetic activity, and improved outcomes of quality of life reduced rate of death, heart transplantation, or implant of a ventricular assist device.[61,237] ASV is a type of positive pressure ventilation that varies the pressure based on algorithmic detection of apneas during sleep, although there are cautions for using ASV in symptomatic HF patients with central sleep apnea and left ventricular ejection fraction (LVEF) less than or equal to 45.[237] A small study showed that ASV may improve the prognosis of heart failure with protected ejection fraction (HFpEF) patients with SDB, with favorable effects such as improvement of symptoms, cardiac diastolic function, and arterial stiffness,[252] however no clear recommendations are available, and further studies of ASV are underway. A small nurse-led study compared ASV with a control group for HF patients with CSA or mixed apneas and reported improved quality of life in the intervention versus the control group after 3 months.[253]

Behavioral interventions in HF patients are few and have been of small samples.

However those that have reported positive results include cognitive behavioral therapy for insomnia (CBT-I) which led to improved sleep-related cognition and reduced insomnia and fatigue,[254] and a 12-week nurse-led tailored education support program which led to greater self-reported sleep quality, lower daytime sleepiness, and improved symptoms of anxiety and depression.[255]

Sleep and Hypertension

SRBD, particularly OSA, continues to be studied as a risk factor for hypertension with a preponderance of evidence from epidemiologic studies indicating a positive relationship when controlling for confounders such as BMI and age.[256] Epidemiologic studies show that approximately 40% of hypertensive patients have SRBD, and this number rises to over 70% among drug-resistant hypertension.[257] Recent studies have also established a dose–response relationship between severity of OSA and hypertension, independent of age, body mass index, gender, alcohol consumption, and smoking.[256] The biologic reasons for the link between OSA and hypertension involve multiple pathways with intermittent hypoxia, negative intrathoracic pressure, and vasoactive factors triggering excessive sympathetic activity which persist during the day.[258] These changes may be reversible with adherent CPAP therapy, and modest reduction of systolic blood pressure has been observed in those with hypertension with greater impact in resistant hypertension.[258]

OSA is also a secondary cause of pulmonary arterial hypertension[256] with sleep disturbances contributing to reduced quality of life in this population.[259] These studies have been conducted with prior definitions of hypertension of 140/90 mm Hg, and the percentages may change when analysis are rerun with newer ACC/AHA definitions specified as SBP greater than or equal to 130 to 139 and/or DBP greater than or equal to 80 to 90 mm Hg.[260]

Sleep duration is another factor to consider when assessing sleep in persons with hypertension or at risk for hypertension. Short sleep, frequently defined as less than 5 hours per night, has been linked to the risk of hypertension and elevated mean 24-hour blood pressure.[261] Important differences may be present in the relationship between OSA and hypertension in special populations. In a cross-sectional adjusted analysis of sleep time reported by over 700,000 adults, increased risk of hypertension was observed in those with short sleep (less than 6 hours) and longer sleep (greater than 9 hours).[262] Short sleep was most important for both sexes and ethnicities across the lifespan, but significantly higher risk was observed at younger ages and in women across the life span. Long sleep was important for those of age less than 24 and greater than 74 years but not as important by ethnicity.[262]

Higher overall sleep efficiency has been associated with lower blood pressure.[215]

Elevated nocturnal blood pressure (referred to as nondipper patterns) during sleep may be a marker of underlying sleep apnea, even among normotensive individuals and should be evaluated further. Higher nocturnal blood pressure, independent of daytime hypertension, places the individual at greater risk for end-organ damage, particularly renal damage, myocardial ischemia, cerebrovascular insults, hypertrophy, cardiovascular morbidity, and mortality.[260,263,264]

Sleep and Stroke

There is growing evidence that both short sleep durations and sleep disorders can increase the risk for cerebrovascular accident (CVA), and that CVAs may cause or exacerbate sleep disorders.[265] In addition, the consequences of untreated sleep disorders, (for example, cognitive dysfunction, altered mood, sleepiness, and fatigue) may also impede stroke rehabilitation, lengthen hospital stay, and influence outcomes and the risk of stroke recurrence.[266,267] The mechanisms underlying these often-bidirectional relationships are unknown.

Numerous studies have documented the high prevalence of SRBDs among patients who have experienced a stroke or transient ischemic attack (TIA),[265,266,268] with estimates of sleep apnea prevalence as high as 91% among stroke patients.[269] Because few patients have been diagnosed and treated prior to their stroke the most recent Guidelines for the Prevention of Stroke in Patients with Stroke and Transient Ischemic Attack,[270] recommend that all patients with ischemic strokes and TIAs have a sleep study and begin treatment with nasal CPAP if OSA is diagnosed.

Although most of the research has focused on the relationship of SRBDs and stroke, insomnia, short sleep durations, RLS and PLMs have also been associated with an increased risk for stroke and increased incidence after stroke.[265,267] Insomnia, which can play a role in the development of CVD can also dramatically increase the risk of stroke. In one study, it was shown that patients with insomnia demonstrated that patients with insomnia had a 54% greater likelihood of developing a stroke compared to those who didn't have insomnia.[266] Those with persistent insomnia had the highest risk of stroke, followed by individuals with relapsing insomnia. Even patients with insomnia in remission had a greater risk for stroke than those without insomnia.[271] Insomnia is also quite common after a CVA, and may be attributable to multiple factors including complications of the stroke and complications associated with hospitalization and/or medications.[272] Sleep-related movement disorders, which include RLS and PLM disorders, are associated with higher risk of stroke, particularly among males and those under 45 years of age.[273] At present, it is not known if increasing sleep durations by treating insomnia and sleep-related movement disorders decreases the risk of stroke.

Sleep and Diabetes Mellitus

Given the high prevalence of diabetes mellitus (DM) in patients with cardiac conditions, it is prudent to note that sleep SDB and sleep loss have been associated with glucose intolerance and insulin resistance.[274] More specifically, incident DM is significantly associated with a habitual sleep duration of 6 hours or less, sleep apnea, and self-reports of troubled sleep.[275] When confounding risk factors are rigorously controlled in studies, sleep-related hypoxemia was also associated with glucose intolerance independent of age, gender, body mass index, and waist circumference and may lead to type 2 DM.[276,277]

While recent epidemiologic, biologic, and behavioral evidence suggests that sleep disorders may contribute to the development of DM, conversely, diabetes itself may contribute to sleep disorders.[278] In patients with diabetes, short sleep duration or oversleeping may contribute to elevations in HgA1c, and symptoms resulting from diabetes, such as nocturia and neuropathic pain, may in turn contribute to sleep disturbance and exacerbate sleep deprivation.[279,280]

Sleep and Chronic Obstructive Pulmonary Disease

Cardiac patients may have **chronic obstructive pulmonary disease** (COPD) as a comorbidity, and approximately 10% of COPD patients experience OSA with some studies seeing prevalences as high as 66%.[281,282] The term "Overlap Syndrome" describes the relationship between COPD and OSA.[283] Patients with overlap syndrome are characterized by having lower Pa_{O2} during wakefulness, greater nocturnal oxygen desaturation (reduced mean peripheral capillary oxygen saturation and greater percentage of sleep time with Sa_{O2} less than 90%), and worse sleep quality than sleep apnea patients without COPD.[284,285] COPD and sleep apnea are recognized to have a detrimental influence on the respiratory physiology of patients, overall health status, and poor quality of life.[286,287]

Patients with COPD who are hypoxic during wakefulness become more hypoxic during sleep.[288] Many patients with COPD complain of poor sleep quality which often worsens as disease severity increases.[286] In addition, they experience difficulty initiating and maintaining sleep, reduced REM sleep, reduced sleep efficiency with delayed time for sleep onset, a reduction in total sleep time, and periods of wakefulness often prolonged.[288] Poor sleep quality in patients with COPD is likely multifactoral and includes nocturnal coughing and dyspnea, effects of medications (i.e., corticosteroid), and aging.[289] The cornerstone of treatment for COPD remains smoking cessation, bronchodilation, inhaled steroids, and pulmonary rehabilitation.[290]

Long-term conventional home O_2 therapy has shown to improve survival and decrease hypoxia in patients with COPD (greater than 15 hr/day).[291]

Sleep and Depression

Sleep is an essential component of the pathophysiology of depression.[292] The majority of people with depressive disorders experience SDB, and most diagnostic criteria for depression include sleep disturbances.[293] While the likelihood of developing a mood disorder is not simply a consequence of having a SPD, longitudinal studies document that insomnia is a risk factor for onset of depressive disorder[294] and may increase the risk for relapse in patients with recurrent illness.[295] Whereas sleep onset problems and frequent awakenings accompany almost any kind of insomnia in the general population, lifetime prevalence of depression is approximately 16%.[296] However, among patients with CVD, these rates of depression are two to three times higher.[297] Major depression affects approximately 15% to 20% of patients with CVD, and minor depression is present in another 20%.[297] Similar prevalence rates are reported for sleep disturbances in CVD.[298,299] As far as mechanisms linking sleep disorder to depression, studies hypothesize that altered dopaminergic function and altered kynurenine metabolism may play a role in both sleep and depression.[300,301]

Most individuals who are depressed exhibit one or more alterations in sleep architecture.[302] Multiple disturbances in PSG recordings have been reported in depressed patients during sleep.[303,304] The most common sleep disturbances in depression include decreased sleep efficiency, nocturnal and early-morning awakening, decreased SWS, reduced REM latency, an increased number of eye movements during REM periods, and increased REM intensity.[293,305]

Major depression and SRBD, particularly CSR and central sleep apnea, are well-established risks for poor clinical outcomes and death in patients with CVD.[297,306] Multiple mechanisms linking depression, sleep disturbances, and heart disease have been proposed.[307–309] Depression lowers adherence to prescribed medications and increases unhealthy lifestyle behaviors among cardiac patients.[310] Similar underlying hypothalamic–pituitary–adrenal axis, neuroendocrine, and immune dysregulation have been reported in both depression and sleep disturbances, further leading to a heightened risk for arrhythmias and sudden death.[311–316]

CARDIAC EVENTS IN SLEEP

Angina

Nocturnal anginal chest pain results from myocardial ischemia, an imbalance between coronary blood flow and myocardial requirements. For the patient prone to cardiac ischemia, nocturnal angina and events are most likely to occur during REM sleep when metabolic demands increase due to surges in sympathetic activity and heart rate.[264] Sleep is generally a time of reduced myocardial demand because of decreased blood pressure and heart rate. During NREM sleep, myocardial ischemia may occur due to decreased coronary flow and volume, reducing coronary perfusion pressure and increasing likelihood of thrombi and embolic events as well as ventricular arrhythmias.[264] Nocturnal hypoxemia occurring in OSA confers a poor prognosis for patients after MI, and it has been suggested that nocturnal oximetry may be practical approach to stratify risk in post-MI patients.[317]

Classic (effort) angina and the full spectrum of cardiac ischemic syndromes including unstable angina, non-Q-wave MI, and variant angina occur more often in the morning hours and early after awakening than at night.[318] These early morning hours reflect a combination of the stress of circadian patterns and behavioral stressors including increased mental activity and stress.[319] Beta adrenergic blocking agents are the primary therapy to reduce morning surges in sympathetic activity and cardiac events. On the contrary, patients with lower ventricular ejection fraction, diabetes, or advanced age are at higher risk for MIs during the night.[264]

Sleep and Arrhythmias

Sinus bradycardia and sinus arrhythmia are the most frequent changes in heart rhythm during sleep in healthy people, consistent with the dominance of parasympathetic activity.

Bradycardia during sleep is more common in men than in women, and the difference between daytime and nighttime heart rates decreases with age. In patients with CVD, SDB is independently associated with nocturnal cardiac arrhythmias, and increased severity of SDB is associated with risk for any cardiac arrhythmia.[320] Obesity increases the risk for OSA, specifically the magnitude of nocturnal O_2 desaturation, and both are independent risk factors for incident AF in patients under the age of 65 years.[321] OSA contributes to atrial remodeling and function and subsequent AF.[322,323] Disruptions in sleep, increased nighttime activity and restlessness, daytime sleepiness, and fatigue are present in conditions of AF and ventricular arrhythmias including those treated with implantable defibrillators and contribute to a reduced quality of life.[324–326] Patients with implantable cardioverter defibrillators and atrial defibrillators may experience sleep disruption initially after implant due to incisional pain and increased awareness of the device. Sleep disruptions may be due to device activations, and appropriate and inappropriate shocks.

The impact of SDB in cardiac patients on arrhythmogenesis cannot be overemphasized. In more recent and the classic Sleep Heart Health Study, individuals with severe SDB had two- to fourfold higher odds of complex arrhythmias including AF, ventricular tachycardia, and ventricular ectopy than those without cardiac disease, even after adjusting for potential confounding factors.[327,328] Appropriate treatment with CPAP in OSA patients is associated with lower recurrence of AF and ventricular ectopy, arrhythmia symptoms, and improved quality of life.[329,330]

NURSING CARE GOALS

After evaluating the subjective and objective data related to sleep noted earlier in the chapter, a nursing assessment may indicate that a patient is experiencing sleep difficulties. A nursing diagnosis of impaired sleep is made when patients experience or are at risk of experiencing a change in the quantity or quality of sleep that causes discomfort or interferes with daily life. The general nursing management plan focuses on promoting adequate, restful sleep for patients with cardiovascular disorders. This can be accomplished first by preventing or reducing the factors that are disturbing the patient's sleep. Depending on the patient's symptoms this might involve encouraging the patient to reduce their intake of caffeine and alcohol, turn off all electronic devices (including the television) several hours before bedtime, and/or controlling environmental noise. A second goal is to provide bedtime routines, comfort measures, and a setting conducive to sleep. A final goal is to detect alterations in physiologic function that are caused by or may accentuate the underlying health problem. Referral to a sleep disorders' specialist is often needed if symptoms of insomnia, OSA, restless legs, or EDS are present.

SLEEP PROMOTING INTERVENTIONS

Nonpharmacologic Outpatient Interventions for the Management of Sleep Disturbances in Patients With Cardiovascular Disease

Nonpharmacologic therapies, including behavioral, cognitive, and physiologic approaches for insomnia are often effective but underutilized by healthcare providers.

Controlled trials and systematic reviews have demonstrated that 70% to 80% of patients with persistent insomnia benefit from CBT-I, and that half of these patients achieve complete remission of their symptoms.[331] Cognitive and behavioral therapies may be used alone or in combination, and are more effective and safer for the long-term management of sleep disturbances than medications. Although complementary and alternative medicine

Table 7-2 • BEHAVIORS AND HABITS NONCONDUCIVE TO SLEEP

Spending too much time in bed
Frequent daytime napping
Too few daytime activities
Late evening exercise
Use of electronic devices , for example, smartphones, tablets, e-readers, computers, and watching television before bedtime
Inadequate morning light exposure
Excessive caffeine, especially in the latter half of the day
Evening alcohol consumption
Smoking in the evening
Late heavy dinner
Anxiety in anticipation of poor sleep
Environmental factors, such as the room being too warm, too noisy, or too bright

(CAM) practices such as yoga, tai chi, and meditation are quite popular, data regarding their efficacy for reducing insomnia in patients with CVD is quite limited, and should not be suggested as first-line therapies.

Sleep Education and Hygiene

Sleep hygiene measures alone are **not** adequate for the treatment of insomnia or other sleep disorders.[332,333] Most of the interventions listed in Table 7-2, were derived from studies done for other purposes, for example, evaluating the effects of moderately large doses of caffeine on the sleep among caffeine naïve young adults,[334] rather than testing whether or not avoiding caffeine improves sleep among those who regularly consume caffeine.[333] Although information about practices that may impair sleep are widely available, and many patients have already tried many of these measures,[332] reviewing them with patients may be helpful.

Relaxation Therapy

Anxiety and related thoughts are often detrimental to sleep and may prevent or delay sleep onset. Relaxation training originally designed to reduce anxiety has also been used successfully for the treatment of sleep onset insomnia. Several relaxation techniques are recommended for the treatment of sleep disturbances. These techniques include progressive muscle relaxation (a deep relaxation technique to control stress and anxiety) and autogenic training. Autogenic training focuses on increasing blood flow to the legs and arms. The sensations of warmth and heaviness are used to promote somatic relaxation. Another effective approach, the constructive worry technique, involves setting aside a specific time several hours before bedtime to complete a worksheet with two columns. Patients are instructed to write down concerns in the first column (Concerns) that are most likely to keep them awake at night, and then write down immediate steps that they can take to decrease their worries in the second column (Solutions). If there are no immediate solutions to the problem, patients are encouraged to write down acceptance-based or self-care strategies that might help reduce their anxiety.[335,336] Once a selected technique is established, the patient must practice it at least twice per day, or nightly if the constructive worry technique is selected. The focus should be on reducing arousal rather than inducing sleep, and practice should be done out of bed, particularly if the patient is also using stimulus control therapy.[331]

Stimulus Control Therapy

To cope with being awake during the night, many individuals with chronic sleep disturbances engage in behaviors in the bedroom that may further contribute to wakefulness. These may include worrying, reading, playing games on their smartphone, and watching television among other behaviors. They may also begin to associate bedtime and the bedroom environment with frustration related to being unable to sleep. Stimulus control therapy is therefore designed to break the relationship between maladaptive behaviors and sleep[337] and to recreate an association between the bedroom environment and sleep.[331] Patients using stimulus control are told to:

- Go to bed only if you are sleepy
- Avoid activities in the bedroom that keep you awake, other than sex
- Only sleep in the bedroom
- Leave the bedroom when awake
- Return to the bedroom only when sleepy
- Get up at the same time each morning, regardless of the amount of sleep
- Avoid napping during the day (although a nap of no more than 60 minutes may be allowed before 3 PM in older adults)

Although these instructions appear quite simple; several visits on a weekly or biweekly basis may been necessary to assist patients in adhering to these guidelines.[331]

Sleep Restriction Therapy

Many individuals who have difficulty falling asleep or staying asleep, increase the time they spend in bed, hoping to obtain more sleep. Although perhaps effective for a short time, this strategy usually results in fragmented and poor quality sleep.[331] Sleep restriction therapy is one of the most effective interventions to consolidate and eventually extend sleep. Sleep restriction therapy causes sleep deprivation, increasing the sleep drive, and shifts the patient's focus from trying to fall asleep to trying to stay up later. Before beginning sleep restriction therapy the individual maintains a sleep log for 2 weeks. This log facilitates estimating the average sleep time versus time spent in bed. The allowed sleep time is the average subjective sleep time, but is never less than 5 hours. The time in bed is adjusted by 15-minute increments or decrements, depending on the sleep efficiency. Sleep efficiency is defined as the average sleep time or time in bed multiplied by 100%. If sleep efficiency is greater than 90%, the time in bed is increased by 15 minutes, and if it is less than 85%, the time is decreased by 15 minutes.[331,337]

Sleep restriction has been shown to increase total sleep time, and improve sleep latency, total wake time, sleep efficiency, and subjective sleep quality.[338–340] The efficacy of sleep restriction therapy alone or in combination with such as stimulus control therapy and cognitive behavioral therapy has also been shown in other controlled trials.[340,341] However, the use of this technique with cardiovascular patients has not been fully tested and should be used only in collaboration with a specialist in sleep disorders medicine.

Cognitive Therapy

Cognitive therapy seeks to alter beliefs, expectations, and excessive self-monitoring that often perpetuate the symptoms of insomnia through Socratic questioning and behavioral experimentation.[331] Because of difficulties sleeping can often trigger negative emotions and thoughts which are incompatible with sleep, and continued difficulties often lead to worries about the consequences of sleep loss on the next day's performance, a vicious cycle develops. Cognitive therapy is thought to short-circuit the self-fulling nature of this cycle by challenging patients to question their unrealistic expectations regarding the necessity of obtaining 8 hours sleep every night, faulty causal attributions (e.g., something is physically wrong with me), and amplification of the consequences of insomnia (e.g., I will get fired if I don't get enough sleep). Patients are encouraged to develop more realistic expectations about sleep (e.g., no everyone needs 8 hours sleep/night and sleep needs change over the lifespan), not to blame all of their daytime difficulties on insomnia, avoid trying to sleep, avoid catastrophizing after a poor night's sleep, and to develop some tolerance for insomnia. Patients may also be encouraged to test out the validity of some of their beliefs, for example, resting in bed the day after a bad night and comparing it to how they feel if they are physically active after a poor night's sleep.

Cognitive therapy usually involves 4 to 6 hours of direct interaction with a skilled therapist, usually a specially trained psychologist, over a period 6 to 8 weeks.[331] Studies have shown that even four individual biweekly sessions can result in significant improvements in the objective wake time and sleep efficiency measures that are sustained for 6 months.[342] Cognitive behavioral therapy can be efficiently provided by masters prepared nurses to individuals[343] and groups.[344] Although face-to-face interactions with a therapist is ideal, the limited number of providers certified in behavioral sleep medicine often prevents patients from accessing CBT-I. To improve patient access to CBT-I, mobile and web-based platforms have been developed by expert clinicians. Both Sleepio (https://www.sleepio.com), developed by Colin Espie PhD and Shut*i* (http://www.myshuti.com), developed by Charles Morin PhD, are available on web-based and mobile platforms; CBT-I Coach, is a smartphone app, originally developed to enhance CBT-I therapy in U.S. Department of Veterans Affairs clinics, is now available for general use. These internet and mobile apps are viewed favorably by patients,[345] and are as effective as in-person therapy for reducing insomnia severity, and improving sleep efficiency and total sleep time.[346]

Complementary and Alternative Medicine

One of the most frequent uses of CAMs is in the treatment of sleep disturbances. While the terms are often used synonymously, a more accurate statement is the National Institutes of Health–National Center for Complementary and Integrative Health (NCCIH) definition that complementary medicines are "used together with conventional medicine," while alternative medicines are "used in place of conventional medicine."[347] The NCCAM lists five broad categories of CAM therapies including: (1) alternative medical systems. These include acupuncture, Ayurveda, or homeopathy; (2) biologically based practices, such as herbal products; (3) mind–body medicine, meditation, Tai Chi, yoga, and biofeedback; (4) manipulative and body-based practices, massage-based therapies; and (5) energy medicine that focuses on the use of energy fields, including bioelectromagnetic-based therapies.

Meditation

While there are several forms of meditation, one of the most commonly studied for insomnia is mindfulness meditation. Stress reduction may be one of the mechanisms by which meditation can exert a beneficial effect on sleep and most of the studies that have demonstrated improved sleep during meditation therapy have been conducted as stress reduction studies. In this regard, it can be used as part of a cognitive therapy approach. Studies among breast cancer patients, insomnia patients, and elderly adults have shown significant decreases in stress, depression symptoms, and sleep disturbances and significant increases in sleep quality after mindfulness meditation practice.[348–351] Few studies have used meditation as a method to improve sleep in patients with CVD but a recent study showed significant reductions in anxiety and depression symptoms, and perceived stress in coronary artery disease patients after mindfulness meditation.[352] However, a recent meta-analysis of six randomized clinical trials revealed that although mindfulness meditation significantly improved perceived sleep quality, there were no significant effects on sleep latency, total sleep time, sleep efficiency, total wake after sleep onset, insomnia severity index scores, or scores on the PSQI.[353]

Aromatherapy

Aromatherapy or essential oil therapy is the use of plant oils and other essential oils from flowers, herbs, or trees to improve an individual's health or mood. Studies have shown some benefit of aromatherapy in reducing anxiety and improving sleep quality. A randomized control study of ICU patients saw a significant improvement in self-measured sleep quality (increased PSQI score) and a significant reduction in anxiety after 15 days of using lavender oil, as compared to the control group.[354] Aromatherapy has been tested in cardiac patients. In a RCT of cardiac patients, Rosa damascene aromatherapy significantly improved sleep quality (measured by PSQI) compared to the control group.[355]

Manipulative and Body-Based Practices

The manipulative and body-based practices include a wide range of hands-on interventions. Massage therapy studies have primarily been conducted for sleep disorders in infants and children. Studies in adult populations focus on patients with specific medical conditions. One study examined the effects of aromatherapy massage for middle-aged women with hypertension. In this study there were statistically significant decreases in systolic and diastolic blood pressure and statistically significant increases in sleep quality after receiving aromatherapy massage compared to a control group.[356] Another study examining the effect of therapeutic massage on insomnia symptoms in postmenopausal women, found a significant reduction in insomnia symptoms after therapeutic massage.[357] Another study investigating the effect of back massage on insomnia symptoms in postpartum women also showed a significant decrease in symptoms after massage.[276] Back massage was also shown to significantly improve quality of sleep in ICU patients.[358] In separate studies examining the effects of message therapy in breast cancer patients and family caregivers of cancer patients respectfully, sleep quality improved.[359,360] Among patients with CVD, studies have shown that massage therapy improves sleep quality.[361,362]

Acupressure

Acupressure, a noninvasive technique that involves stimulation of meridian or acupoints on the body using finger pressing movements has been shown to improve scores on the PSQI and reduce the number of sleeping pills used among chronic hemodialysis patients,[363] and reduce symptoms of insomnia in residents of long-term care facilities.[364,365] Acupressure has had limited use in cardiac patients for sleep, requires further study, and has exhibited little effectiveness for lowering nausea and vomiting following cardiac surgery.[366] Acupressure appears to reduce sleep disturbances and improve self-reported sleep quality in elderly patients with Alzheimer disease or mental disorders.[364,367] It has also shown to be associated with improvements in the self-reported sleep quality and depression symptoms of menopausal women.[368,369] Valerian oil acupressure has shown to improve sleep quality and sleep duration in ICU patients.[296] Acupressure in end-stage renal patients undergoing hemodialysis has been associated with improvements in self-reported sleep quality, sleep latency, sleep efficiency, sleep duration, sleep disturbances, and daytime dysfunction.[363,370] Acupressure in patients with hypertension and patients with acute coronary syndrome has helped improve sleep quality.[371,372]

Yoga

Yoga incorporates the holistic components of physical activity, specific postures, breathing exercises, and a philosophic attitude toward life. It has been shown to reduce anxiety levels and physiologic arousal in cardiac patients,[373] and decrease the severity of both insomnia and climacteric symptoms in postmenopausal women.[374]

Tai chi

Tai Chi is a low- to-moderate-intensity traditional Chinese exercise that includes a meditational component. When compared to CBT-I, and attention control interventions in a randomized clinical trial, CBT-I was more effective for reducing insomnia, than Tai Chi.[375] Although participants assigned to the Tai Chi reported significant improvements in sleep quality, fatigue, and depression, compared to participants assigned to the sleep education group, the severity of their insomnia symptoms remained unchanged. Tai chi appears to be safe and effective for patients with MI and HF, and post-CABG surgery,[376] and may be viewed as an alternative exercise program that may enhance sleep for selected patients with CVDs.

Pharmacologic Interventions to Promote Sleep

The consequences and impact of insomnia (difficulty initiating and/or maintaining sleep, early morning awakenings, or unrefreshing sleep) are associated with a significant negative impact on daytime function including increased fatigue, decreased motivation and vigilance, reduced concentration, and impaired psychomotor function. Chronic sleep problems may also increase the risk of psychiatric disorders, such as depression and anxiety. In addition, poor sleep impacts, not only the patient, but family, friends, and caregivers. In many situations, the judicious use of pharmacologic agents to enhance sleep is indicated—often in conjunction with behavioral therapy.

An assessment of the type and duration of the sleep problem within the context of the underlying cardiac disease should dictate which agent is used. However, before initiating additional pharmacologic therapy, the medications taken by the patient should be carefully examined as many have the potential to disturb sleep. As shown in Table 7-3, many medications have been associated with difficulties falling asleep.

In addition to prescribed medications, some patients with CVD or HF may be taking over-the-counter or herbal medications with stimulant properties. Unless asked specifically about over-the-counter and herbal medications, patients may not volunteer this information. If patients are taking prescribed and/or over-the-counter and herbal medications that interfere with sleep, they should be discontinued whenever possible, or if discontinuing the medication is not possible, advised to take these medications in the morning.

Table 7-3 • MEDICATIONS ASSOCIATED WITH INSOMNIA

Antidepressants
Tricyclics
Amitriptyline
Doxepin
Imipramine
Trimipramine
Desipramine
Nortriptyline
Protriptyline
Selective Serotonin Reuptake Inhibitors
Fluoxetine
Paroxetine
Sertraline
Fluvoxamine
Serotonin and Norepinephrine Reuptake Inhibitors
Venlafaxine
Monoamine Oxidase Inhibitors
Phenelzine
Tranylcypromine
Antihypertensives
β-Blockers (Lipophilic Blockers)
Propranolol
Timolol
Others
Hypolipidemic Drugs
Atorvastatin
Lovastatin
Simvastatin
Nasal Decongestants
Pseudoephedrine
Phenylpropanolamine
Bronchodilators
Theophylline
Antiparkinsonian Medications
Levodopa
Corticosteroids
Prednisone

If pharmacologic therapy is required, the American Academy of Sleep Medicine's most recent treatment guideline[377] recommends that treatment be started with short- or intermediate-acting benzodiazepine receptor agonists such as zolpidem, zaleplon, zopiclone, and eszopiclone. If a patient prefers not to take a United States Drug Enforcement Administration (DEA)-schedule drug, or has a history of substance abuse disorder, ramelteon may be prescribed. If the patient does not respond well to the initial medication, a different agent in the same class may be prescribed. If necessary, a benzodiazepine may be prescribed. When insomnia is accompanied by a comorbid depression, low doses of a sedating antidepressant may be considered next. Finally, a combination of benzodiazepine receptor agonist and a sedating antidepressant, or other medications such as gabapentin may be prescribed.[377] As with all medications, follow-up and further evaluation of patient response to treatment is critical.

Nonbenzodiazepines and Ramelteon

Nonbenzodiazepines recommended as first-line pharmacologic treatment for insomnia include short- and intermediate-acting benzodiazepine receptor agonists and ramelteon.[377,378] The nonbenzodiazepines, often nicknamed the "Z drugs," have similar clinical effects to traditional benzodiazepines, but bind to different receptors, and have a lower potential for misuse.[379] Three nonbenzodiazepine drugs (and their half-lives) are indicated for the treatment of insomnia in the United States—zolpidem (regular formulation 2.5 hours; continued release 2.8 hours), zaleplon (1 hour), and eszopiclone (6 hours in adult; 9 hours in elderly). These medications have demonstrated efficacy in the management of sleep onset and sleep maintenance insomnia, as well as chronic insomnia[377,378] (see Table 7-4). In fact, eszopiclone has been demonstrated to be effective without the development of tolerance for 6 months, and was the first hypnotic approved by the FDA without a limit on the duration of administration.[379]

Benzodiazepines

Polysomnographic studies of sleep indicate that benzodiazepines decrease sleep latency and wake time and increase total sleep time. They also suppress SWS.[379] The benzodiazepines approved for use in insomnia differ primarily based on their half-life; triazolam (2 to 6 hours), temazepam (8 to 20 hours), estazolam (8 to 24 hours), quazepam (48 to 120 hours), and flurazepam (48 to 120 hours).[379] Daytime sedation and dependency may become problematic. Although these medications do not have any significant effects on respiration in patients with normal ventilation, respiratory depression may occur if patients have pre-existing conditions which compromise respiration such as COPD and unrecognized SDB.[379]

Other Drugs Used to Treat Insomnia

Antidepressants

Sedating antidepressant drugs such as amitriptyline, trimipramine, mirtazapine, and trazodone, are frequently prescribed in low doses to treat insomnia despite the absence of methodologically sound studies supporting their use as hypnotic medications in individuals without comorbid depression.[380] Of these medications, trazadone is probably most frequently prescribed, because unlike other traditional antidepressant medications it does not cause anticholinergic side effects (e.g., dry mouth, increased perspiration, constipation, and urinary retention). Trazadone side effects however, include hypotension, lightheadedness, weakness, priapism, weight gain and occasionally ventricular tachyarrhythmias.[380,381] American Academy of Sleep Medicine Guidelines recommend that trazodone not be prescribed for the treatment of sleep onset or sleep maintenance insomnia in adults.[377,378]

Doxepin is the only sedating antidepressant approved by the FDA for treating insomnia. Although less frequently prescribed than trazadone, low doses of doxepin (1, 3, and 6 mg) have been shown in numerous studies to be effective for treating sleep onset and sleep maintenance insomnia in adult and elderly patients.[380,382] The drug is well-tolerated and clinical trials have demonstrated that unlike other tricyclic antidepressants, doxepin is not associated with anticholinergic side effects, memory impairments, next day residual effects, weight gain, rebound insomnia or withdrawal syndrome after the drug was discontinued[382] (Table 7-5).

Over-the-Counter Medications

The major over-the-counter medications used for sleep include antihistamines, melatonin, and herbal therapies, such as valerian. With the exception of melatonin, there are no studies which document the effectiveness of these medications for improving sleep.

Table 7-4 • SELECTED MEDICATIONS USED TO ENHANCE SLEEP

Drug	Half-Life (hours)	Dose (mg)
Quazepam (Doral)	48–120	7.5–15
Flurazepam (Dalmane)	48–120	15–30
Triazolam (Halcion)	2–6	0.125–0.25
Estazolam (ProSom)	8–24	1–2
Temazepam (Restoril)	8–20	15–30
Loprazolam (Dormonoct)	4.6–11.4	1–2
Flunitrazepam (Rohypnol)	10.7–20.3	0.5–1
Lormetazepam (Loramet)	7.9–11.4	1–2 (Elderly: 0.5–1)
Nitrazepam (Alodorm)	25–35	5–10
Zolpidem: Oral tablet	2.5 (1.4–4.5)	5 (age >65 years) 5–10 (age <65 years)
Zolpidem: extended release (Ambien CR)	2.8 (1.6–4.5)	6.25–12.5
Zolpidem: Sublingual (Intermezzo)	2.5 (1.4–3.6)	Women: 1.75; men: 3.5
Zolpidem: Sublingual (Edluar)	2.7 (1.5–6.7)	5–10
Zolpidem: Oral spray (Zolpimist)	2.8 (1.7–8.4)	10
Zopiclone (Imovane)	5–6	3.75 (age >65 years)
Zaleplon (Sonata)	1 (0.8–1.3)	5–10
Eszopiclone (Lunesta)	6 (5–8)	2–3 (age <65 years); 1–2 (age >65 years)
Ramelteon	1–2.6	8
Doxepin	15 (10–30)	3–6 (Silenor)
Suvorexant	12	10–20
Clonazepam (Klonopin)	20–40	0.5–1
Diazepam (Valium)	30–100	2–10
Chlordiazepoxide (Librium)	24–28	10–25
Alprazolam	6–20	0.5–1
Lorazepam	10–20	0.5–1
Quetiapine (Seroquel)	6	25–50
Trazodone (Desyrel)	9 (7–15)	25–50

Table 7-5 • OTHER DRUGS USED TO TREAT INSOMNIA

Drug	Drug Type	Elimination Half-Life	Dosage
Melatonin	Hormone	40–60 minutes	0.2–5 mg
Diphenhydramine	Ethanolamine antihistamine	4–8 hours	25–50 mg
Doxylamine	Ethanolamine antihistamine	10 hours	25 mg
Valerian	Planet extract	Uncertain because of multiple constituents	Unknown
Gabapentin	Anticonvulsant (structural analog of GABA)	5–9 hours	Unknown
Suvorexant	Orexin receptor antagonists	9–12 hours	10–20 mg
Choral hydrate	Two-carbon molecule	5–10 hours (for trichloroethanol)	500 mg

Used with permission from Pak VM, Onen SH, Gooneratne NS, et al. Observation and interview-based diurnal sleepiness inventory for measurement of sleepiness in older adults. *Nat Sci Sleep*. 2017;9(29):241–247.

Adverse effect may include residual daytime sedation and decreased cognitive function in the elderly. Antihistamines may also have anticholinergic side effects (dry mouth, blurred vision, urinary retention, constipation, etc.) and may be contraindicated in patients with cardiac disease. The use of antihistamines should be avoided since these anticholinergic medications have been associated with a statistically significant increased risk for dementia and Alzheimer disease.[383,384] Hepatotoxicity following use of valerian has also been reported.[385,386] And kava, another popular natural product, has been associated with acute liver failure and death.[387,388] More importantly, a recent meta-analysis involving over 1600 participants show there was no significant difference between any herbal medicine for insomnia and placebo, or any herbal medicine and active control, for any of 13 measures of clinical efficacy.[389]

Melatonin

Melatonin is a hormone produced by the pineal gland that is thought to play an important role in regulating the sleep/wake cycle. During the daytime, circulating levels are low with nocturnal levels becoming elevated, which coincide with the sleep phase. Melatonin can alter the timing of the circadian sleep/wake cycle.[115] Melatonin also has exhibited sedative, analgesic, anxiolytic, and anesthetic effects[390–392] and has exhibited positive effects on the cardiovascular system.[393–395] Studies of the effectiveness of melatonin have shown that melatonin significantly reduces sleep latency, significantly increases total sleep time, and significantly improves sleep quality.[393] A study showed that among insomnia patients with hypertension, prolonged-release melatonin improved sleep quality while maintaining the antihypertensive effectiveness of hypertension therapies including calcium channel blockers.[396]

A lack of regulation by the FDA of over-the-counter medications classified as herbal or dietary supplements, for example, melatonin and valerian root, has resulted in variable quality of these preparations. For example, a recent study of 30 melatonin supplements showed that the melatonin content ranged from 83% less to 478% greater amounts than the labelled amount.[397] Lot-to-lot amounts of melatonin within a particular product varied as much as 465%. Finally, the melatonin content did not meet the labelled amount with a 10% margin of the label claim, and 26% contained serotonin (a contaminant).

During the daytime, circulating levels are low with melatonin levels risking at night during darkness.[380] Studies have demonstrated that it can shift circadian rhythms, and can be effective in treating both delayed sleep phase syndrome and insomnia.[118] If administered in the morning, melatonin delays circadian rhythms; if taken in the late afternoon or evening, it advances circadian rhythms, thus encouraging an earlier onset of sleep. Given that studies on the effectiveness of melatonin for the treatment of insomnia have used a range of dosages (e.g., 1 to 80 mg), a variety of dosing schedules, and a variety of outcome measures (e.g., subjective and objective measures of sleep), it is not surprising that findings regarding its utility as a hypnotic are inconsistent. At present, a preponderance of evidence suggests that melatonin may reduce sleep latency and possibly sleep continuity, but does not affect the amount of deep sleep or REM sleep.[380] Melatonin does not have a dose-dependent relationship, for example, larger doses do not have a greater effect on sleep than smaller doses.[118,380] Although melatonin is well tolerated by most individuals in the dose range of 0.1 to 5 mg with few reported adverse events,[380] the American Academy of Sleep Medicine does **not** recommend the use of melatonin for the treatment of sleep onset or sleep maintenance insomnia.[377,378]

SLEEP OF HEALTHCARE PROVIDERS

Hospital nurses, physicians, and others who work the night shift or rotating schedules often experience irregular sleep/wake schedules and insufficient sleep, causing reduced alertness. This reduced alertness is accentuated by the pronounced circadian alertness–sleepiness rhythm, with maximal sleepiness and lowest performance at approximately 4:00 to 5:00 AM, at the low point of the body temperature rhythm.[398] Mental tasks that require sustained visual attention, such as monitoring an ECG oscilloscope or driving home from work, are more affected than are physical tasks. Suggested strategies to improve shift worker's sleep/rest include scheduling one or more nights off after night duty, scheduling no more than three-night shifts in a row, avoidance of extended shifts (no shift greater than 12 hours), fatigue management programs, sleep hygiene education for staff, using rotation schedules that move forward around the clock rather than backward, and taking a nap before going to work. Although night shift workers are often encouraged to remain on a night shift schedule on their days off, there is no evidence to support this often socially undesirable recommendation.[399] Although melatonin may be used to improve circadian adaption to night shift work, its chronobiotic benefits may be counteracted by exposure to daylight during the early morning hours (e.g., typically when the worker is driving home after work).[398,400]

Nurses and other healthcare providers should be routinely screened for depression, anxiety, and sleep disorders since these disorders are common and have an adverse impact on patient safety.[401] For example, one study reported that 20% of hospital staff nurses suffer from depression, a rate that is 2 to 3 times higher than the general population.[402] Insomnia is quite common, with between 18% and 54% of hospital workers reporting symptoms of insomnia.[401,403,404] Finally, a recent study by Weaver et al.,[401] reported that 40.6% of the 295 hospital staff nurses included in their study screened positive for anxiety, depression, insomnia, or some other sleep disorder.

Although extended shifts, for example, shifts of 12 hours or longer, are quite popular among nurses, they have been associated with an increased risk of making errors, increased number of needlestick injuries, increase number of medication errors, difficulties remaining alert on duty, and difficulties remaining alert driving home.[405–408] Research has also shown that even when nurses working 12-hour night shifts obtain the same amount of sleep as nurses working 12-hour day shifts, night shift nurses had decreased reaction times and increased performance lapses.[409] Additional details about the health and safety risks associated with shift work, long work hours, and strategies to mitigate these risks is available at https://www.cdc.gov/niosh/docs/2015-115/.

Summary

Patients with CVD often have disturbed sleep, especially in intensive cardiac care settings, and may be at risk for physiologic changes during sleep that adversely affect their health status. Sleep disorders contribute to risk for cardiac disease and to other cardiac risk factors including metabolic, diabetic, and respiratory conditions. Although beliefs regarding the relationship between sleep and well-being are widely shared, hospital practices are rarely designed to encourage optimal sleep for patients or staff. Research is needed to clarify the role of nighttime sleep and daytime naps in recovery from CVD and surgery (e.g., what are optimal sleep patterns?) and to identify nursing interventions that prevent sleep deprivation, minimize adverse sleep-related physiologic changes, enhance adherence to treatment for OSA, and promote good sleep.

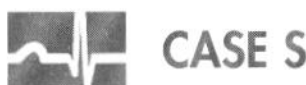

CASE STUDY

Patient Profile

July 8th Initial Visit

Mr. James Gold is a 71-year-old Caucasian male who was referred to the sleep clinic by his cardiologist for evaluation of possible sleep apnea. He goes to bed at 11:00 PM and falls asleep without difficulty in 20 to 30 minutes, and gets out of bed at 8 AM. He reports snoring, witnessed apnea, nonrestorative nocturnal sleep with 2 to 4 awakenings after sleep onset with 60 to 90 minutes of wake time after first falling asleep. He naps 4 to 5 weekly for 1 to 2 hours. Although quite fatigued during the day, his Epworth Sleepiness Scale score is 6/24 suggesting normal daytime vigilance.

Past Medical History

Hypertension, benign prostatic hypertrophy, coronary artery disease poststenting to the right coronary artery in 2011, hypercholesterolemia, and paroxysmal and chronic atrial fibrillation.

Medications

Azor 10 to 40 mg qday, Clopidogrel bisulfate 75 mg q day, Crestor 20 mg q day, Metoprolol 50 mg BID, and Tamsulosin HCL 8 mg q day.

Surgical History

PCI 2011 to RCA.

Social History

The patient is a former pipe smoker of 25 years, consumes two drinks weekly of alcohol within 4 hours of bedtime, and consumes approximately two cups of coffee daily.

Patient Examination

Vital Signs

BP 102/64 mm Hg; PR 84 bpm; RR 17; Ht. 67 in; Wt. 214 lb; BMI 33.02 kg/m^2; neck circumference 17 in.

Physical Examination

Low soft palate and narrow pharyngeal space.

Diagnostic Studies

An overnight sleep study was ordered which revealed moderately severe OSA with an AHI of 25, and a minimum oxygen saturation of 78%, with oxygen saturations less than 90% for 49% of the sleep time.

After an unsuccessful CPAP titration, the patient underwent a BiPAP titration which eliminated most obstructive events at 15/11 cm H_2O pressure. Frequent Cheyne–Stokes respiration was noted and associated with frequent hypoxemia. His minimal oxygen saturation was 75% with saturations less than 89% for 37 minutes. There were 4 obstructive apneas, 132 central apneas, and 15 hypopneas. Atrial fibrillation was noted throughout the recording.

November 2nd

The patient reported that he has been unable to tolerate BiPAP therapy and quit using it after a few nights. The downloaded data verified his nonadherence and the calculated AHI from the limited data available is 12 with a central apnea index of 7 and a hypopnea index of 4 with a pressure of 15/11 cm H_2O. Bilevel at a pressure of 18/8 will be prescribed as well as nocturnal oxygen and a full-face mask to reduce air leaks.

November 15th

The patient reports that his sleep is unchanged since his last visit. He was unable to get oxygen therapy and has not used his machine. He was advised by his vendor to come back to clinic and start over or else nothing would be covered by Medicare.

Echo done on 2/17 shows an EF of 60%. Since the patient is not tolerating BiPAP therapy and his central apneas are persisting, will order an ASV titration to see if this approach will be an effective treatment for his severe obstructive and central sleep apnea. Although ASV can be hazardous in patients with cardiac disease, his myocardial function is adequate to allow this therapy to be used safely.

December 7th

ASV titration revealed a sleep onset latency of 12.5 minutes and a REM latency of 77.0 minutes. Sleep efficiency was 63.3%. On ASV, the AHI was 4.3: the study demonstrated resolution of apneic and hypopnea episodes with an EPAP min 8, IPAP max 25, Ps min 2, Ps max 8, and auto rate was required to obtain the above results. No central apneas or periodic breathing was noted on ASV therapy. Cardiac monitoring was remarkable for PVCs and PACs.

July 15th

The patient returns for follow-up care of his obstructive sleep apnea. Since his last visit, he has consistently used ASV with a nasal mask for 5 to 6 hours nightly, and reports feeling more rested. Daytime napping has been eliminated and his atrial fibrillation controlled with amiodarone 100 mg q day.

KEY READINGS

Mullington JM, Haak M, Toth M, et al. Cardiovascular, inflammatory, and metabolic consequences of sleep deprivation. *Prog Cardiovasc Dis.* 2009;51(4):294–302.

Tietjens JR, Clarman D, Eezirian EJ, et al. Obstructive sleep apnea in cardiovascular disease: A review of the literature and proposted multidisciplinary clinical management strategy. *JAHA.* 2019;8(1):e010440.

REFERENCES

1. Javaheri S, Drager L, Lorenzi-Filho G. Sleep and cardiovascular disease: present and future. In: Kryger M, Roth T, Dement WC, eds. *Principles and Practices of Sleep Medicine.* 6th ed. Philadelphia, PA: Elsevier; 2017:1222–1228.
2. Thorpy MJ. History of sleep and man. In: Thorpy MJ, ed. *The Encyclopedia of Sleep and Sleep Disorders.* New York: Oxford; 1991:ix–xxxiii.
3. Carskadon MA, Dement WC. Normal human sleep: an overview. In: Kryger M, Roth T, Dement WC, eds. *Principles and Practice of Sleep Medicine.* 6th ed. Philadelphia, PA: Elsevier; 2017:15–24.
4. Jike M, Itani O, Watanabe N, et al. Long sleep duration and health outcomes: a systematic review, meta-analysis and meta-regression. *Sleep Med Rev.* 2018;39:25–36.
5. Itani O, Jike M, Watanabe N, et al. Short sleep duration and health outcomes: a systematic review, meta-analysis and meta-regression. *Sleep Med.* 2016;32:246–256.
6. Carroll JE, Stein MS, Seeman TE. Sleep and multisystem biological risk: a population-based study. *PLoS One.* 2015;10(2):e0118467.
7. Nasir U, Shahid H, Shabbir MO. Sleep quality and depression in hospitalized congestive heart failure patients. *J Pak Med Assoc.* 2015;65(3):264–269.
8. Satela M. *The International Classification of Sleep Disorders.* 3rd ed. Darien, IL: American Academy of Sleep Medicine; 2014.
9. Pelayo R, Dement WC. History of sleep physiology and medicine. In: Kryger M, Roth T, Dement WC, eds. *Principles and Practice of Sleep Medicine.* 6th ed. Philadelphia, PA: Elsevier; 2017:3–14.

10. Roehrs T, Carskadon MA, Dement WC, et al. Daytime sleepiness and alertness. In: Kryger M, Roth T, Dement WC, eds. *Principles and Practice of Sleep Medicine*. 6th ed. Philadelphia, PA: Elsevier; 2017:39–48.
11. Feinberg I, Campbell IG. Sleep EEG changes during adolescence: an index of fundamental brain reorganization. *Brain Cogn.* 2010;72(1):56–65.
12. Redline S, Kirchner L, Quan SF, et al. The effects of age, sex, ethnicity and sleep disordered breathing on sleep architecture. *Arch Intern Med.* 2004;164:171–176.
13. Bliwise DL, Ansari FP, Straight LM, et al. Age changes in time and 24-hour distribution of self-reported sleep. *Am J Geriatr Psychiatry.* 2005;13:1077–1082.
14. Bliwise DL, Scullin MK. Normal aging. In: Kryger M, Roth T, Dement WC, eds. *Principles and Practice of Sleep Medicine*. 6th ed. Philadelphia, PA: Elsevier; 2017:25–38.
15. Grandner MA., Chakravorty S, Perlis ML, et al. Habitual sleep duration associated with self-reported and objectively determined cardiometabolic risk factors. *Sleep Med.* 2014;15:42–50.
16. Liu Y, Wheaton AG, Chapman DP, et al. Sleep duration and chronic disease among US adults age 45 years and older: evidence from the 2010 Behavioral Risk Factor Surveillance System. *Sleep.* 2013;36:1421–1427.
17. Gallicchio L, Kalesan B. Sleep duration and mortality: a systematic review and meta-analysis. *J Sleep Res.* 2009;18:148–158.
18. Liu Y, Wheaton AG, Chapman DP, et al. Prevalence of healthy sleep duration among adults-United States 2014. *Morb Mortal Wkly Rep.* 2017;65(6):137–141.
19. Turek FW, Zee PC. Introduction: master circadian clock and master circadian rhythm. In: Kryger M, Roth T, Dement WC, eds. *Principles and Practice of Sleep Medicine*. 6th ed. Philadelphia, PA: Elsevier; 2017:340–342.
20. Fang Z, Rao H. Imaging homeostatic sleep pressure and circadian rhythm in the human brain. *J Thorac Dis.* 2017;9(5):E495–E498.
21. Adan A, Archer SN, Hidalgo MP, et al. Circadian typology: a comprehensive review. *Chronobiol Int.* 2012;29(9):1153–1175.
22. Koskenvuo M, Hublin C, Partien M, et al. Heritability of diurnal type: a nationwide study of 8753 adult twin pairs. *J Sleep Res.* 2007;16:156–162.
23. Gottlieb DJ, O'Conner GT, Wilk JB. Genome-wide association of sleep and circadian phenotypes. *BMC Med Genet.* 2007;8:S9.
24. Chen T, Wilk JB, O'Connor GT, et al. Genetics of sleep phenotypes in the NHLBI's Framingham heart study offspring cohort. *Sleep.* 2009;32:A401.
25. Landolt HP, Dijk DJ. Genetics and genomic basis of sleep in health humans. In: Kryger M, Roth T, Dement WC, eds. *Principles and Practice of Sleep Medicine*. 6th ed. Philadelphia, PA: Elsevier; 2017:310–339.
26. Lack LC, Gradisar M, Van Someren EJW, et al. The relationship between body insomnia and body temperature. *Sleep Med Rev.* 2008;12(4): 307–317.
27. Christensen MA, Bettencourt L, Kaye L, et al. Direct measurement of smartphone screen-time: relationships with demographics and sleep. *PLoS One.* 2016;11(11):e0165331.
28. Chang AM, Aeschbach D, Duffy JF, et al. Impact of light-emitting Ebooks before bed negatively affects sleep, circadian time, and next-morning alertness. *Proc Natl Acad Sci.* 2015;112(4):1232–1237.
29. Fuller-Rowell TE, Curtis DS, El-Sheikh M, et al. Racial disparities in sleep: the role of neighborhood disadvantage. *Sleep Med.* 2016;27–28:1–8.
30. Xiao Q, Hale L. Neighborhood socioeconomic status, sleep duration, and napping in middle-to-old aged US men and women. *Sleep.* 2018;41(7):zsy076.
31. Troxel WM, DeSantis A, Richardson AS, et al. Neighborhood disadvantage is associated with actigraphy-assessed sleep continuity and short sleep duration. *Sleep.* 2018;41:zsy140.
32. Roehrs T, Roth T. Medication and substance abuse. In: Kryger M, Roth T, Dement WC, eds. *Principles and Practice of Sleep Medicine*. 6th ed. Philadelphia, PA: Elsevier; 2017:1380–1389.
33. Ancoli-Isreal S, Roth T. Characteristics of insomnia in the United States: results of the 1991 National Sleep Foundation Survey I. *Sleep.* 2000;22:S347–S353.
34. Roehrs T, Blaisdell B, Cruz N, et al. Tolerance to hynotic effects of ethanol in insomnias. *Sleep.* 2004;27:S352.
35. Brower KJ. Alcohol's effects on sleep in alcoholics. *Alcohol Res Health.* 2001;25:110–125.
36. *In U.S., 45% say they have tried marijuana.* 2017. Available at https://news.gallup.com/poll/214250/say-tried-marijuana.aspx. Accessed July 30, 2018.
37. *Governing: the states and localities. State Marijuana Laws in 2018 map.* 2018. Available at http://www.governing.com/gov-data/state-marijuana-laws-map-medical- recreational.html. Accessed July 30, 2018.
38. Robinson, M, Berke J, Gold S. *This map shows every state that has legalized marijuana.* 2018. Available at https://www.governing.com/gov-data/safety-justice/state-marijuana-laws-map-medical-recreational.html.
39. Rivik RT, Zarcone V, Dement WC, et al. Delta-9-tetrahydrocannabinol and synhex1: effects on human sleep patterns. *Clin Pharmacol Ther.* 1972;13(3):426–435.
40. Feinberg I, Jones R, Walker JM, et al. Effects of high dosage delta-9-tetrahydrocannabinol on sleep patterns in man. *Clin Pharmacol Ther.* 1975;17(4):458–466.
41. Barratt ES, Beaver W, White R. The effects of marijuana on human sleep patterns. *Biol Psychiatry.* 1974;8(1):47–54.
42. Feinberg, I, Jones R, Walker J, et al. Effects of marijuana extract and tetrahydrocannabinol on electroencephalographic sleep patterns. *Clin Pharmacol Ther.* 1976;19(6):782–794.
43. Chait LD. Subjective and behavioral effects of marijuana the morning after smoking. *Psychopharmacology (Berl).* 1990;100(3):328–333.
44. Freemon FR. The effect of chronically administered delta-9-tetrahydrocannabinol upon the polygraphically monitored sleep of normal volunteers. *Drug Alcohol Depend.* 1982;10(4):345–353.
45. Karacan I, Fernandez-Salas A, Coggins WJ, et al. Sleep electroencephalographic-electrooculographic characteristics of chronic marijuana users: part I. *Ann N Y Acad Sci.* 1976;282:348–374.
46. Gates PJ, Albertella L, Copeland J. The effects of cannabinoid administration on sleep: a systematic review of human studies. *Sleep Med Rev.* 2014;18:477–487.
47. Babson KA, Sottile J, Morabito D. Cannabis, cannabinoids, and sleep: a review of the literature. *Curr Psychiatry Rep.* 2017;19:23.
48. Budney AJ, Moore BA, Vandrey RG, et al. The time course and significance of cannabis withdrawal. *J Abnorm Psychol.* 2003;112(3): 393–402.
49. Bolla KI, Lasage SR, Gamaldo CE, et al. Polysomnogram changes in marijuana users who report sleep disturbances during prior abstinence. *Sleep Med.* 2010;11(9):882–889.
50. Ogeil RP, Phillips JG. Commonly used stimulants: sleep problems, dependence and psychological distress. *Drug Alcohol Depend.* 2015;153:145–151.
51. Zhang L, Samet J, Caffo B, et al. Cigarette smoking and nocturnal sleep architecture. *Am J Epidemiol.* 2006;164:529–537.
52. Jaehne A, Loessi B, Barkai Z, et al. Effects of nicotine on sleep during consumption, withdrawal and replacement therapy. *Sleep Med Rev.* 2009;13:363–377.
53. Cano-Marquina A, Tarin JA, Cano A. The impact of coffee on health. *Maturitas.* 2013;75(1):7–21.
54. Clark I, Landoit HP. Coffee, caffeine, and sleep: a systematic review of epidemiological studies and randomized controlled trials. *Sleep Med Rev.* 2017;31:70–78.
55. Savard J, Savard MH, Ancoli-Isreal S. Sleep and fatigue in cancer patients. In: Kryger M, Roth T, Dement WC, eds. *Principles and Practice of Sleep Medicine*. 6th ed. Philadelphia, PA: Elsevier; 2017:1286–1293.
56. Savard J, Ivers H, Villa J, et al. Natural course of insomnia comorbid with cancer: an 18 month longitudinal study. *J Clin Oncol.* 2011;29:3580–3586.
57. Armbruster SD, Song J, Gatus L, et al. Endometrial cancer survivors' sleep patterns before and after a physical activity intervention: a retrospective cohort analysis. *Gynecol Oncol.* 2017;149(1):133–139.
58. Gooneratne NS, Dean GE, Rogers AE, et al. Sleep and quality of life in long-term lung cancer survivors. *Lung Cancer.* 2007;58:403–410.
59. Sanz de Burgoa Y, Rejas J, Ojeda P; Investigators of the Coste Asma study. Self-perceived sleep quality and quantity in adults with asthma: findings from the CosteAsma Study. *J Investig Allergol Clin Immunol.* 2016;26(4):256–262.
60. Luyster FS, Teodorescu M, Bleecker E, et al. Sleep quality and asthma control and quality of life in non-severe and severe asthma. *Sleep Breath.* 2012;16(4):1129–1137.
61. Javaheri S. Heart failure. In: Kryger M, Roth T, Dement WC, eds. *Principles and Practice of Sleep Medicine*. 6th ed. Philadelphia, PA: Elsevier; 2017:1271–1285.
62. Won C, Kirsch D. Fibromyalgia and chronic fatigue syndromes. In: Kryger M, Roth T, Dement WC, eds. *Principles and Practice of Sleep Medicine*. Philadelphia, PA: Elsevier; 2017:1294–1299.
63. Park JG, Ramar K. Sleep and chronic kidney disease. In: Kryger M, Roth T, Dement WC, eds. *Principles and Practice of Sleep Medicine*. Philadelphia, PA: Elsevier; 2017:1323–1328.
64. Grandner MA., Seixas A, Shetty S, et al. Sleep duration and diabetes risk: population trends and potential mechanism. *Curr Diab Rep.* 2016;16(11):106.

65. Minkle JD, Krystal, Benca AD, et al. Unipolar major depression. In: Kryger M, Roth T, Dement WC, eds. *Principles and Practice of Sleep Medicine*. Philadelphia, PA: Elsevier; 2017:1352–1362.
66. Harvey AG, Soehner AM, Buysse DJ. Fibromyalgia and chronic fatigue syndromes. Bipolar depression. In: Kryger M, Roth T, Dement WC, eds. *Principles and Practice of Sleep Medicine*. Philadelphia, PA: Elsevier; 2017:1363–1369.
67. Won C, Kirsch D. Fibromyalgia and chronic fatigue syndromes. In: Kryger M, Roth T, Dement WC, eds. *Principles and Practice of Sleep Medicine*. Philadelphia, PA: Elsevier; 2017:1294–1299.
68. Cirelli C, Bushey D. Sleep and wakefulness in Drosophila melanogaster. *Ann N Y Acad Sci*. 2008;1129:335–349.
69. Sheth BR, Janvelyan D, Khan M. Practice makes imperfect: restorative effects of sleep on motor learning. *PLoS One*. 2008;3(9):e3190.
70. Crespuglio R, Colas D, Gautier-Sauvigne S. Energy processes underlying the sleep-wake cycle. In: Parmeggiani L, Velluti RA, eds. *The Physiologic Nature of Sleep*. London: Imperial College Press; 2005:3–21.
71. Schmidt MH, Swang TW, Hamilton IM, et al. State-dependent metabolic partitioning and energy conservation: a theoretical framework for understanding the function of sleep. *PLoS One*. 2017;12(10):e0185746.
72. Muto V, Shaffil-le Bourdiec A, Matarazzo L, et al. Influence of acute sleep loss on neural correlates of alerting, orientating and executive attention components. *J Sleep Res*. 2012;21(6):648–658.
73. Laperchia C, Imperatore R, Azeez IA, et al. The excitatory/inhibitory input to orexin/hypocretin neuron soma undergoes day/night reorganization. *Brain Struct Funct*. 2017;222:3847–3859.
74. Puentes-Mestril C, Aton SJ. Linking network activity to synaptic plasticity during sleep: hypotheses and recent data. *Front Neural Circuits*. 2017;11:61.
75. Peigneux P, Fogel S, Smith C. Memory processing in relation to sleep. In: Kryger M, Roth T, Dement WC, eds. *Principles and Practice of Sleep Medicine*. 6th ed. Philadelphia, PA: Elsevier; 2017:229–238.
76. Lowe CJ, Safati A, Hall PA. The neurocognitive consequences of sleep restriction: a meta-analytic review. *Neurosci Biobehav Rev*. 2017;80:586–604.
77. Vriend J, Davidson F, Rusak B, et al. Emotional and cognitive impact of sleep restriction in children. *Sleep Med Clin*. 2015;10(2):107–115.
78. Drummond SP, Anderson DE, Straus LD, et al. The effects of two types of sleep deprivation on visual working memory capacity and filtering efficiency. *PLoS One*. 2012;7(4):e35653.
79. Reddy R, Palmer CA, Jackson C, et al. Impact of sleep restriction versus idealized sleep on emotional experience, reactivity and regulation in healthy adolescents. *J Sleep Res*. 2017;26(4):516–524.
80. Banks S, Dinges DF. Behavioral and physiological consequences of sleep restriction. *J Clin Sleep Med*. 2007;3(5):519–528.
81. Mignot E. Why we sleep: the temporal organization of recovery. *PLoS Biol*. 2008;6:e106.
82. Mancia G, Grassi G. The autonomic nervous system and hypertension. *Circ Res*. 2014;114(11):1804–1814.
83. Parati G, Esler M. The human sympathetic nervous system: its relevance in hypertension and heart failure. *Eur Heart J*. 2012;33(9):1058–1066.
84. Shen MJ, Zipes DP. Role of the autonomic nervous system in modulating cardiac arrhythmias. *Circ Res*. 2014;114(6):1004–1021.
85. Tsioufis C, Kordalis A, Flessas D, et al. Pathophysiology of resistant hypertension: the role of sympathetic nervous system. *Int J Hypertens*. 2011;2011:642416.
86. Reyes del Paso GA, Langewitz W, Mulder LJ, et al. The utility of low frequency heart rate variability as an index of sympathetic cardiac tone: a review with emphasis on a reanalysis of previous studies. *Psychophysiology*. 2013;50(5):477–487.
87. Tobaldini E, Nobili L, Strada S, et al. Heart rate variability in normal and pathological sleep. *Front Physiol*. 2013;4:294.
88. Viola AU, Tobaldini E, Chellappa SL, et al. Short-term complexity of cardiac autonomic control during sleep: REM as a potential risk factor for cardiovascular system in aging. *PLoS One*. 2011;6(4):e19002.
89. Hye Khan MA, Pavlov TS, Christain SV, et al. Epoxyeicosatrienoic acid analogue lowers blood pressure through vasodilation and sodium channel inhibition. *Clin Sci (Lond)*. 2014;127(7):463–474.
90. Wehrwein EA, Joyner MJ. Regulation of blood pressure by the arterial baroreflex and autonomic nervous system. In: *Handbook of Clinical Neurology*. Vol 117. Amsterdam, the Netherlands: Elsevier; 2013:89–102.
91. Liu J, Wang Y, Chen Y, et al. Tracking vital signs during sleep leveraging off-the-shelf WiFi. In: *Proceedings of the 16th ACM International Symposium on Mobile Ad Hoc Networking and Computing*. 2015.
92. Azarbarzin A, Ostrowski M, Hanly P, et al. Relationship between arousal intensity and heart rate response to arousal. *Sleep*. 2014;37(4):645–653.
93. Parashar R, Amir M, Pakhare A, et al. Age related changes in autonomic functions. *J Clin Diagn Res*. 2016;10(3):CC11–CC15.
94. Okada Y, Galbreath MM, Shibata S, et al. Morning blood pressure surge is associated with arterial stiffness and sympathetic baroreflex sensitivity in hypertensive seniors. *Am J Physiol Heart Circ Physiol*. 2013;305(6):H793–H802.
95. Shaffer F, McCraty R, Zerr CL. A healthy heart is not a metronome: an integrative review of the heart's anatomy and heart rate variability. *Front Psychol*. 2014;5:1040.
96. Boudreau P, Yeh WH, Dumont GA, et al. A circadian rhythm in heart rate variability contributes to the increased cardiac sympathovagal response to awakening in the morning. *Chronobiol Int*. 2012;29(6):757–768.
97. Chokroverty S, Provini C. Sleep, breathing, and neurologic disorders. In: Chokroverty S, ed. *Sleep Disorders Medicine*. 4th ed. NY, NY: Springer; 2017.
98. McSharry DG, Saboisky JP, DeYoung P, et al. A mechanism for upper airway stability during slow wave sleep. *Sleep*. 2013;36(4):555–563.
99. Mokhlesi B, Punjabi NM. "REM-related" obstructive sleep apnea: an epiphenomenon or a clinically important entity? *Sleep*. 2012;35(1):5–7.
100. McGinty DSR. Neural control of sleep in mammals. In: Roth T, ed. *Principles and Practice of Sleep Medicine*. 6th ed. Philadelphia, PA: Elsevier; 2017:62–77.
101. Okamoto-Mizuno K, Mizuno K. Effects of thermal environment on sleep and circadian rhythm. *J Physiol Anthropol*. 2012;31(1):14.
102. Saini C, Morf J, Stratmann M, et al. Simulated body temperature rhythms reveal the phase-shifting behavior and plasticity of mammalian circadian oscillators. *Genes Dev*. 2012;26(6):567–580.
103. Kräuchi K, DeboerT. Body temperatures, sleep, and hibernation. In: Kryger M, Roth T, and William C. Dement WC, eds. *Principles and Practice of Sleep Medicine*. 5th ed. St. Louis, Missouri: Elsevier Saunders; 2011;323–334.
104. Duffy JF, Zitting KM, Chinoy ED. Aging and circadian rhythms. *Sleep Med Clin*. 2015;10(4):423–434.
105. Franzini C. *Cardiovascular Physiology: The Peripheral Circulation*. Philadelphia, PA: Elsevier Saunders; 2005.
106. Maquet P, Degueldre C, Delfiore G, et al. Functional neuroanatomy of human slow wave sleep. *J Neurosci*. 1997;17(8):2807–2812.
107. Maquet P, Phillips C. Functional brain imaging of human sleep. *J Sleep Res*. 1998;7(suppl 1):42–47.
108. Ma N, Dinges DF, Basner M, et al. How acute total sleep loss affects the attending brain: a meta-analysis of neuroimaging studies. *Sleep*. 2015;38(2):233–240.
109. Firsov D, Tokonami N, Bonny O. Role of the renal circadian timing system in maintaining water and electrolytes homeostasis. *Mol Cell Endocrinol*. 2012;349(1):51–55.
110. Stow LR, Gumz ML. The circadian clock in the kidney. *J Am Soc Nephrol*. 2011;22(4):598–604.
111. Mill J, da Silva A, Baldo M, et al. Correlation between sodium and potassium excretion in 24- and 12-h urine samples. *Braz J Med Biol Res*. 2012;45(9):799–805.
112. Buxton OM, Spiegel K, Van Cauter E. *Modulation of Endocrine Function and Metabolism by Sleep and Sleep Loss*. Philadelphia, PA: Hanley & Belfus; 2002.
113. Kim TW, Jeong JH, Hong SC. The impact of sleep and circadian disturbance on hormones and metabolism. *Int J Endocrinol*. 2015;2015:591729.
114. Gamble KL, Berry R, Frank SJ, et al. Circadian clock control of endocrine factors. *Nat Rev Endocrinol*. 2014;10(8):466–475.
115. Burke TM, Markwald RR, Chinoy ED, et al. Combination of light and melatonin time cues for phase advancing the human circadian clock. *Sleep*. 2013;36(11):1617–1624.
116. Touitou Y, Reinberg A, Touitou D. Association between light at night, melatonin secretion, sleep deprivation, and the internal clock: health impacts and mechanisms of circadian disruption. *Life Sci*. 2017;173:94–106.
117. Ong JC, Arnedt T, Gehrman PR. Insomnia, diagnosis, assessment and evaluation. In: Kryger M, Roth T, Dement WC, eds. *Principles and Practice of Sleep Medicine*. 6th ed. Philadelphia, PA: Elsevier; 2017:785–793.
118. Abbott SM, Reid KJ, Zee PC. Circadian disorders of the sleep wake cycle. In: Kryger M, Roth T, Dement WC, eds. *Principles and Practice of Sleep Medicine*. 6th ed. Philadelphia, PA: Elsevier; 2017:414–423.
119. Buysse DJ, Reynolds CF, Monk TH, et al. The Pittsburgh sleep quality index: a new instrument for psychiatric practice and research. *Psychiatry Res*. 1989;28(2):193–213.

120. Spira AP, Beaudreau, SA, Stone, KL, et al. Reliability and validity of the Pittsburgh sleep quality index and the Epworth sleepiness scale in older men. *J Gerontol A Biol Sci Med Sci.* 2012;67A(4):433–439.
121. Ellis BW, Johns MW, Lancaster R, et al. The St. Mary's Hospital sleep questionnaire: a study of reliability. *Sleep.* 1981;4(1):93–97.
122. Arora T, Broglia E, Pushpakumar D, et al. An investigation into the strength of association and agreement levels between subjective and objective sleep duration in adolescents. *PLoS One.* 2013;8(8):e72406.
123. Van Den Berg JF, Van Rooij F JA., Vos H, et al. Disagreement between subjective and actigraphic measures of sleep duration in a population-based study of elderly persons. *J Sleep Res.* 2008;17(3):295–302.
124. Johns MW. A new method for measuring daytime sleepiness: the Epworth sleepiness scale. *Sleep.* 1991;14:540–545.
125. Johns MW. Reliability and factor analysis of the Epworth sleepiness scale. *Sleep.* 1992;15:376–381.
126. Johns MW. Sensitivity and specificity of the multiple sleep latency test (MSLT), the maintenance of wakefulness test and the Epworth sleepiness scale: failure of the MSLT as a "gold standard". *J Sleep Res.* 2000;9(1):5–11.
127. van der Heide A, van Schie MKM, Lamers GJ, et al. Comparing treatment effect measurements in narcolepsy: the sustained attention to response task, Epworth sleepiness scale and maintenance of wakefulness test. *Sleep.* 2015;38(7):1051–1058.
128. Mihăicută S, Ardelean C, Ursoniu S, et al. Excessive daytime somnolence as a predictor for sleep apnea syndrome-a multivariate analysis. *J Cogn Behavioral Psychother.* 2013;13:183–195.
129. Sanford SD, Lichstein KL, Durrence HH, et al. The influence of age, gender, ethnicity and insomnia on Epworth sleepiness scores: a normative US population. *Sleep Med.* 2006;7:319–325.
130. Keenan S, Hirshkowitz M. Sleep stage scoring. In: Kryger M, Roth T, Dement WC, eds. *Principles and Practice of Sleep Medicine.* 6th ed. Philadelphia, PA: Elsevier; 2017:1567–1575.
131. Penzel T. Home sleep testing. In: Kryger M, Roth T, Dement WC, eds. *Principles and Practice of Sleep Medicine.* Philadelphia, PA: Elsevier; 2017:1610–1614.
132. Collop NA, Tracey SL, Kapur V, et al. Obstructive sleep apnea devices for Out-of-Center (OOC) Testing: technology evaluation. *J Clin Sleep Med.* 2011;7:531–548.
133. Qassem A, Dallas P, Owens DK, et al. Clinical guidelines committee of the American College of Physicians, diagnosis of obstructive sleep apnea in adults: a clinical practice guideline from the American College of Physicians. *Ann Intern Med.* 2014;161(3):210–220.
134. Hirshkowitz M, Sharafkhaunch A. Evaluating sleepiness. In: Kryger M, Roth T, Dement WC, eds. *Principles and Practice of Sleep Medicine.* Philadelphia, PA: Elsevier; 2017:1651–1658.
135. Stone JL, Ancoli-Israel S. Actigraphy. In: Kryger M, Roth T, Dement WC, eds. *Principles and Practice of Sleep Medicine.* 6th ed. Philadelphia, PA: Elsevier; 2017:1671–1178.
136. Bhat S, Ferraris A, Gupta D, et al. Is there a clinical role for smartphone sleep apps? Comparison of sleep cycle detection by a smartphone app to polysomnography. *J Clin Sleep Med.* 2015;11(7):709–715.
137. Morgenthaler T, Alessi C, Friedman L, et al. Practice parameters for the use of actigraphy in the assessment of sleep and sleep disorders: an update for 2007. *Sleep.* 2007;30(4):519–529.
138. Blackwell T, Ancoli-Israel S, Redline S, et al. Osteoporotic Fractures in Men (MrOS) Study Group. Factors that many influence the classification of sleep-wake by wrist actigraphy: the MrOS Sleep Study. *J Clin Sleep Med.* 2011;7(4):357–367.
139. Ko PT, Kientz JA, Choe M, et al. Consumer sleep technologies: a review of the landscape. *J Clin Sleep Med.* 2015;11:1455–1461.
140. Lee-Tobin PA, Ogeil RP, Savic M, et al. Rate my sleep: examining the information, function and basis in empirical evidence within sleep applications for mobile devices. *J Clin Sleep Med.* 2017;13(11):1349–1354.
141. Cook JD, Prairie ML, Plante DT. Ability of multisensory Jawbone UP# to quantify and classify sleep in patients with suspected central disorders of hypersomnolence: a comparison against polysomnography and actigraphy. *J Clin Sleep Med.* 2018;14(5):841–848.
142. Khosla S, Deak MC, Gault D, et al. American Academy of Sleep Medicine Board of Directors. Consumer sleep technology: an American Academy of Sleep Medicine position statement. *J Clin Sleep Med.* 2018;14(5):877–880.
143. Thorpy MJ. Classification of sleep disorders. *Neurotherapeutics.* 2012; 9(4):687–701.
144. Buysse DJ. Sleep health: can we define it? Does it matter? *Sleep.* 2014; 37(1):9–17.
145. Sateia MJ. International Classification of Sleep Disorders-third edition: highlights and modifications. *Chest.* 2014;146(5):1387–1394.
146. Medic G, Wille M, Hemels ME. Short- and long-term health consequences of sleep disruption. *Nat Sci Sleep.* 2017;9:151–161.
147. O'Connor M, Hanlon A, Mauer E, et al. Identifying distinct risk profiles to predict adverse events among community-dwelling older adults. *Geriatr Nurs.* 2017;38(6):510–519.
148. McCoy JG, Strecker RE. The cognitive cost of sleep lost. *Neurobiol Learn Mem.* 2011;96(4):564–582.
149. Walia HK, Mehra R. Overview of common sleep disorders and intersection with dermatologic conditions. *Int J Mol Sci.* 2016;17(5):E654.
150. Chen X, Gelaye B, Williams MA. Sleep characteristics and health-related quality of life among a national sample of American young adults: assessment of possible health disparities. *Qual Life Res.* 2014;23(2):613–625.
151. Watson NF, Badr MS, Belenky G, et al. Joint consensus statement of the American Academy of Sleep Medicine and Sleep Research Society on the recommended amount of sleep for a healthy adult: methodology and discussion. *Sleep.* 2015;38(8):1161–1183.
152. Slater G, Steier J. Excessive daytime sleepiness in sleep disorders. *J Thorac Dis.* 2012;4(6):608–616.
153. Roehrs TCM, Dement W, Roth T. Daytime sleepiness and alertness. In: Kryger M, Roth T, Dement WC, eds. *Principles and Practice of Sleep Medicine.* 6th ed. Philadelphia, PA: Elsevier; 2017.
154. Fernandez-Mendoza J, Vgontzas AN, Kritikou I, et al. Natural history of excessive daytime sleepiness: role of obesity, weight loss, depression, and sleep propensity. *Sleep.* 2015;38(3):351–360.
155. Kim J, Cho SJ, Kim WJ, et al. Excessive daytime sleepiness is associated with an exacerbation of migraine: a population-based study. *J Headache Pain.* 2016;17(1):62.
156. Nakakubo S, Doi T, Makizako H, et al. Sleep duration and excessive daytime sleepiness are associated with incidence of disability in community-dwelling older adults. *J Am Med Dir Assoc.* 2016;17(8):768.e1–768.e5.
157. Vashum KP, McEvoy MA, Hancock SJ, et al. Prevalence of and associations with excessive daytime sleepiness in an Australian older population. *Asia Pac J Public Health.* 2015;27(2):NP2275–NP2284.
158. Leng Y, Wainwright NWJ, Cappuccio FP, et al. Daytime napping and the risk of all-cause and cause-specific mortality: a 13-year follow-up of a British population. *Am J Epidemiol.* 2014;179(9):1115–1124.
159. Zhong G, Wang Y, Tao T, et al. Daytime napping and mortality from all causes, cardiovascular disease, and cancer: a meta-analysis of prospective cohort studies. *Sleep Med.* 2015;16(7):811–819.
160. da Silva AA, de Mello RG, Schaan CW, et al. Sleep duration and mortality in the elderly: a systematic review with meta-analysis. *BMJ Open.* 2016;6(2):e008119.
161. Franklin KA, Lindberg E. Obstructive sleep apnea is a common disorder in the population—a review on the epidemiology of sleep apnea. *J Thorac Dis.* 2015;7(8):1311–1322.
162. Dudley KA, Patel SR. Disparities and genetic risk factors in obstructive sleep apnea. *Sleep Med.* 2016;18:96–102.
163. Pranathiageswaran S, Badr MS, Severson R, et al. The influence of race on the severity of sleep disordered breathing. *J Clin Sleep Med.* 2013;9(4):303–309.
164. Jordan AS, McSharry DG, Malhotra A. Adult obstructive sleep apnoea. *Lancet North Am Ed.* 2014;383(9918):736–747.
165. McCarra MB, Owens RL. Obstructive sleep apnea: can the downward spiral be reversed—a summary of John Stradling's ATS keynote speech. *J Thorac Dis.* 2016;8(suppl 7):S539–S541.
166. Kolla BP, Foroughi M, Saeidifard F, et al. The impact of alcohol on breathing parameters during sleep: a systematic review and meta- analysis. *Sleep Med Rev.* 2018;42:59–67.
167. McEntire DM, Kirkpatrick DR, Kerfeld MJ, et al. Effect of sedative-hypnotics, anesthetics and analgesics on sleep architecture in obstructive sleep apnea. *Expert Rev Clin Pharmacol.* 2014;7(6):787–806.
168. Pak VM, Grandner MA, Pack AI. Circulating adhesion molecules in obstructive sleep apnea and cardiovascular disease. *Sleep Med Rev.* 2014;18(1):25–34.
169. Filgueiras-Rama D, Arias MA, Iniesta A, et al. Atrial arrhythmias in obstructive sleep apnea: underlying mechanisms and implications in the clinical setting. *Pulm Med.* 2013;9:426758.
170. Rossi VA, Stradling JR, Kohler M. Effects of obstructive sleep apnoea on heart rhythm. *Eur Respir J.* 2013;41(6):1439–1451.
171. Daoulah A, Ocheltree S, Al-Faifi SM, et al. Sleep apnea and severe bradyarrhythmia – an alternative treatment option: a case report. *J Med Case Rep.* 2015;9:113.
172. Pak VM, Keenan BT, Jackson N, et al. Adhesion molecule increases in sleep apnea: beneficial effect of positive airway pressure and moderation by obesity. *Int J Obes (Lond).* 2015;39(3):472–479.

173. Gordon A, Wu SJ, Munns N, et al. Untreated sleep apnea: an analysis of administrative data to identify risk factors for early nonadherence. *J Clin Sleep Med.* 2018;14(8):1303–1313.
174. Bidarian-Moniri A, Nilsson M, Rasmusson L, et al. The effect of the prone sleeping position on obstructive sleep apnoea. *Acta Otolaryngol.* 2015;135(1):79–84.
175. Mitchell LJ, Davidson ZE, Bonham M, et al. Weight loss from lifestyle interventions and severity of sleep apnoea: a systematic review and meta-analysis. *Sleep Med.* 2014;15(10):1173–1183.
176. Tuomilehto H, Seppa J, Uusitupa M. Obesity and obstructive sleep apnea—clinical significance of weight loss. *Sleep Med Rev.* 2013;17(5):321–329.
177. Rodriguez JC, Dzierzewski JM, Alessi CA. Sleep problems in the elderly. *Med Clin North Am.* 2015;99(2):431–439.
178. Ngiam J, Balasubramaniam R, Darendeliler MA, et al. Clinical guidelines for oral appliance therapy in the treatment of snoring and obstructive sleep apnoea. *Aust Dent J.* 2013;58(4):408–419.
179. Sutherland K, Vanderveken OM, Tsuda H, et al. Oral appliance treatment for obstructive sleep apnea: an update. *J Clin Sleep Med.* 2014; 10(2):215–227.
180. White DP. Pharmacologic approaches to the treatment of obstructive sleep apnea. *Sleep Med Clin.* 2016;11(2):203–212.
181. Zaghi S, Holty JEC, Certal V, et al. Maxillomandibular advancement for treatment of obstructive sleep apnea: a meta-analysis. 2016;142(1):58–66.
182. Park CY, Hong JH, Lee JH, et al. Clinical effect of surgical correction for nasal pathology on the treatment of obstructive sleep apnea syndrome, *PLoS One.* 2014;9(6):e98765.
183. Camacho M, Certal V, Brietzke SE, et al. Tracheostomy as treatment for adult obstructive sleep apnea: a systematic review and meta-analysis. *Laryngoscope.* 2014;124(3):803–811.
184. Mechcatie E. Implantable sleep apnea fighter wins FDA approval. *Caring for the Ages.* 2014;15(6):16.
185. Stark CD, Stark RJ. Sleep and chronic daily headache. *Curr Pain Headache Rep.* 2015;19(1):468.
186. Strollo PJ, Gillespie MB, Soose RJ, et al. Upper airway stimulation for obstructive sleep apnea: durability of the treatment effect at 18 months. *Sleep.* 2015;38(10):1593–1598.
187. Brack T, Randerath W, Bloch KE. Cheyne-Stokes respiration in patients with heart failure: prevalence, causes, consequences and treatments. *Respiration.* 2012;83(2):165–176.
188. Costanzo MR, Khayat R, Ponikowski P, et al. Mechanisms and clinical consequences of untreated central sleep apnea in heart failure. *J Am Coll Cardiol.* 2015;65(1):72–84.
189. Momomura S. Treatment of Cheyne–Stokes respiration–central sleep apnea in patients with heart failure. *J Cardiol.* 2012;59(2):110–116.
190. Kasai T, Kasagi S, Maeno K, et al. Adaptive servo-ventilation in cardiac function and neurohormonal status in patients with heart failure and central sleep apnea nonresponsive to continuous positive airway pressure. *JACC Heart Fail.* 2013;1(1):58–63.
191. Ekbom KA. Restless legs. *Acta Medica Scandinavia.* 1945;158:1–123.
192. Willis T. *De Animae Brutorum.* London: Wells and Scott; 1672.
193. Amara AW, Maddox MH. Epidemiology of sleep medicine. In: Kryger M, Roth T, Dement WC, eds. *Principles and Practice of Sleep Medicine.* Philadelphia, PA: Elsevier; 2017:627–637.
194. International Restless Legs Syndrome Study Group. *2012 Revised IRLSSG diagnostic criteria for RLS.* 2012. Available at http://irlssg.org/diagnostic-criteria
195. Allen RP, Montplaisir J, Walters AS, et al. Restless legs syndrome and periodic limb movements during sleep. In: Kryger M, Roth T, Dement WC, eds. *Principles and Practice of Sleep Medicine.* 6th ed. Philadelphia, PA: Elsevier; 2017:923–934.
196. Yeh P, Walters A, Tsuang JW. Restless legs syndrome: a comprehensive overview on its epidemiology, risk factors, and treatment. *Sleep Breath.* 2012;16(4):987–1007.
197. Wittom S, Dauvilliers Y, Pennestri MH, et al. Age-at-onset in restless legs syndrome: a clinical and polysomnographic study. *Sleep Med.* 2007;9(1):54–59.
198. Allen RP, Walters AS, Montplaisir J, et al. Restless legs syndrome prevalence and impact: REST general population study. *Arch Intern Med.* 2005;165(1):1286–1292.
199. Picchietti D, Allen RP, Walters AS, et al. Restless legs syndrome: prevalence and impact in children and adolescents-the Peds REST study. *Pediatrics.* 2007;120(2):253–266.
200. Symonds CP. Nocturnal myoclonus. *J Neurol Neurosurg Psychiatry.* 1953;16(3):166–171.
201. Lugaresi E, Coccagna G, Tassinari C, et al. Partigularites cliniques et polygraphiques du syndrome d'impatience des membres inferieurs. *Rev Neurol (Paris).* 1965;113:545–555.
202. Coleman R. Periodic movements in sleep (nocturnal myoclonus) and restless legs syndrome. In: Guilleminault C, ed. *Sleep and Waking Disorders: Indications and Techniques.* Menlo Park, CA: Addison-Wesley; 1982:265–295.
203. Xion L, Montplaisir J, Desautels A, et al. Family study of restless legs syndrome in Quebec, Canada: clinical characterization of 671 family cases. *Arch Neurol.* 2010;67(5):617–622.
204. Allen RP, Auerbach S, Bahrain H, et al. The prevalence and impact of restless legs syndrome on patients with iron deficiency anemia. *Am J Hematol.* 2013;88(4):261–264.
205. Hubner A, Krafft A, Gradient S, et al. Characteristics and determinants of restless legs syndrome in pregnancy: a prospective study. *Neurology.* 2013;80(8):738–742.
206. Sarberg M, Josefsson A, Wirehn AB, et al. Restless legs syndrome during and after pregnancy and its relation to snoring. *Acta Obstet Gynecol Scand.* 2012;91:850–855.
207. Li Y, Walkters AS, Chiuve SE, et al. Prospective study of restless legs syndrome and coronary heart disease among women. *Circulation.* 2012; 126(14):1689–1694.
208. Winkelman J, Finn L, Young T. Prevalence and correlates of restless legs syndrome symptoms in the Wisconsin Sleep Cohort. *Sleep Med.* 2006; 7(7):545–552.
209. Winkelman JW, Shahar E, Sharief I, et al. Association of restless legs syndrome and cardiovascular disease in the sleep heart health study. *Neurology.* 2008;70(2):35–42.
210. Silvestri R, Gagliano A, Arico I, et al. Sleep disorders in children with attention deficit/hyperactivity disorder (ADHD) recorded overnight by video-polysomnography. *Sleep Med.* 2009;10(10):1132–1138.
211. Cortese S, Konofal E, Lecendreus M, et al. Restless legs syndrome and attention-deficit/hyperactivity disorder: a review of the literature. *Sleep.* 2005;28(8):1007–1013.
212. Wetter TC, Stiasny K, Winkelmann J, et al. A randomized controlled study of pergolide in patients with restless legs syndrome. *Neurology.* 1999;52(5):944–950.
213. Allen RP, Chen C, Garcia-Borreguero D, et al. Comparison of pregabalin with pramipexole for restless legs syndrome. *N Engl J Med.* 2014; 370:621–631.
214. Montplasir J, Karrasch J, Haan J, et al. Ropinirole is effective in the long term management of restless legs syndrome: a randomized controlled trial. *Mov Disord.* 2006;21:1627–1635.
215. Benjamin EJ, Muntner P, Alonso A, et al. Heart disease and stroke statistics—2019 update: a report from the American Heart Association. *Circulation.* 2019;139(10):e56–e528.
216. Catalan-Serra P, Campos-Rodriguez F, Reyes-Nunez N, et al. Increased incidence of stroke, but not coronary heart disease, in elderly patients with sleep apnea. *Stroke.* 2019;50(2):491–494.
217. Konishi T, Kashiwagi Y, Funayama N, et al. Obstructive sleep apnea is associated with increased coronary plaque instability: an optical frequency domain imaging study. *Heart Vessels.* 2019;34(8):1266–1279.
218. Koren D, Taveras EM. Association of sleep disturbances with obesity, insulin resistance and the metabolic syndrome. *Metabolism.* 2018;84: 67–75.
219. Deng HB, Tam T, Zee BC, et al. Short sleep duration increases metabolic impact in healthy adults: a population-based cohort study. *Sleep.* 2017;40(10).
220. Lavie L. Oxidative stress in obstructive sleep apnea and intermittent hypoxia–revisited– the bad ugly and good: Implications to the heart and brain. *Sleep Med Rev.* 2015;20:27–45.
221. von Kanel R, Princip M, Schmid JP, et al. Association of sleep problems with neuroendocrine hormones and coagulation factors in patients with acute myocardial infarction. *BMC Cardiovasc Disord.* 2018;18(1):213.
222. Khan NA, Daskalopoulou SS, Karp I, et al. Sex differences in prodromal symptoms in acute coronary syndrome in patients aged 55 years or younger. *Heart.* 2017;103(11):863–869.
223. Cole CS, McSweeney JC, Cleves MA, et al. Sleep disturbance in women before myocardial infarction. *Heart Lung.* 2012;41(5):438–445.
224. McSweeney JC, Cody M, O'Sullivan P, et al. Women's early warning symptoms of acute myocardial infarction. *Circulation.* 2003; 108(21):2619–2623.
225. Lamers F, Milaneschi Y, Smit JH, et al. Longitudinal association between depression and inflammatory markers: results from the Netherlands study of depression and anxiety. *Biol Psychiatry.* 2019;85(10):829–837.

226. Shpilsky D, Erqou S, Patel SR, et al. Association of obstructive sleep apnea with microvascular endothelial dysfunction and subclinical coronary artery disease in a community-based population. *Vasc Med.* 2018; 23(4):331–339.
227. Seo MY, Lee JY, Hahn JY, et al. Association of obstructive sleep apnea with subclinical cardiovascular disease predicted by coronary artery calcium score in asymptomatic subjects. *Am J Cardiol.* 2017;120(4):577–581.
228. Ding Q, Redeker NS, Pisani MA, et al. Factors influencing patients' sleep in the intensive care unit: perceptions of patients and clinical staff. *Am J Crit Care.* 2017;26(4):278–286.
229. Richards KC, Bairnsfather L. A description of night sleep patterns in the critical care unit. *Heart Lung.* 1988;17(1):35–42.
230. Knauert MP, Redeker NS, Yaggi HK, et al. Creating naptime: an overnight, nonpharmacologic intensive care unit sleep promotion protocol. *J Patient Exp.* 2018;5(3):180–187.
231. Mason M, Hernandez Sanchez J, Vuylsteke A, et al. Association between severity of untreated sleep apnoea and postoperative complications following major cardiac surgery: a prospective observational cohort study. *Sleep Med.* 2017;37:141–146.
232. Redeker NS, Hedges C. Sleep during hospitalization and recovery after cardiac surgery. *J Cardiovasc Nurs.* 2002;17(1):56–68; quiz 82–83.
233. Bruni A, Garofalo E, Pelaia C, et al. Patient-ventilator asynchrony in adult critically ill patients. *Minerva Anestesiol.* 2019;85(6):676–688.
234. Caruana N, McKinley S, Elliott R, et al. Sleep quality during and after cardiothoracic intensive care and psychological health during recovery. *J Cardiovasc Nurs.* 2018;33(4):E40–E49.
235. Simeone S, Pucciarelli G, Perrone M, et al. Delirium in ICU patients following cardiac surgery: an observational study. *J Clin Nurs.* 2018;27 (9–10):1994–2002.
236. Delaney L, Litton E, Van Haren F. The effectiveness of noise interventions in the ICU. *Curr Opin Anesthesiol.* 2019;32(2):144–149.
237. Vazir A, Sundaram V. Management of sleep apnea in heart failure. *Heart Fail Clin.* 2018;14(4):635–642.
238. Redeker NS, Conley S, Anderson G, et al. Effects of cognitive behavioral therapy for insomnia on sleep, symptoms, stress, and autonomic function among patients with heart failure. *Behav Sleep Med.* 2018;1–13.
239. Kanno Y, Yoshihisa A, Watanabe S, et al. Prognostic significance of insomnia in heart failure. *Circ J.* 2016;80(7):1571–1577.
240. Lee KS, Lennie TA, Heo S, et al. Prognostic importance of sleep quality in patients with heart failure. *Am J Crit Care.* 2016;25(6):516–525.
241. Moon C, Yoon JY, Bratzke LC. The role of heart failure, daytime sleepiness, and disturbed sleep on cognition. *West J Nurs Res.* 2017;39(4):473–491.
242. Riegel B, Ratcliffe SJ, Weintraub WS, et al. Double jeopardy: the influence of excessive daytime sleepiness and impaired cognition on health-related quality of life in adults with heart failure. *Eur J Heart Fail.* 2012;14(7):730–736.
243. Redeker NS, Adams L, Berkowitz R, et al. Nocturia, sleep and daytime function in stable heart failure. *J Card Fail.* 2012;18(7):569–575.
244. Fritschi C, Redeker NS. Contributions of comorbid diabetes to sleep characteristics, daytime symptoms, and physical function among patients with stable heart failure. *J Cardiovasc Nurs.* 2015;30(5):411–419.
245. Song EK, Wu JR. Associations of vitamin D intake and sleep quality with cognitive dysfunction in older adults with heart failure. *J Cardiovasc Nurs.* 2018;33(4):392–399.
246. Johansson P, Brostrom A, Sanderman R, et al. The course of sleep problems in patients with heart failure and associations to rehospitalizations. *J Cardiovasc Nurs.* 2015;30(5):403–410.
247. Redeker NS, Jeon S, Muench U, et al. Insomnia symptoms and daytime function in stable heart failure. *Sleep.* 2010;33(9):1210–1216.
248. Mazzotti DR, Keenan BT, Lim DC, et al. Symptom subtypes of obstructive sleep apnea predict incidence of cardiovascular outcomes. *Am J Respir Crit Care Med.* 2019;200(4):493–506.
249. Pak VM, Strouss L, Yaggi HK, et al. Mechanisms of reduced sleepiness symptoms in heart failure and obstructive sleep apnea. *J Sleep Res.* 2019; 28(5):e12778.
250. Byun E, Kim J, Riegel B. Associations of subjective sleep quality and daytime sleepiness with cognitive impairment in adults and elders with heart failure. *Behav Sleep Med.* 2017;15(4):302–317.
251. Riegel B, Moelter ST, Ratcliffe SJ, et al. Excessive daytime sleepiness is associated with poor medication adherence in adults with heart failure. *J Card Fail.* 2011;17(4):340–348.
252. Yoshihisa A, Suzuki S, Yamaki T, et al. Impact of adaptive servo-ventilation on cardiovascular function and prognosis in heart failure patients with preserved left ventricular ejection fraction and sleep-disordered breathing. *Eur J Heart Fail.* 2013;15(5):543–550.
253. Olseng MW, Olsen BF, Hetland A, et al. Quality of life improves in patients with chronic heart failure and Cheyne-Stokes respiration treated with adaptive servo-ventilation in a nurse-led heart failure clinic. *J Clin Nurs.* 2017;26(9–10):1226–1233.
254. Redeker NS, Jeon S, Andrews L. Effects of cognitive behavioral therapy for insomnia on sleep-related cognitions among patients with stable heart failure. *Behav Sleep Med.* 2019;17(3):342–354.
255. Chang YL, Chiou AF, Cheng SM, et al. Tailored educational supportive care programme on sleep quality and psychological distress in patients with heart failure: a randomised controlled trial. *Int J Nurs Stud.* 2016;61:219–229.
256. Nieto F, Young T, Peppard P, et al. Systemic and pulmonary hypertension in obstructive sleep apnea. In: Kryger M, Roth T, Dement WC, eds. *Principles and Practices of Sleep Medicine.* 6th ed. Philadelphia, PA: Elsevier; 2017:1253–1263.
257. Sarkar P, Mukherjee S, Chai-Coetzer CL, et al. The epidemiology of obstructive sleep apnoea and cardiovascular disease. *J Thorac Dis.* 2018;10(suppl 34):S4189–S4200.
258. Van Ryswyk E, Mukherjee S, Chai-Coetzer CL, et al. Sleep disorders, including sleep apnea and hypertension. *Am J Hypertens.* 2018;31(8):857–864
259. Matura LA, McDonough A, Hanlon AL, et al. Sleep disturbance, symptoms, psychological distress, and health-related quality of life in pulmonary arterial hypertension. *Eur J Cardiovasc Nurs.* 2015;14(5): 423–430.
260. Whelton PK, Carey RM, Aronow WS, et al. 2017 ACC/AHA/AAPA/ABC/ACPM/AGS/APhA/ASH/ASPC/NMA/PCNA guideline for the prevention, detection, evaluation, and management of high blood pressure in adults: A report of the American College of Cardiology/American Heart Association Task Force on Clinical Practice Guidelines. *Hypertension.* 2018;71(6):e13–e115.
261. Shulman R, Cohen DL, Grandner MA, et al. Sleep duration and 24-hour ambulatory blood pressure in adults not on antihypertensive medications. *J Clin Hypertens (Greenwich).* 2018;20(12):1712–1720.
262. Grandner M, Mullington JM, Hashmi SD, et al. Sleep duration and hypertension: analysis of >700,000 adults by age and sex. *J Clin Sleep Med.* 2018;14(6):1031–1039.
263. Fernandez-Llama P, Pareja J, Yun S, et al. Cuff-based oscillometric central and brachial blood pressures obtained through ABPM are similarly associated with renal organ damage in arterial hypertension. *Kidney Blood Press Res.* 2017;42(6):1068–1077.
264. Verrier R, Mittleman M. Sleep-related cardiac risk. In: Kryger M, Roth T, Dement WC, eds. *Principles and Practices of Sleep Medicine.* 6th ed. Philadelphia, PA: Elsevier; 2017:1229–1236.
265. Mims KN, Kirsch D. Sleep and stroke. *Sleep Med Clin.* 2016;11:39–51.
266. Hermann DM, Bassetti CL. Sleep-related breathing and sleep-wake disturbances in ischemic stroke. *Neurology.* 2009;73:1313–1322.
267. Culebras A. Sleep and stroke. *Semin Neurol.* 2009;29:438–445.
268. Schipper MH, Jellema K, Thomassen BJW, et al. Stroke and other cardiovascular events in patients with obstructive sleep apnea and the effect of continuous positive airway pressure. *J Neurol Neurosurg Psychiatry.* 2017;264(6):1247–1253.
269. Johnson K, Johnson D. Frequency of sleep apnea in stroke and TIA. *J Clin Sleep Med.* 2010;6:131–137.
270. Kernan WN, Ovbiagele B, Black HR, et al. Guidelines for the prevention of stroke in patients with stroke and transient ischemic attack: a guideline for healthcare professionals from the American Heart Association/American Stroke Association. *Stroke.* 2014;45:2160–2236.
271. Wu MP, Lin HJ, Weng SF, et al. Insomnia subtypes and the subsequent risks of stroke: report from a nationally representative cohort. *Stroke.* 2014;45(5):1349–1354.
272. Ferre A, Ribo M, Rodriguez-Luna D, et al. Strokes and their relationship with sleep and sleep disorders. *Neurologia.* 2013;28(2):103–118.
273. Chou CH, Yin JH, Chen SY, et al. The potential impact of sleep-related movement disorders on stroke risk: a population-based longitudinal study. *QJM.* 2017;110(10):649–655.
274. Kent BD, McNicholas WT, Ryan S. Insulin resistance, glucose intolerance and diabetes mellitus in obstructive sleep apnoea. *J Thorac Dis.* 2015;7(8):1343–1357.
275. Boyko EJ, Seelig AD, Jacobson IG, et al. Sleep characteristics, mental health, and diabetes risk: a prospective study of US military service members in the millennium cohort study. *Diabetes Care.* 2013;36(10):3154–3161.
276. Tanno S, Tanigawa T, Saito I, et al. Sleep-related intermittent hypoxemia and glucose intolerance: a community-based study. *Sleep Med.* 2014;15(10):1212–1218.

277. Lesser DJ, Bhatia R, Tran WH, et al. Sleep fragmentation and intermittent hypoxemia are associated with decreased insulin sensitivity in obese adolescent Latino males. *Pediatr Res.* 2012;72(3):293.
278. Aurora RN, Punjabi NM. Obstructive sleep apnoea and type 2 diabetes mellitus: a bidirectional association. *Lancet Respir Med.* 2013;1(4): 329–338.
279. Ohkuma T, Fujii H, Iwase M, et al. Impact of sleep duration on obesity and the glycemic level in patients with type 2 diabetes mellitus: the Fukuoka Diabetes Registry. *Diabetes Care.* 2012;36(3):611–617.
280. Surani S, Brito V, Surani A, et al. Effect of diabetes mellitus on sleep quality. *World J Diabetes.* 2015;6(6):868–873.
281. Agarwal A, Zhang W, Kuo YF, et al. A population based study of prevalence of OSA in patients with COPD: the overlap syndrome. *Chest.* 2016;150(4):843A.
282. Soler X, Gaio E, Powell FL, et al. High prevalence of obstructive sleep apnea in patients with moderate to severe chronic obstructive pulmonary disease. *Ann Am Thorac Soc.* 2015;12(8):1219–1225.
283. McNicholas WT. Chronic obstructive pulmonary disease and obstructive sleep apnoea—the overlap syndrome. *J Thorac Dis.* 2016;8(2):236–242.
284. Shawon MS, Perret JL, Senaratna CV, et al. Current evidence on prevalence and clinical outcomes of co-morbid obstructive sleep apnea and chronic obstructive pulmonary disease: a systematic review. *Sleep Med Rev.* 2017;32:58–68.
285. Lacedonia D, Carpagnano GE, Aliani M, et al. Daytime PaO2 in OSAS, COPD and the combination of the two (overlap syndrome). *Respir Med.* 2013;107(2):310–316.
286. Akinci B, Aslan GK, Kiyan E. Sleep quality and quality of life in patients with moderate to very severe chronic obstructive pulmonary disease. *Clin Respir J.* 2018;12(4):1739–1746.
287. Yosunkaya S, Kutlu R, Cihan FG. Evaluation of depression and quality of life in patients with obstructive sleep apnea syndrome. *Niger J Clin Pract.* 2016;19(5):573–579.
288. McNicholas WT, Verbraecken J, Marin JM. Sleep disorders in COPD: the forgotten dimension. *Eur Respir Soc.* 2013;22(129):365–375.
289. Chang CH, Chuang LP, Lin SW, et al. Factors responsible for poor sleep quality in patients with chronic obstructive pulmonary disease. *BMC Pulm Med.* 2016;16(1):118.
290. Mayo Clinic. *COPD diagnosis and treatment 2017.* 2019. Available at https://www.mayoclinic.org/diseases- conditions/copd/diagnosis-treatment/drc-20353685
291. Branson RD. Oxygen therapy in COPD. *Respir Care.* 2018;63(6): 734–748.
292. Boakye PA, Olechowski C, Rashiq S, et al. A critical review of neurobiological factors involved in the interactions between chronic pain, depression, and sleep disruption. *Clin J Pain.* 2016;32(4):327–336.
293. Murphy M, Peterson MJ. Sleep disturbances in depression. *Sleep Med Clin.* 2015;10(1):17–23.
294. Fernandez-Mendoza J, Shea S, Vgontzas AN, et al. Insomnia and incident depression: role of objective sleep duration and natural history. *J Sleep Res.* 2015;24(4):390–398.
295. Chen PJ, Huang CLC, Weng SF, et al. Relapse insomnia increases greater risk of anxiety and depression: evidence from a population-based 4-year cohort study. *Sleep Med.* 2017;38:122–129.
296. Kessler RC, Petukhova M, Sampson NA, et al. Twelve- month and lifetime prevalence and lifetime morbid risk of anxiety and mood disorders in the United States. *Int J Methods Psychiatr Res.* 2012;21(3): 169–184.
297. Dhar AK, Barton DA. Depression and the link with cardiovascular disease. *Front Psychiatry.* 2016;7:33.
298. Bradley SM, Rumsfeld JS. Depression and cardiovascular disease. *Trends Cardiovasc Med.* 2015;25(7):614–622.
299. Aziz M, Ali SS, Das S, et al. Association of subjective and objective sleep duration as well as sleep quality with non-invasive markers of sub-clinical cardiovascular disease (CVD): a systematic review. *J Atheroscler Thromb.* 2017;24(3):208–226.
300. Cho HJ, Savitz J, Dantzer R, et al. Sleep disturbance and kynurenine metabolism in depression. *J Psychosom Res.* 2017;99:1–7.
301. Finan PH, Smith MT. The comorbidity of insomnia, chronic pain, and depression: dopamine as a putative mechanism. *Sleep Med Rev.* 2013;17(3):173–183.
302. Wichniak A, Wierzbicka A, Jernajczyk W. Sleep as a biomarker for depression. *Int Rev Psychiatry.* 2013;25(5):632–645.
303. Ilanković A, Damjanović A, Ilanković V, et al. Polysomnographic sleep patterns in depressive, schizophrenic and healthy subjects. *Psychiatr Danub.* 2014;26(1):20–26.
304. Augustinavicius JL, Zanjani A, Zakzanis KK, et al. Polysomnographic features of early-onset depression: a meta-analysis. *J Affect Disord.* 2014;158:11–18.
305. Lovato N, Gradisar M. A meta-analysis and model of the relationship between sleep and depression in adolescents: recommendations for future research and clinical practice. *Sleep Med Rev.* 2014;18(6):521–529.
306. Khayat R, Jarjoura D, Porter K, et al. Sleep disordered breathing and post-discharge mortality in patients with acute heart failure. *Eur Heart J.* 2015;36(23):1463–1469.
307. Huffman JC, Celano CM, Beach SR, et al. Depression and cardiac disease: epidemiology, mechanisms, and diagnosis. *Cardiovasc Psychiatry Neurol.* 2013;2013:695925.
308. Halaris A. Inflammation, heart disease, and depression, *Curr Psychiatry Rep.* 2013;15(10):400.
309. Grandner MA, Sands-Lincoln MR, Pak VM, et al. Sleep duration, cardiovascular disease, and proinflammatory biomarkers. *Nat Sci Sleep.* 2013;5:93–107.
310. Bauer LK, Caro MA, Beach SR, et al. Effects of depression and anxiety improvement on adherence to medication and health behaviors in recently hospitalized cardiac patients. *Am J Cardiol.* 2012;109(9): 1266–1271.
311. Lok A, Mocking RJT, Ruhé HG, et al. Longitudinal hypothalamic–pituitary–adrenal axis trait and state effects in recurrent depression. *Psychoneuroendocrinol.* 2012;37(7):892–902.
312. Karaca Z, Ismailogullari S, Korkmaz S, et al. Obstructive sleep apnoea syndrome is associated with relative hypocortisolemia and decreased hypothalamo–pituitary–adrenal axis response to 1 and 250μg ACTH and glucagon stimulation tests. *Sleep Med.* 2013;14(2):160–164.
313. Kim YK, Na KS, Myint AM, et al. The role of pro-inflammatory cytokines in neuroinflammation, neurogenesis and the neuroendocrine system in major depression. *Prog Neuropsychopharmacol Biol Psychiatry.* 2016;64:277–284.
314. Inutsuka A, Yamanaka A. The physiological role of orexin/hypocretin neurons in the regulation of sleep/wakefulness and neuroendocrine functions. *Front Endocrinol.* 2013;4:18.
315. Boorman E, Zajkowska Z, Ahmed R, et al. Crosstalk between endocannabinoid and immune systems: a potential dysregulation in depression? *Psychopharmacology (Berl).* 2016;233(9):1591–1604.
316. Irwin MR, Opp MR. Sleep health: reciprocal regulation of sleep and innate immunity. *Neuropsychopharmacology.* 2017;42(1):129–155.
317. Xie J, Sert Kuniyoshi FH, Covassin N, et al. Nocturnal hypoxemia due to obstructive sleep apnea is an independent predictor of poor prognosis after myocardial infarction. *J Am Heart Assoc.* 2016;5(8):e003162.
318. Mann D, Zipes DP, Libby P, et al. *Braunwald's Heart Disease: A Textbook of Cardiovascular Medicine.* 10th ed. Philadelphia, PA: Elsevier Health Sciences; 2015.
319. Scheer F, Chellappa SL, Hu K, et al. Impact of mental stress, the circadian system and their interaction on human cardiovascular function. *Psychoneuroendocrinology.* 2019;103:125–129.
320. Selim BJ, Koo BB, Qin L, et al. The association between nocturnal cardiac arrhythmias and sleep-disordered breathing: the DREAM study. *J Clin Sleep Med.* 2016;12(6):829–837.
321. Gami AS, Hodge DO, Herges RM, et al. Obstructive sleep apnea, obesity, and the risk of incident atrial fibrillation. *J Am Coll Cardiol.* 2007;49(5):565–571.
322. Anter E, Di Biase L, Contreras-Valdes FM, et al. Atrial substrate and triggers of paroxysmal atrial fibrillation in patients with obstructive sleep apnea. *Circ Arrhythm Electrophysiol.* 2017;10(11):e005407.
323. Kendzerska T, Gershon AS, Atzema C, et al. Sleep apnea increases the risk of new hospitalized atrial fibrillation: a historical cohort study. *Chest.* 2018;154(6):1330–1339.
324. Drager LF, McEvoy RD, Barbe F, et al. Sleep apnea and cardiovascular disease: lessons from recent trials and need for team science. *Circulation.* 2017;136(19):1840–1850.
325. Randolph TC, Simon DN, Thomas L, et al. Patient factors associated with quality of life in atrial fibrillation. *Am Heart J.* 2016;182: 135–143.
326. Berg SK, Higgins M, Reilly CM, et al. Sleep quality and sleepiness in persons with implantable cardioverter defibrillators: outcome from a clinical randomized longitudinal trial. *Pacing Clin Electrophysiol.* 2012;35(4):431–443.
327. Salama A, Abdullah A, Wahab A, et al. Is obstructive sleep apnea associated with ventricular tachycardia? A retrospective study from the National Inpatient Sample and a literature review on the pathogenesis of obstructive sleep apnea. *Clin Cardiol.* 2018;41(12):1543–1547.

328. Mehra R, Benjamin EJ, Shahar E, et al. Association of nocturnal arrhythmias with sleep-disordered breathing: the Sleep Heart Health Study. *Am J Respir Crit Care Med.* 2006;173(8):910–916.
329. Abumuamar AM, Newman D, Dorian P, et al. Cardiac effects of CPAP treatment in patients with obstructive sleep apnea and atrial fibrillation. *J Interv Card Electrophysiol.* 2019;54(3):289–297.
330. Yaeger A, Cash NR, Parham T, et al. A nurse-led limited risk factor modification program to address obesity and obstructive sleep apnea in atrial fibrillation patients. *J Am Heart Assoc.* 2018;7(23):e010414.
331. Morin CM, Davidson JR, Beaulieu-Bonneau S. Cognitive behavioral therapies for insomnia I: approaches and efficacy. In: Kryger M, Roth T, Dement WC, eds. *Principles and Practice of Sleep Medicine.* Philadelphia, PA: Elsevier; 2017:804–813.
332. Posner D, Gehrman PR. Sleep hygiene. In: Perlis M, Aloia M, Kuhn B, eds. *Behavioral Treatments for Sleep Disorders.* Philadelphia, PA: Elsevier; 2011:31–43.
333. Irish LA, Kline CE, Gunn HE, et al. The role of sleep hygiene in promoting public health: a review of empirical evidence. *Sleep Med Rev.* 2015;22:23–36.
334. Roehrs T, Roth T. Caffeine: sleep and daytime sleepiness. *Sleep Med Rev.* 2008;12:153–162.
335. Edinger JD, Leggett MK, Carney CE, et al. Psychological and behavioral treatments for insomnia II: implementation and specific populations. In: Kryger M, Roth T, Dement WC, eds. *Principles and Practice of Sleep Medicine.* Philadelphia, PA: Elsevier; 2017:814–831.
336. Jansson-Frojmark N, Lind M, Sunnhed M. Don't worry, be constructive: a randomized controlled feasibility study comparing behavioral therapy singly and combined with constructive worry for insomnia. *Br J Clin Psychol.* 2012;51:142–157.
337. Joshi S. Nonpharmacological therapy for insomnia in the elderly. *Clin Geriatr Med.* 2008;24:107–119.
338. Fernando A 3rd, Arroll B, Falloon K. A double-blind randomized controlled study of brief intervention of bedtime restriction for adult patients with primary insomnia. *J Prim Health Care.* 2013;5:5–10.
339. Kyle SD, Miller CB, Rogers Z, et al. Sleep restriction therapy for insomnia is associated with objectively-impaired vigilance: implications for the clinical management of insomnia disorder. *Sleep.* 2014;37(2):229–237.
340. Epstein DR, Sidani S, Bootzin RR, et al. Dismantling multicomponent behavioral treatment for insomnia in older adults: a randomized controlled trial. *Sleep.* 2012;35:797–805.
341. Miller CB, Espie CA, Epstein DR, et al. The evidence base of sleep restriction therapy for treating insomnia disorder. *Sleep Med Rev.* 2014;18:415–424.
342. Edinger JD, Wohlgemuth WK, Radtke RA, et al. Dose- response effects of cognitive behavioral insomnia therapy: a randomized clinical trial. *Sleep.* 2007;30(2):203–212.
343. Buysse DJ, Germain A, Mould DE, et al. Efficacy of brief behavioral treatment for chronic insomnia in older adults. *Arch Intern Med.* 2011;171(10):887–895.
344. Espie CA, MacMahon KMA, Kelly HL, et al. Randomized clinical effectiveness trial of nurse-administered small-group cognitive behavior therapy for persistent insomnia in general practice. *Sleep.* 2007;30(5):574–584.
345. Kuhn E, Weiss BJ, Taylor KL, et al. CBT-I Coach: a description and clinician perceptions of a mobile app for cognitive behavioral therapy. *J Clin Sleep Med.* 2016;12(4):597–606.
346. Seyffert M, Lagisetty P, Landgraf J, et al. Internet-delivered cognitive behavioral therapy to treat insomnia: a systematic review and meta-analysis. *PLoS One.* 2016;11(2):e0149139.
347. National Center for Complementary and Integrative Health (NIH). *Complimentary, alternative, or integrative health: What's in a name?* 2016. Available at https://nccih.nih.gov/health/integrative-health. Accessed September 1, 2018.
348. Andersen SR, Würtzen H, Steding-Jessen M, et al. Effect of mindfulness-based stress reduction on sleep quality: results of a randomized trial among Danish breast cancer patients. *Acta Oncol.* 2013;52(2):336–344.
349. Black DS, O'reilly GA, Olmstead R, et al. Mindfulness meditation and improvement in sleep quality and daytime impairment among older adults with sleep disturbances: a randomized clinical trial. *JAMA Intern Med.* 2015;175(4):494–501.
350. Bower JE, Crosswell AD, Stanton AL, et al. Mindfulness meditation for younger breast cancer survivors: a randomized controlled trial. *Cancer.* 2015;121(8):1231–1240.
351. Ong JC, Manber R, Segal Z, et al. A randomized controlled trial of mindfulness meditation for chronic insomnia. *Sleep.* 2014;37(9):1553–1563.
352. Parswani MJ, Sharma MP, Iyengar SS. Mindfulness-based stress reduction program in coronary heart disease: a randomized control trial. *Int J Yoga.* 2013;6(2):111–117.
353. Gong H, Ni CX, Liu YZ, et al. Mindfulness meditation for insomnia: a meta-analysis of randomized clinical trials. *J Psychosom Res.* 2016;89:1–6.
354. Karadag E, Samancioglu S, Ozden D, et al. Effects of aromatherapy on sleep quality and anxiety of patients. *Nurs Crit Care.* 2017;22(2):105–112.
355. Hajibagheri A, Babaii A, Adib-Hajbaghery M. Effect of Rosa damascene aromatherapy on sleep quality in cardiac patients: a randomized controlled trial. *Complement Ther Clin Pract.* 2014;20(3):159–163.
356. Ju MS, Lee S, Bae I, et al. Effects of aroma massage on home blood pressure, ambulatory blood pressure, and sleep quality in middle-aged women with hypertension. *Evid Based Complement Alternat Med.* 2013;2013:403251.
357. Oliveira DS, Hachul H, Goto V, et al. Effect of therapeutic massage on insomnia and climacteric symptoms in postmenopausal women. *Climacteric.* 2012;15(1):21–29.
358. Shinde MB, Anjum S. Effectiveness of slow back massage on quality of sleep among ICU patent's. *IJSR.* 2014;3(3):292–298.
359. Kashani F, Kashani P. The effect of massage therapy on the quality of sleep in breast cancer patients. *Iranian J Nurs Midwifery Res.* 2014;19(2):113–118.
360. Pinar R, Afsar F. Back massage to decrease state anxiety, cortisol level, blood pressure, heart rate and increase sleep quality in family caregivers of patients with cancer: a randomised controlled trial. *Asian Pac J Cancer Prev.* 2015;16(18):8127–8133.
361. Oshvandi K, Abdi S, Karampourian A, et al. The effect of foot massage on quality of sleep in ischemic heart disease patients hospitalized in CCU. *Iran J Crit Care Nurs.* 2014;7(2):66–73.
362. Shafiee Z, Babaee S, Nazari A, et al. The effect of massage therapy on sleep quality of patients after coronary artery bypass graft operation. *Iran J Cardiovasc Nurs.* 2013;2(2):22–29.
363. Wu Y, Zou C, Liu X, et al. Auricular acupressure helps improve sleep quality for severe insomnia in maintenance hemodialysis patients: a pilot study. *J Altern Complement Med.* 2014;20(5):356–363.
364. Simoncini M, Gatti A, Quirico PE, et al. Acupressure in insomnia and other sleep disorders in elderly institutionalized patients suffering from Alzheimer's disease. *Aging Clin Exp Res.* 2015;27(1):37–42.
365. Sun JL, Sung MS, Huang MY, et al. Effectiveness of acupressure for residents of long-term care facilities with insomnia: a randomized controlled trial. *Int J Nurs Stud.* 2010;47(7):798–805.
366. Klein AA, Djaiani G, Karski J, et al. Acupressure wristbands for the prevention of postoperative nausea and vomiting in adults undergoing cardiac surgery. *J Cardiothorac Vasc Anesth.* 2004;18(1):68–71.
367. Lu MJ, Lin ST, Chen KM, et al. Acupressure improves sleep quality of psychogeriatric inpatients. *Nurs Res.* 2013;62(2):130–137.
368. Ozgoli G, Armand M, Heshmat R, et al. Acupressure effect on sleep quality in menopausal women. *Complementary Med J.* Arak University of Medical Sciences: 2012;2(3):212–224.
369. Abedian Z, Eskandari L, Abdi H, et al. The effect of acupressure on sleep quality in menopausal women: a randomized control trial. *Iran J Med Sci.* 2015;40(4):328–334.
370. Shariati A, Jahani S, Hooshmand M, et al. The effect of acupressure on sleep quality in hemodialysis patients. *Complement Ther Med.* 2012;20(6):417–423.
371. Zheng LW, Chen Y, Chen F, et al. Effect of acupressure on sleep quality of middle-aged and elderly patients with hypertension. *Int J Nurs Sci.* 2014;1(4):334–338.
372. Nesami MB, Gorji MAH, Rezaie S, et al. The effect of acupressure on the quality of sleep in patients with acute coronary syndrome in cardiac care unit. *Iran J Crit Care Nurs.* 2014;7(1):7–14.
373. Mamtani R. Ayurveda and yoga in cardiovascular disease. *Cardiol Rev.* 2005;13:155–162.
374. Afonso RF, Hachul H, Kozasa EH, et al. Yoga decreases insomnia in post-menopausal women: a randomized clinical trial. *Menopause.* 2012;19(2):186–193.
375. Irwin MR, Olmstead R, Carrillo C, et al. Cognitive behavioral therapy vs tai chi for late life insomnia and inflammatory risk: a randomized controlled comparative efficacy trial. *Sleep.* 2014;37(9):1543–1552.
376. Yeh GY, Wayne PM, Phillips RS. Tai chi exercise in patients with chronic heart failure. *Med Sport Sci.* 2008;52:195–208.
377. Schutte-Rodin S, Broch L, Buysse D, et al. Clinical guideline for the evaluation and management of chronic insomnia in adults. *J Clin Sleep Med.* 2008;4(5):487–504.

378. Sateia MJ, Buysse DJ, Krystal AD, et al. Clinical practice guideline for the pharmacologic treatment of chronic insomnia in adults: an American Academy of Sleep Medicine clinical practice guideline. *J Clin Sleep Med.* 2017;13(2):307–349.
379. Kilduff TS, Mendelson WB. Hypnotic medications: mechanisms of action and pharmacolotic effects. In: Kryger M, Roth T, Dement WC, eds. *Principles and Practice of Sleep Medicine*. Philadelphia, PA: Elsevier; 2017:424–431.
380. Buysse DJ, Tyagi S. Clinical Pharmacology of other drugs used as hypnotics. In: Kryger M, Roth T, Dement WC, eds. *Principles and Practice of Sleep Medicine*. 6th ed. Philadelphia, PA: Elsevier; 2017:432–445.
381. Golden RN, Dawkins K, Nicholas L. Trazadone and nefazodone. In: Schatzberg A, Nemeroff C, eds. *The American Psychiatric Publishing Textbook of Psychopharmacology*. Washington, DC: American Psychiatric Publishing; 2009:315–325.
382. Katwala J, Kumar AK, Sejpal JJ, et al. Therapeutic rationale for low dose doxepin in insomnia patients. *Asian Pac J Trop Dis.* 2013;3(4):331–336.
383. Gray SL, Anderson ML, Dublin S, et al. Cumulative use of strong anticholinergic medications and incident dementia. *JAMA Intern Med.* 2015;175(3):401–407.
384. Gray SL., Hanlon JT. Anticholinergic medication use and dementia: latest evidence and clinical indications. *Ther Adv Drug Saf.* 2016;7(5):217–224.
385. Vassiliadis T, Anagnostis P, Patsiaoura K, et al. Valeriana hepatotoxicity. *Sleep Med.* 2009;10:935.
386. Cohen DL, Del Toro Y. A case of valerian-associated hepatotoxicity. *J Clin Gasteroenterol.* 2008;42(8):961–962.
387. Brauer RB, Stangl M, Stewart JR, et al. Acute liver failure after administration of the herbal tranquilizer kava-kava (piper methysticum). *J Clin Psychiatry.* 2003;64(2):216–218.
388. Gow PJ, Connelly NJ, Hill RL, et al. Fatal fulminant hepatic failure induced by a natural therapy containing kava. *Med J Aust.* 2003; 178(9):442–443.
389. Leach MJ, Page AT. Herbal medicine for insomnia: a systematic review and meta- analysis. *Sleep Med Rev.* 2015;24:1–12.
390. Marseglia L, D'Angelo G, Manti S, et al. Analgesic, anxiolytic and anaesthetic effects of melatonin: new potential uses in pediatrics. *Int J Mol Sci.* 2015;16(1):1209–1220.
391. Mistraletti G, Umbrello M, Sabbatini G, et al. Melatonin reduces the need for sedation in ICU patients: a randomized controlled trial. *Minerva Anestesiol.* 2015;81(12):1298–1310.
392. Vidor LP, Torres IL, de Souza ICC, et al. Analgesic and sedative effects of melatonin in temporomandibular disorders: a double-blind, randomized, parallel-group, placebo-controlled study. *J Pain Symptom Manage.* 2013;46(3):422–432.
393. Ferracioli-Oda E, Qawasmi A, Bloch MH. Meta-analysis: melatonin for the treatment of primary sleep disorders. *PLoS One.* 2013;8(5):e63773.
394. Paredes SD, Forman KA, García C, et al. Protective actions of melatonin and growth hormone on the aged cardiovascular system. *Horm Mol Biol Clin Investig.* 2014;18(2):79–88.
395. Simko F, Paulis L. Antifibrotic effect of melatonin—perspective protection in hypertensive heart disease. *Int J Cardiol.* 2013;168(3):2876–2877.
396. Lemoine P, Wade AG, Katz A, et al. Efficacy and safety of prolonged-release melatonin for insomnia in middle-aged and elderly patients with hypertension: a combined analysis of controlled clinical trials. *Integr Blood Press Control.* 2012;5:9–17.
397. Erland LAE, Saxena PK. Melatonin natural health products and supplements: presence of serotonin and significant variability of melatonin content. *J Clin Sleep Med.* 2017;13(2):275–281.
398. Drake CL, Wright KP. Shift work, shift-work disorder, and jet lag. In: Kryger M, Roth T, Dement WC, eds. *Principles and Practice of Sleep Medicine*. Philadelphia, PA: Elsevier; 2017:714–725.
399. Folkard S. Do permanent night shift workers show circadian adjustment? A review based on endogenous melatonin rhythm. *Chronobiol Int.* 2008;25:215–224.
400. Wright KP, Rogers NL. Endogenous versus exogenous effects of melatonin. In: Pandi-Perumal S, Cardinali D, eds. *Melatonin: From Molecules to Therapy*. New York: Nova Science Publishers; 2007:547–569.
401. Weaver MD, Vetter C, Rajaratnam SMW, et al. Sleep disorders, depression and anxiety are associated with adverse safety outcomes in healthcare workers: a prospective cohort study. *J Sleep Res.* 2018;27:e12772.
402. Letvak S, Ruhm CJ, McCoy T. Depression in hospital-employed nurses. *Clin Nurse Spec.* 2012;26:177–182.
403. Eldevik MF, Flo E, Moen E, et al. Insomnia, excessive sleepiness, excessive fatigue, anxiety, depression, and shift work disorder in nurses having less than 11 hours in-between shifts. *PLoS One.* 2013;8:e70882.
404. Flo E, Pallesen S, Mageroy N, et al. Shifts work disorders in nurses-assessment, prevalence, and related health problems. *PLoS One.* 2012;7: e33981.
405. Scott L, Rogers A, Hwang WT, et al. The effects of critical care nurse work hours on vigilance and patient safety. *Am J Crit Care.* 2006; 15(4):30–37.
406. Scott LD, Hwang WT, Rogers AE, et al. The relationship between nurse work schedules and drowsy driving. *Sleep.* 2007;30(12):1801–1807.
407. Rogers AE, Hwang WT, Scott LD, et al. The working hours of hospital staff nurses and patient safety. *Health Aff (Millwood).* 2004;23(4): 202–212.
408. Olds DM, Clarke SP. The effects of work hours on adverse events and errors in health care. *J Safety Res.* 2010;41:153–162.
409. Wilson M, Permito R, English A, et al. Performance and sleepiness in nurses working 12-hour day shifts or night shifts in a community hospital. *Accid Anal Prev.* 2019;126:43–46.

8 Physiologic Adaptations With Aging

Janet Fredal Wyman

OBJECTIVES

1. Identify changes that occur in cardiac structure and function that predispose the elderly to heart failure (increase in LV stiffness, hypertrophy and enlargement, amyloid deposition, LA enlargement, decrease in predicted maximum heart rate).
2. Describe the impact that fibrosis creates on the cardiac electrical conduction system during aging.
3. Describe changes in the respiratory system that may increase susceptibility and vulnerability to pulmonary disease.
4. Describe changes in renal function with aging and their impact on the selection of medication and treatments.
5. Describe changes in drug pharmacokinetics that occur with aging and their impact on the selection of medications and assessment of patient symptoms.

KEY QUESTIONS

1. How do the pathophysiologic adaptations of aging affect the cardiovascular system?
2. What specific cardiopulmonary assessment findings are expected in the elderly?
3. What knowledge and skills must the cardiac nurse possess in order to care for the aging population?

BACKGROUND

Aging is a series of biologic, physiologic, and psychological changes that take place over the lifespan. Aging is initially directed by genetic makeup, yet there is a wide variation in the aging process based on environmental factors, social relationships, and health status. Studies have suggested that 25% of longevity is genetically determined and 50% by environmental factors[1] such as nutrition, activity, infection, trauma, contaminants, and radiation exposure. At later ages genetic makeup plays a greater role.[1] The longest-living humans, the super-centenarians, live between 116 and 122 years. The worldwide average life expectancy in 2015 was 70.5 years.[2] Environmental impact, however, is reflected by the variations reported by continent with life expectancy: at the low end, only 60 years in Africa with its numerous emerging populations, and at the high end up to 79 years in Northern America within more developed societies.[2]

The lifespan is divided into phases, with the commonly used periods for these phase being infancy (birth to 1 year), early childhood (1 to 6 years), late childhood (7 to 10 years), adolescence (11 to 18 years), young adulthood (19 to 35 years), early middle age (36 to 49 years), late middle age (50 to 64 years), young-old (65 to 74 years), old (75 to 85 years), and old-old (86 years and older). In the United States, between 2010 and 2050, there is projected a rapid growth in the elderly population with the group of people over the age of 65 projected to double from 40.2 million in 2010 to 88.5 million in 2050 (Fig. 8-1). Older age groups typically have an increased prevalence of chronic disease and decreased functional status. This has far reaching implications for the health care system.

There is no single theory of aging; biologic theories of aging fall into two main categories: "programmed" theories and "damage or error" theories.[3] Programmed aging theories are based on the concept that aging proceeds along a timetable, a continuation of the variables that impact childhood development into adulthood. Programmed aging theories include: "programmed longevity" theories: genes turning on-and-off impact system function[4]; "endocrine" theories: hormonal regulation determines the rate of aging and "immunologic" theories: declining immune systems lead to increased susceptibility to disease which leads to decline and death.[5]

There are numerous "damage or error" theories, all which focus on the environmental factors causing cumulative damage impacting the aging process. They include "wear and tear" theories: cells and tissue wear out from use; "rate of living" theories: higher metabolism results in shorter lifespan; accumulation of "cross-linked proteins" leading to decline and aging; "free radical accumulation" results in progressive damage of cellular DNA. Regardless of the theory, aging is characterized by a progressive decline in tissue and organ function, increased risk of disease and mortality.

The two general types of aging theories are founded on the concept that aging is a time-dependent process based on the accumulation of cellular damage and an inability to prevent natural deterioration. Current research has identified nine hallmarks of aging which impact the process. These hallmarks include: genome instability, telomere attrition, epigenetic alterations, loss of proteostasis,

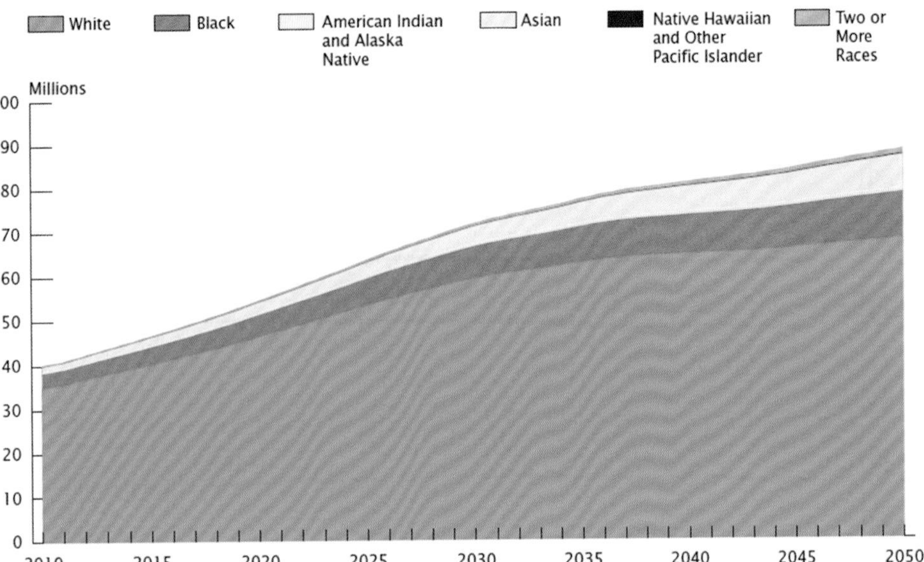

Figure 8-1. The projected population for people over 65 in the United States: 2010–2050. (From Vincent GK, Velkoff VA. The next four decades, the older population in the United States: 2010 to 2050. Current Population Reports. Washington, DC: U.S. Census Bureau; 2010:25–1138.)

deregulation of nutrient sensing, mitochondrial dysfunction, cellular senescence, stem cell exhaustion, and altered intercellular communication.[6] Each of these hallmarks contributes to a progressive loss of physiologic function and connectivity, leading to increased susceptibility to disease and death. These hallmarks are the current areas of research focusing on understanding the mechanisms of aging and improving longevity.

The nurse needs to be aware of several concepts in addressing the health care needs of older adults:

1. Age-related changes are gradual and individual, and different systems age at different rates within an individual. There is more intra-individual variability among older people than there is among younger people.
2. Complex functions that require multisystem coordination show the most obvious decline and require the greatest compensation and support.
3. Vulnerability to disease increases with age.
4. Stressful situations (physiologic or psychosocial) produce a more pronounced reaction in the elderly and require longer period of time for readjustment.

Although statistically, humans are living longer, the increase in longevity does not necessarily mean an increase in healthy living. Lifespan is the number of years lived whereas "health span" is defined as "the period of life spent in good health, free from the chronic diseases and disabilities of aging."[7,8] Aging is the predominant risk factor for most diseases that limit health span. Chronic illnesses, such are arthritis, cardiac and vascular diseases, and diabetes generally occur together. In 2017, 81% of Americans over the age of 65 had at least one chronic illness[9] (Fig. 8-2), and over 65% had two or more (Figs. 8-3 and 8-4). Yet a significantly higher percentage reported being in "excellent health" (Fig. 8-5) which supports the concept "good health" reaches beyond the presence or absence of chronic disease.

Over the last 20 years there has been an emphasis on lifestyle changes and the prevention and management of the diseases that cause heart disease. These public health efforts have resulted in a progressive decline in the incidence of cardiovascular diseases (CVDs) in older adults in the United States, however, despite these efforts it still remains the leading cause of death (Fig. 8-6).

General Physiologic Changes

Aging is a continuous process, beginning at conception, evolving through life, and ending with death. The process involves generation and degeneration of organ systems, tissues and cells and is associated with increased susceptibility to many diseases as time passes. The first two decades of life the process involves development and maturation while the remaining years are comprised of a progressive decline in organ system function and structure.

The aging process falls into three general physiologic process types. First are changes that occur on the cellular level, these are changes that impact homeostatic mechanisms such as body temperature, blood components, and fluid volumes. Second are changes that involve a decrease in organ mass, such as loss of nephrons; and the third which have the greatest impact, involve a decline in and loss of functional capacity and reserve of body systems. In reviewing the age-related changes in selected systems, the changes in structure and function of each system are discussed along with the clinical implications of the changes.

Cardiovascular Changes

One of the challenges in discussing aging of any system is that of separating those changes that can be attributed only to age from changes related to disease. Aging is recognized as a major risk factor for CVD, consequently, it is important to understand the physiology and pathophysiology of aging, separate from that which occurs with CVD.

Cardiac Structural Changes

The heart is comprised of numerous cell types: myocytes, fibroblasts, vascular smooth muscle cells (VSMCs), and endothelial cells. The aging heart shows a progressive decrease in number of myocytes from death through both apoptosis and necrosis, but

90
80
70
60
50
40
30
20
10
0
Percentage of adults with multiple chronic conditions
81%
65 years and older
50%
45–64 years
42%
Overall
18%
18–44 years
2008
2009
2010
2011
2012
2013
2014
Year

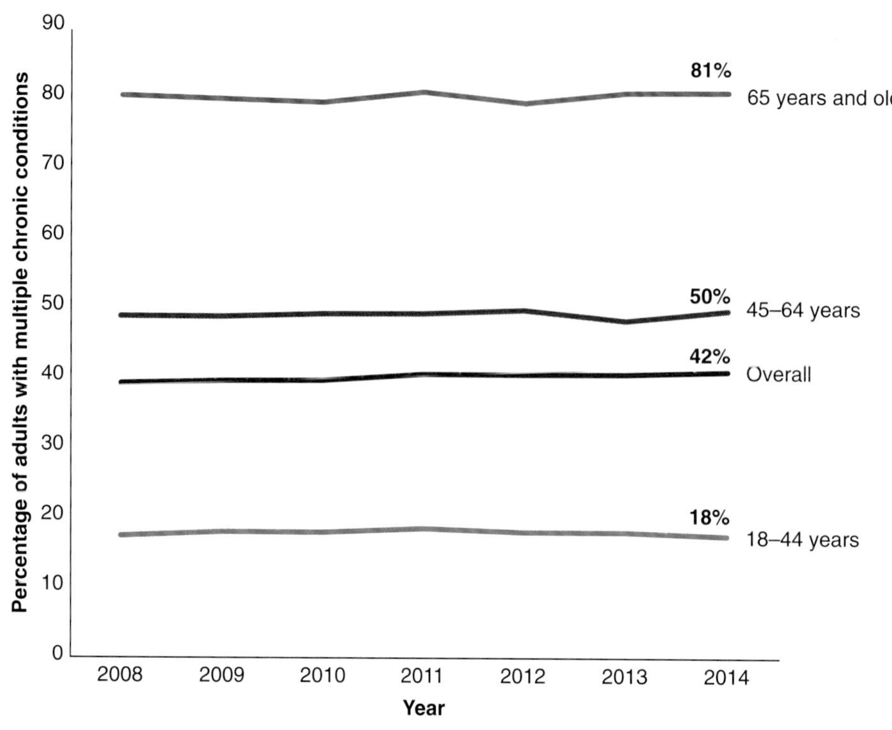

Figure 8-2. Prevalence of multiple chronic conditions by age (2008–2014). (From Buttorff C, Ruder T, Bauman M. *Multiple Chronic Conditions in the United States.* Santa Monica, CA: RAND Corporation; 2017:TL221.)

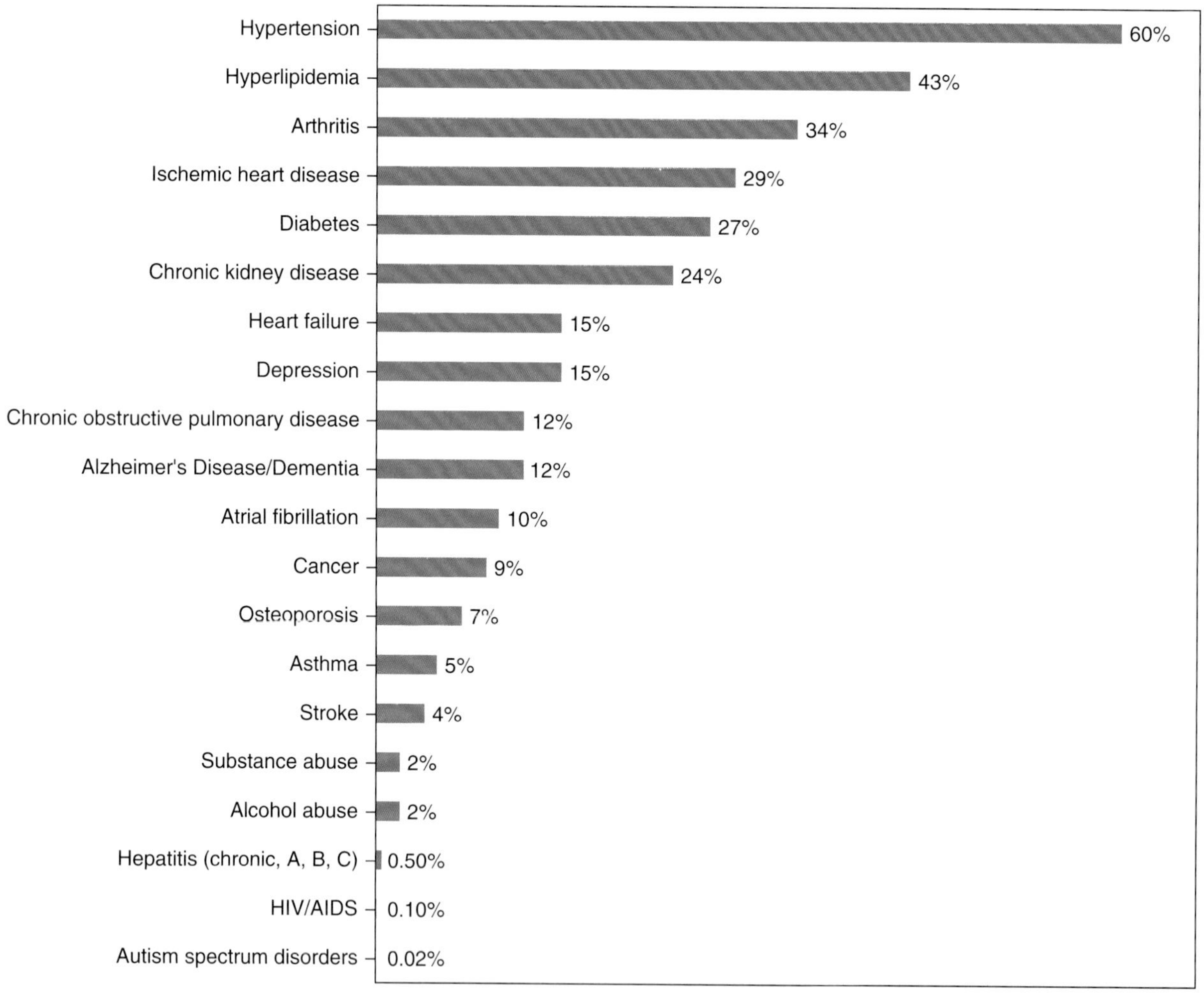

Hypertension 60%
Hyperlipidemia 43%
Arthritis 34%
Ischemic heart disease 29%
Diabetes 27%
Chronic kidney disease 24%
Heart failure 15%
Depression 15%
Chronic obstructive pulmonary disease 12%
Alzheimer's Disease/Dementia 12%
Atrial fibrillation 10%
Cancer 9%
Osteoporosis 7%
Asthma 5%
Stroke 4%
Substance abuse 2%
Alcohol abuse 2%
Hepatitis (chronic, A, B, C) 0.50%
HIV/AIDS 0.10%
Autism spectrum disorders 0.02%

Figure 8-3. 2017 Prevalence of Chronic Conditions in Medicare Beneficiaries Age ≥65. (From CMS.gov. Last modified 4/9/2019 10:46 AM; U.S. Centers for Medicare & Medicaid Services. https://www.cms.gov/Research-Statistics-Data-and-Systems/Statistics-Trends-and-Reports/Chronic-Conditions/Chartbook_Charts.)

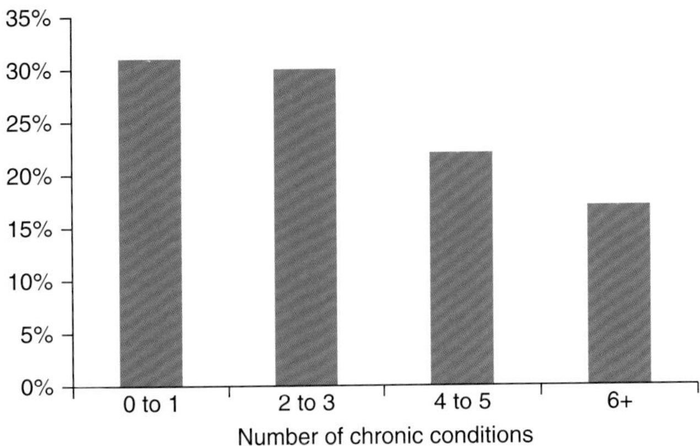

Figure 8-4. 2017 Prevalence of Multiple Chronic Conditions in Medicare Beneficiaries Age ≥65. (From CMS.gov. Last modified 4/9/2019 10:46 AM; U.S. Centers for Medicare & Medicaid Services. https://www.cms.gov/Research-Statistics-Data-and-Systems/Statistics-Trends-and-Reports/Chronic-Conditions/Chartbook_Charts.)

increase in size of the remaining cells. Concurrently, there is an increase in the number of cardiac fibroblasts, which cause interstitial fibrosis and a decrease in myocardial compliance which translates to ventricular stiffening.[10,11] The changes in myocardial cell types result in an increase in left ventricular volume.[10] In healthy individuals without CVD, the development of left ventricular hypertrophy, enlargement, and stiffening occurs with aging.[10,12] These changes take place regardless of exposure to risk factors for CVD such as hypertension, diabetes, smoking, etc. Alterations in vascular compliance which increase afterload results in a greater workload on the left ventricle contributing to the ventricular hypertrophy and remodeling.[11] This change is called "ventricular-vascular-coupled stiffening." Recent discoveries have been made regarding regeneration of myocytes by cardiac stem cells. Previously, myocytes were believed to be terminally differentiated, however advances in stem cell therapy for myocardial infarction and heart failure are ongoing.[13] They offer promise in the long-term treatment of heart failure.

Another change that occurs with aging on a cellular level is an increase in deposition of amyloid. Aggregates of starch-like proteins fold into shapes that allow multiple copies to stick together creating fibrils. Amyloid is known to impact contractility and conduction. Progressive deposition of amyloid can eventually result in heart failure. Accumulation of amyloid occurs in both the atria and ventricle. Atrial samples of people with atrial fibrillation contain higher amounts of amyloid than those with normal heart rhythms.[14]

Aging changes in the valves are characterized by increases in fibrosis, collagen degeneration, lipid accumulation, and calcification. Calcific aortic valve (AV) disease is the most common valvular heart disease in the aging population of the developed world with projected disease burden expected to increase from 2.5 million in 2000 to 4.5 million in 2030.[15] The AV experiences the highest pressure and flow transitions of the four heart valves. The AV cusps thicken from fibrosis and develop plaque-like lesions, as the valve disease progresses, calcified masses gradually build on the surface of the cusps and along the closure edges decreasing leaflet motion over time. As the valve opening narrows, pressures increase in the left ventricle leading to progressive left ventricular hypertrophy.[16]

Percentage of people age 65 and over with respondent-assessed good to excellent health status, by age group and race and Hispanic origin, 2012–2014

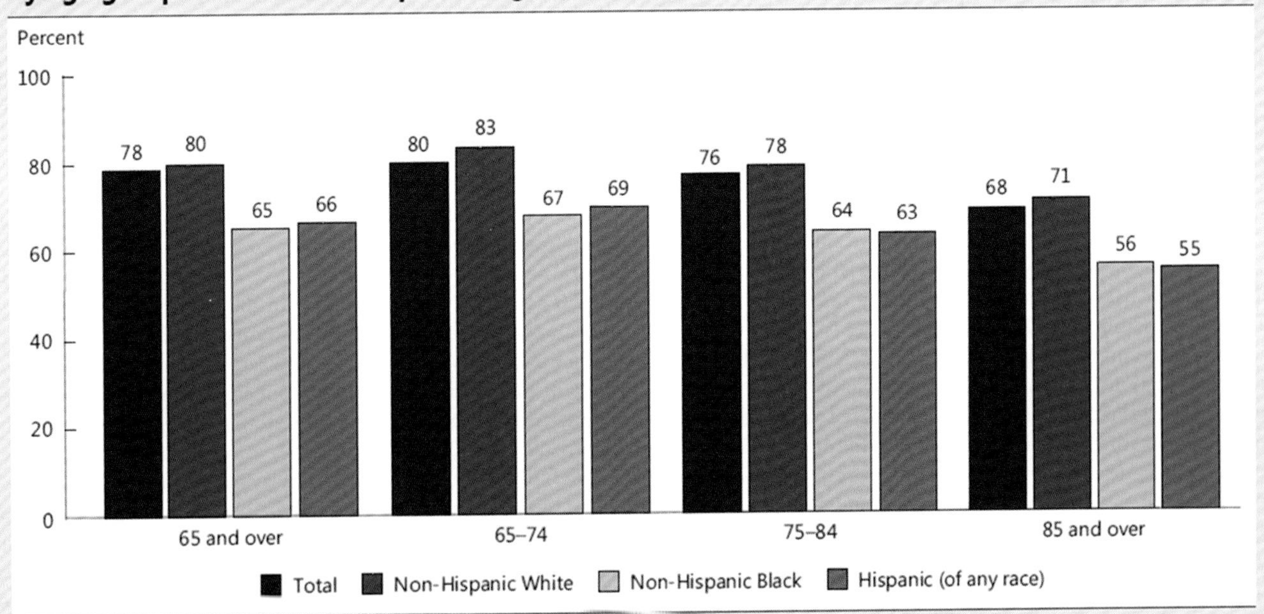

Figure 8-5. Reports of excellent health status. (From CMS.gov. Last Modified: 05/10/2017 10:32 AM; U.S. Centers for Medicare & Medicaid Services. 7500 Security Boulevard, Baltimore, MD 21244.)

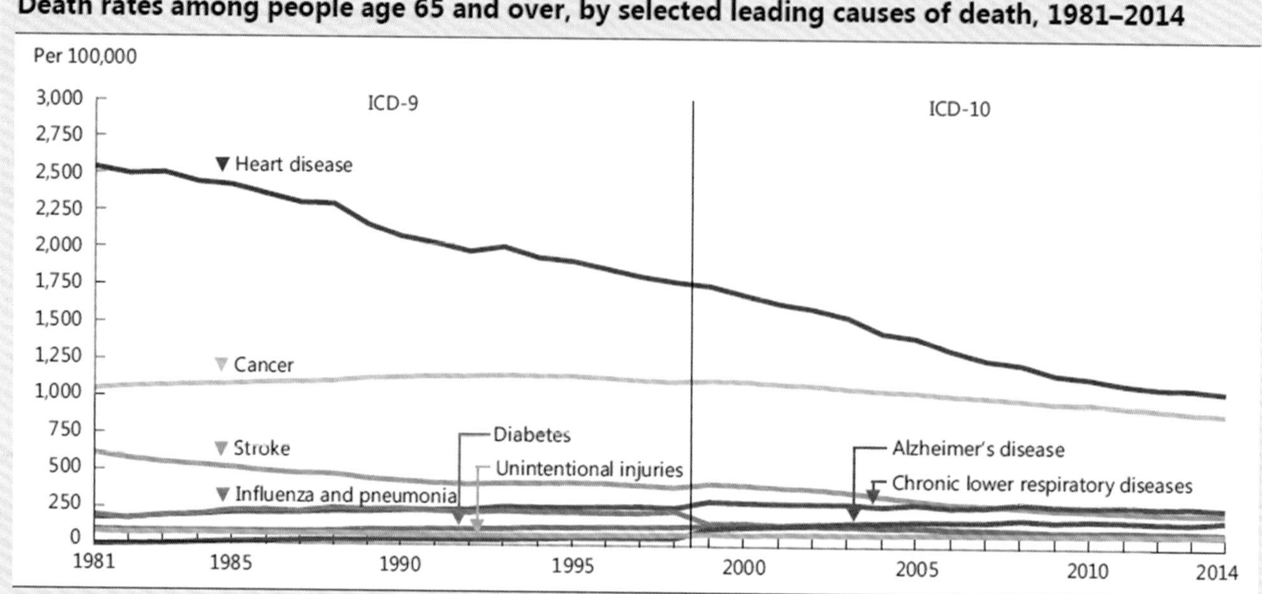

Figure 8-6. Death rates among people 65 years and older by selected leading causes of death, 1981–2014. (From CMS.gov. Last Modified: 05/10/2017 10:32 AM; U.S. Centers for Medicare & Medicaid Services. 7500 Security Boulevard, Baltimore, MD 21244.)

Cardiac Functional Changes. Cardiac function is divided into two phases: diastole and systole. The most significant change that occurs with aging is a decrease in left ventricular diastolic function. Diastole is divided into two phases: early diastole associated with passive filling and late diastole associated with active filling from atrial contraction. The increase in left ventricular stiffness and hypertrophy that occurs with aging, impairs early diastolic filling, resulting in the left atrial contraction contributing a greater portion of cardiac output. Stiffness and hypertrophy also increase the LV workload as it attempts to overcome higher pressures. The increase in left atrial work is accompanied by left atrial enlargement, and left atrial size has been associated with the occurrence of atrial fibrillation.[17] Clinical implications of these age-related changes in diastolic function are linked to an increase in heart failure with preserved ejection fraction or HFpEF. Previously called diastolic heart failure, HFpEF is associated with delayed ventricular relaxation, cardiac stiffening, and reduced LV filling. The increased dependence on atrial contraction for cardiac output is particularly problematic in the setting of atrial fibrillation which occurs at an increasing rate with aging. In atrial fibrillation there is a loss of late LV filling from atrial contraction which reduces cardiac output, and leads to increased risk of heart failure.[14]

Systolic function and myocardial mass remain relatively constant with aging, however during exercise systolic function becomes impaired and maximum heart rate declines with aging.[11,18] The predicted maximum heart rate (PMHR) during dynamic exercise decreases with age (PMHR = 220 – age). This age-related decrease in maximum heart rate explains the age-related decrease in maximum cardiac output in healthy people. Maximum cardiac output reserve is approximately 3.5-fold in younger and 2.5-fold in older people.[19]

Cardiac Electrical System Changes. The increased fibrosis that occurs with aging also impacts cardiac electrical conduction. Fatty and fibrous tissue deposition occurs in the sinoatrial node and throughout the conduction system. The intrinsic rate of the sinoatrial node decreases with aging. The sympathetic and parasympathetic (PS) systems maintain balance so resting heart remains stable, however, the maximal heart rate response to exercise decreases by 0.7 beats/min/yr after the age of 20.[20] The reduction of SA node cells is associated with an increase in the prevalence of sinus node dysfunction after the age of 60. Also called sick sinus or bradycardia–tachycardia syndrome, it is associated with dizziness and syncope. It may include an inability to increase heart rate in response to exercise, a condition called chronotropic incompetence. Atrioventricular (AV) block also increases in the fifth and sixth decades of life.[21] First-degree AV block, a delay in conduction from the SA node to the AV node, is considered a benign arrhythmia however it is associated with an increase in atrial fibrillation, left ventricular dysfunction, and mortality.[22] Second-degree block involves disease of the AV node/His–Purkinje system and is classified as two types, type 1 and type 2. Second-degree type 1, also called Wenkebach, is generally left untreated unless symptomatic, in which case permanent pacing is indicated. Second degree type 2 block involves disease further down the His-Purkinje system. Third-degree block, or complete heart block, is considered an advanced form of conduction disorder. Implantation of a permanent cardiac pacemaker is indicated for both second-degree type 2 and third-degree heart block. The increase incidence of conduction abnormalities accounts for the high pacemaker rates in the elderly with 70% to 80% of all devices being implanted in those who are 65 years or older.[14]

The most common electrical conduction abnormality in the elderly is atrial fibrillation, showing a progressive increase in incidence after the age of 55, with a rise to nearly 1 in 10 after the age of 80, more often in men than women.[23] Atrial fibrillation is associated with an increased risk of stroke, heart failure, and a decline in physical and cognitive function.[21]

A study from the Netherlands of 13,354 electrocardiograms (ECG) of cardiac healthy individuals from four populations showed there are ECG changes that occur based on age and gender.[24] The median heart rate after the age of 20 was approximately 65 for men, and approximately 67 for women, both showing an increase during the ninth decade of life to 74 and 72, respectively. The P wave hardly varies with age. The QRS duration lengthens until around 20 years then plateaus. The remodeling that occurs with aging also impacts the QRS complex with the R wave in the inferior leads, II, III and aVf decreasing and the S wave increasing. There is a tendency to develop a left axis deviation with age, which is consistent with the development of left ventricular hypertrophy. As the cardiac conduction system ages, oxidative stress, cardiomyocyte apoptosis, fibrosis, and disease all contribute to the potential for conduction abnormalities, atrial, and ventricular arrhythmias.

Vascular System

The structural, functional, and mechanical changes that occur in the vasculature begin during infancy yet do not become apparent until middle age.[25]

Vascular Structural Changes. Both mechanical and humoral stress on the arteries promote cellular aging and structural changes resulting in vascular remodeling. These age-associated vascular changes include luminal dilation, increased stiffness, and diffuse intimal and medial thickening.[10]

Repeated mechanical stress causes elastin in the media to fragment, allowing prediction of vascular fatigue that becomes apparent at approximately 40 years of age.[25] Studies have shown the more elastic central arteries, aorta, and carotid, dilate leading to an increase in luminal diameter.[26] Fracturing and depletion of elastin and deposition of collagen cause stiffening of the media layer and ultimately the vessel wall.[12] With increasing age there is also decrease in the VSMCs found in the media which produce elastin, further contributing to vascular stiffening. VSMCs normally found in the media, migrate to the intima, thickening the intimal layer. Increased intimal-to-media thickness (IM) has been observed in aging vasculature, IM thickness of the carotid artery increases two- to threefold between 20 and 90 years of age.[12,26] Thickening of the IM, strongly associated with aging, is used as an indicator of subclinical coronary disease[27] and is considered a predictor of cardiovascular events.[12]

Calcium deposition in vessels, once thought to be a passive process, is now recognized as complex and highly regulated that involves pro-calcifying conditions. VSMCs undergo differentiation to bone marrow stem cells when exposed to cellular and/or systemic processes that facilitate vascular calcification.[10,28] Vascular calcification is correlated with age, described in 5% of individuals less than 50 years of age to greater than 12% in individuals over 80 years of age.[29]

Vascular Functional Changes. The structural changes that occur in the vasculature during aging including the decrease in elastin, increase in collagen, and thickening of the IM, lead to changes in vessel behavior. In early life, the backward deflection of the arterial pulse wave returns to the central aorta during diastole and acts to maintain diastolic perfusion pressure in the coronary artery circulation.[30] With age, the increase in central arterial stiffness and reduced elasticity from changes in the media layer result in increased aortic impedance and are associated with a general increase in systolic pressure. The return of reflected pulse wave is shifted to an earlier time during systole resulting in augmentation of the central systolic and pulse pressures and decrease in coronary perfusion pressure. Pulse pressure is an independent indicator for CV events.[31] The majority of uncontrolled systolic hypertension in Americans over the age of 50 is attributed to isolated systolic hypertension.[32]

The endothelium, part of the intima, is a layer of cells lining the blood vessels. A healthy endothelium has vasodilatory, anti-inflammatory, and anti-thrombotic characteristics. Independent of other changes that occur with aging, studies suggest that endothelial function declines with age.[29] The primary mechanism contributing to the age-related endothelial dysfunction is a reduction in the production of the relaxing factor: nitric oxide (NO). Nitric oxide plays crucial roles in regulating vascular tone, cellular proliferation, leukocyte adhesion, and platelet aggregation.[33] Circulating angiotensin II (AII) during aging, stimulates an increase in the production of proinflammatory and a decrease in anti-oxidant substances in the vascular walls which leads to oxidative stress. Oxidative stress is a potent inducer of pathways that contribute to the inflammation and vascular damage that occurs with age.[29]

The structural, mechanical, and functional changes of the vascular associated with aging, closely resemble those that occur with hypertension. Large and small vessels undergo remodeling, inflammation, calcification, endothelial dysfunction, and increased stiffness with increased blood pressure.[29] These normal physiologic processes that occur with aging are accelerated with hypertension creating "early vascular aging" (EVA).[34] Traditional risk factors for CVD are associated with acceleration of age-related vascular changes. Current risk assessment tools that assess for gender, blood pressure, lipids, smoking, and diabetes are recognized as potential factors impacting vascular health and cardiovascular risk. There is ongoing work exploring other factors that are linked with EVA such as prenatal and early postnatal life, birth weight, early life hypertension and pregnancy experience.[34–36]

Cardiovascular Autonomic Nervous System Modulation

Optimal cardiovascular function involves communications between the cardiovascular system and autonomic nervous system. Under stress the sympathetic component of the autonomic nervous system dominants and the PS system recedes, producing vasoconstriction while increasing heart rate and contractility. At rest, the PS system ascends, slowing the heart rate. Heart rate variability (HRV) is an index of the balance between the sympathetic and PS nervous system. The PS activity of the heart declines with aging. Since PS tone is responsible for modulating or slowing the heart rate, a decrease in PS activity results in a decrease in the component that slows the heart, resulting in a decrease in HRV.[37,38] A reduction in HRV has been associated with an increase in CVD, increased PS activity has protective effects and increased sympathetic activity is associated with increased cardiac events.[38]

The normal sympathetic response to exercise and stress is an increase in sympathetic activity producing an increase in heart rate, myocardial contractility, reduction of afterload, and vascular changes that increase blood flow to the working muscles.[38]

During aging, there is a decreased response to β-adrenoceptor stimulation, resulting in diminished LV contractility, modulation of HR, and arterial afterload.[38] Decreased responsiveness is not caused by a decreased number of β-receptors, but to a decrease in affinity of β-agonists for the receptors and decreased efficacy of post receptor intercellular coupling responsible for muscle contraction.[19] Additionally, the higher the end-diastolic volume, the greater the cardiac contractility (Frank–Starling mechanism). If the ventricular response to β_1-receptor stimulation is reduce in the aging heart, the ventricles are more dependent on adequate filling. Respiratory activity influences venous return to the heart, with increasing depth and rate of respiration increasing ventricular filling. Consequently, the aging heart is less tolerant of hypoventilation. Decreased β-receptor responsiveness in the vasculature produces less vasodilation and higher resting blood pressure. The combined effect of changes in autonomic function is decreased baroreflex function and response to physiologic stressors. Research has shown that exercise may reduce the decline in baroreflex function and the abnormalities of autonomic regulation seen in the elderly. Thus, the positive effects of regular exercise may reduce the cardiac risks specific to aging, as well as overall cardiac risk.[39]

Respiratory Changes

Throughout life, despite progressive changes in pulmonary structure and function overall respiratory performance is sufficient to support normal activities. Normal gas exchange is maintained however a narrowing of protective mechanisms occurs that allows the environmental and life experience "assaults" render the elderly more susceptible to disease.

Structural Changes

Over the lifespan morphologic changes in chest, immune system function, and muscle strength impact pulmonary function and reduce defenses. Narrowing of the intervertebral discs that occurs with aging, results in progressive kyphosis or curving of the spine. As the curvature worsens the space between the ribs narrows and chest cavity size decreases.[40] The intercostal muscle mass and strength decline after the age of 50, and although diaphragmatic muscle area remains the same there is a decrease in strength. These skeletal and muscular changes result in increased compliance and decrease in air exchange, reducing vital capacity (VC), volume of gas expired with maximal expiration, and ability to exhale.[40,41]

Pulmonary immune mechanisms decline with age. Basal levels of circulating proinflammatory cells increase while microphages decrease creating a chronic low-grade respiratory inflammation, a phenomenon called "inflamm-aging." These factors contribute to reduced elasticity and destruction of the lung and airways.[40–42] Concurrently there is a blunted immune response to pathogenic threat or injury, known as "immunosenescence." The increased basal level of inflammation contributes to a reduction in cytokine production in response to an infectious threat.[40] These two processes, "inflamm-aging" and "immunosenescence" create a proinflammatory environment, in which innate and adaptive immune responses are diminished.

There is a decline in airway defenses. The upper and lower airways are lined with ciliated cells which beat in synchrony, capturing foreign particles, continuously clearing air passages. With aging there is decreased clearance by this mucociliary elevator, allowing foreign particles to remain in airways for longer periods of time. The earlier described decline in intercostal and diaphragmatic muscle strength impacts the ability to generate force to cough and clear airways. Declining muscle strength, "inflamm-aging," "immunosenescence," and the diminished mucociliary elevator are all factors that contribute increased susceptibility to respiratory disease with the aging process.

Functional Changes

Changes that occur with aging in chest cavity size and shape, alveolar enlargement and respiratory muscle strength impact respiratory performance. The decrease in compliance, elastic recoil and decrease in strength all contribute to changes in pulmonary function, respiratory mechanics, and gas exchange. Key changes are described based on pulmonary function measurements and the mechanics of breathing (Fig. 8-7).

Total lung capacity (TLC), the volume of gas in the lungs after a maximal inspiration, remains the same over the lifespan. The lungs become less elastic and more compliant, in essence stiffer. The loss of connective tissue in around the small airways allows earlier collapse, impairing airflow and preventing alveoli from emptying. The aging alveoli enlarge and coalesce, trapping more air and increasing fixed lung volume. The decline in muscle strength and loss of lung recoil result in an increase in *residual volume* (RV) of 1% to 3% per decade and a decrease in forced vital capacity (FVC), a measure of maximal expiratory flow rate[41]. The *expiratory reserve volume* (ERV), the volume of

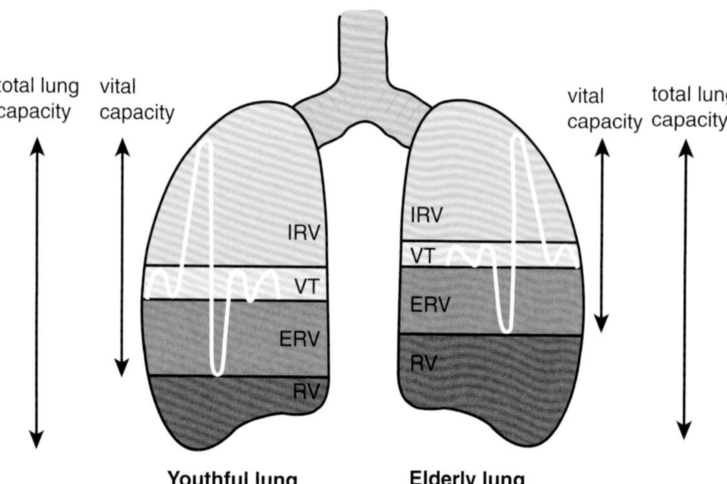

Figure 8-7. Changes in lung volumes with age. With aging note particularly the decrease in vital capacity (VC) and the increase in residual volume (RV). IRV, inspiratory research volume; VT, tidal volume; ERV, expiratory reserve volume; RV, reserve volume; total lung capacity (TLC) = IRV = VT + ERV + RV; vital capacity (VC) = IRV + VT + ERV. (Reproduced from Timiras PS, ed. *Physiological Basis of Aging and Geriatrics.* 3rd ed. 2003:324.)

gas expired with a maximal expiration after a normal expiration, decreases with age. As chest wall compliance and muscle strength decrease, and there is a greater tendency for small airways to collapse. Two tests used to assess dynamic lung function are the forced expiratory flow rate over one second (FEV_1), and the FEV_1/FVC ratio. The FEV_1, peaks between ages 20 and 36 then declines with age.[40] The FEV_1/FVC ratio is used to assess for airway obstruction.

Renal Changes

The kidney is an elegant organ with complex functions that are intimately related with other organ systems, including the cardiovascular, endocrine, and neurologic systems. In discussing the aging kidney, changes are discussed as they relate to intrinsic changes in the kidney as well as those adaptive changes that result due to the effects of other systems.

Structural Changes

Kidney mass progressively increases from birth through the fourth decade of life reaching a maximum size between 250 and 270 g (8.5 to 9.5 oz) then declines at a rate of 10% per decade.[43] There is a 10% to 30% decrease in kidney weight by the seventh to eighth decades of life.[44] Determinants of the number of glomeruli at birth are race, gender, and birth weight. As the kidney size declines with aging, the renal cortex decreases in size more than the medulla. As the cortex declines, the number of functioning glomeruli decreases while the number of sclerotic and hyaline infiltrated glomeruli increases. The changes in the renal vasculature are consistent with those occurring systemically showing intimal and medial hypertrophy, sclerosis, and the development of arteriosclerotic lesions.[43] There is a decline in vascular flow with aging that is linked to the structural changes in the renal vasculature.

Functional Changes

There is a linear relationship between aging and the decline in renal function. Renal blood flow remains constant at 600 mL/min until the fourth decade then declines approximately 10% per decade. The decline in kidney size and renal blood flow correlate with a decline in the glomerular filtration rate (GFR). GFR achieves adult levels by the second year of life (140 mL/min/1.73 m^2), is maintained until the fourth decade when an average decline of 8 mL/min/1.73 m^2 per decade occurs.[45] Formulas have been derived using endogenous markers to estimate glomerular filtration. Creatinine, a breakdown product from muscle, is the endogenous marker most commonly used. Due to the decline in muscle mass, decrease in protein and fluid intake that occurs with age, creatinine clearance (C_{cr}) should be used to assess renal function instead of direct creatinine levels. Various serum creatinine (S_{cr})-based equations have been developed to estimate C_{cr}. The Cockcroft–Gault (C–G) formula is not adjusted for body surface area, the "modification of diet in renal disease" formula (eGFR-MDRD) does include adjustment for body surface area and the more recent CKD-EPI[46] uses the same variables as the MDRD formula but was developed using a more diverse population. Inclusion of age and gender in equations helps to adjust for the anticipated decline in creatinine production rate associated with a declining muscle mass. The various equations for eGFR are shown in Table 8-1.

Table 8-1 • ESTIMATED GLOMERULAR FILTRATION RATE FORMULAS

CKD-EPI Formula[46]

$$GFR = 141 \times \min(S_{cr}/\kappa, 1)^{\alpha} \times \max(S_{cr}/\kappa, 1)^{-1.209} \times 0.993^{Age} \times 1.018 \text{ (if female)} \times 1.159 \text{ (if black)}$$

S_{cr} is serum creatinine in mg/dL, κ is 0.7 for females and 0.9 for males, α is –0.329 for females and –0.411 for males, min indicates the minimum of S_{cr}/κ or 1, and max indicates the maximum of S_{cr}/κ or 1

GFR-eMDRD Formula

$$eGFR = 175 \times (S_{cr})^{-1.154} \times (age)^{-0.203} \times 0.742 \text{ (if female)} \times 1.212 \text{ (if black)}$$

S_{cr} (standardized serum creatinine) = mg/dL, age = years

Cockroft–Gault Formula

$$CreatClear = ((140 - Age)/(SerumCreat)) \times (Weight/72) \times Sex$$

Sex: Male = 1.0; Female = 0.85

Accurate estimation of renal function and glomerular filtration has clinical implications in the aging patient with cardiac disease. Chronic kidney disease is assessed in stages based on eGFR, beginning with an eGFR less than or equal to 60 mL/min. Because many medications are cleared through the kidneys, accurate measurement of renal function is indicated for calculating doses and in determining appropriate clinical treatment pathways. Declining renal function impacts the clearance rate of medications, requiring dosage adjustments or medication class changes. Many cardiac diagnostic tests involve the use of nephrotoxic agents that require additional measures for renal protection with decreased renal function.

Tubular changes in length and volume, atrophy and scarring along with changes in antidiuretic hormone (ADH) regulation impact the aging kidney's ability to manage salt and water. In the nephron, there is greater proximal tubule sodium reabsorption along with decreased distal tubule reabsorption which allows a normal sodium balance under steady-state conditions. However, this sodium activity rearrangement impacts their ability to conserve sodium in the setting of low salt intake or excrete excess sodium when there is a salt-load.[43]

With aging there is a deceased ability to concentrate and dilute urine. ADH suppression is essential to prevent reabsorption of water in the collecting ducts. Studies of aging rats, suggest changes in vasopressin (ADH) receptor activity impact the age-related decline in ability to concentrate urine, including the number of receptors and responsiveness to vasopressin.[47]

Limited synthesis and release of renin occurs with aging, there is approximately 50% decrease in plasma renin activity and aldosterone which predisposes the elderly to fluid and electrolyte abnormalities.[43] These lower renin and aldosterone levels in the older populations are associated with an impaired response of the renin-angiotensin system (RAS) activity to changes in posture, periods of sodium depletion or excess of potassium.[48] With a decrease in RAS activity comes changes in response to attempts as RAS blockade. When the elderly are treated with ACE inhibitors, there is a decrease in antihypertensive response when compared to younger populations.[48]

The elderly are at increased risk for development of vitamin D deficiency from both internal and external factors. Diet and exposure to sunshine are the primary sources for vitamin D in its inactive form. Due to the decline in renal function, there is a decrease in the kidneys ability to hydroxylate vitamin D to its active form, calcitriol. In individuals with impaired renal function, levels of calcitriol are independent predictors of progression to dialysis and death. In studies of postmenopausal women over the age of 80 with preserved renal function, higher vitamin D levels were associated with exposure to sunshine and active lifestyles.[43] Erythropoietin (EPO), produced in the kidney, promotes the formation of red blood cells. In healthy elderly EPO levels are increased, understood to occur as a response to the higher RBC turnover, as well as EPO resistance.[43]

Hepatic Changes

The liver has remarkable ability to regenerate, however, aging is associated with gradual changes in hepatic structure and function. These progressive changes impact its ability to respond to acute and chronic injury as well as diminish its ability to clear drugs.

Structural Changes

During the aging process, there is a decrease in the volume and blood flow of the liver. From studies that use ultrasound assessments, the liver volume decreases by 20% to 40% related to the decline in blood flow. Individuals over the age of 65 show approximately 35% decrease in blood volume compared to 40-year-olds. However, studies that use radioisotope assessments find that there is a decrease in the mass of functional liver cells.[49] With aging there is an increase in oxidative stress. Liver cells show an increase in lipofuscin, an undegradable protein aggregate formed when protein is damaged and denatured by oxidative stress. Increases in lipofuscin are associated with decrease in cell survivability.[49] Polyploidy occurs with hepatocyte aging, as multiple chromosome chains develop in the cells, there is a decrease in mitochondrial number and function. The many age-related changes that impact the liver, including increased oxidative stress, increased inflammatory response, accelerated cellular senescence, and progressive organ dysfunction impact the liver's ability to respond to acute and chronic injuries.[50]

Functional Changes

Despite changes in liver volume and changes at the cellular level, liver function tests do not show dramatic changes with aging. Albumin levels slightly decrease or remain unchanged, aminotransferase remains normal, while serum γ-glutanyl transferase and alkaline phosphatase levels show an increase with aging.[49] Metabolism of low-density lipoprotein cholesterol decreases by 35% while total blood cholesterol, high-density lipoprotein, and triglycerides increase with aging.[49] There is a decrease in the activity of some but not all of the cytochrome P450 enzymes which impacts drug metabolism that are dependent on those cytochrome P450 families.

EFFECTS OF AGING ON PHARMACOKINETICS

Drug Absorption

Gastric acid secretion and splanchnic blood flow both decrease with aging resulting a decrease in absorption of some medications. At the same time there is a decrease in gastrointestinal motility resulting in longer transit times which can increase absorption.[51] Drug absorption may be further impacted by the increase use of proton pump inhibitors (PPIs) in the elderly which elevates gastric pH and modifies release of drugs which are pH-dependent.[52]

Drug Distribution

With aging there are significant changes in body composition which impacts the concentration of drug available at target sites. There is a decrease in lean body mass and total body water with an increase in body fat. This allows elimination of lipophilic (fat-soluble) drugs to be prolonged, exerting influence over a longer period of time. The decrease in total body water means hydrophilic (water-soluble) drugs tend to have a smaller distribution.

A decrease in serum albumin concentration is associated with changes protein-binding ability. Drugs that are protein bound are inactive, unbound or free and the drug is able to exert its therapeutic effect. There is a higher-free fraction in plasma of some highly protein-bound acidic drugs allowing greater functionality of the drugs in the elderly.

Drug Metabolism and Excretion

The effects of aging on drug metabolism depend on the phase of metabolism in the liver. There is reduced clearance of drugs that undergo Phase I mandatory oxidative/reduction processes due to reduced activity of some sub-families of the cytochrome P450 enzymes. Decreased Phase I metabolism leads to increased half-life which gives rise to drug toxicity. Whereas, aging does not show significant impact on Phase II metabolism which involves conjugative reactions. Multiple drug, genetic, epigenetic, and environmental factors also affect the P450 system and explain observed decreases in drug metabolism in older adults.[52–55]

Summary

"Successful aging" is a term used to describe individuals who continue to function into old age, without physical or cognitive limitations, and are free from chronic disease. Yet aging is marked by progressive changes in structure and decline in function of cells, organs, and systems. Cardiovascular function declines progressively with age, and because of the inter-relatedness of the major systems, it is affected by and affects other systems as well. The challenge for health care providers is to differentiate the normal decline in function that occurs with aging, decline that can be attenuated through promotion of healthy behaviors and problems that result from CVDs.

Future Considerations and Implications

"Success" in the treatment of diseases and a focus on healthier living has resulted in a greater percentage of people reaching "older age." Yet CVD remains the leading cause of death in developing nations. In the United States, over 70% of individuals between 60 and 79 years of age and over 80% over 80 years suffer from some form of CVD and more than two thirds develop non-CVD diseases.[58]

Physical resilience, a characteristic which determines one's ability to resist or recover from functional decline following stressors, has gained increasing attention as a construct that is highly relevant to successful aging.[59] The future challenges for health care providers will be working with patients to focus on those factors which impact ability to achieve more than a longer lifespan but also a successful "healthspan." Identifying and modifying factors that not only impact debilitating aspects of aging and disease but also facilitate and maintain health and function across the lifespan.

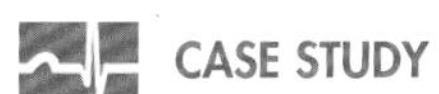

CASE STUDY

Patient Profile

History of Present Illness

Mrs. Oleander is an 86-year-old female who presents to clinic describing a progressive decline in exercise tolerance over the last year. Due to fatigue, the furthest distance she can walk is across a room. Last month her son took her to the emergency room for shortness of breath that worsened over the course of a day. During the hospital admission she was told that she has a "tight valve" was treated with intravenous medication to get rid of the "extra water." She discharged to assisted living a few weeks ago and was referred to Cardiology.

Currently, she reports swelling in her ankles that worsens over the course of the day but is improved in the morning. She is distressed that her regular trips to the casino have decreased in frequency. In fact, she has not been there for 2 months.

Past Medical History/Problem List

Hypothyroidism
Hypertension
Aortic stenosis
Coronary artery disease: (significant but nonobstructive by catheterization)
Sick sinus syndrome
Paroxysmal atrial fibrillation
Chronic diastolic heart failure

Social History

Widowed, lives in assisted living facility, enjoys a weekly trip with her son to the local casino where she likes to play the "slot machines": reports she has "a system."

Family History

Mother: Cancer (deceased), Father (deceased), Daughter: Diabetes, Heart Disease, Cancer (alive)

Medications

apixaban 2.5 mg twice daily
amlodipine 5 mg daily
furosemide 20 mg daily
levothyroxine 150 mcg daily
atorvastatin 20 mg daily

Allergies

Penicillins

Patient Examination

Vital Signs

BP 110/60 left; HR 73; RR 18; SaO_2 99%; Temp 98.6; Wt. 174 lb; Ht. 5′2″

Physical Examination

- *HEENT:* No scleral icterus
- *Endocrine:* No thyromegaly
- *Neuro:* Alert and oriented ×3. Moves all extremities. Cranial nerves grossly intact, no sensory or motor deficits appreciated.
- *Musculoskeletal:* Gait stable, able to complete 5 chair rises in 23 seconds.
- *Cardiovascular:* Delayed carotid upstrokes bilaterally without bruits. Estimated CVP is 7 cm H_2O at 20 degrees. Negative hepatojugular reflux. Regular rhythm with normal S1 and diminished S2; no S3, S4. Systolic murmur II/VI at 2nd right ICS with soft radiation to carotids. 2+ pulses. bilaterally radial, brachial, carotid, DP and PT.
- *Pulmonary:* Clear anteriorly
- *GI:* Abdomen soft, nondistended, no tenderness; no hepatomegaly.
- *Skin:* Warm, well perfused; lower extremities (1+) edema.
- *Psychiatric:* Appropriate affect.

Diagnostic Studies

Select Labs: Creatinine: 1.2, Hemoglobin: 12.3, Albumin: 4.1
Echocardiogram (key findings): Ejection fraction 57%; Pulmonary artery systolic pressure (PASP): 29 mm Hg

- Right atrial size: normal; right ventricle: normal size and function.
- Left atrial size: enlarged.
- Left ventricle (LV): cavity size is normal, wall thickness increased.
- Spectral Doppler shows (Grade I) mild LV diastolic dysfunction.
- Aortic Valve: Peak/mean gradients: 68 mm Hg/41 mm Hg; Velocity 4.0 m/sec; AVA 1.0 cm^2

Assessment and Plan

Mrs. Oleander is showing hallmark signs of cardiovascular disease influenced by aging.

Hospitalized with acute on chronic heart failure, the echocardiogram at that time demonstrated multiple characteristics consistent with diastolic dysfunction: increased LV thickness (hypertrophy), impaired relaxation (diastolic dysfunction Stage I), and left atrial enlargement. Guideline-based therapy would suggest changing the amlodipine, which was used for hypertension treatment, to beta-blocker therapy as tolerated. A renal-angiotensin system (RAS) inhibitor, a mainstay of guideline-directed medical therapy for heart failure, holds a relative contraindication in the patient with moderate to severe aortic stenosis.

To that end, the echocardiogram demonstrates another diagnosis of aging: senile, calcific aortic stenosis, which is a progressive disease; based on the American Heart Association (AHA)/American College of Cardiology (ACC) guidelines she would be classified as having ACC/AHA Stage D3 valve disease: symptomatic and severe by echocardiographic criteria.[56] As the valve becomes calcified and thickened the opening decreases in size, the ventricle sustains further increases in afterload, leading to the progressive hypertrophy. Since Mrs. Oleander has been hospitalized recently for, and continues to show signs of, heart failure, it is appropriate to refer her for valve intervention.

The left atrial enlargement shown in the echocardiogram is also consistent with paroxysmal atrial fibrillation. Guideline-based treatment may recommend beta-blocker therapy for rate management for when episodes of atrial fibrillation occur.[57] However, the history of sick sinus syndrome or sinus node disease would suggest proceeding with caution as episodes of bradycardia may occur.

On furosemide 20 mg daily, she complains of increased ankle swelling as the day progresses. Assessment of renal function shows a glomerular filtration rate (GFR) of 43, which is consistent with chronic kidney disease Stage 3a. Furosemide dosing may be increased to twice-daily dosing or alternate day twice-daily dosing to help alleviate the swelling with repeat labs indicated if pursued as a long-term therapy or if renin-angiotensin-aldosterone system (RAAS) is needed.

She is mentally active, living in an assisted living facility. Exercise rehabilitation has been shown to have cardiovascular benefits. Discussion with Mrs. Oleander regarding exploring exercise activities at the assisted living facility may help her further increase her activity tolerance and help engage in social interaction.

Key Takeaways

This case highlights many of the physiologic changes of aging. These changes carry specific considerations for the cardiac nurse (Display 8-1), which must be attended to in the care of this specific patient population.

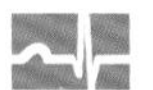

DISPLAY 8-1

Physiologic Changes With Aging and Considerations for the Cardiac Nurse

1. General approach to patient management
   a. Determine patient's goals for quality life and incorporate into treatments.
   b. Focus on patient's definition of "successful aging."
   c. Incorporate the balance of normal decline in function with treatments for abnormalities in which side effects may negatively impact function.
   d. Encourage "healthy lifestyle" to lower risk of developing disability.
2. Screening
   a. Cognitive function: Include screening for memory declines and dementia. Impairments impacts patient safety and behavioral issues.
   b. Functional and geriatric: Include "get up and go" and strength testing. Deficits reflect falls risks and safety issues.
   c. Depression: Include screening, as late life depression negatively impacts quality of life, outcomes of disease, use of health care resources, morbidity and mortality.
   d. Social Support: Include assessment, as social isolation, lack of relatives and friends impact independence and well-being.
3. Functional Changes
   a. Cardiac: Decline in predicted maximal heart rate and systolic function may impact ability to exercise. Encourage patients to continue active lifestyle and exercise. Exercise to maintain and increase muscle strength and flexibility.
   b. Renal: Recall that a decline in GFR may impact dosing of medications. Review renal function status prior prescribing or administering that are renally excreted. Protective measures may be indicated for cardiac diagnostic testing that involve nephrotoxic agents.
   c. Respiratory: Assess for progressive decline in muscle strength, immune system function and morphologic changes increase susceptibility. Encourage regular exercise to maintain respiratory and postural strength.
   d. Pharmacologic: Assess for changes in body composition, hepatic, renal, and gastric clearance of medications all impact dosing requirement and drug interactions.
      i. Review weight and renal-adjusted dosing
      ii. Drug–drug interactions: overload of same metabolic pathways
      iii. Poly-pharmacy:
         1. Keep regimens simple
         2. Once- or twice-daily dosing
      iv. Engage pharmacist when regimens increase in complexity.
4. Clinical Pearls
   a. Pursue collaboration and communication between multiple care providers.
   b. Engage family and social support, incorporate into care planning and goals.
   c. Emphasis on education to support self-care and independence, patient preferences and goals.
   d. Utilize social support resources: home care, meals on wheels, ride assistance and social networking.

KEY READINGS

Brubaker PH, Kitzman DW. Chronotropic incompetence: causes, consequences, and management. *Circulation*. 2011;123(9):1010–1020. doi:10.1161/CIRCULATIONAHA.110.940577. Available at https://www.ncbi.nlm.nih.gov/pubmed/21382903

Forman DE, Rich MW, Alexander KP, et al. Cardiac care for older adults: time for a new paradigm. *J Am Coll Cardiol*. 2011;57(18):1801–1810. Available at https://doi.org/10.1016/j.jacc.2011.02.014

Lopez-Otin C, Blasco MA, Partridge L, et al. The hallmarks of aging. *Cell*. 2013;153(6):1194–1217.

Paneni F, Cañestro CD, Libby P, et al. The aging cardiovascular system: understanding it at the cellular and clinical levels. *J Am Coll Cardiol*. 2017;69(15):1952–1967. https://doi.org/10.1016/j.jacc.2017.01.064

Steenman M, Lande G. Cardiac aging and heart disease in humans. *Biophys Rev*. 2017;9:131–137. Available at https://doi.org/10.1007/s12551-017-0255-9

Strait JB, Lakatta EG. Aging-associated cardiovascular changes and their relationship to heart failure. *Heart Fail Clin*. 2012;8(1):143–164. doi:10.1016/j.hfc.2011.08.011.

REFERENCES

1. Hjelmborg J, Iachine I, Skytthe A, et al. Genetic influence on human lifespan and longevity. *Hum Genet*. 2006;119(3):312–321.
2. *World Population Prospects: The 2015 Revision, Volume I: Comprehensive Tables*. In: Department of Economic and Social Affairs PD, ed. New York: 2015.
3. Jin K. Modern biological theories of aging. *Aging Dis*. 2010;1(2):72–74.
4. Deelen J, Beekman M, Capri M, et al. Identifying the genomic determinants of aging and longevity in human population studies: progress and challenges. *Bioessays*. 2013;35(4):386–396.
5. Salvioli S, Monti D, Lanzarini C, et al. Immune system, cell senescence, aging and longevity—inflamm-aging reappraised. *Curr Pharm Des*. 2013; 19(9):1675–1679.
6. Lopez-Otin C, Blasco MA, Partridge L, et al. The hallmarks of aging. *Cell*. 2013;153(6):1194–1217.
7. Burch JB, Augustine AD, Frieden LA, et al. Advances in geroscience: impact on healthspan and chronic disease. *J Gerontol A Biol Sci Med Sci*. 2014;69(suppl 1):S1–S3.
8. Kaeberlein M. How healthy is the healthspan concept? *Geroscience*. 2018;40(4):361–364.
9. Buttorff C, Ruder T, Bauman M. *Multiple Chronic Conditions in the United States*. Santa Monica, CA: RAND Corporation; 2017:TL221.
10. Maruyama Y. Aging and arterial-cardiac interactions in the elderly. *Int J Cardiol*. 2012;155(1):14–19.
11. Horn MA. Cardiac physiology of aging: extracellular considerations. *Compr Physiol*. 2015;5(3):1069–1121.
12. Lakatta EG, Levy D. Arterial and cardiac aging: major shareholders in cardiovascular disease enterprises: Part I: aging arteries: a "set up" for vascular disease. *Circulation*. 2003;107(1):139–146.
13. Carvalho E, Verma P, Hourigan K, et al. Myocardial infarction: stem cell transplantation for cardiac regeneration. *Regen Med*. 2015;10(8): 1025–1043.
14. Steenman M, Lande G. Cardiac aging and heart disease in humans. *Biophys Rev*. 2017;9(2):131–137.
15. Aikawa E, Schoen FJ, Stone J, et al. Calcific and degenerative heart valve disease. In: Willis M, Homeister J, Stone J, eds. *Cellular and Molecular Pathobiology of Cardiovascular Disease*. Elsevier; 2014:161–181.
16. Yutzey KE, Demer LL, Body SC, et al. Calcific aortic valve disease: a consensus summary from the Alliance of Investigators on Calcific Aortic Valve Disease. *Arterioscler Thromb Vasc Biol*. 2014;34(11):2387–2393.
17. Lam CS, Rienstra M, Tay WT, et al. Atrial fibrillation in heart failure with preserved ejection fraction: association with exercise capacity, left ventricular filling pressures, natriuretic peptides, and left atrial volume. *JACC Heart Fail*. 2017;5(2):92–98.
18. Chiao YA, Rabinovitch PS. The aging heart. *Cold Spring Harb Perspect Med*. 2015;5(9):a025148.

19. Lakatta EG. Arterial and cardiac aging: major shareholders in cardiovascular disease enterprises: Part III: cellular and molecular clues to heart and arterial aging. *Circulation.* 2003;107(3):490–497.
20. Chow GV, Marine JE, Fleg JL. Epidemiology of arrhythmias and conduction disorders in older adults. *Clin Geriatr Med.* 2012;28(4):539–553.
21. Curtis AB, Karki R, Hattoum A, et al. Arrhythmias in patients ≥80 years of age: pathophysiology, management, and outcomes. *J Am Coll Cardiol.* 2018;71(18):2041–2057.
22. Kwok CS, Rashid M, Beynon R, et al. Prolonged PR interval, first-degree heart block and adverse cardiovascular outcomes: a systematic review and meta-analysis. *Heart.* 2016;102(9):672–680.
23. Go AS, Hylek EM, Phillips KA, et al. Prevalence of diagnosed atrial fibrillation in adults: national implications for rhythm management and stroke prevention: the AnTicoagulation and Risk Factors in Atrial Fibrillation (ATRIA) Study. *JAMA.* 2001;285(18):2370–2375.
24. Rijnbeek PR, van Herpen G, Bots ML, et al. Normal values of the electrocardiogram for ages 16–90 years. *J Electrocardiol.* 2014;47(6):914–921.
25. Collins JA, Munoz JV, Patel TR, et al. The anatomy of the aging aorta. *Clin Anat.* 2014;27(3):463–466.
26. Lakatta EG. Cardiovascular regulatory mechanisms in advanced age. *Physiol Rev.* 1993;73(2):413–467.
27. Madhavan MV, Gersh BJ, Alexander KP, et al. Coronary artery disease in patients ≥ 80 years of age. *J Am Coll Cardiol.* 2018;71(18):2015–2040.
28. Leopold JA. Vascular calcification: mechanisms of vascular smooth muscle cell calcification. *Trends Cardiovasc Med.* 2015;25(4):267–274.
29. Harvey A, Montezano AC, Touyz RM. Vascular biology of ageing—Implications in hypertension. *J Mol Cell Cardiol.* 2015;83:112–121.
30. Sugawara J, Hayashi K, Tanaka H. Distal shift of arterial pressure wave reflection sites with aging. *Hypertension.* 2010;56(5):920–925.
31. Franklin SS, Khan SA, Wong ND, et al. Is pulse pressure useful in predicting risk for coronary heart Disease? The Framingham heart study. *Circulation.* 1999;100(4):354–360.
32. Paneni F, Diaz Canestro C, Libby P, et al. The aging cardiovascular system: understanding it at the cellular and clinical levels. *J Am Coll Cardiol.* 2017;69(15):1952–1967.
33. Forstermann U, Munzel T. Endothelial nitric oxide synthase in vascular disease: from marvel to menace. *Circulation.* 2006;113(13):1708–1714.
34. Laurent S. Defining vascular aging and cardiovascular risk. *J Hypertens.* 2012;30(suppl):S3–S8.
35. Nilsson PM, Lurbe E, Laurent S. The early life origins of vascular ageing and cardiovascular risk: the EVA syndrome. *J Hypertens.* 2008;26(6):1049–1057.
36. Minissian MB, Kilpatrick S, Eastwood JA, et al. Association of spontaneous preterm delivery and future maternal cardiovascular disease. *Circulation.* 2018;137(8):865–871.
37. Lakatta EG, Levy D. Arterial and cardiac aging: major shareholders in cardiovascular disease enterprises: Part II: the aging heart in health: links to heart disease. *Circulation.* 2003;107(2):346–354.
38. Droguett VS, Santos Ada C, de Medeiros CE, et al. Cardiac autonomic modulation in healthy elderly after different intensities of dynamic exercise. *Clin Interv Aging.* 2015;10:203–208.
39. La Rovere M, Pinna G. Beneficial effects of physical activity on baroreflex control in the elderly. *Ann Noninvasive Electrocardiol.* 2014;19(4):303–310.
40. Lowery EM, Brubaker AL, Kuhlmann E, et al. The aging lung. *Clin Interv Aging.* 2013;8:1489–1496.
41. Lalley PM. The aging respiratory system–pulmonary structure, function and neural control. *Respir Physiol Neurobiol.* 2013;187(3):199–210.
42. Tran D, Rajwani K, Berlin DA. Pulmonary effects of aging. *Curr Opin Anaesthesiol.* 2018;31(1):19–23.
43. Bolignano D, Mattace-Raso F, Sijbrands EJ, et al. The aging kidney revisited: a systematic review. *Ageing Res Rev.* 2014;14:65–80.
44. Glassock RJ, Rule AD. The implications of anatomical and functional changes of the aging kidney: with an emphasis on the glomeruli. *Kidney Int.* 2012;82(3):270–277.
45. Karam Z, Tuazon J. Anatomic and physiologic changes of the aging kidney. *Clin Geriatr Med.* 2013;29(3):555–564.
46. Levey AS, Stevens LA, Schmid CH, et al. A new equation to estimate glomerular filtration rate. *Ann Intern Med.* 2009;150(9):604–612.
47. Sands JM. Urine concentrating and diluting ability during aging. *J Gerontol A Biol Sci Med Sci.* 2012;67(12):1352–1357.
48. Yoon HE, Choi BS. The renin-angiotensin system and aging in the kidney. *Korean J Intern Med.* 2014;29(3):291–295.
49. Kim IH, Kisseleva T, Brenner DA. Aging and liver disease. *Curr Opin Gastroenterol.* 2015;31(3):184–191.
50. Poulose N, Raju R. Aging and injury: alterations in cellular energetics and organ function. *Aging Dis.* 2014;5(2):101–108.
51. Ayan M, Pothineni NV, Siraj A, et al. Cardiac drug therapy-considerations in the elderly. *J Geriatr Cardiol.* 2016;13(12):992–997.
52. Blume H, Donath F, Warnke A, et al. Pharmacokinetic drug interaction profiles of proton pump inhibitors. *Drug Saf.* 2006;29(9):769–784.
53. Wedemeyer RS, Blume H. Pharmacokinetic drug interaction profiles of proton pump inhibitors: an update. *Drug Saf.* 2014;37(4):201–211.
54. Yu AM, Ingelman-Sundberg M, Cherrington NJ, et al. Regulation of drug metabolism and toxicity by multiple factors of genetics, epigenetics, lncRNAs, gut microbiota, and diseases: a meeting report of the 21(st) International Symposium on Microsomes and Drug Oxidations (MDO). *Acta Pharm Sin B.* 2017;7(2):241–248.
55. Rendic S, Guengerich FP. Update information on drug metabolism systems. *Curr Drug Metab.* 2010;11(1):4–84.
56. Nishimura RA, Otto CM, Bonow RO, et al. 2014 AHA/ACC guideline for the management of patients with valvular heart disease: a report of the American College of Cardiology/American Heart Association Task Force on Practice Guidelines. *J Am Coll Cardiol.* 2014;63(22):e57–e185.
57. January CT, Wann LS, Alpert JS, et al. 2014 AHA/ACC/HRS guideline for the management of patients with atrial fibrillation: a report of the American College of Cardiology/American Heart Association Task Force on Practice Guidelines and the Heart Rhythm Society. *J Am Coll Cardiol.* 2014;64(21):e1–e76.
58. Dunlay SM, Chamberlain AM. Multimorbidity in older patients with cardiovascular disease. *Curr Cardiovasc Risk Rep.* 2016;10:3.
59. Whitson HE, Duan-Porter W, Schmader KE, et al. Physical resilience in older adults: systematic review and development of an emerging construct. *J Gerontol A Biol Sci Med Sci.* 2016;71(4):489–495.

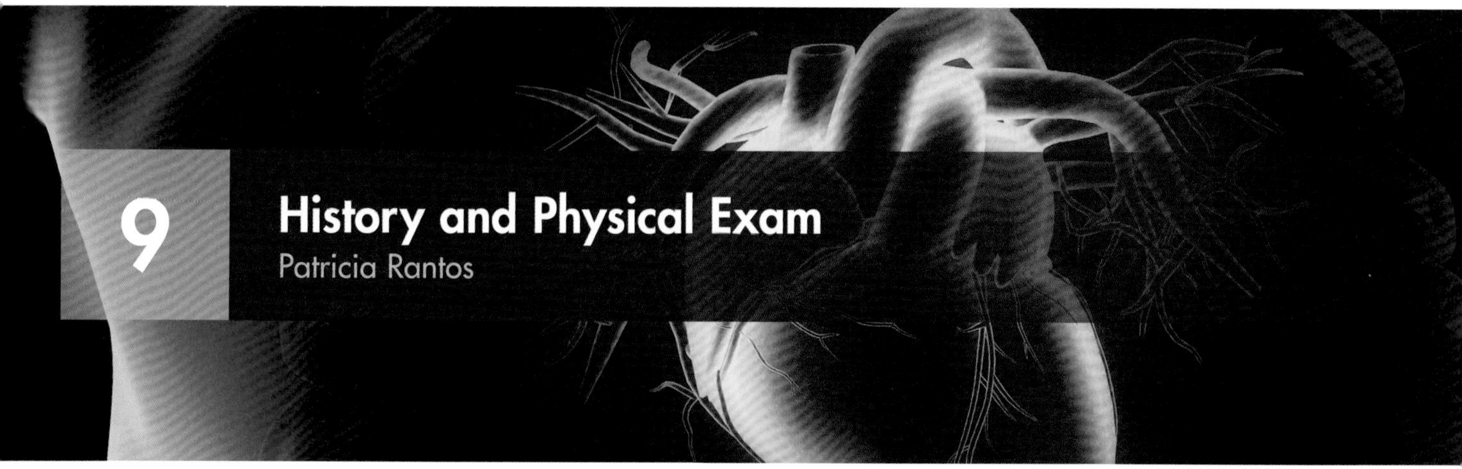

9 History and Physical Exam

Patricia Rantos

OBJECTIVES

1. Describe the steps in conducting a detailed cardiovascular history and physical examination.
2. Develop a plan to incorporate the information obtained from the history and physical examination into nursing care.
3. Identify the elements of a problem-focused cardiovascular examination for a patient experiencing chest pain.
4. Identify the auscultation points for normal systolic and diastolic heart sounds.
5. Describe the events in the cardiac cycle and auscultation findings associated with each event.
6. Describe the location for auscultation of and timing of systolic and diastolic murmurs.
7. Describe the timing of S3 and S4 in the cardiac cycle and causes of these sounds.
8. Identify noncardiac areas of focus on a physical examination in a patient presenting with chest pain.

KEY QUESTIONS

1. What are the data obtained from the patient history, physical examination and diagnostic tests used for?
2. In a patient presenting with chest discomfort, what are the key elements of the history and physical exam to obtain?
3. Assessment of the peripheral vascular system includes inspection, palpation and auscultation of what areas?
4. What are the goals of auscultating the precordium?
5. What physical assessment competencies and skills are required for the cardiac nurse?

BACKGROUND

Assessment data, which are obtained from the patient's history, physical examination, and diagnostic tests, are used to formulate clinical diagnoses, establish patient goals, plan care, and evaluate patient outcomes. A complete history and physical examination includes the same content areas, whether elicited by nurses or physicians. A complete history and physical examination is impractical in most clinical situations. Most hospitals and clinics are using an electronic health record that establishes which data are included in the history and physical. The electronic health record assures systematic assessment but may constrain the kinds of data that are obtained. With freeform records the inclusion of appropriate content areas is determined by the patient's clinical condition, the purpose and context of the clinical encounter, and the clinician. Specific content areas may be investigated in greater detail by clinicians from different disciplines, and the data may be used in different ways. Nurses must be able to incorporate historical data into the nursing assessment so the interdependent nursing and medical responsibilities are completed in the correct priority sequence. Conversely, physicians need to be aware of the data elicited by nurses so the complete database is the foundation for the total plan of care.

The provision of culturally appropriate care requires understanding of and sensitivity to differences in health beliefs and practices that reflect cultures or subcultures. The challenge is to be sensitive to cultural influences that may affect the clinical encounter without stereotyping the patient based on limited knowledge of the culture of origin. Three overarching concepts that are influenced by culture and affect the clinical encounter are perception of illness or explanatory model, patterns of kinship and decision making, and comfort with touch.[1]

This chapter focuses on history taking and physical examination of the patient with heart disease. Emphasis is placed on those sections of the health history and physical examination that are affected by heart disease. General assessment techniques, with their rationale, are described. Competence in obtaining a history and in performing a physical examination cannot be achieved simply by reading the material presented. It is vitally important to become actively involved in clinical assessment, ideally with a qualified preceptor. Many hours of practice are required before the beginning student becomes skilled in assessment techniques.

HISTORY

Cardiovascular History

Patient acuity, presentation, and history determine the extent of cardiovascular history obtained. Cardiac patients who are acutely ill require a different initial history than do cardiac patients with stable or chronic conditions. A patient experiencing a myocardial infarction requires immediate, and possibly life-saving, medical and nursing interventions (e.g., relief of chest discomfort and treatment of arrhythmia) rather than an extensive interview. For this patient, asking a few, well-chosen questions regarding chest discomfort using the patient's descriptors are important. In addition, associated symptoms (such as shortness of breath or palpitations), drug allergies and reactions, current medications, history of cardiac and other major illnesses, and smoking history should be determined while assessing vital signs (heart rate and rhythm and blood pressure) and starting an intravenous line. As the patient's condition stabilizes, a more extensive history should be obtained. Cardiac patients who are not acutely ill benefit from a more detailed history and physical examination.

A comprehensive history includes the following areas:

- Identifying information
- Chief complaint or presenting problem
- History of the present illness
- Past history
- Review of systems
- Family history
- Personal and social history
- Perceived health status
- Functional patterns

The responsibility for obtaining particular portions of the health history varies with practice model and setting. In traditional, hospital-based practice models, the first six areas of the history are usually obtained by a physician, some data related to personal and social history are obtained by a physician and some by a nurse, and data related to perceived health status and functional patterns are obtained by a nurse. In collaborative practice models, all data may be obtained by an advanced-practice provider (nurse practitioner or physician assistant), or responsibility for all areas of data collection may be shared by the physician, advanced-practice provider, nurse, and other members of the health care team. The cardiac nurse uses the data to make informed clinical judgments, to monitor change over time, to identify patient and family learning needs, and to coordinate care across settings.

Health History

The health history is the patient's story of his or her diseases, symptoms, illness experiences, and responses to actual and potential health problems. Because concepts of health and healing are rooted in culture, it is essential to elicit information about the person's beliefs about the causes, symptoms, and treatment of illness. Empathy, openness, and interest communicated by the clinician will enable patients to share their perspectives and beliefs.

The history-taking process may be the first phase in establishing a therapeutic relationship. The history is a precise, concise, chronologic description of the patient's current health status. The patient is the primary source of historical data; however, questioning of family members or close friends may provide essential information about symptoms and the impact of heart disease on family members. For example, the bed partner is more likely than the patient to provide a history of periodic respiration or sleep apnea. Review of records from previous encounters is a valuable secondary source of historical data.

The primary symptoms of heart disease include chest discomfort, dyspnea, syncope, palpitations, edema, cough, hemoptysis, and excess fatigue. Heart disease develops slowly, and the patient may have a long period of asymptomatic disease and may present initially with acute collapse. To describe the health history, a sample symptom, chest discomfort, is used throughout this chapter. A systematic approach is useful in differentiating chest discomfort due to serious, life-threatening conditions from those conditions that are less serious or would be treated in a different manner.[2] Table 9-1 summarizes conditions associated with chest discomfort.

Identifying Information

The patient's name, the name by which he or she prefers to be called, his or her age and birth date, and date and time of the interview are all recorded under identification of the patient. Country of origin, religious or cultural group, education, and socioeconomic level constitute optional information that may be

Table 9-1 • DIFFERENTIAL DIAGNOSIS OF EPISODIC CHEST PAIN RESEMBLING ANGINA PECTORIS

Diagnosis	Duration	Quality	Provocation	Relief	Location	Comment
Effort angina	5–15 minutes	Visceral (pressure)	During effort or motion	Rest, nitroglycerin	Substernal radiates	First episode vivid
Rest angina	5–15 minutes	Visceral (pressure)	Spontaneous	Nitroglycerin	Substernal radiates	Often nocturnal
Mitral prolapse	Minutes to hours	Superficial (rarely visceral)	Spontaneous (no pattern)	Time	Left anterior	No pattern, variable character
Esophageal reflux	10–60 minutes	Visceral	Recumbency, lack of food	Food, antacid	Substernal epigastric	Rarely radiates
Esophageal spasm	50–60 minutes	Visceral	Spontaneous, cold liquids, exercise	Nitroglycerin	Substernal radiates	Mimics angina
Peptic ulcer	Hours	Visceral (burning)	Lack of food, "acid" foods	Food, antacids	Epigastric substernal	
Biliary disease	Hours	Visceral (wax and wane)	Spontaneous, food	Time, analgesia	Epigastric radiates	Colic
Cervical disc	Variable (gradually subsides)	Superficial	Head and neck movement	Time, analgesia	Arm, neck	Not relieved by rest palpation
Hyperventilation	2–3 minutes	Visceral	Emotion tachypnea	Stimulus removal	Substernal	Facial paresthesia
Musculoskeletal	Variable	Superficial	Movement, palpation	Time, analgesia	Multiple	Tenderness
Pulmonary	30+ minutes	Visceral (pressure)	Often spontaneous	Rest, time, bronchodilator	Substernal	Dyspneic

Reprinted with permission from Christie LG Jr, Conti CR. Systematic approach to the evaluation of angina-like chest pain. *Am Heart J.* 1981;102(5):897–912.

included. It is assumed that all data in the history are obtained from the patient; when this is not the case, secondary data sources (e.g., family member, clinical records) should be identified. The use of an interpreter should also be recorded.

Chief Complaint or Presenting Problem

The chief complaint or presenting problem is the reason the person has sought health care and represents his or her priority for treatment. It should be recorded within quotation marks exactly as stated. The chief complaint also should indicate duration, such as "chest discomfort for 2 hours."

An asymptomatic patient may present because of a community screening activity (e.g., "high blood cholesterol discovered on finger-stick last month") or because of a positive diagnostic result (e.g., "positive calcium score on electron beam CT last week").

A patient may have more than one chief complaint. Some complaints are closely related and may be listed together, such as "chest discomfort and weakness for 2 hours." If complaints are unrelated, they should be listed separately in the order of importance to the patient. In general, "the greater the number of symptoms, the less the significance of each."[3]

There are four important points to remember when evaluating chest discomfort.[4]

1. For a patient who has a history of or who is at risk for development of coronary heart disease, always assume that the chest discomfort is secondary to ischemia until proven otherwise. This practice is important because unrelieved myocardial ischemia is immediately life threatening and can extend infarct size, resulting in serious complications such as lethal arrhythmia or cardiogenic shock. Chest discomfort related to other conditions, such as pulmonary emboli, usually is not as immediately life threatening.
2. There may be little correlation between the severity of the chest discomfort and the gravity of its cause. That is, pain is a subjective experience and depends, in part, on a lifetime of learned reactions to it. A stoic person may not admit to having much discomfort and yet may be having a large myocardial infarction. Another person may express extreme pain and yet may be experiencing stable angina rather than an acute myocardial infarction. Stress can increase pain. Taking into account the patient's usual response to pain (often obtained from a family member) may help the nurse interpret the patient's pain response better. In addition, older adults or people with diabetes may have altered sensory perception and little or no discomfort in the presence of severe disease.[5] When present, positive objective signs, such as ST segment shifts on the electrocardiogram, are clear indicators of the significance of the subjective symptom. It is important to realize that the absence of electrocardiographic criteria for ischemia or infarction does not eliminate the clinical significance of the chest discomfort.
3. There is a poor correlation between the location of chest discomfort and its source because of the concept of "referred pain," which is pain originating in one location but being interpreted by the patient as occurring in another location. Commonly, cardiac discomfort is perceived as being in the arm, jaw, neck, or epigastric area rather than in the chest.
4. The patient may have more than one clinical problem occurring simultaneously, particularly if he or she has delayed seeking medical assistance.

History of Present Illness

For the symptomatic patient, obtaining the history of the present illness starts with a more detailed discussion of the chief complaint. Begin with an open-ended question, such as "Tell me more about your chest discomfort." There is a wide range in patients' abilities to express thoughts accurately, chronologically, and succinctly. Some patients need guidance more than others. Listen to the patient. It is best to let patients tell their stories in a comfortable manner. However, patients who appear to be rambling need to be redirected by clarifying or leading questions. The information that must be obtained when describing any symptom is the time and manner of onset, frequency and duration, location, quality, quantity, setting, associated symptoms, alleviating or aggravating factors, pertinent negative responses, impact of the symptom on usual or desired activities, and the meaning attributed to the symptom by the patient.

The *time of onset* should be recorded, when possible, with both the date and time (e.g., "9 PM on December 22nd"). When the patient presents with chest discomfort, it is essential to know how long the discomfort has been present and if it has been present continuously since onset. The *manner of onset* is the way in which the symptom began. For example, discomfort may begin suddenly and reach maximum intensity immediately, or there may be a growing awareness of the discomfort over time. *Frequency and duration* should be stated specifically rather than generally (e.g., "once a week," "once a day," or "more than three times a day"). Likewise, patients should be assisted to express the duration of the discomfort, as in "2 minutes," "15 minutes," or "1 hour." For patients with a history of angina, it is also important to determine if there has been any change in frequency or duration of chest discomfort, which suggests worsening of the underlying disease.

Ask the patient to describe the exact *location* of the symptom by pointing to it. Cardiac pain is diffuse, and the patient often rubs a hand over the sternum and precordium. Chest pain that can be precisely located with a fingertip is usually related to chest wall abnormalities.[6] If the pain radiates, the patient should trace its path with a fingertip. The *quality* of a symptom refers to its unique characteristics, such as color, appearance, and texture. It is important to use various descriptive terms when questioning a patient about chest discomfort. They may describe the discomfort as a pressure, heaviness or squeezing sensation. Chest discomfort is so subjective that its quality is particularly difficult to describe. Thus, whenever possible, it is important to use the patient's own words (in quotation marks). *Angina* means tightening, and the discomfort associated with angina may be described as "pressing," "squeezing," "tightening," "strangling," or "constricting."[6] The patient's response to the symptom also should be recorded (e.g., "It makes me stop what I'm doing and sit down," or "I can continue my activities without stopping").

Quantity refers to the size, extent, or amount of the symptom. The quantity of the chest discomfort is described in terms of its severity. Again, quantity is extremely subjective and might be rated best on a 10-point scale, ranging from "barely noticeable" (1) to "the worst pain ever" (10). The severity of pain should be recorded as a fraction (e.g., 2/10 or 10/10).

Ask patients to describe the *setting* and if they were alone or with someone when the symptom occurred. If the symptom has occurred before, ascertain if the setting, circumstances, or the presence of another person is consistent during symptom onset. This information may be useful later in counseling or helping a patient gain insight into the development of his or her symptoms.

Chest discomfort that is reliably associated with activity (e.g., walking up hill) is a specific indicator of cardiac ischemia.

The patient should be asked to describe any *associated symptoms* that always accompany the chief complaint. For example, palpitations and dizziness might always precede the chest discomfort. If the patient mentions associated symptoms, these should be described in the same manner as the chief complaint (i.e., quality, quantity, onset, duration). It is important to note whether these associated symptoms occur consistently with the chief complaint or occur independently at other times.

Alleviating factors, such as resting, changing position, or taking medication, should be noted. Change in the time it takes for alleviating factors to be effective should be identified. For example, if, in the past, the chest discomfort resolved with 5 minutes of rest and now requires 10 minutes, worsening or a new pathologic process is suggested. *Aggravating factors*, such as eating, exercising, or being in a cold climate, also must be recorded. These factors can provide helpful diagnostic information. To complete the present illness history, it is also important to record any *pertinent negative responses* to the interviewer's questions, such as "The chest discomfort is not made worse by strenuous exercise." The patient should be specifically asked about palpitations, dizziness, syncope, dyspnea, orthopnea, and paroxysmal nocturnal dyspnea, if these symptoms have not already been described.

Impact of the symptom on usual or desired activities should be explored. Some people with recurrent chest discomfort reduce their activity over time to try and prevent chest discomfort. It is essential that clinicians understand how the symptom or disease has affected the patient's activity and perceived quality of life.

Throughout the interview, the nurse observes the patient carefully and may begin to understand the meaning the illness has for the patient. The personal meaning of the illness can amplify or reduce the symptom experience and course of action. When interviewing members of a culture not one's own, ask "Can you tell me what caused your illness?" and about the use of home remedies, foods, or traditional healers.[7]

The results of diagnostic or laboratory testing specifically related to heart disease are included in the *history of present illness.* Prior cardiac events (e.g., coronary artery bypass surgery or myocardial infarction) are included also.

Cardiovascular risk factors and current activity may be added in a separate paragraph to the conventional content of the history of present illness. Risk factors for coronary heart disease are described in detail elsewhere in this textbook.

Sample questions that may be used in assessing the patient with acute or recurrent chest discomfort are listed below. Similar questions may be generated to assess patients with other symptoms. However, it is important to phrase the questions according to the appropriateness of the situation and logically to pursue areas where further clarification is necessary.

- When exactly do you get the discomfort? Are you having discomfort now?
- What were you doing when the chest discomfort occurred?
- Exactly how often does the chest discomfort occur?
- How many minutes does it usually last?
- Can you point to the exact location where it starts?
- Does the discomfort move anywhere else?
- If so, can you trace its path with your fingertip?
- What words would you use to describe how the discomfort feels?
- What do you do when you have the chest discomfort?
- Quantify your discomfort on a 1-to-10 scale.
- Where were you when the discomfort occurred?
- If the chest discomfort has occurred before, have you always been in the same place?
- Were you alone at the time or with someone?
- Did you notice any other symptoms that occurred at the same time?
- If yes, does this other symptom ever occur by itself?
- What can you do to make the chest discomfort better?
- What can you do to make it worse?
- Are you taking any medication, botanical medications, supplements, foods or home remedies to improve your chest discomfort?
- If yes, what is the medication, botanical medication, supplement, food, or home remedy?
- Does any medication you are taking affect your chest discomfort?
- If yes, what is the medication?
- What time of day do you prefer to take your medication?
- Are you doing anything else to improve your chest discomfort, for example yoga or meditation?
- What activities have you given up because of your chest discomfort?
- What do you think this chest discomfort means?
- Do you know anyone else who has had this kind of discomfort?

Past History

The past history includes past illnesses and interventions not directly related to the present illness. For a patient with chest discomfort, the history of a previous myocardial infarction, coronary artery bypass surgery, or cholecystectomy belongs in the *history of present illness*, whereas a remote appendectomy does not. Major elements of the *past history* include childhood and adult illnesses, accidents and injuries, current health status, current medications, allergies, and health maintenance. Always ask about major illnesses such as chronic obstructive airway disease, diabetes mellitus, bleeding disorders, and acquired immunodeficiency syndrome (AIDS).

Allergic reactions (e.g., to drugs, food, environmental agents, or animals) also should be noted. Always ask if the patient has an allergy to penicillin or to commonly used emergency drugs, such as lidocaine hydrochloride and morphine sulfate. Allergy to shellfish has previously been suggested as representing an iodine sensitivity. Documented allergies to contrast media or shellfish should be noted; but do not necessarily imply that the patient is allergic to iodine.[8] Both the allergen and the reaction should always be noted, because some patients confuse an allergic reaction with a drug's side effect.

Medication history includes all prescription and over-the-counter drugs, including botanical medicines, supplements, and home remedies. Over-the-counter preparations, botanical medications, and supplements that increase heart rate or afterload may precipitate or worsen symptoms. If the patient has brought medications with him or her, these should be reviewed by the nurse and then sent home or to the appropriate area for safekeeping.

Psychosocial History

Family History

The major purpose of the family history is to assess risk factors affecting the patient's current or future health. Notations regarding the age and health status of each first-degree family member are made: living and well, deceased, and the possible or confirmed diagnosis now or at death. Family occurrences of diabetes, kidney disease, tuberculosis, cancer, arthritis, asthma, allergies, mental illness, alcoholism, and drug addiction are included. A family history of coronary heart disease, myocardial infarction, or sudden death would be included in the history of present illness for a patient presenting with chest discomfort.

Personal and Social History

The personal and social history includes important and relevant information about the patient as a person. A person's response to illness is determined in part by his or her cultural background, socioeconomic standing, education, and beliefs about the illness. Major elements include health habits, home situation, and supports and resources. Occupational history may be included here or in the past history. *Health habits* include alcohol, drug, or tobacco use; nutrition; sleep; and physical activity. Use of alcohol and the amount per time period (day, week, year) should be recorded. The use of recreational drugs, especially cocaine and its derivative "crack," should also be assessed. The cigarette smoking history should be recorded as the number of pack-years (packs per day multiplied by the number of years) the patient has smoked. For ex-smokers, approximate quit date should be recorded. Other tobacco use, such as pipe or cigar smoking or chewing tobacco, should be recorded. Special diets, such as low-sodium, low-fat, low-carbohydrate, or high-protein diets, should be identified, and the patient's usual eating pattern should be described. The usual number of hours the patient sleeps and circumstances that impair or facilitate sleep should be assessed.

Current Living Circumstances. These circumstances include marital status, number of children, occupation, financial resources, and hobbies. Patients should also be asked about their current living arrangements; single family home, apartment, with roommate or alone, or shelter or homeless.

Perceived Health and Coping Challenges. The patient's perception of his or her current health status as either good or bad is helpful in assessing how he or she views its effect on daily living. For example, a 42-year-old man with an old anterior myocardial infarction is seen in the clinic. His chief complaint is extreme fatigue that prevents him from working a full day at the office. Initial investigation focuses on ruling out any new process affecting the adequacy of cardiac output, such as a left ventricular aneurysm or decreased left ventricular function. Nonpathophysiologic causes for fatigue must be considered also, such as fear of overstressing his heart and sudden death, changes in the work situation, family difficulties, or depression.

Being aware of patients' goals in terms of health and lifestyle is important in determining whether their expectations are realistic. "What do you see yourself doing 3 months from now?" is a good way to ask the patient to define the goal. Another approach is ascertaining what changes the patient would be willing to make in life if the goal could not be achieved.

Assessing the patient's and family's expectations of health care has implications for teaching. For example, is the patient with unstable angina pectoris who has been admitted after "cardiac catheterization" able to explain what the test was and why it resulted in admission? Communication among the health care team members is essential before planning any teaching.

Resources and Support System. It is important to consider the patient's strengths and support system when planning care across the continuum: environmental resources, such as the proximity to the hospital; personal—social support, such as a spouse to provide home care; and economic support, such as adequate insurance, are all examples. Needed resources that are not readily available also must be considered. Knowledge of the patient's health benefits and financial status assists the health care team in designing an affordable therapeutic regimen (e.g., the avoidance of expensive combination or sustained-release medications when other drugs and dosage forms that are as effective and less costly are available).

Review of Systems

To ensure that all important areas have been considered, a systematic review of all body systems is conducted. Lists of major symptoms associated with each body system are included in health assessment textbooks.[8] Some clinicians prefer to conduct the review of systems simultaneously with the physical examination. For the patient with chest discomfort, the review of the cardiac, pulmonary, and gastrointestinal systems is logically included in the history of present illness.

Functional Patterns

Clinical information related to function is collected in the following areas[9]:

- Health perception–health management
- Nutrition–metabolism
- Elimination
- Activity–exercise
- Cognitive–perceptual
- Sleep–rest
- Self-perception–self-concept
- Roles and relationships
- Sexuality
- Coping–stress
- Values–beliefs

Information collected within these functional patterns does not duplicate information collected within other areas of the health history. The sequence of data gathered in the functional assessment is determined by the patient's clinical condition and the purpose of the encounter. Relevant data obtained earlier in the history should not be repeated.

For the acutely ill cardiac patient who is admitted to the hospital, areas that affect the hospital experience are assessed first. As the patient is able, all functional patterns are assessed. To facilitate the gathering of subjective information for the functional assessment, examples of questions, using the sample symptom of chest discomfort, are listed below. Functional assessment is an ongoing process that evaluates the effect of intervention on patient outcome.

Health Perception–Health Management. Collect the following information:

- What concerns do you have about your health or hospitalization?
- What things are important to you while you are hospitalized? How can we make this experience as easy as possible for you?
- What do you think caused this illness (symptom)?
- Compared with others your age, how would you rate your general health?
- What things do you believe are important to maintain your health?

Nutrition–Metabolism. Collect the following information:

- What do you like to eat (including cultural or ethnic favorites)?
- How are your foods prepared (canned or commercially prepared foods vs. fresh foods)?
- Do you usually eat in a restaurant, fast-food outlet, or at home?

- Who shops for groceries?
- Who prepares the meals?
- Are you on a special diet?

Elimination. Collect the following information:

- Is the amount that you urinate normal for you?
- Do you ever get up at night to use the bathroom? If so, how many times?
- If there was a change in elimination pattern, when did you notice it?
- Do you sometimes lose urine or find that you cannot quite make it to the bathroom?
- Do you take a diuretic? If so, when do you take it?
- What is your usual frequency of bowel movements? When was your last movement?
- Are there things you do to maintain that pattern?

Activity–Exercise. Collect the following information:

- Have you noticed a change in your usual or desired activity level?
- Do you have sufficient energy for your desired activities?
- What is the most strenuous activity you perform on a regular basis? How often and how long? What stops you?
- What leisure or recreational activities do you enjoy? Are you currently able to participate in these activities? What prevents your participation?
- Are you satisfied with your current level of activity?

Cognitive–Perceptual. Collect the following information:

- Do you have any difficulty with seeing or hearing? Glasses or hearing aid?
- Do you think as fast as you used to? As clearly?
- In general, what is the easiest way for you to learn new material? Any learning difficulties?
- Do you understand why you are in the hospital?
- What does your diagnosis mean to you?
- What is your understanding of the treatment plan?
- Do you understand the risk factors for heart disease and how to modify them?
- Do you understand how long you will be in the hospital and when you can return to your usual activities of daily living?

Sleep–Rest. Collect the following information:

- How many hours do you usually sleep? What hours?
- Do you have difficulty falling asleep or staying asleep? Has this been a change for you or have you always had this difficulty?
- Do you follow a specific bedtime routine or ritual?
- Do you snore loudly?
- Do you feel rested when you wake up in the morning?[10]
- Are you tired and excessively sleepy during daytime hours?[10]

Self-Perception–Self-Concept. Collect the following information:

- How would you describe yourself? Your personality? Your approach to life?
- Most of the time, do you feel good about yourself?
- Have you noticed changes in yourself or your body? Do these changes concern you?

Roles and Relationships. Collect the following information:

- Do you live alone? With whom do you live?
- Do you have a close friend or confidant?
- How do you and those close to you feel about your illness?
- Do you often feel lonely? Do you feel part of the neighborhood in which you live?

Sexuality. Collect the following information:

- Have you experienced any changes in your sexuality? Problems in sexual relationships?
- For women: are you still menstruating? Are you taking hormone replacements? Do you have menopausal symptoms (such as hot flashes and sleep disturbances)?

Coping–Stress. Collect the following information:

- Do you feel tense or anxious much of the time? What helps? Do you use medicines for anxiety?
- When you feel stressed, who is most helpful to you?
- When you have big problems in your life, how do you handle them? Does that usually work for you?

Values–Beliefs. Collect the following information:

- Are you generally satisfied with your life?
- Is religion important to you?
- Do you hold religious or other beliefs that you wish to observe here?

Functional and Therapeutic Classification

After the history is completed, it may be possible to categorize the patient according to the New York Heart Association's Functional and Therapeutic Classification (Table 9-2).[11] This classification may be helpful in assessing symptom severity and monitoring effects of treatment over time. The patient's functional classification may improve as recovery from an acute event, such as myocardial infarction, occurs or as intervention is optimized. Conversely, it may decline with worsening or additional disease.

PHYSICAL ASSESSMENT

Assessment of physical findings confirms or expands data obtained in the health history. Baseline information is obtained at the initial encounter, and frequency of subsequent assessments is based on the clinical encounter. Change in the data over time documents progression of, or recovery from, acute disease; new disease; the effectiveness of current interventions; and the patient's current functional status. The type, degree, and rate of change assist the nurse in identifying or predicting immediate or long-term problems, formulating nursing diagnoses, planning care, and establishing individual patient outcome criteria.

In the acutely ill cardiac patient, segments of the physical examination are performed every 2 to 4 hours or more frequently if indicated. Although some data may be available from monitoring devices, physical examination assists in evaluating the accuracy of those data. As the acutely ill patient improves, assessments are routinely done once per shift or more frequently if indicated. If a rapid change in patient condition occurs, the initial assessment is problem focused and the complete assessment is done at a later time. Because nurses spend 24 hours per day with the hospitalized patient, they are in the best position to identify any changes that occur. It is to the patient's benefit for changes to be detected early, before serious complications develop. Any changes observed in the examination should be documented in the patient's record and reported to the physician. To collect, correlate, and interpret

Table 9-2 • FUNCTIONAL AND THERAPEUTIC CLASSIFICATION OF PATIENTS WITH DISEASES OF THE HEART

Functional	Classification	Therapeutic	Classification
Class I	Patients with cardiac disease but without resulting limitations of physical activity. Ordinary physical activity does not cause undue fatigue, palpitation, dyspnea, or anginal pain	Class A	Patients with cardiac disease whose physical activity need not be restricted in any way
Class II	Patients with cardiac disease resulting in slight limitation of physical activity. They are comfortable at rest. Ordinary physical activity results in fatigue, palpitation, dyspnea, or anginal pain	Class B	Patients with cardiac disease whose ordinary physical activity need not be restricted, but who should be advised against severe or competitive efforts
Class III	Patients with cardiac disease resulting in marked limitation of physical activity. They are comfortable at rest. Less than ordinary physical activity causes fatigue, palpitation, dyspnea, or anginal pain.	Class C	Patients with cardiac disease whose ordinary physical activity should be moderately restricted and whose more strenuous efforts should be discontinued
Class IV	Patients with cardiac disease resulting in inability to carry on any physical activity without discomfort. Symptoms of cardiac insufficiency or of the anginal syndrome may be present even at rest. If any physical activity is undertaken, discomfort is increased	Class D	Patients with cardiac disease whose ordinary physical activity should be markedly restricted
		Class E	Patients with cardiac disease who should be at complete rest, confined to bed or chair

Reprinted with permission from New York Heart Association Criteria Committee. *Diseases of the Heart and Blood Vessels: Nomenclature and Criteria for Diagnosis.* 9th ed. Boston, MA: Little, Brown; 1994.

the data accurately, a thorough understanding of the cardiac cycle is essential. A cardiac physical assessment should include an evaluation of:

- The heart as a pump—reduced pulse pressure, cardiac enlargement, and presence of murmurs and gallop rhythms
- Filling volumes and pressures—the degree of jugular venous pressure and the presence or absence of crackles, peripheral edema, and postural changes in blood pressure
- Cardiac output—heart rate, blood pressure, pulse pressure, systemic vascular resistance, urine output, and central nervous system manifestations
- Compensatory mechanisms—increased filling volumes, peripheral vasoconstriction, and elevated heart rate

The order and techniques of examination proceed logically. The precise order may vary with the setting and the condition of the patient. With practice, the focused cardiovascular examination can be done in approximately 10 minutes:

- General appearance
- Head
- Arterial pulse
- Jugular venous pressure
- Blood pressure
- Peripheral vasculature
- Heart
- Lungs
- Abdomen

General Appearance

Observe the general appearance of the patient while the history is being obtained.[6] The patient's appearance and responses provide cues to the cardiovascular status. Note general build, skin color, presence of shortness of breath, and distention of neck veins. Assess the patient's level of distress. If he or she is in pain, the patient's response to it may assist in the differential diagnosis. For example, moving about is a characteristic response to the pain of myocardial infarction, whereas sitting quietly is more characteristic of angina, and leaning forward is more characteristic of pericarditis.[12] Some abnormalities of the arterial pulses may be observed unobtrusively. For example, patients with severe aortic insufficiency may have bounding pulses that cause the head to bob. Note appropriateness of weight; malnutrition and cachexia are associated with chronic, severe heart failure.[6] Skeletal manifestations of Marfan syndrome, tall stature, and arachnodactyly, may be observed. Level of consciousness should be described. Appropriateness of thought content, reflecting the adequacy of cerebral perfusion, is particularly important to evaluate. Family members who are most familiar with the patient can be of help in alerting the examiner to subtle behavior changes. The nurse also should be aware of the patient's anxiety level, not only to attempt to put the patient more at ease, but to realize its effects on the cardiovascular system.

Height, Weight, and Waist Circumference

Height and weight are best measured using a standing platform scale with a height attachment. Weak, immobile, or critically ill patients may require a bed or chair scale for weighing, and it may be necessary to rely on the patient's self-reported height. Weight is an indicator of nutritional and fluid status; excessive weight indicates increased cardiovascular risk.

Body mass index (BMI) describes relative weight for height. BMI is calculated as weight in kilograms (kg) divided by the square of the height in meters (m^2). In adults, obesity is defined as a BMI of 30 kg/m^2 or more; overweight is a BMI of 25 kg/m^2 or more.[13]

Larger BMI and abdominal fat distribution are associated with increased cardiovascular risk.[14] In overweight people, waist circumference of 102 cm (40 in) in men or 88 cm (35 in) in women indicates increased risk of cardiovascular disease, Type II diabetes mellitus, and metabolic syndrome.

Head

The examination of the head includes assessment of facial characteristics, color, temperature, and eyes. Advanced practice nurses may examine the fundi and retinal vasculature.

Facial Characteristics

Examination of the facial characteristics may aid in the recognition of disorders affecting the cardiovascular system.[6] *Coronary heart disease* may be suggested by the presence of an earlobe crease. *Rheumatic heart disease* with severe mitral stenosis is associated with a malar flush, cyanotic lips, and slight jaundice from hepatic congestion. With severe aortic regurgitation, head bobbing with each heartbeat (de Musset sign) may be present. Infective endocarditis is associated with a "café au lait" complexion. *Constrictive pericarditis* and *tricuspid valve disease* tend to cause facial edema. *Pheochromocytoma* is associated with episodic facial flushing, as well as severe hypertension and tachyarrhythmia.

Systemic conditions may affect or reflect cardiovascular function or treatment.[6] *Systemic lupus erythematosus* may present with a butterfly rash on the face and may suggest inflammatory heart disease. *Myxedema* is characterized by dry, sparse hair; loss of lateral eyebrows; a dull, expressionless face; and periorbital puffiness. Because a myocardial effect of hypothyroidism is reduced cardiac output, heart failure may develop in these patients. *Cushing syndrome* is characterized by moon facies, hirsutism, acne, and centripetal obesity with thin extremities. High blood pressure frequently occurs with Cushing syndrome.

Color

Cyanosis is the bluish discoloration seen through the skin and mucous membranes when the concentration of reduced hemoglobin exceeds 5 g/100 mL of blood. *Peripheral cyanosis* implies reduced blood flow to the periphery. Because more time is available for the tissues to extract oxygen from the hemoglobin molecule, the arteriovenous oxygen difference widens. Cyanosis of the nose, lips, and earlobes is considered peripheral. Peripheral cyanosis may occur physiologically with the vasoconstriction associated with anxiety or a cold environment, or pathologically in conditions that reduce blood flow to the periphery, such as cardiogenic shock.

Central cyanosis, as observed in the buccal mucosa, implies serious heart or lung disease and is accompanied by peripheral cyanosis. In severe heart disease, a right-to-left shunt exists in which blood passes through the lungs without being fully oxygenated, as happens in severe heart failure with interstitial pulmonary edema. In severe lung disease, changes produced by chronic obstructive airway disease or fibrosis impede oxygenation. *Pallor* can denote anemia (with concomitant decreased oxygen-carrying capacity) or an increased systemic vascular resistance. *Jaundice* can be associated with hepatic engorgement from right ventricular failure.

Temperature

Temperature reflects the balance of heat production and dissipation in the body. Normal oral temperature is considered to be 37°C (98.6°F). However, there is a diurnal pattern of temperature fluctuation, with temperatures as low as 35.8°C (96.4°F) orally in the early morning to as high as 37.3°C (99.1°F) orally in the late afternoon or evening. Oral temperatures average 0.5°C (1.0°F) lower than rectal temperatures, but this difference is quite variable.[8] Normal body temperature may be less than 37°C in older adults because of reduced heat production (lower metabolic activity, less muscle mass and activity) and conservation (less insulation).[15]

In hospitalized patients, body temperature usually is measured on admission and then every 4 hours or more often if indicated. After cardiac surgery, temperature is measured every 15 to 30 minutes until rewarming is complete, and every 1 to 4 hours until normothermia is achieved. Measure the temperature orally unless the patient is unconscious or unable to close his or her mouth. Body temperatures also may be measured rectally, by means of a pulmonary artery catheter equipped with a thermistor, by means of a thermistor-equipped urinary bladder catheter, or with a device that measures temperature in the insulated auditory meatus close to the tympanic membrane or temporal artery. Pulmonary artery, urinary bladder, tympanic, and rectal temperatures are all considered to be core temperatures; however, they actually measure somewhat different things, and simultaneous measurements may not agree, especially during hypothermia. Pulmonary artery temperature measures the mean blood temperature that results from core thermogenesis and peripheral heat loss or gain. Because urine is a filtrate of blood, urinary bladder temperature also reflects mean blood temperature, but may be falsely low in the setting of low-output renal failure. During hypothermia after cardiac surgery, rectal temperatures reflect peripheral, rather than core, temperatures.[16]

Eyes

The eyes are examined for vision and appearance. A funduscopic examination may be performed.

Vision. Vision is assessed to determine if defects exist that may affect activities of daily living. The examination is as simple as having the patient read a name tag or identify an object.

Appearance. *Corneal arcus*, a thin, grayish-white circle around the iris, may occur normally with aging (Fig. 9-1A). When seen in white people younger than age 40 years, corneal arcus suggests hyperlipidemia. *Xanthelasmas* are slightly raised, yellowish plaques of cholesterol in the skin that appear along the nasal side of one or both eyelids (Fig. 9-1B). They are associated with hyperlipidemia but also may occur normally. *Ophthalmitis* and *petechial* and *subconjunctival hemorrhages* of the upper and lower eyelids may be seen with bacterial endocarditis.

A Corneal Arcus

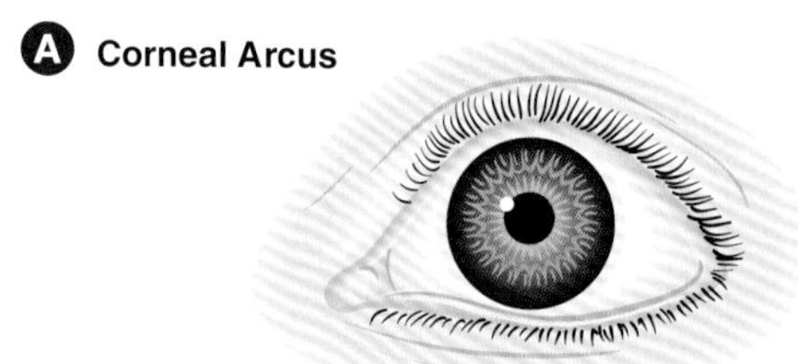

A corneal arcus is a thin grayish white arc or circle not quite at the edge of the cornea. It accompanies normal aging but may also be seen in younger people, especially African Americans. In young people, a corneal arcus suggests the possibility of hyperlipoproteinemia but does not prove it. Some surveys have revealed no relationship.

B Xanthelasmas

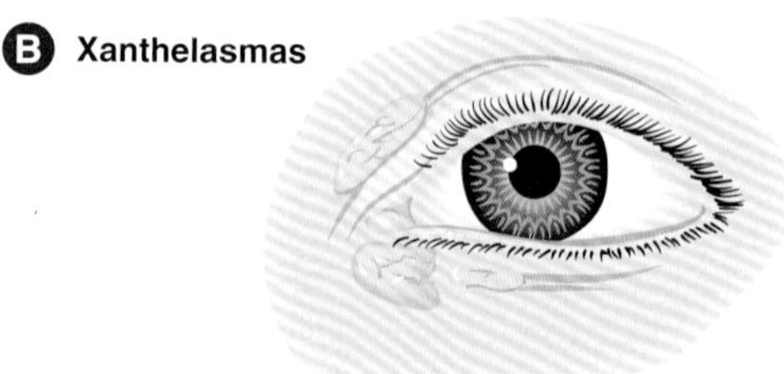

Slightly raised, yellowish, well circumscribed plaques in the skin, xanthelasmas appear along the nasal portions of one or both eyelids. They may accompany lipid disorders (e.g., hypercholesterolemia), but may also occur independently.

Figure 9-1. Eye changes suggestive of hyperlipoproteinemia. **(A)** Corneal arcus. **(B)** Xanthelasmas.

Fundi. Examination of the ocular fundi provides the only opportunity for direct visualization of blood vessels. Vascular changes from high blood pressure and diabetes mellitus can be detected in the arteries and small veins of the retina. In general health care, funduscopic examination is conducted without pharmacologic dilation of the pupils. Physiologic dilation may be maximized by darkening the room and asking the patient to gaze off in the distance. Photographs printed in books are taken through a maximally dilated pupil with a special camera. The view through the ophthalmoscope is only a small portion of the retina. It is necessary to direct the ophthalmoscope in varying directions, following blood vessels and observing the retinal structures and background.

The *funduscopic examination technique* is as follows[8]:

- Darken the room.
- Turn on the ophthalmoscope light; select the large round beam of white light.
- Adjust the lens disc to 0 diopter. Keep your index finger on the lens disc throughout the examination.
- Use your right hand and right eye to examine the patient's right eye; use your left hand and left eye to examine the patient's left eye.
- Place your opposite thumb over the patient's eyebrow to gain proprioceptive guidance as you move closer to the patient.
- Ask the patient to look straight ahead and to fix his or her gaze on a distant point.
- Brace the ophthalmoscope firmly against your face, with your eye directly behind the sight hole.
- Position yourself 15 in away from the patient and 15 degrees lateral to his or her line of vision. Shine the light beam on the patient's pupil and note the *red reflex.* Absence of a *red reflex* suggests a lens opacity, such as a cataract.
- With both of your eyes open and keeping the light beam focused on the red reflex, move horizontally at a 15-degree angle slowly toward the patient. When you are approximately 1.5 to 2 in (3 to 5 cm) from the patient, the optic disc or blood vessels should come into view (Fig. 9-2). Rotate lenses with your index finger until fundic structures are as clearly visible as possible.
- To overcome corneal reflection (light reflected back into the examiner's eye), direct the light beam toward the edge of the pupil rather than through its center.
- Examine the *optic disc,* a yellowish-orange to creamy pink oval or round structure. If you do not see the disc, follow a blood vessel centrally (by noting the angles of vessel branching and the progressive enlargement of vessel size toward the disc) until it is visible. Assess disc border clarity (nasal margin may be normally somewhat blurred) and color.
- Identify the *retinal arteries* and *veins* using the differential criteria of color, size, and light reflex (or reflection; Fig. 9-3A). Arteries and veins appear to originate from the *physiologic cup,* a small, white depression in the optic disc. Arteries are light red, are two thirds to four fifths the diameter of veins, and have a bright light reflex. Veins are dark red, are larger than arteries, and have an inconspicuous or absent light reflex. Follow the vessels peripherally in all directions, noting the character of the arteriovenous crossings. To examine the extreme periphery, instruct the patient to look up, down, temporally, and nasally.
- Assess the retina for any *lesions,* noting size, shape, color, and distribution. *Optic disc edema* (swollen optic disc with blurred margins) is present in patients with increased intracranial pressure, retinal venous outflow obstruction, inflammation, or ischemia (Fig. 9-4).[8] *Beading* (abnormal constriction) of a retinal vein is common in diabetic retinopathy. With high blood pressure, thickening of the walls and narrowing of the lumen of retinal arteries develop. These changes are observed as *focal narrowing,* a *narrowed column of blood,* and a *narrowed light reflex* (Fig. 9-3B). If opacity is such that no blood column is visible, the artery appears as a *silver wire artery* (Fig. 9-3C). With increased filling and tortuosity, arteries closest to the optic disc manifest an increased light reflex and are known as *copper wire arteries* (Fig. 9-3D). Arteriovenous crossings also are affected by thickening of the artery walls, demonstrated by *tapering* of the vein on either side of the artery (Fig. 9-3E), *arteriovenous nicking* (abrupt cessation of the vein on either side of the artery; Fig. 9-3F), or *banking* of the vein (venous twisting distal to the artery, forming a dark, wide knuckle; Fig. 9-3G).[8,17]

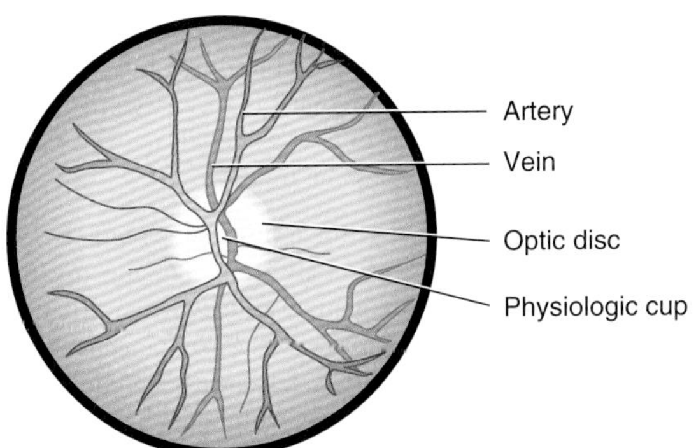

Figure 9-2. Funduscopic examination of retinal structures.

Red spots in the retina may be due to hemorrhage or microaneurysms, which can be associated with hypertension, diabetes, or a number of other conditions.[8,17] *Roth spots,* hemorrhages with white centers, occur with subacute bacterial endocarditis, hypertensive retinopathy, diabetes, intracranial haemorrhage and leukemia.[8,17] *Cotton wool patches* are white or gray and have large irregular shapes and fuzzy borders (Fig. 9-5A). They occur with hypertension and are seen frequently in patients with diabetes, HIV infection and severe anemia. *Hard exudates* are small, creamy white or yellow lesions with well-defined borders (Fig. 9-5B). They occur frequently in clusters and are indicative of diabetes, hypertension, and other conditions.[8] Abnormalities of the fundi are difficult to see, require much practice, and may require eye drops to dilate the pupil.

Arterial Pulse

Information about pulse rate, rhythm, amplitude and contour, and obstruction to blood flow is obtained from palpation of the arterial pulse. Pulses should be evaluated at baseline, before and after vascular procedures that might impair blood flow, and with the onset of any symptom associated with reduced peripheral flow or ischemia. On initial examination, both carotid, both radial, both femoral, both tibial, and both dorsal pulses should be assessed.

Pulse Rate and Rhythm

Pulse rate and rhythm commonly are assessed in the radial artery. However, in certain clinical situations, such as shock (with very low-amplitude or absent peripheral pulses) or during cardiac arrest (when information about central blood flow is essential), pulses should be assessed in the more centrally located carotid artery.

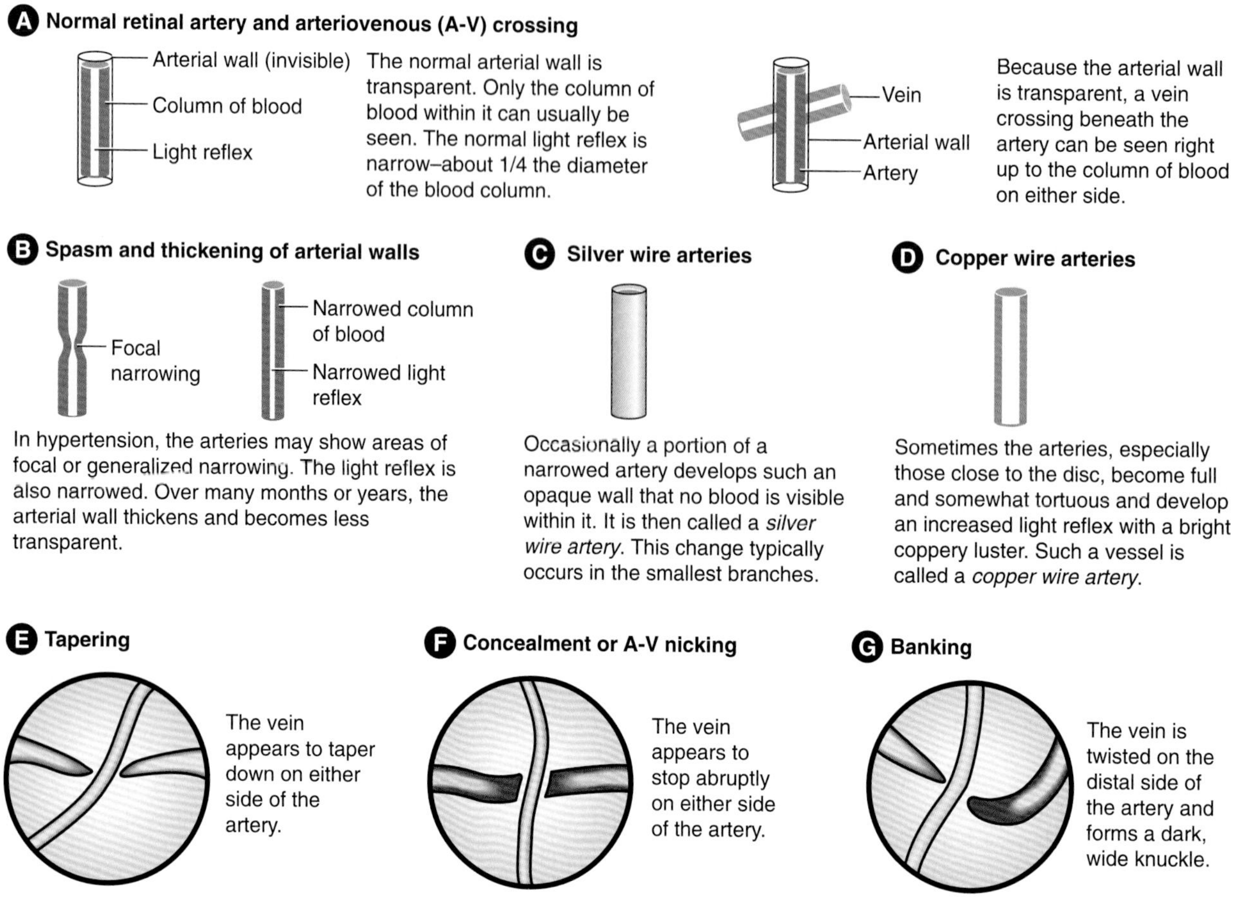

A Normal retinal artery and arteriovenous (A-V) crossing

Arterial wall (invisible)
Column of blood
Light reflex

The normal arterial wall is transparent. Only the column of blood within it can usually be seen. The normal light reflex is narrow–about 1/4 the diameter of the blood column.

Vein
Arterial wall
Artery

Because the arterial wall is transparent, a vein crossing beneath the artery can be seen right up to the column of blood on either side.

B Spasm and thickening of arterial walls

Focal narrowing
Narrowed column of blood
Narrowed light reflex

In hypertension, the arteries may show areas of focal or generalized narrowing. The light reflex is also narrowed. Over many months or years, the arterial wall thickens and becomes less transparent.

C Silver wire arteries

Occasionally a portion of a narrowed artery develops such an opaque wall that no blood is visible within it. It is then called a *silver wire artery.* This change typically occurs in the smallest branches.

D Copper wire arteries

Sometimes the arteries, especially those close to the disc, become full and somewhat tortuous and develop an increased light reflex with a bright coppery luster. Such a vessel is called a *copper wire artery.*

E Tapering

The vein appears to taper down on either side of the artery.

F Concealment or A-V nicking

The vein appears to stop abruptly on either side of the artery.

G Banking

The vein is twisted on the distal side of the artery and forms a dark, wide knuckle.

Figure 9-3. Vascular changes associated with high blood pressure. **(A)** Normal. **(B)** Spasm and thickening of arteriolar walls. **(C)** Silver wire arterioles. **(D)** Copper wire arterioles. **(E)** Venous tapering. **(F)** Arteriovenous nicking. **(G)** Venous banking.

Pulse Rate. The pulse rate at rest usually is between 60 and 100 (average of approximately 70) pulsations per minute. A lower resting heart rate is common in athletes. Conditions or activities such as exercise, fever, and stress increase the pulse rate. Hypothermia, certain drugs, and heart blocks, for example, decrease the pulse rate. Each pulse wave is indicative of a cardiac contraction. However, each cardiac contraction does not necessarily result in a peripheral pulse. In patients with heart disease, pulse rate may be slower than heart rate because not all cardiac contractions perfuse the periphery. Extremely fast heart rates, such as atrial fibrillation with a rapid ventricular response or premature supraventricular or ventricular contractions, have shortened diastolic filling times, resulting in reduced stroke volume and, therefore, diminished or absent pulses. For this reason, pulse rate should not be recorded from the heart rate display on the cardiac monitor or counted from an electrocardiographic strip.

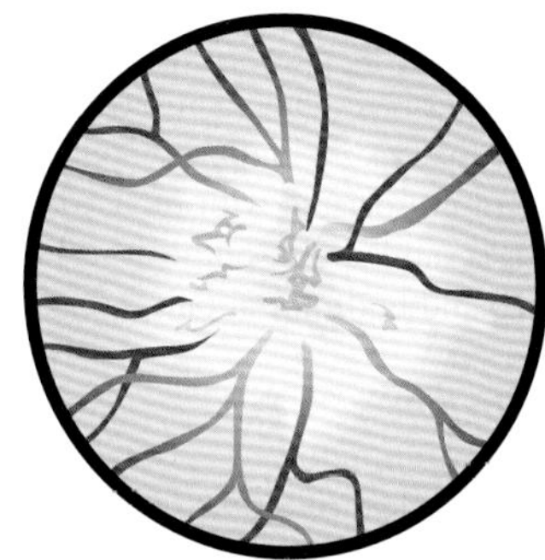

Figure 9-4. Papilledema. The optic disc is swollen, its margins are blurred, and the physiologic cup is not visible.

Using the pads of the index and middle fingers, compress the artery until maximum pulsation is detected. Count the rate. If regular, count for 15 seconds and multiply by 4; if irregular, count for a full minute, noting the variations in rhythm and amplitude.

In all cardiac patients and in any patient with an irregular heart rate, simultaneously auscultate the apical rate and palpate the peripheral rate (*apical–radial rate*); record both rates. It is important that the apical–radial rates be counted during the *same* minute. If the apical–radial difference is very large, if the rate is very fast, or if the examiner is not yet skilled, it may be helpful to have two people count for the same minute.

Pulse Rhythm. Pulse rhythm is normally regular. Physiologic variation can occur with respiration. During inspiration, blood flow to the right heart is increased, right ventricular output is enhanced, and pulmonary venous capacitance is increased. Consequently, blood flow to the left heart is reduced, causing a drop in left ventricular stroke volume. Cardiac output is maintained by a compensatory increase in heart rate (mediated by the baroreceptors). During expiration, the large amount of

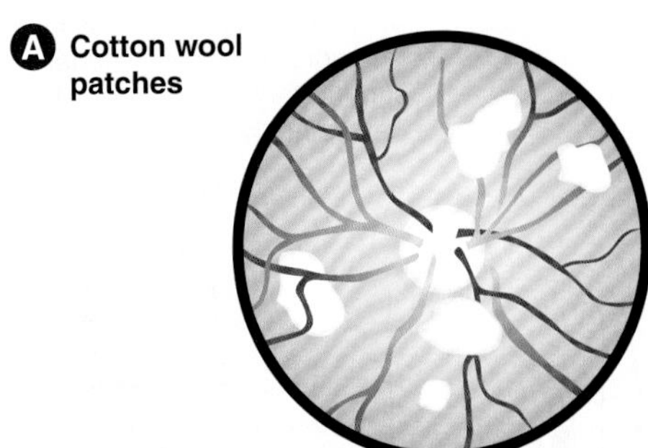

Cotton wool patches are white or grayish, ovoid lesions with irregular (thus "soft") borders. They are moderate in size but usually smaller than the disc. They result from infarcted nerve fibers and are seen with hypertension and many other conditions.

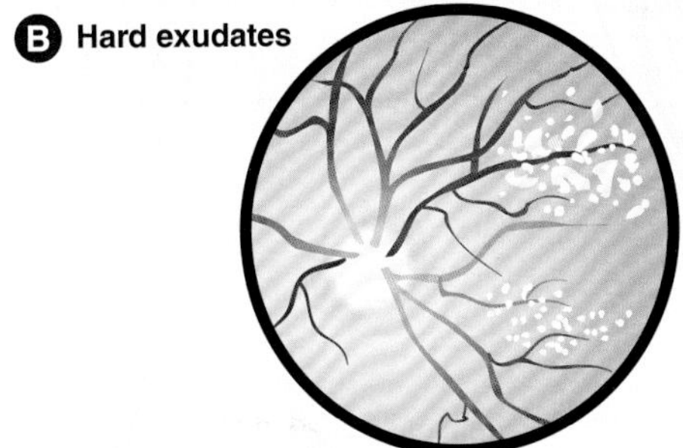

Hard exudates are creamy or yellowish, often bright lesions with well defined (thus "hard") borders. They are small and round (as shown in the lower group of exudates) but may coalesce into larger irregular spots (as shown in the upper group). They often occur in clusters or in circular, linear, or star-shaped patterns. Causes include diabetes and hypertension.

Figure 9-5. Light-colored spots in the retina. **(A)** Cotton wool patches. **(B)** Hard exudates.

blood residing in the pulmonary vascular bed during inspiration reaches the left heart. Left ventricular contractility is enhanced by means of the Frank–Starling mechanism, increasing left ventricular stroke volume. Because an increased heart rate is no longer needed to maintain cardiac output, the heart rate returns to baseline. This physiologically irregular rhythm is termed *sinus arrhythmia*. It is common in people younger than 40 years of age. Other irregular rhythms are not normal. The irregularity should be described as regularly irregular (e.g., every other pulse wave is early) or irregularly irregular (e.g., atrial fibrillation). Occasional, early pulsations that are perceived as transient skips or breaks in an otherwise regular rhythm are common and are not necessarily abnormal.

Pulse Amplitude and Contour

Pulses are described in a variety of ways. The simplest classification is absent, present, and bounding. A 0-to-4 scale is often used, and pulses are graded as follows: absent (0), diminished (1+), normal (2+), moderately increased (3+), and markedly increased (4+).[18] This scale is fairly subjective, and, although an individual tends to be internally consistent over time, different people may grade the same pulse differently. There are also other scales in which the numbers are defined differently.

The amplitude of an arterial pulse is a function of the pulse pressure, which is related to stroke volume, elasticity of the arterial tree, and velocity of left ventricular ejection. Increased stroke volume, as occurs with exercise or excitement, results in increased amplitude and a bounding arterial pulse.

Small, weak pulses (Fig. 9-6B) have a diminished pulse pressure, which is indicative of a reduced stroke volume and ejection fraction and of increased systemic vascular resistance.

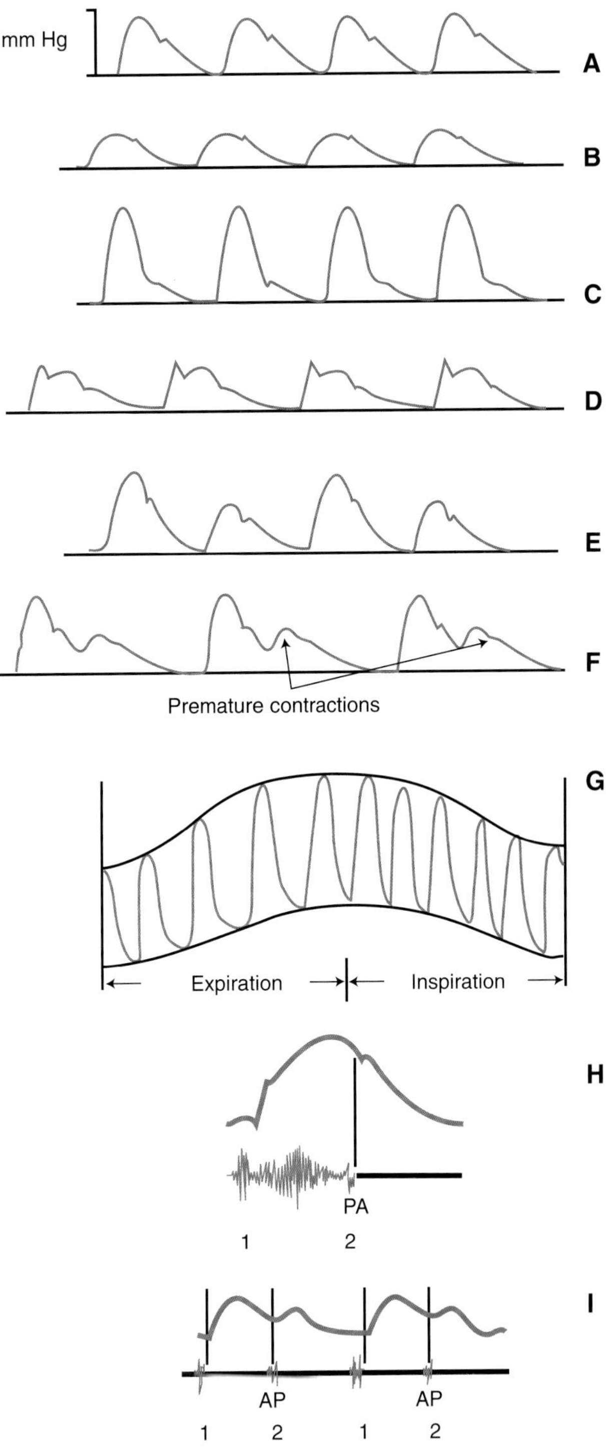

Figure 9-6. Normal and abnormal pulses. **(A)** Normal. **(B)** Small and weak. **(C)** Large and bounding. **(D)** Bisferiens. **(E)** Pulsus alternans. **(F)** Bigeminal. **(G)** Pulsus paradoxus. **(H)** Parvus et tardus. **(I)** Dicrotic.

Large, bounding pulses result from an increased pulse pressure (Fig. 9-6C). Increased pulse pressure is caused by increased stroke volume and ejection velocity and by diminished peripheral vasoconstriction. *Corrigan pulse* is a bounding pulse visible in the carotid artery. It occurs with aortic regurgitation.

The amplitude of a pulse contributes to its contour, but contour refers to the rate of rise and the shape of the arterial pulse. Because of the distortion that occurs when the pulse wave is transmitted peripherally, pulse contour is best assessed in the carotid arteries. The *normal pulse contour* has a rapid and smooth upstroke. The dicrotic notch is not palpable (Fig. 9-6A), although the dicrotic wave (Fig. 9-6I) may be palpable in heart failure and in febrile states.[18] Usually it is palpable only in the peripheral arteries.

Pulsus bisferiens (Fig. 9-6D) is characterized by a rapid upstroke and double systolic peak. This pulse may be present in idiopathic hypertrophic subaortic stenosis, aortic stenosis with regurgitation, and pure aortic insufficiency.

Pulsus alternans (Fig. 9-6E) is a regular rhythm in which strong pulse waves alternate with weak ones. It is an ominous sign when it occurs at normal heart rates and suggests serious heart disease. The difference in amplitude may be slight and difficult to palpate. The presence of pulsus alternans can be confirmed with a sphygmomanometer. The cuff is inflated above systolic pressure and slowly released until the first heart sound is audible. Cuff pressure is held at this point, and the pulse is palpated to determine if every pulse is audible.

Bigeminal pulses (Fig. 9-6F), which should not be confused with pulsus alternans, are caused by a bigeminal, premature ectopic rhythm. Note that every other pulse wave is not only diminished but is early.

Pulsus paradoxus (Fig. 9-6G) is the reduction in strength of the arterial pulse that can be felt during abnormal inspiratory decline of left ventricular filling. However, it is more apparent and can be quantified if sphygmomanometry is used. (Refer to the discussion of the determination of paradoxical blood pressure below.)

Pulsus parvus et tardus (Fig. 9-6H) is found in severe aortic stenosis. It resembles the double systolic beat in pulsus bisferiens, but its upstroke is more gradual and the pulse pressure is smaller. Usually it is palpable only in the carotid artery.

Carotid Pulse. The carotid artery is best for assessing pulse-wave amplitude and contour. Observe the neck for pulsations. Carotid pulsations are visible bilaterally just medial to the sternocleidomastoid muscle. Place your fingertips along the medial border of the sternocleidomastoid muscle in the lower half of the neck. Press posteriorly to feel the artery. Palpate well below the upper border of the thyroid cartilage to avoid compressing the carotid sinus, which might result in a reflex drop in heart rate or blood pressure. Compare one side with the other, but do not palpate both sides simultaneously because brain blood flow might be interrupted. Using the side with the strongest pulsations, assess the amplitude and contour of the pulse wave and determine whether it occurs in early systole or has a delayed upstroke.

Peripheral Circulation. In the legs, assess femoral, popliteal, dorsalis pedis, and posterior tibial pulses (Fig. 9-7). Palpation of the popliteal pulse may be difficult because the artery is deeper and the examiner is not palpating over a bone. Pedal pulses should be assessed in a dependent position before determining that they are absent.[18] In the arms, assess brachial, radial, and ulnar pulses. When assessing peripheral circulation, always compare one side with the other. An *Allen test* should be performed before radial arterial cannulation to evaluate radial and ulnar arterial patency.

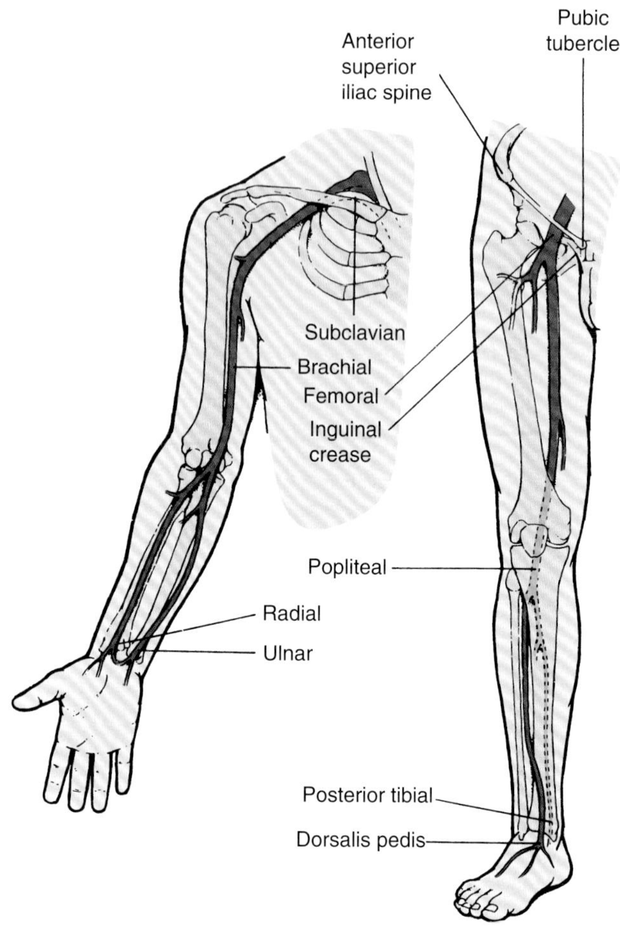

Figure 9-7. Peripheral arteries and their landmarks.

Simultaneously compress the radial and ulnar arteries and ask the patient to make a fist. The hand blanches. Ask the patient to open his or her fist. Release the pressure from the ulnar artery while maintaining pressure on the radial artery. The hand color returns to normal within 5 to 15 seconds if the ulnar artery is patent. Repeat the process releasing pressure from the radial artery. If dual circulation to the hand is not present, do not attempt radial arterial puncture or cannulation.

In shock states associated with reduced cardiac output and elevated systemic vascular resistance, or with arterial insufficiency, pulses may not be palpable in the periphery. In this case, *Doppler ultrasound* should be used to evaluate arterial flow. Using light pressure so that the artery is not occluded, place the Doppler probe (with conducting gel) over the general area of the artery to be assessed. Move the probe until the arterial signal is audible. Mark the location of the pulse with indelible ink.

Bruits

Bruits are arterial sounds, similar to cardiac murmurs that occur with turbulence of blood flow. Bruits in the carotid arteries may indicate a partial obstruction to cerebral blood flow, whereas bruits in the femoral arteries suggest partial obstruction to blood flow to the legs. When listening for carotid bruits, instruct the patient to inhale and then hold his or her breath during the examination to prevent bruits from being obscured by respiratory sounds. Auscultate for bruits with the diaphragm of the stethoscope over the carotid, renal, iliac, and femoral arteries.

Jugular Venous Pulse

Inspection of the jugular venous pulse can reveal important information about right heart hemodynamics. The level of the jugular venous pressure reflects the right atrial pressure and, in most instances, reflects the right ventricular diastolic pressure (filling pressure). The pattern of the jugular venous pulse can reveal abnormalities of conduction and abnormal function of the tricuspid valve.[6] Assess the right side of the neck because right heart hemodynamics are transmitted more directly to the right, rather than to the left, jugular vein. It is important to inspect the skin for evidence of previous cannulation of the vessel that may result in thrombosis and affect the accuracy of pressure measurement. Oblique light may assist in visualizing the jugular veins.

Jugular Venous Pressure

Jugular venous pressure reflects filling volume and pressure on the right side of the heart. Jugular veins act like manometers; blood in the jugular veins assumes the level that corresponds to the right atrial (central venous) pressure. The normal jugular venous pressure is less than 9 cm H_2O.[8] The right internal jugular vein provides the most accurate reflection of right heart hemodynamics because it is in an almost straight line with the innominate vein and the superior vena cava.[8] It lies deep to the sternocleidomastoid muscle; however, the pulsations are usually transmitted to the skin. The top level of skin pulsation is recorded as the jugular venous pressure. If the right internal jugular vein is not visible, the right external jugular vein may be used to measure jugular venous pressure, although it is more subject to thrombosis or compression, and the presence of venous valves may make the data less reliable.[19] To measure the jugular venous pressure, follow these below-mentioned steps (Fig. 9-8).

- Begin with the patient supine; the head and trunk should be in a straight line without significant flexion of the neck.
- Position the patient's backrest so that the jugular meniscus can be seen in the lower half of the neck. Elevating the backrest 15 to 30 degrees above horizontal is usually sufficient. The hypovolemic patient may need to be lower than 15 degrees and the hypervolemic patient may need to be elevated more than 30 degrees to visualize the level of peak excursion.
- Visualize the right internal jugular vein and identify the level of peak excursion. If the external jugular vein is used, identify the level at which it appears collapsed.
- Place a ruler vertically on the sternal angle (angle of Lewis). Position a straight edge (e.g., tongue blade) horizontally at the highest point of the jugular vein so that it intersects the ruler at a right angle, and measure the vertical distance above the sternal angle.

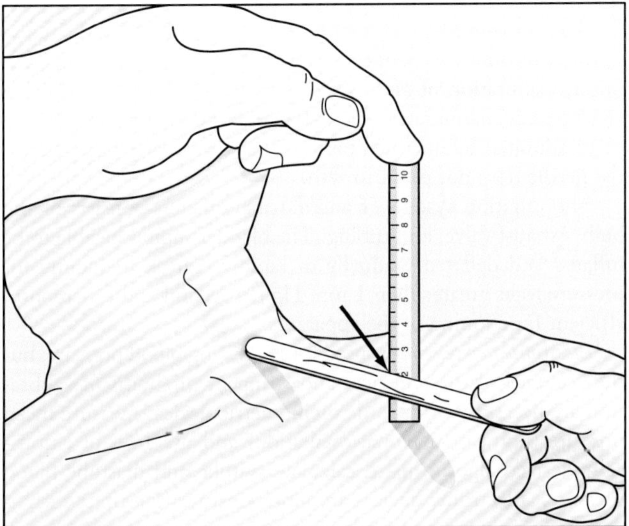

Figure 9-8. Assessment of jugular venous pressure.

If the top of the neck veins is more than 3 cm above the sternal angle, venous pressure is abnormally elevated. Elevated venous pressure reflects right ventricular failure (and is a late finding in left ventricular failure), reduced right ventricular compliance, pericardial disease, hypervolemia, tricuspid valve stenosis, and obstruction of the superior vena cava.[18] During inspiration, the jugular venous pressure normally declines, although the amplitude of the *a* wave may increase.[6] With the patient in the horizontal position, if the neck veins collapse on deep inspiration (intrathoracic pressure of −5 cm H_2O), the central venous pressure is less than 5 cm H_2O.

Abdominojugular reflux occurs in right ventricular failure. It can be demonstrated by pressing the periumbilical area firmly for 30 to 60 seconds and observing the jugular venous pressure. If there is a rise in the jugular venous pressure by 3 cm or more that is sustained throughout pressure application, abdominojugular reflux is present.[3] *Kussmaul sign* is a paradoxical elevation of jugular venous pressure during inspiration and may occur in patients with chronic constrictive pericarditis, heart failure, or tricuspid stenosis.

Patterns of the Venous Pulse

Before evaluating the venous pulse, it is important to discriminate between venous and carotid pulsations. Venous pulse waves are observed more readily than they are palpated. The descents are often more easily seen than the peaks and are inward movements.[3] The carotid pulsation is a brisk, outward movement. Palpation of the jugular vein obliterates the pulsations except in extreme venous hypertension.[19] Palpation of the carotid does not obliterate the observable pulsation in the neck.

Right atrial systole increases right atrial pressure and causes venous distention and the resultant a wave (Fig. 9-9). Atrial emptying and relaxation, and descent of the atrial floor during ventricular systole, result in the *x* descent. The c wave occurs simultaneously with the carotid arterial pulse, interrupting the *x* descent. The c wave may be related to tricuspid valve closure and bulging into the right atrium or it may be an artifact from the adjacent carotid pulse. The v wave reflects the rise in right atrial pressure from atrial filling during ventricular contraction while the tricuspid valve is closed. The *y* descent results from

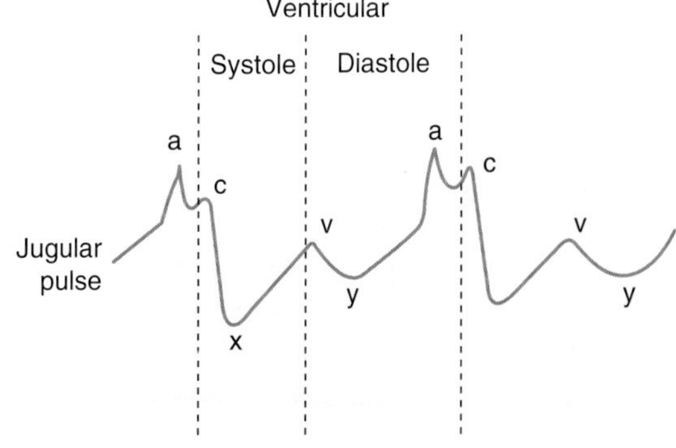

Figure 9-9. Patterns of the venous pulse.

reduction in right atrial volume and pressure when the tricuspid valve opens.[19]

Timing of the venous pulse can be appreciated by auscultating the heart or palpating the carotid artery on the opposite side of the neck. The a wave occurs just before the first heart sound or carotid pulse and has a sharp rise followed by the rapid *x* descent. The v wave occurs immediately after the arterial pulse and has a slower, undulating pattern. The *y* descent is less steep than the *x* descent. Consistently large a waves are seen in tricuspid stenosis, pulmonary hypertension, and right ventricular failure. *Cannon* a waves are seen in patients with atrioventricular dissociation as the right atrium contracts against the closed tricuspid valve.[3] The a wave is absent in atrial fibrillation because of the absence of coordinated atrial contraction. Elevated v waves and rapid *y* descents suggest tricuspid regurgitation or increased intravascular volume. Blunting of the *y* descent suggests impaired atrial emptying in early ventricular diastole, such as occurs in tricuspid stenosis, pericardial disease, or cardiac tamponade.

Blood Pressure

Systemic arterial blood pressure can be measured indirectly or directly. Indirect measurement of blood pressure is most common and is described in this section. Direct measurement of blood pressure, an invasive technique requiring placement of an arterial catheter, may be necessary in certain conditions, such as clinical shock. Direct measurement of blood pressure is described in detail elsewhere in this textbook

Blood pressure should be measured at each health encounter. The auscultatory method of measurement with a properly calibrated and validated instrument should be used. Patients should be seated quietly in a chair, with feet on the floor and arm supported for at least 5 minutes before measurement.[20]

Evaluate the patient's current blood pressure. If it differs greatly from the usual, immediate intervention may be required. Normal blood pressure in people 18 years of age or older is defined as less than 120/80 mm Hg, and prehypertension is defined as systolic pressure of 120 to 139 mm Hg or diastolic pressure of 80 to 89 mm Hg. Patients with prehypertension are at increased risk for progression to hypertension.[20] Stage 1 hypertension is defined as systolic blood pressure of 140 to 159 mm Hg, diastolic blood pressure of 90 to 99 mm Hg, or taking antihypertensive medication.[20] In western societies, blood pressure tends to increase with increasing age. This increase is not biologic, and there is clear evidence that lowering blood pressure in older adults reduces the risk of stroke, cardiac disease, and all-cause mortality.[21] The higher the blood pressure, the greater the increase in the heart's work and oxygen consumption. Blood pressures less than 90/60 mm Hg may decrease blood and oxygen delivery to an already compromised myocardium. Taking into account symptoms of myocardial ischemia and adequacy of cerebral and peripheral perfusion may enable the examiner to judge more accurately the clinical significance of blood pressure changes in the cardiac patient.

Sphygmomanometer

Blood pressure is measured indirectly using a sphygmomanometer (inflatable bladder inside a pressure cuff, a manometer, and an inflation system) and stethoscope. Stethoscopes are described later in this chapter.

Bladder and Cuff. The inflatable bladder fits inside a nondistensible covering, termed the *cuff.* Size and placement of the bladder (rather than the cuff) are crucial in obtaining accurate blood pressure measurements. The bladder width should be 40% of the circumference of the limb (usually the arm) to be used. Bladders that are too narrow for the size of the limb reflect a falsely elevated blood pressure, whereas bladders that are too wide reflect an erroneously low blood pressure. Bladder length, which also affects accuracy of measurement, should be approximately twice that of width, or 80% of the limb circumference. Inflatable bladders and cuffs are available in various sizes. Table 9-3 summarizes recommended bladder dimensions for blood pressure cuffs. It is important to remember that cuff size is determined by patient size, not patient age.[22]

Table 9-3 • ACCEPTABLE BLADDER DIMENSIONS (IN CM) FOR ARMS OF DIFFERENT SIZES[a]

Cuff	Bladder Width (cm)	Bladder Length (cm)	Arm Circumference Range at Midpoint (cm)
Newborn	3	6	≤6
Infant	5	15	6–15[b]
Child	8	21	16–21[b]
Small adult	10	24	22–26
Adult	13	30	27–34
Large adult	16	38	35–44
Adult thigh	20	42	45–52

[a]There is some overlapping of the recommended range for arm circumferences to limit the number of cuffs; it is recommended that the larger cuff be used when available.

[b]To approximate the bladder width:arm circumference ratio of 0.40 more closely in infants and children, additional cuffs are available.

Reprinted with permission from Perloff D, Grim C, Flack J, et al. *Human Blood Pressure Determination by Sphygmomanometry.* Dallas, TX: American Heart Association; 2001.

Manometers. There are two types of manometers: mercury and aneroid. In response to efforts by the Environmental Protection Agency to reduce potential mercury spills and exposure, clinical facilities are transitioning to aneroid gauges or electronic monitoring devices,

Aneroid manometers have round gauges calibrated in millimeters of mercury, or torr (1 torr = 1 mm Hg), and affixed to the blood pressure cuff. Advantages of the aneroid manometer are that it is easily seen, is conveniently portable, and, with the cuff, composes one unit. Unfortunately, the calibration of the dial frequently becomes inaccurate. It is important before each use to check that the indicator needle is pointing to the zero mark on the dial. If the needle is either below or above this mark, the blood pressure reading will be incorrect and the scale may no longer be linear. Calibration of an aneroid manometer is performed using an electronic manometer (Fig. 9-10). Aneroid manometers should be recalibrated by qualified personnel at least yearly or whenever the needle does not point to zero.

The inflation system of aneroid manometers consists of the bulb, exhaust valve, and tubing. The bladder should be able to be inflated and deflated gradually or rapidly. Check frequently for pressure leaks greater than 1 mm Hg per second and for smooth, efficient functioning of the apparatus.

Electronic devices can be used for measuring blood pressure, but the accuracy of these devices and stringent programs of calibration are necessary. Electronic oscillometric devices measure mean pressure (point of maximal oscillation) and use a set of empirically derived algorithms to calculate systolic and diastolic blood pressure.[6] Electronic devices are more sensitive to artifact such as patient movement or muscle contraction than are mercury and aneroid devices. Cardiac arrhythmias and low pulse pressure also

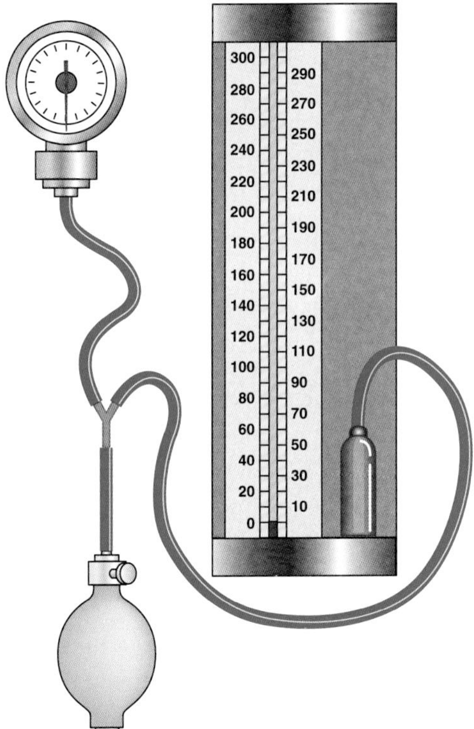

Figure 9-10. Calibration of an aneroid manometer. Disconnect the cuffs from both the aneroid and reference manometers. Attach a bulb to a Y connector and the Y connector to the tubes to each of the manometers. Inflate the bulb and observe the pressure at several points over the entire range on both manometers. The pressures should be equal on both manometers.

reduce the accuracy of electronic devices. Electronic devices do not require use of a stethoscope and may be used by patients for self-monitoring of blood pressure.

Technique

On initial examination, blood pressure should be recorded in both arms and, in infants, in one leg as well. Subsequently, the arm with the higher blood pressure should be used. Indicate whether the blood pressure was taken on the right arm or left arm. Avoid possible development of lymphedema after mastectomy by always taking the patient's blood pressures on the arm *opposite* the affected side. Avoid taking blood pressure on an arm with an arteriovenous shunt or fistula, as well as those with subclavian stenosis.[24]

Differences in blood pressure between the arms or between the arms and the legs have important diagnostic implications. In patients with occlusive arterial disease of the subclavian artery, the blood pressure is lower in the affected arm. In patients with coarctation of the aorta or dissecting aortic aneurysm, depending on the location of the lesion, the blood pressure may be higher in one arm than the other, or in both arms (proximal) compared with the legs (distal).

Bladder and Cuff Position. The deflated cuff is placed snugly around the arm, with the bladder covering the inner aspect of the arm and the brachial artery. The lower margin of the cuff should be 2.5 cm above the antecubital space.

Arm Position. As long as the patient's arm is at heart level, the blood pressure can be determined with the patient in any

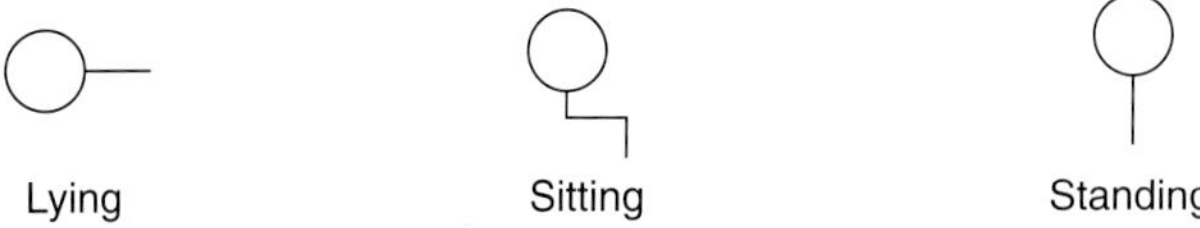

Figure 9-11. Symbols used to record a patient's position during blood pressure determination.

position. Errors up to 10 mm Hg, both systolic and diastolic, can be made if the arm is not at the correct level. Falsely elevated pressures are obtained if the arm is lower than the heart; falsely low pressures are measured if the arm is higher than the heart. The arm must be supported during pressure determination.

Patient Position. The patient's position during blood pressure measurement always should be recorded. Use the symbols or drawings shown in Figure 9-11.

Palpation. After the cuff is in place, the brachial artery is palpated continuously. Once the brachial or radial pulse is obtained, the cuff is inflated rapidly. The pressure at which the pulse disappears should be noted, but the cuff inflation should continue for another 30 mm Hg before the actual measurement of the blood pressure begins. For example, if the brachial pulse disappears when the cuff pressure is 110 mm Hg, the cuff should be pumped to 140 mm Hg before starting. The cuff should not be inflated further than necessary, because high cuff pressures are uncomfortable, create undue anxiety in the patient, and tend to raise the patient's blood pressure. The pressure in the cuff should be reduced gradually by 2 to 3 mm Hg per second. The point at which the brachial pulse is first detected on expiration is the systolic blood pressure. Diastolic blood pressure cannot be determined accurately by palpation. Once measurement is made, the cuff should be deflated rapidly. If possible, allow a minimum of 1 to 2 minutes before the blood pressure is measured again to release venous blood.

Systolic blood pressure is measured by palpation in patients whose blood pressures cannot be heard (e.g., patients in shock). It is also useful when checking blood pressures frequently (e.g., every 1 to 2 minutes). Palpated blood pressures are charted using "P" as diastolic pressure (e.g., 90/P).

Auscultation. Preparation of the patient and use of the blood pressure equipment are identical in the auscultatory method. After the brachial pulse has been located, the stethoscope is applied over the artery using light pressure. Heavy pressure might partially occlude the artery, creating turbulence in the blood flow, prolonging phase IV, and falsely lowering the diastolic blood pressure. Care must be taken to avoid causing extraneous noise, such as from the stethoscope touching the cuff or any other material.

Korotkoff sounds are the sounds created by turbulence of blood flow within the vessel caused by constriction of the blood pressure cuff (Fig. 9-12). The five Korotkoff sounds are summarized in Table 9-4.

Systolic blood pressure is the highest point at which initial tapping (phase I) is heard in two consecutive beats (to ascertain that the sound is not extraneous) during expiration. Systolic blood pressure is higher in the expiratory phase compared to the inspiratory phase of the respiratory cycle (see "Measurement of Paradoxical Blood Pressure" section). Systolic blood pressure should be read to the nearest 2 mm Hg mark on the manometer.

Diastolic blood pressure is equated with disappearance of Korotkoff sounds (phase V) in adults. Phase V most closely approximates intra-arterial diastolic pressure. Muffling of sounds (phase IV) usually occurs at pressures 5 to 10 mm Hg higher

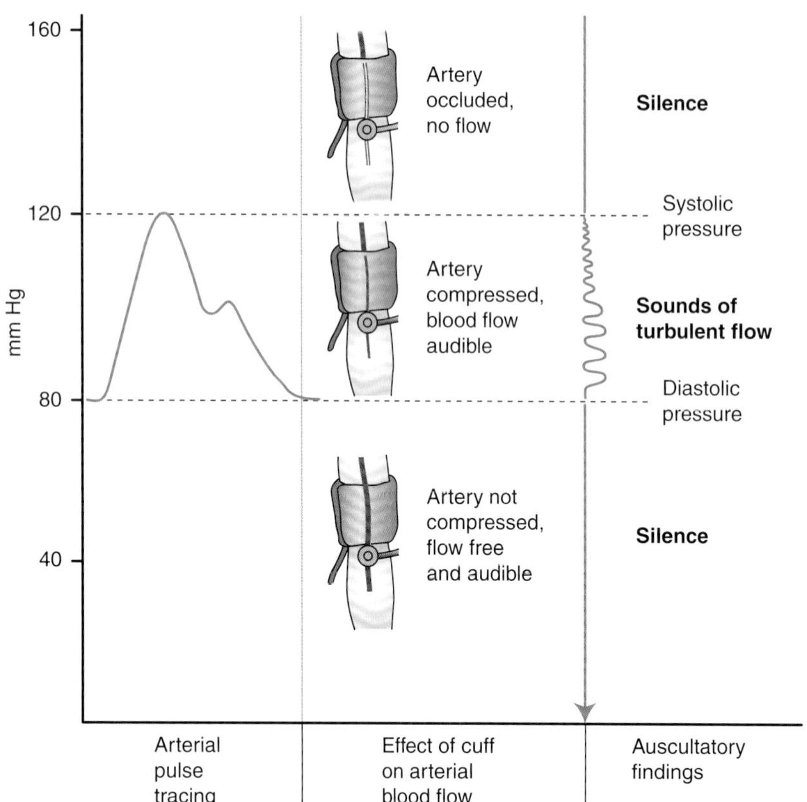

Figure 9-12. Auscultation of the blood pressure.

than intra-arterial diastolic pressures and, therefore, is not a good indicator of diastolic blood pressure in adults. However, muffling, rather than disappearance of sounds, is a better index of intra-arterial diastolic pressure in children and in adults with hyperkinetic states. Hyperkinetic conditions, including hyperthyroidism, aortic insufficiency, and exercise, increase the rate of blood flow, resulting in disappearance of sounds (absence of turbulence) far below intra-arterial diastolic pressure. In children and adults with hyperkinetic states, sounds can be detected below muffling for much longer than normal.[22] As with systolic blood pressure, read diastolic pressure to the nearest 2 mm Hg mark on the manometer. If there is a difference of 10 mm Hg or more between disappearance and muffling of sounds, record both diastolic pressures (e.g., 140/56/20 mm Hg).[22]

Table 9-4 • PHASES OF THE KOROTKOFF SOUNDS[a]

Phase I
The pressure level at which the first faint, consistent tapping sounds are heard. The sounds gradually increase in intensity as the cuff is deflated. The first of at least two of these sounds is defined as the *systolic pressure.*

Phase II
The time during cuff deflation when a murmur of swishing sounds is heard.

Phase III
The period during which sounds are crisper and increase in intensity.

Phase IV
The time when a distinct, abrupt, muffling of sound (usually of a soft blowing quality) is heard. This is defined as the *diastolic pressure* in anyone in whom sounds continue to zero.

Phase V
The pressure level when the last regular blood pressure sound is heard and after which all sound disappears. This is defined as the *diastolic pressure* unless sounds are heard to zero.

[a]To avoid error, the observer must be prepared to recognize two normal Korotkoff sound variations associated with blood pressure (BP) readings. The auscultatory gap is a period of silence occurring during Korotkoff phases I and II. This disappearance of sound is temporary and is usually short, but the gap can occur over a period of 40 mm Hg. It seems to be associated with higher BP readings. An absent Korotkoff phase V occurs when sounds are heard to zero. When this is the case, phase IV should be recorded along with phase V. In this case, phase IV is the best reference for diastolic pressure.

Reprinted with permission from Grim CM, Grim CE. Blood pressure measurement. In: Izzo JL, Black HR, eds. *Hypertension Primer.* 3rd ed. Dallas, TX: American Heart Association; 2003.

In some patients, Korotkoff sounds may be soft and could result in falsely low blood pressure values. To augment the loudness of Korotkoff sounds, increase brachial flow by having the patient open and clench a fist; quickly inflate cuff to a value 30 mm above the palpable systolic blood pressure.

Auscultatory gap is a temporary disappearance of sound that occurs during the latter part of phase I and phase II (Fig. 9-13). It is particularly common in patients with high blood pressure, venous distention, or reduced velocity of arterial flow (e.g., severe aortic stenosis).[18] The auscultatory gap can be as wide as 40 mm Hg. Serious errors in blood pressure measurement can be made if the cuff is not inflated high enough to exceed true systolic pressure. Systolic blood pressure would be underestimated if the second appearance of the Korotkoff sounds were recorded as phase I. Diastolic blood pressure would be overestimated if the first muffling of sounds was considered to be phase IV. The auscultatory gap can be avoided if a preliminary palpable blood pressure is obtained before auscultation.

Measurement of Pulse Pressure

Pulse pressure is the difference between the systolic and diastolic blood pressures, expressed in millimeters of mercury. For example, if the blood pressure is 120/80 mm Hg, the pulse pressure is 40 mm Hg. Pulse pressure reflects stroke volume, ejection

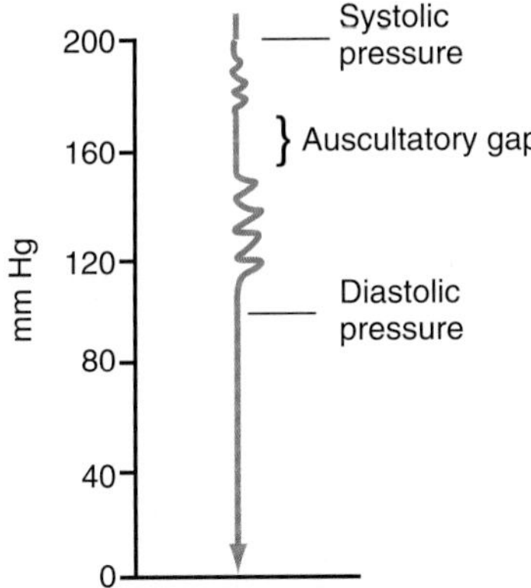

Figure 9-13. Auscultatory gap.

velocity, and systemic vascular resistance. Use pulse pressure as a noninvasive indicator of the patient's ability to maintain cardiac output.

Pulse pressure is increased in many situations. A widened pulse pressure is seen in sinus bradycardia, complete heart block, aortic regurgitation, anxiety, exercise, and catecholamine infusion, which are examples of situations characterized by increased stroke volume. Examples of conditions that increase pulse pressure by reducing systemic vascular resistance are fever, hot environment, and exercise. Conditions such as atherosclerosis, aging, and high blood pressure widen the pulse pressure because of decreased distensibility of the aorta, arteries, and arterioles. A narrowed pulse pressure also can be caused by many factors: reduced ejection velocity in heart failure, shock, and hypovolemia; mechanical obstruction to systolic outflow in aortic stenosis, mitral stenosis, and mitral insufficiency; peripheral vasoconstriction in shock and with certain drugs; and artifactually from an auscultatory gap.[6,18] If the pulse pressure in the cardiac patient falls below 30 mm Hg, further assessment of the patient's cardiovascular status may be indicated.

Measurement of Postural Blood Pressure

Postural (orthostatic) hypotension occurs when the blood pressure drops after an upright posture is assumed. It usually is accompanied by dizziness, lightheadedness, or syncope. Although there are many causes of postural hypotension, the three most commonly seen in the cardiac patient are (1) intravascular volume depletion, which often results from aggressive diuretic therapy, inadequate intake, or intravascular to extravascular fluid shift; (2) inadequate vasoconstrictor mechanisms, which may be a primary pathologic process but also result from immobility; and (3) autonomic insufficiency, which is often related to the sympathetic blocking drugs used in the cardiac patient. Postural changes in blood pressure, along with the appropriate history, can help the clinician differentiate between them.[25,26] Postural changes in blood pressure and pulse should be measured in patients who are older than 65 years of age, diabetic, receiving antihypertensive therapy, or who complain of dizziness or syncope. Important points to remember are the following:

- Position the patient supine and as flat as symptoms permit for 10 minutes before the initial measurement of blood pressure and heart rate.
- Always check supine measurements before upright measurements.
- Always record both heart rate and blood pressure at each postural change.
- Do not remove the blood pressure cuff between position changes, but do check to see that it remains placed correctly.
- Safety considerations may require assessment of blood pressure and pulse with the patient seated with legs in the dependent position before standing. Measurement of blood pressure and pulse in this position is not sufficient to rule out orthostasis.[26]
- Have the patient assume a standing position. Measure the blood pressure and pulse immediately and after 2 minutes. If orthostasis is strongly suspected and not apparent after 2 minutes, continue to monitor blood pressure and pulse every 2 minutes for 10 minutes. If the purpose of collecting the data is to assess the risk of falling, another approach is to ask the patient to get out of bed as he or she normally does and evaluate the change in pulse rate and blood pressure and associated symptoms at the patient's rate of position change.
- Be alert for any signs or symptoms of patient distress, including dizziness, weakness, blurring of vision, and syncope. When the patient returns to a recumbent position, these symptoms should reverse and the blood pressure and pulse return to normal.
- Record any signs or symptoms that accompany the postural change.

Normal postural responses are a transient increased heart rate of 5 to 20 beats per minute (to offset reduced stroke volume and to maintain cardiac output), a drop in systolic pressure of less than 10 mm Hg, and an increase in diastolic pressure of approximately 5 mm Hg. *Orthostasis* is defined as a drop in systolic pressure of 20 mm Hg or greater or a drop in diastolic pressure of at least 10 mm Hg within 3 minutes of standing,[26] although any drop in diastolic pressure may be cause for concern. The change from lying to sitting position is not sufficient to make a diagnosis of orthostasis; it may be used as a screening test because decreased blood pressure, increased pulse, or symptoms in the sitting position presage similar events in the erect position. Often, the change in blood pressure does not meet the criteria for orthostasis, but it is accompanied by a significant change in heart rate or associated symptoms, or both. These circumstances identify people at risk and should prompt further investigation by the cardiac nurse of the patient's present volume status and vasodilatory or cardioinhibitory drug regimen.

The presence of intravascular volume depletion (such as with diuretic therapy) should be suspected when, in response to sitting or standing, the heart rate increases and the systolic pressure decreases by 15 mm Hg and the diastolic blood pressure drops by 10 mm Hg.[26] It is difficult to differentiate intravascular volume loss from inadequate vasoconstrictor mechanisms solely by changes in vital signs accompanying postural changes. With intravascular volume depletion, reflexes to maintain cardiac output (increased heart rate and peripheral vasoconstriction) function correctly, but, because of reduced intravascular fluid volume, these reflexes are not adequate to maintain systemic arterial pressure and the blood pressure falls. With inadequate vasoconstrictor mechanisms, the heart rate responds appropriately also, but blood pressure drops because of diminished peripheral vasoconstriction. Differentiation, therefore, depends in part on the patient's history. However, intravascular depletion and inadequate vasoconstrictor mechanisms are not mutually exclusive. The following is an example of postural blood pressure recordings showing either saline depletion or inadequate vasoconstrictor mechanisms:

Blood Pressure (mm Hg)	Heart Rate (bpm)	Patient Position
120/70	70	
100/55	90	
98/52	94	

Measurement of Paradoxical Blood Pressure

Paradoxical blood pressure is an exaggerated decrease in the systolic blood pressure during inspiration. The mechanism is complex and controversial. Normally, during inspiration, blood flow into the right heart is increased, right ventricular output is enhanced, and pulmonary venous capacitance is increased. Consequently, less blood reaches the left ventricle, which reduces left ventricular stroke volume and arterial pressure.[27]

During cardiac tamponade, effects of respiration on both right and left ventricular filling appear to be greater than normal, causing a reduction of 10 mm Hg or more in systolic pressure during normal inspiration (Fig. 9-14).[27] In addition, echocardiography has demonstrated a shift of the intraventricular septum to the left, further impairing left ventricular filling and stroke volume. With high intrapericardial pressures, the thin-walled right ventricle may collapse during diastole, further impairing venous return and cardiac output.[27] Chronic obstructive airway disease, constrictive pericarditis, pulmonary emboli, restrictive cardiomyopathy, and cardiogenic shock have also been associated with an abnormal inspiratory decline of blood pressure. Echocardiographic studies of patients with emphysema demonstrate both an augmented inspiratory filling of the right ventricle and an exaggerated inspiratory decline of left ventricular filling.[5]

The patient should breathe normally and must not exaggerate respiratory effort during an examination for a paradoxical blood pressure. As before, the nurse should inflate and gradually deflate the cuff until the first systolic sound is heard on expiration and continue slowly releasing the cuff pressure until sounds are heard both on inspiration and expiration. The difference between the two is termed the *paradox*, and it normally is less than 10 mm Hg.[27] For example, if the first systolic sound occurs at 140 mm Hg during expiration and Korotkoff sounds begin appearing with both inspiration and expiration at 120 mm Hg, the paradox is 20 mm Hg. Paradoxical blood pressures should be determined as a baseline in all patients on the cardiac care unit and routinely in all patients with pericarditis or with heart catheters, such as a temporary pacing wire.

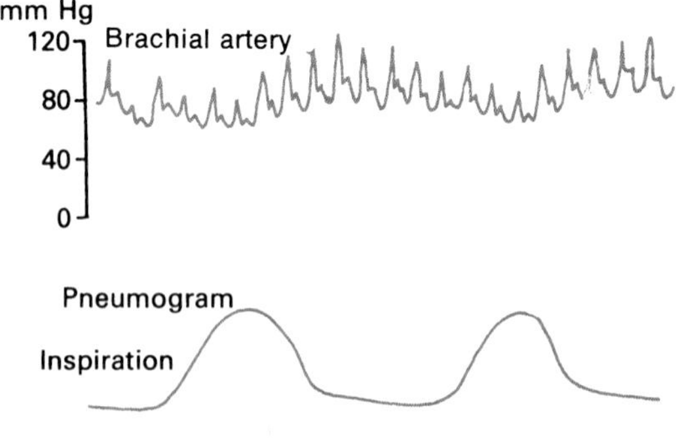

CARDIAC TAMPONADE

Figure 9-14. Paradoxical blood pressure in cardiac tamponade. The paradox is greater than 20 mm Hg. (Reprinted with permission from Fowler NO. *Examination of the Heart, Part 2: Inspection and Palpation of Arterial and Venous Pulses.* New York: American Heart Association with permission of the American Heart Association, Inc; 1972:33.)

Blood Pressure Measurement Under Special Conditions

Arrhythmia. With very irregular rhythms, accurate assessment of blood pressure is difficult because of the beat-to-beat variation in both stroke volume and blood pressure. Systolic blood pressure is related directly to the stroke volume and duration of the preceding cycle. Pulse pressure is related inversely to pulse cycle duration. A short cycle (reduced ventricular filling time) increases the diastolic blood pressure of that cycle and reduces systolic blood pressure during the next cycle. A long pulse cycle (increased ventricular filling time) causes a decreased diastolic blood pressure in that cycle but an increased systolic blood pressure in the next cycle.[3]

Any arrhythmia that alters stroke volume and cardiac output can be detected during blood pressure measurement. Always record the presence of an irregular cardiac rhythm along with the blood pressure.

Premature ectopic beats (either ventricular or supraventricular) have a short cycle followed by a long cycle (postextrasystolic beat). If they occur only occasionally, they have minimal effects on blood pressure. In *bigeminal rhythms*, as the blood pressure cuff is deflated, Korotkoff sounds of the alternate strong beats are heard first and are half as fast as the heart rate. Further reduction in cuff pressure enables the listener to hear the alternating weaker sounds produced by the ectopic impulses as well.

Pulsus alternans, indicative of severe organic heart disease and left heart failure, also is manifested by alternating strong and weak pulses but with a regular cadence. Pulsus alternans can occur with ectopic bigeminal rhythms that are interpolated rather than premature, but, in this instance, it does not necessarily indicate severe organic heart disease.

Because pulse cycle length changes constantly in *atrial fibrillation*, both systolic and diastolic blood pressures must be approximated.[24] For systolic blood pressure, average a series of readings (three to five) of phase I pressures. For diastolic blood pressure, average the pressure readings obtained in phase IV and phase V.

Atrioventricular dissociation can be detected during auscultation of blood pressure. Examples of rhythms with atrioventricular dissociation include *ventricular tachycardia*, *high-grade* or *complete atrioventricular block*, and *asynchronous ventricular pacing*. In atrioventricular dissociation, an occasional, well-timed atrial contraction contributes to diastolic ventricular filling. This "atrial kick" augments the stroke volume for that beat. As the cuff bladder is deflated, phase I sounds periodically are increased.

Clinical Shock. In shock states associated with reduced cardiac output and elevated systemic vascular resistance, Korotkoff sounds may not be generated in the periphery. Direct measurement of blood pressure may be required to manage these critically ill patients. When indirect cuff measurements are compared with direct (femoral arterial) pressure measurements, direct pressures are higher than auscultated pressures. In hypotensive states, when direct measurement of blood pressure is not feasible, *Doppler ultrasound* may provide a more reliable indirect measurement of systolic blood pressure than the auscultatory method. Place the Doppler probe (with conducting gel) over the patient's artery. As in auscultatory measurement, inflate the cuff and listen for the arterial signal as the bladder is deflated. Cuff widths of 50% of the arm circumference have been recommended for the Doppler technique.[24]

Obesity. Cuff size and bladder size frequently are too small for use in the obese patient. If a proper-sized cuff cannot be used, apply a standard cuff to the forearm 13 cm from the elbow and auscultate the radial artery to obtain the blood pressure measurement.

Thigh Blood Pressure Measurement. Blood pressures are measured in the thigh if the arms cannot be used or to confirm or rule out certain conditions that alter circulation, such as coarctation of the aorta or dissecting aortic aneurysm.

For thigh blood pressure measurement, use a cuff and bladder that are both longer and wider than an arm cuff. The bladder of the cuff should be about 40% of the circumference of the thigh. The length should be about 75% to 80% of the circumference. With the patient in the prone position, apply the compression bladder over the posterior aspect of the mid-thigh. Place the stethoscope over the artery in the popliteal fossa and auscultate in the same manner as described previously. If the patient is unable to tolerate the prone position, have the patient remain supine with the knee slightly flexed. Apply the stethoscope over the popliteal artery. When cuffs of the correct size are used for both arms and legs, pressures should vary by only a few millimeters of mercury. (The arm cuff, incorrectly used on the thigh, produces a falsely high value.)

Community Blood Pressure Readings. Blood pressures taken in the patient's home may provide a better indication of basal blood pressure than those obtained in an office or clinic setting. However, if the patient takes his or her own blood pressure, readings may be elevated because of the isometric exercise required to inflate the cuff and because of the concentration necessary. Newer devices for home use inflate the cuff automatically and some maintain a record of recent measurements. Many fire stations and hospital auxiliaries provide blood pressure measurement as a community service. Alternately, a fully automated system that measures blood pressure at preset intervals over the 24-hour period may be used.

Pseudohypertension. Misleadingly high systolic blood pressure values may be obtained in older adults because of excessive vascular stiffness.[28] Pseudohypertension should be suspected in the presence of high systolic blood pressure values and the absence of target organ damage. To confirm suspected pseudohypertension, inflate the cuff above systolic pressure and palpate the radial artery. Presence of a palpable, pulseless radial artery provides additional evidence of pseudohypertension.

Peripheral Vascular System

Adequacy of both arterial and venous circulation is assessed when examining the extremities. Always make arm-to-arm and leg-to-leg comparisons. Careful examination of the lower extremities is impossible without removing shoes and stockings.

Inspection and Palpation

Inspection and palpation are the primary techniques used in examining the peripheral vasculature (see "Bruits" section).

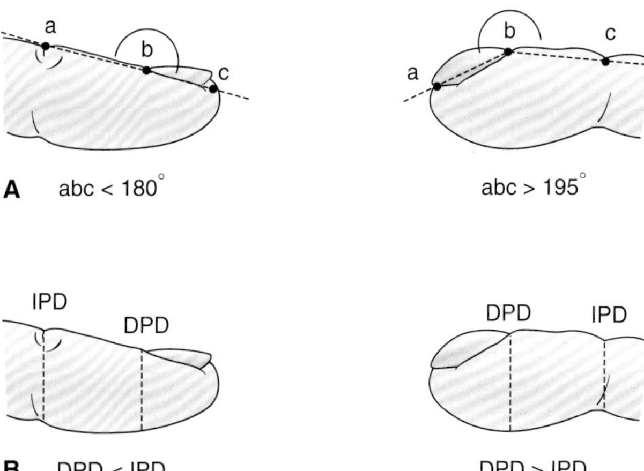

Figure 9-15. Clubbing is diagnosed from the angle between the base of the nail and the skin next to the cuticle and by phalangeal depth. **(A)** In healthy adults, the hyponychial angle is 180 degrees (*left*); with clubbing, the angle increases above 195 degrees (*right*). **(B)** The ratio of distal phalangeal depth (DPD) to interphalangeal depth (IPD) is normally less than 1 (*left*). In clubbing, it exceeds 1.0 (*right*). (After Hansen-Flaschen J, Nordberg J. Clubbing and hypertrophic osteoarthropathy. *Clin Chest Med.* 1987;8:291.)

Observe and compare (right to left) size, temperature, symmetry, swelling, venous pattern, pigmentation, scars, and ulcers. Palpate the superficial lymph nodes, noting their size, consistency, discreteness, and any tenderness.

Clubbing

Clubbing is a pathologic sign that is defined as focal enlargement of the terminal phalanges. Two diagnostic findings are present in clubbing: change in the angle between the base of the nail and the phalangeal skin, and "floating" nails. When viewed from the side, the base angle normally is less than 180 degrees and the distal phalangeal diameter is less than the interphalangeal diameter. In clubbing, the base angle becomes 195 degrees or greater and the distal phalangeal diameter becomes greater than the interphalangeal diameter (Fig. 9-15).[29] Floating nails can be detected by palpating the base of the nail while moving the tip of the nail. Rather than a firm anchor, the base of the nail appears to float or move under the palpating finger. Clubbing may develop in a variety of conditions, including congenital heart disease and lung abscess; its cause is unknown.

Arterial Circulation

Adequacy of peripheral arterial circulation is assessed by arterial pulse; skin color, temperature, and moistness; and capillary refill time. Pulse-wave analysis and skin color are described earlier in this chapter under the "Arterial Pulse" and the "Head" section, respectively.

Temperature and Moistness. Temperature and moistness are controlled by the autonomic nervous system. Normally, hands and feet are warm and dry. Under stress, the periphery may be cool and moist. In cardiogenic shock, skin becomes cold and clammy.

Capillary Refill Time. Capillary refill time provides an estimate of the rate of peripheral blood flow. When the tip of the fingernail is depressed, the nail bed blanches. When the pressure is released quickly, the area is reperfused and becomes pink.

Normally, reperfusion occurs almost instantaneously. More sluggish reperfusion indicates a slower peripheral circulation, such as in heart failure.

Peripheral Atherosclerosis. Risk factors for peripheral atherosclerosis include advancing age, diabetes mellitus, hyperlipidemia, and tobacco use. Peripheral atherosclerosis may present with pain or fatigue in the muscles (intermittent claudication) that occurs with exercise and resolves with rest. Physical findings of chronic arterial insufficiency include decreased or absent pulses, reduced skin temperature, hair loss, thickened nails, smooth shiny skin, and pallor or cyanosis. Elevation of the feet and repeated flexing of the calf muscles may produce pallor of the soles of the feet. Returning the feet to a dependent position may produce rubor secondary to reactive hyperemia. If the ankle–brachial systolic pressure index (calculated by dividing the ankle systolic pressure by the brachial systolic pressure) is less than 0.8, it is highly probable (greater than 95%) that arterial insufficiency is present. When vascular ulcers associated with arterial insufficiency occur, they are more commonly located near the lateral malleolus. Acute arterial occlusion produces sudden cessation of blood flow to an extremity. It is characterized by the 6 P's: pallor, pain, paresthesia, paralysis, pulselessness, and poikilothermia. Severe pain, numbness, and coldness develop in the affected extremity quickly (within 1 hour). Physical findings include loss of pulse distal to the occlusion, decreased skin temperature, loss of sensation, weakness, and absent deep tendon reflexes.

Venous Circulation

Edema. Edema is an abnormal accumulation of fluid in the interstitium. Causes include right-sided heart failure, hypoalbuminemia, excessive renal retention of sodium and water, venous stasis from obstruction or insufficiency, lymphedema, orthostatic edema, or increased capillary permeability.[6] In the cardiac patient, peripheral edema frequently occurs because of sodium and water retention and right-sided heart failure. Bilateral edema of the lower extremities suggests a systemic etiology; unilateral edema is usually the result of a local etiology. A weight gain of 10 lb (indicative of 5 L of extracellular fluid volume) precedes visible edema in most patients. Interstitial edema occurs in the most dependent part of the body, its location varying with the patient's posture. With sitting or standing, edema develops in the lower extremities. With bedrest, edema forms in the sacrum. Because the distribution of edema fluid varies with position, daily weights provide the best serial assessment of edema. *Pitting edema* is a depression in the skin from pressure. To demonstrate the presence of pitting edema, the nurse presses firmly with his or her thumb over a bony surface such as the sacrum, medial malleolus, the dorsum of each foot, and the shins. When the thumb is withdrawn, an indentation persists for a short time. The severity of edema is described on a five-point scale, from none (0) to very marked (4). *Pigmentation, reddening, induration,* and *fibrosis* of the skin and subcutaneous tissues of the lower extremities may result from long-standing edema.[30,31] *Skin mobility* is decreased by edema.

Thrombophlebitis. Thrombophlebitis is inflammation of the vein associated with a clot. Diagnosis is made using subjective and objective data.

In *superficial thrombophlebitis,* the affected vein is hard, red, sensitive to pressure, warm to touch, and engorged. *Deep vein thrombosis* may be asymptomatic or associated with pain, warmth, and mottling of the leg. With severe edema, the leg may be cool and cyanotic. Deep vein thrombosis can cause thromboembolism, resulting in a pulmonary embolus.[32] Among hospitalized patients, hip surgery is the most common precipitant of deep venous thrombosis.[31] Elicitation of pain with dorsiflexion of the foot (*Homans sign*) is an unreliable diagnostic sign. Noninvasive imaging with duplex venous ultrasonography or plethysmography is required for diagnosis.[32]

Varicose Veins. Varicose veins are tortuous dilations of the superficial veins that result from defective venous valves, intrinsic weakness of the vein wall, high intraluminal pressure, or arteriovenous fistulas. Patients may be concerned about the appearance of their legs or may complain of a dull ache that is present with standing and relieved by elevation. Visual inspection of the legs with the patient in the standing position confirms the presence of varicose veins.

Chronic Venous Insufficiency. Chronic venous insufficiency (incompetence of venous valves) may follow deep venous thrombosis or may occur without previous thrombosis. It may be unilateral, but more commonly is bilateral. Patients complain of a dull ache in the legs that is present with standing and relieved by elevation. Physical examination reveals increased leg circumference, edema, and superficial varicose veins. Erythema, dermatitis, and hyperpigmentation may develop in the distal lower extremity.[30,31] When venous ulcers occur, they are more common near the medial malleolus.

Heart

The precordium should be assessed in an orderly fashion using the techniques of inspection, palpation, and auscultation. Careful inspection and palpation provide better information on heart size than does percussion. Percussion is most useful in the rare instance where dextrocardia is suspected.[6] The room should be quiet and permit privacy. Both the patient and the examiner should be in comfortable positions before beginning the examination.

Topographic Anatomy

Knowledge of the topographic anatomy of the cardiac and vascular structures is essential to understanding the clinical findings. The *left ventricle* is primarily a posterior structure and is evaluated on the anterior chest wall at the cardiac apex, which is normally in the fifth intercostal space (ICS) at, or slightly medial to, the midclavicular line (MCL). The *right ventricle* is anterior to the left ventricle and underlies the sternum and the lower left sternal border at the fourth and fifth ICS. The *right atrium* is just lateral to the lower right sternal border. The outflow tracts of both ventricles underlie the third left ICS (Erb point). The main *pulmonary artery* underlies the second left ICS, and the *ascending aorta* underlies the second right ICS (Fig. 9-16).[8,33]

Inspection

Inspect the precordium with the patient supine, the chest exposed, and the backrest slightly elevated. Stand at the foot or right side of the bed or examining table. Tangential lighting allows the examiner to detect chest wall movements more easily.

Note any *pulsations* (outward movement) or *retractions* (inward movement) and describe the location by ICS and distance in centimeters from the sternum or the MCL. Determine whether it occurs in systole or diastole by timing it with the carotid pulse or the heart sounds. In general, retractions are more easily seen, and pulsations are more easily palpated.

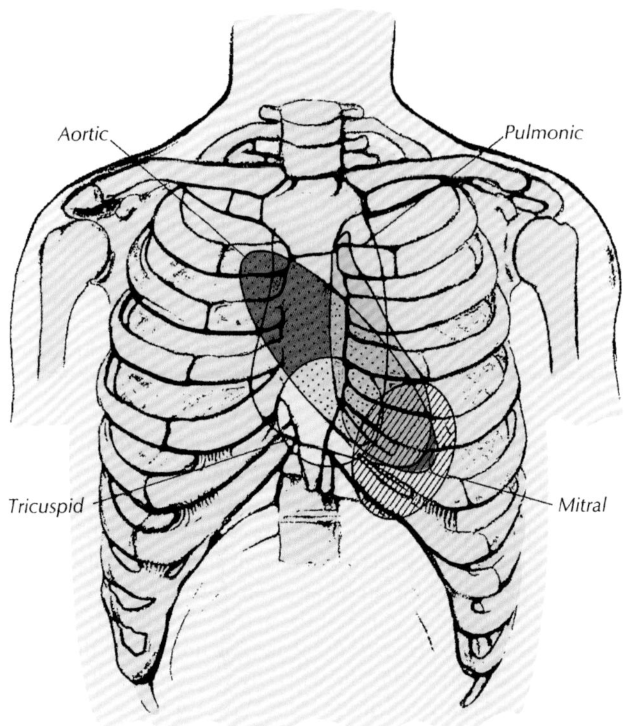

Figure 9-16. Areas to be assessed in the precordial examination. (Drawn from Leatham A. *An Introduction to the Examination of the Cardiovascular System.* 2nd ed. Oxford: Oxford University Press; 1979:20.)

When visible, the normal *apex impulse* can be seen within the fifth ICS at or just medial to the MCL. It is an early systolic pulsation with a rapid upstroke and downstroke. A late systolic retraction, 1 to 2 cm long, in the fourth or fifth ICS may also be normally seen and is produced by ventricular emptying. The apex impulse cannot be seen in every patient. It is easily detected in thin patients, whereas it may not be visible in those who are obese or have large breasts or barrel chests. An apex impulse that is below the fifth ICS, lateral to the MCL, or seen in more than one ICS represents left ventricular enlargement.

Slight movement over the sternum or the epigastrium can be normal in thin people and in those with fever or anemia who may have hyperdynamic heartbeats. A *sternal rise* that is sustained after systole begins usually indicates right ventricular enlargement. Pulsations in other areas are abnormal. For example, pulsation over the second right ICS may represent an aortic aneurysm, and pulsation over the second left ICS can represent increased filling pressure or flow in the pulmonary artery.

Paradoxical movement of the left anterior precordium is suggestive of a left ventricular aneurysm. With paradoxical movement, as the apex contracts, the aneurysmic area bulges. This ectopic impulse usually is seen above the apex impulse. The visibility of abnormal pulsations can be enhanced by balancing a tongue depressor on the chest over the pulsation.

Palpation

Movement that was not visible on inspection may be detected by palpation. All areas should be palpated using either the ball of the palm (at the base of the fingers) or the fingertips. In general, the palm surface is more sensitive to *thrills* (vibrations), whereas fingertips are more sensitive to *pulsations.* Thrills indicate turbulence of blood flow and are associated with murmurs. Impulses are described in terms of *location, size, amplitude, duration,* and *time in the cardiac cycle* (systole or diastole). To facilitate measurement of the horizontal location in centimeters from the MCL, or the size of the impulse, it is helpful for the examiner to measure his or her hand and use it as a "ruler." For example, the distance from the tip of the finger to the first joint, the second joint, and the third joint can be used.

Assess the apex impulse for location, size, amplitude, and duration. The apex impulse is, by definition, the furthest point leftward and downward at which a cardiac pulsation can be seen or felt.[3] The normal apex impulse is felt as a light tap, extending over 3 cm or less. The apex impulse is felt immediately after the first heart sound and lasts halfway through systole. An impulse that is diffuse (felt over two ICSs), increased in amplitude, or laterally or inferiorly displaced suggests increased volume load and left ventricular dilatation, such as occurs in mitral insufficiency or left ventricular failure. An impulse that is sustained, enlarged, and, sometimes, laterally displaced suggests obstruction to outflow with increased ventricular pressure load and concentric hypertrophy of the muscle, such as occurs in aortic stenosis or systemic hypertension.[6] If the apex impulse cannot be felt with the patient lying supine, examine the patient in the left lateral position, which brings the apex of the heart against the chest wall; the quality of the apex beat still can be determined even though its size and position may be slightly altered. A diastolic outward pulsation indicates impaired ventricular filling and corresponds to an S_3 (early to mid-diastole) or S_4 (late diastole) heard on auscultation.

Next, palpate the right ventricular area. The presence of a pulsation suggests right ventricular enlargement. Palpation of the epigastrium, by placing the palmar surface of the hand over the area and sliding the fingers toward the xiphoid, can also detect right ventricular enlargement. Pulsations beating down on the fingertips indicate right ventricular movement. Pulsations pushing upward against the hand originate in the aorta. An increased aortic pulse could indicate abdominal aortic aneurysm or aortic regurgitation. Hepatic pulsations may be felt in the epigastrium but also over the right upper abdomen. The liver may pulsate with tricuspid valve disease, severe right ventricular failure, or pulmonary hypertension.[3] A thrill at the lower left sternal border suggests tricuspid valve disease.

Then, palpate the third left ICS and the second left and right ICSs. Systolic pulsations in the second left or right ICS suggest increased pressure or enlargement of the pulmonary artery or the aorta, respectively; thrills suggest pulmonary or aortic valve abnormalities.

Auscultation

Stethoscope. A good-quality stethoscope is required for cardiac auscultation. Although the human ear is able to hear sounds ranging in frequency from 20 cycles per second, or Hertz (Hz), to 20,000 Hz, it is most sensitive to 1000 to 5000 Hz. The frequency of most heart sounds is less than 1000 Hz. The stethoscope must transmit these low-frequency sounds to the ear.

The parts of the stethoscope are the ear pieces, tubing, and chest pieces. The ear pieces should fit comfortably into the ear canal and be snug enough so that extraneous sound cannot enter. They also must be kept free of ear wax. Double tubing with a small internal diameter (3 mm) should extend from the ear pieces to the chest pieces. In addition, the tubing should be reasonably short (25 to 30 cm) so the sound is not diluted and should be thick to minimize room noise.[33]

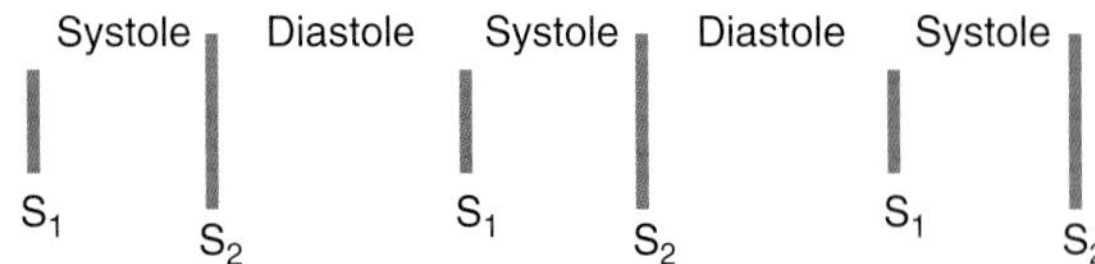

Figure 9-17. Normal heart sounds.

There are two classic types of chest pieces, the diaphragm and the bell. The *diaphragm*, which brings out higher frequencies and filters out the lower ones, is useful for listening to the first and second heart sounds (S_1 and S_2), high-frequency murmurs, and lung sounds. The diaphragm should be pressed firmly against the chest wall. The *bell* filters out high-frequency sounds and accentuates the low-frequency ones. Diastolic filling sounds and the low-frequency murmurs of mitral and tricuspid stenosis are heard best with the bell.[33] The bell should rest lightly on the chest; if firm pressure is applied, the skin becomes taut and acts like a diaphragm. When auscultating heart sounds, the nurse stands on the patient's right side so that, as he or she places the bell of the stethoscope on the patient's chest, the chest piece is balanced. Because the bell does not have to be held in place, the possibilities of creating extraneous sounds and filtering out low frequencies are reduced. Some stethoscopes have a single chestpiece with tunable diaphragm. Very light skin contact is used to listen to low-frequency sounds and firm pressure is used to listen to high-frequency sounds.

As part of a cardiac examination, all areas identified in Figure 9-17 should be auscultated except the epigastrium. The listener's goals when auscultating the precordium are to identify normal heart sounds, the heart rate, and rhythm; extra diastolic and systolic sounds; murmurs; and pericardial friction rubs.

Technique. The stethoscope is placed directly on the chest wall; adequate auscultation of the heart and lungs through clothing is impossible. The room should be quiet; the patient and examiner should be comfortable. Cardiac auscultation should be performed with the patient in three positions: supine, lying partially on the left side, and sitting up, leaning forward. The examiner can begin listening either at the cardiac apex or at the base. Beginning at the apex allows the examiner to focus initially on the first heart sound, clearly identify systole and diastole, and think through the cardiac cycle while listening at each site. The apex is the location of the apex impulse identified by palpation. Remember that left ventricular enlargement shifts the apex from the normal location. The timing of extra sounds in the cardiac cycle, the location in which they are best heard, and the quality of the sound are used to differentiate one from another.

It is important to proceed in a systematic manner. Inching the stethoscope up and down the chest wall is a useful technique and allows the examiner to focus on specific events in the cardiac cycle (Table 9-5). At each location, listen sequentially to four events: S_1, systole (interval between S_1 and S_2), S_2, and diastole (interval between S_2 and S_1). For example, begin at the apical area with the diaphragm of the stethoscope and focus on S_1 and S_2 (Note, a description of the heart sounds follow.). Normally, S_1 is louder than or equal to S_2 at the apex. Listen carefully during systole and during diastole for clicks, murmurs, or other extra sounds. Inch the stethoscope toward the sternum to the right ventricular area and listen for a split S_1. Continue to move the stethoscope up the left sternal border to the second left ICS and note the change in relative intensity of the heart sounds. Normally, S_2 is louder than S_1 at the base. Continue to listen for splitting of the second heart sound and, if present, determine whether it is physiologic or abnormal. Move the stethoscope to the second right ICS and listen for an ejection sound in early systole after S_1. Listen with the bell along the lower left sternal border for right ventricular S_3 and S_4. Move the bell to the apical area and listen for left ventricular S_3 and S_4. An opening sound of the mitral valve (high frequency) can be distinguished from an S_3 by pressing firmly with the bell to stretch the skin. Stretching the skin causes it to act as a diaphragm and filters out low-frequency sounds. When using a stethoscope with a tunable diaphragm one can alternate listening with light (bell) and firm (diaphragm) pressure at each site.

Table 9-5 • AUSCULTATORY TECHNIQUE

Location	Chest Piece	Sounds
Apex	Diaphragm	S_1 intensity; opening sounds; murmurs from aortic and mitral valve
	Bell	Left S_3, S_4; murmurs
Left sternal border	Diaphragm	S_2 intensity; split S_1; murmurs from tricuspid and pulmonic valves and from atrial septal defects
	Bell	Right S_3, S_4
Base	Diaphragm	Split S_2; ejection sounds; murmurs from aortic valve
	Bell	Murmurs from aortic valve or dilated aorta

Normal Heart Sounds. Normal heart sounds consist of the first and second heart sounds, S_1 and S_2. Both are of relatively high frequency and can, therefore, be heard clearly with the diaphragm of the stethoscope. Systole is normally shorter than diastole; with slow heart rates (less than 100 beats/min), the two sounds are easily distinguished by the cadence of the rhythm (Fig. 9-17). However, in more rapid rhythms, diastole shortens so that systole and diastole are of equal duration or, as the rate increases further, diastole becomes shorter than systole. To identify systole and diastole properly in this instance, the examiner should palpate the carotid artery while listening to the heart; the carotid upstroke immediately follows S_1.

Phonocardiograms or echocardiograms can be used to validate the auscultatory findings. In a phonocardiogram, heart sounds, electrocardiogram, and carotid pulse tracings are recorded simultaneously. Phonocardiograms are most often used for research or teaching. Echocardiograms are used clinically to demonstrate abnormalities of valve structure and cardiac function.

The *first heart sound* is due primarily to closure of the mitral and tricuspid valves and is, therefore, heard loudest at the apex of the heart. Phonetically, if the heart sounds are "lub-dup," S_1 is the "lub." Mitral and tricuspid closure usually is heard as a single sound.

The intensity of the S_1 depends on leaflet mobility, position of the atrioventricular valves at the onset of systole, and the rate of ventricular upstroke. A loud S_1 is noted clinically in mitral stenosis when the cusps are mobile; with a short PR interval (0.08 to 0.13 second) because the leaflets are wide open when systolic contraction begins; in tachycardia, hyperthyroidism, or exercise because of an increased rate of pressure rise in the ventricle; and in the presence of a mechanical prosthetic mitral valve. Most commonly, a soft S_1 is due to poor conduction of sound through the chest wall, but other causes include a fixed or immobile valve; a long PR interval (0.20 to 0.26 second) or a slow heart rate, which allows the atrioventricular valves to float back into position before the onset of ventricular systole; low flow at the end of diastole;

and β-adrenergic or calcium-channel blockers that reduce the rate of rise of ventricular pressure. The intensity of S_1 varies from beat to beat in atrial fibrillation because diastolic filling time is not constant. In a regular rhythm with a variable S_1 intensity, complete heart block should be suspected.[34] Variation in the intensity of S_1 can be evaluated by listening carefully to the relative intensity of S_1 and S_2 at the apex and the base. For example, when the intensity of S_1 is increased, it may be equal to or louder than S_2 at the base.[34] When assessing variation in S_1, it is helpful to have the patient hold his or her breath because respiratory movements may cause variation in the intensity of heart sounds.

Splitting of the first heart sound occurs when tricuspid closure is delayed and is best heard at the lower left sternal border. Pathologic splitting of S_1 results from right bundle branch block, tricuspid stenosis, and atrial septal defect.[34] Splitting of S_1 helps to differentiate supraventricular from ventricular tachycardia. In supraventricular rhythms, S_1 is normal; in ventricular rhythms, S_1 is split.[3] When supraventricular rhythms are conducted aberrantly, S_1 is split.

The *second heart sound* results primarily from closure of the aortic and pulmonic valves and is loudest at the base of the heart. Phonetically, the "dup" of the "lub-dup" is the S_2. The intensity of S_2 is determined by the pressure in the receiving vessels, the mobility of the valve leaflets, the degree of apposition of the leaflets, and the size of the aortic root. Intensity is increased with systemic or pulmonary hypertension, ascending aortic aneurysm, and in the presence of a mechanical prosthetic aortic valve. Intensity may be diminished in heart failure, myocardial infarction, pulmonary embolism, clinical shock, and stenosis of the aortic or pulmonic valve.[34]

Physiologic (normal) *splitting* of S_2 occurs during inspiration. During inspiration, an increased amount of blood is returned to the right side of the heart and a decreased amount of blood is returned to the left side of the heart due to trapping in the expanded lung. Pulmonic valve closure (P_2) is delayed because of the extra time needed for the increased blood volume to pass through the pulmonic valve, and aortic valve closure (A_2) occurs slightly early because of the relatively smaller amount of blood ejected from the left ventricle. In addition, the time of closure of P_2 is affected by the "hang out" interval, which is inversely related to pulmonary vascular impedance. During inspiration, the pulmonary vascular impedance decreases and P_2 is delayed; on expiration the opposite occurs.[34] If the two components are fairly close together, it is difficult to appreciate two distinct and separate sounds. A physiologic split S_2 may seem muffled or sound like a short drum roll on inspiration compared with expiration. On expiration, the split sounds merge (Fig. 9-18A). Normal splitting should be evaluated during quiet respiration and may be better heard with the patient sitting.[3] In pathologic splitting of S_2 (wide or fixed splits), the second sound is split during both inspiration and expiration, although there may be some respiratory variation in the amount of the split.

Paradoxical (abnormal) *splitting* of S_2 also can occur. Paradoxical splitting is due to any mechanism that causes late aortic valve closure (A_2), such as electrical delay (left bundle branch block, right ventricular pacing, or right ventricular ectopy), mechanical obstruction (aortic stenosis or systolic hypertension), or impaired left ventricular contractile function (left ventricular failure or left ventricular ischemia; see Fig. 9-18B). Because P_2 is soft and A_2 is comparably loud and easily transmitted, a split S_2 is heard best in the second left ICS (pulmonary outflow tract). In paradoxical splitting, the second component (aortic closure) is louder than the first component (pulmonic closure).

Normally, A_2 is louder than P_2, even in the pulmonic area, and P_2 is not well heard, if at all, in other areas of the precordium. In pulmonary hypertension, the intensity of P_2 increases so that A_2 is less than or equal to P_2. The loud P_2 can be heard in other areas of the precordium, particularly the lower left sternal border and the cardiac apex.[8]

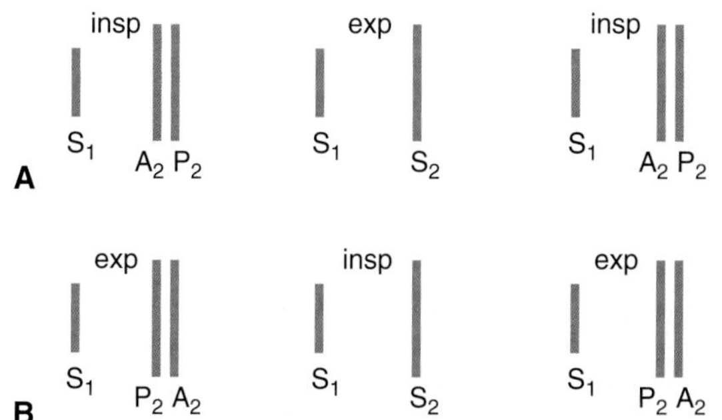

Figure 9-18. Splitting of the S_2. **(A)** Physiologic splitting. During inspiration (*insp*), the P_2 sound is delayed. **(B)** Paradoxical splitting. During expiration (*exp*), A_2 is delayed.

Extra Diastolic Sounds. Extra diastolic sounds consist of diastolic filling sounds and opening snaps. *Diastolic filling sounds* (S_3 and S_4) occur as blood enters a noncompliant ventricle during the two phases of rapid ventricular filling: the end of the early rapid filling phase, as active ventricular relaxation ceases (S_3); and, with atrial contraction, the active, rapid filling phase (S_4). Three theories have been proposed to explain the generation of the third and fourth heart sounds: the mitral valve theory, the chest wall theory, and the ventricular wall vibration theory. The last is the most widely accepted theory. Sound is produced within the ventricle by the abrupt decrease in wall motion (S_3) or with rapid filling of a noncompliant ventricle that causes a rapid deceleration of blood flow.[35] Diastolic filling sounds can arise from either or both ventricles. The cadence suggests the sound of a galloping horse, and these sounds are sometimes called diastolic gallops.

A *physiologic S3* can be heard in healthy children or young adults but usually disappears by 40 years of age. Its disappearance with advancing age has been attributed to decreased ventricular wall compliance with reduced early ventricular filling.[3] An S_3 in people older than age 40 years is usually pathologic and signals impaired systolic function.[35] It is one of the first clinical findings associated with cardiac decompensation, such as left ventricular heart failure (left ventricular S_3), primary pulmonary hypertension and cor pulmonale (right ventricular S_3), or insufficiency of the mitral, aortic, or tricuspid valves. An S_3 follows the S_2 in a "lub-dup-*ta*" cadence (Fig. 9-19). Using the bell of the stethoscope, listen for a left ventricular S_3 over the apex of the heart; for a right ventricular S_3, listen over the lower left sternal border. By having the patient in the left lateral position, the apex is brought forward against the chest wall, making the left ventricular S_3 louder and, therefore, easier to hear.

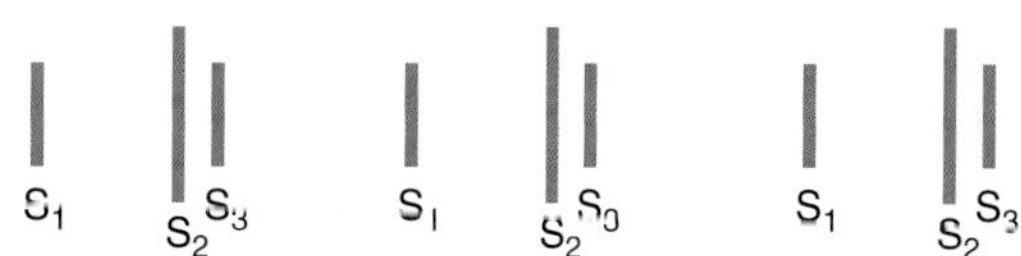

Figure 9-19. An S_3 gallop immediately follows the S_2.

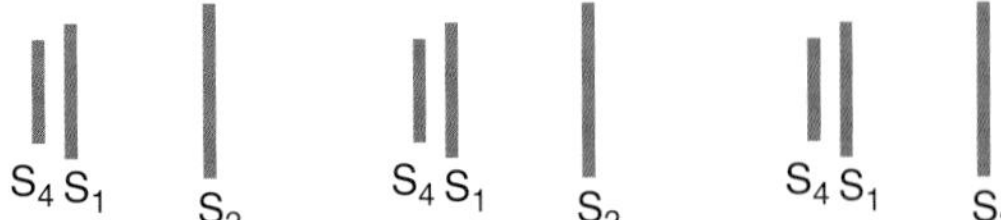

Figure 9-20. An S_4 gallop immediately precedes the S_1.

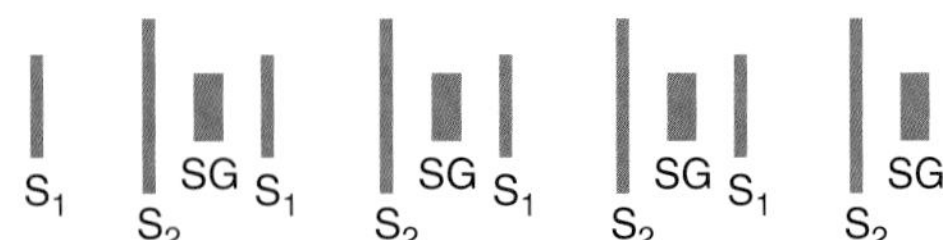

Figure 9-22. Summation gallop.

The S_4 occurs after atrial contraction as the blood is ejected into a noncompliant ventricle, producing a rapid elevation of ventricular pressure, and signals diastolic dysfunction. Although it is the fourth heart sound, because the S_4 occurs at the end of ventricular diastole, it is heard immediately before S_1 and sounds like "*ta*-lub-dup" (Fig. 9-20). The S_4 is heard in most patients who have had a myocardial infarction, in a large number of patients experiencing angina pectoris, and in patients with coronary heart disease. It is also heard in patients with left ventricular hypertrophy due to hypertension, hypertrophic cardiomyopathy, or aortic stenosis. It is common in older adults because of the decreased compliance of the ventricle that occurs with age and the prevalence of hypertension and aortic stenosis in this population. An S_4 does not necessarily imply cardiac failure in people with ventricular hypertrophy. Because atrial contraction is necessary to produce an S_4, it is not heard in patients with atrial fibrillation. As with the S_3, listen for an S_4 using the bell of the stethoscope. A left ventricular S_4 is heard best at the apex, with the patient lying in the left lateral position; right ventricular S_4 is loudest over the lower left sternal border. Inching the stethoscope from the apex to the lower left sternal border can be helpful in differentiating right- and left-sided sounds. Left-sided sounds fade and right-sided sounds get louder as the stethoscope approaches the sternum.

A *quadruple rhythm* may be heard in patients with severe cardiac failure and both systolic and diastolic dysfunctions. If the heart rate is slow enough, four distinct heart sounds (S_1, S_2, and both S_3 and S_4) can be heard (Fig. 9-21). However, if a patient is ill enough to have a quadruple rhythm, tachycardia also usually is present. In this case, a *summation gallop* is heard, in which the S_3 and S_4 gallops fuse in mid-diastole to one loud diastolic sound. The summation gallop resembles the sound of a galloping horse (Fig. 9-22).

It stands to reason that in a noncompliant ventricle there should be more resistance to active ventricular filling than to passive ventricular filling; therefore, an S_4 gallop should be generated more easily than an S_3 gallop. Therefore, one would expect all patients with normal sinus rhythm who have an S_3 gallop to have an S_4 gallop as well. However, patients with normal sinus rhythm frequently have only an S_3. The cause for this finding is unknown, although one possibility may be an absence of actual mechanical atrial contraction in spite of electrical atrial activity.

Opening snaps are associated with the opening of a stenotic mitral valve. Opening sounds are not heard with normal valves. The sound is heard in very early diastole, medial to the cardiac apex. The sound can be loud and transmitted throughout the precordium (Fig. 9-23). Unlike an S_3, an opening snap has a high-pitched, snapping quality and is heard best with the diaphragm of the stethoscope.[33]

Extra Systolic Sounds. Extra systolic sounds consist of early systolic ejection sounds and systolic clicks. *Early ejection sounds* (Fig. 9-24) coincide with the opening of the aortic and pulmonic valves. They are heard shortly after S_1 and are high-pitched and clicking in quality. An *aortic ejection sound* is heard at the base or apex and accompanies a dilated aorta or aortic stenosis. *Pulmonic ejection sounds* are heard loudest in the second or third left ICSs and occur with pulmonary artery dilatation, pulmonary hypertension, and pulmonary stenosis.[33] *Mid- to late-systolic clicks* are associated with mitral valve prolapse; they occur from tensing of the leaflet or chordae when the limit of excursion is reached, and frequently they are followed by a murmur (Fig. 9-25).

Murmurs. Heart murmurs are sounds produced in the heart or great vessels by turbulent blood flow. Turbulent blood flow can be produced by[33]:

- Increased rate of flow across a normal valve (exercise, pregnancy, anemia)
- Flow across a partial obstruction (valvular stenosis, pulmonary or systemic hypertension)
- Flow across an irregularity without obstruction (bicuspid aortic valve, thickening of aortic cusps with aging)
- Flow into a dilated vessel (dilation of the aortic root)
- Backward flow across an incompetent valve or through a ventricular septal defect

Murmurs are classified according to systolic or diastolic *timing* (Fig. 9-26); *intensity* (Table 9-6); *location* (where the murmur is heard loudest); *radiation,* such as to the back, neck, or axilla; *configuration* (Fig. 9-27); *quality,* such as harsh, rough, rumbling, blowing, squeaking, or musical; and *duration* (Fig. 9-26).[6,33] Murmurs may be organic (due to intrinsic cardiovascular disease), functional (produced by circulatory disturbances such as anemia, pregnancy), or innocent (occur in the absence of disease).[3]

In adults, the most common systolic murmurs are produced by semilunar valve stenosis (ejection murmurs), atrioventricular valve insufficiency (regurgitant or holosystolic murmurs), and ventricular septal defect (early systolic murmurs) secondary to myocardial infarction. In older adults, the murmur of aortic sclerosis (thickening of aortic valve leaflets) is common. The most common diastolic murmurs are produced by the reverse set of circumstances: insufficiency of semilunar valves (early regurgitant murmurs) and stenosis of the atrioventricular valves (mid- to

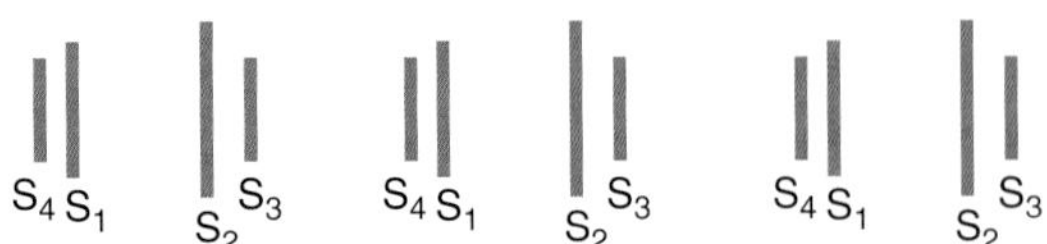

Figure 9-21. Quadruple rhythm.

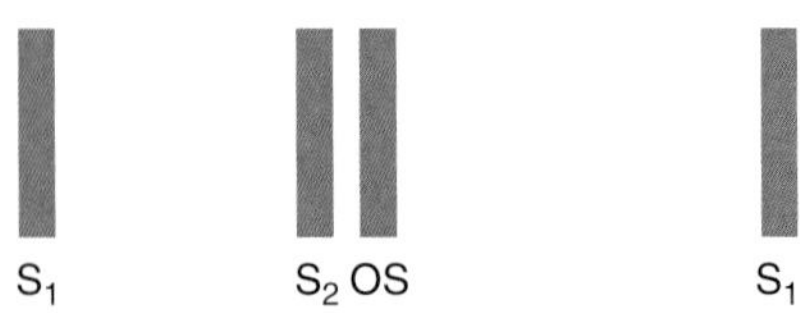

Figure 9-23. Opening snap (OS).

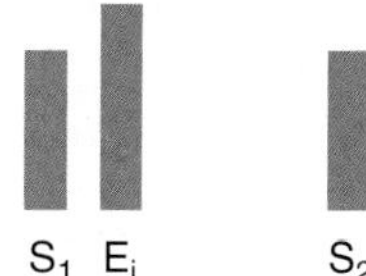

Figure 9-24. Early systolic ejection sound.

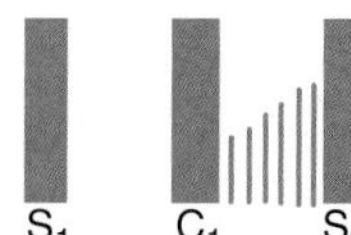

Figure 9-25. Mid- to late-systolic click.

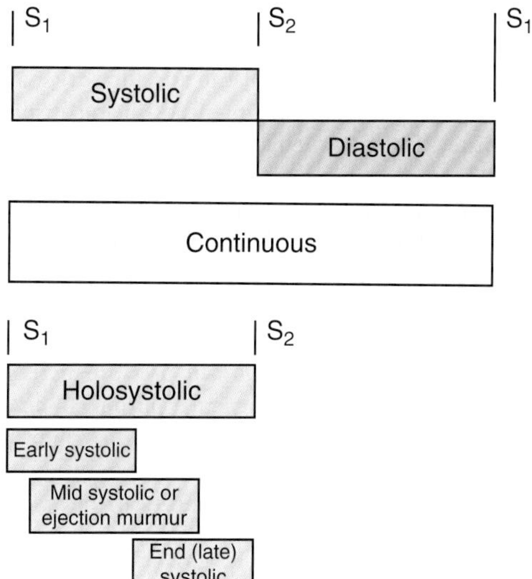

Figure 9-26. Classification of murmurs by timing. (From Tilkian A, Conover M. *Understanding Heart Sounds and Murmurs.* 3rd ed. Philadelphia, PA: Saunders; 1993:99.)

Table 9-6 • GRADATIONS OF MURMURS

Grade	Description
Grade 1	Very faint, heard only after listener has "tuned in"; may not be heard in all positions
Grade 2	Quiet, but heard immediately after placing the stethoscope on the chest
Grade 3	Moderately loud
Grade 4	Loud, with palpable thrill
Grade 5	Very loud, with thrill. May be heard when the stethoscope is partly off the chest
Grade 6	Very loud, with thrill. May be heard with stethoscope entirely off the chest

Reprinted with permission from Bickley LS, Szilagyi PG. *Bates' Guide to Physical Examination and History Taking.* 10th ed. Philadelphia, PA: Lippincott Williams & Wilkins; 2009.

Figure 9-27. Configuration of murmurs. **(A)** Crescendo. **(B)** Decrescendo. **(C)** Crescendo-decrescendo (diamond). **(D)** Plateau (even). **(E)** Variable (uneven). (From Perloff JK. *Physical Examination of the Heart and Circulation.* Philadelphia, PA: WB Saunders; 1990:208.)

late-diastolic rumbles). The loudness of the murmur may not correlate with the severity of the valvular lesion (e.g., a patient with a grade 5 to 6 murmur in whom cardiogenic shock develops actually may have reduced intensity of the murmur because of diminished cardiac blood flow).

Recognizing an innocent murmur is an important and difficult skill. The innocent murmur can often be diagnosed by its clinical features and the absence of other clinical abnormalities. Clinical features of innocent murmurs include the following: always systolic, soft, short, modified by change in posture, normal S_2, and most common at left sternal border.[3] Echocardiography may be needed to confirm its innocence, and follow-up is essential. The precordial "whoop" or "honk" may be an innocent finding in patients without organic heart disease or may represent an exaggerated phase of an organic murmur.[3,33]

In the cardiac care unit, nurses are most often concerned with changes in murmurs rather than in their diagnosis. However, it is important to diagnose accurately the onset of murmurs of papillary muscle dysfunction and aortic insufficiency.

Normally, papillary muscle contraction allows for complete closure of the atrioventricular valves. However, when the papillary muscles are ischemic (most often in the left ventricle), they are unable to contract properly, preventing the chordae tendineae from being held tautly and, in turn, from holding the mitral valve leaflets closed during left ventricular contraction. Blood is, therefore, allowed to flow backward through the mitral valve (mitral regurgitation) during systole. The murmur of mitral regurgitation secondary to papillary muscle dysfunction is systolic (occurring in early- to mid-systole) and usually soft, high pitched, and crescendo–decrescendo in configuration. In the presence of heart failure or angina, the murmur may become holosystolic.

A new murmur of *papillary muscle dysfunction* in the patient with acute myocardial infarction must be recognized immediately because interventions must be instituted to relieve the papillary muscle ischemia and prevent progression to papillary muscle infarction. Should the papillary muscles infarct, they also may rupture; there is a high mortality rate associated with papillary muscle rupture because of the development of sudden and profound heart failure.

In the setting of acute aortic dissection, coronary artery bypass grafting with a friable aorta, or aortic valve replacement, *new-onset aortic insufficiency* indicates retrograde dissection of the aorta, or valve dehiscence. The murmur of aortic insufficiency is an early diastolic, decrescendo murmur, heard at the second right or third left ICS that radiates toward the apex. In acute aortic

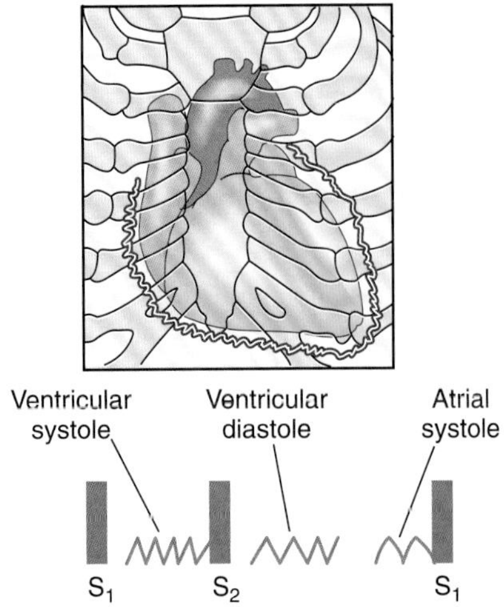

Timing	May have three short components, each associated with cardiac movement: (1) atrial systole, (2) ventricular systole, and (3) ventricular diastole. Usually the first two components are present; all three make diagnosis easy; only one (usually the systolic) invites confusion with a murmur.
Location	Variable, but usually heard best in the 3rd left ICS
Radiation	Little
Intensity	Variable. May increase when the patient leans forward, exhales, and holds breath (in contrast to pleural rub)
Quality	Scratchy, scraping
Pitch	High (heard better with a diaphragm)

Figure 9-28. Pericardial friction rub.

insufficiency, the intensity of S_1 is frequently diminished because of the increase in ventricular volume, and P_2 may be accentuated because of the rapid rise in pulmonary vascular pressure.[33] Acute left ventricular failure may result from volume overload alone or, in the case of continued retrograde dissection, from myocardial infarction secondary to dissection of the coronary arteries.

Pericardial Friction Rubs. Pericardial friction rubs are characteristic of pericarditis, which occurs in more than 15% of patients with acute myocardial infarction. A pericardial friction rub develops in approximately 7% of patients with myocardial infarction, commonly by the fourth day after myocardial infarction. Rubs may be transient, lasting only several hours. The rub occurs with heart movement; each movement creates its own short, scratchy sound (Fig. 9-28). Pericardial friction rubs are classified as three-component (atrial systole, ventricular systole, and ventricular diastole), two-component (ventricular systole and diastole), or one-component (ventricular systole) rubs. One-component rubs may be difficult to differentiate from a murmur. Rubs are best heard either with the patient sitting upright and leaning forward with the breath expelled (most appropriate for the patient with an acute myocardial infarction) or with the patient on his or her hands and knees in bed or on the examination table (useful in a nonacute situation). A pericardial friction rub can be heard with or without a pericardial effusion. Pericardial friction rubs can be differentiated from pleural friction rubs by having the patient hold his or her breath.

Pericardial friction rubs are common in postoperative cardiac patients. Also, a respirophasic squeak may be heard that is related to mediastinal or pleural tubes. Air in the mediastinum produces a crunching sound (Hamman sign) during auscultation of the precordium.

Dynamic Auscultation. Dynamic auscultation can be used to aid in the interpretation of heart sounds and murmurs. A variety of physiologic or pharmacologic maneuvers can be used to alter circulatory dynamics: respiration, postural changes, the Valsalva maneuver, postextrasystolic beats, isometric exercise, and vasoactive agents.[8] Table 9-7 summarizes the auscultatory effects of these maneuvers.

Respiration affects blood flow. *Inspiration* increases venous return to the right heart, increasing right ventricular diastolic pressure, stroke volume, and ejection time. Pulmonary vascular impedance is reduced, with increases in pulmonary vascular capacitance. With a normal respiratory rate, blood return to the left ventricle is reduced, resulting in decreased left ventricular diastolic pressure, stroke volume, and ejection time. Transmission of the augmented right ventricular volume to the left ventricle is delayed by three to four cardiac cycles in the pulmonary vasculature. All of the auscultatory events generated by the right heart are augmented during inspiration.[33] The use of the Müller maneuver (sustained inspiratory effort against a closed glottis) further augments the auscultatory effects of inspiration. *Expiration* increases venous return to the left heart, increasing left ventricular diastolic pressure, stroke volume, and ejection time.[6]

The *Valsalva maneuver* (forced expiration against a closed glottis) has variable effects associated with each of its four phases. In *phase I*, the *initial* phase, intrathoracic pressure increases, causing a transient elevation in left ventricular output. In *phase II*, the *straining* phase, venous return is decreased; first right, then left ventricular filling is reduced; stroke volume, mean arterial pressure, and pulse pressure are reduced; and heart rate is increased. In *phase III*, the *release* phase, venous return is increased, with subsequent increases in right, then left, ventricular filling. In *phase IV*, the *overshoot* phase, right ventricular filling and stroke volume return to baseline or may be elevated briefly. The return to baseline of left ventricular hemodynamics is delayed for six to eight beats and also may be elevated briefly.[6,33] During phase II, all murmurs diminish except those of hypertrophic cardiomyopathy and mitral valve prolapse. The Valsalva maneuver should not be held for more than 10 seconds because it reduces cardiac output.

Postural change from sitting or standing to lying down increases venous return first to the right and then to the left ventricle. Recumbence and passive leg raising cause most auscultatory cardiac events to increase except the murmurs of idiopathic hypertrophic subaortic stenosis and mitral valve prolapse. Sudden standing has the opposite effect; it reduces venous return and causes most murmurs, except hypertrophic cardiomyopathy and mitral valve prolapse, to decrease. Squatting simultaneously increases venous return and systemic vascular resistance.[6]

Postextrasystolic beats, if followed by a pause, increase ventricular filling and cardiac contractility. Similar hemodynamic changes occur with diastolic pauses in atrial fibrillation and sinus arrhythmia.[6]

Isometric exercise increases systemic vascular resistance, arterial pressure, heart rate, cardiac output, left ventricular filling

Table 9-7 • AUSCULTATORY EFFECTS OF PHYSIOLOGIC AND PHARMACOLOGIC MANEUVERS

Maneuver	Effect	Maneuver	Effect
Inspiration	Physiologically splits S_2	Valsalva maneuver	
	Attenuates left ventricular S_3 and S_4, mitral opening snap, and pulmonic ejection sound	Phase II (strain)	Attenuates S_3 and S_4
			Narrows A_2–P_2 interval
	Accentuates right ventricular S_3 and S_4, tricuspid opening snap, and right heart murmurs	Phase III (release)	Widens A_2–P_2 interval
		Phase IV (overshoot)	Returns to baseline or transiently accentuates S_3 and S_4
	Hastens and accentuates click-murmur of mitral valve prolapse	Postextrasystolic beats	Augments murmurs of aortic and pulmonic stenosis, tricuspid and aortic regurgitation, and hypertrophic obstructive cardiomyopathy
Expiration	Paradoxically splits S_2 opening snap, and left heart murmurs		Delays click-murmur of mitral valve prolapse
	Accentuates left ventricular S_3 and S_4, and murmur of mitral regurgitation		
	Attenuates right ventricular S_3 and S_4, and tricuspid opening snap	Isometric exercise	Accentuates left ventricular S_3 and S_4 and murmurs of aortic regurgitation, rheumatic mitral regurgitation
Lying down	Widens split S_2 in all respiratory phases		Ventricular septal defect, mitral stenosis
	Augments first right, then left, ventricular S_3 and S_4		Attenuates murmur of aortic stenosis
	Augments most systolic murmurs		Delays click-murmur of mitral valve prolapse
	Diminishes systolic murmur of hypertrophic obstructive cardiomyopathy	Amyl nitrate	Augments opening snaps; S_3; and murmurs of aortic, pulmonic, mitral, and tricuspid stenosis, and tricuspid regurgitation
	Delays and attenuates click-murmur of mitral valve prolapse		Diminishes murmurs of mitral and aortic regurgitation, ventricular septal defect, and Austin Flint
Sudden standing	Narrows split S_2 in all respiratory phases		Hastens click-murmur of mitral valve prolapse
	Diminishes first right, then left, ventricular S_3 and S_4		
	Diminishes most systolic murmurs		
	Accentuates systolic murmur of hypertrophic obstructive cardiomyopathy		
	Hastens and accentuates click-murmur of mitral valve prolapse	Methoxamine and phenylephrine	Accentuates murmurs of aortic and mitral regurgitation, and ventricular septal defect
Squatting	Augments right and left ventricular S_3 and S_4, and most murmurs		Diminishes murmurs of hypertrophic obstructive cardiomyopathy and aortic stenosis
	Delays click-murmur of mitral valve prolapse		Delays click-murmur of mitral valve prolapse

Adapted from Braunwald E. The physical examination. In: Braunwald E, ed. *Heart Disease: A Textbook of Cardiovascular Medicine.* 2nd ed. Philadelphia, PA: WB Saunders; 1984:35–38.

pressure, and heart size. Using a calibrated handgrip device, the patient sustains the handgrip for 20 to 30 seconds. The handgrip enhances S_3 and S_4 and aortic regurgitant murmurs. Avoid isometric exercise in patients with myocardial ischemia or ventricular arrhythmia. The patient should not perform the Valsalva maneuver simultaneously with isometric exercise.

Pharmacologic agents used in dynamic auscultation are amyl nitrate, methoxamine, and phenylephrine.[6] Inhalation of *amyl nitrate* for 10 to 15 seconds causes marked vasodilatation, reducing systemic arterial pressure and producing a reflex tachycardia, followed by an increase in stroke volume and venous return. *Methoxamine* and *phenylephrine* increase systemic vascular resistance. Both cause a reflex drop in heart rate and decrease contractility and cardiac output. Methoxamine, 3 to 5 mg intravenously, results in blood pressure elevation of 20 to 40 mm Hg, lasting 10 to 20 minutes. Phenylephrine, 0.5 mg intravenously, elevates blood pressure 30 mm Hg for 3 to 5 minutes.

Lungs

The respiratory assessment described in this chapter is elementary and is designed to assist the cardiac nurse in identifying respiratory manifestations seen in patients with heart disease. The room should be quiet and the patient's chest exposed. Proceed in a systematic manner: inspect, palpate, percuss, and auscultate. Always compare one side with the other; always place the stethoscope in direct contact with the chest wall. Begin with examination of the posterior chest, if possible, with the patient sitting upright and arms folded across the chest. Follow with assessment of the anterior chest with the patient lying down. Only the upper and lower lobes of the lung are accessible by posterior chest examination; to assess the right middle lobe, the lateral and anterior chest must be examined (Fig. 9-29).[8]

Inspection

Respiratory Rate, Depth, Rhythm, and Effort. Normally, the respiratory rate is less than 16 breaths per minute and the rhythm is regular (Fig. 9-30A). *Tachypnea*, rapid, shallow breathing, may be noted in patients who have heart failure, pain, or anxiety (Fig. 9-30B). *Bradypnea,* slow breathing, can be noted during sleep or after administration of respiratory depressant agents, such as morphine sulfate or anesthesia (Fig. 9-30C). *Cheyne–Stokes respirations*, characterized by periods of alternating deep breathing and apnea, occur in patients with severe left ventricular failure (Fig. 9-30D). Of particular concern is the duration of the apneic period. Use of accessory muscles of respiration, an upright, forward-leaning position, and pursed-lip breathing are visible signs of increased respiratory effort. Retraction of the ICSs is seen in severe asthma or upper airway obstruction.[8] A prolonged expiratory phase is associated with early airway obstruction.

Cough and Sputum. A dry, hacking *cough* from irritation of small airways is common in patients with pulmonary congestion from heart failure or patients taking angiotensin-converting

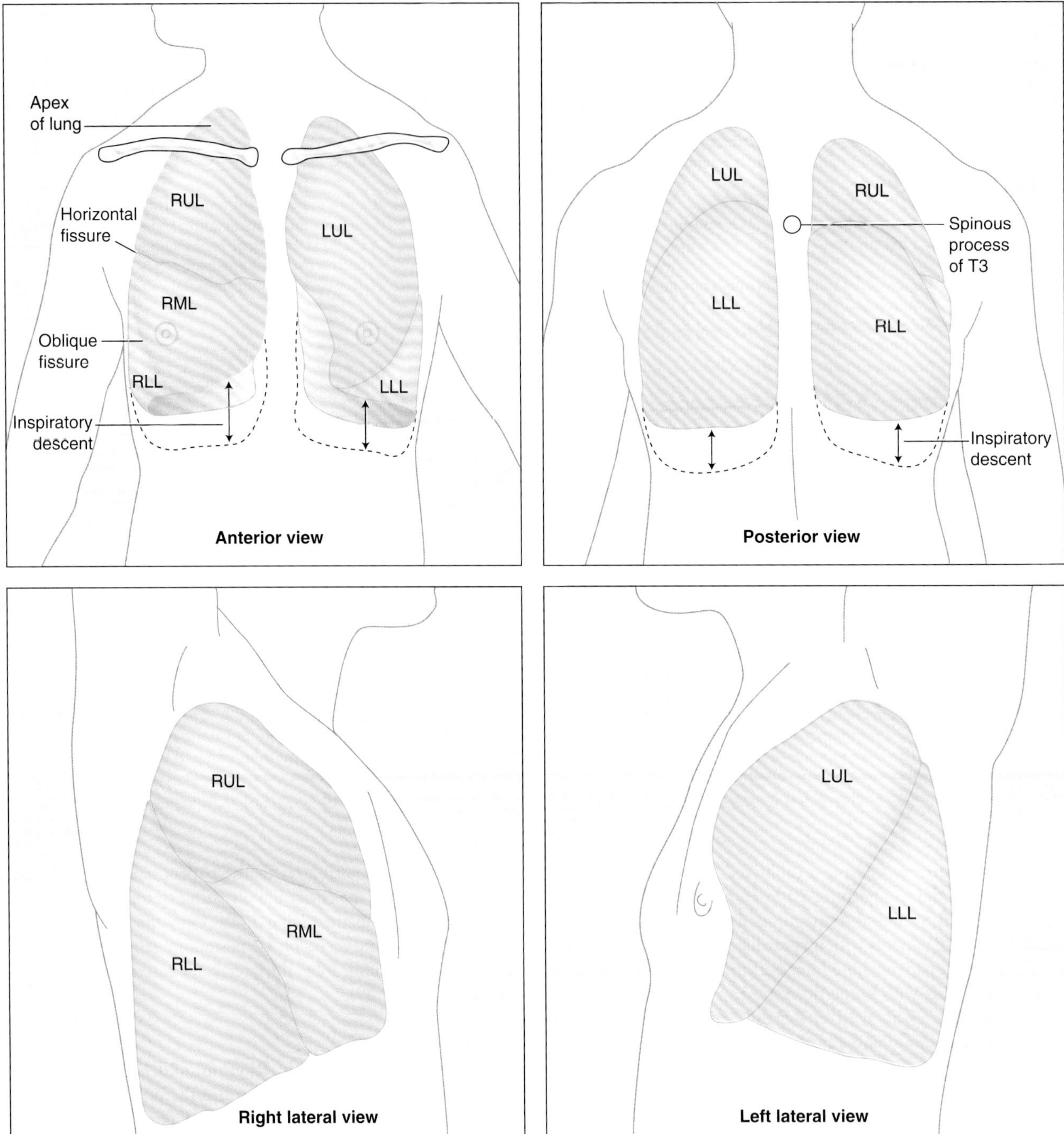

Figure 9-29. Respiratory assessment: Lobar localization. RUL, right upper lobe; RML, right middle lobe; RLL, right lower lobe; LUL, left upper lobe; LLL, left lower lobe.

enzyme inhibitors (ACE-Is). *Pink, frothy sputum* is indicative of pulmonary edema. Although an occasional cough may be normal, sputum production is always abnormal.

Chest Configuration. With *normal* chest configuration, the anteroposterior to lateral diameter ratio ranges from 1:2 to 5:7 (Fig. 9-31A). With a *barrel chest*, associated with pulmonary emphysema and aging, the anteroposterior to lateral diameter ratio increases to 1:1 or more (Fig. 9-31B). *Kyphoscoliosis*, an abnormal spinal curvature, may prevent the patient from fully expanding his or her lungs (Fig. 9-31C).

Posterior Chest

Palpation. Palpation is performed to identify areas of tenderness, respiratory excursion, and any observed abnormality and to elicit tactile fremitus. To assess *respiratory excursion*, the examiner places his or her thumbs slightly to either side of the spine and parallel to the 10th ribs (Fig. 9-32). As the patient inhales deeply, the examiner evaluates the depth and symmetry of the patient's breath by the movement of his or her thumbs.

Fremitus is the palpable vibration transmitted to the chest wall through the bronchopulmonary system when the patient speaks. The patient is asked to repeat the word "ninety-nine," and the

A

Inspiration Expiration

Normal
The respiratory rate is about 14–20 per min in normal adults and up to 44 per min in infants.

B

Rapid shallow breathing (*Tachypnea*)
Rapid shallow breathing has a number of causes, including restrictive lung disease, pleuritic chest pain, and an elevated diaphragm.

C

D

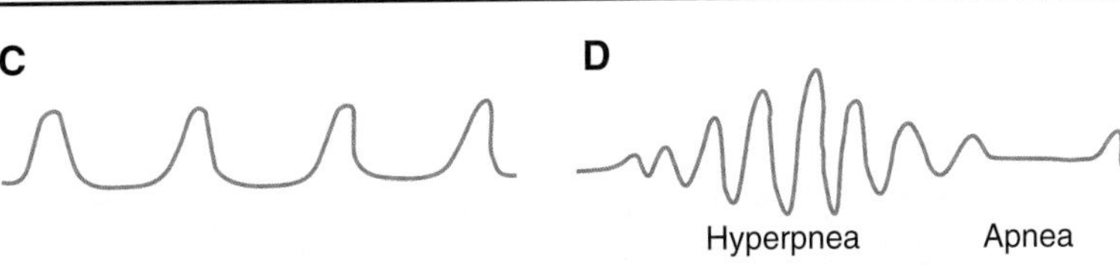

Slow breathing (*Bradypnea*)
Slow breathing may be secondary to such causes as diabetic coma, drug-induced respiratory depression, and increased intracranial pressure.

Cheyne–Stokes breathing
Periods of deep breathing alternate with periods of apnea (no breathing). Children and older adults normally may show this pattern in sleep. Other causes include heart failure, uremia, drug-induced respiratory depression, and brain damage (typically on both sides of the cerebral hemispheres or diencephalon).

Figure 9-30. Respiratory rate and rhythm. **(A)** Normal. **(B)** Tachypnea. **(C)** Bradypnea. **(D)** Cheyne–Stokes.

nurse uses the ball of his or her hand to palpate and compare areas over the posterior chest. Fremitus is decreased with air or fluid in the pleural space and by an obstructed bronchus; it is increased by lung consolidation. To estimate the level of the diaphragm bilaterally, the examiner places the ulnar surface of his or her hand parallel to its expected level and progressively moves the hand downward until fremitus is no longer felt. Posteriorly, the diaphragm is located between the 10th and 12th (with deep inspiration) ribs. An abnormally high diaphragm suggests a pleural effusion or atelectasis.

Percussion. Percussion causes vibrations in the underlying tissues, resulting in sounds that indicate if the tissues are solid or filled with fluid or air (Table 9-8). The technique of percussion involves the examiner placing the passive finger firmly over the area to be percussed and striking the distal interphalangeal joint of the middle finger of that hand with the middle finger of the opposite hand (Fig. 9-33). Percuss across both shoulders and then at 5-cm intervals down the back (Fig. 9-34), making side-to-side comparisons. Normal lung tissue (air-filled) produces *resonance*. *Dullness* replaces resonance when fluid or solid tissue

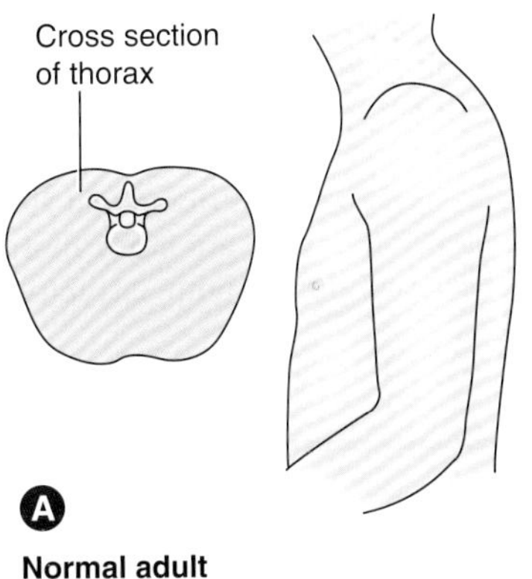

Normal adult
The thorax in the normal adult is wider than it is deep. Its lateral diameter is larger than its anteroposterior diameter.

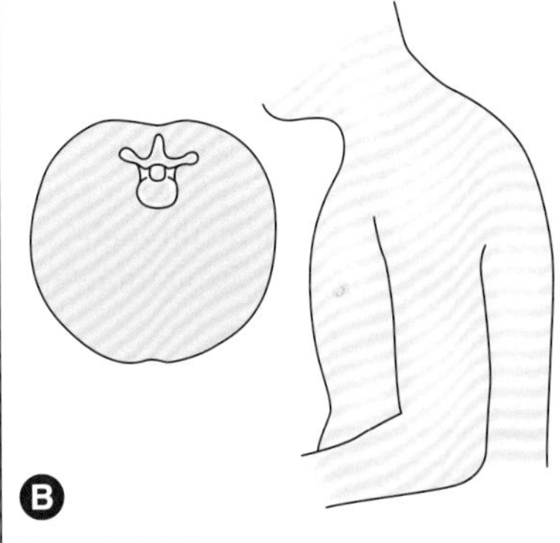

Barrel chest
A barrel chest has an increased antero-posterior diameter. This shape is normal during infancy, and often accompanies normal aging and chronic obstructive pulmonary disease.

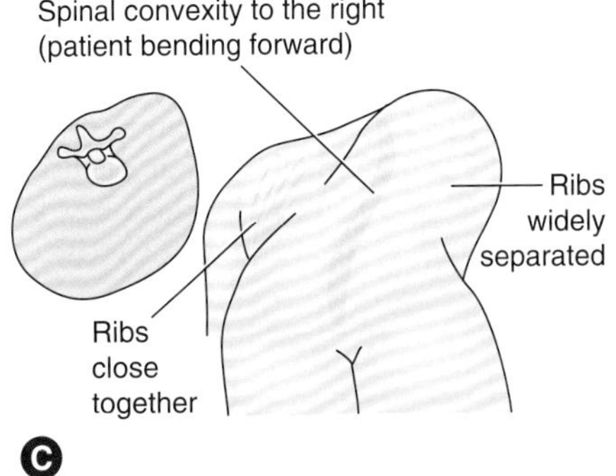

Thoracic kyphoscoliosis
In thoracic kyphoscoliosis, abnormal spinal curvatures and vertebral rotation deform the chest. Distortion of the underlying lungs may make interpretation of lung findings very difficult.

Figure 9-31. Chest wall configurations. **(A)** Normal. **(B)** Barrel chest. **(C)** Kyphoscoliosis.

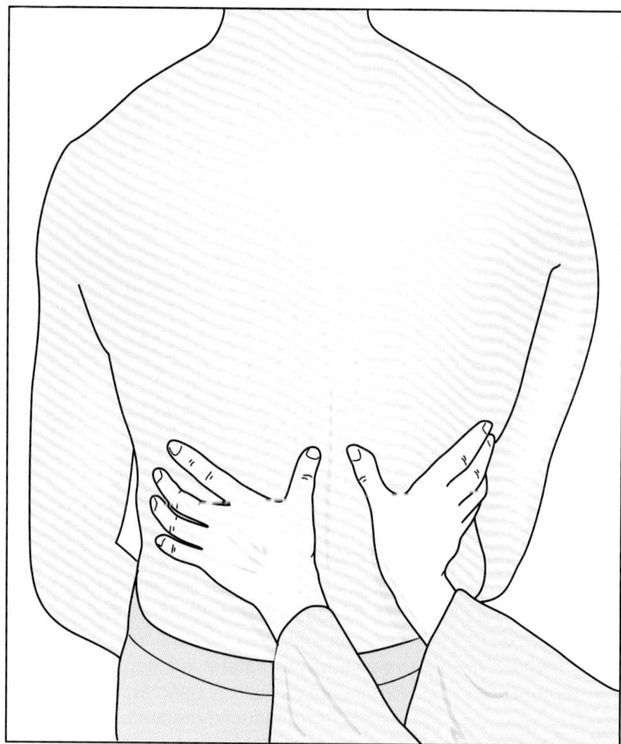

Figure 9-32. Assessment of respiratory excursion.

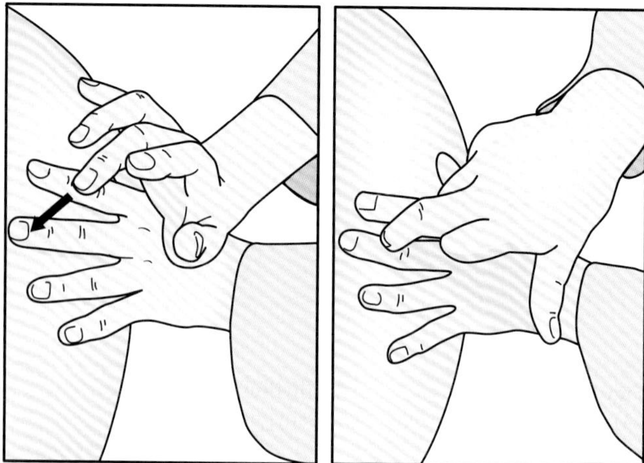

Figure 9-33. The technique of percussion.

replaces air-filled tissue. In patients with emphysema and air trapping, *hyper-resonance* replaces resonance. *Diaphragmatic excursion* can be ascertained by percussion of the border between resonance (lung tissue) and dullness (muscle) in expiration and inspiration. Normal excursion is 5 to 6 cm.

Auscultation. Airflow, obstruction, and the condition of the lungs and pleural space can be assessed with auscultation. Use the diaphragm of the stethoscope pressed firmly on the skin in the sequence illustrated in Figure 9-34. Ask the patient to breathe slowly and deeply through his or her mouth because nose breathing changes the pitch of the sounds. Listen through one full breath in each location for pitch, intensity, and duration of inspiration and expiration.

Normal breath sounds (vesicular) are heard in peripheral lung tissue away from large airways. They are soft, low-pitched, blowing sounds. The inspiratory–expiratory time ratio is 5:2. Normal breath sounds are diminished at the bases. The sounds are decreased in obese patients and with shallow breathing or pleural effusion, and they are increased with exercise.

Bronchovesicular sounds are heard normally in the areas around the mainstem bronchi (below the clavicles and between the scapulae). They have moderate pitch and intensity, with an inspiratory–expiratory time ratio of 1:1. These sounds are abnormal if heard in the lung periphery.

Bronchial sounds, heard normally over the bronchial areas, are loud and high pitched. Expiratory time is greater than inspiratory time. If heard in the lung periphery, bronchial sounds are abnormal.

Adventitious breath sounds are superimposed over normal breath sounds. There are two categories of adventitious sounds: discontinuous (crackles) and continuous (wheezes and pleural friction rubs). When adventitious breath sounds are heard, note loudness, pitch, duration, number, timing (phase of respiratory cycle), location on the chest wall, and persistence from breath to breath. Have the patient cough, and note any change in adventitious sounds.

Crackles are discrete, discontinuous sounds that are similar to the sound generated by rubbing hairs together in front of the ears (Fig. 9-35A). Crackles are attributed to fluid in the alveoli or to explosive reopening of alveoli. Heart failure or atelectasis associated with bed rest, splinting from ischemic or incisional pain, or the effects of pain medication and sedatives often result in development of crackles. Typically, crackles are noted first at the bases (because of gravity's effect on fluid accumulation and decreased ventilation of basilar tissue), but may progress to all portions of the lung fields.

Wheezes are continuous, musical sounds from rapid air movement through constricted airways. They are heard most often on expiration but can be heard during both inspiration and

Table 9-8 • PERCUSSION NOTES AND THEIR CHARACTERISTICS

	Relative Intensity	Relative Pitch	Relative Duration	Example of Location
Flatness	Soft	High	Short	Thigh
Dullness	Medium	Medium	Medium	Liver
Resonance	Loud	Low	Long	Normal lung
Hyperresonance	Very loud	Lower	Longer	None normally
Tympany	Loud	High[a]	[a]	Gastric air bubble or puffed-out cheek

[a]Distinguished mainly by its musical timbre.
Bickley LS, Szilagyi PG. *Bates' Guide to Physical Examination and History Taking.* 10th ed. Philadelphia, PA: Lippincott Williams & Wilkins; 2009.

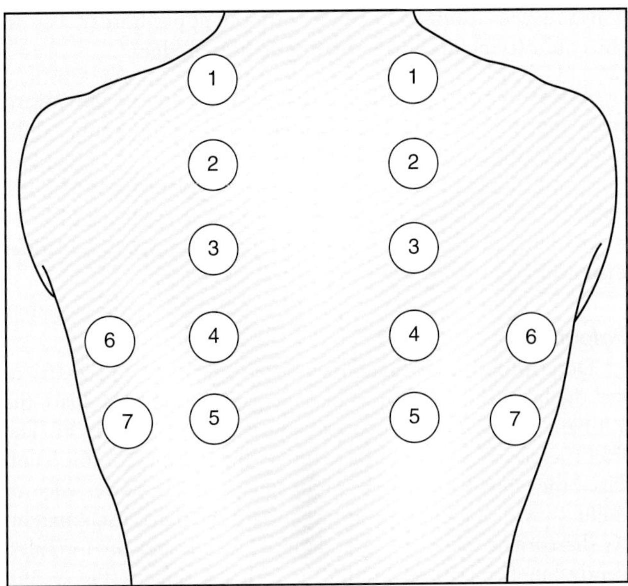

Figure 9-34. Sequence of posterior percussion and auscultation.

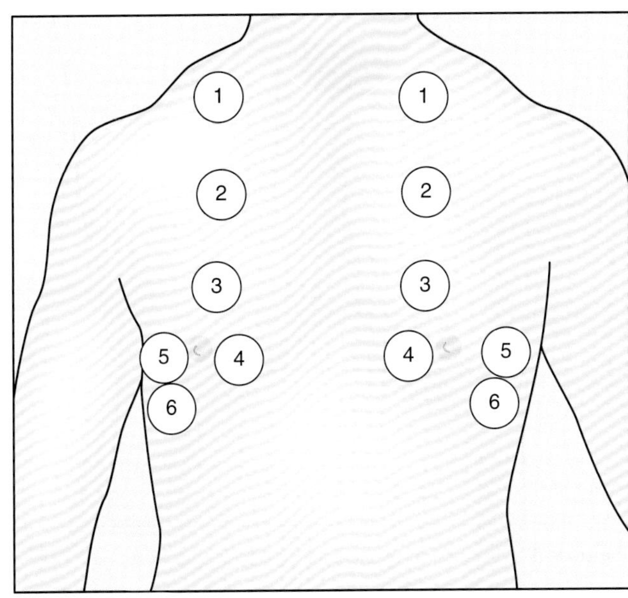

Figure 9-36. Sequence of anterior percussion and auscultation.

expiration (Fig. 9-35B). Although wheezes are characteristic of obstructive lung disease, they can be caused by interstitial pulmonary edema compressing small airways. Nonselective β-Adrenergic blocking agents, such as propranolol, may precipitate airway narrowing, especially in patients with underlying reactive airway disease. A fixed wheeze is characteristic of an endobronchial mass or tumor.

Transmitted voice sounds may be louder and clearer than normal (bronchophony, whispered pectoriloquy) when heard through the chest wall. The quality of voice sounds may have a nasal or bleating character (egophony). Transmitted voice sounds suggest consolidation of lung tissue.

Pleural friction rubs result from inflamed pleura rubbing together. A pleural friction rub, characteristic of pleuritis, is a coarse, grating sound that can be heard on inspiration and expiration (Fig. 9-35C).

Anterior Chest

Palpation. Tenderness of the pectoral muscles or costal cartilage suggests a musculoskeletal origin of chest pain. Respiratory excursion is assessed in the same manner as on the posterior chest, except that the examiner's thumbs are placed along each costal margin. Assess vocal or tactile fremitus. Fremitus normally is diminished over the precordium.

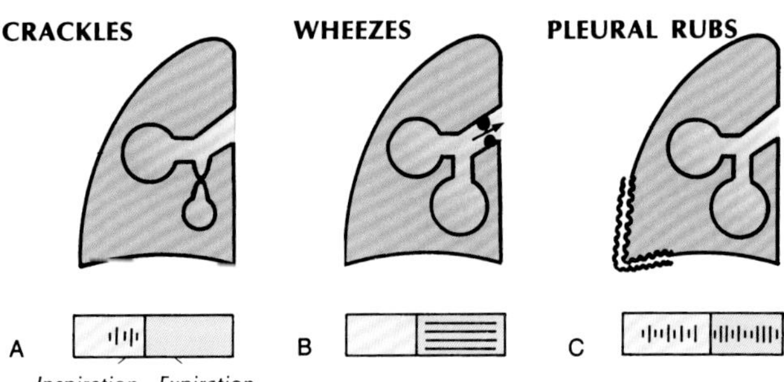

Figure 9-35. Adventitious breath sounds. (A) Crackles. (B) Wheezes. (C) Pleural friction rubs.

Percussion. The pattern for percussion of the anterior chest is diagrammed in Figure 9-36. Gently displace a female patient's breast before percussion. The heart produces dullness between the third and fifth ICSs. Note and mark the upper border of liver dullness.

Auscultation. Listen for breath sounds over the patient's anterior and lateral chest. Place the stethoscope in the sequence illustrated in Figure 9-36. If indicated, assess for transmitted voice sounds.

Abdomen

The abdominal examination presented here has a narrow focus. Purposes include evaluation of bowel tones, determination of liver size, assessment of bladder distention, and auscultation for bruits. After anesthesia, resumption of bowel tones must be confirmed before initiating a diet. Liver engorgement occurs because of decreased venous return secondary to right ventricular failure. Urine output is an important indicator of cardiac output. In a patient who is unable to void (e.g., secondary to strict bed rest or after atropine sulfate administration) or who has not voided despite adequate fluid intake, always assess for bladder distention before initiating other measures.

Inspection

Observe the abdomen for symmetry and visible peristalsis. Note the presence of abdominal distention. Abdominally localized obesity (waist circumference greater than 35 in for women or greater than 40 in for men) is associated with coronary artery disease, type 2 diabetes, and metabolic syndrome.

Auscultation

Auscultate the abdomen after observation because palpation and percussion can either increase or diminish bowel sounds. Gently

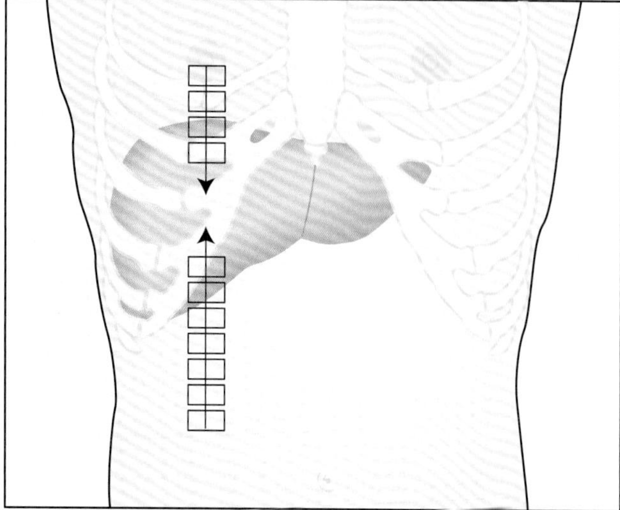

Figure 9-37. Percussion of the liver.

place the diaphragm of the stethoscope on the abdomen. Listen over all quadrants. Normal bowel sounds consist of clicks and gurgles, at a frequency of 5 to 34 per minute. It is necessary to listen for 2 minutes or more to determine that bowel sounds are absent. Borborygmi (prolonged gurgles of hyperperistalsis) also may be heard. Bowel sounds are increased with diarrhea and early intestinal obstruction, and they are decreased or absent with paralytic ileus and peritonitis.[8] Listen for bruits over the renal, ischial, and femoral arteries.

Percussion

Determination of Liver Size. Percussion of the liver (Fig. 9-37) should start in the right MCL, at or below the umbilicus, and proceed upward from an area of tympany (intestine) to an area of dullness (liver). Identify the lower edge of the liver in the MCL. Next, percuss downward at the MCL from resonance (lung) to dullness (liver). Measure the distance from the upper to the lower liver edge at the MCL; the normal liver span is 6 to 12 cm (Fig. 9-38). A right pleural effusion or lung consolidation (dullness) may obscure the upper border. Gas in the colon (tympany) may obscure the lower edge.

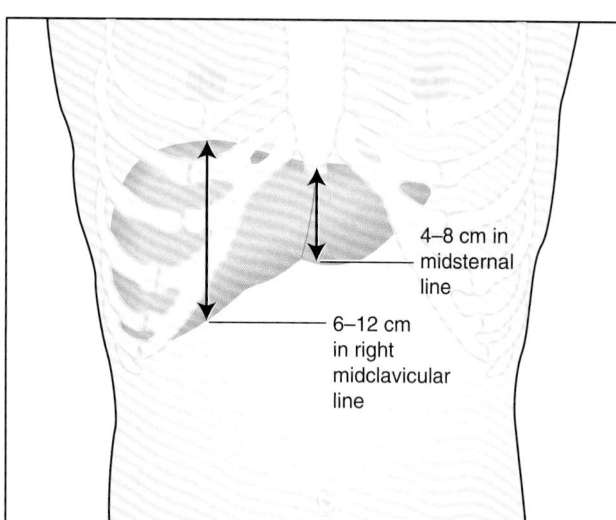

Figure 9-38. Measurement of liver span.

Assessment of Bladder Distention. Percuss downward from the umbilicus to the symphysis pubis. Suprapubic dullness may indicate a distended urinary bladder. If percussion does not confirm suspicions of a distended urinary bladder, palpate gently above the symphysis pubis. If ascites is present, neither abdominal percussion nor palpation may reveal bladder distention.

Palpation

Determination of Liver Size. Deep palpation is necessary to feel the liver. It is imperative that the patient is relaxed. Place the left hand under the patient's 11th and 12th ribs for support. The liver is easier to palpate if the examiner pushes up with this hand. Place the right hand on the abdomen below the lower edge of dullness, with the fingers pointing toward the right costal margin. As the patient takes a deep abdominal breath and then exhales, gently but firmly push in and up with the fingers (Fig. 9-39). With each exhalation, move the hand further toward the liver. The liver edge should come down to meet the fingers. Normally, it feels firm with a smooth edge. It should not be tender. With venous engorgement from right heart failure, the liver is enlarged, firm, tender, and smooth (Table 9-9).

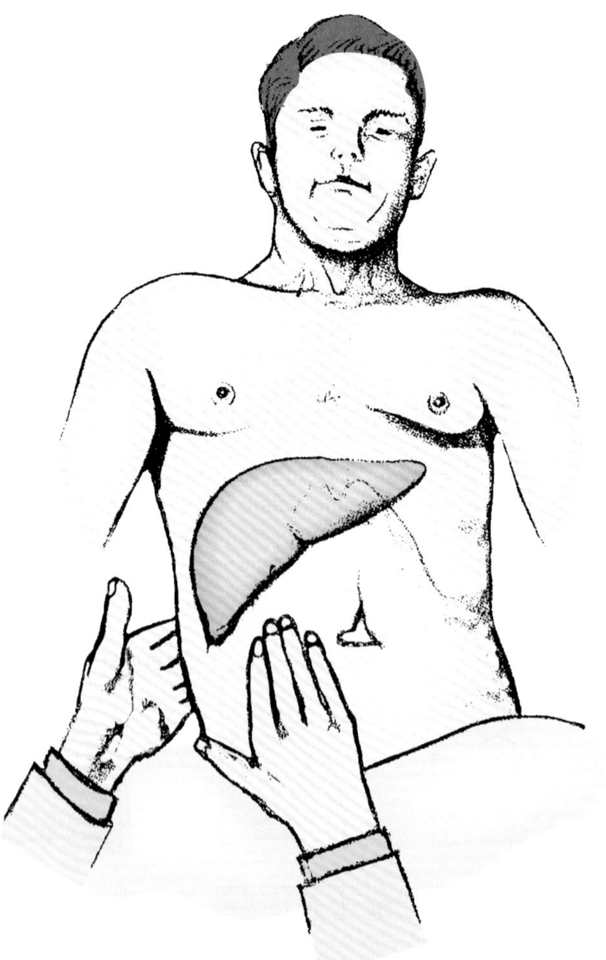

Figure 9-39. Palpation of the liver.

Table 9-9 • SUMMARY OF CARDIAC NURSING PEARLS FOR HISTORY TAKING AND PHYSICAL EXAMINATION

Patient Assessment

1. Remember patient privacy. Ask the patient if friends or family should be asked to leave the room before beginning your assessment.
2. Make sure you have a quiet environment for history taking and physical exam.
3. Keep an open mind when beginning your assessment.
4. Talk to the patient before beginning the physical exam. Hear their story; listen for key bits of information, which may help guide your physical assessment.
5. Use various words to ask about symptoms; such as chest pressure or shortness of breath. Patients may not describe their chest discomfort as "pain." It may be described as a heaviness, uncomfortable sensation or other term. Shortness of breath may be described by the patient as breathlessness or some other descriptor.
6. Use the level of terminology that the patient uses when speaking. Avoid using acronyms. When using medical terminology, use teach-back strategies to confirm with the patient that the terms used are indeed understood.
7. Remember that patients' generally do not have the same level of medical knowledge or knowledge of human physiology that you do.
8. Use the patient's own words when asking more about specific symptoms.
9. Complete a review of symptoms in an organized manner, such as head to toe. Develop your own format and use it for every patient. This can vary in length depending on assessment type; comprehensive or focused
10. There is a therapeutic value for the patient to the history and physical exam. They should be conducted in a professional manner.
11. Patients with cardiovascular disease tend to have the same quality of discomfort with recurrent episodes.
12. Cardiac discomfort does not move from spot to spot and is not pinpoint, localized with one finger.
13. Never be hesitant or avoid admitting you do not know or understand a medical treatment or concept or physical finding
14. Never assume anything!

Performing the Physical Exam

1. Remember patient privacy when conducting your physical exam. Make sure doors or curtains are closed.
2. Never miss an opportunity to practice. With repetition abnormal findings will become easier to identify.
3. When time permits, if an abnormal physical finding has been noted by another medical staff and you do not see or hear it, ask them to help you identify the finding.
4. Inspection begins when you first encounter the patient. Completion of inspection should occur before palpation and auscultation.
5. You should have a quality stethoscope.
6. If you are not performing pediatric auscultation the pediatric diaphragm should be removed, unless you have a model with a closed bell, thus providing a diaphragm and a bell.
7. Know how to use your stethoscope and what sounds are best heard with the diaphragm and the bell.
8. Auscultation should be performed with the stethoscope placed on bare skin.
9. When performing auscultation it can be helpful to close your eyes when listening for quiet sounds such as murmurs, bruits or diastolic filling sounds
10. Auscultation with the bell should be done with the stethoscope placed lightly on the chest. Pressing firmly with the bell causes the taught underlying skin to become a diaphragm.
11. Know what findings are associated with each phase of the cardiac cycle. (See Figs. 9-17 to 9-28 and Tables 9-5 and 9-7)
12. Cardiac auscultation should be done in a systematic manner, beginning in the aortic area at the right 2nd intercostal space close to the sternum then proceed to the pulmonic area in the left 2nd intercostal space close to the sternum, then the 3rd interspace; the tricuspid area and finally the left 4th and 5th interspaces in the mitral area at the apex. (See Fig. 9-16)
13. Focus on listening to one heart sound at a time; starting with S_1 followed by S_2 then listen for murmurs in systole followed by murmurs and gallops in diastole.
14. Always check blood pressure in both arms in acute chest pain patients. A finding of markedly lower reading in one arm is an indication of aortic dissection. If the subclavian artery is involved this will be the the left arm.

Physical Exam Findings

1. Assessing JVP can be difficult. Practice. (See Fig. 9-8)
2. A laterally displaced PMI, identified on palpation, indicates an increased likelihood of increased left ventricular size and possibly decreased left ventricular ejection fraction.
3. Wheezes may be found in left heart failure. This is typically expiratory wheezing. Inspiratory and expository wheezing is more likely to be caused by intrinsic lung disease.
4. Palpating the carotid pulse during auscultation of the heart can aid in identification of heart sounds. S_1 occurs just prior to the palpated carotid upstroke and S_2 follows the carotid pulse.
5. Palpation and auscultation combined can be helpful in identifying cardiac lifts, heaves and thrills.
6. Causes of increased intensity of the S_1 heart sound include short PR interval, fast heart rate and mild mitral stenosis.
7. Causes of decreased intensity of the S_1 heart sound include long PR interval, slow heart rate and severe mitral stenosis.
8. A fixed split of S2 may be from an atrial septal defect.
9. S_3, S_4 and the murmur of mitral stenosis are best heard with the patient in the left lateral decubitus position.
10. S_3 and S_4 are diastolic sounds. S_3 is an early diastolic sound and S_4 late diastolic sound. Timing is S_4, S_1, S_2, S_3
11. S_3 can be the most difficult heart sound to hear.
12. An S_3 heart sound cannot be present in the setting of severe mitral stenosis due to the reduced blood flow through the mitral valve during diastole.
13. An S_3 heart sound may be present in athletes, pregnant females and other young healthy individuals or may indicate severe systolic heart failure.
14. An S_3 gallop or pulses alternans are early signs of heart failure decompensation and is seen before crackles, edema, liver engorgement or JVD.
15. An S_4 cannot be heard in a patient in atrial fibrillation, as it is caused by blood flow of atrial contraction; which is absent in atrial fibrillation.
16. An S_4 heart sound is frequently pathologic and may indicate diastolic heart failure, left ventricular hypertrophy or active myocardial ischemia.
17. Large systolic jugular venous pulsations may be V waves seen in severe tricuspid regurgitation.
18. A holosystolic murmur at the left lower sternal border which becomes louder with inspiration is due to tricuspid regurgitation (Carvallo sign).
19. The aortic stenosis murmur can radiate to the cardiac apex where it sounds holosystolic and can mimic the murmur of mitral regurgitation (Galiveriden phenomenon).
20. A palpable rumble may be felt in mitral stenosis indicating the best site for auscultation.
21. The decrescendo diastolic murmur of aortic insufficiency is heard best with the patient leaning forward in full expiration in a quiet room.
22. Cheyne–Stokes respiration is a manifestation of decompensated heart failure.
23. Acute pulmonary edema can occur with a conversion from sinus rhythm to atrial fibrillation.

CONCLUSIONS

Obtaining the patient history and performing a physical examination is the foundation of cardiac nursing. The techniques of history taking and physical exam have remained relatively constant over many years. This chapter has been updated to include current recommendations, although the majority of techniques for obtaining a patient history and performing a physical examination stand the test of time.

Nursing practice has evolved dramatically as patients and health care have become increasingly complex. To contribute their valuable assessment findings to patient care, the nurse must apply the knowledge and practice the skills and techniques learned in this chapter, which better equip the cardiac nurse to share and receive clinical information with members of the multidisciplinary medical team. As the clinician who typically has with the greatest proximity and longest duration of time with the patient, the cardiac nurse is often first to identify changes in a patient which indicate a change in health status, which may prevent clinical deterioration or catastrophic events.

Nursing is both an art and a science. On the one hand, obtaining an accurate and relevant patient history relies upon understanding the clinical context and using patient engagement, empathy, and listening skills. On the other hand, performing a physical examination combines technical skills, science, and cultural competence. Taken together, cardiac nurses must develop the skills needed to assess the patient's status, collaborate with the care team, and provide timely intervention to optimize patient outcomes.

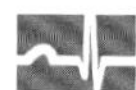

CASE-BASED LEARNING 1

Patient Profile

History of Present Illness

Felicia Drake is an 80-year-old female who presented to the local Urgent Care today with complaints of increasing dyspnea on exertion. She also reported new onset of lightheadedness and dizziness with exertional activity. It has been about a year since she was last seen by her primary care physician. She tells you that her blood pressure and cholesterol were under "good" control at her last visit. She reports having had an "ultrasound" of her heart about 5 years ago. She thinks this was to investigate a heart murmur. She has never seen a cardiologist and denies a prior cardiac history. Mrs. Drake acknowledges that she may experience some exertional chest pressure; but is somewhat vague in her reply.

Past Medical History/Problem List

Hypertension
Hyperlipidemia
Hypothyroidism
Osteoporosis

Family History

Father—CAD died of a myocardial infarction age 71
Mother—Dementia

Social History

Married to "Ron." Retired secretary. She has no siblings. One daughter. Occasional alcohol intake. 30 year smoking history, quit 20 years ago. No recreational drug use.

Medications

Current medications:
Lisinopril/HCTZ 20/12.5 mg daily
Rosuvastatin 5 mg daily
Alendronate 70 mg weekly
Levothyroxine 75 mcg daily

Allergies

No known food or drug allergies

Considerations

Clinical Questions

1. What would be the first area of question focus for Mrs. Drake, with a history of HTN, hyperlipidemia, tobacco use and a family history of CAD?
2. Once you have determined that she is stable and not currently experiencing chest discomfort what might be the type of question you would be interested in asking this woman regarding past medical history and current symptoms?
3. What might you expect to find on physical exam?
4. Mrs. Drake mentions a previously noted cardiac murmur. What valvular abnormality might you expect to see in an 80-year-old patient? What is/are the auscultation points where you might expect to hear the murmur most clearly?
5. Given her presenting symptoms, what additional diagnostic examinations might you expect to be ordered?

Clinical Review

1. Upon initial questioning it is important to understand Mrs. Drake's medical history and whether this may be associated with her current presentation. She is at risk for coronary artery disease. She denies a prior history of coronary artery disease. She thinks she has a heart murmur. She has no history of valvular heart disease, to her knowledge. She has no history of rheumatic fever.
2. If her ECG and initial troponin are within normal limits, there is a low likelihood that she is having an acute myocardial infarction. Nevertheless, Mrs. Drake should be questioned about the severity and quality of her chest discomfort.
   - Location: Where is her pain? Cardiac discomfort is described as a pressure, heaviness, squeezing, burning or choking sensation. The discomfort tends to be localized and may present at the sternum, epigastrium, back, neck, jaw or shoulders.
   - Duration and Precipitating/Alleviating Factors: How long does the pain last? How many days or months has this been occurring? What makes this pain better or worse? Angina generally lasts 1 to 5 minutes and is precipitated by exertion, eating, exposure to cold, or emotional stress. The intensity of the pain does not change with respiration, cough, or change in position. The pain does remit with rest, which decreases myocardial oxygen demand.
   - Associated Symptoms: What other symptoms does she notice with this pain? Dyspnea on exertion and lightheadedness and dizziness were reported. She may not be able to separate her symptoms into subgroups of dyspnea with exertion and lightheadedness as both may occur together. Mrs. Drake states that she has noted a gradual onset over the last 6 months with progression now to the point where she becomes short of breath and lightheaded just getting dressed. Her husband assists her in dressing by bringing her clothes from the closet. She is no longer able to complete grocery shopping, now relying on her daughter to purchase groceries.
   - Recurring Event(s): Has this happened to her before? Mrs. Drake conveys that she has had these symptoms before and she was informed the cause was valvular heart disease. She tells you that the prior "ultrasound" of

CASE-BASED LEARNING 1 (*Continued*)

her heart, echocardiogram, was ordered by her primary care physician to investigate a heart murmur heard on routine exam. She was told that "everything was fine" and that the exam would be repeated "in a few years."

Patient Examination

Vital Signs

BP 130/90 mm Hg; pulse pressure 30 mm Hg; PR 78; RR 14; Temp 37°C

Physical Examination

Given Mrs. Drake's age and history of smoking, a delayed and plateaued peak in the carotid arterial pulse is not observed, due to rigid carotid vessels. Auscultation of her carotids does however reveal bilateral carotid bruits. Jugular venous pressure is not elevated. Visual exam of her chest is unremarkable. Palpation of her chest reveals a sustained and slightly laterally displaced apical impulse. Proceeding to cardiac auscultation you hear a regular S1, S2. Normal physiologic splitting of S2 on inspiration is absent. There is no S3 or S4. A crescendo–decrescendo murmur is appreciated during auscultation. It is loudest at the second intercostal space along the right sternal border.

Diagnostic Studies

ECG: No acute ST segment or T wave changes and reveals sinus rhythm with LV hypertrophy indicated by Q wave height. Laboratory Studies: Troponin I, drawn in the ED, is less than 0.04 ng/mL.

Assessment and Plan

Based on her symptoms and physical exam, it is determined that Mrs. Drake likely has aortic stenosis. Review of her chart, after having been seen by the hospitalist team, reveals orders for a transthoracic echocardiogram. Orders have also been written for serial troponin I, chemistry panel, CBC and thyroid function testing. A cardiology consultation has been ordered.

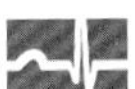

CASE-BASED LEARNING 2

Patient Profile

Michael Thomas is a 56-year-old who presents to the ED of his local hospital. He is complaining of recent onset of anterior chest pressure and exertional dyspnea. He is currently pain free; but reports an episode of discomfort this AM while out for a brisk walk. He recently decided to begin a regular walking program on the advice of his primary care physician. He was diagnosed with Type II diabetes mellitus (DM) 2 years ago. At that time his hemoglobin A1C (HbA1c) was 11.5. Most recent labs, one month ago, revealed a HbA1c of 5.6%. Fasting glucose was 126 mg/dL; renal function was normal. Total cholesterol was 199 mg/dL, triglycerides 200 mg/dL, HDL 38 mg/dL, and LDL 121 mg/dL. He denies prior cardiac history.

Past Medical History/Problem List

Type II diabetes mellitus
Hypertriglyceridemia
Diabetic retinopathy with hx laser surgery

Family History

Father—Type II DM, PVD, Mitral valve disease with hx MVR. Sudden cardiac death age 80.
Mother—Type II DM. Alive at age 79.

Social History

Divorced. Currently in a stable relationship with Mary. Works as a private seller on Amazon. History of no regular exercise. One younger sister, who is in good health. Two sons, both in good health. Occasional alcohol intake. No smoking history. No recreational drug use.

Medications

Metformin 500 mg twice daily
Omega 3 fish oil, over the counter, recently started

Allergies

No known food or drug allergies

Considerations

1. What would be the first area of question focus for Mr. Thomas given his complaint of exertion chest discomfort and a history of type II DM hyperlipidemia and hypertriglyceridemia?
2. Once you have determined that he is stable and not currently experiencing chest discomfort what will be the focus of questions asked in obtaining a history.
3. What might you expect to find on physical exam? Are there certain areas of increased focus?
4. Given his presenting symptoms, what additional diagnostic examinations might you expect to be ordered?

Clinical Course

In the Emergency Department Mr. Thomas denied current chest discomfort. He reported 6/10 anterior chest pressure this AM while out walking. He stopped to rest and the discomfort resolved after approximately five minutes. He reports similar episodes occurring regularly over the last five to seven days while out walking. He describes the discomfort at starting when he walks up an incline or climbs a flight of stairs. The discomfort is located in his mid sternal area and "feels like a weight is sitting on his chest." There is no radiation to his neck, jaw or arm. There is no associated nausea or diaphoresis. Upon reaching the top of the hill or stairs he must stop and rest 3 to 5 minutes before the discomfort resolves. This AM his discomfort was more severe and lasted longer prompting his presentation to the ED. He denies any current chest discomfort.

Ischemic Symptoms

Angina pectoris is usually described as a discomfort (not necessarily pain) in the chest or adjacent areas. It is variably described as tightness, heaviness, pressure, squeezing, or a smothering sensation. In some patients, particularly those with diabetes, the symptom may be a more vague discomfort, a numbness, or a burning sensation. Alternatively, so-called anginal equivalents such as dyspnea, faintness, or fatigue may occur. The location is usually substernal and radiation may occur to the neck, jaw, arms, back, or epigastrium. Isolated epigastric discomfort or pain in the lower mandible may rarely be a symptom of myocardial ischemia. The typical episode of angina pectoris begins gradually and reaches its maximum intensity over a period of minutes. Typical angina pectoris is precipitated by exertion or emotional stress and is relieved within

(*continued*)

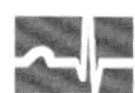

CASE-BASED LEARNING 2 (*Continued*)

minutes by rest or nitroglycerin. Because of the variation in symptoms that may represent myocardial ischemia, the clinical scenarios are presented using the broad term "ischemic symptoms" to capture this concept.

He is admitted from the Emergency Department to the telemetry unit with a diagnosis of Rule out MI. Upon arrival to your unit his vital signs are stable and his ECG shows no acute findings.

Patient Examination

Vital Signs

Ht. 172.72 cm; Wt. 82.3 kg; BMI 27.6 kg/m^2; BP 128/70 mm Hg–prehypertension; PR 74; RR 12; SaO_2 98%; Temp 37°C

Physical Examination

General appearance, unremarkable. Mood/affect: Somewhat anxious. Eyes, clear, arterial pulse is regular and 1+ in all areas of palpation. Palpation of the carotid pulse reveals no abnormality. There are no noted bruits on auscultation. Jugular venous pressure is normal. Inspection of his extremities shows no clubbing, normal capillary refill time and no edema. Careful assessment of the lower extremity pulses reveals no evidence of peripheral vascular disease. All lower extremity pulses are 1+, hair distribution is normal and skin shows no discoloration. Given his diabetic history, this should be an area of focus on physical exam. There is no edema, varicosities or evidence of chronic venous insufficiency. Inspection of the chest reveals no paradoxical movement. An apex movement is not visualized. Palpation reveals an apex beat at the 5th intercostal space just lateral to the midclavicular line. Auscultation of the chest reveals a regular rhythm without murmurs, rubs or gallops. S1 is heard loudest at the apex. S2 is physiologically split and heard loudest at the 2nd intercostal spaces along the right and left sternal border. His chest contour is normal and auscultation of the lung fields reveals clear lungs. Abdominal inspection reveals obesity. Auscultation reveals normal bowel sounds. Findings of percussion and palpation of the abdomen reveal no abnormalities.

Diagnostic Studies

ECG: No acute ST segment or T wave changes

Laboratory Studies: Initial Troponin I was negative; repeat is Troponin I <0.04 ng/mL. Nonfasting blood glucose is 200 mg/dL.

Chest x-ray: Normal.

Assessment and Plan

Rule out unstable angina/acute coronary syndrome in a 56 yo male with poorly controlled Type II DM. The admitting hospital team has ordered serial cardiac enzymes, lipid profile and HbA1c. There is an order for a STAT ECG if he develops recurrent chest discomfort, as needed sublingual nitroglycerin, aspirin 81 mg daily and atorvastatin 10 mg daily. Mr. Thomas' third Troponin I is again negative at <0.04 ng/mL. A cardiology consultation has been ordered. Further diagnostic testing and/or risk stratification according to current guidelines will commence per the cardiology service.

CAD, coronary artery disease; HCTZ, hydrochlorothiazide; HTN, hypertension; ECG, electrocardiogram; ED, emergency department; MI, myocardial infarction.

KEY READINGS

Benner P. *From Novice to Expert, Excellence and Power in Clinical Nursing Practice.* Menlo Park, CA: Addison-Wesley Publishing Company; 1984.

Harvey WP. Heart sounds and murmurs. *Circulation.* 1964;30:262–271.

Runge MS, Ohman EM, Stouffer GA. The history and physical examination. In: Runge MS, Stouffer G, Patterson C, eds. *Netter's Cardiology.* 2nd ed. Philadelphia, PA: Saunders; 2010:3–14.

REFERENCES

1. Abbott PD, Short E, Dodson S, et al. Improving your cultural awareness with culture clues. *Nurse Pract.* 2002;27(2):44–47, 51.
2. Braunwald E, Goldman L. *Primary Cardiology.* 2nd ed. Philadelphia, PA: WB Saunders; 2002.
3. Marriott HJL. *Bedside Cardiac Diagnosis.* Philadelphia, PA: J.B. Lippincott; 1993.
4. Underhill SL. Assessment of cardiovascular function. In: Bruner LS, Suddarth DS, eds. *Textbook of Medical–Surgical Nursing.* 5th ed. Philadelphia, PA: J.B. Lippincott; 1984:457–563.
5. Chatterjee K. The history. In: Parmley W, Chatterjee K, eds. *Cardiology.* Vol 1. 2nd ed. Philadelphia, PA: J.B. Lippincott; 1991:3.2–3.10.
6. Fang JC, O'Gara PT. The history and physical examination: an evidence-based approach. In: Libby PP, Bonow RO, Mann DL, et al., eds. *Heart Disease: A Textbook of Cardiovascular Medicine.* 8th ed. Philadelphia, PA: Saunders-Elsevier; 2008:125–148.
7. Staff Development Workgroup, Patient and Family Education Committee. Culture cuesTM: communicating with your Latino patient. 1999. Available at http//depts.washington.edu/pfes/cultureclues.html
8. Bickley LS, Szilagyi PG. *Bates' Guide to Physical Examination and History Taking.* 9th ed. Philadelphia, PA: Lippincott Williams & Wilkins; 2007.
9. Gordon M. *Nursing Diagnosis, Process, and Application.* New York: McGraw-Hill; 1994.
10. Spieker ED, Motzer SA. Sleep-disordered breathing in patients with heart failure: pathophysiology, assessment, and management. *J Am Acad Nurse Pract.* 2003;15(11):487–493.
11. New York Heart Association Criteria Committee. *Diseases of the Heart and Blood Vessels: Nomenclature and Criteria for Diagnosis.* 6th ed. Boston, MA: Little, Brown; 1964.
12. Chatterjee K. Bedside evaluation of the heart: the physical examination. In: Parmley W, Chatterjee K, eds. *Cardiology.* Vol 1. 2nd ed. Philadelphia, PA: J.B. Lippincott; 1991:3.11–13.53.
13. U.S. Department of Health and Human Services. *Healthy People 2010: Understanding and Improving Health.* 2nd ed. Washington, DC: U.S. Government Printing Office; 2000.
14. Poirier P, Despres JP. Waist circumference, visceral obesity, and cardiovascular risk. *J Cardiopulm Rehabil.* 2003;23(3):161–169.
15. Kenney WL. Thermoregulation at rest and during exercise in healthy older adults. *Exerc Sport Sci Rev.* 1997;25:41–76.
16. Ponte J. Warming the core after cardiac surgery. *J Cardiothorac Vasc Anesth.* 1998;12(4):496.
17. Frank RN. The eye in hypertension. In: Izzo JL, Black HR, eds. *Hypertension Primer.* 3rd ed. From the Council on High Blood Pressure Research, American Heart Association, Philadelphia, PA: Lippincott Williams & Wilkins; 2003.
18. O'Rourke RA, Silverman ME, Shaver JA. The history, physical examination and cardiac auscultation. In: Fuster V, Alexander RW, O'Rourke RA, et al., eds. *Hurst's the Heart.* 11th ed. New York: McGraw-Hill; 2004: 217–274.
19. McGee SR. Physical examination of venous pressure: a critical review. *Am Heart J.* 1998;136(1):10–18.
20. Chobanian AV, Bakris GL, Black HR, et al. The Seventh Report of the Joint National Committee on Prevention, Detection, Evaluation, and Treatment of High Blood Pressure: the JNC 7 report. *JAMA.* 2003; 289(19):2560–2572.
21. Insua JT, Sacks HS, Lau TS, et al. Drug treatment of hypertension in the elderly: a meta-analysis. *Ann Intern Med.* 1994;121(5):355–362.
22. Grim CM, Grim CE. Blood pressure measurement. In: Izzo JL, Black HR, eds. *Hypertension Primer.* 3rd ed. From the Council on High Blood Pressure Research, American Heart Association, Philadelphia, PA: Lippincott Williams & Wilkins; 2003:321–324.
23. Jones DW, Frohlich ED, Grim CM, et al. Mercury sphygmomanometers should not be abandoned: an advisory statement from the Council for

High Blood Pressure Research, American Heart Association. *Hypertension.* 2001;37(2):185–186.
24. Perloff D, Grim C, Flack J, et al. Human blood pressure determination by sphygmomanometry. *Circulation.* 1993;88(5 Pt 1):2460–2470.
25. Calkins H, Zipes DP. Hypotension and syncope. In: Libby PP, Bonow RO, Mann DL, et al., eds. *Heart Disease: A Textbook of Cardiovascular Medicine.* 8th ed. Philadelphia, PA: Saunders-Elsevier; 2008:975–984.
26. Robertson D. Treatment of orthostatic disorders and baroreflex failure. In: Izzo JL, Black HR, eds. *Hypertension Primer.* 3rd ed. From the Council on High Blood Pressure Research, American Heart Association, Philadelphia, PA: Lippincott Williams & Wilkins; 2003:479–482.
27. LeWinter MM. Pericardial diseases. In: Libby PP, Bonow RO, Mann DL, et al., eds. *Heart Disease: A Textbook of Cardiovascular Medicine.* 8th ed. Philadelphia, PA: Saunders-Elsevier; 2008:1829–1854.
28. Franklin SS, Izzo JL. Aging, hypertension, and arterial stiffness. In: Izzo JL, Black HR, eds. *Hypertension Primer.* 3rd ed. From the Council on High Blood Pressure Research, American Heart Association, Philadelphia, PA: Lippincott Williams & Wilkins; 2003:170–175.
29. Charan NB, Carvalho P. Cardinal symptoms and signs in respiratory disease. In: Pierson DJ, Kacmarek RM, eds. *Foundations of Respiratory Care.* New York: Churchill-Livingston; 1992:672–674.
30. Fahey VA. Clinical assessment of the vascular system. In: Fahey VA, ed. *Vascular Nursing.* 4th ed. Philadelphia, PA: WB Saunders; 2004: 49–71.
31. Kerr KA, Watson WC, Dalsing MC. Chronic venous disease. In: Fahey VA, ed. *Vascular Nursing.* 4th ed. Philadelphia, PA: WB Saunders; 2004:399–425.
32. Walsh ME, Rice KL. Venous thromboembolic disease. In: Fahey VA, ed. *Vascular Nursing.* 4th ed. Philadelphia, PA: WB Saunders; 2004:365–397.
33. Tilkian A, Conover M. *Understanding Heart Sounds and Murmurs With an Introduction to Lung Sounds.* 4th ed. Philadelphia, PA: WB Saunders; 2001.
34. Ronan JA Jr. Cardiac auscultation: the first and second heart sounds. *Heart Dis Stroke.* 1992;1(3):113–116.
35. Ronan JA Jr. Cardiac auscultation: the third and fourth heart sounds. *Heart Dis Stroke.* 1992;1(5):267–270 contd.

10 Laboratory Tests Using Blood

Pamela L. Patel, Patricia A. Keegan

OBJECTIVES

1. Identify nursing role in laboratory testing and interpretation.
2. Recognize common laboratory tests used to confirm or diagnose cardiac conditions.
3. Describe nursing interventions utilized with laboratory testing.

KEY QUESTIONS

1. How does patient position affect laboratory results?
2. What role does point-of-care testing (POCT) play in patient care?
3. What is the importance of myocardial proteins in diagnosing myocardial infarction (MI)?

Diagnosis, treatment, and management of patients require a multimodal, multidisciplinary approach. Along with an in-depth history and physical, the clinician frequently depends on test results to complete the assessment picture. The laboratory plays an essential role in health care, and by one estimate nearly 70% of all medical decisions are based on laboratory results.[1] The purpose of the laboratory is to provide healthcare professionals with information to (1) detect disease; (2) confirm or reject a diagnosis; (3) establish prognosis; (4) guide patient management; and (5) monitor efficacy of therapy.[2] One of the most frequently used testing modalities is laboratory testing of blood specimens and due to recent advancements, blood specimens can now reveal information that once required special imagining or invasive surgery. The nurse has a key role in maximizing the conditions under which specimens are collected, thereby controlling for as many variables as possible.

BLOOD SPECIMEN COLLECTION

Blood specimen collection requires three phases: patient preparation, collection of the blood sample, and interpretation of results.[2] Any errors in this process can create additional work or added investigation to the patient, therefore adding extra costs to the healthcare system. By some estimates, specimen collection errors cost the average 400-bed hospital about $200,000/yr in recollection costs.[2]

Patient Preparation

While preparing the patient for phlebotomy, the nurse should take into account several variables that can influence the laboratory readings. These variables include fasting, diet, nicotine use, timing of testing, and drug ingestion. Patients and their families should receive a thorough explanation of the purpose of the lab test and when the results are predicted to be available.[2]

Universal Precautions

All blood is considered a source of potential infection. Universal precautions, as well as institution-specific phlebotomy policies and procedures should be followed when collecting and transporting specimens. Centers for Disease Control and Prevention (CDC) developed standard precautions to help protect both healthcare workers and patients from infection with blood-borne pathogens in the healthcare setting.[3] Standard precautions apply to blood; all body fluids, secretions, and excretions (except sweat). The core elements of standard precautions comprise of hand washing after patient contact, the use of barrier precautions (gloves, gowns, and facial protection) to prevent mucocutaneous contact, and minimal manual manipulation of sharp instruments and devices and disposal of these items in puncture-resistant containers.[3]

Blood Sample Collection

General guidelines for blood sample collection have been developed that help to ensure patient and clinician safety and maximize interpretation of results. The clinician should consider the organizational policies and procedures with regard to blood specimen collection, as well as standards for professional, national, and international organizations.[2] Control of variability can be enhanced by the use of proper technique during collection and processing of the specimen. Venipuncture is performed using a needle/adapter assembly attached to an evacuated plastic test tube with a rubber stopper.[4] During specimen collection through venipuncture, the use of a tourniquet produces changes within the vein. Once a tourniquet is placed on the arm, veins dilate because of their inability to drain. Cellular injury and hemolysis can be caused by the prolonged use of a tourniquet, described as 3 minutes or longer. Under these conditions, return of fluid and electrolytes to the vein are decreased or prohibited, resulting in a hemoconcentrated specimen. To avoid problems with hemoconcentration or hemodilution, the patient should be seated in a supine position for 15 to 20 minutes before the blood is drawn. Hemolysis refers to the lysis of red blood cells (RBCs). This can be caused by using a needle that is too small, pulling a syringe plunger back too fast, expelling the blood vigorously, or performing blood collection before the alcohol has dried at the collection site. Hemolysis can falsely increase blood constituents such as potassium, magnesium, iron, lactic acid dehydrogenase, phosphorus, ammonium, and total protein. Because of the extremely important role of potassium in cardiac excitation, elevations due to hemolysis can be problematic, especially for emergency room patients who are at risk of hemolysis during frantic blood collection.[4] Hemolysis can also occur in hemolytic disease states, such as transfusion reactions and with the use of some drugs.

Blood specimens can be contaminated in several ways. During collection, contamination may occur from intravenous (IV) fluids. Blood draws should not be done on the same arm as an infusion. If the infusion arm cannot be avoided, a tourniquet may be placed between the IV site and the phlebotomy site. Slowing the IV to keep-open rate (if not contraindicated) for 3 to 5 minutes before the draw may help to reduce contamination of the blood sample. In any event, concomitant infusions should be noted on the laboratory slip that the sample was obtained under these conditions.

Contamination may also be introduced by improper use of blood tubes. Most specimen collection tubes contain some form of anticoagulant. If blood has been mistakenly collected in one tube containing anticoagulant, it should never be poured into a different tube. Also, blood entering one tube should never be allowed to contaminate remaining blood that will be introduced into another tube.

Another source of contamination is introduced when routine samples are drawn from arterial lines, vascular catheters, or ports. The use of an indwelling intravascular catheter provides ready access to the patient's circulation, eliminating multiple phlebotomies, and is especially useful in critical care and surgical situations. Blood specimens drawn from catheters may be contaminated with previously administered or infused medications or fluids given via catheter. The solution used to maintain patency of the vein must be cleared before blood for analysis is collected. Sufficient blood (minimum of 2 to 5 mL) must be withdrawn to clear the line, so laboratory data are reliable.

The diameter and length of the catheter are important determinants when collecting blood specimens. The institution's policy and procedure manual should be consulted for recommended withdrawal and discard from vascular devices. Additional resources, such as professional nursing society standards, may assist in making decisions about recommended discard volumes.

Whether sampling from a pulmonary artery catheter, center venous line, arterial catheter, or other intravascular catheter, attention should be paid to the feasibility of interruption of the system. The pulmonary artery catheter presents particular problems. Both the right atrium (RA) port and venous infusion port (VIP) are useful for administration of drugs and fluids. Although the RA port allows access to the central circulation, use of this port for thermodilution cardiac output calculations makes it difficult to infuse drugs or fluids (a large amount of the infusate might be delivered during delivery of the cardiac output injectate). Consequently, the VIP is often chosen for fluid and drug infusion. In this situation, the use of the RA port may be preferable for blood withdrawal. If vasoactive drugs are not infusing through the VIP, it may also be used for blood sampling. The proximal opening into the RA is upstream of any drugs or fluid infusing through the RA port; therefore, the possibility of contamination of the blood sample by infusates is minimized. Typically the distal port of the pulmonary artery catheter is only used for blood sampling when measuring a mixed venous blood gas from the pulmonary artery where venous blood mixes after circulating through the superior and inferior vena cava, coronary sinuses, and the chambers of the right side of the heart.

Many institutions have shifted to the use of saline in lieu of heparin in IV lines and pressure tubing, however, questions persist about appropriate discard from vascular catheters (instilled with heparin) when drawing blood for coagulation studies. Inconsistent results may increase the cost to the patient through repeated testing, wasted blood, or erroneous treatment decisions. Again, the nurse should refer to policy and procedure manuals or professional organization standards for guidance. In any event, coordination in obtaining multiple blood specimens decreases the amount of blood that is eventually discarded and the number of times that the sterile system is invaded, thus reducing risk of introducing infection.

Sepsis has been associated with intravascular monitoring equipment including stopcocks and pressure transducers, which may be the most frequent reservoirs for endemic contamination. The incidence of local infection and bacteremia has been reduced by the use of disposable transducers and the percutaneous sheath systems used to introduce pulmonary artery catheters. The withdrawal of blood from an IV catheter should be considered a sterile procedure. Once removed, caps used to cover stopcock openings should be replaced with a sterile cap. The person performing the procedure should be gloved. Syringes, once used, should be discarded.

Types of Specimens

When blood is withdrawn from the body, it eventually clots. The fluid that separates from the clot is called *serum*. Many blood tests are done on serum, and therefore require use of a tube that allows blood to clot.[4] Plasma is the clear, watery portion of the blood in which several types of blood cells are suspended. Plasma is composed of serum and clotting factor. Blood collection tubes have color-coded stoppers that distinguish the presence of a specific anticoagulation or additive. Red-top tubes can be used for most chemistry, blood bank, and immunology assays. Lavender-top tubes, which contain ethylenediaminetetraacetic acid (EDTA), are usually used for hematology and certain other chemistries. Green-top tubes contain heparin. Heparin accelerates the action of antithrombin III, neutralizing thrombin and preventing the formation of fibrin. These tubes can be used for chemistries, arterial blood gases, hormone level, and some immune function studies. For coagulation testing, a light blue-top tube containing sodium citrate is commonly used because it preserves the coagulation factors. Gray-top tubes are generally used for glucose measurements because they contain a preservative, sodium fluoride, which prevents glycolysis for 3 days.

When multiple blood samples are drawn at the same time, the preferred order is as follows: blood culture tubes, tubes with no preservatives (red top); tubes with mild anticoagulants (blue then green-top tubes); tubes with EDTA (lavender top); and oxalate/fluoride tubes (gray top) should be collected last. Blood for coagulation studies should never be drawn first because tissue injury can initiate the clotting process and result in falsely low levels of coagulation factors. Specimens in tubes with additives should be rotated gently to mix the anticoagulant with the blood and should never be shaken.[4]

All specimens must be collected, labeled, transported, and processed according to hospital procedure. An incorrect sample collection may harm the patient, especially in the case of a mislabeled specimen. Misidentification of patients during sample collection for transfusion, or at the time of transfusion can be a life-threatening error. The incidence of patient misidentification at the time of specimen collection has been reported to be approximately 1 in 1000, with 1 in 12,000 patients receiving a unit of blood that was not intended for that individual.[5]

Interpretation of Results

Inherent physiologic variability exists based on the patients age, sex, ethnicity, and health status (such as pregnancy or post-myocardial infarction [MI]). These physiologic differences affect interpretation of results. Physiologic changes associated with the aging process bring concomitant changes in some expected laboratory results. Because men usually have more muscle mass than women, gender differences are seen in substances related to muscle function or metabolism, such as creatinine. There may be significant differences among European, African, and Asian populations in testing for cholesterol, enzymes, and hormones. Various physiologic states, such as pregnancy, stress obesity, and endurance exercise, also introduce situational changes in expected results.[6]

Cyclic variability produces daily, monthly, or yearly patterns in the physiologic states.[6] These cycles are often taken into consideration in the collection or interpretation of laboratory results. As a result, most routine specimens, at least in the hospital setting, are drawn in the early morning to control any circadian variability.

Blood tests are sometimes affected by the ingestion of food or fluids. Not only are results affected by the absorption of dietary components into the blood after a meal, but hormonal and metabolic changes occur as well. Partial control for the variability introduced by food or fluid ingestion can be achieved either by drawing early morning or premeal specimens.[5]

Patient position may affect laboratory results. Patient positioning prior to and during sampling can affect results. In the upright position, there may be a shift in extracellular fluid volume into the tissues. With the resulting increased concentration of proteins and protein-bound substances in the vascular space, samples for proteins, enzymes, hematocrit (Hct), hemoglobin (Hb), calcium, iron, hormones, and several drugs may show an average 5% to 8% increase. Redistribution of extracellular fluid volume and electrolytes within the vascular space does not stabilize until a patient has assumed the sitting position for at least 15 minutes (from the standing position), and in some cases 20 to 30 minutes. In some settings, such as the hospital, it is not difficult to stabilize the patient's position and thus reduce variability. In other settings, such as ambulatory care, significant variability is introduced if the patient is not made to sit for at least 15 minutes before the blood draw. Because control over sitting time is not usually feasible or practical, care should be taken in the interpretation of results.[7] Exercising immediately before blood sample collection frequently produces significantly erroneous results, especially with enzyme evaluation.[8]

The timing of blood sampling should include consideration of the effect of medications on the interpretation of results. Medications affect results of many specimens drawn for chemistry, hematology, coagulation, hormonal, and enzyme studies. Knowledge of the effect of the drug assists in the proper timing or subsequent interpretation of the results. Consideration should also be given to the effects of other influences, including over-the-counter medications, caffeine, nicotine, ethanol, home remedies, and herbal therapies.

In therapeutic drug monitoring, blood drug levels are monitored to evaluate the effects of the drug therapy, make decisions regarding dosage, prevent toxicity, and monitor patient adherence. Timing of the blood sample usually depends upon the half-life of the drug; samples drawn at projected peak level assist in monitoring toxicity, whereas levels drawn at trough help to verify the minimum satisfactory therapeutic level for that patient. Regardless of the purpose of the blood sample, drugs that may affect interpretation of results should be noted on the laboratory slip. For therapeutic drug monitoring, it is important to note the date and time of the last dose as well.

Different laboratories utilize different equipment and methods by which to test specimens. Specific reference ranges are usually reported alongside the patient's results on the laboratory report. In an effort to establish a standard for communicating laboratory results, the World Health Organization has recommended that the medical and scientific community throughout the world adopt the use of the International System of Units (ISU). An international unit is defined as the number of moles of substrate converted per second under defined conditions. Thus, many laboratories may report results in different ways, depending on their accepted standard of practice. Most laboratories also report critical values. These values should be reported promptly to the provider so that results may be evaluated and decisions made in light of the patient's condition.

Most reference ranges have been established utilizing venous blood samples. Because arterial blood has higher concentrations of glucose and oxygen, and lower concentrations of waste products (i.e., ammonia, potassium, and lactate), an arterial source should be noted on the laboratory slip. Capillary samples yield results that are closer to arterial blood than venous.

Critical evaluation of laboratory results should take into account how the reference values are determined. Patients, who have been seen for extended time by the same provider, or those who have been seen within the same healthcare organization, sometimes establish their own reference range. Reference ranges for a specific disease are sometimes established through large-scale clinical trials.

In most circumstances, each laboratory establishes its own reference values by testing a group. It is possible, however that this technique may not reflect the usual values or range of values of the group that the organization serves.[9] When samples are taken from volunteers, such as those who agree to give a blood sample for reference testing in exchange for free cholesterol screening, bias may be introduced because those who are likely to volunteer may be those who have or suspect they have illness already. When reference samples are taken from patient who is undergoing routine physical examination or elective surgery, results may reflect a mix of the surrounding population. Again, these reference values need to be considered in light of who was included or excluded from testing. Usually, those who drink alcohol, smoke, or take certain medications are excluded from reference range testing. However, this exclusion is likely to establish a narrow range of "normal" values, thereby increasing the number of people in the served population who fall outside the established range. Additional care should be taken in interpreting results if the laboratory reports only one set of reference values.[9]

Healthcare professionals who are aware of how reference ranges are obtained are in a better position to interpret laboratory results accurately for their patients. In all situations, interpretations of results should be done in light of all factors that introduce variability, and in light of the clinical condition, remembering that "normal" values do not necessarily indicate absence of disease; just as "abnormal" values do not necessarily establish a pathologic state.

Sensitivity and Specificity of Laboratory Tests

The ability of a laboratory test to identify a particular disease is quantified by two measurements: sensitivity and specificity. Sensitivity is the frequency of a positive (abnormal) test result among all patients with a particular disease or the likelihood that a diseased patient has a positive test. If all patients with given disease have a positive test, the test sensitivity is 100%. Sensitivity is calculated by testing a population of patients who have been found to have a particular disease by some "gold standard" method (a procedure that defines the true disease state of the patients).[10]

Specificity is the frequency of a negative (normal) test among all persons who do not have the disease or the likelihood that a healthy patient has a negative test. If all patients who do not have a particular disease have a negative test, the test specific is 100%. A test with a high specificity is helpful to confirm a diagnosis, because a highly specific test will have few results that are falsely positive. Specificity is calculated by testing a population of patients who have been found to have a particular disease by some gold standard method.[10]

Under the best of circumstances, no blood test is perfect and results may be misleading. Sensitivity and specificity may be altered by the coexistence of other diseases or complications from the primary disease. The most sensitive tests are used to rule out suspected disease so that the number if false-negative tests in minimal; thus, a negative test tends to exclude the disease. The most specific tests are used to confirm or exclude a suspected disease and minimize the number of false-positive results.[11]

Point-of-Care Testing

Point-of-care testing (POCT) also known as bedside testing or alternative site testing, is the testing of blood that is performed outside of a central laboratory. POCT testing is essential for the rapid detection of analytes in proximity to the patient, which facilitates rapid disease diagnosis, monitoring, and management. It enables quick medical decisions, as the diseases can be diagnosed at a very early stage, leading to improved health outcomes for patients by enabling the early start of treatment.[12] The global POCT market was estimated as $13.87 billion in 2017 and is estimated to grow over $23.92 billion by 2026. POCT provides high-quality biomarkers in an array of clinical settings including acute care, outpatient clinics, clinic research centers, homes, rural areas, and the developing world. POCT can improve the efficiency of care by enabling rapid assessment and triage of patients with chest discomfort. Cardiac troponin (cTn), a highly sensitive and specific biomarker of myocardial injury, guides triage and management of patients presenting with symptoms suggestive of acute coronary syndrome. Cardiac marker POCT reduced length of stay in the emergency department and allowed for accurate triaging of chest pain patient within 90 minutes of presentation to the emergency department.[13]

Central laboratories typically measure two key coagulation parameters: prothrombin time (PT) and activated prothromboplastin time. Yet, delays of ~1 hour limit the utility of central laboratory measurements for acute care settings such as the ICU or operating room, where thrombotic risk can vary moment to moment due to administration of anticoagulant boluses and pharmacologic reversal agents. In these setting, activated clotting time (ACT), a whole blood measurement that integrates intrinsic and extrinsic coagulation with platelet function, commonly serves to quantify thrombotic potential. In the case of ACT measurements, nurses within steps of the patient can perform POCT independent of the central laboratory. This goes to show how real-time POCT can be integrated into acute clinical workflow.[14]

POCTs have great potential to advance cardiovascular care. To ensure accuracy of data, POCT system requires that there be upfront training of nonlaboratory personnel on how to use new equipment, continued proficiency testing of staff, and assurance that electronic quality control requirements are met. It is important that POCT systems are linked to hospital or laboratory systems by radiofrequency and infrared to ensure that information handling, storage, and billing are done properly.

Administration of a POCT system includes designating someone to be responsible for the POCT service, which would include: knowing who is performing POCT and which test they are performing, maintaining quality control documentation, selecting appropriate equipment, troubleshooting all aspects of POCT, coordinating training, and serving as a liaison between nursing and other services.

Possible limitations of using POCT system include its use by personnel with limited training in laboratory technology and the lack of understanding of quality control. POCT is considered to me more expensive than traditional laboratory analysis because the cost of cartridges is more expensive. Cost analysis needs to include the decreased labor by nursing and laboratory personnel plus the ability to make rapid decisions about acutely ill patients that may alter their course of illness.[15]

BIOCHEMICAL MARKERS OF MYOCARDIAL INJURY

The internal environment of the health person is in a state of balance with respect to water, electrolytes, energy storage and use, and metabolic end products.[16] Stability is maintained through homeostatic mechanisms that regulate the activities of cells and organs. During periods of critical illness, a disruption in cell membrane stability may cause chemical substances that are responsible for intracellular homeostatic mechanisms to appear in the blood. Frequent evaluation of blood results is a means by which the status of the internal environment and the extent and nature of tissue damage can be monitored. These blood tests can be run expeditiously and require small sample volumes, and provide important information concerning the diagnosis and management of patients.[17]

Certain intracellular enzymes and proteins are rarely found in measurable amounts in the blood or healthy people. However, after an event leading to cellular injury or death, these substances may leak into the blood. Because of the importance of the timing of the appearance (and disappearance) of enzymes and proteins in the blood, it is crucial that ordered tests are drawn on time. It is equally important that the date and time of the blood draw are noted on the laboratory slip so the temporal sequence of the rise and fall can be established by those interpreting the results.

Table 10-1 • COMPARISON OF SENSITIVITY AND SPECIFICITY OF VARIOUS TESTS FOR MYOCARDIAL INFARCTION

Test	Sensitivity at Peak (%)	Specificity (%)
Electrocardiogram	63–84	100
AST increased	89–97	48–88
CK increased	93–100	57–88
CK-MB increased	94–100	93–100
LDH increased	87	88
Myoglobin	75–95	70
Troponin-I	>98	95
Troponin-T	>98	80

AST, aspartate aminotransferase; CK, creatine kinase; LDH, lactate dehydrogenase. Range of values provided because different studies used various methods, periods after onset of symptoms, serial tests, benchmarks for establishing the diagnosis, and so forth.
From Wallach J. Cardiovascular diseases. In: *Interpretation of Diagnostic Tests*. 8th ed. Philadelphia, PA: Lippincott Williams & Wilkins; 2007.

Over the years more specific biochemical markers of myocardial injury have become available and detecting myocardial injury has become more accurate. The original marker, glutamine-oxaloacetic transaminase was replaced by lactate dehydrogenase (LDH) and later by creatine kinase (CK) and creatine kinase-MB (CK-MB). Troponin has now become the preferred laboratory testing for diagnosing MI and other markers are becoming obsolete.[16] Initial diagnosis of MI, reinfarction, or other types of myocardial damage is made through evaluation of clinical signs and symptoms, 12-lead electrocardiogram (ECG), and biochemical markers including myocardial proteins (troponins). If troponins are not available cardiac enzymes are used. A comparison of the sensitivity and specificity of various tests to detect myocardial injury is in Table 10-1.

Myocardial Proteins

Troponins

Troponins are protein complexes that regulate the calcium-dependent interaction of myosin with actin in the muscle contractile apparatus of striated muscle. They are found in both cardiac and skeletal muscle. Three isotypes have been identified: troponin-I (cTnl), troponin-T (cTnT), and troponin-C (cTnC). Troponins T and I are both found in the myocardium. cTnT binds the troponin complex to tropomyosin, and cTnl inhibits the muscle contractions in the absence of calcium and cTnC.[4] cTnC lacks cardiac specificity; therefore, it is the least studied of the troponins and has no assay available in the clinical setting.

Because of the high specificity and sensitivity for detecting myocardial injury, troponin is the gold-standard biomarker for risk stratification and diagnosis of acute MI. It has become the most important addition to clinical laboratory testing for assessment of biochemical marker in the early diagnosis of MI because it is either low or undetectable in healthy people, but in an event of an MI, is detectable as early as 2 to 3 hours after injury.[17]

According to specific criteria for diagnosis of acute MI it is recommended that sampling take place at time 0 (presentation), followed by repeat sampling 6 to 9 hours later, with a rise or fall of troponin with at least one value exceeding the 99th percentile.[18] A troponin level greater than the 99th percentile of normal reference population is indicative of myocardial necrosis.[19] Guidelines were recently updated in 2012 shortening the marker sampling interval to 3 to 6 hours, reflecting the improved Troponin assay sensitivity. An additional sample may be measured between 12 and 24 hours if biochemical markers have not shown elevation and MI is still suspected.[19] Because most troponin is so tightly bound to muscle, it is released slowly and may remain detectable for 1 to 2 weeks post-MI.[19] See Table 10-2 and Figure 10-1 for typical appearance, peak, and disappearance of various biochemical markers and enzymes.

Table 10-2 • TIMING OF APPEARANCE AND DISAPPEARANCE OF COMMONLY USED CARDIAC BIOMARKERS AND ENZYMES IN RELATION TO ONSET OF CARDIAC SYMPTOMS

Marker or Enzyme	Starts to Rise (h)	Peaks (h)	Returns to Normal (days)
AST	6–12	18–24	7
Total CK	2–6	18–36	3–6
CK-MB	4–8	18–24	3
Myoglobin	2–3	6–9	1–2
Troponin-I	3	10–24	7–10
Troponin-T	3	10–24	10–14

In patients with ST-segment MI, percutaneous coronary intervention (PCI) or fibrinolytic therapy should not be delayed waiting for biochemical marker evaluation.[16] For other patients with suspected cardiac symptoms, troponin is used along with clinical signs and symptoms and 12-lead ECG to make treatment decisions concerning emergency angiogram versus fibrinolytic therapy.

High-sensitivity troponin (HscTn) assays measure cTn concentrations fivefold to 100-fold lower than conventional assays and should be able to detect cTn concentrations below the 99th percentile in greater than 50% of normal individuals.[20] Clinicians must be aware that the rise is more rapid than the fall and take that into account when evaluating those who present more than 12 hours after the possible onset of symptoms.[21]

In the setting of acute coronary syndrome and MI, rapid reperfusion through coronary intervention, a rapid peak or "washout" of cTnl may be seen indicating reperfusion of the ischemic muscle tissue. This elevation is considered a favorable prognostic indicator.[4,22]

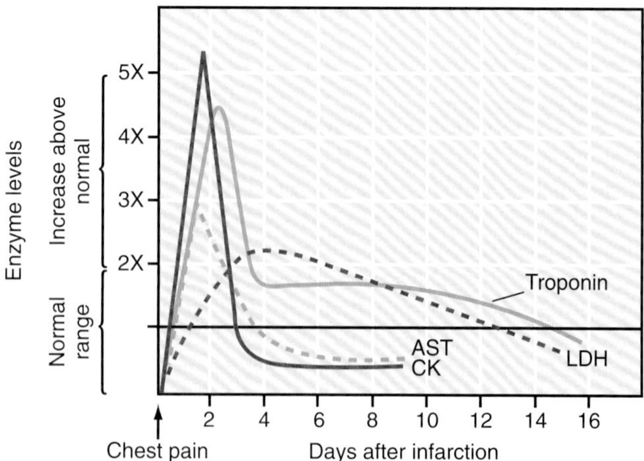

Figure 10-1. Patterns and timing of elevation for aspartate aminotransferase (AST), creatine kinase (CK), lactate dehydrogenase (LDH), and troponin. (From Pagana KD, Pagana TJ. *Mosby's Diagnostic and Laboratory Test Reference*. 8th ed. St. Louis, MO: Mosby Elsevier; 2007.)

Patients whom the MI diagnosis was missed by a less-sensitive assay are at the highest risk of adverse clinic outcomes. When results of the more sensitive assay were clinically available, this group, which previously would have been missed by the less-sensitive assay had the greatest improvement in outcomes. The APACE study which looked at the triage of patients with suspected acute coronary syndrome in the emergency room found that the utilization of HscTns helped reduce cardiac stress testing from 29% to 19%. It also decreased median emergency room length of stay by 79 minutes and mean costs were lowered by 20%.[23]

Troponins are not just elevated in the presence of coronary ischemia. Other conditions that may release troponin include: tachycardia, pericarditis, heart failure, and strenuous exercise. In addition, a mismatch between myocardial oxygen supply and demand may result in troponin release. Sepsis, hypotension, extracellular fluid volume deficit, and atrial fibrillation may increase the oxygen demand of the heart and cause troponin to leak into the bloodstream in patients with no evidence of coronary artery disease.[24] See Display 10-1 for elevations for troponin in the absence of overt ischemic heart disease.

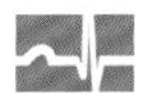 DISPLAY 10-1

Elevations of Troponin in the Absence of Overt Ischemic Heart Disease

Trauma (including contusion, ablation, pacing, implantable cardioverter-defibrillator firings including atrial defibrillators, cardioversion, endomyocardial biopsy, cardiac surgery, after interventional closure of atrial septal defects)
Congestive heart failure, acute and chronic
Aortic valve disease and hypertrophic obstructive cardiomyopathy with significant left ventricular hypertrophy
Hypertension
Hypotension, often with arrhythmias
Postoperative noncardiac surgery patients who seem to do well
Renal failure
Critically ill patients, especially with diabetes, respiratory failure
Drug toxicity, for example, Adriamycin, 5-fluorouracil, Herceptin, snake venoms
Hypothyroidism
Apical ballooning syndrome
Coronary vasospasm
Inflammatory disease, for example, myocarditis, Parvovirus B10, Kawasaki disease, sarcoid, smallpox vaccination, or myocardial extension of bacterial endocarditis
Postpercutaneous coronary intervention patients who seem to have no complications
Pulmonary embolism, severe pulmonary hypertension
Sepsis
Burns, especially if total body surface area is >30%
Infiltrative disease including amyloidosis, hemachromatosis, sarcoidosis, and scleroderma
Acute neurologic disease, including cerebrovascular accident, subarachnoid bleeds
Rhabdomyolysis with cardiac injury
Transplant vasculopathy
Vital exhaustion

Jaffe AS, Babuin L, Apple FS. Biomarkers in acute cardiac disease—The present and the future. *J Am Coll Cardiol.* 2006;48(1):1–11.

Troponin elevation may also be seen in patients with pulmonary diseases. This elevation is usually associated with right heart strain. Of patients diagnosed with moderate to large pulmonary emboli, 30% to 50% have elevated troponin levels. This elevation may be from the acute right heart overload and has been associated with significant increase in mortality.[16,25]

Assessing for myocardial damage after blunt cardiac trauma may be difficult given the high rate of false-positive and false-negative results when using CK-MB. cTnl along with ECG has emerged as an accurate test for confirming presence of myocardial damage after cardiac contusion.[22,26]

Although we have witnessed great strides in the utilization of HscTn, it is important to recognize that troponin in not infallible. All laboratory assessments should be completed in the context of a thorough evaluation of 12-lead ECG in conjunction with the patient presentation.

Cardiac Enzymes

Enzymes are protein substances that catalyze chemical reactions in cells but do not themselves enter into the reaction. Substrates in the cells bind to the enzymes and form products. After the reaction, the enzyme molecule is free to undergo the same reaction with other substrate molecules. Specific enzymes are responsible for nearly every chemical reaction in the body. Some enzymes are present in almost all cells; others are specific to cells of certain organs.

Creatine Kinase

CK is an enzyme specific to cells of the brain, myocardium, and skeletal muscle, but also is found in minimal amounts in other tissues, such as smooth muscle. In these organ systems, the function of CK is primarily that of energy production, where it serves as a catalyst in the phosphorylation of adenosine diphosphate (ADP) to creatine and adenosine triphosphate (ATP). In this manner, CK is responsible for the transfer of an energy-rich bond to ADP. This reaction provides a rapid means of forming ATP for contractile activity in muscle as well as for energy requirements in nonmuscle tissue. The reaction is reversible, and ATP can phosphorylate creatine to form creatine phosphate and ADP during periods of rest.

In an acute MI, inadequate oxygen delivery to the myocardium causes cell injury. An acidic environment promotes the activity of lysosomal enzymes, which are responsible for cell membrane damage or destruction. CK is among the cellular enzymes that diffuse from the damaged cell into the blood. CK is released after irreversible injury. The appearance of CK in the blood indicates cardiac, cerebral, or skeletal muscle necrosis or injury and follows a predictable rise and fall over a specified time.[27]

Age, sex, race, physical activity, lean body mass, medications, and other unidentified factors are known to affect total CK. A patient's baseline CK level is related to his or her overall muscle mass. Adults have lower values than children. Serum CK declines with age and older adults have very low values. CK values measured in women are lower than those of men; European Americans have lower values than African Americans. Chronic exercise raises serum CK levels; however, there is a training effect, and well-trained athletes have smaller increases in CK after physical exertion. Medications that may increase CK include anticoagulants, aspirin, furosemide, captopril, lidocaine, propranolol, and morphine. In addition, high-intensity lipid- lowering therapy with lipophilic statins (i.e., simvastatin or lovastatin) have been found to increase CK.[28] Early and abnormally high increases in CK are sometimes seen after reperfusion by PCI or thrombolytic agents.[4,5]

The importance of monitoring the concentration of serum CK is related to its specificity in the organ in which it functions. Slightly different molecular forms (isoenzymes or *isozymes*) of CK have different tissues of origin. The three CK isoenzymes are combinations of the protein subunits, named for their primary sites of isolation—the muscle (M) and brain (B). CK-MM is the predominant muscle isoenzyme, found in cardiac and skeletal muscle. It also can be detected in normal serum. The myocardium is primarily responsible for the CK-MB form. CK-BB is present in the brain, lung, stomach, prostate, and smooth muscle of the gastrointestinal tract and bladder. Diagnostic precision depends on laboratory analysis of CK isoenzymes and may well be imperative in critically ill patients with multiple-organ system involvement.

Because of the wide range in baseline values among "healthy" people, and various enzyme assay techniques, there are no uniform reference values for CK and CK isoenzymes. Consequently, the practice of reporting the isoenzyme as a percentage of the total CK, as well as in U/L has been encouraged.

Creatine Kinase-BB. The brain fraction CK-BB (CK-1) is seen infrequently in serum. Its rare appearance has been associated with brain trauma, cerebral contusions, and cerebrovascular accidents. The presence of CK-BB in association with cancer has been reported. Other causes of serum CK-BB activity include malignant hyperthermia, renal failure, and after central nervous system surgery.[5] With the significant improvement in diagnostic imaging techniques, CK-BB is now rarely evaluated.

Creatine Kinase-MM. CK-MM constitutes almost the entire CK total in healthy people. Skeletal muscle injury or severe muscle exertion is the most frequent source of high serum CK-MM (CK-3) levels. Specific examples include myopathy, vigorous exercise, multiple intramuscular (IM) injections, electroconvulsive therapy, cardioversion, surgery, muscular dystrophy, convulsions, and delirium tremens. Elevations in CK-MM fractions have also been noted in conditions producing less obvious effects on muscle, such as hypokalemia and hypothyroidism.[5]

Creatine Kinase-MB. Prior to the discovery of troponin, CK-MB (CK-2) isoenzyme analysis had been an accepted means for diagnosis of an acute MI. Although troponin has superseded CK-MB in the diagnosis of MI, most institutions continue to evaluate CK, CK-MB, and troponin if MI is suspected.

When CK-MB is released from myocardial tissue, it has a biologic half-life in blood of hours-to-days. Total CK and CK-MB rise within 2 to 8 hours after an acute MI. Peak levels are seen within 18 to 36 hours and are more than six times their normal value. If no additional myocyte necrosis occurs, levels return to normal within 3 to 4 days.

Elevated CK-MB levels have also been reported after myocardial damage from unstable angina, cardiac surgery, coronary angioplasty, after defibrillation, in vigorous exercise, and after IM injections, trauma, and surgery. Early and abnormally high increases in CK are sometimes seen after reperfusion by PCI or thrombolytic agents. By 6 to 8 hours post angioplasty, 20% of patients have a mild increase in CK-MB. Elevations are occasionally seen in pericarditis, myocarditis, viral myositis, and sustained tachyarrhythmias. An increase in CK-MB may occur after cardioversion, but that time course for increase is different for that of MI, with the mild increase of CK-MB peaking within 4 hours of cardioversion.

Myoglobin

Myoglobin is a low–molecular-weight, oxygen-binding protein found in the myocardium and skeletal muscle. Myoglobin is released into the circulation after damage to the heart or skeletal muscle.[2] Because of its release from other muscle tissues, troponin rather than myoglobin is the biomarker of choice for diagnosing MI. After MI, myoglobin levels increase in 2 to 3 hours, peak in 6 to 9 hours, and return to normal (undetectable) as early as 12 hours but more typically after 24 to 36 hours.[29]

Elevated myoglobin levels are seen after MI, reinfarction, cocaine use, skeletal muscle injury, trauma, exercise, IM injections, severe burns, electrical shock, polymyositis, alcoholic myopathy, delirium tremens, metabolic disorders (e.g., myxedema), malignant hyperthermia, systemic lupus erythematosus, muscular dystrophy, rhabdomyolysis, and seizures.[4,5] Myoglobin may not be excreted in renal failure, so caution should be used when interpreting results.[4] Further, very high levels of myoglobin are toxic to the kidneys and thus, careful monitoring of renal function is warranted.

Biochemical Marker Activity After PCI

After elective PCI for stable angina, biomarker elevation is fairly common. CK and CK-MB elevation occurs in 5% to 30% of patients. These elevations have been associated with increased risk of death, MI, and need for repeat revascularization.[30] Prasad et al.[31] found that troponin elevation is frequent after elective PCI. Of the patients in their study, 19% had an elevated troponin level. These patients had more complex angiographic characteristics and had undergone multivessel PCI. They found that an elevated troponin level was associated with increased morbidity and mortality. Miller et al.[32] measured troponin before (baseline) and after PCI and found that prognosis was most often related to the baseline troponin level and not the biomarker response after the procedure. Nallamothu et al.[33] analyzed 1157 patients who underwent elective PCI and found that cTnl elevation was common after the procedure (29%), and that large troponin elevations, up to eight times normal, were associated with decreased long-term survival. Taken together, these studies demonstrate that continued use and evaluation of biochemical markers is essential after coronary intervention.

Biochemical Marker Activity After Cardiac Surgery

All types of cardiac surgery involve considerable injury to the myocardium. However, differentiating between ischemic alterations associated with surgery and perioperative MI may be difficult. The evaluation of troponin and cardiac enzymes is common after cardiovascular surgery. Researchers have focused on the prognostic implication of elevated troponin and cardiac enzymes measurements after surgery. Klatte et al.[34] and Costa et al.[35] found that elevated levels of CK-MB in serial measurements after coronary artery bypass graft (CABG) surgery were associated with increased mortality, and that the higher the level of CK-MB, the higher risk of mortality in the immediate to long-term postoperative period. With troponin evaluation becoming more common, Januzzi et al.[36] determined cTnT levels offered a superior predictor of complications from cardiac surgery than CK-MB. Kathiresan et al.[37] and Croal et al.[38] found similar results; the higher the troponin, I or T, the increased risk of mortality after CABG surgery. These studies demonstrate that biomarker evaluation postoperatively also is important and should not be considered inconsequential.

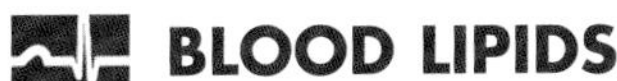

BLOOD LIPIDS

An accumulation of lipids within the arterial wall is considered a part of the process of atherogenesis. Alteration of blood lipid levels has been identified as a coronary heart disease (CHD) risk factor. Certain lipoproteinemias have been identified as contributing to total plasma cholesterol levels. Plasma normally contains insoluble lipid elements: free fatty acids; exogenous triglycerides; endogenous triglycerides, which are manufactured in the liver; cholesterol; and phospholipids. To be transported, each is attached to a protein. Distinguishing lipoprotein abnormalities is useful because therapy is based on an understanding of the origin of the problem.

Blood Lipid Laboratory Measurement

Elevated lipid levels are considered a risk factor for cardiovascular disease. Cholesterol and the protein components of high-density lipid (HDL), low-density lipid (LDL), and triglycerides are evaluated by electrophoresis when hyperlipoproteinemia is suspected.[29] See Table 10-3 for recommended levels of cholesterol and its components. In most people, the cholesterol values remain constant over 24 hours; a nonfasting blood sample for measurement of total blood cholesterol is acceptable. However, a nonfasting sample for HDL, LDL, and triglyceride levels is of less value. National Cholesterol Education Program 2001 guidelines on cholesterol *screening* recommend everyone over age 20 have a fasting lipoprotein profile (total cholesterol, LDL, HDL, and triglycerides) every 5 years.[39] Lipoprotein electrophoresis is necessary to evaluate serum for hyperlipoproteinemia. LDL is more difficult to isolate and measure. Therefore, if LDL is not measured in a screening lipoprotein test, it may be calculated using the Friedewald formula. The Friedewald formula is inaccurate if the triglycerides are greater than 400 mg/dL (see Display 10-2).[40]

Table 10-3 • LIPID PROFILE REFERENCE RANGES

Lipid Profile	
Total blood cholesterol	
Desirable	<200 mg/dL
Borderline high	200–239 mg/dL
High	≥240 mg/dL
HDL-C-cholesterol	
Low—A major risk factor for CHD	<40 mg/dL
Better	40–59 mg/dL
High—Considered protective against heart disease	≥60 mg/dL
LDL-C-cholesterol	
Goal for very high-risk patients	<70 mg/dL
Optimal	<100 mg/dL
Near or above optimal	100–129 mg/dL
Borderline high	130–159 mg/dL
High	160–189 mg/dL
Very high	>190 mg/dL
LDL-C-cholesterol treatment goals	
No CHD or DM with one or no risk factors	<160 mg/dL
No CHD or DM with two or more risk factors	<130 mg/dL
Very high-risk patients—CHD or DM patients	<70 mg/dL
Triglyceride	
Normal	<150 mg/dL
Borderline high	150–199 mg/dL
High	200–499 g/dL
Very high	≥500 mg/dL

CHD, coronary heart disease; DM, diabetes mellitus.
From Expert Panel on Detection, Evaluation, and Treatment of High Blood Cholesterol in Adults (Adult Treatment Panel III), by National Cholesterol Education Program. Executive Summary of The Third Report of The National Cholesterol Education Program (NCEP). *JAMA.* 2001;285:2486–2497; and Grundy SM, Cleeman JI, Merz NB, et al. Implications of recent clinical trials for the National Cholesterol Education Program Adult Treatment Panel III Guidelines. *Circulation.* 2004;110:227–239.

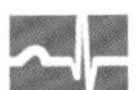

DISPLAY 10-2

Computation Formulas

Computation of LDL Cholesterol
Friedewald formula[a]
LDL cholesterol = total cholesterol − HDL cholesterol − (triglycerides divided by 5)

Computation of Ionized Calcium
Serum calcium can be presumed to be normal if:

(4.5 − albumin level) × (0.8) + lab value for total calcium = 8.8 to 11.0 mEq/L

1. Obtain total calcium level (normal = 8.8 to 10.5 mEq/L). If it is less than normal (e.g., <8.8 mEq/L), follow the steps below.
2. Obtain serum albumin level (normal = 4.5 g/dL).
3. If serum albumin level is decreased, subtract the decreased level from normal value for albumin (e.g., albumin level is measured at 3.0; 4.5 [normal] − 3.0 [measured] = 1.5).
4. For every 1.0 decrease in albumin, add 0.8 to calcium level (for above example, 1.5 × 0.8 = 1.2).
5. Add the calculated figure to the total calcium level (e.g., 7.8 + 1.2 = 9 mEq/L, calcium is within normal range).
6. One half of this level (9/2) is 4.5, within the normal range for ionized calcium (normal ionized calcium = 4.5–5.0).

Computation of Anion Gap
Anion gap = (sodium [140] + potassium [4.0]) − (bicarbonate [24] + chloride [110]) = 10 to 12 mEq/L

Computation of Serum Osmolality
Two times the serum sodium + serum glucose (Glu) divided by 18 + blood urea nitrogen (BUN) divided by 1.8 = serum osmolality ([2 × sodium] + [glucose/18] + [BUN/1.8]) = 280 to 300 mOsm/kg
(e.g., [2 × 122] + [198/2] + [18/1.8] = 265 mOsm [water or intracellular fluid excess]; [2 × 155] + [108/2] + [5.4/1.8] = 318 mOsm [water or intracellular fluid deficit])

[a]Formula valid for estimating LDL cholesterol if the triglyceride level is <400 mg/dL.

ADDITIONAL LABORATORY TESTS ASSOCIATED WITH CARDIAC DISEASE

Nearly half of all patients with known CHD have no established coronary risk factors (i.e., hypertension, hypercholesterolemia, cigarette smoking, diabetes mellitus, marked obesity, and physical inactivity). Atherosclerosis is now considered an inflammatory disease, with cytokines and other bioactive molecules involved in most steps of the atherogenesis process.

With the knowledge that atherosclerosis is an inflammatory disease, researchers are studying different markers to determine if there are other independent risk factors for the disease and if these markers can be used to identify high-risk individuals for CHD that may not have traditional risk factors. Markers being studied include but are not limited to adhesion molecules, C-reactive protein (CRP), cytokines, fibrinogen, homocysteine (Hcy), lipoprotein-associated phospholipase A_2, serum amyloid A, tissue-type plasminogen activator, and white blood cell (WBC) count. Hcy is being researched extensively and is utilized as a possible risk factor for CHD. CRP is showing promise from a clinical chemistry perspective and research perspective as a risk factor for CHD.[41] See Figure 10-2 for risk of future MI related to baseline labs.

C-Reactive Protein

CRP is an acute-phase reactant protein that is produced primarily by the liver during the acute inflammatory process. CRP is a nonspecific but sensitive indicator of inflammation, bacterial infection, or acute injury. CRP is a more sensitive indicator of inflammation and responds more rapidly to inflammation than erythrocyte sedimentation rate (ESR). CRP was discovered approximately 70 years ago and has been used for decades to monitor the effectiveness of treatment for patients with lupus erythematosus, rheumatoid arthritis, and other immune-related conditions. Patients with acute MI or sepsis, or post surgery have elevated CRP levels.

Mounting evidence shows that CRP levels are associated with various aspects of the cardiovascular risk spectrum. Elevated CRP levels were noted among people who are physically inactive with worse cardiorespiratory fitness. CRP was also elevated in the obese and in those with metabolic syndrome.[42]

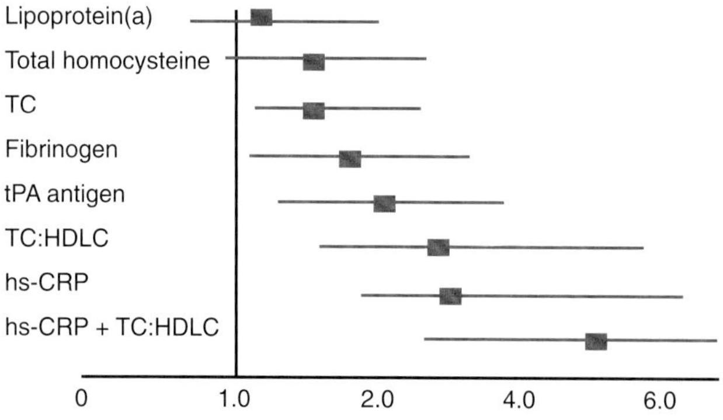

Figure 10-2. Relative risk for future myocardial infarction among apparently healthy middle-aged men in the Physician's Health Study according to baseline levels of lipoprotein(a), total plasma homocysteine, total cholesterol (TC), fibrinogen, tissue-type plasminogen activator (tPA) antigen, the ratio of total cholesterol to high-density lipoprotein cholesterol (HDLC), and high-sensitivity C-reactive protein (hs-CRP). (From Ridker PM. Evaluating novel cardiovascular risk factors: Can we better predict heart attacks? *Annals of Internal Medicine.* 1999;130:933–937.)

Rost et al.[43] also found elevated plasma CRP levels to be an independent risk for future ischemic strokes and transient ischemic attack in older adults. Other studies have continued to demonstrate a link between elevated CRP levels and increased risk of CHD in healthy middle-aged men,[44] healthy but high-risk men,[45] women,[46] and older adults.[47] Ridker et al.[48] demonstrated that CRP was a stronger predictor of cardiovascular events than LDL level in 15,745 women participants in the Women's Health Study.

Increased body mass index, insulin resistance, hypertension, an intrauterine device, cigarette smoking, chronic infections (e.g., gingivitis, bronchitis), or chronic inflammation (e.g., rheumatoid arthritis) can increase CRP levels.[41] Exogenous hormones may cause an increase in CRP. Increased activity, weight loss, and moderate alcohol consumption decrease CRP levels. Drugs that decrease CRP levels include fibrates, HMG-CoA reductase inhibitors (statins), nicotinic acid (niacin), nonsteroidal anti-inflammatory agents, salicylates, and steroids.[41] Many laboratories offer a routine CRP level or a high-sensitivity CRP (hs-CRP) level.

Homocysteine

Hcy is an intermediate amino acid formed during protein catabolism by the conversion of methionine to cysteine. Vitamins B_6, folic acid, B_{12}, and riboflavin, are all required for this metabolism. Epidemiologic studies first showed an association of high levels of Hcy with an increased incidence of atherosclerotic disease.[48] Elevated Hcy is considered a risk factor for CVD and may also be associated with hypertension.[48] Levels of Hcy increase with aging and are also seen in patients who smoke or in those with poor diets. There is an inverse correlation of Hcy levels with folate concentration. Further investigation is indicated to determine if elevated Hcy levels is an independent risk factor for CVD or just linked to other modifiable risks factors.[49] Patients who have multiple risk factors for CVD may benefit from Hcy screening. Patients should also be encouraged to eat a diet in multiple nutrients, including B vitamins, to lower Hcy levels within the blood.

Hcy levels can be genetic or acquired. Hyperhomocysteinemia can be caused by a genetic defect in Hcy metabolism. Children with this disease have very premature and accelerated atherosclerosis during childhood. Hcy testing should be performed when there is a strong familial predisposition for atherosclerotic disease or with a progressive or an early onset of atherosclerotic disease is suspected.[50]

Lipoprotein-Associated Phospholipase A_2

Lipoprotein-associated phospholipase A_2 also known as platelet-activating factor acetylhydrolase or Lp-PLA$_2$ is presently being studied as an inflammatory marker of cardiovascular risk. Lp-PLA$_2$ is an enzyme regulated by inflammatory cytokines and is found predominately on LDL cholesterol. Lp-PLA$_2$ plays a role in the inflammation of blood vessels and is thought to contribute to CAD. Some recent studies have shown that Lp-PLA$_2$ is an independent risk marker for CVD. In these studies, increased concentrations of Lp-PLA$_2$ were seen in many people who were diagnosed with CHD and ischemic stroke, regardless of other risk factors.[51]

Lp-PLA$_2$ may contribute directly to atherogenesis by hydrolyzing oxidized phospholipids into proatherogenic fragments and by generating lysolecithin, which has proinflammatory properties.[52] Studies by Caslake et al.[52] and Packard et al.[53] showed a strong correlation between Lp-PLA_2 levels and risk of CHD in men. By contrast, results from the Women's Health Study showed Lp-PLA_2 was not a strong predictor of future cardiovascular risk in females.[54] Further research is needed to assess Lp-PLA_2 ability to predict cardiovascular risk and establish plasma levels.

Cardiac Natriuretic Peptide Markers

The natriuretic peptide system is part of the neurohormonal system that participates in cardiovascular homeostasis.[55] Investigators have identified three natriuretic peptides; type-A and type-B originate in the cardiac myocyte and type-C originates in the endothelial and renal epithelial cells. A-type natriuretic peptide (ANP) originates in the atrium and is released into the bloodstream when the atrium is stretched beyond normal capacity. BNP (also known as brain natriuretic peptide because it was first identified in small amounts in the brain) is produced and stored in the ventricles of the heart and is released when ventricular diastolic pressure rises.[56] Researchers believe that ANP is released as an acute response to increased volume in the heart, whereas BNP acts as a backup hormone only activated after prolonged volume overload.[54] Both hormones act in a similar manner to increase the loss of water and sodium through the kidneys. Renin and aldosterone are suppressed by the hormones. Glomerular filtration rate is increased by renal vasculature dilation. ANP and BNP have diuretic and antihypertensive effects.

BNP has emerged as the laboratory marker of choice for evaluating dyspnea and heart failure since it is synthesized and secreted by the left ventricle. BNP testing is available as a rapid POCT or can be performed in a centralized laboratory. Plasma BNP concentrations can vary with the assay used, age, sex, and body mass index. Normal values tend to increase with age and to be higher in women than in men. BNP levels are often elevated in patients with renal insufficiency and renal failure whether they have heart failure or not. A low BNP level in these patients may be useful to exclude left ventricular dysfunction. Levels may also be elevated in patients with atrial fibrillation, pulmonary hypertension, and sepsis.

Normally, circulating BNP and NT-proBNP levels are quite low, but in the setting of heart failure (HF), their concentrations rise dramatically. BNP concentrations have been correlated with the New York Heart Association Functional Classification of severity of heart failure, as well as prognosis in heart failure.[56–59] Fonarow et al.[58] found that admission BNP levels along with elevated troponin levels were independent predictors of inhospital mortality in patients with acutely decompensated heart failure. The patients with BNP levels greater than 840 pg/mL and increased troponin were at particular risk for mortality.

Some conditions are associated with lower than expected natriuretic peptide levels: HF with preserved ejection fraction (HFpEF) compared with HF with reduced ejection fraction (HFrEF) and obesity. Obesity has been associated with lower than expected BNP or NT-proBNP values, likely due to the suppression of natriuretic peptide synthesis or release. However elevated BNP and NT-proBNP can still diagnose acute HF regardless of body mass index accurately, but with a lower sensitivity.[60]

MR-ProADM and Copeptin

One of the first responses to cardiac dysfunction is the activation of the sympathetic nervous system. Midregional proadrenomedullin (MR-proADM) is elevated in patients with acute and chronic HF and is a strong predictor of clinical outcomes such as mortality and HF hospitalization.[60] Copeptin is a stable C-terminal propeptide fragment of arginine vasopressin (AVP). In the Biomarkers in Acute Heart Failure (BACH) trial, elevated copeptin level strongly predicted mortality.[61]

Genetic Testing in Cardiac Disease. Genetic testing is a valuable component of managing and diagnosing inherited cardiovascular disease in patients and their families. Examples of conditions include: hypertrophic, dilated, and arrhythmogenic cardiomyopathies as well as inherited arrhythmias.[61] Incorporating genetic testing into clinical practice involves multiple components. Five components are included in the decision to perform genetic testing. First, there needs to be recognition that an inherited cardiovascular disease may be present. Second, there should be proper identification of family members for indicated genetic testing. Next, the provider should select the appropriate genetic test. The provider, or care team, should understand the complexities of genetic result interpretation.[62] Lastly, effective communication of results and implications of the results should be shared with the patient and the family.[61]

Genetic testing is most frequently used as diagnostic testing to identify an underlying genetic etiology in a patient with known or suspected inherited cardiovascular disease. Genetic testing is also helpful in the case of apparently healthy relatives to determine potential at risk for development of an inherited disease. Genetic testing can establish a specific, etiology-based diagnosis.[62] In the case of most inherited cardiovascular disease the inheritance pattern is autosomal dominant, with a 50% chance of transmission to each offspring regardless of sex.

Patients who are newly diagnosed with an inherited cardiovascular disease should be offered a complete evaluation inclusive of phenotypic assessment, family history assessment, genetic counseling, and a coordinated family evaluation.[61] It is essential to perform pretest and posttest genetic counseling. Pretest counseling provides necessary information to obtain informed consent, yield of testing, how the results may affect the patient management, as well as implications for family members. Posttest education can be performed with the care team as well as genetic counselors as indicated. Treating the family as a unit is imperative and a key component of genetic testing. Genetic testing is a powerful tool in the diagnosis of inherited cardiovascular diseases and in the identification of at-risk healthy relatives.[62]

HEMATOLOGIC STUDIES

Cells in the circulating blood are responsible for oxygen and carbon dioxide transport and the body's immune response. Erythrocytes (RBCs), leukocytes (WBCs), and platelets are formed in the bone marrow and are suspended in the plasma). Blood is also the transport system for electrolytes, products of metabolism, hormones, and plasma proteins. An appreciation of the roles of erythrocytes, leukocytes, and other hematologic parameters is an important prerequisite to understanding deviations from normal. This approach is helpful in planning care based on an assessment of the demands of daily living. Each of the aspects of a hematologic study has meaning for patients in terms of their ability to withstand the effects of a cardiac event.

Complete Blood Cell Count

A complete blood cell (CBC) count is important for evaluating the oxygen-carrying capacity of the blood and the response of the body to invasion by foreign cells such as bacteria. Because excessive bleeding, bone marrow disease, hemolytic disorders, some drugs, and infections can alter the number of leukocytes, erythrocytes, or platelets in the blood, the CBC of the patient with cardiac disease is closely monitored. A baseline study can be compared with subsequent studies to evaluate bleeding, the effects of treatment, or the presence of infection.

Red Blood Cell Count

RBCs are formed in the bone marrow and constitute the majority of peripheral cells. The RBCs contain Hb and are responsible for transporting oxygen to the tissues as well as carbon dioxide from tissues. The average life span of an RBC is 120 days, after which it is removed from the blood by the liver, spleen, or bone marrow.[4]

When the RBC count is more than 10% below the expected normal value, the patient is said to be anemic. Conditions under which there are a decreased number of RBCs include cirrhosis, hemorrhage, presence of prosthetic valves, renal disease, chronic illnesses, and various malignancies of the bone marrow.[4] Anemia from any cause must be looked for in the patient with cardiac disease because it may precipitate angina, aggravate heart failure, or contribute to a diagnosis of subacute bacterial endocarditis.

An RBC increase is seen in congenital heart disease, severe chronic obstructive pulmonary disease, and polycythemia vera. It is falsely high in extracellular fluid deficit (volume contraction) and falsely low with extracellular fluid excess.[4]

Hematocrit. Hct is the volume of packed RBCs found in 100 mL of blood, expressed as a percent. As an indirect measure of the RBC count, Hct increases and decreases with the RBC count. Abnormalities in RBC size may alter Hct values.[4] Normal ranges for Hct differ by sex and age group.

Hemoglobin. The RBCs contain a complex protein compound called *hemoglobin*. Hb is the oxygen-carrying protein of the RBC and is an important component of the acid–base buffer system. Insufficient amounts of Hb place a strain on the cardiovascular system, and may cause MI, angina, congestive heart failure, or stroke.

Corpuscular Indices. With the RBC count, the quantity of Hb, and the Hct, the characteristics of individual RBCs can be described in terms of cell size (mean corpuscular volume [MCV]), amount of Hb present in a single cell (mean corpuscular Hb [MCH]), and the proportion of each cell occupied by Hb (mean corpuscular Hb concentration [MCHC]). The indices are calculated by these formulas:

$$\text{MCV} = \text{Hematocrit (as \%)} \times \frac{10}{\text{RBC count}} \text{ (millions/mm}^3\text{)}$$

$$\text{MCH} = \text{Hemoglobin (g/100 mL)} \times \frac{10}{\text{RBC}} \text{ (millions/mm}^3\text{)}$$

$$\text{MCHC} = \text{Hemoglobin (g/dL)} \times \frac{10}{\text{Hematocrit}} \text{ (\%)}$$

White Blood Cells

The WBCs, or leukocytes, work to defend against foreign matter and cells in the body. There are five types of WBCs: neutrophils, eosinophils, basophils, monocytes, and lymphocytes. Elevated WBC counts in the patient with cardiac disease may be due to MI, bacterial endocarditis or other infections, some medications, or Dressler syndrome. After MI, the elevation may be a result of the body's normal response to stress. After an acute MI, WBCs may be elevated. Leukocytosis occurs as the infarcted site is invaded by leukocytes and macrophages that engulf and phagocytose necrotic tissue.

Although an elevated temperature after MI may be expected, an elevated WBC count should always suggest the possibility of concomitant infection. A urinary or respiratory tract infection or an infection secondary to an invasive procedure is a possibility during an extended illness.

White Cell Differential. The differential count is a descriptive list of the types of WBCs. The differential for each of the five leukocyte types is usually expressed as a percentage of the total leukocyte count; the total should add up to 100.

Erythrocyte Sedimentation Rate

The ESR measures the speed at which anticoagulated erythrocytes settle in a long, narrow tube. The speed depends on the size of the clumps into which the cells aggregate in the presence of blood fibrinogen. The ESR is a nonspecific indicator of inflammatory disease. It may be elevated in MI, pericarditis, and bacterial endocarditis as well as many other diseases but it is usually low in heart failure.[5] The degree of increase of the ESR does not correlate with severity or prognosis.

Laboratory Measurement of Complete Blood Cell Values

The RBC and WBC counts are performed by an automated counter that directly measures all parameters, including Hct, corpuscular indices, and platelets. The precision of the Hct analysis is ±2 points. Consequently, a change in measurement by as much as 4 points may not indicate a change in the true Hct.

Activity and change in position may raise Hct and Hb levels; Hb may be higher by 8% in the morning than in the evening. The usual precautions should be taken to avoid hemolysis and ensure accuracy. The specimen should be rapidly transported to the laboratory to avoid changes in distribution of the cells within the plasma. RBC tests can be done using capillary blood, but massage of the fingertip or earlobe can lead to cell destruction and alter the sample. If difficulty is encountered in locating a vein, the tourniquet should be removed long enough to allow restoration of circulation to avoid a hemoconcentrated sample. A blood smear should also be examined if there is an abnormality in one or more of the CBC parameters to evaluate the size, shape, and color of the RBCs, WBCs, and platelets.[4,5]

Complete Blood Count After Cardiac Surgery

The CBC including the Hb and Hct levels are monitored after cardiac surgery to evaluate blood loss. Immediately after cardiac surgery, there are rapid shifts in extracellular fluid volume status because of the hemodilutional effects of cardiopulmonary bypass and the rewarming that follows induced hypothermia. This fluid shift may be reflected in a reduced Hb or Hct level. Frequent monitoring of the WBC count helps identify any leukocytosis and infection. Cardiopulmonary bypass results in a period of reduced phagocytic activity that renders the patient more at risk for infection.

COAGULATION STUDIES

Drug-induced anticoagulation is a routine procedure in the cardiac care unit and requires close monitoring of blood coagulation mechanisms. Anticoagulation is used after thrombolytic therapy, during cardiac surgery, to prevent formation of venous thrombus associated with prolonged bed rest and hemostasis, to prevent formation of intracardiac thrombus, and in treatment for established thrombus and embolus.

The prevention and treatment of blood coagulation is complex and involves a number of hemostatic functions that play roles in the body's homeostasis. Therapy involves interference with this homeostatic mechanism. An understanding of the laboratory tests used to evaluate the effectiveness of treatment is vital to prevent undesired outcomes of anticoagulation therapy. The normal ranges for the coagulation factors and the methods used depend on the laboratory.

Platelet Count

Platelets are elements of the blood that promote coagulation and are produced by the bone marrow. They contribute to blood clotting by clumping or sticking to rough surfaces and injured sites. Platelet counts are useful for monitoring the course of a disease or treatment. Thrombocytopenia (low platelet count) is a common cause of abnormal bleeding. There is a serious risk of hemorrhage when the platelet count is less than 30,000 to 50,000/mm^3, and a spontaneous bleed may occur when platelets are less than 20,000/mm^3. Bleeding due to thrombocytopenia is characterized by petechiae, bleeding from the gums or tongue, or epistaxis. Thrombocytopenia may occur by several mechanisms: reduced platelet production, sequestration of platelets, accelerated platelet destruction, loss from hemorrhage, and dilution from massive blood transfusions that contain few platelets.

Specific conditions that may cause a decrease in platelets include hemorrhage, hypersplenism, leukemia, lymphoma, prosthetic heart valves, heparin-induced thrombocytopenia, idiopathic thrombocytopenic purpura, disseminated intravascular coagulation (DIC), systemic lupus erythematosus, hemolytic anemia, and infection. Medications that decrease the platelet count include acetaminophen, aspirin, chemotherapy, histamine-blocking agents, heparin, hydralazine, quinidine, and thiazide diuretics. Nonsteroidal anti-inflammatory drugs may cause a decrease in platelet aggregation. The concurrent use of heparin with antiplatelet agents increases the risk of bleeding. After a large number of blood transfusions (14 units or more) and after extracorporeal circulation, the platelet count is typically low.[4,5]

Aspirin has been incorporated into the treatment plan after MI to prevent hypercoagulability due to platelet aggregation. Antiplatelet agents prevent platelet aggregation by inhibiting fibrinogen binding and platelet–interaction. Antiplatelet agents are included in most treatment plans to prevent arterial thrombus including post-MI, PCI/stent placement, cardiovascular surgery, and other vascular surgeries. Patients receiving antiplatelet drugs may have a normal platelet count but have increased bleeding due to the drug. The drug alters the platelets for the life of platelets; therefore, increased bleeding may be seen for 7 to 14 days after discontinuation of treatment. Glycoprotein (GP) IIb/IIIa agents are also used to decrease platelet aggregation in acute MI and post-PCI/stent placement patients. Patients who receive GPIIb/IIIa agents should be monitored for signs of bleeding and thrombocytopenia.

Increased amounts of platelets may be seen in malignant disorders including, polycythemia vera, postsplenectomy syndrome, and rheumatoid arthritis. Platelet counts may also be increased in those who live at high altitude or exercise strenuously.[4]

Prothrombin Time

The PT is used to evaluate the extrinsic system and common pathway in the clotting mechanism. Specifically, it measures the activity of prothrombin, fibrinogen, and factors V, VII, and X. Prothrombin is synthesized by the liver. PT may be prolonged in heart failure, vitamin K deficiency, liver disease, bile duct obstruction, DIC, massive blood transfusion, salicylate intoxication, and alcohol use. Severe liver damage may prolong PT. Drugs that may prolong PT include but are not limited to some antibiotics, allopurinol, amiodarone, warfarin, heparin, many nonsteroidal anti-inflammatory drugs, and aspirin. Decreased PT is seen in thyroid dysfunction, thrombophlebitis, MI, and pulmonary embolus. Medications that may decrease PT include but are not limited to antacids, diuretics, diphenhydramine, and oral contraceptives.[4,5]

The PT is used mainly for monitoring patients on warfarin. Warfarin inhibits vitamin K–dependent synthesis of clotting factors II, VII, IX, and X. Therapeutic PTs are considered to be 1.5 to 2 times normal, or a 15% to 50% change in the normal value. If the PT is allowed to prolong greater than 2.5 times the control value, there is a risk of bleeding.

The international normalized ratio (INR) has been adopted for reporting PT. The INR is calculated from the observed PT ratio. The INR is equivalent to the PT ratio that would have been obtained if the patient's PT had been compared to a PT value obtained using the International Reference Preparation, a standard human brain thromboplastin prepared by the World Health Organization. With the INR, standardized PT results are available for healthcare providers in different parts of the country and the world. These standardized results are independent of the reagents used and adjust for the type of instrument used. The therapeutic INR in most situations ranges from 2.0 to 3.5. However, different ranges have been established for deep vein thrombosis prophylaxis (1.5 to 2.0), deep vein thrombosis (2.0 to 3.0), prevention of embolus in atrial fibrillation (2.0 to 3.0), pulmonary embolism (PE) (2.5 to 3.5), and prosthetic valve prophylaxis (2.5 to 3.5).[2] The INR should not be used to initiate warfarin therapy; it should be used only once the patient is thought to be on a stable dose.

Partial Thromboplastin Time and Activated Partial Thromboplastin Time

The partial thromboplastin time (PTT) and activated partial thromboplastin time (aPTT) measure the intrinsic coagulation system and are used in assessing patients receiving unfractionated heparin. With low–molecular-weight heparin, neither the PTT nor aPTT changes, so laboratory monitoring is not required. The PTT measures deficiencies in all factors except factors VII and XIII, whereas the aPTT measures all coagulation factors except platelet factor III, XIII, and VII. The aPTT is measured by adding test reagents to PTT to shorten clotting time. When clotting time is shortened, minor clotting defects can be detected.

The therapeutic range for both PTT and aPTT is maintained at 1.5 to 2.5 times the patient's baseline value. The PTT and aPTT is usually drawn 30 to 60 minutes before the patient's next dose of heparin. For PTT and aPTT results less than 50 seconds, an increase in the heparin dose should be considered. Conversely, a decrease in dose should be considered for PTT and aPTT values greater than 100 seconds.

The PTT and aPTT are prolonged in heparin administration, congenital clotting factor deficiencies, cirrhosis of the liver, vitamin K deficiency, and DIC. Antihistamines, ascorbic acid, chlorpromazine, and salicylates may also cause an increase.[5]

Activated Clotting Time

The ACT is used during cardiac surgery and cardiac catheterization to monitor heparinization. The time it takes whole blood to clot reflects the activity of the intrinsic clotting mechanism. During extracorporeal heparin therapy, the ACT is kept at four to six times the baseline value.

Tests to measure ACT are simple and easy to use at the bedside. The use of ACT rather than aPTT to monitor heparin therapy in patients with unstable angina or acute MI may result in much steadier levels of anticoagulation and prevent ischemic recurrences.[4]

Fibrinogen Level

Fibrinogen is a plasma protein synthesized by the liver. This test measures the conversion of fibrinogen to fibrin by thrombin. Fibrinogen levels are elevated in acute infections, collagen disease, inflammatory diseases, and hepatitis. Decreased levels are seen in severe liver disease, DIC, leukemia, and obstetric complications. Thrombolytic therapy may also affect fibrinogen levels.[5]

Protein C and Protein S

Protein C, with cofactor protein S, is a natural anticoagulant protein whose function is to degrade activated factors V and VIII. Deficiency in either protein C or S can lead to a hypercoagulable state, which may cause venous thrombosis. In order for protein C to be activated, it needs to interact with the thrombin–thrombomodulin complex on the surface of endothelial calls. Protein C is vitamin K dependent and indirectly promotes fibrinolysis.[5] Hereditary protein C deficiency accounts for approximately 3% to 9% of patients with venous thrombosis. Hereditary protein S deficiency accounts for 2% to 7% of patients with venous thrombosis.[6]

Acquired conditions that cause protein C or protein S deficiency include liver disease, vitamin K deficiency or warfarin use, or consumption of protein C or protein S from thrombosis, DIC, or surgery. Protein S deficiency may also be acquired by use of estrogen, including oral contraceptives or estrogen replacement therapy, or pregnancy. Protein S may also be decreased in nephrotic syndrome, HIV infection, or varicella infection. A rapid fall in protein C or protein S can be caused by initiating warfarin therapy without first reducing other coagulation factors with heparin. This rapid fall in protein C or protein S can cause hypercoagulability and cause warfarin-induced skin necrosis. Warfarin-induced skin necrosis causes thrombosis of skin vessels, which can lead to infarction and necrosis. Treatment requires discontinuation of warfarin and vitamin K administration.[4–6]

Warfarin should be discontinued for at least 10 days prior to testing for protein C or protein S. Reference range for protein C or protein S is reported as a percentage of the amount expected in normal plasma. The reference range is approximately 70% to 140%.[6]

D-Dimer (Fibrin Degradation Fragment)

D-dimer is an assay used to measure the amount of clot breakdown products specific for cross-linked fragments derived from fibrin. A positive test indicates that thrombus is forming. This test is most useful in the inpatient and outpatient setting, along with compression ultrasound and chest computed tomography for the diagnosis of deep vein thrombosis or PE. D-dimer may also be used along with fibrin degradation products in the diagnosis of DIC.[4]

For the diagnosis of PE, D-dimer has a good sensitivity and negative predictive value, but poor specificity. D-dimer levels are abnormal in 95% of patients with PE; however, they are abnormal in only 50% of patients with subsegmental PE.[5] Patients with normal D-dimer levels have a 95% likelihood of not having PE, and therefore the test offers an excellent negative predictive value. In the outpatient setting when deep vein thrombosis is suspected, if the D-dimer test is negative, compression ultrasound of the legs is not necessary.[4,63] D-dimer levels are normal in only 25% of patients without PE and so have low specificity. Among patients without PE, D-dimer levels are commonly abnormal in hospitalized patients, particularly those with malignancy or recent surgery.

A normal D-dimer level can exclude recurrent PE in patients with prior venous thrombosis and/or PE. However, fewer patients with prior events will have a normal D-dimer level, thus limiting the test's usefulness. D-dimer testing has been studied to help determine the length of time needed for anticoagulation therapy. Palareti et al.[64] found that patients with an abnormal D-dimer level 1 month after discontinuing anticoagulation therapy had a significantly higher risk of recurrent venous thromboembolism than patients who continued anticoagulation since they had an abnormal D-dimer level.

ARTERIAL BLOOD GASES

Arterial blood gases are frequently assessed in the patient with cardiac disease. Tissue oxygenation, carbon dioxide removal, and acid–base status are analyzed through the assay of arterial blood gases. Arterial blood gas results guide treatment decisions in ventilated patients and critically ill, nonventilated patients. Knowledge of the normal blood gas values and the meaning of deviation from normal are essential to treatment decisions.

The arterial oxygen saturation (SaO_2) and the mixed venous oxygen saturation (SvO_2) reflect the relation between oxygen supply and demand and the extent of overall tissue utilization of O_2. Continuous monitoring of SaO_2 (oxygen supply) can be achieved through pulse oximetry; laboratory analysis, however, is useful in distinguishing the SaO_2 at partial pressure of oxygen (PaO_2) levels above 65 mm Hg. A fiberoptic pulmonary artery catheter is capable of evaluating SvO_2 levels continuously. This information is useful in determining the ideal mode of respiratory intervention, the effect of nursing care on tissue O_2 demands, physiologic alterations requiring increased supply of O_2, and the reflection of physiologic changes on cardiac output. Calibration of the SvO_2 catheter oximeter should be performed every 24 hours by laboratory co-oximeter saturation analysis.

BLOOD CHEMISTRIES

The body's homeostatic mechanisms are responsible for a stable internal environment. The chemical regulation of cellular and plasma metabolites is among the most precise mechanisms in the body. During periods of critical illness, these mechanisms may be inadequate or dramatically altered. The functional alterations that result from altered values are sometimes life threatening. An awareness of the factors affecting blood chemistry homeostasis, as well as the consequences of elevated or decreased levels, aids the nurse in making appropriate patient care decisions.

Some blood chemistry tests are drawn routinely on admission to the hospital to establish the patient's baseline. Other tests are performed frequently over a day and may indicate the need for intervention in the form of altered therapy and treatment modalities. "Normal" or reference values may differ between laboratories or among populations.

Serum Electrolytes

Sodium

Sodium is the major cation in the extracellular space. It has several major functions: maintenance of osmotic pressure, regulation of acid–base balance (by combining with chloride or bicarbonate ions), and transmission of nerve impulses by the sodium pump. Sodium balance is regulated by aldosterone, atrial natriuretic hormone, and antidiuretic hormone (ADH). Aldosterone causes sodium conservation (and water retention) by stimulating the kidneys to reabsorb sodium. Aldosterone is secreted in response to low extracellular sodium levels, an increase in intracellular potassium, low blood volume or cardiac output, and physical or emotional stress. When serum sodium levels are too high, atrial natriuretic hormone is secreted from the atrium and acts as an antagonist to renin and aldosterone. ADH, secreted by the posterior pituitary gland, controls serum sodium by regulation of the amount of intracellular fluid reabsorbed at the distal tubules.[4,5]

Potassium

Potassium is the major intracellular cation in concentrations of approximately 150 mEq/L. It is regulated in a very tight range in the extracellular fluid. Potassium plays a crucial role in initiating and sustaining cardiac and skeletal muscle contraction. It is also important for acid–base balance and maintenance of oncotic pressure.

Maintenance of potassium within the normal range is crucial in the care of a patient with cardiac disease. Failure to do so results in dangerous sequelae for the patient. In general, potassium levels in patients with cardiac disease are maintained above 4.0 mEq/L. Special care should be taken in patients with cardiac disease receiving potassium-sparing diuretics or angiotensin-converting enzyme inhibitors (ACE-Is), especially in light of decreased renal blood flow. Potassium levels are falsely elevated by analysis of hemolyzed specimens. Prolonged use of a tourniquet, having the patient clench and unclench a fist before blood draw, or delayed processing of the specimen all may cause hemolysis.[4,5]

Chloride

Chloride is the major extracellular anion. It helps to maintain electrical neutrality and acts as an acid–base buffer. The rise and fall of chloride levels follows sodium and bicarbonate shifts. When carbon dioxide increases, chloride shifts to the intracellular space as bicarbonate goes extracellular. Along with sodium, chloride also helps to maintain osmotic pressure. Found primarily in hydrochloric acid in stomach secretions, chloride also provides the acid medium for digestion and enzyme activation.[4,5]

Calcium

Calcium is found mainly in the bones and teeth, with only approximately 10% found in the blood. Calcium is essential for the formation of bones and for blood coagulation. Calcium ions affect neuromuscular excitability and cellular and capillary permeability. It is essential for nerve transmission and cardiac and skeletal muscle contraction. Calcium also contributes to anion–cation balance. Calcium can be found ionized (free) in the serum or bound to serum albumin. The ionized calcium, which is approximately one half of the total calcium, is the fraction important to cardiac and neuromuscular excitability. In acidosis, more calcium appears in the ionized form; in alkalotic environments, most of the calcium remains protein bound.

Calcium levels in the blood follow a diurnal variation, with the lowest values occurring in the early morning, and highest values occurring at midevening. Ionized calcium is difficult to measure, so total calcium is reported in most hospitals. In some situations, the measured calcium level may be low, but by estimating the amount bound to protein, the ionized calcium may be found to be normal. The formula for the computation of ionized calcium is shown in Display 10-2. Decreased serum sodium (less than 120 mEq/L) increases protein-bound calcium and consequently increases the total calcium; the opposite is true of increased serum sodium.[4,5]

Magnesium

Magnesium is essential for over 300 enzymatic activities involving lipid, carbohydrate, and protein metabolism. It is the second most predominant intracellular cation. Most of the body's magnesium is stored in the bones in an insoluble state; one third is bound to protein, and approximately 1% is found in the serum. Because of its importance in phosphorylation of ATP, magnesium is seen as a critical component of almost all metabolic processes. Its importance in the care of patients with cardiac disease stems from its role in neuromuscular regulation.[4,5]

Ventricular arrhythmias after MI have been associated with magnesium deficiency. Magnesium sulfate 1 to 2 g IV should be considered in ventricular fibrillation or ventricular tachycardia for patients who have alcoholism or malnutrition with suspected low levels of magnesium (hypomagnesemia). It is recommended that magnesium sulfate should be administered to patients with ventricular fibrillation or ventricular tachycardia with a torsades de pointes pattern.[65]

Hypomagnesemia may precipitate cardiac arrhythmias, including atrial fibrillation, because of enhanced myocardium excitability. Hypomagnesemia is very common after cardiovascular surgery and has been found to be an independent risk factor for atrial fibrillation following cardiac surgery, most likely due to hemodilution, elevated epinephrine levels, increased loss through the urine, or due to the use of diuretics. Atrial fibrillation is a common complication after cardiovascular surgery occurring in approximately 30% to 50% of cases.[66] Research on the administration of magnesium sulfate before and/or after cardiovascular surgery has shown mixed results. However, a recent meta-analysis demonstrated a significant reduction in postoperative atrial fibrillation from 28% in the control group to 18% in the treatment group without a significant change in length of hospital stay.[67] Administration of magnesium sulfate after CABG surgery is considered a frontline strategy in the prevention of atrial fibrillation.[68]

Hypermagnesemia results in depressed neuromuscular conduction, and consequent slowing of conduction in the heart. The most common cause of hypermagnesemia is renal failure.

Carbon Dioxide

Measurement of carbon dioxide assists the clinician in evaluation of electrolyte status and acid–base balance. Because approximately

80% of carbon dioxide is found as bicarbonate, it is a good reflection of the bicarbonate level. The carbon dioxide level should not be confused with the PCO_2 obtained from blood gas readings.[4,5]

Anion Gap

The anion gap measures the normal balance between positive and negative electrolytes in the serum. It describes the relation between serum sodium (a cation) and bicarbonate and chloride (anions). A normal anion gap is 12 mEq/L. A value greater than 12 mEq/L is considered abnormal. This test is useful in determining whether an acid–base imbalance is due to an increase in organic acid (increased lactic acid or ketoacids, or ingestion of acid such as salicylic acid). In this case, the anion gap increases. With mineral acid problems (decreased bicarbonate or increased hydrochloric acid), the anion gap is normal.[4,5] A formula for computation of the anion gap is given in Display 10-2.

Serum Osmolality

Serum osmolality reflects the osmotic property of the blood. It is an important parameter in determining whether water excess or deficit exists. Either of these problems can present in the cardiac care unit, where fluid management is often a problem. The osmolality can be measured in the laboratory or calculated with a simple formula (see Display 10-2).

Serum Electrolytes After Cardiac Surgery

Fluid volume shifts and changes in electrolytes and serum osmolality is common after cardiac surgery. The examination of serum electrolytes frequently during the first 24 hours after surgery has been recommended. Potassium changes may be rapid, sodium may be increased, total calcium and magnesium may be decreased, and total circulating volume may be increased. The hemodilutional effects of cardiopulmonary bypass are responsible for these changes as well as changes in renal function that, in turn, may affect fluid volume and electrolyte status. During and after cardiac surgery, changes in plasma potassium concentration may develop. There appears to be a decrease in potassium during hypothermia and an increase during rewarming, which has been attributed to washout of ischemic areas or to a direct effect of temperature on the transmembrane distribution of potassium. Serum sodium does fall after surgery if large amounts of glucose-containing fluids have been infused. In this situation, glucose is metabolized slowly and draws fluid from the cells by its osmotic effect. Consequently, the sodium is diluted.

Errors in measurement can be costly to the patient in terms of safety, health status, and cost-effective practice. Changes in potassium and other electrolytes must be closely monitored and treatment initiated to keep levels within a very narrow range. Potassium replacement during rewarming must be handled cautiously.

SELECTED CHEMISTRIES

Alkaline Phosphatase

Alkaline phosphatase is an enzyme released in liver and bone disease. An increased serum level suggests an abnormality in the liver or bones, but can be associated with chronic therapeutic use of anticonvulsant drugs such as phenobarbital or phenytoin. In addition, lipid-lowering agents such as bile acid resins, HMG-CoA reductase inhibitors (statins), and nicotinic acid can alter alkaline phosphatase and other liver tests.[4] Alkaline phosphatase along with other liver enzymes (i.e., alanine aminotransferase [ALT], aspartate aminotransferase [AST]) is typically measured before initiation of lipid-lowering therapy, every 4 to 6 weeks at the start of therapy, every 6 to 12 weeks for the first year of therapy, and then every 6 months throughout treatment.

Alanine Aminotransferase

ALT, formerly known as serum glutamic-pyruvic transaminase (SGPT), is found predominantly in liver tissue but is also present in kidneys, heart, and skeletal muscle tissue. This hepatocellular enzyme is released into the bloodstream when there is injury or disease affecting liver parenchyma making ALT a specific and sensitive laboratory test. In hepatocellular disease other than viral hepatitis, the ALT/AST ratio is less than 1. In viral hepatitis, the ratio is greater than 1.[4]

ALT may be elevated with hepatitis, hepatic necrosis, hepatic ischemia, cholestasis, hepatic tumor, hepatotoxic drugs, obstructive jaundice, severe burns, myositis, pancreatitis, infectious mononucleosis, and shock. Drugs that may increase ALT levels include acetaminophen, allopurinol, ampillicin, cephalosporins, chlordiazepoxide, clofibrate, codeine, nicotinic acid, nonsteroidal anti-inflammatory drugs, oral contraceptives, phenytoin, procainamide, propranolol, and salicylates.[4] In addition, high-intensity lipid-lowering therapy with hydrophilic statins (i.e., pravastatin or atorvastatin) have been shown to increase ALT.[28]

Aspartate Aminotransferase

AST, formerly known as serum glutamic-oxaloacetic transaminase (SGOT), is located in the cell cytoplasm and in the mitochondria, where it catalyzes amino acid activity. This enzyme, although not specific to myocardial tissue, was the first to be used extensively to confirm an MI.[69] The enzyme is widely distributed, with high concentrations in the liver, skeletal muscle, kidneys, RBCs, and myocardium. It is found in lesser amounts in the lungs, pancreas, and brain. The presence of AST in so many organ systems reduces its specificity for MI. With its reduced specificity and newer, more specific and sensitive tests, AST is no longer used to diagnosis MI. AST is now used to evaluate, diagnose, and monitor hepatocellular diseases.[4]

AST may be elevated with cardiac surgery, cardiac catheterization and angioplasty, severe angina, acute pulmonary embolus, renal infarction, acute pancreatitis, musculoskeletal diseases, trauma, and strenuous exercise. In alcoholic hepatitis, AST is usually elevated but rarely greater than 300 U/L, but AST is almost invariably twice as high as ALT. Drugs that may increase AST levels include antihypertensives, digitalis preparations, salicylates, verapamil, theophylline, and lipid-lowering agents such as bile acid resins and nicotinic acid (niacin). In addition, high-intensity lipid-lowering therapy with hydrophilic statins (i.e., pravastatin or atorvastatin) have been shown to increase AST.[28] False elevations are seen in pyridoxine deficiency (beriberi, pregnancy), uremia, or diabetic ketoacidosis. Levels are slightly increased in older adults. In chronic conditions, such as severe, long-standing liver disease, the elevation is usually persistent.[4,5]

Bilirubin

Bilirubin is a product of Hb breakdown and is removed from the body by the liver. Elevated direct bilirubin is the result of obstructive jaundice due to extrahepatic (stones or tumor) or intrahepatic (damaged liver cells) causes. Increases in indirect bilirubin occur with hepatocellular dysfunction or an increase in RBC destruction (e.g., transfusion reaction or hemolytic anemia). Care should be taken not to hemolyze the sample. The sample should also be protected from bright light because bilirubin levels are reduced after 1 hour of such exposure.[4,5]

Catecholamines

Epinephrine and norepinephrine are elevated in pheochromocytoma, a tumor of the adrenal medulla. Pheochromocytoma is a cause of high blood pressure.

Creatinine

Creatinine is a waste product formed during muscle protein metabolism. Serum creatinine is a reflection of the excretory function of the kidneys. It is evaluated in conjunction with BUN, but is a more sensitive indicator of renal function. People with large muscle mass have higher serum creatinine levels than do those with less muscle, such as older adults, amputees, and patients with muscle disease.[4,5]

Glucose

Glucose is elevated whenever endogenous epinephrine is mobilized. Hyperglycemia in the hospital setting is common and may result from a variety of reasons including stress, administration of glucocorticoids and vasopressors, decompensation of diabetes mellitus types 1 and 2, chronic renal failure, acute pancreatitis, acute MI, congestive heart failure, extensive surgery, and infections.

Bedside glucose monitoring is the most common POCT available in the hospital. It is recommended that diabetic patients who are eating have glucose testing before their meals and at bedtime. Diabetic patients who are not eating should be tested every 4 to 6 hours unless they are controlled with IV insulin, which typically requires testing every hour until levels are stable and then every 2 hours.[70]

Studies have shown an association between hyperglycemia and increased mortality in hospitalized patients with and without diabetes mellitus. A variety of populations, including medical and surgical patients, acute MI patients, and cardiac surgery patients, have been studied demonstrating more intensive glucose control decreased mortality, reduced length of stay, and decreased infection rates.[71–75] These studies have led to changes in protocols for the monitoring and treatment of glucose while in the hospital.[70]

Glycated Hemoglobin or HbA_{1C}

Glycated hemoglobin (GHb), also referred to as glycohemoglobin, glycosylated hemoglobin, HbA_{1C}, or HbA_1 are terms used to describe a series of stable minor Hb components formed slowly and nonenzymatically from Hb and glucose.[76] The rate at which GHb is formed is proportional to the concentration of blood glucose.[76] Because RBCs survive an average of 120 days, the measurement of GHb provides an index of a person's average blood glucose concentration during a 2- to 3-month period.[70]

GHb comprises a chemically heterogeneous group of substances formed by the reaction between sugars and Hb. In adults, approximately 98% of the Hb in the RBC is hemoglobin A. About 7% of hemoglobin A consists of a type called HbA_1 that can combine strongly with glucose in a process called "glycosylation." Once glycosylation occurs, it is not easily reversible. HbA_{1C} is one of three components of HbA_1 and combines most strongly with glucose. HbA_{1C} is a specific form of GHb that has become the most accurate laboratory blood test in assessing long-term glycemic control in diabetics.[70]

HbA_{1C} can be used to diagnose diabetes. The American Diabetes Association (ADA) recommends: (1) the test is performed using a method that is certified and standardized (2) testing should be evaluated for discordant results for Hb variants (3) in conditions with altered relationship between A1c and glycemia (sickle cell, pregnancy, HIV, hemodialysis, hemodialysis, or recent blood loss/transfusion) only the plasma blood glucose criterion should be used to diagnose diabetes.[77]

HbA_{1C} has a number of advantages as a diagnostic test for diabetes. No fasting is required, has greater preanalytical stability, and less influence from stress or illness. For the A1c test the diagnostic threshold is ≥6.5% (48 mmol/mol).[78] It should be noted that this test only diagnoses approximately 30% of diabetic patients.[79] In nondiabetic patients, increased levels of HbA_{1C} may be seen with an acute stress response, Cushing syndrome, pheochromocytoma, corticosteroid therapy, and acromegaly. HbA_{1C} levels may be decreased in patients with hemolytic anemia, chronic blood loss, and chronic renal failure.[4]

Lactate Dehydrogenase

LDH is an enzyme that catalyzes the reversible conversion of lactate to pyruvate, providing ATP for energy during periods of anaerobic metabolism. LDH is present in nearly all metabolizing cells and is released during tissue injury. LDH is widely distributed in the body. It can be found in skeletal muscle, RBCs, kidneys, liver, pancreas, lungs, and brain. Because of its presence in multiple organs throughout the body, evaluation of LDH is used to help establish many diagnoses. LDH has become obsolete in its use as a diagnostic aid in MI due to the more specific and sensitive troponin markers. Drugs that may cause an elevated LDH include clofibrate, codeine, meperidine, morphine, procainamide, and lipid-lowering agents such as HMG-CoA reductase inhibitors (statins) and nicotinic acid.[2,3] The normal reference range for LDH is listed in Table 10-4.

Protein

Total protein measurement includes albumin (53%) and globulin (15% α, 12% β, and 20% γ). These protein components can be quantified with the use of protein electrophoresis. Albumin (4 to 5.5 g/dL) contributes to the balance of osmotic pressure between blood and tissues. Globulins (2 to 3 g/dL) influence osmotic pressure and include the immunoglobulins (antibodies). Because albumin is produced in the liver, a low serum albumin level is seen in liver disease. Low serum albumin also reflects poor nutritional status, and the finding should prompt a complete nutritional assessment. The half-life of albumin is 18 days. If albumin is reduced, edema results because albumin accounts for 90% of the serum colloid osmotic pressure. Albumin is reduced in heart failure because of hypervolemic dilution. The α- and β-globulins tend to decrease with abnormal liver function. The γ-globulins, the body's antibodies, increase with chronic disease.[4,5]

Urea Nitrogen

Urea nitrogen is the end product of protein metabolism. It is produced by the liver and excreted by the kidneys. BUN is used

Table 10-4 • NORMAL REFERENCE RANGES FOR LABORATORY BLOOD TESTS[a]

Blood Test	Reference Range
Hematologic Studies	
Red blood cell count	
Males	4.7–6.1 mil/mm^3
Females	4.2–5.4 mil/mm^3
Hematocrit	
Males	40–50%
Females	38–47%
Hemoglobin	
Males	13.5–18.0 g/dL
Females	12.0–16.0 g/dL
Corpuscle indices	
Mean corpuscular volume (MCV)	82–98 fL
Mean corpuscular hemoglobin (MCH)	27–31 pg
Mean corpuscular hemoglobin concentration (MCHC)	32–36%
White blood cell count	
Total	4500–11,000/mm^3
Differential (in number of cells/mm^3 blood)	
Total leukocytes	5000–10,000 (100%)
Total neutrophils	3000–7000 (60–70%)
Lymphocytes	1500–3000 (20–30%)
Monocytes	375–500 (2–6%)
Eosinophils	50–400 (1–4%)
Basophils	0–50 (0.1%)
Sedimentation rate	0–30 mm/h
Coagulation Studies	
Platelet count	250,000–500,000/mm^3
Prothrombin time	12–15 s
Partial thromboplastin time	60–70 s
Activated partial thromboplastin time	35–45 s
Activated clotting time	75–105 s
Fibrinogen level	160–300 mg/dL
Blood Chemistries	
Serum electrolytes	
Sodium	135–145 mEq/L
Potassium	3.3–4.9 mEq/L
Chloride	97–110 mEq/L
Carbon dioxide	22–31 mEq/L
Blood gases	
pH	7.35–7.45
$PaCO_2$	35–45 mm Hg
PaO_2	80–105 mm Hg
Bicarbonate	22–29 mEq/L
Base excess, deficit	0 ± 2.3 mEq/L

Blood Test	Reference Range
SvO_2	60–80%
Alkaline phosphatase	35–125 IU/L
Alanine aminotransferase (ALT)	0–40 IU/L
Aspartate aminotransferase (AST)	5–40 IU/L Bilirubin
Total	0.2–1.3 mg/dL
Direct	0–0.4 mg/dL
Calcium	
Total	8.9–10.3 mg/dL
Free (ionized)	4.6–5.1 mg/dL
Creatinine	
Males	0.9–1.4 mg/dL
Females	0.8–1.3 mg/dL
Glucose (fasting)	70–99 mg/dL
LDH	20–200 IU/L
Magnesium	1.3–2.2 mEq/L
Phosphorus	2.5–4.5 mg/dL
Protein (total)	6.5–8.5 g/dL
Urea nitrogen	8–26 mg/dL
Uric acid	
Males	4.0–8.5 mg/dL
Females	2.8–7.5 mg/dL
Serum Enzymes	
CK-MM	95–100%
CK-MB	0–5%
Myocardial Proteins	
Troponin-I	0–1.6 ng/mL
Troponin-T	0–0.1 ng/mL
Myoglobin	
Males	20–90 ng/mL
Females	10–75 ng/mL
High-sensitivity C-reactive protein (hs-CRP)	
Low	<1.0 mg/L
Average	1.0–3.0 mg/L
High	>3.0 mg/L
Homocysteine (Hcy)	
Optimal	<12 μmol/L
Borderline	12–15 μmol/L
High Risk for cardiovascular disease	>15 μmol/L
B-type natriuretic peptide (BNP)	
Most diagnostic of heart failure	>100 pg/mL

[a]Examples: Regional laboratory techniques and methods may result in variations.

with creatinine to evaluate renal function. Increases in BUN are referred to as *azotemia*. Prerenal azotemia occurs whenever a disease or condition affects urea nitrogen before the kidneys are actually damaged or diseased including congestive heart failure, salt and water depletion from vomiting, diarrhea, diuresis, sweating, or shock.[2] Postrenal azotemia is the result of any condition that affects BUN after it has cleared the kidneys, such as in ureteral and urethral obstruction. BUN levels in older adults may be slightly higher because the number of nephrons tends to decrease in the aging process. The BUN may be higher in hospitalized patients because of their increased catabolic state.[80]

Uric Acid

Uric acid is synthesized in the liver and intestinal mucosa and is the end product of purine metabolism. Uric acid may be increased in a variety of conditions but the most common cause in an increase in blood levels is gout. Levels are monitored during the diagnosis and treatment of gout. Levels may also be increased in patients with atherosclerosis, hypertension, and elevated triglycerides. Severe renal disease results in a high level of serum uric acid because excretion is reduced. Levels are very labile and show day-to-day and seasonal variation within the same person. Levels are also increased by emotional stress, total fasting, and increased body weight. Large doses of salicylates may interfere with accurate test results.[80]

BLOOD CULTURES

Blood cultures are indicated when a fever of unknown origin is present. Blood cultures aid in identifying specific bacterial organisms in the blood (bacteremia), and when combined with antibiotic sensitivity tests, can provide information to clinicians about which antibiotic works best against that particular species of bacteria. Policies differ with regard to the number and timing of cultures considered adequate for diagnosis; the policy and procedure of the institution should be followed. Regardless of the number of cultures recommended and the timing between them, collection of blood cultures requires meticulous technique to protect the specimen from contamination. Sampling should be done while the patient's temperature is still elevated and before treatment with antibiotics. Both Beutz et al.[81] and Martinez et al.[82] determined that, although blood cultures may be obtained from a central IV catheter, they are considered less sensitive than through venipuncture but offer an excellent negative predictive value in diagnosing bacteremia. With either method of blood draw, the blood is placed into a specialized culture media. Preliminary results should be available within 24 hours, but final results may not be available for a week or more.[4,5]

SERUM CONCENTRATION OF SELECTED DRUGS

Serum levels of cardiac drugs may be obtained for multiple reasons including determining the effectiveness of drug therapy, especially for drugs with narrow therapeutic ranges or with wide variabilities in metabolism between patients, and confirming cause of organ toxicity. Usual ranges of therapeutic and toxic serum concentrations of selected cardiac drugs are given in Table 10-5.

The serum concentrations must always be interpreted in the context of the clinical data. For example, digitalis intoxication may occur within the usual range of therapeutic serum concentrations if the patient has hypokalemia, hypercalcemia, hypomagnesemia, acid–base imbalances, increased adrenergic tone, hypothyroidism, hypoxemia, or myocardial ischemia.[83]

Serum concentrations of drugs can be altered by many mechanisms including influences on pharmacokinetics such as half-life, time to peak, time to steady state, protein binding, and excretion. For example, a number of factors are known to alter digoxin concentration when the dosage is kept constant, including altered absorption, impaired renal excretion, drug interaction, and impaired metabolism. Theophylline concentration is increased in neonates, in older adults, with obesity, with high carbohydrate diets, and with some comorbid conditions. Theophylline concentration is reduced in children, with a low carbohydrate diet, with eating charcoal-cooked meats, and with some drugs. There is as much as a 50-fold difference in plasma concentration of phenytoin among patients taking the same dosage; altered metabolism and altered protein binding account for the large individual variation in the disposition of phenytoin.

The blood specimen to determine serum concentration of a drug usually is drawn 1 to 2 hours after an oral drug is given because absorption and distribution are usually complete by this time; however, blood should be drawn at a time specified by that laboratory (e.g., 1 hour before the next dose is due to be administered). The route of administration and sampling time after last dose of drug must be known for proper interpretation.[84]

Table 10-5 • COMPARISON BETWEEN SPECIFIC HBA_{1C} LEVELS AND SPECIFIC MEAN PLASMA GLUCOSE LEVELS

	Mean Plasma Glucose	
HbA_{1C} (%)	mg/dL	mmol/L
6	135	7.5
7	170	9.5
8	205	11.5
9	240	13.5
10	275	15.5
11	310	17.5
12	345	19.5

From Rohlfing CL, Wiedmeyer HM, Little RR, et al. Defining the relationship between plasma glucose and HbA1C: Analysis of glucose profiles and HbA1C in the diabetes control and complications trial. *Diabetes Care*. 2002;25:276.

Summary

Laboratory testing plays an essential part in the delivery of quality health care. A physician or other clinician orders lab tests to diagnose, treat, manage, or monitor a patient's condition. The process begins with the preparation for collection of a sample of blood, tissue, or other biologic matter from the patient. The sample is then sent to the laboratory where it is uniquely identified and examined to make certain that it is appropriate for the testing ordered by the healthcare provider. Many factors can affect laboratory testing. It is essential for the nurse to be aware of these factors as well as functionality of testing and implications for patient treatment.

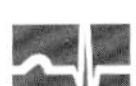

CASE STUDY

Patient Profile
Name/Age/Sex: **Mary Withers, 88-year-old female**

History of Present Illness
Mrs. Withers is an 88-year-old African American female who presented to the Structural Heart Clinic for evaluation of her severe, symptomatic aortic stenosis (AS). She presents with shortness of breath as well as peripheral edema. Her symptoms have been worsening over the past 2 months.

Past Medical History
Hypertension, AS, carpal tunnel syndrome

Surgical History
Carpal tunnel repair, hysterectoma

Family History
Mother with hypertension, father killed during WWII.

Social History
Denies alcohol, tobacco, or illicit drug use

Medications
HCTZ 12.5 mg po q daily, lisinopril 10 mg po q daily

Allergies
NKDA

Patient Examination

Vital Signs
BP 130/68; Resp 16; Temp 37.0°C; HR 75; Ht. 160 cm; Wt. 48 kg

(continued)

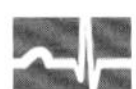 CASE STUDY (*Continued*)

Physical Examination

General: Awake, alert and oriented. No distress noted.

Skin: Clean, dry, intact

Cardiac: Systolic ejection murmur, harsh in quality, III/VI at left upper sternal border. Bilateral lower extremity edema 1+

Respiratory: No respiratory distress. Lung sounds are clear in all lobes bilaterally without rales, rhonchi, or wheezes.

Abdominal: Abdomen is soft, symmetric, and nontender without distention. No masses, hepatomegaly, or splenomegaly are noted.

Psychiatric: Appropriate mood and affect. Good judgement and insight. No visual or auditory hallucinations. No suicidal or homicidal ideation.

Testing: Echocardiogram shows ejection fraction 65%, aortic valve area (AVA) 0.6 cm^2, aortic mean gradient 31 mm Hg, Vmax 3.6 m/s (consistent with a paradoxical low-flow, low-gradient AS.)

Considerations

Key Questions

1. Does Ms. W have a true AS?
2. What are considerations for additional testing in these patients?

Evidence

1. A few interventions should occur at this time. Patient should be evaluated for any potential echocardiogram measurement errors, treat hypertension, and consider obtaining an aortic calcium score.[85]
2. Patient can be considered for transcatheter or surgical aortic valve replacement.[86]
3. The prevalence of calcific AS and of cardiac amyloidosis (CA) increases with age, and their association is not uncommon in the elderly. The identification of CA is particularly challenging in patients with AS because these two conditions share several features. It is estimated that ≤15% of the AS population and ≤30% of the subset with low-flow, low-gradient pattern may have CA.[87]
   a. Testing in this patient is indicated given her low-flow, low-gradient AS, hypertension under control, and her repeat echocardiogram showing similar results.
   b. Patient undergoes genetic testing for Transthyretin (TTR) V122I which is associated with amyloidosis. The gene is found almost exclusively in those of African descent.[88] Patient can also undergo cardiac magnetic resonance imaging (CMR) to confirm diagnosis.
   c. Patient testing returns positive for cardiac amyloid and presence of TTR. In this case patient is not a candidate for treatment of her amyloid, but her family members should be screened. If positive for this gene they should start treatment for cardiac amyloid.

REFERENCES

1. Badrick T. Evidence based laboratory medicine. *Clin Biochem Rev.* 2013;34(2):43–46.
2. McPherson RA, Pincus MR. Markers of myocardial damage. In: *Henry's Clinical Diagnosis and Management by Laboratory Methods.* Philadelphia, PA: WB Saunders Company; 2007.
3. Centers for Disease Control and Prevention (CDC). Standard Precautions. https://www.cdc.gov/oralhealth/infectioncontrol/summary-infection-prevention-practices/standard-precautions.html Updated June 18, 2018. Accessed January 5, 2020.
4. Pagana KD, Pagana TJ. *Mosby's Diagnostic and Laboratory Test Reference.* 8th ed. St. Louis, MO: Mosby Elsevier; 2007.
5. Chernecky CC, Berger BJ. *Laboratory Tests and Diagnostic Procedures.* 5th ed. Philadelphia, PA: Saunders Elsevier; 2008.
6. Jacobs DS, DeMott WR. *Laboratory Test Handbook.* 5th ed. Hudson, OH: Lexi-Comp/NC; 2001.
7. Kost GJ, Tran NK. Point-of-care testing and cardiac biomarkers: the standard of care and vision for chest pain centers. *Cardiol Clin.* 2005;23:467–490.
8. Ng SM, Krishnaswamy P, Morissey R, et al. Coronary artery disease: accelerated pathway for chest pain evaluation. *Am J Cardiol.* 2001;88:611–617.
9. Katayev A, Balciza C, Seccombe DW. Establishing reference intervals for clinical laboratory test results: is there a better way? *Am J Clin Pathol.* 2010;133(2):80–186.
10. Oxley DK, Garg U, Olsowka ES. Maximizing the information from laboratory tests—The Ulysses syndrome: Tests in search of disease. In: Jacobs DS, DeMott WR, eds. *Laboratory Test Handbook.* Hudson, OH: Lexi-Comp/NC; 2001:15–23.
11. Wallach J. Introduction to normal values (reference ranges). In: *Interpretation of Diagnostic Tests.* Philadelphia, PA: Lippincott Williams & Wilkins; 2007.
12. Vashist S. Point of care diagnostics: recent advances and trends. *Biosensors.* 2017;7(4):E62.
13. Amsterdam E, Kirk J, Bluemke D, et al. Testing of low-risk patients presenting to the emergency department with chest pain. A scientific statement from the American heart Association. *Circulation.* 2010;122(17);1756–1776.
14. Shaw J. Practical changes related to point of care testing. *Pract Lab Med.* 2016;1(4):22–29.
15. Giuliano KK, Grant ME. Blood analysis at the point of care: Issues in application for use in critically ill patients. *AACN Clinical Issues.* 2002;13(2):204–220.
16. Jaffe AS, Babuin L, Apple FS. Biomarkers in acute cardiac disease: the present and the future. *J Am Coll Cardiol.* 2006;48(1):1–11.
17. Saenger AK, Jaffe AS. The use of biomarkers for the evaluation and treatment of patients with acute coronary syndromes. *Med Clin North Am.* 2007;45(6):587–591.
18. Hachey B, Kontos MC. Trends in use if biomarkers protocols for the evaluation of possible myocardial infarction. *J Am Heart Assoc.* 2015;10(1):117–122.
19. Thygesen K, Alpert J, White HD, et al. Universal definition of myocardial infarction. *Circulation.* 2007;116:2634–2653.
20. Apple FS. A new season for cardiac troponin assays: it's time to keep a scorecard. *Clin Chem.* 2009;55:1303–1306.
21. Vasile V, Jaffe A. High-Sensitivity Cardiac Troponin in the Evaluation of Possible AMI. https://www.acc.org/latest-in-cardiology/articles/2018/07/16/09/17/high sensitivity-cardiac-troponin-in-the-evaluation-of-possible-ami. Updated July 16, 2018. Accessed Oct 10, 2019.
22. Sarko J, Pollack CV Jr. Cardiac troponins. *J Emerg Med.* 2002;23(1):57–65.
23. Newby K, Lowenstern A. Implications of high-sensitivity troponin testing. *J Am Coll Cardiol.* 2018;71(2):2625–2627.
24. Januzzi J. Causes of Non ACS related Troponin Elevations. https://www.acc.org/latest-in-cardiology/articles/2014/07/18/13/16/causes-of-non-acs-related-troponin-elevations. Updated September 8, 2010. Accessed October 10, 2019.
25. Roongsritong C, Warraich I, Bradley C. Common causes of troponin elevations in the absence of acute myocardial infarction: incidence and clinical significance. *Chest.* 2004;125:1877–1884.
26. Velmahos GC, Karaiskakis M, Salim A, et al. Normal electrocardiography and serum troponin I levels preclude the presence of clinically significant blunt cardiac injury. *J Trauma.* 2003;54:45–50; discussion 50–51.
27. Kress T, Krueger D, Ziccardi S. Creatine kinase: an assay with muscle. *Nursing.* 2008;38(10):62–64.
28. Dale KM, White CM, Henyan NN, et al. Impact of statin dosing intensity on transaminase and creatine kinase. *Am J Med.* 2007;120:706–712.
29. Dugan L, Leech L, Speroni KG, et al. Factors affecting hemolysis rates in blood samples drawn from newly placed IV sites in the emergency department. *J Emerg Nurs.* 2005;31(4):338–345.

30. Califf RM, Abdelmeguid AE, Kuntz RE, et al. Myonecrosis after revascularization procedures. *J Am Coll Cardiol.* 1998;31(2):241–251.
31. Prasad A, Singh M, Lerman A, et al. Isolated elevation in troponin T after percutaneous coronary intervention is associated with higher long-term mortality. *J Am Coll Cardiol.* 2006;48(9):1765–1770.
32. Miller WL, Garratt KN, Burritt MF, et al. Baseline troponin level: key to understanding the importance of post-PCI troponin elevation. *Eur Heart J.* 2006;27:1061–1069.
33. Nallamothu BK, Chetcuti S, Mukherjee D, et al. Prognostic implication of troponin I elevation after percutaneous coronary intervention. *Am J Cardiol.* 2003;91:1272–1274.
34. Klatte K, Chaitman BR, Theroux P, et al. Increased mortality after coronary artery bypass graft surgery is associated with increased levels of postoperative creatine kinase-myocardial band isoenzyme release. *J Am Coll Cardiol.* 2001;38:1070–1077.
35. Costa MA, Carere RG, Lichtenstein SV, et al. Incidence, predictors, and significance of abnormal cardiac enzyme rise in patients treated with bypass surgery in the arterial revascularization therapies study (ARTS). *Circulation.* 2001;104:2689–2693.
36. Januzzi JL, Lewandrowski K, MacGillivray TE, et al. A comparison of cardiac troponin T and creatine kinase-MB for patient evaluation after cardiac surgery. *J Am Coll Cardiol.* 2002;39:1518–1523.
37. Kathiresan S, Servoss SJ, Newell JB, et al. Cardiac troponin T elevation after coronary artery bypass grafting is associated with increased one-year mortality. *Am J Cardiol.* 2004;94:879–881.
38. Croal BL, Hillis GS, Gibson PH, et al. Relationship between postoperative cardiac troponin I levels and outcome of cardiac surgery. *Circulation.* 2006;114:1468–1475.
39. Expert Panel on Detection, Evaluation, and Treatment of High Blood Cholesterol in Adults. Executive summary of the third report of the National Cholesterol Education Program (NCEP) Expert Panel on detection, evaluation, and treatment of high blood cholesterol in adults (Adult Treatment Panel III). *JAMA.* 2001;285(19):2486–2497.
40. Wallach J. Cardiovascular diseases. In: *Interpretation of Diagnostic Tests.* Philadelphia, PA: Lippincott Williams & Wilkins; 2007.
41. Pearson TA, Mensah GA, Alexander RW, et al. Markers of inflammation and cardiovascular disease: application to clinical and public health practice. *Circulation.* 2003;107:499–511.
42. Bisoendial RJ, Boekholdt SM, Vergeer M, et al. C-reactive protein is a mediator of cardiovascular disease. *Eur Heart J.* 2010;31(17):2087–2091.
43. Rost NS, Wolf PA, Kase CS, et al. Plasma concentration of c-reactive protein and risk of ischemic stroke and transient ischemic attack: the Framingham study. *Stroke.* 2001;32:2575–2579.
44. Koenig W, Sund M, Frohlich M, et al. C-reactive protein, a sensitive marker for inflammation, predicts future risk of coronary heart disease in initially healthy middle-aged men: results from the MONICA (Monitoring Trends and Determinants in Cardiovascular Disease) Augsburg Cohort Study, 1984 to 1992. *Circulation.* 1999;99:237–242.
45. Kuller LH, Tracy RP, Shaten J, et al. Relation of C-reactive protein and coronary heart disease in the MRFIT nested case-control study. Multiple risk factor intervention trial. *Am J Epidemiol.* 1996;144:537–547.
46. Ridker PM, Hennekens CH, Buring JE, et al. C-reactive protein and other markers of inflammation in the prediction of cardiovascular disease in women. *N Engl J Med.* 2000;342:836–843.
47. Tracy RP, Lemaitre RN, Psaty BM, et al. Relationship of C-reactive protein to risk of cardiovascular disease in the elderly. Results from the Cardiovascular Health Study and the Rural Health Promotion Project. *Arterioscler Thromb Vasc Biol.* 1997;17:1121–1127.
48. Ridker PM, Cushman M, Stampfer MJ, et al. Inflammation, aspirin, and the risk of cardiovascular disease in apparently healthy men. *N Engl J Med.* 1997;336:973–979.
49. Dinavahl R, Falkner B. Relationship of homocysteine with cardiovascular disease and blood pressure. https://www.medscape.com/viewarticle/489518_7. Accessed on October 10, 2019.
50. Lily LS. Ischemic heart disease. In: Noble J, ed. *Textbook of Primary Care Medicine.* St. Louis, MO: Mosby; 2001:545–570.
51. Madjid M, Ali M, Willerson J. Lipoprotein-associated phospholipase A2 as a novel risk marker for cardiovascular disease: a systematic review of the literature. *Tex Heart Inst J.* 2010;37(1):25–39.
52. Caslake MJ, Packard CJ, Suckling KE, et al. Lipoprotein-associated phospholipase A(2), platelet-activating factor acetylhydrolase: A potential new risk factor for coronary artery disease. *Atherosclerosis.* 2000;150(2):413–419.
53. Packard CJ, O'Reilly DS, Caslake MJ, et al. Lipoprotein-associated phospholipase A2 as an independent predictor of coronary heart disease. West of Scotland Coronary Prevention Study Group. *N Engl J Med.* 2000;343(16):1148–1155.
54. Blake GJ, Dada N, Fox JC, et al. A prospective evaluation of lipoprotein-associated phospholipase A(2) levels and the risk of future cardiovascular events in women. *J Am Cardiol.* 2001;38(5):1302–1306.
55. Grantham JA, Burnett JC. BNP: increasing importance in the pathophysiology and diagnosis of congestive heart failure. *Circulation.* 1997;96:388–390.
56. Maisel AS, Krishnaswamy P, Nowak RM, et al. Rapid measurement of B-type natriuretic peptide in the emergency diagnosis of heart failure. *N Engl J Med.* 2002;347(3):161–167.
57. Wieczorek SJ, Wu AH, Christenson R, et al. A rapid B-type natriuretic peptide assay accurately diagnoses left ventricular dysfunction and heart failure: a multicenter evaluation. *Am Heart J.* 2002;144:834–839.
58. Fonarow GC, Peacock WF, Horwich TB, et al. Usefulness of B-type natriuretic peptide and cardiac troponin levels to predict in-hospital mortality from ADHERE. *Am J Cardiol.* 2008;101:231–237.
59. Berger R, Huelsman M, Strecker K, et al. B-type natriuretic peptide predicts sudden death in patients with chronic heart failure. *Circulation.* 2002;105:2392–2397.
60. Gaggin H, Januzzi J. Cardiac Biomarkers and Heart Failure. https://www.acc.org/%2Flatest-in-cardiology%2Farticles%2F2015%2F02%2F09%2F13%2F00%2Fcardiac-biomarkers-and-heart-failure. Updated February 10, 2015. Accessed on January 5, 2020.
61. Maisel A, Xue Y, Shah K, et al. Increased 90-day mortality in patients with acute heart failure with elevated copeptin: secondary results from the Biomarkers in Acute Heart Failure (BACH) study. *Circ Heart Fail.* 2011;4:613–620.
62. Cirino AL, Ho CY. Genetic testing for inherited heart disease. *Circulation.* 2013;128(1):e4–e8.
63. Kearon C, Ginsberg JS, Douketis J, et al. An evaluation of D-dimer in the diagnosis of pulmonary embolism: a randomized trial. *Ann Intern Med.* 2006;144:812–821.
64. Palareti G, Cosmi B, Legnani C, et al. D-dimer testing to determine the duration of anticoagulation therapy. *N Engl J Med.* 2006;355:1780–1790.
65. American Heart Association. Part 7.2: management of cardiac arrest. *Circulation.* 2005;112:IV-58–IV-66.
66. Echahidi N, Pibarot P, O'Hara G, et al. Mechanisms, prevention, and treatment of atrial fibrillation after cardiac surgery. *J Am Coll Cardiol.* 2008;51:793–801.
67. Miller S, Crystal E, Garfinkle M, et al. Effects of magnesium on atrial fibrillation after cardiac surgery: a meta analysis. *Heart.* 2005;91:618–623.
68. Naghipour B, Faridaalaee G, Shadvar K, et al. Effect of prophylaxis of magnesium sulfate for reduction of postcardiac surgery arrhythmia: randomized clinical trial. *Ann Card Anaesth.* 2016;19:662–667.
69. LaDue JS, Wroblewski F, Karmen A. Serum glutamic oxaloacetic transaminase activity in human acute transmural myocardial infarction. *Science.* 1954;120:497–499.
70. American Diabetes Association. Standards of medical care in diabetes-2007. *Diabetes Care: American Diabetes Association: Clinical Practice.* 2007;30:S4–S41.
71. Van den Berghe G, Wouters P, Bouillon R, et al. Outcome benefit of intensive insulin therapy in the critically ill: insulin dose versus glycemic control. *Crit Care Med.* 2003;31:359–366.
72. Van den Berghe G, Wilmer A, Hermans G, et al. Intensive insulin therapy in the critically ill: Insulin dose versus glycemic control. *N Engl J Med.* 2006;354:449–461.
73. Zerr KJ, Furnary AP, Grunkemeier GL, et al. Glucose control lowers the risk of wound infection in diabetes after open heart operations. *Ann Thorac Surg.* 1997;63:356–361.
74. Furnary AP, Gao G, Grunkemeier GL, et al. Continuous insulin infusion reduces mortality in patient with diabetes undergoing coronary artery bypass surgery. *J Thorac Cardiovasc Surg.* 2003;125:1007–1021.
75. Malmberg K, Ryden L, Wedel H, et al. Intense metabolic control by means of insulin in patients with diabetes mellitus and acute myocardial infarction (DIGAMI 2): effects on mortality and morbidity. *Eur Heart J.* 2005;26:650–661.
76. American Diabetes Association. Standards of medical care for patients with diabetes mellitus. *Diabetes Care.* 2003;26(90001):33S–50S.
77. Rohlfing CL, Wiedmeyer HM, Little RR, et al. Defining the relationship between plasma glucose and HbA1c: analysis of glucose profiles and HbA1c in the Diabetes Control and Complications Trial. *Diabetes Care.* 2002;25(2):275–278.
78. American Diabetes Association. 2. Classification and diagnosis of diabetes: Standards of Medical Care in Diabetes—2019. *Diabetes Care.* 2019:42(Suppl 1):S13–S28.

79. Cowie CC, Rust KF, Byrd-Holt DD, et al. Prevalence of diabetes and high risk for diabetes using A1C criteria in the U.S. population in 1988–2006. *Diabetes Care*. 2010;33:562–568.
80. Wallach J. Core blood analytes: alterations by diseases. In: *Interpretation of Diagnostic Tests*. Philadelphia, PA: Lippincott Williams & Wilkins; 2007.
81. Beutz M, Sherman G, Mayfield J, et al. Clinical utility of blood cultures drawn from central vein catheters and peripheral venipuncture in critically ill medical patients. *Chest*. 2003;123:854–861.
82. Martinez JA, DesJardin JA, Aronoff M, et al. Clinical utility of blood cultures drawn from central venous or arterial catheters in critically ill surgical patients. *Crit Care Med*. 2002;30:7–13.
83. Wallach J. Therapeutic drug monitoring and drug effects. In: *Interpretation of Diagnostic Tests*. Philadelphia, PA: Lippincott Williams & Wilkins; 2007.
84. Sliwa CM Jr. A comparative study of hematocrits drawn from a standard venipuncture and those drawn from a saline lock device. *J Emerg Nurs*. 1997;23(3):228–231.
85. Annabi MS, Clisson M, Clavel MA, et al. Workup and management of patients with paradoxical low-flow, low-gradient aortic stenosis. *Curr Treat Options Cardiovasc Med*. 2018;20:49.
86. Ribeiro H, Lerakis S, Gilard M, et al. Transcatheter aortic valve replacement in patients with low-flow, low-gradient aortic stenosis: the TOPAS-TAVI Registry. *J Am Coll Cardiol*. 2018;71(12):1297–1308.
87. Ternacle J, Krapf L, Mohty D, et al. Aortic stenosis and cardiac amyloidosis. *J Am Coll Cardiol*. 2019;74(21):2638–2651.
88. Jacobson D, Alexander A, Tagoe C, et al. Prevalence of the amyloidogenic transthyretin (TTR) V122I allele in 14333 African Americans. *Amyloid*. 2015;22(3):171–174.

11 Radiologic Examination of the Chest

Melissa Long

OBJECTIVES

1. Identify the major anatomical structures of the chest.
2. Identify accepted indications for obtaining a chest x-ray.
3. Identify strengths and weaknesses of chest x-ray.
4. Identify common clinical presentations in acute care and radiologic findings.
5. Identify radiologic appearances of invasive lines and devices.

KEY QUESTIONS

1. How do chest x-rays work?
2. How is a chest x-ray interpreted?
3. How are invasive lines and devices identified and their placement/position assessed by their radiologic appearance?
4. What are key findings on the chest x-ray for different cardiovascular diseases?

BACKGROUND

Chest radiography is one of the most common diagnostic tools used in the evaluation of cardiovascular disease and the critically ill. Although a variety of other imaging modalities are available, chest radiography remains fundamental because of its ready availability in most settings, relatively low cost, and the ability to interpret films by a wide variety of healthcare providers.

The cardiac care nurse may be the first healthcare professional to see the chest radiograph of a patient in acute distress. Valuable time may be saved if the nurse is able to recognize the presence of an abnormality. Knowledge of chest radiograph interpretation and the disease processes that an abnormal film indicate can help the nurse in understanding disease pathophysiology, thereby allowing for better patient care; dual reading of radiographs significantly increases diagnostic accuracy and decreases the incidence of missed abnormalities.

HOW X-RAYS WORK

X-rays are radiant energy, like light, except that these waves are shorter and can pass through opaque objects. They are produced by bombarding a tungsten target with an electron beam and are channeled so that a narrow but diverging beam is emitted from the tube. When an x-ray exposure is taken, the tube is usually aimed so that the rays pass through the subject to the x-ray film in either a posterior to anterior (posteroanterior) or anterior to posterior (anteroposterior) direction. Because the x-rays are diverging and subject to reflection (scatter), structures more distant from the film are magnified and less distinctly outlined. Standard chest x-rays are obtained with the patient standing, facing an x-ray film. The x-ray tube is placed behind the patient. In general, chest radiographs are taken in the posteroanterior (PA) direction because this places the heart, an anterior structure, closer to the film, resulting in less magnification and allowing the cardiac outline to be seen clearly.

If the patient cannot stand, an anteroposterior (AP) chest radiograph is obtained with the patient lying down. These single view "bedside" x-rays are often taken in cardiac care units (CCUs) and intensive care units (ICUs) because the patient is lying down or sitting in bed and it is difficult to put the x-ray tube behind the patient. The x-ray film is therefore placed behind the patient and the x-ray tube is positioned in front of the patient. Because the heart is relatively far away from the x-ray film, its outline is somewhat less distinct and the heart size is magnified. Moreover, the distance between the tube and the patient is shorter than usual to cut down x-ray scatter, which also results in greater magnification.

The standard two-view chest x-ray is comprised of a PA and a lateral chest radiograph. The lateral chest view is a projection utilized to diagnose small pleural effusions, pneumothorax, and air trapping due to inhaled foreign bodies.

When using conventional radiology methods, the chest x-ray is recorded on a film that is chemically processed. Computerized digital chest radiology utilizes a special phosphor plate instead of traditional film. The digital x-ray image is produced by scanning the phosphor plate with a laser beam that causes light to be released from the phosphor plate. This image is then digitized and converted to an image by computer.[2] The computer image is then viewed from monitors and can also be converted to radiographic film providing a hard copy. Digital images afford many advantages over traditional chest x-rays. Digital images are easily stored and transferred making them more accessible from a variety of remote viewing stations. Digital images can be easily manipulated by changing magnification or relative density, which may add substantial information to the examination without exposing the patient to repeated imaging.[3]

The degree of darkness of the x-ray film depends on how much x-ray energy traverses the patient and exposes the film. This depends on the density of the material through which the x-ray beam passes. The chest has four major types of tissue densities through which rays must pass: bone, water, fat, and air. Because bone is the densest of these tissues, fewer and less energetic x-rays pass through bone. Thus, the shadow on the x-ray film cast by bone is light. (An x-ray image is like a photographic negative, with white color indicating lack of exposure and black color indicating intense exposure.) The lung, which is largely air, is least dense; therefore, it appears black on a chest radiograph. Soft tissues and blood are largely water, with similar densities, between those of bone and air. Fat is usually visibly less dense than other soft tissues. Thus, a chest radiograph is actually a shadowgraph.

The reason a structure can be outlined is that the shadow of one density contrasts with that of an adjacent density. If two structures are of equal density and adjacent to each other, then a single combined shadow results. If two structures of similar density are in different planes or are separated by a structure of a different density, then the two structures are seen on x-ray film separately. This property of the x-ray shadowgraph is helpful in determining where a certain density lies. For example, if a density on a posteroanterior chest radiograph is inseparable from and therefore adjacent to the descending thoracic aorta, then the observer knows that this abnormal density is in the posterior chest; if the density is inseparable from the right heart border, then the density is in an anterior position, because the heart is an anterior structure.

INTERPRETATION OF CHEST RADIOGRAPHS

It is important to understand normal anatomy on a chest x-ray in order to identify and interpret abnormalities. First, identify the patient by name and date of birth and confirm the date of the chest x-ray. The chest radiograph is read as though the reader were looking at the patient. Traditionally, the x-ray film is placed on a view box or light box that allows the radiograph to be backlit so it can be viewed and interpreted. More recently, digital imaging technology is used increasingly in radiology allowing for rapid viewing of films on monitors rather than on light boxes. Computerized radiographs can be viewed immediately on monitors on the CCU and stored images allow the provider to readily compare current films with previous images.[4]

A systematic approach to reviewing a CXR is also important. One systematic approach introduced here is the ABCDE approach.[5]

Airway

First, assess the trachea to determine if it's positioned midline or shifted to the right or left. If the trachea is shifted or deviated this could indicate improper patient positioning, thyroid enlargement, or a tension pneumonothorax. The second step is to examine the carina, which is the area where the trachea bifurcates into the right and left bronchi. This should lie between T4 and T6.

Bones

With maximum inspiration, 9 to 10 posterior ribs should be visualized. Posterior ribs slope downward to form the costovertebral angle. The anterior ribs appear more horizontal. Examine the clavicles, ribs, scapulae, and vertebrae for any fractures.

Circulation

Evaluate the size and shape of the cardiac silhouette. The heart should be approximately 50% the size of the thorax. An enlarged cardiac silhouette suggests cardiomegaly or a possible pericardial effusion. If the mediastinum appears enlarged this could be concerning for aortic aneurysm.

Diaphragm

Determine if the diaphragmatic line is clearly demarcated. The right hemidiaphragm should be higher than the left because of the liver. A depressed or flattened diaphragm is often seen in patients who have COPD or a pneumothorax.

Everything Else

Table 11-1 lists invasive lines, tubes, and devices commonly seen on chest x-ray.

Figure 11-1A is a normal posteroanterior chest radiograph; Figure 11-1B is a normal lateral chest radiograph. Figure 11-2A shows the location of the lung lobes on the frontal chest radiograph. Because some lobes are anterior and some are posterior, an abnormality in a certain area on a frontal chest radiograph can be in one of two lobes. Obtaining a lateral film or noticing whether an anterior or posterior structure is obliterated by an abnormal density can help with localization. Figure 11-2B shows the location of the lung lobes on a lateral radiograph. Abnormalities of the right middle lobe and lingula would go undetected with posterior chest auscultation.

CHEST FILM FINDINGS IN ACUTE CARE DETERMINING LINE, TUBE, AND CATHETER PLACEMENT

In the past, "routine" daily chest x-rays were frequently obtained in critical care, but this practice has been largely abandoned due to diagnostic efficacy. Chest x-rays should be ordered on the basis of clinical evaluation. Bedside radiographs are used not only to assess for cardiopulmonary abnormalities, but also to evaluate placement of lines, tubes, and devices used in acute care. Chest films not only provide valuable information regarding the patient's cardiopulmonary status, but also enable the early recognition of complications related to incorrect line placement and positioning. Evaluation of therapeutic results of after interventions such as drainage of a pleural effusion via chest tube placement are also determined by chest x-ray. Table 11-1 lists invasive lines, tubes, and devices commonly used in acute cardiovascular care, and describes radiologic findings. Figures 11-3 to 11-10 demonstrate radiologic appearance of a variety of invasive lines and devices.

(*text continues on page 282*)

Table 11-1 • RADIOLOGIC APPEARANCE OF INVASIVE LINES AND DEVICES IN CARDIOVASCULAR CARE

Invasive Line or Device	Description of Radiologic Appearance for Correct Position
Central venous pressure catheter (CVP) or peripherally inserted central catheter (PICC)	Ideal position is in the superior vena cava. The CVP line tip should always be above the level of the right atrium or the catheter tip may slip into the right atrium or ventricle and produce arrhythmias, or rarely, cardiac perforation. Central lines can be misplaced into the subclavian artery or misdirected up into the internal jugular vein. Trace the central line from its point of vascular entry to the tip to insure appropriate placement.
Pulmonary artery catheter (PAC)	The PAC tip should be within the main right or left pulmonary arteries and should extend no more than 2–4 cm beyond the vertebral midline. If the catheter tip is beyond this point there is increased risk of pulmonary artery occlusion, infarction, and rupture. The course of the PAC should be traced from its entry point to ensure that there is no looping in the ventricle. If the catheter tip is in the right ventricle, ventricular tachycardia may result from endocardial irritation.
Endotracheal tube (ETT)	The ETT should be visible as a radiopaque line within the trachea. The distal tip of the ETT should be a minimum of 4 cm above the main carina to avoid accidental right or left mainstem intubation. The ETT distal tip should be no higher than the level of the clavicles to avoid accidental extubation. Position of the head affects the location of the ETT tip. Flexion of the head toward the chest pulls the ETT up the trachea, while extension pushes the tube tip further into the trachea.
Chest tube	Chest tubes are used to drain air or fluid from the pleural cavity. Chest tubes inserted for pneumothorax are inserted toward the apex where gas or air collects and chest tubes inserted to drain fluid are inserted toward dependent areas around the base of the lungs. All of the islets that promote drainage (positioned along the proximal portion of the chest tube) need to be projected within the chest wall.
Intra-aortic balloon pump (IABP)	The tip of the IABP should be located in the distal aortic arch, just below the aortic knob and distal to the left subclavian artery. The oblong radiopaque IABP tip has the appearance of a large grain of rice.
Transvenous pacer (TVP)	Pacemaker leads extend from their point of entry in the right or left brachiocephalic veins into the right atrium (atrial lead) and the trabeculae of the right ventricle (ventricular lead). If the pacer is malfunctioning, the chest x-ray (CXR) may show fractured or misplaced leads.
Feeding tube (FT)	The entire FT is radiopaque. One should be able to trace the FT through the esophagus, stomach, and into the duodenum.
Tracheostomy tube	The tracheostomy tube should be midline within the trachea with the tip several centimeters above the main carina.

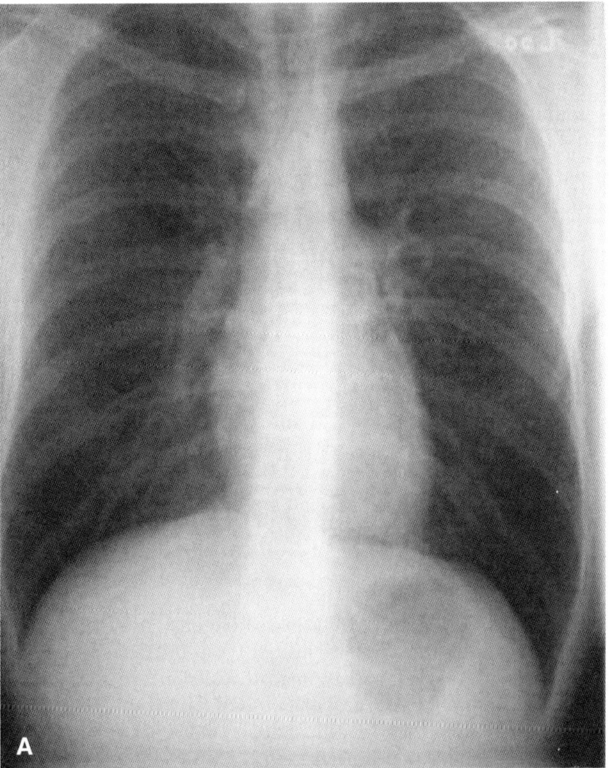

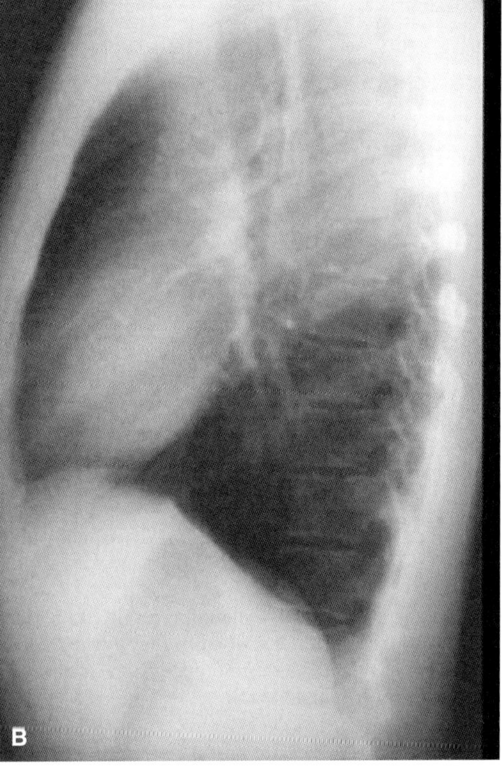

Figure 11-1. **(A)** Normal posteroanterior chest radiograph. **(B)** Normal lateral chest radiograph. The spine is posterior and the heart is anterior.

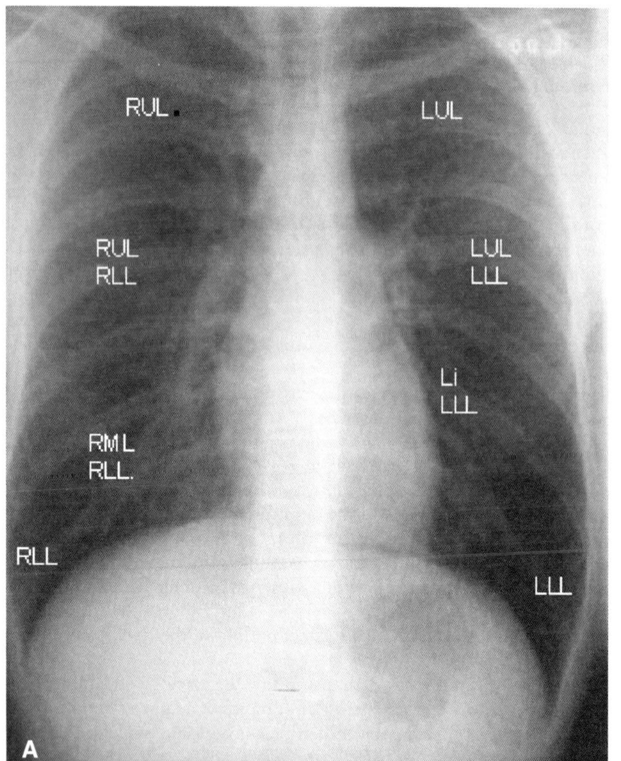

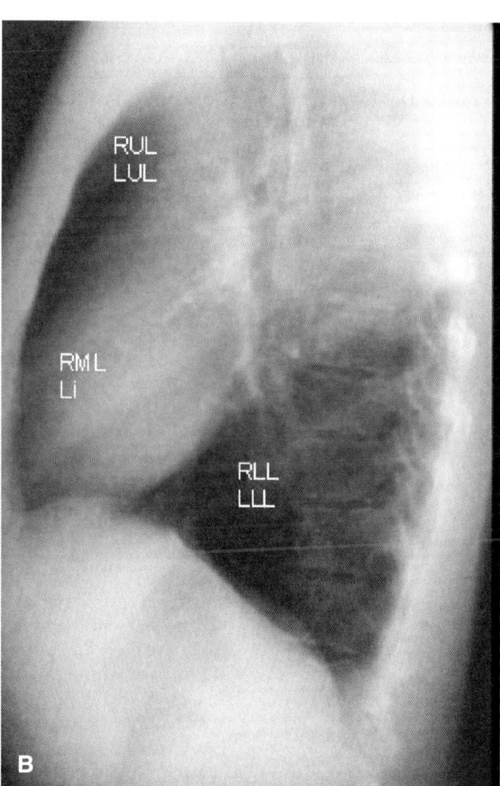

Figure 11-2. **(A)** Location of the lung lobes on the frontal chest radiograph. Because some lobes are anterior and some are posterior, an abnormality in a certain area on a frontal chest radiograph can be in one of two lobes. Obtaining a lateral film or noticing whether an anterior or posterior structure is obliterated by an abnormal density can help with localization. RUL, right upper lobe; RLL, right lower lobe; LLL, left lower lobe; RML, right middle lobe; LUL, left upper lobe; Li, lingula. **(B)** Location of the lung lobes on a lateral radiograph. Abnormalities of the right middle lobe and lingula would go undetected with posterior chest auscultation.

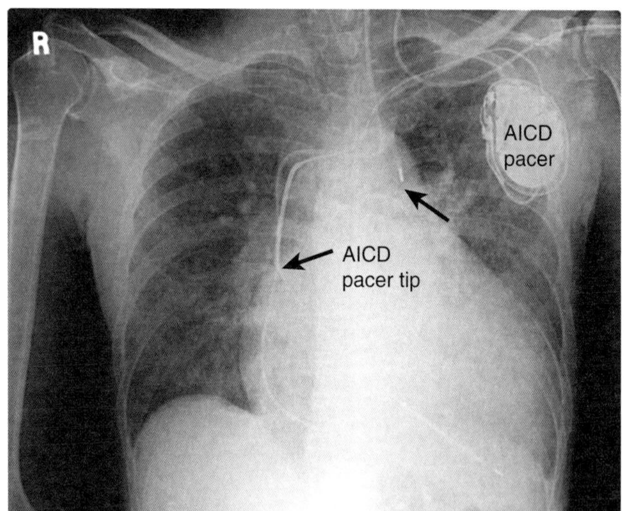

Figure 11-3. Correct intra-aortic balloon pump (IABP) placement in aortic knob. The IABP tip is just distal to the left subclavian artery. The patient has significant cardiomegaly and also has an implantable defibrillator (AICD) pacer.

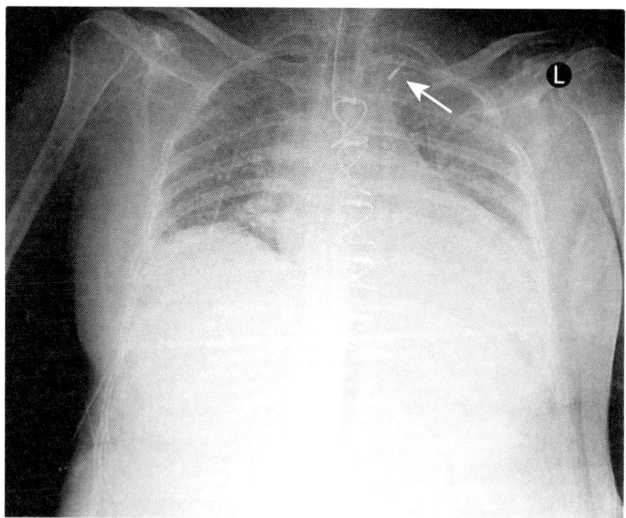

Figure 11-4. The IABP is placed too high into the left subclavian artery (see *white arrow*). This IABP was inserted at the bedside for a cardiac transplant patient in acute rejection and cardiogenic shock. The tip is above the aortic knob into the left subclavian artery. On examination, the patient had no left radial or brachial pulse until the IABP was pulled back 4 cm.

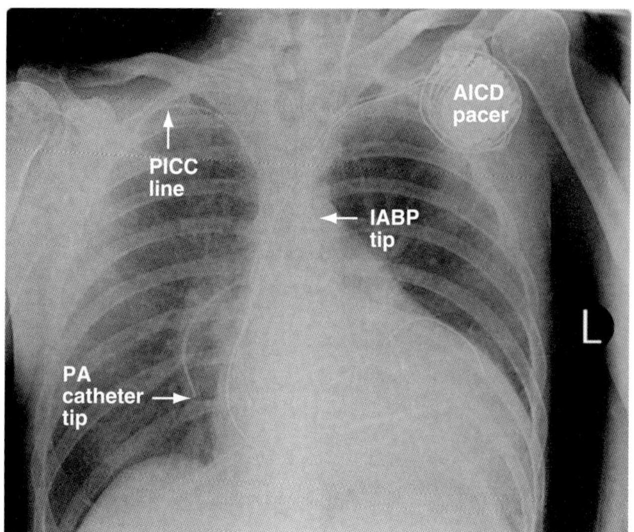

Figure 11-5. The pulmonary artery (PA) catheter tip is out too far. The tip of the PA catheter lies several centimeters beyond the hilum and is at risk for spontaneous wedge and pulmonary infarction. The patient also has an automatic implantable cardioverter defibrillator (AICD), peripherally inserted central catheter (PICC) line, and IABP.

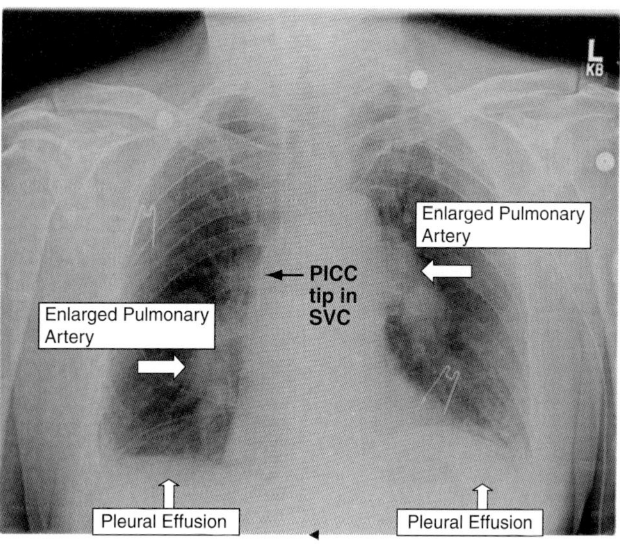

Figure 11-7. PICC line placement in a 56-year-old man with history of severe pulmonary hypertension secondary to chronic thromboembolic disease. He was postoperative after a pulmonary thromboendarterectomy. The tip of the PICC inserted into his left antecubital vein is correctly positioned in the superior vena cava (SVC). Note that, in addition to bilateral pleural effusions (see blunted costal phrenic angles), this individual also has very large pulmonary arteries extending from his hilum.

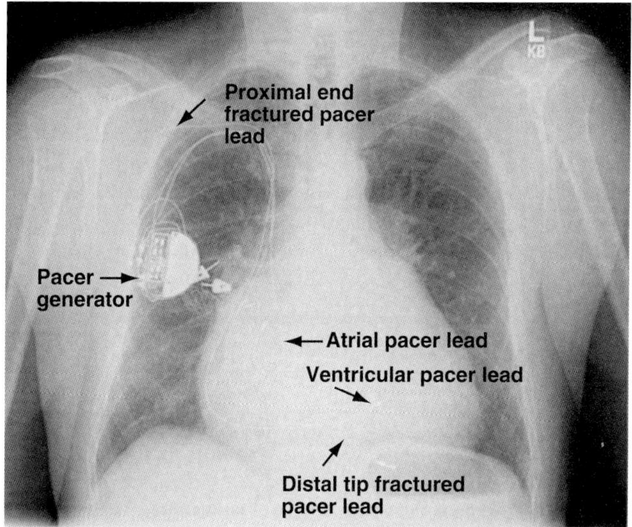

Figure 11-6. Pacemaker in a patient with cardiomegaly. Patient is a 27-year-old man with congenital heart disease. He had a previous pacer, but his original leads fractured and a new device and leads were placed. New leads can be seen in both the right atrium and right ventricle. A second ventricular lead can be seen in the right ventricle; if you trace this lead back, you will find it is fractured at the proximal end.

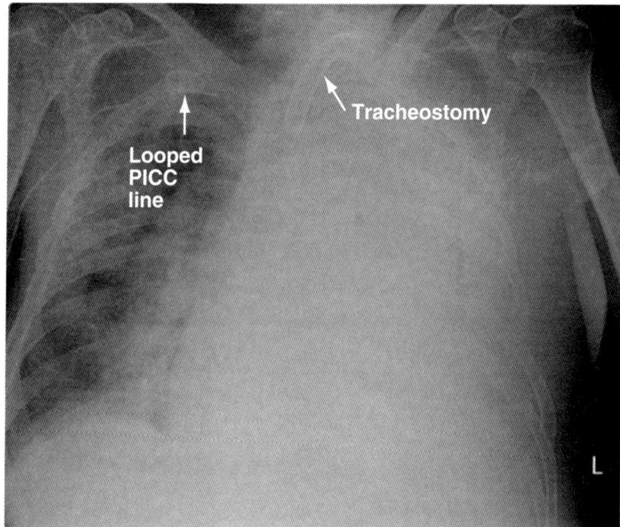

Figure 11-8. The PICC is looped in the right subclavian vein. Patient is a 55-year-old man who had multiple complications after emergency repair of a ruptured descending aortic aneurysm. The white-out on the patient's left is a massive hemothorax, which is pushing the mediastinum including the tracheostomy tube to the right.

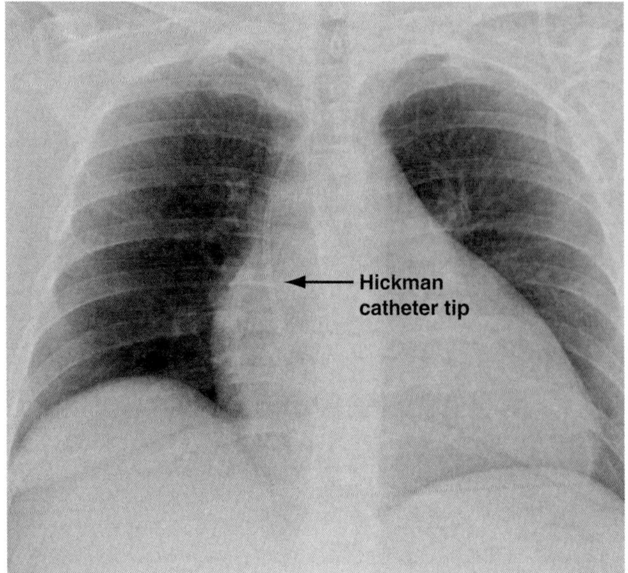

Figure 11-9. Hickman central line placement. There is a tunneled central line with correct position into the superior vena cava.

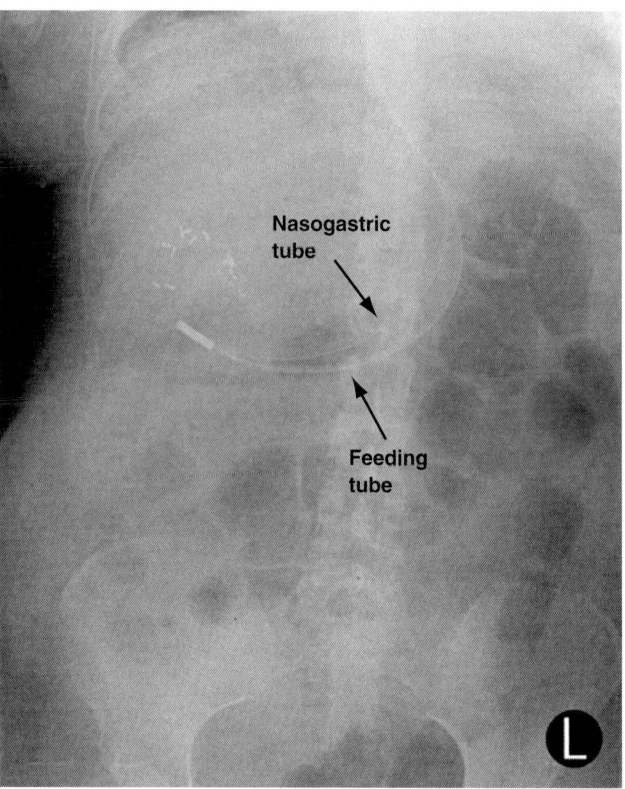

Figure 11-10. Feeding tube placement. The abdominal radiograph shows both the feeding tube and the nasogastric tube in the duodenum.

CHEST FILM FINDINGS IN CARDIOVASCULAR DISEASE

The chest radiograph provides useful data that aid in the complete assessment of the patient with acute chest pain and suspected acute coronary syndrome in the CCU and/or emergency department. Chest radiography aids in evaluating other etiologies of chest pain including pneumothorax, rib fractures, pneumonia, and aortic dissection.[6] Computerized axial tomography angiography is used for the diagnosis of aortic dissection and pulmonary embolism. Table 11-2 lists common cardiovascular clinical diagnoses and their associated radiologic findings. Figures 11-11 to 11-21 illustrate a variety of radiologic findings associated with cardiovascular pathophysiology.

Chest radiographs may also be used to identify cardiac devices used to treat cardiovascular diseases, such as structural and valvular heart disease. Figures 11-22 to 11-24 depict a sampling of the numerous cardiac devices that may be seen on the chest radiographs of patients with a history of open heart surgery or catheter-based intervention for structural and valvular heart disease.

Table 11-2 • COMMON CLINICAL PRESENTATIONS IN ACUTE CARE AND RADIOLOGIC FINDINGS

Clinical Diagnosis	Radiologic Findings
Pericardial effusion	Enlarged cardiac silhouette with a "water bottle" appearance. May look very similar to cardiomegaly. Diagnosis of pericardial effusion should be verified with echocardiography.
Congestive heart failure (CHF)	In chronic CHF the heart is usually enlarged; in acute heart failure the heart may be of normal size. May have cephalization of blood vessels (increased size and number of blood vessels near the lung apices). May have interstitial fluid that begins at the lung bases and extends upward. Frank pulmonary edema and pleural effusions may develop.
Aortic aneurysm	Ascending and/or descending aorta are enlarged. Widened mediastinum. New pleural effusion if leak or rupture.
Pneumothorax	Frontal, full upright CXR shows the visceral pleura as a thin white line. There is a hyperlucent area where there are no bronchovascular or lung markings. Pneumothorax is more difficult to see in supine film.
Pleural effusion	Fluid moves to dependent areas of pleural space and is best seen on upright or decubitus (side-lying) CXR views. At least 200 to 300 cc must be present in the pleural space to cause costophrenic blunting. By doing decubitus views (side lying), one may determine if the effusion is free flowing and amenable to thoracentesis.
Pneumonia	Alveolar or interstitial pattern of white opacity. May be localized to a single lobe or be more diffused. Air bronchograms are frequently present in lobar pneumonia.
Acute respiratory distress syndrome (ARDS)	Diffuse bilateral patchy infiltrates, "ground glass" appearance. May be confused with CHF.

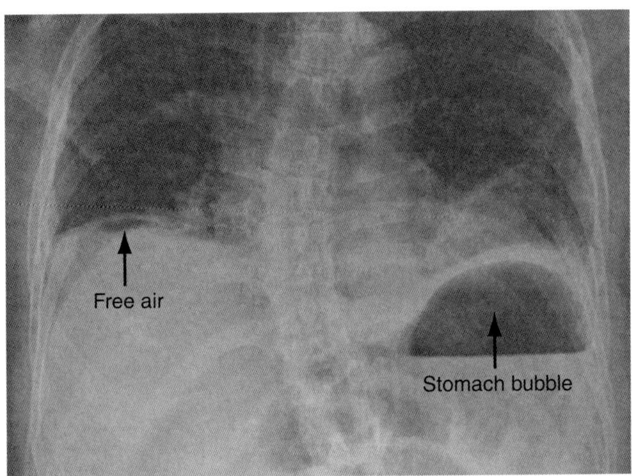

Figure 11-11. Free air under the diaphragm. This patient had epigastric pain and diaphoresis. The admission radiograph showed free air under the diaphragm consistent with a perforated viscus. (Film courtesy of Julie Takasugi, MD.)

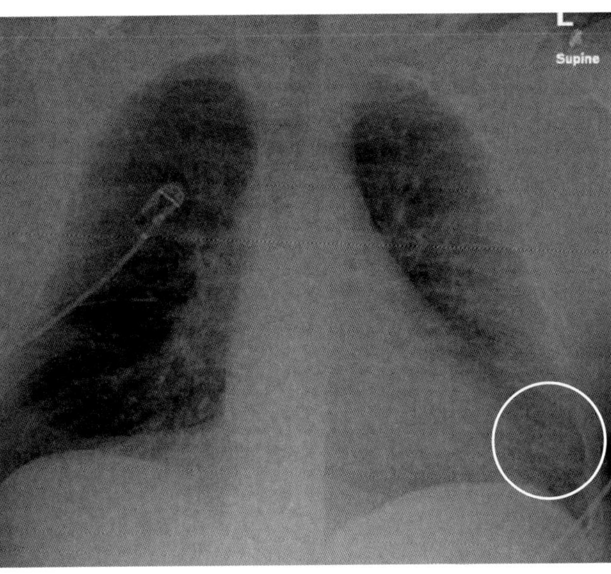

Figure 11-13. Cardiogenic pulmonary edema with cardiomegaly. In this radiograph, Kerley B lines are seen as tiny horizontal lines in the lung periphery. These lines represent dilated pulmonary lymph vessels, which facilitate pulmonary edema removal from the alveolar spaces. (Film courtesy of Julie Takasugi, MD.)

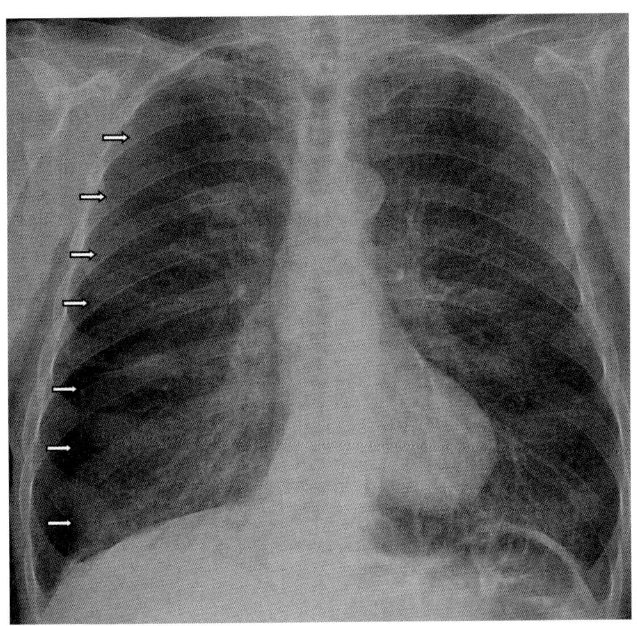

Figure 11-12. Pneumothorax. The patient may have acute chest pain and shortness of breath. Physical findings include absent or reduced breath sounds on the side of the pneumothorax and tympany or a hollow sound on chest percussion, with possibly a shift of the trachea to the side away from the pneumothorax. The *arrows* indicate the outer border of the right lung. The remainder of the right chest cavity is filled with air in the pleural space. (Film courtesy of Julie Takasugi, MD.)

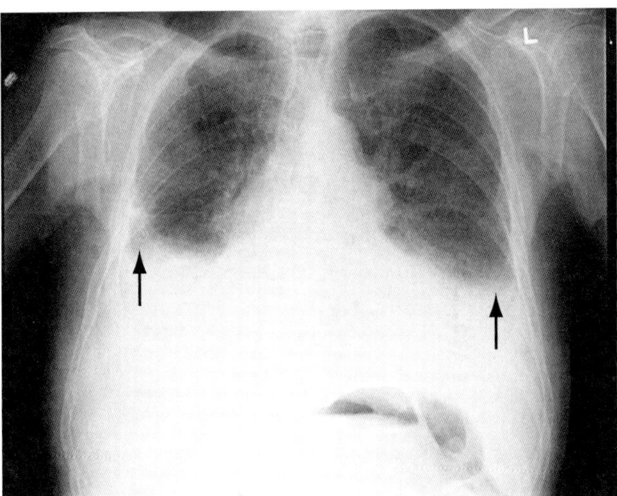

Figure 11-14. Congestive heart failure with bilateral pleural effusions. The *arrows* show that the normal diaphragmatic contour is obliterated. This 88-year-old man with severe aortic stenosis was admitted with severe shortness of breath and worsening heart failure.

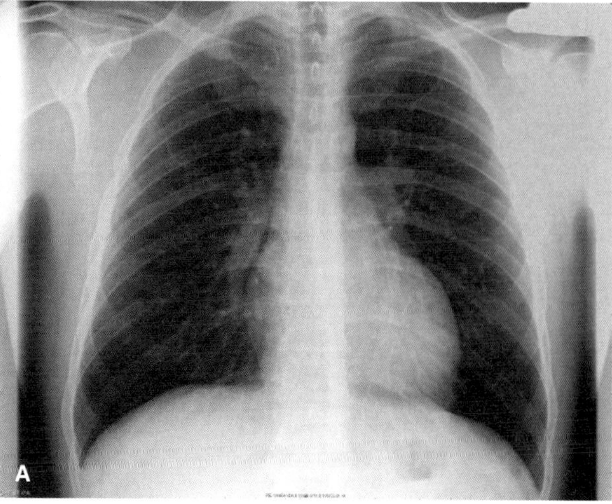

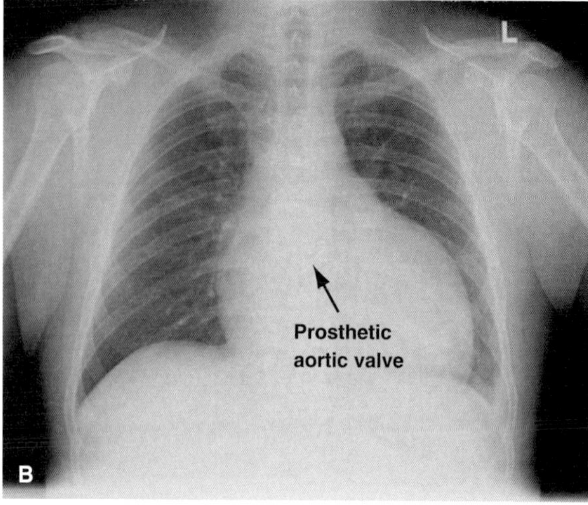

Figure 11-15. **(A)** Preoperative patient with aortic regurgitation. **(B)** Same patient 3 weeks after aortic valve replacement. Patient now has a large pericardial effusion (note enlarged cardiac silhouette) creating tamponade physiology.

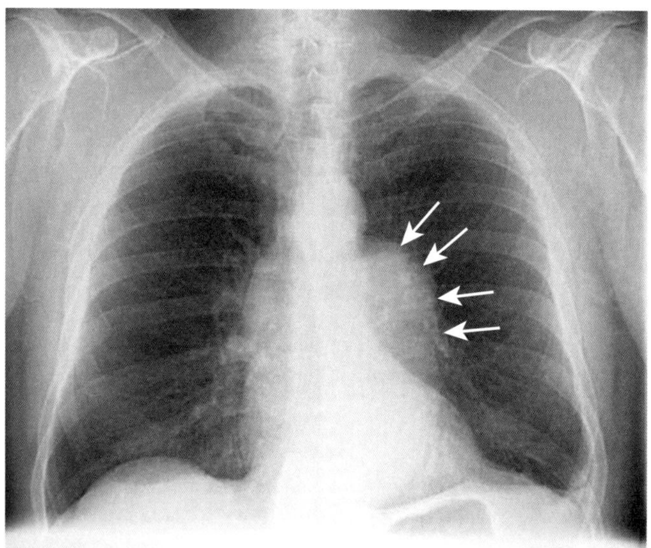

Figure 11-16. Descending thoracic aortic aneurysm. "Bulging" of the descending aorta noted by *arrows* in a 57-year-old man with history of blunt trauma to chest as well as hypertension.

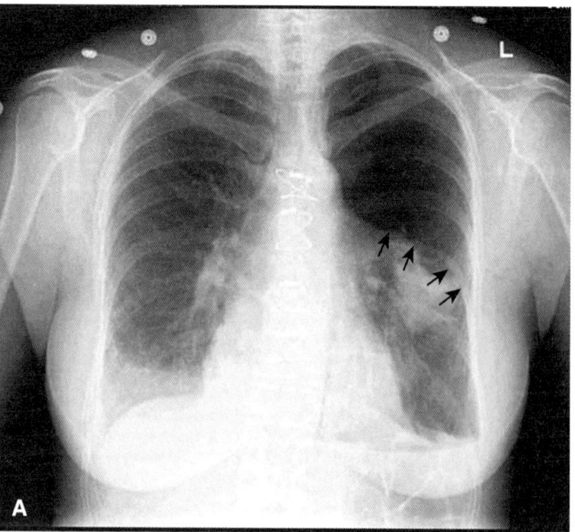

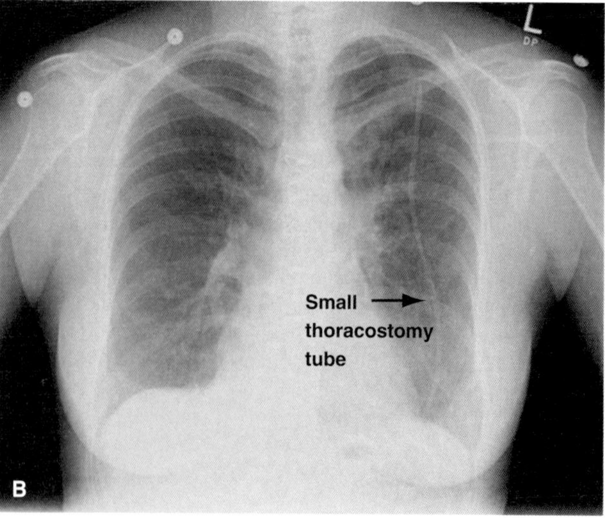

Figure 11-17. **(A)** Large left pneumothorax after surgical repair of a patent foramen ovale. The *arrows* indicate the border of the collapsed lung. **(B)** Re-expansion of left lung after placement of small thoracostomy tube in interventional radiology department.

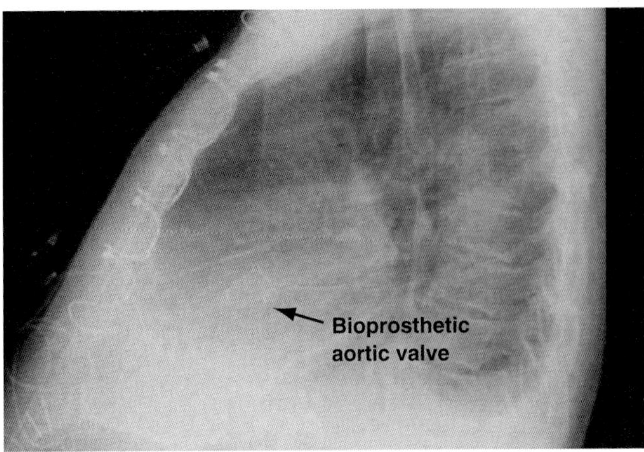

Figure 11-18. Radiologic appearance of stented bioprosthetic aortic valve replacement in lateral chest x-ray (CXR) view. Stents point toward blood flow.

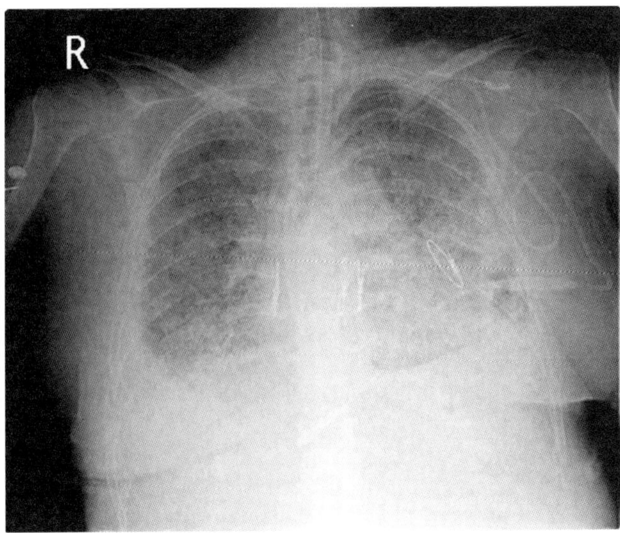

Figure 11-20. Acute respiratory distress syndrome, as evidenced by diffuse bilateral opacities in patient postoperatively after bilateral lung transplantation.

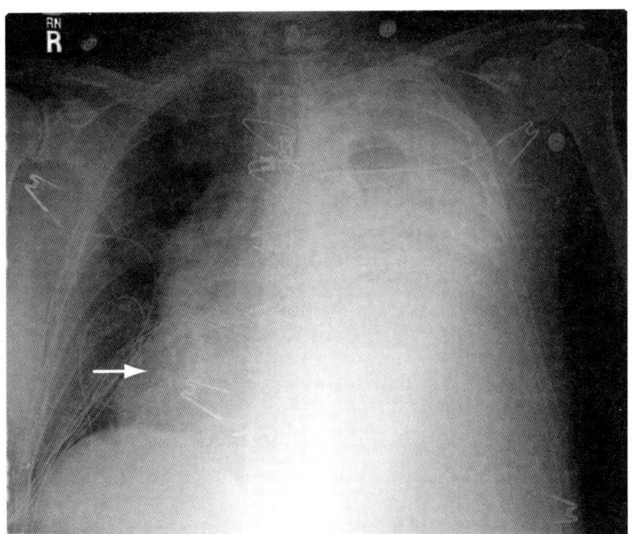

Figure 11-19. Massive left pleural effusion (the patient's left side of chest is whited out) with mediastinal shift, where the right heart border is shifted into the patient's right chest (*arrow*). This 62-year-old man had massive left pleural effusion causing severe orthopnea and shortness of breath. Patient underwent thoracentesis three times in a 24-hour period to drain a total of 3500 cc of serosanguineous fluid.

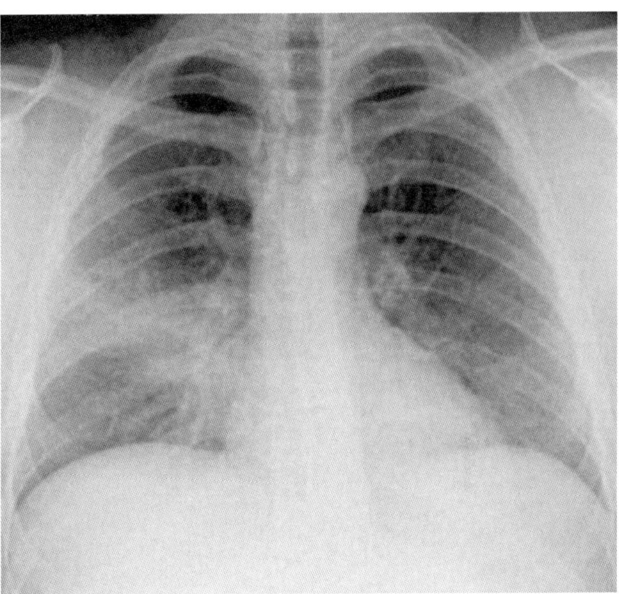

Figure 11-21. Right lower lobe pneumonia. Signs of consolidation (bronchial breathing, crackles, and dullness to percussion) are heard over the right lower chest. In pneumonia, egophony is heard over areas of consolidated lung. The patient is instructed to say the letter "e," and the lung is auscultated to demonstrate this finding. Normally the "e" sound is heard, but consolidated lung changes the "e" to an "a" that sounds like the "bleating of a goat." This sign is also known as "an e-to-a change." (Film courtesy of Julie Takasugi, MD.)

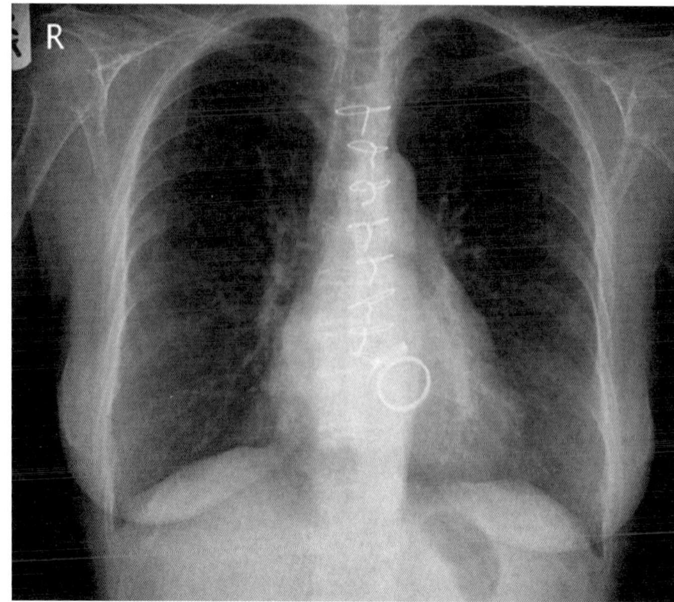

Figure 11-22. Chest radiograph of a patient with a history of open heart surgery for aortic and mitral valve replacement.

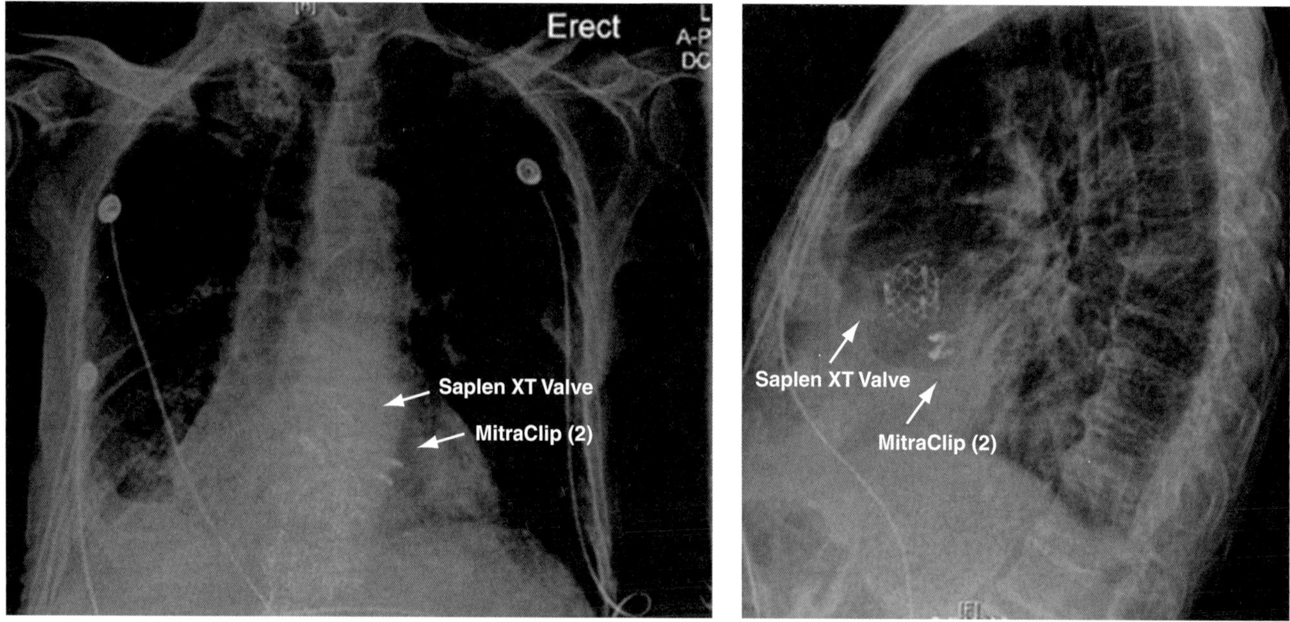

Figure 11-23. Chest radiograph of a patient with a history of transcatheter aortic valve replacement (Sapien XT, Edwards Lifesciences) and transcatheter mitral valve repair (MitraClip, Abbott Vascular) for severe aortic stenosis and mitral regurgitation. (Reprinted with permission from Cressman S, Rheinboldt M, Klochko C, et al. Chest radiographic appearance of minimally invasive cardiac implants and support devices: what the radiologist needs to Know. *Curr Probl Diagn Radiol.* 2019;48(3):274–288.

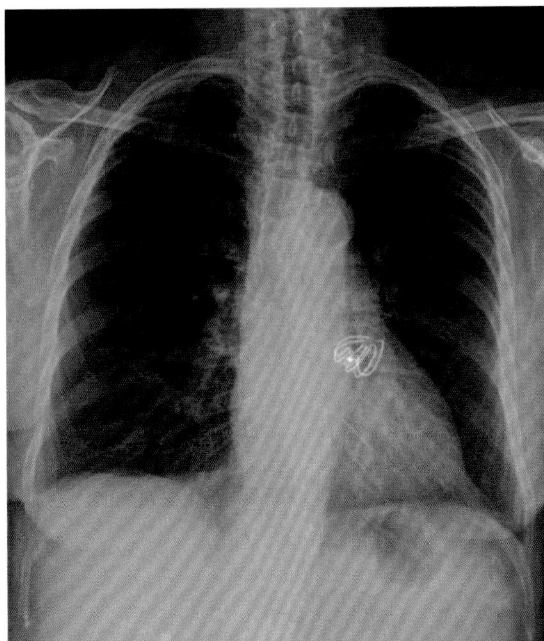

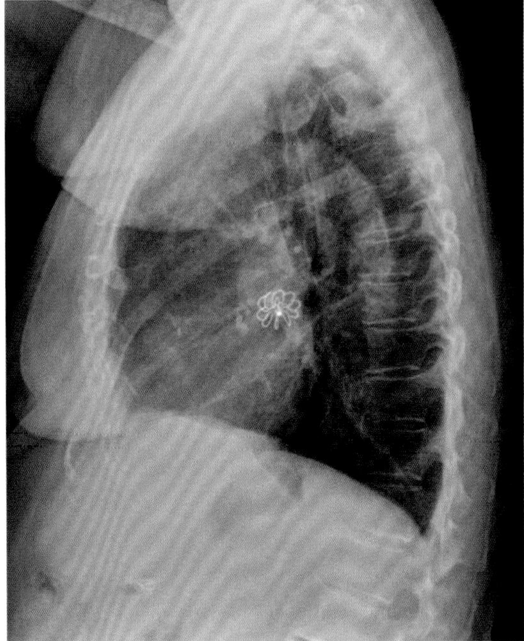

Figure 11-24. Chest radiograph of a patient with a history of transcatheter left atrial appendage occlusion with a Watchman device, as an alternative to long-term anticoagulation for stroke prevention in atrial fibrillation. (Reprinted with permission from Cressman S, Rheinboldt M, Klochko C, et al. Chest radiographic appearance of minimally invasive cardiac implants and support devices: what the radiologist needs to Know. *Curr Probl Diagn Radiol.* 2019;48(3):274–288.)

Summary

Knowledge of (1) a simple, systematic approach to basic chest x-ray interpretation and (2) common cardiovascular diagnoses and devices assessed using chest x-ray, is important for the nurse caring for cardiology patients. Particularly in the acute care setting, the nurse must rapidly identify symptoms and signs that may suggest a change in a patient's cardiopulmonary status, and whether there may be a concern for the positioning and functioning of invasive lines and devices. The chest x-ray provides fundamental information for the cardiac nurse, who is often the front-line caregiver for patients evaluated for cardiovascular disease.

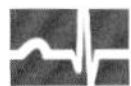

CASE STUDY 1

Patient Profile

History of Present Illness

Mr. Scott is an 88-year-old male who lives alone and recently presented to the emergency with shortness of breath, lower extremity edema, and chest pain. While providing his health history he mentions his wife passed away a few months ago. Upon further assessment he mentions that he has been eating microwaveable dinners or going to the local diner for most of his meals. He states that at one time he was on a "water pill but that medicine ran out" without a refill.

Patient Examination

Vital Signs

BP 140/87 mm Hg; HR 90 bpm; RR 28; Temp 97.9°F; SaO_2 88% on room air

Physical Examination

Lungs are notable for bilateral crackles. 3+ bilateral lower extremity edema.

Diagnostic Studies

Laboratory Studies: BNP 1800, creatinine 0.75 mg/dL, potassium 3.8 mg/dL
Chest x-ray (Fig. 11-14)

Considerations

There are pleural effusions (Fig. 11-14). Costophrenic blunting is noted. At least 200 to 300 cc must be present in the pleural space to cause costophrenic blunting.

- What diagnosis most likely fits this clinical scenario?
- What testing, medications, and labs do you anticipate the provider to order?

This clinical scenario fits a patient with heart failure exacerbation. There are several common chest x-ray findings with congestive failure.

- The size of the heart may be enlarged with patients who have chronic heart failure. In patients with new onset heart failure, the heart size may be normal
- May have interstitial fluid that begins at the lung bases and extends upward
- May have cephalization of blood vessels (increased size and number of blood vessels near the lung apices)
- Pulmonary edema and pleural effusions often may be seen

Assessment and Plan

Mr. Scott was admitted for his heart failure exacerbation. He was treated with 80 mg IV Lasix and 40 mEq potassium. The next morning his weight was down 3 lb and his shortness of breath has improved. He will be transitioned to oral diuretics and educated on the importance of medication compliance and dietary restrictions before discharge.

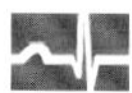

CASE STUDY 2

Patient Profile

History of Present Illness

Mr. Richard is a 60-year-old male who presents to the emergency department with a harsh, productive cough that started 4 days ago. He notes fever, chills, and malaise along with the cough. He became alarmed with his symptoms this morning when he developed pain in his right chest that is worse with inspiration.

Patient Examination

Vital Signs

BP 150/90 mm Hg; HR 110 bpm; RR 22 and labored; Temp 103°F; SaO_2 91%

Physical Examination

Lungs are notable for bilateral rhonchi and crackles, and right-sided dullness to percussion.

Diagnostic Studies

Chest x-ray (Fig. 11-21)

Considerations

- What diagnosis most likely fits this clinical scenario?
- What testing, medications, and labs do you anticipate the provider to order?

This chest x-ray shows right lower lobe pneumonia. This clinical scenario fits a patient with pneumonia. Common chest x-ray findings with pneumonia include:

- Alveloar or interstitial pattern of white opacity
- May be localized to a single lobe or be more diffused
- Air bronchograms are frequently present in lobar pneumonia

Assessment and Plan

Mr. Richard was admitted with a diagnosis of pneumonia. His labwork showed WBC 18,000/mm^3. Sputum sample was obtained for culture, sensitivity, and Gram stain. He was started on a 10-day course of oral antibiotics. He was given analgesic for pain, antipyretics for temp, and a bronchodilator. He will follow up with his primary care provider in 10 days with a repeat chest x-ray.

BP, blood pressure; HR, heart rate; RR, respiratory rate; Temp, temperature; SaO_2, arterial oxygen saturation; BNP, B-type naturietic peptide; IV, intravenous; WBC, white blood cells.

KEY READINGS

Agladioglu K, Serinken M, Dal O, et al. Chest x-rays in detecting injuries caused by blunt trauma. *World J Emerg Med.* 2016;7(1):55–58.

Bettman MA. The chest radiograph in cardiovascular disease. In: Libby P, Bonow RO, Mann DL, et al., eds. *Braunwald's Heart Disease.* 8th ed. Philadelphia, PA: Elsevier; 2008:327–343.

Erkonen WE. Radiography, computerized tomography, magnetic resonance imaging, and ultrasonography: principles and indications. In: Erkonen WE, Smith WL, eds. *Radiology 101. The Basics and Fundamentals of Imaging.* Philadelphia, PA: Lippincott Williams & Wilkins; 2005:3–15.

REFERENCES

1. McAdams HP, Samei E, Dobbins J, et al. Recent advances in chest radiology. *Radiology.* 2006;241(3):663–683.
2. Erkonen WE. Radiography, computerized tomography, magnetic resonance imaging, and ultrasonography: principles and indications. In: Erkonen WE, Smith WL, eds. *Radiology 101. The Basics and Fundamentals of Imaging.* Philadelphia, PA: Lippincott Williams & Wilkins; 2005: 3–15.
3. Bettman MA. The chest radiograph in cardiovascular disease. In: Libby P, Bonow RO, Mann DL, et al., eds. *Braunwald's Heart Disease.* 8th ed. Philadelphia, PA: Elsevier; 2008:327–343.
4. Connolly MA. Black, white, and shades of gray: common abnormalities in chest radiographs. *AACN Clin Issues.* 2001;12(2):259–269.
5. Tarrac SE. A systematic approach to chest x-ray interpretation in the perianesthesia unit. *J Perianesth Nurs.* 2009;24(1):41–47.
6. Stanford W. Radiologic evaluation of acute chest pain-suspected myocardial ischemia. *Am Fam Physician.* 2007;76(4):533–537.

12 Electrocardiography and Cardiac Rhythm

Tao Zheng

OBJECTIVES

1. Review electrocardiographic features of various cardiac conditions, and how these conditions or other disease processes contribute to electrocardiogram (ECG) changes.
2. Describe a systematic method of interpreting both basic and 12-lead ECG.
3. Identify ECG changes associated with myocardial infarction (MI), atrial and ventricular enlargement, medications, and electrolytes imbalance.
4. Examine major mechanisms and causes of cardiac arrhythmias.
5. Discuss evidence-based guidelines and recommendations for cardiac arrhythmias management.

KEY QUESTIONS

1. What are the electrical and mechanical events depicted by the electrocardiogram (ECG)?
2. What foundational knowledge must clinicians acquire to quickly and accurately recognize ECG changes?
3. What are the ECG changes associated with pathologic conditions?

BACKGROUND

Electrocardiogram (ECG) is a graphic display of the cardiac electrical activities captured by the electrodes placed on the body surface. Basic ECG (3 or 5 lead) and 12-lead ECG are frequently used procedures that provide valuable information about the function and structure of the heart. Compared to basic ECG, 12-lead ECG provides more views of the heart from different angles, which provides further diagnostic information to differentiate arrhythmias and identify underlying pathophysiology.

The technology and clinical utilization of ECG has advanced for the past two centuries. ECG is the standard of care for diagnosis of cardiac arrhythmias and conduction abnormalities. ECG is a useful evaluation tool for functionality of implanted devices such as pacemakers and implantable cardioverter defibrillators (ICDs). ECG monitoring is easy to use, cost effective, noninvasive, and can be used across the care continuum.

Clinical conditions that involve electrical disturbances (e.g., myocardial ischemia or infarction, condition abnormalities associated with acid–base and electrolyte imbalance, and drug intoxication) will produce ECG changes. ECG plays a pivotal role in determining the presence and severity of myocardial ischemia and infarction, and localizing regions of cardiac muscle associated with these conditions. ECG provides early detection of myocardial infarction (MI) and arrhythmias, and lead to early revascularization and interventions. Incorrectly used or interpreted ECG can simulate or conceal abnormalities and delay treatment.[1] Fast and appropriate interventions can save myocardial muscle, prevent clinical deterioration, and improve patient outcomes.[2] Therefore, it is important for clinicians to have in-depth knowledge of ECG and its utilization and application.

ELECTRICAL CONDUCTION THROUGH THE HEART

Cardiac Conduction System

The cardiac conduction system is made of specialized electrical cells arranged in a system of pathways, which ensures the heart chambers contract in a coordinated fashion. The spread of this wave of depolarization through the heart produces the classic surface ECG, which can be recorded by an ECG machine or monitored continuously on a bedside cardiac monitor. The conduction system includes the following structures (Fig. 12-1).

Sinus Node

The sinus node or sinoatrial (SA) node is comprised of a small group of dominant pacemaker cells located in the upper part of the right atrium. The SA node typically fires at an intrinsic rate of 60 times per minute. The autonomic nervous system affects the rate of the SA node. Sympathetic stimulation, such as catecholamine release and the fight or flight response will increase the rate of the SA node. Parasympathetic stimulation, such as carotid massage to stimulate the vagus nerve, will decrease the SA node rate. The blood supply of the SA node comes from the right coronary artery (RCA) 55% to 60% of the time or left circumflex 40% to 45% of the time; thus, occlusion of these coronary arteries will decrease the rate of the SA node.[3]

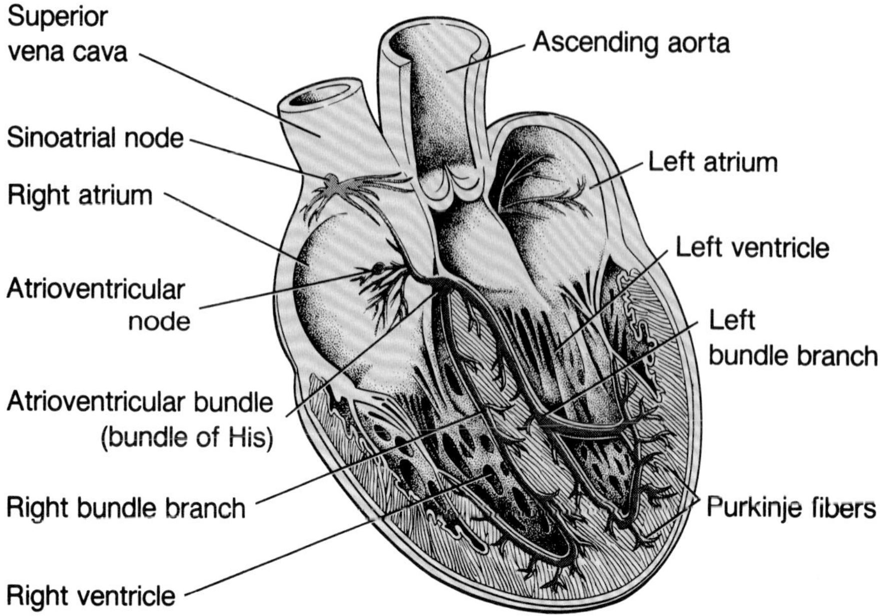

Figure 12-1. Cardiac conduction system. (From Jacobson C. Cardiac arrhythmias and conduction abnormalities. In: Patrick ML, Woods SL, Craven RF, et al., eds. *Medical Surgical Nursing*. 2nd ed. Philadelphia, PA: JB Lippincott; 1991:648–693.)

AV Node

The atrioventricular (AV) node is a group of specialized conducting cells located in the lower right atrium immediately posterior to the tricuspid valve. When the electrical impulse is transmitted to the AV node, the AV node creates a physiologic delay to allow the atria to completely contract and empty before the ventricular contraction begins. The contribution of the atria to ventricular filling is called "atrial kick." The AV node also prevents rapid impulses from traveling to the ventricles, thereby delaying rapid depolarization of the ventricles. The AV node fires at a rate of 40 to 60 times per minute and serves as a backup pacemaker should the SA node fail.[4] The blood supply of the AV node comes from the RCA in 85% to 90% of the population. For others, the blood supply comes from the circumflex coronary artery.[3]

Bundle of His

The Bundle of His is also known as the common bundle or the AV bundle. This short bundle of fibers is the continuation of the AV node. The Bundle of His connects the AV node to the left and right bundle branches.[5]

Bundle Branches

The bundle branches transmit the electrical impulse into the right and left ventricle. The right bundle transmits the electrical current through the interventricular septum to the right ventricle. The left bundle branch is a complex structure divided into three major fascicles: the septal fascicle depolarizes the interventricular septum, and the anterior and posterior fascicles carry the impulse to the left ventricle via anterior and posterior wall of the ventricle.[6]

Purkinje Fibers

Once the electrical impulse leaves the bundle branches, the impulse is transmitted to smaller branches then to a hair-like fibrous network called Purkinje fibers. Purkinje fibers, spread along the endocardial surface of the ventricles, are the final structure through which an impulse is transmitted before it reaches the myocardium and a contraction is initiated. The intrinsic rate of the Purkinje fibers is 20 to 40 times per minute; it will take over as a pacemaker when both SA node and AV node fail.[3]

WAVES, COMPLEXES, AND INTERVALS OF THE CARDIAC CYCLE

P Wave

The P wave is the first waveform in the cardiac cycle and represents atrial depolarization. The normal P wave is smooth and rounded. It is no more than 2.5 mm in height and 0.12 second in duration. In a heart with normal conduction, each P wave precedes each QRS complex.[6] Following the P wave is a short isoelectric line that represents a conduction delay at the AV node.[6]

PR Interval

The PR interval is the measurement from the onset of atrial depolarization to the beginning of ventricular depolarization. The PR interval is measured at the beginning of the P wave to the beginning of QRS complex. Normal PR interval ranges from 0.12 to 0.20 second.[6]

QRS Complex

QRS complex represents ventricular myocardial depolarization which triggers ventricular contraction. Compared to the P wave, the QRS complex has a higher amplitude due to the larger muscle mass of the ventricles. The shape of the QRS complex depends on the lead being recorded and the ventricular activation sequence; not all leads record all waves of the QRS complex. A

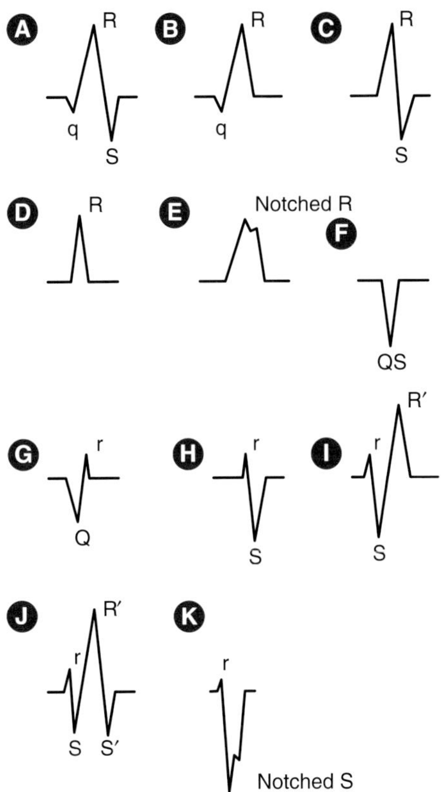

Figure 12-2. QRS variations. Example **A:** A normal QRS complex. Example **B:** A QRS complex with a Q and an R wave but no S wave. Example **C:** An R and Save without a Q wave. Example **D:** An R wave without a Q wave or an S wave. Example **E:** A notched R wave. Example **F:** The entire complex is negative, it is termed QS complex. Example **G:** A large Q wave with a small r wave. Example **H:** A small r wave with a large S wave. Example **I:** More than one R wave. Example **J:** More than one S wave. Example **K:** A notched S wave.

Q wave is an initial negative deflection from baseline and should be less than 0.03 second in duration and less than 25% of the R-wave amplitude. An R wave is the first positive deflection from baseline. An S wave is a negative deflection that follows an R wave. When a complex is entirely positive, it is just an R wave; when it is entirely negative, it is called a QS. Regardless of the shape of the complex, ventricular depolarization waves may be referred to as QRS complexes (Fig. 12-2). The width of the QRS complex represents intraventricular conduction time and is measured from the point at which it first leaves the baseline to the end of the last appearing wave. Normal QRS width is 0.04 to 0.10 second.[7]

T Wave

The T wave represents ventricular repolarization, which follows the QRS complex and it is normally in the same direction as the QRS complex.[7] The absolute refractory period (ARP) is still present during the beginning of the T wave. At the peak of the T wave, the relative refractory period (RRP) has begun. RRP is considered a vulnerable period of the T wave; a stronger than normal stimulus transmitted during this period may produce ventricular dysrhythmias. The normal T wave is rounded and slightly asymmetric: the peak of waveform is closer to its end than to the beginning, and the first half has a more gradual slope than the

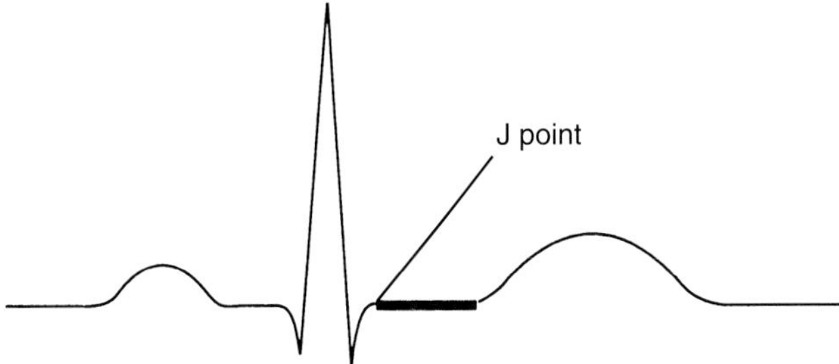

Figure 12-3. The ST segment.

second half.[5] T waves are not normally taller than 5 mm in any limb lead or 10 mm in any precordial lead.[7]

ST Segment

The ST segment is the flat isoelectric line between the QRS complex and the T wave. It represents early repolarization of the ventricles. Normal ST segment begins at the isoelectric line and extends from the end of the S wave. During this period, the heart is in diastole and coronary arteries actively supply blood to the myocardium. The ST segment is important in the evaluation of pathologic abnormalities (Fig. 12-3); deviations from the isoelectric baseline (i.e., ST elevation or depression) indicate compromised myocardial perfusion.

J Point

J (junction) point it is the point where the QRS complex and the ST segment meets (see Fig. 12-3). The J point may be used as a reference point for ST-segment deviation. The ST segment is considered elevated if the segment is deviated above the baseline and is considered depressed if the segment is deviated below the baseline.[5,8]

QT Interval

The QT interval represents one full cycle of ventricular activity (depolarization and repolarization). The QT interval is measured from the beginning of the QRS complex to the end of the T wave, and, because it varies inversely with the heart rate, must be corrected to a heart rate of 60 beats per minute (bpm). Because the QT interval adjusts gradually to a change in heart rate, accurate measurement of the corrected QT interval (QTc) can be done only after several regular and equal cardiac cycles. A slower heart rate results in a prolonged QT interval, and a faster heart rate shortens the QT interval.[5,8] The normal QTc is usually less than half of the preceding R-R interval at normal heart rates, but a more accurate evaluation can be done using Bazett formula: $QTc = QT/\sqrt{R\text{-}R}$ interval, where QT and R-R intervals are in seconds.[9] Normal QT interval is between 0.39 and 0.45 second. The QTc accounts for heart rate. The upper limit of normal QTc is generally considered to be less than 0.44 second in adult men and less than 0.45 second in adult women.[10] A prolonged QT interval may be due to myocardial ischemia, electrolyte disorders, sudden decreases in heart rate, acute neurologic events, and medications (e.g., sotalol, amiodarone, and Haldol).[5]

U Wave

The U wave is a small, rounded wave that sometimes follows the T wave and is most prominent in leads V_2 to V_4 (Fig. 12-4). The

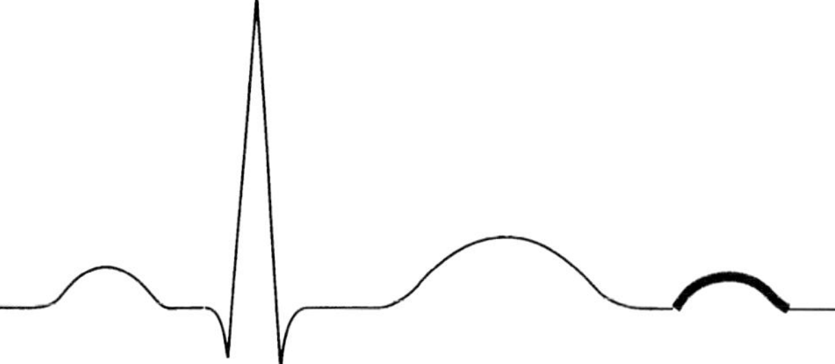

Figure 12-4. The U wave.

deflection of the U wave is normally in the same direction as the T wave but is only approximately 10% of its amplitude.[7] Negative U waves sometimes appear with positive T waves; this abnormal finding has been noted in left ventricular hypertrophy (LVH) and myocardial ischemia.[11] The U wave is thought to be part of ventricular repolarization process and may represent repolarization of the Purkinje network or certain cells in the deep subepicardial layer of the ventricle (M cells), or the summation of ventricular afterdepolarizations.[7]

The amplitude of the normal U wave is usually less than 0.1 mV. Possible causes of prominent U waves include central nervous system disease, electrolyte imbalance, hyperthyroidism, long QT syndrome (LQTS), and medications.[5]

Neither the presence nor absence of U wave is considered abnormal. In a clinical condition of low potassium level (hypokalemia), a large U wave can be observed. A large U wave may be mistaken for a P wave. Comparison of the morphology of both waveforms will help to differentiate the U wave from P wave. If there are two P waves, the P waves will look the same in size, shape, and direction (see Fig. 12-4).[8]

R-R and P-P Intervals

The R-R (R wave-to-R wave) and P-P (P wave-to-P wave) intervals may be used to determine the rate and regularity of ECG. To evaluate the regularity of the atrial rhythm, the interval between two consecutive P waves is measured and compared to the subsequent P-P interval. The same process can be used to evaluate the R-R interval to assess regularity of the ventricular rhythm.[5] Figure 12-5 illustrates waves, complexes, and intervals of the cardiac cycle in both leads II and V_1.

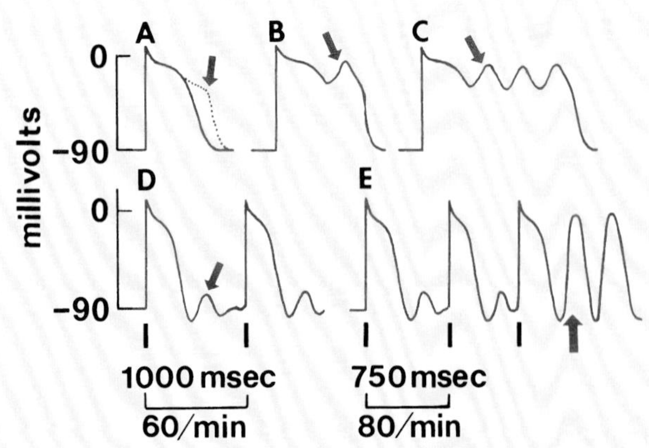

Figure 12-5. Waves, complexes, and intervals of the cardiac cycle in leads II and V1.

BASIC ELECTROCARDIOGRAPHY

ECG is a graphic recording of the cardiac electrical activities. When the electrodes placed on the body surface are connected to the electrocardiography, the ECG machine captures the voltage between the electrodes and the recording is made on ECG paper.

The ECG paper consists of series of small boxes and large boxes vertically and horizontally. Each small box is 1 mm wide and 1 mm high (Fig. 12-6). There are five small boxes in one big box. The vertical boxes measure voltage (or amplitude) of the ECG waveforms (or deflections) using millivolt (mV). Each vertical box represents 0.1 mV and each big box equals to 0.5 mV. The horizontal boxes measure time using second. Each small box is measured 1 mm, and it represents 0.04 second and each big box (five small boxes) equals to 0.2 second. The horizontal boxes are used to measure the duration of time required for electrical impulse to travel through the heart, which provides important information on the function of cardiac conduction system and cardiac muscle itself.[5]

The waveforms of the cardiac cycle can be recorded by a bedside cardiac monitor and displayed continuously on an oscilloscope or recorded on a rhythm strip, which consists of the same grid as described previously. The standard 12-lead ECG simultaneously records 12 different views of electrical activity as it travels through the heart and displays all 12 views on a full-page layout, which consists of the same grid. The 12 leads of the ECG are described in detail in following sections.

Determining Heart Rate on the ECG

It is important to determine the heart rate; changes in heart rate may affect blood pressure and cardiac output. In general, the

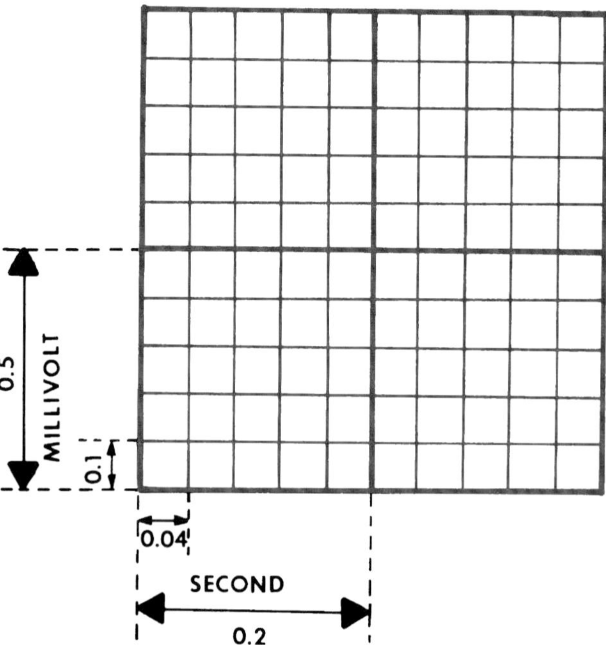

Figure 12-6. Time and voltage lines on ECG paper at standard paper speed of 25 mm/s. Horizontal axis measures time: each small box = 0.04 second, one large box = 0.20 second. Vertical axis measures voltage: each small box = 1 mm or 0.1 mV, one large box = 5 mm or 0.5 mV.

atrial and ventricular rates are the same with exceptions of some dysrhythmias. Thus, it is important to evaluate both atrial and ventricular rates which may be performed using several different methods.

Six-Second Method

Most ECG paper has 3-second or 6-second markers at the top of the paper (see Fig. 12-7); thus, calculating the heart rate using the 6-second method is easily performed. Without the 3-second or 6-second markers, clinicians can measure a 6-second strip by calculating a total of 30 large boxes (5 large boxes = 1 second, 30 large boxes ÷ 5 large boxes = 6 seconds). To determine the atrial rate, count the number of P waves on the 6-second strip and multiple by 10. The same process applies to calculate the ventricular rate, counting the number of QRS complexes. The 6-second method can be used for both regular and irregular rhythms.[5,7]

Large Box Method

There are 300 large boxes (30 large boxes/6 seconds × 10) in 1 minute. To determine the ventricular rate, count the number of large boxes in one R-R interval and divide into 300. The same principle applies to calculating the atrial rate using the P-P interval. The large box method is best applied to a regular rhythm. Using the large box method for an irregular rhythm will depend upon the given heart rate range.[5,7] Table 12-1 provides a quick reference for calculating heart rate using large box method.

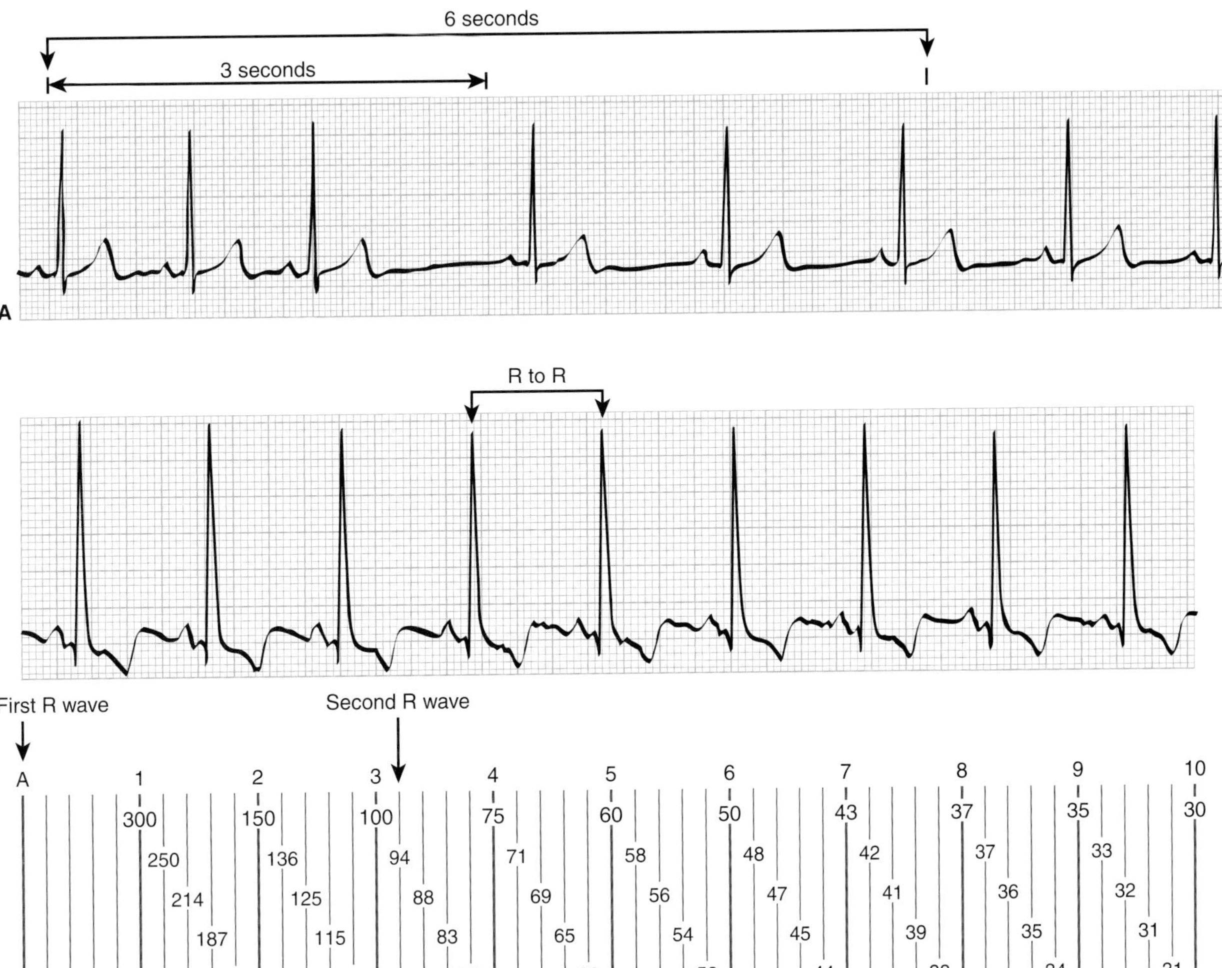

Figure 12-7. A: Heart rate determination for an irregular rhythm. Count the number or R-R intervals in a 6-second strip and multiply by 10. In **(A)** there are five complete R-R intervals in a 6-second strip; the heart rate is about 50 beats per minute. **B:** Heart rate determination for a regular rhythm using the rate ruler. Count the number of large and small boxes between R waves on the rhythm strip. In **(B)** there are three *large boxes* and one small box between the R waves marked on the strip. On the rate ruler, the first R wave is represented by the thick line marked "A." Each large box on the ECG paper is represented by a thick line on the rate ruler and is numbered at the top; each small box on the strip is represented by a *thin line* on the ruler. The number on the line on the ruler that corresponds to the second R wave on the strip represents the heart rate. In **(B)**, count three *large boxes* at the top of the ruler and then one *small box*; the heart rate is 94 beats per minute. (Rate ruler in B, from Marriott HJL. *Practical electrocardiography*. 8th ed. Baltimore: Williams & Wilkins; 1988:15.)

Table 12-1 • CALCULATE HEART RATE USING LARGE BOX METHOD

Calculate Heart Rate Using Large Box Method	
Number of Large Boxes	**Heart Rate (Bpm)**
1	300
2	150
3	100
4	75
5	60
6	50
7	43
8	38
9	33
10	30

Small Box Method

The principles of calculating heart rate using the large box method can also be applied to the small box method. There is a total of 1500 small boxes in 1 minute (60 s/min divided by 0.04 s/box = 1500 boxes/min). To calculate the ventricular rate, count the number of small boxes between the R-R intervals and divide into 1500. The same concept applies to calculating the atrial rate using the P-P interval. Counting the small boxes can be time consuming; however, it provides an accurate calculation of the heart rate. Table 12-2 provides a quick reference for calculating heart rate using small box method. Figure 12-7 demonstrates heart rate determination using a heart rate ruler.

Determining the Cardiac Rhythm on the ECG

The first step in interpreting an ECG is to determine the cardiac rhythm. A rhythm strip should be analyzed in a systematic manner

Table 12-2 • CALCULATE HEART RATE USING SMALL BOX METHOD

Calculate Heart Rate Using Small Box Method			
Number of Small Boxes	**Heart Rate (Bpm)**	**Number of Small Boxes**	**Heart Rate (Bpm)**
5	300	28	54
6	250	29	52
7	214	30	50
8	188	31	48
9	167	32	47
10	150	33	45
11	136	34	44
12	125	35	43
13	115	36	42
14	107	37	41
15	100	38	40
16	94	39	39
17	88	40	38
18	83	41	37
19	79	42	36
20	75	43	35
21	71	44	34
22	68	45	33
23	65	46	33
24	62	47	32
25	60	48	31
26	58	49	31
27	56	50	30

to aid in rhythm interpretation. With experience, arrhythmias may be identified by scanning the strip. The following steps provide a systematic approach to rhythm interpretation. The rhythm is determined based on an analysis of the information obtained in these steps.

Step 1: Regularity. First determine if the rhythm is regular or irregular; this information determines the method of heart rate calculation.

1. Is the rhythm regular? Do the P-P and R-R intervals "march out" (i.e., are the P-P intervals the same duration throughout? Are the R-R intervals the same throughout?)?
2. If the rhythm is irregular, does it have a pattern? In other words, is the rhythm regularly irregular or irregularly irregular?

Step 2: Rate. Calculate the heart rate using the methods described. Examine both the atrial and ventricular rate to determine if these are the same.

Step 3: P Wave. Evaluate the P waves for morphology and relationship to the QRS complex.

1. Are there P waves?
2. Do all the P waves look the same (i.e., are they morphologically identical? Does the morphology suggest that they originate from the SA node?)?
3. Is each P wave followed by a QRS complex (i.e., did each atrial depolarization result in ventricular depolarization?)?
4. Does the P wave occur before or after the QRS complex?
5. If not all the P waves are followed by a QRS complex, is there a pattern? For example, is there a QRS complex missing after every other P wave?

Step 4: PR Interval. Measure the PR interval of several complexes in a row to determine if it is of normal duration and consistent for all QRS complexes.

1. Is the PR interval within the defined normal range (0.12 to 0.2 second)?
2. Are all PR intervals the same length?

Step 5: QRS Characteristics. Examine the QRS width to determine if it is normal or wide (normal 0.04 to 0.10 second).[5,7]

12-LEAD ECG

The ECG summarizes the cardiac electrical activity of the heart in three dimensions. A 12-lead ECG records electrical activity as it spreads through the heart from 12 different leads that are recorded through electrodes placed on the arms, legs, and specific spots on the chest. Each lead represents a different view of the heart and consists of two electrodes with opposite polarity (bipolar), or one electrode and a reference point (unipolar). A bipolar lead has a positive pole and a negative pole, with each contributing equally to the recording. A unipolar lead has one positive pole and a reference pole in the center of the chest that is algebraically determined by the ECG machine. The reference pole represents the center of the electrical field of the heart and has a zero potential, so only the positive pole of a unipolar lead contributes to the tracing. One electrode is connected to the positive input of the ECG machine and the other to the negative input.[12] As compared to basic 3- or

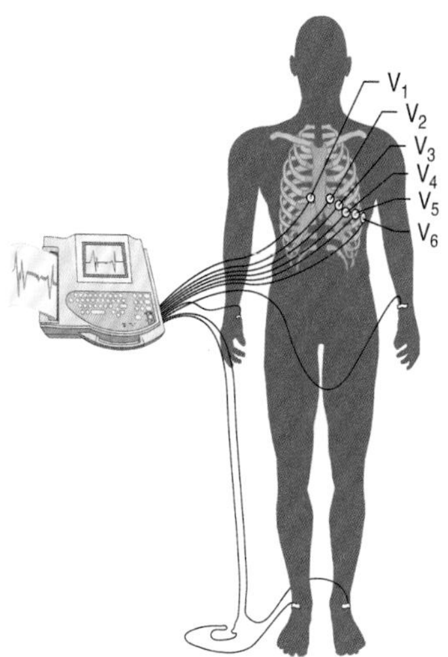

Figure 12-8. 12-lead electrodes placement. Electrode placement for limb leads and precordial leads. Limb electrodes can be placed anywhere on the arms and legs. Chest electrodes are placed as follows: V_1 = fourth intercostal space at right sternal border; V_2 = fourth intercostal space at left sternal border; V_3 = halfway between V_2 and V_4 in a straight line; V_4 = fifth left intercostal space at midclavicular line; V_5 = fifth left intercostal space at anterior axillary line; V_6 = fifth left intercostal space at midaxillary line. (Courtesy of T. Eric Goffier.)

5-lead ECG, the 12-lead ECG has additional electrodes, placed to provide supplementary views by recording the voltage difference between positive and negative electrodes. Thus, the 12-lead ECG enhances the sensitivity to a specific region of the heart by providing more diagnostic information.[6]

The standard 12-lead ECG consists of six limb leads and six precordial leads. The limb leads can be placed anywhere on all four extremities. The limb leads view the heart from the frontal plane and record the associated electrical activities: Electrical impulse travels up and down and right to left of the heart. For convenience in continuous bedside monitoring, arm electrodes can be placed on the shoulders and leg electrodes on the lower part of the rib cage rather than on the limbs without significantly altering the signals recorded. The precordial leads are placed on the chest (Fig. 12-8). The precordial leads view the heart from the horizontal plane and capture the associated electrical activities: electrical current travels from anterior to posterior, and right to left of the body.[7]

A camera analogy makes the 12-lead ECG easier to understand (Fig. 12-9). Each lead of the ECG represents a picture of the electrical activity in the heart taken by a camera. In any lead, the positive electrode is the recording electrode or the camera lens. The negative electrode tells the camera which way to "shoot" its picture and determines the direction in which the positive electrode records. When the positive electrode detects electrical activity traveling toward it, it records an upright deflection on the ECG. When the positive electrode detects electrical activity traveling away from it, it records a negative deflection. If a positive electrode is positioned where electrical activity travels toward it and then away from it, a diphasic deflection is recorded. If the electrical activity travels perpendicular to a positive electrode, no activity is recorded. The 12-lead ECG records three bipolar frontal plane leads—lead I, lead II, and lead III; three unipolar frontal plane leads—aVR, aVL, and aVF; and six unipolar precordial leads: V_1, V_2, V_3, V_4, V_5, and V_6.[5–7]

Standard Limb Leads

Figure 12-10 demonstrates the orientation of standard limb leads. In each lead, the camera represents the recording electrode (positive electrode) of the lead, and the arrow represents the direction of ECG recording. In lead I, the positive electrode (camera lens) is located on the left arm, and it records the potential difference between left arm and the right arm. Lead I views the lateral surface of the left ventricle, and the normal depolarization usually produces a positive waveform in lead I. In lead II, the positive electrode is located on the left leg and looks toward the right arm. Lead II records the potential difference between left leg and right arm. Lead II looks at the bottom (inferior) surface of the left ventricle and the normal depolarization produces a positive waveform in lead II. Lead II is commonly used for cardiac monitoring because the position of lead II electrodes most closely resembles the normal electrical flow in the heart. In lead III, the camera is located in the left leg and looks toward the left arm and it records the potential difference in between left leg and left arm. Lead III views the inferior surface of the left ventricle.[5,7,13]

Augmented Limb Leads

Figure 12-11 demonstrates the orientation of augmented limb leads on the frontal plane. The camera represents the location of the positive electrode, and the direction of the lens represents the direction of the recording of the electrical activity. Lead

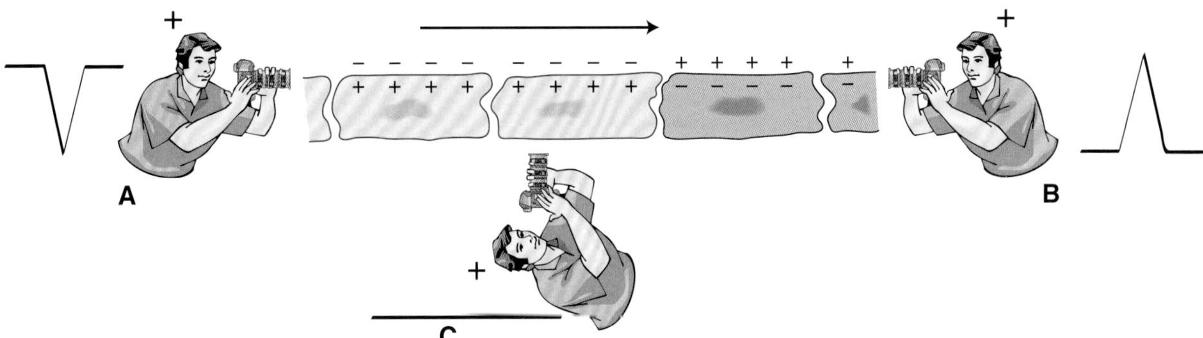

Figure 12-9. A strip of cardiac muscle depolarizing in the direction of the arrow. A positive electrode at **B** sees depolarization coming toward it and records an upright deflection. A positive electrode at **A** sees depolarization going away from it and records a negative deflection. A positive electrode at **C** records a flat line because depolarization is traveling perpendicular to the electrode's view.

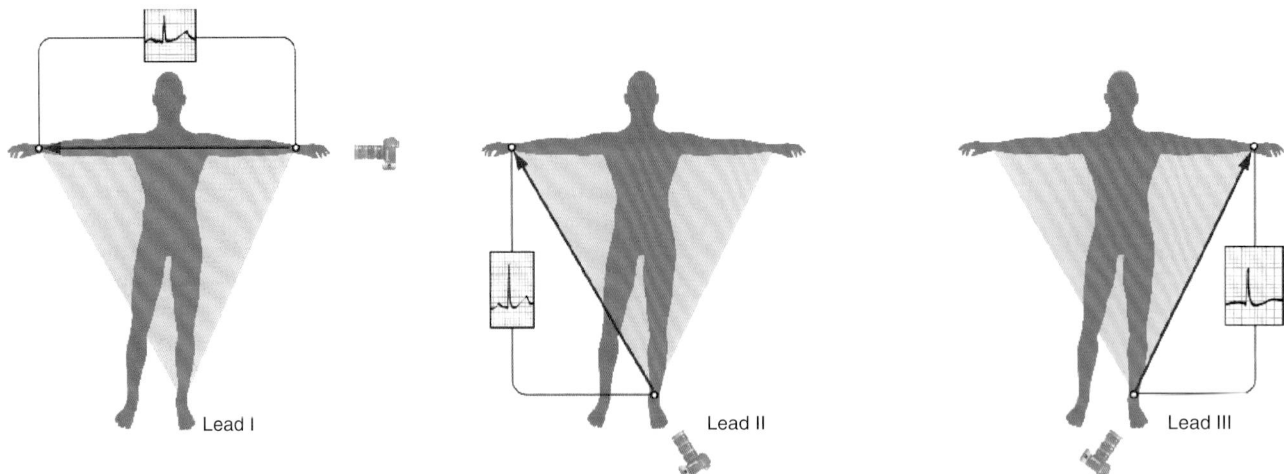

Figure 12-10. Standard limb leads. The camera represents the location of the positive electrode (recording electrode) looking toward the direction of the *red arrow head.* (Courtesy of T. Eric Goffier.)

aVR (think of R as "right") combines the view from the left arm and the left foot. The camera is located on the right shoulder and looks toward the center terminal. The wave of depolarization is moving away from the camera. Thus, the waveforms in this lead are typically negative. Lead aVL (think of L as "left"), combines the views from right arm and left leg. The camera is located on the left shoulder and oriented to the lateral wall of the left ventricle. Waveforms observed in lead aVL are usually positive (the wave of depolarization is moving toward the camera) but can be biphasic. Lead aVF (think of F as "foot") combines views from right arm and left arm toward left leg. The camera is located at the left foot and looks toward the bottom (inferior) portion of left ventricle. Waveforms observed in this lead are usually positive but may be biphasic.[7] The red arrow head in Figure 12-11 presents direction of recording of the electrical activity.

Precordial Leads

Figure 12-12 shows the six chest leads recording locations on the chest and the "shooting" direction toward the center of the chest. Lead V_1 is placed in the fourth intercostal space to the right of the sternum, and it views the interventricular septum of the heart. Lead V_2 is placed in the further intercostal space to the left of the sternum, it views the interventricular septum. Lead V_3 is placed on the midway between the lead V_2 and V_4, and lead V_4 is placed in the left midclavicular line in the fifth intercostal space. Both lead V_3 and V_4 provide the view of anterior surface of heart. Lead V_5 and V_6 are located in the left anterior axillary line at the same level of lead V_4. Both lead V_5 and V_6 look at the lateral surface of the heart. Table 12-3 shows "which leads look where" in the heart, and the coronary artery supplying that particular area.

Right-Side and Posterior ECG

Right-side ECG provides further diagnostic information on right ventricular hypertrophy (RVH) and right ventricular infarction. To perform right-side ECG, simply place V_3 to V_6 to the right side of the chest (Fig. 12-13A). A posterior ECG can be performed when there are suspicions of posterior infarction. Additional leads V_7 to V_9 are placed on the same horizontal line as

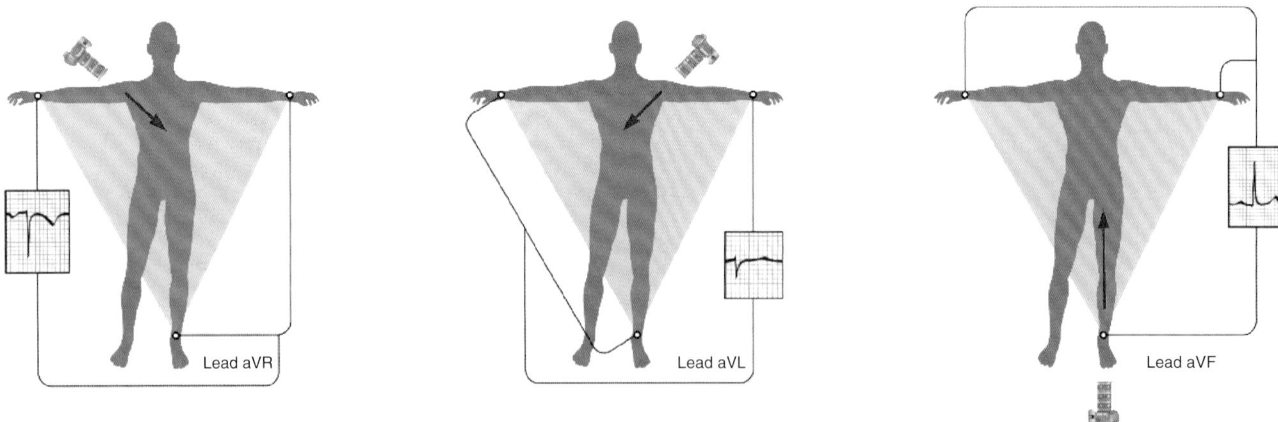

Figure 12-11. Augmented limb leads. The camera represents the location of the positive electrode (recording electrode), looking toward center terminal (the direction of the *red arrow head*). Waveforms in both lead aVL and aVF can be biphasic, because of the direction of ventricular depolarization. (Courtesy of T. Eric Goffier.)

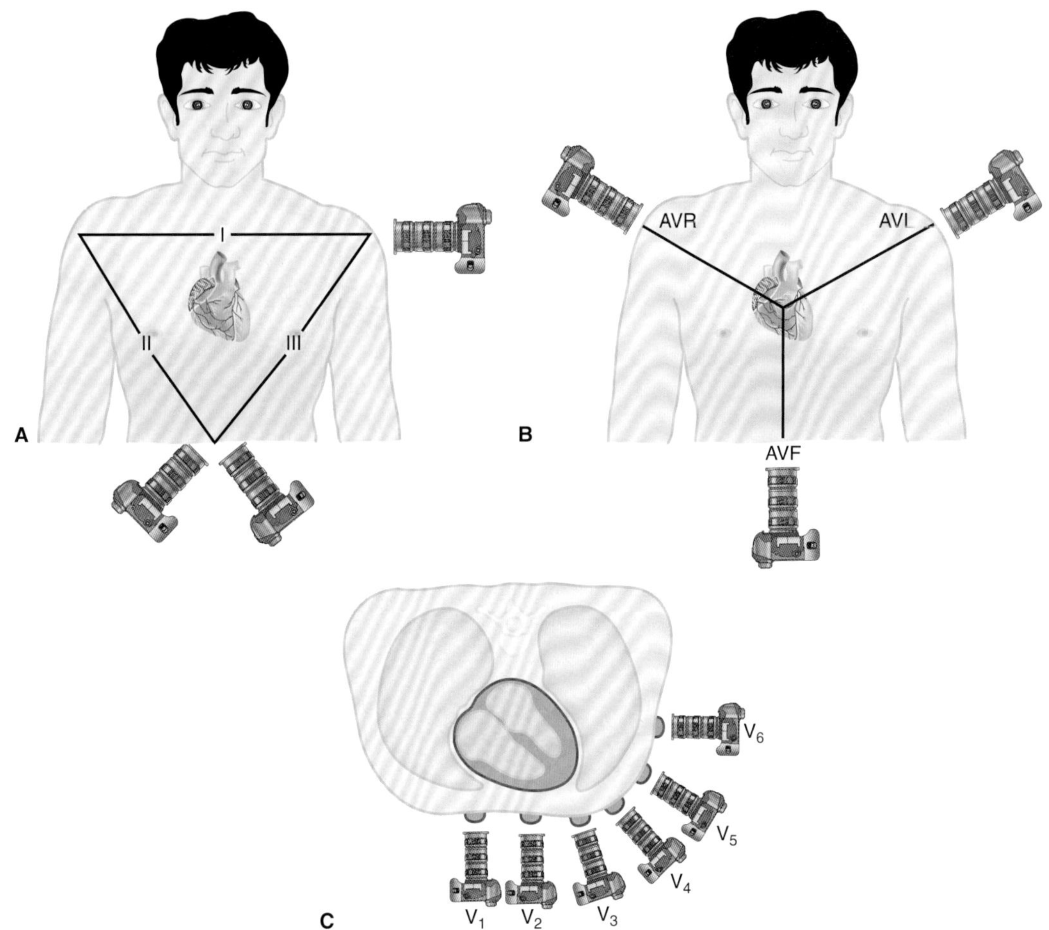

Figure 12-12. The camera represents the location of the positive, or recording, electrode in each lead. **A:** Bipolar frontal plane leads I, II, and III. **B:** Unipolar frontal plane leads aVR, aVL, and aVF. **C:** Unipolar precordial leads V_1–V_6.

V_4 to V_6 and further left toward the back (Figure 12-13B shows the placement of additional leads for posterior ECG recording).[7]

The Hexaxial Reference System

The hexaxial reference system, also known as cardiac axis wheel, refers to the mean direction of the electrical wave of ventricular depolarization in the vertical plane (Fig. 12-14).[14] The axis wheel measures from zero reference point, aligning with the same viewpoint as lead I. The axis above the zero reference point is labeled as negative numbers, and what below the zero reference point is labeled as positive numbers. The axis wheel demonstrates the angle and viewpoint of each lead.[7,14]

Table 12-3 • ANATOMICAL RELATIONSHIPS BETWEEN ECG LEADS AND AREAS OF THE HEART

I: Circumflex	aVR: None	V_1 Septum		V_4: LAD
II: RCA	aVL: Circumflex	V_2 Septum		V_5: Circumflex
III: RCA	aVF: RCA	V_3: LAD		V_6: Circumflex

Lateral Wall I, aVL, V_5, V_6
Inferior Wall II, III, aVF
Anterior Wall V_1 to V_4
Septum V_1, V_2

The 12 Views of the Heart

In a normal conduction system, the electrical impulse originates from the SA node, spreads downward toward the AV node and leftward to the left atrium. In lead I and aVL, the positive

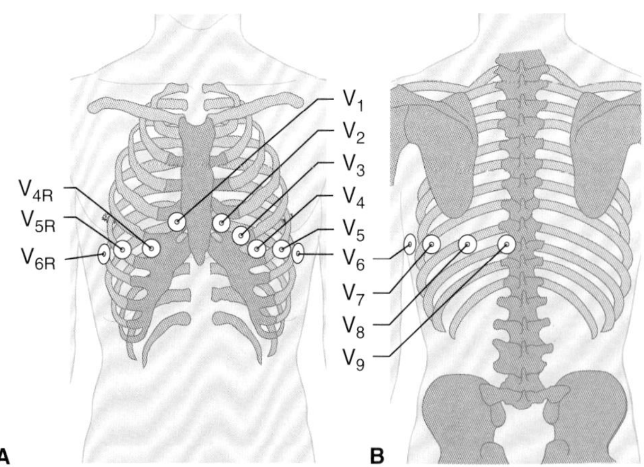

Figure 12-13. **A:** Electrode placement for standard precordial and right precordial leads. Only three right-sided leads are needed: V_{4R}, right fifth intercostal space at midclavicular line; V_{5R}, right fifth intercostal space at anterior axillary line; V_{6R}, right fifth intercostal space at midaxillary line. **B:** Electrode placement for posterior leads: V_7, left posterior axillary line; V_8, tip of left scapula; V_9, left border of spine. All three are in the same horizontal plane of V_4 to V_6.

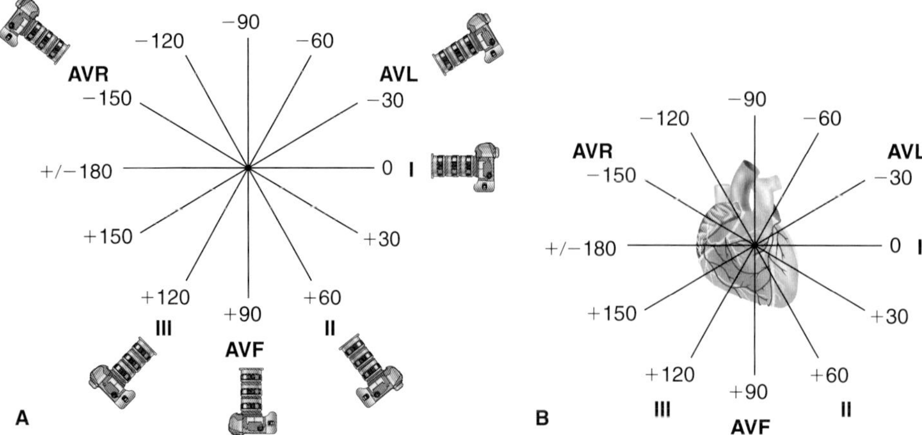

Figure 12-14. Hexaxial reference system (or axis wheel). Each lead is labeled at its positive end in both examples. **A:** All six frontal plane leads bisect each other. The degrees of the axis wheel are shown. **B:** The axis wheel superimposed on the heart to demonstrate each lead's view of the heart. Leads I and aVL face the left lateral wall, leads II, III, and aVF face the inferior surface. Lead aVR does not face a ventricular surface.

electrodes (camera lens) located on the left side of the body look at atrial depolarization moving toward them. Thus, both lead I and aVL capture an upright P wave. In lead aVR, the camera lens located on the right arm looks at the electrical impulse travel away from it and captures a downward deflection of P wave. In leads II, III, and aVF, the positive electrode located in the bottom of the heart, looks upward at the electrical impulse traveling toward them, and records a positive P wave. Figure 12-15A demonstrates normal sequence of depolarization through the heart as recorded by each of the frontal plane leads.

No electrical activity is recorded when the impulse travels through AV node due to small size of the AV node. When the electrical impulse exits the AV node, it spreads through the bundle of His before entering the left and right bundle branches. The Purkinje fibers bring the impulse into the septum and cause septum to depolarize first in the left-to-right direction. The impulse then arrives at the Purkinje system of both ventricles concurrently and initiates the depolarization from endocardium to epicardium (a small arrow in Figure 12-15B demonstrates the depolarization direction). The main direction of averaged electrical impulses is downward, leftward, and posterior toward left ventricle. The larger arrow in Figure 12-15B represents the net direction of the ventricular depolarization and it is known as mean axis.[7]

During ventricular depolarization, a small negative (downward) deflection (Q wave) is observed in lead I and aVL because the septum depolarizes away from their positive electrodes. Then the large left ventricular wall depolarization results in an upright deflection (R wave). In leads II, III and aVF, they may or may not capture the septal activity. When these leads see the downward septal activities toward them, they will produce positive deflections. The left ventricle then moves the electrical force toward them and results in any positive (upright) deflection. Lead aVR sees all the electrical activities moving away from it and register a downward negative deflection.[7]

The precordial leads capture the electrical activity spreading through the horizontal plane. Figure 12-15B shows the orientation of precordial leads and how they record the electrical activities as they travel through the ventricles. Septal depolarization from left to right results in a small R wave in lead V_1. As the left ventricle depolarizes (electrical current spread away), lead V_1 records a deep downward S wave.[7]

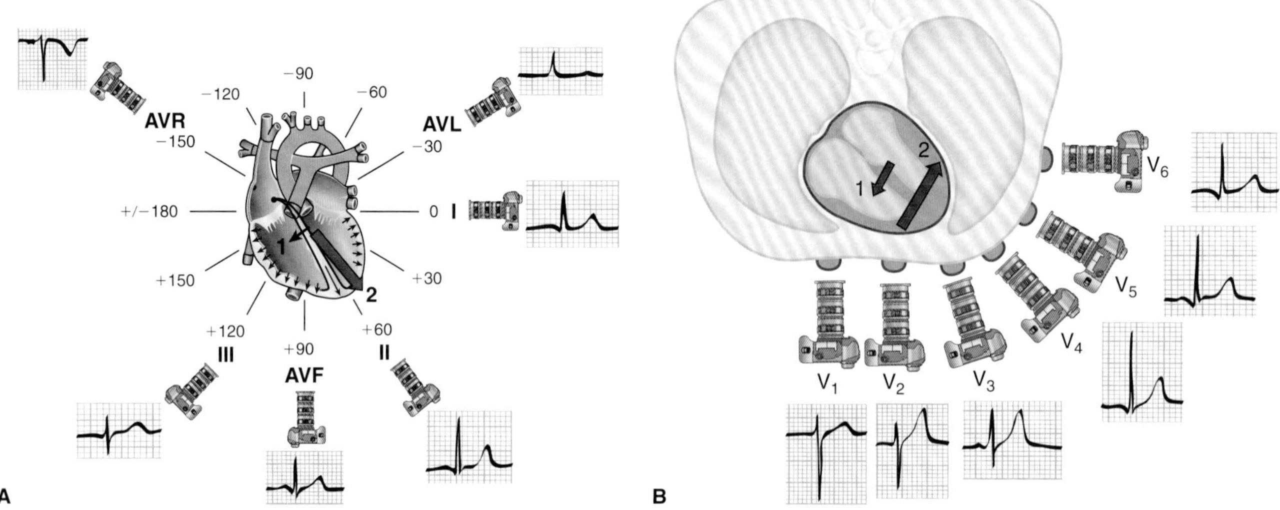

Figure 12-15. **A:** Normal sequence of depolarization through the heart as recorded by each of the frontal plane leads. **B:** Cross section of the thorax illustrating how the six precordial leads record the normal ECG. In both examples, the *small arrow* (*1*) shows the initial direction of depolarization through the septum, followed by the mean direction of ventricular free wall depolarization, *larger arrow* (*2*).

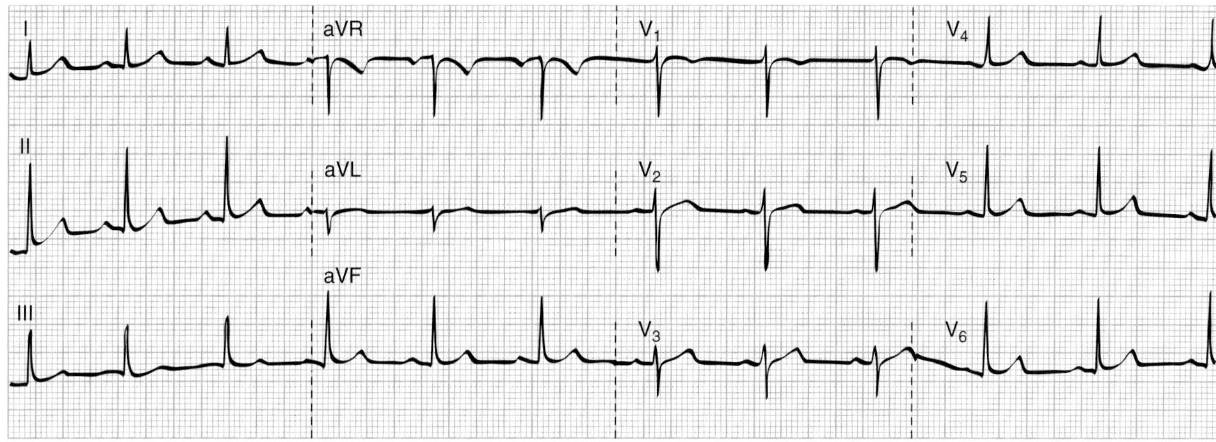

Figure 12-16. Normal 12-lead ECG.

Precordial leads allow for the assessment of R wave progression: in the normal heart, the R wave in these leads typically becomes progressively larger from V_1 to V_6. Compared to the S wave, the R wave in lead V_6 is predominant in lead V_6. Poor R-wave progression in the precordial leads has been associated with various cardiac conditions, such as acute MI, LVH, RVH, and a variant of normal with diminished anterior forces.[15–17]

Figure 12-16 shows a normal 12-lead ECG. Normal sinus rhythm is present at a rate of 70 bpm, and the axis is approximately +60 degrees. P waves are normal (flat P waves in aVL is a normal variant), and T waves are normal (flat or slightly inverted in lead aVL and V_1 is a normal variant). The QRS complex is normal (0.08 second wide), there are no abnormal Q waves, and R-wave progression is normal across the precordium. The ST segment is at baseline in all leads. This ECG can be used for comparison as abnormalities are discussed throughout this chapter.[7]

AXIS DETERMINATION

Figure 12-17A illustrates the sequential instantaneous vectors generated by ventricular depolarization. The eight instantaneous vectors are only representations of thousands of electrical potentials moving in multiple directions. The electrical charge of more than 80% of these electrical potentials are "canceled out" by the similar instantaneous vectors travelling in the opposite directions. The mean vector represents an average of all the instantaneous vectors. The direction of the mean vector (Fig. 12-17B), known as mean electrical axis, represents the sum of all of the mean electrical vectors occurring during ventricular depolarization. This section will only discuss the QRS axis determination.[7,18]

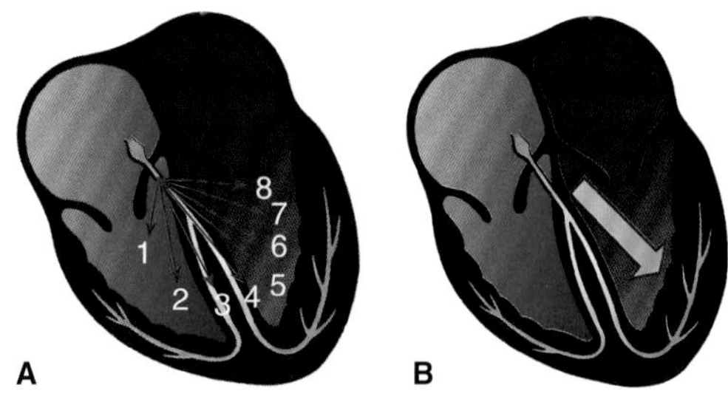

Figure 12-17. A: Eight sequential instantaneous vectors represent ventricular depolarization. In this figure, we only show only instantaneous vectors as a representation. **B:** The single vector (*big yellow arrow*) summarizes all the instantaneous vectors and it represents the mean vector and. The direction of the *arrow* represents the axis of ventricular depolarization.

The average of electrical force flow travels leftward and inferiorly during the entire ventricular depolarization. In Figure 12-18, the mean electrical axis is depicted by a green arrow. In this example, the mean electrical axis is approximately +40 degrees. The normal QRS axis ranges from −30 to +90 degrees. Left axis deviation (LAD) is defined as −31 to −90 degrees, at which most of the electrical currents travels in a leftward and upward direction. The right axis deviation (RAD) is defined as +91 to +180 degrees, under which most of the electrical force moves rightward. Table 12-5 shows the potential causes of LAD and RAD.[7]

Indeterminate axis or extreme axis is defined as the electrical current travels upward and rightward between −91 and −180 degrees. This deviation can occur in ventricular tachycardia (VT) and occasionally bifascicular block.[7] Figure 12-19 displays the axis wheels separated into its normal, LAD, RAD, and indeterminate sections.

The most accurate method to determine frontal QRS axis deviation is to average the electrical forces moving right and left with those moving up and down. Lead I and aVF can be used to define QRS axis deviation, because lead I represents the most direct right/left lead and lead aVF is the most direct up/down lead. Figure 12-20A demonstrates an example of frontal leads in 12-lead ECG. Figure 12-20B shows the enlarged leads I and aVF along with axis wheels and small hash marks representing the electrical force: each hash mark equals to 1-mV box on the ECG paper. Below are the steps to determine the mean QRS axis.

Step 1: Examine Lead I. Determine the number of positive and negative boxes on the QRS complex in lead I. Lead I is predominantly positive and has no significance of negative deflection. There is a total of eight positive boxes in lead I. Count 8 hash marks toward the positive end of lead I and marks the spot on the axis wheel.

Table 12-4 • ECG LOCALIZATION OF MYOCARDIAL ISCHEMIA/INFARCTION

I: Lateral	aVR: none	V_1: Septum/Anterior	V_4: Anterior
II: Inferior	aVL: Lateral	V_2: Septum/Anterior	V_5: Lateral
III: Inferior	aVF: Inferior	V_3: Anterior	V_6: Lateral

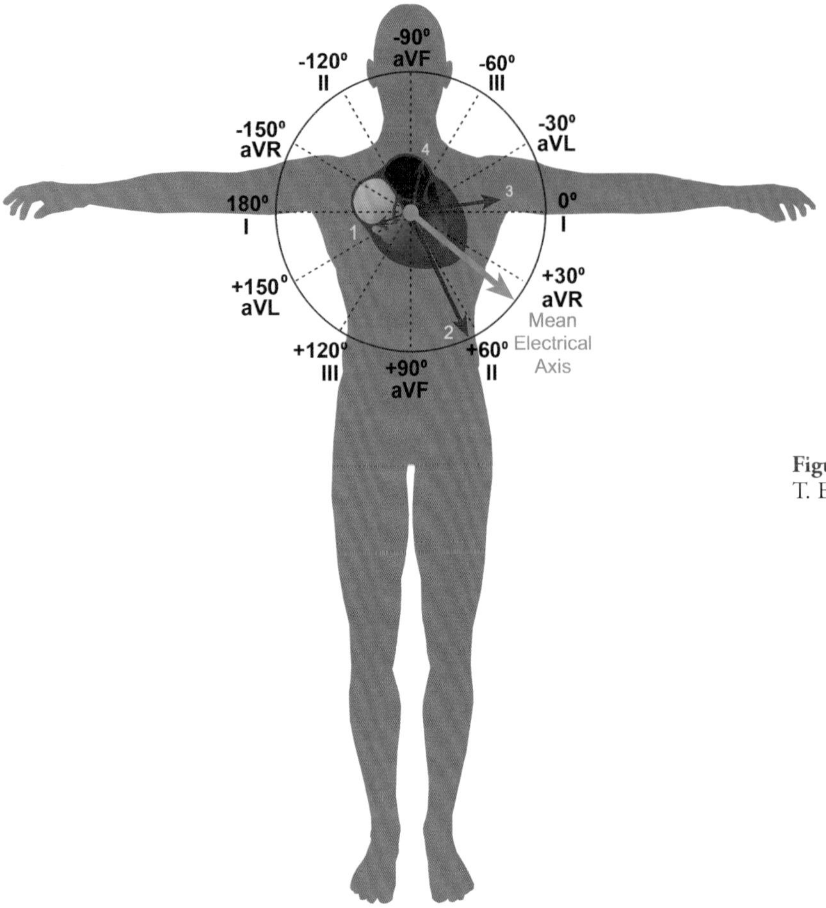

Figure 12-18. Axis in 12-lead ECG. (Courtesy of T. Eric Goffier.)

Step 2: Examine Lead aVF. Determine the number of positive and negative boxes on the QRS complex in lead aVF. Lead aVF is predominantly positive and shows no significance of negative deflection. There is a total of 14 positive boxes in lead aVF. Count 14 hash marks toward the positive end of aVF axis and marks the spot on the axis wheel.

Step 3: Examine Lead I and Lead aVF. Draw a perpendicular line down from the mark on the lead I axis and a perpendicular line from the mark on the lead aVF axis.

Step 4: Mean of the QRS Axis. Draw a line from the center of the axis wheel to the point where these two perpendicular lines meet. This line is the mean QRS axis—approximately +60 degrees. There is no axis deviation when the mean value lies within the normal zone of the axis wheel.

Table 12-5 • POSSIBLE CAUSES OF LAD AND RAD

Possible Causes of LAD	Possible Causes of RAD
Left ventricular hypertrophy	Right ventricular hypertrophy
Left anterior fascicular block	Left posterior fascicular block
Inferior myocardial infarction	Right bundle branch block
Left bundle branch block	Dextrocardia
Congenital defects	Ventricular tachycardia
Arrhythmias (ventricular tachycardia, Wolff–Parkinson–White syndrome)	Wolff–Parkinson–White syndrome

A quick but less accurate method to determine axis deviation is to place the axis in its proper quadrant of the axis wheel by looking at leads I and aVF, because these leads divide the wheel into four quadrants. If the QRS in both of these leads is positive, the axis falls in the normal quadrant, 0 to +90 degrees. If the QRS in lead I is positive and the QRS in aVF is negative, the axis falls in the left quadrant, 0 to −90 degrees; this is LAD. If the QRS in lead I is negative and the QRS in aVF is positive, the axis falls in the right quadrant, +90 to +180 degrees; this is RAD. This may be summarized by the mnemonic "left apart, right together" (Fig. 12-21). When the Q wave

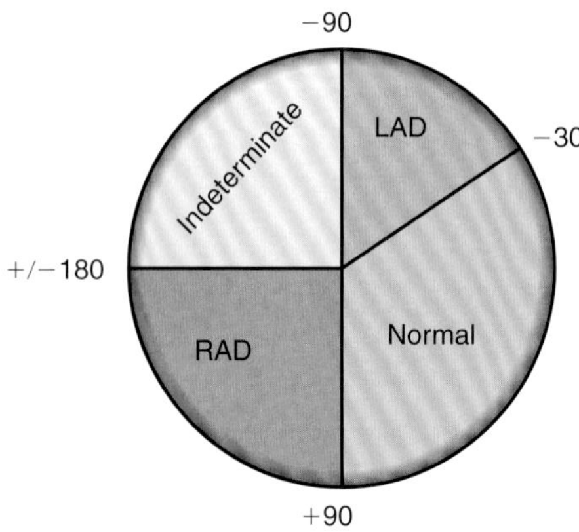

Figure 12-19. Normal axis = −30° to +90°, LAD = −31° to −90°, RAD = +91° to +180°, indeterminate axis = −91° to −180°.

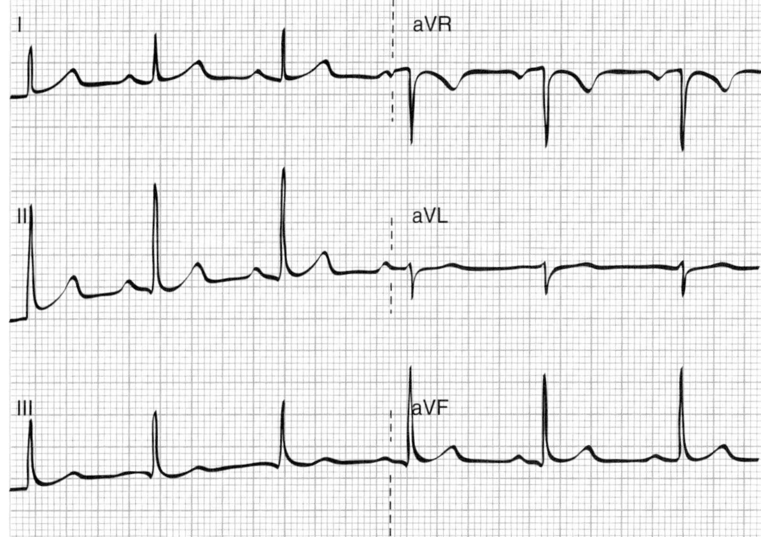

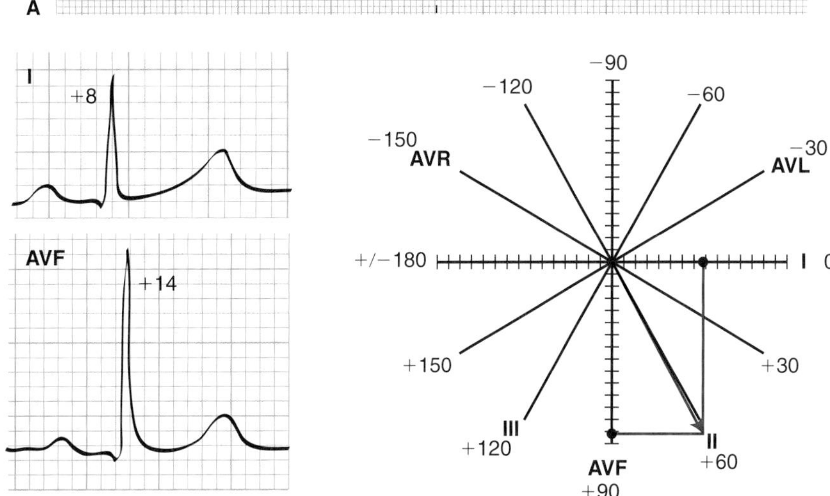

Figure 12-20. Calculating the mean QRS axis. **A:** The six frontal plane leads of an ECG. **B:** Lead I and lead aVF enlarged. See text for instructions on calculating the axis using leads I and aVF on the axis wheel.

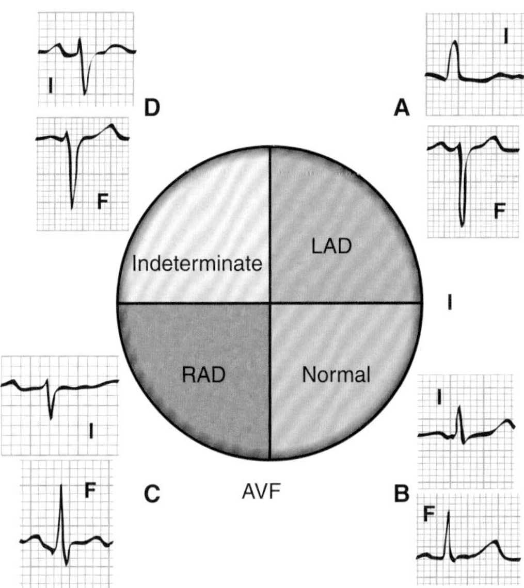

Figure 12-21. The four quadrants of the axis wheel. **A:** If the QRS in lead I is positive and the QRS in aVF is negative, the axis is in the left quadrant. **B:** If the QRS is positive in both leads I and aVF, the axis is normal. **C:** If the QRS in lead I is negative and the QRS in aVF is positive, the axis is in the right quadrant. **D:** If the QRS is negative in both leads I and aVF, the axis is indeterminate.

points downward in lead I and upward in lead aVF, the electrical current is traveling in the same direction ("right" together) and there is a RAD. When the Q wave points upward in lead I and downward in aVF, the electrical current is traveling in opposite directions ("left" apart) and there is a potential LAD.[19] If the QRS complexes in lead I and aVF (double negative) point downward, the axis falls in the indeterminate quadrant or "no-man's land," −90 to −180 degrees. This is an indeterminate axis deviation.[19,20]

Locating the correct quadrant is often adequate for the determination of QRS axis. However, because the section of the left quadrant between 0 and −30 degrees is considered normal, it is necessary to define whether the axis is less or greater than −30 degrees. To do this quickly, look at lead II: if the QRS in lead II is positive, meaning the electrical activity travels toward the positive electrode of lead II, the axis is less than −30 degrees; if the QRS in lead II is negative, representing electrical activity travels away from the positive electrode of lead II, the axis is more negative than −30 degrees indicating LAD.[19,20]

INTRAVENTRICULAR CONDUCTION ABNORMALITIES

The intraventricular conduction system is viewed to include three major fascicles separate from the bundle of His: right bundle

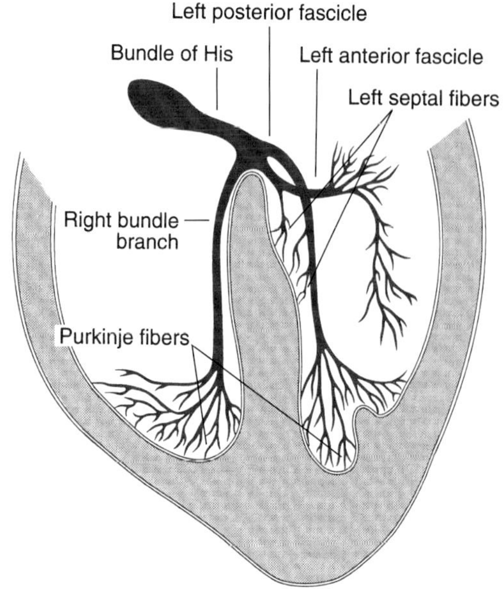

Figure 12-22. Intraventricular conduction system. Right bundle branch carries impulse into right ventricle. Left main bundle branch divides into anterior and posterior fascicles, which carry impulse into left ventricle.

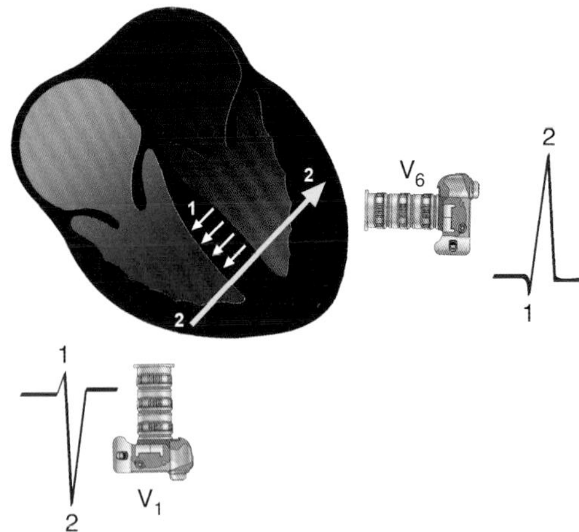

Figure 12-23. Normal ventricular depolarization. The number *1* represents the small electrical current generated by a septal depolarization, which is reflected as a small R wave in lead V_1. Then the number *2* represents the main current moves away from the positive electrode of lead V_1 and creates a large negative S wave, which results in an rS complex in V_1. In lead V_6, a small negative Q wave is generated due to the septum is depolarized away from the positive electrode. A tall R wave in lead V_6 represents the electrical current travel toward left ventricle, which results in a normal qR complex in lead V_6. (Courtesy of T. Eric Goffier.)

branch, left anterior fascicle, and posterior fascicle. Conduction block can occur in any section of the intraventricular conduction system. Monofascicular block is defined as block in only one of the three fascicles. Bifascicular block is referred to as the combination of right bundle branch block (RBBB) and either left anterior fascicular block (LAFB) or left posterior fascicular block (LPFB). Trifascicular block is the block to all three major fascicles Figure 12-22 illustrates the intraventricular conduction system.[7]

Bundle Branch Block

Bundle branch block (BBB) is defined as a disturbance in electrical impulse conduction from bundle of His across either right or left bundle branch to the Purkinje fiber. The conduction delay results in abnormal spread of electrical activity through the affected ventricle and asynchronous ventricular depolarization.[7,20] BBB produces a widening QRS complex (a duration equal to 0.12 second or greater). The widened QRS characteristic can be best identified in precordial leads V_1 and V_6 and limb leads I and aVL.[7]

In the normal conduction system, the electrical current passes through the AV node and down the left bundle branch into the interventricular septum. The electrical impulse activates the septum by left posterior fascicle and results in a septal depolarization in left-to-right direction. Then both ventricles continue to depolarize from right to left.[7] Figure 12-23 illustrates normal ventricular depolarization recorded with lead V_1 and V_6.

Right Bundle Branch Block

When there is a RBBB, the electrical impulse travels through AV node and down left bundle branch into the interventricular septum. The septum is depolarized from left-to-right direction by the left posterior fascicle. As the left bundle continues to conduct the impulse, the left ventricle is depolarized from right-to-left direction. Then the impulse that depolarizes the left ventricle is conducted through the myocardial cells and depolarizes the right ventricle.[20] Figure 12-24 illustrates the spread of electrical impulses in the ventricles when the right bundle branch is blocked.

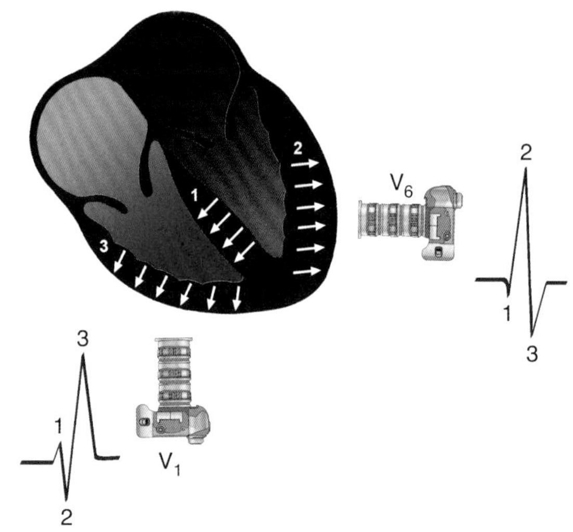

Figure 12-24. Ventricular depolarization in RBBB. *1*. Septal depolarization occurs first from left to right, resulting in the normal small R wave in V_1 and small Q wave in V_6.[7] *2*. The left ventricle is activated next through the normally functioning left bundle branch. Depolarization spreads normally through the Purkinje fibers in the left ventricle, causing an S wave in V_1 as the impulse travels away from its positive electrode and an R wave in V_6 as the impulse travels toward the positive electrode of lead V_6.[7] *3*. The right ventricle depolarizes late and abnormally. This abnormal activation causes a wide second R1 wave (called Rprime) in V_1 as it travels toward the positive electrode in V_1, and a wide S wave in V_6 as it travels away from the positive electrode in V_6. Because muscle cell-to-cell conduction is much slower than conduction through the Purkinje system, the QRS complex widens to 0.12 second or greater.[7] (Courtesy of T. Eric Goffier.)

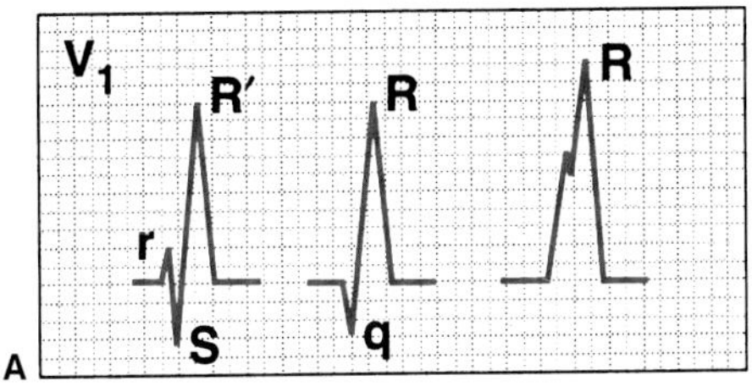

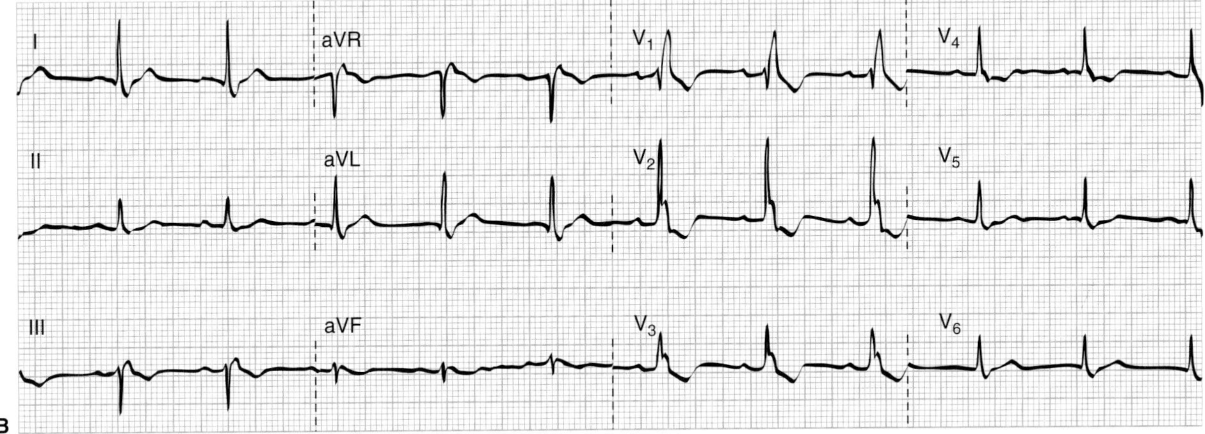

Figure 12-25. A: Three commonly seen variations of RBBB pattern. **B:** 12-lead ECG illustrating RBBB.

Typical uncomplicated RBBB can be recognized by a wide rSR' pattern in V_1 and a wide qRs pattern in V_6 and in leads I and aVL, because the positive electrodes in these two limb leads are located on the left side of the body. Figure 12-25B illustrates three variations of the RBBB pattern most commonly seen. If a patient with RBBB has a septal MI, the initial small R wave usually seen in lead V_1 in RBBB disappears because the septum no longer depolarizes normally from left to right, resulting in a qR pattern as seen in the second example in Figure 12-25B. Sometimes RBBB presents as a wide R wave in lead V_1 that may or may not be notched, as shown in the third example of Figure 12-25B. The ECG in Figure 12-25C is an example of typical RBBB.[7]

Left Bundle Branch Block

When there is a left bundle branch block (LBBB), the septum does not depolarize from left to right due to the obstructed impulse above the Purkinje fibers, which normally activate the septal depolarization. Instead, the septal depolarization is initiated by the right bundle branch, and electrical current travels from right to left, away from the positive electrode of lead V_1, thus a negative deflection is recorded in V_1 initially.[7]

Right ventricular depolarization then occurs, in which electrical current moves toward the positive electrode in V_1 and generates an upright notch in QRS complex on lead V_1. As the remainder of the left ventricle depolarizes from right to left through myocardial cells, a deep negative deflection (an S wave) is captured in lead V_1 due to large muscle mass of the left ventricle (Fig. 12-26).[7,20,21] Lead V_6 shows a wide, tall, entirely positive (R) wave due to the electrical current goes toward the positive electrode of lead V_6. With LBBB, the QS wave in lead V_1 sometimes shows a small notching at its point, giving the wave a characteristic W shape. Similarly, the broad R wave in lead V_6 may show a notching at its peak, giving it a distinctive M shape. (Figure 12-27 demonstrates two commonly seen patterns in LBBB).[22]

Differentiating Right and Left Bundle Branch Block

As previously discussed, BBB results in sequential ventricular depolarization. The last ventricle that depolarizes is the ventricle with blocked bundle branch. To elaborate, when the left bundle branch is blocked, the impulse will travel down the right bundle branch first and depolarize the right ventricle. The impulse then travels down the left ventricle and depolarize the left ventricle. When the right bundle branch is blocked, the impulse will travel down the left bundle branch first and depolarize the left ventricle. The impulse then travels down the right ventricle and depolarize the right ventricle. Based on this electrical conduction characteristic, if the morphology of last ventricular depolarization is identified, then it is possible to identify which bundle branch is blocked.[20]

The direction of the QRS complex represents the direction of electrical current, and the last portion of the QRS complex is identified as the terminal force, indicating the ventricle depolarizing

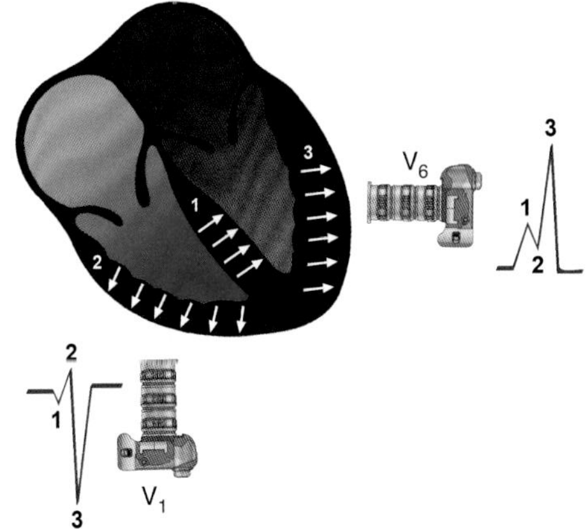

Figure 12-26. Ventricular depolarization in LBBB. (Courtesy of T. Eric Goffier.)

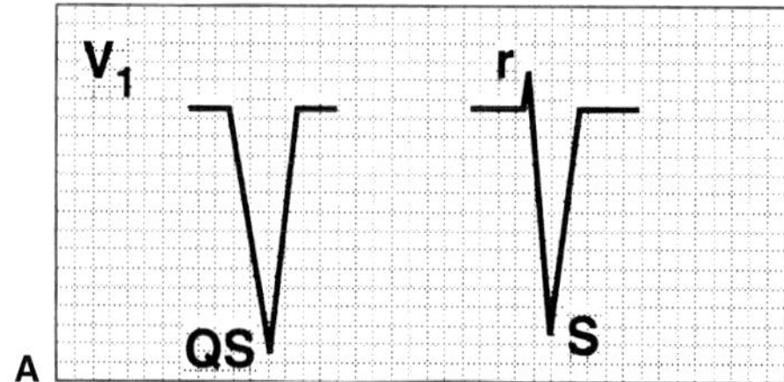

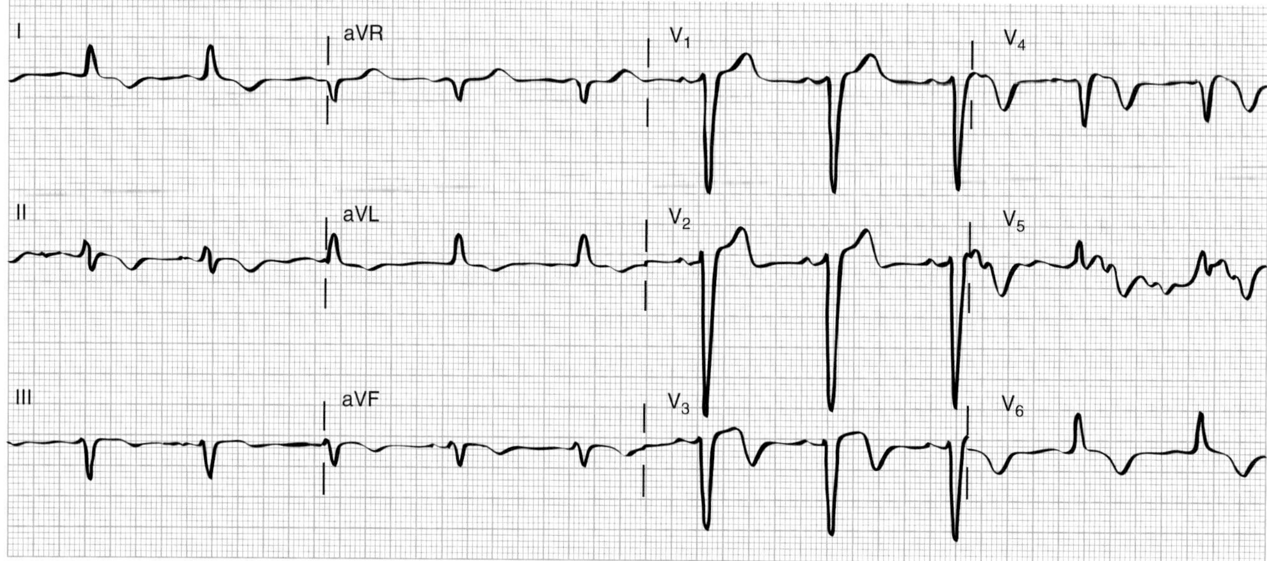

Figure 12-27. A: Two commonly seen patterns of LBBB. **B:** 12-lead ECG illustrates LBBB.

last. To examine the direction of electrical force, first locate the J point on the QRS in lead V_1. Then trace backward to the QRS to identify the positive or negative deflection of the QRS wave. If the right ventricle depolarizes last (the right bundle branch is blocked), the QRS will be an upward positive deflection due to the current travels from the left ventricle to the right ventricle toward the positive electrode of the lead V_1. If the left ventricle depolarizes last (the left bundle branch is blocked), the QRS will be a negative deflection due to the current travels from right to left ventricle and away from the positive electrode of lead V_1.[20] The rule of determining the terminal force of the QRS complex has been described in a simpler way using "turning signal" theory. To indicate a right turn, the arm of the turning signal needs to lift up. Likewise, the terminal force of the QRS complex points up when there is presence of RBBB. Conversely, with left turn, the terminal force of the QRS complex points downward.[20]

Fascicular Block

Fascicular block, also known as hemiblock, is defined as block in either division of the left bundle branch. Hemiblock commonly occurs with MI and is associated with diminished blood supply to anterior or posterior division of left bundle branch.[23] Both ventricles depolarize concurrently in fascicular block. Thus, the QRS complex remains narrow. Understanding axis deviation in lead I and aVF and typical patterns of fascicular block in lead I and III are particularly useful for recognizing fascicular block.[7]

When the left ventricular free wall is activated normally, the anterior fascicle carries the electrical impulse in a superior and leftward direction, and the posterior fascicle carries the electrical impulse downward and rightward. Because free wall activation proceeds in both directions simultaneously, most of the forces cancel each other and result in the normal QRS shape seen in leads I and III, and a normal QRS axis as the combined forces proceed downward and leftward through the left ventricle (Fig. 12-28A). When fascicular block occurs, left ventricular activation proceeds from one site instead of both simultaneously, removing the cancellation and altering the shape of the QRS in leads I and III. Because the left ventricle is depolarized in an abnormal direction, an axis deviation IS always a result from fascicular block, but the QRS duration remains normal or is very slightly prolonged.[7]

Left Anterior Fascicular Block

LAFB is also known as anterior hemiblock. Similar to BBB, the electrical impulse travels to the fascicle that is not blocked first, then to the blocked fascicle (Fig. 12-28B). Thus, in LAFB, the current depolarizes the ventricle in an inferior and rightward direction, then it travels through the left ventricular free wall in a superior and leftward direction and results in a LAD.[2] Figure 12-29 is an ECG example of RBBB and LAFB. The ECG characteristics of LAFB are described as the following.[24]

1. LAD (−45 degrees or more)
2. Small Q in lead I, large S in lead III (QI, SIII), or an rS pattern in leads II, III, and aVF
3. QRS duration not prolonged more than 0.11 second
4. Increased QRS voltage in limb leads due to loss of cancellation of forces in left ventricle

Left Posterior Fascicular Block

In LPFB, all the electrical current travels down the left anterior fascicle and depolarizes the ventricular myocardium in a

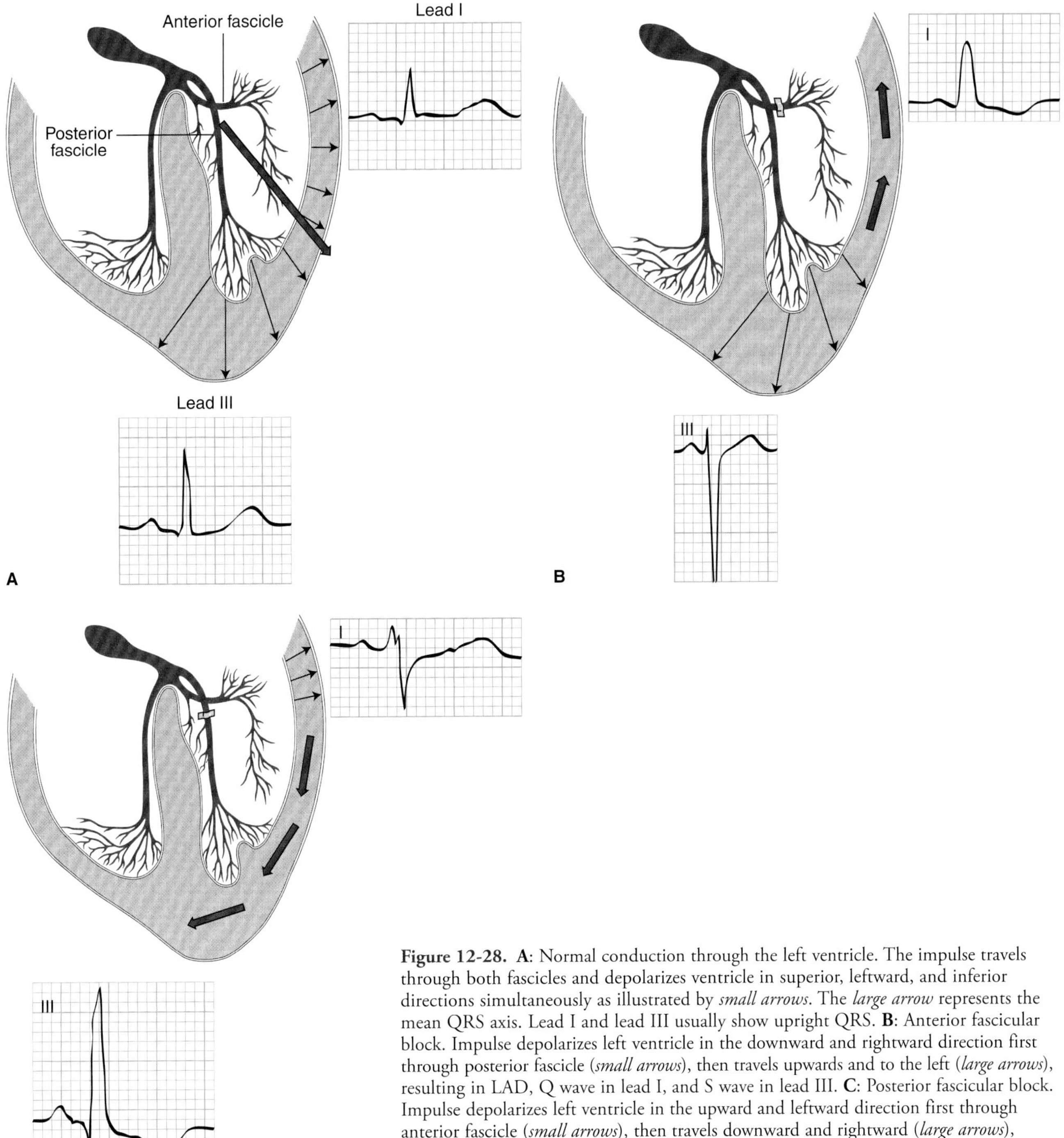

Figure 12-28. **A**: Normal conduction through the left ventricle. The impulse travels through both fascicles and depolarizes ventricle in superior, leftward, and inferior directions simultaneously as illustrated by *small arrows*. The *large arrow* represents the mean QRS axis. Lead I and lead III usually show upright QRS. **B**: Anterior fascicular block. Impulse depolarizes left ventricle in the downward and rightward direction first through posterior fascicle (*small arrows*), then travels upwards and to the left (*large arrows*), resulting in LAD, Q wave in lead I, and S wave in lead III. **C**: Posterior fascicular block. Impulse depolarizes left ventricle in the upward and leftward direction first through anterior fascicle (*small arrows*), then travels downward and rightward (*large arrows*), resulting in RAD, S wave in lead I, and Q wave in lead III.

superior-to-inferior and left-to-right direction (Fig. 12-28C). The axis of depolarization is directed downward and rightward, resulting in tall R waves in inferior leads, deep S waves in left lateral leads, and RAD. The QRS complex will be negative in lead I and positive in lead aVF.[21] Figure 12-30 is an ECG example of RBBB and LPFB. The ECG characteristics of LPFB are outlined.

1. RAD (greater than or equal to +100 degrees)
2. Small R in leads I and aVL, small Q in leads II, III, and aVF (SI, QIII), or an rS pattern in leads I and aVL
3. Normal QRS duration (not greater than 0.11 second)
4. Increased QRS voltage in limb leads due to loss of cancellation of QRS forces
5. No evidence of RVH

Bifascicular Block

Bifascicular block is defined as the two of the three main fascicles are blocked. Block to both anterior and posterior fascicles results in a complete LBBB, thus the term bifascicular block usually refers to the block in the right bundle branch along with block in

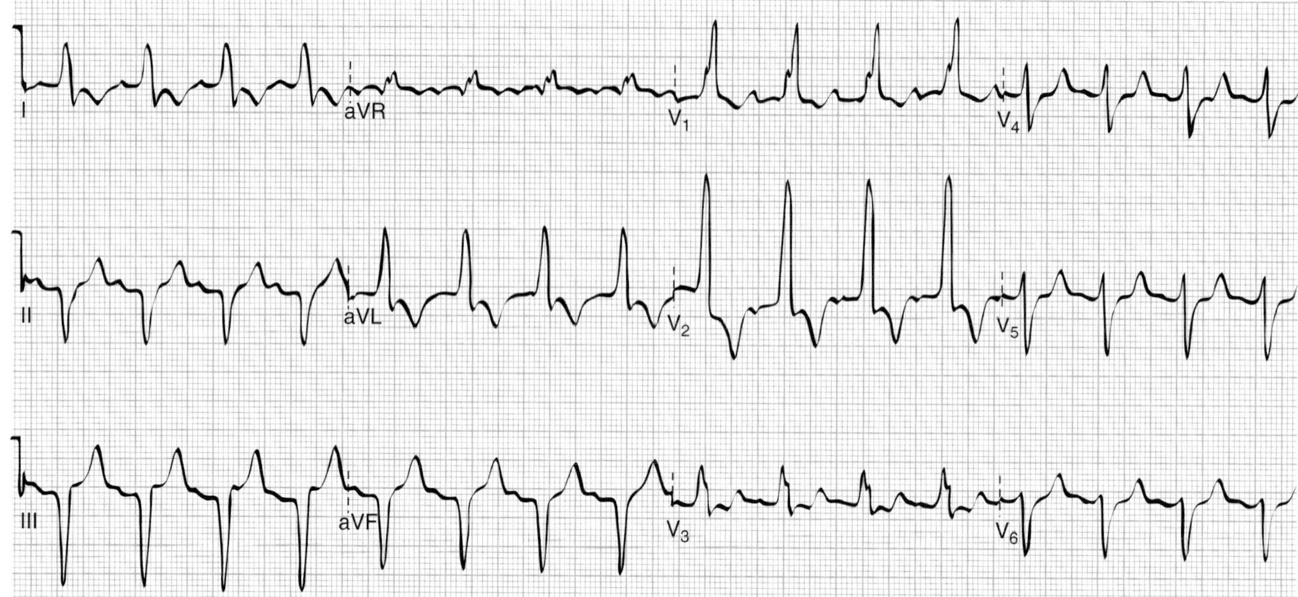

Figure 12-29. ECG of RBBB and LAFB. Rhythm is sinus, QRS width is 0.14 second, there is LAD (−70°) due to LAFB, and V_1 shows the wide notched R-wave variation of RBBB.

left anterior or posterior fascicle. The ECG characteristics would demonstrate RBBB and axis deviation consistent with the fascicular block.[7]

ACUTE CORONARY SYNDROME

The pathophysiologic continuum of acute coronary syndrome (ACS) begins with rupture of atherosclerotic plaque in a coronary artery, resulting in subsequent platelet aggregation and intracoronary thrombus formation. The thrombus ultimately obstructs or blocks the blood flow, leading to imbalance of myocardium oxygen demand and blood flow. When the blood flow is not restored relatively soon, myocardium ischemia occurs. Prolonged ischemia leads to cell injury and eventually necrosis (cell death). Coronary artery spasm can also alter coronary blood flow and cause myocardial ischemia. The ACS consists of three distinct phases: unstable angina (UA), non–ST-elevation acute coronary syndrome (NSTE-ACS), and ST-elevation myocardial infarction (STEMI). The UA and NSTE-ACS are closely associated with partial occlusive thrombus.[25,26] Table 12-6 lists the distinguishing features of ACS.

Table 12-6 • DISTINGUISHING FEATURES OF ACUTE CORONARY SYNDROME

	Features of Acute Coronary Syndrome		
		Myocardial Infarction	
Feature	**Unstable Angina**	**NSTE-ACS**	**STEMI**
Typical symptoms	Crescendo, rest, or new	Prolonged "crushing" chest pain, more severe	Onset severe angina and wider radiation than usual angina
Serum biomarkers	No	Yes	Yes
ECG initial findings	ST depression and/or T-wave inversion	ST depression and/or T wave inversion	ST elevation (and Q waves later)

NSTE-ACS, non–ST-elevation myocardial infarction; STEMI, ST-elevation myocardial infarction.
Adapted from Rhee JW, Sabatine MS, Lilly LS. Acute coronary syndromes. In: Lilly LS, ed. *Pathophysiology of Heart Disease: A Collaborative Project of Medical Students and Faculty*. 5th ed. Baltimore, MD.

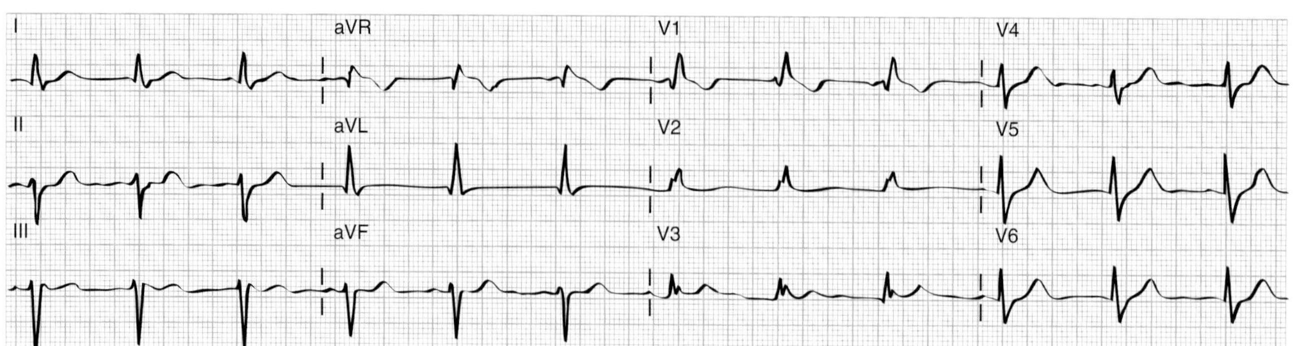

Figure 12-30. ECG of RBBB and LPFB. Rhythm is atrial fibrillation, QRS width is 0.12 second, there is RAD (about +150°) due to LPFB, and V_1 shows the wide R wave variation of RBBB.

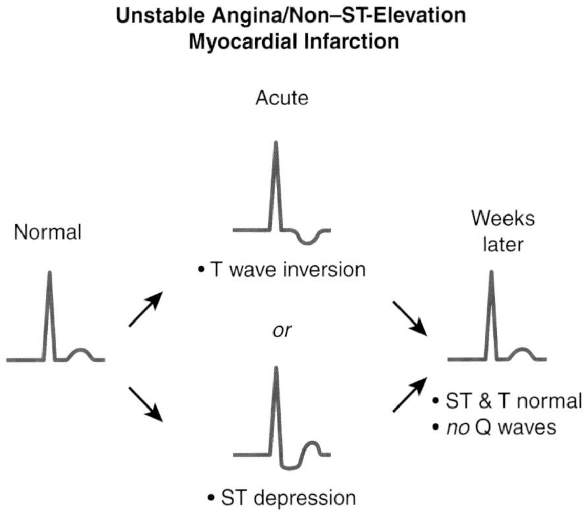

Unstable Angina/Non–ST-Elevation Myocardial Infarction

Normal

Acute

• T wave inversion

or

• ST depression

Weeks later

• ST & T normal
• *no* Q waves

Figure 12-31. ECG abnormalities in unstable angina and non–ST-elevation myocardial infarction.

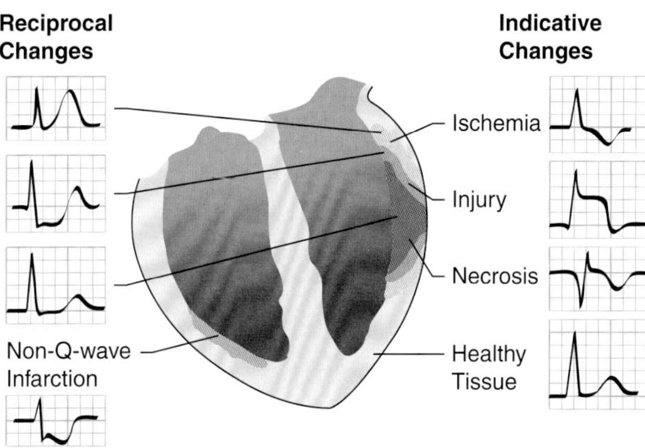

Figure 12-33. Zones of ischemia, injury, and infarction with associated ECG changes. Indicative changes of ischemia, injury, and necrosis are seen in leads facing the injured area. Reciprocal changes are often seen in leads not directly facing the involved area. Non–Q-wave MI causes reduced R-wave height, ST-segment depression, and T-wave inversion. Ischemia can also present this way.

STEMI is associated with presence of myocardial necrosis indicated with elevated biochemical cardiac markers, and sometimes presence of a Q wave on the ECG. Approximately 30% to 40% of patients with ACS will present with STEMI.[25] Historically, STEMI is identified as Q wave or non–Q-wave MI based on the presence or absence of Q wave.[7,27,28] A Q wave MI is typically associated with full-thickness damage of the myocardium. Q waves are the first negative deflections of the QRS complex. The Q waves are considered pathologic when they are greater than 25% of the size of the R wave, or equal or greater than 0.04 second in duration. Pathologic Q waves indicate distorted depolarization due to necrotic tissue.[29]

ECG changes or abnormalities reflect the disturbed electrical current during ACS. ST depression and/or T wave inversion are seen in UA and NSTE-ACS. These ECG abnormalities may be transient during episodes of chest pain in UA, or they may persist in patients with NSTE-ACS (Fig. 12-31) or in patients with STEMI, which is associated with tissue necrosis. The ECG would demonstrate a sequence of abnormalities: initial ST elevation, inverted T wave for the course of several hours, and Q wave development. Figure 12-32 illustrates ECG patterns associated with acute myocardial injury.[27]

ECG DIAGNOSIS OF STEMI

12-lead ECG is a classic diagnostic tool in STEMI. ST-segment elevation, Q waves, and T-wave inversion are considered indicative changes of MI. Immediate reperfusion is required for patients with ST elevation at J point in at least two contiguous leads of greater than or equal to 2 mm (0.2 mV) in men, or greater than or equal to 1.5 mm (0.15 mV) in women in leads V_{2-3}, and/or of greater than or equal to 1 mm in more than two other contiguous chest or limb leads.[30,31] These ECG changes can be captured in leads whose positive electrodes face the infarcted myocardium. The positive electrodes of some leads do not face the involved myocardium; however, the ECG of these leads is affected by the disrupted electrical current in the damaged tissue. These mirrored ECG changes in these leads are called reciprocal changes, demonstrated as ST-segment depression and/or T-wave inversion on the ECG (Fig. 12-33).[7] Table 12-7 lists ECG characteristics in myocardial ischemia/injury. Table 12-8 lists ECG changes associated with STEMI.

The location of blood flow occlusion and coronary artery circulation determines the area of myocardial ischemia/injury and the subsequent ECG changes. Most individuals (70% to 80%) have right-dominant coronary circulation, in which the posterior descending branch (PDA) of the RCA supplies blood to the posterior wall of the left ventricle. Approximately 5% to 10% of the population has left-dominant coronary circulation, with the PDA originating from the left circumflex artery. About 10% to 20% of the population has codominant coronary circulation, in which the PDA is supplied by both the left circumflex artery and RCA.[32]

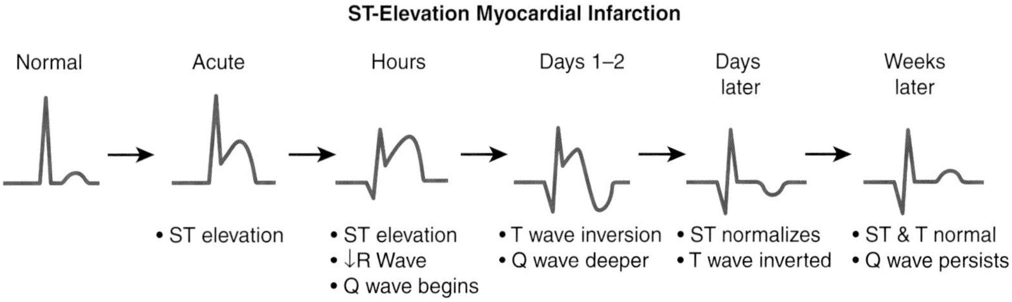

ST-Elevation Myocardial Infarction

Normal → Acute → Hours → Days 1–2 → Days later → Weeks later

Acute: • ST elevation

Hours: • ST elevation • ↓R Wave • Q wave begins

Days 1–2: • T wave inversion • Q wave deeper

Days later: • ST normalizes • T wave inverted

Weeks later: • ST & T normal • Q wave persists

Figure 12-32. ECG evolution during ST-elevation myocardial infarction.

Table 12-7 • ECG CHARACTERISTIC IN MYOCARDIAL ISCHEMIA/INJURY

Myocardial Ischemia[33–35]	Myocardial Injury[33–35]
Horizontal or down-sloping ST depression of 0.5 mm or more	ST-segment elevation of 1 mm or more above the baseline in leads with positive electrodes facing the infracted area
An ST segment forms a sharp angle with the upright T wave	A straightening of the ST segment that slopes up to the peak of the T wave without spending anytime in baseline
Tall, wide-based T waves	Tall, peaked T waves
Inverted U waves	Symmetric T-wave inversion

Anterior MI

Anterior wall MI is associated with occluded blood flow to the left anterior descending (LAD) artery, one of the primary branches of the left main coronary artery. An occlusion of the LAD artery can lead to widespread myocardial damage and complications. Coined the "widow maker," a blockage in the proximal portion of the LAD artery may result in cardiogenic shock and sudden death. Because the LAD artery supplies blood to the anterior surface of left ventricle, indicative changes of anterior MI can be observed in anterior leads (lead V_3 and V_4). Anteroseptal MI is used to describe an infarction that involves both anterior wall and septum. ECG indicative changes of anteroseptal MI can be seen in leads V_{1-4}. Figure 12-34 is an ECG example of anterior MI.[7,20]

Symptoms associated with anterior MI are due to sympathetic nervous system activation: tachycardia, and/or hypertension to compensate a decreased cardiac output, which may worsen myocardial ischemia. Septal occlusion leads to BBBs, second-degree AV block type II, and third-degree AV block.[7,20]

Inferior MI

Inferior MI can be caused by the occlusion of RCA or circumflex, based on the artery of origin for the PDA (i.e., whether coronary circulation is right or left dominant). ECG changes (ST segment and T wave) indicative of an occlusion of the RCA occur in leads II, III, and aVF, and reciprocal ECG changes occur in lead I, aVL, or the V leads. When an occlusion occurs in the circumflex, ST-segment elevation in lead II is greater than that in lead III, and ST in lead I is either isoelectric or elevated (Fig. 12-35).[7,20]

Symptoms of inferior MI are associated with parasympathetic nervous system activation: bradydysrhythmias, conduction delays such as first-degree AV block, second-degree AV block type I.[7,20]

Table 12-8 • ELECTROCARDIOGRAPHIC CHANGES ASSOCIATED WITH STEMI

Location of MI	Indicative Changes: ST Elevation, Q Waves, T-Wave Inversion	Reciprocal Changes: ST Depression, Tall R Waves, Upright T Waves
Anterior	V_1 to V_4	I, aVL, II, III, aVF
Septal	V_1, V_2	I, aVL
Inferior	II, III, aVF	I, aVL in V_1 to V_3 suspect posterior MI
Posterior	None in standard 12 leads Posterior leads V_7–V_9	V_1 to V_4
Lateral	I, aVL, V_5, V_6	II, III, aVF in V_1, V_3 suspect posterior MI
Right ventricle	II, III, aVF (inferior MI) right chest leads V_4R–V_6R	

Adapted from Jacobson C. Electrocardiography. In: Woods SL, Sivarajan Froelicher ES, Motzer SA, et al., eds. *Cardiac Nursing*. 6th ed. Philadelphia, PA: LWW; 2009.

Lateral MI

The blood that supplies the lateral wall may come from the circumflex artery, the LAD artery, or a branch of the RCA; thus, a lateral MI may be associated with an anterior, inferior, or posterior infarction. ECG indicative changes of lateral MI are observed in in lead I, aVL, V_5, and V_6. Reciprocal ECG changes are reflected in the inferior and anterior leads (Fig. 12-36). Figure 12-37 shows examples of anterolateral MI.

Posterior MI

Posterior MI (PMI) is usually associated with inferior or lateral wall MI. Because electrodes of a standard 12-lead ECG are placed on the anterior chest, additional leads V_{7-9} may be placed on the back of the chest to view posterior surface of the heart. Lead V_7 is placed at the level of lead V_6 at the posterior axillary line. Lead V_8 is placed at the tip of the left scapula. Lead V_9 is placed at the left border of the spine (see Figure 12-13B: Electrode placement for posterior leads).[7,32] ST-segment elevation of greater than 1 mm in the posterior leads are indicative changes of PMI.[36]

Left ventricular dysfunction is a complication associated with PMI. Dysrhythmias involving the SA node, AV node, and bundle of His are complications when the posterior wall is supplied by the RCA.[20] Figure 12-38 shows ECG examples of PMI.

Right Ventricular MI

About 50% of inferior wall MI cases are associated with right ventricular MI (RVMI).[37] ECG changes indicative of RVMI are seen in inferior leads II, III, and aVF; ST-segment elevation can also be seen in lead V_1, which has the closest position for viewing the right ventricle. ST-segment elevation in lead V_1 and the inferior leads indicate potential RVMI. Discordance in ST segment in lead V_1 and V_2 can be another clue of RVMI: ST-segment elevation in lead V_1, while lead V_2 has a normal or depressed ST segment.[7] The standard 12-lead ECG is not sufficient assessing right ventricle involvement; right side precordial leads (V_{4R-6R}) must be included to diagnose RVMI (see Figure 12-13A for electrode placement for right precordial leads).[37] ST-segment elevation in precordial leads is a transient event, and it may be absent within 12 hours of onset of chest pain. Thus, right-sided ECG needs to be performed as soon as possible.[12,38,39] ST-segment elevation in lead V_{4R} greater than or equal to 1.0 mm is diagnostic of RVMI with 100% sensitivity, 87% specificity, and 92% predictive accuracy.[40,41]

Patients with RVMI are often preload dependent; hypotension is common in these patients. Avoiding medications that further reduce preload is crucial (e.g., morphine, nitrates, and diuretics). Other complications associated with RVMI include bradycardias, AV blocks, and ventricular dysrhythmias.[20] See Figure 12-39 for ECG example of RVMI. Figure 12-40 depicts the ECG pattern associated with myocardial injury.

(*text continues on page 313*)

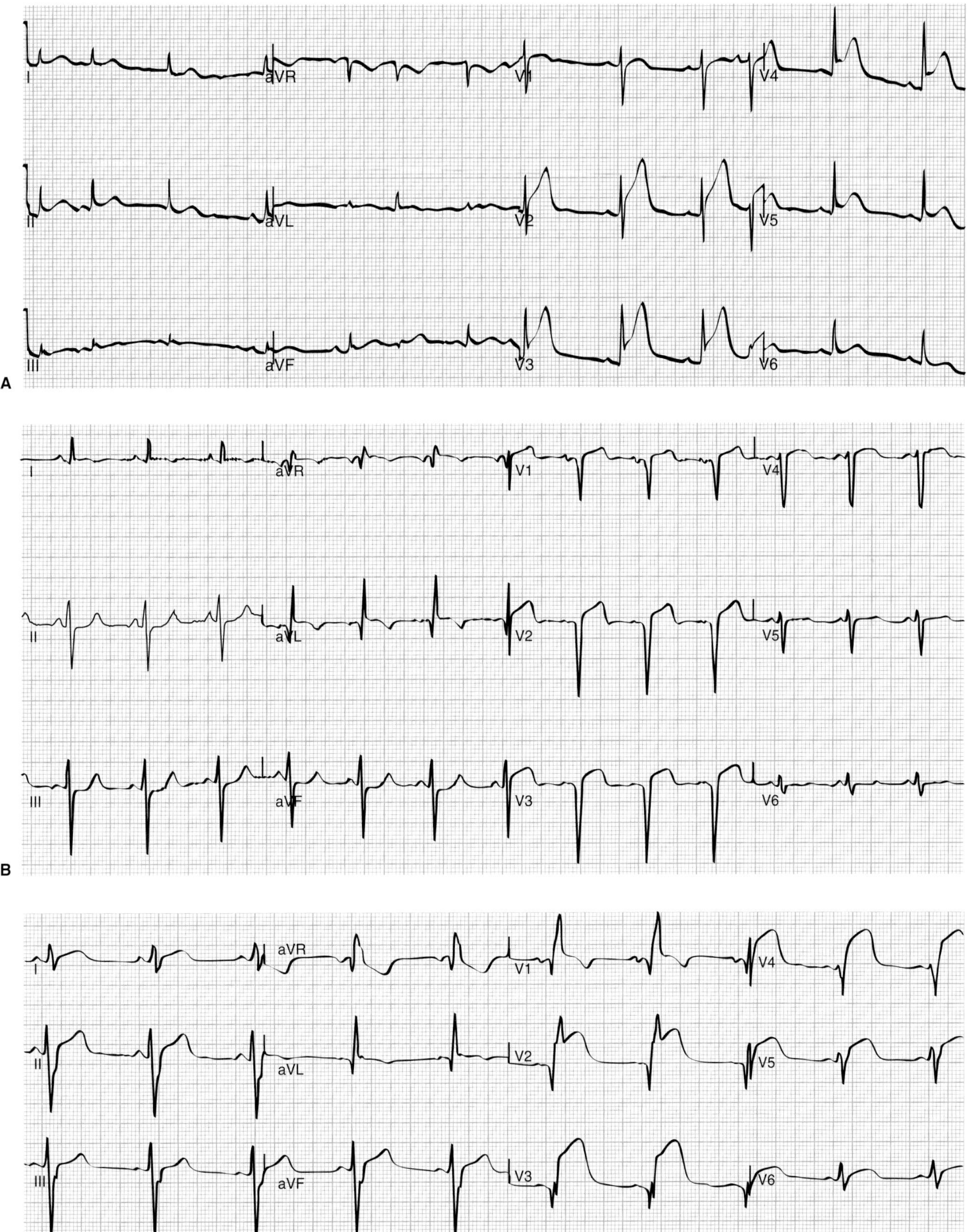

Figure 12-34. **A:** Early acute anterior wall MI. Note ST elevation most pronounced in leads V_2–V_5 indicating acute injury and intact R-wave progression in the V leads indicating that no necrosis has yet occurred. **B:** Anterior wall MI. ST elevation is present in V_1–V_4 and there is a loss of R-wave progression across the precordium resulting in Q waves in V_1–V_3. The QRS axis is about −50 degrees indicating probable LAFB. **C:** Same patient as in **(B)** an hour later. Now there is RBBB and the axis is further left at about −80 degrees: bifascicular block. ST elevation is now present in the lateral leads I, and V_4–V_6 indicating extension to the lateral wall.

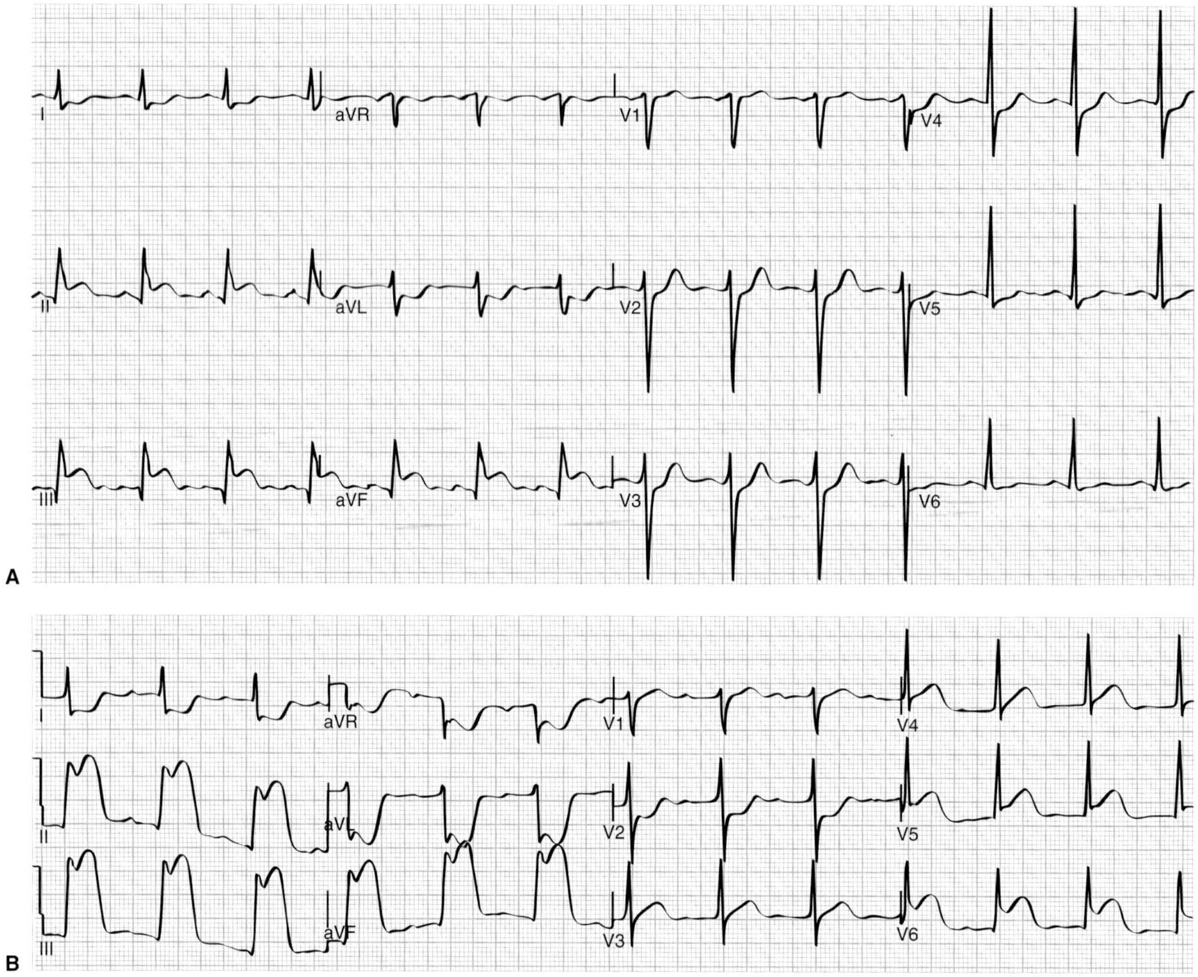

Figure 12-35. **A:** Inferior wall MI. Note ST elevation in leads II, III, and aVF and reciprocal ST depression in leads V_2–V_4, I, and aVL. **B:** Acute inferolateral MI. "Hyperacute" ST elevations in leads II, III, and aVF, with ST elevation also in V_4–V_6 indicating lateral involvement. Reciprocal ST depression is present in leads I, aVL, aVR, and V_2.

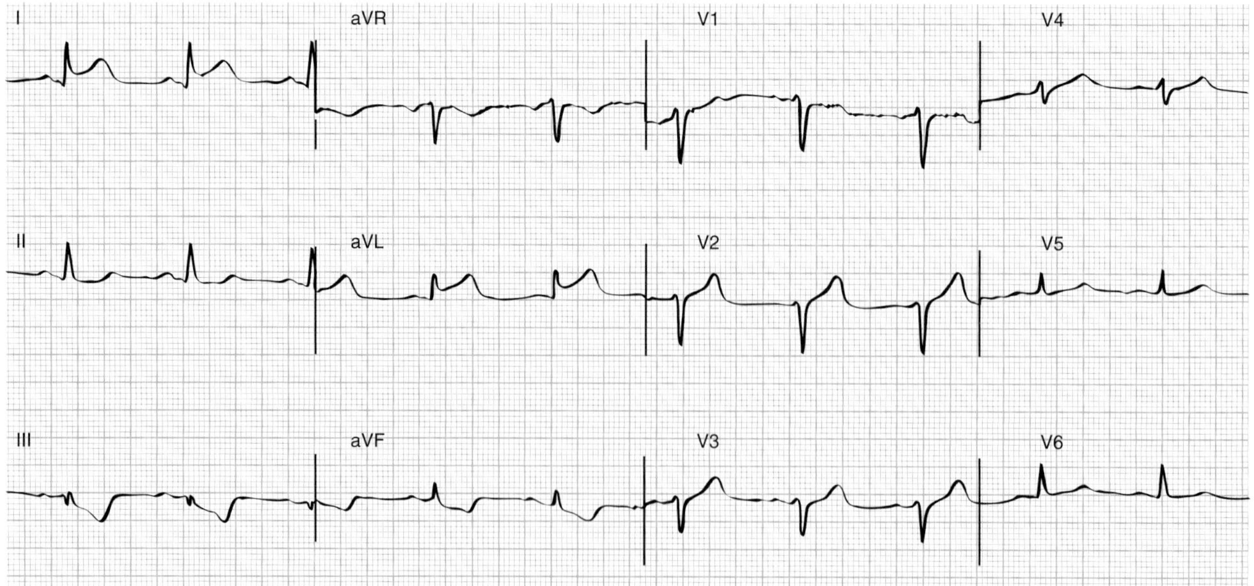

Figure 12-36. Lateral wall infarction. ST elevation is present in leads I and aVL with reciprocal depression in inferior leads. The absence of ST elevation in V_4 and V_5 indicates that the high lateral wall is involved but not the lower portion. R-wave progression is not normal in V_1–V_3, indicating potential anterior involvement.

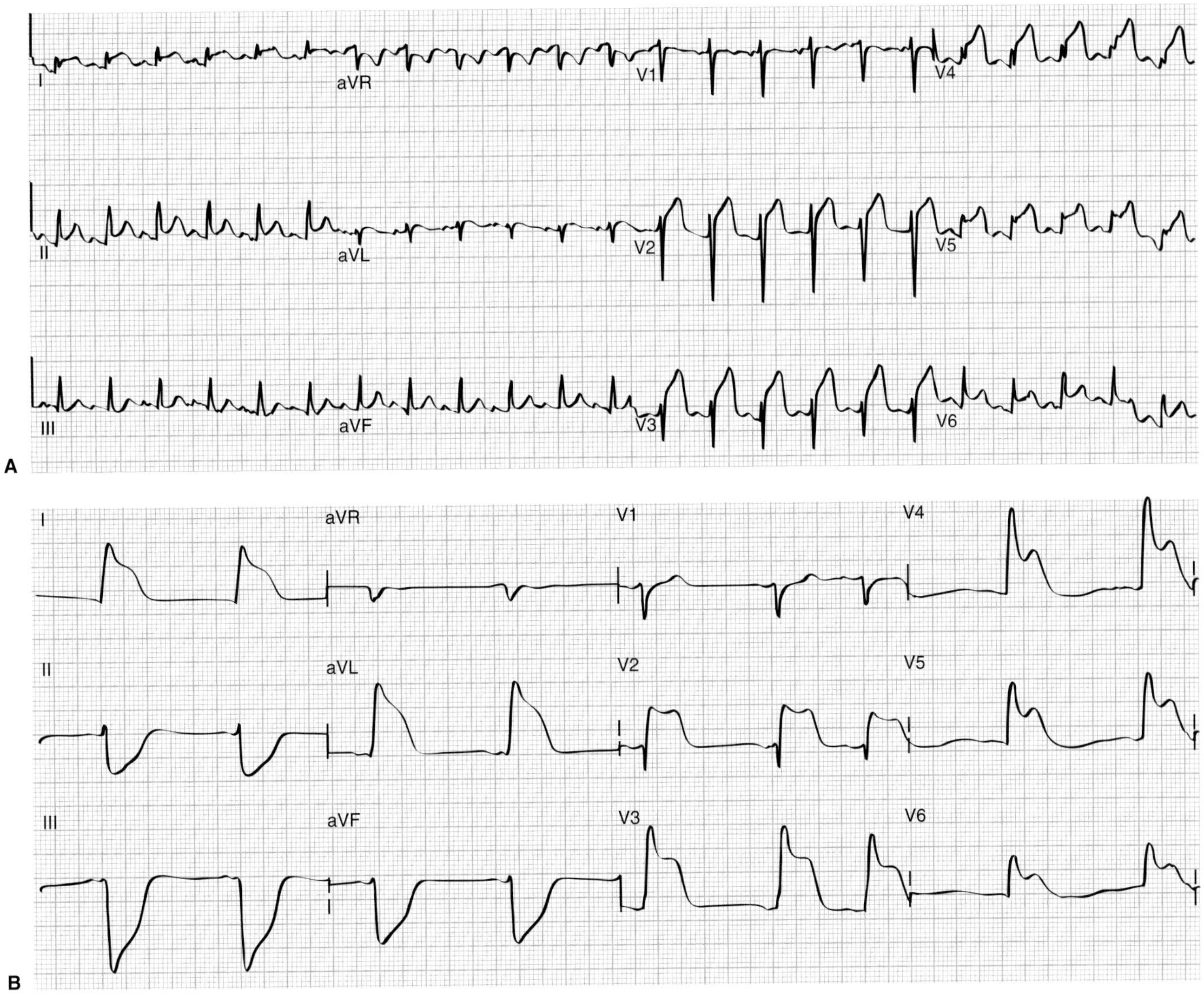

Figure 12-37. **A:** Acute anterolateral wall MI. ST elevation is present in leads I, aVL, and V_2–V_6. Reciprocal ST depression is present in leads III, aVF, and aVR. **B:** Acute anterolateral MI. Dramatic ST elevation in leads I, aVL, and V_2–V_6 with equally dramatic reciprocal ST depression in inferior leads. This is sometime called a "huge current of injury."

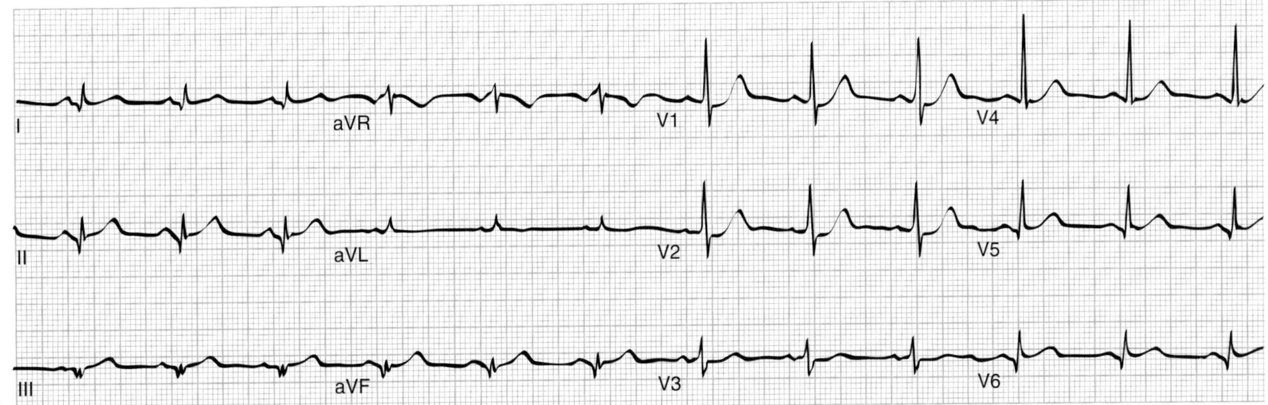

Figure 12-38. **A:** Posterior wall MI. Large R waves and ST depression are present in V_1 and V_2. There are Q waves in the inferior leads but no ST elevation, probably due to old inferior MI. (*continued*)

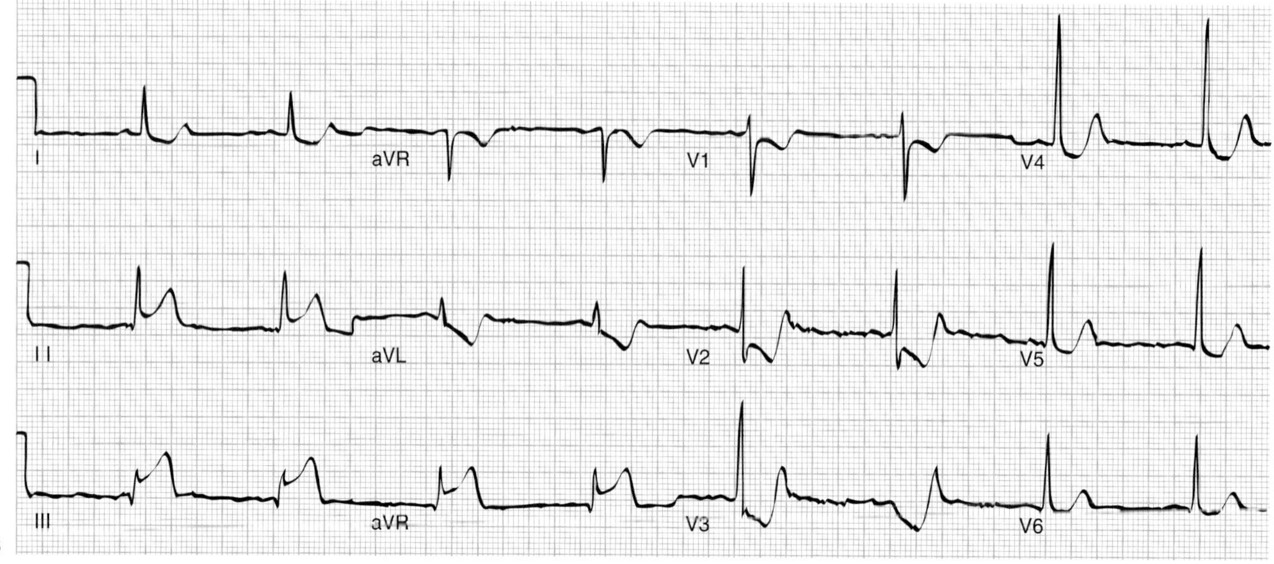

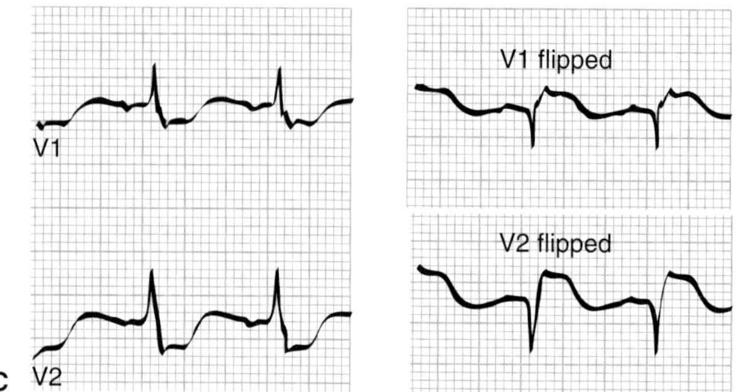

Figure 12-38. (*Continued*) **B:** Inferior–posterior MI. Leads II, III, and aVF show ST elevation of inferior MI with reciprocal ST depression in most other leads. The very tall R waves in V_2 and V_3 raise suspicion of posterior involvement. **C:** Verification of posterior MI by flipping leads V_1 and V_2. On the **left**, standard V_1 and V_2 showing large R waves and ST depression suspicious of posterior MI. On the **right**, these leads are shown flipped vertically and now demonstrate Q waves and ST elevation typical of MI. This is what posterior leads would show if they were recorded.

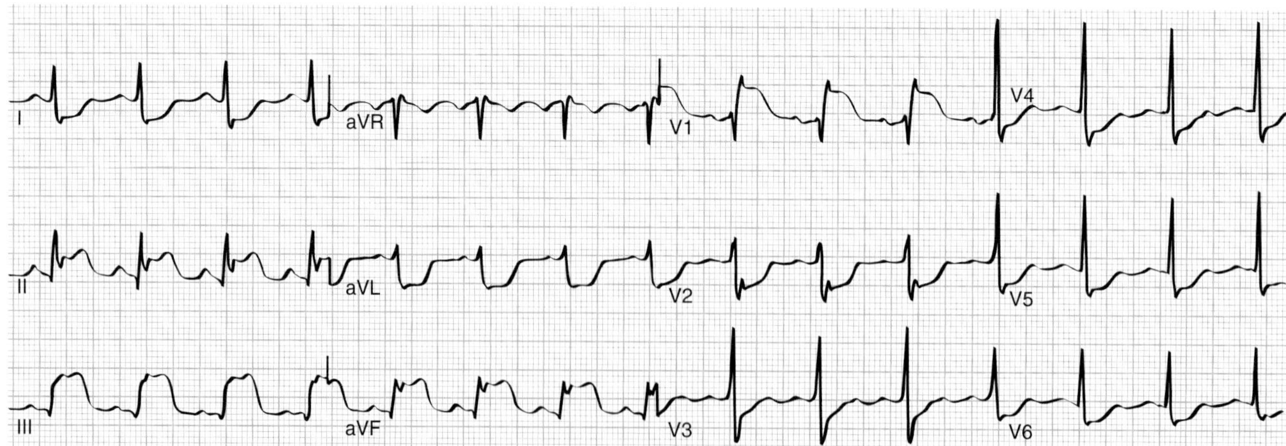

Figure 12-39. Acute RVMI. ST elevation is present in leads II, III, aVF, and V_1; reciprocal ST depression in all other leads. Note the discordant ST elevation in V_1 and depression in V_2.

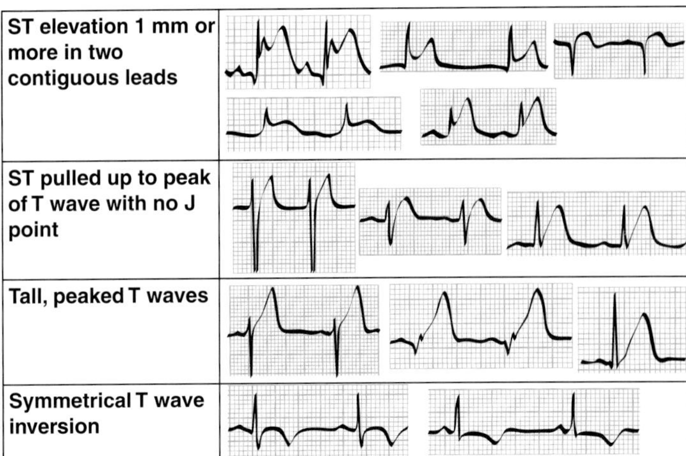

Figure 12-40. ECG patterns associated with myocardial injury.

ECG DIAGNOSIS OF UA/NSTE-ACS

The ECG characteristics associated with UA/NSTE-ACS are ST-segment depression and T-wave inversion. The presence or absence of cardiac biomarkers is the differentiate diagnosis of UA and NSTE-ACS. UA occurs with ischemia without myocardium injury, thus there is no release of cardiac biomarker. Conversely, NSTE-ACS is associated with more severe ischemia that results in cardiac biomarker release. NSTE-ACS is previously referred as "NSTEMI" or "non–Q wave MI" due to ST-T wave abnormalities and necrosis of the subendocardial layer of the ventricle and not the entire thickness of ventricular wall.[1] UA and NSTEMI share the same ECG characteristics.[7]

Figure 12-41 demonstrates ECG patterns associated with myocardial ischemia. Figure 12-42 are some ECG examples of NSTE-ACS. Table 12-7 lists the ECG characteristics associated with myocardial ischemia/injury.

ATRIAL AND VENTRICULAR HYPERTROPHY/ENLARGEMENT

The terms hypertrophy and enlargement are often used interchangeably; however, they do not mean the same thing. Hypertrophy usually refers to increased muscle mass, and the underlying cause is mostly because of pressure overload. For example, in the setting of aortic stenosis, the left ventricle pumps blood against an increased resistance and the cardiac muscle will become thicker (hypertrophy) as a result.[18] Enlargement refers to the dilation of a cardiac chamber, mostly due to volume overload or dilated cardiomyopathy. The chamber dilates to compensate increased amount of blood. For example, in mitral valve insufficiency, increased volume back into the left atria overtime leads to left atrial enlargement.[18]

When there is hypertrophy or enlargement, specific ECG changes may be present: (1) an increase in duration of the ECG wave due to prolonged depolarization due to size of the chamber; (2) an increase in amplitude due to more current and larger voltage generated by the chamber; (3) electrical axis shift due to an increased percentage of total electrical current passing through expanded chamber.[18]

Atrial Enlargement

Atrial enlargement is reflected as a change in size of P wave and morphology. The first half of the P wave represents the right atrial depolarization, and second half the P wave represents left atrial depolarization. Lead II and V_1 are the most optimal leads to examine atrial enlargement. Lead II is parallel to the direction of the current traveling through the atria; therefore, lead II records the largest positive deflection. Lead V_1 is perpendicular to the direction

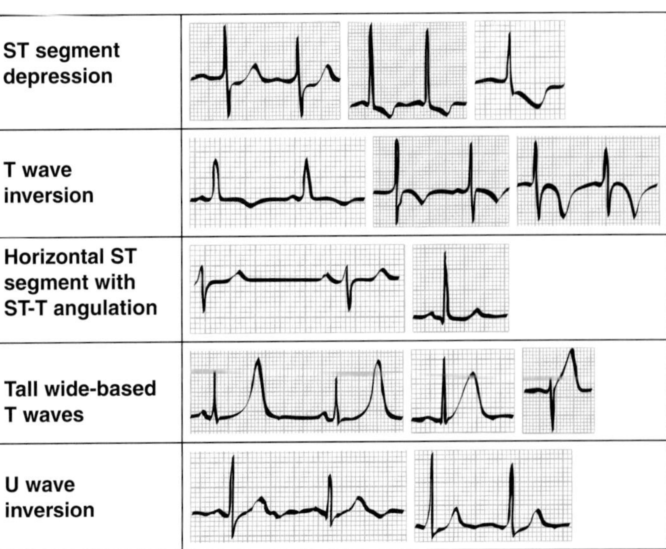

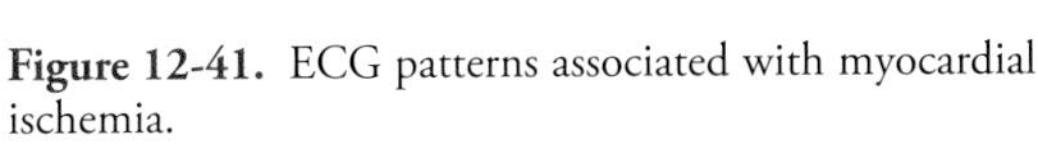

Figure 12-41. ECG patterns associated with myocardial ischemia.

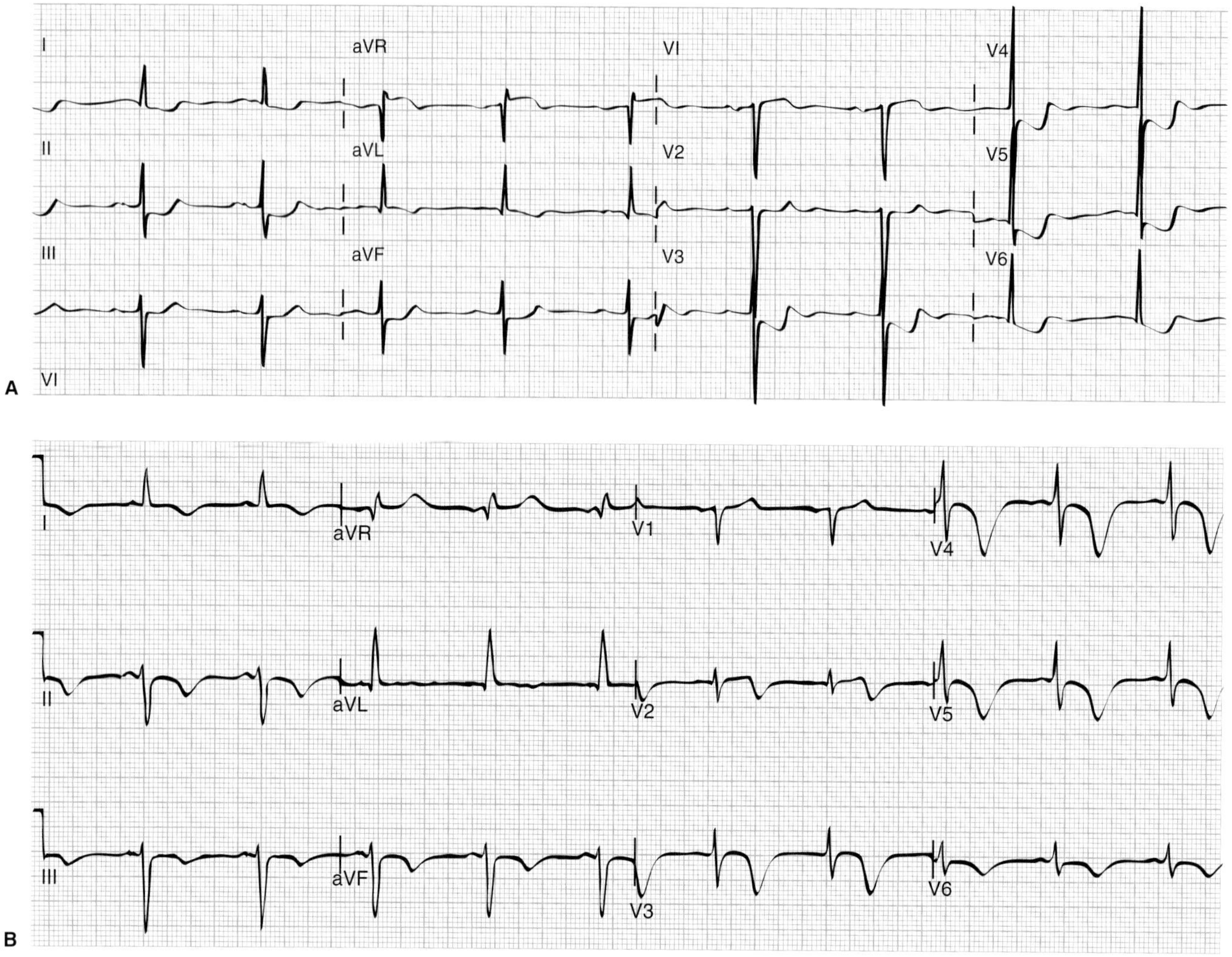

Figure 12-42. **A:** NSTEMI. Note widespread ST depression in leads I, II, III, aVF, and V_{2-6}. The ST-segment elevation in aVR and V_1 along with ischemic changes in all other leads is suggestive of left main or significant triple-vessel coronary artery disease. This patient's troponin and CK-MB were elevated, leading to the diagnosis of NSTEMI. **B:** NSTEMI. There is T-wave inversion in several leads, especially deep in V_3–V_5, but no significant Q waves in any lead. Cardiac biomarkers were elevated.

of the atrial current, and it records a biphasic P wave to allow easy differentiation of right and left atrial components (Fig. 12-43).[18]

Right Atrial Enlargement

Right atrial enlargement is commonly associated with overwork of the right atrium, which can be due to increased volume (e.g., tricuspid stenosis or regurgitation, and atrial septal defect) or pressure (e.g., chronic pulmonary hypertension).[7,18] ECG changes indicative of right atrial enlargement (Fig. 12-44) include: (1) The P waves are tall and peaked (greater than 2.5 mm) in leads II, III, and aVF (termed *P pulmonale*); (2) P waves in leads V_{1-3} are sharp and pointed, increasing the area under the positive portion of the P wave; (3) Rightward shift of P wave axis to greater than +75 degrees.[7,18]

Left Atrial Enlargement

Similar to right atrial enlargement, left atrial enlargement is caused by either increased pressure or volume to the left atrium (e.g., mitral stenosis or regurgitation, systemic hypertension, and left-sided heart failure [HF]).[7,18] ECG changes indicative of left atrial enlargement (see Fig. 12-44) include: (1) The P wave is wider than 0.12 second and often notched in leads I, II, aVL, and V_{4-6} (termed *P mitrale*); (2) The interval between the notches is greater than 0.04 second, and the P wave may encroach into the PR segment, making the PR segment appear shorter than normal;

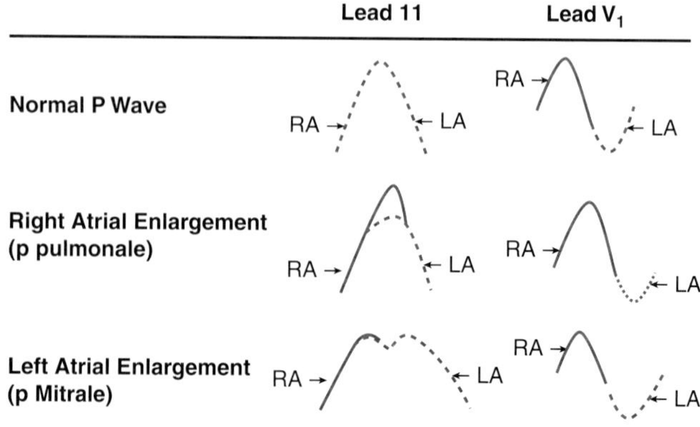

Figure 12-43. Illustration of P waves in leads II and V_1, showing normal, right atrial enlargement, and left atrial enlargement.

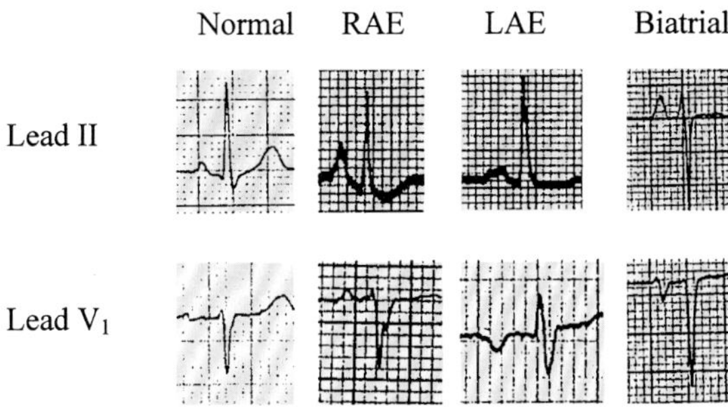

Figure 12-44. Normal P waves compared to those of left atrial enlargement, right atrial enlargement, and biatrial enlargement in leads II and V_1. Left atrial enlargement causes widening and notching of P waves in many leads, and enlargement of the terminal negative portion of the P wave in V_1. Right atrial enlargement causes tall peaked P waves in many leads and enlargement of the initial upright portion of the P wave in V_1. Biatrial enlargement can make the entire P wave wider and taller than normal and vary its configuration in many leads.

(3) Increased width and depth of the terminal negative component of the P wave in lead V_1 or V_2; leftward shift of P-wave axis to between −30 and +45 degrees.[7,18]

Biatrial Enlargement

Both atria can become enlarged in some clinical conditions (e.g., mitral valve disease, atrial septal defect, valvular disease, and biventricular failure). In biatrial enlargement, there is an increase in both amplitude and duration in P wave: P wave is taller than 2.5 mm and wider than 0.11 second in lead II. Enlargement in both positive and negative components of the P wave may be seen in lead V_1.[7,18]

Ventricular Enlargement

Ventricular enlargement/hypertrophy and remodeling are results of cardiac compensatory processes overtime in response to either increased pressure (afterload) or increased volume (preload). Chronic cardiac chamber dilation (increased chamber radius) is due to volume overload (e.g., chronic mitral or aortic regurgitation). Chronic pressure overload can be caused by hypertension or aortic stenosis.[42] Ventricular enlargement/hypertrophy of the affected chamber produces greater electrical current during depolarization, reflecting on an increase in the size of the QRS complex, and subsequent ST-segment and T-wave changes.[7,43]

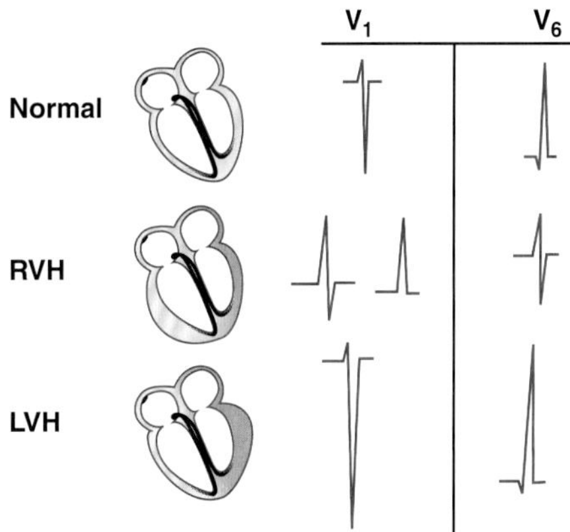

Figure 12-45. Normal ventricular size results in a dominant S wave in V_1, a dominant R wave in V_6, and a normal QRS axis. RVH increases the amplitude of forces directed rightward and anteriorly through the enlarged right ventricle, causing large R waves in V_1 (usually R, rS, or qR pattern) and deep S waves in V_6. LVH increases the amplitude of forces directed to the left and posteriorly toward the enlarged left ventricle, resulting in large voltage S waves in V_1 and R waves in V_6, and shifting the axis leftward.

Figure 12-45 demonstrates ECG characteristics of normal ventricular size, RVH, and LVH.

Right Ventricular Enlargement/Hypertrophy

RVH may be caused by any condition that produces a sufficient load on the right ventricle, such as pulmonary disease or congenital or acquired heart disease, particularly mitral valve disease. In normal ventricles without enlargement, the left ventricle is electrically dominant; the electrical events of the right ventricle are normally masked by the events taking place nearly simultaneously in the dominant left ventricle. When there is right ventricular remodeling, these right-sided forces are revealed and may become the dominant force, resulting in RAD. The normal sequence of depolarization is altered, resulting in ECG changes in axis (RAD, between +90 and +180 degrees), QRS morphology and voltage, and ST-T waves.[7,18,43]

The most obvious ECG change with RVH is a reversal of normal R-wave progression in precordial leads. R waves become dominant and the S wave shrinks in right chest leads, whereas R waves shrink and S waves dominate in left-sided leads (the R wave is larger than the S wave in lead V_1; the S wave is larger than the R wave in lead V_6 (Fig. 12-46). The same "strain" pattern

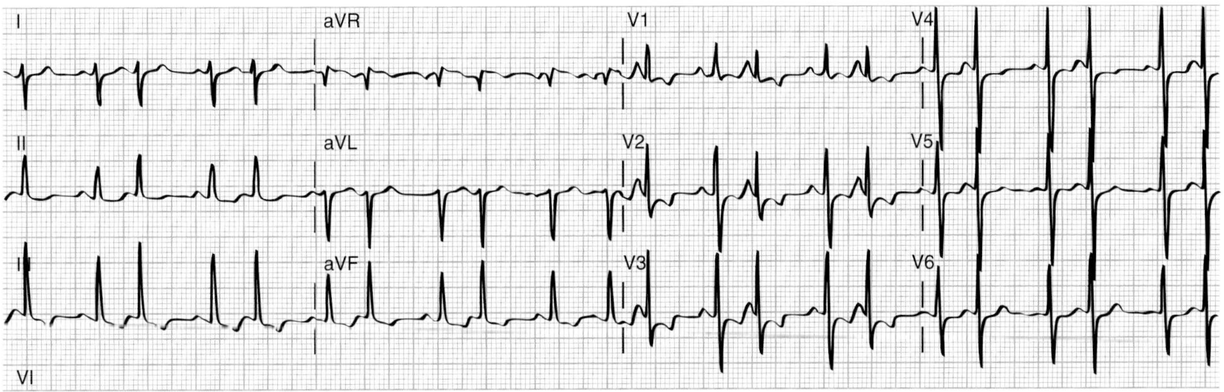

Figure 12-46. RVH in a patient with primary pulmonary hypertension. Note RAD of +120 degrees with large R waves in V_1–V_3 and ST-T wave changes of RV strain. (Courtesy of Dr. William Nelson, Denver, Colorado.)

described previously with ST-segment depression and T-wave inversion occurs in right chest leads and in leads II, III, and aVF. ECG features commonly seen with RVH are listed in Figure 12-45.[7,18,43]

Left Ventricular Enlargement/Hypertrophy

Left ventricular enlargement caused by increased volume (diastolic overload or increased preload) or hypertrophy due to increased pressure (systolic overload or increased afterload) can be expressed on the ECG. The most characteristic effect of LVH is an increase in R-wave amplitude in leads facing the left ventricle (leads I, aVL, V_5, and V_6) as more forces travel through the thickened left ventricle. There is a concurrent decrease in R-wave amplitude and increase in S-wave amplitude in leads facing the right ventricle (leads V_1 and V_2). The intrinsicoid deflection (the time from the beginning of the QRS complex to the peak of the R wave) is slightly delayed in leads facing the left ventricle, and the QRS width approaches the upper limit of normal because of the increased time required for electrical forces to travel through the thick left ventricular muscle. Figure 12-47 is an example of LVH.[7,18,43]

The ST-T–wave changes that occur reflect repolarization abnormalities and may be due to hypertrophy or may be secondary consequences of dilation or ischemia. The term *strain* is often used to describe the ST-T–wave changes that commonly occur with LVH. ST-segment depression, often downsloping, with T-wave inversion commonly develops in left chest leads. Increased T-wave amplitude may be found in leads that show large R waves, and ST segments may be elevated in leads that show deep S waves. A variety of methods have been proposed to help diagnose LVH on the ECG (Table 12-9).

ELECTROLYTE IMBALANCES

Electrolytes imbalance may lead to electrical conduction abnormalities, increased cardiac irritability, and cardiac arrhythmias. Some ECG characteristics are associated with electrolytes

Table 12-9 • METHODS TO DIAGNOSE LEFT VENTRICULAR ENLARGEMENT ON THE ECG

Author/Method	ECG Criteria Favoring Left Ventricular Enlargement	
Dubin, 1988	R wave in lead I + S wave in lead III >26 mm	
	S wave in lead V_1 + R wave in lead V_5 or V_6 >35 mm	
Sokolow and Lyon, 1949	R wave in VL ≥11 mm	
	S wave in lead V_1 + R wave in lead V_5 or V_6 >35 mm	
	R wave in V_5 or V_6 >26 mm	
Estes scorecard	*Criteria*	Points[a]
	1. R or S wave in limb lead 20 mm or more	
	S wave in lead V_1, V_2, or V_3 25 mm or more	3
	R wave in lead V_4, V_5, or V_6 25 mm or more	
	2. Any ST shift (without digitalis)	3
	Typical ST strain (with digitalis)	1
	3. LAD—30 degrees or more	2
	4. QRS interval 0.09 s or more	1
	5. Intrinsicoid deflection in V_5 and V_6 0.05 second or more	1
	6. P-wave terminal force in V_1 >0.04 s	3
	Total possible	14
Scott criteria	Limb leads	
	R in 1 + S in 3 >25 mm	
	R in aVL >7.5 mm	
	R in aVF >20 mm	
	S in aVR >14 mm	
	Chest leads	
	S in V_1 or V_2 + R in V_5 or V_6 >35 mm	
	R in V_5 or V_6 >26 mm	
	R + S in any V lead >45 mm	
Cornell index	Women: R in aVL + S in V_3 >20 mm	
	Men: R in aVL + S in V_3 >28 mm	

[a]5 = Left ventricular enlargement; 4 = probable left ventricular enlargement.

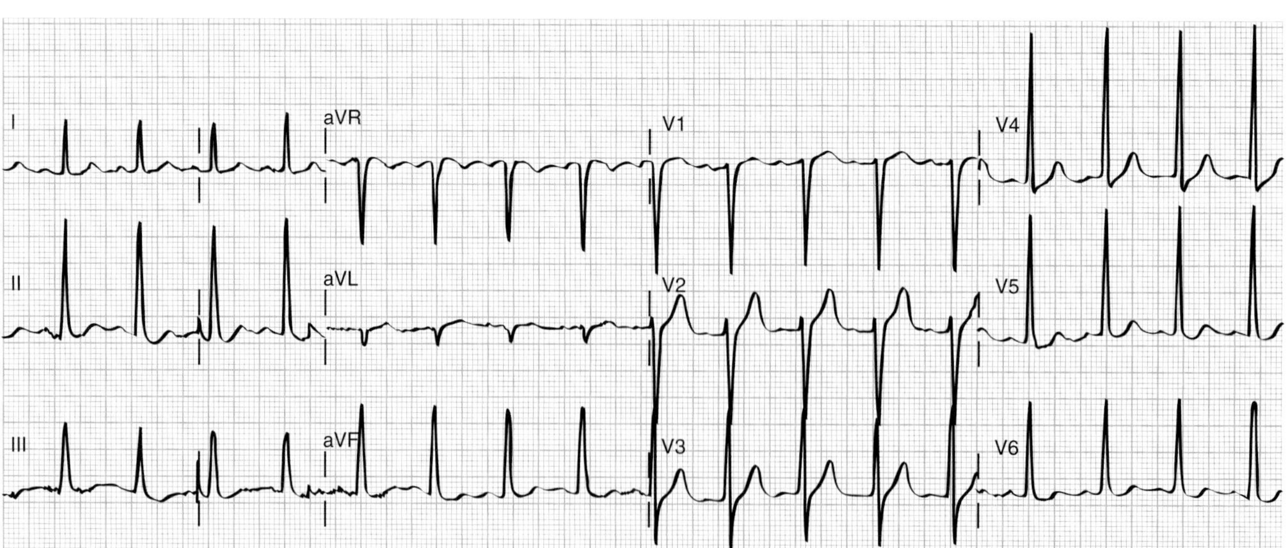

Figure 12-47. LVH with deep S waves in V_{1-2} and large voltage R waves in V_{4-6}. ST depression and T-wave inversion (strain pattern) are seen in V_{4-6}.

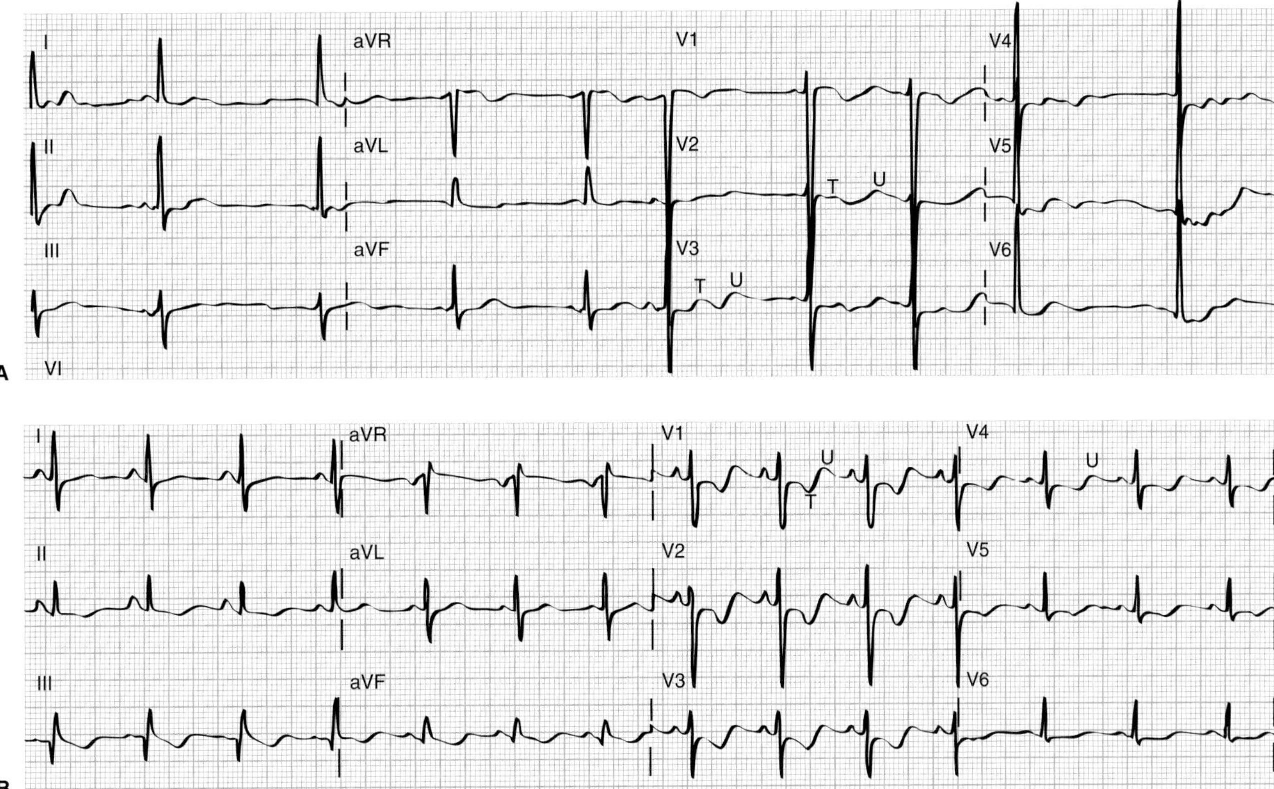

Figure 12-48. ECG effects of hypokalemia. **A:** T waves are flattened in many leads; large U waves are best seen in the V leads. **B:** Large U waves of hypokalemia. This ECG also shows the typical pattern of acute cor pulmonale with S wave in lead I, Q-wave and T-wave inversion in lead III (the S1, Q3, and T3 pattern of cor pulmonale). (Courtesy of Dr. William Nelson, Denver, Colorado.)

imbalance. Early identification of these ECG changes will facilitate correction of electrolyte imbalance and prevent potential life-threatening complications.[7]

Hypokalemia

Hypokalemia (potassium deficit) is defined as serum potassium level of less than 3.5 mEq/L or 3.5 mmol/L. Hypokalemia can be a result of prolonged diuretic therapy, inadequate dietary intake of potassium, severe gastrointestinal loss of potassium associated with gastric suction or lavage, vomiting and diarrhea, or use of laxative. Electrophysiologic changes associated with hypokalemia include hyperpolarization of myocardial cell membranes and increased action potential duration (Fig. 12-48). The ECG characteristics of hypokalemia include ST-segment depression with flatten T waves; T-wave inversion; prominent U wave; prolonged QT interval (which may lead to lethal arrhythmias including VT, ventricular fibrillation (VF), and Torsade de Pointes [TdP]). [7,18,43,44]

Hyperkalemia

Hyperkalemia (potassium excess) is defined as serum potassium level of greater than 5.5 mEq/L or 5.5 mmol/L. Hyperkalemia is often associated with decreased renal function, due to the kidneys' role in potassium excretion. Other causes for hyperkalemia include potassium overdose (intravenous potassium or salt substitutes), and metabolic acidosis. A number of cardiac medications can cause an elevated serum potassium level: angiotensin-converting enzyme inhibitors (ACE-Is), angiotensin receptor blockers (ARBs), spironolactone (potassium-sparing diuretics), and nonsteroidal anti-inflammatory drugs. ECG characteristics of hyperkalemia include: increased T-wave amplitude ("peaked" or "tented" T waves); prolonged PR interval; decreased P-wave amplitude or loss of P wave; widened QRS complex; and lethal arrhythmias (e.g., VF and asystole) (Fig. 12-49).[7,18,43,44]

Hypocalcemia

Hypocalcemia (calcium deficit) is defined as serum calcium of less than 8.5 mEq/L, or 8.5 mmol/L, which may result from the following mechanisms: increased renal loss of calcium, increased binding of ionized calcium to protein, decreased parathyroid hormones, and inadequate intake of calcium. Hypocalcemia is often found in renal patients due to their phosphate-retention tendency: calcium and phosphate have an inverse relationship. When level of phosphate increases, the level of calcium decreases, and vice versa. Prolonged QTc interval is a common ECG characteristic associated with hypocalcemia due to long ST segment. T waves are usually unchanged, but sometimes T waves might be flat or sharply inverted (Fig. 12-50). Complications of hypocalcemia include ventricular dysrhythmias and TdP.[7,20,43,44]

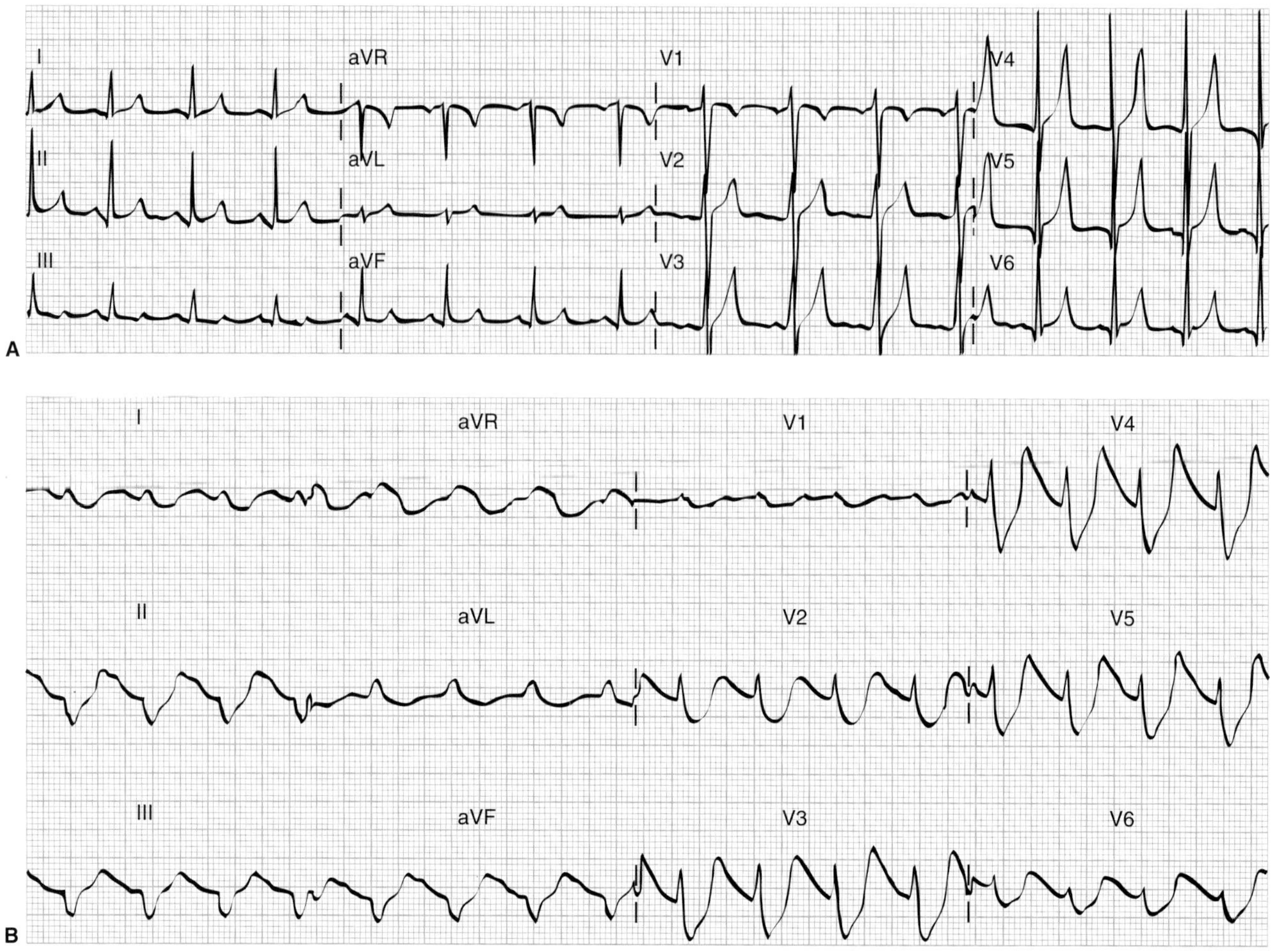

Figure 12-49. ECG effects of hyperkalemia. **A:** Tall, peaked, narrow-based T waves typical of hyperkalemia. **B:** Advanced hyperkalemia (K = 9.2 mEq/L). Note very wide QRS and almost sine-wave look in leads I and aVR.

Hypercalcemia

Hypercalcemia (calcium excess) is defined as a serum calcium level of greater than 12 mEq/L or 12 mmol/L. Hypercalcemia is more common than hypocalcemia, and is commonly associated with cancers and hyperparathyroidism. Other causes of hypercalcemia include chronic or acute renal failure, excessive vitamin D or vitamin A intake, adrenal insufficiency, and excessive of calcium-containing antacids and calcium supplement. Shortened ST segment and decreased QTc interval can be seen with hypercalcemia. Bradydysrhythmias are frequently associated with hypercalcemia (Fig. 12-51).[7,20,43,44]

Hypomagnesemia and Hypermagnesemia

Hypomagnesemia (magnesium deficit) is defined as a serum magnesium level of less than 1.5 mg/dL (0.62 mmol/L). Hypermagnesemia (magnesium excess) is defined as a serum magnesium level of greater than 2.3 mg/dL (0.95 mmol/L). While hypomagnesemia and hypermagnesemia do not demonstrate specific ECG

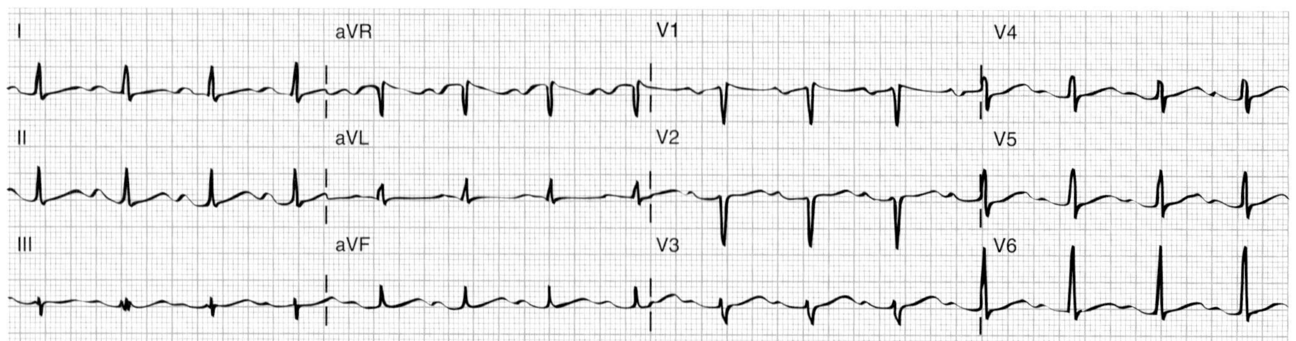

Figure 12-50. ECG effects of hypocalcemia. Note the long ST segment that contributes to a prolonged QT interval.

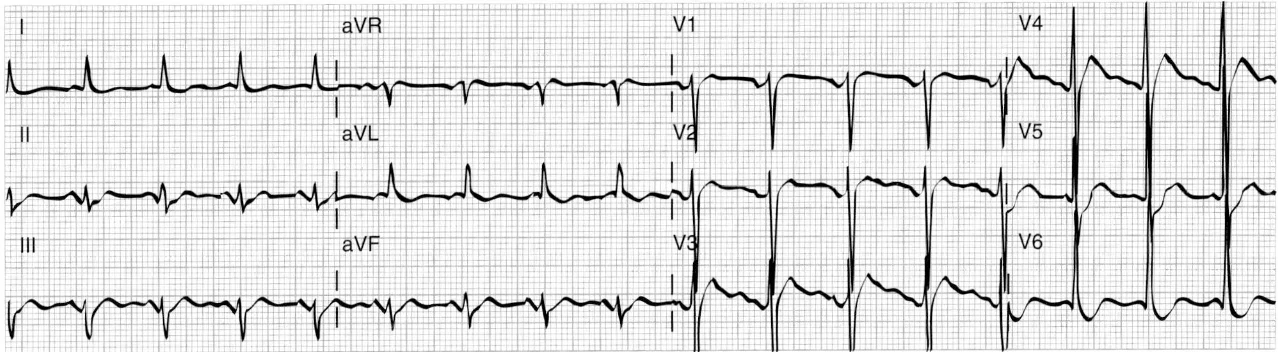

Figure 12-51. ECG effects of hypercalcemia. Note the short QT interval and how the T wave seems to take off from the end of the QRS in the V leads, especially V_3 and V_4.

changes, both are often associated with calcium abnormalities. Hypomagnesemia can be a result of excess diuretic therapy, excess calcium or vitamin intake, lack of magnesium replacement, alcoholism, protein–calories' malnutrition, and excess renal or gastrointestinal excretion. Hypomagnesemia may contribute arrhythmias with digitalis toxicity, ischemia, drugs, and potassium imbalance, and it has been implicated as a potential cause of TdP. Hypermagnesemia is common in patients with renal insufficiency or renal failure. Severe hypermagnesemia can lead to AV block and intraventricular conduction abnormalities.[7,20,43,44]

DRUG EFFECTS AND LONG QT SYNDROMES

Many medications may affect myocardium depolarization and repolarization, which may subsequently affect the ECG (e.g., ST segment, T wave, U wave, and QT interval). As a result, the changes in ECG may lead to conduction disturbances and arrhythmias.[7]

Digitalis

Digitalis is recognized for its proarrhythmic effects, which vary based on serum blood levels of digoxin level. Arrhythmia is the most common cardiac manifestation. Digitalis induces vagal activation which can lead to bradyarrhythmias (e.g., AV block) (Fig. 12-52).[45,46]

Drugs That Prolong QT Interval

Many medications may prolong the QT interval: antihistamines, antimicrobials, tricyclic antidepressants, antipsychotics, neuroleptics, prokinetics.[47,48] Antiarrhythmic medications may also prolong the QT interval. Quinidine is the most commonly implicated agent. Prolonged QT interval is often associated with lethal arrhythmias (e.g., TdP, also known as polymorphic VT). Rapid or prolonged TdP can lead to VF and sudden cardiac death.

Long QT Syndromes

The signature characteristic of LQTS is delayed myocardium repolarization. LQTS induce prolongation of the QT interval and increase the risk for TdP, syncope, seizure, and sudden cardiac death.[49] Further discussion about LQTS can be found later this chapter under section *Genetics of Channelopathies.*

MECHANISM OF ARRHYTHMIAS

Cardiac depolarization and repolarization are controlled by movement of ions across channels embedded on individual cell membrane of cardiomyocytes. The movement of ions is crucial for generation and propagation of cardiac electric impulse and is influenced by the activity of autonomic nervous system.[50–52] Normal cardiac function is dependent upon the flow of electrical impulse through the heart in intricately coordinated fashion.[53] Abnormal activity of these ionic movements is important in cardiac arrhythmogenesis.[50–52] Abnormalities of cardiac rhythm are called cardiac arrhythmias, also known as cardiac dysrhythmias. Cardiac arrhythmias can be a result of abnormal impulse initiation, abnormal impulse conduction, or a combination of both mechanisms.[53] The mechanisms of cardiac arrhythmias can be divided into two major categories: (1) enhanced or abnormal impulse formation, and (2) reentry.

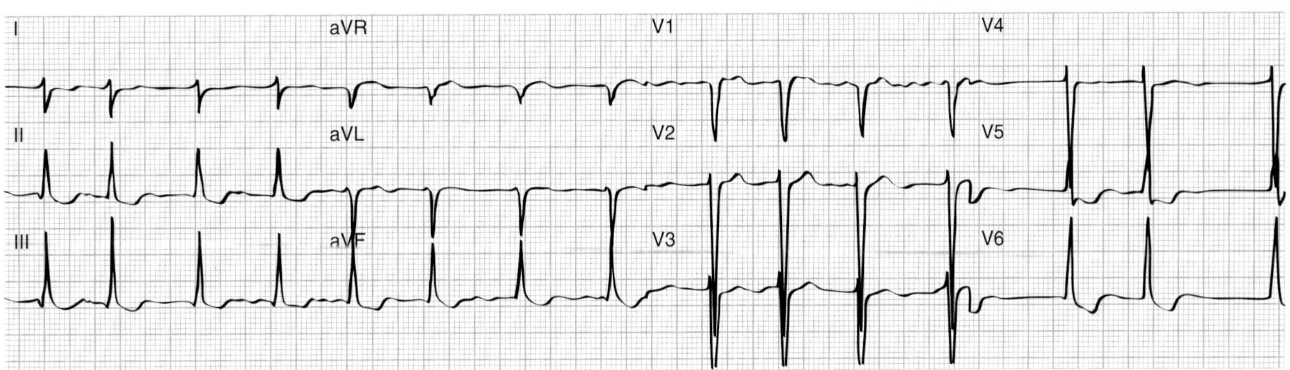

Figure 12-52. ECG effects of digitalis. Note sagging type ST depression in inferior leads and in V_5 and V_6.

Abnormal Impulse Initiation

Cardiac cells have the ability to spontaneously initiate an electrical impulse and depolarize, and this is known as automaticity. The SA node is the primary pacemaker of the heart as it has the fastest rate of automaticity. Other cells within the conduction system may act as pacemaker cells if necessary; these cells are referred to as latent pacemaker (ectopic pacemaker) or subsidiary pacemaker cells. Latent pacemaker cells will take over the pacemaker responsibilities when the SA node fails to generate impulses or when the impulses fail to propagate. Subsidiary pacemakers have their intrinsic rates that have normal automaticity: atrial pacemakers have faster intrinsic rates at than AV junctional pacemakers, and AV junctional pacemakers have faster rates than ventricular pacemakers. Arrhythmias may occur from altered impulse formation at the SA node or other sites. The abnormal impulse initiation can be a result of altered automaticity, abnormal automaticity, and triggered activity.[53]

Increased/Decreased Sinus Node Activity

Abnormal automaticity includes both reduced automaticity that results in bradycardia, and increased automaticity that causes tachycardia. Autonomic nervous system is an important modulator for normal sinus node automaticity. Sympathetic activities stimulate sinus node (during the time of stress) by increasing both heart rate and causing action potential to be more negative. Parasympathetic nervous system decreases SA node automaticity and it becomes the regulator of the heart rate at rest.[53] Alterations in sinus rate can occur when there is a shift of origin of the dominant pacemaker within the sinus node or subsidiary pacemaker sites elsewhere in the atria.[54]

Enhanced Normal Automaticity

Impulse initiation can be shifted from the SA node to other parts of the heart, if a latent pacemaker assumes control of impulse formation and develops an intrinsic rate of depolarization faster than that of the SA node. Impulse originates from other sites of the heart rather than the SA is called an ectopic beat; a sequence of similar ectopic beats is called an ectopic rhythm. High concentration of catecholamine can enhance automaticity of latent pacemaker and produce ectopic beats. Common inducers of ectopic beats include hypoxemia, ischemia, electrolyte disturbances, and drug toxicities (e.g., digitalis). Increased vagal tone, drugs, electrolyte abnormalities, or disease of the SA node can decrease its rate of automaticity or cause exit block of its impulse.[55]

Examples of clinical arrhythmias due to shifting of pacemaker from the SA node include atrial, junctional, or ventricular escape rhythms that occur due to sinus bradycardia or AV block. Such "escape" pacemaker activity cannot be considered abnormal because it is a manifestation of the normal automaticity of these cells. Sinus tachycardia is due to enhanced normal automaticity, and accelerated ventricular rhythm following MI may be due to enhanced automaticity.[55]

Subsidiary pacemaker activity can be enhanced by factors that decrease the transmembrane resting potential (TRP), decrease the threshold potential, or increase rate of diastolic phase 4 depolarization of the subsidiary pacemaker cells. Figure 12-53 illustrates how these mechanisms can change the rate of firing of pacemaker cells.[55]

Enhanced normal automaticity can occur with enhanced sympathetic activity; drugs such as digitalis and sympathomimetic agents; ischemia; stretch that occurs in HF, cardiomyopathy,

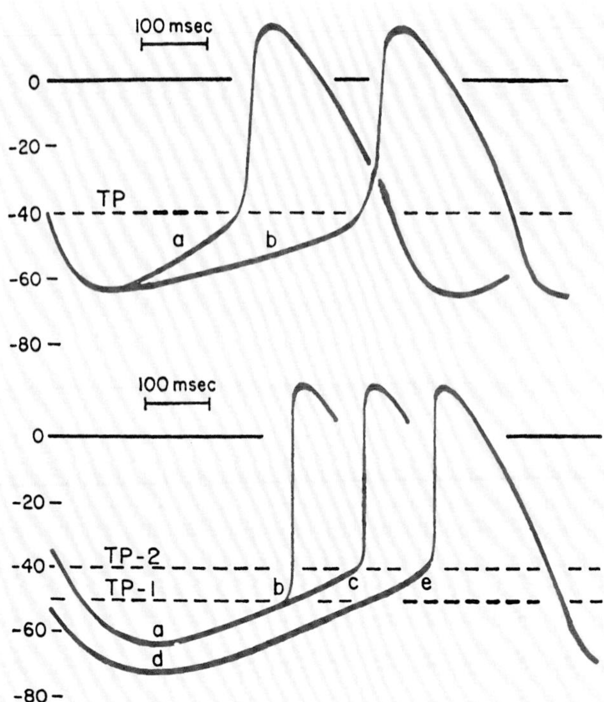

Figure 12-53. Diagram illustrating the principal mechanisms underlying changes in the frequency of discharge of a pacemaker fiber. The upper diagram shows a reduction in rate caused by a decrease in the slope of diastolic, or pacemaker, depolarization from a to b, and thus an increase in the time required for the membrane potential to decline to the threshold potential (TP) level. The lower diagram shows the reduction in the rate associated with a shift in the level of the threshold potential from TP-1 to TP-2, and a corresponding increase in cycle length (b to c); also illustrated is a further reduction in rate due to an increase in the maximal diastolic potential level (Compare a with c and d with e). (From Hoffman BF, Cranefield PF. *Electrophysiology of the Heart.* New York: McGraw-Hill; 1960, used with permission of the McGraw-Hill Book Company.)

and ventricular aneurysms; and with genetic mutations that alter the function of ion channels in the cardiac membrane. Clinical arrhythmias that may be due to enhanced normal automaticity include sinus tachycardia, some atrial tachycardias (ATs), junctional tachycardia, accelerated ventricular rhythm, and ventricular parasystole. Automaticity is not the mechanism of most rapid tachycardias, but it can precipitate or trigger reentrant tachycardias that can occur at very rapid rates.[55]

Abnormal Automaticity

Atrial and ventricular myocardial cells do not normally have spontaneous diastolic depolarization and do not initiate spontaneous impulses, even when they are not excited for long periods of time by propagating impulses.[56] However, under conditions when the TRP is reduced, atrial and ventricular cells can develop abnormal automaticity, which is referred to as depolarization-induced automaticity.[55,56] Similarly, cells in the Purkinje system show abnormal automaticity when the TRP is reduced. Abnormal automaticity is distinguished by membrane potentials reduced from their normal level. The intrinsic rate of a focus with abnormal automaticity is a function of the membrane potential. The more positive the membrane potential, the faster the automatic rate.[56]

When resting potential of a cell is reduced (e.g., from −90 to −70 mV), the cell can partially be depolarized by anything that increases the extracellular potassium concentration, decreases the intracellular potassium concentration, increases the permeability of the membrane to sodium, or decreases the membrane permeability to potassium. Ischemia, hypoxia, acidosis, hyperkalemia, digitalis toxicity, chamber enlargement or dilation, stretch, and other metabolic abnormalities or drugs can reduce the resting potential and result in abnormal automaticity.[55]

Hypoxia and ischemia affect the TRP by decreasing the amount of oxygen available to supply adenosine triphosphate in amounts sufficient to operate the sodium–potassium pump efficiently. Anything that interferes with proper operation of this pump (e.g., digitalis) reduces normal resting ionic gradients across the cell membrane and results in reduction of the resting potential. When TRP is reduced at rest, the cell is partially depolarized, and the time required for spontaneous diastolic depolarization to reach threshold is reduced; thus, pacemaker activity is increased (see Fig. 12-53). For the same reason, automaticity is increased when the threshold potential is reduced (e.g., from −40 to −50 mV) by ischemia or drug effects, because less time is required for phase 4 depolarization to reach the lower threshold. The rate of phase 4 depolarization can be increased by several factors, including local norepinephrine release at ischemic sites, systemic catecholamine release, reduced vagal tone, and drugs.[55]

Cardiac arrhythmias that may be due to abnormal automaticity include some ATs, accelerated junctional or ventricular rhythm, parasystole, and some VTs associated with acute MI. The rate of a rhythm due to abnormal automaticity is related to the membrane potential from which it arose: the less negative the membrane potential (i.e., the greater the depolarization), the faster the rate. Rhythms due to abnormal automaticity tend to occur at faster rates than rhythms due to normal automaticity.[55]

Triggered Activity Due to Afterdepolarizations

An action potential can be triggered and produce abnormal depolarization that lead to extra heart beats or rapid arrhythmias. Afterdepolarization is a process of a transient depolarization of the cell membrane that occurs at some time during or right after repolarization. This type of automaticity is stimulated by a preceding action potential. Early afterdepolarizations (EADs) occur during the repolarization phase of an action potential. Delayed afterdepolarization (DAD) occurs right after repolarization is complete but before the next action potential is due to occur. In either EADs or DADs, abnormal potentials are triggered if the afterdepolarization reaches a threshold potential.[53,55]

Early Afterdepolarizations

EADs are the changes of the membrane potential in the positive direction that interrupt the normal repolarization.[53] The plateau of the action potential is a time of high membrane resistance when there is little current flow. EADs can occur either during the plateau of the action potential (phase 2) or during rapid repolarization (phase 3). Normally, during phases 2 and 3, the net membrane current is outward. Any factor that transiently shifts the net current in the inward direction can potentially overcome and reverse repolarization and lead to EADs.[56]

EADs develop more often in Purkinje fibers and midmyocardial M cells in the ventricles. Cardiac tissues exposed to injury, altered electrolytes, hypoxia, acidosis, catecholamines, and pharmacologic agents (including antiarrhythmic drugs) are susceptible to develop EADs. Individuals with ventricular hypertrophy and HF are also at risk for developing EADs.[54] Gene mutations that alter sodium and potassium ion channel activity and result in prolonged action potential duration have been identified and shown to cause EADs. EADs appear to be the initiating mechanism of the polymorphic VT (TdP), due to genetic mutations that affect ion channel function and prolong repolarization.

Triggered activity due to EADs occurs at slow heart rates, and arrhythmias thought to be due to EADs often occur during bradycardia or after a pause in rhythm. The proarrhythmic effects of many drugs, especially class IA and class III antiarrhythmics, are due to their ability to prolong repolarization in cardiac cells and cause EADs. Cardiac arrhythmias attributed to EADs include both the acquired and congenital types of TdP, and many arrhythmias that occur with hypertrophy and HF.[55]

Delayed Afterdepolarizations

DADs occur shortly after repolarization is complete and before the next propagated impulse. Subthreshold afterdepolarizations do not result in triggered activity, but if the DADs is large enough to reach threshold, a triggered impulse arises. This triggered impulse may also be followed by its own afterdepolarization, leading to trains of triggered beats. Again, the mechanism differs from automaticity in that afterdepolarizations depend on and arise as a result of preceding action potentials.[55] DADs commonly develop in the states of high intracellular calcium (e.g., digitalis intoxication, marked catecholamine stimulation).[53]

Catecholaminergic polymorphic ventricular tachycardia (CPVT) is an example of arrhythmia induced by DADs. DADs may also contribute significantly to arrhythmogenesis in common arrhythmias. HF is associated with structural and electrophysiologic remodeling, leading to tissue heterogeneity that enhances arrhythmogenesis and the propensity of sudden cardiac death.[54]

Abnormal Impulse Conduction

Altered impulse conduction can lead to bradyarrhythmias (slow, abnormal cardiac rhythm) or aberrancy when impulses are blocked, or premature beats and tachyarrhythmias (fast abnormal cardiac rhythm) when reentrant excitation occurs.[53,55]

Conduction Block

The electrical impulse can be prevented from propagating through the heart for a variety of reasons.[55] The conduction block can be either transient or permanent and unidirectional (i.e., conduction proceeds when the involved region is stimulated from one direction but not when stimulated from the opposite direction) or bidirectional (conduction is blocked in both directions). The causes of conduction block include ischemia, fibrosis, inflammation, and certain medications. A propagating impulse may arrive late but be conducted, and this is known as functional block, for example, block caused by antiarrhythmic drugs that prolong action potential duration. When the conduction block is caused by a barrier such as fibrosis or scarring that replaces myocytes, the conduction block is known as fixed conduction block.[53]

If the propagating impulse is not strong enough to excite the tissue ahead of it, conduction will fail (i.e., decremental conduction). If an impulse arrives at an area where the tissue is still refractory after a previous depolarization, it will not be able to conduct further (i.e., phase 3 block). If an impulse reaches tissue that is abnormally depolarized due to ischemia, disease, or drugs, it may not be able to conduct at all or will conduct with delay (i.e., phase

4 block). Scar tissue from previous MI, surgery, or catheter ablation also prevents conduction.[55]

Decremental Conduction

Decremental conduction is the progressive decrease in conduction velocity of an impulse as it travels through a region of myocardium and occurs when an action potential loses its ability to stimulate the tissue ahead of it. Decremental conduction is a normal function of the AV node, delaying the impulse in the AV node long enough for atrial contraction to contribute to ventricular filling. Decremental conduction normally occurs in areas of the heart where resting potentials are low and action potentials depend on slow channels, such as the AV and SA nodes. It can also occur in areas where resting potentials are low due to ischemia, disease, or drugs. Under such circumstances, conduction velocity is slow because of the slower rate of rise of the action potential that occurs when cells are stimulated at reduced resting potentials. At times, decremental conduction can be so pronounced that the impulse fails to conduct, thus leading to block. This failure of conduction can occur in the SA node, leading to sinus exit block; in the AV node, leading to AV block; or in the bundle branch system, causing BBB.[55]

Phase 3 Block

The more negative the membrane potential is, the more sodium channels are available for activation, the greater the influx of sodium into the cell during phase 0, and the greater the conduction velocity.[57] When a cell is stimulated during phase 3 of the action potential, before full recovery and at less negative potentials of the cell membrane, conduction is impaired because a portion of sodium channels remains refractory and unavailable for activation.[57] In another word, the membrane has not yet returned to its resting level. Whenever a cell is stimulated at a less negative membrane potential, the rate of rise of the action potential, and thus conduction velocity, is slow because most sodium channels are inactivated at reduced membrane potentials. Figure 12-54 illustrates phase 3 block occurring in the right bundle branch, resulting in aberrant conduction of the impulse with a RBBB pattern.[55]

Phase 3 block, also called short-cycle aberrancy or tachycardia-dependent block,[57] can occur in normal hearts if impulses are premature enough to reach fibers during their normal refractory period, resulting in aberrant conduction of premature beats. It is also responsible for rate-dependent BBBs and for the aberration that commonly occurs when cycle lengths are very irregular, as in atrial fibrillation (AF). Phase 3 block can occur pathologically if the refractory period is abnormally prolonged by drugs or disease.[55]

Phase 4 Block

Phase 4 block, also called long-cycle aberrancy or bradycardia-dependent block, occurs when conduction of an impulse is blocked in tissues well after their normal refractory periods have ended.[57] In this case, the membrane has begun to depolarize spontaneously during its normal phase 4. By the time a stimulus arrives, the resting potential has been reduced enough to cause slow conduction. Phase 4 block is governed by the same physiologic principles as those for phase 3 block: Whenever a cell is stimulated at a less negative membrane potential, the availability of the Na^+ channels is reduced, and slow conduction results. Figure 12-55 shows a normal right bundle branch action potential followed by spontaneous phase 4 depolarization. By the time the second impulse arrives in that bundle, membrane potential has been reduced enough to cause slow conduction and RBBB.[55]

Phase 4 block is responsible for abnormal conduction that occurs only at the end of long cycles or for so-called bradycardia-dependent BBB. Phase 4 block is uncommon and is considered pathologic when it occurs.[55]

Reentry

Reentry occurs when a propagating impulse fails to die out after normal activation of the heart and continues to reexcite the heart after end of the refractory period.[54] Reentry is a type of conduction abnormality that leads to the occurrence of premature beats or sustained tachycardias rather than to a block.[55] Reentry has a fundamentally different mechanism of arrhythmogenesis than automaticity or triggered activity. The circus movement reentry

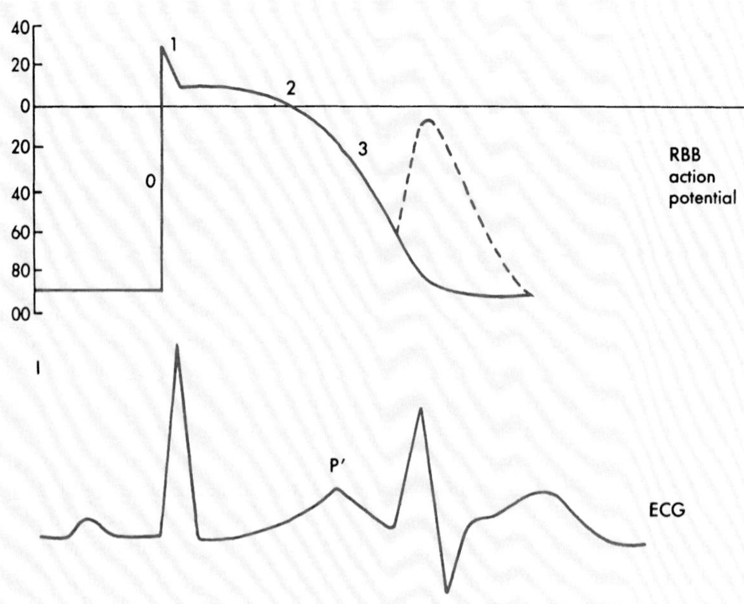

Figure 12-54. Phase 3 block. The ECG on the bottom shows a normal beat followed by a premature atrial beat that conducts with RBBB. The action potentials on top illustrate that the early beat entered the right bundle during phase 3, when the membrane potential was still reduced. The resulting action potential is a slow channel response and conduction fails. (From Conover M. *Understanding Electrocardiography*. 8th ed. St. Louis, MO: CV Mosby; 2003:172.)

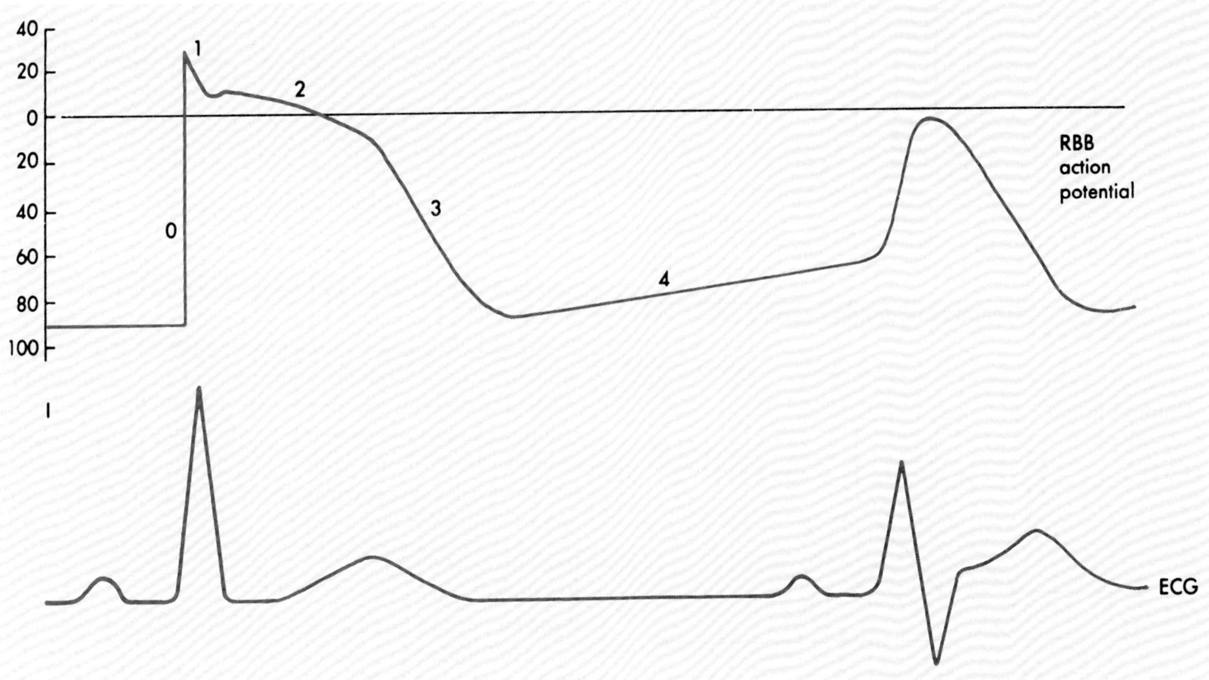

Figure 12-55. Phase 4 block. The ECG on the bottom shows a normal beat followed by a pause and a second beat that conducts with RBBB. The action potential on top illustrates that the pause after the first normal action potential allowed sufficient time for spontaneous phase 4 depolarization to occur in the RBBB. The impulse after the pause enters the RBBB at a time when its membrane potential is reduced, resulting in conduction failure. (From Conover M. *Understanding Electrocardiography*. 8th ed. St. Louis, MO: CV Mosby; 2003:173.)

occurs when an activation impulse propagates around an anatomical or functional core and reexcites the site of origin.[54] In order for the mechanism of reentry to occur, the propagating impulse must continuously encounter the excitable site. Thus, the time of impulse traveling around the reentrant loop must be greater than the time required for recovery (known as refractory period) of the tissue. If the conduction time is shorter than the recovery time, the impulse will reach the refractory tissue and stop (Fig. 12-56C). If the conduction velocities are slow, a shorter reentry circuit is possible (Fig. 12-56D). In summary, two conditions need to exist when for a reentry to occur: 1) unidirectional block and 2) slow conduction through the reentry path.

Based on these general concepts, three main types of reentry have been described. *Anatomic reentry* (Fig. 12-56) involves an anatomic obstacle around which the circulating wave of depolarization can travel. *Functional reentry* does not require an anatomic obstacle but depends on local differences in conduction velocity and refractoriness among neighboring fibers that allow an impulse to circulate repeatedly around the area. *Anisotropic reentry* is caused by structural differences among adjacent fibers that cause variations in conduction velocity and repolarization between these fibers. An impulse conducts more rapidly when it travels along the length of fibers than it does when it travels in the transverse direction across fibers. These differences in conduction velocity can result in unidirectional block and slow conduction, leading to reentry.[55]

When the impulse travels the reentry loop only once, a single premature beat occurs. If conduction velocity is slow enough and the refractory period of normal tissue is short enough, a single impulse could travel the loop numerous times, resulting in a run of premature beats or in a sustained tachycardia.[55] Reentry around distinct anatomic pathways usually appears as a monomorphic tachycardia on the ECG.[53] Reentry that occurs in small loops of tissue, such as the AV node or Purkinje tissue, is called *microreentry*. If the reentry loop involves large tracts of tissue, such as AV bypass tracts or the bundle branch system in the ventricles, it is called *macroreentry*.[55]

Many arrhythmias are thought to be due to reentry, including most VT, AF, atrial flutter, and some AT. Arrhythmias that are known to involve discrete reentry circuits are atrial flutter, atrioventricular nodal reentry tachycardia (AVNRT), circus movement tachycardia (CMT) using an accessory pathway in Wolff–Parkinson–White (WPW) syndrome, and bundle branch reentry VT.[55]

Arrhythmias and Conduction Disturbances

Arrhythmias can be a result of abnormal impulse initiation, and it can be originated from the SA node or a site other than the SA node, or abnormal impulse conduction in any part of the heart. This section will focus on arrhythmias originate from the SA node, atria, AV junction, and ventricles, and AV junction disturbance.

Rhythms Originating in the SA Node

SA is the primary pacemaker of the heart, and its intrinsic rate is 60 to 100 bpm. The arrhythmias originating from SA include sinus bradycardia, sinus tachycardia, sinus arrhythmias, sinus arrest, sinus exit block, and sick sinus syndrome (SSS).

Normal Sinus Rhythm

Normal sinus rhythm is sometimes called sinus rhythm. In normal sinus rhythm, an electrical impulse initiates from the SA node

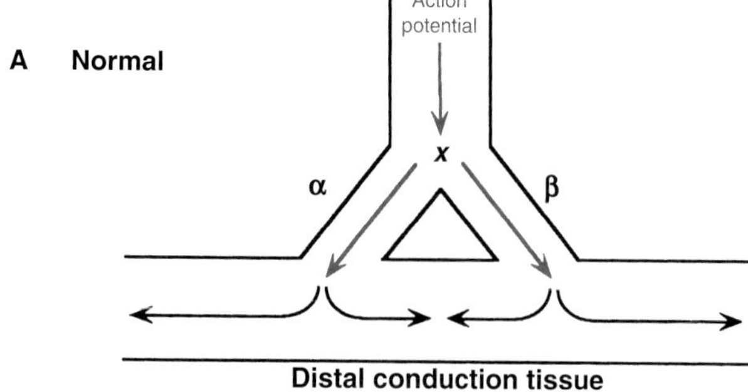

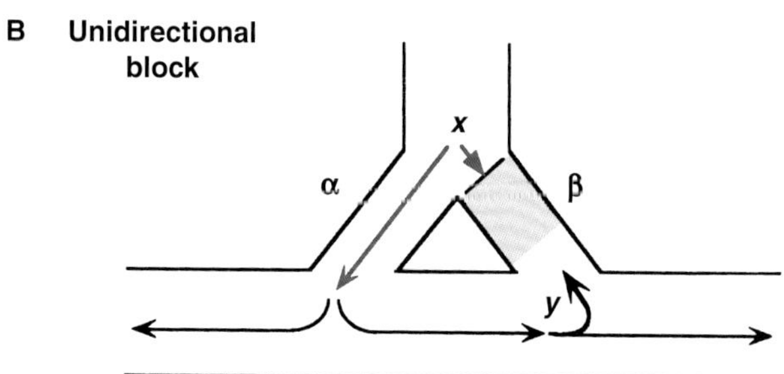

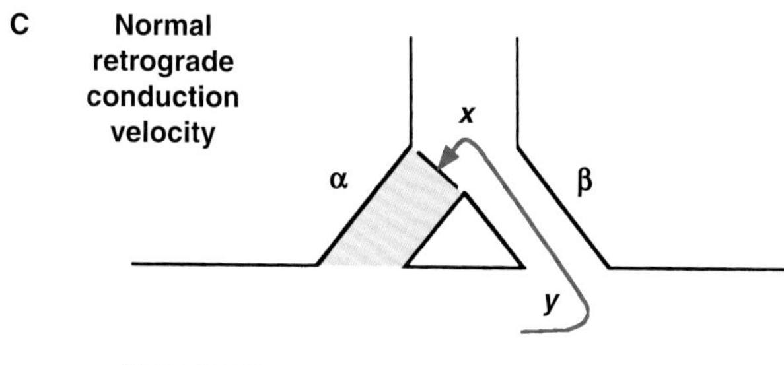

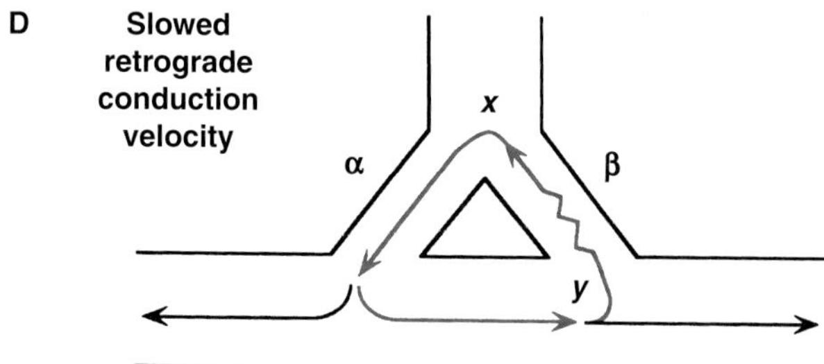

Figure 12-56. Mechanism of reentry. **A:** Normal conduction. When an action potential (AP) reaches a branch in the conduction pathway (point x), the impulse travels down both pathways (α and β) to excite distal conduction. **B:** Unidirectional block. The impulse is blocked in one limb of the pathway (β). Thus, the impulse only propagates down the α pathway. However, the AP can enter β from below and conduct in a retrograde fashion. **C:** When the impulse is able to propagate retrogradely and reach point x again, if the α pathway has not had sufficient time to repolarize, then the impulse stops. **D:** β represents a diseased pathway that the conduction is sufficiently slow (*jagged line*). When the impulse reaches point x after the α pathway has recovered, the impulse will be able to reexcite the α pathway and a reentrant loop is formed.

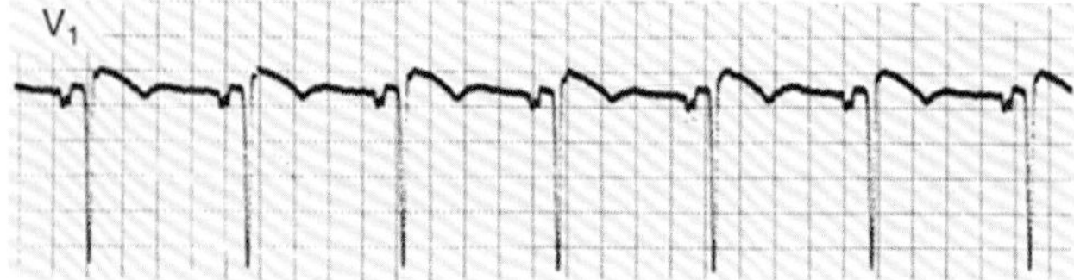

Figure 12-57. Example of normal sinus rhythm.

(intrinsic rate at 60 to 100 bpm) and travels to the AV node, which produces a slight delay to allow ventricles to completely fill. The impulse then goes through the bundle of His before it goes into right and left bundle branches, and then Purkinje fiber to depolarize the ventricles. In normal sinus rhythm, each P wave is followed by one QRS complex. In addition, the rhythm is defined as regular based on the consistent P-P interval and R-R interval (regular atrial and ventricular rhythm).The ECG characteristics of normal sinus rhythm are listed.[55,58]

Rate: 60 to 100 bpm
Rhythm: Regular
P waves: Positive (upright) in lead II. Precede each QRS complex and are consistent in shape
PR interval: 0.12 to 0.20 second, constant
QRS complex: 0.04 to 0.10 second
Example: Normal sinus rhythm. Rate: 65 bpm; PR interval: 0.14 second; QRS interval: 0.06 second (Fig. 12-57)

Sinus Bradycardia

In sinus bradycardia, the impulse originates from the SA at a slower rate: less than 60 bpm. The rhythm of sinus bradycardia is regular (consistent P-P interval and R-R interval). Each P wave is followed by one QRS complex.[55,58]

Sinus bradycardia can occur in athletes and in adults during sleep. Vagal nerve stimulation can result in sinus bradycardia, such as carotid massage, ocular pressure, coughing, vomiting, and straining to have a bowel movement. In inferior MI, the obstructed blood flow the SA node can also lead to slowing of the HR. Other conditions that cause sinus bradycardia include hypothyroidism, hypothermia, sleep apnea, increased intracranial pressure, glaucoma, myxedema, hypoxia, infections, and SSS. Medications such as beta-blocker, calcium channel block, digitalis, and antiarrhythmics can also cause sinus bradycardia. The ECG characteristics of sinus bradycardia are listed.[55,58]

Rate: Less than 60 bpm
Rhythm: Regular
P waves: Positive (upright) in lead II. Precede every QRS, consistent shape
PR interval: Usually normal
QRS complex: Usually normal
Conduction: Normal through atria, AV node, bundle branches, and ventricles
Example: Sinus bradycardia (Fig. 12-58)

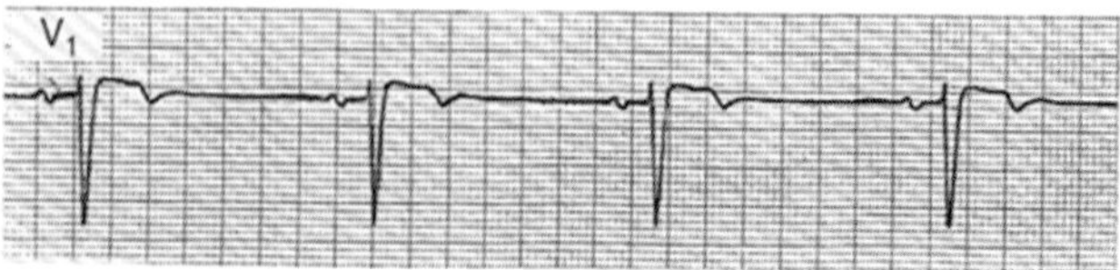

Figure 12-58. Example of sinus bradycardia.

Asymptomatic patients with sinus bradycardia do not require treatment. Atropine is the drug of choice to treat symptomatic or hemodynamically significant sinus bradycardia. Atropine increases the heart rate by blocking acetylcholine at the endings of the vagus nerves allowing more activities from the sympathetic division of the autonomic nervous system. The dose of atropine is 0.5 mg intravenously.

Sinus Tachycardia

In sinus tachycardia, the impulse originates from the SA node at a faster rate: more than 100 bpm. The rhythm of sinus tachycardia is regular with consistent P-P interval and R-R interval. Each P wave is followed by one QRS complex.[55,58]

Sinus tachycardia is a normal response to stimulation of sympathetic nervous system (e.g., exercise, pain, fear, and anxiety, etc.), and it is also a compensatory mechanism when there is a decrease in cardiac output. Drugs that cause sinus tachycardia include sympathomimetic drugs, atropine, isoproterenol, epinephrine, dopamine, dobutamine, norepinephrine, nitroprusside, and caffeine. The ECG characteristics of sinus tachycardia are listed.[55,58]

Rate: Greater than 100 bpm
Rhythm: Regular
P waves: Positive (upright) in lead II. Precede every QRS; have consistent shape; may be buried in the preceding T wave
PR interval: Usually normal, may be difficult to measure if P waves are buried in T waves
QRS complex: Usually normal
Conduction: Normal through atria, AV node, bundle branches, and ventricles
Example: Sinus tachycardia (Fig. 12-59)

Sinus tachycardia is usually associated with an underlying cause, and it is important to identify the cause and treat the cause. For example, administer intravenous fluid to correct dehydration; blood transfusion to correct anemia; medications or relaxation technique to reduce anxiety. When sinus tachycardia is a clinical indication of possible decreased cardiac output, it is crucial to intervene and optimize cardiac function.[55,58]

Sinus Arrhythmia

Sinus arrhythmia is a result of irregular initiation of impulse from the SA node. The electrical impulse follows the normal conduction pathway and leads to atrial and ventricular depolarization. Sinus arrhythmia can be associated with phases of respiration and fluctuations of intrathoracic pressure: faster rate during inspiration, and slower rate during expiration. Thus, it is called respiratory sinus arrhythmia. When sinus arrhythmia is isolated from ventilatory cycle, it is called nonrespiratory sinus arrhythmia. ECG characteristics of sinus arrhythmia are listed.[55,58]

Rate: 60 to 100 bpm
Rhythm: Irregular; phasic increase and decrease in rate, which may be related to respiration

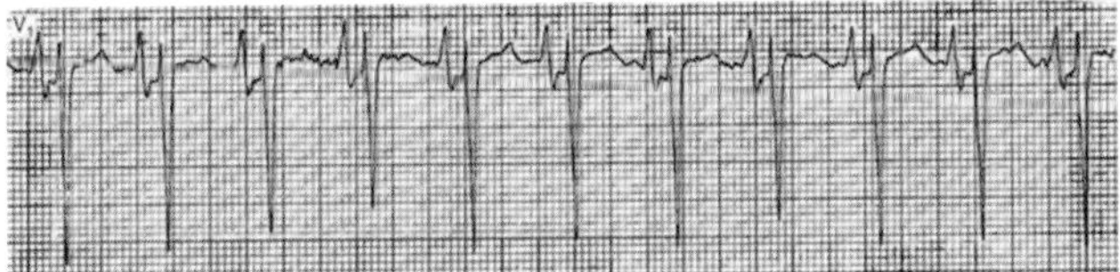

Figure 12-59. Example of sinus tachycardia.

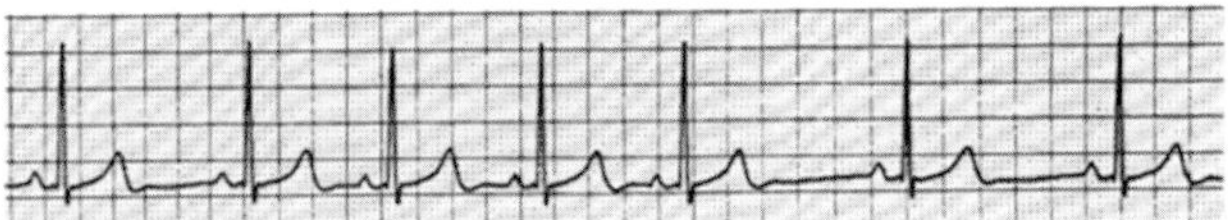

Figure 12-60. Example of sinus arrhythmia.

P waves: Positive (upright) in lead II. Precede every QRS; have consistent shape
PR interval: Usually normal
QRS complex: Usually normal
Conduction: Normal through atria, AV node, bundle branches, ventricles
Example: Sinus arrhythmia (Fig. 12-60)

Sinus arrhythmia does not require a treatment unless it causes hemodynamic changes, and it is common in children and young adults.[55,58]

Sinus Arrest

Sinus arrest is also known as SA arrest. Sinus arrest occurs when the automaticity of SA node is depressed and the SA node fails to initiate an electrical impulse, resulting in the absence of PQRST complex on the ECG. When only one sinus impulse fails to be initiated, the term sinus pause is used. The causes of sinus arrest include vagal stimulation, carotid sinus sensitivity, acute MI obstructing blood flow to the SA node, rheumatic disease, sudden increased parasympathetic activities, and reaction to medications (e.g., digitalis, beta-blocker, and calcium channel blockers). ECG characteristics of sinus arrest are listed.[55,58]

Rate: Atrial—usually within normal range but may be in bradycardic range if one more than one sinus impulse fails to form. Ventricular—usually within normal range but may be in bradycardic range if more than one sinus impulse fails to form and there are no junctional or ventricular escape beats. Occasionally, the ventricular rate may be faster than the atrial rate because of junctional or ventricular escape beats that occur during the period of sinus arrest.
Rhythm: Irregular due to the absence of one or more SA node impulse
P waves: Present when SA node is firing and absent during periods of sinus arrest. When present, they precede every QRS complex and are consistent in shape. If junctional escape beats occur, P waves may be inverted either before or after the junctional QRS
PR interval: Usually normal when P waves are present. If junctional escape beats occur, the PR interval is short when the P wave precedes the QRS.
QRS complex: Usually normal when SA node is functioning and absent during periods of sinus arrest unless escape beats occur. If ventricular escape beats occur, QRS complex is wide
Conduction: The impulse travels through the normal conduction pathway when the SA node is firing. When the SA node fails to initiate an impulse, there is no conduction through the atria. If a junctional escape beat occurs, ventricular conduction is usually normal. Whereas if a ventricular escape beat occurs, the ventricular conduction is abnormally slow.

Example: (A) Sinus pause and (B) sinus arrest with a junctional escape beat (fifth beat) (Fig. 12-61)

The signs and symptoms of sinus arrest are dependent upon the number of absent impulses. The treatment for sinus arrest should focus on the underlying causes. Observation is the only

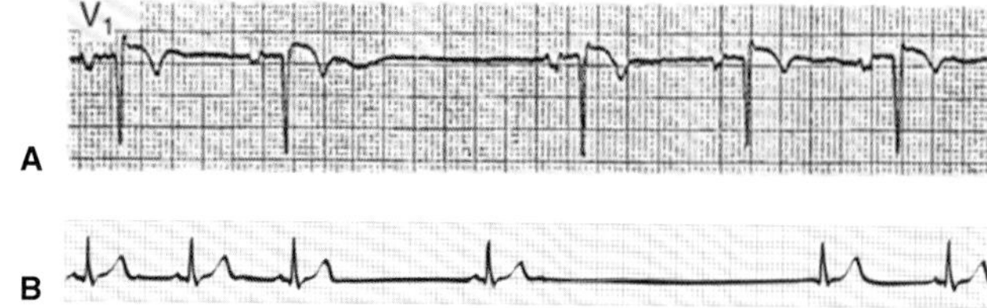

Figure 12-61. Example of sinus arrest.

necessary measure if the episodes of sinus arrest are transient. If episodes of sinus arrest are a result of medications, the offending agents should be discontinued. Avoid vagal stimulation if the cause of sinus arrest is due to carotid sinus sensitivity. Intravenous atropine 0.5 mg can be used to increase the ventricular rate.[55,58]

Sinus Exit Block

Sinus exit block occurs when an electrical impulse initiated in the SA node but fails to exit the node to depolarize the atrial tissue. There are three different types of sinus exit block: type I, type II, and complete. Wenckebach is type I sinus exit block, which will be discussed later in this chapter. Type II sinus exit block appears exactly like the sinus arrest except for the P-P intervals, which are the multiples of the basic sinus cycle length. No impulses reach the atria in complete exit block; thus, there is absence of P waves. A junctional or ventricular pacemaker will take over the pacing duties, otherwise asystole may occur. The ECG characteristics of sinus exit block are listed.[55,58]

Rate: Atrial—usually within normal range however can be in bradycardic range if more than one sinus impulse fails to exit the SA node. Ventricular—usually in normal range however can be in bradycardic range if no junctional or ventricular escape beats occur during episodes of sinus exit block

Rhythm: Irregular due to pauses caused by sinus exit block

P waves: Present except when impulse fails to exit SA node. When present, they precede every QRS and are consistent in shape. The P-P interval is an exact multiple of the sinus cycle because impulses are formed regularly but occasionally fail to exit the SA node

PR interval: Usually normal when P waves are present but may be prolonged if AV node conduction is slow

QRS complexes: Usually normal when sinus impulse conducts and absent when exit block occurs. If ventricular escape beats occur, QRS is wide

Conduction: Normal through atria, AV node, bundle branches, and ventricles when impulse exits SA node normally

Example: Sinus exit block. The length of the pause is exactly double the sinus rate (Fig. 12-62)

Treatment for sinus exit block depends on the signs and symptoms. If episodes of sinus exit block are transient, and patient has no significant signs and symptoms, further observation is adequate. If sinus exist block causes hemodynamic instability, or it is a result of medications, offending agents should be discontinued. Intravenous atropine, temporary pacing, or permanent pacemaker can be considered if the episodes of sinus exit block are frequent.[55,58]

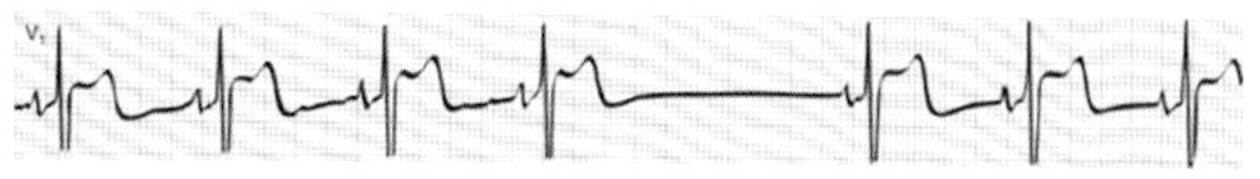

Figure 12-62. Example of sinus exit block.

Sick Sinus Syndrome

SSS is sometimes referred as brady-tachy syndrome due to its characteristics: sinus bradycardia, sinus pauses, or period of sinus arrest alternating with paroxysms of rapid atrial arrhythmias (atrial flutter or AF). SSS is common in elderly patients, and it can be a result of atrial fibrosis which impairs the function of SA node and predisposes AF and atrial flutter. Junctional escape rhythm usually takes over during the episodes of sinus bradycardia or arrest. The ECG characteristics of SSS are listed.[55,58]

Rate: Varies, can be bradycardic to tachycardic rates. It depends on SA node function, rate of escape pacemakers, and presence of atrial tachyarrhythmias

Rhythm: Irregular; pauses of 3 seconds or more can occur during periods of sinus arrest. Regularity of rhythm depends on reliability of SA node and escape pacemakers, and on the type of tachyarrhythmia present (e.g., AF is very irregular)

P waves: Usually normal during periods of sinus rhythm. Absent during periods of sinus arrest or AF or inverted with junctional rhythms. Flutter waves are present during periods of atrial flutter

PR interval: May be normal or prolonged depending on state of AV conduction. During the episodes of AF or atrial flutter, the PR interval cannot be measured

QRS complex: Usually normal unless there is associated BBB or ventricular escape rhythms

Conduction: Normal through the atria when the SA node is in control; abnormal through atria during periods of atrial tachyarrhythmias. AV conduction may be normal or abnormal depending on the degree of AV node disease. Conduction through ventricles is normal unless BBBs are present, or a ventricular escape rhythm occurs

Examples: (A) SSS presenting with extreme variation in sinus rate. (B) Brady-tachy syndrome. Rhythm changes back and forth from atrial flutter to sinus (Fig. 12-63)

Treatment options for SSS include atropine or pacing for bradyarrhythmias. Antiarrhythmics can be used for tachyarrhythmias. Medications used for tachyarrhythmias can further depress SA node and exacerbate bradycardia. Thus, a permanent pacemaker might become necessary.

Rhythms Originating in the Atria

Ectopic impulse or reentry circuits can originate in the atrial myocardium and lead to atrial arrhythmias: premature atrial contractions, wandering atrial pacemaker (WAP), AT, multifocal atrial tachycardia (MAT), atrial flutter, and AF. Atrial arrhythmias are results of abnormal electrical impulse formation and conduction in the atria.

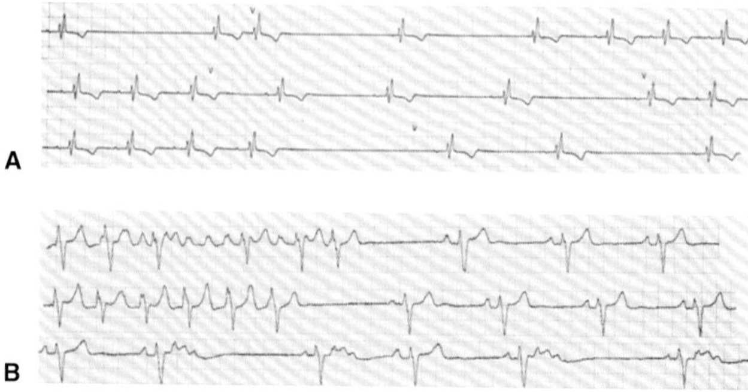

Figure 12-63. Examples of (**A**) sick sinus syndrome (**B**) and brady-tachy syndrome.

Premature Atrial Complex

A premature atrial complex (PAC) is also known as atrial premature depolarization. A premature atrial impulse may or may not travel to the ventricle and produce ventricular depolarization. When there is an atrial contraction, but no ventricular contraction (absence of a QRS complex follows the P wave), it is called a nonconducted PAC. A PAC occurs when an irritable area (site/focus) within the atria fires before the next SA node impulse is expected to fire. The characteristics of premature P wave are dependent upon the location of the impulse. The P wave will look very similar to P wave initiated by the SA node if the irritable focus is near the SA node. The P wave of a PAC may be biphasic, flattened, notched, pointed, or lost in the preceding T wave. The causes of PACs include caffeine, alcohol, nicotine, atrial distention (stretch), interruption of blood flow due to myocardial ischemia or infarction, anxiety, and hypermetabolic states. The ECG characteristics of PAC are listed.[55,58]

Rate: Usually within normal range

Rhythm: Usually regular except the PACs. PACs often have a noncompensatory pause (interval between the complex before and that after the PAC is less than two normal R-R intervals) because premature depolarization of the atria by the PAC also causes premature depolarization of the SA node, thus causing the SA node to "reset" itself

P waves: Positive (upright) in lead II. Precede every QRS except when there is a nonconducted PAC. The configuration of the premature P wave differs from the P waves initiated from the SA because the premature impulse originates in a different part of the atria and depolarizes the atria in a different way. Very early P waves may be buried in the preceding T wave

PR interval: May be normal or long depending on the prematurity of the beat. Very early PACs may find the AV junction still partially refractory and unable to conduct at a normal rate, resulting in a prolonged PR interval

QRS complex: May be normal, aberrant (wide), or absent, depending on the prematurity of the beat. If the bundle branches have repolarized completely, they are able to conduct the early impulse normally, resulting in a normal QRS complex. If the PAC occurs during the RRP of the bundle branches or ventricles, the impulse conducts aberrantly and the QRS is wide. If the PAC occurs very early during the complete refractory period of the AV node or both bundle branches, the impulse does not conduct to the ventricles and the QRS is absent

Conduction: PACs travel through the atria differently from sinus impulses because they originate from a different spot. Conduction through the AV node, bundle branches, and ventricles is usually normal unless the PAC is very early (see previous discussion of PR interval and QRS complex)

Examples: (A) Sinus rhythm with PAC. (B) Sinus rhythm with a nonconducted PAC (Fig. 12-64)

PACs may occur in patterns.[55,58]

- Couplet: two PACs in a row
- Runs or bursts: three or more PACs in a row
- Bigeminy: every other beat is a PAC
- Trigeminy: every third beat is a PAC
- Quadrigeminy: every fourth beat is a PAC

Treatments for PACs are not required if the PACs are infrequent and do not cause hemodynamic instability. Patients may feel the skipped beats or palpitation with PACs. Treat underlying causes when PACs become frequent and cause hemodynamic

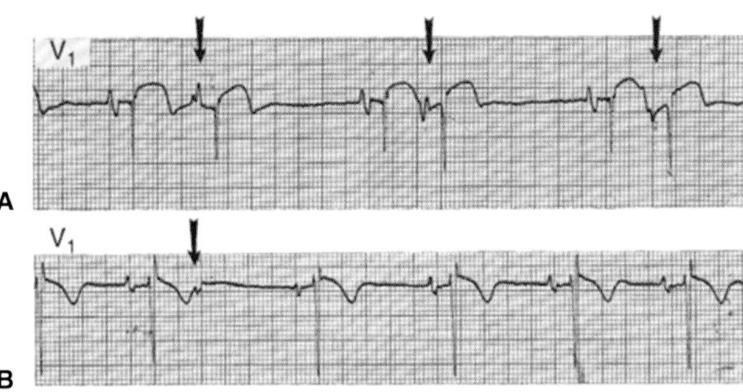

Figure 12-64. Examples: **A:** Sinus rhythm with PAC. **B:** Sinus rhythm with a nonconducted PAC.

compromises: stop stimulant-like caffeine, alcohol, and smoking; replace electrolytes, etc.[55,58]

Multiform Atrial Rhythm

Multiform atrial rhythm is also known as WAP. The P waves in WAP demonstrate varied morphology: size, shape, and direction of the P waves can vary from beat to beat. The difference in the look of the P waves is dependent upon the location of initiated impulse origin: the SA node, the atria, and/or the AV junction. A minimum of three different P waves is required for the diagnosis of WAP.[55,58]

The ECG characteristics of WAP are as the following:[55,58]

Rate: Normal or slow. 60 to 100 bpm

Rhythm: Usually irregular

P waves: Exhibit varying shapes (upright, flat, inverted, biphasic, rounded, pointed, notched) depend on the location of originated impulse: different parts of the atria or junction and as atrial fusion occurs. P waves can also be buried in QRS complexes. At least three different P-wave configurations should be seen

PR interval: May vary depending on proximity of the dominant pacemaker to the AV node

QRS complex: Usually normal

Conduction: Conduction through the atria varies as it is depolarized from different spots.

Conduction through the bundle branches and ventricles is usually normal

Example: WAP (Fig. 12-65)

WAP is usually transient. Thus, treatment is usually not necessary. WAP can be a result of underlying heart disease and digitalis toxicity. Treat the underlying cause or withhold medications. When patient is symptomatic with WAP, atropine can be given.[55,58]

Multifocal Atrial Tachycardia

MAT is also known as chaotic AT. MAT is a WAP rhythm associated with rapid chaotic firing of several ectopic atrial sites at a faster than 100 bpm, and rapid ventricular response. MAT is the most commonly seen in elderly patients and is associated with chronic obstructive pulmonary disease. MAT also occurs in the

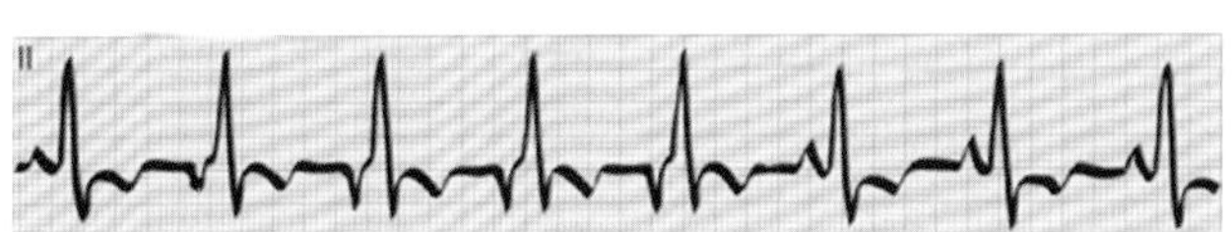

Figure 12-65. Example of WAP.

setting of HF, hypokalemia, hypomagnesemia, hypoxia, acute MI, and mitral stenosis. MAT may be a precursor of AF, and it often misdiagnosed as AF due to similar ECG characteristics. ECG characteristics of MAT are listed.[55,58]

Rate: Usually 100 to 130 bpm
Rhythm: Usually irregular, as the pacemaker site can be from SA node, ectopic atrial locations, or AV junction
P waves: One P wave precedes each QRS complex, but varies in shape because they originate in different spots in the atria. At least three different P waves are seen. Sometimes some P waves may be blocked in the AV node
PR interval: Varies depending on proximity of each ectopic atrial focus to the AV node and the prematurity of atrial impulses
QRS complex: Usually normal unless it is abnormally conducted
Conduction: Usually normal through the AV node and ventricles. Aberrant ventricular conduction may occur if an impulse is conducted into the ventricles while they are partially refractory
Example: MAT (Fig. 12-66)

The treatment for MAT aims to eliminate the underlying causes, such as hypoxia, and electrolytes imbalance. Beta-blockers, verapamil, flecainide, amiodarone, and magnesium have been reported as successful treatments for MAT. Beta-blockers need to be used with caution due to the association of MAT and pulmonary disease. Radiofrequency ablation of the AV can be an option when MAT becomes chronic and unresponsive to drug therapy. Permanent pacemaker can be used to control rapid ventricular rate.[55,59]

Atrial Tachycardia

AT is a regular atrial rhythm that arises from an ectopic site in the right and left atrium at a rate of 100 to 250 bpm. AT is often precipitated by a PAC, especially when there are three or more PACs in a row at a rate of more than 100 bpm. AT can be a result of caffeine, tobacco, alcohol, mitral valve disease, rheumatic heart disease, chronic obstructive pulmonary disease, acute MI, theophylline administration, hypokalemia, and digitalis toxicity.[59]

Atrial to ventricular conduction is usually 1:1 in AT unless the atrial rate is rapid. In a healthy heart with normal conduction, the AV node can usually conduct each atrial impulse up to a rate of 180 bpm or more. The AV node is not able to conduct each impulse in patients with cardiac disease or who take drugs to slow AV conduction, resulting in AT with block. The presence of AT with block can be a sign of digitalis toxicity.[59] ECG characteristics of AT are listed.[55]

Rate: Atrial rate is 100 to 250 bpm (quite often in the range of 140 to 180 bpm). The ventricular rate depends on the amount of block at the AV node and may be the same as the atrial rate or slower.
Rhythm: Regular unless there are blocks at the AV node
P waves: One P wave precedes each QRS complex, and P waves might be hidden in the preceding T waves. Differ in configuration from sinus P waves because they are ectopic. When block is present, more P waves appear before each QRS complex
PR interval: Usually in the normal range, sometimes can be shorter or longer than normal. It is often difficult to measure because of hidden P waves
QRS complex: Usually normal but may be wide if aberrant conduction is present
Conduction: Usually normal through the AV node and into the ventricles. In AT with block, some atrial impulses do not conduct into the ventricles. Aberrant ventricular conduction may occur if atrial impulses are conducted into the ventricles while the bundle branches are still partially refractory
Examples: AT. Both strips are from the same patient. (A) AT at a rate of 187 bpm. (B) AT with block, occurring after administration of propranolol (Fig. 12-67)

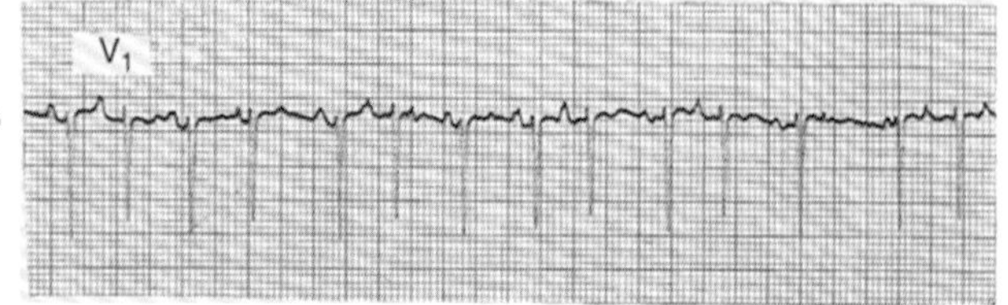

Figure 12-66. Example of MAT.

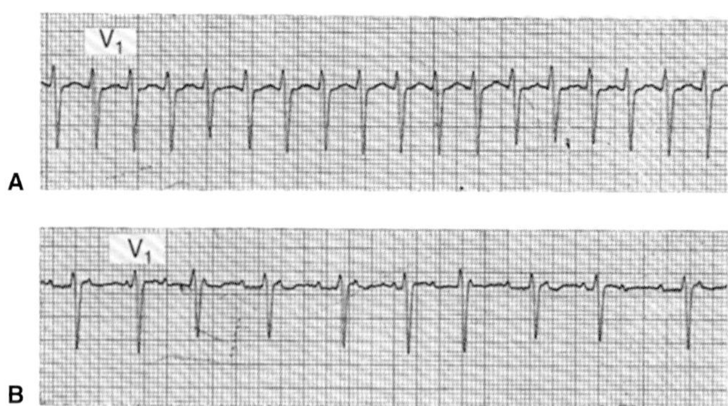

Figure 12-67. AT. Both strips are from the same patient. **A:** AT at a rate of 187 beats per minute. **B:** AT with block, occurring after administration of propranolol.

AT can lead to hemodynamic instability, and prolonged AT along with other supraventricular tachycardias (SVTs) can result in tachycardia-mediated cardiomyopathy. Left ventricular dilation can result in dilated cardiomyopathy and systolic dysfunction. Thus, it is required to treat chronic tachycardia to prevent the development of cardiomyopathy.[55] Treatment for AT is directed at eliminating the underlying cause, decreasing the ventricular rate and preventing recurrences of tachycardia. Vagal stimulation, such as carotid massage and Valsalva maneuver can terminate AT. Adenosine can be beneficial to restore sinus rhythm (if AT is persistent and cause hemodynamic compromise) or diagnose mechanism of tachycardia in patients with suspected focal AT.[60] Beta-blockers and calcium channel blockers can be used to slow down the ventricular rate.[55,60] If patient cannot tolerate beta-blockers and calcium channel blockers, intravenous amiodarone can be used for ventricular rate control and convert AT to sinus rhythm.[55] Synchronized cardioversion can be performed as a treatment option.[60] Radiofrequency catheter ablation of the ectopic focus or reentry circuit is the primary treatment for AT.[55]

Atrial Fibrillation

AF is the most common dysrhythmia treated in clinical practice and the most common dysthymia for which that patients are hospitalized.[61] AF is an extremely rapid and disorganized atrial depolarization. AF occurs when atrial tissue is altered by structural and/or electrophysiologic abnormalities promoting abnormal impulse formation and/or propagation[61]: abnormal automaticity in one or several rapidly firing sites in the atria or reentry involving one or more circuits in the atria.[59] Clinical conditions alter atrial tissue include the presence of atherosclerotic or rheumatic heart disease, thyrotoxicosis, HF, cardiomyopathy, valve disease, pulmonary disease, MI, congenital heart disease, electrolyte imbalance, and cardiac surgery.[29]

AF is typically classified as following: *Paroxysmal* refers to AF that terminates spontaneously in less than 7 days. *Persistent* refers to AF that remains for more than 7 days and fails to terminate within 7 days. *Permanent* refers to AF that is persistent for longer than 1 year and cardioversion has either not been attempted or has failed to restore or maintain sinus rhythm. Patients may start out with paroxysmal AF that then becomes persistent or permanent. Lone AF refers to AF occurring in people younger than 60 years without any evidence of structural heart disease, pulmonary disease, or hypertension. Patients with lone AF are at lower risk for thromboembolic complications. ECG characteristics of AF are listed.[61]

Rate: Atrial rate is 400 to 600 bpm or faster. Ventricular rate variable depends on the amount of block at the AV node. In new-onset AF, the ventricular response is usually rapid, 110 to 160 bpm; in treated AF, the ventricular rate is controlled in the normal range of 60 to 100 bpm

Rhythm: Irregular. One of the distinguishing features of AF is the marked irregularity of the ventricular response because of concealed conduction in the AV junction. If the ventricular response is ever regular in the presence of AF, AV dissociation should be suspected

P waves: No identifiable P waves. Atrial activity is chaotic, with no formed atrial impulses visible. Irregular fibrillation waves are often seen and vary in size from coarse to very fine

PR interval: Not measurable because there are no identifiable P waves

QRS complex: Usually normal; aberration is common, especially at faster ventricular rates

Conduction: Intra-atrial conduction is disorganized and irregular. Most of the atrial impulses are blocked in the AV junction; those impulses that are conducted through the AV junction are usually conducted normally through the ventricles. If an atrial impulse reaches the bundle branch system during its refractory period, aberrant intraventricular conduction can occur.

Examples: (A) AF. (B) Alternating coarse and fine AF (sometimes called *atrial fib-flutter*). (C) Fine AF. (D) AF with a slow and regular ventricular response, most likely due to complete AV block (Fig. 12-68)

AF is associated with an approximately fivefold increase in risk of stroke and twofold increase in the risk for all-cause mortality.[61] AF also leads to peripheral thromboembolism.[61] Atria become quivering in AF, and as a result, there is a loss of atrial kick and a subsequent decrease in cardiac output. Coronary blood flow can be impaired due to decreased diastolic coronary perfusion time. Stasis of blood in the atria could lead to mural thrombus formation, leading to pulmonary or systemic embolization. Sustained rapid ventricular response can lead to tachycardia-mediated cardiomyopathy with ventricular dilation and reduced LV function.[55]

Treatment for AF focuses on ventricular rate control, prevention of thrombus formation, and eliminating the underlying causes. Emergent or urgent electrical cardioversion may be necessary when AF with rapid ventricular response cause hemodynamic instability. Cardioversion is more likely to be successful if AF has been present for less than 24 hours.[55]

Two main management strategies are available for managing patients with AF: rate control or rhythm control. Rate control is using drug therapy to control ventricular rate (usually less than 100 bpm) without intention of restore sinus rhythm. Rhythm control has a goal of restoring and maintaining sinus rhythm. It has been thought that the benefit of rhythm would be superior with restored atrial kick, improved cardiac output, and possible reduced incidence of stroke and bleeding. Studies have not demonstrated rhythm control is a more superior management strategy than rate control.[55]

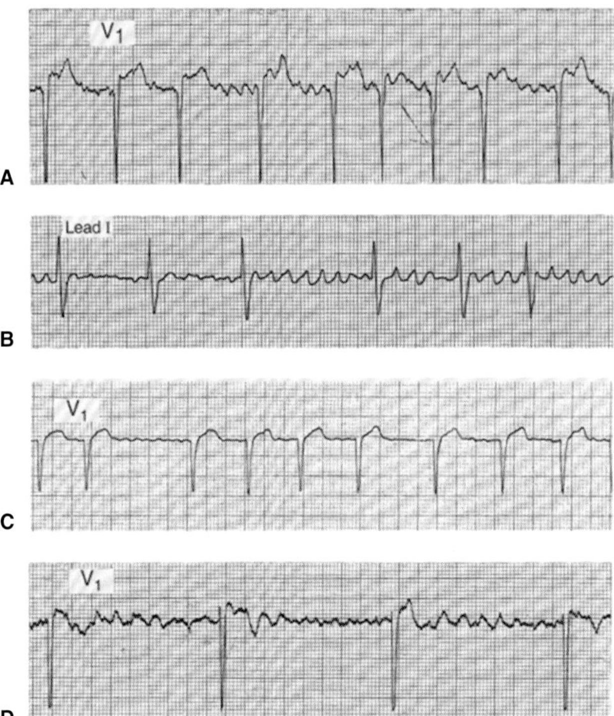

Figure 12-68. A: AF. **B:** Alternating coarse and fine AF (sometimes called *atrial fib-flutter*). **C:** Fine AF. **D:** AF with a slow and regular ventricular response, most likely due to complete AV block.

Approximately 90% of left atrial thrombi form in the atrial appendage. Thus, successful excision or closure of the left atrial appendage should reduce the risk for thromboembolic complications in patients with AF.[61] Closure of left atrial appendage can be achieved with surgery or percutaneous techniques. Percutaneous Closure of the Left Atrial Appendage Versus Warfarin Therapy for Prevention of Stroke in Patients With Atrial Fibrillation (PROTECT AF) was a randomized clinical trial conducted by Holmes et al.[62] The investigators compared the efficacy of a percutaneous closure device versus warfarin to prevent thromboembolic complications in 707 eligible patients who had at least one of the following: previous stroke or transient ischemic attack, congestive HF, diabetes, hypertension, or were 75 years or older. The percutaneous device was found to be noninferior than warfarin. Alli et al.[63] assessed quality of life parameters in a subset of patients enrolled in the PROTECT AF trial; it was found that patients with nonvalvular AF treated with left atrial appendage closure have favorable quality of life changes at 12 months versus patients treated with warfarin.

Atrial Flutter

Atrial flutter is an organized atrial rhythm, caused by reentry in which the impulse initiated from an irritable site circles within the atria and depolarizes the atria regularly at a very rapid rate

(240 to 320 bpm).[64,65] Atrial flutter is characterized by a saw-tooth pattern of regular atrial activation called flutter (F) waves on the ECG. Classic or typical atrial flutter (type I) is due to fix reentry circuit in the right atrium around which the impulse circulates in a counterclockwise direction, which results in F waves inverted (negative) in ECG leads II, III, and aVF and upright (positive) in lead V_1. When the direction of impulse is reversed, it leads to F waves that are upright (positive) in leads II, III, and aVF and inverted (negative) in lead V_1. Atrial flutter commonly occurs with 2:1 AV block (see Fig. 12-69 example A: Atrial flutter with 2:1 conduction), resulting in a regular or irregular ventricular rate of 120 to 160 bpm (most characteristically about 150 bpm). Atrial flutter and AF may revert back and forth, which fluctuates on the ECG.[65] Type II A flutter is more rapid (greater than 340 bpm)[61] and less stable than type I, and it is more likely to revert to AF.[55] The underline mechanism of type II A flutter remained undefined.[64]

The ECG characteristics of atrial flutter are as the following[55]:

Rate: Atrial rate varies between 240 and 320 bpm, most commonly 300 bpm. Ventricular rate depends on AV blockage, and it usually will not exceed 180 bpm due to the intrinsic rate of the AV junction. Ventricular rates can be within the normal range when atrial flutter is treated with appropriate drugs. Rarely, 1:1 conduction results in a ventricular rate of 300 bpm
Rhythm: Atrial rhythm is regular. Ventricular rhythm may be regular or irregular because of varying AV block
P waves: F waves are seen, characterized by a regular, biphasic saw-tooth pattern with no isoelectric segment between waves. One F wave is usually hidden in the QRS complex, and when 2:1 conduction occurs, F waves may not be readily apparent. Flutter waves are best seen in the inferior leads (II, III, and aVF) and may appear more like individual P waves in lead V_1
PR interval: Not measurable
QRS complex: Usually normal; aberration can occur
Conduction: Usually normal through the AV node and ventricles
Examples: Atrial flutter. All strips are from the same patient. (A) Atrial flutter with 2:1 conduction. (B) Ventricular rate slows momentarily, and flutter waves are clearly visible at a rate of 300 bpm. (C) Atrial flutter with variable conduction (Fig. 12-69)

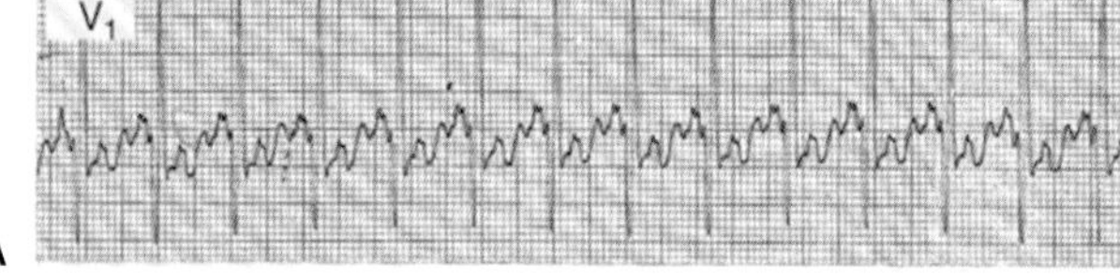

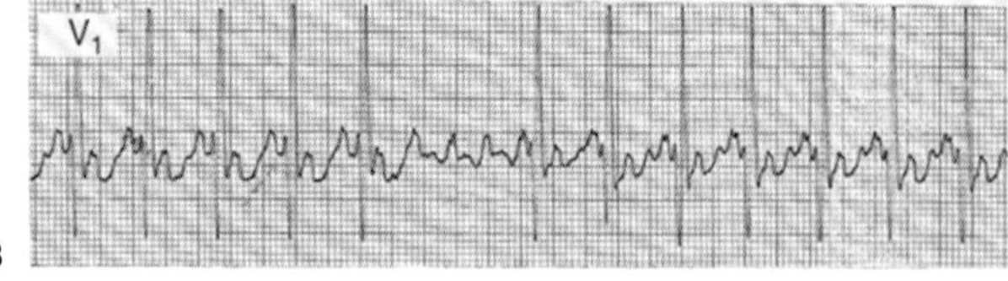

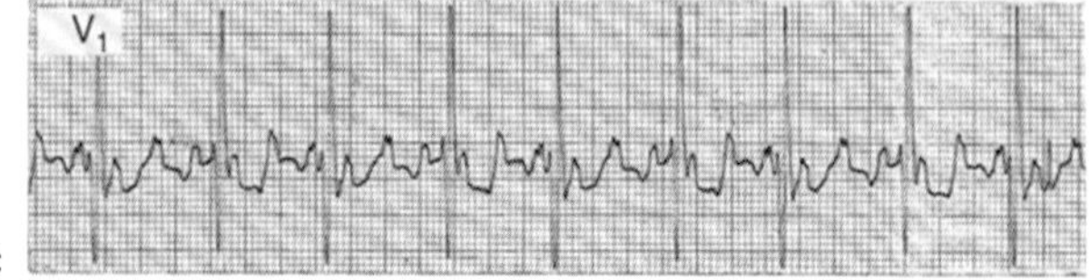

Figure 12-69. Atrial flutter. All strips are from the same patient. **A:** Atrial flutter with 2:1 conduction. **B:** Ventricular rate slows momentarily, and flutter waves are clearly visible at a rate of 300 beats per minute. **C:** Atrial flutter with variable conduction.

Atrial flutter may cause hemodynamic compromise due to rapid ventricular response resulting in decreased cardiac output. Thrombi formation may occur in atria due to lack of strong atrial contraction and the presence of blood stasis. Ventricular rate control is the primary goal of treatment. Anticoagulation is required prior to electrical or chemical cardioversion if atrial flutter has been present for 48 hours or more, or unknown onset. Radiofrequency is treatment of choice for chronic or recurrent atrial flutter, and it is an alternative for chronic drug therapy[55,59]

Table 12-10 for guidelines of rate control and rhythm control in patients with AF

Table 12-11 Guidelines for management of AF and atrial flutter: Preventing Thromboembolism.

Table 12-12 Guidelines for management of AF and atrial flutter: Electrical and Pharmacologic Cardioversion for AF: Prevention of Thromboembolism

Table 12-13 Guidelines for management of AF and atrial flutter: Maintenance of Sinus Rhythm

Supraventricular Tachycardia

The term SVT can be used to describe any rhythm which originates above the ventricle at a rate of faster than 100 bpm at rest[60]: the impulse can begin in the SA node, atrial tissue, or the AV junction.[55] Based on this definition, sinus tachycardia, AT, atrial flutter, AF, junctional tachycardia, AVNRT, and CMT utilizing an accessory pathway in WPW syndrome can all be named SVT. If the type of tachycardia is clear from the ECG, it should then be called by its appropriate name and the term SVT should be reserved for regular, narrow QRS tachycardias in which the exact mechanism cannot be identified from the ECG.[55] ECG characteristics of SVT are listed[55]:

Rate: Faster than 100 bpm; can be as fast as 280 bpm
Rhythm: Regular
P waves: Usually not visible, making the exact mechanism of the tachycardia uncertain
PR interval: Not measurable due to invisible P waves
QRS complex: Usually narrow; may be wide if aberrant ventricular conduction occurs
Conduction: Conduction through the atria varies depending on the mechanism of tachycardia. Atria may depolarize in a retrograde direction when the mechanism is AVNRT or CMT. Conduction through ventricles is normal unless BBB is present or there is anterograde conduction through an accessory pathway
Examples: Two examples of SVT. (A) SVT at a rate of 187 bpm, found to be AVNRT during electrophysiology study. (B) Narrow QRS tachycardia at a rate of 187 bpm, mechanism is unknown (Fig. 12-70)

Treatment options for SVT depend on patient's tolerance to SVT. If the rapid ventricular rate causes hemodynamic

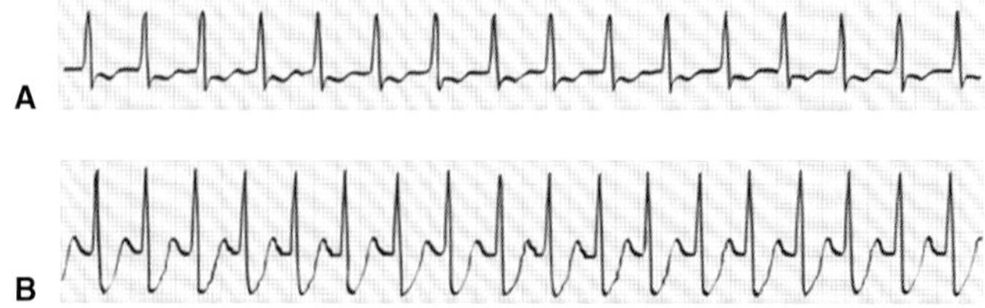

Figure 12-70. Two examples of SVT. **A:** SVT at a rate of 187, found to be AVNRT during electrophysiology study. **B:** Narrow QRS tachycardia at a rate of 187, mechanism is unknown.

Table 12-10 • GUIDELINES FOR MANAGEMENT OF AF AND ATRIAL FLUTTER: PHARMACOLOGIC RATE CONTROL DURING AF

Class	Indication	LOE
Class I	Control ventricular rate using a beta-blocker or nondihydropyridine calcium channel antagonist for paroxysmal, persistent, or permanent AF	B
	IV beta-blocker (esmolol, metoprolol, or propranolol) or nondihydropyridine calcium channel blocker (verapamil, diltiazem) is recommended to slow ventricular heart rate in the acute setting in patients without pre-excitation. Exercise caution in patients with hypotension and HF. In hemodynamically unstable patients, electrical cardioversion is indicated	B
	For AF, assess heart rate control during exertion, adjusting pharmacologic treatment as necessary	C
	Measurement of the heart rate at rest and control of the rate using pharmacologic agents (either a beta-blocker or nondihydropyridine calcium channel antagonist, in most cases) are recommended for patients with persistent or permanent AF	B
	Intravenous administration of digoxin or amiodarone is recommended to control the heart rate in patients with AF and HF who do not have an accessory pathway	B
	In patients who experience symptoms related to AF during activity, the adequacy of heart rate control should be assessed during exercise, adjusting pharmacologic treatment as necessary to keep the rate in the physiologic range	C
	Digoxin is effective following oral administration to control the heart rate at rest in patients with AF and is indicated for patients with HF, LV dysfunction, or for sedentary individuals	C
Class IIa	A heart rate control (resting heart rate <80 bpm) strategy is reasonable for symptomatic management of AF	B
	IV amiodarone can be useful for rate control in critically ill patients without pre-excitation	B
	AV nodal ablation with permanent ventricular pacing is reasonable when pharmacologic therapy is inadequate and rhythm control is not achievable	B
	A combination of digoxin and either a beta-blocker or nondihydropyridine calcium channel antagonist is reasonable to control the heart rate both at rest and during exercise in patients with AF. The choice of medication should be individualized, and the dose modulated to avoid bradycardia	B
	It is reasonable to use ablation of the AV node or accessory pathway to control heart rate when pharmacologic therapy is insufficient or associated with side effects	B
	Intravenous amiodarone can be useful to control the heart rate in patients with AF when other measures are unsuccessful or contraindicated	C
	When electrical cardioversion is not necessary in patients with AF and an accessory pathway, intravenous procainamide or ibutilide is a reasonable alternative	C
Class IIb	A lenient rate-control strategy (resting heart rate <110 bpm) may be reasonable when patients remain asymptomatic and LV systolic function is preserved	B
	Oral amiodarone may be useful for ventricular rate control when other measures are unsuccessful or contraindicated	C
	When the ventricular rate cannot be adequately controlled both at rest and during exercise in patients with AF using a beta-blocker, nondihydropyridine calcium channel antagonist, or digoxin, alone or in combination, oral amiodarone may be administered to control the heart rate	C
	Intravenous procainamide, disopyramide, ibutilide, or amiodarone may be considered for hemodynamically stable patients with AF involving conduction over an accessory pathway	B
	When the rate cannot be controlled with pharmacologic agents or tachycardia-mediated cardiomyopathy is suspected, catheter-directed ablation of the AV node may be considered in patients with AF to control the heart rate	C
Class III	AV nodal ablation should not be performed without prior attempts to achieve rate control with medications	C
	Nondihydropyridine calcium channel antagonists should not be used in decompensated HF	C
	With pre-excitation and AF, digoxin, nondihydropyridine calcium channel antagonists, or amiodarone should not be administered	B
	Dronedarone should not be used to control ventricular rate with permanent AF	B
	Digitalis should not be used as the sole agent to control the rate of ventricular response in patients with paroxysmal AF	B
	Catheter ablation of the AV node should not be attempted without a prior trial of medication to control the ventricular rate in patients with AF	C
	In patients with decompensated HF and AF, intravenous administration of a nondihydropyridine calcium channel antagonist may exacerbate hemodynamic compromise and is not recommended	C
	Intravenous administration of digitalis glycosides or nondihydropyridine calcium channel antagonists to patients with AF and a pre-excitation syndrome may paradoxically accelerate the ventricular response and is not recommended	C

Class I: strong/indicated; Class IIa: moderate/reasonable; Class IIb: weak/may be considered; Class III: no benefit or harm/not indicated or may be harmful.
Adapted from January CT, Wann LS, Alpert JS, et al. 2014 AHA/ACC/HRS guideline for the management of patients with atrial fibrillation. *J Am Coll Cardiol.* 2014;64(21):e1–e76.

compromise, cardioversion may be required. Medications such as adenosine, beta-blockers, and calcium channel blockers can be used to slow down ventricular rate or terminate SVTs.[55]

Rhythms Originating in the AV Junction

AV node is a group of cells located in the lower part of right atrium above tricuspid valve.[66] The cells in AV node have automaticity (intrinsic rate of 40 to 60 bpm), and they are capable of initiating impulses and regulating heart rhythm.[55] Junctional arrhythmias can include premature junctional complex (PJC), junctional rhythm, and junctional tachycardia.[55]

Based on the location of the junctional pacemaker and speed of conduction through the atria and ventricle, junctional beats and rhythms may have different ECG characteristics[55]:

1. Inverted P wave occurs when a junctional focus fires, the wave of depolarization spreads backward (retrograde) into

Table 12-11 • GUIDELINES FOR MANAGEMENT OF AF AND ATRIAL FLUTTER: PREVENTING THROMBOEMBOLISM

Class	Indication	LOE
Class I	Antithrombotic therapy to prevent thromboembolism is recommended for all patients with AF, except those with lone AF or contraindications.	A
	The selection of the antithrombotic agent should be based upon the absolute risks of stroke and bleeding and the relative risk and benefit for a given patient.	A
	For patients without mechanical heart valves at high risk of stroke, chronic oral anticoagulant therapy with a vitamin K antagonist is recommended in a dose adjusted to achieve the target intensity INR of 2.0–3.0, unless contraindicated. Factors associated with highest risk for stroke in patients with AF are prior thromboembolism (stroke, TIA, or systemic embolism) and rheumatic mitral stenosis.	A
	Anticoagulation with a vitamin K antagonist is recommended for patients with more than one moderate risk factor. Such factors include age 75 yr or greater, hypertension, HF, impaired LV systolic function (ejection fraction 35% or less or fractional shortening less than 25%), and diabetes mellitus.	A
	INR should be determined at least weekly during initiation of therapy and monthly when anticoagulation is stable.	A
	Aspirin, 81–325 mg daily, is recommended as an alternative to vitamin K antagonists in low-risk patients or in those with contraindications to oral anticoagulation.	A
	For patients with AF who have mechanical heart valves, the target intensity of anticoagulation should be based on the type of prosthesis, maintaining an INR of at least 2.5.	B
	Antithrombotic therapy is recommended for patients with atrial flutter as for those with AF.	C
Class IIa	For primary prevention of thromboembolism in patients with nonvalvular AF who have just one of the following validated risk factors, antithrombotic therapy with either aspirin or a vitamin K antagonist is reasonable, based upon an assessment of the risk of bleeding complications, ability to safely sustain adjusted chronic anticoagulation, and patient preferences: age greater than or equal to 75 yr (especially in female patients), hypertension, HF, impaired LV function, or diabetes mellitus.	A
	For patients with nonvalvular AF who have one or more of the following less well-validated risk factors, antithrombotic therapy with either aspirin or a vitamin K antagonist is reasonable for prevention of thromboembolism: age 65–74 yr, female gender, or CAD. The choice of agent should be based upon the risk of bleeding complications, ability to safely sustain adjusted chronic anticoagulation, and patient preferences.	B
	It is reasonable to select antithrombotic therapy using the same criteria irrespective of the pattern (i.e., paroxysmal, persistent, or permanent) of AF.	B
	In patients with AF who do not have mechanical prosthetic heart valves, it is reasonable to interrupt anticoagulation for up to 1 wk without substituting heparin for surgical or diagnostic procedures that carry a risk of bleeding.	C
	It is reasonable to reevaluate the need for anticoagulation at regular intervals.	C
Class IIb	In patients 75 yr of age and older at increased risk of bleeding but without frank contraindications to oral anticoagulant therapy, and in other patients with moderate risk factors for thromboembolism who are unable to safely tolerate anticoagulation at the standard intensity of INR 2.0–3.0, a lower INR target of 2.0 (range 1.6–2.5) may be considered for primary prevention of ischemic stroke and systemic embolism.	C
	When surgical procedures require interruption of oral anticoagulant therapy for longer than 1 wk in high-risk patients, unfractionated heparin may be administered, or low–molecular-weight heparin given by subcutaneous injection, although the efficacy of these alternatives in this situation is uncertain.	C
	Following percutaneous coronary intervention or revascularization surgery in patients with AF, low-dose aspirin (less than 100 mg per day) and/or clopidogrel (75 mg per day) may be given concurrently with anticoagulation to prevent myocardial ischemic events, but these strategies have not been thoroughly evaluated and are associated with an increased risk of bleeding.	C
	In patients undergoing percutaneous coronary intervention, anticoagulation may be interrupted to prevent bleeding at the site of peripheral arterial puncture, but the vitamin K antagonist should be resumed as soon as possible after the procedure and the dose adjusted to achieve an INR in the therapeutic range. Aspirin may be given temporarily during the hiatus, but the maintenance regimen should then consist of the combination of clopidogrel, 75 mg daily, plus warfarin (INR 2.0–3.0). Clopidogrel should be given for a minimum of 1 mo after implantation of a bare metal stent, at least 3 mo for a sirolimus-eluting stent, at least 6 mo for a paclitaxel-eluting stent, and 12 mo or longer in selected patients, following which warfarin may be continued as monotherapy in the absence of a subsequent coronary event. When warfarin is given in combination with clopidogrel or low-dose aspirin, the dose intensity must be carefully regulated.	C
	In patients with AF younger than 60 yr without heart disease or risk factors for thromboembolism (lone AF), the risk of thromboembolism is low without treatment and the effectiveness of aspirin for primary prevention of stroke relative to the risk of bleeding has not been established.	C
	In patients with AF who sustain ischemic stroke or systemic embolism during treatment with low-intensity anticoagulation (INR 2.0–3.0), rather than add an antiplatelet agent, it may be reasonable to raise the intensity of anticoagulation to a maximum target INR of 3.0–3.5.	C
Class III	Long-term anticoagulation with a vitamin K antagonist is not recommended for primary prevention of stroke in patients below the age of 60 yr without heart disease (lone AF) or any risk factors for thromboembolism.	C

AF, atrial fibrillation; INR, international normalized ratio; CAD, coronary artery disease; TIA, transient ischemic attack.
Adapted from January CT, Wann LS, Alpert JS, et al. 2014 AHA/ACC/HRS guideline for the management of patients with atrial fibrillation. *J Am Coll Cardiol.* 2014;64(21):e1–e76.

the atria as well as forward (anterograde) into the ventricles. If the impulse arrives in the atria before it arrives in the ventricles, the ECG shows a P wave followed immediately by a QRS complex. Thus, the PR interval is shorter than normal. P wave is inverted in inferior leads because the atria are depolarized from the bottom to top.

2. No visible P wave observed when the junctional impulse reaches both the atria and ventricles at the same time. Only a QRS is seen on the ECG because larger muscle mass of the ventricles and only the ventricular depolarization is seen.
3. When the junctional impulse reaches the ventricles before it reaches the atria, and the QRS precedes the P wave on the

Table 12-12 • GUIDELINES FOR MANAGEMENT OF AF AND ATRIAL FLUTTER: ELECTRICAL AND PHARMACOLOGIC CARDIOVERSION FOR AF: PREVENTION OF THROMBOEMBOLISM

Class	Indication	LOE
Class I	With AF or atrial flutter for ≥48 hr, or unknown duration, anticoagulate with warfarin for at least 3 wk before and 4 wk after cardioversion.	B
	With AF or atrial flutter for >48 hr or unknown duration, requiring immediate cardioversion, anticoagulate as soon as possible and continue for at least 4 wk.	C
	With AF or atrial flutter <48 hr and high stroke risk, IV heparin or LMWH, or factor Xa or direct thrombin inhibitor, is recommended before or immediately after cardioversion, followed by long-term anticoagulation.	C
	Following cardioversion of AF, long-term anticoagulation should be based on thromboembolic risk.	C
Class IIa	With AF or atrial flutter for 48 hr or unknown duration and no anticoagulation for preceding 3 wk, it is reasonable to perform TEE before cardioversion and then cardiovert if no LA thrombus is identified, provided anticoagulation is achieved before TEE and maintained after cardioversion for at least 4 wk.	B
	With AF or atrial flutter >48 hr or unknown duration, anticoagulation with dabigatran, rivaroxaban, or apixaban is reasonable for 3 wk before and 4 wk after cardioversion.	C
Class IIb	With AF or atrial flutter <48 hr and low thromboembolic risk, IV heparin, LMWH, a new oral anticoagulant, or no antithrombotic may be considered for cardioversion.	C
Direct Current Cardioversion		
Class I	Cardioversion is recommended for AF or atrial flutter to restore sinus rhythm. If unsuccessful, cardioversion attempts may be repeated.	B
	Cardioversion is recommended for AF or atrial flutter with RVR that does not respond to pharmacologic therapies.	C
	Cardioversion is recommended for AF or atrial flutter and pre-excitation with hemodynamic instability.	C
Class IIa	It is reasonable to repeat cardioversion in persistent AF when sinus rhythm can be maintained for a clinically meaningful time period between procedures.	C
Pharmacologic Cardioversion		
Class I	Flecainide, dofetilide, propafenone, and IV ibutilide are useful for cardioversion of AF or atrial flutter, provided contraindications to the selected drug are absent.	A
Class IIa	Amiodarone is reasonable for pharmacologic cardioversion of AF.	A
	Propafenone or flecainide ("pill-in-the-pocket") to terminate AF out of hospital is reasonable once observed to be safe in a monitored setting.	B
Class III	Dofetilide should not be initiated out of hospital.	B

Class I: strong/indicated; Class IIa: moderate/reasonable; Class IIb: weak/may be considered; Class III: no benefit or harm/not indicated or may be harmful.
LOE, level of recommendation; LMWH, low molecular weight heparin; TEE, transesophageal echocardiogram; RVR, rapid ventricular response; LA, left atrium.
Adapted from January CT, Wann LS, Alpert JS, et al. 2014 AHA/ACC/HRS guideline for the management of patients with atrial fibrillation. *J Am Coll Cardiol.* 2014;64(21):e1–e76.

Table 12-13 • GUIDELINES FOR MANAGEMENT OF AF AND ATRIAL FLUTTER: MAINTENANCE OF SINUS RHYTHM

Class	Recommendation	LOE
Class I	Before initiating antiarrhythmic drug therapy, treatment of precipitating or reversible causes of AF is recommended.	C
	The following antiarrhythmic drugs are recommended in patients with AF to maintain sinus rhythm, depending on underlying heart disease and comorbidities. a. Amiodarone b. Dofetilide c. Dronedarone d. Flecainide e. Propafenone f. Sotalol	A
	The risks of the antiarrhythmic drug, including proarrhythmia, should be considered before initiating therapy with each drug.	C
	Because of its potential toxicities, amiodarone should only be used after consideration of risks and when other agents have failed or are contraindicated.	C
Class IIa	A rhythm-control strategy with pharmacologic therapy can be useful in patients with AF for the treatment of tachycardia-induced cardiomyopathy.	C
Class IIb	It may be reasonable to continue current antiarrhythmic drug therapy in the setting of infrequent, well-tolerated recurrences of AF when the drug has reduced the frequency or symptoms of AF.	C
Class III	Antiarrhythmic drugs for rhythm control should not be continued when AF becomes permanent including dronedarone (level of evidence: C), including dronedarone (level of evidence: B).	
	Dronedarone should not be used for treatment of AF in patients with New York Heart Association class III and IV HF or patients who have had an episode of decompensated HF in the past 4 wk.	B

Class I: strong/indicated; Class IIa: moderate/reasonable; Class IIb: weak/may be considered; Class III: no benefit or harm/not indicated or may be harmful.
LOE, level of evidence; AF, atrial fibrillation; HF, heart failure.
Adapted from January CT, Wann LS, Alpert JS, et al. 2014 AHA/ACC/HRS guideline for the management of patients with atrial fibrillation. *J Am Coll Cardiol.* 2014;64(21):e1–e76.

ECG. P wave is inverted in inferior lead due to retrograde atrial depolarization, and the RP interval (distance from the beginning of the QRS to the beginning of the following P wave) is short, 0.10 second or less.

Premature Junctional Complexes

PJCs occur when there is an irritable site in the AV junction. The irritability can be a result of coronary artery disease, HF, rheumatic heart disease, valvular heart disease, or ACS disrupt blood flow to the AV junction. The irritation can also be caused by electrolyte imbalance, stimulants (e.g., nicotine, caffeine, and cocaine), catecholamines, or drugs such as digitalis. ECG characteristics of PJCs are listed[55]:

Rate: Usually within the normal range 60 to 100 bpm, or the rate of underline rhythm
Rhythm: Irregular because of the premature beats
P waves: May occur before, during, or after the QRS complex; if visible, the P waves are inverted in the inferior leads II, III, and aVF

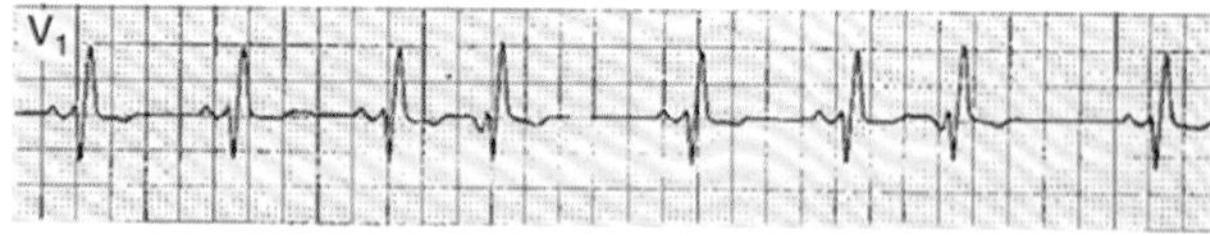

Figure 12-71. Sinus rhythm with two PJCs.

PR interval: If a P wave is present, the PR is usually short, 0.10 second or less when P waves precede the QRS
QRS complex: Usually normal but may be aberrant if the PJC occurs very early and conducts into the ventricles during the refractory period of a bundle branch
Conduction: Retrograde through the atria, usually normal through the ventricles
Example: Sinus rhythm with two PJCs (Fig. 12-71)

Treatments are not necessary for PJCs as long as the patient is asymptomatic.

Investigating the underlying stimulants or digitalis toxicity might be necessary if these are the potential causes.[55]

Junctional Rhythm and Junctional Tachycardia

Impulse of junctional rhythm comes from AV junction when the SA node rate falls below the automatic rate of AV junctional pacemaker (40 to 60 bpm). Junctional rhythm can also be a result of digitalis toxicity. Based on the rate, the rhythms can be classified into three different categories: junctional rhythm is used when the rate is between 40 and 60 bpm; accelerated junctional rhythm is used when the rate is between 60 and 100 bpm; junctional tachycardia is used to define the rhythm when the rate is between 100 and 250 bpm. Junctional tachycardia is rare but common in pediatric patients undergoing surgical repair of congenital defects. Junctional rhythm can be a result of digitalis toxicity or effects of medication (e.g., beta-blockers, digitalis, diltiazem, quinidine, or verapamil). Decreased blood supply to the SA after an inferior wall MI can be another cause of junctional rhythm. Other causes include hypoxia, cardiac surgery, increased parasympathetic tone, rheumatic heart disease, SA node disease, and valvular disease. ECG characteristics of junctional rhythm are listed[55,66]:

Rate: Usually 40 to 60 bpm; accelerated junctional rhythm, 60 to 100 bpm; junctional tachycardia, 100 to 250 bpm
Rhythm: Regular
P waves: May occur before, during or after the QRS; if visible, the P wave is inverted in lead II, III, and aVF
PR interval: Short, 0.10 second or less when a P wave occurs before the QRS
QRS complex: Usually normal unless abnormally conducted.
Conduction: Retrograde through the atria, normal through the ventricles
Examples: (A) Junctional rhythm (rate, 43 bpm). (B) Accelerated junctional rhythm (rate, 84 bpm) (Fig. 12-72)

Treatment is usually not necessary for junctional rhythm unless the rate is too slow and causes decreased cardiac output. Atropine can be given to increase sinus rate and override the junctional focus or increase the rate of firing of the junctional pacemaker. Treat underlying causes like withholding digoxin until serum drug level return to normal. Medications like beta-blockers, propafenone, flecainide, and amiodarone can be given to slow down the rate or terminate the rhythm when rapid rate causes hemodynamic instability. Synchronized cardioversion can also be used when cardiac output is severely limited.[55,66]

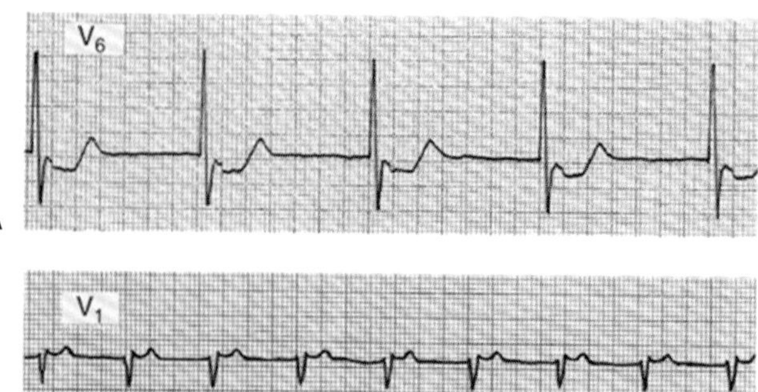

Figure 12-72. A: Junctional rhythm (rate, 43 beats per minute). **B:** Accelerated junctional rhythm (rate, 84 beats per minute).

Rhythms Originating in the Ventricles

Ventricular arrhythmia is considered more dangerous than other arrhythmias due to the potential severely limited cardiac output. Ventricular arrhythmias usually originate in the ventricular muscle or Purkinje system. The ventricles are an ineffective pacemaker however they will assume the responsibility of pacing the heart at 20 to 40 bpm when both the SA node and AV node fail. Ventricular arrhythmias include premature ventricular contractions (PVC), accelerated ventricular rhythm, VT, ventricular flutter, VF, and ventricular asystole.[55]

Premature Ventricular Contractions

Premature ventricular contractions (PVCs) are known as ventricular premature beats or premature ventricular depolarizations. The PVCs arise from an irritable site in either ventricle causing premature depolarization of cells in the ventricular myocardium or Purkinje system.[55]

PVCs can occur in individuals with healthy heart or individuals with structure heart disease. The causes of PVCs include acid–base imbalance (acidosis), acute coronary syndromes, cardiomyopathy, digitalis toxicity, electrolyte imbalance, HF, hypoxia, stimulants (e.g., caffeine, tobacco), increased levels of circulating catecholamines and sympathetic tone (e.g., emotional stress, anxiety), medications (sympathomimetic drugs), valvular heart disease, and ventricular aneurysm. ECG characteristics of PVCs are listed[40,55]:

Rate: 60 to 100 bpm or the rate of the basic rhythm
Rhythm: Irregular because of the early/premature beats
P waves: Not related to the PVC. Sinus rhythm is often not interrupted, so sinus P waves can frequently be seen occurring regularly throughout the rhythm. P waves may follow a PVC because of retrograde conduction from the ventricle backward through the atria; these P waves are inverted in the inferior leads (II, III, aVF)
PR interval: None with the PVC because the ectopic beat originates from the ventricles. If a P wave happens, by coincidence, to precede a PVC, the PR interval is short
QRS complex: Wide and bizarre, usually greater than 0.12 second in duration. May vary in morphology if PVCs originate from more than one focus in the ventricles. T waves are usually in the opposite direction from the QRS complex
Conduction: Impulses originating in the ventricles conduct through the ventricular myocardium from muscle cell to muscle cell rather than through Purkinje fibers, resulting in wide QRS complexes. Some PVCs may conduct retrograde into the

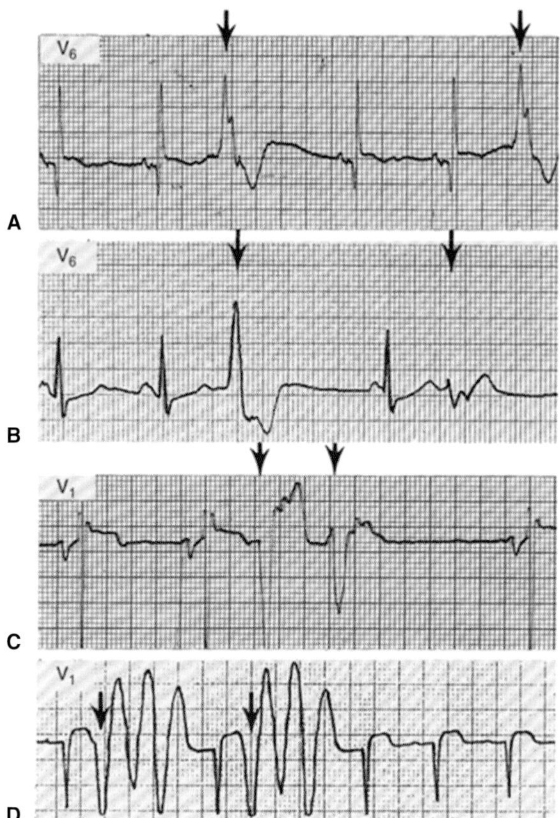

Figure 12-73. Examples of PVCs. **A:** Normal sinus rhythm with a PVC. **B:** Sinus rhythm with multifocal PVC. **C:** Paired PVC. **D:** R-on-T PVC, resulting in short runs of VT.

atria, resulting in inverted P waves that follow the PVC. When the sinus rhythm is undisturbed by PVCs, the atria depolarize normally

Examples: (A) Normal sinus rhythm with a PVC. (B) Sinus rhythm with multifocal PVC. (C) Paired PVC. (D) R-on-T PVC, resulting in short runs of VT (Fig. 12-73)

The significance of PVCs is dependent upon the frequency of the PVCs and whether the PVCs affect cardiac output. Many individuals have chronic PVCs and remain asymptomatic; thus, treatment is not necessary. Goal of treating PVCs is to search the potential reversible causes. For example, avoid stimulants if they are the potential cause. Antiarrhythmics may be used to treat PVCs. However due to their proarrhythmic effect, antiarrhythmics may cause serious adverse effects like sustained ventricular tachydysrhythmia. PVCs can potentially lead to lethal ventricular arrhythmias, especially when they occur near the apex of the T wave (R-on-T PVC).[55,67]

Accelerated Idioventricular Rhythm

Accelerated idioventricular rhythm (AIVR) occurs when three or more ventricular beats occur in a row at a rate of 41 to 100 bpm. Some cardiologists consider the ventricular rate of AIVR range from 41 to 120 bpm.[55,67] AIVR is usually considered a benign escape rhythm, and commonly occurs with inferior MI and during reperfusion thrombolytic therapy. ECG characteristics of accelerate ventricular rhythm[55,67]:

Rate: 41 to 100 bpm
Rhythm: Usually regular
P waves: May be seen but are dissociated from the QRS. If retrograde conduction from the ventricle to the atria occurs, P waves follow the QRS complex
PR interval: Not present
QRS complex: Wide and bizarre
Conduction: If sinus rhythm is the basic rhythm, atrial conduction is normal. Impulses originating in the ventricles conduct through the ventricular myocardium by cell-to-cell conduction, resulting in the wide QRS complex
Example: Sinus rhythm with accelerated ventricular rhythm at a rate of 70 bpm. Note sinus P waves that continue uninterrupted during the period of accelerated ventricular rhythm (an example of AV dissociation). (*N* = arrhythmia computer's interpretation of normal beat, *V* = computer's interpretation of ventricular beat) (Fig. 12-74)

Treatment for AIVR is usually not necessary, because the rhythm is usually benign, protective, and transient. AIVR usually spontaneously resolves on its own. The loss of atrial kick might cause hemodynamic compromise or symptoms in patients with AIVR, and atropine can be used in this situation. Suppressive therapy is rarely used because abolishing the ventricular rhythm may leave an even less desirable heart rate.[55,67]

Ventricular Tachycardia

VT is a rapid ventricular rhythm, and it occurs when three or more sequential PVCs occur at a rate of more than 100 bpm. VT is most likely due to reentry in the ventricles. VT can be classified base on (1) duration—*nonsustained* (greater than or equal to three beats, terminating spontaneously), *sustained* (lasts greater than 30 seconds or requiring termination due to hemodynamic compromise in less than 30 seconds), *incessant* (VT present most of the time); (2) morphology—*monomorphic* (stable single QRS morphology from beat to beat. VT most likely originate from one ectopic focus in either ventricle), *polymorphic* (changing or multiform QRS morphology from beat to beat, VT originate from varied focuses in either ventricle), *bidirectional* (VT with a beat-to-beat alternation in the QRS frontal plane axis, often seen in the setting of digitalis toxicity or catecholaminergic polymorphic VT).[68] The terms *salvos* and *bursts* are often used to describe short runs of VT (i.e., five to ten or more beats in a row). Patient may be stable or unstable with VT, and they may have a pulse or without a pulse.[55,67]

VT can be a result of disorders of impulse formation and can be associated with underlying heart disease. The possible causes of VT include acid–base imbalance, ACS, cardiomyopathy, cocaine abuse, digitalis toxicity, electrolyte imbalance (e.g., hypokalemia,

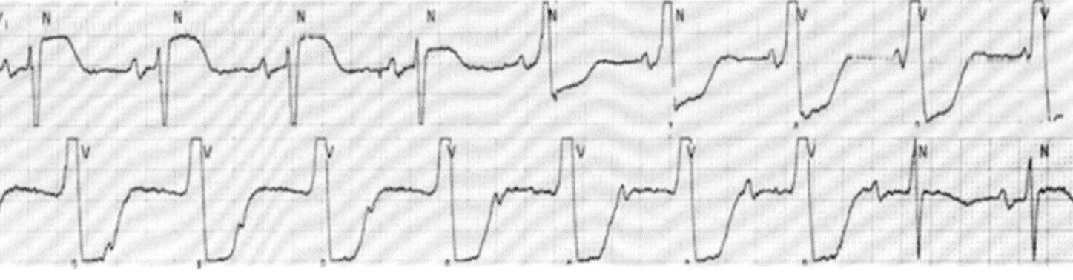

Figure 12-74. Example of accelerated ventricular rhythm. Sinus rhythm with accelerated ventricular rhythm at a rate of 70 beats per minute. Note sinus P waves that continue uninterrupted during the period of accelerated ventricular rhythm (an example of AV dissociation). (*N* = arrhythmia computer's interpretation of normal beat, *V* = computer's interpretation of ventricular beat.)

hyperkalemia, hypomagnesemia), mitral valve prolapse, trauma (e.g., myocardial contusion, invasive cardiac procedures), tricyclic antidepressant overdose, and valvular heart disease. ECG characteristics of monomorphic VT are listed[55,67]:

Rate: Ventricular rate is usually 150 to 300 bpm
Rhythm: Usually regular but may be slightly irregular
P waves: Usually not seen, as P waves are often buried in QRS complexes or T waves. If sinus rhythm is the underlying basic rhythm, regular P waves may be seen but are not related to QRS complexes. P waves are often buried in QRS complexes or T waves. VT may conduct retrograde to the atria with P waves visible after each QRS
PR interval: Not measurable because of dissociation of P waves from QRS complexes
QRS complex: Wide and bizarre, greater than 0.12 second in duration
Conduction: Impulse originates in one ventricle and spreads by muscle cell-to-cell conduction through both ventricles. There may be retrograde conduction through the atria, but often the SA node continues to fire regularly and depolarizes the atria normally. Rarely, one of these sinus impulses may conduct normally through the AV node and into the ventricle before the next ectopic ventricular impulse fires, resulting in a normal QRS complex, called a *capture beat.* Occasionally, a *fusion beat* may occur as the ventricles are depolarized by a descending sinus impulse and the ventricular ectopic impulse simultaneously, resulting in a QRS complex that looks different from both the normal beats and the ventricular beats
Examples: (A) Sinus rhythm with a PVC and a run of monomorphic VT. (B) AV dissociation is evidenced by independently occurring P waves. (C) VT with a fusion beat (fourth complex) (Fig. 12-75)

Immediate treatment of VT may be required depending on how well the patient tolerates the rhythm. The ventricular rate and patient's underlying ventricular function are the two major determinants of patient tolerance. Cardiac output can be severely depressed when there is a poor underlying ventricular function or very rapid ventricular rate. Cardiopulmonary resuscitation (CPR) and defibrillation are used to treat pulseless VT. Oxygen (if indicated) and ventricular antiarrhythmics are used to treat stable but symptomatic patients. Oxygen (if indicated), sedation, and synchronized cardioversion are used for unstable patients (usually with a sustained heart rate of 150 bpm).[67]

Beta-blockers are often first-line antiarrhythmic therapy because of their excellent safety profile and effectiveness in treating ventricular arrhythmias.[69,70] In the setting of polymorphic VT after MI, beta-blockers reduce mortality in patient with polymorphic VT after MI.[71] Beta-blockers suppress ventricular arrhythmias in some patients with structurally normal hearts.[72] When used in combination with membrane-stabilizing antiarrhythmic medications, beta-blockers can enhance antiarrhythmic efficacy.[73] Amiodarone can reduce the risk of sudden cardiac death and all-cause mortality.[74] Intravenous amiodarone has a role in reducing recurrent VF/VF during resuscitation.[75–78] Long-term administration of amiodarone is associated with complex medication interactions and adverse effects involve multiple organ systems. For this reason, chronic treatment of young patients with amiodarone should be reserved as a bridge to more definitive treatment options such as catheter ablation.[68] Sotalol is effective in suppressing ventricular arrhythmias. In addition, sotalol has significant proarrhythmic effects and has not been shown to improve survival.[79]

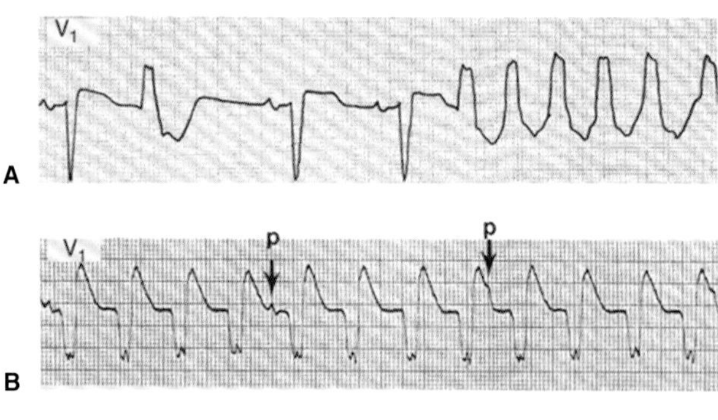

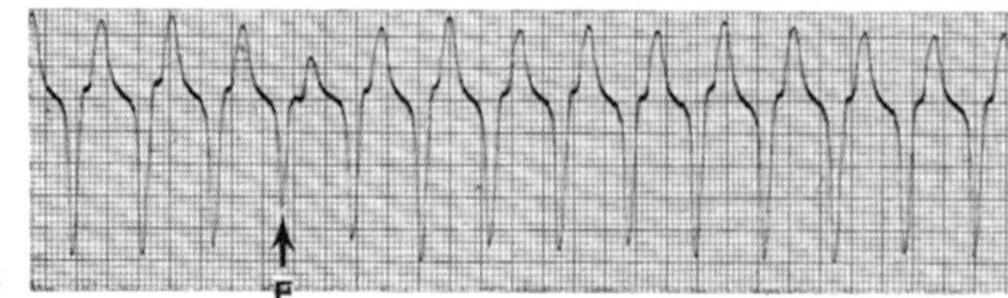

Figure 12-75. A: Sinus rhythm with a PVC and a run of monomorphic VT. **B:** AV dissociation is evidenced by independently occurring P waves. **C:** VT with a fusion beat (fourth complex).

Ventricular Flutter

Ventricular flutter is similar to VT with faster rate: it is defined as monomorphic VT with a ventricular rate of 150 to 300 bpm.[80] Compared to VT, ventricular flutter is more dangerous due to a lack of cardiac output. ECG characteristics of ventricular flutter are listed[55]:

Rate: Ventricular rate is usually 220 to 400 bpm
Rhythm: Usually regular
P waves: None seen
PR interval: None measurable
QRS complex: Very wide, regular, sine-wave type of pattern
Conduction: Originates in the ventricle and spreads through muscle cell-to-cell conduction, resulting in very wide, bizarre complexes
Example: Ventricular flutter (Fig. 12-76)

Ventricular flutter can be fatal and needs to be treated immediately by defibrillation. If a defibrillator is not immediately available, CPR should be started. When the rhythm is converted, antiarrhythmic therapy should be initiated to prevent recurrence. Drug therapy is similar to that used for VT.[55]

Ventricular Fibrillation

VF is a chaotic rhythm that origins in the ventricle. The ventricles are rapidly quivering and produce no cardiac output. CPR and electrical defibrillation should be performed immediately, as VF can be fatal and it is the most frequent cause of sudden cardiac death. ECG characteristics are listed[68]:

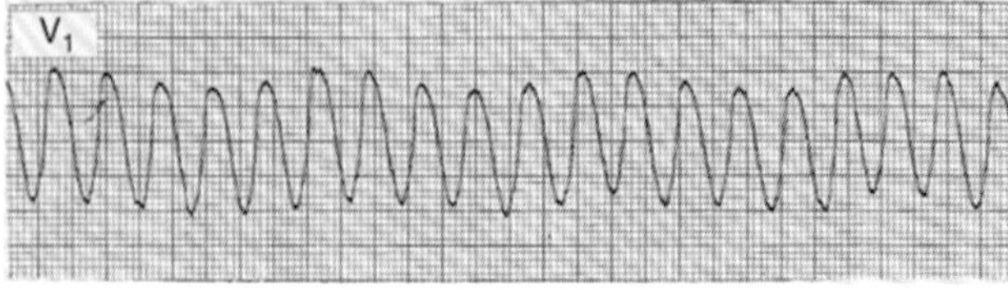

Figure 12-76. Ventricular flutter.

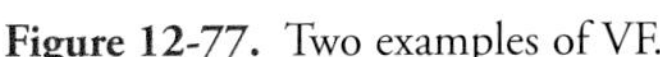
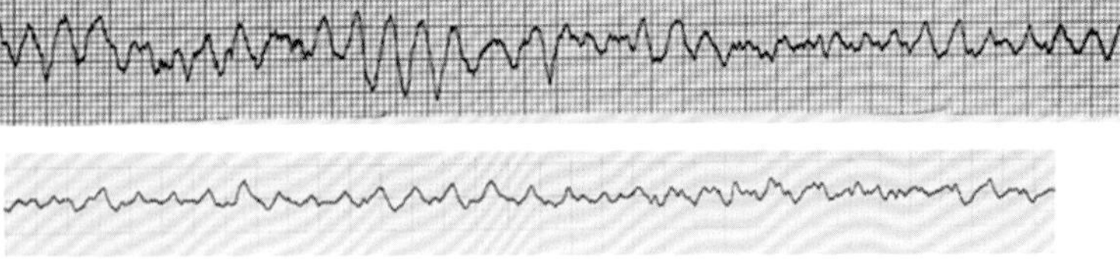

Figure 12-77. Two examples of VF.

Rate: Rapid, uncoordinated, ineffective. Ventricular rate is usually greater than 300 bpm
Rhythm: Chaotic, no pattern or regularity
P waves: None seen
PR interval: None
QRS complex: No formed QRS complexes seen; rapid, irregular undulations without any specific pattern. This erratic electrical activity can be coarse or fine
Conduction: Random electrical activity in ventricles depolarizes them irregularly and without any organized pattern. There is no organized conduction and the ventricles do not contract
Examples: Two examples of VF (Fig. 12-77)

VF and pulseless VT are considered shockable rhythms, and they are treated in similar fashion. According to American Heart Association Advanced Cardiac Life Support (ACLS) 2018 guidelines, shock should be the first intervention in treating patients with VF followed by immediate CPR for 2 minutes. If a defibrillator is not immediately available, CPR should be initiated. When using a biphasic defibrillator with VF, start with the dose recommended by the manufacturer. If the manufacturer-recommended shock dose is unknown, start with the maximum available dose. Every shock after the initial shock should be of equal or greater dose strength. Increase the dosing in a stepwise fashion as needed (e.g., 120 J, 200 J, 300 J to 360 J).[81]

IV Amiodarone 300 mg bolus is recommended for VF arrest (class III recommendation). After the bolus is administered, continue the amiodarone IV infusion at 1 mg/min for 6 hours, then 0.5 mg/min for 18 hours.[68]

Ventricular Asystole

Ventricular asystole is a total absence of ventricular electrical activity. There is no QRS on ECG, no pulse, and the heart produces no cardiac output. "Ventricular standstill" is used when atrial electrical activity is present but there is an absence of ventricular activity. Both situations are fatal and need to be treated immediately. ECG characteristics of ventricular asystole are listed[68]:

Rate: None
Rhythm: None
P waves: May be present if the SA node is functioning
PR interval: None
QRS complex: None
Conduction: Atrial conduction may be normal if the SA node is functioning. There is no conduction into the ventricles
Example: Ventricular asystole. Two P waves are seen at the beginning of the strip (Fig. 12-78)

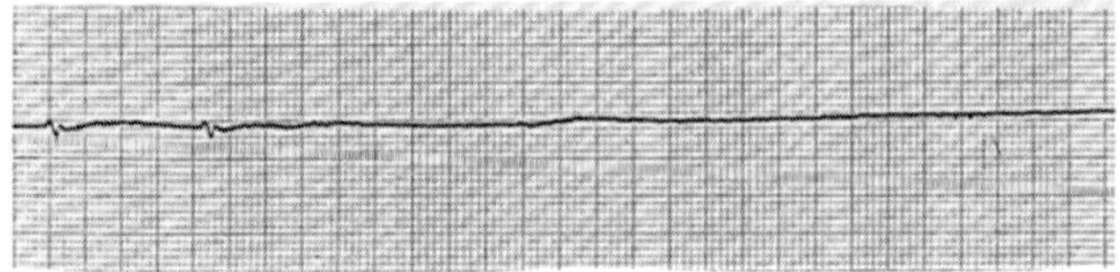

Figure 12-78. Ventricular asystole. Two P waves are seen at the beginning of the strip.

High-quality CPR should be performed immediately for patient with ventricular asystole. IV epinephrine is used for its vasoconstriction effects to increase blood flow to the heart and brain. Administration of epinephrine should not delay the initiation and continuation of CPR. After the initial CPR, epinephrine can be given every 3 to 5 minutes.[82]

Conduction Abnormalities

The term AV block is used to describe dysrhythmia, in which the impulse conduction from the atria to the ventricles is delayed or interrupted due to a transient or permanent anatomic or functional impairment.[83] The AV blocks are classified into three categories based on the location of the block and severity of the conduction abnormality: (1) first-degree AV block (2) second-degree AV block (type I, type II, and 2:1 conduction) (3) third-degree AV block.[55,83]

When the AV blocks occur at the level of AV node, junctional pacemaker can take over as a primary pacemaker at a rate of 40 to 60 bpm. When AV blocks occurs below the AV junction, the ventricles as pacemakers will only fire at a rate of 20 to 40 bpm. Ventricular pacemakers are not as reliable as junctional pacemaker due to their slow rate and they are prone to long pauses.[55,83]

First-Degree AV Block

First-degree AV block is defined as a conduction delay within the AV node: the time of the impulse travelling from the SA node to the ventricles is prolonged. The impulses are not blocked. In a first-degree AV block, all components of the cardiac cycle are usually within the normal limits with the exception of the PR interval (greater than 0.20 second).[83,84]

First-degree AV block may be a normal finding in individual without history of cardiac disease. Mild prolonged PR interval may be a normal variant with sinus bradycardia during rest or sleep. The causes of first-degree AV block include the following: acute MI resulting in decreased blood supply to the conduction system; acute myocarditis or endocarditis; cardiomyopathy; degenerate fibrosis and sclerosis of the conduction system; drug effect (e.g., beta-blockers, calcium channel blockers, and digoxin); hyperkalemia; increased vagal tone (e.g., inferior infarction, vomiting, carotid stimulation); ischemia or injuring to the AV node or AV bundle; rheumatic heart disease; valvular heart disease. ECG characteristics of first-degree AV block are listed[83]:

Rate: Can occur at any sinus rate, usually 60 to 100 bpm
Rhythm: Regular
P waves: Normal in size and shape, each P wave is followed by a QRS complex
PR interval: Constant and prolonged, greater than 0.20 second
QRS complex: Usually normal unless abnormally conducted or BBBs exist. Impulses are only delayed and no blocked, thus no dropping of QRS
Conduction: Normal through the atria, delayed through the AV node, normal through the ventricles
Example: First-degree AV block (PR interval, 0.44 second) (Fig. 12-79)

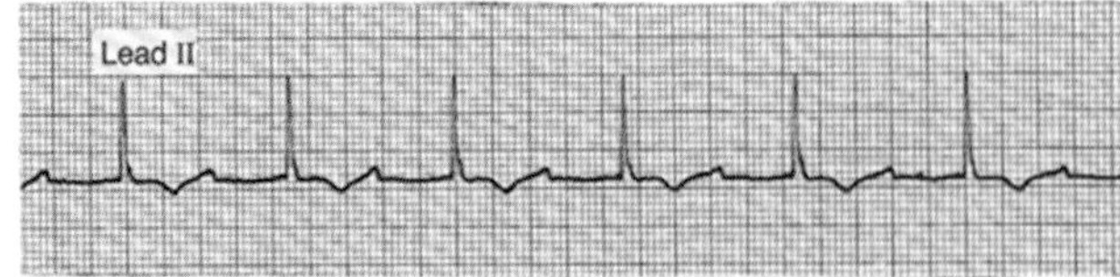

Figure 12-79. First-degree AV block (PR interval, 0.44 second).

First-degree AV block does not require any specific treatment because patients often are asymptomatic. ECG should be observed for progression to more serious and higher degree of AV block especially in the setting of acute MI.[85]

Second-Degree AV Block

Second-degree AV block is defined as one or more, but not all, atrial impulses fail to be conducted to the ventricles. The impulses from the SA node are generated normally, and each P wave will occur at a regular interval. Since not all P waves are conducted through the ventricle, there are more P waves than the QRS complexes on the ECG. Second-degree AV block is subclassified into type I (Wenckebach or Mobitz type I), type II (Mobitz type II) based on pattern of the PR intervals.[83,84]

Type I (Wenckebach)

Second-degree AV block type I is also known as Wenckebach or Mobitz I. The PR intervals in Wenckebach demonstrate a progressive lengthening pattern, and eventually an impulse fails to be conducted to the ventricles resulting in a dropping of a ventricular beat (a missing QRS complex).[83,84]

Because the RCA supplies the right ventricle and the inferior wall of the left ventricle in most individuals, blockage of the RCA will lead to an inferior MI or right ventricular infarction resulting in conduction delays such as first-degree AV block and second-degree AV block type I.[83] Some athletes may have second-degree AV block type I condition; it is probably due to an increased resting vagal tone.[80] Second-degree AV block type I can also occur in healthy individual during sleep. Other causes of second-degree AV block type I include aortic valve disease, atrial septal defect, medications (e.g., beta-blockers, digoxin, and calcium channel blockers), mitral valve prolapse, and rheumatic heart disease. ECG characteristics of second-degree AV block type I are listed.[83,84]

Rate: Can occur at any sinus or atrial rate, however the atrial rate is greater than the ventricular rate (more Ps than the QRSs) due to conduction failure

Rhythm: Ventricular rate is irregular, and atrial rate is regular

P waves: Normal. Some P waves are not conducted to the ventricles, but only one at a time fails to conduct

PR interval: Gradually lengthens in consecutive beats until a P wave appears without a QRS complex. The PR interval preceding the pause is longer than that following the pause. When 2:1 conduction is present, PR intervals are constant

QRS complex: Usually normal unless there is associated BBB

Conduction: Normal through the atria, progressively delayed through the AV node until an impulse fails to conduct. Ventricular conduction is normal. Wenckebach conduction ratios describe the number of P waves to QRS complexes: 6:5 conduction means six P waves resulted in five QRS complexes, or every sixth P wave is blocked. Conduction ratios can vary from low (e.g., 2:1, 3:2) to high (e.g., 12:11, 15:14)

Examples: (A) Second-degree AV block, type I (Wenckebach) with 3:2 conduction. (B) Second-degree AV block, type I. Note that the PR interval preceding the pause is longer than the PR interval after the pause (Fig. 12-80)

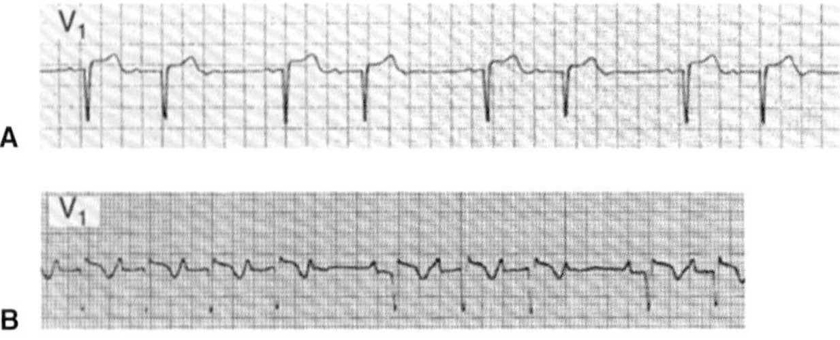

Figure 12-80. A: Second-degree AV block, type I (Wenckebach) with 3:2 conduction. **B:** Second-degree AV block, type I. Note that the PR interval preceding the pause is longer than the PR interval after the pause.

The patient with second-degree AV block type I is usually asymptomatic as the ventricular rate often remains normal. The patient may become symptomatic when the ventricular rate is too low and cardiac output is significantly reduced as a result. Atropine can be used to increase the sinus rate and speed conduction through the AV node. If the block is a result of drug therapy, it is necessary to decrease dose or discontinue the drug. If drug therapy must be continued, pacemaker implantation may be required. Second-degree AV block type I is usually transient and benign. Temporary pacing may be needed when the ventricular rate is slow and atropine is not effective.[55]

Type II

Second-degree AV block type II is also known as Mobitz II. The PR intervals in Mobitz II are constant, and the failure of conduction of an atrial impulse to the ventricles is sudden. Mobitz II is less common than type I. However, Mobitz II is more serious and has greater potential to progress to a third-degree AV block.[55,83]

The site of second-degree AV block type II is almost always below the AV node, occurring in bundle of His about 30% of the time and in the bundle branch about 70% of the time.[84] Blood that supplies the bundle branches and the anterior wall of the left ventricle comes from a branch of the left coronary artery. Thus, diseases of the left coronary artery or an interior MI are often the cause of conduction abnormalities within the bundle branches. Second-degree AV block type II may also be a result of acute myocarditis, aortic valve disease, cardiomyopathy, fibrosis of the conduction system, or rheumatic heart disease. ECG characteristics of second-degree AV block type II are listed[83]:

Rate: Atrial rate is greater than the ventricular rate (more P waves than the QRs complexes)

Rhythm: Atrial rate is regular; ventricular rate irregular due to blocked beats unless 2:1 conduction is present

P waves: Normal size and shape. Some P waves are not followed by a QRS complex

PR interval: Constant before all conducted beats. The PR interval preceding the pause is the same as that after the pause

QRS complex: Can be wide when the block occurs below the bundle of His; can be narrow when block occurs above or within the bundle of His

Conduction: Normal through the atria and through the AV node but intermittently blocked in the bundle branch system and fails to reach the ventricles. Conduction through the ventricles is abnormally slow because of associated BBB. Conduction ratios can vary from 2:1 to only occasional blocked beats

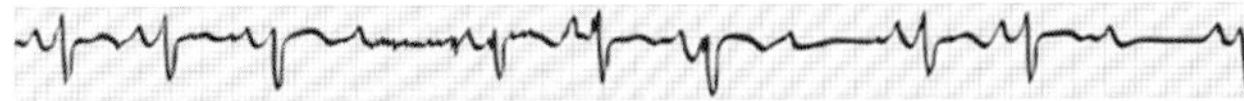

Figure 12-81. Second-degree AV block, type II. All PR intervals are constant.

Example: Second-degree AV block, type II. All PR intervals are constant (Fig. 12-81)

Ventricular rate will determine if the patient is symptomatic of second-degree AV block type II. Patient may be asymptomatic if the ventricular rate is within normal limit. When the ventricular rate is significantly reduced and there is an increased number of nonconducted beats, second-degree AV block type II will lead to more severe symptoms due to decreased cardiac output. Second-degree AV block type II is more dangerous than type I due to its greater potential to progress to third-degree AV block. Temporary or permanent pacing may be necessary in second-degree AV block type II: external pacing can be used until transvenous pacing can be initiated. Atropine is not recommended because of its potential of further slowing the ventricular rate by increasing the number of impulses conducting through the AV node and bombarding the diseased bundles with more impulses resulting in further conduction failure.[83]

Conduction

In second-degree AV block with 2:1 conduction, there is a failure of conduction of every other beat: one conducted P wave followed by a blocked P wave. In another word, two P waves occur for every QRS complex. Because there are no two PQRST cycles in a row, the PR interval pattern cannot be determined, and 2:1 AV block cannot be classified as type I or type II.[83]

If the QRS complex is normal or narrow, site of the block is located within the AV node and it is a form of second-degree AV block type I. If the QRS complex is wide, site of the block is below the AV node and it is usually a type II block.[83]

Specific ECG characteristics of 2:1 conduction block will be helpful in determining the type of block.[83]

PR interval: Often longer than normal (more than 0.20 second) in type I and normal in type II. Sometimes, the PR in type I is normal on conducted beats because the blocked P wave allows enough time for the AV node to recover so that it is able to conduct every other P wave with a normal PR interval. If there are any periods of typical Wenckebach conduction with progressive lengthening of the PR interval on consecutively conducted P waves (even if it only happens once), it is type I block.

QRS complex: Usually narrow in type I and almost always wide in type II. Exceptions can occur in type I when there is a coincidental BBB that widens the QRS, and in type II when the block is in the His bundle (still below the AV node, thus type II), resulting in a narrow QRS. Type II block is rare compared with type I, and intra-His type II block is even more rare, so the odds are in favor of type I block when the QRS is narrow.

Examples: (A) Top strip shows 2:1 conduction that can be assumed to be type I because of the narrow QRS complex. Second strip proves that it is type I when consecutive P waves conduct with increasing PR intervals. (B) Top strip shows 2:1 conduction that can be assumed to be type II because of wide QRS. Second strip proves that it is type II when consecutively conducted PR intervals remain constant (Fig. 12-82)

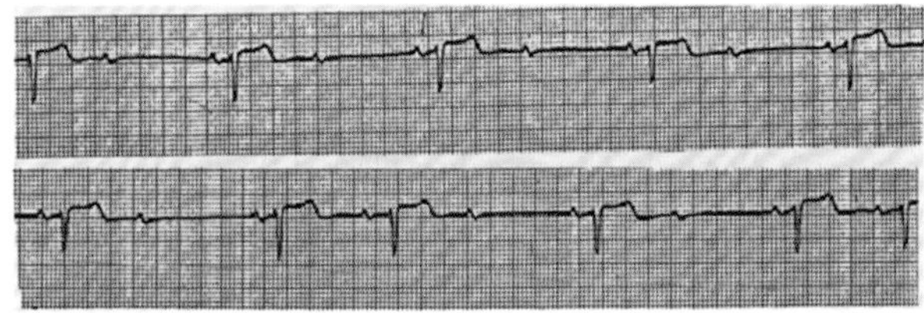

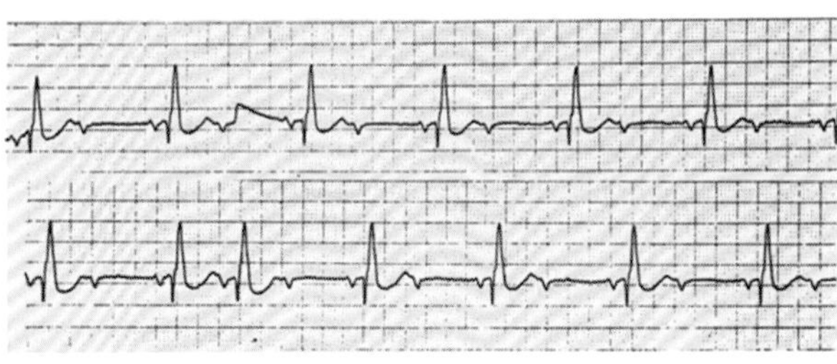

Figure 12-82. A: Top strip shows 2:1 conduction that can be assumed to be type I because of the narrow QRS complex. Second strip proves that it is type I when consecutive P waves conduct with increasing PR intervals. **B:** Top strip shows 2:1 conduction that can be assumed to be type II because of wide QRS. Second strip proves that it is type II when consecutively conducted PR intervals remain constant.

High-Grade AV Block

High-grade AV block is also known as advanced second-degree AV block, in which there is a failure of conduction of two or more consecutive P waves. Similar to 2:1 AV block, high-grade AV block cannot be classified as a type I or type II as there are no consecutive two PQRST cycles and the pattern of PR interval cannot be determined.[55,83,84]

The site of block can be in the AV node or below the AV node in the Purkinje system. When the block occurs in the AV node, QRS complexes of the conducted beats are usually narrow. Wenckebach periodicity can also be seen in high-grade AV block, and atropine is effective in lessening degrees of AV block. However, atropine is not effective when the block is in the Purkinje system.[84]

Third-degree AV block can be a progression of first-degree AV block or second-degree AV block type I. Other causes of third-degree AV block include acute MI (inferior MI, an anterior or an anteroseptal MI), acute myocarditis, congenital heart disease, drug effect, fibrosis of the conduction system, and increased parasympathetic tone. When third-degree AV block is associated with an inferior MI, it is thought to be the result of a block above the bundle of His.[83] Third-degree AV block associated with an anterior or an anteroseptal MI is often preceded by second-degree AV block type II or an intraventricular conduction delay. ECG characteristics of high-grade AV block are listed[55,83,84]:

Rate: Atrial rate less than 135 bpm
Rhythm: Regular or irregular, depending on conduction pattern
P waves: Normal, present before every conducted QRS, but several P waves may not be followed by QRS complexes
PR interval: Constant before conducted beats; may be normal or prolonged
QRS complex: Normal unless BBB is present
Conduction: Normal through the atria. Two or more consecutive atrial impulses fail to conduct to the ventricles. Conduction through the ventricles is normal if block occurs in the AV node and slow if block occurs in the bundle branches
Example: High-grade (advanced) AV block. There are three blocked P waves in a row and the ventricular rate is about 25 bpm. PR intervals before conducted QRS complexes are constant at 0.32 second (Fig. 12-83)

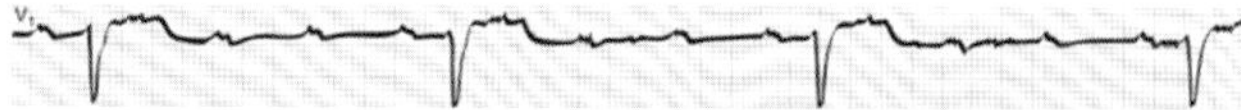

Figure 12-83. Example of high-grade AV block. High-grade (advanced) AV block. There are three blocked P waves in a row and the ventricular rate is about 25 beats per minute. PR intervals before conducted QRS complexes are constant at 0.32 second.

Because the ventricular rate tends to be low, the patient is often symptomatic due to decreased cardiac output. Atropine can be given but usually is more effective when block located in the AV node. External pacing can be used until a temporary transvenous pacemaker can be inserted or permanent pacemaker can be implanted.[55,83,84]

Third-Degree AV Block

Third-degree AV block is also known as complete heart block, in which there is a complete failure of conduction of all atrial impulses to the ventricles and AV disassociation (atria and ventricles are firing at their own pacemaker rates). The site of third-degree AV block can be located in the AV node, the bundle of His, or distal to the bundle of His. The secondary pacemaker can be the AV junction or the ventricles. Thus, the ventricular rate can vary but is usually less than 45 bpm. The QRS may be narrow or wide depending on the location of the escape pacemaker: the QRS complexes will be narrow with junctional escape rhythm; the QRS complexes will be wide when the impulses come from distal bundle of His. ECG characteristics of third-degree AV block are listed[84]:

Rate: Atrial rate is normal when sinus rhythm is present; ventricular rate is usually less than 45 bpm
Rhythm: Regular
P waves: Normal but dissociated from QRS complexes
PR interval: PR intervals cannot be determined because there is no true relation between P waves and QRS complexes
QRS complex: Normal if ventricles controlled by a junctional pacemaker, wide if controlled by a ventricular pacemaker
Conduction: Normal through the atria. All impulses are blocked at the AV node or in the bundle branches, so there is no conduction to the ventricles. Conduction through the ventricles is normal if a junctional escape rhythm occurs and is abnormally slow if a ventricular escape rhythm occurs
Examples: (A) Third-degree AV block with (most likely) a junctional pacemaker at a rate of 36 bpm. (B) Third-degree AV block with a ventricular pacemaker at a rate of 32 bpm. (C) AF with third-degree block and ventricular escape pacemaker at rate of 25 bpm (Fig. 12-84)

Patient may become symptomatic with third-degree AV block with slow ventricular rate and associated decreased cardiac output. Atropine may be effective if the disruption in AV nodal conduction is caused by increased parasympathetic tone by reversing excess vagal tone and improving AV node conduction. Other treatment options include epinephrine or dopamine IV infusion and transcutaneous pacing. Permanent pacemaker may be indicated for third-degree AV block.[84]

Complex Arrhythmias and Conduction Disturbances

Abnormality of cardiac rhythm can range from simple to complex. This section will discuss advanced concepts in arrhythmia interpretation and provides clues to aid in the recognition of selected advanced arrhythmias.

Ventricular Pre-Excitation Syndromes

In normal conduction system, the AV node serves as a "filter" that produces a delay to prevent the ventricles from depolarizing prematurely. Ventricular pre-excitation occurs when the electrical impulse bypasses the AV node, conducted to the ventricles more quickly (via accessory pathways) than usual resulting early activation of the ventricular myocardium. The result of ventricular pre-excitation is a portion of ventricle is depolarized early. Patients with pre-excitation syndrome have alternative tracts or accessary connection. A number of accessory pathways have been discovered. The most common accessory pathway is an AV bypass tract, the bundle of Kent, which originates in the atrium and inserts in the ventricle, bypassing the entire conduction system. Other accessory pathways include AV nodal bypass tracts, which carry the impulse from the atrium into the distal or compact AV node or from the atrium to the bundle of His (sometimes called James fibers or atriohisian fibers), and nodoventricular connections, which originate in or below the AV node and carry the impulse directly into the ventricular myocardium (Mahaim fibers).[55] The accessory pathway may exist in normal healthy heart, or they may exist in conjunction with mitral valve prolapse, hypertrophic cardiomyopathies, and various congenital disorders.[86]

Figure 12-85 illustrates the possible locations of the accessory pathways: around the valve rings, the septum, and the free walls of both ventricles. The table in Figure 12-85 demonstrates localizing the accessory pathway using ECG characteristics.

Wolff–Parkinson–White Syndrome

The most common type of pre-excitation syndrome is WPW syndrome, in which the impulse is transmitted down the bundle of

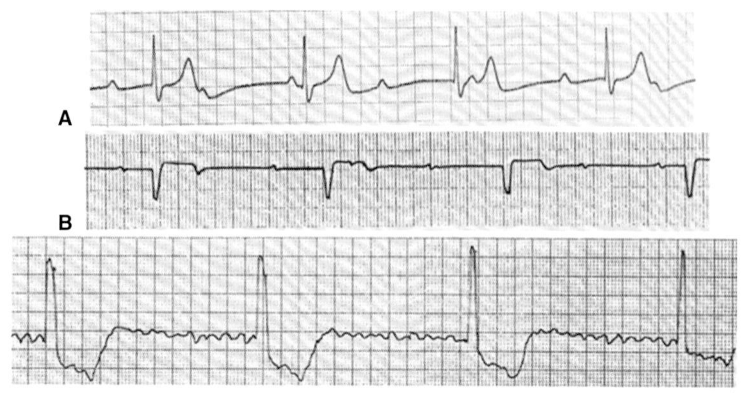

Figure 12-84. Examples of third-degree AV block. **A:** Third-degree AV block with most likely a junctional pacemaker at a rate of 36 beats per minute. **B:** Third-degree AV block with a ventricular pacemaker at a rate of 32 beats per minute. **C:** AF with third-degree block and ventricular escape pacemaker at rate of 25 beats per minute.

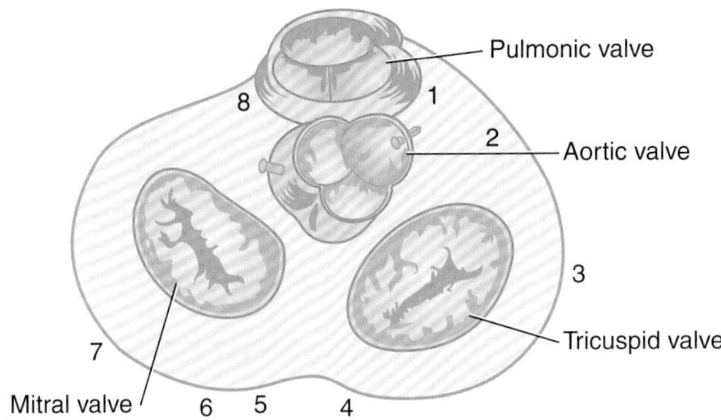

Delta wave polarity

	I	II	III	aV_R	aV_L	aV_R	V_1	V_2	V_3	V_4	V_5	V_6
1	+	+	+	−		+			+	+	+	+
2	+	+	−	−	+	−		+	+	+	+	+
3	+		−	−	+			+	+	+	+	+
4	+	−	−	−	+	−		+	+	+	+	+
5	+	−	−	−	+	−	+	+	+	+	+	+
6	+	+		−		+	+	+	+	+	+	+
7	−		+		−	+	+	+	+	+	+	+
8	−	+	+	−	−	+	+	+	+	+	+	+

Figure 12-85. Locating the accessory pathway from delta wave polarity on the ECG. Numbers on the diagram at top indicate potential sites of accessory pathways. The table at the bottom shows delta wave polarity (+ = positive; − = negative) in each lead of the ECG for each site. (From Conover M. *Understanding Electrocardiography*. 8th ed. St. Louis, MO: Mosby; 2003:278.)

Kent directly from the atrium into the ventricles, bypassing the AV node. In WPW, the ventricles are activated prematurely due to the impulse enter accessory pathway (the Kent bundle) and is conducted through normal His–Purkinje conduction system.[55,86] In WPW, the bypass pathway can be left sided (connecting the left atrium and left ventricle) or right sided (connecting the right atrium and right ventricle). The accessory pathway provides a shortcut and allows the impulse to bypass the AV node and activate the ventricles prematurely.[86] Early activation of ventricles results in a shorter PR interval. Premature ventricular stimulation induces upstroke of the initial portion of the QRS complex called delta wave. The QRS complex is widened due to the ventricle is depolarized through muscle cell-to-cell conduction. The majority of ventricular myocardium is activated through normal conduction pathway (the Purkinje system); thus, the remainder of the QRS complex is normal (Fig. 12-86).[55]

The length of PR interval and the size of the delta wave are dependent upon the degree of pre-excitation (how much of the ventricle is depolarized through the bypass connection), which depends on the relative rates of conduction through the bypass connection and the AV node. Extremely short PR interval and uniformly wide QRS complex are results of maximal excitation during which the ventricles are activated by the accessory pathway. When less than maximal pre-excitation occurs, the impulse enters the ventricle through both pathways simultaneously.[55] Figure 12-86 demonstrates the mechanism of pre-excitation and the characteristic short PR interval and delta waves that occur. WPW syndrome can be diagnosed easily based on ECG characteristics (Fig. 12-87):

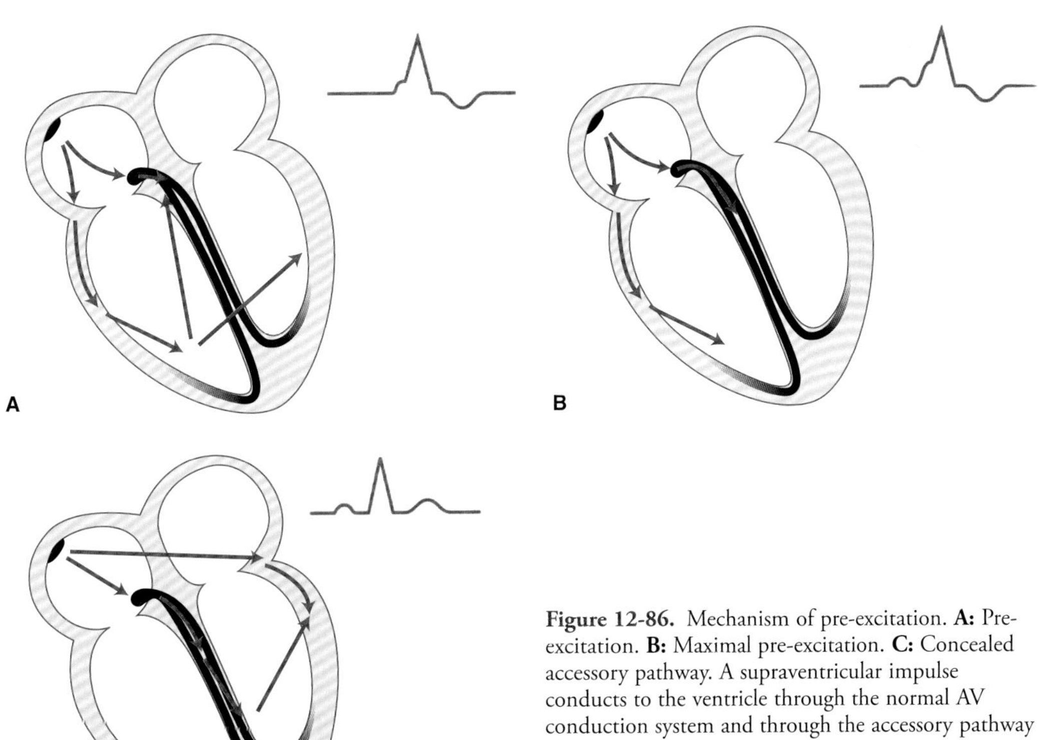

Figure 12-86. Mechanism of pre-excitation. **A:** Pre-excitation. **B:** Maximal pre-excitation. **C:** Concealed accessory pathway. A supraventricular impulse conducts to the ventricle through the normal AV conduction system and through the accessory pathway simultaneously. The impulse reaches the ventricle first through the accessory pathway and pre-excites it, causing a delta wave and short PR interval on the ECG.

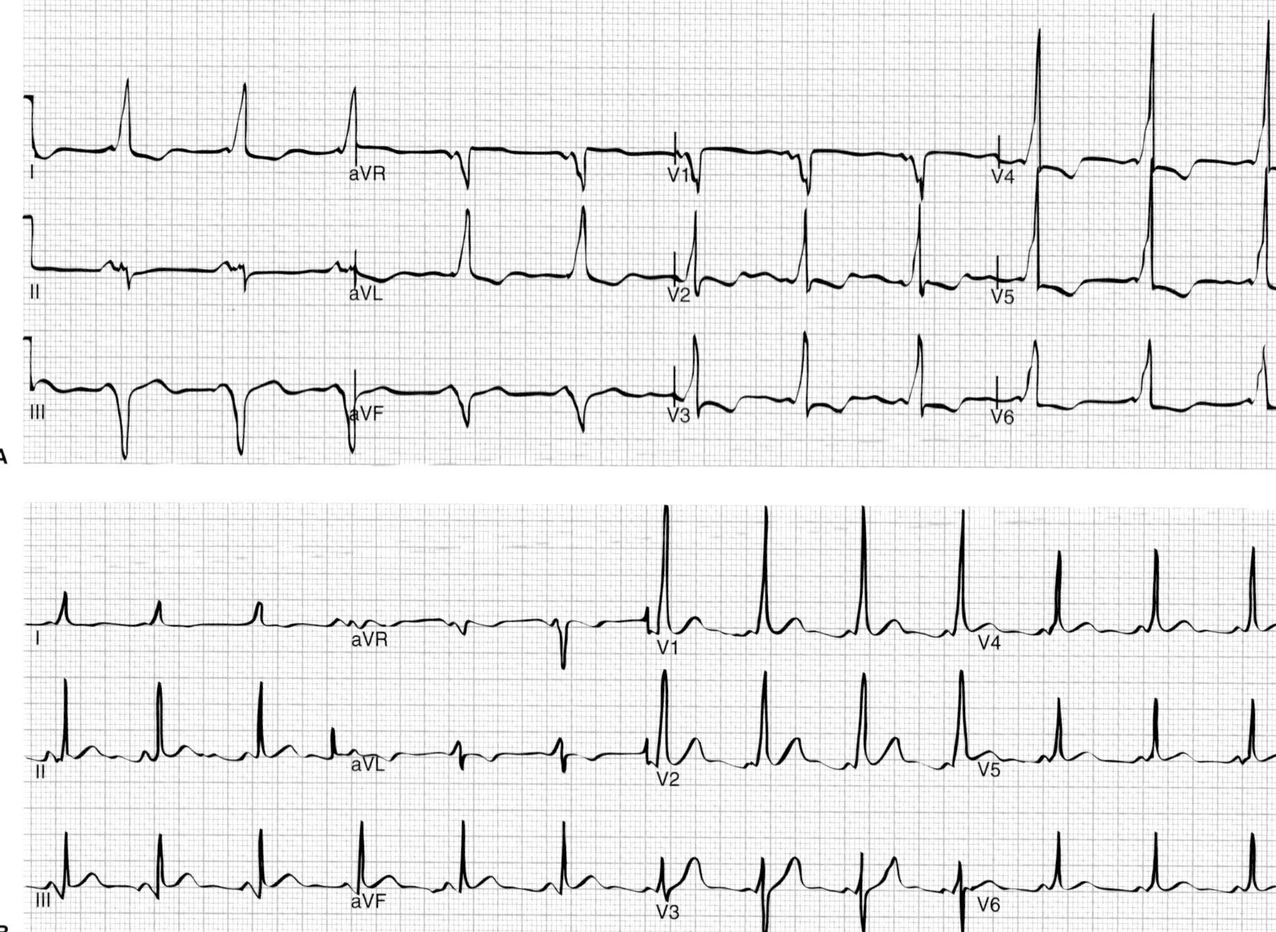

Figure 12-87. Wolff–Parkinson–White syndrome. **A:** The PR interval is very short and prominent delta waves are present. Delta waves are positive in all leads except aVR and V_1 where they are negative. **B:** The PR interval is short and there are positive delta waves in all leads except III and aVF where they are negative and lead II where it is isoelectric. Note how the negative delta waves in III and aVF simulate Q waves of MI.

1. A shortened PR interval. The electrical impulse travels from atrium via the accessary pathway to the ventricle directly, bypassing the AV node which shortens the time from the start of atrial depolarization to the start of ventricular depolarization.[7,86]
2. The faster speed of the electrical impulse travels to the ventricle produces an initial slurring upstroke of the QRS complex called a delta wave. The last part of the QRS complex is usually normal, however the overall QRS complex is widened to more than 0.1 second due to the presence of a delta wave.[7,86]

Some patients develop symptoms associated with WPW (e.g., palpitation, shortness of breath, and tachycardia). When both symptoms and classic WPW ECG presentations exist, the term WPW syndrome is used. The two most commonly seen tachyarrhythmias in WPW are SVT and AF. See subsection titled "Supraventricular Tachycardia" for information on re-entrant arrhythmias associated with accessory pathways.[55]

In AF with WPW, the accessory pathway provides a free conduit for the chaotic atrial activity. Without AV node working as filter, the ventricular rate can go up to 300 bpm which may lead to devastating hemodynamic compromises. Very rapid AF is also known to induce VF which may result in sudden cardiac death.[86] ECG characteristics of AF with anterograde conduction through an accessory pathway are listed (Fig. 12-88)[55]:

Rate: Ventricular rates up to 300 bpm
Rhythm: Irregular. Often appears as groups of very short R-R intervals alternating with groups of longer R-R intervals. The longest R-R intervals are often more than twice the shortest R-R intervals
P waves: None, because atria are fibrillating
PR interval: None
QRS complex: Wide, bizarre due to abnormal depolarization of ventricles through accessory pathway
Conduction: Disorganized and chaotic through atria. Atrial impulses conduct into ventricles through accessory pathway, resulting in muscle cell-to-cell conduction through ventricles

Immediate treatment may be required if the ventricular rate is rapid and patient has poor tolerance to AF with anterograde conduction through an accessory pathway. Cardioversion is treatment of choice if there is severe hemodynamic instability. The goal of drug treatment is to slow down the conduction rate and maintain sinus rhythm.[55]

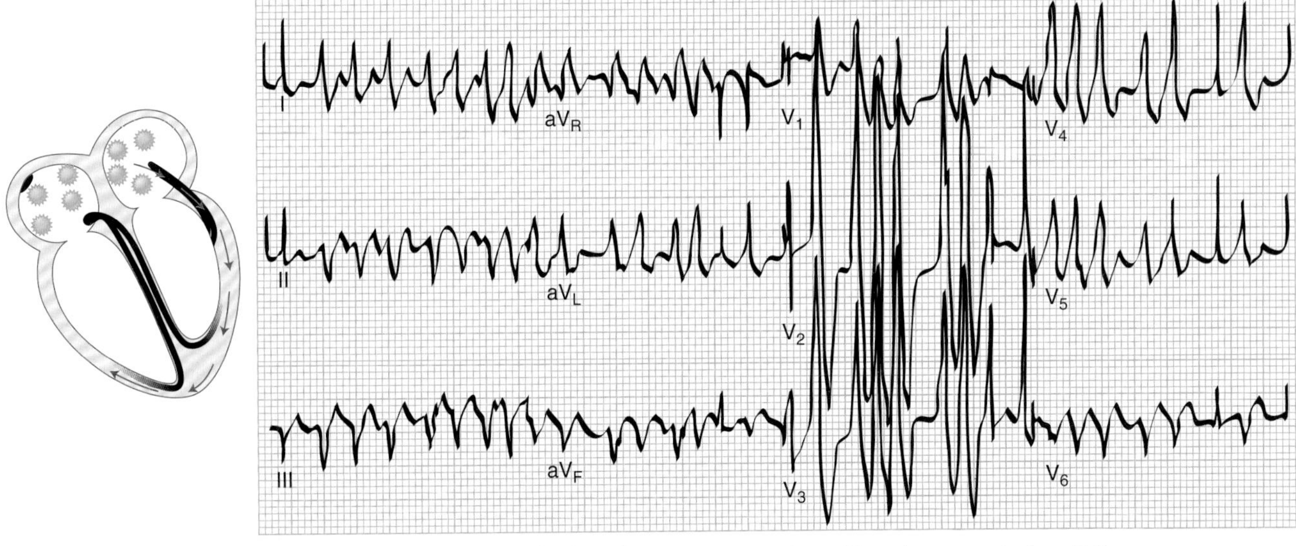

Figure 12-88. AF conducting anterograde through an accessory pathway. Note the extremely short R-R intervals in leads V_1 to V_3. QRS is fast, wide, and irregular.

Supraventricular Tachycardia

The term supraventricular arrhythmias is used to describe arrhythmias that originate above the bundle of His, including rhythms that originate from the SA node, atrial tissue, or the AV junction.[59] The term SVT is used for all tachycardias that either originate from supraventricular tissue (i.e., SA node reentry, atrial flutter, junctional tachycardia) or incorporate supraventricular tissue in a reentry circuit (i.e., AV nodal reentry tachycardia and complex movement tachycardia using an accessory pathway).[55] When the impulses are conducted through the normal intraventricular conduction pathway, the QRS complex in SVT will be narrow. When the impulses are conducted with BBB, the QRS complexes will be wide.[55]

SVT can be classified as AV nodal passive or AV nodal active. In AV nodal passive SVT, the AV node does not participate in maintaining the tachycardia but only conducts the supraventricular impulses into the ventricles. In AV nodal active SVT, the AV node plays a part in sustaining the rhythm. The two most common causes of a regular, narrow QRS tachycardia are AVNRT and CMT, and these two rhythms will be discussed below.

Atrioventricular Nodal Reentry Tachycardia

AVNRT is the most common type of SVT.[87] Patients with AVNRT have dual AV nodal pathways that conduct the impulses at different speed and recover at different rates: a fast conducting pathway with a long refractory period and a slow conducting pathway with a short refractory period.[55,59] in AVNRT, a reentry circuit or loop can be formed. As one side of the loop is recovering, the other is firing.[59]

It is estimated that 80% of AVNRT are slow-fast tachycardias that result from a single or multiple PACs.[87] When a PAC occurs during the refractory period of the fast pathway, the impulses will be conducted to the ventricles by the slow pathway resulting in a long PR interval on ECG. The long conduction time allows the fast pathway to recover. When the impulses reach the end of slow pathway and the fast pathway has recovered, the impulses will be conducted retrograde up the fast pathway and depolarize the atria. The impulse can then reenter the slow pathway to conduct again. If this conduction pattern continues, it will lead to AVNRT with a very rapid and regular ventricular rhythm ranging from 150 to 250 bpm. Figure 12-89 illustrates the most common mechanism of AVNRT. In AVNRT, the QRS complexes are normal as the activation of ventricles is through the normal His–Purkinje system. The P waves are either inverted (due to retrograde conduction) or seen peeking out at the end of the QRS complex (Fig. 12-90).[55,59]

A less common type of AVNRT is atypical AVNRT, and it is also known as fast-slow tachycardia (about 5% of cases of AVNRT).[87] In atypical AVNRT, the premature complex conducts down the fast pathway and returns via the slow pathway. Thus, there is a long R-P pattern due to delay in atrial activation and P waves are inverted in inferior leads due to retrograde depolarization.[55,59]

Treatment for AVNRT is based on the duration of tachycardia and the severity of patient's response to AVNRT. Because AVNRT is an AV nodal active SVT, vagal maneuver can be affective as long as there is no contraindication. Adenosine is the drug of choice, and beta-blockers and calcium channel blockers can also be considered.[55,59,87] However, it is estimated that 80% to 98% of stable patients with SVT respond to pharmacologic therapy with adenosine, diltiazem, or verapamil.[60] Radiofrequency catheter ablation can be an option for patients who are resistant to drug therapy and do not wish to remain on lifelong medications. The success rate of radiofrequency ablation for AVNRT is up to 98%.[88]

Circus Movement Tachycardia

CMT, also known as atrioventricular reentrant tachycardia (AVRT), is next most common type of SVT and occurs in individuals who have accessory pathways. AVRT has underlying pre-excitation ideology, because the rhythm originates above the ventricles and the accessory pathways allow the impulses travel from atria to ventricles directly.[55,59]

In AVRT, the reentry circuit involves four components: the atria, AV node, ventricle, and an accessory pathway. There are two types of AVRT: The most common type is called orthodromic (accounts for approximately 90% to 95% of AVRT),[60] and the rare form is called antidromic which is a pre-excited AVRT (accounts for approximately 5% of AVRT).[60]

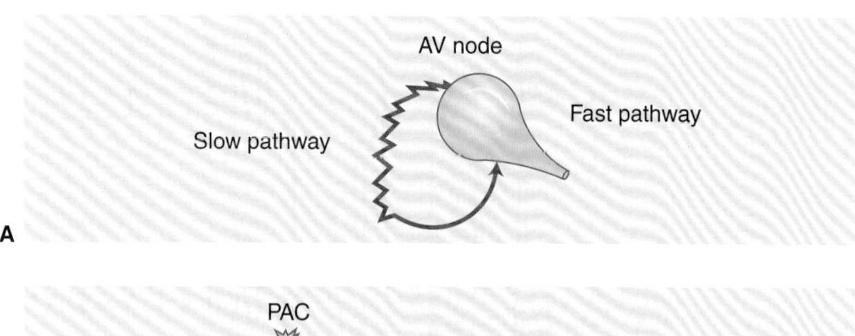

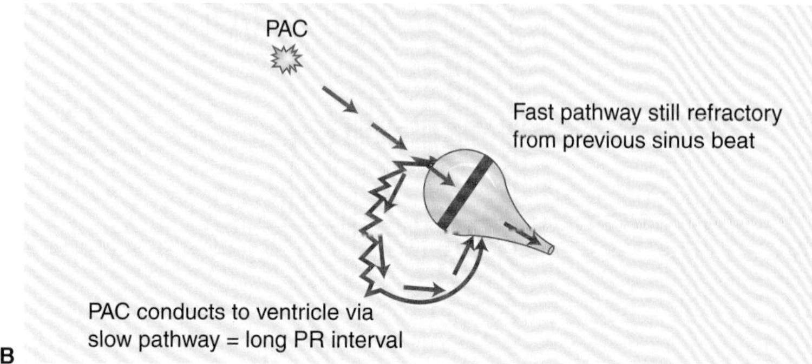

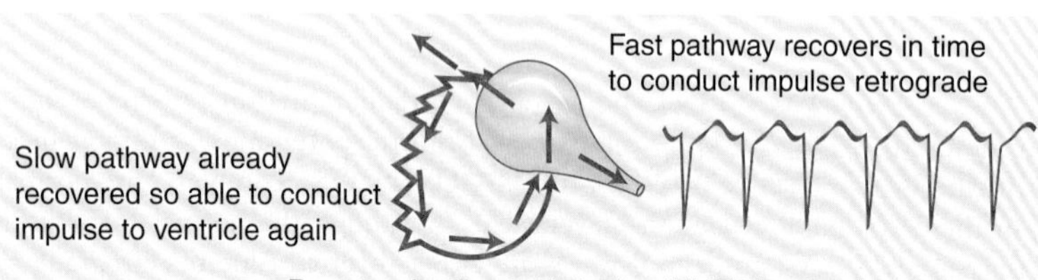

Figure 12-89. Mechanism of AVNRT. **A:** The dual AV nodal pathways responsible for AVNRT. The normal AV node is the fast conducting pathway with a long refractory period; the slow conducting pathway lies outside the AV node and has a shorter refractory period. **B:** A PAC finds the fast pathway still refractory but is able to conduct through the slow pathway. **C:** When the impulse arrives at the end of the slow pathway it finds the AV node recovered and ready to conduct retrograde to the atria. The slow pathway has already recovered due to its short refractory period and is able to conduct the same impulse back into the ventricle. This sets up the reentry circuit and causes AVNRT.

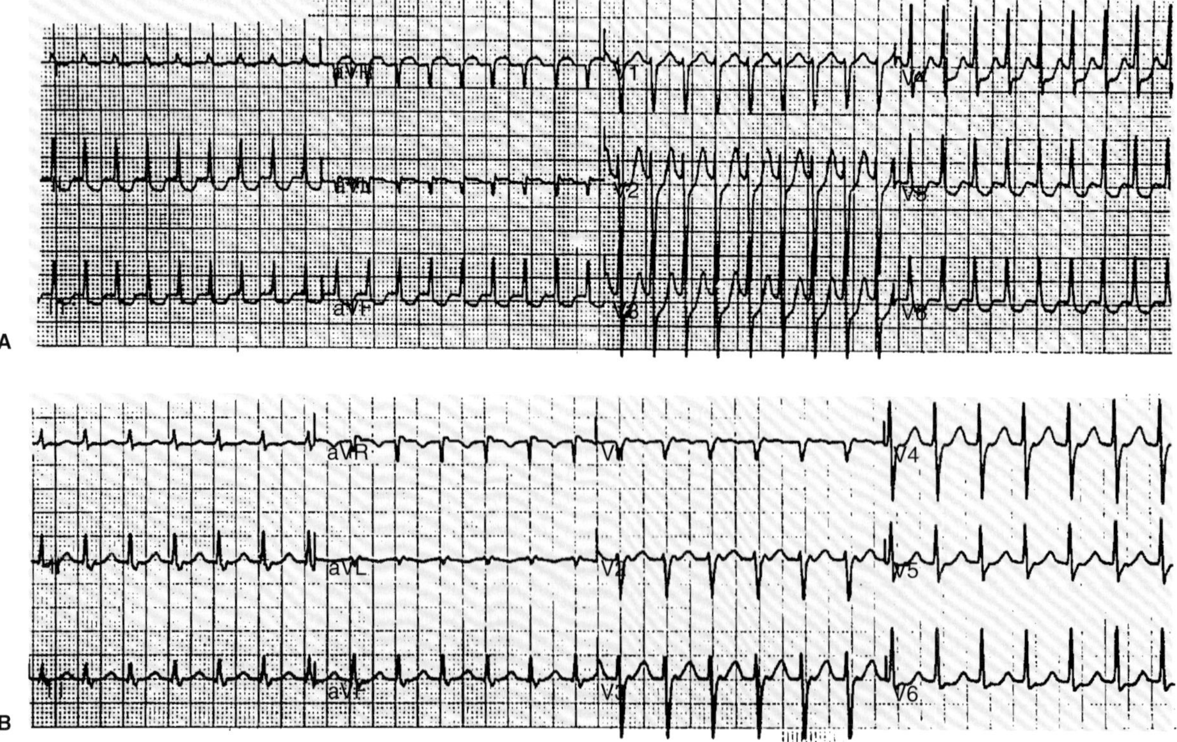

Figure 12-90. **A:** AVNRT; rate—214 beats per minute. No P waves are visible. **B:** AVNRT; rate—150 beats per minute. P waves distort the end of the QRS complex in leads II, III, aVF, and V_{1-3}.

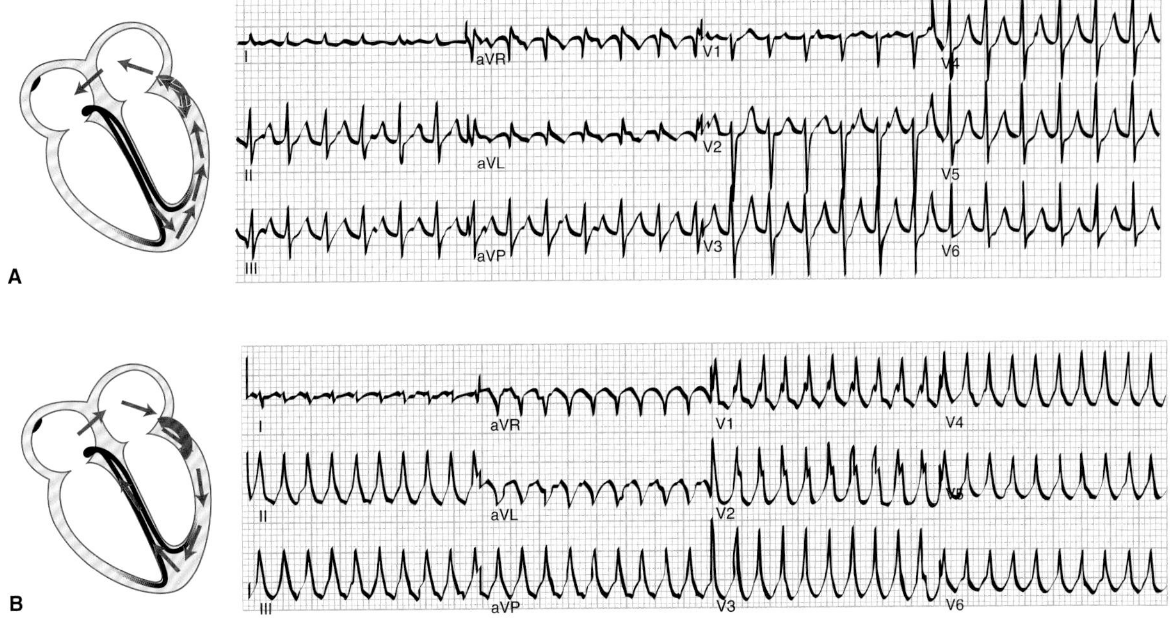

Figure 12-91. A: Orthodromic CMT using the AV node as anterograde limb and accessory pathway as retrograde limb of the reentry circuit. P waves are visible in the ST segment in most leads. **B:** Antidromic CMT using the accessory pathway as the anterograde limb and the AV node as the retrograde limb of the reentry circuit.

In orthodromic AVRT, the AV node is used as the anterograde limb and the accessory pathway is used as the retrograde limb of the circuit, which results in a narrow QRS tachycardia due to normal depolarization of ventricles through the His–Purkinje system. The QRS will be wide with the presence of BBB because the atria and ventricles depolarize separately. The P waves in CMT, if visible, are often seen in the ST segment or between the QRS complexes, usually closer to the preceding QRS than the following QRS (Fig. 12-91A).[55]

In antidromic AVRT, the accessory pathway is used as the anterograde limb of the circuit and the AV node is used as the retrograde limb. Antidromic AVRT has a wide QRS tachycardia due to abnormal depolarization of the ventricles through the accessory pathway, and it is often indistinguishable from VT (Fig. 12-91B).[55] In rare cases of antidromic AVRT, the return conduction occurs through a second accessory AV pathway. AF can occur in patients with accessory pathways, which may lead to extremely rapid conduction to the ventricle over a manifest pathway, which increases the risk of inducing VF and sudden cardiac death (SCD).[60]

CMT is an AV nodal active tachycardia. Thus, vagal maneuvers such as carotid massage or Valsalva maneuver, or adenosine may terminate the arrhythmia by causing the AV conduction delay (class I recommendation). Synchronized cardioversion should be performed if AVRT causes hemodynamic instability and if vagal maneuvers or adenosine is ineffective or not feasible. Ibutilide or intravenous procainamide is beneficial for acute treatment in patients with pre-excited AF who are hemodynamically stable (class I recommendation). Intravenous diltiazem, verapamil, or beta-blockers can be effective for acute treatment in patients with orthodromic AVRT who do not have pre-excitation on their resting ECG during sinus rhythm (class IIa recommendation).[60]

Ventricular Tachycardia

VT is defined as three or more consecutive PVCs that occur at a rate of more than 100 bpm. Nonsustained VT is defined as a short run of VT for less than 30 seconds and terminate spontaneously. This rhythm occurs in up to 3% of healthy individuals.[89] Sustained VT lasts for more than 30 seconds. Sustained VT can cause a significant decrease in cardiac output especially in patients with decreased ventricular function.[67,90] VT is one of the most serious arrhythmias and can progress to VF. VT often requires immediate treatment to prevent CLINICAL deterioration. VTs can be classified into three different types based on QRS complexes morphology: monomorphic VT, polymorphic VT, and TdP.[55,67,90]

The sequence of ventricular activation determines the QRS morphology of the arrhythmia. The QRS complex will be wide when the impulse is conducted through the ventricular myocardium, because the conduction through ventricular myocardium is slower than the activation through the Purkinje system. The QRS is typically more than 0.12 second. When VT is caused by repetitive activation from the same site, the QRS complexes are of the same shape and amplitude from beat to beat, and VT is monomorphic. A continually changing activation sequence produces polymorphic VT with a changing QRS morphology.[90]

Monomorphic VT

Monomorphic VT with a ventricular rate of 150 to 300 bpm is also known as ventricular flutter (Fig. 12-92). Sustained monomorphic VTs are associated with underlying cardiac diseases. When VT occurs in patients with underlying heart disease, there is an increased risk of sudden cardiac death.[80] Other possible causes of VT include acid–base imbalance, acute coronary syndromes, cardiomyopathy, cocaine abuse, digitalis toxicity, electrolyte imbalance (e.g., hypokalemia, hyperkalemia, hypomagnesemia), mitral valve prolapse, trauma (e.g., myocardial contusion, invasive cardiac procedures), tricyclic antidepressant overdose, and valvular heart disease.[67]

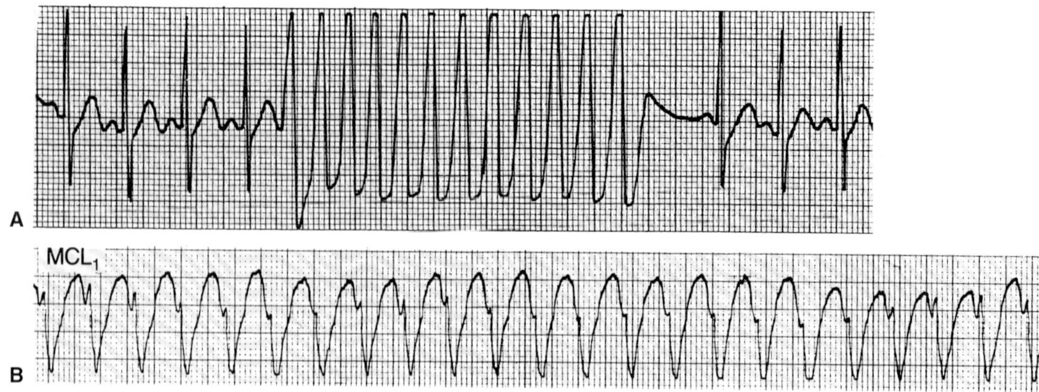

Figure 12-92. Monomorphic VT. Tracings show two different examples, each with QRS complexes of one morphology.

The most common mechanism of monomorphic VT is reentry, and its presentation ranges from asymptomatic to sudden cardiac death. Signs and symptoms associated with VT are determined by the ventricular rate and underlying ventricular function. Patients may be able to tolerate sustained monomorphic VT and be stable for a long period of time. The more rapid ventricular rate and the lower the ejection fraction, the more symptomatic the patient is. ECG characteristics of monomorphic VT are listed[55,67]:

Rhythm: Regular ventricular rhythm
Rate: Ventricular rate 150 to 300 bpm
P waves: Not seen
PR interval: Cannot be measured due to a lack of P waves
QRS Complex: 0.12 second or greater; often difficult to differentiate the QRS and T wave

The term idiopathic VT refers to VT that occurs in individuals with structurally normal heart. The two main clinical entities of idiopathic VT include "outflow tract" VT and "idiopathic left ventricular" VT (also known as fascicular VT or verapamil-sensitive VT). "Outflow tract" VT is often provoked by exercise and emotional stress and occurs frequently in young to middle-aged patients without structural heart disease. The right ventricular outflow tract (RVOT) is the most common site of origin of idiopathic VT. The ECG characteristics of idiopathic VT originating from RVOT are a LBBB pattern in V_1 and tall, monophasic R waves in the inferior leads (II, III, and aVF). RVOT tachycardia presents in two different forms: (1) no sustained, repetitive monomorphic VT characterized by frequent repetitive salvos VT or (2) paroxysmal, sustained monomorphic VT induced by exercise. Approximately, 25% of idiopathic VTs originate from other sites (coronary cusps, mitral annulus, left ventricular summit, or within or adjacent to the epicardial coronary venous structures).[91]

Idiopathic left VT is characterized by a RBBB pattern with a left superior axis and narrow QRS complex on a 12-lead ECG. The site of origin of the tachycardia is usually in the region of the left posterior fascicle (inferior posterior LV septum).[91] Reentry is thought to be the mechanism for this arrhythmia.[92,93] The reentrant circuit encompasses the distal Purkinje network of the left posterior fascicle, which results in the relatively narrow QRS.[94]

Idiopathic VT is associated with an excellent prognosis, and treatment is aimed at the relief of symptoms.[95] Beta-blockers and calcium channel blockers are usually treatment of choice for symptomatic VT. Beta-blockers are effective in approximately 25% to 50% of patients, whereas calcium channel blockers are effective in approximately 25% to 30%.[96,97] Radiofrequency ablation can be an option for idiopathic VT and it has successful rate of 75% to 100%.[96]

Polymorphic VT

Polymorphic VT has clearly defined QRS complexes, but the QRS complexes are constantly changing and varied in shape and amplitude. The ventricular rate of polymorphic VT is approximately 200 bpm (Fig. 12-93). Polymorphic VT has intermediate severity between monomorphic VT and VF, and it can degenerate into VF and lead to sudden cardiac death.[55] Coronary artery disease and resultant MI is the most common etiology of polymorphic VT. Other causes of polymorphic VT include dilated cardiomyopathy, hypertrophy cardiomyopathy, myocarditis, valvular heart disease, congenital heart disease, proarrhythmia from drugs, acid–base and electrolyte abnormalities, inherited arrhythmia syndromes, and AF in a patient with WPW syndrome with an anterograde rapidly conducting bypass tract.[95]

Polymorphic VT can occur in the setting of long QT interval and short QT interval. Polymorphic VT that occurs in the presence

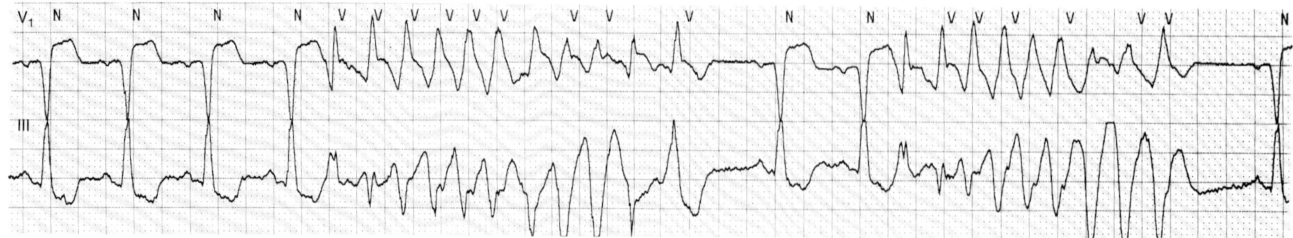

Figure 12-93. PVT recorded in two leads (V_1 and III). Note the normal QT interval and the ST elevation in lead V_1 with reciprocal ST depression in lead III due to anterior MI. (*N* = arrhythmia computer's determination of a normal beat; *V* = computer determination of ventricular beat.)

of a long QT interval (typically 0.45 second or more and often 0.50 second or more) is called TdP. Polymorphic VT can also occur with abnormally short QT interval (typically less than 0.32 second). ECG characteristics of polymorphic VT are listed[67]:

Rhythm: Regular or irregular ventricular rhythm
Rate: Ventricular rate 150 to 300 bpm; typically, 200 to 250 bpm
P waves: Not seen
PR interval: Cannot be measured due to a lack of P waves
QRS Complex: 0.12 second or greater; there is an alternation in amplitude and direction of the QRS complexes

Torsade de Pointes

TdP means "twisting of the points." TdP is polymorphic VT with a prolonged QT interval, and it is often self-terminating. TdP is characterized by a rapid polymorphic VT that is constantly changing cycle length, axis, and morphology, in a pattern that appears to twist around a central axis.[95] TdP often has a characteristic initiation sequence of PVCs that induces a pause, followed by a sinus beat that has prolonged QT interval and interruption of the T wave by a PVC that is the first beat of the polymorphic VT.[90] Ventricular rate during TdP is commonly 200 to 250 bpm. TdP is usually self-terminating and occurs in repeated episodes, but it can deteriorate into VF.[55] The underlying cause of TdP is abnormally prolonged QT interval. A long QT can be acquired, congenital, or idiopathic.[67] This subsection will focus on the acquired long QT interval.

The acquired type is most often due to repolarization abnormalities precipitated by drugs, including antiarrhythmic drugs (sotalol, dofetilide, and ibutilide), other medications used for noncardiac diseases: macrolide antibiotics, antifungals, antipsychotic and antidepressant drugs, some antihistamines, some gastric motility agents, and many others. Haloperidol (Haldol) has been known for its risks of QT prolongation, especially when it is given intravenously or in doses higher than recommended. QT prolongation is often associated with electrolytes abnormalities (e.g., hypokalemia and hypomagnesemia). The risk of developing TdP from drugs increases in the presence of hypokalemia, hypomagnesemia, or when taking other drugs that also prolong the QT interval or slow drug metabolism, or drug interactions that elevate levels of the offending agent. Grapefruit juice can slow metabolism of many drugs and can also increase the QT interval directly. Other factors that can lead to delayed repolarization include cerebral events such as cerebral vascular accidents and subarachnoid hemorrhage and liquid protein weight loss diets or starvation.[55,90]

Characteristic ECG findings of TdP include (1) markedly prolonged QT intervals with wide T and U waves; (2) initiation of the arrhythmia by an R-on-T PVC with a long coupling interval; and (3) wide, bizarre, multiform QRS complexes that change direction frequently, appearing to twist around the isoelectric line (Figs. 12-94 and 12-95). The acquired type of TdP is usually associated with bradycardia and is "pause dependent," meaning that it tends to occur after pauses produced by a PVC or sudden slowing of the heart rate. TdP is often initiated by a "long–short" cycle sequence in which episodes begin on the T wave of a beat that terminates a long cycle.[55]

The differentiation of TdP from PVT and VF is extremely important because TdP does not respond to conventional antiarrhythmic therapy and is usually made worse by the drugs used to treat ordinary VT. Treatment of TdP is aimed at shortening the refractory period and unifying repolarization by increasing the heart rate and correcting any contributing factors: removing of all medications that prolong the QT interval and correcting electrolyte abnormalities. Cardiac pacing at rates of 100 to 110 bpm can be instituted until the underlying cause is corrected. Magnesium can suppress the arrhythmia in both the acquired and congenital forms by reducing the amplitude of afterdepolarizations thought to cause TdP. Patients with history of a PVT induced by QT prolongation should be considered to have a susceptibility to the arrhythmia, and medications known to prolong the QT interval (e.g., quinidine, procainamide, disopyramide, sotalol, and amiodarone) are contraindicated.[55,90]

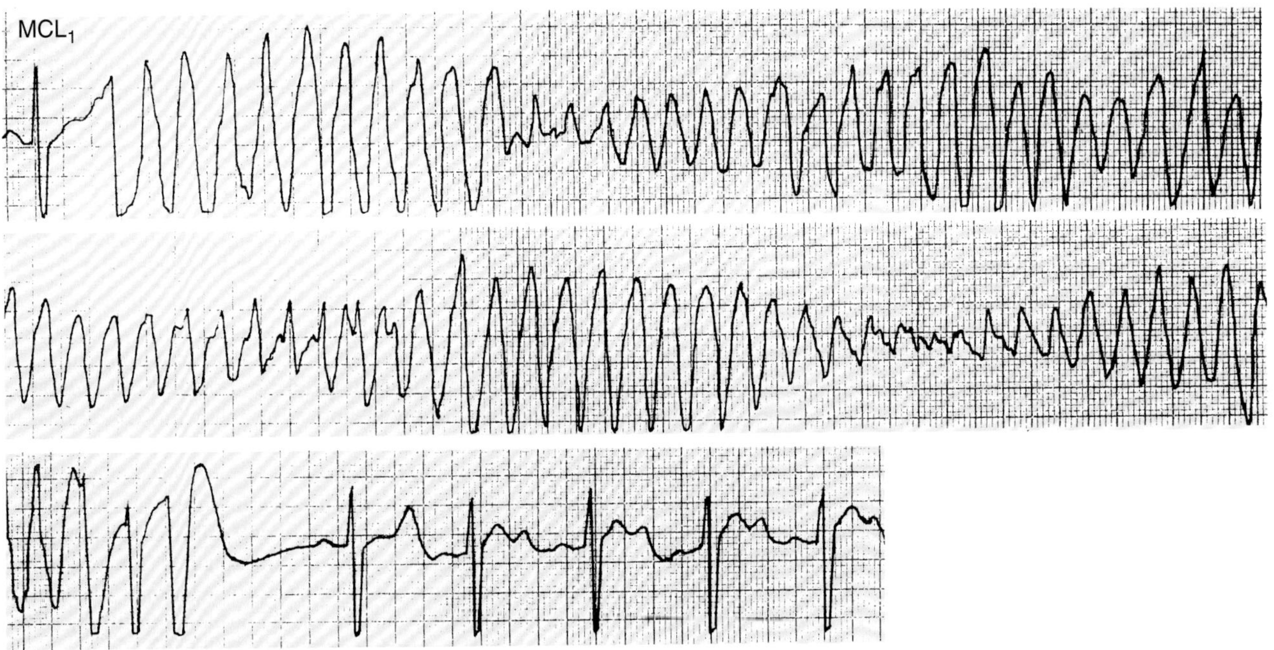

Figure 12-94. Note characteristic features: (1) multiform QRS complexes that twist and around the baseline, (2) initiation by a PVC with a long coupling interval, and (3) associated long QT interval and wide TU waves during sinus rhythm.

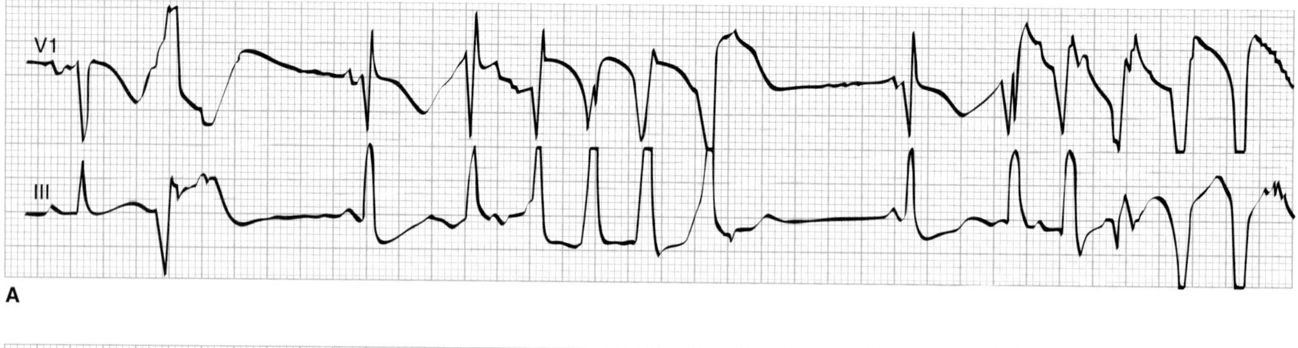

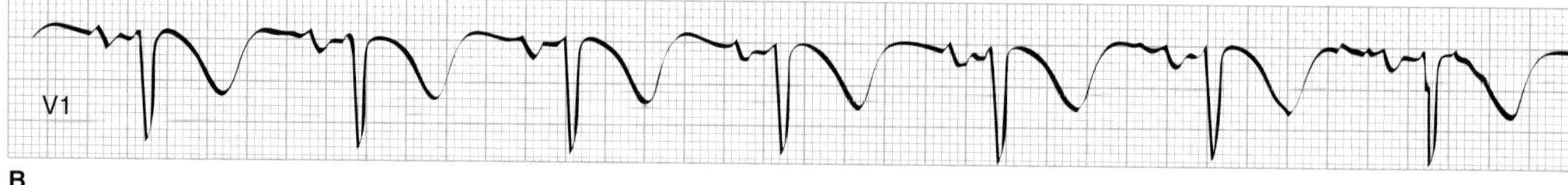

Figure 12-95. **A:** Short runs of TdP. Note that the episodes of TdP occur following a pause: the first pause follows a PVC; the second pause is due to termination of the first TdP episode and initiates the next episode. **B:** Same patient in normal sinus rhythm. Note: prolonged QT interval measuring about 520 milliseconds.

GENETICS OF CHANNELOPATHIES

The term cardiac channelopathies refers to a group of genetic diseases in which the primary dysfunction is an abnormal electrophysiologic substrate creating susceptibility to arrhythmias in the setting of a substantially normal cardiac structure. Channelopathies are also referred to as *inherited arrhythmogenic diseases* (IADs).[98] This section will review the clinical and genetic features of the most epidemiologically relevant cardiac channelopathies: catecholaminergic ventricular tachycardia, short QT syndrome (SQTS), LQTS, and Brugada syndrome.

Catecholaminergic Polymorphic Ventricular Tachycardia

CPVT was first described in 1978. It is genetic disorder characterized by a typical reproducible pattern of bidirectional adrenergic-dependent VT (one QRS pointing up, the next pointing down in alternating fashion) that occurs in individuals with structurally normal heart (Fig. 12-96). CPVT usually occurs in children or adolescents and is associated with exercise or emotional stress. Individuals that experience CPVT usually have unremarkable resting ECG with the exception of sinus bradycardia and a prominent U wave reported in some cases, which create diagnostic challenge and potential delay diagnosis. CPVT causes high incidence of sudden cardiac death. Syncope, triggered by exercise or acute emotion, is the typical manifestation of the disease.[98,99] Beta-blockers are the drugs of choice for treating CPVT and are indicated for genetically positive family members. Despite the use of beta-blockers, there is a 25% to 35% risk of recurrent cardiac events.[100,101] Current guidelines recommend the use of ICD, in addition to beta-blockers with or without flecainide, in patients with a diagnosis of CPVT who experience cardiac arrest, recurrent syncope, or polymorphic/bidirectional VT despite optimal therapy.[98]

Short QT Syndrome

SQTS is also known as short-coupled TdP; it is a rare genetically determined disorder causing arrhythmias and sudden death in healthy children and young adults with structurally normal hearts.[55,98] The shortened QT interval represents the shortened ventricular repolarization, which is a marker of action potential shortening in the cellular level (Fig. 12-97).[98] This results in a short cardiac refractory period and increases tissue temporal vulnerability for initiating reentry.[102] SQTS can be diagnosed in the presence of QTc less than 340 milliseconds (class Ic) and can also be considered (class IIa) in the presence of a QTc less than or equal to 360 milliseconds and one or more of the following: (1) confirmed pathogenic mutation; (2) family history of SQTS; (3) family history of sudden death at age less than 40 years; or (4) survival from a VT/VF episode in the absence of heart disease.[98] With a lack of drugs with documented efficacy, ICD is recommended as primary prevention of VF in all patients. Quinidine can be effective in normalizing the QT interval prolonging the ventricular refractory period, but more data is needed to determine whether quinidine can impact mortality in SQTS.[98]

Long QT Syndrome

LQTS is an inherited condition with abnormally prolonged QT interval, and it is associated with TdP and SCD.[55] It typically occurs in children and teenagers. Fifteen genes have been associated with LQTS, which disrupt one or more ionic currents contributing to the generation of cardiac action potential. For example, an excess of sodium flow into the cell causes LQTS.[98] LQTS can be diagnosed under the following conditions: (1) either QTc greater than or equal to 480 milliseconds in repeated 12-lead ECGs or LQTS risk score greater than 3; (2) confirmed pathogenic LQTS mutation, irrespective of the QT duration; or (3) a QTc greater than or equal to 460 milliseconds in repeated 12-lead ECGs in patients with unexplained syncope in the absence of secondary causes for QT prolongation.[103] Treatments for LQTS include avoidance of QT-prolonging drugs, correction of electrolyte disturbances (especially hypokalemia), and the avoidance of genotype-specific triggers have a class I indication.[104] Beta-blockers are recommended in all patients with a diagnosis of LQTS.[105]

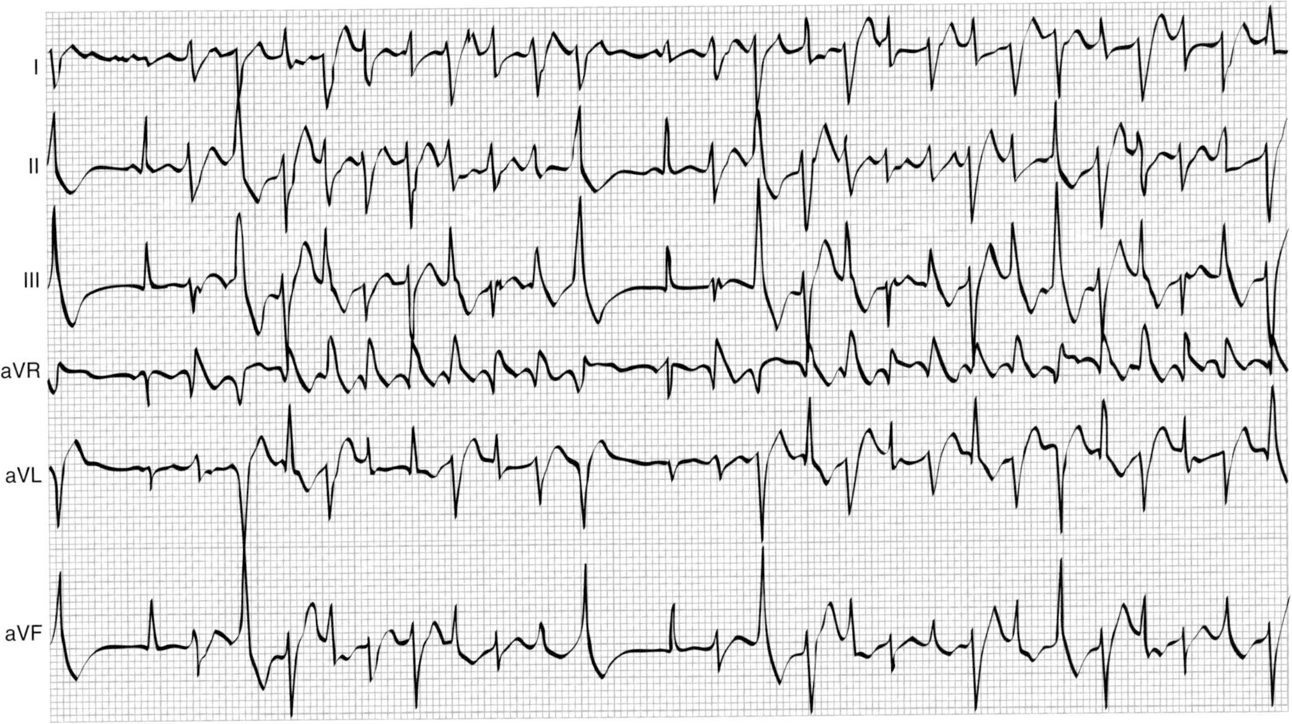

Figure 12-96. Catecholaminergic PVT in a 12-year-old patient during exercise. (From Wellens HJJ, Conover M. *The ECG in emergency decision making*. 2nd ed. St. Louis, MO: Saunders; 2006:224.)

Brugada Syndrome

Brugada syndrome was first described in 1992 and it is characterized as RBBB and persistent ST-elevation in right precordial leads (lead V_1 to V_3) in the absence of signs of acute myocardial ischemia. Brugada syndrome is associated with increased risk for sudden cardiac death: it is responsible for 12% of sudden cardiac death cases, and 20% of sudden cardiac death with structurally normal hearts.[105,106] Three ECG repolarization patterns of Brugada syndrome are described[107,108]:

1. A coved ST-segment elevation greater than or equal to 2 mm is followed by a negative T-wave, with little or no isoelectric separation in more than one right precordial leads (V_1 to V_3)
2. A ST-segment elevation followed by a positive or biphasic t-wave that results in a saddle-back configuration
3. A right precordial ST-segment elevation less than or equal to 1 mm either with a coved-type or a saddle-back morphology.

The definite diagnosis of Brugada syndrome is based on one of the above ECG characteristics (see Fig. 12-98) and presence of one of the following criteria[109]:

1. Family history: sudden cardiac death in a family member less than 45 years or ECG repolarization pattern type 1 in relatives
2. Arrhythmia-related symptoms: syncope, seizures, or nocturnal agonal respiration
3. Ventricular arrhythmias: PVT or VF

Implantation of an internal cardioverted-defibrillator (ICD) is the only effective therapy to prevent sudden cardiac death and reduce mortality in patient with Brugada syndrome. Most antiarrhythmic drugs are contraindicated with the possible exception of quinidine. Class IA antiarrhythmic drugs (mainly quinidine) have shown excellent protective effective during electrophysiologic testing and an excellent clinical outcome in patients treated with these medications. However, quinidine is currently indicated only for the treatment of electrical storm (Class IIa) or in patients with contraindications to ICD (Class IIa).[104]

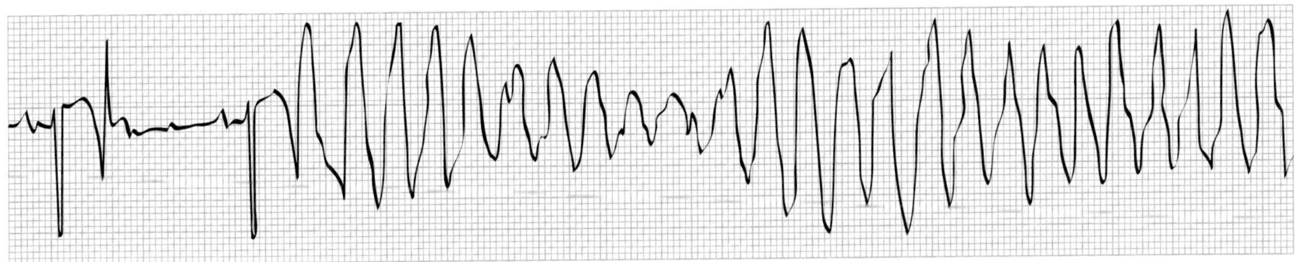

Figure 12-97. Short-coupled PVT. Note the very short coupling interval of about 240 milliseconds between the normal beat and the first beat of VT. This PVT has characteristics of TdP but the QT interval is short.

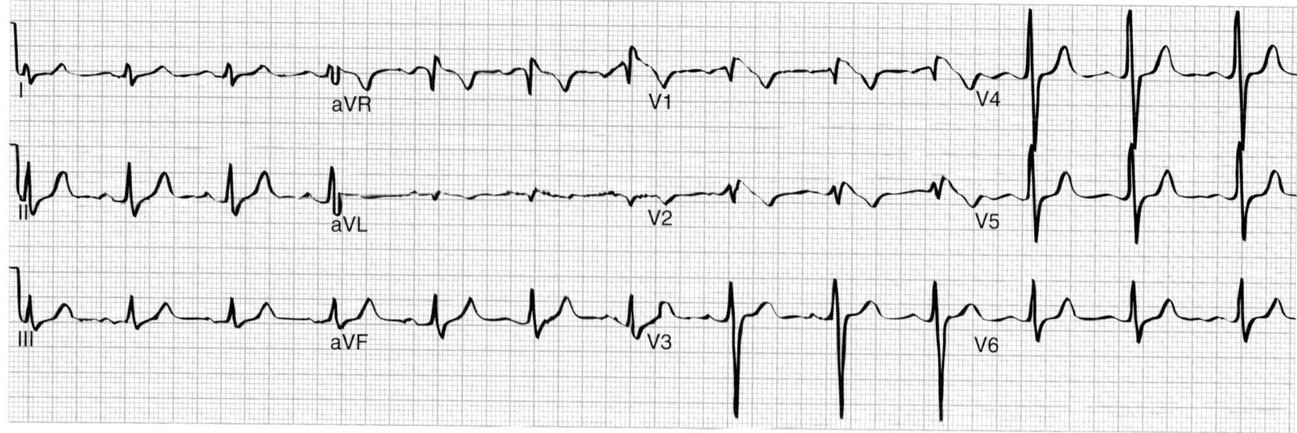

Figure 12-98. **Brugada syndrome.**

DIFFERENTIAL DIAGNOSIS OF WIDE QRS BEATS AND TACHYCARDIAS

Both VT and SVT can cause wide QRS complex and it can be difficult to differentiate the two based on ECG characteristics. Aberrantly conducted supraventricular beats and tachycardias can look almost identical to ventricular ectopic beats or VT, it is sometimes impossible to tell them apart. Correct diagnosis of rhythm will lead to immediate therapy for acute event as well as determine long-term therapy for the arrhythmia.[55,103]

There are three major causes of wide QRS complex tachycardia (WCT): (1) ventricular origin of the beat or rhythm, VT is the most common cause of WCT, which accounts for up to 80% of cases; (2) SVT with aberrant conduction (SVT-A). The widening of the QRS complex results from conduction delay or block or both along the bundle branches or fascicles (temporary or permanent BBB). SVT-A accounts for 15% to 25% of WCT cases[110]; (3) pre-excitation of the ventricle through an accessory pathway. Other conditions that can also cause the QRS to widen include antiarrhythmic drugs; electrolyte imbalance, especially hyperkalemia; and ventricular paced rhythms.[55,110] These causes along with pre-excitation SVT account for only 1% to 5% of WCTs. Because the vast majority (95%) of WCTs are either VT or SVT-A, the main differential diagnosis for WCT is to distinguish VT from SVT-A.[110]

Although many criteria have been proposed to aid in differentiating wide QRS beats and rhythms, this section concentrates only on selected criteria that seem to be the most helpful in the everyday clinical situation. Table 12-14 lists the ECG characteristics most helpful for differentiating wide QRS rhythms.[55]

Mechanism of Aberration

Aberrancy can occur whenever the His–Purkinje system is still partly or completely refractory when a supraventricular impulse attempts to traverse it. The refractory period of the conduction system is directly proportional to preceding cycle length. Long cycles (slow heart rates) are followed by long refractory periods, whereas short cycles (fast heart rates) are followed by short refractory periods. Supraventricular beats that occur early in the cycle, like a PAC, may enter the conduction system during its refractory period and be conducted aberrantly. Similarly, beats that follow a sudden lengthening of the cycle may be conducted

Table 12-14 • ELECTROCARDIOGRAPHIC CLUES FOR DIFFERENTIATING WIDE QRS RHYTHMS

ECG Feature	Aberrancy	Ventricular Ectopy
P waves	Precede QRS complexes (may be hidden in T waves)	Dissociated from QRS or occur at rate slower than that of QRS. If 1:1 ventriculoatrial conduction is present, retrograde P waves follow every QRS
RBBB QRS morphology	Triphasic rSR' in V_1 Triphasic qRs in V_6	Monophasic r wave or diphasic qR complex in V_1
LBBB QRS morphology	Narrow R wave (<0.04 s) in V_1 Straight downstroke of S wave in V_1 (often slurs or notches on upstroke) Usually no Q wave in V_6	Left "rabbit ear" taller in V_1 Monophasic QS or diphasic rS in V_6 Wide R wave (>0.03 s) in V_1 Slurring or notching on downstroke of S wave in V_1 Delay of >0.06 s to nadir of S wave in V_1 Any Q wave in V_6
Precordial QRS concordance	Positive concordance may occur with WPW	Negative concordance favors VT Positive concordance favors VT if WPW ruled out
Fusion or capture beats	Often normal	Strong evidence in favor of VT
QRS axis QRS width	May be deviated to right or left Usually <0.14 s unless pre-existing bundle branch block	Indeterminate axis favors VT Often deviated to left or right QRS >0.16 s favors VT

RBBB, right bundle branch block; LBBB, left bundle branch block; WPW, Wolfe Parkinson White; VT, ventricular tachycardia.

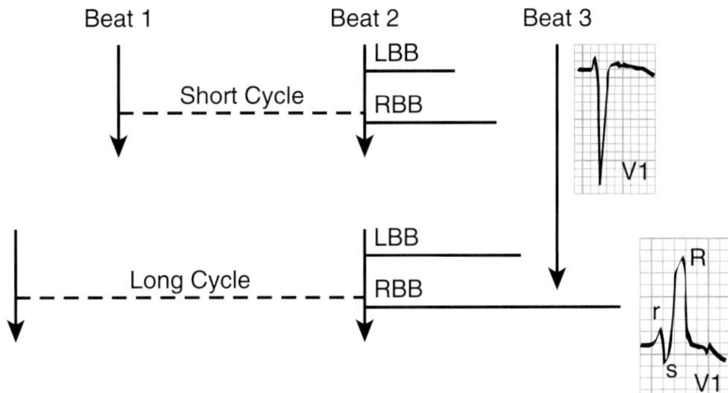

Figure 12-99. Diagram of the effect of cycle length on conduction. Beats 1, 2, and 3 are consecutive beats. The refractory periods of the left bundle branch (LBB) and the right bundle branch (RBB) are shown following beat 2 (note the longer refractory period in the RBB). In the **top** panel, the basic cycle length from beat 1 to beat 2 is short, resulting in short refractory periods after beat 2 and allowing beat 3 to conduct normally even though it is premature. In the **bottom** panel the basic cycle lengthens, resulting in longer refractory periods. Beat 3 is no earlier here than it was in the **top** panel, but it now conducts with RBBB because of the longer refractory periods following the longer cycle. The QRS complexes are recorded in lead V_1 and illustrate normal conduction (**top**) and RBBB (**bottom**).

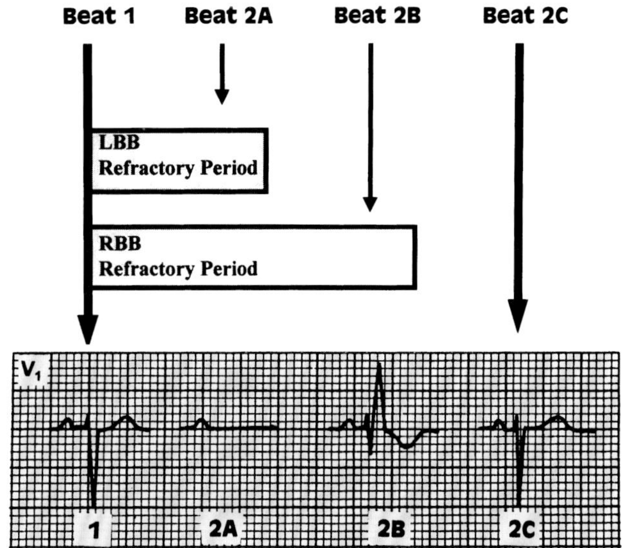

Figure 12-100. Diagram of refractory periods in the bundle branches and the effect of prematurity on conduction. The right bundle has a longer refractory period than the left. Beat 2A occurs so early that it cannot conduct through either bundle branch, resulting in the blocked P wave illustrated in the strip below. Beat 2B encounters a refractory right bundle and conducts with RBBB. Beat 2C falls outside the refractory period of both bundles and is able to conduct normally.

aberrantly because of the increased length of the refractory period that occurs when the cycle lengthens. There are three situations in which aberration is likely to occur: (1) early supraventricular beats (e.g., PAC), (2) rapid heart rates where the supraventricular focus conducts into the intraventricular conduction system so rapidly that the bundles do not have time to repolarize completely, and (3) irregular rhythms where cycle lengths are constantly changing (e.g., AF). Because the right bundle branch has a longer refractory period than the left, aberrant beats tend to be conducted most often with an RBBB pattern. Figures 12-99 and 12-100 illustrate these principles of refractory periods and cycle lengths.[55]

Electrocardiographic Criteria

P Waves. When trying to make the distinction between aberrancy and ventricular ectopy, a helpful first step is to search for P waves and note their relation to QRS complexes. Atrial activity (represented by a P wave) preceding a wide beat or a run of tachycardia strongly favors a supraventricular origin of that beat or tachycardia. Figure 12-101 illustrates an early ectopic P wave initiating three beats of a wide QRS rhythm that could easily be mistaken for PVCs.[55]

An exception to the preceding P wave rule is the case of end-diastolic PVCs that occur after the sinus P wave has occurred. Figure 12-102 shows sinus rhythm with an end-diastolic PVC occurring immediately after the sinus P wave. In this case, the P wave preceding the wide QRS is merely a coincidence and does not represent aberrant conduction; the PR interval is much too short to have conducted that beat. In addition, the P wave preceding the wide QRS is not early; it is the regularly scheduled sinus beat coming on time. Thus, early P waves that precede early wide QRS complexes are usually related to those QRS, whereas "on time" P waves in front of end-diastolic PVCs are not early and do not cause the wide QRS, although they may result in ventricular fusion beats.[55]

P waves seen during a wide complex tachycardia can be very helpful in making the differential diagnosis between SVT with aberration and VT. It is common for the SA node to continue to fire regularly and independent of the ventricular focus when VT occurs. The relationship between P waves and QRS complexes sometimes demonstrates AV dissociation, which means that the atria and ventricles are under the control of separate pacemakers (Fig. 12-103). Therefore, the presence of independent P waves in a wide QRS tachycardia indicates AV dissociation and is diagnostic of VT, whereas P waves seen before each QRS complex indicate a supraventricular origin of the rhythm. Figure 12-104 illustrates how P waves can be useful in differentiating two similar wide QRS tachycardias due to two different mechanisms.[55]

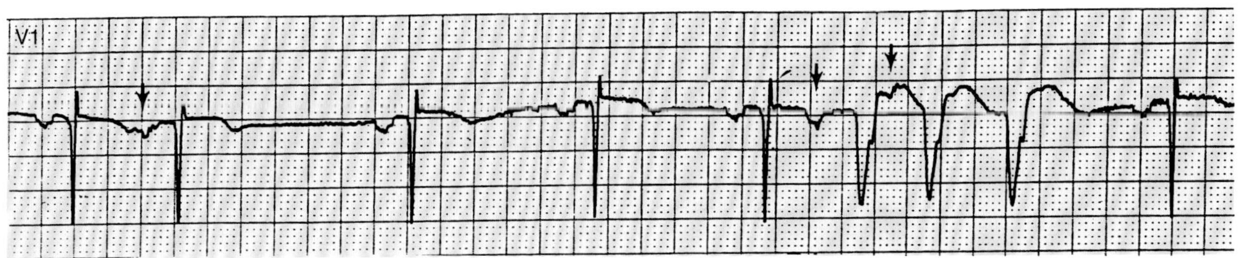

Figure 12-101. Sinus rhythm with PACs and three wide QRS beats that could be mistaken for VT. The second beat in the strip is a PAC that conducts normally. Note the P waves preceding the wide QRS complexes, indicating aberrant conduction (PACs with LBBB aberration).

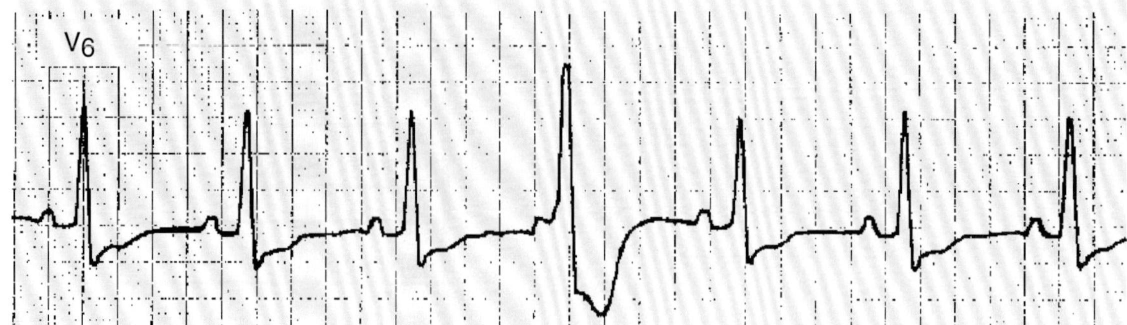

Figure 12-102. Sinus rhythm with one end-diastolic PVC. The P wave preceding the PVC is the sinus P wave that coincidentally occurred just before the PVC.

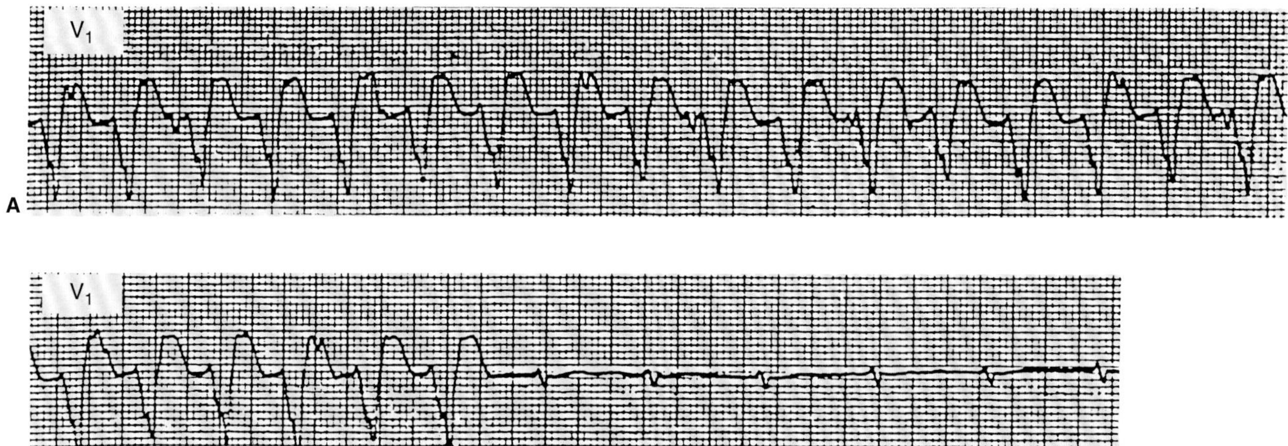

Figure 12-103. **A:** VT at a rate of 136 beats per minute. Independent P waves can be seen throughout the strip. **B:** Sudden termination of VT, revealing the underlying sinus rhythm at a rate of 94 beats per minute.

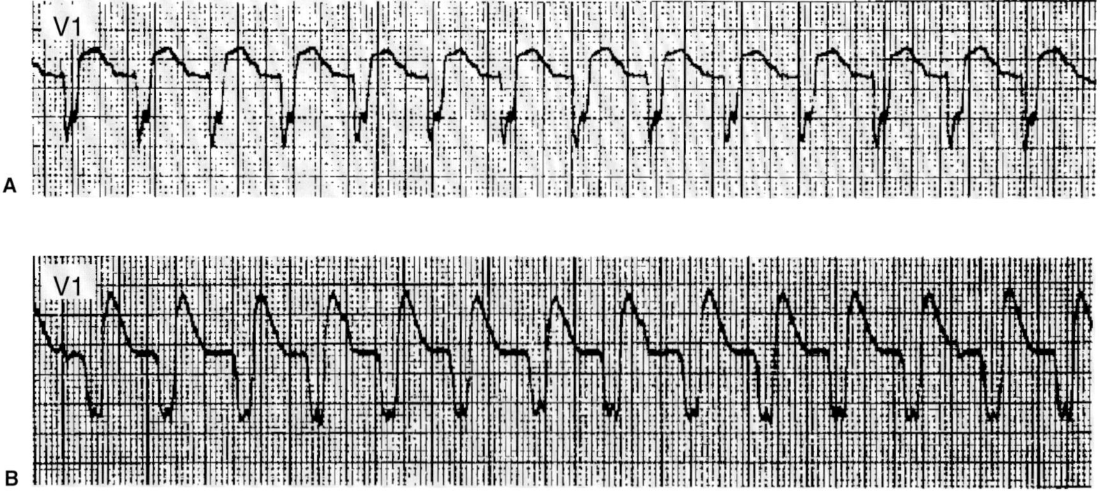

Figure 12-104. Two similar wide QRS tachycardias. **A:** Sinus tachycardia; rate—115 beats per minute. P waves can be seen preceding each QRS, indicating a supraventricular origin of the tachycardia. **B:** P waves are independent of QRS complexes, indicating AV dissociation that favors VT.

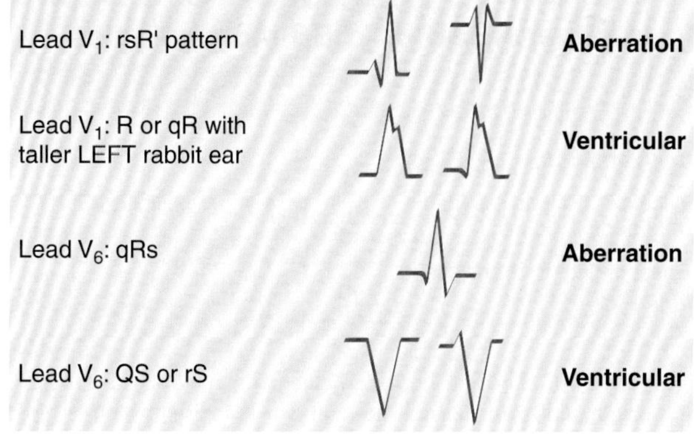

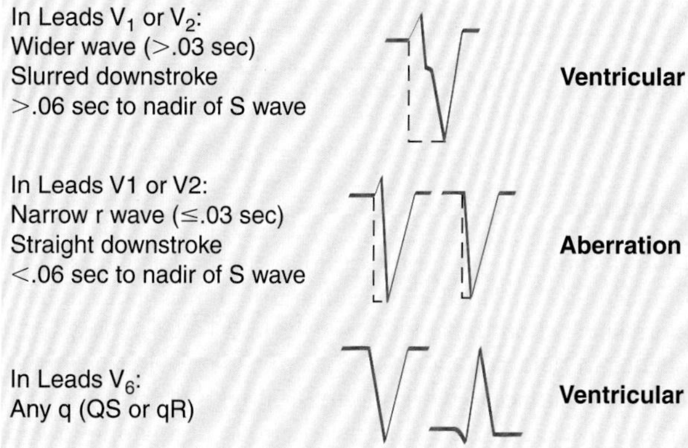

Figure 12-105. Morphology clues for wide QRS beats and rhythms with RBBB morphology and LBBB morphology.

QRS Morphology. The shape of the QRS complexes in a wide QRS tachycardia can be helpful in determining the mechanism of the arrhythmia. The following sections discuss the morphologic clues for wide complex tachycardias with RBBB and LBBB morphologies.[55]

RBBB Pattern (QRS Wide and Upright in V_1). Because the right bundle has a longer refractory period than the left, an impulse entering the conduction system early or at very rapid rates is more likely to encounter a still-refractory right bundle branch; therefore, most (80% to 85%) aberrantly conducted beats conduct with RBBB. However, approximately 60% of ventricular ectopic beats simulate an RBBB pattern.[111] During normal ventricular depolarization, the septum depolarizes from left to right and creates a small initial r wave in V_1 (see section *Intraventricular Conduction Abnormalities*). In the absence of septal infarction, the initial forces remain undisturbed during RBBB and beats that conduct with RBBB aberration have the same initial r wave in V_1 as during normal intraventricular conduction. Studies have shown that, of those beats presenting with an RBBB pattern in lead V_1, most aberrantly conducted supraventricular beats show a triphasic rSR' pattern, whereas almost all ectopic ventricular beats show a monophasic (R) or biphasic (qR) pattern in V_1.[111,112] Therefore, a wide QRS complex with a triphasic pattern of RBBB in lead V_1 strongly favors aberrancy, whereas a monophasic or biphasic complex of RBBB type favors ventricular ectopy.[55]

Other morphologic clues are presented in Figure 12-105. A monophasic or biphasic complex of RBBB type in lead V_1 with a taller left "rabbit ear" favors ectopy, whereas a taller right "rabbit ear" favors neither. Often V_6 is as helpful as V_1; a triphasic qRs complex in V_6 favors RBBB aberrancy, whereas a monophasic QS complex or a biphasic rS complex favors ventricular ectopy. Figure 12-106A shows VT with RBBB morphology.[55]

LBBB Pattern (QRS Negative in V_1). Leads V_1 or V_2 and V_6 also offer morphologic clues for tachycardias with LBBB

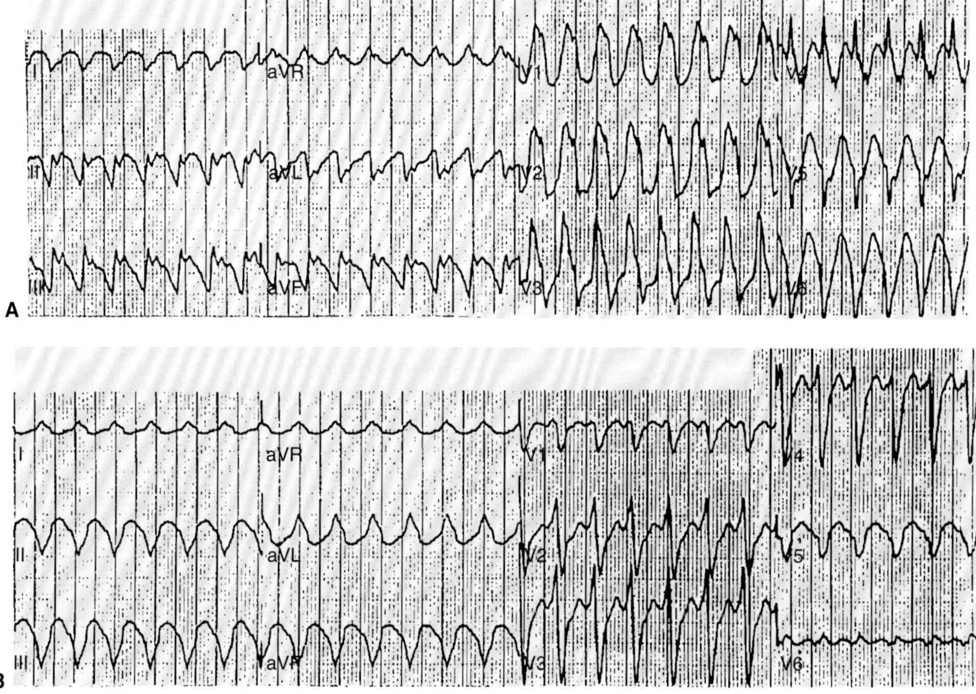

Figure 12-106. A: Twelve-lead ECG of VT with RBBB morphology. Note monophasic R wave with taller left rabbit ear in V_1 and QS complex in V_6. The indeterminate QRS axis also favors VT. **B:** Twelve-lead ECG of VT with LBBB morphology. Note wide R waves in V_1 and V_2, and qR pattern in V_6.

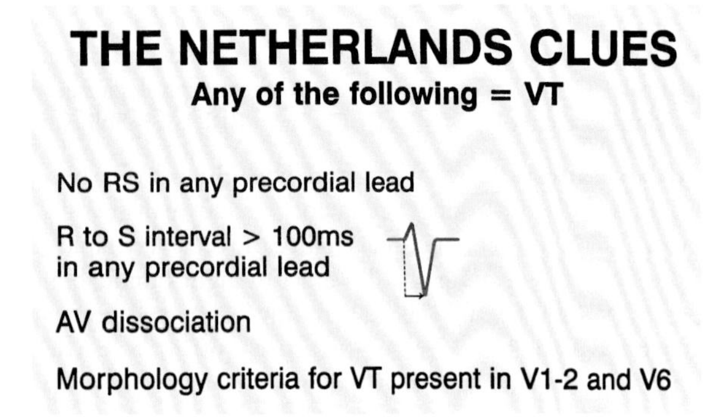

THE NETHERLANDS CLUES

Any of the following = VT

No RS in any precordial lead

R to S interval > 100ms in any precordial lead

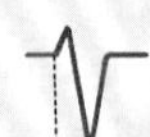

AV dissociation

Morphology criteria for VT present in V1-2 and V6

Figure 12-107. The Netherlands clues (so named because these clues originated in the Netherlands from research done by Brugada et al.[112]). In a wide QRS tachycardia, if no precordial lead displays an RS complex, or if any precordial lead displays an RS complex that measures greater than 100 milliseconds from onset to nadir, VT is the favored diagnosis. AV dissociation and the morphology clues favoring VT in V_{1-2} and V_6 are also helpful.

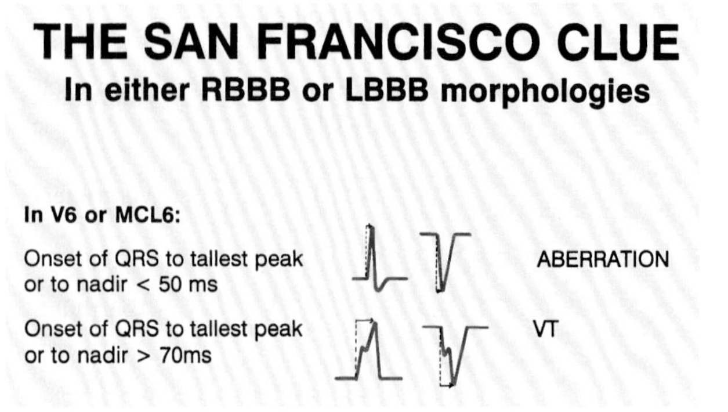

THE SAN FRANCISCO CLUE

In either RBBB or LBBB morphologies

In V6 or MCL6:

Onset of QRS to tallest peak or to nadir < 50 ms — ABERRATION

Onset of QRS to tallest peak or to nadir > 70ms — VT

Figure 12-108. The San Francisco clue (so named because these clues originated from research done in San Francisco by Drew and Scheinman). In wide QRS tachycardias of either right or LBBB morphology, if measurement from beginning of QRS to tallest peak or to nadir of S wave is less than 50 milliseconds in V_6 or MCL_6, aberration is favored. If the measurement is more than 70 milliseconds, VT is favored.

morphology.[103,113] Three characteristics of the QRS complex in V_1 or V_2 favor a ventricular origin: a wide initial R wave of greater than 0.03 second, slurring or notching on the downstroke of the S wave, and a delay of 0.06 second or more from the beginning of the QRS to the nadir (deepest part) of the S wave. In addition, any Q wave (qR or QS) in V_6 favors a ventricular origin. Figure 12-106B shows VT with LBBB morphology.[55]

Brugada et al.[104] suggest that additional morphologic clues in the precordial leads V_1 through V_6 can also be helpful. They suggest that a helpful first step in diagnosing a wide QRS rhythm is to scan the precordial leads to see if any lead shows an rS complex. If no precordial lead shows an rS pattern, VT is the likely diagnosis. If any precordial lead displays an rS pattern in which the measurement from onset of the R wave to nadir of the S wave exceeds 100 milliseconds (0.10 second), it favors the diagnosis of VT. They also emphasize that the presence of AV dissociation or any of the morphologic clues found in leads V_1, V_2, or V_6 discussed previously favor the diagnosis of VT (Fig. 12-107).

Lead V_6 or MCL_6 can be useful in differentiating supraventricular rhythms with aberrancy from ventricular ectopy.[105,106] In wide QRS rhythms of either RBBB or LBBB pattern, an interval of 50 milliseconds (0.05 second) or less from the onset of the QRS to the tallest peak of the R wave or nadir of the S wave favors a supraventricular origin, whereas an interval of 70 milliseconds (0.07 second) or more favors a ventricular origin (Fig. 12-108).

Summary

ECG is a clinical tool capturing cardiac electrical activities to provide diagnostic information on cardiac arrhythmias and conduction abnormalities. Both basic ECG and 12-lead ECG are easy to use, cost effective, and noninvasive. Because ECG uses electrodes placed on the body surface to detect electrical currents of the heart, incorrect lead placement (applying the electrode in a wrong location, connecting the cable to the wrong electrode, or both) can lead to inaccurate ECG waveform and potential misdiagnosis. It is important for clinicians to understand the fundamental electrophysiologic principles to recognize why ECG shapes go up and down. To further understand the underlying pathophysiology and alternations of clinical condition associated with ECG changes, and to provide differential diagnoses, it is crucial to compare current ECG with patient's baseline waveforms. The principles of ECG interpretation remain relatively constant. However, recommendations of arrhythmias management change as research evolves, technology improves, and new medications, procedures, and devices are developed. As a result, it is essential to follow the most current literature and resuscitation guideline.

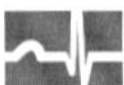

CASE STUDY

Patient Profile

Ms. Shah, a 45-yr-old female, came to the emergency room because she has been feeling palpitations for 2 days. This morning, Ms. Shah felt like her heart was beating even faster than before, and she almost "fainted" after taking a shower. Ms. Shah said that she had "fast and irregular" heart rhythm in the past, and "they had to shock me to get me to normal." Ms. Shah also said she was sent home with some medications to control her heart rate at the time, and she just came back from visiting family on the east coast and "will need to refill medications."

History

Atrial fibrillation (AF)

Allergies

Dilaudid

Social History

Alcohol use: two to three glasses of wine every wk
Smoking: 20 packs of cigarettes a week for 10 yr
Diet: no restriction, "trying to use less salt"
Exercise: a walk to the parking lot after work; that is about it
Occupation: cashier in a local grocery store

Current Medical Diagnoses

Hyperlipidemia
Hypertension

Current Home Medications

Lisinopril 10 mg tablet, one tablet by mouth daily
Simvastatin 40 mg tablet, one tablet by mouth at night
Metoprolol 25 mg tablet, twice daily
Multivitamin, one tablet by mouth daily

(continued)

CASE STUDY (*Continued*)

Physical Examination
Wt. 230 lb; Ht. 5'4"; BP 110/40 mm Hg; MAP 63 mm Hg; HR 140 bpm; Respiration 22 breaths/min; Temperature 37.6°C; O_2 Sat 92%; Heart sounds irregular

Admission Laboratory Data
Sodium 138 mmol/L; potassium 4.0 mmol/L; hemoglobin 15.5 g/dL; hematocrit 35%; chloride 105 mmol/L; BUN 25 mg/dL; Creatinine 1.3 mg/dL; WBC 10,000 mm^3

Diagnostics
12-lead ECG STAT (Fig. 12-109)

ECG Interpretation
AF with rapid ventricular response
Ventricular rate 142 bpm
Marked ST abnormality, possible inferior subendocardial injury

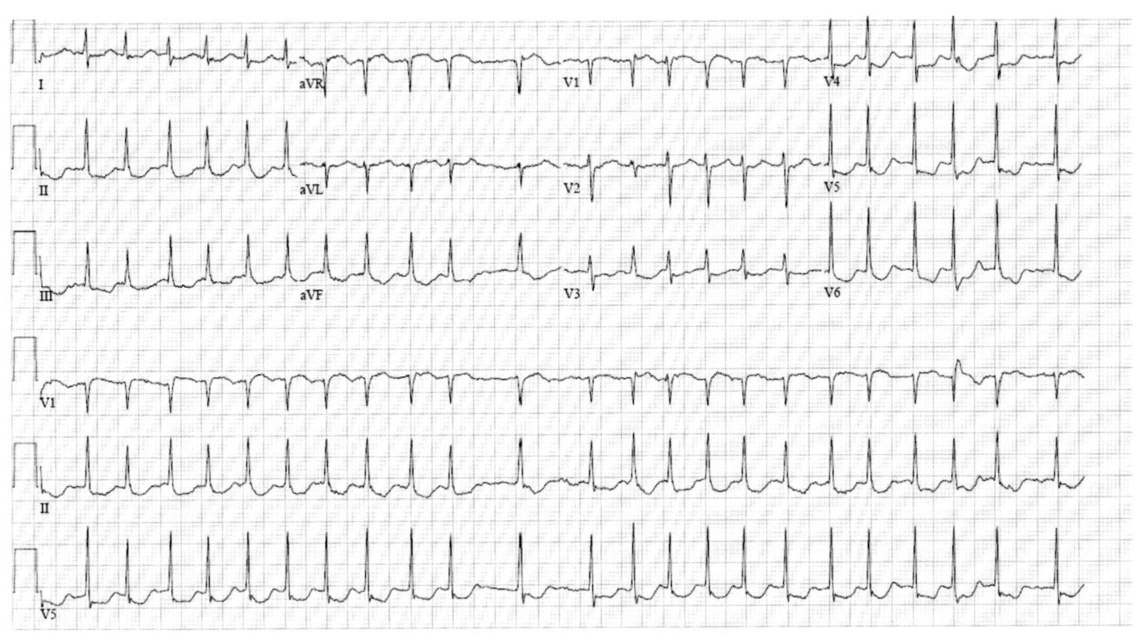

Figure 12-109. Atrial fibrillation with rapid ventricular response.

Treatment
Metoprolol 5 mg IV push over 2 to 3 min.
Upon administration of metoprolol, Ms. Shah heart rate decreased to 90 bpm. She was admitted to cardiology medicine unit for overnight observation. The plan of care was to resume her home medications and to discharge her in the morning if no recurrence of AF overnight.

Hospital Course
At 2300 in the evening, Ms. Shah's telemetry alarmed for high heart rate. The on-call resident was paged, and another 12-lead ECG was ordered (Fig. 12-110).

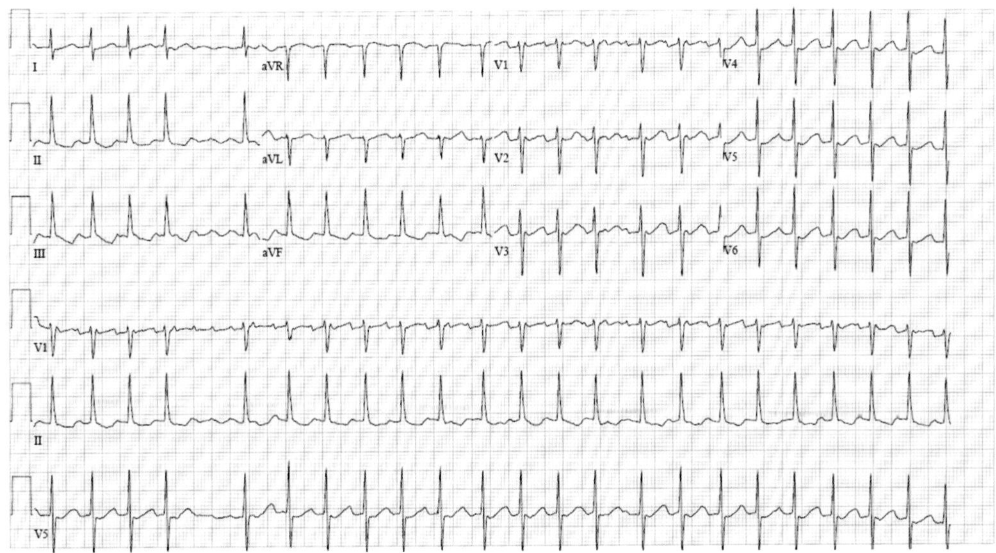

Figure 12-110. Atrial flutter.

(continued)

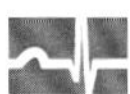

CASE STUDY (*Continued*)

ECG Interpretation

Atrial flutter with variable block
Ventricular rate 135 bpm
Compared to admission ECG
ST was no longer depressed in anterior leads.
T wave inversion was no longer evident in anterior-lateral leads.

Treatment

Metoprolol 5 mg IV push over 2 to 3 min.
Ms. Shah continued to respond favorably to metoprolol, and her heart rate decreased to 95 bpm.
At 0645 in the morning, Ms. Shah called the nurse to the bedside and complained about severe chest pain. Ms. Shah described that she felt so some heaviness on top of her chest and felt like having some horrible gas pain as well.
Resident was called to the bedside and another 12-lead ECG was performed (Figs. 12-111 and 12-112).

ECG Interpretation

Acute inferior MI with probable right ventricular involvement.
Large ST elevations in leads II, III, and aVF with reciprocal depression in I and aVL indicates the inferior MI.
Note minor ST elevation in V_1 with minor ST depression in V_2, raising suspicion about right ventricular involvement.
Cardiology was paged immediately. Rapid response team was called to assist the nurse.
A right-sided ECG was performed.

ECG Interpretation

Right-sided leads showed ST elevation in $V_4R–V_6R$, confirming RVMI.
Code STEMI was then activated. Ms. Shah was transported to cardiac cath lab for reperfusion therapy.

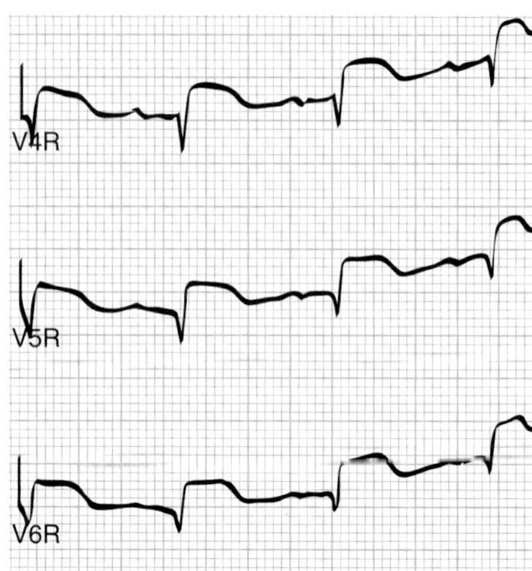

Figure 12-112. Right-sided leads from the patient in Figure 12-98 showing ST elevation in $V_4R–V_6R$, confirming RVMI.

Take Home Points

- Atrial flutter and AF may revert back and forth.
- When there is a suspicion of MI with right ventricular involvement, a right-sided ECG can be performed to confirm RVMI.
- Time is cardiac muscle. Follow STEMI guidelines to limit myocardial ischemia and infarct.
- Reperfusion including antiplatelet/anticoagulation therapy and early repercussion with percutaneous coronary intervention can prevent myocardial injury.

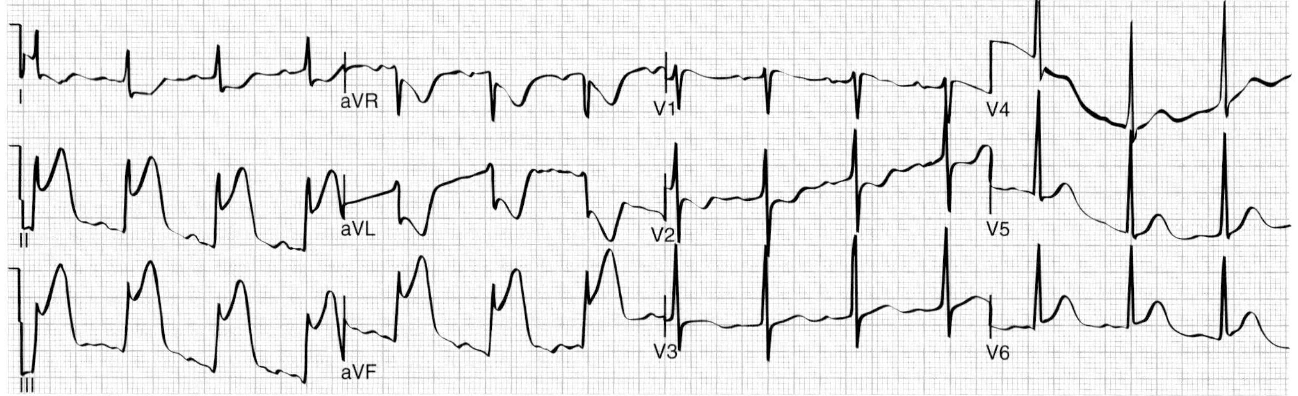

Figure 12-111. Acute inferior MI with probable right ventricular involvement. Large ST elevations in leads II, III, and aVF with reciprocal depression in I and aVL indicates the inferior MI. Note minor ST elevation in V_1 with minor ST depression in V_2, raising suspicion about right ventricular involvement.

KEY READINGS

Aehlert B. *ECGs Made Easy*. 6th ed. St. Louis, MO: Elsevier; 2017:336.
Fuster V, Harrington RA, Narula J, et al, eds. *Hurst's The Heart*. 14th ed. New York, NY: McGraw-Hill Education; 2017.
Issa ZF, Miller JM, Zipes DP. *Clinical Arrhythmology and Electrophysiology a Companion to Braunwald's Heart Disease*. 2nd ed. Elseiver/Saunders; 2012.
Kudenchuk PJ, Brown SP, Daya M, et al. Amiodarone, lidocaine, or placebo in out-of-hospital cardiac arrest. N Engl J Med. 2016;374(18):1711–1722.

REFERENCES

1. Khunti K. Accurate interpretation of the 12-lead ECG electrode placement: A systematic review. *Health Educ J*. 2014;73(5):610–623.
2. Amsterdam EA, Wenger NK, Brindis RG, et al. 2014 AHA/ACC guideline for the management of patients with non–ST-elevation acute coronary syndromes. *J Am Coll Cardiol*. 2014;64(24):e139–e228.
3. Mann DL, Zipes DP, Libby P, et al. Genesis of cardiac arrhythmias: electrophysiologic considerations. In: *Braunwald's Heart Disease E-Book:*

A Textbook of Cardiovascular Medicine. London, United States: Elsevier Health Sciences Division; 2014.
4. Hwang HJ, Ng FS, Efimov. Mechanism of atrioventricular nodal excitability and propagation. In: Zipes DP, Jalife J, eds. *Cardiac Electrophysiology: From Cell to Bedside*. 6th ed. Philadelphia, PA: Elsevier/Saunders; 2014.
5. Aehlert B. Basic electrophysiology. In: *ECGs Made Easy*. 6th ed. St. Louis, MO: Elsevier; 2017:336.
6. Thaler M. The basics. In: *The Only EKG Book You'll Ever Need*. 9th North American ed. Philadelphia, PA: LWW; 2018.
7. Jacobson C. Electrocardiography. In: Woods SL, Sivarajan Froelicher ES, Motzer SA, et al., eds. *Cardiac Nursing*. 6th ed. Philadelphia, PA: LWW; 2009.
8. Huff J. Waveforms, intervals, segments and complexes. In: *ECG Workout: Exercises in Arrhythmia Interpretation*. 7th ed. Philadelphia, PA: LWW; 2016.
9. Dubin D. Basic principles. In: *Rapid Interpretation of EKG's*. 6th ed. Tampa, FL: Dubin COVER Publishing Company; 2000.
10. Drugs That Prolong the QT Interval. Medscape. http://www.medscape.org/viewarticle/704202. Accessed August 23, 2018.
11. Goldberger AL, Goldberger ZD, Shvilkin A. ECG basics: Waves, intervals, segments. In: *Goldberger's Clinical Electrocardiography a Simplified Approach*. 8th ed. Philadelphia, PA: Elsevier/Saunders; 2013.
12. Wagner GS, Macfarlane P, Wellens H, et al. AHA/ACCF/HRS recommendations for the standardization and interpretation of the electrocardiogram: Part VI: Acute ischemia/infarction. *J Am Coll Cardiol*. 2009;53(11):1003–1011.
13. Klabunde RE. Electrical activity of the heart. In: *Cardiovascular Physiology Concepts*. 2nd ed. Philadelphia, PA: LWW; 2011.
14. Meek S, Morris F. Introduction. I—Leads, rate, rhythm, and cardiac axis. *BMJ*. 2002;324(7334):415–418.
15. DePace NL, Colby J, Hakki AH, et al. Poor R wave progression in the precordial leads: Clinical implications for the diagnosis of myocardial infarction. *J Am Coll Cardiol*. 1983;2(6):1073–1079.
16. Kurisu S, Iwasaki T, Watanabe N, et al. Poor R-wave progression and myocardial infarct size after anterior myocardial infarction in the coronary intervention era. *Int J Cardiol Heart Vasc*. 2015;7:106–109.
17. Zema MJ, Kligfield P. ECG poor R-wave progression: review and synthesis. *Arch Intern Med*. 1982;142(6):1145–1148.
18. Thaler M. Hypertrophy and enlargement of the heart. In: *The Only EKG Book You'll Ever Need*. 9th North American ed. Philadelphia, PA: LWW; 2018.
19. Knippa SM. *12 lead ECG: Tips and tricks for nurses who want to understand why the shapes go up and down*. Presented at the American Association of Critical-Care Nurses National Teaching Institute and Critical Care Exposition; May 23, 2018; Boston, MA.
20. Aehlert B. Introduction to the 12-lead ECG. In: *ECGs Made Easy*. 6th ed. New York, NY: Elsevier; 2017:336.
21. Thaler M. Conduction blocks. In: *The Only EKG Book You'll Ever Need*. Ninth, North American ed. Philadelphia, PA: LWW; 2018.
22. Goldberger AL, Goldberger ZD, Shvilkin A. Ventricular conduction disturbances: Bundle branch blocks and related abnormalities. In: *Goldberger's Clinical Electrocardiography a Simplified Approach*. 8th ed. Philadelphia, PA: Elsevier/Saunders; 2013.
23. Dubin D. Infarction. In: *Rapid Interpretation of EKG's*. 6th ed. Tampa, FL: Cover Pub Co; 2000.
24. Thaler M. The cells of the heart. In: *The Only EKG Book You'll Ever Need*. 9th North American ed. Philadelphia, PA: LWW; 2018.
25. Mottillo S, Filion KB, Genest J, et al. The metabolic syndrome and cardiovascular risk. *J Am Coll Cardiol*. 2010;56(14):1113–1132.
26. Birnbaum Y, Wilson JM, Fiol M, et al. ECG diagnosis and classification of acute coronary syndromes. *Ann Noninvasive Electrocardiol*. 2014;19(1):4–14.
27. Rhee JW, Sabatine MS, Lilly LS. Acute coronary syndromes. In: Lilly LS, ed. *Pathophysiology of Heart Disease: A Collaborative Project of Medical Students and Faculty*. 5th ed. Baltimore, MD: Wolters Kluwer/Lippincott Williams & Wilkins; 2011.
28. Makki N, Brennan TM, Girotra S. Acute coronary syndrome. *J Intensive Care Med*. 2015;30(4):186–200.
29. Jacobson C, Marzin K, Webner C. Coronary artery disease and acute coronary syndrome. In: *Cardiovascular Nursing Practice: A Comprehensive Resource Manual and Study Guide for Clinical Nurses*. 2nd ed. Burien, WA: Cardiovascular Nursing Education Associates; 2015.
30. O'Gara PT, Kushner FG, Ascheim DD, et al. 2013 ACCF/AHA guideline for the management of ST-elevation myocardial infarction. *J Am Coll Cardiol*. 2013;61(4):e78–e140.
31. Ibanez B, James S, Agewall S, et al. 2017 ESC Guidelines for the management of acute myocardial infarction in patients presenting with ST-segment elevation. *Eur Heart J*. 2018;39(2):119–177.
32. Shahoud JS, Tivakaran VS. Cardiac dominance. In: *StatPearls*. Treasure Island, FL: StatPearls Publishing; 2019. http://www.ncbi.nlm.nih.gov/books/NBK537207/. Accessed April 16, 2019.
33. Mrivis DM, Goldberger AL, Libby P, et al. Electrocardiography. In: *Braunwald's Heart Disease E-Book: A Textbook of Cardiovascular Medicine*. London, United States: Elsevier—Health Sciences Division; 2014.
34. Wagner GS. Myocardial infarction. In: *Marriott's Practical Electrocardiography*. 10th ed. Philadelphia, PA: Lippincott Williams & Wilkins; 2001.
35. Antman EM. ST-segment myocardial infarction: pathology, pathophysiology, and clinical features. In: *Braunwald's Heart Disease E-Book: A Textbook of Cardiovascular Medicine*. London, United States: Elsevier – Health Sciences Division; 2014.
36. Brady WJ. Acute posterior wall myocardial infarction: Electrocardiographic manifestations. *Am J Emerg Med*. 1998;16(4):409–413.
37. Ondrus T, Kanovsky J, Novotny T, et al. Right ventricular myocardial infarction: from pathophysiology to prognosis. *Exp Clin Cardiol*. 2013;18(1):27–30.
38. Andersen HR, Nielsen D, Lund O, et al. Prognostic significance of right ventricular infarction diagnosed by ST elevation in right chest leads V3R to V7R. *Int J Cardiol*. 1989;23(3):349–356.
39. Shiraki H, Yokozuka H, Negishi K, et al. Acute impact of right ventricular infarction on early hemodynamic course after inferior myocardial infarction. *Circ J*. 2010;74(1):148–155.
40. Somers MP, Brady WJ, Bateman DC, et al. Additional electrocardiographic leads in the ED chest pain patient: right ventricular and posterior leads. *Am J Emerg Med*. 2003;21(7):563–573.
41. Fijewski TR, Pollack ML, Chan TC, et al. Electrocardiographic manifestations: right ventricular infarction. *J Emerg Med*. 2002;22(2):189–194.
42. Chatterjee NA, Fifer MA. Heart failure. In: Lilly LS, ed. *Pathophysiology of Heart Disease: A Collaborative Project of Medical Students and Faculty*. 5th ed. Baltimore, MD: Wolters Kluwer/Lippincott Williams & Wilkins; 2011.
43. Pomedli SR, Lilly LS. The electrocardiogram. In: Lilly LS, ed. *Pathophysiology of Heart Disease: A Collaborative Project of Medical Students and Faculty*. 5th ed. Baltimore, MD: Wolters Kluwer/Lippincott Williams & Wilkins; 2011.
44. Kupchik N. Electrolyte emergencies. In: Good VS, Kirkwood PL, eds. *Advanced Critical Care Nursing*. 2nd ed. St. Louis, MO: Elsevier; 2017.
45. Agarwal A, Amsterdam EA. Too much of a good thing: Digitalis toxicity. *Am J Med*. 2015;128(3):257–259.
46. Ziff OJ, Kotecha D. Digoxin: the good and the bad. *Trends Cardiovasc Med*. 2016;26(7):585–595.
47. Nachimuthu S, Assar MD, Schussler JM. Drug-induced QT interval prolongation: mechanisms and clinical management. *Ther Adv Drug Saf*. 2012;3(5):241–253.
48. Yap YG, Camm AJ. Drug induced QT prolongation and Torsades de Pointes. *Heart*. 2003;89(11):1363–1372.
49. Tester DJ, Ackerman MJ. Genetics of long QT syndrome. *Methodist Debakey Cardiovasc J*. 2014;10(1):29–33.
50. Shen MJ, Zipes DP. Role of the autonomic nervous system in modulating cardiac arrhythmias. *Circ Res*. 2014;114(6):1004–1021.
51. Abriel H, Rougier JS, Jalife J. Ion channel macromolecular complexes in cardiomyocytes: Roles in sudden cardiac death. *Circ Res*. 2015;116(12):1971–1988.
52. Antzelevitch C, Yan GX. J wave syndromes. *Heart Rhythm*. 2010;7(4):549–558.
53. Rhee JW, Hu R, Stevenson WG, et al. Mechanisms of cardiac arrhythmias. In: Lilly LS, ed. *Pathophysiology of Heart Disease: A Collaborative Project of Medical Students and Faculty*. 5th ed. Baltimore, MD: Wolters Kluwer/Lippincott Williams & Wilkins; 2011.
54. Chen PS, Antzelevitch C. Mechanisms of cardiac arrhythmias and conduction. In: Fuster V, Harrington RA, Narula J, et al., eds. *Hurst's The Heart*. 14th ed. New York: McGraw-Hill Education; 2017.
55. Jacobson C. Arrhythmias and conduction disturbance. In: Woods SL, Sivarajan Froelicher ESSF, Motzer SA, et al, eds. *Cardiac Nursing*. 6th ed. Philadelphia, PA: LWW; 2009.
56. Issa ZF, Miller JM, Zipes DP. Electrophysiological mechanisms of cardiac arrhythmias. In: *Clinical Arrhythmology and Electrophysiology a Companion to Braunwald's Heart Disease*. 2nd ed. Philadelphia, PA: Elseiver/Saunders; 2012.

57. Issa ZF, Miller JM, Zipes DP. Intraventricular conduction abnormalities. In: *Clinical Arrhythmology and Electrophysiology a Companion to Braunwald's Heart Disease*. 2nd ed. Philadelphia, PA: Elseiver/Saunders; 2012.
58. Aehlert B. Sinus mechanisms. In: *ECGs Made Easy*. 6th ed. New York, NY: Elsevier; 2017:336.
59. Aehlert B. Atrial rhythms. In: *ECGs Made Easy*. 6th ed. New York, NY: Elsevier; 2017:336.
60. Page RL, Joglar JA, Caldwell MA, et al. 2015 ACC/AHA/HRS Guideline for the Management of Adult Patients With Supraventricular Tachycardia: Executive Summary: A Report of the American College of Cardiology/American Heart Association Task Force on Clinical Practice Guidelines and the Heart Rhythm Society [published correction appears in Circulation. 2016 Sep 13;134(11):e232–3]. *Circulation*. 2016;133(14):e471–e505.
61. Morady F, Zipes DP. Atrial fibrillation: Clinical features, mechanisms, and management. In: *Braunwald's Heart Disease E-Book: A Textbook of Cardiovascular Medicine*. London, United States: Elsevier – Health Sciences Division; 2014.
62. Holmes DR, Reddy VY, Turi ZG, et al. Percutaneous closure of the left atrial appendage versus warfarin therapy for prevention of stroke in patients with atrial fibrillation: a randomised non-inferiority trial. *Lancet*. 2009;374:534–542.
63. Alli O, Doshi S, Kar S, et al. Quality of life assessment in the randomized PROTECT AF (percutaneous closure of the left atrial appendage versus warfarin therapy for prevention of stroke in patients with atrial fibrillation) trial of patients at risk for stroke with nonvalvular atrial fibrillation. *J Am Coll Cardiol*. 2013;61(17):1790–1798.
64. January CT, Wann LS, Alpert JS, et al. 2014 AHA/ACC/HRS guideline for the management of patients with atrial fibrillation. *J Am Coll Cardiol*. 2014;64(21):e1–e76.
65. Fuster V, Rydén LE, Cannom DS, et al. 2011 ACCF/AHA/HRS focused updates incorporated into the ACC/AHA/ESC 2006 guidelines for the management of patients with atrial fibrillation. *J Am Coll Cardiol*. 2011;57(11):e101–e198.
66. Aehlert B. Junctional rhythm. In: *ECGs Made Easy*. 6th ed. New York, NY: Elsevier; 2017:336.
67. Aehlert B. Ventricular rhythms. In: *ECGs Made Easy*. 6th ed. New York, NY: Elsevier; 2017:336.
68. Al-Khatib SM, Stevenson WG, Ackerman MJ, et al. 2017 AHA/ACC/HRS guideline for management of patients with ventricular arrhythmias and the prevention of sudden cardiac death: a report of the American College of Cardiology/American Heart Association Task Force on Clinical Practice Guidelines and the Heart Rhythm Society. *Circulation*. 2018;138(13):e272–e391.
69. Reiter MJ, Reiffel JA. Importance of beta blockade in the therapy of serious ventricular arrhythmias. *Am J Cardiol*. 1998;82(4 Suppl 1):9I–19I.
70. Ellison KE, Hafley GE, Hickey K, et al. Effect of beta-blocking therapy on outcome in the Multicenter UnSustained Tachycardia Trial (MUSTT). *Circulation*. 2002;106(21):2694–2699.
71. Nademanee K, Taylor R, Bailey WE, et al. Treating electrical storm : sympathetic blockade versus advanced cardiac life support-guided therapy. *Circulation*. 2000;102(7):742–747.
72. Krittayaphong R, Bhuripanyo K, Punlee K, et al. Effect of atenolol on symptomatic ventricular arrhythmia without structural heart disease: A randomized placebo-controlled study. *Am Heart J*. 2002;144(6):1–5.
73. Hirsowitz G, Podrid PJ, Lampert S, et al. The role of beta blocking agents as adjunct therapy to membrane stabilizing drugs in malignant ventricular arrhythmia. *Am Heart J*. 1986;111(5):852–860.
74. Claro JC, Candia R, Rada G, et al. Amiodarone versus other pharmacological interventions for prevention of sudden cardiac death. *Cochrane Database Syst Rev*. 2015;(12):CD008093.
75. Kudenchuk PJ, Cobb LA, Copass MK, et al. Amiodarone for resuscitation after out-of-hospital cardiac arrest due to ventricular fibrillation. *N Engl J Med*. 1999;341(12):871–878.
76. Kudenchuk PJ, Brown SP, Daya M, et al. Amiodarone, lidocaine, or placebo in out-of-hospital cardiac arrest. *N Engl J Med*. 2016;374(18):1711–1722.
77. Dorian P, Cass D, Schwartz B, et al. Amiodarone as compared with lidocaine for shock-resistant ventricular fibrillation. *N Engl J Med*. 2002;346(12):884–890.
78. Levine JH, Massumi A, Scheinman MM, et al. Intravenous amiodarone for recurrent sustained hypotensive ventricular tachyarrhythmias. *J Am Coll Cardiol*. 1996;27(1):67–75.
79. Kühlkamp V, Mewis C, Mermi J, et al. Suppression of sustained ventricular tachyarrhythmias: a comparison of d,l-sotalol with no antiarrhythmic drug treatment. *J Am Coll Cardiol*. 1999;33(1):46–52.
80. Olgin JE, Zipes DP. Specific arrhythmias: diagnosis and treatment. In: Mann DL, Zipes DP, Libby P, et al., eds. *Braunwald's Heart Disease E-Book: A Textbook of Cardiovascular Medicine*. London, United States: Elsevier—Health Sciences Division; 2014.
81. Ventricular Fibrillation and Pulseless Ventricular Tachycardia | Learn & Master ACLS/PALS. https://acls-algorithms.com/vfpulseless-vt/. Accessed September 14, 2018.
82. ACLS Algorithm Asystole | Learn & Master ACLS/PALS. https://acls-algorithms.com/asystole/. Accessed September 14, 2018.
83. Aehlert B. Atrioventricular blocks. In: *ECGs Made Easy*. 6th ed. New York, NY: Elsevier; 2017:336.
84. Issa ZF, Miller JM, Zipes DP. Atrioventricular conduction abnormalities. In: *Clinical Arrhythmology and Electrophysiology a Companion to Braunwald's Heart Disease*. 2nd ed. Philadelphia, PA: Elseiver/Saunders; 2012.
85. Blank AC, Loh P, Vos MA. Atrioventricular block. In: Zipes DP, Jalife J, eds. *Cardiac Electrophysiology: From Cell to Bedside*. 6th ed. Philadelphia, PA: Elsevier/Saunders; 2014.
86. Thaler M. Preexcitation syndromes. In: *The Only EKG Book You'll Ever Need*. 9th North American ed. Philadelphia, PA: LWW; 2018.
87. Mani BC, Pavri BB. Dual atrioventricular nodal pathways physiology: a review of relevant anatomy, electrophysiology, and electrocardiographic manifestations. *Indian Pacing Electrophysiol J*. 2014;14(1):12–25.
88. Miller JM, Zipes DP. Therapy for cardiac arrhythmias. In: Mann DL, Zipes DP, Libby P, et al., eds. *Braunwald's Heart Disease E-Book: A Textbook of Cardiovascular Medicine*. London, United States: Elsevier—Health Sciences Division; 2014.
89. Camm AJ, Zareba W, Katritsis D. Nonsustained ventricular tachycardia. In: Saksena S, Camm AJ, eds. *Electrophysiological Disorders of the Heart*. St. Louis, MO: Elsevier; 2014.
90. Cecil RL, Goldman L, Schafer AI. Ventricular arrhythmias. In: *Goldman's Cecil Medicine*. 24th ed. Philadelphia, PA: Elsevier/Saunders; 2012:359–368.
91. Nogami A, Naito S, Tada H, et al. Demonstration of diastolic and presystolic Purkinje potentials as critical potentials in a macroreentry circuit of verapamil-sensitive idiopathic left ventricular tachycardia. *J Am Coll Cardiol*. 2000;36(3):811–823.
92. Okumura K, Matsuyama K, Miyagi H, et al. Entrainment of idiopathic ventricular tachycardia of left ventricular origin with evidence for reentry with an area of slow conduction and effect of verapamil. *Am J Cardiol*. 1988;62(10):727–732.
93. Okumura K, Yamabe H, Tsuchiya T, et al. Characteristics of slow conduction zone demonstrated during entrainment of idiopathic ventricular tachycardia of left ventricular origin. *Am J Cardiol*. 1996;77(5):379–383.
94. Andrade FR, Eslami M, Elias J, et al. Diagnostic clues from the surfacee ECG to identify idiopathic (fascicular) ventricular tachycardia: correlation with electrophysiologic findings. *J Cardiovasc Electrophysiol*. 1996;7(1):2–8.
95. Bradfield JS, Boyle NG, Shivkumar K. Ventricular arrhythmias. In: Fuster V, Harrington RA, Narula J, et al., eds. *Hurst's The Heart*. 14th ed. New York: McGraw-Hill Education; 2017.
96. Hoffmayer KS, Gerstenfeld EP. Diagnosis and management of idiopathic ventricular tachycardia. *Curr Probl Cardiol*. 2013;38(4):131–158.
97. Gill JS, Mehta D, Ward DE, et al. Efficacy of flecainide, sotalol, and verapamil in the treatment of right ventricular tachycardia in patients without overt cardiac abnormality. *Br Heart J*. 1992;68(4):392–397.
98. Priori SG, Napolitano C. Genetics of channelopathies and clinical implications. In: Fuster V, Harrington RA, Narula J, et al., eds. *Hurst's The Heart*. 14th ed. New York: McGraw-Hill Education; 2017.
99. Cerrone M, Napolitano C, Priori SG. Genetic diseases. In: Saksena S, Camm AJ, eds. *Electrophysiological Disorders of the Heart*. St. Louis, MO: Elsevier; 2014.
100. Roston TM, Vinocur JM, Maginot KR, et al. Catecholaminergic polymorphic ventricular tachycardia in children: an analysis of therapeutic strategies and outcomes from an international multicenter registry. *Circ Arrhythm Electrophysiol*. 2015;8(3):633–642.
101. Priori SG, Napolitano C, Memmi M, et al. Clinical and molecular characterization of patients with catecholaminergic polymorphic ventricular tachycardia. *Circulation*. 2002;106(1):69–74.
102. Deo M, Ruan Y, Pandit SV, et al. KCNJ2 mutation in short QT syndrome 3 results in atrial fibrillation and ventricular proarrhythmia. *Proc Natl Acad Sci U S A*. 2013;110(11):4291–4296.
103. Miller JM, Das MK. Differential diagnosis of narrow and wide complex tachycardias. In: Zipes DP, Jalife J, eds. *Cardiac Electrophysiology: From Cell to Bedside*. 6th ed. Philadelphia, PA: Elsevier/Saunders; 2014.

104. Brugada P, Brugada J, Mont L, et al. A new approach to the differential diagnosis of a regular tachycardia with a wide QRS complex. *Circulation.* 1991;83(5):1649–1659.
105. Drew BJ, Scheinman MM. Value of electrocardiographic leads MCL1, MCL6and other selected leads in the diagnosis of wide QRS complex tachycardia. *J Am Col Cardiol.* 1991;18(4):1025–1033.
106. Drew BJ, Scheinman MM, Dracup K. MCL1 and MCL6 compared to V1 and V6 in distinguishing aberrant supraventricular from ventricular ectopic beats. *Pacing Clin Electrophysiol.* 1991;14(9):1375–1383.
107. Brugada R, Campuzano O, Sarquella-Brugada G, et al. Brugada syndrome. *Methodist Debakey Cardiovasc J.* 2014;10(1):25–28.
108. Sheikh AS, Ranjan K. Brugada syndrome: a review of the literature. *Clin Med.* 2014;14(5):482–489.
109. Canty JMJ. Coronary blood flow and myocardial ischemia. In: *Braunwald's Heart Disease E-Book: A Textbook of Cardiovascular Medicine.* London, United States: Elsevier—Health Sciences Division; 2014.
110. Vereckei A. Current algorithms for the diagnosis of wide QRS complex tachycardias. *Curr Cardiol Rev.* 2014;10(3):262–276.
111. Marriott HJL, Sandler IA. Criteria, old and new, for differentiating between ectopic ventricular beats and aberrant ventricular conduction in the presence of atrial fibrillation. *Prog Cardiovasc Dis.* 1966;9(1):18–28.
112. Wylie JV, Garlitski AC. Brugada syndrome: Clinical presentation, diagnosis, and evaluation. UpToDate. https://www-uptodate-com. Published 2018. Accessed October 14, 2018.
113. Kindwall KE, Brown J, Josephson ME. Electrocardiographic criteria for ventricular tachycardia in wide complex left bundle branch block morphology tachycardias. *Am J Cardiol.* 1988;61(15):1279–1283.

13 Echocardiography

Russell Brandwein, Elizabeth M. Perpetua

OBJECTIVES

1. Understand the basic concepts of echocardiography.
2. Identify the nurse's role in patients undergoing echocardiography.
3. Learn the clinical applications of echocardiography.

KEY QUESTIONS

1. What are the indications for echocardiography?
2. What are the patient care considerations for transthoracic echocardiography (TTE), transesophageal echocardiography (TEE), and stress echocardiography?
3. How are echocardiography findings assimilated into nursing assessment and care planning?

BACKGROUND

Echocardiography (echo) is ultrasound technology as applied to imaging the heart and the associated great vessels.[1] As cardiac catheterization and invasive angiography transformed our understanding of the structure and function of the heart, echo allowed clinicians the same opportunities noninvasively. Clinical experience utilizing echo for patient care is vast and spans many decades. Echo is one of the most widely used imaging modalities today within cardiology because of the following attributes: safe, fast, lacks exposure to ionizing radiation, noninvasive, and portable.

In the United States, the acquisition of echo images is most commonly performed by sonographers (individuals who have completed specialized training programs in ultrasound), echocardiographers (cardiologists with training in echo), or cardiovascular anesthesiologists. As the field has expanded, other physicians including those who practice emergency medicine, primary care, or critical care have received training in image acquisition.

This chapter will focus on four general topics: (1) principles and techniques of echo, (2) echo examination, (3) echo applications, and (4) the nurse's role in echo.

PRINCIPLES AND TECHNIQUES OF ECHO

Sound Waves

Ultrasound is sound with a frequency above 20,000 Hz (cycles per second) or 20 kHz. This sound is outside of the range of the human ear. Diagnostic ultrasound for cardiovascular imaging uses frequencies ranging from 2 to 30 MHz: adult transthoracic frequencies range from 2 to 4 MHz, transesophageal frequencies from 5 to 7 MHz, and intravascular ultrasound frequencies (coronary artery) from 20 to 30 MHz.

Sound waves are generated at the transducer, the hand-held probe that is applied to the body part of interest. Today, transducers contain a piezoelectric crystal, which when applied to an electric current, will cause the crystal to deform. This deformation results in the generation of a sound wave, which is transmitted to the body. Returning sound waves can also deform the crystal and thus be detected by the transducer.[2] The transducer receives sound waves that are generated from the interaction of the transmitted sound waves and the tissues of the body. The transducer generates and receives reflected sound waves. Interestingly, the time the transducer is in receiver mode (i.e., listening mode) is far greater than when in transmitting mode (i.e., generating sound waves) with one exception—continuous wave Doppler, which will be explained further in a subsequent section.

Sound moves through media in the form of waves and may interact with the tissues in different ways. This chapter presents two of the more common interactions, reflection and attenuation. Reflection occurs when a transmitted sound wave interacts with tissues of different density within the body. For example, there is a different density of the blood than of the myocardium. The boundary between the two tissues causes reflection of the transmitted sound wave, which is then detected by the transducer. Depending upon the time it took for the transducer to emit the sound wave and detect the reflected sound wave, it will place that object at a certain distance (depth) on the image.[2]

Attenuation is degradation of the sound wave as it propagates from the transducer. Sound waves pass through tissues and attenuate with greater distances from the transducer. This attenuation results in a finite ability of the transducer to capture reflected sound waves from greater depths. The greater the distance the transducer is from the heart, the greater the number of sound waves that will be attenuated, and the result will be poor image quality. Examples of sound wave attenuation for echo caused by greater depth (distance) include obesity and breast tissue. But depth is not the only cause of sound wave attenuation in echo. Bone and air also result in considerable attenuation. Because the heart is surrounded by the sternum and ribs, imaging can be performed only in the rib spaces. In patients with smaller rib spaces, imaging can be particularly challenging. Because the heart is in close proximity to the lungs and trachea, these structures must also be avoided. In patients with enlarged lung spaces (i.e., chronic obstructive pulmonary disease), imaging can be difficult. Pneumomediastinum, pneumothorax, and subcutaneous air will all result in signal attenuation.

A clinical pearl for the cardiac nurse is to recognize that challenges in echo image acquisition may be described as "poor echo windows," or "technically challenging study." To summarize, challenges to obtaining quality images include limited acoustic windows due to extremes in body habitus (e.g., obesity or cachexia), depth and location of the cardiac structure in relation to the ultrasound probe (e.g., left atrial appendage is deeper in the chest and cannot be visualized by TTE), and the size/position of anatomical structures (e.g., lung tissue in a patient with chronic obstructive pulmonary disease) that prevent the reflective transmission of ultrasound waves necessary to perform an echo.

Experienced echocardiographers and sonographers should possess a thorough understanding of the impact of image artifacts. Inability to recognize artifacts could lead to false interpretation, some with significant consequences. Ultrasound can cause several different types of artifacts and an explanation of each is beyond the scope of this chapter. To reduce misdiagnosing artifacts, abnormalities should be visualized in more than one imaging window, thus reducing the likelihood of false interpretation.

M-Mode

M-mode (motion) echo displays a narrow ultrasound beam of information within the heart along the *y*-axis (vertical axis) and displays it according to time on the *x*-axis (horizontal axis). Heart structures are displayed with respect to motion and time. M-mode echo provides high temporal resolution and provides information regarding both the structure and function of the heart. M-mode echo predated the existence of two-dimensional (2D) echo and although it is not as commonly used as in the past, M-mode can still be useful to describe motion of structures of the heart with respect to the cardiac cycle (Fig. 13-1).

2D

2D echo was developed from similar concepts of M-mode. Because M-mode only allowed a very narrow and focused area of interrogation of the heart, it was limited. 2D echo provided a wider area investigation into the structure and function of the heart within a 90-degree scanning sector.[1] Thus, 2D echo provides a more complete investigation of the entire structure and function of the heart (Figs. 13-2 to 13-6).

Doppler

Doppler affords clinicians a powerful and integral tool for assessing heart function. This is based on the Doppler principle, first described by Christian Johann Doppler in the 19th century. It describes the change in reflected sound wave frequency compared with the transmitted sound wave frequencies generated from the transducer. These sound waves are reflected off of moving red blood cells. This change in frequency (transmitted to reflected sound waves) is related to the velocity of moving red blood cells

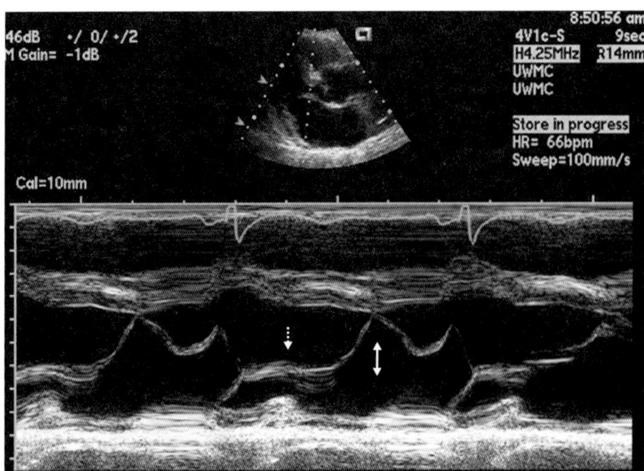

Figure 13-1. Example of 2D guide M-mode. At the center, top of the image, there is a 2D image of the heart in still frame. The *dashed line* going through the center of the 2D image represents the narrow beam of ultrasound. Motion of the heart structures as they move through this beam is displayed in the bottom of the image. The *x*-axis represents time, which is associated with the ECG tracing. The *y*-axis represents motion of the structures with respect to time. The specific structure of most interest in this image is the motion of the mitral leaflets during the cardiac cycle. The *arrowhead* represents the two mitral leaflets in the closed position as is appropriate in systole. The *double-headed arrow* represents the separation of the two leaflets in diastole. Notice how there are two distinct waves for mitral valve opening. The first wave is the E wave, which represents early passive filling of the left ventricle. The second wave is the "A" wave, which represents atrial contraction. (Echo courtesy of University of Washington Medical Center, Seattle, Washington.)

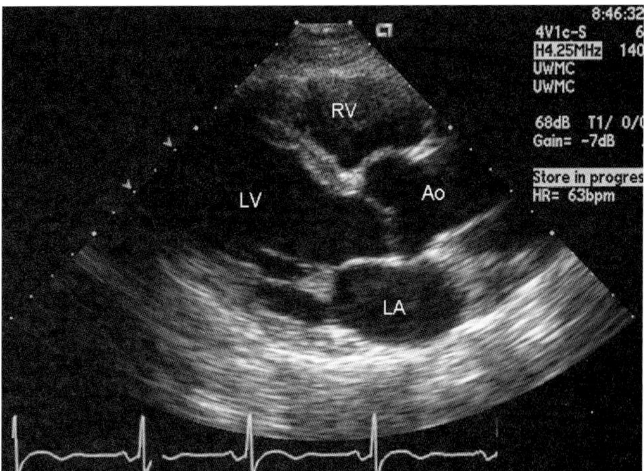

Figure 13-2. 2D image of the heart. The image is displayed so that the top of the image represents structures closest to the transducer (i.e., closest to the chest wall in this case) and the bottom of the image represents structures farthest away from the transducer. The image displays structures within a 90-degree scanning sector. This image nicely demonstrates that the right ventricle is an anterior structure. LV, left ventricle; RV, right ventricle; Ao, aorta; LA, left atrium. (Echo courtesy of University of Washington Medical Center, Seattle, Washington.)

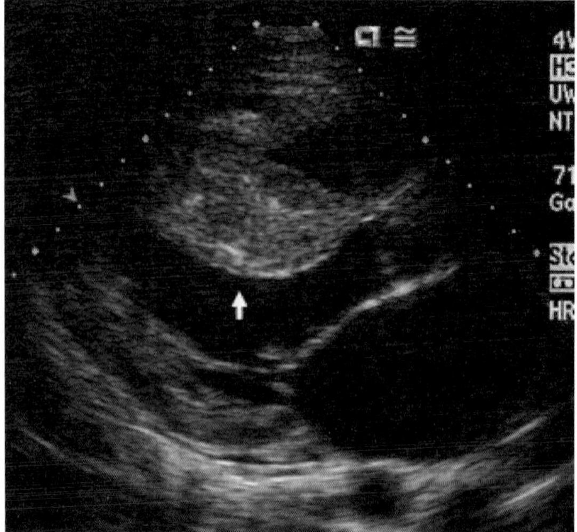

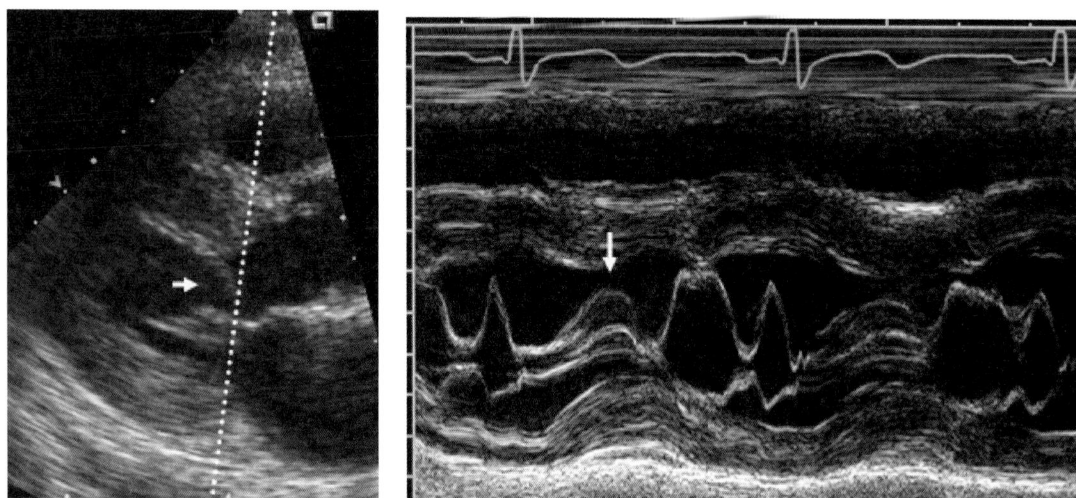

Figure 13-3. **Top:** 2D image in a patient with hypertrophic cardiomyopathy showing significant asymmetric hypertrophy of the anterior septum (*arrow*). Evidence of systolic anterior motion of the mitral valve apparatus (*arrow*) with 2D echo (**bottom, left**). In this same 2D image, the *dashed line* represents the area of the narrow beam of ultrasound with M-mode echo and that information is displayed in the next image (**bottom, right**) with time (cardiac cycle) on the *x*-axis and motion on the *y*-axis. The *arrow* represents systolic anterior motion of the mitral valve apparatus resulting in obstruction of blood flow in the left ventricular outflow tract. (Echo courtesy of University of Washington Medical Center, Seattle, Washington.)

through the heart, which can be used to describe the hemodynamics of blood flow through the heart.

One important feature of Doppler interrogation is the angle of the transmitted frequency as compared to blood flow. To achieve the most accurate estimate of the velocity of blood flow, the angle of interrogation (angle of the transmitted sound wave) should be parallel to blood flow. As the angle increases, so does the error, which results in underestimation (never overestimation) of blood flow velocity.

A clinical pearl to assist the cardiac nurse in conceptualizing this feature of Doppler interrogation is to understand how it works in the evaluation of a prevalent diagnosis such as aortic stenosis (AS). Recall that the severity of AS is evaluated by the peak velocity of blood through the aortic valve. The severity of AS based on the peak velocity can never be overestimated (i.e., a higher peak velocity than the true peak velocity). However, AS severity can be underestimated (i.e., a lower peak velocity than the true peak velocity) if the transducer is off-axis. When AS is truly severe but underestimated due to the transducer being off-axis, the patient may be misdiagnosed to have moderate AS, which may result in delayed and/or inadequate treatment. The risk of underestimating AS severity is why great attention is paid to accurately obtaining the peak velocity. The echosonographer may spend a lot of time confirming that the transducer is not off-axis, which the echocardiologist (e.g., interpreting or "reading" cardiologist") will verify when officially reading the study.

Because air (lung) and bones (ribs and sternum) limit the number of imaging spaces that can be used to interrogate blood flow through the heart, Doppler interrogation should be performed from multiple locations to minimize this error. The highest velocity obtained should be interpreted then as the sound wave most parallel to blood flow.[1–3]

There are three types of Doppler techniques: pulsed wave, continuous wave, and color. Pulsed wave Doppler is used for the assessment of blood flow at specific locations and is useful for velocities less than 2 m/s (Fig. 13-7).

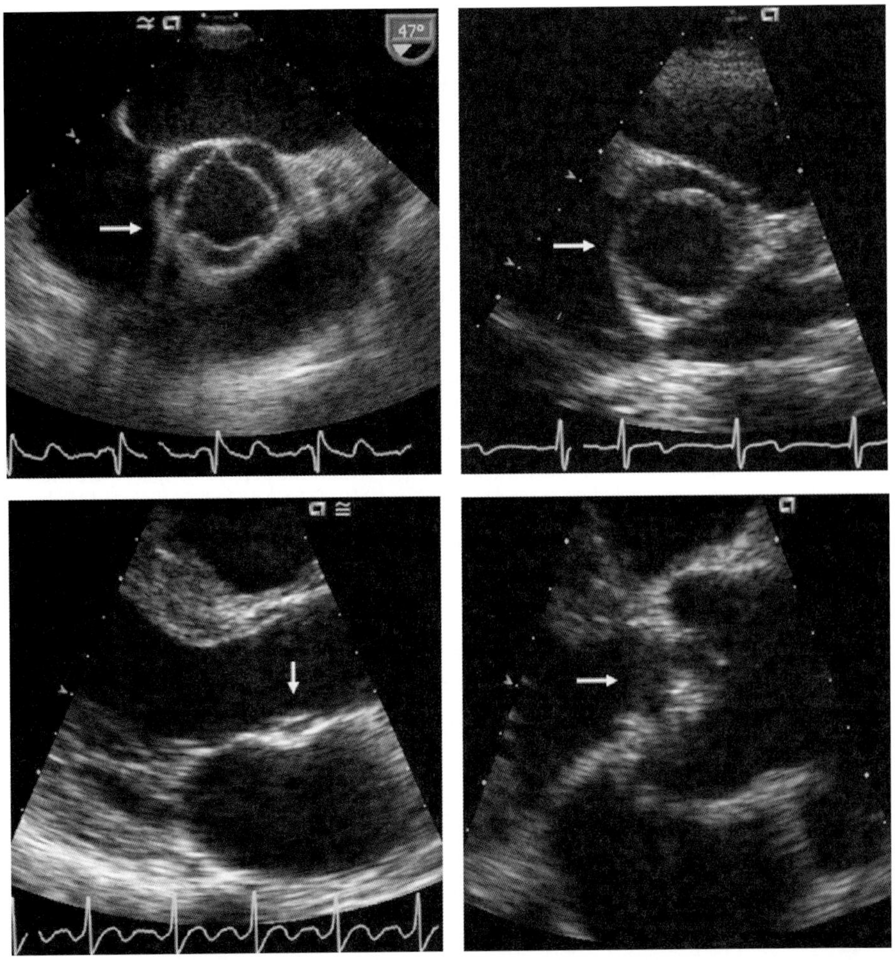

Figure 13-4. 2D images can also be used for imaging valve leaflets. **Top:** Systolic frame of a normal trileaflet aortic valve (**left**) and a bicuspid aortic valve (**right**). **Bottom:** Normal trileaflet aortic valve in systole with the leaflets fully opened (**left**); a comparison image of a patient with calcific aortic stenosis showing reduced aortic valve leaflet opening in systole (**right**). (Echo courtesy of University of Washington Medical Center, Seattle, Washington.)

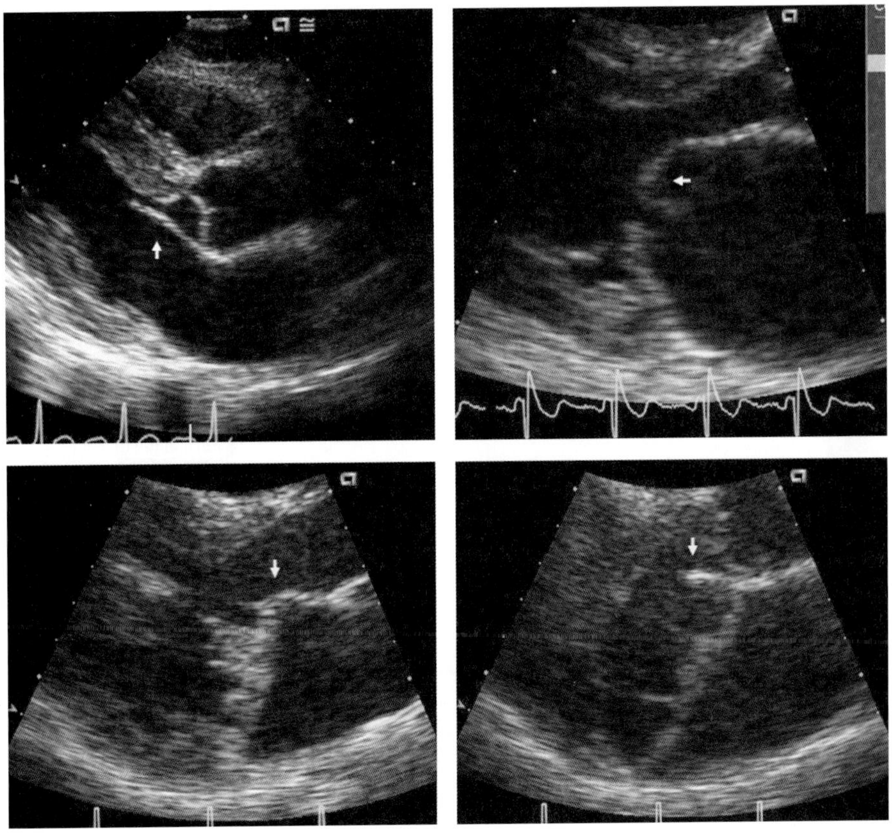

Figure 13-5. **Top:** Normal mitral valve in diastole with the leaflets fully open (**left**); a comparison image of a patient with rheumatic mitral stenosis demonstrates significant reduction in leaflet opening in diastole (**right**). **Bottom:** Myxomatous mitral valve disease. In early systole, the valve leaflets are thickened and redundant (**left**). In late systole, there is bileaflet mitral valve prolapse (**right**). The *arrow* marks the mitral valve annulus. Notice the difference of the leaflets to the annulus compared with early and late systole. (Echo courtesy of University of Washington Medical Center, Seattle, Washington.)

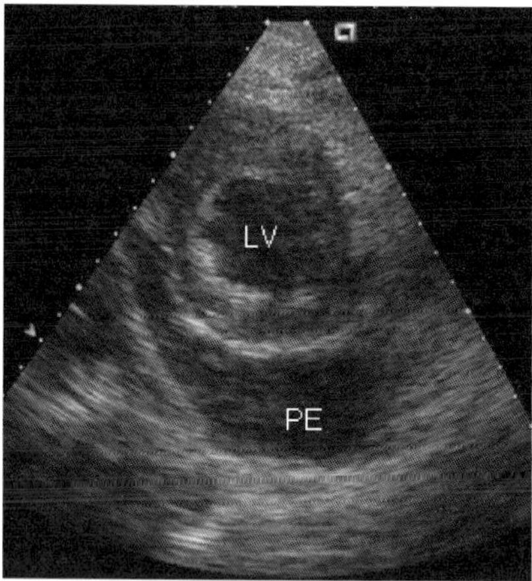

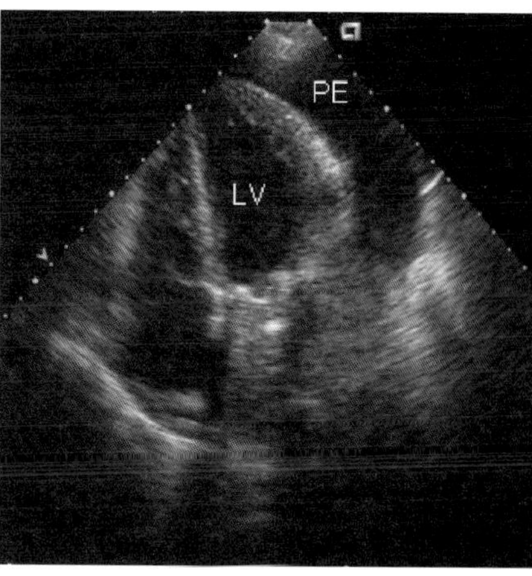

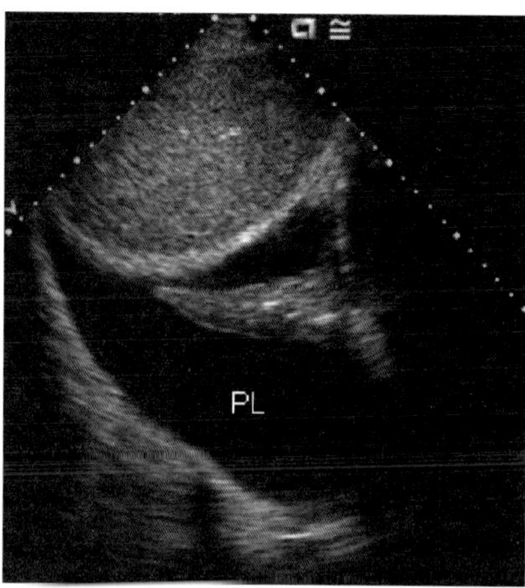

Figure 13-6. Echolucent (*black*) spaces within the pericardial space (**left** and **middle**) represent pericardial effusions. Echolucent spaces (**right**) outside of the pericardium but within the pleural space represent a right-sided pleural effusion. LV, left ventricle; PE, pericardial effusion; PL, pleural effusion. (Echo courtesy of University of Washington Medical Center, Seattle, Washington.)

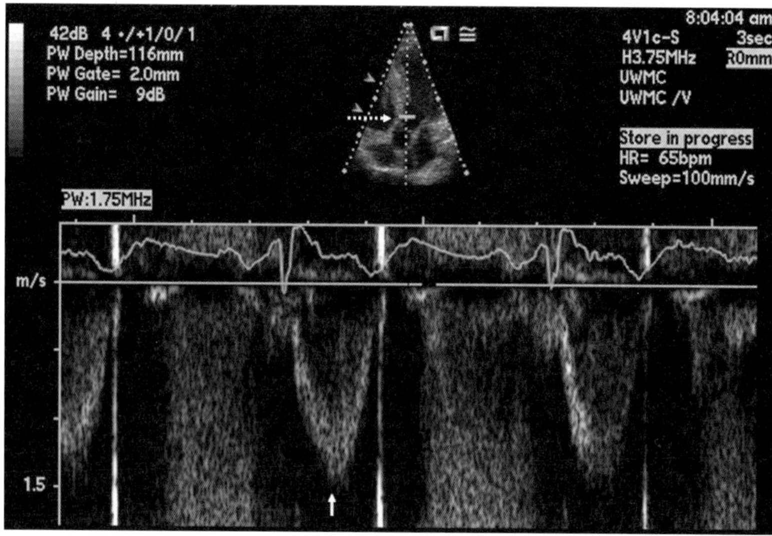

Figure 13-7. With pulsed wave Doppler, a 2D image (**top**) is used to localize the specific area (*dashed arrow*) of the heart in which velocity is measured. Time (cardiac cycle) is displayed on the *x*-axis and velocities on the *y*-axis (m/s). Systole and diastole can be distinguished based on the ECG signal. The *arrow* represents the peak velocity seen in the left ventricular outflow tract in this patient. (Echo courtesy of University of Washington Medical Center, Seattle, Washington.)

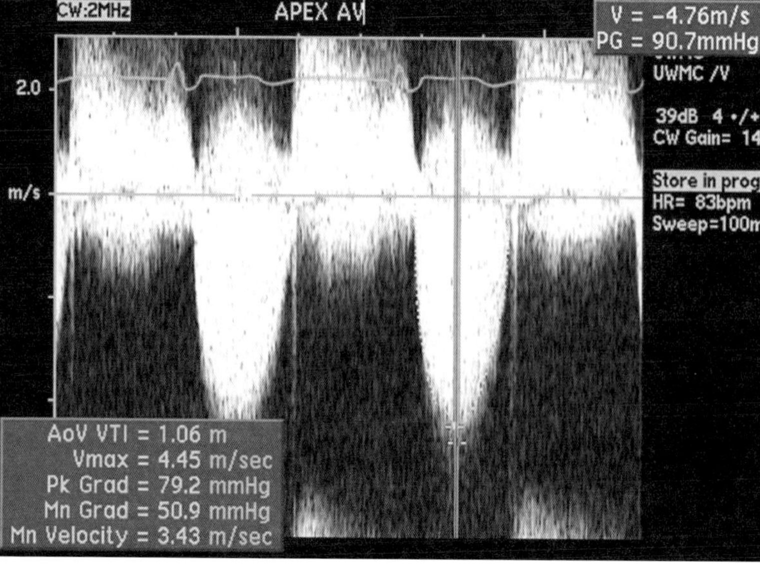

Figure 13-8. Continuous wave Doppler image acquired from the apical window in a patient with severe aortic stenosis. The white signal below the baseline (marked m/s) represents blood away from the transducer, which is located at the apex of the heart. The white signal during systole (see ECG tracing) represents the velocities of red blood cells along the entire wave pathway. In this example, the peak velocity is very high at 4.5 m/s, which translates into a peak gradient of 79 mm Hg. This is interpreted as the velocity of red blood cells which are crossing the aortic valve. By integrating the velocities under the entire spectral curve during systole, one can obtain the mean gradient, which in this case is 51 mm Hg. (Echo courtesy of University of Washington Medical Center, Seattle, Washington.)

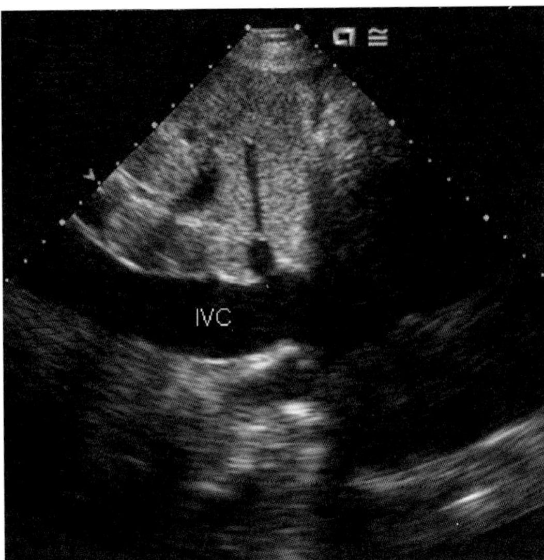

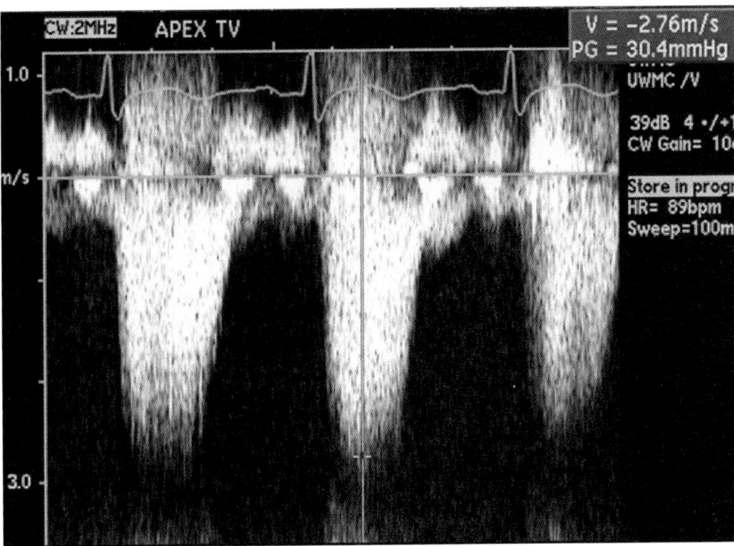

Figure 13-9. The right atrial pressures can be determined noninvasively by imaging the inferior vena cava (IVC) (**left**). The degree of dilatation and collapse of the IVC are used to determine the right atrial pressures. The right ventricular systolic pressures can be determined by the peak velocity of tricuspid valve regurgitation jet with continuous wave Doppler (**right**). In the absence of pulmonary stenosis, the addition of the right atrial pressures plus the right ventricular systolic pressure should equal the pulmonary artery systolic pressure. (Echo courtesy of University of Washington Medical Center, Seattle, Washington.)

Continuous wave Doppler is used for assessing velocities along the entire pathway of the sound wave and is used for velocities up to 8 m/s (Figs. 13-8 and 13-9). Continuous wave Doppler as its name suggests is continuously transmitting and receiving sound waves using separate crystals. This technique is unlike all other echo techniques, such as 2D echo, pulsed wave Doppler, and color Doppler, which all use the same crystal to transmit and receive sound waves and predominantly spend the majority of time receiving sound waves.

Color Doppler is a pulsed wave technique in which multiple points in a specified sector are sampled. Depending upon the direction and turbulence of blood flow, a color is encoded upon a 2D image (Fig. 13-10). This technique is useful for visualizing the presence of blood flow, the presence of turbulent blood flow, and shunts. A clinical pearl for the cardiac nurse is to remember that color Doppler is the assessment used for regurgitant valve lesions. Color Doppler waves are red when blood is flowing toward the transducer, and blue when blood is flowing away from the transducer.

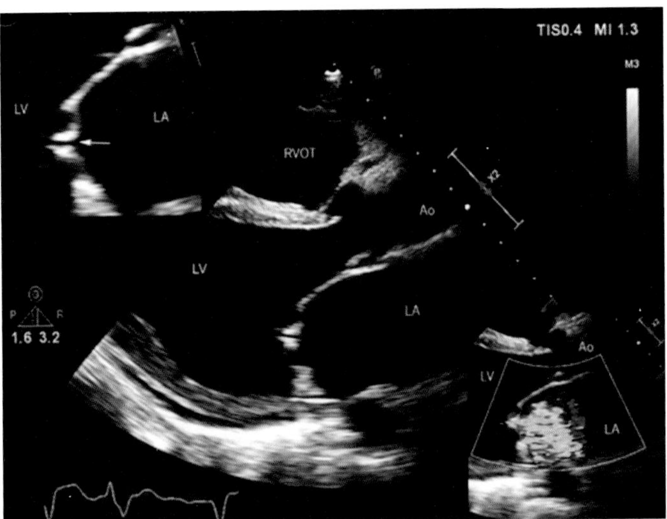

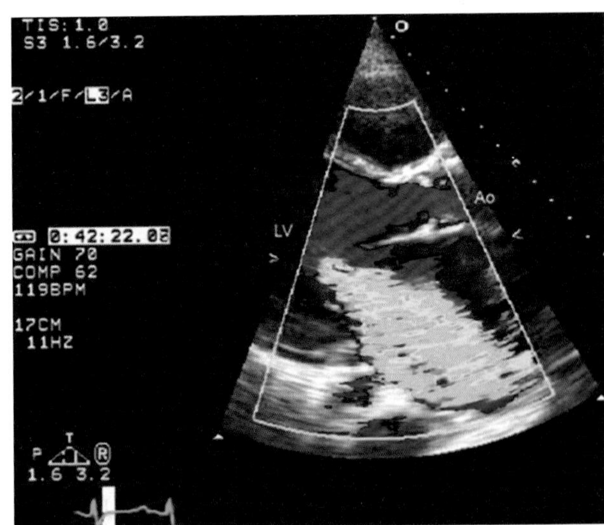

Figure 13-10. 2D image of an abnormal mitral valve. A chordae tendineae to the anterior mitral leaflet is no longer attached to the valve leaflet, which results in the anterior leaflet prolapsing into the left atrium in systole (**left**). The posterior and anterior leaflets do not completely oppose each other, which results in a regurgitant orifice area. Color Doppler superimposed on a 2D image (**right**) shows the regurgitation of blood flow through this area in systole. (Echo courtesy of University of Washington Medical Center, Seattle, Washington.)

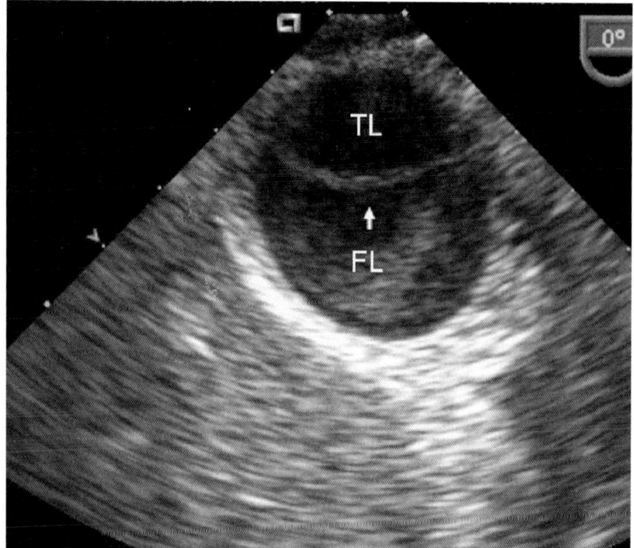

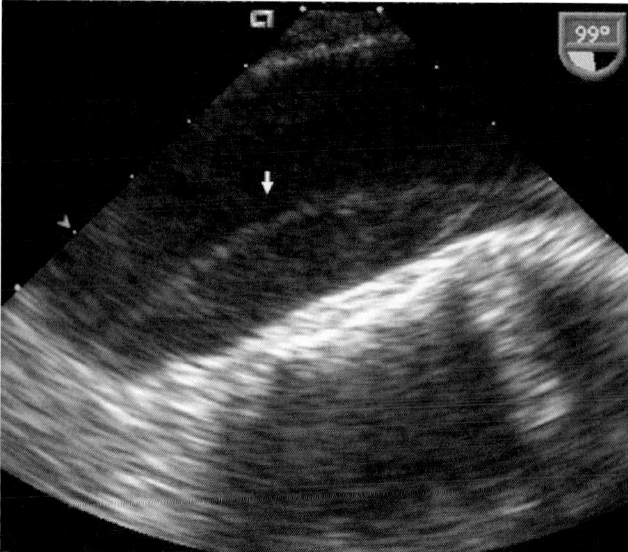

Figure 13-11. Transesophageal echo image of the descending thoracic aorta demonstrating a dissection flap (*arrow*), which creates a true lumen (TL) and false lumen (FL) in the short axis (**left**) and long axis (**right**). (Echo courtesy of University of Washington Medical Center, Seattle, Washington.)

3D

Three-dimensional (3D) echo displays a volume of data within three spatial orientations.[2] The first ever use of 3D echo was in 1974.[4] However, the equipment was not practical, and the images were not suitable for clinical use. Due to the poor image quality, time-consuming acquisition, and offline reconstruction, 3D echo use was once limited. The field has since evolved rapidly in response to the need for improved 3D imaging, especially with transesophageal echo (TEE), detailed in a subsequent section.

3D echocardiography has many applications and provides clinicians with critical information required to accurately diagnose heart disease. A few of these applications include left and right ventricle chamber quantification, now described in the current American Society of Echocardiography (ASE) chamber quantification guideline recommendations. In addition, 3D echocardiography is proven to be an essential tool to localize specific regurgitant valvular lesions. Furthermore, 3D for the guidance of catheter placement during interventional procedures such as balloon valvuloplasty, transcatheter aortic valve replacement (TAVR), and transcatheter mitral valve repair has increased significantly in recent years.[5] This demand has driven major advances in 3D imaging with TEE.[5]

Transesophageal Echo

TEE uses an imaging crystal placed on the end of a flexible probe that is inserted into the esophagus and stomach to image the heart. A clinical pearl for the cardiac nurse is to recall that the esophagus lies immediately posterior to the heart, thereby decreasing image attenuation and increasing image quality. Because the distance between the transducer and the heart is reduced, the spatial resolution of TEE is much improved for some (but not all) structures of the heart, resulting in superior image quality. Image quality with transthoracic echo (TTE) is not always of diagnostic quality and can be improved by TEE.[5,6] For certain clinical circumstances, TTE cannot provide the diagnostic accuracy needed and TEE is recommended. The specific clinical circumstances may suggest whether TEE is needed but some indications include aortic dissection, valvular endocarditis, prosthetic valve malfunction, left atrial appendage thrombus, interatrial septal defect, and patent foramen ovale (Figs 13-11 to 13-13).

The first ever 3D TEE was performed in 1992.[6] It was thought to allow a better understanding of spatial relationships of the cardiac structures and of the mitral valve.[7] However, the quality of the 3D images were dependent upon the 2D images, and minor patient movement (usually from ventilation) or cardiac movement (arrhythmias) resulted in artifact which rendered the 3D images useless.

One of the major challenges in ultrasound interpretation is the ability to mentally visualize a 3D structure based on 2D images. The complexity of the cardiac anatomy, along with the learning curve in interpreting cardiac ultrasound images created a desire to display "live" cardiac images.[8] The ability to perform real-time (RT) 3D TEE and "live" display the images have increased the use and ease of performing a 3D echo.[9]

Similar to the creation of a 2D image, a 3D ultrasound image of the heart involves a four-step process consisting of: data acquisition, data storage, data processing, and image display.

One of the major differences between 2D and 3D echo is how the images are acquired and displayed. While a full in-depth discussion about the physics of 3D TEE is beyond the scope of this text, a primer for 3D TEE imaging is provided in Figure 13-14.

ECHO EXAMINATION

Patient Preparation

Imaging is most ideally performed on special examination beds that allow for ideal placement of the imaging transducer. This simple feature improves the quality of the examination. In circumstances where the patient cannot be transported safely to the echo laboratory (i.e., ICU level of care, emergency), the ultrasound machine can be brought to the patient's bedside. The portability of echo is unique among cardiovascular imaging modalities.

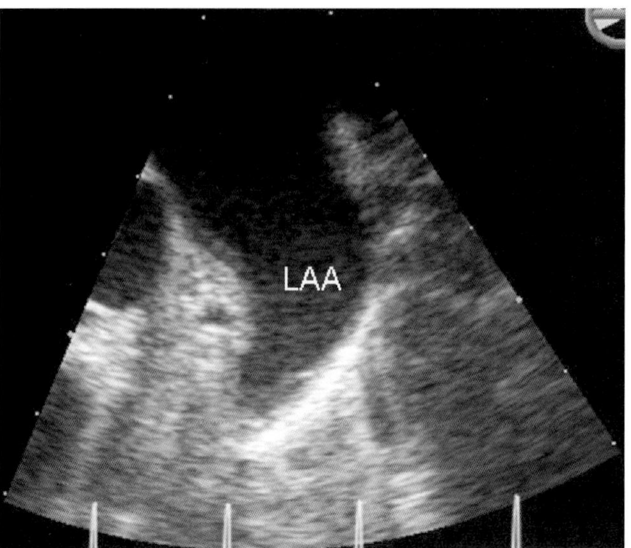

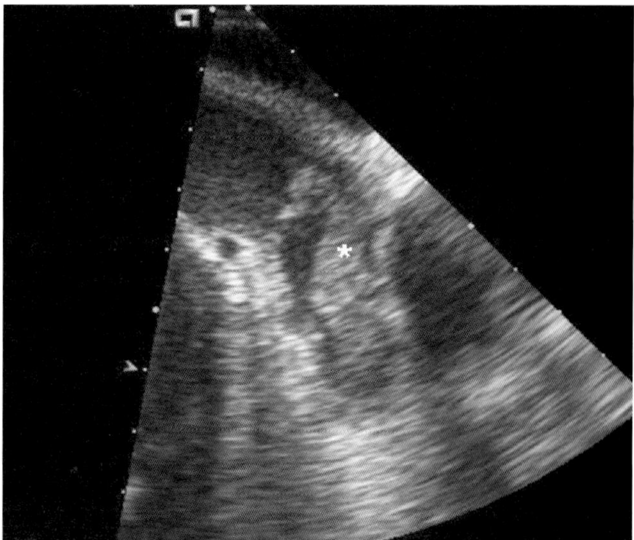

Figure 13-12. Left: A normal left atrial appendage (LAA) is a pouch-like structure arising from the left atrium. This LAA does not contain thrombus. Mitral stenosis and atrial fibrillation are risk factors for thrombus formation in the LAA. **Right:** Large thrombus (*asterisk*) within the LAA. This patient had atrial fibrillation. (Echo courtesy of University of Washington Medical Center, Seattle, Washington.)

Transthoracic Echo

TTE is performed by placing an ultrasound transducer on the patient's chest and images are obtained through the chest wall. The patient is positioned in the left lateral decubitus position for the first part of the examination and then is moved to the supine position to complete the image set. Occasionally, the patient is positioned in the right lateral decubitus position. Electrocardiogram (ECG) electrodes are placed on the patient's skin to acquire a continuous ECG rhythm. The timing of events to the cardiac cycle is important. The blood pressure and heart rate should always be recorded at the time of the examination as these measurements affect cardiovascular hemodynamics. A clinical pearl for the cardiac nurse is to recall that in the heart, an electrical event precedes a mechanical event; thus, a continuous ECG strip is recorded along with the echo images. The interpreting cardiologist uses the ECG strip to reference the cardiac rhythm (electrical activity) along with the echo images (mechanical activity) in the cardiac cycle.

The transducer is the part of the echo machine that is placed on the patient's skin to acquire images. Because ultrasound waves have significant attenuation through air, a coupling gel is used between the transducer and the patient's skin to eliminate any air.

Transesophageal Echo

TEE is usually performed by physicians (cardiologists or anesthesiologists) with the help of sonographers who aid in image acquisition. Depending upon the risk of conscious sedation, a nurse or anesthesiologist is also present to monitor the patient during the procedure.

A detailed patient history should be obtained as there are contraindications (absolute and relative) to TEE. Dysphagia,

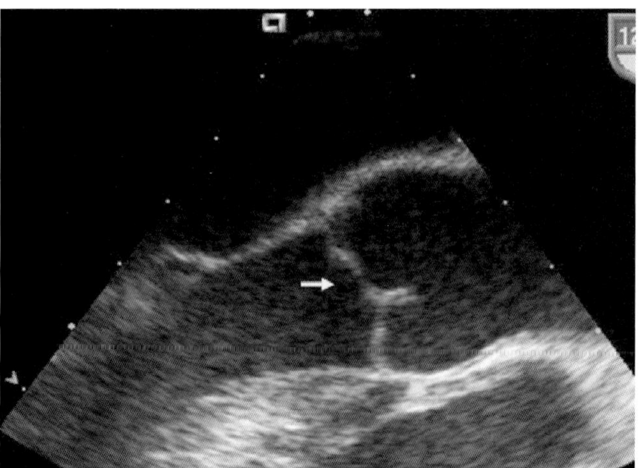

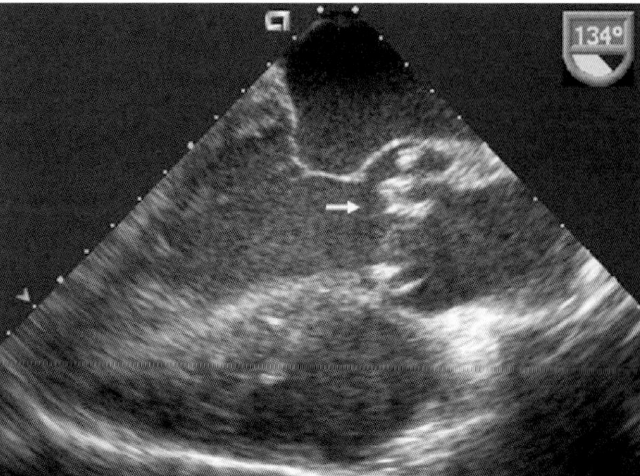

Figure 13-13. Left: Transesophageal echo image demonstrating normal aortic valve leaflets (*arrow*) in diastole. **Right:** Thickened aortic valve leaflets with masses attached, all consistent with infectious endocarditis. (Echo courtesy of University of Washington Medical Center, Seattle, Washington.)

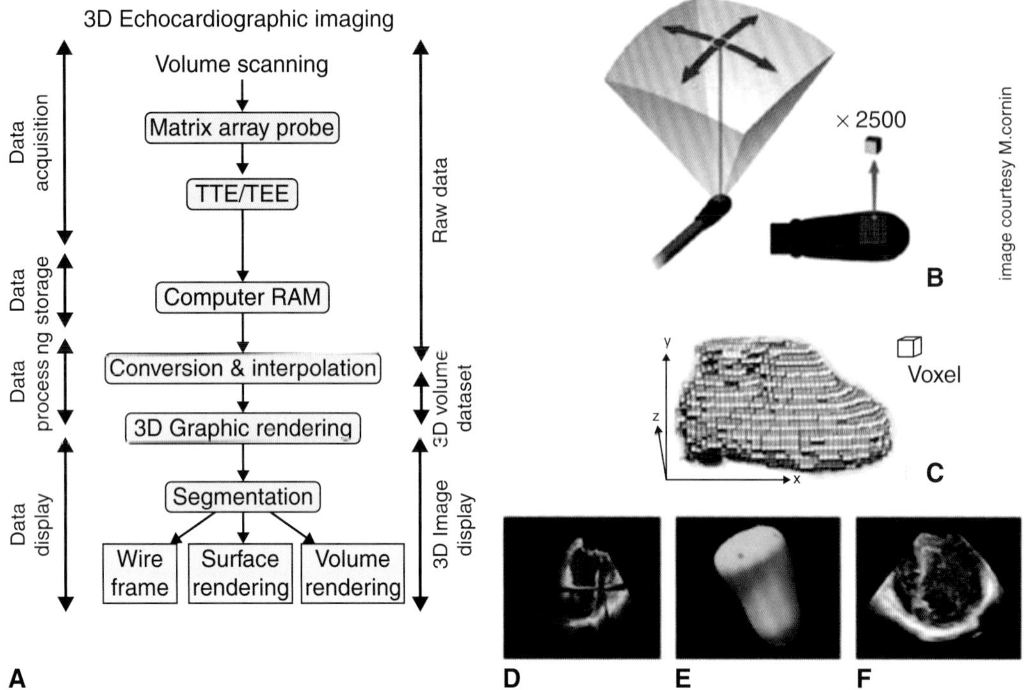

Figure 13-14. A: Algorithm of three-dimensional (3D) imaging. 3D echocardiographic imaging includes four stages for data handling: acquisition, storage, processing, and display. **B:** A matrix array transesophageal echocardiography probe is comprised 2500 piezoelectric crystals for which each can be independently activated to volume scan and acquire raw three-dimensional data. **C:** Data processing in two-dimensional (2D) scanning. After initial raw data acquisition, data processing is shown here using the linear 2D scanning technique. Interpolation fills the gaps (*gray cubes*) between known acquired data points in space to generate a 3D dataset. 3D datasets can be rendered and displayed as (**D**) wire frame, (**E**) surface, or (**F**) volume as shown here for the left ventricle. (Reprinted from Vargas A, Meineri M. Three-dimensional transesophageal echocardiography is a major advance for intraoperative clinical management of patients. *Anesth Analg.* 2010;110(6): 1548--1573.)

esophageal strictures or webs, esophageal or gastric cancer, upper gastrointestinal bleeding, cervical neck trauma, thrombocytopenia, or coagulopathy are some contraindications that may require consultations with a gastroenterologist first.

A clinical pearl for the cardiac nurse is to understand the rationale for this screening: the TEE ultrasound probe is passed from the oral cavity through the esophagus and to the stomach. Frequently, a patient with dysphagia who requires a TEE will undergo an esophogram (e.g., "Barium swallow test"). The esophogram provides images of the esophagus and confirms there are no strictures that would hinder the TEE probe. In more complex cases, or with prior esophageal injury or varices, an esophagoduodenoscopy (EGD) may need to be performed prior to proceeding with a TEE. Assessing for relative and absolute contraindications, and coordinating the necessary consultations or studies if indicated, serves to prevent complications and adverse events due to a TEE.

Anticoagulation (e.g., warfarin, direct oral anticoagulants, heparin) is not an absolute contraindication to TEE but the internationalized normalized ratio and partial thromboplastin time should be checked beforehand to ensure that supratherapeutic levels are not present. The patient should be fasting for 6 hours and the patient should remain fasting postprocedure until there is an appropriate level of consciousness and the local anesthetic of the posterior pharynx has dissipated.

For the procedure, the patient is positioned in the left lateral decubitus position to minimize the risk of aspiration. A topical anesthetic agent is used on the posterior pharynx to suppress the gag reflex, allowing easier passage of the probe into the esophagus. Typically, TEEs are performed under conscious sedation. Therefore, supervision by nurses with experience and training in sedative and analgesic administration, and in oral airway management is necessary. Conscious sedation requires that heart rate, blood pressure, respiration, and arterial oxygen saturation are monitored throughout the procedure. This monitoring is routinely performed by the nurse. However, clinical circumstances may exist where an anesthesiologist should be present during the procedure. An intravenous catheter is needed to administer analgesics and sedatives. Medicines to reverse analgesics (naloxone for opioids) and sedatives (flumazenil for benzodiazepines) should be readily available. Suctioning should always be available to manage excess oral secretions. Risks of TEE include, but are not limited to, aspiration, bronchospasm, respiratory depression, or hypotension from sedation, bleeding, and trauma to the teeth, esophagus, or stomach such as perforation.[2]

Axis of the Heart

The heart is situated obliquely in the chest with the apex toward the left. Imaging is not therefore performed in a straight axial or sagittal orientation. Instead, most of the cardiovascular imaging is performed along the axis of the heart and not the axis of the body. There are two standard axes of the heart: long and short. In the long axis views, the heart is imaged from the base to the apex. The short axis of the heart is perpendicular to this axis.

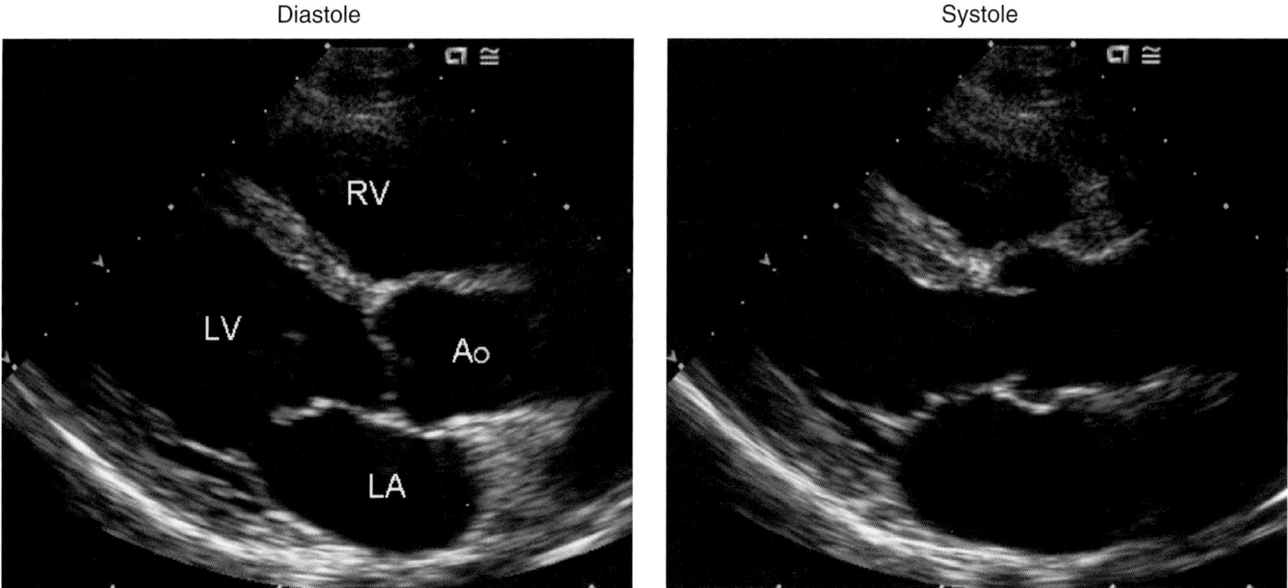

Figure 13-15. 2D images in the parasternal long axis in diastole and systole in a patient with normal ventricular function. LV, left ventricle; RV, right ventricle; LA, left atrium; Ao, aorta. (Echo courtesy of University of Washington Medical Center, Washington.)

Imaging Windows

Ultrasound waves have significant attenuation through air and bone and therefore, care must be taken to avoid the areas over the sternum, ribs, and lungs. Imaging is thereby limited to the spaces between the ribs. There are four standardized anatomic windows for the echo examination and are usually acquired in the following order: parasternal, apical, subcostal, and suprasternal. Standard nomenclature used in echo is to first identify the window in which the images were obtained and then whether the long or short axis is used. Multiple windows are used to maximize imaging of heart structures, likewise attempts are made to image most structures from at least two windows. For a standard and complete echo examination, all four windows should be utilized. 2D echo and Doppler (pulsed wave, continuous wave, and color) are typically performed in each window.

Parasternal Window

The patient is positioned in the left lateral decubitus position and imaging is performed in the rib spaces left of the sternum. Imaging is performed in the long axis and short axis (Figs. 13-15 and 13-16).

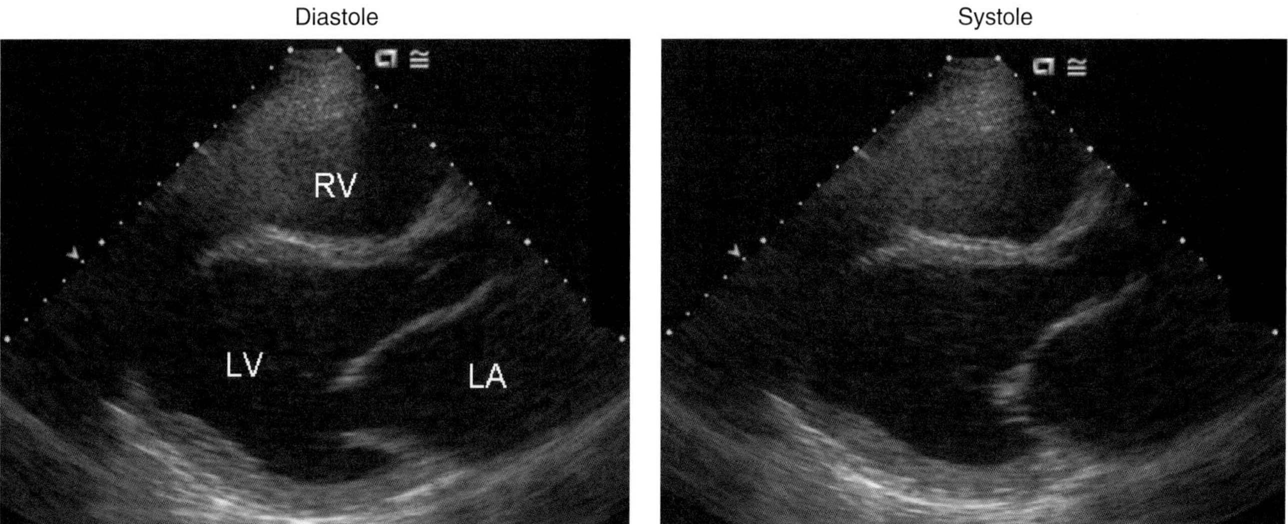

Figure 13-16. Parasternal long axis images in diastole and systole in a patient with a severe dilated cardiomyopathy. There is not much difference in the size of the left ventricle between diastole and systole, indicating poor systolic function. RV, right ventricle; LV, left ventricle; LA, left atrium. (Echo courtesy of University of Washington Medical Center, Seattle, Washington.)

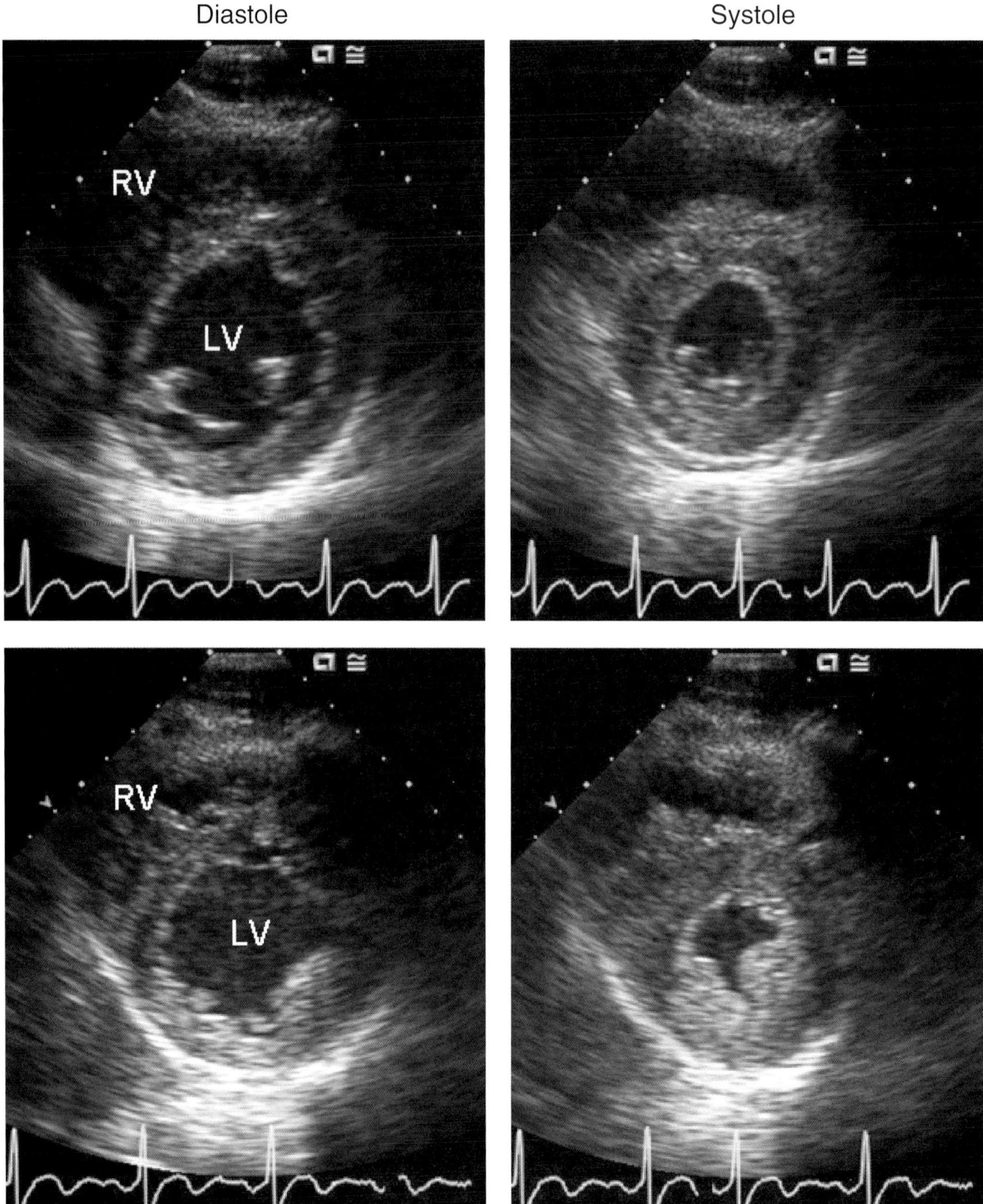

Figure 13-17. **Top:** Parasternal basal short axis at the level of the mitral annulus. **Bottom:** Parasternal mid short axis at the level of papillary muscles. RV, right ventricle; LV, left ventricle. (Echo courtesy of University of Washington Medical Center, Seattle, Washington.)

The short axis can be obtained at multiple levels of the heart from base to apex (Fig. 13-17).

Apical Window

The patient is positioned in the left lateral decubitus position and imaging is performed in the rib spaces overlying the apex of the heart. In this window, imaging is performed only along the long axis of the heart. By rotating the transducer, multiple different orientations of the long axis of the heart are produced so that each wall of the left ventricle can be visualized (Fig. 13-18).

Subcostal Window

The patient is positioned in the supine position with the knees bent. The transducer is placed just below the xiphoid process of the sternum and images are obtained through the diaphragm. In this window, imaging is performed in the long and short axis of the heart (Fig. 13-19).

Suprasternal Window

The patient is positioned in the supine position with the chin tilted upward and rightward. In this window, imaging is performed in the long and short axis (Fig. 13-20).

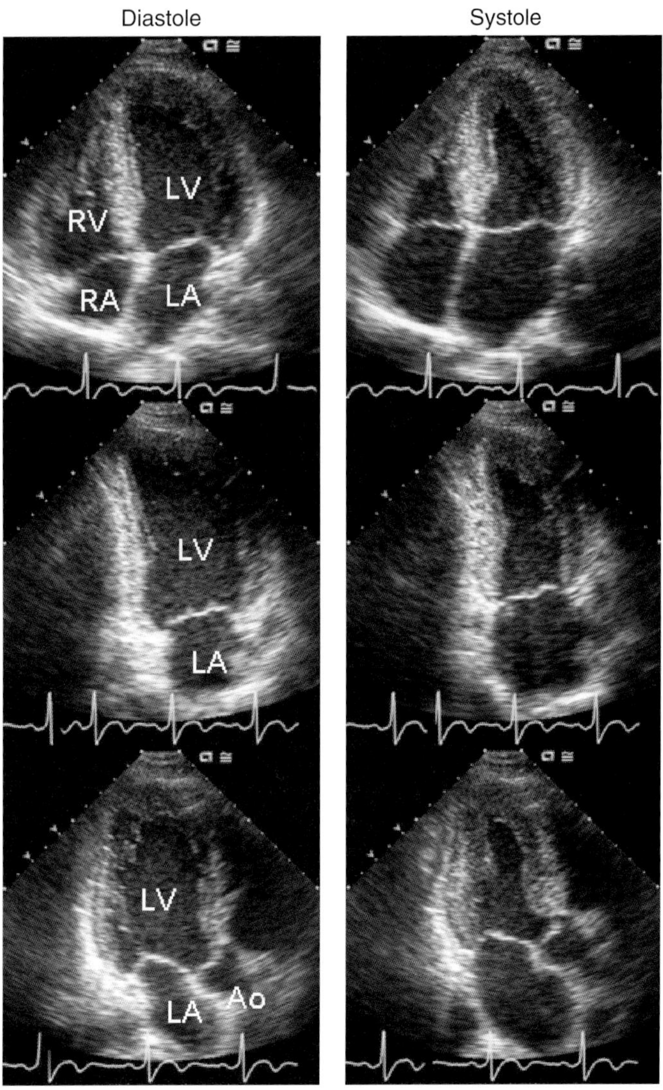

Figure 13-18. **Top:** Apical four-chamber view. **Middle:** Apical two-chamber view. **Bottom:** Apical long axis view. RV, right ventricle; LV, left ventricle; RA, right atrium; LA, left atrium; Ao, aorta. (Echo courtesy of University of Washington Medical Center, Seattle, Washington.)

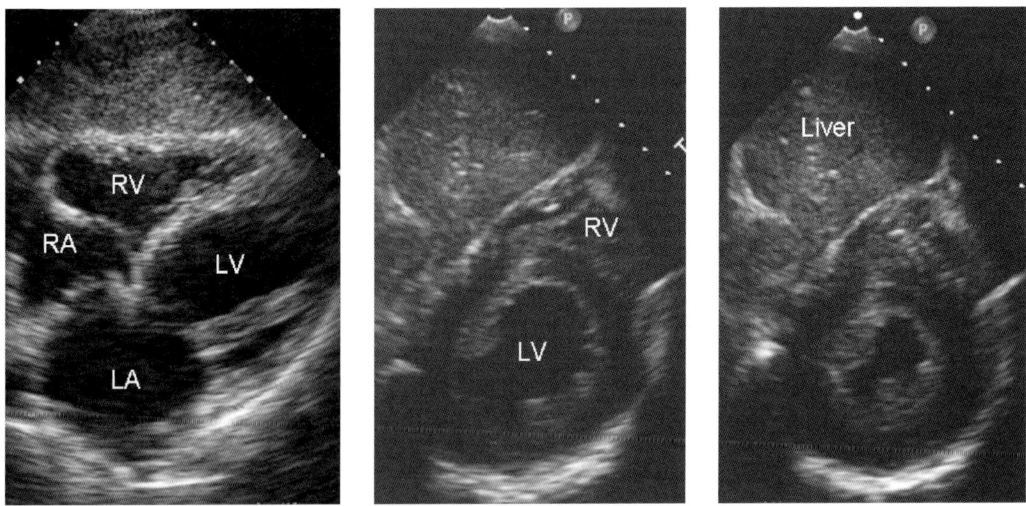

Figure 13-19. These images are from the subcostal window as evidenced by the liver at the top of images. **Left:** Subcostal long axis. **Middle:** Subcostal short axis in diastole. **Right:** Subcostal short axis in systole. RA, right atrium; RV, right ventricle; LA, left atrium; LV, left ventricle. (Echo courtesy of Harborview Medical Center, Seattle, Washington.)

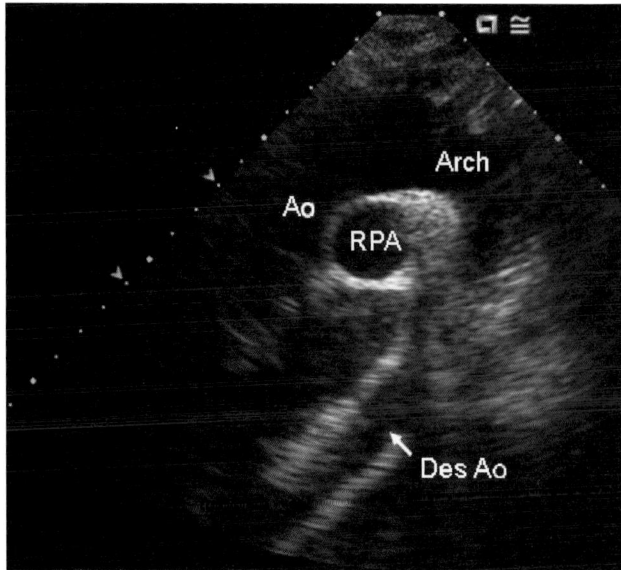

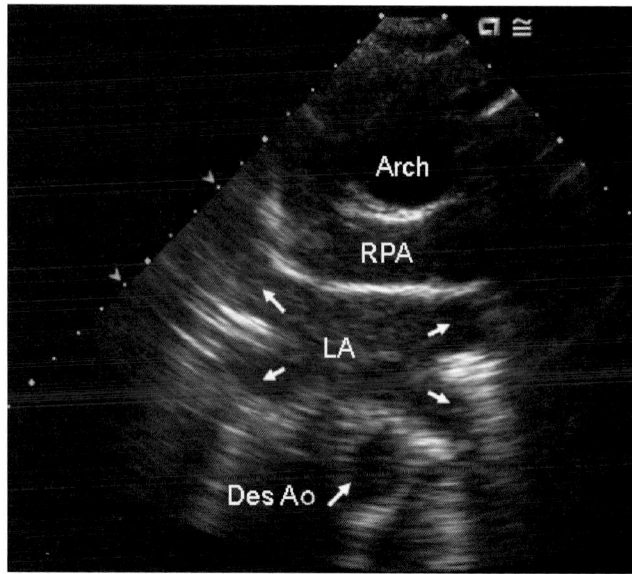

Figure 13-20. **Left:** Suprasternal long axis. **Right:** Suprasternal short axis. Ao, aorta; RPA, right pulmonary artery; Des Ao, descending thoracic aorta; LA, left atrium. Four *arrows* in left atrium identify each pulmonary vein. (Echo courtesy of University of Washington Medical Center, Seattle, Washington.)

ECHO APPLICATIONS

Contrast Echo

There are several purposes for the use of contrast in echocardiography. The diagnostic indication will dictate the specific type of contrast. One simple classification system of echo contrast agents is whether the contrast agent crosses the pulmonary vasculature microcirculation. Some contrast agents remain in the venous circulation (right heart structures) while others will be in the venous and arterial circulation (right and left heart structures). Echo contrast agents are composed of bubbles. The size of the bubbles determines whether they will cross the pulmonary vasculature microcirculation. Red blood cells cross the pulmonary capillaries and are 6 to 8 mcm in diameter.

Saline microbubbles (agitated saline) are commonly used for detection of shunts, primarily because the bubbles are too large to cross the pulmonary vasculature microcirculation (Fig. 13-21). Saline microbubbles are injected into an intravenous catheter and opacify the right side of the heart. Because the microbubbles are larger (greater than 8 mcm) than red blood cells, they cannot cross the pulmonary vasculature and are absorbed by the lungs. Therefore, they should not opacify the left heart structures. Saline microbubbles that do appear in the left side of the heart are indicative of a right-to-left shunt (i.e., atrial septal defect, patent foramen ovale, pulmonary arterial venous malformation). Saline microbubbles are created by connecting a two-way stopcock to an intravenous catheter with two 10-cc syringes. One syringe is filled with 9 cc of normal saline and 1 cc of air and then transferred to the empty syringe back and forth. This action makes bubbles of air throughout the saline. The full 10 cc is then *quickly* injected into the intravenous catheter. Emphasis is placed on *quickly*, so as to achieve bolus opacification of saline microbubbles and not streaming of the saline microbubbles of the right heart structures.

Lipid (Definity) or albumin (Optison) microspheres are commercially available contrast agents. These agents have a diameter of 1.1 to 4.5 mcm and contain a gas (perfluoropropane) within their shell,[10,11] permitting opacification of the left ventricle because the microspheres are small enough to cross the pulmonary capillaries (Fig. 13-22). Opacification of the left ventricle allows improved endocardial definition, which enhances the diagnostic accuracy of global and regional wall motion assessment. Contraindications to the use of these contrast agents include: cardiac shunts, unstable congestive heart failure, acute myocardial infarction, ventricular arrhythmias, respiratory failure, pulmonary hypertension, intra-arterial injection, hypersensitivity to perflutren, or hypersensitivity to albumin (Optison).[10,11] Adverse effects are uncommon but can include back/chest pain, headache, dizziness, nausea, flushing, altered taste sensation, palpitations, urticaria, or anaphylaxis.[10,11]

Stress Echo

Stress echo is performed in combination with continuous 12-lead ECG monitoring to improve the diagnostic accuracy of coronary artery detection or risk stratification of patients with known coronary artery disease (CAD). Image acquisition is performed in the same standard views, as described previously and optimal endocardial definition is necessary. Sometimes, contrast is needed to provide endocardial definition to visualize wall motion. Global and regional wall motion is compared from rest to stress periods. A normal finding: a myocardial segment has normal function at rest and hyperdynamic function at stress. An abnormal finding suggestive of obstructive CAD: a myocardial segment has normal function at rest and becomes hypokinetic or akinetic at stress (Fig. 13-23).[12]

The preferred method of stress testing is exercise, provided the patient is able. Exercise is usually done on a treadmill or supine bicycle. For treadmill exercise, rest images are performed while the patient is lying on the examination bed. The patient then exercises on the treadmill with continuous ECG monitoring. When peak exercise is achieved, the patient is quickly moved from the treadmill back to the examination bed and imaging is repeated. This sequencing requires practice and coordination. The longer it takes to perform the imaging after peak exercise, the heart rate decreases and so does the sensitivity of the test. Image acquisition should

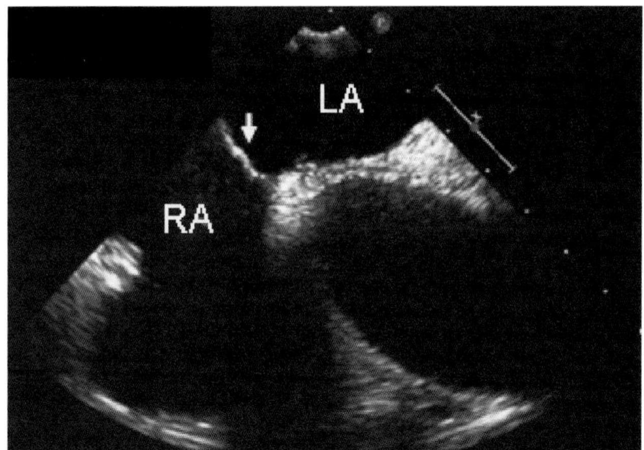

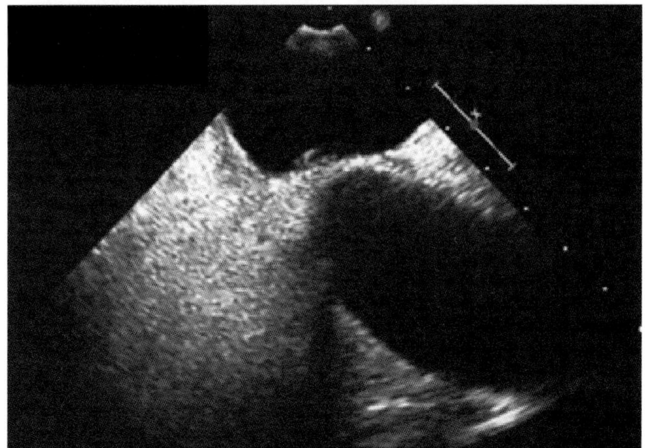

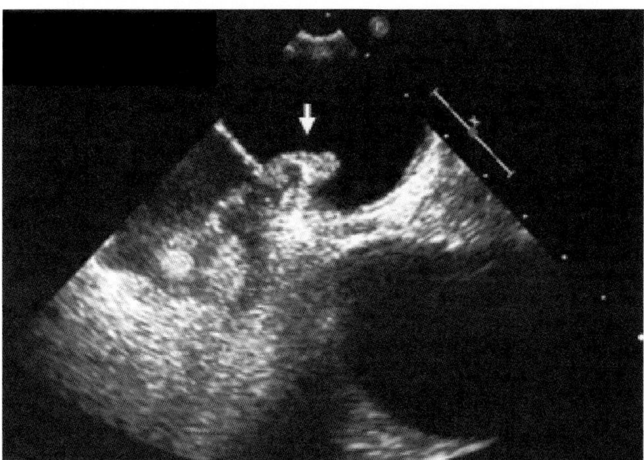

Figure 13-21. **Top:** Transesophageal echo image demonstrating the right atrium (RA), left atrium (LA), and the interatrial septum (*arrow*). **Middle:** Same view as described above during the injection of saline microbubbles via an intravenous catheter. Notice that the right atrium is filled with the bubbles (*white*). **Bottom:** The next cardiac cycle demonstrates shunting of the microbubbles (*arrow*) through the interatrial septum into the left atrium, consistent with a patent foramen ovale. (Echo courtesy of Harborview Medical Center, Seattle, Washington.)

occur within 60 seconds of the termination of peak exercise. With supine bicycle stress, imaging can be performed *throughout* the exercise period. With treadmill stress, imaging can only be performed *after* exercise is complete. However, the physiologic workload with bicycle stress is not the same as treadmill. Some studies have shown that patients are more apt to achieve their peak aerobic capacity with treadmill stress as opposed to bicycle stress.[12] During exercise stress, a physician, nurse practitioner, or physician assistant is usually present and responsible for supervising the test (i.e., taking blood pressures, examining the ECG). A sonographer is present for image acquisition; an ECG technician may also be present.

For those patients who cannot exercise, dobutamine is the most common stress agent used; however, it should be understood that dobutamine does not completely simulate the physiologic state of exercise. A nurse should be present during dobutamine infusion since medications need to be given intravenously. Starting doses are between 5 and 10 mcg/kg/min, increasing by 10 mcg/kg/min increments every 3 minutes to a peak of 40 mcg/kg/min. Doses of atropine can be given and physical maneuvers can be performed in addition to dobutamine infusion to achieve 85% of the maximally predicted heart rate.[12]

Stress echo is also utilized in the assessment of valve disease. The increase in catheter-based valve procedures has increased the awareness of valve disease. As a result, more patients are being evaluated for valve disease. Stress echo may be indicated to determine whether the patient is truly asymptomatic with severe valve disease, or whether the valve disease is indeed severe. For the evaluation of valve disease, a stress echo is performed in the same manner as the assessment for CAD (described above); however, the emphasis is on evaluating the presence of exercise-induced symptoms, severity of valve disease (i.e., mean and peak gradients and velocities), and the increase in pulmonary artery pressures with exercise.

Dobutamine stress echo is also used in the assessment of patients with AS. In patients with a depressed ejection fraction (EF) and severe aortic stenosis, a dobutamine stress echo is indicated to confirm the severity of AS and to differentiate it from pseudosevere AS.

Periprocedural Transesophageal Echocardiography

From a clinical perspective, intraoperative TEE has become commonplace during cardiac surgery reflecting the mounting complexity of surgical technique and patient pathology. Advances in technology presently permit RT 3D echocardiography using a transthoracic (TTE) or transesophageal matrix array ultrasound probe that provides detailed online 3D images.[9] The use of 3D TEE has redefined the way we image, diagnose, and treat a variety of cardiac conditions, including valve disease, especially AS and mitral regurgitation; congenital heart disease; cardiac masses; and hypertrophic obstructive cardiomyopathy.

3D TEE can image multiple cardiac structures to aid in planning surgical and catheter-based interventions. Importantly, 3D TEE is increasingly used in addition to fluoroscopy for periprocedural guidance of transcatheter procedures.[13] Some of these catheter-based interventions include TAVR, transcatheter mitral valve repair (e.g., MitraClip), transcatheter mitral valve replacement (TMVR), transcatheter tricuspid valve repair (TTVR), left atrial appendage occlusion (LAAO), and bioprosthetic paravalvular leak (PVL) repair. Examples of these images are provided in Figures 13-24 to 13-26.

Typically, guidance of these catheter-based procedures is performed using fluoroscopy and 2D TEE. Both of these imaging modalities have significant limitations. Fluoroscopy is limited by its 2D projections of a 3D heart, and its inability to delineate soft structures precisely; 2D TEE, because of its tomographic nature, needs multiple planes and adjustments to visualize the course of intracardiac catheters and their complex relationship with cardiac structures.

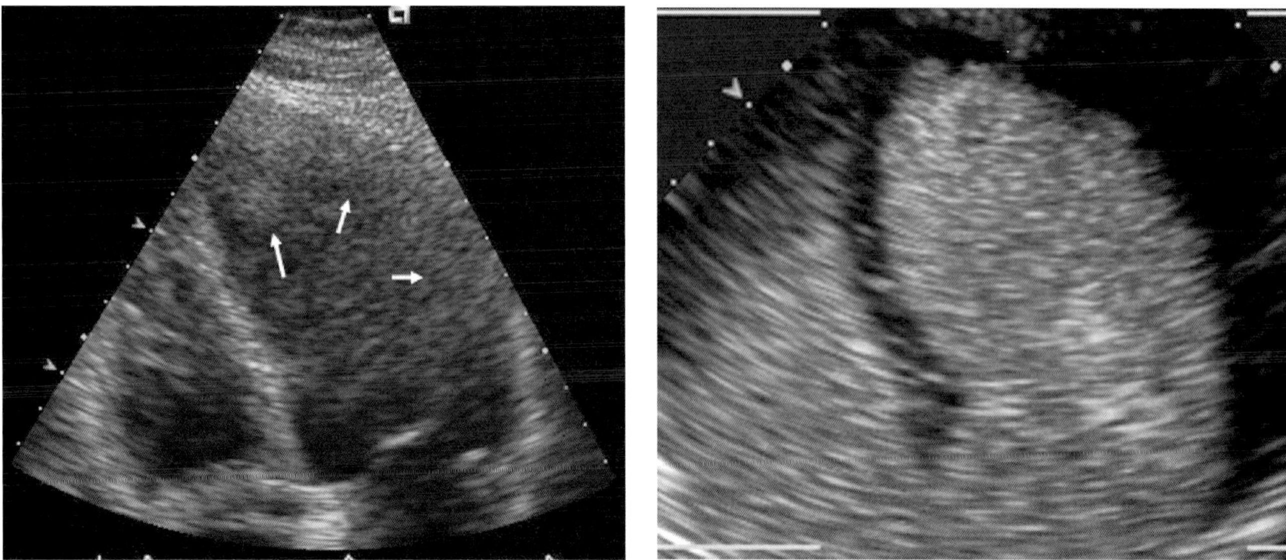

Figure 13-22. Left: Apical four-chamber view in a patient with poor endocardial definition and thus suboptimal image quality. **Right:** The same patient with improved image quality with the administration of a transpulmonary contrast agent (Definity). Notice the endocardial definition is now of diagnostic quality. (Echo courtesy of University of Washington Medical Center, Seattle, Washington.)

The 3D TEE is useful in both pre- and postprocedural assessment, as well as to guide intraprocedural device placement, including transseptal puncture for procedures that require it.[14,15] The TEE can assess cardiac function, in addition to structural and valvular anatomy. It can help determine the severity of the condition being assessed as well as the appropriateness of the anatomy for a structural intervention. During the procedure, it can help with device placement and immediately assess the efficacy of the device placement. The use of periprocedural 3D TEE helps to obtain the appropriate diagnosis, anticipate potential problems and adjust strategy accordingly, maximize procedural success, and minimize complications.

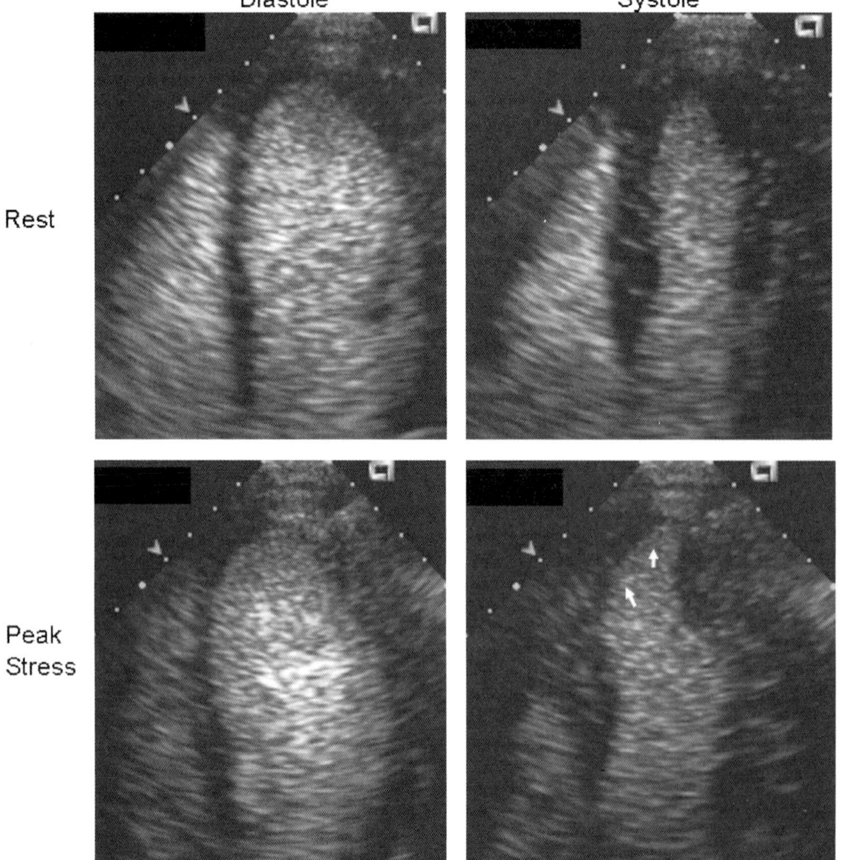

Figure 13-23. Apical four-chamber view of patient undergoing a dobutamine stress echo. **Top:** At rest, there is normal wall motion and the left ventricular cavity is noticeably smaller in systole. **Bottom:** During peak stress, the left ventricular cavity is smaller in systole but there is a noticeable wall motion abnormality in the apical septum and apex (*arrows*), which would be consistent with obstructive epicardial disease in the left anterior descending coronary artery. (Echo courtesy of Harborview Medical Center, Seattle, Washington.)

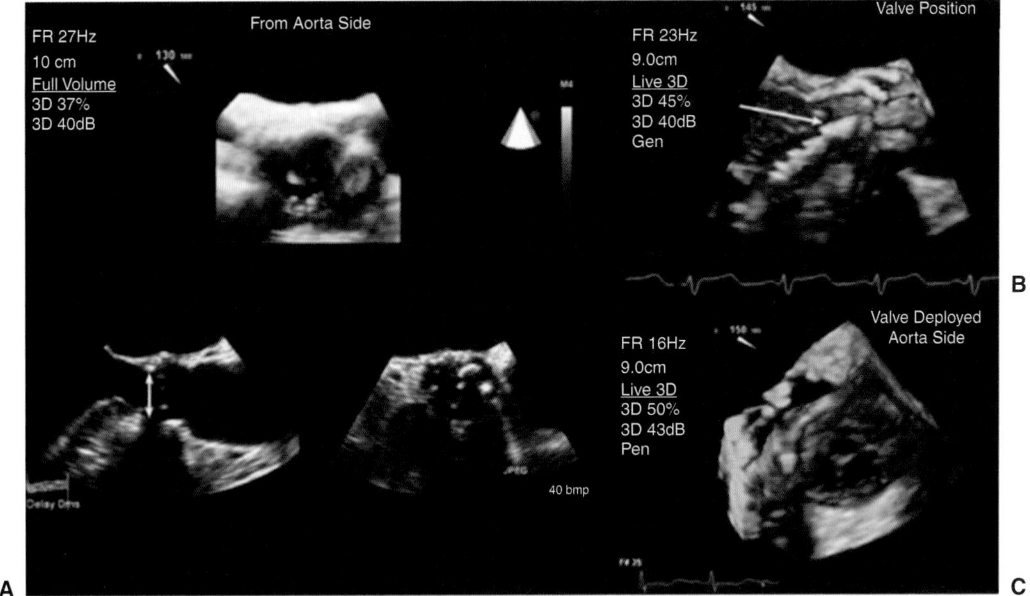

Figure 13-24. Three-dimensional (3D) transesophageal echo (TEE) in transcatheter aortic valve replacement. **A:** Shown is a full volume dataset of a calcified aortic valve (AV) from the aorta with 2D AV LAX and AV SAX views for reference. Measurement of the calcific AV annulus is more easily performed in 2D. **B:** During TAVR procedures, 3D TEE can provide real-time information about positioning of various wires, catheters, and the prosthetic valve (*arrow*). Correct alignment of the prosthetic valve equator is slightly below the native AV annulus. **C:** Post valve deployment in zoom of a well-functioning Edwards Sapien transcatheter heart valve from the aorta during diastole. (Reprinted with permission from Perrino AC, Reeves ST, eds. *A Practical Approach to Transesophageal Echocardiography.* 3rd ed. Philadelphia, PA: Wolters Kluwer Health (LWW PE); 2013.)

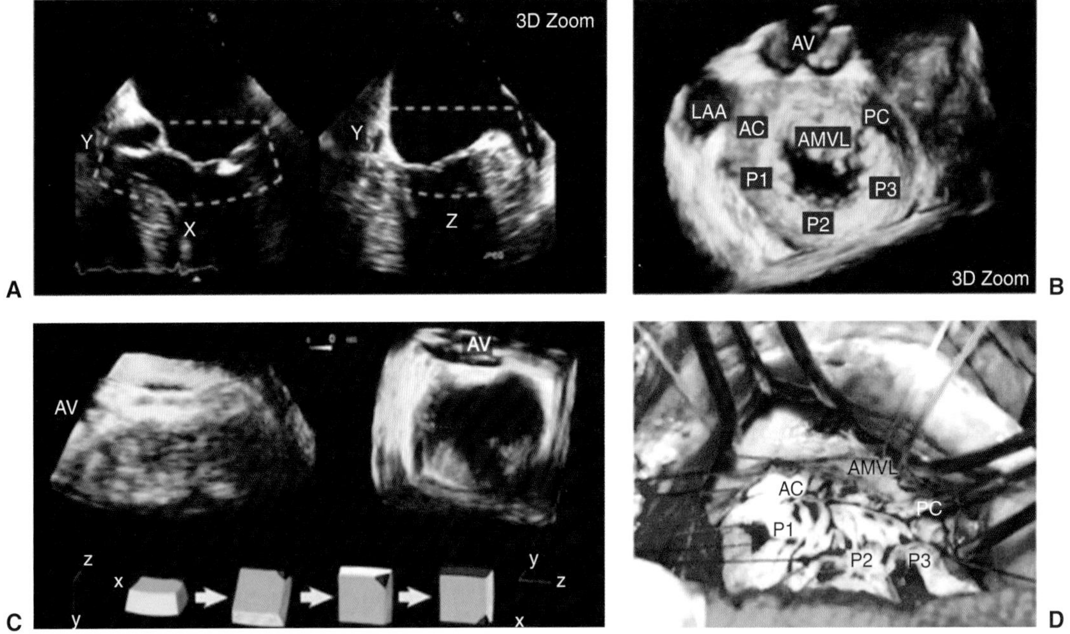

Figure 13-25. Three-dimensional (3D) echo zoom of the mitral valve. **A:** Acquisition of a zoom dataset for the mitral valve (MV) begins with positioning two boxes to encompass the MV. It is useful to include a portion of the aortic valve (AV) to aid orientation of the 3D image. **B:** The initial 3D volume needs to be rotated and optimized by reducing the gain to display (**C**) an enface view of the MV. This orientation is comparable to (**D**) the surgeon's intraoperative view of the MV through the left atrium. The commissures (anterior, AC and posterior, PC) and individual scallops of the posterior MV leaflet (P1, P2, P3) are easily identifiable. AMVL, anterior mitral valve leaflet; LAA, left atrial appendage. (Reprinted from Vegas A, Meineri M. Three-dimensional transesophageal echocardiography is a major advance for intraoperative clinical management of patients undergoing cardiac surgery: a core review. *Anesth Analg.* 2010;110:1548–1573, with permission.)

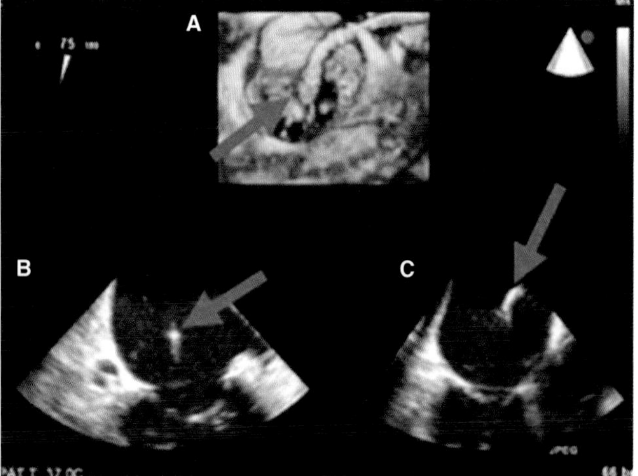

Figure 13-26. Examples of three-dimensional echocardiography (3D) images obtained during guidance of structural heart disease procedures. **Top**, from left to right: Transseptal puncture showing tenting of the foramen ovale; atrial septal defect (ASD) closure using an Amplatzer device, where 3D echocardiography depicted the correct position of both disks on the two sides of the interatrial septum; balloon valvuloplasty in a patient with severe mitral stenosis depicting the trajectory of the balloon catheter; left atrial appendage (LAA) closure depicting the device in a correct position. **Bottom**, from left to right: Mitral valve clip deployment with 3D echocardiography depicting the clip positioned perpendicular to the closing line of the valve and an "Alfieri"-type repair after clip insertion; paravalvular leak (PVL) closure device seen in the 1 o'clock position. (The two images on the right are courtesy of Dr. Luigi Badano.). (Reprinted with permission from Roberto M, Addetia K, Narang A, et al. 3-Dimensional echocardiography. *J Am Coll Cardiol Img.* 2018;11(12):1854–1878.)

NURSING ROLE IN ECHOCARDIOGRAPHY

Foundational Literacy

Echo literacy encompasses comprehension of fundamental terminology and its corresponding significance for the patient's clinical presentation and nursing care needs. The cardiac nurse must understand the patient's cardiovascular history, whether an echo has already been performed or may be indicated, and how to locate and apply key information from an echo report. To illustrate: A cardiac nurse may care for a patient with syncope in the clinic or telemetry unit. The nurse must understand that in order to determine whether the structure and/or function of the heart is a cause or contributing factor for syncope, echo is frequently a guideline-recommended part of the evaluation. Upon review of the chart the nurse peruses the medical history, providers' progress notes, and reports of diagnostic studies. If an echo has been performed, the nurse reviews the report's conclusions and understands the clinical relevance of terms such as EF. If the patient's EF is documented to be 25% as per a recent echo report, the nurse anticipates arrhythmias or hypovolemia as possible contributing factors for syncope in the patient with heart failure due to reduced EF (HFrEF), managed with aggressive diuretics and a fluid restriction. If fluids are given and diuretics are held, the nurse knows to assess for signs and symptoms of hypervolemia, cognizant that it is challenging for the patient with an EF less than 30% to attain euvolemia and/or remain compensated for their HFrEF. If an echo has not been performed for a patient with syncope, the nurse seeks to understand the care team's rationale.

Patient Preparation and Surveillance

The nurse may be involved in preparing and monitoring the patient for an echo. The nurse must have knowledge of the required preparation for various echo studies. For a TTE, the nurse must educate the patient on the indication for the study; however, no specific patient preparation is required. Conversely, if a TEE is ordered, the nurse may be screening for absolute and relative contraindications to TEE (e.g., esophageal strictures, achalasia, or varices; ability to tolerate moderate sedation), and risks of intravenous sedation given the patient (e.g., reduced EF less than 30%, severe AS, pulmonary hypertension, severe pulmonary disease, obstructive sleep apnea) and practice setting (i.e., echo lab in a clinic vs. bedside in the critical care unit will have different criteria for administering sedation). The nurse may also screen the preprocedural laboratory data and alerting the performing physician should a laboratory value (e.g., prothrombin time and international normalized ratio) fall outside of the set parameters.[16]

The nurse may also provide or ensure adherence to preprocedure instructions including when the patient must discontinue oral intake (NPO). Based on nursing and institutional licensure and scope of practice, the nurse may administer intravenous sedation (e.g., fentanyl, midazolam) during a TEE. For stress echo, the nurse will provide similar pre- and periprocedural care and education, targeted to ensure safety with exercise or pharmacologic agents such as intravenous dobutamine. For both TEE and stress echo, the nurse provides postprocedure physical assessment and monitoring until the patient returns to his or her baseline status.

Specialization and Advanced Practice

Nurses, especially advanced practice nurses and nurses in specific settings (e.g., echo lab, cardiothoracic intensive care) or specialties (e.g., structural and valvular heart disease; advanced heart failure/mechanical circulatory support/cardiac transplant) may have advanced education and training in echocardiography. Advanced practice nurses may also interpret study images. Roles and responsibilities may range from the nurse monitoring stress echo, to the nurse practitioner performing bedside TTE in critical care, to the nurse anesthetist initiating or performing intraoperative TTE/TEE. Some institutions (e.g., Mayo Clinic Scottsdale, University of Washington) offer specialized fellowships for cardiac advanced practice nurses. Professional societies, licensing bodies, and institutional policies provide guidance on these competencies and the required education/training.

CONCLUSION

For the cardiac nurse, the high prevalence of cardiovascular disease and the numerous indications to evaluate the structure and function of the heart (e.g., syncope, palpitations, cardiac arrhythmias, ischemic heart disease, structural and valvular heart disease, heart failure) warrants a basic understanding of echocardiography. This competency is not unique to practice setting. It is imperative that the cardiac nurse understands the indications, findings, and patient education needs of echocardiography for patients with cardiovascular disease.

CASE-BASED LEARNING 1

Patient Profile

History of Present Illness

Nancy Albert is a 68-year-old female who presents to the emergency room with a "fluttering" in her chest which started approximately 4 hours ago. Associated symptoms include shortness of breath and lightheadedness with activity. She denies experiencing these symptoms in the past.

Medical History

Hypertension, hypothyroidism, known "heart murmur" but denies any diagnostic evaluation such as an echocardiogram, dysphagia due to history of pill-induced esophagitis, 30–pack year history of smoking, and chronic obstructive pulmonary disease (COPD)

Surgical History

Appendectomy, tonsillectomy

Allergies

None

Medications

Synthroid 125 mcg daily, Vitamin D 2000 IU daily, and albuterol inhaler as needed

Physical Examination

Vital Signs

Temp 98.4°F; BP 100/70 mm Hg; HR 138 bpm; RR 24

Diagnostic Studies

ECG: Atrial fibrillation with rapid ventricular response, HR range 100 to 140 bpm
QRS 80 msec; QT 320 msec
Normal axis
No STT changes
Labs: Complete blood count, complete metabolic panel, thyroid-stimulating hormone, prothrombin and partial thromboplastin time all within normal limits

Considerations

- Guidelines specify interventions for atrial fibrillation based on whether then onset is less than or greater than 48 hours. Thrombus development in the left atrial appendage is more likely after 48 hours of decreased left atrial emptying with loss of atrial kick secondary to atrial fibrillation. Is it possible to confirm that the onset of atrial fibrillation is indeed less than 48 hours?
- If it is determined that the onset of atrial fibrillation was indeed less than 48 hours ago, what interventions would be expected? What important role would echocardiography play in this scenario?
- Past medical history is notable for a heart murmur. What additional considerations would be relevant for this patient?
- Guidelines for atrial fibrillation specify evaluation and treatment based on the patient history and presentation.
- This patient would be prescribed anticoagulation to prevent a thromboembolic stroke and pharmacologic therapy to control the heart rate.
- Because Mrs. Albert is symptomatic, it is likely that she would be admitted for cardioversion. An antiarrhythmic agent would be initiated along with cardioversion, after it was determined that there was no left atrial appendage thrombus, as restoration of sinus rhythm could result in possible thrombus ejection from the left atrium. If thrombus is ejected from the left atrium into the left ventricle, upon systole the thrombus could enter the systemic circulation and cause a thromboembolic stroke.
- A TTE in this patient would evaluate the structure and function of the heart and its structures, including the left ventricle and any significant valvular or structural abnormalities to which the known "heart murmur" could be attributed. Specific valvular abnormalities, such as severe mitral stenosis or regurgitation, influence the management of atrial fibrillation, and warrant further evaluation and treatment.
- A TEE in this patient would evaluate whether there is any thrombus in the left atrium or left atrial appendage to contraindicate cardioversion and/or an antiarrhythmic medication.

Assessment/Plan

Mrs. Albert is a 68-year-old female with symptomatic, new-onset atrial fibrillation with rapid ventricular response and symptom onset reported to be approximately 4 hours ago.

1. Admission to telemetry
2. Cardiology consultation has been requested with plan to initiate anticoagulation and antiarrhythmic therapy
3. Transthoracic echocardiography
4. NPO in anticipation of possible cardioversion per cardiology

Interval Course

The cardiologist reads the TTE which shows normal left ventricular size and function, left atrial enlargement, mitral valve prolapse with moderate mitral regurgitation, normal aortic valve with no stenosis or insufficiency, and normal tricuspid valve with no stenosis or insufficiency (Fig. 13-27). Pulmonary artery systolic pressure is elevated at 40 mm Hg. A TEE is performed with plan for cardioversion.

- What is the significant finding seen in this TEE image?
- How does this finding impact Mrs. Albert's treatment plan?

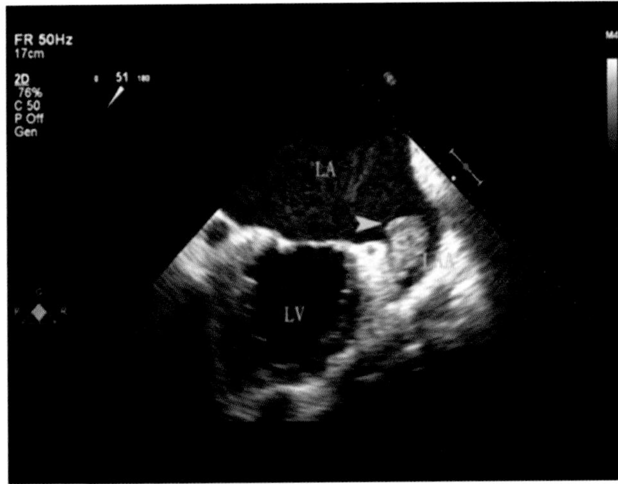

Figure 13-27. Transesophageal echocardiogram depicting a left atrial appendage thrombus (*yellow arrow*). LA, left atrium; LV, left ventricle; LAA, left atrial appendage. (Image used with permission via Creative Common License for Gan L, Yu L, Xie M, et al. Analysis of real-time three dimensional transesophageal echocardiography in the assessment of left atrial appendage function in patients with atrial fibrillation. *Exp Ther Med.* 2016;12(5):3323–3327.)

(continued)

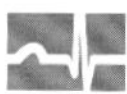

CASE-BASED LEARNING 1 (*Continued*)

Conclusion

The cardiologist does not proceed with cardioversion due to the left atrial appendage thrombus seen on the TEE. Mrs. Albert is started on oral anticoagulation, continued on rate control medications, and discharged to home when she is symptom-free and hemodynamically stable. She will return in 4 to 6 weeks for an elective outpatient TEE and cardioversion.

Key Takeaways

- In this patient with new-onset atrial fibrillation, history of a heart murmur, and hypertension, the TTE provided vital information about the structure and function of the heart. Mitral valve prolapse with moderate mitral regurgitation was diagnosed. Guidelines for valvular heart disease specify how frequently a patient with mitral regurgitation should be evaluated, based on symptoms and disease severity.
- The TEE was indicated to assess for left atrial appendage thrombus. The left atrial appendage is highly trabeculated, and when the atrium does not contract normally in atrial systole, as with atrial fibrillation, thrombus may develop. Should thrombus enter the systemic circulation, a thromboembolic stroke may result. Left atrial appendage thrombus is a risk for stroke, and a contraindication for cardioversion and antiarrhythmic therapy. A patient in atrial fibrillation with left atrial appendage thrombus would require anticoagulation for typically 4 to 6 weeks, followed by a plan of care that may include (1) a repeat TEE to determine if the thrombus had resolved, (2) initiation of antiarrhythmic therapy, and (3) cardioversion.
- In this patient with mitral valve prolapse and moderate mitral regurgitation diagnosed by TTE, a TEE would allow for further investigation of the mitral valve apparatus. The pathoanatomical changes of the mitral valve and mechanism of mitral regurgitation may be evaluated by 3D TEE. During the TEE to exclude left atrial appendage thrombus, the mitral valve apparatus may be assessed.

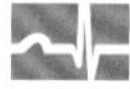

CASE-BASED LEARNING 2

Patient Profile

Mr. Smith is a 76-year-old man who presents to valve clinic with complaints of worsening angina and shortness of breath.

Medical History

Hypertension and diabetes

Surgical History

Coronary artery bypass graft surgery

Diagnostic Studies

- Echocardiogram demonstrated an ejection fraction of 45% with moderate to severe aortic stenosis and a possible bicuspid aortic valve.
- Coronary and graft angiography showed native triple vessel disease (i.e., left anterior descending [LAD] coronary artery, left circumflex coronary artery, and right coronary artery [RCA]) with patent bypass grafts to the LAD and circumflex and an occluded graft to the RCA, with excellent left-to-right collateral flow. No intervention was required for his CAD. The aortic valve was also assessed at the time of cardiac catheterization; the mean gradient was 40 mm Hg, consistent with severe aortic stenosis.

Considerations

- A low ejection fraction (less than 50%) can decrease the flow of blood, thereby underestimating the pressure gradient and velocity across the aortic valve when the valve may indeed be severely stenotic. This is known as low-flow, low-gradient severe aortic stenosis.

Assessment and Plan

Mr. Smith is a 77-year-old man with symptomatic, suspected low-flow, low-gradient severe aortic stenosis.

1. Dobutamine stress echocardiography to confirm the severity of aortic stenosis (i.e., whether Mr. Smith has low-flow, low-gradient severe aortic stenosis).
2. If low-flow, low-gradient severe aortic stenosis is confirmed, guidelines for valvular heart disease deem that a patient with symptomatic, severe aortic stenosis should be referred for valve replacement, which may be performed via surgical aortic valve replacement (sAVR) or transcatheter aortic valve replacement (TAVR). To make this decision, the patient is at the center of a shared decision-making process that evaluates the patient's values and goals, benefits, and risks.
3. Should Mr. Smith decide to proceed with further evaluation and treatment, characteristics such as anatomy of the aortic valve and risk of mortality and morbidity with sAVR versus TAVR are considered. A key diagnostic test to evaluate these characteristics is ECG-gated cardiac CT angiography (CTA).

Interval Course

- Dobutamine stress echocardiography found that the aortic valve mean pressure gradient increased from 26 to 44 mm Hg, consistent with severe aortic stenosis.
- ECG-gated cardiac CTA confirmed a trileaflet aortic valve. Calcium score on the cardiac CTA was 2356. The calcium score value was also consistent with severe aortic stenosis (greater than 2000 for men, 1200 for women).

Conclusion

Mr. Smith underwent a successful TAVR procedure and is currently doing well without symptoms.

Key Takeaways

- When evaluating a patient with valve disease, several diagnostic studies may be indicated. Multiple imaging modalities may be used to confirm valve disease severity and to help guide the best therapy.

CASE-BASED LEARNING 2 (*Continued*)

- Some of these modalities involve the use of echocardiography (TTE, dobutamine stress echo, 3D TEE). TTE is an invaluable tool for determining severity of valve disease. The dobutamine stress echo is the standard for assessment of low-flow, low-gradient severe aortic stenosis. A TEE is often a valuable tool for evaluating valve anatomy; however, in the patient with severe aortic stenosis, particularly low-flow, low-gradient severe aortic stenosis (i.e., low ejection fraction), a TEE carries an increased risk of hemodynamic stability arising from sedation-induced hypotension. Thus, other imaging modalities including CT or MRI may be used, each having their own advantages and disadvantages (see Table 13-1).

Table 13-1 • COMPARISON OF CARDIAC IMAGING MODALITIES

	Advantages	Disadvantages
3D TEE	• Readily available • Portable • No risk for renal compromise • No radiation • Excellent temporal resolution • Good spatial resolution • Hemodynamic information	• Somewhat invasive • Sedation required • No vascular assessment • Potentially more skill required for 3D and annular assessment (not widely performed) • Lack of automated tools • Acoustic shadowing • Looks fuzzy to nonimagers • Lateral resolution issues
CT	• Excellent spatial resolution • Noninvasive • Vascular assessment • Fast • Easy to use/familiarity • Automated tools available	• IV contrast (risk of allergy or renal compromise) • Radiation • Poor temporal resolution • Suboptimal with increased HR/arrhythmia • Not portable • Calcification can be overestimated ("blooming" artifacts)
MRI	• Good temporal resolution • Infinite imaging planes • Minimal effect of body habitus • No radiation • Noninvasive • Can assess annulus without IV gadolinium (bright blood) • Vascular assessment • Hemodynamic information	• Spatial resolution inferior to CT and 3D TEE (thick slices) • Long examination (not tolerated easily) • Claustrophobia • Incompatible with cardiac pacemakers and implantable cardioverter-defibrillators • Suboptimal with increased HR/arrhythmia • Cannot accurately assess calcium

IV, intravenous; CT, computerized tomography; HR, heart rate.

KEY READINGS

American College of Cardiology Foundation Appropriate Use Criteria Task Force; American Society of Echocardiography; American Heart Association, et al. ACCF/ASE/AHA/ASNC/HFSA/HRS/SCAI/SCCM/SCCT/SCMR 2011 appropriate use criteria for echocardiography. A report of the American College of Cardiology Foundation Appropriate Use Criteria Task Force, American Society of Echocardiography, American Heart Association, American Society of Nuclear Cardiology, Heart Failure Society of America, Heart Rhythm Society, Society for Cardiovascular Angiography and Interventions, Society of Critical Care Medicine, Society of Cardiovascular Computed Tomography, Society for Cardiovascular Magnetic Resonance American College of Chest Physicians. *J Am Soc Echocardiogr*. 2011;24:229–267.

Gilman G, Nelson JM, Murphy AT. The role of the nurse in clinical echocardiography. *J Am Soc Echocardiogr*. 2005;18(7):773–777.

Otto CM. *Textbook of Clinical Echocardiography*. 5th ed. London: Elsevier; 2014.

REFERENCES

1. Feigenbaum H, Armstrong WF, Ryan T, eds. *Feigenbaum's Echocardiography*. 6th ed. Philadelphia, PA: Lippincott Williams & Wilkins; 2005.
2. Otto CM. *Textbook of Clinical Echocardiography*. 3rd ed. Philadelphia, PA: W.B. Saunders; 2004.
3. Weyman AE. *Principles and Practice of Echocardiography*. 2nd ed. Philadelphia, PA: Lea & Febiger; 1994.
4. Dekker DL, Piziali RL, Dong E Jr. A system for ultrasonically imaging the human heart in three dimensions. *Comput Biomed Res*. 1974;7(6):544–553.
5. Kruse EJ, Lang RM. Demystifying three-dimensional echocardiography: keeping it simple for the sonographer. *J Indian Acad Echocardiogr Cardiovasc Imaging*. 2017;1:206–213.
6. Pandian NG, Nanda NC, Schwartz SL, et al. Three-dimensional and four-dimensional transesophageal echocardiographic imaging of the heart and aorta in humans using a computed tomographic imaging probe. *Echocardiography*. 1992;9(6):677–687.
7. Levine RA, Handschumacher MD, Sanfilippo AJ, et al. Three-dimensional echocardiographic reconstruction of the mitral valve, with implications for the diagnosis of mitral valve prolapse. *Circulation*. 1989;80(3):589–598.
8. Gill EA, Klas B. Three-dimensional echocardiography: a historical perspective. *Cardiol Clin*. 2007;25:221–229.
9. Vegas A, Meineri M. Core review: three-dimensional transesophageal echocardiography is a major advance for intraoperative clinical management of patients undergoing cardiac surgery: a core review. *Anesth Analg*. 2010;110(6):1548–1573.
10. Definity®. *Perflutren Lipid Microsphere [Package Insert]*. Billerica, MA: Bristol-Myers Squibb Medical Imaging; 2007.

11. Optison™. *Perflutren Protein-Type A Microspheres [Package Insert]*. Princeton, NJ: Amersham Health; 2003.
12. Ellestad MH. *Stress Testing: Principles and Practice*. 4th ed. New York: Oxford University Press; 1996.
13. Faletra FF, Pedrazzini G, Pasotti E, et al. 3D TEE during catheter-based interventions. *JACC Cardiovasc Imaging*. 2014;7(3):292–308.
14. Ho SY, McCarthy KP, Faletra FF. Anatomy of the left atrium for interventional echocardiography. *Eur J Echocardiogr*. 2011;12:i11–i15.
15. Earley MJ. How to perform a transseptal puncture. *Heart*. 2009;95:85–92.
16. Gilman G, Nelson JM, Murphy AT, et al. The role of the nurse in clinical echocardiography. *J Am Soc Echocardiogr*. 2005;18(7):773–777.

14 Cardiac Stress Testing—Physiologic Evaluation With Exercise and Pharmacologic Agents

Adam M. Diesi, Angela D. Pal

OBJECTIVES

1. Understand cardiac stress testing and how its data are used to improve outcomes.
2. Identify indications and contraindications for performing a cardiac stress test.
3. Determine the cardiac stress test that is most appropriately suited for the patient's cardiac history.
4. Understand the current guidelines for performing a successful cardiac stress test.
5. Understand test results in order to guide care.
6. Identify reasons a cardiac stress test may be terminated.
7. Determine the risks associated with performing a cardiac stress test.

KEY QUESTIONS

1. What are the most common types of cardiac stress testing?
2. What are the primary responsibilities of the nurse before, during, and after cardiac stress testing?
3. What are the key components of patient education prior to and after the completion of a cardiac stress test?
4. Should the patient continue taking their cardiac medications prior to performing their test?
5. What nursing interventions might be appropriate if a patient develops chest pain during cardiac stress testing?

BACKGROUND

Historical State and Context

Cardiac stress testing has been around for many decades. Scherf and Boyd realized specific changes were noted on electrocardiogram (ECG) after exercise during an angina episode and published these findings in 1933. Exercise testing was based on the premise that patients with coronary artery disease (CAD) may have a normal ECG at rest without pain due to a balance in myocardial oxygen supply and demand. When myocardial oxygen demands are increased, such as with exercise and stress, and there is a lack of coronary flow due to an atherosclerotic lesion, cardiac muscle becomes ischemic. This in turn may cause changes in the ECG and possibly anginal pain. It was soon realized that exercise testing did not confirm the presence of anginal pain, but instead provided a newer diagnostic tool to assess for the existence of CAD.[1]

CURRENT STATE AND CONTEXT

Cardiac stress testing is a widely used, noninvasive approach that provides diagnostic, prognostic, and functional information for a wide spectrum of patients with cardiovascular, pulmonary, and other disorders. Graded exercise tests are used to assess a patient's ability to tolerate increased physical activity, while electrocardiographic, hemodynamic, and symptomatic responses are monitored in a controlled environment. Graded, progressive exercise can produce abnormalities that are not present at rest, the most important of which are manifestations of myocardial ischemia including ST-segment changes on the ECG, symptoms, and electrical instability. The test is also commonly used to evaluate other system disorders, such as gas exchange abnormalities in patients with pulmonary disease or chronic heart failure, symptoms associated with peripheral vascular disease, and even neurologic disorders.

In cardiovascular medicine, the cardiac stress test is commonly used for evaluating the efficacy of medical therapy, for the assessment of interventions, and as a first-choice diagnostic tool in patients with suspected CAD. In these patients, the cardiac stress test functions as risk stratification of the likelihood of a cardiac event, and as a "gatekeeper" to more expensive and invasive procedures such as cardiac catheterization.[2,3] In the latter role, the test has become even more important in the current era of healthcare cost containment. Although originally developed as a diagnostic tool, recent studies have established the role of the exercise test in the selection of patients for cardiac transplantation, risk stratification after a myocardial infarction (MI), and the assessment of disability.[4–8]

Because of the need to standardize the implementation and interpretation of the exercise test, professional organizations such as the American Heart Association (AHA), the American College of Cardiology (ACC),[5] the American College of Sports Medicine (ACSM),[9] the American Thoracic Society,[4] and the European Society of Cardiology (ESC)[10] have developed guidelines designed to optimize the safety, methodology, and objectives of the test.

This chapter describes the applications, methodology, and principles of cardiac stress testing for the cardiovascular nurse and the professional standards for exercise testing in the aforementioned guidelines.

INDICATIONS AND GUIDELINES

Indications for Cardiac Stress Testing

There are many indications for cardiac stress testing. Understanding why the patient has been referred for this testing, in order to evaluate the response of the heart, is of major importance. These indications may include, but are not limited to:

- Assessment for CAD in patients with chest pain or other symptoms suspicious for CAD or myocardial ischemia
- Assessment of physiologic response of post-MI and postrevascularization patients
- Determination of functional capacity prior to starting an exercise program (for the purpose of exercise/activity prescription)
- Examination for the presence and severity of arrhythmias
- Evaluation of the efficacy of medical, surgical, or pharmacologic treatment
- Evaluation of preoperative physiologic status, for example, valvular dysfunction
- Evaluation of potential causes of syncopal episodes
- Measurement of exercise capacity in children, adolescents, or adults with congenital heart disease
- Evaluation of functional classification of disability
- Evaluation of perioperative risk for noncardiac surgery[5,11–17]

Patients may be referred for cardiac stress testing for many reasons for assessment and evaluation of the previously mentioned conditions, particularly, if they report chest pain or any equivocal symptoms that may indicate myocardial ischemia. Additionally, providers may consider stress testing for patients with known CAD for worsening of symptoms to assess the functional severity of CAD.[5,12,13,15] For patients who may be referred for cardiac rehabilitation or would like to begin an exercise program, cardiac stress testing may be appropriate prior to beginning these activities, especially in older individuals to determine the level of activity tolerance.[5,14] If patients report symptoms that might indicate exercise-induced cardiac arrhythmias, then a provider may order the noninvasive cardiac stress test prior to more invasive tests.[14,16] For patients with valvular heart disease, cardiac stress testing may allow providers to better understand the patient's exercise tolerance, symptoms, disease severity, and need for surgical intervention.[5,15] Cardiac stress testing may be used in the evaluation of syncope or syncopal episodes.[17] Additionally, providers may recommend cardiac stress testing for newly diagnosed heart failure or cardiomyopathy to assess the functional status of the patient and/or the patient's response to pharmacologic treatment.[5,11,15]

Contraindications to Cardiac Stress Testing

A patient's medical history is fundamental to determining if the patient is an appropriate candidate or has a contraindication to testing or a specific modality of cardiac stress testing. Factors that need to be taken into account include past medical history; recent and past symptoms, specifically cardiopulmonary symptoms; vital signs; age; physical activity or physical inactivity/limitations; chemistry and hematology lab profiles; and physical examination. Specifically, providers should ask the patient if they a history of cardiac disease, or other significant condition (Table 14-1). Tables 14-2 and 14-3 list the absolute and relative contraindications of cardiac stress testing.[14]

Ultimately, it is the role of the provider to assess the risks and benefits of cardiac stress testing for each individual patient. While these tests are noninvasive and commonly used for many indications, there are certain risks of cardiac stress testing, related to the contraindications as listed previously.

Guidelines of Cardiac Stress Testing

Since 1980, the AHA, ACC, and ESC among other societies have published many cardiovascular guidelines on various cardiovascular conditions, evaluation and treatment. In 1997, Gibbons et al.[5,15] revised the 1986 exercise testing guidelines to include newer studies

Table 14-1 • PATIENT ASSESSMENT FOR CARDIAC STRESS TESTING

History	Physical Examination
• Medical diagnoses and past medical history: A variety of diagnoses should be reviewed, including cardiovascular disease (known existing coronary artery disease [CAD], previous myocardial infarction, or coronary revascularization); arrhythmias, syncope or presyncope; pulmonary disease, including asthma, emphysema, and bronchitis or recent pulmonary embolism; cerebrovascular disease, including stroke; peripheral artery disease; current pregnancy; and musculoskeletal, neuromuscular, or joint disease • Symptoms: Angina; chest, jaw, or arm discomfort; shortness of breath; and palpitations, especially if associated with physical activity, eating a large meal, emotional upset, or exposure to cold • Risk factors for atherosclerotic disease: Hypertension, diabetes, obesity, dyslipidemia, and smoking • If patient is without known CAD, determine the pretest probability of CAD • Recent illness, hospitalization, or surgical procedure • Medication dose and schedule • Ability to perform physical activity	• Pulse rate and regularity • Resting blood pressure sitting and standing • Auscultation of the lungs, with specific attention to uniformity of breath sounds in all areas, particularly in patients with shortness of breath, a history of heart failure, or pulmonary disease • Auscultation of the heart, particularly in patients with heart failure or valvular disease • Examination related to orthopedic, neurologic, or other medical conditions that might limit exercise

From Balady GJ, Morise AP. Exercise electrocardiographic testing. In: Zipes D, Libby P, Bonow R, eds. *Braunwald's Heart Disease: A Textbook of Cardiovascular Medicine.* 11th ed. Philadelphia, PA: Elsevier; 2019.

Table 14-2 • ABSOLUTE CONTRAINDICATIONS TO CARDIAC STRESS TESTING

Acute myocardial infarction (within 2 days)
Ongoing unstable angina
Uncontrolled cardiac arrhythmia with hemodynamic compromise
Active endocarditis
Symptomatic severe aortic stenosis
Decompensated heart failure
Acute pulmonary embolism, pulmonary infarction, or deep vein thrombosis
Acute myocarditis or pericarditis
Acute aortic dissection
Physical disability (that precludes safe and adequate testing)

From Fletcher GF, Ades PA, Kligfield P, et al. Exercise standards for testing and training: a scientific statement from the American Heart Association. *Circulation.* 2013;128(8):873–934.

that added to the evidence of predicting outcomes in both asymptomatic and symptomatic patients, as well as the use of oxygen consumption measurements with exercise testing in patients who potentially were candidates for heart transplantation. Furthermore, the 1997 guidelines included evidence of cost-effectiveness of exercise testing as compared to other more expensive cardiovascular imaging. However, these guidelines from 1997 referred to exercise testing with the use of a treadmill or bicycle with electrocardiographic and blood pressure monitoring. New modalities of cardiac stress testing were not included in the 1997 guidelines.[15]

In 2002, Gibbons et al.[5] updated the 1997 guidelines to reflect the more current evidence available, but still did not include newer modalities of cardiac stress testing, including pharmacologic stress testing and the use of radionuclide imaging and echocardiography testing. The 2002 ACC/AHA guidelines on exercise testing including 10 modifications, including revisions on confounders of stress ECG interpretation, risk stratifications with exercise testing, use of exercise testing after MI, as well as modifications on special populations, including asymptomatic patients without known CAD, in those with valvular heart disease, cardiac conduction disorders, and patients with hypertension.[5] For a full listing of the recommendations and modifications on exercise testing, please refer to the 1997 and 2002 guidelines.

Table 14-3 • RELATIVE CONTRAINDICATIONS TO CARDIAC STRESS TESTING

Known obstructive left main coronary artery stenosis
Moderate to severe aortic stenosis (with uncertain relation to symptoms)
Tachyarrhythmias with uncontrolled ventricular rates
Acquired advanced or complete heart block
Hypertrophic obstructive cardiomyopathy (with severe resting gradient)
Recent stroke or transient ischemic attack
Mental impairment (with limited ability to cooperate)
Resting hypertension (with systolic or diastolic blood pressures >200/110 mm Hg)
Uncorrected medical conditions • Severe anemia • Important electrolyte imbalances • Hyperthyroidism

From Fletcher GF, Ades PA, Kligfield P, et al. Exercise standards for testing and training: a scientific statement from the American Heart Association. *Circulation.* 2013;128(8):873–934.

Because the 1997 and 2002 ACC/AHA guidelines on exercise testing do not include newer modalities of cardiac stress testing, some of the guidelines for specific conditions providers may consider cardiac stress testing for are included in the chapter. While the chapter does not cover all of the published guidelines in which cardiac stress testing may be warranted, the recommendations and indications germane to the role of the cardiac nurse are detailed.

The systems used for classes of recommendations (COR) and levels of recommendations (LOR) will vary based on the guideline publication year and the disease state/condition, and may differ from those introduced in Chapter 1 of this text. It must be noted that the cardiac nurse must also stay apprised of guideline updates, new research, and local health system standards of care.

Coronary Artery Disease

The evaluation and risk stratification of CAD is a primary indication for cardiac stress testing. Figure 14-1 illustrates recommendations for patients with suspected ischemic heart disease. Figure 14-2 illustrates recommendations for patients with *known* ischemic heart disease. Figure 14-3 describes the American College of Cardiology Foundation (ACCF)/AHA COR and level of evidence (LOE) used in the 2012 guidelines.

Arrhythmias

The ACC, AHA, and Heart Rhythm Society (HRS) have published guidelines for various cardiac arrhythmias, including atrial fibrillation, bradycardia and cardiac conduction delays, supraventricular tachycardia, and ventricular tachycardia. Exercise testing has been recommended in these cardiac arrhythmic conditions with various COR and LOEs (Table 14-4). It is important to note that the COR system changed in 2015 with the supraventricular tachycardia guidelines (Fig. 14-4).[18]

Syncope

For evaluation of patients with syncope due to an unknown etiology, the 2017 ACC/AHA/HRS guidelines describe that exercise stress testing may assist in establishing the cause of syncope in a subset of patients who have syncope or presyncope during exertional activity (Class IIa, LOE C-LD). Figure 14-5 illustrates the recommendations from ACCF/AHA. Highlighted areas correspond to the ACC/AHA Recommendation System in Figure 14-4.

SELECTION AND TYPES OF STRESS TESTS

Pretest Considerations

Before a cardiac stress test, all patients should undergo a complete medical evaluation and a physical examination to identify contraindications to exercise testing. The medical history should include any remote or recent medical problems, symptoms, medication use, and findings from previous examinations and tests. Major CAD risk factors and signs and symptoms suggesting cardiopulmonary disease should be identified on the medical history. Physical activity patterns, vocational requirements, physical limitations, and family history of cardiopulmonary and metabolic disorders should also be assessed and documented in the medical history. Identification of absolute contraindications (Table 14-2) should result in cancellation of the test and referral of the patient to the primary physician or cardiology for further medical management. Patients with relative contraindications (Table 14-3) may be tested only after careful evaluation of the risk-to-benefit ratio as assessed on the individual patient.

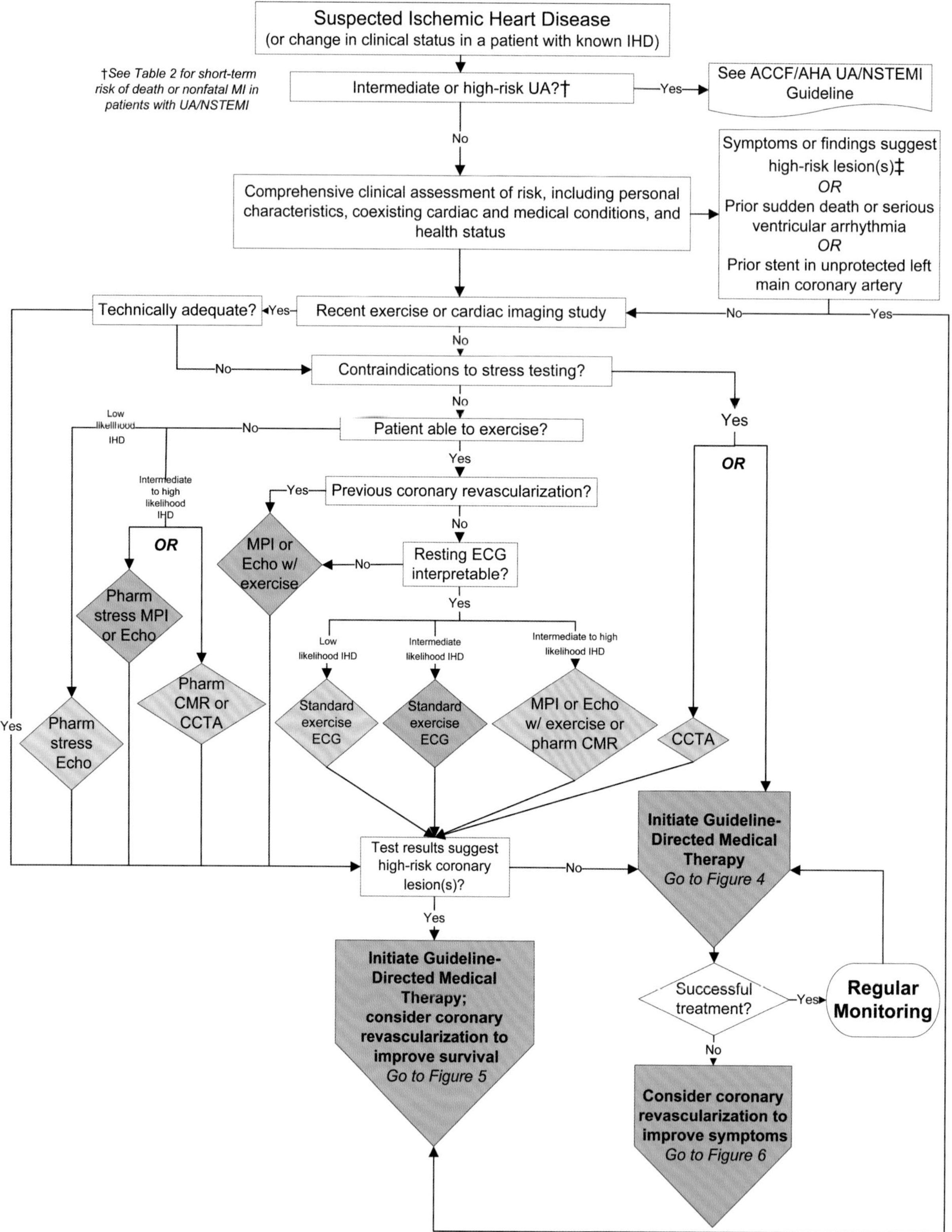

Figure 14-1. Diagnosis of patients with suspected ischemic heart disease. **Colors correspond to the class of recommendations in the ACCF/AHA Guidelines, see* Figure 14-3. The algorithms do not represent a comprehensive list of recommendations (see full guidelines for all recommendations). CCTA, computed coronary tomography angiography; CMR, cardiac magnetic resonance; ECG, electrocardiogram; Echo, echocardiography; IHD, ischemic heart disease; MI, myocardial infarction; MPI, myocardial perfusion imaging; pharm, pharmacologic; UA, unstable angina; UA/NSTEMI, unstable angina/non–ST-elevation myocardial infarction. (Used with permission from Fihn SD, Gardin JM, Abrams J, et al. ACCF/AHA/ACP/AATS/PCNA/SCAI/STS Guideline for the diagnosis and management of patients with stable ischemic heart disease: executive summary. *Circulation.* 2012;126(25):3097–3137.)

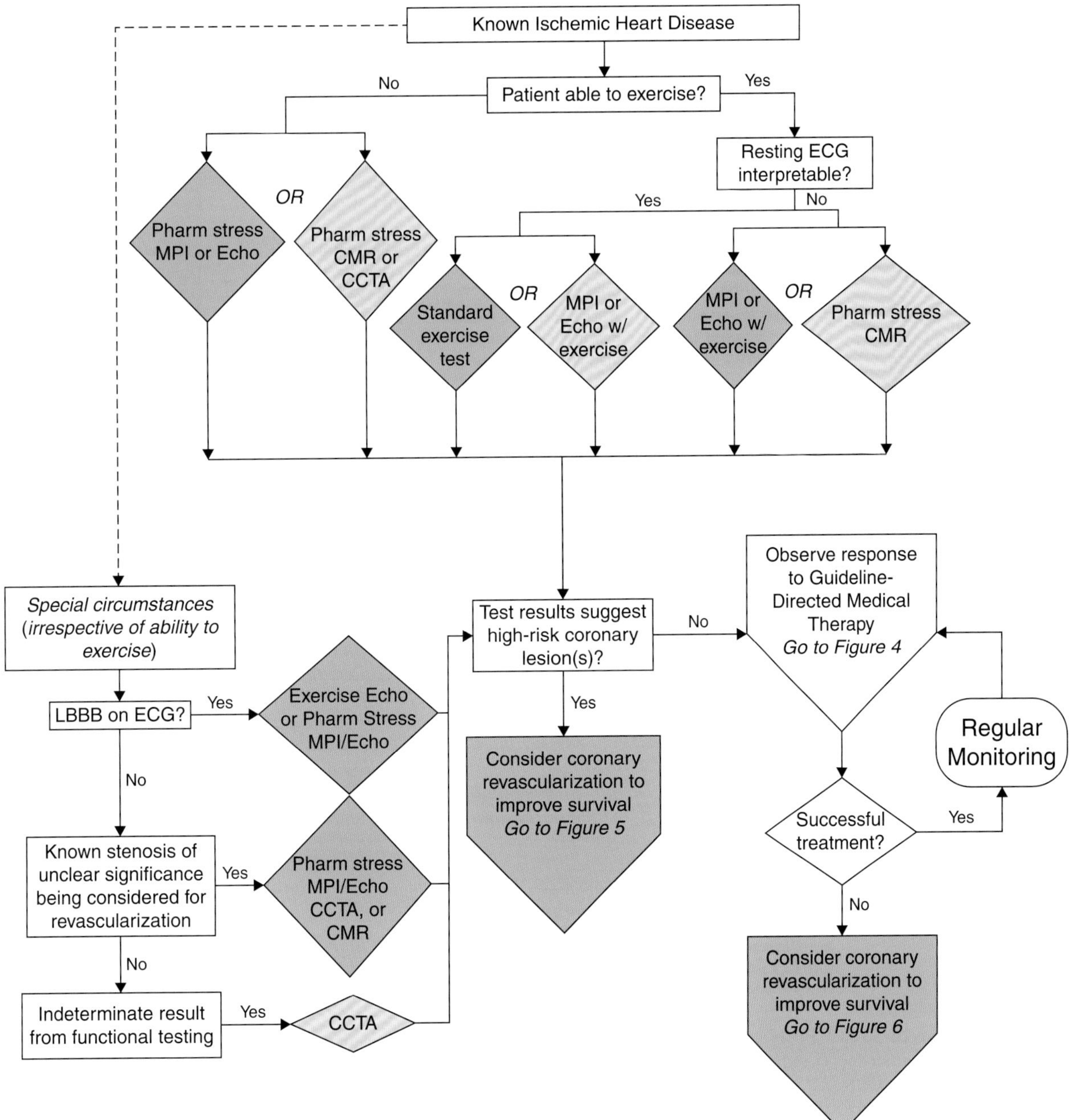

Figure 14-2. Algorithm for risk assessment of patients with known ischemic heart disease. **Colors correspond to the class of recommendations in the ACCF/AHA Guidelines, see* Figure 14-3. CCTA, computed coronary tomography angiography; CMR, cardiac magnetic resonance; ECG, electrocardiogram; Echo, echocardiography; IHD, ischemic heart disease; MI, myocardial infarction; LBBB, left bundle branch block; MPI, myocardial perfusion imaging; pharm, pharmacologic; LBBB, left bundle-branch block. (Used with permission from Fihn SD, Gardin JM, Abrams J, et al. ACCF/AHA/ACP/AATS/PCNA/SCAI/STS Guideline for the diagnosis and management of patients with stable ischemic heart disease: executive summary. *Circulation.* 2012;126(25):3097--3137.)

Detailed verbal and written instructions, provided to the patient in advance, should include a request that the patient refrain from ingesting food, alcohol, or using tobacco products within 3 hours of testing and caffeine products within 24 hours of testing as it may interfere with some pharmacologic testing.[14] It is important to enquire about risk of pregnancy or breastfeeding prior to testing due to the effect some medications may have on the fetus or breast milk. Patients should be well rested and avoid vigorous activity the day of the test such that undue fatigue does not impact their activity tolerance. Clothing should be comfortable and provide freedom of movement as well in order to allow access for electrode, blood pressure cuff, and intravenous access if necessary. Properly fitting shoes with rubber soles should be worn to ensure good traction, particularly if a treadmill is the mode of testing. A thorough explanation of the potential risks and discomforts associated

SIZE OF TREATMENT EFFECT

ESTIMATE OF CERTAINTY (PRECISION) OF TREATMENT EFFECT

	CLASS I *Benefit >>> Risk* Procedure/Treatment **SHOULD** be performed/administered	CLASS IIa *Benefit >> Risk* *Additional studies with focused objectives needed* **IT IS REASONABLE** to perform procedure/administer treatment	CLASS IIb *Benefit ≥ Risk* *Additional studies with broad objectives needed; additional registry data would be helpful* Procedure/Treatment **MAY BE CONSIDERED**	CLASS III *No Benefit* or CLASS III *Harm* (Procedure/Test / Treatment) COR III: No benefit — Not Helpful — No Proven Benefit COR III: Harm — Excess Cost w/o Benefit or Harmful — Harmful to Patients
LEVEL A Multiple populations evaluated* Data derived from multiple randomized clinical trials or meta-analyses	■ Recommendation that procedure or treatment is useful/effective ■ Sufficient evidence from multiple randomized trials or meta-analyses	■ Recommendation in favor of treatment or procedure being useful/effective ■ Some conflicting evidence from multiple randomized trials or meta-analyses	■ Recommendation's usefulness/efficacy less well established ■ Greater conflicting evidence from multiple randomized trials or meta-analyses	■ Recommendation that procedure or treatment is not useful/effective and may be harmful ■ Sufficient evidence from multiple randomized trials or meta-analyses
LEVEL B Limited populations evaluated* Data derived from a single randomized trial or nonrandomized studies	■ Recommendation that procedure or treatment is useful/effective ■ Evidence from single randomized trial or nonrandomized studies	■ Recommendation in favor of treatment or procedure being useful/effective ■ Some conflicting evidence from single randomized trial or nonrandomized studies	■ Recommendation's usefulness/efficacy less well established ■ Greater conflicting evidence from single randomized trial or nonrandomized studies	■ Recommendation that procedure or treatment is not useful/effective and may be harmful ■ Evidence from single randomized trial or nonrandomized studies
LEVEL C Very limited populations evaluated* Only consensus opinion of experts, case studies, or standard of care	■ Recommendation that procedure or treatment is useful/effective ■ Only expert opinion, case studies, or standard of care	■ Recommendation in favor of treatment or procedure being useful/effective ■ Only diverging expert opinion, case studies, or standard of care	■ Recommendation's usefulness/efficacy less well established ■ Only diverging expert opinion, case studies, or standard of care	■ Recommendation that procedure or treatment is not useful/effective and may be harmful ■ Only expert opinion, case studies, or standard of care
Suggested phrases for writing recommendations	should is recommended is indicated is useful/effective/beneficial	is reasonable can be useful/effective/beneficial is probably recommended or indicated	may/might be considered may/might be reasonable usefulness/effectiveness is unknown/unclear/uncertain or not well established	COR III: No Benefit is not recommended is not indicated should not be performed/administered/other is not useful/beneficial/effective COR III: Harm potentially harmful causes harm associated with excess morbidity/mortality should not be performed/administered/other
Comparative effectiveness phrases†	treatment/strategy A is recommended/indicated in preference to treatment B treatment A should be chosen over treatment B	treatment/strategy A is probably recommended/indicated in preference to treatment B it is reasonable to choose treatment A over treatment B		

Figure 14-3. ACCF/AHA classification of recommendations and level of evidence, stable ischemic heart disease guideline. (Used with permission from Fihn SD, Gardin JM, Abrams J, et al. ACCF/AHA/ACP/AATS/PCNA/SCAI/STS Guideline for the diagnosis and management of patients with stable ischemic heart disease: executive summary. *Circulation.* 2012;126(25):3097–3137.)

with exercise testing should be provided to the patient and family. Written informed consent has important ethical and legal implications and ensures the patient knows and understands the purposes and risks associated with the exercise test. A demonstration of how to get on and off the testing apparatus should be performed. Expectations of the patient should be described (reporting of symptoms, level of exertion, and testing endpoints). Adequate time to address patient's questions should be provided.

Patients should remain on all prescribed medications unless the ordering provider has specifically given instructions to stop said cardiac or antianginal medications for testing purposes. A list of current medications, including any over-the-counter medications or herbal supplements, should be brought to the stress test. If the patient has asthma, they should bring their inhaler in case of a respiratory episode. Furthermore, diabetic patients may have to adjust insulin dosing depending on the amount of exercise that they perform.

Cardiac Stress Test Selection

The purpose of the test, the physical health and fitness of the patient, the exercise modality, and the test protocol are fundamental considerations when selecting the appropriate test for a given patient. In many exercise testing laboratories, these issues are determined by evidence-based policies and the availability of equipment, but each can have a profound effect on the response to the stress test. For example, a treadmill test may be inappropriate for patients who have difficulty with balance or gait, severe peripheral vascular disease, a permanent pacemaker, or a left bundle-branch block[19]; therefore an alternative approach would be a more appropriate choice for such patients.

Exercise Stress Testing

An ideal exercise mode increases total body and myocardial oxygen demand to its highest level safely and in moderate, measurable,

Table 14-4 • GUIDELINES FOR CARDIAC ARRHYTHMIAS

Class I
Exercise treadmill testing is useful to assess for exercise-induced ventricular arrhythmias in patients with **ventricular arrhythmias** and symptoms with exertion, suspected IHD, or **catecholaminergic** polymorphic VT
Findings of an abrupt loss of conduction over a manifest pathway during exercise testing in sinus rhythm in asymptomatic patients with **pre-excitation** (LOE: B-NR) are useful, in addition to **intermittent loss of pre-excitation** in ECG or ambulatory monitoring (LOE: C-LD), to identify patients at low risk of rapid conduction over the pathway
Findings of an abrupt loss of conduction over a manifest pathway during exercise testing in sinus rhythm in symptomatic patients with pre-excitation (LOE: B-NR) are useful, in addition to intermittent loss of **pre-excitation** in ECG or ambulatory monitoring (LOE: C-LD), to identify patients at low risk of rapid conduction over the pathway
Class IIa
Exercise ECG testing can be reasonable to diagnose and provide information on prognosis in patients for suspected **chronotropic incompetence** (LOE: B-NR)
Exercise ECG testing can be reasonable for patients with exercise-related symptoms that may be suspicious for **bradycardia or other conduction disorders** (LOE: C-LD)
Exercise ECG testing can be reasonable to determine whether patients with exertional symptoms (chest pain, shortness of breath, etc.) who have **first-degree atrioventricular block or second-degree Mobitz type I atrioventricular block** at rest (LOE: C-LD)
Exercise treadmill testing can be reasonable for establishing a diagnosis and monitoring for response to therapy in patients with suspected **long QT syndrome**, in addition to ambulatory ECG monitoring, and/or recording ECG in a lying position and immediately upon standing (LOE: B-NR)
Class IIb
Class III
Routine cardiac imaging is not indicated in the evaluation of patients with **SB or first-degree AV block** without symptoms and evidence of structural heart disease (LOE: B-NR)
No Class of Recommendation or LOE Noted
Exercise testing can be useful in patients with **atrial fibrillation** if adequacy of rate control is in question, to reproduce exercise-induced atrial fibrillation, or to exclude ischemia before treatment of selected patients with a type IC antiarrhythmic agent
For patients with **ventricular arrhythmias**, exercise testing can be used to assess rhythm burden, response to therapy, and risk stratification
For patients with **arrhythmogenic right ventricular cardiomyopathy**, exercise testing can be used to assess the adequacy of beta-blocking dosing

IHD, ischemic heart disease; LOE, level of evidence; SB, sinus bradycardia; VT, ventricular tachycardia.
From Al-Khatib SM, Stevenson WG, Ackerman MJ, et al. 2017 AHA/ACC/HRS guideline for management of patients with ventricular arrhythmias and the prevention of sudden cardiac death: a report of the American College of Cardiology/American Heart Association Task Force on Clinical Practice Guidelines and the Heart Rhythm Society. *Circulation*. 2018;138:e272–e391; January CT, Wann LS, Alpert JS, et al. 2014 AHA/ACC/HRS guideline for the management of patients with atrial fibrillation a Report of the American College of Cardiology/American Heart Association Task Force on practice guidelines and the Heart Rhythm Society. *Circulation*. 2014.130:e199–e267; Kusumoto FM, Schoenfeld MH, Barrett C, et al. 2018 ACC/AHA/HRS Guideline on the evaluation and management of patients with bradycardia and cardiac conduction delay: Executive Summary: a Report of the American College of Cardiology/American Heart Association Task Force on clinical practice guidelines, and the Heart Rhythm Society. *Circulation*. 2019;74(7):932–987; and Page RL, Joglar JA, Caldwell MA, et al. 2015 ACC/AHA/HRS guideline for the management of adult patients with supraventricular tachycardia: a Report of the American College of Cardiology/American Heart Association Task Force on clinical practice guidelines and the Heart Rhythm Society. *Circulation*. 2016;133:e471–e505.

continuous, and equal increments. This requires a dynamic exercise or pharmacologic approach that uses major muscle groups, permits large increases in cardiac output, oxygen delivery, and gas exchange. Many modalities have been used for exercise diagnostic testing, including cycle ergometers, treadmills, arm ergometers, and steps. Isometric exercise, or static exercise, which involves muscle contraction without movement of the corresponding joint, causes a greater increase in systolic blood pressure and heart rate (HR) in relation to total body oxygen uptake and therefore a greater pressure load on the heart compared with dynamic exercise. Thus, it is not preferred for diagnostic exercise testing.

The bicycle ergometer and the treadmill are the most commonly and preferred used dynamic exercise devices with pharmacologic approaches increasing in popularity. The bicycle is usually less expensive, occupies less space, and is quieter. Upper body motion is decreased, making blood pressure and electrocardiography easier for recording results. The workload administered by simple, mechanically braked bicycle ergometers is not always accurate and depends on pedaling speed, causing variations in the work performed. These have been replaced by electronically braked bicycle ergometers, which maintain the workload at a specified level over a wide range of pedaling speeds and are therefore more accurate. Bicycle ergometer work is commonly expressed in kilogram-meters per minute (kg m/min) or watts. The treadmill is usually more expensive than the cycle ergometer, is relatively immobile, makes more noise, and is harder to acquire ECG data due to potential artifact. Study authors comparing treadmill and bicycle ergometer exercise tests have reported the maximal oxygen uptake to be approximately 10% to 20% higher and maximal HR 5% to 20% higher on the treadmill.[20–24] Significant ST-segment changes have been reported to be more frequent and angina is elicited more frequently during treadmill testing compared with the cycle ergometer.[23,24] In addition, exercise-induced myocardial ischemia by thallium scintigraphy was reported to be greater after treadmill testing than after cycle ergometry.[21] Although most of these differences are minor, if assessing the functional limits of the patient and eliciting subjective or objective signs of ischemia are important goals of the test, the treadmill may be preferable.

Pharmacologic Stress Testing

A pharmacologic stress test may be ordered after an exercise stress test to further evaluate any findings. Furthermore, in patients who are unable to exercise for reasons such as deconditioning, peripheral vascular disease, orthopedic disabilities, neurologic disease, or other concomitant illnesses, several pharmacologic agents can be used to induce mismatch of myocardial oxygen supply and demand in lieu of exercise testing. These pharmacologic agents may also be used to unmask locally limited capacity

CLASS (STRENGTH) OF RECOMMENDATION

CLASS I (STRONG) — **Benefit >>> Risk**

Suggested phrases for writing recommendations:
- Is recommended
- Is indicated/useful/effective/beneficial
- Should be performed/administered/other
- Comparative-Effectiveness Phrases†:
  - Treatment/strategy A is recommended/indicated in preference to treatment B
  - Treatment A should be chosen over treatment B

CLASS IIa (MODERATE) — **Benefit >> Risk**

Suggested phrases for writing recommendations:
- Is reasonable
- Can be useful/effective/beneficial
- Comparative-Effectiveness Phrases†:
  - Treatment/strategy A is probably recommended/indicated in preference to treatment B
  - It is reasonable to choose treatment A over treatment B

CLASS IIb (WEAK) — **Benefit ≥ Risk**

Suggested phrases for writing recommendations:
- May/might be reasonable
- May/might be considered
- Usefulness/effectiveness is unknown/unclear/uncertain or not well established

CLASS III: No Benefit (MODERATE) — **Benefit = Risk**
(Generally, LOE A or B use only)

Suggested phrases for writing recommendations:
- Is not recommended
- Is not indicated/useful/effective/beneficial
- Should not be performed/administered/other

CLASS III: Harm (STRONG) — **Risk > Benefit**

Suggested phrases for writing recommendations:
- Potentially harmful
- Causes harm
- Associated with excess morbidity/mortality
- Should not be performed/administered/other

LEVEL (QUALITY) OF EVIDENCE‡

LEVEL A
- High-quality evidence‡ from more than 1 RCT
- Meta-analyses of high-quality RCTs
- One or more RCTs corroborated by high-quality registry studies

LEVEL B-R — **(Randomized)**
- Moderate-quality evidence‡ from 1 or more RCTs
- Meta-analyses of moderate-quality RCTs

LEVEL B-NR — **(Nonrandomized)**
- Moderate-quality evidence‡ from 1 or more well-designed, well-executed nonrandomized studies, observational studies, or registry studies
- Meta-analyses of such studies

LEVEL C-LD — **(Limited Data)**
- Randomized or nonrandomized observational or registry studies with limitations of design or execution
- Meta-analyses of such studies
- Physiological or mechanistic studies in human subjects

LEVEL C-EO — **(Expert Opinion)**

Consensus of expert opinion based on clinical experience

COR and LOE are determined independently (any COR may be paired with any LOE).

A recommendation with LOE C does not imply that the recommendation is weak. Many important clinical questions addressed in guidelines do not lend themselves to clinical trials. Although RCTs are unavailable, there may be a very clear clinical consensus that a particular test or therapy is useful or effective.

* The outcome or result of the intervention should be specified (an improved clinical outcome or increased diagnostic accuracy or incremental prognostic information).

† For comparative-effectiveness recommendations (COR I and IIa; LOE A and B only), studies that support the use of comparator verbs should involve direct comparisons of the treatments or strategies being evaluated.

‡ The method of assessing quality is evolving, including the application of standardized, widely used, and preferably validated evidence grading tools; and for systematic reviews, the incorporation of an Evidence Review Committee.

COR indicates Class of Recommendation; EO, expert opinion; LD, limited data; LOE, Level of Evidence; NR, nonrandomized; R, randomized; and RCT, randomized controlled trial.

Figure 14-4. ACC/AHA recommendation system, stable ischemic heart disease guideline. (Used with permission from Fihn SD, Gardin JM, Abrams J, et al. ACCF/AHA/ACP/AATS/PCNA/SCAI/STS Guideline for the diagnosis and management of patients with stable ischemic heart disease: executive summary. *Circulation.* 2012;126(25):3097–3137.)

for coronary vasodilatation. Paired with advanced imaging and echocardiography, these medications will also be able to show any ventricular wall motion abnormalities, coronary narrowing, or functional deficits. Medications used for pharmacologic stress testing include dobutamine, vasodilators, or radioactive isotopes that will be visible upon scanning using specific equipment such as single-photon emission computed tomography (SPECT) (Table 14-5).[14,19]

Protocols of Cardiac Stress Testing

Protocols of cardiac stress testing have not changed much over the last decade. Their tried and true approaches have proven successful and repeatable. The purpose of the test and the person tested are important considerations in selecting the protocol. Cardiac stress testing may be performed for diagnostic purposes, for functional assessment, or for risk stratification. An often ignored but

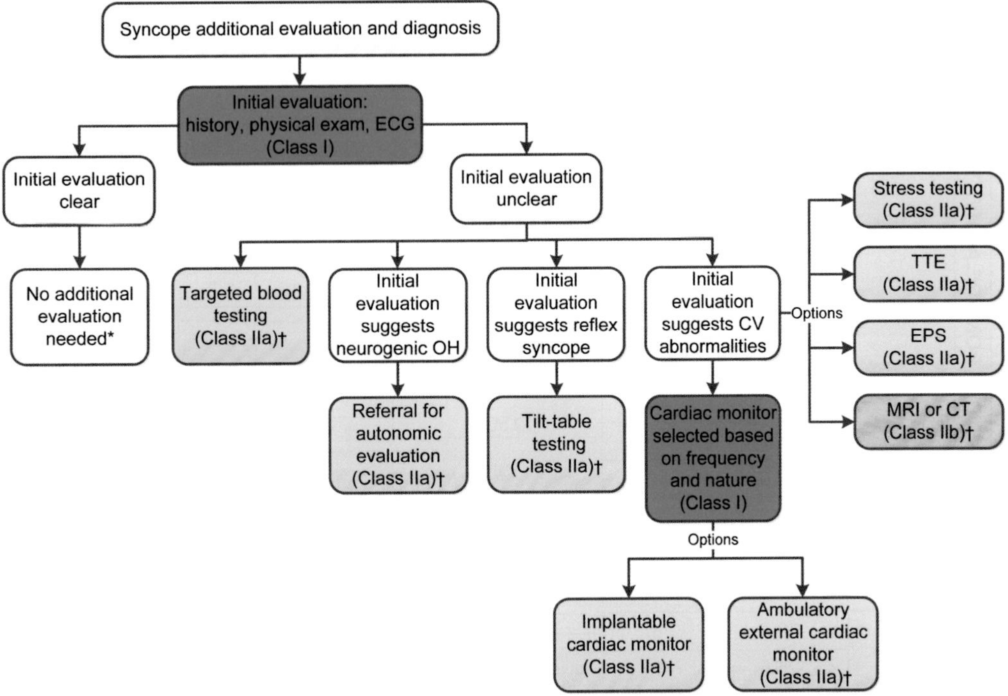

Figure 14-5. ACCF/AHA additional evaluation of syncope guidelines. Additional evaluation and diagnosis for syncope. *Applies to patients after a normal initial evaluation without significant injury or cardiovascular morbidities; patients followed-up by primary care physician as needed. †In selected patients (see full guidelines for description). CT, computed tomography; CV, cardiovascular; ECG, electrocardiogram; EPS, electrophysiologic study; MRI, magnetic resonance imaging; OH, orthostatic hypotension; TTE, transthoracic echocardiography. (Used with permission from Fihn SD, Gardin JM, Abrams J, et al. ACCF/AHA/ACP/AATS/PCNA/SCAI/STS Guideline for the diagnosis and management of patients with stable ischemic heart disease: executive summary. *Circulation.* 2012;126(25):3097–3137.)

Table 14-5 • CHOICE OF PHARMACOLOGIC STRESS TESTS

Factors That Favor Vasodilator Stress Myocardial Perfusion Imaging

- Peripheral vascular disease
- Muscular disorders
- Skeletal disorders
- Neurologic disorders
- Left bundle-branch block
- Electronically paced rhythm
- Chronotropic incompetence
- Inability to achieve exercise endpoints
  - Limited exercise capacity
  - Morbid obesity
  - Poor motivation
  - Poor physical conditioning
  - Pulmonary disease
  - Diabetes mellitus
- Presence of large abdominal aneurysm
- Acute myocardial infarction (within 72 h)
- Percutaneous coronary intervention (within 48–72 h)

Factors that Favor Dobutamine Stress MPI When Exercise Is Not Indicated

- Bronchospasm
- Second- or third-degree heart block without a functioning pacemaker
- Use of dipyridamole, aspirin/dipyridamole (Aggrenox), or aminophylline within the past 24 hours
- Sick sinus syndrome
- Systolic blood pressure <90 mm Hg

Adapted with permission from Iskandrian AE, Garcia EV. *Atlas of Nuclear Cardiology: An Imaging Companion to Braunwald's Heart Disease.* Philadelphia, PA: Elsevier/Saunders; 2012.

nevertheless consistent recommendation in the recent guidelines is that the protocol be individualized for the patient being tested and not standardized across the board.[5,9,25,26] For example, a maximal, symptom-limited test on a relatively demanding protocol would not be appropriate or very informative for a patient with severe limitations. Likewise, a very gradual protocol might not be useful for an apparently healthy, active person. Use of submaximal testing, gas exchange techniques, the presence of a physician or nurse, and the exercise mode and protocol should be determined by considering the person being tested and the goals of the test.

Commonly used exercise protocols, their stages, and the metabolic equivalent task (MET) level (metabolic equivalent is defined as an estimated value representing a multiple of the resting metabolic rate) for each stage is outlined in Figure 14-6. The most suitable protocols for physical clinical testing should include a low-intensity warm-up phase followed by progressive, continuous exercise in which the demand is elevated to a patient's maximal level within a total duration of 8 to 12 minutes.[4,5,9,20,23,25] In the absence of gas exchange techniques, it is important to report exercise capacity in METs rather than exercise time, so that exercise capacity can be compared uniformly between protocols. METs can be estimated from any protocol using standardized equations that have been put into tabular form.[5,9,27] In general, 1 MET represents an increment on the treadmill of approximately 1.0 mph or 2.5% grade. On a cycle ergometer, 1 MET represents an increment of approximately 20 W (120 kg m/min) for a person weighing 70 kg. The assumptions necessary for predicting MET levels from treadmill or cycle ergometer work rates (including not holding the handrails, that oxygen uptake is constant

FUNCTIONAL CLASS	CUNICAL STATUS	O_2 COST ml/kg/min	METS	BICYCLE ERGOMETER	TREADMLL PROTOCOLS: BRUCE MODIFIED 3 min Stages MPH	%GR	BRUCE 3 min Stages MPH	%GR	NAUGHTON 2 mln Stages MPH	%GR	METS
				1 WATT = 6.1 Kpm/min FOR 70 KG BODY WEIGHT kpm/min	6.0	22	6.0	22			
					5.5	20	5.5	20			
					5.0	18	5.0	18			
NORMAL AND I	HEALTHY.DEPENDENT ON AGE.ACTIVITY	56.0	16								16
		52.5	15								15
		49.0	14								14
		45.5	13	1500	4.2	16	4.2	16			13
		42.0	12	1350							12
		38.5	11	1200							11
	SEDENTARY HEALTHY	35.0	10	1050	3.4	14	3.4	14			10
		31.5	9								9
		28.0	8	900					2	17.5	8
	LIMITED	24.5	7	750	2.5	12	2.5	12	2	14.0	7
II	SYMPTOMATIC	21.0	6	600					2	10.5	6
		17.5	5	450	1.7	10	1.7	10	2	7.0	5
III		14.0	4	300	1.7	5			2	3.5	4
		10.5	3						2	0	3
		7.0	2	150	1.7	0			1	0	2
IV		3.5	1								1

Figure 14-6. Relation of exercise workload ($\dot{V}O_2$ and metabolic equivalents [METs]) to stages of the standard Bruce protocol and other treadmill protocols and to stationary bicycle ergometry. Completion of Stage 4 of the Bruce protocol (4.2 mph at a 16% grade) approximates 1500 kpm/min on the bicycle. Functional class refers to New York Heart Association (NYHA) class. Kpm, kilopond-meters; MPH, miles per hour; %GR, percent grade. (Reproduced with permission from Fletcher GF, Balady GJ, Amsterdam EA, et al. Exercise standards for testing and training: a statement for healthcare professionals from the American Heart Association. *Circulation.* 2001;104:1694–1740.)

[i.e., steady-state exercise is performed], that the subject is healthy, and that all people are similar in their walking efficiency) raise uncertainties as to the accuracy of estimating the work performed for an individual patient. For example, the steady-state requirement is rarely met for most patients on most exercise protocols. Most clinical testing is performed among patients with varying degrees of cardiovascular or pulmonary disease; and people vary widely in their walking efficiency.[27] It has therefore been recommended that a patient be ascribed a MET level only for stages in which all or most of a given stage duration has been completed.[28] During pharmacologic testing, dobutamine is infused intravenously at doses that increase every 3 minutes until a maximal dose is reached or a subjective or objective endpoint has been achieved. ECG, HR, and blood pressure are monitored during each stage.[6]

Bruce Treadmill Protocol

The Bruce protocol remains the most widely used method of cardiac stress testing in North America.[29,30] An advantage of using this test is that a great deal of functional and prognostic data have been generated over several decades using the Bruce protocol, and many published normative values have been derived from it. For example, some of the most robust databases on the use of the exercise test for assessing prognosis, such as those from the Coronary Artery Surgery Study (CASS)[31] and the Duke Treadmill Score,[32] were generated from patients who underwent exercise testing using the Bruce protocol. Numerous study authors have shown that participants who are unable to complete the first stage of this protocol (approximately 5 METs) have an extremely poor prognosis, and may need follow-up pharmacologic stress testing.[31,33,34] However, the disadvantages of the Bruce protocol include its large and unequal increments in work, which have been shown to result in less accurate estimates of exercise capacity, particularly for patients with cardiac disease. Investigations have demonstrated that work rate increments that are too large or rapid result in a tendency to overestimate exercise capacity, less reliability for studying the effects of therapy, and possibly even lowered sensitivity for detecting coronary disease.[20,23,25,35,36]

Balke Treadmill Protocol

The Balke protocol and its modifications have been widely used for clinical exercise testing. This protocol uses constant walking speeds (2.0 or 3.0 mph) and modest increments in grade (2.5% or 5.0%), and it has been used particularly often in studies assessing anginal responses. Modifications of the original Balke treadmill protocol have become widespread. One modification, developed by the United States School of Aerospace Medicine (Balke–Ware)[37] consists of 5% grade increases every 2 minutes and a constant brisk walking speed of 3.3 mph (after an initial warm-up of 2.0 mph), which has been considered the most efficient speed for walking. The constant speed is advantageous in that it requires only an initial adaptation in stride. Departing from the standard protocol may hamper reproducible results if the test needed to be repeated.

Naughton Treadmill Protocol

The Naughton treadmill protocol is a low-level test that has become common for multicenter trials in participants with chronic heart failure. The test begins with 2-minute stages at 1 and 2 mph and 0% grade, then continually increases grade in approximately 1-MET increments at a constant speed of 2 mph for the next 8 minutes. As per this protocol, speed then increases to 3 mph with a slight decrease in grade, followed by increases in grade equivalent to approximately 1 MET. The Naughton protocol provides reasonable and gradual work rate increases for patients with more advanced heart disease. Because this protocol has been used extensively in patients with chronic heart failure, it provides a substantial amount of functional and prognostic comparative data. The Naughton test, however, can result in tests of excessive duration among more fit subjects.[38]

Bicycle Ergometer Protocols

Although there are specific bicycle protocols named after early researchers in Europe, such as Astrand and Rodahl,[39] bicycle ergometer protocols tend to be more generalized than those for the treadmill. For example, 15- to 25-Watt increments per 2-minute stage are commonly used for patients with cardiovascular disease, whereas for apparently healthy adults or athletic individuals, appropriate work rate increments might typically be between 40 and 50 Watts per stage. Most modern, electronically braked cycle ergometers have controllers that permit ramp testing in which the work rate increments can be individualized in continuous fashion. A metronome is sometimes used in order to standardize pedal rate in order to not overpedal.

Ramp Testing Protocol

An approach to exercise testing that has gained interest in recent years is the ramp protocol, in which work increases constantly and continuously. In 1981, Whipp et al.[40] first described cardiopulmonary responses to a ramp test on a cycle ergometer. Many of the gas exchange equipment manufacturers now include ramp software. Treadmills have also been adapted to conduct ramp tests.[23,41,42] The ramp protocol uses a constant and continuous increase in metabolic demand that replaces the "staging" used in conventional exercise tests. The uniform increase in work allows for a steady increase in cardiopulmonary responses and permits a more accurate estimation of oxygen uptake.[23] The recent call for "optimizing" exercise testing would appear to be facilitated by the ramp approach, because large work increments are avoided and increases in work are individualized, permitting test duration to be targeted.[5,20,25,28] Because there are no stages per se, the number of errors associated with predicting exercise capacity alluded to previously are lessened.[5,9,23]

Submaximal Testing Protocol

In general, maximal, symptom-limited tests are not considered appropriate until 1 month after MI or surgery. Submaximal tests have been shown to be important in risk stratification[43–45] for making appropriate activity recommendations, for recognizing the need for modification of the medical regimen, or for further interventions in patients who have sustained a cardiac event. Thus, submaximal exercise testing has an important role clinically for predischarge, post-MI, or after coronary artery bypass surgery (CABG) evaluations. A submaximal, predischarge test appears to be as predictive for future events as a symptom-limited test among patients less than 1 month after MI. Submaximal testing is also appropriate for patients with a high probability of serious arrhythmias. The testing endpoints for submaximal testing have traditionally been arbitrary but should always be based on clinical judgment. Since achieving a specific HR may be difficult for some populations, 220 minus the patient's age is often used to assess maximal HR response during testing. Failure to achieve 85% of this rate is considered chronotropic incompetence.[6] For those using beta blocker (β-blockers) pharmacologic therapy, a Borg perceived exertion level in the range of 7 to 8 (1 to 10 scale) or 15 to 16 (6 to 20 scale) are conservative endpoints (Fig. 14-7).[46] The initial onset of symptoms, including fatigue, shortness of breath, or angina, are also indications to stop testing. A low-level protocol should be used, that is, one that uses no more than 1-MET increments per stage. The Naughton protocol[38,47] is commonly used for submaximal testing. Ramp testing is also ideal for this purpose because the ramp rate (such as 5 METs achieved over a 10-minute duration) can be individualized depending on the patient tested.[23]

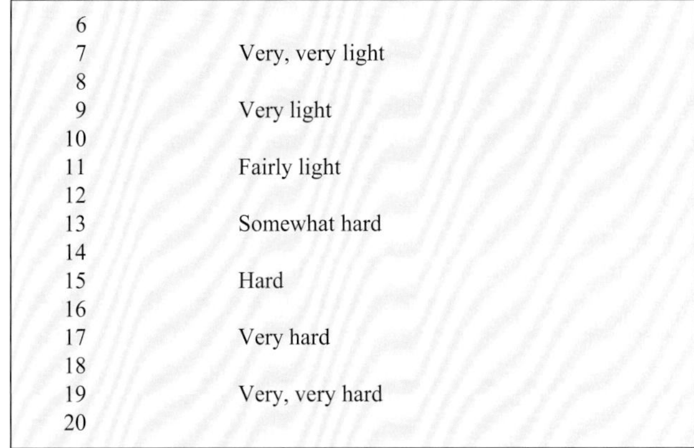

6	
7	Very, very light
8	
9	Very light
10	
11	Fairly light
12	
13	Somewhat hard
14	
15	Hard
16	
17	Very hard
18	
19	Very, very hard
20	

Figure 14-7. Borg rating of perceived exertion scale. (Reproduced with permission from Borg GE. *An Introduction to Borg's RPE-Scale.* Ithaka, NY: Movement Publication; 1985.)

Ancillary Methods for the Detection of CAD

Radionuclide Angiography

The most commonly used technique to evaluate myocardial perfusion is the application of the radionuclide thallium-201. When thallium-201 is injected intravenously at maximal exercise, it is rapidly extracted from the blood by living cells in the myocardium. Uptake of thallium-201 is similar to that of potassium in living cells. Radiologic images are then taken, which reveal areas of absent, poor, or moderately poor uptake of thallium-201. When exercise images are compared with resting images, the differences in uptake of thallium-201 indicate areas of decreased blood flow. At the same time, if areas absent of thallium-201 uptake occur at rest, it can be assumed that this represents areas of myocardial scarring and not ischemia with exercise. This information, along with the exercise test, can be more definitive in the evaluation of the extent and localization of ischemia and prevascularization interventions.[48]

Perfusion imaging with technetium-99m sestamibi has become common practice after an abnormal exercise stress test. This imaging agent permits higher dosing with less radiation exposure than thallium, resulting in improved images that are sharper and have less artifact and attenuation. Sestamibi is the preferred imaging agent for obtaining tomographic images of the heart SPECT imaging. SPECT images are obtained with a gamma camera, which rotates 180 degrees around the patient, stopping at preset angles to record the image. Cardiac images are then displayed in slices from three different axes to allow visualization of the heart in three dimensions (3D). Thus, multiple myocardial segments can be viewed individually, without the overlap of segments that occurs with planar imaging.[49,50] As with thallium-201 imaging, perfusion defects that are present during exercise but not seen at rest suggest ischemia or malperfusion. Perfusion defects that are present during exercise and persist at rest suggest previous MI or scarring of the tissue. In this manner, the extent and distribution of ischemic myocardium can be identified. Because of a very high sensitivity of abnormal stress nuclear imaging studies for detecting patients at risk for perioperative cardiac events, the negative predictive value of a normal scan has remained uniformly high at approximately 99% for MI or cardiac death.[51]

This modality also permits the localization of ischemia, which is not possible with ST-segment depression on the ECG. This technique is especially helpful in patients with equivocal exercise ECGs, those using digoxin, or those with left bundle-branch block, in whom the interpretation of electrocardiographic changes is more problematic.[5,52] Figures 14-8 and 14-9 illustrate an example of the color imaging of SPECT.[53]

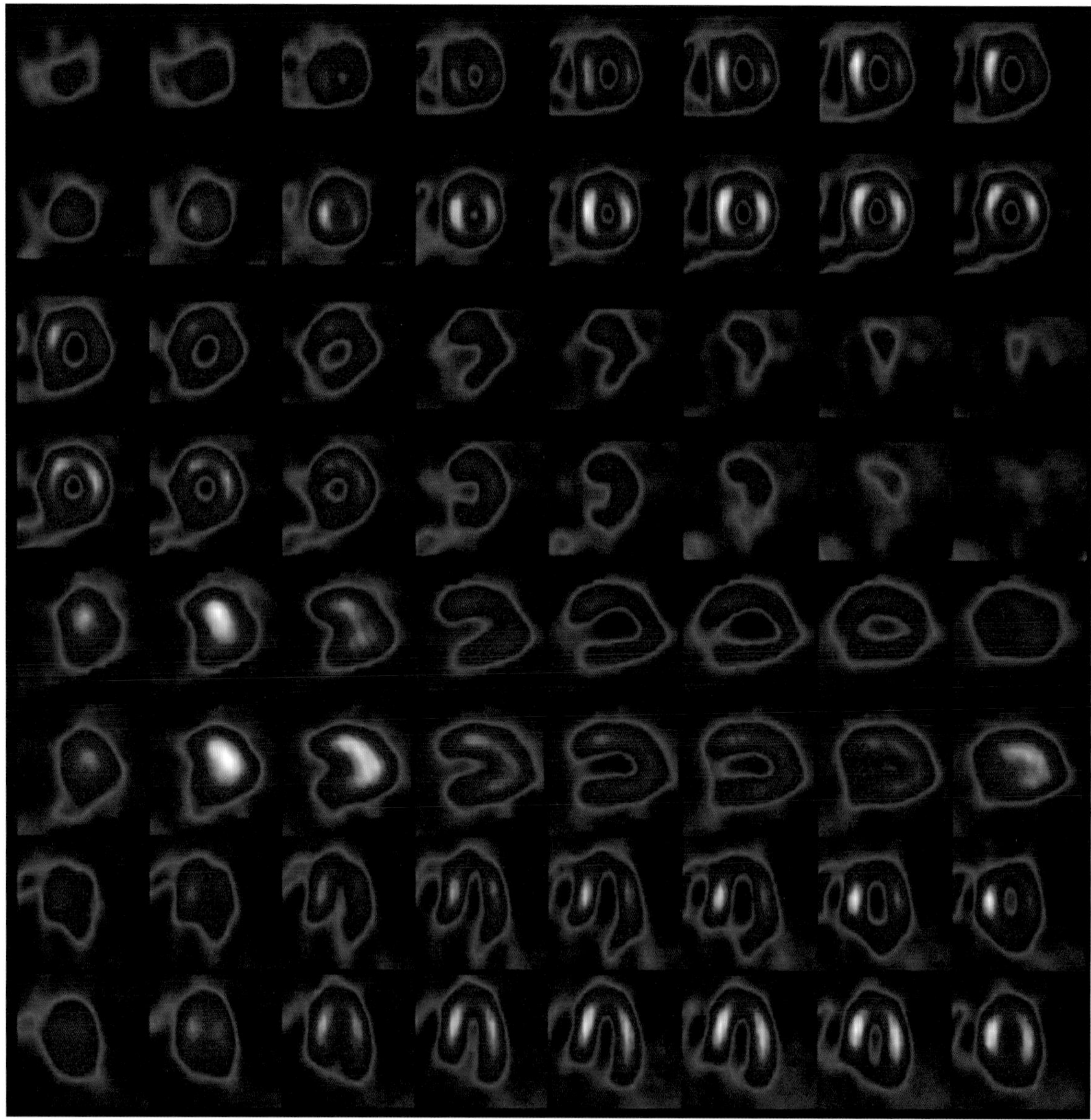

Figure 14-8. SPECT images. The SPECT images show reversible perfusion abnormality in the three vascular territories in image labeled C. (Reproduced with permission from Zoghbi GJ, Iqbal FM, Iskandrian AE. Choice of stress test. In: Iskandrian AE, Garcia EV, eds. *Atlas of Nuclear Cardiology.* Philadelphia, PA: Elsevier Saunders; 2012.)

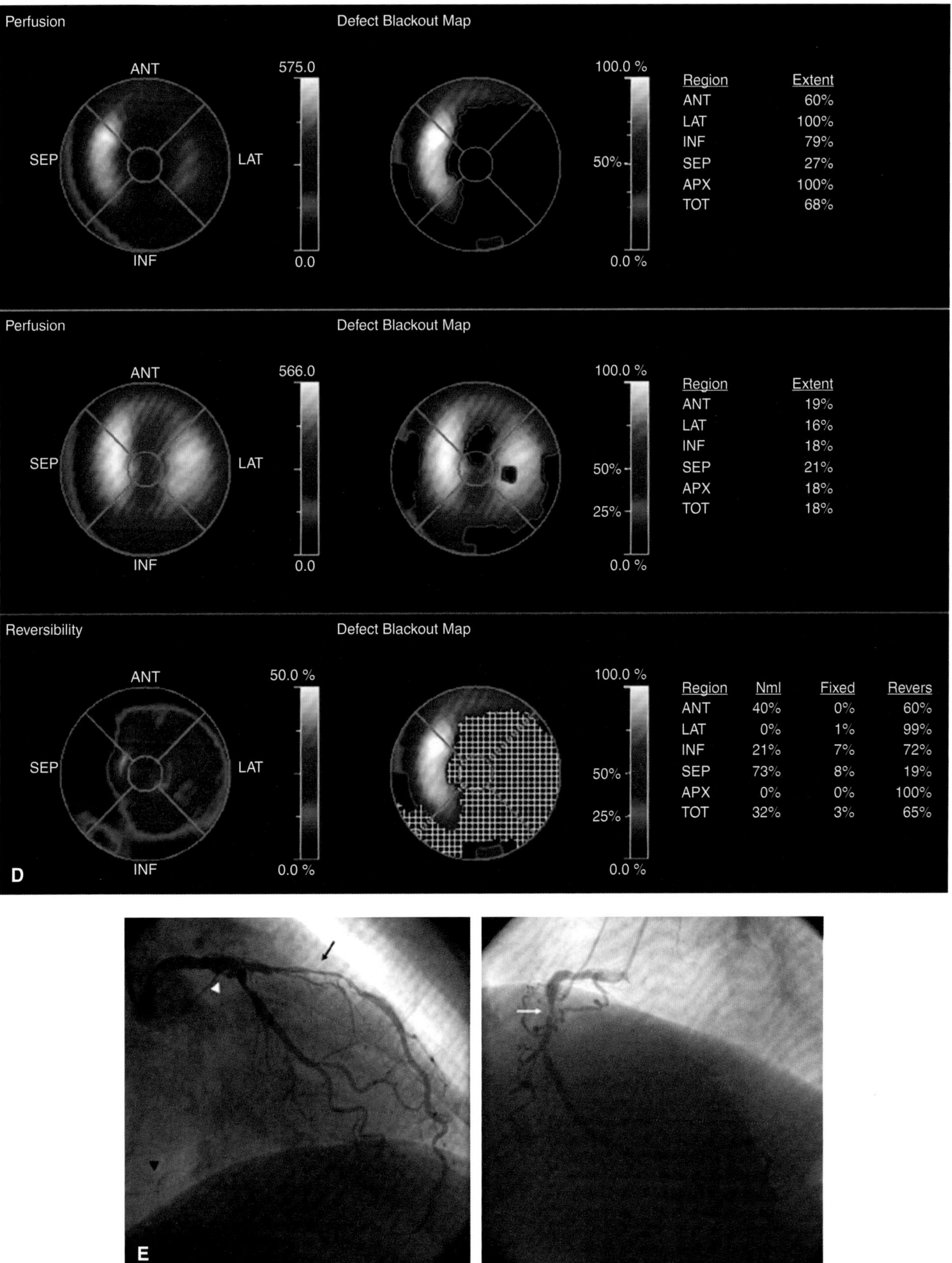

Figure 14-9. SPECT images. SPECT imaging shows the LVEF is normal. The polar maps show a large abnormality in image **D**. Coronary angiography shows severe left anterior descending coronary artery (**LAD**) (*black arrow*), left circumflex coronary artery (**LCX**) (*white arrowhead*), and right coronary artery (**RCA**) stenoses (*white arrow*). Image **E** shows the presence of left-to-right collaterals (*black arrowhead*). (Reproduced with permission from Zoghbi GJ, Iqbal FM, Iskandrian AE. Choice of stress test. In: Iskandrian AE, Garcia EV, eds. *Atlas of Nuclear Cardiology*. Philadelphia, PA: Elsevier Saunders; 2012.)

Pharmacologic Stress Techniques

It is advantageous to use pharmacologic stress techniques for patients who are unable to exercise on a treadmill or cycle ergometer to an adequate level. These include patients who have orthopedic limitations, peripheral vascular disease, and chronic obstructive pulmonary disease (COPD), or other limiting pulmonary diseases; elderly patients with low functional capacity; diabetic patients with severe neuropathy; and patients with neuromuscular conditions.[5,6,8] For these patients, pharmacologic methods can be extremely useful for evaluating coronary blood flow and myocardial function.

Two types of pharmacologic stress agents have been used: (1) those that increase coronary blood flow through coronary vasodilation and (2) those that increase myocardial oxygen demand by increasing the HR. The commonly used coronary vasodilators are adenosine, dipyridamole (Persantine), and Regadenoson (CVT-3146 or Lexiscan). The vasodilators cause greatly increased endocardial and epicardial blood flow in normal coronary arteries but not in stenotic segments. The primary pharmacologic stress agent used to increase myocardial oxygen demand by increasing HR is dobutamine. Dobutamine can create an imbalance between myocardial oxygen supply and demand by increasing HR, as well as contractility. These drugs are administered intravenously and, when associated with an imaging technique such as thallium-201 scintigraphy, sestamibi, or echocardiography, can provide important information about coronary artery stenosis. The disadvantages of dipyridamole and adenosine stress testing include side effects of headache, dizziness, and nausea (40% to 50% of patients have minor side effects) and lack of cardiovascular response (approximately 10% of patients). The main side effects of dobutamine are arrhythmogenicity and hypertension (5% of patients), which are generally well tolerated and self-limiting.[54,55]

Ventricular Function Studies

Ventricular function is commonly evaluated with the use of the radioisotope technetium-99m. This radioisotope is administered as an intravenous bolus, and its transit through the ventricles is measured by special cameras. Technetium-99m is also used to "tag" red blood cells for equilibrium gated blood pool studies in order to evaluate efficacy of cardiac medications as well as assessing atrioventricular sequencing in suspected arrhythmias. Both methods have been used extensively in the evaluation of left and right ventricular function after acute MI and other cardiac events. This technique can be performed at rest as well as at maximal exercise. When performed at maximal exercise, it has the capability of determining decreased ventricular function compared with rest measures. This can help in the diagnosis of ischemic abnormalities as well as exercise-induced ventricular dysfunction. In addition to measures of ejection fraction, measures of specific regional wall motion can also be taken.[49,50,56]

The limitations of thallium, sestamibi, and technetium SPECT imaging include higher cost and exposure of the patient to ionizing radiation. Additional equipment and personnel are also required for image acquisition and interpretation, including a nuclear technician to administer the radioactive isotope and acquire the images and a physician trained in nuclear medicine to reconstruct and interpret the images.

Exercise Echocardiographic Imaging

Echocardiographic imaging of the heart is being increasingly used during exercise and pharmacologic stress testing. This technique is frequently combined with an exercise ECG to increase the sensitivity and specificity of exercise testing. Typically, a two-dimensional image is taken at rest, and repeat images are obtained at peak exercise or immediately afterward. If images are taken after exercise, they must be obtained within 1 to 2 minutes because abnormal wall motion begins to normalize after this point. Rest and stress images are compared side by side in a cine-loop display that is gated during systole from the QRS complex. Myocardial contractility normally increases with exercise, whereas ischemia causes hypokinesis, akinesis, and dyskinesis of the affected segments. Therefore, a test is considered positive if wall motion abnormalities develop in previously normal territories with exercise or worsen in an already abnormal segment.[57]

Some advantages of exercise echocardiography over nuclear imaging include the absence of exposure to ionizing radiation and a shorter amount of time required for testing. Like standard exercise testing and radionuclide techniques, the diagnostic accuracy of echocardiography depends primarily on the specific methodology used and the pretest probability of CAD in the subjects tested. The accuracy of echocardiographic testing also depends on observer experience. Reviews of studies published since the advent of exercise echocardiography in the early 1980s suggest that the average sensitivity and specificity of this technique for detecting coronary disease are both approximately 85%.[58] The limitations of exercise echocardiography include dependence on the operator for obtaining adequate, timely images, and some variation exists in image interpretation. In addition, as many as 20% of patients have inadequate echocardiographic windows secondary to body habitus or lung interference.[59]

Gas Exchange Techniques

Because of the inaccuracies associated with estimating oxygen uptake and METs from work rate (i.e., treadmill speed and grade), many laboratories directly measure expired gases. The measurement of gas exchange and ventilatory responses provides an added dimension to the exercise test by increasing the information obtained concerning a patient's cardiopulmonary function. The direct measurement of $\dot{V}O_2$ has been shown to be more reliable and reproducible than estimated values from treadmill or cycle ergometer work rate.[27] Peak $\dot{V}O_2$ is the most accurate measurement of functional capacity and is a useful reflection of overall cardiopulmonary health. Measurement of expired gases is not considered necessary for all clinical exercise testing, but the additional information provides important physiologic data. Heart and lung diseases frequently manifest themselves through gas exchange abnormalities during exercise, and the information obtained is increasingly used in clinical trials to objectively assess the response to interventions. Moreover, a growing body of literature suggests that exercise capacity measured directly by gas exchange techniques provides superior prognostic information relative to exercise time or estimated METs.[8,27,60] Recent studies have demonstrated that indices of ventilatory inefficiency (e.g., ventilatory equivalents for oxygen ($VE/\dot{V}O_2$) slope, oscillatory breathing patterns, oxygen kinetics) are very powerful predictors of risk for adverse outcomes in patients with heart failure.[8,60] Gas exchange measurements are appropriate in specific scenarios[5,9]:

1. When a precise response to a specific therapeutic intervention is needed for a particular patient
2. When a research question is being addressed
3. When the cause of exercise limitation or dyspnea is uncertain
4. To evaluate exercise capacity in patients with heart failure to assist in the estimation of prognosis and assess the need for transplantation

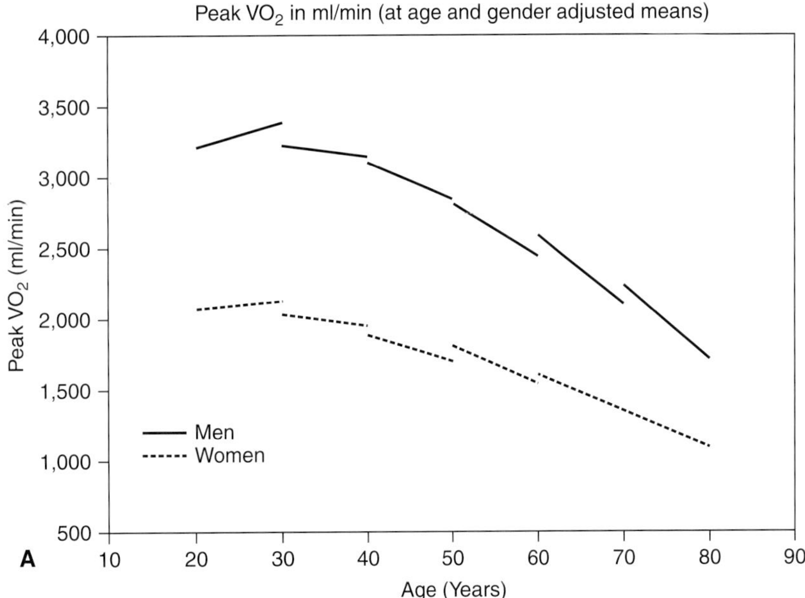

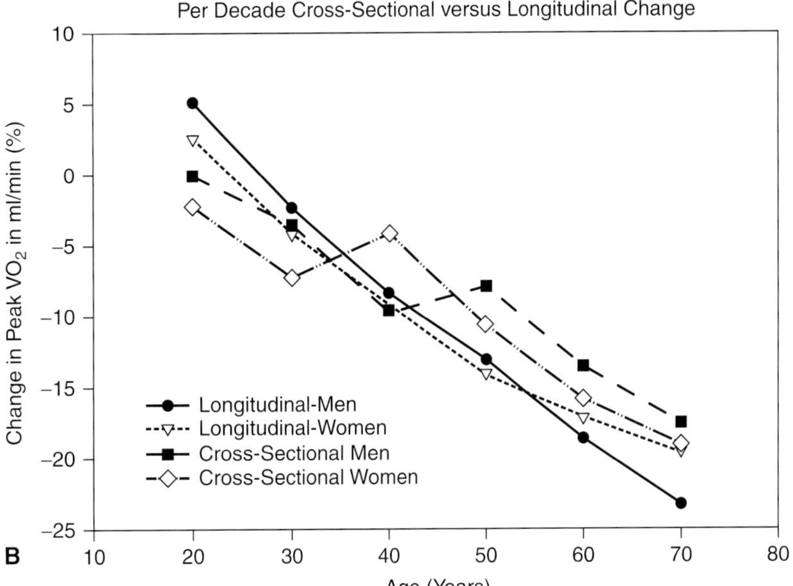

Figure 14-10. Cross-sectional and longitudinal changes in peak $\dot{V}O_2$ in milliliters per minute by gender and age decade. **A:** The per-decade longitudinal change in peak $\dot{V}O_2$ for age decades from the 20s through the 70s, predicted from a mixed-effects linear regression model. Note the progressively steeper decline in peak $\dot{V}O_2$ with successive age decades, particularly in men, leading to near convergence of peak $\dot{V}O_2$ in men and women at extreme old age. **B:** Per-decade percent cross-sectional and longitudinal changes in peak $\dot{V}O_2$ by gender and age decade, derived from the mixed-effects model. Note that both longitudinal and cross-sectional declines in peak $\dot{V}O_2$ steepen with age. However, from the 50s onward, longitudinal declines in peak $\dot{V}O_2$ are substantially larger than cross-sectional declines. (Reproduced with permission from Fleg JL, Morrell CH, Bos AG, et al. Accelerated longitudinal decline of aerobic capacity in healthy older adults. *Circulation*. 2005;112[5]:674–682.)

5. To assist in the development of an appropriate exercise prescription for cardiac rehabilitation

The use of these techniques, however, requires added attention to detail and a working knowledge of the equipment and basic physiology. This is particularly important given advances in automation for the collection and calculation of expired gases. Figure 14-10 illustrates the cross-sectional and longitudinal changes in peak $\dot{V}O_2$ in milliliters per minute by gender and age decade.[61]

TEST INTERPRETATION

The important exercise test responses that should be monitored and recorded are HR, blood pressure, electrocardiographic changes, exercise capacity, and subjective responses, including chest discomfort, undue fatigue, shortness of breath, leg pain, and rating of perceived exertion (RPE). Each of these responses should be described in a comprehensive test report following stress testing. Useful programs have been developed that automatically summarize the test responses and apply published regression equations that report pretest and posttest risks of CAD, and some provide mortality estimates.[62] An example of one such report is presented in Table 14-6.

Heart Rate

HR increases linearly with oxygen uptake during exercise. Of the two major components of cardiac output, HR and stroke volume, HR is responsible for most of the increase in cardiac output during exercise, particularly at higher levels of exertion. Thus, maximal HR achieved is a major determinant of exercise capacity.[52,63,64] The inability to appropriately increase HR during exercise (chronotropic incompetence) has been associated with the presence of

Table 14-6 • EXAMPLE OF AN AUTOMATED EXERCISE TEST SUMMARY REPORT WITH DIAGNOSTIC AND PROGNOSTIC PROBABILITIES GENERATED FROM A COMPUTER PROGRAM

Pretest Information

This patient is a 74-year-old active, White, male outpatient 70-in tall, weighing 180 lb, who underwent a treadmill test on April 12, 2001. This exercise test was performed to evaluate symptoms/signs of possible heart disease or elevated risk factors.

Current Cardiac Medications

The patient is not taking any cardiac medications.

Medical History

The patient has the following symptoms: uncertain chest pain. The patient has no history of dysrhythmias.

Risk Factors

The patient is currently not smoking but has 15 pack year history of smoking. The patient is 8 lb over the average appropriate body mass index. Other risk factors include low high-density lipoprotein level (31 mg/dL) and noninsulin-dependent diabetes mellitus.

History of Cardiac Events

No previous MI. No bypass surgery performed. No percutaneous transluminal coronary angioplasty performed. No catheterization performed.

Resting ECG

The resting ECG is abnormal because of the following: left ventricular hypertrophy. The ejection fraction is approximately 45% based on the resting ECG.

Pulmonary Function

Forced vital capacity was 3.4 L (90.4% of expected), and the forced expiratory volume in 1 s was 76.2% of expected (normal is >75%).

Exercise Test Information

Exercise Capacity

The patient achieved 4.3 estimated METs and 4.1 measured METs at a perceived exertion level of 18 of 20 on the Borg scale. The test was terminated because of ST changes.

Hemodynamic Data	*Heart Rate (bpm)*	*Blood Pressure (mm Hg)*	*Double Product (× 1000)*
Resting:	65	146/70	9.5
At Max Exercise:	116	122/70	14.1

Chest Pain

Typical angina occurred during exercise.

Exercise ECG Response

The resting ECG shows no ST depression in V_5.

At maximal exercise, the ST-segments showed 3.0 mm of downsloping depression in the lateral and inferior leads. In recovery, the ST segments showed 3.0 mm of downsloping depression in the lateral and inferior leads. No significant dysrhythmias occurred in response to exercise. No bundle-branch blocks or conduction defects were present at rest or developed during exercise.

Conclusions

ST segments exhibited abnormal depression during exercise and abnormal depression in recovery (abnormal ST response).

Exertional hypotension occurred (systolic blood pressure dropped below pretest standing SBP).

The exertional hypotension could be due to ischemia (ST depression).

The patient achieved 66% of normal exercise capacity for age and 80% of normal maximal heart rate for age.

The patient has a high probability of having severe CAD.

Estimated prognosis from treadmill scores may be worse than expected for age, sex, and race.

Prognostic Addendum

Cardiovascular Mortality Prediction

The Framingham score (age, sex, cholesterol, diabetes, smoking, left ventricular hypertrophy, SBP) estimates a 5-yr incidence of cardiovascular events (angina, MI, or death) of 11% (as expected for age and gender). For comparison with the treadmill scores, the age-expected annual mortality rate from any cause is 5.1% (National Center for Health Statistics, 1990).

The Duke score (METs, ST depression, and angina) estimates an annual cardiovascular mortality of 9.5% (approximately two times the age-expected mortality). The VA score (METs, congestive heart failure, SBP rise, and ST depression) estimates an annual cardiovascular mortality of 15.7% (three times the age-expected mortality).

Angiographic CAD Prediction

The patient has no recorded history of coronary disease. Pretest probabilities for any significant coronary disease are 50% (CASS, 1981 [chest pain, age, gender]), 71% (Morise, 1992), and 51% (Do/Froelicher, 1997,1998). Pretest probabilities for severe coronary disease are 22% (Pryor, 1993), 52% (Morise, 1992), and 17% (Do/Froelicher, 1997,1998).

The posttest probabilities for any clinically significant CAD are 99% (Detrano, 1992), 98% (Morise, 1992), and 94% (Do/Froelicher, 1997,1998) due to age, diabetes mellitus, symptoms, and abnormal ST depression.

The probabilities of having severe CAD are 75% (Detrano, 1992) due to abnormal ST depression, 91% (Morise, 1992) due to age abnormal ST depression, and 74% (Do/Froelicher, 1997,1998) due to abnormal ST depression.

Operative Mortality Prediction

If the patient would be selected for nonemergent bypass surgery and no renal dysfunction was present, the estimated operative morality rates are 9% (Parsonnet, 1989), 2% (NY State Department of Health, 1992), and 3% (VA, 1993). This is partially based on an estimated EF of 45%, so compare with measured EF.

Disclaimer: This report was computer generated and the results are dependent on rules and correct data entry. It must be overread by a physician.

EF, ejection fraction; ECG, electrocardiographic; METs, metabolic equivalents; SBP, systolic blood pressure.

From Froelicher VF. *Exercise Test Reporting Aid (EXTRA) Software*. St. Louis, MO: Mosby-Year Book; 1996.

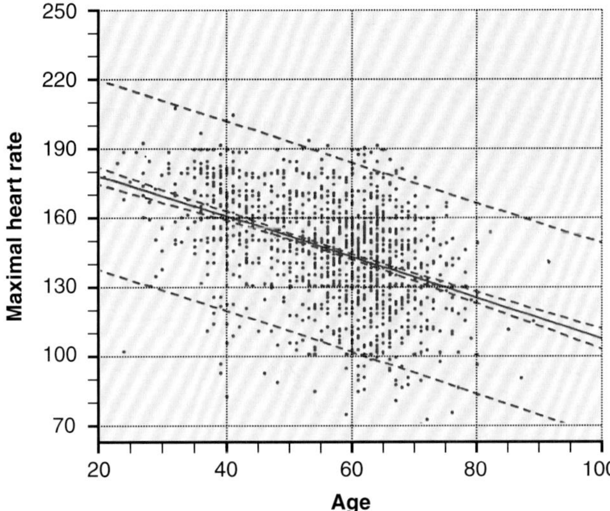

Figure 14-11. The relationship between maximal heart rate and age among patients referred for exercise testing. *Inner lines* represent the standard error; *outer lines* represent 95% confidence limits. (Reproduced with permission from Morris CK, Myers J, Froelicher VF, et al. Nomogram based on metabolic equivalents and age for assessing aerobic exercise capacity in men. *J Am Coll Cardiol.* 1994;22:175–182.)

heart disease and a worse prognosis.[63–65] Although maximal HR has been difficult to explain physiologically,[66] it is affected by age, gender, health, type of exercise, body position, blood volume, and environment. Of these factors, age is the most important. There is an inverse relationship between maximal HR and age. However, the scatter around the regression line is quite large, with standard deviations ranging from 10 to 15 beats per minute (bpm) (Fig. 14-11).[67] Thus, age-predicted "target" maximal HR is a limited measurement for clinical purposes and should not be used as an endpoint for exercise testing.[5,9,52,64]

Blood Pressure

Assessment of systolic and diastolic blood pressure at rest and during the exercise test is important for patient safety and can provide important diagnostic and prognostic information. Properly trained personnel can obtain accurate and reliable blood pressures using noninvasive auscultatory techniques, and guidelines have been developed for this purpose.[66] Blood pressure should be measured at rest before the test in both the supine and standing positions. Blood pressure at rest, when measured before an exercise test, may be elevated compared with normal resting conditions because of pretest anxiety. Uncontrolled hypertension is a relative contraindication to exercise testing.[5,6,9] However, if blood pressure is elevated because of anxiety, it is not uncommon or of concern to observe a slight decrease in blood pressure during the initial stage of an exercise test when the workloads are light.

The increase in systolic blood pressure during exercise reflects the inotropic reserve of the left ventricle. Systolic and diastolic blood pressure should be assessed during the last minute of each exercise stage and more frequently if hypotensive or hypertensive responses are observed. Normally, systolic blood pressure increases in parallel with an increase in work rate, and it is not uncommon in healthy people to exceed 200 mm Hg. In general, a value above 250 mm Hg is an indication to terminate the exercise test.[5,9] Diastolic pressure normally stays the same or increases slightly during exercise. The fifth Korotkov sound, however, can be frequently heard all the way to zero in a young, healthy person.[68] A diastolic blood pressure exceeding 115 mm Hg is an indication to terminate the exercise test.[5,9] A decrease in systolic blood pressure with progressive exercise suggests cardiac output is unable to increase in accordance with the work rate and is usually a reflection of severe ischemia. If systolic blood pressure appears to decrease, it should be remeasured immediately. If the decrease in systolic blood pressure is confirmed, the test should be terminated. The clinical consequences of abnormal blood pressure responses to exercise range from moderate to severe in which decreases in systolic blood pressure have been associated with ventricular fibrillation in the laboratory.[44,69,70] Dubach et al.[71–73] have observed that systolic blood pressure must drop below the standing resting value to be prognostically valuable, whereas others have suggested that more modest decreases, in the order of 10 to 20 mm Hg, are associated with severe ischemia, left ventricular impairment, a high incidence of future cardiac events, or all three.

Troponin

Circulating troponin is a quantifiable predictor of cardiac stress during testing. This lab value may be obtained if a person has had a symptomatic or objective response to stress testing. These values should be obtained while the patient is resting after testing is complete. If a person's troponin level continues to rise as well as there is a marked change in ST-segments, cardiac catheterization may be the next reasonable intervention for this patient as active ischemia may be occurring.[5,51]

Exercise Capacity

Exercise capacity can be an extremely important test response to document because it has important implications concerning the efficacy of current therapies, the assessment of disability, and risk stratification. A patient's exercise capacity says a great deal about overall cardiovascular health. Although subjective, the Borg Perceived Exertion Scale is helpful for assessing exercise effort (Fig. 14-7),[46] good judgment on the part of the physician remains the most effective criterion for terminating exercise.

The most accurate method of measuring exercise capacity is with the use of ventilatory gas exchange techniques, but this requires specialized equipment and is not available in many clinical testing sites. Exercise capacity is therefore usually objectively expressed as exercise duration, watts achieved (on a bicycle ergometer), maximal exercise stage, or METs. In the absence of gas exchange techniques, it is preferable to express exercise capacity in METs rather than exercise time. This is because a MET value can be ascribed to any speed and grade on a treadmill or workload achieved on a cycle ergometer; therefore, exercise capacity can be compared uniformly between protocols.

As mentioned previously in the discussion on protocols, there can be a great deal of uncertainty in predicting a person's energy cost from the treadmill or cycle ergometer workload. How accurately a MET level predicts a person's true oxygen uptake depends on several factors. For most patients with cardiovascular or pulmonary disease, there is a substantial overprediction of the MET level.[9,23,27,74] The error associated with this prediction is accentuated when rapidly incremented protocols are used, when patients are unaccustomed to walking on a treadmill or pedaling a cycle ergometer, and when patients are allowed to use handrail support.[9,27,74]

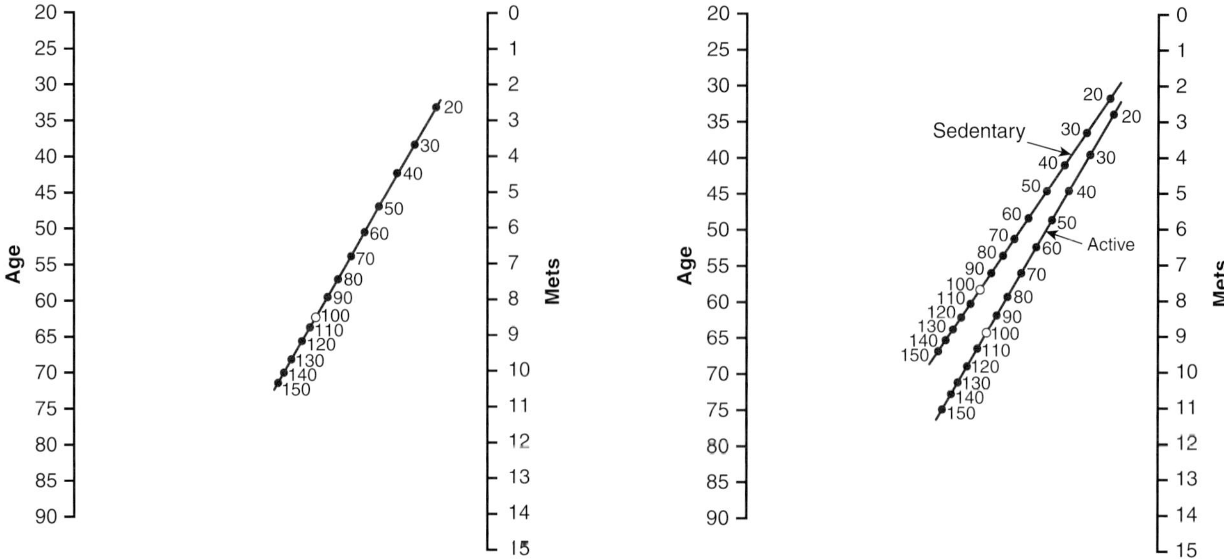

Figure 14-12. Nomogram of percentage normal exercise capacity for age in 1388 male veterans referred for exercise testing (based on metabolic task equivalents [METs]). (Reproduced with permission from Morris CK, Myers J, Froelicher VF, et al. Nomogram based on metabolic equivalents and age for assessing aerobic exercise capacity in men. *J Am Coll Cardiol.* 1994;22:175–182.)

Figure 14-13. Nomogram of percentage normal exercise capacity for age among active and sedentary men referred for exercise testing (based on metabolic equivalents [METs]). (Reproduced with permission from Morris CK, Myers J, Froelicher VF, et al. Nomogram based on metabolic equivalents and age for assessing aerobic exercise capacity in men. *J Am Coll Cardiol.* 1994;22:175–182.)

Exercise capacity should be expressed as both an absolute value and as a relative percentage of normal reference values for age and gender. The latter can be important because exercise capacity declines with increasing age and higher values are observed in men. Thus, when measuring or estimating oxygen uptake or MET levels, it is useful to have reference values for comparison. Normal reference values can facilitate communication with patients and between physicians regarding levels of exercise capacity in relation to a given patient's peers. Figures 14-12 and 14-13 are illustrations of nomograms for male patients referred for exercise testing. Expressing relative exercise capacity using a nomogram is advantageous because it offers a simple visual method of classifying a patient's response, without having to make cumbersome calculations from a particular regression equation. However, there are numerous available regression equations for "normal." All are population specific, and numerous factors affect a person's exercise tolerance other than age and gender, including height, weight, body composition, activity status, and exercise test mode used, in addition to many clinical factors such as smoking history, heart disease, and medications.[27,75]

Electrocardiographic Responses

In patients with CAD, exercise can cause an imbalance between myocardial oxygen supply and demand (ischemia), which can result in an alteration (decrease or elevation relative to the baseline) in the ST segment of the ECG. These changes are the foundation of the exercise test clinically. Normal and abnormal ST-segment responses to exercise are illustrated in Figure 14-14. Ever since electrocardiographic changes were first associated with myocardial ischemia in the 1920s, the diagnostic electrocardiographic criteria and leads that exhibit abnormalities during exercise have been the

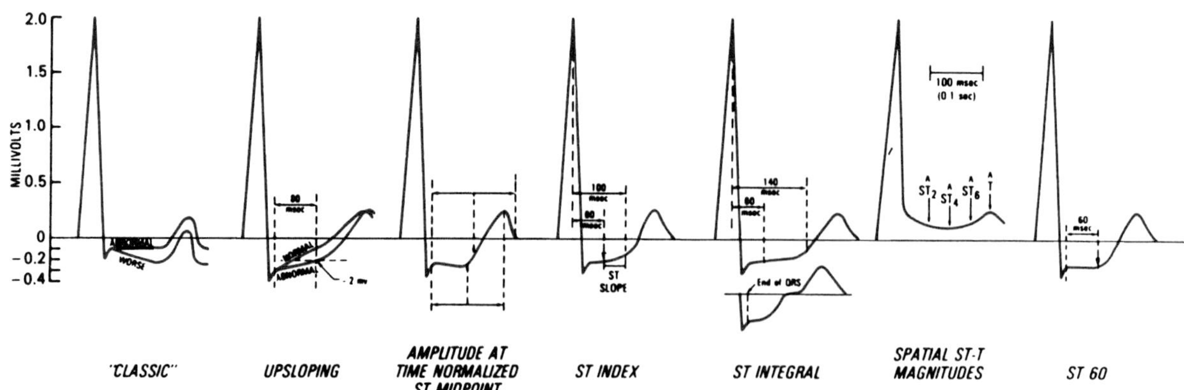

Figure 14-14. Normal and abnormal ST-segment responses to exercise and the various criteria for ST-segment depression. (Reproduced with permission from Froelicher VF, Myers J. *Exercise and the Heart.* 5th ed. Philadelphia, PA: W.B. Saunders; 2006.)

Figure 14-15. Example of exercise-induced ST-segment elevation when the resting electrocardiogram is normal (*left*) and when the resting ECG has a diagnostic Q wave (*right*).

source of significant debate. Numerous electrocardiographic criteria, including complex mathematical constructs, combined scores, and ST areas during exercise and recovery have been proposed to optimally diagnose the presence of CAD. Few of these studies, however, have followed accepted rules for evaluating a diagnostic test.[76] Virtually every edition of exercise testing guidelines that has been published suggests the application of a traditional diagnostic criterion that dictates: 1.0 mm or greater ST-segment depression that is horizontal or downsloping 60 to 80 milliseconds after the J-point (a "positive" response). ST-segment depression greater than 1.0 mm that is downsloping is generally indicative of more severe CAD. Most (approximately 90%) ischemic ST changes occur in the lateral precordial leads.[5] Although it has historically been thought that the diagnostic performance of the test was incomplete without all 12 leads, some evidence suggests that ST-segment changes isolated to the inferior leads frequently may be causes for false-positive responses.[77]

The significance of ST-segment elevation depends on the presence or absence of Q waves. When ST elevation occurs in the presence of a normal resting ECG, it is usually indicative of severe transmural ischemia, it can be arrhythmogenic, and it localizes the ischemia. Conversely, exercise-induced ST-segment elevation occurring in leads with Q waves is more common and is related to the presence of dyskinetic areas. This response is relatively common in patients after an MI and is of much less concern. Examples of these two responses are illustrated in Figure 14-15.

There are several important nuances concerning the proper measurement of exercise-induced ST-segment changes. ST-segment depression is measured as a change from the isoelectric line (PR segment) and is considered abnormal if the next 60 to 80 milliseconds after the J-point are flat or downsloping (see Fig. 14-14). However, in patients who exhibit ST-segment depression at rest, exercise-induced ST-segment depression is measured from the baseline (resting) level (Fig. 14-16). In contrast, ST-segment elevation is measured from the level at which the ST segment starts, and slope is not considered. The significance of upsloping or horizontal ST-segment depression with T-wave inversion has been debated in the literature. Infarction, ventricular aneurysm, bundle-branch block, hypokalemia, ventricular hypertrophy, abnormal oxygen-carrying capacity of blood caused by anemia, pulmonary disease, and drugs such as digoxin and quinidine may all influence the ST-segment response. These and other conditions may cause exercise-induced ST-segment depression that is not caused by CAD (see section titled "False-Positive and False-Negative Responses"). An example of an ECG obtained during stress testing is depicted in Figure 14-17.

Arrhythmias During Exercise Testing

Arrhythmias can occur during the exercise test or recovery period and can range in severity from life threatening to benign. There has been a great deal of debate about the importance of arrhythmias during exercise. The occurrence of "serious" arrhythmias during exercise, although rare, is an indication to terminate the exercise test. Arrhythmias may be overt, such as ventricular tachycardia, or subtle, such as unifocal premature

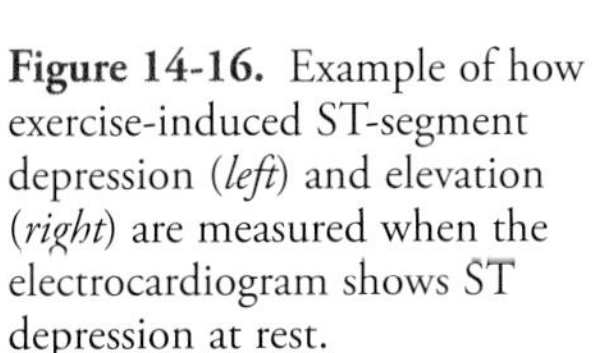

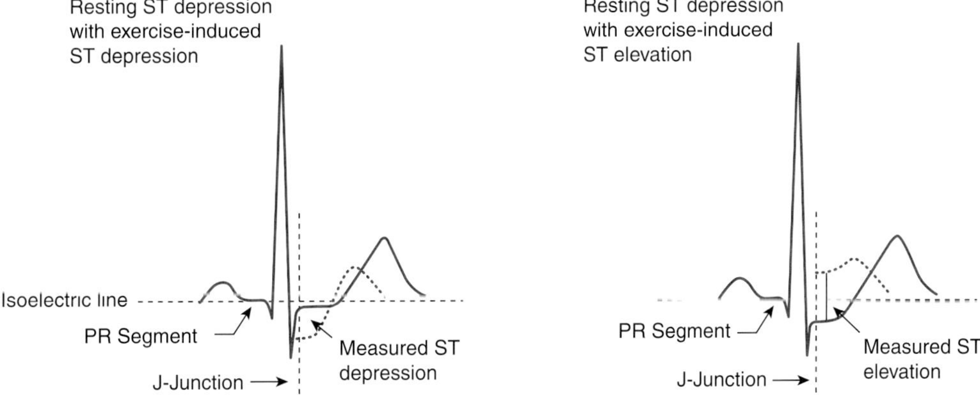

Figure 14-16. Example of how exercise-induced ST-segment depression (*left*) and elevation (*right*) are measured when the electrocardiogram shows ST depression at rest.

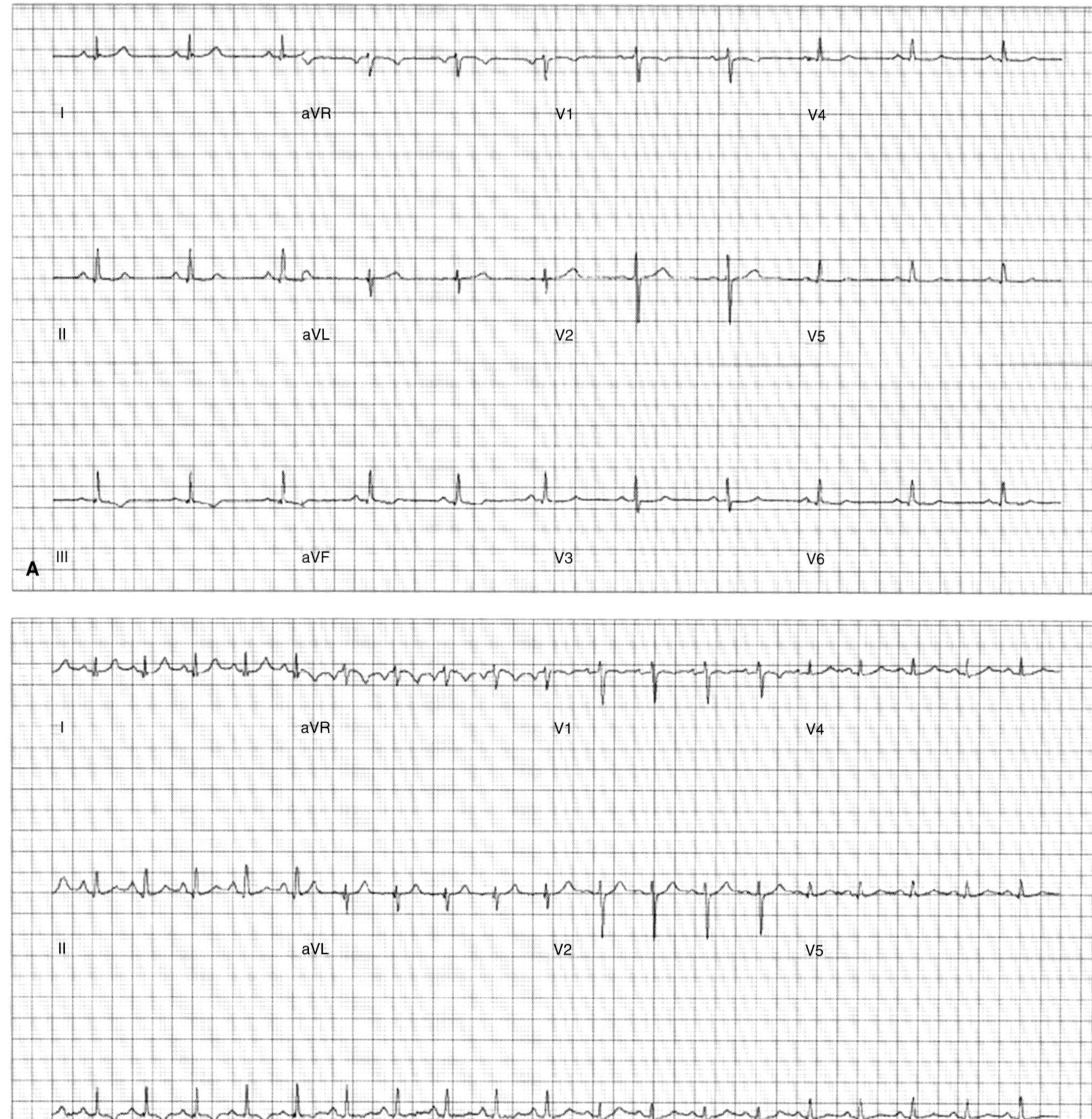

Figure 14-17. ECG. **Image A** shows a patient's ECG at rest. **Image B** shows the ECG at peak exercise with a normal response with no ST changes. Therefore, this ECG did not show any ischemia. (Reproduced with permission from Zoghbi GJ, Iqbal FM, Iskandrian AE. Choice of stress test. In: Iskandrian AE, Garcia EV, eds. *Atlas of Nuclear Cardiology*. Philadelphia, PA: Elsevier Saunders; 2012.)

ventricular contractions (PVCs) increasing in frequency, or a period of supraventricular tachycardia. Arrhythmias for which there should be no debate about stopping the test include second- or third-degree heart block and ventricular tachycardia of any duration. Other arrhythmias that have been generally classified as "significant" or "complex" include R-on-T PVCs, frequent unifocal or multifocal PVCs (constituting 30% or more of the bpm), and coupling of PVCs (two in succession).[5,9] On rare occasion, any of these complex arrhythmias can be a precursor to a life-threatening sustained rhythm disturbance. When there is doubt as to the nature or origin of the arrhythmia, the test should be stopped. Electrophysiologic testing is commonly used to more fully evaluate complex arrhythmias and direct appropriate treatment.

The prognostic significance of exercise-induced PVCs, even when they occur frequently, has varied widely in the literature. This variation is most likely due to differences in how exercise-induced arrhythmias have been defined. Some studies have demonstrated that the occurrence of PVCs during an exercise test has minimal prognostic impact and should be interpreted in the context of "the company they keep,"[5,78] such that the decision to terminate the test should be made on the basis of the patient's history and whether the patient remains hemodynamically stable or the arrhythmias are accompanied by symptoms. Other studies have shown a clear association between PVCs that occur during exercise, recovery, or both, and increased mortality.[52,79–81] An example of an ischemic ECG is depicted in Figure 14-18.

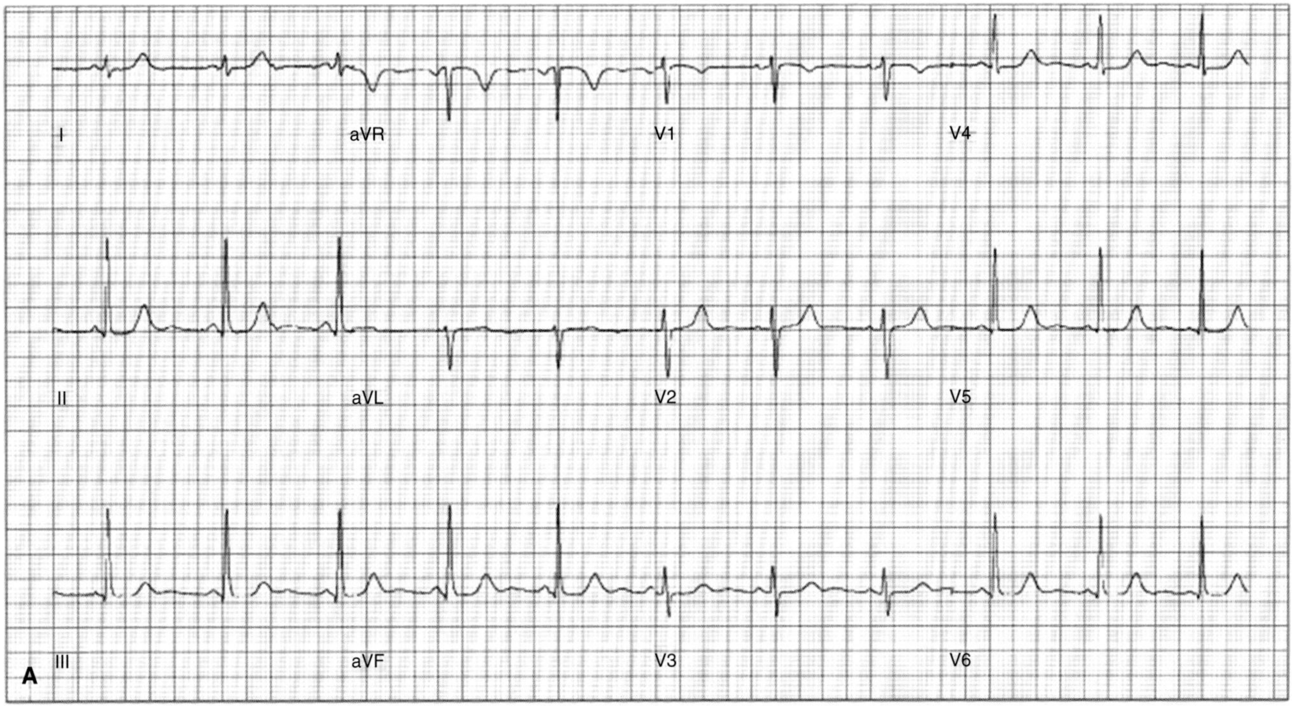

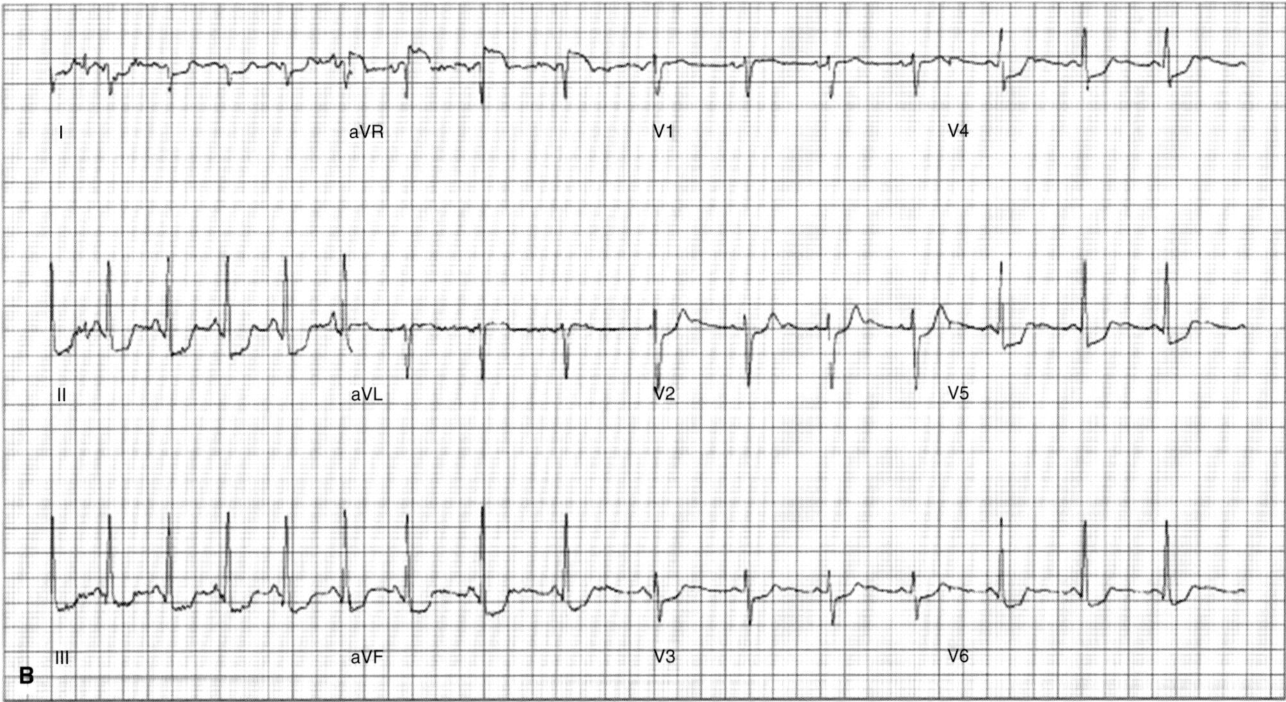

Figure 14-18. ECG. **Image A** shows a patient's ECG at rest. **Image B** shows the ECG at peak exercise with ST depression indicative of an ischemic response. (Reproduced with permission from Zoghbi GJ, Iqbal FM, Iskandrian AE. Choice of stress test. In: Iskandrian AE, Garcia EV, eds. *Atlas of Nuclear Cardiology*. Philadelphia, PA: Elsevier Saunders; 2012.)

Table 14-7 • ANGINA AND DYSPNEA SCALES

Angina Scale	
1+	Onset of discomfort
2+	Moderate, bothersome
3+	Moderately severe
4+	Severe; most pain ever experienced
Dyspnea Scale	
1+	Mild, noticeable to patient but not observer
2+	Mild, some difficulty, noticeable to observer
3+	Moderate difficulty, but can continue
4+	Severe difficulty, patient cannot continue

Subjective Responses

Assessment of symptoms and perception of effort during the exercise test are important to maximize safety, and these subjective measures yield valuable diagnostic information. Obtaining careful assessments of subjective measures during the stress test requires thorough explanations to ensure that the patient understands what is expected and how to communicate these responses to those conducting the test. Angina and dyspnea are the most common cardiopulmonary symptoms elicited during exercise and each is typically evaluated using a four-point scale (Table 14-7).[9,82] These scales should be carefully explained to the patient before the exercise test. Patients should be encouraged to report any and all symptoms during the test.

It is important to distinguish between typical and atypical angina, because they have quite different diagnostic implications. Typical angina tends to be consistent in its presentation and location, is brought on by physical or emotional stress, and is relieved by rest or nitroglycerin. Atypical angina refers to pain that has an unusual location, prolonged duration, or inconsistent precipitating factors that are unresponsive to nitroglycerin. Exercise-induced chest discomfort that has the characteristics of stable, typical angina provides better confirmation of the presence of significant CAD than any other test response. A patient exhibiting the combination of typical angina and an abnormal ST response has a 98% probability of having significant CAD. An important indication to stop the exercise test is moderately severe angina (level 3 on a scale of 1 to 4; see Table 14-7), which should correspond with pain that would normally cause the patient to stop daily activities or take a sublingual nitroglycerin pill.[25,82]

Dyspnea may be the predominant symptom in some patients with CAD, but it is more often associated with reduced left ventricular function or COPD. In both conditions, it may be the predominant factor causing poor exercise capacity. Dyspnea is also commonly quantified using a scale of 1 to 4 (Table 14-7). Claudication is indicative of peripheral vascular disease. If peripheral vascular disease is known or suspected, pretest determination of the presence and strength of peripheral pulses should be made so that posttest comparisons are possible. Leg fatigue not related to claudication is often experienced at maximum exercise; a careful distinction should be made between these two symptoms.

Dizziness and light-headedness may reflect cerebral hypoxia and may coincide with a feeling of exhaustion at maximum exercise. Light-headedness can also be a sign of left ventricular dysfunction or hypotension. Dizziness may be accompanied by signs of gray or ashen pallor, diaphoresis, ataxic gait, dyspnea, and strained appearance as blood is maximally shunted to the exercising muscles. These signs and symptoms may also be observed during pharmacologic stress testing as the cardiopulmonary system is being taxed via a different method. Trained observers should be able to recognize these responses and make a determination as to when the test should be stopped.

Termination of Exercise Testing

The usual goal of the exercise test in patients with known or suspected disease is to achieve a maximal level of exertion. This permits the greatest information yield from the test. However, achieving a maximal effort should be superseded by any of the clinical indications to stop the test (Table 14-8), by clinical judgment, or by the patient's request to stop. The reason for stopping the test should be carefully recorded because the symptoms or signs manifested by exercise often relate to the mechanism of impairment. Determining the endpoint of an exercise test can be problematic. It requires integration of objective physiologic data and termination criteria with subjective judgment based on clinical experience. Some patients may be unable or unwilling to exercise to an adequate level. In patients with suspected coronary disease, a symptom-limited, maximal test is usually more diagnostic. Thus, patients should be instructed to exercise to the point at which they can no longer continue because of fatigue, dyspnea, or other symptoms. They should be informed that the test will be terminated if abnormal responses are observed by the test proctors. Although patients should be encouraged to exercise as long as possible, they should not be pushed beyond their capacity and any request to stop the test should be honored. Inability to fully

Table 14-8 • INDICATIONS FOR STOPPING AN EXERCISE TEST

Absolute

- Drop in systolic blood pressure of >10 mm Hg from baseline despite an increase in workload, when accompanied by other evidence of ischemia
- Moderate to severe angina
- Increasing nervous system symptoms (e.g., ataxia, dizziness, or syncope)
- Signs of poor perfusion (cyanosis or pallor)
- Technical difficulties in monitoring electrocardiogram or systolic blood pressure
- Subject's desire to stop
- Sustained ventricular tachycardia
- ST elevation (≥1.0 mm) in leads without diagnostic Q waves (other than V_1 or aVR)

Relative

- Drop in systolic blood pressure of ≥10 mm Hg from baseline blood pressure despite an increase in workload, in the absence of other evidence of ischemia
- ST or QRS changes such as excessive ST depression (>2 mm of horizontal or downsloping ST-segment depression) or marked axis shift
- Arrhythmias other than sustained ventricular tachycardia, including multifocal PVCs, triplets of PVCs, supraventricular tachycardia, heart block, or bradyarrhythmias
- Fatigue, shortness of breath, wheezing, leg cramps, or claudication
- Development of bundle-branch block or intraventricular conduction delay that cannot be distinguished from ventricular tachycardia
- Increasing chest pain
- Hypertensive response[a]

[a]In the absence of definitive evidence, the Committee suggests systolic blood pressure of >250 mm Hg or a diastolic blood pressure of 115 mm Hg.
From Gibbons RJ, Balady GJ, Bricker JT, et al. ACC/AHA 2002 guideline update for exercise testing: summary article. A Report of the ACC/AHA Task Force on practice guidelines (committee to update 1997 exercise testing guidelines). *J Am Coll Cardiol.* 2002;40:1531–1540.

monitor the patient's responses because of technical difficulties should result in immediate termination of the test. Most problems can be avoided by having an experienced physician, nurse, or exercise physiologist standing next to the patient, measuring blood pressure and assessing patient appearance during the test. The exercise technician should operate the recorder and treadmill, take appropriate tracings, enter data on a form, and alert the physician to any abnormalities that may appear on the monitor.

Although many efforts have been made to objectify maximal effort, such as age-predicted maximal HR, a plateau in oxygen uptake, exceeding the ventilatory threshold, or a respiratory exchange ratio greater than unity, all have considerable measurement error and intersubject variability.[64,83–86] This variability occurs regardless of the population tested. The 95% confidence limits for maximal HR based on age, for example, range considerably (Fig. 14-11); therefore, this endpoint is maximal for some and submaximal for others.[52] The classic index of a person's cardiopulmonary limits, a plateau in oxygen uptake, is not observed in many patients, is poorly reproducible, and has been confused by the many different criteria applied.[83–86]

Recovery Period

Some debate exists as to whether the postexercise recovery period should be an active or passive process. This decision should be made on the basis of the purpose of the exercise test. If the test is performed for diagnostic purposes, then it appears to be of value to place the patient in the supine position immediately after stopping exercise, especially if imaging will be taken immediately after the test. The increase in venous return to the heart observed in the supine position results in increases in ventricular volume, wall stress, and, consequently, myocardial oxygen demand. Several studies have shown that ST-segment abnormalities are enhanced in the supine position and that an active recovery may attenuate the magnitude of these changes.[5,87] Once thought to be false-positive responses, ST-segment changes 2 to 4 minutes into recovery are now known to be particularly important for the detection of ischemia. Patients with symptom-limiting angina or dyspnea may become more uncomfortable in the supine position and should recover in a seated upright or semi-recumbent position. If the test is performed for nondiagnostic purposes such as for a fitness evaluation in a healthy or athletic person, then an active recovery (cool-down phase) may be safer and more comfortable.

Typically, an active recovery period consists of walking on the treadmill at a speed of 1.5 to 2.0 mph or continuing to pedal the cycle ergometer slowly at a work rate ranging from 0 to 25 W. An active recovery decreases the risk of hypotension and may minimize the risk of dysrhythmias secondary to elevated catecholamines in the postexercise period. Standing recovery should be avoided because of potential complications associated with venous pooling. Regardless of the method of recovery, patients should be monitored for at least 6 to 8 minutes into the postexercise period. Blood pressure, the ECG, and symptoms should be monitored and recorded at 2-minute intervals for the duration of the recovery period. The recovery period should be extended as long as necessary to resolve symptoms or abnormal hemodynamic or electrocardiographic responses. After completion of the recovery portion of the test, patients should be given posttest instructions that include avoidance of long, hot showers or baths due to systemic vasodilation. In addition, patients should be told they may experience fatigue and muscle soreness and to avoid any heavy exertion that day. Any pain or discomfort during the day after the test should be reported to the physician immediately.

Assessing Test Accuracy

All diagnostic tests misclassify patients a certain percentage of the time. In the context of the exercise test, this is not a trivial issue, because people who are inaccurately identified as having disease may be subjected unnecessarily to additional, more invasive, and costly procedures. When the test is performed properly, it commonly serves the very important purpose of screening those who should or should not undergo these additional procedures. However, a patient with significant CAD who is incorrectly classified as normal may not receive appropriate medical therapy. How accurately the exercise test distinguishes people with disease from those without disease depends on the population tested, the definition of disease, and the criteria used for an abnormal test.

Sensitivity and Specificity

The most common terms used to describe test accuracy are sensitivity and specificity. Sensitivity is the percentage of times a test correctly identifies those with CAD. Specificity is the percentage of times a test correctly identifies those without cardiovascular disease. Sensitivity and specificity are inversely related and are affected by the choice of discriminant value for abnormal, the definition of disease, and, most importantly, by the prevalence of disease in the population tested. For example, if the population has a greater prevalence or severity of disease (such as coronary disease in multiple vessels) the test will have a higher sensitivity. Alternatively, the test will have a higher specificity (and low sensitivity) when performed in a group of younger, healthier subjects.

Meta-analysis of the exercise testing literature indicates that the exercise test has, on the average, a sensitivity of approximately 68% and a specificity of approximately 77%.[88] However, these values range widely in the various studies; sensitivity can be as low as 40% among patients with single-vessel disease, but greater than 90% among those with triple-vessel disease. Conversely, the specificity of the test is usually quite low (i.e., 50% to 60%) in patients who have more severe CAD but is quite high in populations that are relatively healthy. These values reported in the literature and the inverse relationship between sensitivity and specificity underscore the importance of considering the patient's pretest characteristics (chest pain and CAD risk factors) before beginning the test. No test result can be interpreted accurately without considering the patient in the context of his or her pretest characteristics.

Predictive Value

Another important term that helps define the diagnostic value of a test is the predictive value. The predictive value of an abnormal test (positive predictive value) is the percentage of people with an abnormal test result who have disease. Conversely, the predictive value of a normal test (negative predictive value) is the percentage of people with a normal test result who do not have disease. The predictive value of a test cannot be determined directly from the sensitivity and specificity but is strongly associated with the prevalence of disease in the population tested. The calculations used to determine sensitivity, specificity, and predictive value are presented in Table 14-9.

False-Positive and False-Negative Responses. The factors associated with false-positive or false-negative responses should also be considered before deciding on the most appropriate cardiac stress test. A false-positive response is defined as an abnormal exercise test response in a person *without* significant heart disease and causes the specificity to be decreased. A false-negative response

Table 14-9 • TERMS USED TO DEMONSTRATE THE DIAGNOSTIC VALUE OF A TEST

Sensitivity	$\frac{TP}{TP + FN} \times 100$
Specificity	$\frac{TN}{TN + FP} \times 100$
Positive predictive value	$\frac{TP}{TP + FP} \times 100$
Negative predictive value	$\frac{TN}{TN + FN} \times 100$

TP, true positives, or those with abnormal test results and with disease; FN, false negatives, or those with normal test results with disease; FP, false positives, or those with abnormal test results and no disease; TN, true negatives, or those with normal test results and no disease.

occurs when the test is normal in a person *with* disease and causes the sensitivity of the test to be reduced. Factors associated with false-positive and false-negative responses are listed in Table 14-10. In people in whom the probability of a false-positive or false-negative test is high, an alternative procedure (exercise or pharmacologic echocardiogram or radionuclide test) may be appropriate.

Prognosis

The exercise test has been shown to be of value for estimating prognosis in patients with a wide range of severity of cardiovascular diseases.[5,8,32–34,52,60,89,90] One of the most important clinical applications of the exercise test is the identification of low-risk patients in whom catheterization (and revascularization) can be safely deferred. There are several reasons why accurately establishing prognosis is important. An estimate of prognosis provides answers to patients' questions regarding the probable outcome of their illness, which may be useful to the patient in planning return to work or making decisions regarding disability, recreational activities, and finances. A second reason to estimate prognosis is to identify patients for whom interventions might improve outcome. Combining clinical and exercise test information into scores has been shown to improve the estimation risk among men and women undergoing exercise testing.[32,43,91,92]

Table 14-10 • CAUSES OF FALSE-NEGATIVE AND FALSE-POSITIVE TEST RESULTS

False Positive

1. Resting repolarization abnormalities (e.g., left bundle-branch block)
2. Cardiac hypertrophy
3. Accelerated conduction defects (e.g., Wolff–Parkinson–White syndrome)
4. Digitalis
5. Nonischemic cardiomyopathy
6. Hypokalemia
7. Vasoregulatory abnormalities
8. Mitral valve prolapse
9. Pericardial disease
10. Coronary spasm in absence of CAD
11. Anemia
12. Female gender

False Negative

1. Failure to reach ischemic threshold secondary to medications (e.g., β-blockers)
2. Monitoring an insufficient number of leads to detect electrocardiographic changes
3. Angiographically significant disease compensated by collateral circulation
4. Musculoskeletal limitations preceding cardiac abnormalities

Although there are many exercise test variables known to be of value for estimating prognosis, including exercise capacity, maximal HR, a hypotensive response, ST depression, and symptoms, the most powerful predictor of risk appears to be exercise capacity. It has also been recently demonstrated that the rate in which HR recovers from exercise, long empirically associated with better cardiovascular health, is an important risk marker among patients undergoing exercise testing.[93–95] For example, patients who fail to decrease HR more than 12 bpm, 1 minute after completing the exercise test have four times the risk of mortality over the subsequent 6 years.[93]

Exercise Testing—Special Populations

Women

The interpretation of exercise testing results in women is more challenging than that in men.[5,96,97] Exercise-induced ST-segment depression is less sensitive among women as compared to men.[98,99] Test specificity is also thought to be lower among women, although there is a wide variation in the reported studies.[5] Some of these differences may be explained by differences in the meaning of chest pain presentation between men and women, although typical angina is as meaningful in women older than 60 years as it is in men. Nearly half the women with anginal symptoms in the CASS (who were younger than 65 years) had normal coronary arteries.[100] Other possible explanations for the lower test accuracy in women include lower disease prevalence, higher incidence of mitral valve prolapse and syndrome X (chest pain without coronary disease), differences in microvascular function, and possibly hormonal differences.[5,101]

The accuracy for diagnosing CAD in women has been shown to be improved by the use of multivariate methods[102] and by the addition of nuclear or echocardiographic imaging techniques.[101,103,104] Thus, when exercise testing is performed in women, factors that may affect test accuracy should be carefully considered; if the exercise test results are uncertain or when otherwise appropriate, a radionuclide imaging procedure should be considered. The optimal strategy for circumventing false-positive test results in women remains to be defined. Nevertheless, the current AHA/ACC guidelines suggest that there are insufficient data to justify routine radionuclide imaging procedures as the initial test for CAD in women.[5]

The Elderly

The prevalence of CAD increases with increasing age, and the exercise test can be an extremely useful tool for diagnosing CAD in the elderly. However, exercise testing in the elderly can be problematic given their frequently compromised ability to exercise in the context of an increased prevalence of CAD. The occurrence of fatigue and light-headedness caused by muscle weakness and deconditioning, vasoregulatory abnormalities, and difficulties with gait are important concerns in these patients. Thus, a test modality and protocol should be chosen that provides the highest degree of safety. For instance, cycle ergometry may be more appropriate for elderly patients who have a residual deficit from a cerebral vascular accident. In addition, the testing protocol should be modified considering the expected levels of exercise tolerance. More gradually incremented protocols, such as the Balke, ramp, or Naughton, are usually more suitable in the elderly population. The elderly are more likely to present with more complex medication regimens, more comorbidities, and increased prevalence of aortic stenosis and other valvular diseases, in addition to more severe CAD.

For these reasons, the elderly require particularly close evaluation before clearance for exercise testing, a modified testing protocol, and particular attention to appropriate endpoints.[5,96]

Interpretation of the exercise test in the elderly can also differ significantly from that in younger people. Resting electrocardiographic abnormalities, including previous MI, left ventricular hypertrophy, and intraventricular conduction delays, may compromise the diagnostic accuracy of the exercise test. Nevertheless, the application of standard ST-segment criteria among elderly subjects has been shown to have similar diagnostic characteristics as in younger subjects.[98] No doubt because of the higher prevalence of CAD in the elderly, test sensitivity has even been shown to be comparatively higher among the elderly (84%), although specificity is somewhat lower when compared with younger populations (70%).[105] Thus, despite several problems posed by elderly subjects that require additional attention, exercise testing is not contraindicated in this group.[5]

Patients After Cardiac Transplantation

Over the past two decades, transplantation has become a widely used and successful treatment option for patients with end-stage heart failure. The 1-year survival rate for patients who have undergone this procedure is now approximately 85%.[106] The hemodynamic response to exercise in patients who have undergone cardiac transplantation has been characterized since the early 1970s.[107–109] Because the heart is denervated, some intriguing hemodynamic responses are observed. Orthotopic transplantation removes the nervous system connections to the heart. Thus, the heart is not responsive to the normal actions of the parasympathetic and sympathetic systems. The absence of vagal tone explains the high resting HRs in these patients (100 to 110 bpm) and the relatively slow adaptation of the heart to a given amount of submaximal work.[109] This slows the delivery of oxygen to the working tissue, contributing to an earlier than normal metabolic acidosis and hyperventilation during exercise.[107,108,110–112] Although transplantation significantly improves the hemodynamic and ventilatory response to exercise, the transplanted patient still exhibits many of the responses typical of the patient with chronic heart failure.[112] These include heightened ventilatory responses attributable to uneven matching of ventilation to perfusion and an increase in physiologic dead space. Maximal HR is lower in transplant recipients compared with normal subjects, which contributes to a reduction in cardiac output and peak $\dot{V}O_2$; the arteriovenous oxygen difference widens as a compensatory mechanism.

The exercise test in patients who have undergone cardiac transplantation is less a diagnostic and more a functional tool. In the latter role, it is useful for assessing and modifying therapy in these patients, in addition to evaluating the appropriateness of daily activities and return to work. Although rare cases of chest pain associated with accelerated graft atherosclerosis have been reported in transplant recipients, decentralization of the myocardium usually eliminates anginal symptoms. Exercise electrocardiography is also inadequate in terms of assessing ischemia, as evidenced by its low sensitivity (21% or less).[113] Thus, radionuclide testing may be more useful for assessing ischemia in these patients.

Patients With Congenital Cardiac Disorders

Cardiac stress testing can be useful for those who have congenital cardiac disorders. With the advent of radionuclide angiography (RNA) and pharmacologic stress testing, these patients are able to be assessed for functional cardiac flow and exercise tolerance. This population should be followed up with after any repair of the great vessels, coarctation, or septal defect. Congenital patients should reveal any major cardiac surgeries with their doctor or nurse prior to being scheduled for a cardiac stress test. If a cardiac defect remains the patient may not be able to achieve full exercise capacity which might skew the purpose of the cardiac stress test.[114]

CONCLUSIONS

Although there have been advances in technologies related to the diagnosis of CAD, the numerous applications and widespread availability of the exercise test continue to make it one of the more important tools in cardiovascular medicine. The test is increasingly being supervised by nonphysicians,[115] and the cardiovascular nurse's role has expanded in many centers to include exercise test supervision. The cost-effectiveness of this test should not be abused. Only patients that would truly benefit from this type of testing should be tested. It is also worth mentioning that the cardiac stress test is only one test used to assess a patient with chest pain, post MI, or arrhythmias. The indication, selection, results and interpretation of these tests should be included in the entire patient's clinical picture and integrated into the care plan accordingly by the cardiac nurse.

ACKNOWLEDGMENT

We would like to thank Dr. Jonathan Myers, Ph.D. for his exceptional lifelong work in the study of cardiac and exercise stress testing.

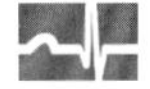 CASE STUDY

Patient Profile

Mr. Ron Sanchez, 67-year-old Hispanic male

Past Medical History

Diabetes type II, chronic kidney disease, and hyperlipidemia

Family History

(Father) Acute myocardial infarction (age 59, deceased from event)

Social History

40 pack year history of smoking and has been quit since he was 56 years old

Medications

Metformin 1,000 mg orally twice daily, atorvastatin 40 mg orally daily at bedtime, aspirin 81 mg orally daily

Allergies

No known drug allergies

Case Scenario

Mr. Sanchez reports to clinic to see his primary care physician because he has recently started experiencing occasional chest tightening during activity with his grandchildren. The chest pressure resolves once the activity has ceased. His primary care provider recommends he

(*continued*)

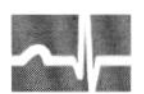

CASE STUDY (*Continued*)

undergo a cardiac stress test. Mr. Sanchez is capable of performing a traditional treadmill stress test due to no physical limitations.

Mr. Sanchez is scheduled to receive a cardiac stress test at the local testing facility. Mr. Sanchez's ECG at baseline is normal with no indications of ST-segment changes. The patient is not experiencing any chest pain prior to the beginning of the test.

Clinical Considerations

- **What protocol would be most appropriate for Mr. Sanchez?** Mr. Sanchez is how to rate his perceived level of exertion using the Borg Rating of Perceived Exertion (RPE) Scale. He is at a 7 while the treadmill is at 0.0% grade and 1.7 mph. HR and BP are within normal limits. The treadmill is then placed on 5.0% grade but still at 1.0 mph. His RPE is now 10.
- **What is the next phase in the Bruce protocol?** 1.7 mph and 10% grade is the next phase in the Bruce protocol.

Diagnostic Studies

The protocol is followed and Mr. Sanchez's HR tops out at 145 bpm with a BP of 160/90 mm Hg. His RPE is 19. The test is concluded, and the patient is asked to rest. He is assessed for chest pain, dizziness, nausea, or ST-segment changes. Mr. Sanchez does not have any chest pain and does not exhibit any ST-segment changes.

Assessment and Plan

- **Would this test be considered positive or negative?** Negative, if no signs or symptoms of ischemia occur during the testing the test is deemed negative. If chest pain occurs, ST-segments change, or wall motion abnormalities are seen the test would be deemed positive.
  Mr. Sanchez is then discharged home on his previous dose of cardiac medications and asked to follow up in 1 year.

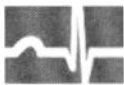

CASE-BASED LEARNING

Patient Profile

Mr. William Smith, 65-year-old Caucasian male

Physical Examination

Normal

Past Medical History

Hyperlipidemia s/p STEMI, s/p percutaneous transluminal coronary angioplasty (PTCA); inferior MI

Medications

Aspirin; clopidogrel; esomeprazole, fenofibrate, levothyroxine, lisinopril, metoprolol; nitroglycerin tablets

Allergies

Simvastatin

Case Scenario

Mr. Smith had a myocardial infarction within the past year. He is status-post PTCA. Mr. Smith's physical examination is normal with no physical deficits and normal range of motion in all extremities.

- **What modality would be most appropriate for Mr. Smith?** Exercise stress test

Diagnostic Studies

Mr. Smith arrives for his stress test and is explained what to subjectively look for while conducting the test. He is hooked up to an ECG monitor to establish some baseline vital signs which are as follows:

- HR (resting/supine): 59 bpm
- BP (resting/supine): 106/66 mg Hg
- O_2% (resting/supine): 93% saturation
- ECG monitor noted right bundle branch block (RBBB) and some T-wave inversions in leads V1-2

Mr. Smith begins his treadmill test and the Bruce protocol is followed. Mr. Smith completes the warm-up phase with an RPE of 9. The test is continued to the next phase of where his RPE increases to 11. Finally, Mr. Smith begins the third phase (3.1 mph and 13.3% grade). Mr. Smith's vitals are as follows:

- HR (exercise/standing): 113 bpm
- BP (exercise/standing): 168/70 mm Hg
- O_2% (exercise/standing): 93% saturation

Mr. Smith asks the provider to stop the examination due to fatigue. A dynamic cool-down phase is initiated. No chest pain was experienced, and no signs of ischemia were noted although the patient did experience rare PVCs and a six-beat run of atrial tachycardia on the ECG during recovery.

- **Was this a conclusive test? No, the patient's HR only achieved 75% of predicted maximal heart rate (PMHR) therefore his ECG is nondiagnostic.**

Mr. Smith was asked to come back again in order to perform a pharmacologic stress test. He is now complaining of right-sided chest pain. All baseline vitals are similar to the previous test. He is attached to the ECG machine and the same RBBB is present on ECG (Figure 14-19). An abbreviated BRUCE PROTOCOL is followed for 4 minutes and 25 seconds. The test was terminated due to 5 out of 10 chest pain and ST-segment depression. His maximal HR was 99 bpm which is 65% (suboptimal) of the PMHR, his BP increased to 158/72 mm Hg with hypotension in early recovery.

- **What would the cardiac nurse recommend at this time?** Admission to the hospital for coronary angiography.

CASE-BASED LEARNING (*Continued*)

Case Conclusion

Technetium Tc99m Sestamibi (Cardiolite) was injected during ST-segment depressions and images were taken by a nuclear scanning camera. Mr. Smith was recommended to be admitted to the hospital for coronary angiography. He was found to have a 90% occlusion to his left main coronary artery.

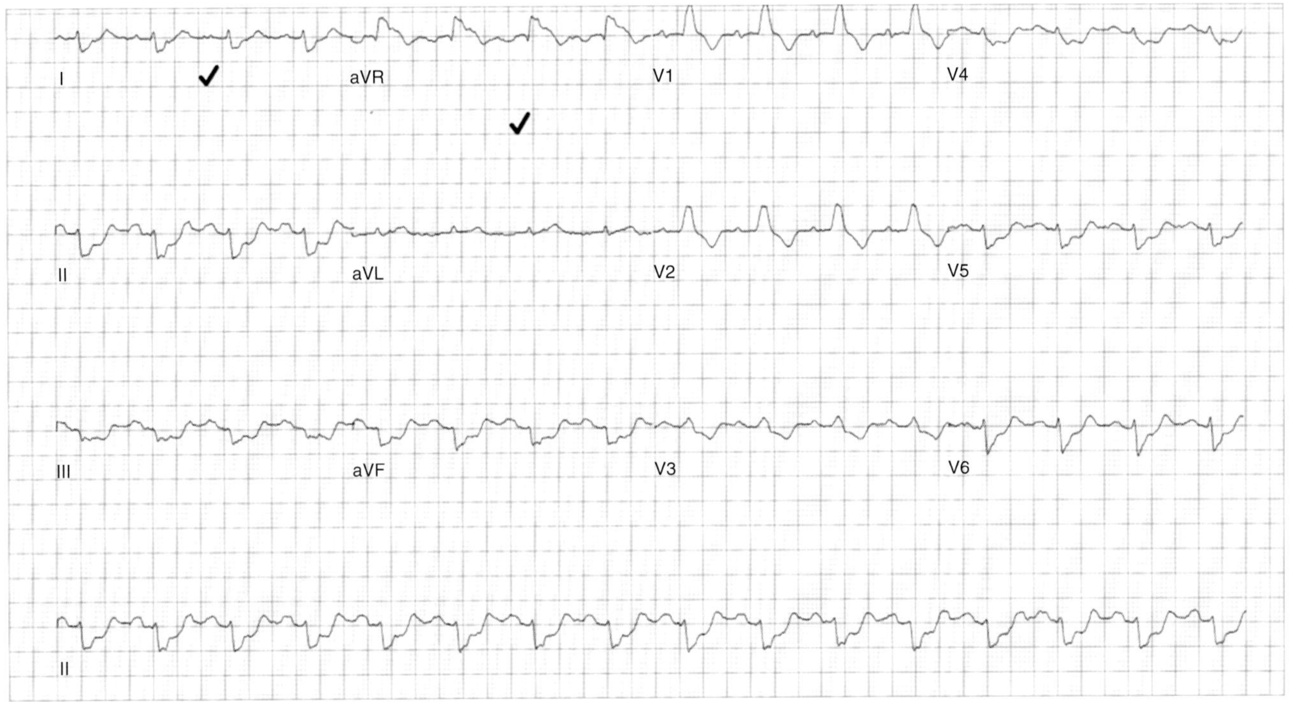

Figure 14-19. ECG. Image shows patient with RBBB that experienced 5/10 chest pain and ST-segment changes during exercise testing. This patient was referred to the cardiac catheterization lab for coronary angiography.

KEY READINGS

American Heart Association Subcommittee on Exercise; Cardiac Rehabilitation, and Prevention of the Council on Clinical Cardiology; Council on Lifestyle and Cardiometabolic Health, et al., Myers J, Forman DE, Balady GJ, et al. Supervision of exercise testing by nonphysicians: a scientific statement from the American Heart Association. *Circulation.* 2014;130:1014–1027.

Diagnosing a Heart Attack. https://www.heart.org/en/health-topics/heart-attack/diagnosing-a-heart-attack

Iskandrian AE, Garcia EV. *Atlas of Nuclear Cardiology: An Imaging Companion to Braunwald's Heart Disease.* 1st ed. Philadelphia, PA: Elsevier/Saunders; 2012.

REFERENCES

1. Scherf D. Fifteen years of electrocardiographic exercise test in coronary stenosis. *N Y State J Med.* 1947;47(22):2420–2424.
2. Ashley EA, Myers J, Froelicher V. Exercise testing in clinical medicine. *Lancet.* 2000;356:1592–1597.
3. Marcus R, Lowe R, Froelicher VF, et al. The exercise test as gatekeeper: limiting access or appropriately directing resources? *Chest.* 1995;107(5):1442–1446.
4. American Thoracic Society; American College of Chest Physicians. ATS/ACCP Statement on cardiopulmonary exercise testing. *Am J Respir Crit Care Med.* 2003;167(2):211–277.
5. Gibbons RJ, Balady GJ, Timothy Bricker J, et al. ACC/AHA 2002 guideline update for exercise testing: summary article. A Report of the American College of Cardiology/American Heart Association Task Force on practice guidelines (Committee to update the 1997 exercise testing guidelines). *J Am Coll Cardiol.* 2002;40(8):1531–1540.
6. Mehra MR, Kobashigawa J, Starling R, et al. Listing criteria for heart transplantation: international society for heart and lung transplantation guidelines for the care of cardiac transplant candidates-2006. *J Heart Lung Transplant.* 2006;25(9):1024–1042.
7. Arena R, Myers J, Guazzi M. The clinical and research applications of aerobic capacity and ventilatory efficiency in heart failure: an evidence-based review. *Heart Fail Rev.* 2008;13(2):245–269.
8. Myers J. Applications of cardiopulmonary exercise testing in the management of cardiovascular and pulmonary disease. *Int J Sports Med.* 2005;26(Suppl 1):S49–S55.
9. American College of Sports Medicine. *Guidelines for Exercise Testing and Prescription.* 7th ed. Baltimore, MD: Lippincott Williams & Wilkins; 2006.
10. Working Group on Cardiac Rehabilitation and Exercise Physiology and the Working Group on Heart Failure of the European Society of Cardiology. Recommendations for exercise training in chronic heart failure patients. *Eur Heart J.* 2001;22(2):125–135.
11. Balady GJ, Morise AP. Exercise electrocardiographic testing. In: Zipes D, Libby P, Bonow R, eds. *Braunwald's Heart Disease: A Textbook of Cardiovascular Medicine.* 11th ed. Philadelphia, PA: Elsevier; 2019.
12. Banerjee A, Newman DR, Van den Bruel A, et al. Diagnostic accuracy of exercise stress testing for coronary artery disease: a systematic review and meta-analysis of prospective studies. *Int J Clin Pract.* 2012;66(5):477–492.
13. Fihn SD, Gardin JM, Abrams J, et al. 2012 ACCF/AHA/ACP/AATS/PCNA/SCAI/STS guideline for the diagnosis and management of patients with stable ischemic heart disease. Executive summary: a report

of the American College of Cardiology Foundation/American Heart Association Task Force on Practice Guidelines, and the American College of Physicians, American Association for Thoracic Surgery, Preventive Cardiovascular Nurses. *Circulation.* 2012;126(25):3097–3137.

14. Fletcher GF, Ades PA, Kligfield P, et al. Exercise standards for testing and training: a scientific statement from the American Heart Association. *Circulation.* 2013;128(8):873–934.
15. Gibbons RJ, Balady GJ, Beasley JW, et al. ACC/AHA Guidelines for exercise testing. a report of the American College of Cardiology/American Heart Association Task Force on Practice Guidelines (committee on exercise testing). *J Am Coll Cardiol.* 1997;30(1):260–311.
16. Kusumoto FM, Schoenfeld MH, Barrett C, et al. 2018 ACC/AHA/HRS guideline on the evaluation and management of patients with bradycardia and cardiac conduction delay: a report of the American College of Cardiology/American Heart Association Task Force on clinical practice guidelines and the Heart Rhythm Society. *J Am Coll Cardiol.* 2019;74:932–987.
17. Shen WK, Sheldon RS, Benditt DG, et al. 2017 ACC/AHA/HRS guideline for the evaluation and management of patients with syncope: a Report of the American College of Cardiology/American Heart Association Task Force on clinical practice guidelines and the Heart Rhythm Society. *Circulation.* 2017;136(5):e60–e122.
18. Halperin JL, Levine GN, Al-Khatib SM, et al. Further evolution of the ACC/AHA clinical practice guideline recommendation classification system: a Report of the American College of Cardiology/American Heart Association Task Force on clinical practice guidelines. *Circulation.* 2016;133(14):1426–1428.
19. Iskandrian AE, Garcia EV. *Atlas of Nuclear Cardiology: An Imaging Companion to Braunwald's Heart Disease.* Philadelphia, PA: Elsevier/Saunders; 2012.
20. Buchfuhrer MJ, Hansen JE, Robinson TE, et al. Optimizing the exercise protocol for cardiopulmonary assessment. *J Appl Physiol Respir Environ Exerc Physiol.* 1983;55(5):1558–1564.
21. Hambrecht RP, Schuler GC, Muth T, et al. Greater diagnostic sensitivity of treadmill versus cycle exercise testing of asymptomatic men with coronary artery disease. *Am J Cardiol.* 1992;70(2):141–146.
22. Hermansen L, Saltin B. Oxygen uptake during maximal treadmill and bicycle exercise. *J Appl Physiol.* 1969;26(1):31–37.
23. Myers J, Buchanan N, Walsh D, et al. Comparison of the ramp versus standard exercise protocols. *J Am Coll Cardiol.* 1991;17(6):1334–1342.
24. Wicks JR, Sutton JR, Oldridge NB, et al. Comparison of the electrocardiographic changes induced by maximum exercise testing with treadmill and cycle ergometer. *Circulation.* 1978;57(6):1066–1070.
25. Myers J, Froelicher V. Optimizing the exercise test for pharmacologic studies in patients with angina pectoris. In: Ardissino D, Savonitto S, Opie LH, eds. *Drug Evaluation in Angina Pectoris.* Pavia, Italy: Kluwer Academic; 1994:41–52.
26. Webster MWI, Sharpe DN. Exercise testing in angina pectoris: the importance of protocol design in clinical trials. *Am Heart J.* 1989;117(2):505–508.
27. Myers J. *Essentials of Cardiopulmonary Exercise Testing.* Champaign, IL: Human Kinetics; 1996.
28. Arena R, Myers J, Williams MA, et al. Assessment of functional capacity in clinical and research settings: a Scientific Statement from the American Heart Association Committee on Exercise, Rehabilitation, and Prevention of the Council on Clinical Cardiology and the Council on Cardiovascular Nursing. *Circulation.* 2007;116(3):329–343.
29. Myers J, Voodi L, Umann T, et al. A survey of exercise testing: methods, utilization, interpretation, and safety in the VAHCS. *J Cardiopulm Rehabil.* 2000;20:251–258.
30. Stuart RJ, Ellestad MH. National survey of exercise stress testing facilities. *Chest.* 1980;77(1):94–97.
31. Weiner DA, Ryan TJ, McCabe CH, et al. Value of exercise testing in determining the risk classification and the response to coronary artery bypass grafting in three-vessel coronary artery disease: a Report from the Coronary Artery Surgery Study (CASS) Registry. *Am J Cardiol.* 1987;60(4):262–266.
32. Mark DB, Hlatky MA, Harrell FE Jr, et al. Exercise treadmill score for predicting prognosis in coronary artery disease. *Ann Intern Med.* 1987;106(6):793–800.
33. Myers J, Gullestad L. The role of exercise testing and gas exchange measurement in the prognostic assessment of patients with heart failure. *Curr Opin Cardiol.* 1998;13:145–155.
34. Mark DB, Lauer MS. Exercise capacity: the prognostic variable that doesn't get enough respect. *Circulation.* 2003;108(13):1534–1536.
35. Panza JA, Quyyumi AA, Diodati JG, et al. Prediction of the frequency and duration of ambulatory myocardial ischemia in patients with stable coronary artery disease by determination of the ischemic threshold from exercise testing: importance of the exercise protocol. *J Am Coll Cardiol.* 1991;17(3):657–663.
36. Redwood DR, Rosing DR, Goldstein RE, et al. Importance of the design of an exercise protocol in the evaluation of patients with angina pectoris. *Circulation.* 1971;43(5):618–628.
37. Wolthuis RA, Froelicher VF, Fischer J, et al. New practical treadmill protocol for clinical use. *Am J Cardiol.* 1977;39(5):697–700.
38. Naughton JP, Hayden R. Methods of exercise testing. In: Naughton JP, Hellerstien HK, Mohler LC, eds. *Exercise Testing and Exercise Training in Coronary Heart Disease.* New York: Academic Press; 1973:79–91.
39. Astrand PO, Rodahl K. *Textbook of Work Physiology.* 3rd ed. New York: McGraw-Hill; 1986.
40. Whipp BJ, Davis JA, Torres F, et al. A test to determine parameters of aerobic function during exercise. *J Appl Physiol Environ Exerc Physiol.* 1981;50(1):217–221.
41. Myers J, Buchanan N, Smith D, et al. Individualized ramp treadmill: observations on a new protocol. *Chest.* 1992;101(5 Suppl):236S–241S.
42. Porszasz J, Casaburi R, Somfay A, et al. A treadmill ramp protocol using simultaneous changes in speed and grade. *Med Sci Sports Exerc.* 2003;35(9):1596–1603.
43. Chang J, Froelicher VF. Clinical and exercise test markers of prognosis in patients with stable coronary artery disease. *Curr Probl Cardiol.* 1994;19(9):539–587.
44. Froelicher ES. Usefulness of exercise testing shortly after acute myocardial infarction for predicting 10-year mortality. *Am J Cardiol.* 1994;74(4):318–323.
45. Olona M, Candell-Riera J, Permanyer-Miralda G, et al. Strategies for prognostic assessment of uncomplicated first myocardial infarction: 5-year follow-up study. *J Am Coll Cardiol.* 1995;25(4):815–822.
46. Borg G. *An Introduction to Borg's RPE-Scale.* Ithaca, NY: Movement Publications; 1985.
47. Naughton J, Balke B, Nagle F. Refinements in method of evaluation and physical conditioning before and after myocardial infarction. *Am J Cardiol.* 1964;14(6):837–843.
48. American College of Cardiology Foundation/American Heart Association Task Force on Practice Guidelines; American Society of Echocardiography; American Society of Nuclear Cardiology, et al., Fleisher LA, Beckman JA, Brown KA, et al. 2009 ACCF/AHA focused update on perioperative beta blockade incorporated into the ACC/AHA 2007 guidelines on perioperative cardiovascular evaluation and care for noncardiac surgery. *J Am Coll Cardiol.* 2009;54(22):e13–e118.
49. McGie AI, Gould KL. Nuclear cardiology. In: Willerson JT, Cohn HJ, Wallens HJ, et al., eds. *Cardiovascular Medicine.* 3rd ed. London: Springer-Verlag; 2007:137–160.
50. Gibbons RJ. Nuclear cardiology. In: Giuliani ER, Fuster V, Gersh BJ, et al., eds. *Cardiology: Fundamentals and Practice.* 2nd ed. St. Louis, MO: Mosby-Year Book; 1991:161–180.
51. Fleisher LA, Beckman J, Brown KA, et al. 2009 ACCF/AHA focused update on perioperative beta blockade incorporated into the ACC/AHA 2007 guidelines on perioperative cardiovascular evaluation and care for noncardiac surgery. *J Am Coll Cardiol.* 2009;54(22):13–118.
52. Froelicher VF, Myers J. *Exercise and the Heart.* 5th ed. Philadelphia, PA: W.B. Saunders; 2006.
53. Zoghbi GJ, Iqbal FM, Iskandrian AE. Choice of stress test. In: Iskandrian AE, Garcia EV, eds. *Atlas of Nuclear Cardiology.* Philadelphia, PA: Elsevier Saunders; 2012.
54. Iskandrian AS. Single-photon emission computed tomographic thallium imaging with adenosine, dipyridamole, and exercise. *Am Heart J.* 1991;122(1 Pt 1):279–284; discussion 302–306.
55. Ranhosky A, Kempthorne-Rawson J. The safety of intravenous dipyridamole thallium myocardial perfusion imaging. Intravenous dipyridamole thallium imaging study group. *Circulation.* 1990;81(4):1205–1209.
56. Borges-Neto S. Perfusion and function assessment by nuclear cardiology techniques. *Curr Opin Cardiol.* 1997;12:581–586.
57. Armstrong W, Marcovitz PA. Stress echocardiography. In: Braunwald E, ed. *Heart Disease Updates.* Philadelphia, PA: W. B. Saunders; 1993.
58. Armstrong WF, Zoghbi WA. Stress echocardiography: current methodology and clinical applications. *J Am Coll Cardiol.* 2005;45(11):1739–1747.

59. Schmidt DH, Port SC, Gal RA. Nuclear cardiology and echocardiography: non-invasive tests for diagnosing patients with coronary artery disease. In: Pollack M, Schmidt DH, eds. *Heart Disease and Rehabilitation*. 3rd ed. Champaign, IL: Human Kinetics; 1995:81–94.
60. Arena R, Guazzi M, Myers J. Ventilatory abnormalities during exercise in heart failure: a mini review. *Curr Respir Med Rev*. 2007;3:179–187.
61. Fleg JL, Morrell CH, Bos AG, et al. Accelerated longitudinal decline of aerobic capacity in healthy older adults. *Circulation*. 2005;112(5):674–682.
62. Froelicher VF. *Exercise Test Reporting Aid (EXTRA) Software*. St. Louis, MO: Mosby-Year Book; 1996.
63. Myers J, Tan SY, Abella J, et al. Comparison of the chronotropic response to exercise and heart rate recovery in predicting cardiovascular mortality. *Eur Cardiovasc Prev Rehabil*. 2007;14(2):215–221.
64. Hammond HK, Froelicher VF. Normal and abnormal heart rate responses to exercise. *Prog Cardiovasc Dis*. 1985;27(4):271–296.
65. Lauer MS, Okin PM, Larson MG, et al. Impaired heart rate response to graded exercise prognostic implications of chronotropic incompetence in the Framingham heart study. *Circulation*. 1996;93(8):1520–1526.
66. Bailey RH, Bauer JH. A review of common errors in the indirect measurement of blood pressure: sphygmomanometry. *Arch Intern Med*. 1993;153(24):2741–2748.
67. Morris CK, Myers J, Froelicher VF, et al. Nomogram based on metabolic equivalents and age for assessing aerobic exercise capacity in men. *J Am Coll Cardiol*. 1993;22(1):175–182.
68. Gibbons RJ, Blair SN, Kohl HW, et al. The safety of maximal exercise testing. *Circulation*. 1989;80:846–852.
69. Mazzotta G, Scopinaro G, Falcidieno M, et al. Significance of abnormal blood pressure response during exercise-induced myocardial dysfunction after recent acute myocardial infarction. *Am J Cardiol*. 1987;59(15):1256–1260.
70. Irving JB, Bruce RA. Exertional hypotension and postexertional ventricular fibrillation in stress testing. *Am J Cardiol*. 1977;39(6):849–851.
71. Dubach P, Froelicher VF, Klein J, et al. Exercise-induced hypotension in a male population. Criteria, causes, and prognosis. *Circulation*. 1988;78(6):1380–1387.
72. Sanmarco ME, Pontius S, Selvester RH. Abnormal blood pressure response and marked ischemic ST-segment depression as predictors of severe coronary artery disease. *Circulation*. 1980;61(3):572–578.
73. Weiner DA, McCabe CH, Cutler SS, et al. Decrease in systolic blood pressure during exercise testing: reproducibility, response to coronary bypass surgery and prognostic significance. *Am J Cardiol*. 1982;49(7):1627–1631.
74. Foster C, Crowe AJ, Daines E, et al. Predicting functional capacity during treadmill testing independent of exercise protocol. *Med Sci Sports Exerc*. 1996;28(6):752–756.
75. American College of Sports Medicine. *Resource Manual for Guidelines for Exercise Testing and Prescription*. Baltimore, MD: Lippincott Williams & Wilkins; 2006.
76. Philbrick JT, Horwitz RI, Feinstein AR. Methodologic problems of exercise testing for coronary artery disease: groups, analysis and bias. *Am J Cardiol*. 1980;46(5):807–812.
77. Miranda CP, Liu J, Kadar A, et al. Usefulness of exercise-induced ST-segment depression in the inferior leads during exercise testing as a marker for coronary artery disease. *Am J Cardiol*. 1992;69(4):303–307.
78. Yang JC, Wesley RC Jr, Froelicher VF. Ventricular tachycardia during routine treadmill testing: risk and prognosis. *Arch Intern Med*. 1991;151(2):349–353.
79. Beckerman J, Wu T, Jones S, et al. Exercise test–induced arrhythmias. *Prog Cardiovasc Dis*. 2005;47(4):285–305.
80. Partington S, Myers J, Cho S, et al. Prevalence and prognostic value of exercise-induced ventricular arrhythmias. *Am Heart J*. 2003;145(1):139–146.
81. Frolkis JP, Pothier CE, Blackstone EH, et al. Frequent ventricular ectopy after exercise as a predictor of death. *N Engl J Med*. 2003;348(9):781–790.
82. Myers JN. Perception of chest pain during exercise testing in patients with coronary artery disease. *Med Sci Sports Exerc*. 1994;26(9):1082–1086.
83. Myers J, Walsh D, Buchanan N, et al. Can maximal cardiopulmonary capacity be recognized by a plateau in oxygen uptake? *Chest*. 1989;96(6):1312–1316.
84. Myers J, Walsh D, Sullivan M, et al. Effect of sampling on variability and plateau in oxygen uptake. *J Appl Physiol (1985)*. 1990;68(1):404–410.
85. Noakes TD. Implications of exercise testing for prediction of athletic performance: a contemporary perspective. *Med Sci Sports Exerc*. 1988;20(4):319–330.
86. Midgley AW, McNaughton LR, Polman R, et al. Criteria for determination of maximal oxygen uptake: a brief critique and recommendations for future research. *Sports Med*. 2007;37(12):1019–1028.
87. Lachterman B, Lehmann KG, Abrahamson D, et al. "Recovery only" ST-segment depression and the predictive accuracy of the exercise test. *Ann Intern Med*. 1990;112(1):11–16.
88. Gianrossi R, Detrano R, Mulvihill D, et al. Exercise-induced ST depression in the diagnosis of coronary artery disease. A meta-analysis. *Circulation*. 1989;80(1):87–98.
89. Myers J, Prakash M, Froelicher VF, et al. Exercise capacity and mortality among men referred for exercise testing. *N Engl J Med*. 2002;346(11):793–801.
90. Roger VL, Jacobsen SJ, Pellikka PA, et al. Prognostic value of treadmill exercise testing: a population-based study in Olmsted County, Minnesota. *Circulation*. 1998;98(25):2836–2841.
91. Ashley E, Myers J, Froelicher V. Exercise testing scores as an example of better decisions through science. *Med Sci Sports Exerc*. 2002;34(8):1391–1398.
92. Ashley E, Myers J. New insights into the clinical exercise test. *ACSM's Certified News* 2003;13:1–5.
93. Cole CR, Blackstone EH, Pashkow FJ, et al. Heart rate recovery immediately after exercise as a predictor of mortality. *N Engl J Med*. 1999;341(18):1351–1357.
94. Cole CR, Foody JM, Blackstone EH, et al. Heart rate recovery after submaximal exercise testing as a predictor of mortality in a cardiovascularly healthy cohort. *Ann Intern Med*. 2000;132(7):552–555.
95. Shetler K, Marcus R, Froelicher VF, et al. Heart rate recovery: validation and methodologic issues. *J Am Coll Cardiol*. 2001;38(7):1980–1987.
96. Marolf GA, Kuhn A, White RD. Exercise testing in special populations: athletes, women, and the elderly. *Prim Care*. 2001;28(1):55–72.
97. Giardina A, DeCastro S, Fedele F, et al. Noninvasive testing for coronary artery disease in women. *Minerva Cardioangiol*. 2006;54(3):323–330.
98. Hlatky MA, Pryor DB, Harrell FE, et al. Factors affecting sensitivity and specificity of exercise electrocardiography: multivariable analysis. *Am J Med*. 1984;77(1):64–71.
99. Morise AP, Diamond GA. Comparison of the sensitivity and specificity of exercise electrocardiography in biased and unbiased populations of men and women. *Am Heart J*. 1995;130(4):741–747.
100. Kennedy H, Kilip T, Fischer L, et al. The clinical spectrum of coronary artery disease and its surgical and medical management, 1974–1979. The coronary artery surgery study. *Circulation*. 1982;66(5):16–23.
101. Cerqueira MD. Diagnostic testing strategies for coronary artery disease: special issues related to gender. *Am J Cardiol*. 1995;75(11):52D–60D.
102. Robert AR, Melin JA, Detry JM. Logistic discriminant analysis improves diagnostic accuracy of exercise testing for coronary artery disease in women. *Circulation*. 1991;83(4):1202–1209.
103. Marwick TH, Anderson T, Williams MJ, et al. Exercise echocardiography is an accurate and cost-efficient technique for detection of coronary artery disease in women. *J Am Coll Cardiol*. 1995;26(2):335–341.
104. Morise AP, Diamond GA, Detrano R, et al. Incremental value of exercise electrocardiography and thallium-201 testing in men and women for the presence and extent of coronary artery disease. *Am Heart J*. 1995;130(2):267–276.
105. Kasser IS, Bruce RA. Comparative effects of aging and coronary heart disease on submaximal and maximal exercise. *Circulation*. 1969;39(6):759–774.
106. Khush KK, Cherikh WS, Chambers DC, et al. The international thoracic organ transplant registry of the international society for heart and lung transplantation: thirty-fifth adult heart transplantation report—2018; focus theme: multiorgan transplantation. *J Heart Lung Transplant*. 2018;37(10):1155–1206.
107. Savin WM, Haskell WL, Schroeder JS, et al. Cardiorespiratory responses of cardiac transplant patients to graded, symptom-limited exercise. *Circulation*. 1980;62(1):55–60.
108. Schroeder JS. Hemodynamic performance of the human transplanted heart. *Transplant Proc*. 1979;11:304–308.
109. Stinson EB, Griepp RB, Schroeder JS, et al. Hemodynamic observations one and two years after cardiac transplantation in man. *Circulation*. 1972;45(6):1183–1194.
110. Brubaker PH, Berry MJ, Brozena SC, et al. Relationship of lactate and ventilatory thresholds in cardiac transplant patients. *Med Sci Sports Exerc*. 1993;25(2):191–196.

111. Degre SG, Niset GL, De Smet JM, et al. Cardiorespiratory response to early exercise testing after orthotopic cardiac transplantation. *Am J Cardiol.* 1987;60(10):926–928.
112. Marzo KP, Wilson JR, Mancini DM. Effects of cardiac transplantation on ventilatory response to exercise. *Am J Cardiol.* 1992;69(5): 547–553.
113. Ehrman JK, Keteyian SJ, Levine AB, et al. Exercise stress tests after cardiac transplantation. *Am J Cardiol.* 1993;71(15):1372–1373.
114. Al-Khatib SM, Stevenson WG, Ackerman MJ, et al. 2017 AHA/ACC/HRS Guideline for management of patients with ventricular arrhythmias and the prevention of sudden cardiac death: a Report of the American College of Cardiology/American Heart Association Task Force on clinical practice guidelines and the Heart Rhythm Society. *Circulation.* 2018;138(13):e272–e391.
115. Franklin BA, Gordon S, Timmis GC, et al. Is direct physician supervision of exercise stress testing routinely necessary? *Chest.* 1997;111(2):262–265.

15 Nuclear, Magnetic Resonance, and Computed Tomography Imaging

Jeremy L. Iman, Kevin Widner, Mario Ramos

OBJECTIVES

1. Review basic principles and indications of nuclear imaging, magnetic resonance imaging, and computed tomography imaging studies.
2. Understand the types of images produced by these imaging studies, and how they are used in the evaluation and treatment of patients with cardiovascular disease.
3. Describe nursing considerations and patient education in the care of patients undergoing these imaging studies.

KEY QUESTIONS

1. How is the heart visualized using nuclear imaging, magnetic resonance imaging, and computed tomography?
2. What are the most common indications for these studies? What are their relative and absolute contraindications?
3. What are the advantages, disadvantages, and limitations of each of these imaging studies?
4. Which studies may require administration of intravenous agents such as contrast or medications?
5. What are the nursing and patient care considerations for patients undergoing these studies?

BACKGROUND

The purpose of this chapter is to assist nurses to navigate the complexities of cardiac imaging in Radiology and support patients undergoing cardiac imaging studies. Diagnostic imaging continues to rapidly evolve in many ways, and cardiovascular imaging is a major beneficiary of these advancements. New scanners and protocols have improved the spatial and temporal resolution of cardiac images. New post processing workstations and techniques have improved the ability to measure, interpret, and present the anatomy and physiology of our patients in new, more accurate ways. Through these advancements, nuclear medicine, magnetic resonance imaging (MRI), and computed tomography (CT) are imaging modalities that are able to provide noninvasive answers to providers.

NUCLEAR CARDIOLOGY

Nuclear cardiac imaging refers to cardiac radiologic diagnostic techniques performed with the aid of radiopharmaceuticals.[1] Since 1973 when H. William Straus imaged the heart at stress and rest using a planar gamma (Anger) camera, cardiac nuclear imaging has been a significant part of the field of nuclear medicine.

Radioisotope Pharmaceuticals

Radionuclides are atoms in an unstable form. They have a finite probability of spontaneously converting to a more stable configuration. When they do so, small amounts of energy in the form of rays are emitted. The rate at which atoms in a given sample undergo this conversion is denoted by the half-life, the time required for one half of the sample to undergo the conversion. Half-lives of radioactive substances vary from a fraction of a second to a millennium; the half-life for any given radionuclide is always the same. The characteristics of an ideal radiotracer to assess myocardial blood flow would include: a half-life long enough to allow for convenient imaging, easy combination with biologic substances, 100% myocardial extraction across the entire spectrum of achievable or inducible coronary blood flow states, instantaneous intracellular binding, low extraction and clearance by organs adjacent to the heart, and extraction by only viable cells. Unfortunately, to date, no commercially available radiotracer of myocardial perfusion meets all of these criteria.

Single photon emission computed tomography (SPECT) and positron emission tomography/computed tomography (PET/CT) are the two most common nuclear cardiovascular imaging modalities. The three most common radiotracers used in SPECT imaging are thallium 201 (^{201}Tl) and the two technetium 99m-labeled tracers: ^{99m}Tc-sestamibi (Cardiolite) and ^{99m}Tc-tetrofosmin (Myoview). Nitrogen-13-ammonia, oxygen-15 labeled water, and rubidium-82 are the most common tracers used in PET imaging to assess blood flow; fluorine-18-2-fluoro-2-deoxyglucose (FDG) is used in PET imaging to assess myocardial metabolism.

Injection and detection of these radiotracers allow for the measurement of relative myocardial blood flow. The radiotracers follow blood flow and are extracted from the blood pool by myocytes in proportion to blood flow. The mechanism by which the various radiotracers used in SPECT and PET imaging are extracted from the bloodstream and taken up by myocytes varies. In SPECT imaging, the radioactive decay of tracer is detected outside the body as scintillation (flash of light) by a gamma scintillation camera. The camera functions as a scanning device (large Geiger counter) to detect the distribution of radioactivity emitting from the myocardium through the chest wall, allowing examination of myocardial structure and function. ^{201}Tl is a potassium analog. Because of the dynamic equilibrium of potassium between cells and the blood pool, potassium and therefore ^{201}Tl distribute in the myocardium in proportion to the blood flow. Myocytes with an intact sodium–potassium pump take up ^{201}Tl. However, the relatively low energy (60 keV) emitted by ^{201}Tl makes imaging of this tracer suboptimal in large patients. The technetium 99m-labeled radiotracers passively distribute across sarcolemmal and mitochondrial membranes and remain intracellularly bound. The relatively higher energy (140 keV) emitted by this group of tracers allows for improved transmission through the chest tissue resulting in improved image quality, particularly in large patients.

PET imaging likewise allows for quantitative and tomographic imaging of myocardial perfusion and metabolism without intrinsically altering these processes. A positron-emitting radiotracer travels only a short distance in tissue prior to encountering an electron. This interaction causes annihilation of both particles, producing two high-energy photons that depart at an angle of 180 degrees from each other. PET imaging systems are designed to detect the two photons, which travel in opposite directions at essentially the speed of light (511 keV). By measuring the time that it takes for each photon to encounter the circumferential ring of detectors, localization of the event can be mathematically derived.

Diagnostic Indications for Nuclear Imaging

Table 15-1 summarizes the diagnostic uses of the imaging modalities discussed in this chapter. Stress myocardial perfusion with SPECT and PET imaging is useful clinically for the detection of flow-limiting coronary artery disease and risk stratification for patients with known coronary heart disease.[1] The clinical aim of these studies is to evaluate the physiology of coronary blood flow. Myocardial perfusion images provide the clinician and patient with important predictive and prognostic information, including left ventricular (LV) chamber size, and global and regional LV function; location, size, and extent of impairment of coronary flow reserve (myocardial ischemia); and location, size, and extent of myocardial infarction.[2]

Table 15-1 • CLINICAL APPLICATION OF TOMOGRAPHIC IMAGING MODALITIES

	Nuclear (SPECT/PET)	MRI	CT	Echo
Anatomy				
Chambers	+++	++++	++++	++++
Valves	–	++	++++	++++
Large vessels	–	++++	++++	++
Coronary arteries	–	++	++++	+
Pericardium	–	++++	++++	+
Physiology				
Myocardial perfusion (ischemia)	++++	+++	–	++
Global & regional ventricular function	++++	++++	+	++++
Ventricular volumes	++++	++++	–	+++
Valve function	–	+++	++++	++++
Tissue Characterization				
Myocardial viability/ infarction	++++	++++	–	+++
Masses	++++	++++	++++	++
Larger vessel wall atherosclerosis	++	++	++++	–

++++ Indicates most applicable; – indicates not applicable.

Stress myocardial perfusion imaging (MPI) involves comparing the pattern of myocardial blood flow, as reflected by myocyte uptake of radiotracer, in a resting state and in the hyperemic or stress state. The goals of stress perfusion imaging are creating heterogeneity of myocardial blood flow, marking this effect with a radiotracer, and applying SPECT or PET to obtain images of myocardial uptake.

One method for a stress myocardial perfusion study is using SPECT imaging with a "dual" (two) isotope imaging protocol. This protocol uses ^{201}Tl to evaluate the pattern of myocardial blood flow/viability at rest and a technetium 99m-labeled product to provide better functional information from ECG-gated imaging at stress. However, increasingly low doses of technetium 99m-labeled products are injected at rest followed by higher doses at peak stress. Regardless of the radiotracer used, the premise remains the same—obtaining images of myocardial blood flow at rest and comparing these images to a pattern of radiotracer myocardial uptake in the stressed state. Thus, all patients receive an intravenous (IV) injection of radiotracer while sitting quietly at rest. A gated set of SPECT or PET myocardial perfusion images are then acquired. For sestamibi delays of 45 to 60 minutes for rest, 15 to 20 minutes for exercise and 60 minutes for pharmacologic stress are recommended. For tetrofosmin, minimum delays of 30 to 45 minutes for rest, 10 to 15 minutes for exercise, and 45 minutes for pharmacologic stress are optimal. After acquisition of the images at rest, the patient is "stressed," or rather a hyperemic state of coronary blood flow is created, and this state is marked with a second radiotracer injection. A patient reaches the stress state by exercising on the treadmill, and achieving 85% of the maximal predicted heart rate for age (220 − patient's age × 0.85). In patients with normal coronary arteries, as the heart rate and blood pressure rise in response to exercise, normal coronary arteries dilate. Coronary flow reserve is maintained in arteries with less than 70% stenosis.[3] In contrast, a region of the myocardium supplied by a diseased artery is unable to appropriately dilate in response to increasing myocardial work, resulting in a relative reduction in blood flow/radiotracer uptake compared with normal coronary arteries. Studies of myocardial blood flow have demonstrated that at a heart rate of 85% of maximal predicted for age, blood flow through a normal coronary artery increases approximately twofold. Therefore, at peak exercise, regions of the myocardium supplied by normal coronary arteries receive twofold the amount of radiotracer compared with regions of the myocardium supplied by diseased vessels unable to dilate. In patients unable to exercise adequately, an IV infusion of dipyridamole (0.57 mg/kg infused over 4 minutes) or adenosine (140 mcg/kg/min) reproduce this hyperemic state. The vasodilator agents do not stress the myocardium but rather dilate normal coronary arteries, having little effect on diseased vessels. At the standard infusion doses and rates, these agents dilate normal coronary arteries four- to fivefold.[4] Following the stress study, a second set of gated SPECT or PET images are acquired.

Alternative imaging to the standard 1-day protocol is to perform a 2-day myocardial perfusion examination although on many patients, 2-day imaging is impractical. The advantage to the 2-day protocol is that the stress study can be performed first and if interpreted as normal, the rest study does not need to be performed. Many institutions perform 2-day MPI examinations based on body weight, with larger patients being converted from a 1- to a 2-day protocol.

The rest and poststress gated SPECT images when processed and reconstructed, reflect the pattern of myocardial blood flow in the two states. ECG-triggered images provide an evaluation of LV ejection fraction (LVEF) and evaluation of LV regional wall motion and thickening and diastolic function. The images are reconstructed in standardized views (short, vertical, and horizontal long axes). Patterns of radiotracer uptake are compared between the two data sets. A segmental scoring system has become a widely applied quantitative tool to integrate the extent and severity of perfusion abnormalities.[5] Summed stress score is a quantitative tool used to evaluate the extent and severity of myocardium at risk.[3] The score is determined by dividing the myocardium into 17 segments, scoring the percent reduction in radiotracer uptake, and adding the segments. The 17-segment representation of the myocardium is a standard format used in most myocardial imaging modalities.

A segment or region of the myocardium that has reduced radiotracer uptake on the images obtained at stress state that appears more uniform (improved) on the images obtained at rest is consistent with myocardial ischemia. The severity of the impairment of coronary flow reserve can be qualitatively estimated by the degree of reduction of radiotracer uptake (i.e., mildly reduced, moderately reduced, or severely reduced uptake). A segment or region of the myocardium with a fixed (i.e., present on both rest and stress) reduction in radiotracer uptake on both stress and rest images is most consistent with myocardial injury or infarction. An alternative explanation of an apparent fixed region of reduced radiotracer uptake that thickens and moves normally on gated cines may be attenuation artifact. The most common attenuating structures include breast tissue (anterior wall) and diaphragm (inferior wall). A reversible abnormality (present on stress, not on rest) is consistent with myocardial ischemia (Fig. 15-1).

The summed stress score (extent and severity of ischemia and infarction) when combined with Duke Treadmill Score has been shown to be an independent predictor of cardiac death (Fig. 15-2).[6] In addition to increasing the identification and quantification of coronary artery disease, stress myocardial perfusion data have been shown to be an independent additional predictor of serious cardiac events in the ensuing year in men and women of all ages, as well as patients with diabetes.[2,3]

Stress myocardial perfusion using PET imaging provides a more quantitative measurement of coronary blood flow. By comparing absolute blood flow at rest with absolute flow in a hyperemic state created by a vasodilator infusion, impairment of coronary flow reserve can be more precisely measured. PET imaging allows for precise detection of global impairment in coronary flow reserve and therefore may increasingly be useful in the diagnosis of microvascular disease. Several of the radiotracers used in PET imaging require an on-site cyclotron for radiotracer generation. Thus, widespread application of PET imaging is currently limited by the cost associated with generating the radiotracers.

Myocardial Viability

LV dysfunction and associated heart failure is increasing in both incidence and prevalence in the United States. The mortality and morbidity associated with LV dysfunction and heart failure are high.[7] While dramatic advances in medical therapy have resulted in improved survival and functional capacity, the best and most definitive therapy, when appropriate, is revascularization. Imaging studies to assess myocardial viability help identify patients who may benefit from revascularization. Myocardial

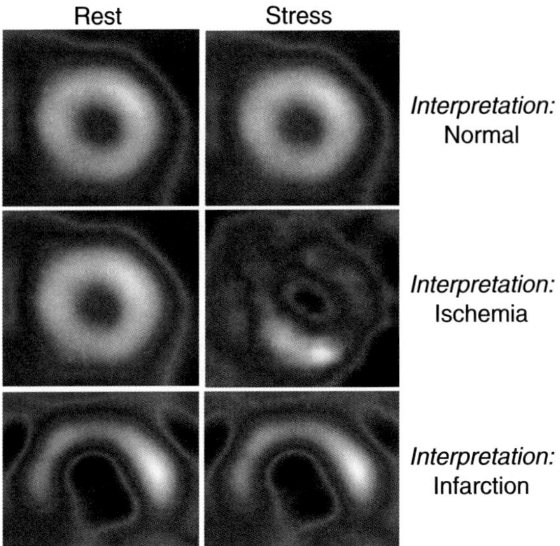

Figure 15-1. Stress and rest SPECT myocardial perfusion images. Top panel demonstrates no abnormalities in radiotracer uptake on either stress or rest image and are normal. Middle panel demonstrates a defect at stress but none at rest, consistent with myocardial ischemia. Lower panel demonstrates a defect at stress and rest, consistent with myocardial infarction. (Images obtained from University of Washington Medical Center, Department of Radiology, Division of Nuclear Medicine, Seattle, Washington.)

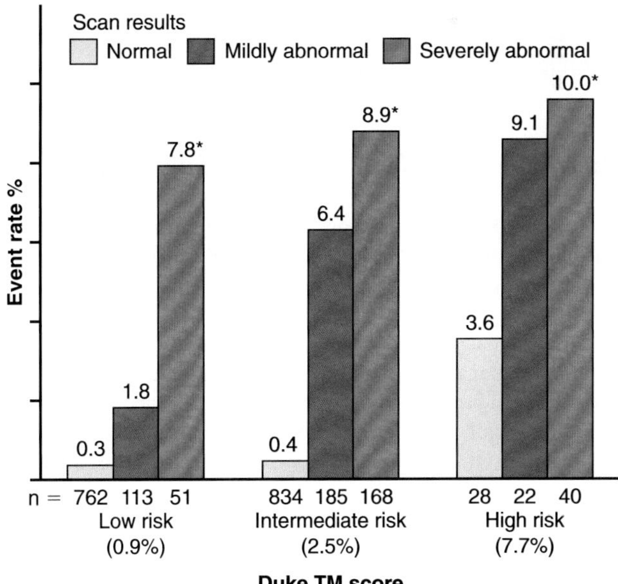

Figure 15-2. SPECT myocardial perfusion scan results add incremental prognostic data when combined with Duke Treadmill (TM) score. Event rates for myocardial infarction or cardiac death are shown in parentheses under Duke TM subgroups. *$p < 05$ across scan. (Adapted from Hachamovitch R, Berman DS, Kiat H, et al. Exercise myocardial perfusion SPECT in patients without known coronary artery disease: incremental prognostic value and use in risk stratification. *Circulation.* 1996;93:905–914.)

viability is described as a condition of chronic sustained abnormal contraction of the myocardium secondary to chronic underperfusion, in patients with known coronary artery disease and in whom revascularization results in recovery of LV function. LV dysfunction may not be the result of irreversible scar but rather caused by impairment in function and energy use of viable myocytes—myocytes that if fueled with adequate blood flow would demonstrate improved function. Chronic myocardial ischemia is associated with a severe reduction in contractile function. Patients with LV dysfunction who have viable myocardium are at highest risk of cardiac death, but at the same time benefit most from revascularization. In contrast to infarct-related scar, dysfunctional but viable myocardium has the potential to regain function.[3]

^{201}Tl combined with SPECT imaging has historically been the most common radionuclide used for distinguishing viable or hibernating myocardium from scar. ^{201}Tl is injected in the resting state; gated SPECT images immediately acquired reflect myocardial perfusion. Delayed images acquired 4 to 24 hours later represent tissue metabolism. A region of the myocardium with reduced perfusion (resting thallium uptake) but preserved metabolism (improved thallium uptake on delay images), defines myocardial viability. Myocardial viability studies with ^{201}Tl are clinically helpful in patients with multivessel coronary artery disease and LV dysfunction. Potential reversibility of LV dysfunction is an important clinical consideration in these patients. Multiple studies have demonstrated that patients with viable myocardium benefit from revascularization versus augmented medical therapy. Alternatively, patients without evidence of viability do not show this same improvement after revascularization.[3]

PET imaging has emerged as a precise method for the detection of myocardial viability. The use of FDG to assess myocardial metabolism and nitrogen-13-ammonia to assess perfusion, results in a highly sensitive study for differentiating viable myocardium from scar. A perfusion–metabolism mismatch pattern has become synonymous with reversible contractile dysfunction and thus prediction of improvement in LV function after revascularization.[8]

Patient Preparation for Myocardial Perfusion Studies

It is recommended that patients fast for 3 to 6 hours before injection of radionuclides. This preparation minimizes gastrointestinal blood flow, resulting in reduced gastric uptake of radionuclides. Consider holding cardiac medications, particularly nitrates, β-blockers, and calcium channel blockers, before stress studies, because these agents have been shown to reduce the sensitivity of the study for the detection of myocardial ischemia.[8] However, medication administration prior to the study depends on the clinical question at hand. If a provider is attempting to establish the diagnosis of coronary artery disease, then it is recommended that cardiac medications be held. In a patient with known disease undergoing risk stratification, continuing medications is a reasonable option. Patients should be warned that they may activate radiation detectors (e.g., at the U.S. border crossings and airports) in the days following injection of radiotracers. A letter is commonly given to a patient planning a trip in the days following SPECT or PET imaging.

Radionuclide Ventriculogram

A radionuclide ventriculogram (RNVG), also known as a MUGA (multiple gated acquisition) study, is a procedure in which a small amount of the patient's blood is withdrawn, labeled with a technetium 99m-labeled radionuclide, and then reinjected. Using the electrocardiogram (ECG) signal for timing (gating), images are acquired throughout the cardiac cycle. Radioactive scintillation counts from corresponding time segments are summed to augment image clarity. In this way, the manner in which radioactivity and hence the blood pool change over the cardiac cycle is demonstrated. This summed cardiac cycle can be played back as a cine loop video display of a normally recurring cardiac cycle. Left ventricular ejection fraction (EF), right ventricular (RV) EF, and segmental wall motion can be precisely calculated. The video display resembles a contrast LV or RV angiogram. Variation in radioactive counts over time is analyzed to provide information about systolic function. Rhythm disturbances, such as atrial fibrillation or frequent premature contractions altering beat-to-beat filling and cycle length, may decrease quantitative accuracy. RNVG is commonly used to evaluate cardiac function in patients with heart failure and valvular heart disease or to monitor the potential cardiotoxic effects of the commonly used chemotherapeutic agents.

First-Pass

A first-pass nuclear cardiac procedure is where a rapid bolus of technetium 99m-labeled red blood cells is reinjected into a patient. The imaging provides calculations for right and left ventricular EF, assesses wall motion abnormalities, measures cardiac output and absolute ventricular chamber volumes, and aids in quantifying left-to-right cardiac shunts. To evaluate a left-to-right shunt, a computer-aided assessment of the first transit pulmonary time–activity curves must be performed. The rapid bolus is administered in a large proximal vein through large-gauge IV access in an antecubital vein.

Patient Preparation for RNVG

There is no special patient preparation for an RNVG study. The patient may continue to take all medications. The entire study usually takes approximately 30 minutes. Patients should be warned that they may activate radiation detectors (e.g., at U.S. border crossings and airports) in the days following injection of radiotracers. A letter is commonly given to a patient planning a trip in the days following an RNVG.

Hybrid Imaging

SPECT/CT is the integration of a SPECT system with a CT scanner to fuse two data sets. Hybrid imaging is seen as synergistic, as the sum of its parts provides more information beyond what's achievable with either data set alone. The CT configuration of these hybrid imaging systems ranges from a low-resolution CT to a 2 to 64 multidetector row CT. The CT scan when combined with the MPI provides an estimation of attenuation and scatter and additional information in regard to calcium scoring. Image quality of MPI studies is affected by attenuation of photons in the body leading to nonuniform distribution of activity; scattering of photons which degrade image contrast; and changes in spatial resolution altering the distribution of activity in the myocardium. The addition of CT to SPECT results can reduce or even eliminate these image quality concerns.

The most common source of artifacts on hybrid imaging comes from misregistration of the CT and/or PET and SPECT. Misregistration can arise from patient motion between the examinations and respiratory cycle movement.

Risks of Radionuclides

In contrast to radioactive substances used for therapeutic (tissue ablation) purposes, radiopharmaceuticals used for imaging have short half-lives (minutes to several hours), contributing to their relatively rapid decay in the body. They are used in very small amounts. Thus, there is no need to isolate patients who have had these studies, and no particular precautions are needed for disposal of body substances (including blood, urine, or stool). The risk to a fetus is small, but it is recommended that patients who are pregnant or breast-feeding not undergo injection of radionuclides. Personnel should remember that radioactivity decreases dramatically with distance from the source. Personnel who work in nuclear medicine departments wear detection badges like those worn by radiology personnel to monitor their exposure.

MAGNETIC RESONANCE IMAGING

MRI is a diagnostic noninvasive imaging modality that does not use ionizing radiation like CT or nuclear imaging. MRI uses a magnet, radiofrequency (RF) emitting coils, gradient coils which can slightly vary the strength of the magnetic field, and receive coils that act as antennae to create an image. Cardiac MRI is usually performed using a superconducting electromagnet which is the most common type of magnet used in MRI. Magnets are described in terms of the density of their field strength, Tesla (T). The most common field strength of clinical magnets used for cardiovascular imaging is 1.5 T. However, 3-T cardiovascular imaging is becoming more common. The lack of ionizing radiation makes MRI appealing for patients that require multiple follow-up examinations and to which exposure to ionizing radiation is of greater concern than the general population.

Clinical MR images are composed of signals received from hydrogen atoms. Outside of the influence of a strong magnetic field, hydrogen atoms are oriented in random directions as they spin on their individual axes. When they are exposed to the magnetic field of an MRI machine, the randomly oriented atoms become aligned with the main magnetic field. The axes of the hydrogen atoms also begin to precess, or rotate, at a known rate based on the strength of the main magnetic field. Coils transmit RF pulses to the atoms within the bore of the magnet at the same frequency at which the atoms are precessing. This energy tilts the orientation of the atoms away from the direction of the main magnetic field. After the RF pulse is stopped, the atoms return to their previous energy states and give off RF energy. This energy is detected by the receive coil and processed to create the image. Gradient coils change the magnetic field during specific points in the process to encode spatial information in the signal.

Artifacts caused by respiratory and cardiovascular motion must be compensated for during cardiac imaging. The most common technique for correcting respiratory motion with a cooperative patient is to acquire images while a patient holds their breath. These breath-holds typically take 10 to 20 seconds and are repeated for the duration of the MRI scan. Other ways to compensate for respiratory motion include acquiring images based on the position of the diaphragm while breathing normally or taking multiple samples and averaging those images together; however, this lengthens scan time and degrades images quality. Acquiring data over multiple cardiac cycles and gating the acquisition to the patient's ECG compensate for artifact caused by cardiovascular motion.

Gadolinium chelates are the most commonly used IV MRI contrast agents. Gadolinium, an extracellular compound, alters the magnetic properties of adjacent protons within the patient. The need for contrast depends on the diagnostic indication for the study. Indications for gadolinium in cardiovascular imaging include but are not limited to myocardial viability, stress perfusion, vessel angiography, and mass perfusion. Gadolinium is not needed for evaluation of ventricular or valve function. Oral contrast agents are not used currently for cardiovascular MRI. Precautions and considerations for gadolinium are discussed later in the chapter.

Indications

Cardiovascular MRI provides diagnostic information on anatomy, physiology, and tissue characterization (Table 15-1). If an echocardiogram or other type of diagnostic imaging is inconclusive, MRI can be used for further evaluation. MRI provides anatomical descriptions of the size, location, and connection of all four cardiac chambers and valves (Fig. 15-3). Ventricular volumes and function, left and right, can be obtained by MRI because of the excellent visualization of endocardial borders.[5–7] Ejection fraction (EF) and valve function can also be evaluated with MRI. The ability of MRI to characterize tissues of the human body is a very important and powerful technique by MRI. Tissue characterization is aided by late gadolinium enhancement (LGE) which is a unique tool possessed by MRI and used in diagnosing multiple diseases involving fibrosis.

Nonischemic Cardiomyopathy

In patients with nonischemic cardiomyopathy, MRI can define the etiology of heart failure. Unlike echocardiography (echo), MRI is able to characterize tissue allowing it to differentiate between diseases such as cardiac sarcoidosis, cardiac amyloidosis, hemochromatosis, myocarditis, and hypertrophic cardiomyopathy (HCM), all of which appear different on MRI. MRI is the

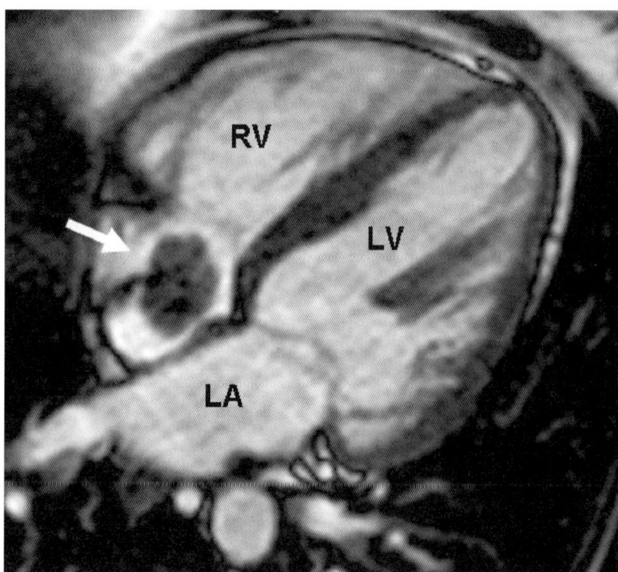

Figure 15-3. Cardiac MRI demonstrating a large mass (*arrow*) located within the right atrium. RV, right ventricle; LV, left ventricle; LA, left atrium. (Images obtained from University of Washington Medical Center, Department of Radiology, Seattle, Washington.)

gold standard for cardiac iron quantification.[9] MRI is preferred for diagnosing cardiac amyloidosis because of the reliability of LGE to determine cardiac involvement in patients with amyloidosis. LGE has been shown to be a valuable tool in diagnosing and differentiating cardiac sarcoidosis and HCM as well. MRI LGE is the reference standard for noninvasive assessment and delineation of fibrosis in patients with HCM.[10–12] MRI is the reference standard for diagnosing left ventricular noncompaction (LVNC) and is able to differentiate between LVNC and HCM which may have similar appearances on echo.[13] Aside from LGE, techniques such as black blood imaging, T1 mapping, and T2* have various roles in differentiating these diseases. T1 mapping can be used to evaluate diffuse fibrosis, T2 black blood imaging is used to evaluate edema, and T2* imaging is used to evaluate for iron overload.

Ischemic Cardiomyopathy

Cardiovascular MRI has many uses in patients with ischemic cardiomyopathy. Myocardial perfusion can be used to assess the presence or absence of flow-limited coronary artery disease.[14,15] Exercise testing is not performed. Instead, perfusion at stress can be assessed with vasodilator agents such as regadenoson.

MRI can identify areas of myocardial infarction by identifying areas of wall thinning and fibrosis. LGE can depict whether hypokinetic areas of myocardial tissue are viable or scar (infarction) and the probability of improvement of ventricular function after revascularization.[16,17] This can determine which areas of myocardium should be revascularized and is often used prior to coronary intervention. Although MRI descriptions of coronary artery stenoses have been performed in research studies, MRI is not commonly performed clinically for that purpose. MRI does allow descriptions of anomalous coronary artery origins and courses of the arteries.

Congenital Heart Disease

Patients with congenital heart disease (CHD) may undergo MRI evaluation (Figs. 15-3 and 15-4) due to complex anatomy and the prevalence of RV pathology. In contrast to echo, MRI can easily provide anatomical information about the RV as well as precise measurements of size and function of the RV. This is important for planning and management of patients with CHD. The RV's anterior location within the thorax makes it especially difficult to visualize with echo. Furthermore, the utility of echo is limited in adult patients with CHD because of the limited acoustic ultrasound windows due to scar tissue from prior surgeries. The limited views with which the RV is seen with echo most commonly means the function is described qualitatively. With MRI, quantitation of RV function can be performed in terms of RV volumes and EF. While echo remains the most common modality to detect and evaluate atrial and ventricular septal defects (ASD/VSD), MRI has been shown to have advantages in some cases. MRI can delineate anatomy more accurately than echo which yields a more precise evaluation of the size and shape of the ASD/VSD. MRI is preferred for indications of atrioventricular septal defect and partial anomalous pulmonary vein return (PAPVR). MRI is commonly used to evaluate and quantify ASD/VSD when echo is inconclusive.[18,19]

Atrial Ablation Planning

MR angiography of the left atrium provides descriptions of the size and locations of the pulmonary veins. This information is used in ablation planning for atrial fibrillation. Recently, ablation planning is an area where MRI and LGE have been shown to have increasing value. Some facilities are currently utilizing MRI LGE to identify fibrosis in the left atrium and pulmonary veins as an indicator of the likelihood of success of an ablation (Fig. 15-5). These techniques require specialized sequences and training.[20,21]

Evaluation of Cardiac Valves

Transvalvular velocities, transvalvular pressure gradients, and valve areas are all measures of the severity of valvular stenosis.[22–25] Typically, these measures are obtained by echo, which is preferred to MRI, but can also be evaluated by MRI. Quantitation of the amount of valvular regurgitation (regurgitant volumes) is more reproducible with MRI than with echo.[26,27] Evaluation of valve regurgitation volumes can be useful when echo is inconclusive.

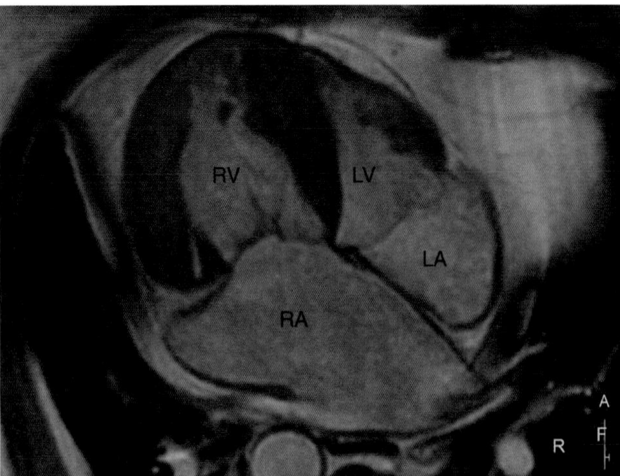

Figure 15-4. Cardiac MRI demonstrating the anatomy of a patient with mirror image dextrocardia with abdominal and atrial situs inversus and physiologically corrected transposition of the great arteries. RA, right atrium; RV, right ventricle; LA, left atrium; LV, left ventricle.

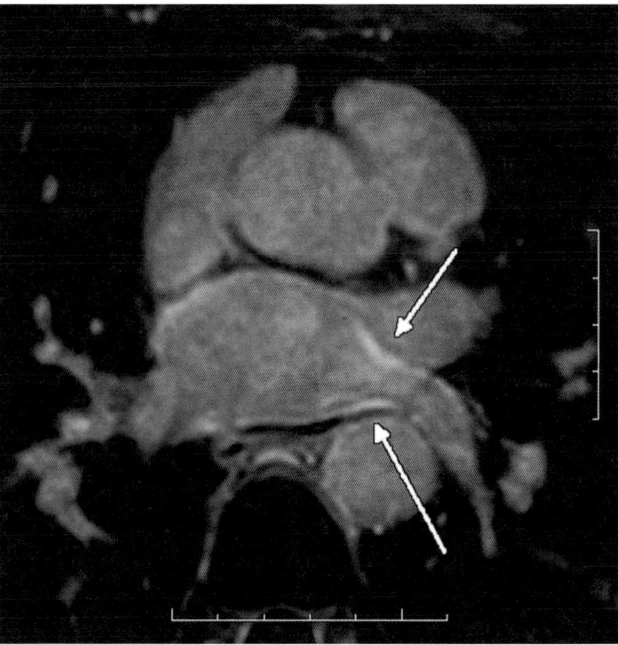

Figure 15-5. MRI LGE imaging showing fibrosis in the left atrium/pulmonary veins.

Arrhythmogenic Right Ventricular Cardiomyopathy

Cardiovascular MRI is the preferred imaging modality used in diagnosing arrhythmogenic RV cardiomyopathy (ARVC). Patients with ARVC have fibrofatty infiltration of the RV. This will typically appear as a dilated RV, often with focal areas of dyskinesia or akinesia. The ability of MRI to characterize tissue and to visualize the RV allows it to identify areas of intramyocardial fat and fibrosis.[28]

Large Vessel Pathology

Aneurysms and aberrant vascular connections can be easily assessed via MRI. MRI is the preferred imaging modality for follow-up examinations for patients with aortic coarctation primarily detected with echo and has the ability to evaluate all segments of the aorta without using ionizing radiation.[29,30] Much of atherosclerosis imaging has been focused on the degree of luminal stenosis by conventional x-ray angiography. Imaging of the actual disease (wall) can be performed in larger vessels such as the carotid artery or aorta with correlations to histology.[31–35] MRI is an effective modality for imaging vasculitis in large and medium vessels with the potential for earlier diagnosis over traditional testing. Cardiovascular MRI can also evaluate treatment response in patients with vasculitis. MRI is the most commonly used imaging modality to diagnose Takayasu arteritis due to its ability to assess for inflammation in the vessel wall as well as evaluate for gadolinium uptake.[36]

Intracardiac Mass

The differential diagnosis of any intracardiac mass includes tumor and thrombus. Tissue characterization, perfusion, and LGE can help differentiate the two and differentiate between tumors.[37] Locations in relation to cardiac structures can also be described. MRI is commonly used to evaluate suspected masses identified on echo. A prominent Coumadin ridge can be misinterpreted as a thrombus on echo, whereas MRI easily recognizes this as normal anatomy. Cardiovascular MRI is considered the preferred imaging modality along with echo for evaluation of intracardiac masses.

Pericardial Effusions

The pericardium can be visualized by MRI, and thus provide descriptions of pericardial thickness and locations of pericardial effusions. Pericardial constriction can be evaluated using MRI.

Patient Preparation

External magnetic fields can cause ferromagnetic metal to move or conduct energy into heat, either of which can cause serious bodily injury. Therefore, all patients undergoing an MRI should first undergo a formalized written screening process by experienced MR personnel. Resources are available regarding the safety of various external and internal objects.[38] One such Web site is http://www.mrisafety.com.[39] Orthopedic implants such as hip replacements, rods in the spine are MRI compatible. Implants in or around blood vessels like stents, inferior vena cava (IVC) filters, aneurysm clips, and heart valves must be cleared by a level 2 MR personnel as do implanted pumps, stimulators, inner ear implants, and metallic foreign bodies such as bullets. Some sites have recently begun scanning cardiac pacemakers and implantable cardioverter-defibrillators but those must go through an extensive screening and monitoring process by qualified personnel and therefore have a large negative impact on image quality. Temporary metallic breast tissue expanders are contraindicated for MRI. It is also important to consider the location of metallic implants and their effect on imaging. Metallic implants influence the spins of the atoms around them and create an area around the implant where imaging by MRI is unobtainable. For example, while imaging near sternal wires is routinely done with minimal effect on image quality, imaging an aorta on a patient with an endovascular aneurysm repair graft is much less likely to produce diagnostic quality images despite the implant being safe for MRI. The size, location, and ferromagnetic properties of the implant dictate its effect on image quality.

While most patients tolerate MRI procedures well, some may experience claustrophobia. Sedation in most cardiovascular MRI procedures is not considered ideal and should be avoided due to the level of cooperation required from the patient. While breath holds during MRI decrease artifact and thereby improve image quality, multiple breath holds may be difficult in the setting of cardiopulmonary disease, particularly in elderly and pediatric patients. Some facilities, such as those that specialize in pediatric imaging, use free-breathing protocols or moderate sedation protocols to address these challenges. Positioning a family member or friend in the same room as the patient may reduce anxiety. The family member or friend must also undergo MRI prescreening because they also are exposed to the external magnet. During imaging, loud noises are emitted from the magnet, so ear protection is required for safety.

To minimize artifact, patients should not move inside of the MRI and may be asked to hold their breath for short periods. Cardiovascular MRI examinations for most indications are done by acquiring a series of angled views planned on previously acquired views. If a patient shifts their body during the MRI, images preceding the patient movement will have to be reobtained to continue with the scan. The typical duration of cardiovascular MRI examinations is approximately 1 hour, which can be difficult for patients who may have pain while lying flat or difficulty holding their breath. It is common to temporarily discontinue diuretic medications prior to a cardiovascular MRI to reduce the likelihood of the patient needing to urinate during the MRI.

Patients are not required to fast prior to a cardiovascular MRI unless necessary for a sedation protocol. It is recommended that patients withhold from consuming caffeine prior to a cardiovascular MRI. Caffeine can artificially increase the heart rate. Irregular heart rhythms can be problematic and lead to reduced image quality of cardiovascular MRI examinations. Blood pressure, heart rate, respirations, pulse oximetry, and an ECG rhythm strip may be monitored. Intubated patients are not contraindicated for MRI.

If IV contrast is anticipated, an IV will need to be placed. Some contrast injections are performed via a power injector, usually for indications that require angiography or perfusion. Specialized, MRI-safe power injectors, IV pumps, ventilators, and vital sign monitoring equipment must be used since all of this equipment is usually within the same room as the magnet.

Gadolinium chelates are generally well tolerated. The most common minor adverse reactions include nausea or a transient metallic taste. More severe reactions are rare and include itchiness, hives, difficulty breathing, and anaphylactoid reactions. Patients with a known allergy to gadolinium can be premedicated with medications such as corticosteroids and antihistamines. Allergic reactions to other iodinated contrast agents do not increase the chance of having an allergic reaction to gadolinium. The Food and Drug Administration warns of an increased risk of nephrogenic systemic fibrosis in patients with acute or chronic renal insufficiency when exposed to gadolinium; the patient's glomerular filtration rate (GFR) should be obtained on patients with these conditions. Gadolinium is excreted from the body by the kidneys and can be removed with dialysis. Gadolinium can be retained in several organs for months or years. The consequences of gadolinium retention are an area of ongoing research and are yet unknown. Clinicians and patients should be informed of this risk when gadolinium use is anticipated; risks and benefits should be weighed on an individual basis.

COMPUTED TOMOGRAPHY

CT System

CT Scanners

CT scanners use an x-ray tube, special radiation detectors, and a moving table to image patient anatomy. The patient is placed on the table, which moves incrementally. The x-ray tube housed in a gantry, rotates around the patient. The detectors measure the energy from the photons as they exit the patient. The energy signal of the photons is measured, and special algorithms are applied to produce an image of the patient's anatomy.

Modern CT Scanner

CT scanners have had many advancements in recent years. Most are able to reconstruct images of approximately 0.625-mm thickness, by half 0.625-mm increments, which allows for superior spatial resolution and is especially advantageous for imaging structures such as coronary arteries, and heart valves. Some CT scanners are capable of imaging whole organs in one rotation, and also able to rotate around the patient in less than 0.25 seconds. The fast rotation and wide coverage is relevant in cardiac imaging because it allows for better temporal resolution which is important when imaging the heart, an organ that is constantly moving.

Cardiac Gating

To image an organ such as the heart, and evaluate anatomical structures such as valves and coronary arteries, the CT scanner has to have the ability to make an exposure during the optimal phase or window of the cardiac cycle to improve temporal resolution. Many modern CT scanners have the ability to gate or time the scan to the patient's heart beat. A cardiac-gated CT scan is accomplished by placing leads on the patient, and triggering the center of the scan at the selected part of the heart rhythm (Fig. 15-6). The x-ray beam can also be kept on for fractions of a second longer to capture the heart structures before and after the center of the selected part of the heart rhythm. This can allow for visualization of cardiac valves in an open versus a closed position, or to find a view of the coronary arteries with no motion. Leaving the beam on for a longer duration however will increase the radiation dose to the patient.

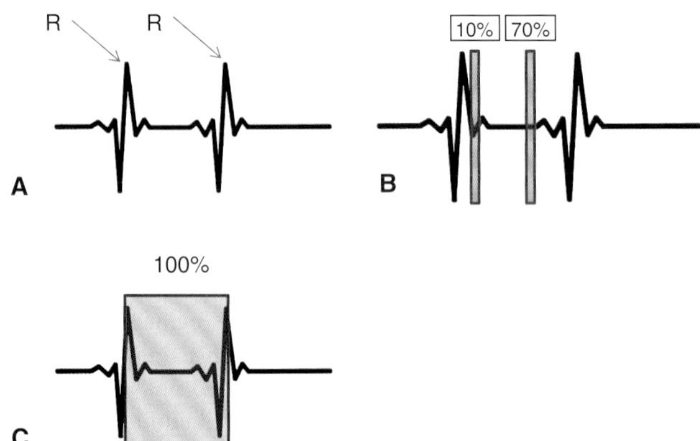

Figure 15-6. A gated cardiac CT is synchronized to the electrocardiogram. **(A)** R to R interval or R-R interval. **(B)** 10% of the R-R interval generally represents peak systole. 70% of the R-R interval generally represents end diastole. **(C)** 100% of the R-R interval is one cardiac cycle.

Contrast

CT scans use IV contrast to help image organs and blood vessels. Contrast mixes and increases the density of the blood or body fluid, and attenuates or reduces the energy of the x-ray. The result is an enhancement or opacification of these organs and blood vessels. All of the IV contrast used for modern CT protocols is nonionic. Nonionic IV CT contrast is less reactive than the ionic IV contrasts of the past, which has allowed for faster injection rates, and better imaging of high blood volume vessels and organs such as the heart. A high concentration of IV contrast appears bright on the CT image. Leveraging the flow in the body, CT protocols have been refined to image most structures based on the anticipated timing for contrast to enhance that specific organ, or blood vessel.

Adverse reactions can occur from the administration of IV contrast. These can range from sneezing and light rashes to anaphylaxis. Patients with prior reactions are more likely to have more severe subsequent reactions from the IV contrast. Premedication protocols typically include a time-released steroid to suppress the response. This is further discussed in a later section.

Protocols

CT protocols for cardiac imaging take advantage of modern scanner's ability to gate or time the scan acquisition to the patient's heart beat. Some scanners even have the ability to make images of the entire heart, and full cardiac cycle in one rotation. This allows for a much better temporal resolution and the potential for motion-free images of the heart and its structures. The scans are also timed to the optimal peak enhancement of the particular organ or vessel. For example, to time for the coronary arteries, a region of interest measurement area is drawn over the aortic root, and the scanner will create a graph to indicate the peak enhancement of the vessel. This can be done either in real time or preplanned time. For the coronary arteries to fully opacify, extra time is added to allow for full contrast circulation to the distal parts of the vessel.

Indications

Cardiovascular CT is most commonly used for anatomical imaging (Table 15-1). The use of CT for cardiovascular imaging has increased significantly in recent years. Modern CT scanners and current protocols allow for the acquisition of excellent images of most of the blood vessels and heart structures. With the use of post processing workstations, CT images are reconstructed in a manner that enables practitioners to accurately and consistently image and measure anatomical structures and features such as coronary arteries, heart valves, and pulmonary veins (Fig. 15-7).

Indications for cardiac CT scans are reviewed.

Coronary Anatomy

A properly performed coronary artery CTA provides an excellent evaluation of the full length of the coronary arteries.[40] Imaging

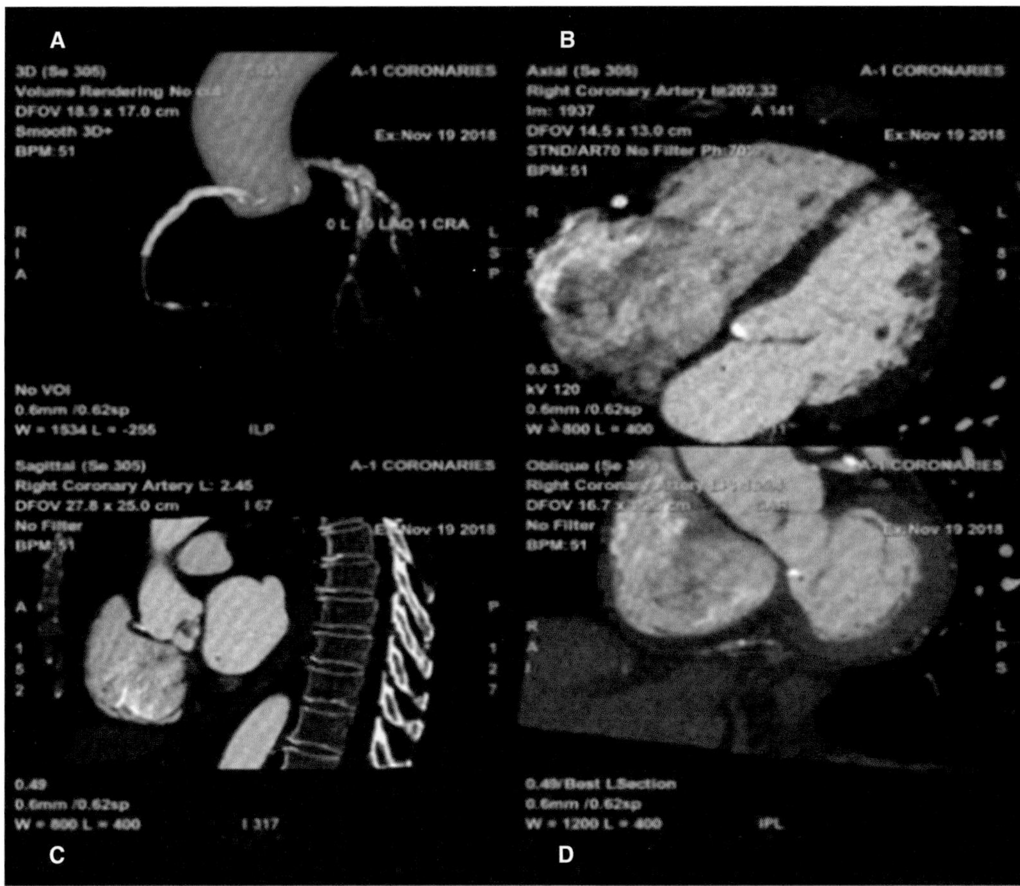

Figure 15-7. CT workstation multiplane view of heart. **(A)** Volume rendered view of aortic root with coronary arteries. **(B)** Oblique four chamber view of the heart showing tricuspid and mitral valves open. **(C)** Sagittal view of the heart. **(D)** Oblique view of the heart with mitral valve open.

of coronary arteries from their origin to vessel termination allows for evaluation of coronary artery stenosis and anomalous coronary artery anatomy (Fig. 15-8). Patency of coronary artery stents may also be verified by coronary CTA. New algorithms to suppress metal artifacts are better able to differentiate the metal lined stents from contrast (Fig. 15-9). The location and patency of coronary artery bypass grafts may also be ascertained by modern CT scanners. Scanning very thin slices improves the spatial resolution of the images and enables clinicians to visualize the entire bypass graft.

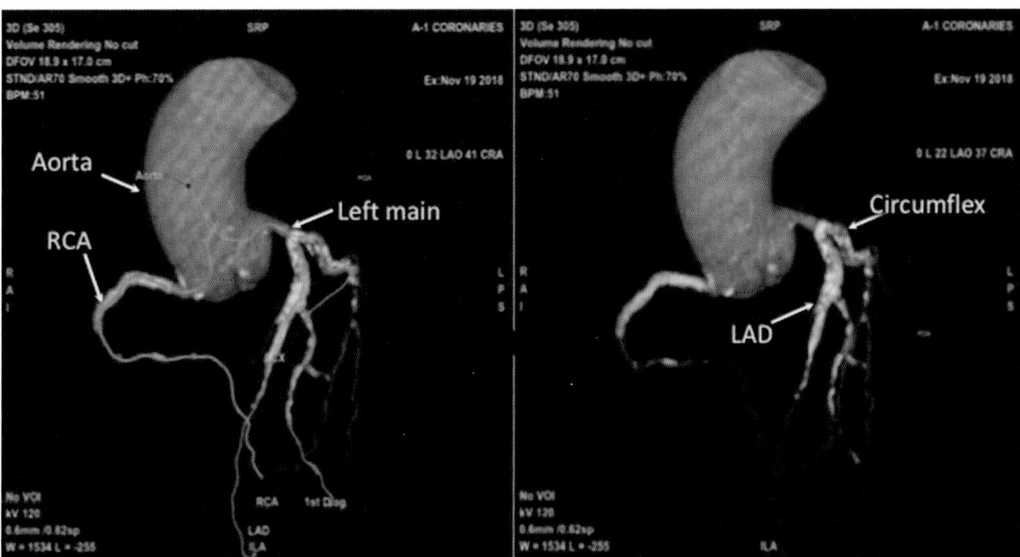

Figure 15-8. Volume rendered CT image of the aortic root with coronary arteries. RCA, right coronary artery; LAD, left anterior descending.

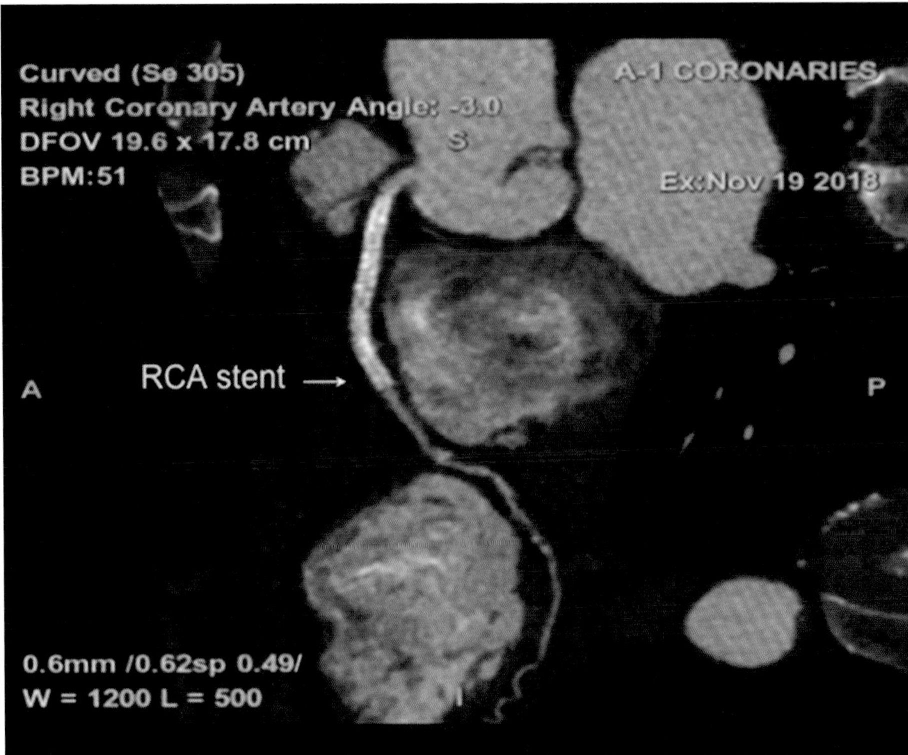

Figure 15-9. Curved reformat CT image of right coronary artery (RCA) with stent.

Although improvements in scanner technology have occurred in the last 5 years, temporal resolution is still a limiting factor. Heart rate and rhythm dramatically affect the resolution of images. At low regular rates, resolution is reasonable. A beta-blocker protocol may be used to slow the heart rate, thereby decreasing the likelihood of motion artifact and improving image quality. Patients who have rhythm disturbances, such as atrial fibrillation, or contraindications to beta blockers pose challenges to coronary CT imaging.[40]

Cardiac Valve Interventions

The patient with congenital heart disease and valvular heart disease requiring evaluation will frequently be referred for CT imaging.[41,42] A cardiac-gated CT scan of the chest and heart is used for obtaining the measurements of the aortic valve for repair or replacement. Properly performed CT imaging of the aortic valve can demonstrate the valve in a motion-free state, enabling accurate and replicable measurements (Figs. 15-10 and 15-11). CT is also used to evaluate the mitral valve for percutaneous

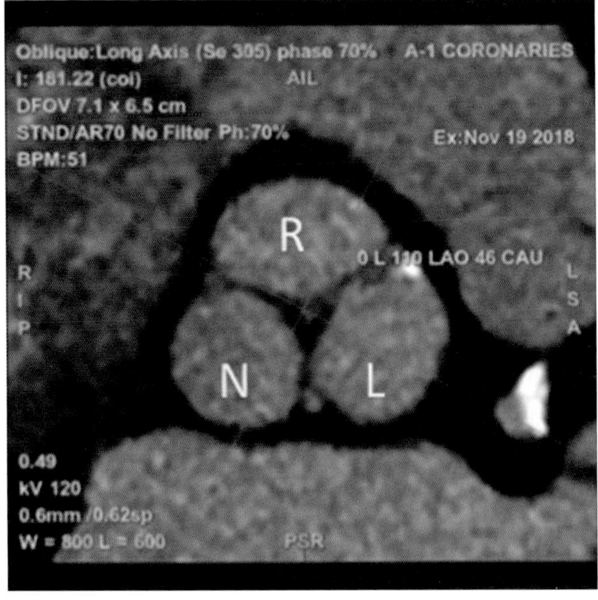

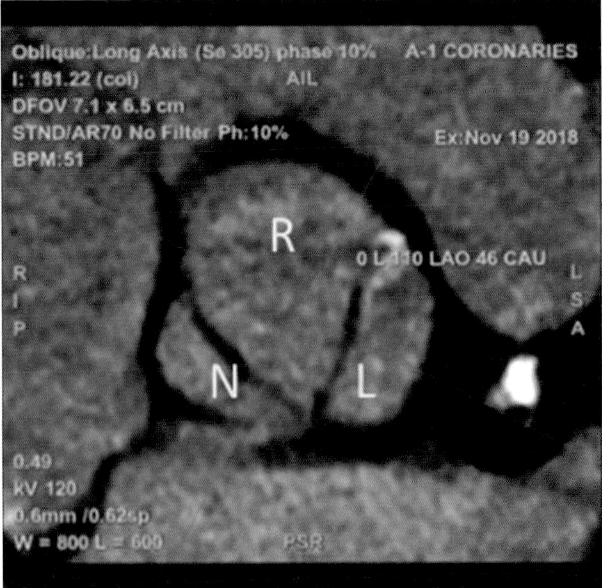

Figure 15-10. Oblique long axis view, cross-sectional plane of the aortic valve. **(A)** Aortic valve is open. **(B)** Aortic valve is closed. R, right; N, non-coronary; L, left.

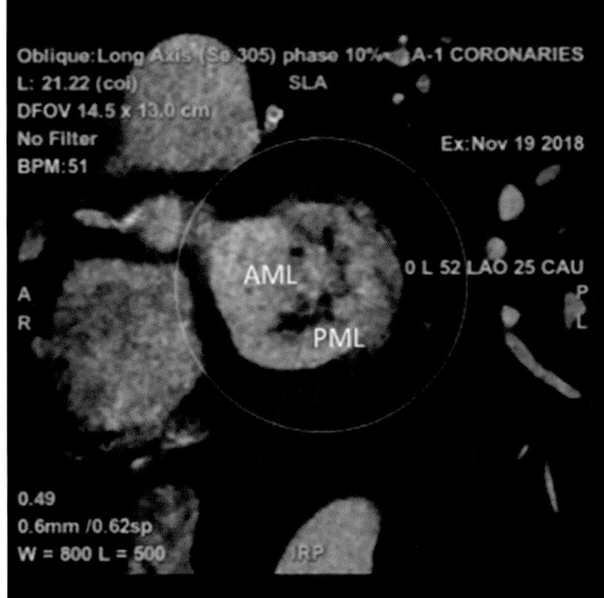

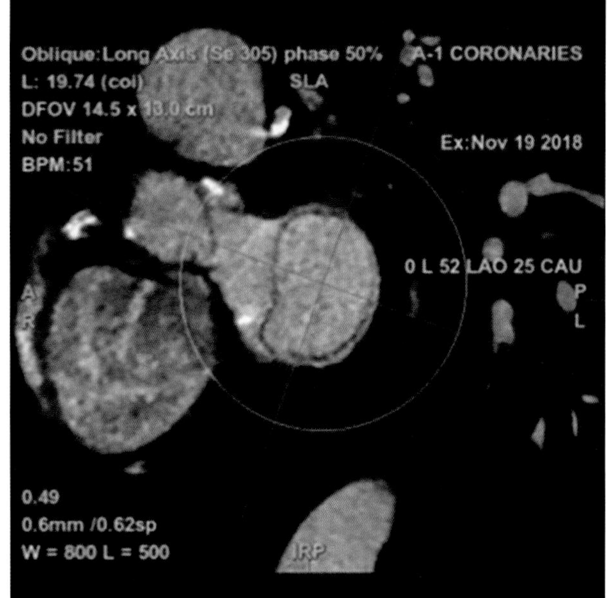

Figure 15-11. Oblique long axis view of the mitral valve. **A**, the mitral valve is open. **B**, the mitral valve is closed. AML, anterior mitral leaflet; PML, posterior mitral leaflet.

and/or surgical repair or replacement. Occasionally, an evaluation of the venous system in the abdomen and lower extremities is obtained in addition to the chest and heart. Contrast timing is optimized to demonstrate the left atrium, LV, and its outflow tract. The lower extremities are then scanned when the contrast is opacifying the IVC and the iliac veins. For tricuspid valve intervention, CT imaging of the right heart may be challenging if pure IV contrast is used. A blended mix of saline and contrast is used to demonstrate the right atrium, tricuspid valve, and RV, as well as the IVC and the hepatic veins. Lastly, the pulmonic valve is one of the most challenging cardiac structures to image; it is very dynamic, and the window of opportunity for optimal IV contrast enhancement is very short (about 2 to 3 seconds). With a modern CT scanner and a distinct protocol, the pulmonic valve and the artery/RV outflow tract can be well visualized and properly measured.

Cardiac Arrhythmia Interventions

Gated cardiac and chest CT is also used for assessment and procedure planning for cardiac arrhythmia interventions. The images produced are an excellent representation of the patient's cardiac anatomy. The CT images are loaded onto a workstation where structures may be measured in detail. The left atrium and the pulmonary veins are imaged for atrial fibrillation (pulmonary vein ablation) (Fig. 15-12). The RV outflow tract is imaged for preprocedural planning of transcatheter and surgical pulmonic valve intervention/replacement using the protocol for the imaging of the pulmonic valve/ pulmonary artery.

The left atrial appendage (LAA) is imaged for LAA occlusion, closure, or ligation.[43] LAA size and shape vary greatly and is best imaged at its most distended form. To get an accurate measurement and description of the LAA, the full cardiac cycle is needed. CT scan coverage begins just above the carina and continues to the apex of the ventricles. To guide the implementation of LAA occlusion devices, a number of parameters are evaluated: orthogonal measurements of the LAA, volume of he appendage, best fluoroscopic angle for deployment, and proposed landing zone for device implantation (Fig. 15-13).

Left Ventricular Assist Devices

Evaluation of left ventricular assist devices (LVADs) is often prompted by pump alarms. CT may be used to verify placement of an LVAD, and to exclude any obstruction to the inflow cannula. With algorithms capable of suppressing metal artifact, and the ability to scan during a full cardiac or pump cycle, modern scanners and scan protocols can rule out whether inflow tract of the LVAD or any portion of the driveline is compromised.

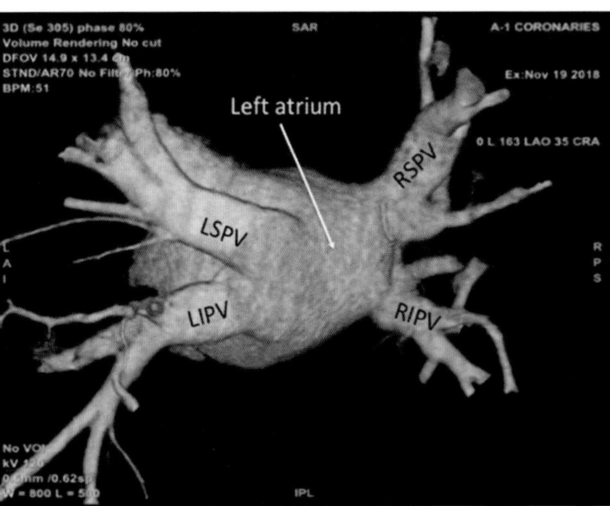

Figure 15-12. Volume rendered CT image of the left atrium and pulmonary veins. LSPV, left superior pulmonary vein; LIPV, left inferior pulmonary vein; RSPV, right superior pulmonary vein; RIPV, right inferior pulmonary vein.

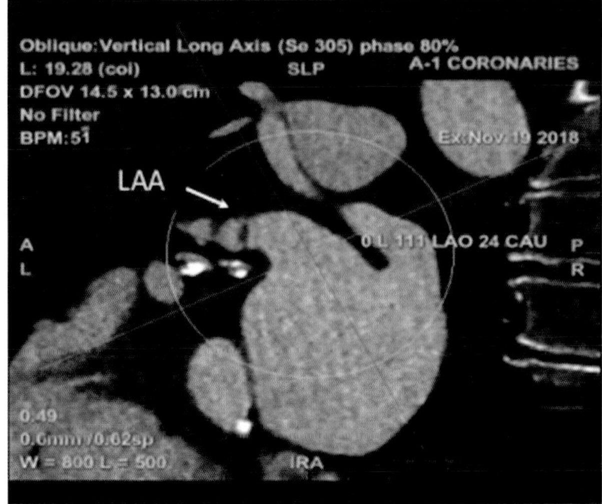

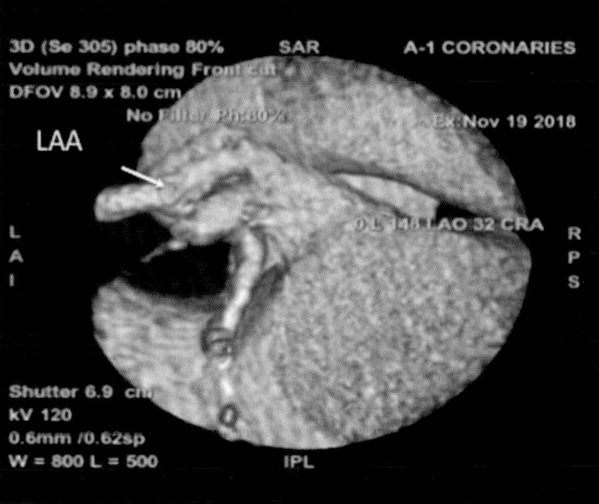

Figure 15-13. CT images of the left atrial appendage (LAA). **(A)** Oblique long axis view. **(B)** Volume rendered image.

Patient Considerations

Patient Preparation

Most CT scans with IV contrast do not require any special preparation for patients. Cardiac-specific CT scans ask that patients not take any stimulants such as caffeine, or any medications that can affect heart rate or blood pressure. Beta blockers, as described, may be given to decrease heart rate. Nitroglycerin may also be given during coronary artery–specific scans to dilate the blood vessels. Depending on the diagnostic indication, the patient is educated on the risks of exposure to ionizing radiation. The provider ordering the procedure must likewise weigh radiation exposure as a patient risk. Pregnancy is a contraindication.

Contrast Reactions

Hypersensitivity reactions to contrast occur and cannot always be predicted. In general, reactions occur within minutes to days, with severity ranging from sneezing or urticaria to angioedema to anaphylaxis. Therefore, a thorough history of prior exposure to contrast agents, asthma, or other allergic or atopic illnesses is required. Premedicate with steroids and antihistamines in patients with a history of a previous hypersensitivity reaction, regardless of the severity. If a patient has contraindications to the IV contrast, such as prior allergic reactions (depending on the severity of the reaction), they may be given a premedication regimen consisting of oral steroids and diphenhydramine. The risk of a contrast reaction versus the benefits of the diagnostic information must be weighed by the ordering provider on an individual basis. It is important to remember that premedication prior to exposure to a contrast agent does not eliminate completely the risk of a hypersensitivity reaction but does reduce it. Minor, usually transient, reactions to contrast include but are not limited to flushing, metallic taste, nausea, or bradycardia, and are not usually hypersensitivity reactions.

The contrast is eliminated from the body mainly via the kidney. Thus, significant renal insufficiency is a contraindication to contrasted cardiovascular CT imaging. Although there is not necessarily a specific GFR at which a study is contraindicated, the risks of worsening renal insufficiency versus the benefits of the diagnostic information must be weighed on an individual basis by the provider ordering the procedure. Before any IV contrast injection is given, the patient's creatinine clearance should be calculated. Laboratory testing to evaluate renal functions may be performed if a patient has a history of kidney disease, dehydration, or is on multiple medications. If renal functions are compromised, prehydration protocols, reduced IV contrast volumes or cancellation of the scan may be recommended. An algorithm for acute reactions to contrast media is depicted in Figure 15-14.

Post Processing

After the scan, the CT image data are loaded onto a workstation for post processing. The workstations can take the slice data to create a volume, and accurately assess any of the structures that are within the field of view. For example, to evaluate the aortic valve annulus for transcatheter aortic valve replacement, the area, diameter, and perimeter of the annulus must be measured at the basal points of valve leaflets insertion or attachment into the aorta, and where the left ventricular outflow tract enters (Fig. 15-15). Once the desired anatomy is rendered and in view, questions regarding the particular structure can be answered with a measurement and/or visual confirmation.

CONCLUSION

Nuclear imaging, MRI, and CT are diagnostic imaging modalities that provide answers in noninvasive ways for some of the most challenging anatomical and physiologic questions in cardiology. The images, measurements, and interpretations provided are increasingly part of the standard of care for the diagnosis and management of cardiovascular disease. With ever-evolving technology, nursing and radiology must partner to provide optimal care for patients.

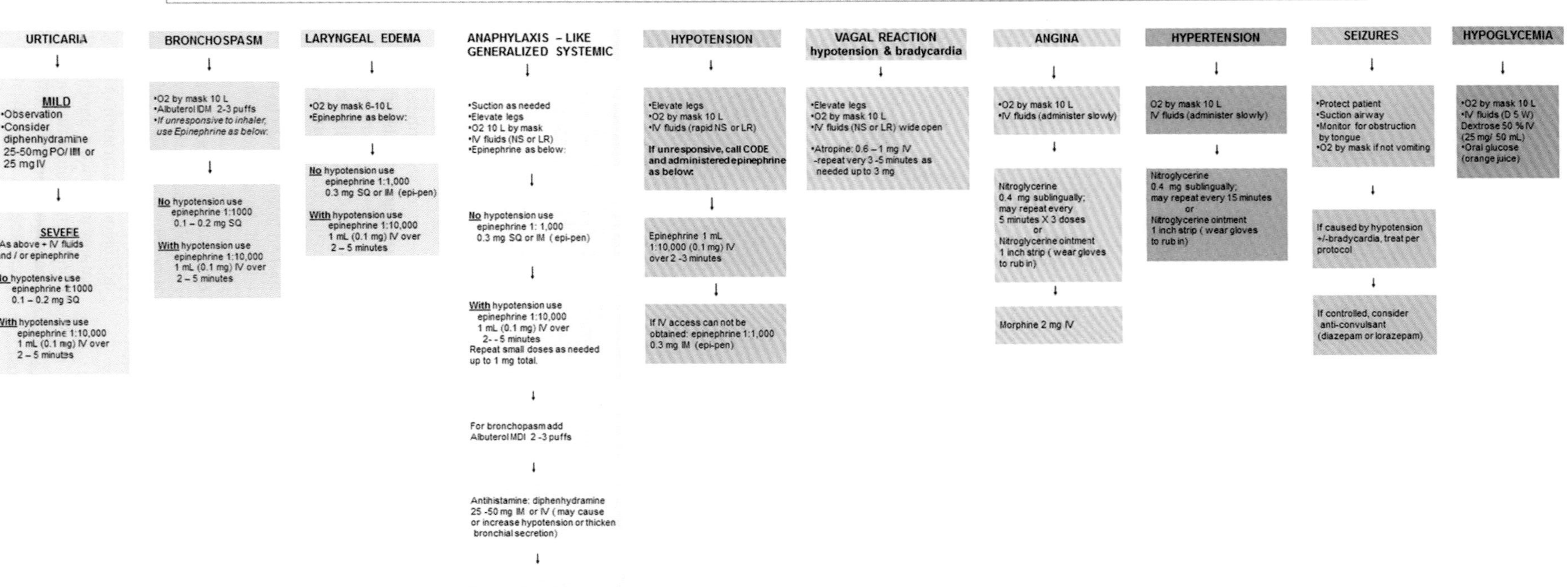

Figure 15-14. Algorithm for acute reaction to contrast media.

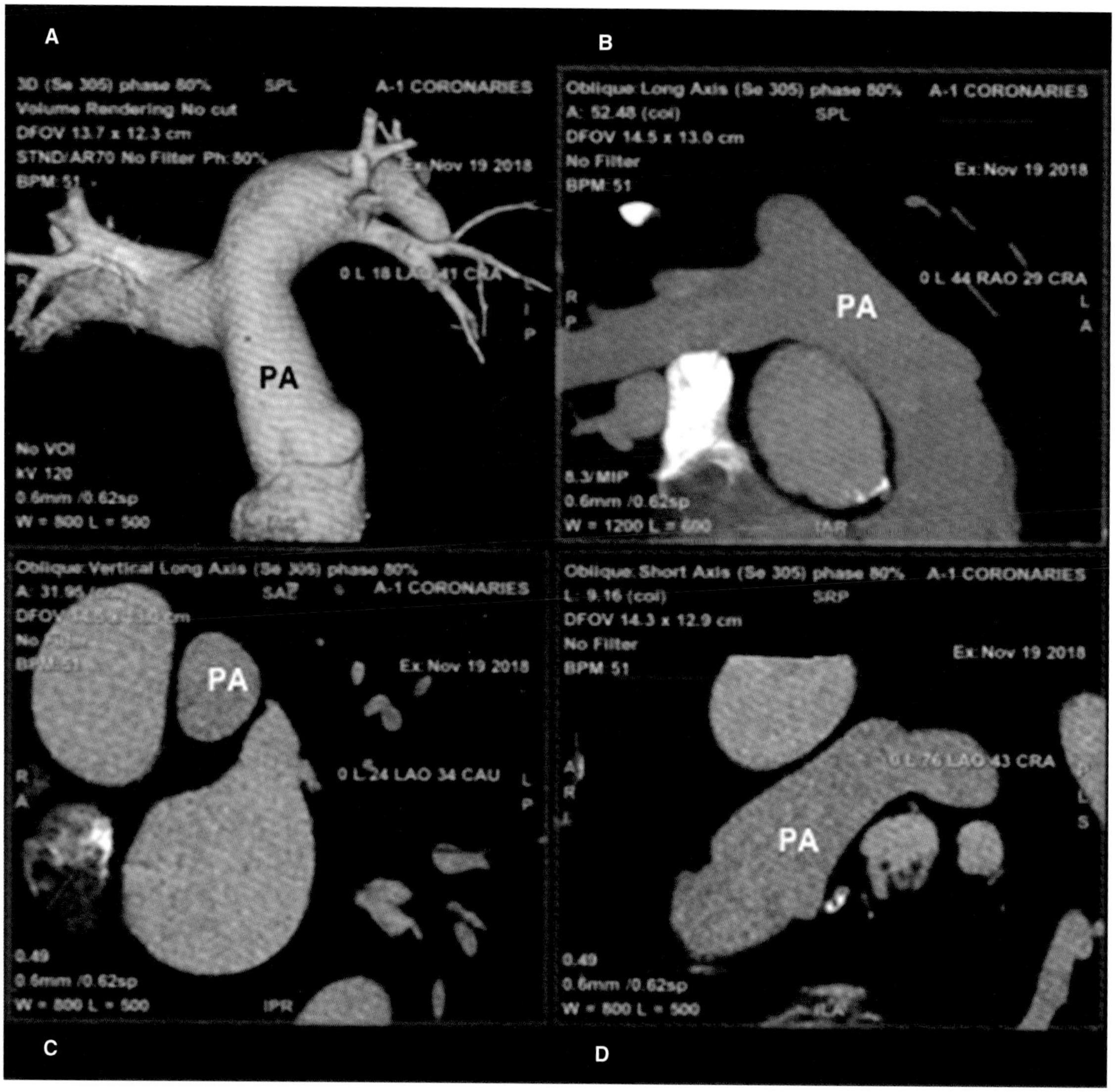

Figure 15-15. Volume data set is loaded onto a post processing workstation to demonstrate multiplanar views of the pulmonary artery. **(A)** Volume rendered view. **(B)** Oblique long axis view. **(C)** Oblique vertical long axis view. **(D)** Oblique short axis view.

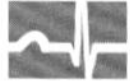

CASE STUDY 1

Patient Profile

Mrs. Katherine White is a 54-year-old female with pulmonary arterial hypertension thought to be related to a history of a pulmonary embolism (chronic thromboembolic pulmonary hypertension), although various studies revealed no ongoing pulmonary emboli or DVT. Past medical history includes pulmonary hypertension, pulmonary emboli, DVT, subclavian artery stenosis, psoriatic arthritis, surgery on salivary gland, surgery on neuroma of right foot, depression with multiple suicide attempts, sleep apnea now using CPAP, endometriosis with total abdominal hysterectomy and bilateral salpingo-oophorectomy. Her medications include apixaban, methotrexate, leucovorin, hydroxychloroquine, and estrogen. Her sister had a ventricular septal defect closure at a very young age and her father has COPD. She has an allergy to iodinated contrast which gives her a rash.

The patient underwent surgery in July of 2017 on one of her salivary glands and on her right foot for a neuroma. In August of that year, she noticed dyspnea after walking a few blocks. Her dyspnea continued until May of 2018. At that time, she had a chest x-ray showing an enlarged pulmonary artery and a transthoracic echocardiogram (TTE) showing a moderately enlarged right atrium with low normal systolic function. In August of 2018, she had a nuclear medicine scan indicating she had an intermediate to high probability of acute pulmonary emboli. An ultrasound found evidence of a DVT. She started on apixaban at this point. CT imaging 3 weeks later showed no evidence of pulmonary embolus while a follow-up TTE showed her pulmonary artery systolic pressure had increased over that time. She then had a right heart catheterization (RHC) with pulmonary angiogram which suggested a probable thrombotic occlusion in a branch of her left pulmonary artery. The patient underwent another CT and TTE and continued to get conflicting results until a second RHC suggested the possibility of a shunt. She underwent a cardiac MRI which confirmed the presence of a small atrial septal defect with a left-to-right shunt.

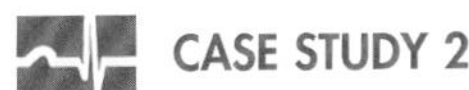

CASE STUDY 2

Patient Profile

Mrs. Laura Frank is a 75-year-old female who underwent LVAD implantation (HeartMate™) due to severe LV dysfunction. HeartMate alarms intermittently. An ECG-gated CT scan of the heart and aorta was recommended.

Medical History

Nonischemic cardiomyopathy, status post LVAD implantation, HeartMate pump

Family History

Significant for nonspecified heart disease; mother died at age 59

Allergies

Ibuprofen, topical iodine

Diagnostic Studies

Cardiac CT scan (heart and aorta) (Figs. 15-16 and 15-17) showed the inflow cannula is pointed and nearly touching the intraventricular septum. During the cardiac cycle, partial ingestion/occlusion is noted over the external opening of the inflow cannula.

Conclusion

Cardiothoracic surgery recommended surgical intervention, and repositioning of the inflow cannula.

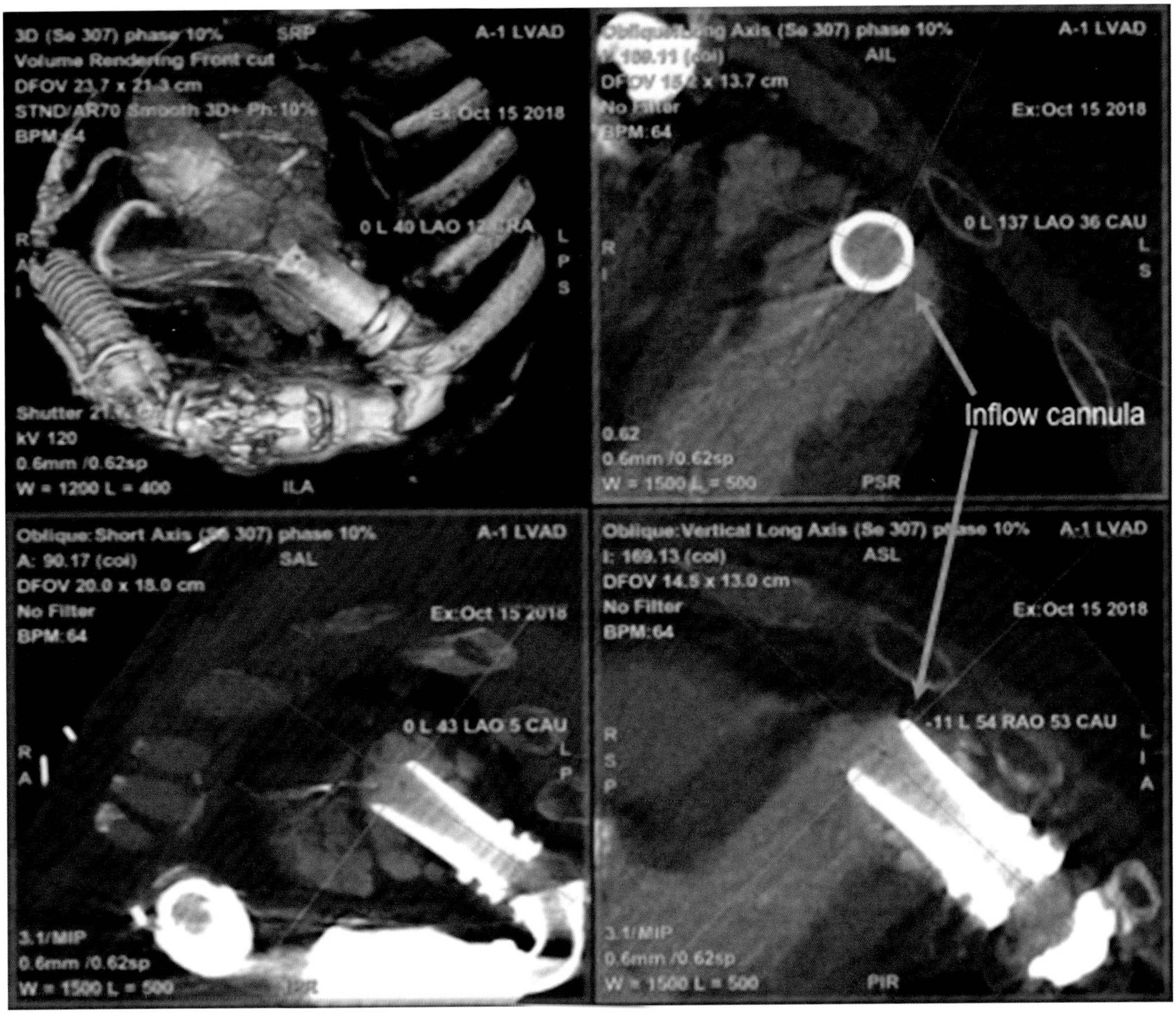

Figure 15-16. Multiplanar views of the heart with a left ventricular access device. LVAD function is not suspended during the acquisition of this image to allow the demonstration of inflow obstruction.

(continued)

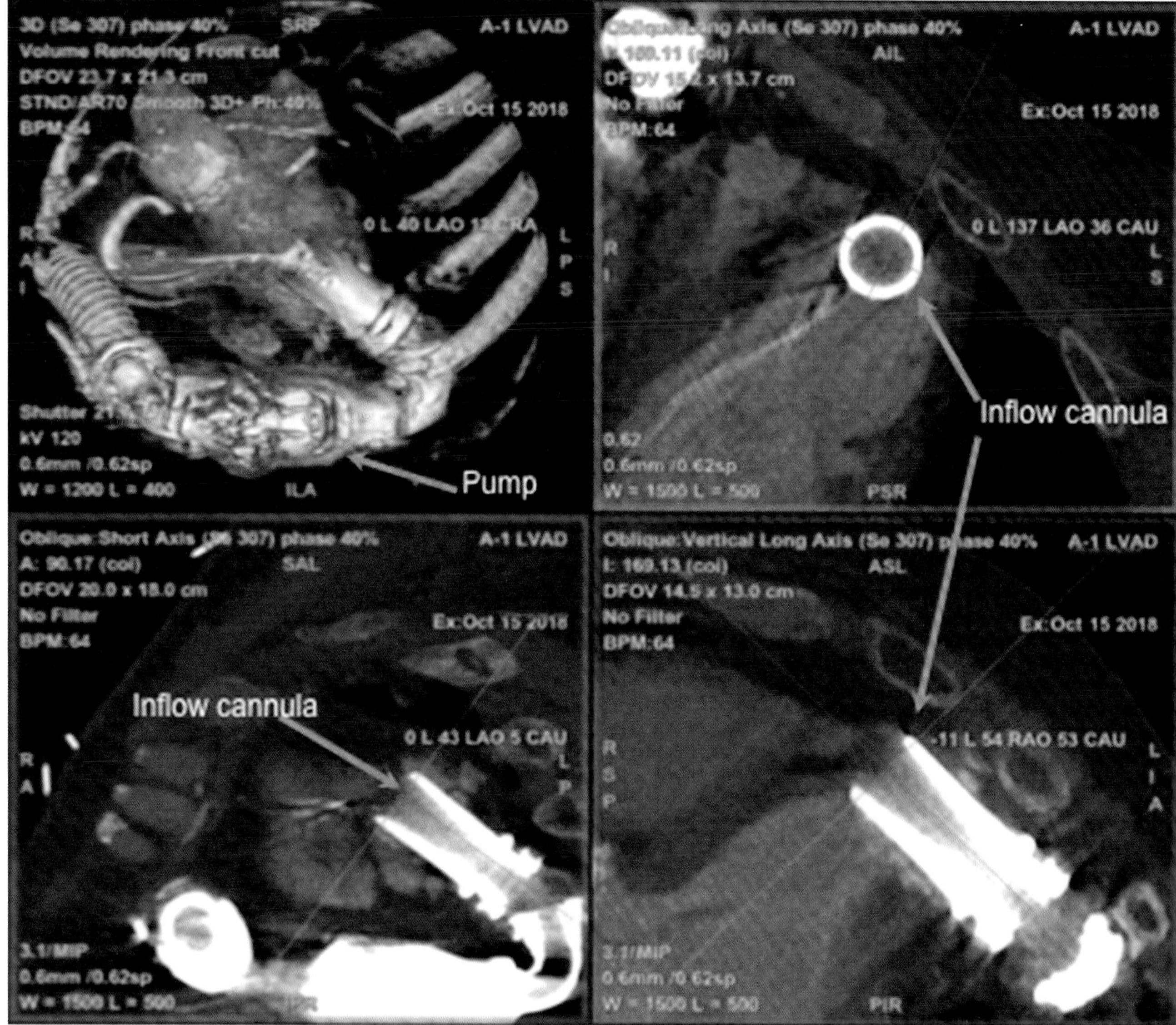

Figure 15-17. Multiplanar views of the heart with a left ventricular access device. LVAD function is resumed during the acquisition of this image. Note that the interventricular septum is being pulled into the left ventricular inflow tract.

KEY READINGS

Doherty JU, Kort S, Mehran R, et al. ACC/AATS/AHA/ASE/ASNC/HRS/SCAI/SCCT/SCMR/STS 2019 appropriate use criteria for multimodality imaging in the assessment of cardiac structure and function in nonvalvular heart disease. A report of the American College of Cardiology Appropriate Use Criteria Task Force, American Association for Thoracic Surgery, American Heart Association, American Society of Echocardiography, American Society of Nuclear Cardiology, Heart Rhythm Society, Society for Cardiovascular Angiography and Interventions, Society of Cardiovascular Computed Tomography, Society for Cardiovascular Magnetic Resonance, and the Society of Thoracic Surgeons. *J Am Coll Cardiol*. 2019;73(4):488–516.

Indik JH, Gimbel JR, Abe H, et al. 2017 HRS expert consensus statement on magnetic resonance imaging and radiation exposure in patients with cardiovascular implantable electronic devices. *Heart Rhythm*. 2017;14(7):e97–e153.

Nishimura RA, Otto CM, Bonow RO, et al. 2017 AHA/ACC focused update of the 2014 AHA/ACC guideline for the management of patients with valvular heart disease: a report of the American College of Cardiology/American Heart Association Task Force on clinical practice guidelines. *Circulation*. 2017;135(25):e1159–e1195.

REFERENCES

1. Ami EI, Ernest VG. *Nuclear Cardiac Imaging: Principles and Applications*. 5th ed. New York, NY: Oxford University Press; 2015.
2. Verberne HJ, Acampa W, Anagnostopoulos C, et al. EANM procedural guidelines for radionuclide myocardial perfusion imaging with SPECT and SPECT/CT: 2015 revision. *Eur J Nucl Med Mol Imaging*. 2015;42(12):1929–1940.
3. Henzlova MJ, Duvall WL, Einstein AJ, et al. ASNC imaging guidelines for SPECT nuclear cardiology procedures: stress, protocols, and tracers. *J Nucl Cardiol*. 2016;23(3):606–639.
4. Wolk MJ, Bailey SR, Doherty JU, et al. ACCF/AHA/ASE/ASNC/HFSA/HRS/SCAI/SCCT/SCMR/STS 2013 Multimodality appropriate use criteria for the detection and risk assessment of stable ischemic heart disease: A report of the American College of Cardiology Foundation Appropriate Use Criteria Task Force, American Heart Association, American Society of Echocardiography, American Society of Nuclear Cardiology, Heart Failure Society of America, Heart Rhythm Society, Society for Cardiovascular Angiography and Interventions, Society of Cardiovascular Computed Tomography, Society for Cardiovascular Magnetic Resonance, and Society of Thoracic Surgeons. *J Am Coll Cardiol*. 2014;63(4):380–406.

5. Longmore DB, Klipstein RH, Underwood SR, et al. Dimensional accuracy of magnetic resonance in studies of the heart. *Lancet.* 1985;1(8442):1360–1362.
6. Rehr RB, Malloy CR, Filipchuk NG, et al. Left ventricular volumes measured by MR imaging. *Radiology.* 1985;156(3):717–719.
7. Benjamin EJ, Muntner P, Alonso A, et al. Heart disease and soke satistics—2019 Update: a report from the American Heart Association. *Circulation.* 2019;139(10):e56–e528.
8. American Society of Nuclear Cardiology and Society of Nuclear Medicine and Molecular Imaging Joint Position Statement on the Clinical Indications for Myocardial Perfusion PET. *J Nucl Cardiol.* 2016;23(5):1227–1231.
9. Jauhiainen T, Jarvinen VM, Hekali PE, et al. MR gradient echo volumetric analysis of human cardiac casts: focus on the right ventricle. *J Comput Assist Tomogr.* 1998;22(6):899–903.
10. Baxi AJ, Restrepo CS, Vargas D, et al. Hypertrophic cardiomyopathy from A to Z: genetics, pathophysiology, imaging, and management. *Radiographics.* 2016;36(2):335–354.
11. Oda S, Kawano Y, Okuno Y, et al. Base-to-apex gradient pattern of cardiac impairment identified on myocardial T1 mapping in cardiac amyloidosis. *Radiol Case Rep.* 2019;14(1):72–74. Available at www.sciencedirect.com/science/article/pii/S1930043318303765. Accessed November 23, 2018.
12. Kouranos V, Tzelepis GE, Rapti A, et al. Complementary role of CMR to conventional screening in the diagnosis and prognosis of cardiac sarcoidosis. *JACC Cardiovasc Imaging.* 2017;10(12):1437–1447.
13. Zuccarino F, Vollmer I, Sanchez G, et al. Left ventricular noncompaction: imaging findings and diagnostic criteria. *Am J Roentgenol.* 2015;204(5):W519–W530.
14. Klem I, Heitner JF, Shah DJ, et al. Improved detection of coronary artery disease by stress perfusion cardiovascular magnetic resonance with the use of delayed enhancement infarction imaging. *J Am Coll Cardiol.* 2006; 47(8):1630–1638.
15. Nagel E, Klein C, Paetsch I, et al. Magnetic resonance perfusion measurements for the noninvasive detection of coronary artery disease. *Circulation.* 2003;108(4):432–437.
16. Kim RJ, Fieno DS, Parrish TB, et al. Relationship of MRI delayed contrast enhancement to irreversible injury, infarct age, and contractile function. *Circulation.* 1999;100(19):1992–2002.
17. Wagner A, Mahrholdt H, Holly TA, et al. Contrast-enhanced MRI and routine single photon emission computed tomography (SPECT) perfusion imaging for detection of subendocardial myocardial infarcts: an imaging study. *Lancet.* 2003;361(9355):374–379.
18. Wang ZF, Reddy GP, Gotway MB, et al. Cardiovascular shunts: MR imaging evaluation. *Radiographics.* 2003;23:S181–S194.
19. Beerbaum P, Parish V, Bell A, et al. Atypical atrial septal defects in children: noninvasive evaluation by cardiac MRI. *Pediatr Radiol.* 2008; 38(11):1188–1194.
20. Njeim M, Yokokawa M, Frank L, et al. Value of cardiac magnetic resonance imaging in patients with failed ablation procedures for ventricular tachycardia. *J Cardiovasc Electrophysiol.* 2016;27(2):183–189.
21. Olsen FJ, Bertelsen L, de Knegt MC, et al. Multimodality cardiac imaging for the assessment of left atrial function and the association with atrial arrhythmias. *Circ Cardiovasc Imaging.* 2016;9(10):e004947. Available at https://doi.org/10.1161/CIRCIMAGING.116.004947. Accessed November 24, 2018.
22. John AS, Dill T, Brandt RR, et al. Magnetic resonance to assess the aortic valve area in aortic stenosis: how does it compare to current diagnostic standards? *J Am Coll Cardiol.* 2003;42(3):519–526.
23. Lin SJ, Brown PA, Watkins MP, et al. Quantification of stenotic mitral valve area with magnetic resonance imaging and comparison with Doppler ultrasound. *J Am Coll Cardiol.* 2004;44(1):133–137.
24. Caruthers SD, Lin SJ, Brown P, et al. Practical value of cardiac magnetic resonance imaging for clinical quantification of aortic valve stenosis: comparison with echocardiography. *Circulation.* 2003;108(18):2236–2243.
25. Djavidani B, Debl K, Lenhart M, et al. Planimetry of mitral valve stenosis by magnetic resonance imaging. *J Am Coll Cardiol.* 2005;45(12): 2048–2053.
26. Hundley WG, Li HF, Willard JE, et al. Magnetic resonance imaging assessment of the severity of mitral regurgitation. Comparison with invasive techniques. *Circulation.* 1995;92(5):1151–1158.
27. Ley S, Eichhorn J, Ley-Zaporozhan J, et al. Evaluation of aortic regurgitation in congenital heart disease: value of MR imaging in comparison to echocardiography. *Pediatr Radiol.* 2007;37(5):426–436.
28. Haugaa KH, Haland TF, Leren IS, et al. Arrhythmogenic right ventricular cardiomyopathy, clinical manifestations, and diagnosis. *Europace.* 2016;18(7):965–972.
29. Karaosmanoglu, AD, Khawaja RD, Onur MR, et al. CT and MRI of aortic coarctation: pre- and postsurgical finding. *Am J Roentgenol.* 2015; 204(3):W224–W233.
30. Dijkema EJ, Leiner T, Grotenhuis HB. Diagnosis, imaging, and clinical management of aortic coarctation. *Heart.* 2017;103(15):1148–1155.
31. Yuan C, Beach KW, Smith LH Jr, et al. Measurement of atherosclerotic carotid plaque size in vivo using high resolution magnetic resonance imaging. *Circulation.* 1998;98(24):2666–2671.
32. Hatsukami TS, Ross R, Polissar NL, et al. Visualization of fibrous cap thickness and rupture in human atherosclerotic carotid plaque in vivo with high-resolution magnetic resonance imaging. *Circulation.* 2000; 102(9):959–964.
33. Yuan C, Mitsumori LM, Ferguson MS, et al. In vivo accuracy of multispectral magnetic resonance imaging for identifying lipid-rich necrotic cores and intraplaque hemorrhage in advanced human carotid plaques. *Circulation.* 2001;104(17):2051–2056.
34. Yuan C, Zhang SX, Polissar NL, et al. Identification of fibrous cap rupture with magnetic resonance imaging is highly associated with recent transient ischemic attack or stroke. *Circulation.* 2002;105(2):181–185.
35. Takaya N, Yuan C, Chu B, et al. Presence of intraplaque hemorrhage stimulates progression of carotid atherosclerotic plaques: a high-resolution magnetic resonance imaging study. *Circulation.* 2005;111(21): 2768–2775.
36. Russo RAG, Katsicas, MM. Takayasu arteritis. *Front Pediatr.* 2018;6:265. Available at https://www.frontiersin.org/article/10.3389/fped.2018.00265. Accessed November 26, 2018.
37. Motwani M, Kidambi A, Herzog B, et al. MR imaging of cardiac tumors and masses: a review of methods and clinical applications. *Radiology.* 2013;268(1):26–43.
38. Expert Panel on MR Safety; Kanal E, Barkovich AJ, Bell C, et al. ACR guidance document on MR safe practices: 2013. *J Magn Reson Imaging.* 2013;37(3):501–530.
39. Shellock FG. MRISafety.com. 2019. Available at http://mrisafety.com/
40. Lepsic J, Abarra S, Achenbach S, et al. SCCT guidelines for the interpretation and reporting of conronary CT angiography. A report of the Society of Cardiovascular Computed Tomography Guidelines Committee. *J Cardiovasc Comput Tomogr.* 2014;8(5):342–358.
41. Stout KK, Daniels CJ, Aboulhosn JA, et al. 2018 AHA/ACC guideline for the management of adults with congenital heart disease: a report of the American College of Cardiology/American Heart Association Task Force on clinical practice guidelines. *Circulation.* 2019;139(14):e698–e800.
42. Otto CM, Kumbhani DJ, Alexander KP, et al. 2017 ACC expert consensus decision pathway for transcatheter aortic valve replacement in the management of adults with aortic stenosis: a report of the American College of Cardiology Task Force on clinical expert consensus documents. *J Am Coll Cardiol.* 2017;69(10):1313–1346.
43. Kavinsky CJ, Kusumoto FM, Bavry AA, et al. SCAI/ACC/HRS institutional and operator requirements for left atrial appendage occlusion. *J Am Coll Cardiol.* 2016;67(19):2295–2305.

16 Cardiac Catheterization

Maureen B. Julien

OBJECTIVES

1. Understand indications for right and left heart catheterization
2. Understand the basic procedures performed in the cardiac catheterization laboratory
3. Understand the care of patients pre- and postcardiac catheterization
4. Understand procedure specific considerations for patients

KEY QUESTIONS

1. What are the implications of radiation exposure in the cardiac catheterization laboratory for patients and staff?
2. What are the hemodynamic data derived from a right heart catheterization?
3. What are the major complications following cardiac catheterization and what should nurses assess to identify complications early?

BACKGROUND

Cardiac catheterization is widely used for diagnostic evaluation and therapeutic intervention in the management of patients with cardiac disease. Nurses have a critical role in precatheterization teaching, intracatheterization, and postcatheterization care. The many nursing responsibilities related to cardiac catheterization are outlined in the Society for Coronary Angiography and Intervention (SCAI) Expert Consensus Statement: 2016 Best Practices in the Cardiac Catheterization Laboratory[1] as well the Society of Invasive Cardiovascular Professionals New 2015 Educational Guidelines for Invasive Cardiovascular Technology Personnel in the Cardiovascular Catheterization Laboratory[2] endorsed by SCAI.

Although noninvasive diagnostic techniques have an important role, cardiac catheterization remains the most definitive procedure for the diagnosis and evaluation of coronary disease. Right heart catheterization (RHC) remains the clinical gold standard for hemodynamic evaluation. Coronary angiography together with adjunctive technologies during angiography, including intravascular ultrasound (IVUS), fractional flow reserve (FFR), and coronary flow reserve (CFR), provide direct quantitative measurements to evaluate significance of coronary lesions. This chapter describes cardiac catheterization procedures and their possible complications. It also describes the nursing care given before and after catheterization and the interpretation of data as they relate to cardiovascular disease (CVD) (Table 16-1).

Historical State and Context

Cardiac catheterization developed as a result of 50 years of clinical effort. Werner Forssman performed the first documented cardiac catheterization in 1929 in Germany. Guided by fluoroscopy, Forssman passed a catheter into his own right heart through an antecubital vein. He then walked upstairs to the radiology department and confirmed the catheter position by radiograph. The techniques of right and left heart catheterization were developed

Table 16-1 • NONINVASIVE TESTS RESULTS PREDICTING HIGH RISK FOR ADVERSE OUTCOME HIGH RISK (>3% ANNUAL DEATH OR MI)

1. Severe resting LV dysfunction (LVEF <35%) not readily explained by noncoronary causes
2. Resting perfusion abnormalities ≥10% of the myocardium in patients without prior history or evidence of MI
3. Stress ECG findings including ≥2 mm of ST-segment depression at low workload or persisting into recovery, exercise-induced ST-segment elevation, or exercise-induced VT/VF
4. Severe stress-induced LV dysfunction (peak exercise LVEF <45% or drop in LVEF with stress ≥10%)
5. Stress-induced perfusion abnormalities encumbering ≥10% myocardium or stress segmental scores indicating multiple vascular territories with abnormalities
6. Stress-induced LV dilation
7. Inducible wall motion abnormality (involving 2 > segments or 2 coronary beds)
8. Wall motion abnormality developing at low dose of dobutamine (≤10 mg/kg/min) or at a low heart rate (<120 beats/min)
9. CAC score >400 Agatston units
10. Multivessel obstructive CAD (≥70% stenosis) or left main stenosis (≥50% stenosis) on CCTA

CAC, coronary artery calcium; CCTA, coronary computed tomography angiography; LV, left ventricular; LVEF, left ventricular ejection fraction; MI, myocardial infarction.
Adapted from Fihn SD, Gardin JM, Abrams J, et al. 2012 ACCF/AHA/ACP/AATS/PCNA/SCAI/STS Guideline for the diagnosis and management of patients with stable ischemic heart disease. *J Am Coll Cardiol.* 2012;60:e44–e164.

during the 1940s and 1950s.[3–5] In 1953, the percutaneous techniques of arterial catheterization were introduced by Seldinger,[6] and, in 1959, selective coronary arteriography was introduced by Sones et al.[7] Important advances related to cardiac catheterization included the development of the Swan–Ganz catheter in 1970 for measuring right heart pressures and the thermodilution method for determination of cardiac output (CO). Catheter-based interventions, pioneered by Andreas Gruentzig in the late 1970s,[8] have led to percutaneous coronary interventions (PCIs), including percutaneous transluminal coronary angioplasty, atherectomy, laser therapy, and stent placement[9]; and noncoronary structural interventions like valvuloplasty,[10] percutaneous mitral valve repair,[11] closure of patent foramen ovale (PFO),[12] atrial septal defect (ASD), and ventricular septal defect (VSD),[13] left atrial appendage occlusion (LAAO),[14] and transcatheter valve replacement.[15]

Epidemiology (Prevalence, Incidence) and Demographics

CVD is a significant public health problem as the leading cause of death in the United States. One study estimates that by 2030 greater than 40% of U.S. adults, or 116 million people, will have one or more forms of CVD.[16] In 2009, approximately 683,000 patients were discharged from U.S. hospitals with a diagnosis of acute coronary syndrome (ACS). With improvements in processes and access to care, mortality from ACS has improved.[17] However, there are disparities in outcomes geographically as well as by gender and race. A review of Centers for Medicare and Medicaid Services (CMS) 2009 acute myocardial infarction (AMI) 30-day mortality metric found a higher mortality in the region of Oklahoma and Arkansas, extending into New Mexico, Texas, Kansas, Louisiana, Mississippi, Alabama, Southern Missouri, and Western Tennessee. Whereas, a lower AMI mortality was found in a smaller, more densely populated region in the Northeast.[18] Early reperfusion with PCI has positively impacted these outcomes. Women represent 30% of all STEMI cases. They are more likely to present later and have less typical symptoms. They are also less likely to receive standard medications like aspirin and beta-blockers and have longer treatment times for fibrinolysis and cardiac catheterization. The 2009 ACTION Registry in quarters 1 and 2 found 13.3% of STEMI patients to be nonwhite. Regional care centers were found to have similar treatment times in both white and non-white patients as well as between women and men.[19]

The incidence of RHC is difficult to quantify. There is no registry or database specific to RHC. Institutions may choose to participate in the National Cardiovascular Data Registry's (NCDR) CathPCI Registry; however, many institutions only provide data related to interventions and not diagnostic catheterization alone. There are studies that look to determine RHC incidence in specific populations. Duarte et al. (2016) found that RHC was performed in 42% of patients within 3 months of initial pulmonary hypertension (pHTN) diagnoses and 60.2% of patients over a 9 year study period.[20] A recent abstract presented at the American Heart Association (AHA) 2017 Annual Scientific Session used the Nationwide Inpatient Sample databases and International Classification of Diseases to determine RHC usage in the United States. They found that between 2003 and 2014, only 1% of all hospitalized patients underwent an RHC.[21] The top 5 admission diagnoses for those undergoing RHC were heart failure (HF) (30.4%), AMI (9.8%), coronary artery disease (CAD) (8.5%), valvular heart disease (6.6%) and pulmonary heart disease (6.1%). In that time period, RHC use increased significantly among males (57.1% to 60.8%), blacks (18.0% to 20.6%), publicly insured (63.6% to 70.1%), Southern U.S. hospitals (28.5% to 34.2%) and urban-teaching facilities (79.2% to 88.2%). RHC usage also increased for hospitalizations related to HF (28.3% to 33.6%), pulmonary heart disease (5.9% to 6.4%) and valvular heart disease (5.2% to 7.3%), while it declined for AMI (11.8% to 9.3%) and CAD (12.2% to 6.2%). In-hospital mortality declined from 8.6% to 7.1%.[21]

Current State and Context

Cardiac catheterization is indicated in a wide variety of circumstances. The most frequent use of cardiac catheterization is to confirm or define the extent of suspected CAD. Anatomical and physiologic severity of the disease is determined, the presence or absence of related conditions is explored, and the need for PCI can be determined. Cardiac catheterization is also used for the evaluation of patients with acquired or congenital heart disease. The American College of Cardiology (ACC), AHA, and SCAI have published guidelines for coronary angiography and indications for right and left cardiac catheterization.[22–27] Indications for coronary angiography are classified for specific clinical presentations, including risk stratification for patients with stable ischemic heart disease (SIHD) and asymptomatic patients with ischemia on noninvasive stress testing, as well as patients with ACS: non–ST-elevation acute coronary syndrome (NSTE ACS) and ST-elevation myocardial infarction (STEMI).[19,22,25–27]

Improvements in cardiac procedures and decline in risk associated with diagnostic cardiac catheterizations have increased the number of outpatient procedures. Advantages include decreased costs and avoidance of an unnecessary overnight hospital stay. Patients considered for outpatient cardiac catheterization are those with stable coronary symptoms. While in the past there were a number of relatively rigid exclusions around same-day discharge (SDD), current consensus statements are primarily focused on the patient's clinical situation.[1]

Patients needing preadmission to the hospital for cardiac catheterization include those who require continuous anticoagulation. Previously those with significant renal insufficiency or brittle diabetes mellitus were admitted, but earlier arrival and management may occur the same day as their procedure. Noninvasive testing may identify patients with high-risk coronary or valvular disease before catheterization. Freestanding cardiac catheterization laboratories that are not physically attached to a hospital facility are available and are used for diagnostic studies. It is the responsibility of each freestanding laboratory to have a formal relationship with a referral hospital for emergency services. Patients studied at freestanding laboratories require thorough screening. High-risk patients must be excluded to avoid complications that require emergency services.

Preprocedure teaching is best done before hospital admission. The content is similar to that for patients undergoing an inpatient procedure. After a diagnostic procedure, the patient spends 2 to 6 hours in a short-stay unit, ambulatory recovery, or similar setting. Postprocedure orders are the same for inpatient and outpatient cardiac catheterization. Vital signs, access site, respiratory and neurologic status should be monitored every 15 minutes for the first 2 hours postprocedure by staff trained in recovery from moderate/conscious sedation as well as access site management.[1]

Telemetry is monitored continuously. After the required period of bed rest, postural blood pressure and heart rate are obtained, and the patient is observed ambulating. During this time, instructions are reviewed. The patient is then permitted to leave or transferred

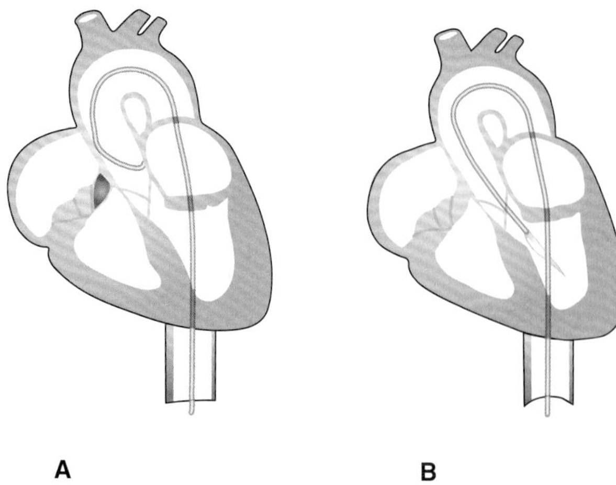

Figure 16-1. (A) Catheterization for coronary arteriography (shown: left main coronary artery catheterization). (B) Left heart catheterization for left ventriculography. (From Deelstra MH, Jacobson C. Cardiac catheterization. In: Woods SL, Sivarajan Froelicher ES, Admas Motzer S, et al., eds. *Cardiac Nursing*. 7th ed. Philadelphia, PA: Lippincott Williams & Wilkins; 2009:446.)

to an inpatient unit. Results of the catheterization are reviewed with the patient and/or family after the procedure by the cardiologist or before discharge. Patients who have had PCI may stay overnight for observation and monitoring, but many institutions have protocols for SDD which are supported by SCAI.[1]

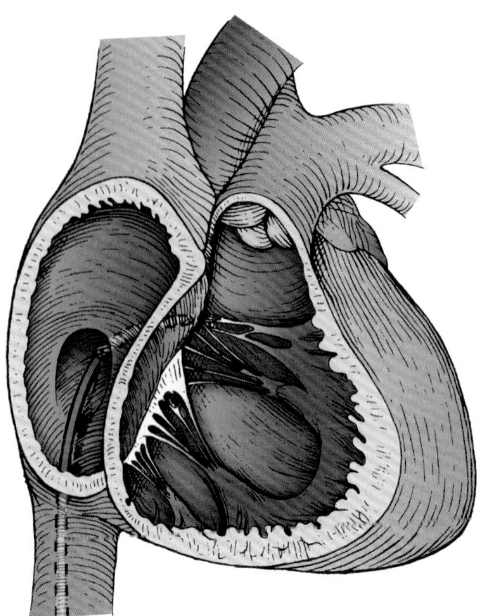

Figure 16-2. Transseptal catheterization. Front of right atrium and ventricle cut away to show the catheter entering the right atrium via the inferior vena cava and crossing the septum into the left atrium. (From Hill JA, Lambert CR, Vuestra RE, et al. Review of techniques. In: Pepine JC, Hill JA, Lambert CR, eds. *Diagnostic and Therapeutic Cardiac Catheterization*. 3rd ed. Baltimore, MD: Williams & Wilkins; 1998:116.)

LEFT HEART CATHETERIZATION

Left heart catheterization is used to perform coronary angiography for the evaluation of coronary anatomy (see Fig. 16-1A), to obtain pressure measurements to evaluate mitral and aortic valve function, left ventricular outflow tract obstruction and pericardial disease, to perform left ventriculography as well as perform structural interventions like mitral valvuloplasty and transcatheter aortic valve replacement (TAVR) (Fig. 16-1B).

The two main approaches into the left heart are retrograde entry through the aortic valve by either the percutaneous radial, femoral, or brachial approach and transseptal entry from the right atrium (Fig. 16-2). The progress of the catheter in both approaches is followed by fluoroscopy and pressure measurement. In the retrograde approach, the catheter is threaded along the aorta and across the aortic valve to the left ventricle.

Indications for Coronary Angiography

Guideline Recommendations

Coronary Angiography as an Initial Testing Strategy to Assess Risk for Stable Ischemic Heart Disease (SIHD): Recommendations[25]

CLASS I

1. Patients with SIHD who have survived sudden cardiac death or potentially life-threatening ventricular arrhythmia should undergo coronary angiography to assess cardiac risk. (Level of Evidence: B)
2. Patients with SIHD who develop symptoms and signs of heart failure should be evaluated to determine whether coronary angiography should be performed for risk assessment. (Level of Evidence: B)

Coronary Angiography to Assess Risk After Initial Workup with Noninvasive Testing for Stable Ischemic Heart Disease: Recommendations[25]

CLASS I

1. Coronary arteriography is recommended for patients with SIHD whose clinical characteristics and results of noninvasive testing indicate a high likelihood of severe IHD and when the benefits are deemed to exceed risk. (Level of Evidence: C)

CLASS IIa

1. Coronary angiography is reasonable to further assess risk in patients with SIHD who have depressed LV function (ejection fraction [EF] <50%) and moderate risk criteria on noninvasive testing with demonstrable ischemia. (Level of Evidence: C)
2. Coronary angiography is reasonable to further assess risk in patients with SIHD and inconclusive prognostic information after noninvasive testing or in patients for whom noninvasive testing is contraindicated or inadequate. (Level of Evidence: C)
3. Coronary angiography for risk assessment is reasonable for patients with SIHD who have unsatisfactory quality of life due to angina, have preserved LV function (EF >50%), and have intermediate risk criteria on noninvasive testing. (Level of Evidence: C)

CLASS III: No Benefit

1. Coronary angiography for risk assessment is not recommended in patients with SIHD who elect not to undergo

revascularization or who are not candidates for revascularization because of comorbidities or individual preferences. (Level of Evidence: B)

2. Coronary angiography is not recommended to further assess risk in patients with SIHD who have preserved LV function (EF >50%) and low-risk criteria on noninvasive testing. (Level of Evidence: B)
3. Coronary angiography is not recommended to assess risk in patients who are at low risk according to clinical criteria and who have not undergone noninvasive risk testing. (Level of Evidence: C)
4. Coronary angiography is not recommended to assess risk in asymptomatic patients with no evidence of ischemia on noninvasive testing. (Level of Evidence: C)

Early Invasive and Ischemia-Guided Strategies for NSTE ACS: Recommendations[26]

CLASS I

1. An urgent/immediate invasive strategy (diagnostic angiography with intent to perform revascularization if appropriate based on coronary anatomy) is indicated in patients (men and women) with NSTE-ACS who have refractory angina or hemodynamic or electrical instability (without serious comorbidities or contraindications to such procedures). (Level of Evidence: A)
2. An early invasive strategy (diagnostic angiography with intent to perform revascularization if appropriate based on coronary anatomy) is indicated in initially stabilized patients with NSTE-ACS (without serious comorbidities or contraindications to such procedures) who have an elevated risk for clinical events (Table 16-2). (Level of Evidence: B)

Table 16-2 • FACTORS ASSOCIATED WITH APPROPRIATE SELECTION OF EARLY INVASIVE STRATEGY OR ISCHEMIA-GUIDED STRATEGY IN PATIENTS WITH NSTE-ACS

Immediate invasive (within 2 hours)	Refractory angina Signs or symptoms of HF or new or worsening mitral regurgitation Hemodynamic instability Recurrent angina or ischemia at rest or with low-level activities despite intensive medical therapy Sustained VT or VF
Ischemia-guided strategy	Low-risk score (e.g., TIMI [0 or 1], GRACE [<109]) Low-risk Tn-negative female patients Patient or clinician preference in the absence of high-risk features
Early invasive (within 24 hours)	None of the above, but GRACE risk score >140 Temporal change in Tn New or presumably new ST depression
Delayed invasive (within 25–72 hours)	None of the above but diabetes mellitus Renal insufficiency (GFR <60 mL/min/1.73 m^2) Reduced LV systolic function (EF <0.40) Early postinfarction angina PCI within 6 months Prior CABG GRACE risk score 109–140; TIMI score ≥2

CABG, coronary artery bypass graft; EF, ejection fraction; GFR, glomerular filtration rate; GRACE, Global Registry of Acute Coronary Events; HF, heart failure; LV, left ventricular; NSTE-ACS, non–ST-elevation acute coronary syndrome; PCI, percutaneous coronary intervention; TIMI, Thrombolysis in myocardial infarction; Tn, troponin; VF, ventricular fibrillation; VT, ventricular tachycardia.
Adapted from Amsterdam EA, Wenger NK, Brindis RG, et al. 2014 AHA/ACC Guideline for the management of patients with non–ST-elevation acute coronary syndromes. *J Am Coll Cardiol.* 2014;64(24):e139–e228.

CLASS IIa

1. It is reasonable to choose an early invasive strategy (within 24 hours of admission) over a delayed invasive strategy (within 25 to 72 hours) for initially stabilized high-risk patients with NSTE-ACS. For those not at high/intermediate risk, a delayed invasive approach is reasonable. (Level of Evidence: B)

CLASS IIb

1. In initially stabilized patients, an ischemia-guided strategy may be considered for patients with NSTE-ACS (without serious comorbidities or contraindications to this approach) who have an elevated risk for clinical events. (Level of Evidence: B)
2. The decision to implement an ischemia-guided strategy in initially stabilized patients (without serious comorbidities or contraindications to this approach) may be reasonable after considering clinician and patient preference. (Level of Evidence: C)

CLASS III: NO BENEFIT

1. An early invasive strategy (i.e., diagnostic angiography with intent to perform revascularization) is not recommended in patients with:
   a. Extensive comorbidities (e.g., hepatic, renal, pulmonary failure; cancer), in whom the risks of revascularization and comorbid conditions are likely to outweigh the benefits of revascularization. (Level of Evidence: C)
   b. Acute chest pain and a low likelihood of ACS who are troponin-negative (Level of Evidence: C), especially women. (Level of Evidence: B)

Primary PCI in STEMI: Recommendations[26]

CLASS I

1. Primary PCI should be performed in patients with STEMI and ischemic symptoms of less than 12 hours' duration. (Level of Evidence: A)
2. Primary PCI should be performed in patients with STEMI and ischemic symptoms of less than 12 hours' duration who have contraindications to fibrinolytic therapy, irrespective of the time delay from first medical contact (FMC). (Level of Evidence: B)
3. Primary PCI should be performed in patients with STEMI and cardiogenic shock or acute severe HF, irrespective of time delay from MI onset. (Level of Evidence: B)

CLASS IIa

1. Primary PCI is reasonable in patients with STEMI if there is clinical and/or electrocardiogram (ECG) evidence of ongoing ischemia between 12 and 24 hours after symptom onset. (Level of Evidence: B)

CLASS III: HARM

1. PCI should not be performed in a noninfarct artery at the time of primary PCI in patients with STEMI who are hemodynamically stable. (Level of Evidence: B)

Coronary Angiography in Patients Who Initially Were Managed with Fibrinolytic Therapy or Who Did Not Receive Reperfusion: Recommendations[26]

CLASS I

1. Cardiac catheterization and coronary angiography with intent to perform revascularization should be performed after STEMI in patients with any of the following:
   a. Cardiogenic shock or acute severe HF that develops after initial presentation. (Level of Evidence: B);
   b. Intermediate- or high-risk findings on predischarge non-invasive ischemia testing. (Level of Evidence: B); or
   c. Myocardial ischemia that is spontaneous or provoked by minimal exertion during hospitalization. (Level of Evidence: C)

CLASS IIa

1. Coronary angiography with intent to perform revascularization is reasonable for patients with evidence of failed reperfusion or reocclusion after fibrinolytic therapy. Angiography can be performed as soon as logistically feasible. (Level of Evidence: B)
2. Coronary angiography is reasonable before hospital discharge in stable patients with STEMI after successful fibrinolytic therapy. Angiography can be performed as soon as logistically feasible, and ideally within 24 hours, but should not be performed within the first 2 to 3 hours after administration of fibrinolytic therapy. (Level of Evidence: B)

Contraindications and Special Considerations for Left Heart Catheterization

Contraindications

Cardiac catheterization has relatively few contraindications. The only absolute contraindication is refusal to informed consent for the procedure by a mentally competent patient. Any correctable illness or condition that, if corrected, would improve the safety of the procedure should be managed before catheterization. These conditions include uncontrolled ventricular irritability, uncorrected hypokalemia or digitalis toxicity, decompensated heart failure, febrile illness, uncontrolled hypertension, severe thrombocytopenia (<40,000–50,000/mcL), anemia, active gastrointestinal bleed, and severe renal insufficiency or anuria unless dialysis is planned after the procedure. Preexisting renal insufficiency, particularly in patients with diabetes, and patients with prior anaphylactic reaction to contrast medium require special treatment before the procedure and will be discussed further under SPECIAL CONSIDERATIONS. Other relative contraindications are recent stroke (within 1 month) and recent major surgery due to the anticoagulation that may be delivered during the catheterization.[28]

Special Considerations

Chronic Oral Anticoagulation. Cardiac catheterization is an invasive procedure and is considered high risk for bleeding when arterial access is required. The decision to hold anticoagulants periprocedurally balances the risk of bleeding risk versus thrombosis. The risk of thrombosis off oral anticoagulation (OAC) is categorized into low, moderate, and high in Table 16-3. Patient-related bleeding risk should also be assessed. The HAS-BLED score is used to identify any modifiable patient risk factors (see Table 16-4). There is some recent data to suggest it is safe to proceed

Table 16-3 • RISK OF THROMBOSIS OFF ORAL ANTICOAGULATION

Low risk: CHA2DS2-VASc[a] <4 or aortic mechanical valve and no prior history of transient ischemic attack/cerebrovascular accident (TIA/CVA), prior VTE >12 months.

Moderate risk: CHA2DS2-VASc of 5–6 or prior history of TIA/CVA, arterial embolism, VTE within 3–12 months, recurrent VTE, nonsevere thrombophilia (e.g., heterozygous factor V Leiden or prothrombin gene mutation), Bileaflet aortic valve prosthesis and one or more of the following risk factors: atrial fibrillation, prior CVA/TIA, Hypertension, diabetes, age >75 years.

High risk: CHA2DS2-VASc ≥7 or recent (<3 months) TIA/CVA, Rheumatic valvular disease, any mechanical mitral valve or any caged ball or tilting disc aortic valve, VTE <3 months, severe thrombophilia (e.g., deficiency of protein C, protein S, or antithrombin; antiphospholipid antibodies; multiple abnormalities).

[a]CHA2DS2-VASc is a risk score to predict the ischemic stroke rate per year in atrial fibrillation.
Adapted from Douketis JD, Spyropoulos AC, Spencer FA, et al. *Perioperative management of antithrombotic therapy: Antithrombotic therapy and prevention of thrombosis,* 9th ed: American College of Chest Physicians Evidence-Based Clinical Practice Guidelines. *Chest.* 2013;141:e326S–e350S.

Table 16-4 • HAS-BLED PATIENT BLEED RISK FACTORS

HAS-BLED parameters[30]
- Hypertension[a]
- Abnormal renal function[b]
- Abnormal liver function[c]
- Prior stroke
- History of or predisposition to (anemia) major bleeding
- Labile INR[d]
- Elderly (>65 years)
- Concomitant use of an antiplatelet agent or nonsteroidal anti-inflammatory drug
- Alcohol or drug usage history (≥8 drinks/wk)[e]

Additional items included in the periprocedural management algorithm:
- Prior bleed event within 3 months (including intracranial hemorrhagic)
- Quantitative or qualitative platelet abnormality
- INR above the therapeutic range at the time of the procedure
- Bleed history from previous bridging
- Bleed history with similar procedure

[a]Defined in HAS-BLED as systolic blood pressure >160 mm Hg.
[b]Defined in HAS-BLED as presence of chronic dialysis, renal transplantation, or serum creatinine ≥200 micromol/L.
[c]Defined in HAS-BLED as chronic hepatic disease (e.g., cirrhosis) or biochemical evidence of significant hepatic derangement (e.g., bilirubin >2× ULN, AST or ALT >3× ULN).
[d]Defined in HAS-BLED as time in the therapeutic range <60%.
[e]Defined in HAS-BLED as >8 U/wk.
Each bullet is counted as 1 point. A HAS-BLED score ≥3 was shown to be highly predictive of bleeding events, with 1 point being given for the presence of each individual parameter.
ALT, alanine transaminase; AST, aspartate transaminase; INR, international normalized ratio; ULN, upper limit of normal.
Adapted from Doherty JU, Gluckman TJ, Hucker WJ, et al. 2017 ACC expert consensus decision pathway for periprocedural management of anticoagulation in patients with nonvalvular atrial fibrillation. *J Am Coll Cardiol.* 2017;69(7):871–898.

Table 16-5 • EXAMPLE OF DOAC HOLD PRECATHETERIZATION DIRECT ORAL ANTICOAGULANTS (DOACs) DAYS TO HOLD ACCORDING TO CREATININE CLEARANCE (CrCl) (mL/min BY COCKROFT–GAULT)

	Dabigatran	Rivaroxaban	Apixaban	Edoxaban
CrCl ≥50	3	2	3	2
30≤ CrCl ≤50	4	2	4	3
15≤ CrCl ≤30	6	2–3	4	4
CrCl <15	Unknown	Unknown	Unknown	Unknown

on warfarin for radial artery access.[29] However, radial access may not always be achieved, and alternative access may be required and therefore necessitate interruption of anticoagulation. There are a range of indications for anticoagulation including nonvalvular and valvular atrial fibrillation (AF), mechanical heart valves, hypercoagulable states and venothromboembolism (VTE). The indication and associated thromboembolic risk should be taken into consideration when deciding to hold anticoagulation for a procedure.

Warfarin has routinely been held for 3 to 5 days before catheterization to achieve an international normalized ratio (INR) below 2.0. The addition of direct oral anticoagulants (DOACs) has created a more complex algorithm as medications have varying half-lives and are often renally excreted requiring tailored hold parameters.[31–33] Table 16-5 shows one example of an approach to holding DOACs precardiac catheterization based on recent studies and guidelines.[31–33]

For patients at high risk for thrombosis off anticoagulation, bridging therapy with heparin or low–molecular-weight heparin (LMWH) can be used while OACs are held. The DOACs have short half-lives that eradicate the need to administer an alternative anticoagulant during medication interruption.[31] Typically, warfarin is held for 4 days precatheterization. As the INR falls, bridging is initiated 2 days preprocedure with the last dose being given 24 hours before the procedure. LMWH may not be used in patients with a creatinine clearance of less than 30 mL/min due to renal excretion and increased bleeding risk. Immediate reversal of prothrombin time can be facilitated by fresh frozen plasma and vitamin K administration for urgent or emergent procedures.[28]

Resuming OACs post catheterization requires consideration of several factors including successful hemostasis and patient-specific factors like bleeding diathesis, platelet dysfunction, and concomitant antiplatelet medications. Warfarin may be initiated following hemostasis as the anticoagulant effect will take 24 to 72 hours to be achieved. INR should be reassessed in 5 to 7 days to ensure a therapeutic goal. Parenteral anticoagulation (Heparin and LMWH) and DOACs may usually be resumed within 24 to 48 hours after hemostasis is achieved and the proceduralist or primary care team has assessed patient specific factors for bleeding risk.[31]

Contrast Allergy. It has been estimated that mild immediate reactions occur in about 0.5% to 3% of patients exposed to radiographic contrast medium.[34] It has become routine to premedicate those with a previous contrast reaction with corticosteroids and antihistamines. However, there are no randomized trials to support this specific practice. SCAI 2016 consensus document on Best Practices suggests a regimen of prednisone 50 mg at 13, 7, and 1 hours preprocedure or 60 mg the night before and morning of the procedure in conjunction with diphenhydramine 50 mg one hour before the procedure.[1] For emergent procedures, the experts recommend 60 mg of methylprednisone but there is limited data on this.[1] Shellfish allergy does not predispose patients to a contrast reaction and does not require pretreatment.[35] Risk factors for allergic reaction to contrast are prior reactions, other hypersensitivities, asthma, female gender, and renal insufficiency.[29]

Those pretreated may suffer a breakthrough reaction. Catheterization laboratory staff must assess for early signs of a reaction that include urticaria and nausea. Most symptoms become apparent within the first 5 minutes of contrast administration.[34] More severe reactions may include respiratory distress and cardiovascular collapse. Emergency care requires ongoing assessment and monitoring of vital signs and airway while administering antihistamines and epinephrine for cardiovascular support.[36]

Chronic Kidney Disease. Patients with baseline renal insufficiency (glomerular filtration rate [GFR] <60 mL/min/1.73 m^2) are at increased risk for contrast-induced nephropathy (CIN). CIN is defined as a 25% decrease in renal function 24 to 72 hours after the administration of contrast. CIN has been shown to increase morbidity, mortality, and healthcare costs.[37] Strategies to reduce the risk of CIN include adequate hydration and limiting the dose of contrast given.[22] Dose of contrast is the largest predictor for CIN leading to dialysis.[38] Hydration protocols recommend isotonic saline at rates of 1 mL/kg for 12 hours pre- and postprocedure.[22] The SCAI 2016 Best Practices consensus document recommends a maximum contrast volume of 3.7 × GFR as the upper limit of acceptable contrast dose during a single procedure.[1] It is important for staff to monitor contrast dose and alert physicians as the upper limit is reached. Randomized trials have shown no improvement with the administration of N-acetylcysteine.[39] Most increases in serum creatinine are mild and transient and not typically associated with oliguria. Creatinine peaks within 2 to 4 days and generally resolves by 7 days.[38] The true incidence of CIN is hard to state as studies have varying patient populations and definitions of CIN. Rates range from 3.3% to 16.5%.[38] SCAI recommends that a CIN risk score be calculated.[1] The Mehran contrast nephropathy risk score was developed in 2004 (see Fig. 16-3).[40] It accounts for 8 variables (hypotension, intra-aortic balloon pump [IABP], congestive heart failure, chronic kidney disease [CKD], diabetes, age greater than 75 years, anemia, and volume of contrast) and assigns a weighted number to each. The sum of which gives a score for risk of CIN.

Radiation Exposure. Ionizing radiation has detrimental effects on human tissue and has the potential to harm both patients and staff. It is important for all staff (physicians, nurses, cardiovascular technologists) to be familiar with techniques to employ radiation safety and management and keep radiation doses as low as reasonably achievable (ALARA). Radiation dosage is measured in millisieverts (mSv). Natural background radiation exposure per person per year in the United States is 3 mSv. The range of radiation dose for diagnostic coronary angiography is 2 to 20 mSv and 5 to 57 mSv for percutaneous coronary angiography.[41] Proceduralists carry the highest risk of exposure due to their location at the table. Nurses and technologists have lower exposure but should take note of their time and location in an active room. Tissue injury may include skin breakdown,

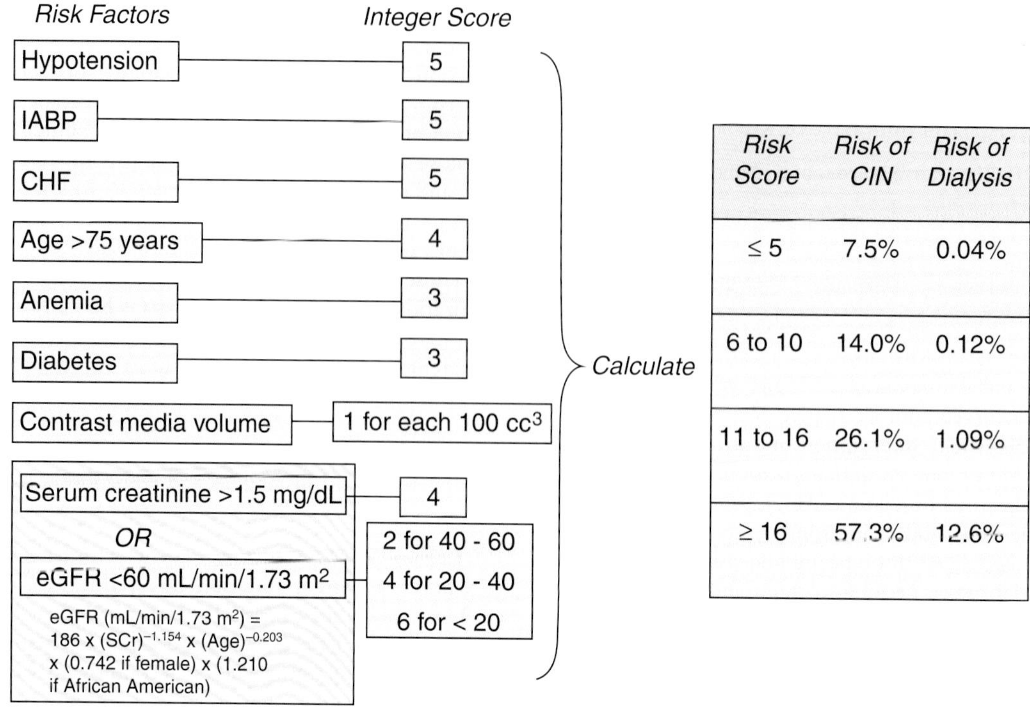

Risk Score	Risk of CIN	Risk of Dialysis
≤ 5	7.5%	0.04%
6 to 10	14.0%	0.12%
11 to 16	26.1%	1.09%
≥ 16	57.3%	12.6%

Figure 16-3. Mehran contrast nephropathy risk score. (From Mehran R, Aymong ED, Nikolsky E, et al. A simple risk score for prediction of contrast-induced nephropathy after percutaneous coronary intervention: development and initial validation. *J Am Coll Cardiol.* 2004;44[7]:1393–1399.)

superficial bone necrosis, and cataracts. SCAI recommends that patients and referring physicians be notified when the threshold for potential harm has been reached in order to be vigilant for skin injury for prompt treatment.[1] There may be an increased life risk of cancer related to radiation exposure.[41] This has been difficult to define and measure given the rates of cancer in the population who have not been exposed to radiation. There are models (BIER VII) to help predict incremental solid organ cancer risk based on age and exposure.[41]

Nonphysician staff are not typically exposed to direct radiation but to radiation scatter as it comes off the patient. Scatter decreases proportionately from the square of distance from the source. Therefore, location within the procedure room is paramount to reducing exposure to scatter. Figure 16-4 depicts how radiation scatters from the patient in all directions. Additionally, shielding with personal protective equipment reduces exposure. Standard shielding equipment for diagnostic x-ray uses lead or another material, such as titanium to absorb the radiation. Aprons should also include neck thyroid shields and humeral shields. Leaded glasses should be worn for staff close to the radiation source. There are some theoretical suggestions to wear lead caps to reduce cranial exposure but are only anecdotal at this time. Overhead mounted shields should be placed between the patient and the operator to decrease scatter exposure.

Staff wear personal radiation monitors (formerly known as "film badges") to measure their radiation exposure. Badges are worn both outside protective garments (at the collar level on the left side) and under protective garments (at waist level). For pregnant staff, a badge should also be worn under the abdominal apron to measure uterine dosage. As the uterus is a deep structure and shielded, females can work in fluoroscopy without excessive harm to the fetus.

Angiographic Contrast Agents. Iodinated radiocontrast agents are either ionic or nonionic and have variable osmolality. First-generation contrast agents are the high-osmolar ionic agents and have osmolalities as high as six times that of blood; second-generation agents are lower-osmolar nonionic agents that have an osmolality approximately two to three times that of blood. The newest nonionic agents are iso-osmolal and have

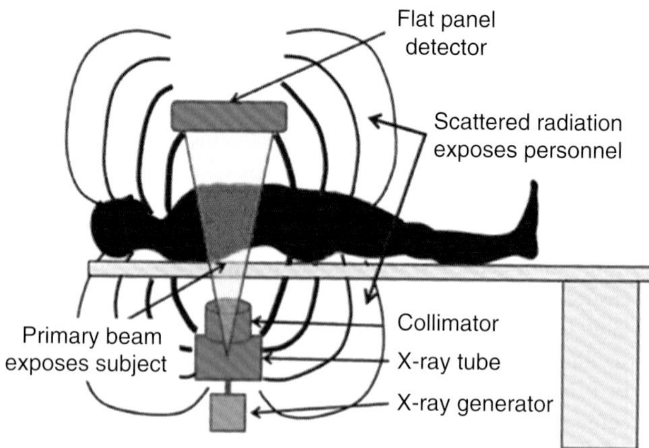

Figure 16-4. Diagramatic representation of the pattern of x-ray scatter from a subject undergoing x-ray fluoroscopy. (From Hirshfeld JW, Ferrari VA, Bengel FM, et al. 2018 ACC/HRS/NASCI/SCAI/SCCT Expert consensus document on optimal use of ionizing radiation in cardiovascular imaging: Best practices for safety and effectiveness: A report of the American College of Cardiology Task Force on Expert Consensus Decision Pathways. *J Am Coll Cardiol.* 2018;71[24]:e283–e351.)

an osmolality similar to that of blood.[42] Contrast agents contain iodine, which absorbs x-rays and, thus, provides their imaging properties. The hemodynamic and other side effects of contrast agents are related to their osmolality and their chemical and pharmacologic differences. Low-osmolal and iso-osmolal nonionic agents are associated with fewer side effects and less dramatic hemodynamic reactions than high-osmolar ionic agents, particularly in high-risk patients. Nonionic agents are more costly than ionic agents.[42] Most catheterization laboratories use nonionic low-osmolar or iso-osmolar agents. It is the recommendation of SCAI that nonionic, low-osmolar contrast (e.g., iohexol, iopamidol, ioversol) should be utilized for the majority of cases. Recent data suggests that iso-osmolar contrast agents (e.g., iodixanol) may have no benefit over low-osmolar agents for patients with CKD.[1] The hemodynamic effects of contrast agents are well documented. These effects vary with the site and volume of the injection as well as with the osmolality, sodium content, and calcium concentration of the agent used. Immediate effects (within 10 to 120 seconds) are seen with both ventriculography and coronary angiography, whereas long-term effects are seen primarily with ventriculography or other injections that require large amounts of contrast medium.[43]

After left ventricular injection, there is depression of left ventricular contractility, an increase in intravascular volume, and a rise in left ventricular end-diastolic pressure. As contrast reaches the systemic arterial system, there is arteriolar vasodilation; this response increases with the osmolality of the agent used. There is a corresponding decrease in arterial pressure. These effects peak within 2 to 3 minutes, and values return to normal within 5 minutes.[43]

With coronary arteriography, immediate effects of contrast may include sinus bradycardia, systemic arterial hypotension, an increase in left ventricular end-diastolic pressure, arrhythmias, myocardial ischemia, and T-wave changes on the ECG. Usually, these changes revert quickly to normal when the catheter is withdrawn from the coronary ostia and the patient coughs, clearing the contrast medium from the coronary arteries.

The high osmolarity of contrast medium raises serum osmolality. In response, plasma volume increases when water moves from the extravascular to the intravascular space. Both hematocrit and hemoglobin levels fall, whereas left atrial and left ventricular end-diastolic pressures increase in response to the increased intravascular volume. Cardiac output (CO) and stroke volume increase as a secondary response to both the reduced systemic vascular resistance (SVR) (afterload) and increased filling volume and pressures (preload).

Contrast agents act as an osmotic diuretic.[43] The diuresis that occurs after catheterization may result in water and saline deficits, which precipitate hypotension. For this reason, patients should be given intravenous (IV) replacement or be encouraged to drink liquids on returning from the laboratory. Hydration is also important for patients with pre-existing renal insufficiency.

Left Heart Catheterization Approaches

Percutaneous Catheterization

Percutaneous catheterization is accomplished using the modified technique initially described by Seldinger (Fig. 16-5). The same technique is used for both arterial and venous entry. Using the modified Seldinger technique, the vessel is located and a local anesthetic is used to numb the puncture area. The percutaneous needle, with fluid-filled syringe attached, is inserted through the skin nearly parallel to the vessel and enters the front wall of the vessel.

Entry of the needle into the vessel is verified by blood return into the syringe with aspiration. The syringe is removed, and a

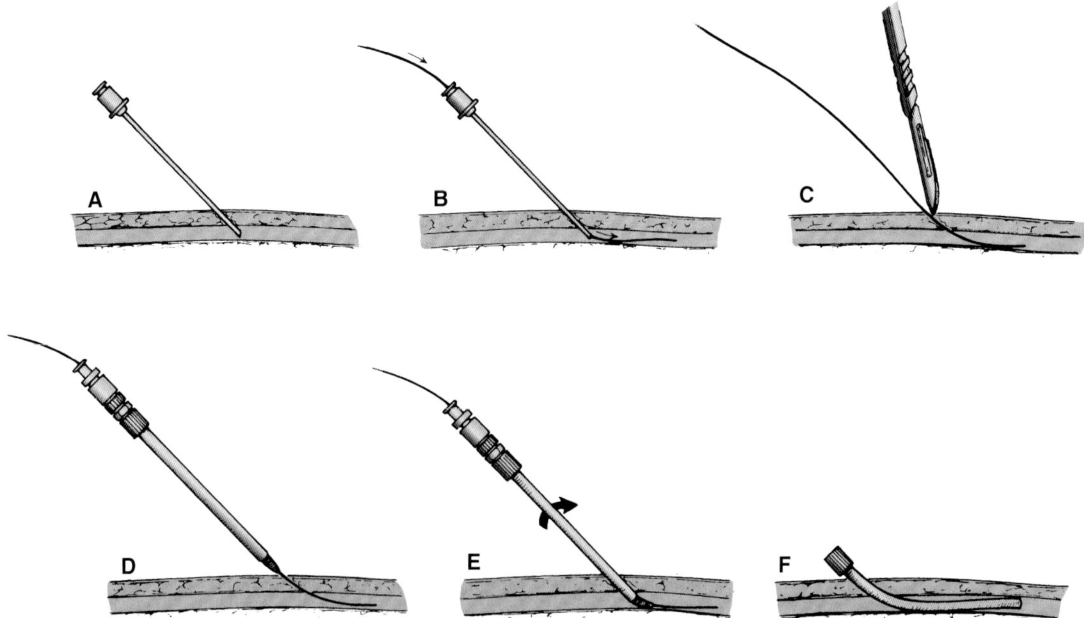

Figure 16-5. Modified Seldinger technique for percutaneous catheter sheath introduction. (**A**) Vessel punctured by needle. (**B**) Flexible guidewire placed in vessel through needle. (**C**) Needle removed, guidewire left in place, and hole in skin around wire enlarged with scalpel. (**D**) Sheath and dilator placed over guidewire. (**E**) Sheath and dilator advanced over guidewire and into vessel. (**F**) Dilator and guidewire removed while sheath remains in vessel. (From In: Bonow RO, Mann DL, Zipes DP, et al., eds. *Braunwald's Heart Disease: A Textbook of Cardiovascular Medicine*. 9th ed. Philadelphia, PA: Elsevier Saunders; 2012:388.)

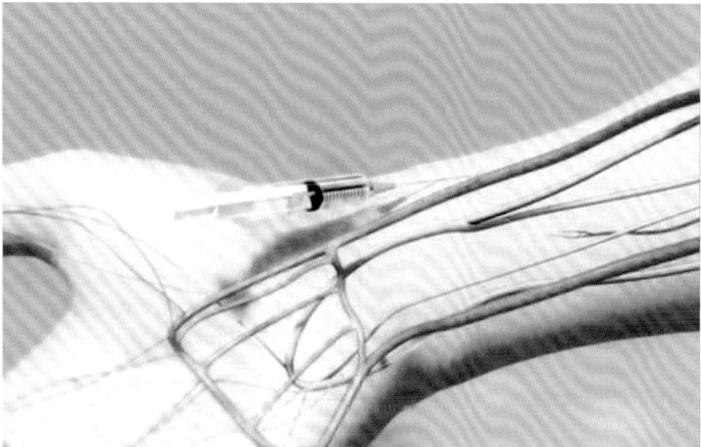

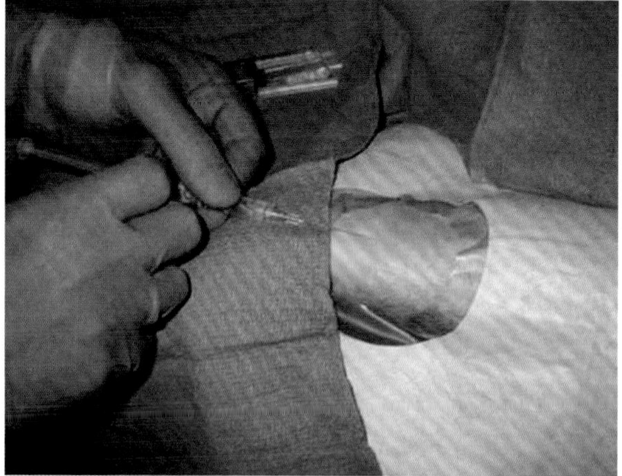

Figure 16-6. Transradial access technique- front wall technique. **1.** A short 2.5 cm 21 gauge needle is used to puncture the radial artery. **2.** The needle is advanced into the radial artery. The blood return indicates the intraluminal position. The blood return is rarely pulsatile or brisk. **3.** A 0.018 in short guidewire is advanced without resistance through the needle into the proximal radial artery. Then the needle is exchanged for a hydrophilic-coated sheath. (From Cohen MG, Rai SV. Radial artery approach. In: Moscucci M, ed. *Grossman and Baim's Cardiac Catheterization, Angiography, and Intervention.* 8th ed. Philadelphia, PA: Lippincott Williams & Wilkins; 2013:174–175.)

guidewire is passed through the needle into the vessel. The needle is then removed, and a nick is made in the skin with a blade to create a hole large enough for a hemostatic introducer sheath to be advanced over the guidewire and placed within the vessel.

Catheters are exchanged by inserting a guidewire into the catheter and inserting the catheter with the guidewire through the introducer sheath, into the vessel. A guidewire is advanced past the distal end of the catheter so the wire leads as the catheter and wire are advanced to the aortic arch. The guidewire is removed from the catheter completely before catheter placement.

Radial Approach. The femoral approach is no longer the preferred site for catheterization as radial access has less vascular complications, allows for earlier ambulation and increased patient satisfaction as well as cost reduction (Fig. 16-6). The first published trial supporting radial artery access was published in 1997.[44] In 2013, the European Society of Cardiology updated its guidelines to affirm that radial arteries should be the default access site for PCI.[45] ACC and SCAI have not published a statement of support in access site to date. However, use is increasing across the United States. In the NCDR CathPCI Registry, national radial artery access for PCI grew from 54.55% to 75.51% over 4 quarters in 2017.[46]

Before using the radial artery, an Allen test is performed to verify patency of the ulnar artery to ensure circulation to the hand. The small caliber of the radial artery sometimes mandates the use of small catheters, but generally the standard 6 French sheath may be used. Injection of lidocaine, nitroglycerin, or calcium channel blocker through the sheath arm is usually necessary to control local spasm in the radial artery. Use of the radial or brachial approach allows for easier control of bleeding at the access site, eliminates the need for bed rest after the procedure, and facilitates earlier discharge of outpatients. Radial artery thrombosis is a potential complication of this approach, but is reduced when compression time is decreased and sheath size is smaller.[47] There are ongoing trials to continue to optimize the practice of radial access.

Femoral Approach. When femoral access is used, the location of the femoral puncture is important to avoid vascular complications. The ideal puncture site should be in the common femoral artery (Fig. 16-7). Puncture of the artery at or above the inguinal ligament makes catheter advancement difficult and predisposes to inadequate compression, hematoma formation, and retroperitoneal bleeding. Puncture of the artery more than 3 cm below the inguinal ligament increases the chance that the femoral artery will divide into its profunda and superficial branches. Puncture into these branches can cause development of a pseudoaneurysm or thrombotic occlusion of a small vessel.[48]

Direct Brachial Approach. The direct brachial approach is rarely used. It requires a cutdown in the antecubital fossa to isolate the brachial artery and vein. A cardiologist trained in brachial cutdown and vascular repair of the artery and vein is required for this procedure. An incision is made over the medial vein for RHC or over both the vein and the brachial artery if right and left heart catheterization is planned. The vein and artery are approached by blunt dissection and are brought to the surface and tagged with surgical tape. Venotomy and arteriotomy are performed using scissors or a scalpel. The distal segment of the artery is flushed with heparinized saline to prevent clotting from distal arterial stasis. The catheterization is performed. After catheterization, the distal brachial artery is aspirated until a forceful backflow is achieved, and heparinized saline is injected. The arterial incision is then sutured. The patient may sit up in chair or bed after the procedure with arm held straight on an arm board. Distal pulses, sensation, and motor function are checked every 15 minutes for 2 hours for all access sites.

Left Heart Catheterization Procedures

Coronary Arteriography

Coronary arteriography is performed most commonly by the percutaneous radial or femoral approach. Preformed polyurethane catheters (most commonly Judkins or Amplatz catheters) are used for catheterization of the right and left coronary arteries (Figs. 16-8 and 16-9). The catheters are guided over a guidewire through the distal aortic arch to the coronary ostium, the guide is withdrawn, and the catheter is filled with contrast medium.

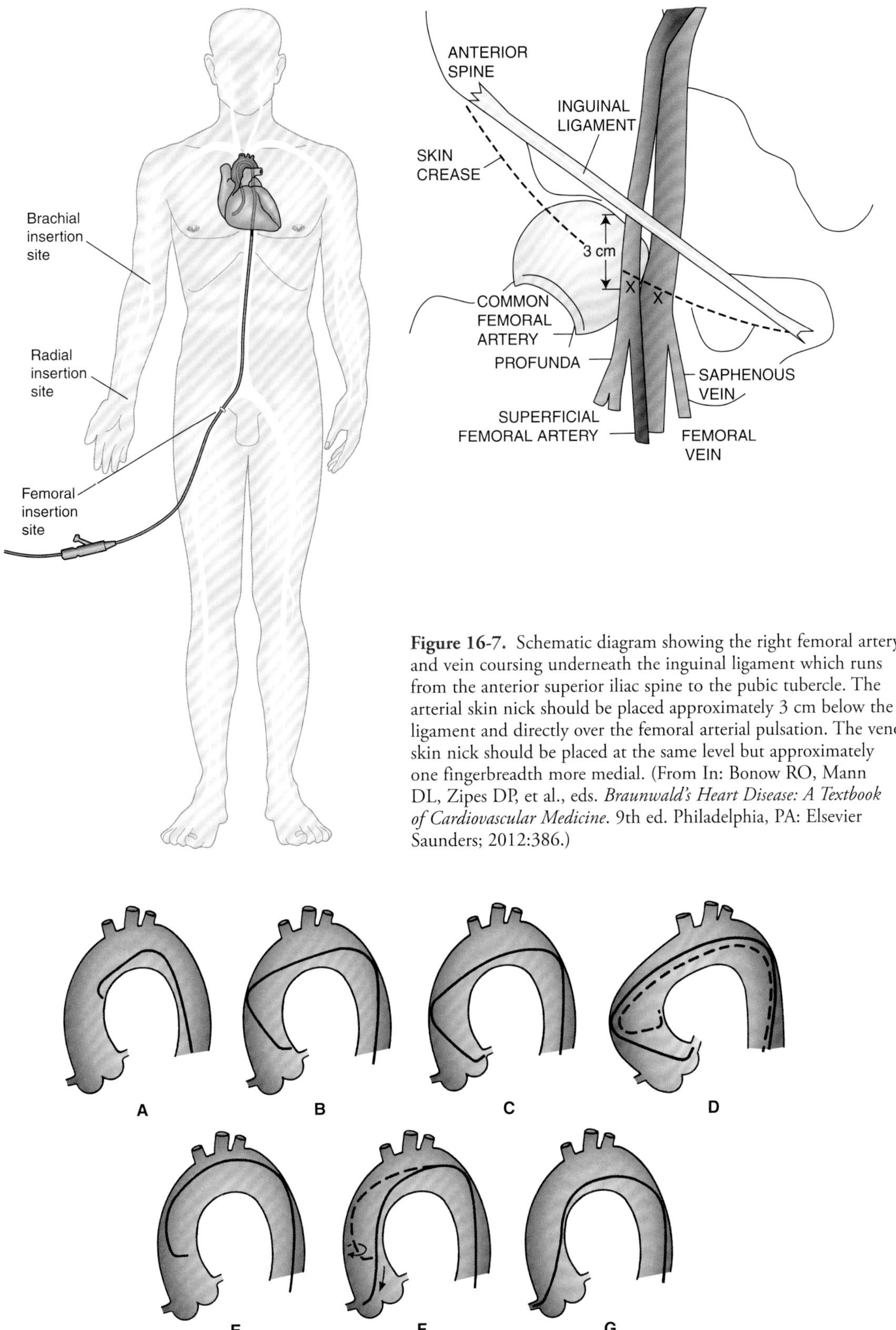

Figure 16-7. Schematic diagram showing the right femoral artery and vein coursing underneath the inguinal ligament which runs from the anterior superior iliac spine to the pubic tubercle. The arterial skin nick should be placed approximately 3 cm below the ligament and directly over the femoral arterial pulsation. The venous skin nick should be placed at the same level but approximately one fingerbreadth more medial. (From In: Bonow RO, Mann DL, Zipes DP, et al., eds. *Braunwald's Heart Disease: A Textbook of Cardiovascular Medicine*. 9th ed. Philadelphia, PA: Elsevier Saunders; 2012:386.)

Figure 16-8. Judkins technique for catheterization of the left and right coronary arteries as viewed in the left anterior oblique (LAO) projection. In a patient with a normal size aortic arch, simple advancement of a JL4 catheter leads to intubation of the left coronary ostium (**A**, **B**, and **C**). In a patient with an enlarged aortic root (**D**) the arm of the JL4 may be too short, causing the catheter tip to point upward or even flip back into its packaged shape (*dotted catheter*). A catheter with an appropriately longer arm (a JL5 or JL6) is required. To catheterize the right coronary ostium, the right Judkins catheter is advanced around the aortic arch with its tip directed leftward, as viewed in the LAO projection, until it reaches a position 2–3 cm above the level of the left coronary ostium (**E**). Clockwise rotation causes the catheter tip to drop into the aortic root and point anteriorly (**F**). Slight further rotation causes the catheter tip to enter the right coronary ostium (**G**). (From Moscucci M. Coronary angiography. In: Moscucci M, ed. *Grossman and Baim's Cardiac Catheterization, Angiography, and Intervention*. 8th ed. Philadelphia, PA: Lippincott Williams & Wilkins; 2013:303.)

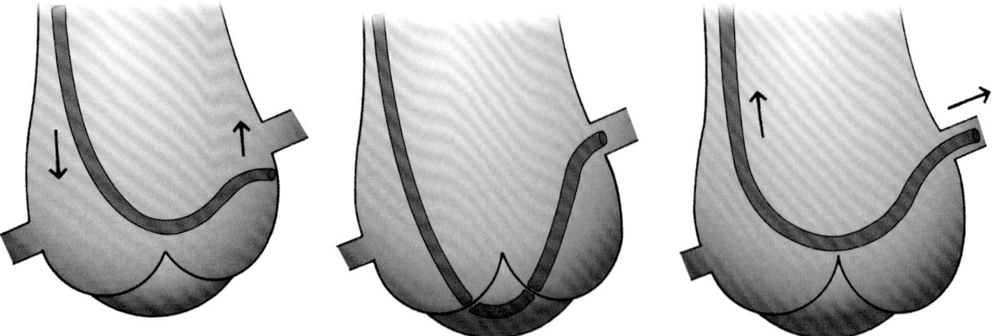

Figure 16-9. Catheterization of the left coronary artery with an Amplatz catheter. The catheter should be advanced into the ascending aorta with its tip pointing downward so that the terminal catheter configuration resembles a diving duck. As the Amplatz catheter is advanced into the left sinus of Valsalva, its tip initially lies below the left coronary ostium *(left)*. Further advancement causes the tip to ride up the aortic wall and enter the ostium *(center)*. Slight withdrawal of the catheter causes the tip to seat more deeply in the ostium *(right)*. (From Moscucci M. Coronary angiography. In: Moscucci M, ed. *Grossman and Baim's Cardiac Catheterization, Angiography, and Intervention*. 8th ed. Philadelphia, PA: Lippincott Williams & Wilkins; 2013:303.)

Figure 16-10 shows the coronary anatomy as viewed from the right anterior oblique (RAO) and left anterior oblique (LAO) projections. Images of both the right and left coronary arteries are recorded in the LAO and RAO views to ensure that all coronary segments are seen. The image intensifier can also be angulated toward the head (cranial) or the foot (caudal) to better visualize specific lesions (Figs. 16-11 and 16-12). A common sequence of angiographic views for the left coronary artery includes:

1. RAO-caudal: to visualize the left main, proximal left anterior descending (LAD) and proximal circumflex coronary arteries
2. RAO-cranial: to visualize the middle and distal LAD without overlap of septal or diagonal branches
3. LAO-cranial: to visualize the middle and distal LAD in an orthogonal projection
4. LAO-caudal: to visualize the left main and proximal circumflex

One or more additional view (posterior-anterior, lateral-cranial, lateral-caudal) may be taken to clarify any areas of uncertainty.

A common sequence of angiographic views for the right coronary includes:

1. LAO: to visualize the proximal and right coronary artery (RCA)
2. LAO cranial: to visualize the distal RCA and its bifurcation into the posterior descending and posterolateral branches
3. RAO-cranial: to visualize the posterior descending and posterolateral branches
4. Lateral: to visualize the middle RCA

The patient is asked to take a deep breath and hold it without bearing down, just before the injection, to clear the diaphragm from the field. After the injection, the patient is told to breathe and cough, which helps clear the contrast medium from the coronary arteries. Imaging of the coronary arteries may also be performed after the administration of nitroglycerin or other vasodilators to evaluate possible vasospasm effects on the coronary circulation, including the collateral vessels.

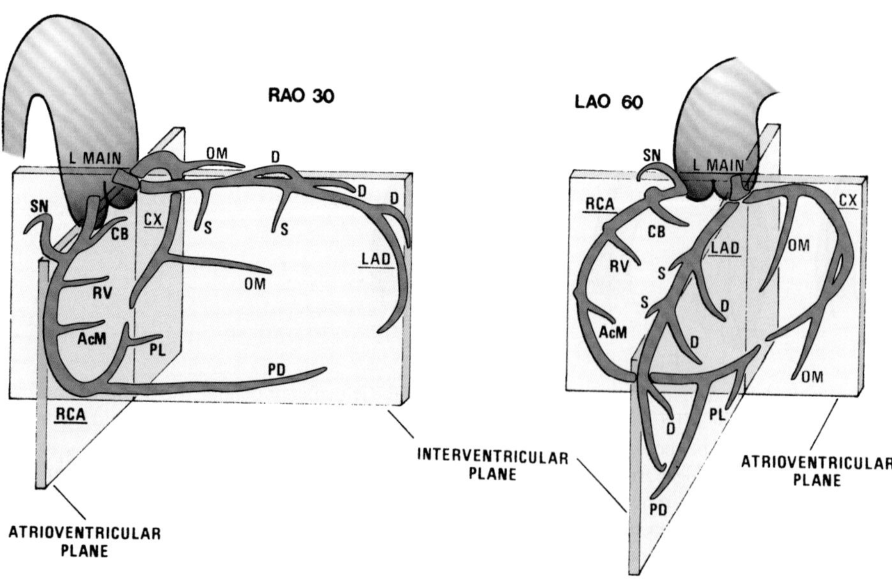

Figure 16-10. Representation of coronary anatomy in relation to the interventricular and atrioventricular valve planes. Coronary branches are as indicated: L Main (left main), LAD (left anterior descending), D (diagonal), S (septal), CX (circumflex), OM (obtuse marginal), RCA (right coronary artery), CB (conus branch), SN (sinus node), AcM (acute marginal), PD (posterior descending), PL (posterolateral left ventricular). (From Moscucci M. Coronary angiography. In: Moscucci M, ed. *Grossman and Baim's Cardiac Catheterization, Angiography, and Intervention*. 8th ed. Philadelphia, PA: Lippincott Williams & Wilkins; 2013:314.)

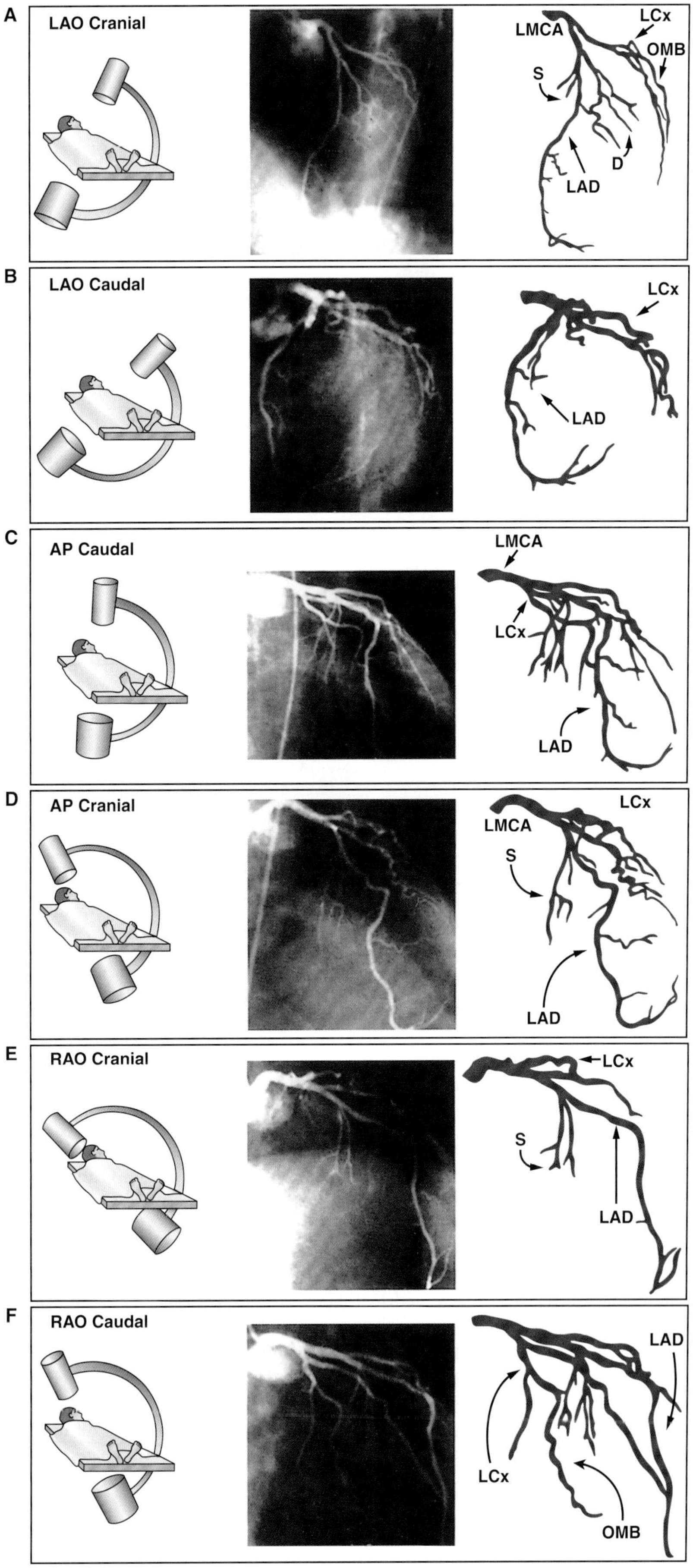

Figure 16-11. Angiographic views of the left coronary artery. The approximate position of the x-ray tube and image intensifier are shown for each of the commonly used angiographic views. (**A**) The 60-degree LAO view with 20 degrees of cranial angulation (LAO cranial) shows the ostium and distal portion of the left main coronary artery (LMCA), the middle and distal portions of the LAD artery, septal perforators (*S*), diagonal branches (**D**), and the proximal left circumflex (LCx) and superior obtuse marginal branch (OMB). (**B**) The 60-degree LAO view with 25 degrees of caudal angulation (LAO caudal) shows the proximal LMCA and the proximal segments of the LAD and LCx. (**C**) Anteroposterior projection with 20 degrees of caudal angulation (AP caudal) shows the distal LMCA and proximal segments of the LAD and LCx. (**D**) Anteroposterior projection with 20 degrees cranial angulation (AP cranial) also shows the midportion of the LAD and its septal (*S*) branches. (**E**) The 30-degree RAO view with 20 degrees of cranial angulation (RAO cranial) shows the course of the LAD and its septal (*S*) and diagonal branches. (**F**) 30-degree RAO with 25 degrees of caudal angulation (RAO caudal) shows the LCx and obtuse marginal branches (OMB). (From Popma JJ. Coronary angiography and intravascular ultrasonography. In: Bonow RO, Mann DL, Zipes DP, et al., eds. *Braunwald's Heart Disease: A Textbook of Cardiovascular Medicine*. 9th ed. Philadelphia, PA: Elsevier Saunders; 2005:432.)

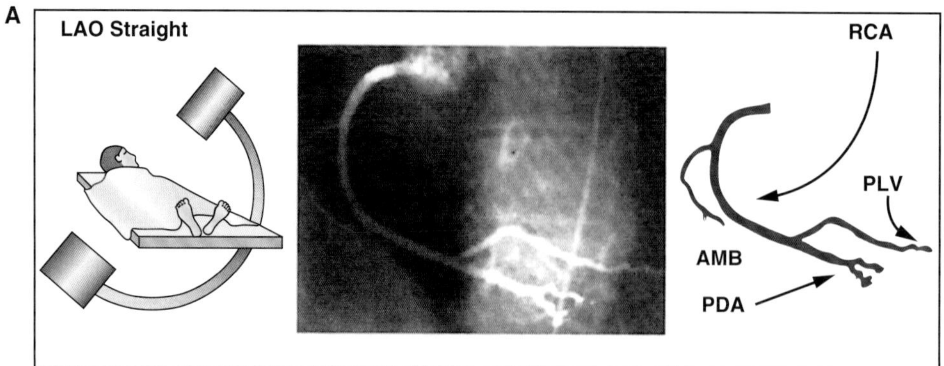

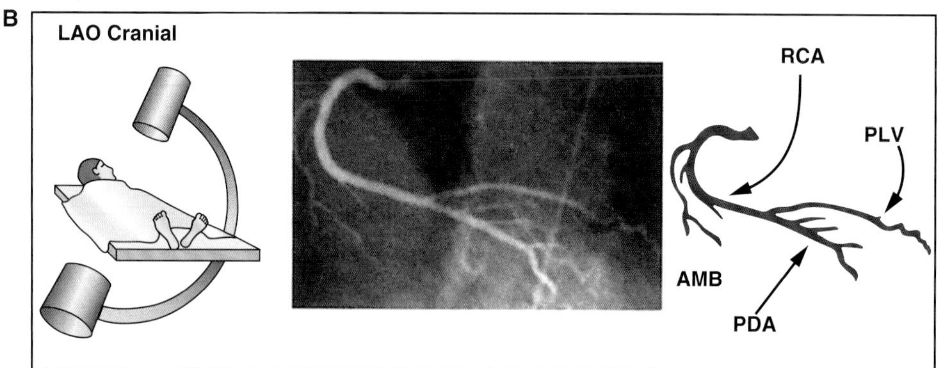

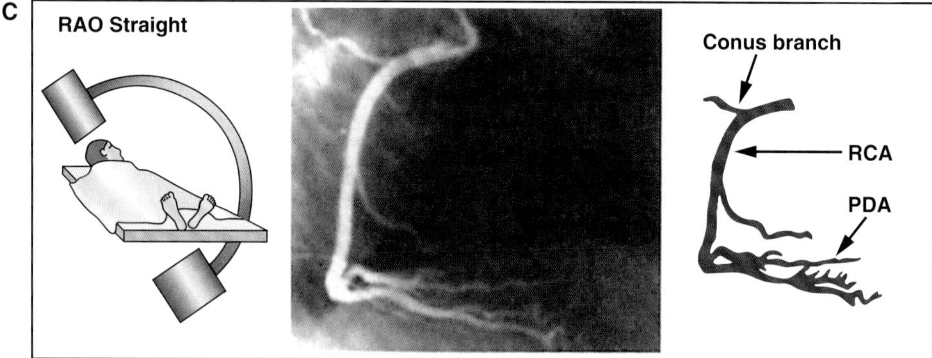

Figure 16-12. Angiographic views of the right coronary artery (RCA). The approximate position of the x-ray tube and image intensifier are shown for each of the commonly used angiographic views. (**A**) The 60-degree left anterior oblique view (LAO straight) shows the proximal and midportions of the RCA as well as the acute marginal branches (AMB) and termination of the RCA in the posterior left ventricular branches (PLV). (**B**) The 60-degree LAO view with 25 degrees of cranial angulation (LAO cranial) shows the midportion of the RCA and the origin and course of the posterior descending artery (PDA). (**C**) The 30-degree RAO view shows the midportion of the RCA, the conus branch, and the course of the PDA. (From Popma JJ. Coronary angiography and intravascular ultrasonography. In: Bonow RO, Mann DL, Zipes DP, et al., eds. *Braunwald's Heart Disease: A Textbook of Cardiovascular Medicine*. 9th ed. Philadelphia, PA: Elsevier Saunders; 2005:433.)

The first step in evaluating the coronary arteriogram is to determine whether the coronaries are unobstructed and free of lesions. Each major artery is traced along its entire length, and branches and collaterals are noted and evaluated for irregularities or narrowing. When occlusion is present, the degree of disease and the suitability of the artery for revascularization are of primary concern.

In addition to grading the occlusion, the condition of the distal artery must be evaluated. The distal artery may be identified by antegrade or collateral flow, and its caliber and suitability as a recipient for bypass grafting are evaluated. Arteries with diffuse atherosclerotic plaquing and small distal targets are less suitable for bypass grafting. The proximity of the occlusion determines the amount of myocardium in jeopardy. A subjective evaluation of the degree of arterial flow is made by observing the time required for perfused arteries to fill and clear.

Contrast medium clears faster with higher flow rates. Intermittent luminal obstruction due to systolic constriction from encircling muscle bands or to coronary artery spasm is also observed, and its degree, distribution, and pattern are evaluated. If bypass grafts have been injected, they are evaluated in the same manner for patency, flow indices, and the condition of the perfused artery.

Quantitative Angiography

Quantitative angiography involves adjunctive imaging with IVUS and measurement of coronary physiology in the catheterization laboratory, enhancing clinical decision making. Determination of the severity of coronary artery stenoses during coronary angiography can sometimes be challenging when the stenosis is indeterminate and appears significant in one planar view but not in other views. When a stenotic lesion is evaluated by angiography the segment is compared to the presumed-normal adjacent segment. The degree of stenosis can be underestimated when there is diffuse narrowing in the artery and can be exaggerated when there is adjacent coronary dilatation.[49,50] As a stenosis develops in an artery, a drop in blood pressure occurs across the stenotic lesion. Maximal stress and increased oxygen consumption cause blood flow to fall when about 70% of the cross-sectional area of an artery is stenosed. Resting blood flow falls when the stenosis

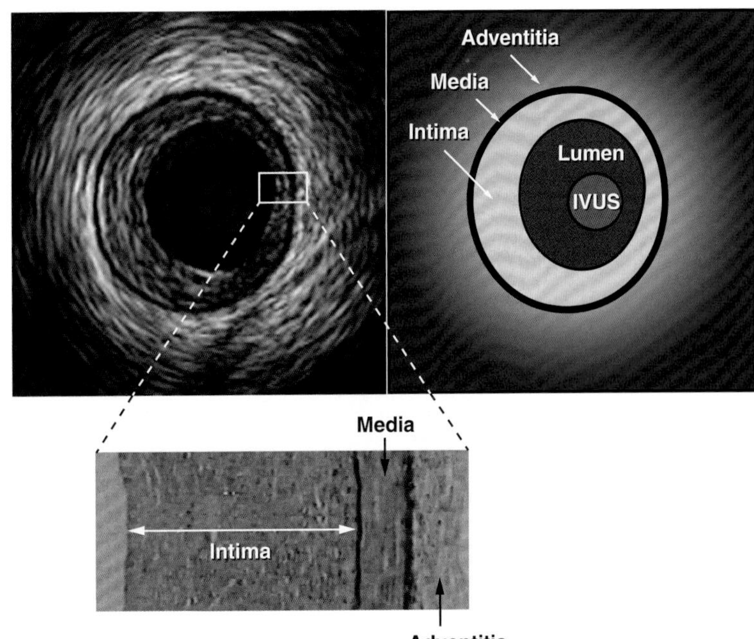

Figure 16-13. Cross-sectional format of a typical IVUS image. The bright-dark-bright, three-layered appearance is seen in the image with corresponding anatomy as defined. "IVUS" represents the imaging catheter in the blood vessel lumen. Histologic correlations with intima, media, and adventitia are shown. The media has lower ultrasound reflectance owing to less collagen and elastin as compared with the neighboring layers. Because the intimal layer reflects ultrasound more strongly than does the media, there is a spillover in the image, which results in a slight overestimation of the thickness of the intima and a corresponding underestimation of the media thickness. (From Honda Y, Fitzgerald PJ, Yock PG. Intravascular imaging techniques. In: Moscucci M, ed. *Grossman and Baim's Cardiac Catheterization, Angiography, and Intervention*. 8th ed. Philadelphia, PA: Lippincott Williams & Wilkins; 2013:520.)

reaches 85% or more.[49] The microvessels dilate to compensate for the reduced distal arterial perfusion pressure to maintain normal resting blood flow. During exercise, the capacity of the microcirculation to dilate further is limited resulting in ischemia. Determination of physiologic significance of a coronary lesion provides information about coronary blood flow (CBF) and the extent of myocardial perfusion impairment at rest and during stress.

The magnitude of the obstruction can be measured as a reduction in CFR, which is the ability of an artery to increase blood flow in response to a physiologic stimulus or as FFR, which is a pressure gradient across the stenotic lesion.

Intravascular Ultrasound Imaging

IVUS imaging provides a transluminal 360-degree scan of the vessel to identify the blood/intima (vessel lumen) border and the media/adventitia interface. IVUS enables cross-sectional measurements of the diameter of the vessel and identification of the distribution of the plaque, either concentric or eccentric, and plaque characteristics such as soft plaque, thrombus, or calcification. Figure 16-13 shows a typical cross-sectional view of the vessel.

IVUS has facilitated improvement in PCI device selection and outcomes. IVUS involves placement of an ultrasound catheter into the coronary artery during left heart catheterization. The catheter is placed distal to the segment of interest and gradually pulled back to visualize the vessel wall. The two-dimensional images are displayed on a monitor that allows evaluation of lesion stenosis, extent of disease and assessment of postintracoronary stent placement.

SCAI Expert Consensus Statement on Use of IVUS[51]

Definitely Beneficial. IVUS is an accurate method for determining optimal stent deployment (complete stent expansion and apposition and lack of edge dissection or other complications after implantation), and the size of the vessel undergoing stent implantation.

Probably Beneficial. IVUS can be used to appraise the significance of LMCA stenosis and, employing a cutoff minimal luminal area (MLA) of 6 mm^2, assess whether revascularization is warranted.

Possibly Beneficial. IVUS can be useful for the assessment of plaque morphology.

No Proven Value/Should Be Discouraged. IVUS measurements for determination of non-LMCA lesion severity should not be relied upon, in the absence of additional functional evidence, for recommending revascularization.

Coronary Flow Reserve

The normal physiologic response to increased myocardial demand is enhanced blood flow by vasodilatation of epicardial and resistance vessels. The ability to increase CBF by reducing vasomotor tone to meet myocardial demand in response to a physiologic stimulus is the CFR. In the presence of a significant lesion, the epicardial artery and microvascular coronary bed compensate by vasodilation. In response to a physiologic or pharmacologic stress, the flow resistance in the coronary vasculature is unable to increase myocardial demand further by vasodilating, causing a state of impaired CFR. Measurement of CFR in the catheterization laboratory is performed by placement of an intracoronary Doppler wire into the coronary artery and administration of an adenosine infusion as a stress agent to evaluate the microcirculation.[52]

Fractional Flow Reserve

The FFR is the fraction of maximal CBF that goes through the stenotic vessel. The FFR calculates a ratio of distal coronary pressure to aortic pressure measured during maximal hyperemia or vasodilatation (when minimal resistance is present across both the epicardial and microvascular beds), reflecting myocardial perfusion. A pressure wire is placed across the suspected lesion and an adenosine infusion is administered. Normal FFR is 1.0; a value less than 0.80 is abnormal and associated with abnormal stress tests and inducible myocardial ischemia. Revascularization is recommended for coronary lesions with an FFR less than 0.80.[53] Figure 16-14 shows tracings and calculations of FFR and CFR.

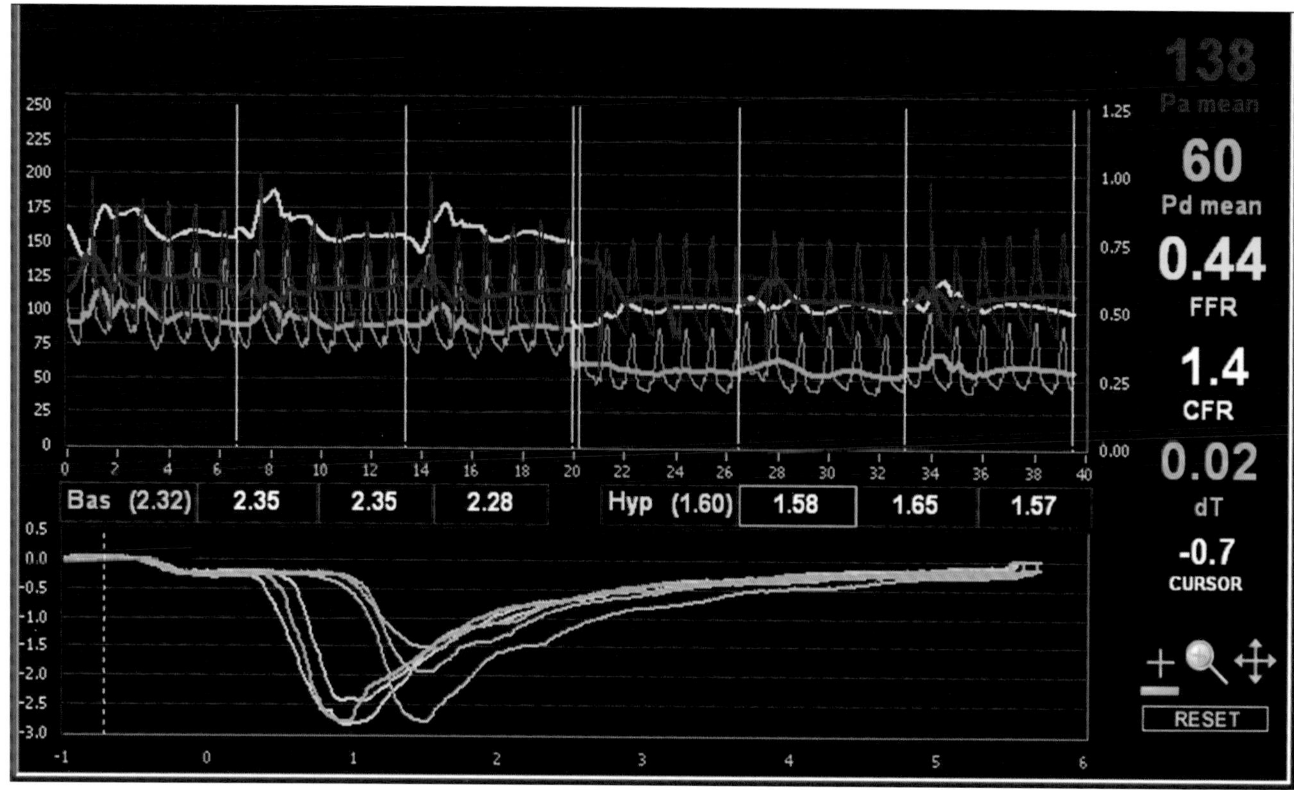

Figure 16-14. Determining coronary flow using the St. Jude Medical pressure wire system. As can be seen in the top panel of the figure, the red signals reflect the guide catheter pressure (*Pa*), the green signals reflect the coronary pressure (*Pd*), and the yellow line represents the calculated FFR for the corresponding pressures. The particulars of the measurement of coronary flow can be seen in the bottom panel of the figure. The curves at the bottom represent the thermodilution temperature changes during rest and subsequently at maximal hyperemia. The numbers just above the curves depict the calculated transit time corresponding to each of the color-coded thermodilution curves. The average of the baseline and hyperemic transit times are then used to calculate the coronary flow reserve (CFR), as shown on the right side of the figure. (From Kern MJ, Lim MJ. Evaluation of myocardial and coronary blood flow. In: Moscucci M, ed. *Grossman and Baim's Cardiac Catheterization, Angiography, and Intervention*. 8th ed. Philadelphia, PA: Lippincott Williams & Wilkins; 2013:547.)

Adjunctive in-laboratory coronary physiologic measurements facilitate clinical decisions to treat or defer PCI or coronary artery bypass graft surgery in patients who have intermediate stenoses. Decisions based on quantitative angiography have shown equivalent clinical outcomes in patients deferred for revascularization without the cost of PCI and the risk of restenosis.[51]

SCAI Expert Consensus Statement on Use of FFR[51]

Definitely Beneficial. In SIHD, when noninvasive stress imaging is contraindicated, discordant, nondiagnostic, or unavailable, FFR should be used to assess the functional significance of intermediate coronary stenoses (50% to 70%) and more severe stenoses (<90%). In patients with multivessel coronary disease, PCI guided by FFR measurement improves outcomes and saves resources when compared to PCI guided by angiography alone. In patients with three-vessel coronary disease, measuring FFR could allow reclassification of number of vessels diseased and/or SYNTAX* score, thereby guiding decisions regarding revascularization by coronary artery bypass grafting (CABG) or PCI.

*SYNTAX score is an angiographic grading tool to determine the complexity of CAD.

In SIHD, PCI of lesions with FFR less than 0.80 improves symptom control and decreases the need for hospitalization requiring urgent revascularization when compared with medical therapy alone.

In SIHD, medical therapy is indicated for an angiographically intermediate stenosis (left main or non-left main coronary artery) of unclear clinical significance when FFR is greater than 0.80.

No Proven Benefit. FFR measurement of the culprit vessel in a patient with an acute ST-segment elevation myocardial infarction or any unstable ACS presentation should not be performed.

Optical Coherence Tomography (OCT). OCT generates tomographic images by the use of scattering and absorption of infrared light. It has very good resolution but less power of penetration than IVUS. OCT can offer unique characterization of plaque morphology by identifying thin fibrous caps, lipid pools, and fibrocalcific plaques and assess the thickness of calcification that IVUS cannot do. This is helpful when determining interventional strategies like rotational atherectomy. Its strength is that it can define specific detail around the lumen and stent edges. However, its lack of penetration through the diseased arterial wall does not allow for assessment of plaque burden or remodeling.

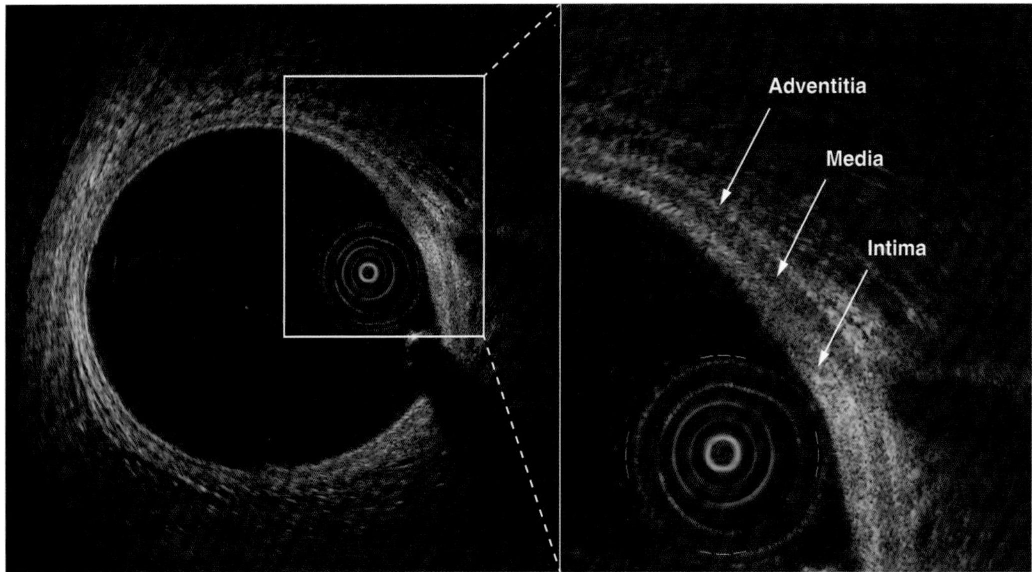

Figure 16-15. Cross-sectional format of a typical OCT image. Similar to that seen by IVUS, the normal vessel wall is characterized by a three-layered architecture, comprising a highly backscattering intima, a media with low backscattering, and a heterogenous and frequently highly backscattering adventitia. The periadventitial tissues may present an appearance consistent with adipocytes, characterized by large clear structures. (From Kern MJ, Lim MJ. Evaluation of myocardial and coronary blood flow. In: Moscucci M, ed. *Grossman and Baim's Cardiac Catheterization, Angiography, and Intervention*. 8th ed. Philadelphia, PA: Lippincott Williams & Wilkins; 2013:557.)

Figure 16-15 shows a cross-sectional image of a typical OCT assessment.

SCAI Expert Consensus Statement on Use of Optical Coherence Tomography[51]

Probably Beneficial. Determination of optimal stent deployment (sizing, apposition, and lack of edge dissection), with improved resolution compared with IVUS.

Possibly Beneficial. OCT can be useful for the assessment of plaque morphology.

No Proven Value/Should Be Discouraged. OCT should not be performed to determine stenosis functional significance.

Transseptal Left Heart Catheterization. The transseptal approach to left heart catheterization involves crossing from the right atrium to the left atrium through the fossa ovalis. This technique is infrequently done for diagnostic angiograms but can be used in the rare situation when retrograde left heart catheterization is not possible due to severe aortic stenosis or a prosthetic valve that cannot be adequately evaluated by transthoracic or transesophageal echocardiography. More common uses of the transseptal approach include mitral valvuloplasty, electrophysiology studies requiring access to the left atrium or left ventricle, LAAO, and transcatheter closure of PFO or ASD.

Transseptal catheterization is traditionally performed through the right femoral vein but can be accomplished via right internal jugular and left femoral veins with more difficulty. The transseptal catheter is threaded into the right atrium over a guidewire, which is then removed.

The transseptal needle, with a blunt stylet extending beyond its tip to prevent the needle from puncturing the catheter (Fig. 16-16), is threaded up the catheter, the stylet is withdrawn, and the needle is connected to a pressure transducer. The catheter and needle are guided together to the fossa ovalis, where the needle is advanced to perforate the atrial septum. After perforation of the septum, left atrial pressure (LAP) is recorded and a blood sample is drawn to confirm the catheter location. The catheter and needle are advanced well into the left atrium, the needle is withdrawn, and the desired studies are performed. The catheter may also be advanced to enter the left ventricle.

The most common reason to assess the mitral valve is in preparation for balloon valvuloplasty or valve replacement surgery. Mitral gradients are influenced greatly by volume status, flow across the valve, and compliance of the left atria. Simultaneous left

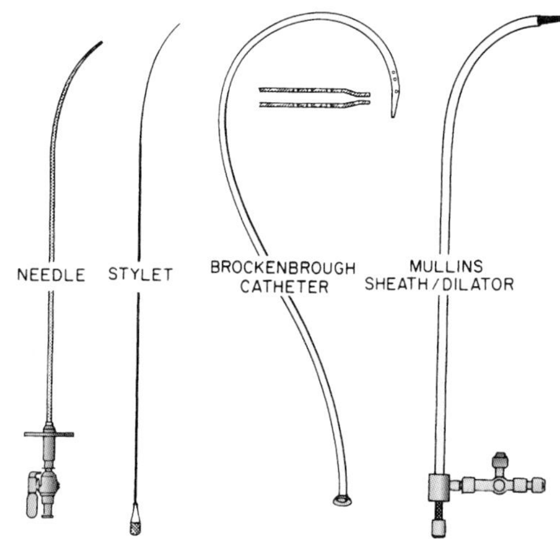

Figure 16-16. Equipment for transseptal puncture. From left to right: the Brockenbrough needle, Bing stylet, Brockenbrough catheter, Mullins sheath/dilator system. (From Hill JA, Lambert CR, Vuestra RE, et al. Review of techniques. In: Pepine JC, Hill JA, Lambert CR, eds. *Diagnostic and Therapeutic Cardiac Catheterization*. 3rd ed. Baltimore, MD: Williams & Wilkins; 1998:116.)

atrial and left ventricular end diastolic pressures are measured. LAP is measured after performing a transseptal puncture from the right to the left atria. Alternatively, some laboratories use the pulmonary capillary wedge pressure (PCWP) as a surrogate for the LAP. Mean gradients less than 5 mm Hg are mild mitral stenosis. Mean gradients of 5 to 10 mm Hg are classified as moderate mitral and those mean gradients greater than 10 mm Hg are severe mitral stenosis.

Transseptal puncture of the fossa ovalis is safe, but the danger in this approach is that the needle or catheter will inadvertently puncture an adjacent structure such as the posterior free wall of the right atrium, the coronary sinus, or the aortic root causing myocardial hemorrhage, tamponade, or death. The risk is higher in patients who are taking anticoagulants. If the patient is not taking anticoagulants and the perforation is limited to the needle puncture, it is usually benign. However, if the catheter is advanced into the pericardium or aortic root, potentially fatal complications can occur. To minimize risk, the operator must have a detailed familiarity of the regional anatomy of the atrial septum, which can be distorted in aortic and mitral valve disease. Transseptal puncture should be reserved for these highly skilled operators particularly in patients who have severe chest and spine deformities, abnormal heart position, marked right or left atrial enlargement, or in those who cannot lie flat, require ongoing anticoagulation, or a have a large left atrial thrombus.[52]

Ventriculography

Ventriculography is performed to evaluate valve structure or function, to define ventricular anatomy, and to evaluate ventricular function. Ventriculography is accomplished by opacifying the ventricular cavity with contrast medium and filming ventricular motion (Fig. 16-17). Digital image acquisition by biplane or single-plane left ventriculography provides information on the location and severity of segmental wall motion abnormalities. It can define the degree of mitral regurgitation by observing for leakage of contrast material from the left ventricle into the left atria in the RAO projection. The ventriculogram may be performed before the coronary arteriogram because intracoronary contrast medium may have a depressant effect on ventricular function. In very sick patients, coronary angiography may be performed first because it is usually better tolerated than ventriculogram. Ventriculography may also be used to define VSDs, mural thrombus, left ventricular aneurysms, abnormalities of the proximal aorta, or to find anomalous coronary arteries or difficult to locate saphenous vein grafts.

Evaluation of myocardial function is an important part of the evaluation of CAD. Patterns of ventricular contraction are evaluated by ventriculography and estimated ejection fraction.

Analysis of ventriculography should be performed after a normal beat and when the ventricle is completely opacified. The anterolateral, apical, inferior, and posterobasal segments of the left

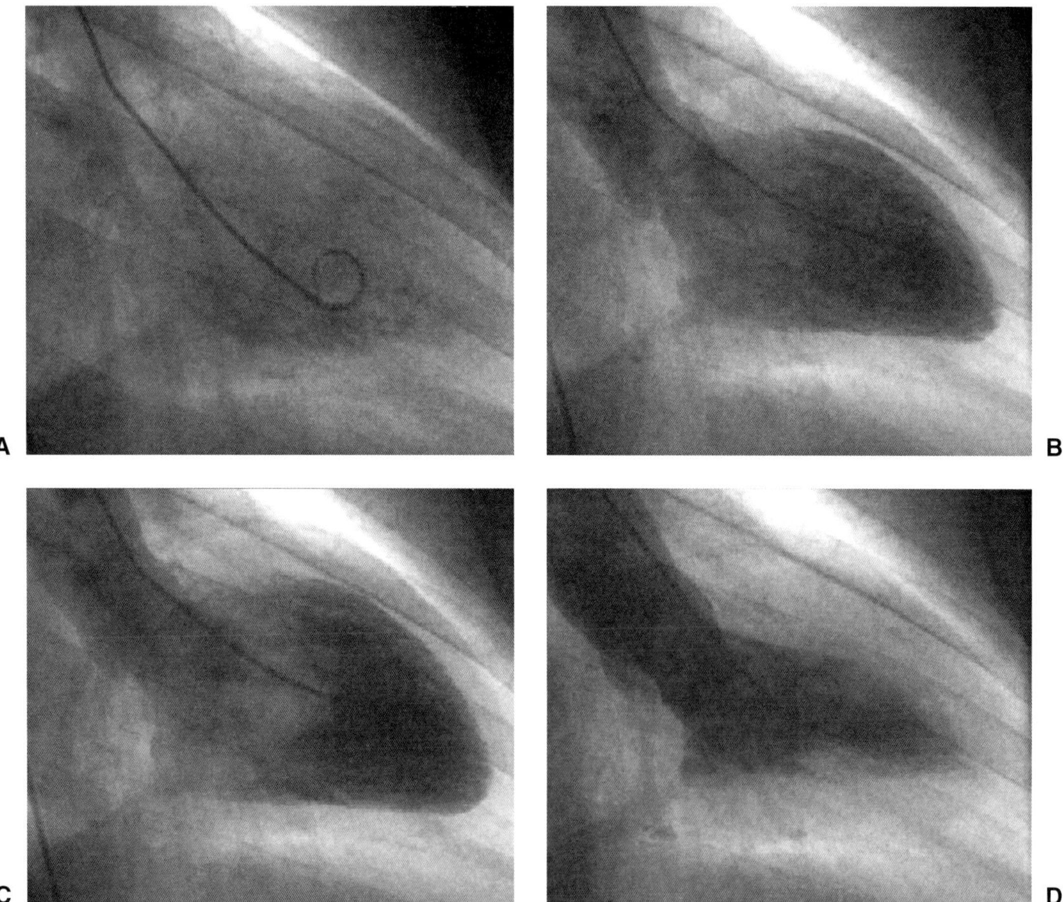

Figure 16-17. Left ventriculogram. Example of midcavitary catheter position for 30 degrees right anterior oblique left ventriculography using an angled pigtail catheter. (**A**) Just before injection of contrast material. (**B**) At the end of rapid filling. (**C**) At end-diastole. (**D**) At end systole. (From Moscucci M, Hendel RC. Cardiac ventriculography. In: Moscucci M, ed. *Grossman and Baim's Cardiac Catheterization, Angiography, and Intervention*. 8th ed. Philadelphia, PA: Lippincott Williams & Wilkins; 2013:357.)

ventricle can be examined in the RAO projection. In the LAO projection, the basal septal, apical septal, apical lateral, and basal lateral segments can be evaluated. Regional contraction may be classified as follows:

1. Normal
2. Mild hypokinesis—mild reduction in myocardial contraction
3. Severe hypokinesis—more severe reduction in myocardial contraction
4. Akinesis—total absence of wall motion in a discrete area
5. Dyskinesis—disturbance causing abnormal movement of left ventricular wall contraction
6. Aneurysm—paradoxical systolic expansion of a portion of the left ventricular wall

The reversibility of myocardial contraction abnormalities is an important consideration in the decision for surgery and long-term prognosis. Improved function is more common with hypokinesis than with akinesis or dyskinesis. The presence of collateral vessels and the lack of Q waves favor the reversibility of hypokinesis.[54]

The catheter used for contrast injection during ventriculography delivers a large amount of contrast medium (30 to 36 mL) in a short period (10 to 12 mL/s). Many types of catheters are available for ventricular injections (Fig. 16-18). Catheters with side holes, with or without an end hole, are preferred to end-hole catheters because they have less tendency to recoil. Catheter stability is also important to minimize the risk of ventricular arrhythmias during injection. Arrhythmias change the quality of contraction and, thus, make it impossible to use ventriculography for studies of ventricular function.[48]

Contrast injection is accomplished by power injection. Before the power injection is performed, it is important to verify that the injection syringe is free of air to prevent air embolism. A low-pressure injection is done to ensure proper catheter placement, then the power injection is done. Patients often feel a hot flash for 30 seconds after injection, resulting from the vasodilatation caused by the contrast agent throughout the arterial system. Occasionally, the patient may experience nausea with the injection, or may vomit. The principal complications of injection are arrhythmias, intramyocardial or endocardial injection of contrast medium, transient left anterior fascicular block, and embolism from injection of air or thrombi.[48]

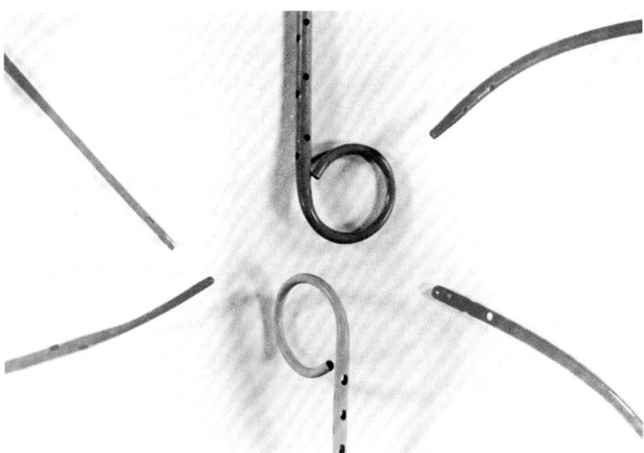

Figure 16-18. Examples of ventriculographic catheters (clockwise from the top): pigtail 8 French (F) (Cook); Gensini 7F; NIH 8F; pigtail 8F (Cordis); Lehman ventriculographic 8F; Sones 7.5F tapering to a 5.5F tip. (From Moscucci M, Hendel RC. Cardiac ventriculography. In: Moscucci M, ed. *Grossman and Baim's Cardiac Catheterization, Angiography, and Intervention.* 8th ed. Philadelphia, PA: Lippincott Williams & Wilkins; 2013:357.)

Gradient Assessment

Gradients or changes in pressure can be measured across the valves to assess for stenosis. The most common valve gradient assessed is the aortic valve. Assessing the aortic valve gradient invasively is usually reserved for when there is discrepancy on noninvasive imaging and degree of symptoms. Typically, two transducers are used with one connected to the sidearm of the arterial sheath and the other to the catheter that crosses the aortic valve and sits in the LV. Simultaneous aortic and LV waveforms are recorded. Three gradients can be obtained from the tracings: peak instantaneous gradient occurring at the peak of LV pressure with the corresponding aortic pressure, and peak and mean gradients derived from the area between the two pressures. Figure 16-19 shows simultaneous LV and aortic pressures illustrating the three gradients. Severe aortic stenosis is defined as a mean gradient greater than 40 mm Hg. Digital imaging may be performed during contrast injection of the left atrium, left ventricle, or aortic root to evaluate valve function further.

RIGHT HEART CATHETERIZATION AND HEMODYNAMICS

Indications for Right Heart Catheterization

RHC (Fig. 16-20) is used to obtain right heart pressures, to evaluate the pulmonic and tricuspid valves, to sample blood oxygen content of right heart chambers for detection of left-to-right shunt, to determine CO, and obtain EMB. Additionally, advanced structural procedures like transcatheter pulmonic valve replacement can be performed via RHC. It should not be performed for routine HF evaluation but reserved for a specific clinical or therapeutic question.

2013 Heart Failure Guidelines for Invasive Evaluation[24]

CLASS I

1. Invasive hemodynamic monitoring with a pulmonary artery catheter should be performed to guide therapy in patients who have respiratory distress or clinical evidence of impaired perfusion in whom the adequacy or excess of intracardiac filling pressures cannot be determined from clinical assessment. (Level of Evidence: C)

CLASS IIa

1. Invasive hemodynamic monitoring can be useful for carefully selected patients with acute HF who have persistent symptoms despite empiric adjustment of standard therapies and:
   a. whose fluid status, perfusion, or systemic or pulmonary vascular resistance (PVR) is uncertain;
   b. whose systolic pressure remains low, or is associated with symptoms, despite initial therapy;
   c. whose renal function is worsening with therapy;
   d. who require parenteral vasoactive agents; or who may need consideration for mechanical circulatory support (MCS) or transplantation. (Level of Evidence: C)

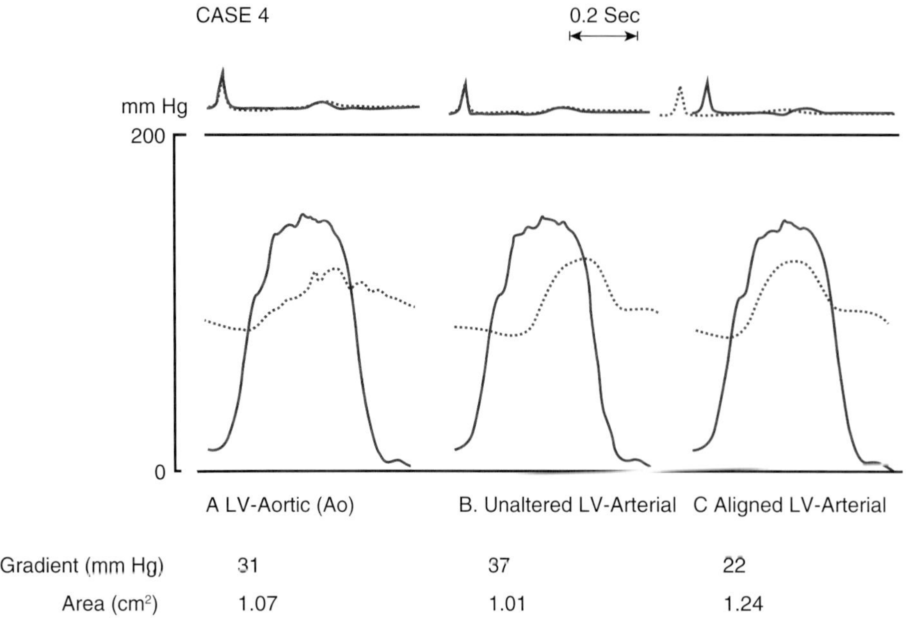

Figure 16-19. Invasive determination of an aortic valve pressure gradient shown with simultaneous aortic (Ao) and left ventricular (LV) waveforms on a 200 mm Hg scale. Three potential gradients can be determined from this tracing: (1) Peak instantaneous gradient occurring at the peak of the LV pressure envelope with the corresponding Ao pressure, (2) peak-to-peak gradient that compares the peak LV pressure to the peak Ao pressure, and (3) mean pressure gradient determined by the area between the two pressures. (From Kern MJ, Lim MJ, Goldstein JA. *Hemodynamic Rounds: Interpretation of Cardiac Pathophysiology from Pressure Waveform Analysis*. 3rd ed. Hoboken, New Jersey: John Wiley & Sons; 2009:74.)

2. When ischemia may be contributing to HF, coronary arteriography is reasonable for patients eligible for revascularization. (Level of Evidence: C)
3. Endomyocardial biopsy (EMB) can be useful in patients presenting with HF when a specific diagnosis is suspected that would influence therapy. (Level of Evidence: C)

CLASS III: No Benefit

1. Routine use of invasive hemodynamic monitoring is not recommended in normotensive patients with acute decompensated HF and congestion with symptomatic response to diuretics and vasodilators. (Level of Evidence: B)

CLASS III: Harm

1. EMB should not be performed in the routine evaluation of patients with HF. (Level of Evidence: C)

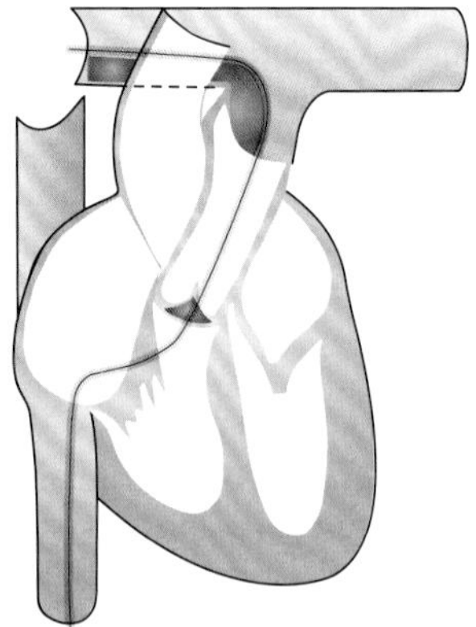

Figure 16-20. Right heart catheterization from the femoral approach. (From Deelstra MH, Jacobson C. Cardiac catheterization. In: Woods SL, Sivarajan Froelicher ES, Motzer SA, et al., eds. *Cardiac Nursing*. 7th ed. Philadelphia, PA: Lippincott Williams & Wilkins; 2009:446.)

Right Heart Catheterization Studies

The right heart can be approached through the femoral, internal jugular, brachial or subclavian veins. Once the inferior vena cava (IVC) or superior vena cava (SVC) is reached, the catheter is advanced through the right atrium (RA), right ventricle (RV), and pulmonary artery (PA) to a distal pulmonary vessel. RV irritability may be noted when the catheter tip passes through the RV. Additionally, nurses should be aware that RV outflow tract placement of the catheter may cause a right bundle branch block. Therefore those patients with pre-existing left bundle branch block may develop complete heart block. The course of the catheter is followed with pressure monitoring through the catheter and with fluoroscopy. When indicated, blood samples are taken, and pressures are recorded as the catheter is advanced. Through these measurements, calculations can determine systemic and PVR. If LHC is planned, the catheter may be left in the distal pulmonary vessel, so that simultaneous left ventricular and pulmonary artery wedge pressure waveforms can be recorded. As the catheter is removed, pull-back pressure can be measured and recorded from the pulmonary artery to the right ventricle and from the right ventricle to the right atrium. These measurements are used to determine valve gradients and to evaluate pulmonic and tricuspid valve function. Blood samples can also be taken as the catheter is withdrawn for detection of left-to-right shunts. If pulmonic or tricuspid valve disease is suspected, contrast can be injected for digital imaging of the right atrium, right ventricle, or pulmonary artery.[48] The most common right heart catheter in use is the Swan–Ganz catheter (see Fig. 16-21).[55] Components of right and left heart catheterization are included in Table 16-6.

Endomyocardial Biopsy

EMB is performed using bioptomes (biopsy forceps) to remove several pieces of RV tissue. The bioptomes are inserted through a sheath and directed at the RV septum under fluoroscopy guidance. Some centers use echocardiography as well. Typically, 3 to 5 specimens are taken. Patients are monitored for several minutes following biopsy for hemodynamic stability and symptoms of

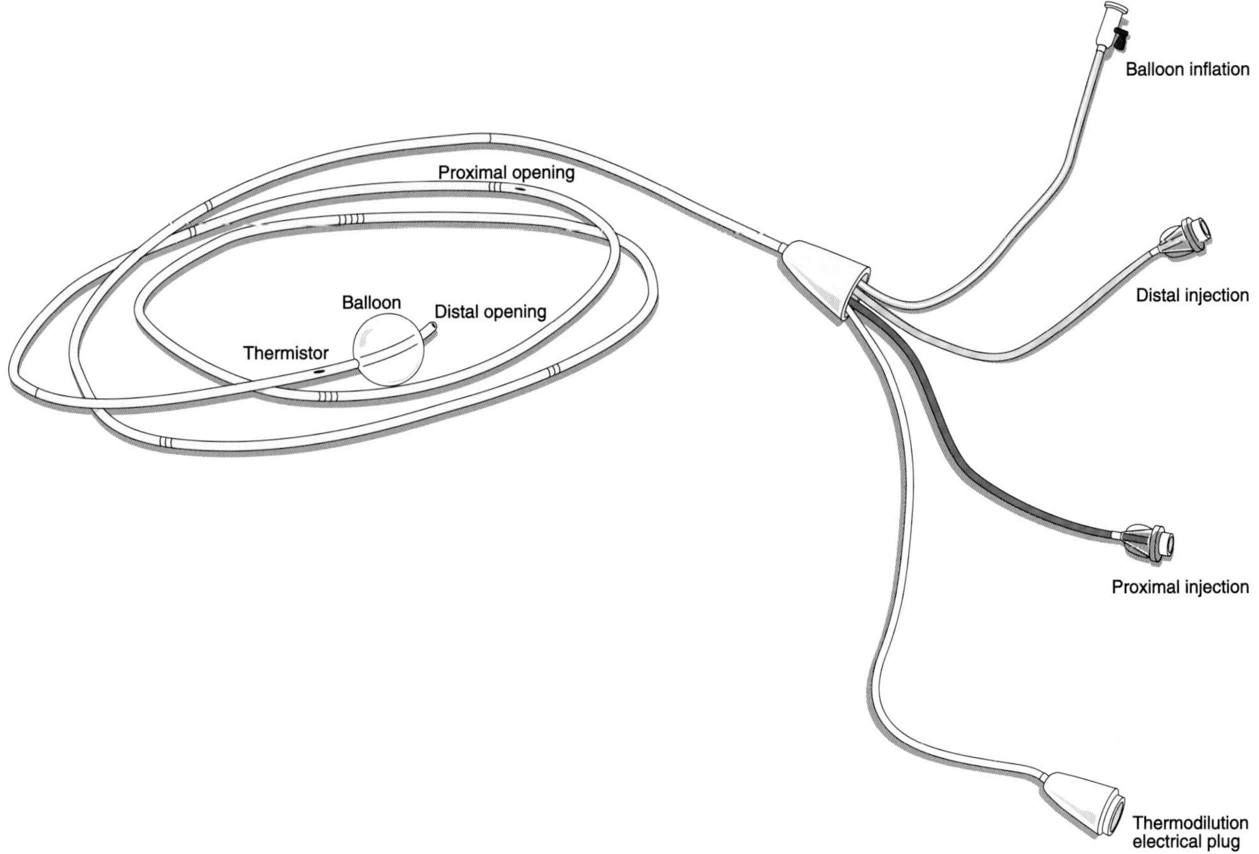

Figure 16-21. The popular Swan–Ganz catheter. This model has 4 ports consisting of the balloon port which inflates the balloon mounted at the tip of the catheter, the distal lumen, proximal lumen, and a thermistor for performance of thermodilution cardiac outputs that connects to the computer via a connecting plug. The catheter has 10-cm increments marked by lines. (Source: LifeArt image copyright © [2019]. Lippincott Williams & Wilkins. All rights reserved.)

chest pain. This procedure is reserved for those with rapidly deteriorating hemodynamics despite optimal medical therapy. Diagnosis of amyloidosis and Giant cell myocarditis can be obtained and then treated. Additionally, EMB is performed following heart transplant when rejection is suspected.

Table 16-6 • COMPONENTS OF A ROUTINE COMPLETE RIGHT AND LEFT HEART CATHETERIZATION

1. Position pulmonary artery (PA) catheter
2. Position aortic (AO) catheter
3. Measure PA and AO pressure
4. Measure thermodilution cardiac output
5. Measure oxygen saturation in PA and AO blood samples to determine Fick output and screen for shunt
6. Enter the LV by retrograde crossing the AO valve
7. Advance PA catheter to PCWP position
8. Measure simultaneous LV-PCWP waveforms
9. Pull back PCWP to PA
10. Pull back from PA to right ventricle (RV) to screen for pulmonic stenosis and record RV
11. Record simultaneous LV–RV waveforms
12. Pull back from RV to RA to screen for tricuspid stenosis and record RA
13. Pull back from LV to AO to screen for aortic stenosis

Adapted from Ragosta M. *Textbook of Clinical Hemodynamics*. Philadelphia, PA: Elsevier/Saunders; 2008.

Hemodynamic Waveform Interpretation

Accurate review of hemodynamics includes ensuring the transducer is at the phlebostatic axis (estimated location of the RA in the midchest at the fourth intercostal space). The stopcock is then opened to air (atmospheric pressure) and set to zero in the hemodynamic system.

Misplacement of the transducer above or below the phlebostatic axis will lead to errors in diagnosis and potentially treatment. Pressures are then recorded with simultaneous EKG tracing. Figure 16-22 notes the interrelationship of electrical and physiologic activity.

Right Atrial Waveform. Normal RA pressure is 2 to 6 mm Hg. The waveform has *a* and *v* waves with *x* and *y* descents. The *a* wave signifies the pressure increase within the RA during atrial contraction. The *a* wave follows the *P* wave on EKG. The *x* descent indicates the decrease in pressure during atrial relaxation and the downward motion of the atrioventricular junction during ventricular systole. The *v* wave correlates to the *T* wave on EKG and represents the passive filling in the RA during atrial diastole. The *y* descent occurs as pressure decreases due to rapid emptying of the RA as the tricuspid valve opens. Figure 16-23 depicts a normal RA waveform.

Right Ventricular Waveform. Normal RV systolic pressure is 20 to 30 mm Hg and normal RV end-diastolic pressure is 0 to 8 mm Hg. The waveform depicts a rapid pressure rise

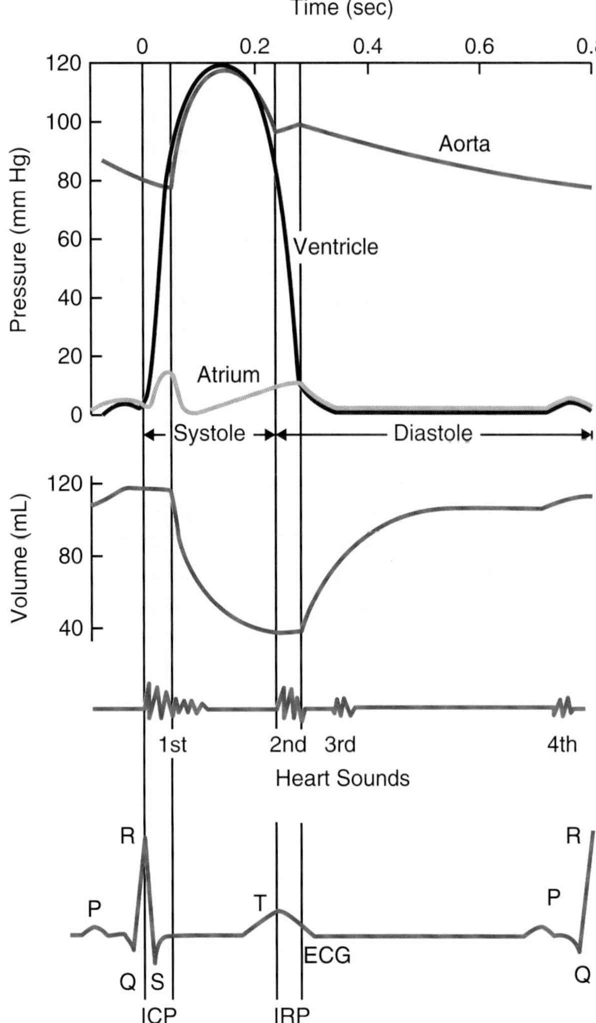

Figure 16-22. Timing of the major electrical and mechanical events during the cardiac cycle. Phase 1 = atrial contraction; Phase 2 = isovolumic contractions; Phase 3 = rapid ejection; Phase 4 = reduced ejection; Phase 5 = isovolumic relaxation; Phase 6 = rapid ventricular filling; Phase 7 = reduced ventricular filling. (From Ragosta M. *Textbook of Clinical Hemodynamics*. Philadelphia, PA: Saunders/Elsevier; 2008:19.)

with ventricular contraction and rapid pressure decrease with ventricular relaxation. Figure 16-24 depicts a normal RV waveform.

Pulmonary Artery Waveform. Normal PA systolic pressure is 20 to 30 mm Hg and normal PA diastolic pressure is 4 to 12 mm Hg. The PA waveform is similar to other arterial waveforms with a rapid rise in pressure, systolic peak, a pressure decrease with a dicrotic notch from pulmonic valve closure and a diastolic trough. Peak systolic pressure occurs with the *T* wave on EKG. The waveform is impacted by changes in respiration and may have respiratory variation. With inspiration, the intrathoracic pressure decreases. Conversely, intrathoracic pressure increases with expiration. It is recommended to measure the PA pressure at end expiration as the intrathoracic pressure is closest to zero. Figure 16-25 depicts a normal PA waveform and Figure 16-26 shows respiratory variation in a PA pressure waveform.

Pulmonary Capillary Wedge Pressure Waveform. The normal PCWP is 2 to 14 mm Hg. It represents the LAP without direct measurement of that chamber. The *a* wave follows the *P* wave and the *v* wave follows the *T* wave in a delayed timeframe as the pressure is transmitted from the pulmonary capillary bed. Figure 16-27 shows a normal PA pressure waveform. This waveform is obtained as the balloon on the distal tip of the catheter is inflated and the catheter moves forward into a capillary. It is imperative that tracings be monitored and assessed to ensure good waveforms. Overwedging the catheter can result in PA rupture and death.

Cardiac Output Studies

The methods of CO determination include the Fick oxygen method, indicator dilution technique, and the thermodilution method.

Direct Fick Method. The direct Fick method, which has historically been used in the catheterization laboratory for calculation of CO determination, is rarely used today in the original technique, but the theoretical principle has been maintained. The Fick method requires measurement of arterial oxygen saturation and mixed venous (pulmonary artery) oxygen saturation. Oxygen consumption ideally is a measured value obtained during catheterization. The methods of measuring oxygen consumption are extremely cumbersome and time consuming and, in general, not routinely employed in modern catheterization laboratories. Alternatively, oxygen consumption can be assumed on the basis of the patient's body surface area (BSA). This is not as accurate a measurement, but it is acceptable. The Fick method of CO determination is helpful in cases where the patient is in atrial fibrillation, has significant tricuspid regurgitation, or a low CO state. It has largely been replaced by the thermodilution method for CO determination. CO is calculated as oxygen consumption divided by the arteriovenous oxygen concentration difference. Calculated assumed oxygen consumption is 125 × the BSA. BSA is calculated as the square root of (body weight [kg] × height [cm]/3600). Oxygen saturation percentages are converted to amount (or content) of oxygen using the following formula: content (1.36 × hemoglobin × O_2 saturation × 10). Therefore, the equation is as follows: CO = (O_2 consumption [mL/min]/A – mixed venous O_2 difference [mL O_2/100 mL blood] × 10).

Thermodilution Method and Indicator Dilution Methods. Indicator dilution method is based on the principle that if a known amount of an indicator is added to an unknown quantity of flowing liquid and the concentration of the indicator is then measured downstream, the time course of its concentration gives a quantitative index of the flow. Applied to the circulatory system, the amount of indicator, its dilution within the circulation, and the time during which the first circulation of the substance occurs can be used to compute CO.[56]

The thermodilution technique using cold or room temperature dextrose or saline injectate solution is the most frequently used CO determination method in cardiac catheterization laboratories. The benefits of the thermodilution technique are that (1) it is performed over a short period and is, therefore, more likely to be recorded during a period of steady state; (2) it is most accurate in patients with normal or high CO; (3) the indicator used is inert and inexpensive; (4) it does not require an arterial puncture; and (5) the computer analysis curve is reasonably simple to interpret.[56] Drawbacks of this method include its unreliability in the presence of atrial fibrillation, significant tricuspid

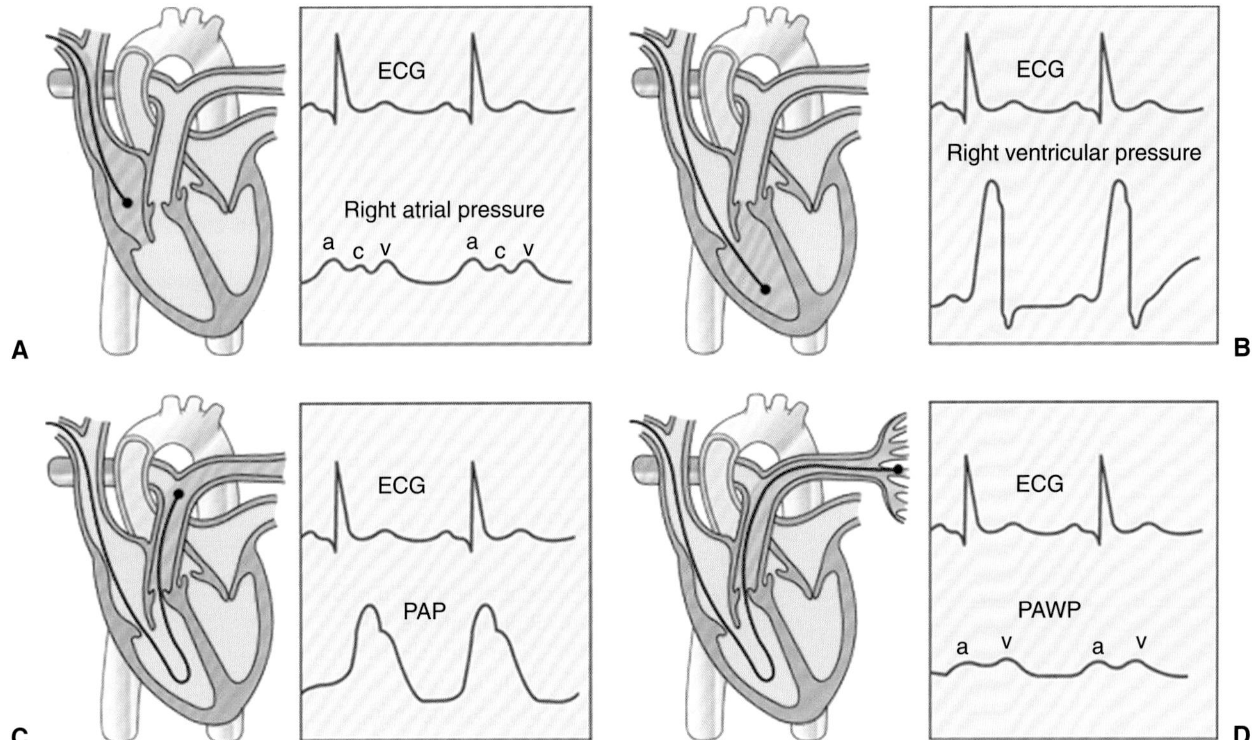

Figure 16-23. Normal right atrial pressure waveform. Note the timing of the electrocardiographic *P* and *T* waves to the hemodynamic *a* and *v* waves, respectively. (From Ragosta M. *Textbook of Clinical Hemodynamics*. Philadelphia, PA: Saunders/Elsevier; 2008:20.)

regurgitation, and its tendency to overestimate CO in patients with low CO.

Cardiac index (CI) is derived from the cardiac output. It takes into account body size through BSA. CI is CO divided by BSA.

Oximetry Runs

Oxygen saturation can be measured in sequential blood samples through the right heart. This will identify and locate a left-to-right shunt if a significant step-up in oxygen saturation is found. A significant step-up exceeds the normal variability that may be observed if multiple samples are taken from one chamber. In 1947, Dexter and colleagues found that the RA can have variable oxygen saturations based on the location of the sampling.[56] This is attributed to the fact that the RA receives blood from the SVC, IVC, and coronary sinus. Systemic and pulmonic blood flow is calculated. When the ratio of pulmonic flow is greater to systemic flow, there is a left to right shunt. The order of sampling is enumerated below. Table 16-7 describes the criteria for significant step-ups and possible etiologies.

An oximetry run takes blood samples from various chambers of the right heart in order to localize a step-up. Two-mL samples should be obtained in the following locations:

1. Left and/or right pulmonary artery
2. Main pulmonary artery

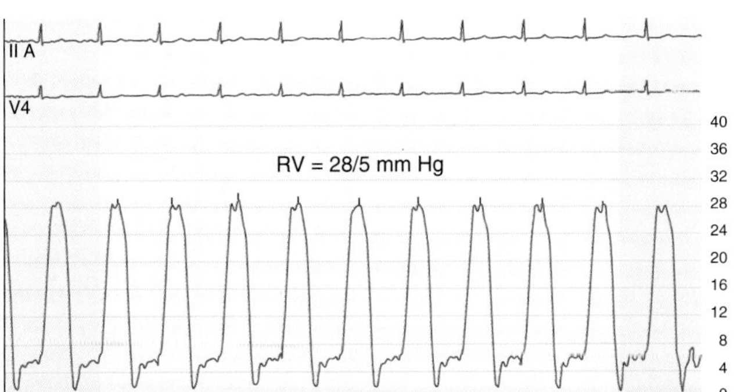

Figure 16-24. Normal right ventricular waveform. (From Ragosta M. *Textbook of Clinical Hemodynamics*. Philadelphia, PA: Saunders/Elsevier; 2008:22.)

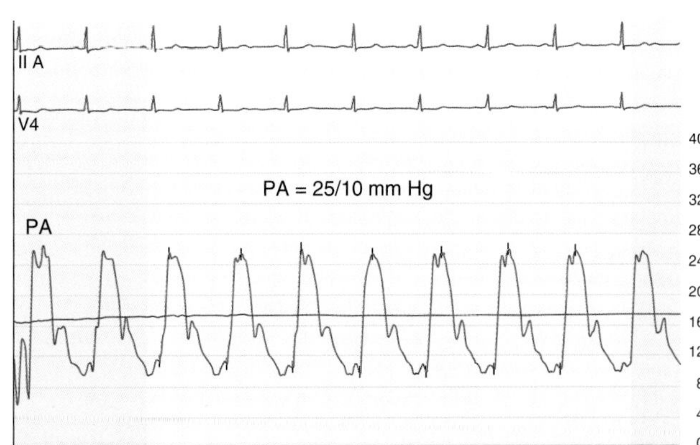

Figure 16-25. Normal pulmonary artery waveform. Note the dicrotic notch. (From Ragosta M. *Textbook of Clinical Hemodynamics*. Philadelphia, PA: Saunders/Elsevier; 2008:22.)

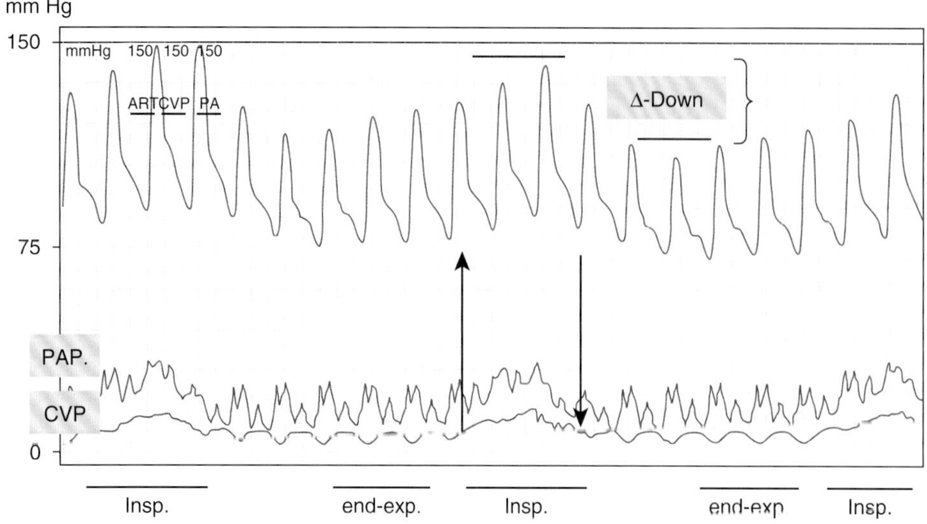

Figure 16-26. Respiratory variation in a PA pressure waveform. (From Ragosta M. *Textbook of Clinical Hemodynamics*. Philadelphia, PA: Saunders/Elsevier; 2008:22.)

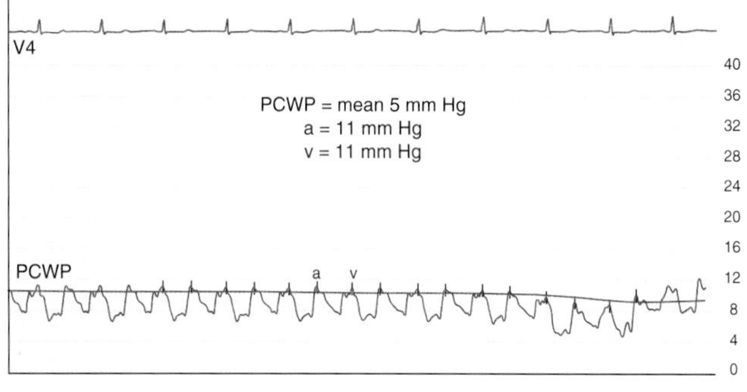

Figure 16-27. Normal pulmonary capillary wedge pressure waveform with distinct *a* and *v* waves. (From Ragosta M. *Textbook of Clinical Hemodynamics*. Philadelphia, PA: Saunders/Elsevier; 2008:22.)

3. Right ventricle, outflow tract
4. Right ventricle, mid
5. Right ventricle, tricuspid valve or apex
6. Right atrium, low or near tricuspid valve
7. Right atrium, mid
8. Right atrium, high
9. Superior vena cava, low (near junction with right atrium)
10. Superior vena cava, high (near junction with innominate vein)
11. Inferior vena cava, high (just at or below diaphragm)
12. Inferior vena cava, low (near L4-L5)
13. Left ventricle
14. Aorta (distal to insertion of ductus)

Table 16-7 • DETECTION OF LEFT TO RIGHT SHUNT BY OXIMETRY

Level of Shunt	Mean of Distal Chamber Samples (O_2% Sat)	Mean of Proximal Chamber Samples (O_2 Vol%)	Highest Value in Proximal Chamber (O_2% Sat)	Highest Value in Distal Chamber (O_2 Vol%)	Approximate Minimal Qp:Qs Required for Detection	Possible Causes of Step Up
Atrial (SVC/IVC to RA)	>7	≥1.3	≥11	≥2.0	1.5–1.9	ASD, partial anomalous pulmonary venous drainage, ruptured Sinus of Valsalva, VSD with TR, coronary fistula to RA
Ventricular (RA to RV)	> 5	≥1.0	≥10	≥1.7	1.3–1.5	VSD, PDA with PR primum ASD, coronary fistula to RV
Great Vessel (RV to PA)	>5	≥1.0	≥5	≥1.0	≥1.3	PD A, aorta-pulmonic window, aberrant coronary artery origin
Any Level (SVC to PA)	≥7	≥1.3	≥8	≥1.5	≥1.5	All of the above

SVC and IVC, superior and inferior vena cava; RA, right atrium; RV, right ventricle; PA, pulmonary artery; VSD, ventricular septal defect; TR, tricuspid regurgitation; PDA, patent ductus arteriosus; PR, pulmonic regurgitation; ASD, atrial septal defect; Qp/Qs, pulmonary to systemic flow ratio.
Adapted from Grossman W, Moscucci M. In: Moscucci M, ed. *Grossman and Baim's Cardiac Catheterization, Angiography, and Interventions*. Philadelphia, PA: Lippincott Williams & Wilkins; 2013:267.

NURSING CARE OF THE CARDIAC CATHETERIZATION PATIENT

Nursing Assessment and Patient Preparation Preprocedure

Nursing assessment and teaching are important parts of patient preparation. The nursing assessment includes the patient's heart rate and rhythm, blood pressure, evaluation of the peripheral pulses of the arms and legs, and assessment of heart and lung sounds. The sites for best palpation of the patient's dorsalis pedis and posterior tibial pulses are marked on the skin. This information will be used for comparison in evaluating peripheral pulses after the catheterization procedure if femoral access is obtained. A procedural sedation assessment is performed, including assessment of the patient's cardiovascular, respiratory, and renal systems. Care is taken to identify characteristics or conditions that may cause the patient to be at greater risk for complications associated with procedural sedation, such as a history of difficult intubation; history of difficulty with sedation; morbid obesity; sleep apnea; extremes of age; severe cardiac, respiratory, renal, hepatic, or central nervous system disease; and history of substance abuse. The nursing assessment also includes an evaluation of the patient's emotional status and attitude toward catheterization.

1. Is this the patient's first cardiac catheterization?
2. What are the patient's apprehensions about the procedure?
3. What has the patient heard about cardiac catheterization? (Patients have sometimes heard "horror stories" from friends or acquaintances about catheterization experiences and may, therefore, need reassurance about the safety of the procedure.)
4. What decisions are being faced? (Patients may be facing good or bad news about the absence or presence and extent of disease. Thus, the period before catheterization most likely is a time of anxiety and fear for a variety of reasons. Discussion and reassurance may help to relieve some of these feelings.)

The catheterization laboratory confronts the patient with new sights, sounds, and experiences that may be intimidating and frightening. Teaching is aimed at preparing the patient for this experience and should begin in the physician's office. In some institutions, patients are given a video to view before the procedure. A printed booklet to which the patient can refer is also helpful. The following points should be covered in patient teaching:

1. The patient is given nothing by mouth for 6 to 8 hours before the catheterization and is asked to void before arriving at the catheterization laboratory.
2. Medication is given before or during the procedure, if prescribed, but the patient is awake during the procedure.
3. The patient should be instructed in deep breathing, how to stop a breath without bearing down, and in coughing on request. With deep inspiration, the diaphragm descends, preventing it from obstructing the view of the coronary arteries in some radiographic projections. Bearing down (Valsalva maneuver) increases intra-abdominal pressure and may raise the diaphragm, obstructing the view. After the injection of contrast medium, coughing is requested to help clear the material from the coronary arteries. The rapid movement of the diaphragm also acts as a mechanical stimulant to the heart and helps prevent the bradycardia that may accompany the injection of contrast medium.[28]
4. The appearance of the laboratory should be explained to the patient, including the general function of the equipment.
5. The patient wears a gown to the laboratory.
6. The patient lies on a table that is hard and narrow.
7. The catheter insertion site is washed with an antibacterial scrub and hair is removed using a shaver. Usually, both groins are prepped to provide easy access to the other side for patients with peripheral vascular disease and obstructive disease preventing catheter advancement or sudden instability during the procedure requiring an IABP. The right groin is generally used because the operator standing on that side of the table has easier access. However, many laboratories use the radial artery for access now. Either side may be used depending on physician preference. For RHC, the right internal jugular vein is commonly used. Femoral veins may also be used as an alternative.
8. The expected length of the procedure should be explained to the patient (approximately 30 minutes for RHC, 1 hour for coronary angiogram and 2 hours for PCI). Complex procedures will be longer.
9. The patient is given a local anesthetic at the catheter entry site. They will feel a pinch and burn. Catheters are placed. They may feel pressure.
10. The patient may have warm sensation or experience nausea during injection of the coronary arteries with contrast medium, most commonly occurring with the injection of the ventricle during ventriculogram.
11. The patient should report angina, SOB, and other symptoms to the staff.
12. The patient should be told the expected length of bed rest after the catheterization.

The physician performing the catheterization explains the procedure and obtains informed consent before the procedure. Precatheterization orders usually include the following:

1. Standard 12-lead ECG.
2. Laboratory tests: complete blood count including platelets and differential, electrolytes, blood urea nitrogen (BUN), creatinine, and coagulation panel if taking warfarin or history of coagulopathy.
3. Patients should be NPO for 6 hours preprocedure. Although some institutions maintain NPO after midnight before the procedure despite lack of evidence to support this practice.[43]
4. Premedication with a mild sedative may be given. During the procedure, a procedural sedation protocol should be followed.
5. Patients with renal insufficiency should be adequately hydrated before and after the procedure and a minimum amount of radiographic low–osmolar-contrast medium should be used.
6. Patients with a history of allergy to previous contrast administration should receive pretreatment with steroids and antihistamine (diphenhydramine).
7. Patients who are fasting should hold their short-acting insulin but continue their long-acting insulin as this accounts for their basal needs. Oral diabetic agents are usually held the morning of the procedure. Metformin is held the day of the procedure and 48 hours after the

catheterization due to the risk of lactic acidosis with contrast administration.

8. Anticoagulation issues are directed by the physician. Acetylsalicylic acid (ASA) and antiplatelet medications are usually given before catheterization. Warfarin is generally discontinued 3 to 4 days before the procedure until the INR is less than 2.0. Warfarin can be reversed with vitamin K or fresh frozen plasma. If the patient is receiving heparin therapy, heparin can be continued during the catheterization and discontinued for sheath removal. See SPECIAL CONSIDERATIONS for information regarding DOACs prior to catheterization.
9. Patient to void before going to catheterization laboratory.
10. There is no evidence-based data to support the prophylactic use of antibiotics.
11. Patients who wear dentures, glasses, or hearing aids should be sent to the laboratory wearing them. The patient is better able to communicate when dentures and hearing aids are in place. Glasses allow the patient to view the angiogram on the monitor and help keep the patient oriented to the surroundings.
12. Do not resuscitate orders are revoked for a minimum of 24 hours following the procedure.[1]
13. Beta-HCG levels should be checked within 2 weeks of the procedure in women of childbearing age.

Nursing Care Intraprocedure

Nurses working in cardiac catheterization laboratories fill many roles. They are part of the multidisciplinary team that may include physicians, advanced practice providers, nurses and certified technologists. The basic roles needed in a catheterization laboratory during a procedure are scrubber, recorder, and circulator. When scrubbing, the nurse usually works with another staff member to assist in the procedure. When tableside, nurses must be familiar with the set-up as well as equipment like wires, catheters, balloons, and pacemakers. It is imperative that the nurse be trained in radiation safety as well as sterile technique to fulfill this role. The nurse will administer moderate sedation when appropriate. They must be vigilant in assessing the patient for changes in the emotional status, alertness, vocal responses, and facial expressions, as well as vital signs. Typically there are 1 to 2 other staff members that are monitoring and recording and are responsible for monitoring pressure and cardiac rhythm. The nurse may visit the patient before the procedure to teach and help in preparing the patient or after the procedure to evaluate puncture site stability. Ideally, the nurse has a background in intensive or coronary care and a thorough knowledge of cardiovascular drugs, arrhythmias, the principles of IV procedural sedation, sterile technique, cardiac anatomy and physiology. The nurse's alertness to these clues and early intervention with reassurance or appropriate medication may help to prevent more serious events. Training in basic and advanced cardiac life support is a requirement for catheterization laboratory nurses and those nurses caring for patients after the procedure.[1]

The cardiac catheterization laboratory is a specially equipped radiologic laboratory for the study of children and adults with known or suspected heart disease. The primary technical focus is the generation, recording, and display of high-quality x-ray images and hemodynamic data during diagnostic and interventional procedures. The technique of imaging has moved away from cineangiographic to digital images in most laboratories. The laboratory usually has the following equipment:

A patient-support table, adjustable height, flat top whose locks can be released to allow the table top to move horizontally head-to-toe and side-to-side for "panning."

1. Equipment for monitoring intracardiac pressures, CO determination, and physiologic recordings.
2. A suspended C-arm that rotates around the patient and allows variable angulations of the x-ray beam.
3. The image chain consists of a generator and cine pulse system, an x-ray tube, an image intensifier, an optical distributor, a 35-mm cine camera, and a television camera and monitor. The image chain produces fluoroscopy, which is the continuous presentation of an x-ray image on a fluorescent screen, allowing the viewing of structures in motion. The image intensifier receives the fluoroscopic image and increases its brightness, permitting filming (cinefluoroscopy) or digital acquisition of motion pictures and viewing of the image with a television camera, television screen, and videotape recorder. Although 35-mm film was originally used for recording, since 1998 all new images are permanently recorded digitally.
4. Single or biplane imaging system can be used. Biplane imaging provides simultaneous viewing of cardiac structures from two angles, which is helpful for congenital heart disease, transseptal punctures, and electrophysiology ablations as well reducing the amount of contrast delivered in patients with CKD.
5. Advanced cardiac life support drugs and equipment with a cardioverter–defibrillator available for emergency treatment.
6. Monitoring electrocardiographic activity with continuous ECG monitor display.
7. A standby pacemaker, either a temporary transvenous electrode and pulse generator system or an external transthoracic pacemaker.
8. IABP.
9. Many advanced laboratories will also have carts with sternotomy and cardiopulmonary bypass equipment.

Nursing Assessment for Complications

The nursing care of patients both during and after cardiac catheterization is directed toward the prevention and detection of complications. Cardiac catheterization is safely performed in experienced laboratories with low risk even in the sickest patients. Major complications from cardiac catheterization have been reported in less than 2% of the population with mortality less than 0.08%.[38] The risk of an adverse event is dependent on individual comorbidities, cardiovascular anatomy, and type of procedure. Therefore, the risk to benefit ratio must always be assessed before proceeding with a procedure. Factors that reduce the incidence of complications include the use of iso-osmolar contrast media, lower profile diagnostic catheters (6Fr or less), measures to reduce the incidence of bleeding and extensive operator experience.

Although complications are rare, they do occur and may be life threatening. Early detection and intervention are essential in prevention. Local vascular problems at the catheter entry site are the most commonly seen complications after cardiac catheterization procedures. These problems include minor or major oozing, ecchymosis, hematoma, or poorly controlled bleeding at the puncture site. Other vascular complications that are less common are vessel thrombosis, distal embolization, or dissection, pseudoaneurysm and arteriovenous fistula. Major postprocedural bleeding and blood transfusions have significant impact on increased length of stay and decreased long-term survival.[57] With the increased adoption of radial access, overall vascular complications are decreasing.[58]

Ventricular arrhythmias occur in response to catheter manipulation or contrast medium injection and tend not to recur after the predisposing stimulus is removed. Atrial and junctional arrhythmias and varying degrees of blocks also occur in response to these stimuli. Bradycardia is common in response to injection of the coronary arteries with contrast. Coughing can help to clear contrast and resolve bradycardia related to this. Vasovagal reactions may also occur during sheath insertion or removal that can lead to significant bradycardia and hypotension. It is important to recognize and treat early to avoid cardiovascular collapse. Other associated signs of vasovagal reactions are nausea, diaphoresis, pallor, and yawning. Incidence has been reported in 3.5 % of patients.[59] Treating underlying pain and anxiety can lessen the reaction or development of bradycardia. Prompt support with intravenous fluid and atropine can prevent further hemodynamic instability.

Cerebrovascular complications are rare but can be devastating. The incidence of stroke is based on contemporary, large registries of diagnostic and invasive coronary procedures. Rates of both ischemic and hemorrhagic stroke have been reported from 0.07% to 0.38%.[60,61] About 50% of postcatheterization strokes are hemorrhagic and those treated with abciximab in addition to heparin may be at higher risk.[61] Embolic strokes may originate from dislodgement of atherosclerotic plaque in the aorta or from thrombus on the catheter tip. Identification of neurologic changes and prompt formal neurology evaluation and imaging is key to improving outcomes. Patients with postcatheterization strokes have longer length of stay and increased mortality.[61] Thrombolysis and mechanical embolectomy are promising treatments to reduce disability.[62,63]

Table 16-8 • POSTCATHETERIZATION PROTOCOLS

General Guidelines

1. Assess vital signs every 15 minutes for 1–2 hours, every 30 minutes for 1 hour, and hourly for 4 hours or until discharge.
2. Assess catheterization site for bleeding, hematoma formation, and swelling. Assess peripheral pulses and neurovascular status every 15 minutes for 1 hour, every 30 minutes for 1 hour, and hourly for 4 hours or until discharge.
3. Resume precatheterization diet and medications (see SPECIAL CONSIDERATIONS regarding anticoagulation and diabetic medications).
4. Administer analgesic agents as needed.
5. Notify physician if any of the following occur:
   a. Decrease in peripheral pulses
   b. New hematoma or increase in size of existing hematoma
   c. Unusually severe catheter insertion site pain or affected extremity pain
   d. Onset of chest discomfort or shortness of breath

Femoral Approach

6. Order bed rest for 4–6 hours depending on sheath size. The head of the bed may be raised to 30 degrees.
7. Instruct patient not to flex or hyperextend the hip joint of the affected leg for 4–6 hours, and to use the bed controls to elevate the head of the bed or lower the foot of the bed.
8. Compression device may be applied. Monitor peripheral pulses as per protocol.

Brachial or Radial Approach

9. The patient may sit up in bed and ambulate once recovered from sedation. Pressure dressing or Ace bandage may be applied to the affected arm.
10. Monitor distal pulses every 15 minutes for 1 hour, every 30 minutes for 1 hour, and hourly for 4 hours until discharge or stable.
11. Instruct patient not to keep the arm in a flexed position for an extended period of time, hyperextend or lie on the affected arm for 24 hours.
12. Instruct patient to observe for bleeding or hematoma. If sutures were used, instruct patient regarding suture removal.

Nursing Care Postprocedure

After the procedure, the patient may be transferred to an observation unit, telemetry unit, interventional cardiology unit, or intensive care unit depending on the type of procedure done and the patient's condition. In most facilities, patients undergoing diagnostic catheterization are cared for in an observational unit, such as an ambulatory care unit or same-day surgery unit, for up to 6 hours and then discharged if stable. Patients who have undergone interventional procedures often stay overnight and are cared for in a telemetry unit or interventional cardiology unit where nurses are specially trained and experienced in postprocedure care and have more in-depth knowledge of cardiovascular drugs, arrhythmia interpretation, advanced cardiac life support skills, and management of access sites. If the patient is hemodynamically unstable or has a complication of the procedure, such as MI, severe respiratory distress, acute or threatened vessel closure post-PCI, tamponade, unstable arrhythmias, or requires close observation or intensive nursing care, he or she is transferred to an intensive care unit.

After a diagnostic procedure, the arterial or venous introducer sheaths are removed and manual or mechanical pressure is applied to the access site until hemostasis is achieved.

Compression devices may be used for either femoral or radial access. Vascular closure devices may be used to achieve hemostasis for femoral access. For interventional procedures in which extensive anticoagulation was used or IV antiplatelet therapy (i.e., glycoprotein IIb/IIIa receptor inhibitors) is to be continued for several hours, the sheath is often left in place until the activated clotting time is below a critical level and then removed by either catheterization laboratory staff or nurses in the postprocedure unit. Nurses caring for patients after cardiac catheterization must be prepared to perform sheath removal according to institutional policies and guidelines and must be able to recognize complications associated with this procedure.[1]

After returning from the laboratory, the patient must be thoroughly assessed. Information about the approach used, the procedures performed, and any complications experienced during the catheterization should be obtained from the physician, nurse, or technician. Table 16-8 lists typical postcatheterization protocols. The elements of the nursing assessment and intervention and potential findings are listed and explained in the following sections.

Psychological Assessment and Patient Teaching

Patients are often tired, hungry, and uncomfortable when they return from the laboratory. They are usually relieved that the procedure is over and may already know the preliminary findings of their study. The nurse caring for the patient should receive a verbal or written report for the patient postprocedure. It is important to find out what the patient has been told and pertinent follow-up. The patient may have questions about surgery or about what to expect next. Some patients are anxious or depressed. Giving patients the

Table 16-9 • PATIENT DISCHARGE INSTRUCTIONS FOR INPATIENT AND OUTPATIENT CATHETERIZATION

1. Report the following symptoms to your physician if they occur:
   a. New bleeding or swelling at the catheterization site. (If marked bleeding occurs, press hand firmly over the area of bleeding and call 911.)
   b. Increased tenderness, redness, drainage, or pain at the catheterization site
   c. Fever
   d. Change in color (pallor), temperature (coolness), or sensation (numbness) in the leg or arm used for catheterization
2. Acetaminophen or other non–aspirin-containing analgesic may be taken every 4 hours as needed for pain unless contraindicated
3. If stitches are present, wear an adhesive bandage and remove as directed by physician. Otherwise, cover site with an adhesive bandage for 24 hours
   a. Patient may shower the day after the procedure
   b. Tub bath should be avoided for 3 days after the procedure
4. Patient to see physician for follow-up appointment
5. For those at risk for CIN, creatinine should be checked in 3 to 5 days
6. Continue prescribed medications as before unless otherwise indicated by your physician
7. Avoid strenuous activity for 48 hours. Do not lift anything heavier than 5 lb for the next 48 hours
8. Limit excessive stair climbing
9. Patient must be driven home and be accompanied by a responsible adult until the next morning
10. If pain or pressure occurs in chest, arms, shoulders, neck, or jaw:
    a. Take nitroglycerin if it is prescribed for the patient
    b. Notify cardiologist of chest pain if it is relieved with nitroglycerin
    c. If chest pain is not relieved, call 911

opportunity to express their feelings about the procedure helps to relieve stress. Reassure the patient by describing the sensations that can be expected, such as thirst and the frequent need to urinate although the patient has had nothing to eat or drink for several hours. Reemphasize the need for bed rest and the need to keep the catheterized limb immobile. Let the patient know that frequent checking of vital signs is routine and not a cause for alarm. Before hospital discharge, the patient should be instructed regarding symptoms for which to call the physician and procedures for site care (Table 16-9).

Circulatory Integrity of Access Site. Careful assessment of the access site and limb is an important element of postcatheterization nursing care. The site should be checked for visible bleeding, swelling, or tenderness. The arterial pulse at the site and at points distal to it should be compared with pulses on the opposite limb and those recorded before the procedure. Capillary filling and the warmth of the limb should also be evaluated. Blanching, cramping, coolness, pain, numbness, or tingling may indicate reduced perfusion and must be carefully evaluated. A diminished or absent pulse is a sign of serious arterial occlusion, which often constitutes a surgical emergency. The first step, if any of these signs occur, is to check the compression device (if used) and release pressure. If symptoms do not resolve, the covering provider should be notified immediately and steps should be taken to preserve the limb.

Manual pressure or pressure with a compression device such as a FemoStop™ (St. Jude Medical) can be used for femoral hemostasis if bleeding continues or recurs after initial hemostasis. When pressure is applied at an arterial site, the pulse distal to the site may be safely occluded for 2 to 5 minutes, and then pressure is released until the pulse returns. Distal pulses should remain palpable during the remainder of pressure application, which continues for 15 to 20 minutes. Similarly, a transradial band may be reinflated for radial artery bleeding. If oozing from the sheath insertion tract continues after initial hemostasis, infiltration of the tract with a solution of lidocaine and epinephrine (1:100,000 strength) followed by 2 to 5 minutes of light manual pressure is usually effective in controlling bleeding.

Blood Pressure. Evaluation of the blood pressure after cardiac catheterization should include comparison of pre- and postprocedure pressures, checking for orthostatic hypotension once the bed rest period is over, and monitoring for paradoxical pulse. Mild systolic hypotension frequently occurs after cardiac catheterization and is usually not of concern. Angiographic contrast medium acts as an osmotic diuretic, and patients frequently return with signs of volume depletion, including orthostatic hypotension. Therefore, patients are kept on bed rest until fluid balance is restored with oral liquids or by IV replacement. *Hypotension* may also be a response to the drugs given during the procedure. If the blood pressure is consistently low, other causes need to be investigated, such as possible bleeding at the insertion site or in the pericardium. Patient assessment needs to be performed and the physician notified. *Paradoxical pulse* suggests pericardial tamponade, which is very rare but may occur as a result of perforation of a coronary artery or the myocardium. In patients with known perforation, this sign should be specifically assessed with each blood pressure measurement, and, if it occurs, the physician should be notified. *Hypertension* can also occur and may contribute to access site bleeding if not controlled. It is important that patients take their regularly scheduled antihypertensive medications.

Heart Rate and Rhythm. Patients who have had an interventional procedure should be on a cardiac monitor for rhythm and ST-segment monitoring. A mild sinus tachycardia (100 to 120 beats/min) is not unusual after catheterization and may be a sign of anxiety or pain, an indication of saline and water loss due to diuresis, or a reaction to medication such as atropine. Fluids, time, and reassurance often bring the heart rate down to more normal levels. Heart rates above 120 beats/min should be evaluated for other causes such as hemorrhage, more severe fluid imbalance, fever, or arrhythmias. Bradycardia may indicate vasovagal responses, arrhythmias, or infarction and should be assessed by 12-lead ECG and correlated with other clinical signs, such as pain and blood pressure. Vasovagal reactions are fairly common and can occur immediately or hours after sheath removal. Cardiac monitoring for ST-segment displacement is useful to detect acute reocclusion of the artery or MI after an interventional procedure.

Temperature. Early increases in temperature may occur because of the fluid loss that occurs with catheterization. More persistent elevations may indicate infection or pyrogenic reactions.

Urinary Output. Because angiographic contrast medium acts as an osmotic diuretic, patients have an increase in urine output for a short time after catheterization. IV fluids are often continued for a variable time after the procedure, and oral fluids should be encouraged unless the patient has been ordered NPO for another reason.

Other Possible Problems. Heart failure may occur after cardiac catheterization with the delivery of IV fluid and contrast. Nurses should be aware of the signs and symptoms of HF and alert the physician or covering provider with any concerns.

CONCLUSIONS

Summary

Table 16-10 lists normal ranges for some of the data gathered during cardiac catheterization. The assessment of CAD involves evaluation of the coronary vasculature and left ventricular function.

Table 16-10 • NORMAL ADULT VALUES FOR DATA COLLECTED DURING CARDIAC CATHETERIZATION

Pressures	mm Hg
Systemic arterial	
Peak-systolic	100–140
End-diastolic	60–90
Mean	70–105
Left ventricular	
Peak-systolic	100–140
End-diastolic	3–12
Left atrial	
Left atrial mean (or PAWP)	1–10
a wave	3–15
v wave	3–12
Pulmonary artery	
Peak-systolic	15–30
End-diastolic	3–12
Systolic mean	9–16
Right ventricular	
Peak-systolic	15–30
End-diastolic	0–8
Right atrial	
Mean	8–10
a wave	2–10
v wave	2–10
Left ventricular volumes	
End-systolic volume (mL/m^2)	20–30
End-diastolic volume (mL/m^2)	70–79
Ejection fraction	.58–.72
Resistance (dynes/s/cm^{-5})	
Total systemic resistance	900–1,440
Pulmonary arteriolar (vascular) resistance	37–97
Flow	
CO (L/min)	4.0–8.0
Cardiac index (L/min/m^2)	2.5–4.0
Stroke index (mL/beat/m^2)	35–70
Stroke volume (mL/beat)	60–130
Oxygen consumption (mL/min/m^2)	125
Oxygen saturation (%)	
Right atrium	60–75
Right ventricle	60–75
Pulmonary artery	60–75
Left atrium	95–99
Left ventricle	95–99
Aorta	95–99

PAWP, pulmonary artery wedge pressure.
From Kucher N, Goldhaber SZ. Pulmonary angiography. In: Baim DS, ed. *Grossman's Cardiac Catheterization, Angiography, and Intervention*. 7th ed. Philadelphia, PA: Lippincott Williams & Wilkins; 2006:236.

CVD is a global health problem that requires invasive assessment through cardiac catheterization to define and treat disorders. Great strides have been made in cardiac catheterization since the early 1900s when the first RHC was performed. The field has advanced to perform detailed diagnostic procedures with advanced imaging and technology to better understand and treat heart disease. It allows for interventional procedures like PCI, ASD/PFO closure, mitral valvuloplasty, and TAVR. Nurses play a pivotal role in the cardiac catheterization laboratory. Astute assessment and monitoring are vital to preventing complications and intervening appropriately before, during, and after procedures. Nursing care ensures efficiency and safety in the cardiac catheterization laboratory. Nurses are able to educate patients and provide emotional support as well. Supportive nursing care promotes positive patient experiences and impacts outcomes. Nursing care and interventions directly impact metrics like bleeding, CIN, and defect free care. Engaging nurses in quality improvement initiatives and project implementation is vital to impacting change and sustaining positive outcomes.

Future Considerations/Implications

As Interventional Cardiology continues to grow and expand, the types of procedures performed and technology used will evolve. Hybrid procedures will continue to advance and develop requiring multidisciplinary teams including cardiac and vascular surgery, interventional cardiology, nursing, and administration. Information technology systems should be leveraged to improve workflow and allow for ease of access to data. Robotic procedures are gaining credibility in clinical trials by reducing radiation exposure for staff. An increase in robotic technology is expected to occur in the future. Computed tomography FFR (CT-FFR) technology is being developed but not yet validated. CT-FFR performs noninvasive angiographic assessment and may be able to determine hemodynamically significant lesions. The technology allows for implant of virtual stents and assessment of flow. This could support a personalized interventional plan for each patient. The addition of 3-D imaging to traditional fluoroscopy is likely to be implemented in future angiography systems. Three-dimensional imaging would allow for live reconstruction of anatomy and potentially help with interventional planning.

Cardiac catheterization nursing will need to maintain competency and knowledge in this evolving field. Association with professional societies like SCAI and the Society for Invasive Cardiovascular Professionals (SICP) will help to support educational efforts and certifications. Nurses may choose to specialize as a Registered Cardiovascular Invasive Specialist (RCIS) through Cardiovascular Credentialing International. Through this certification, curriculum will continue to be updated to support nurses as the field advances at a rapid pace. Locally, catheterization laboratories will need to support staff with ongoing education and exposure and training with new technologies.

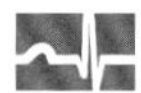

CASE STUDY 1

Patient Profile

Name/Age/Sex: **Mary Green, 77-year-old female**

History of Present Illness

Mrs. Green has no PMH of CAD but has several risk factors including HTN, CVA, DM, dyslipidemia, remote tobacco use, and family history. She told her PCP that she had been getting SOB when carrying laundry upstairs over the past few months. At times, she has felt chest tightness as she gets to top of the stairs. The SOB and chest tightness resolve once she puts the laundry basket down and rests. She has not had any episodes at rest. She has noticed that the symptoms are starting to occur when she climbs the stairs without laundry.

Past Medical History

HTN, CKD, AF, CVA, diabetes mellitus (DM), dyslipidemia

Surgical History

Hysterectomy, Cholecystectomy

Family History

F—CAD with CABG at age 65, deceased at age 80, M—HTN, deceased at age 83

Medications

Aspirin 81 mg daily, carvedilol 12.5 mg twice daily, atorvastatin 40 mg daily, metformin 500 mg twice daily, amlodipine 2.5 mg daily, warfarin 2.5 mg on Monday/ Wednesday/Friday—5 mg on Tuesday/Thursday/Saturday/ Sunday (INR goal 2.0 to 3.0)

Allergies

IV contrast (hives), Sulfa (nausea/vomiting)

Patient Examination

Vital Signs

BP 114/68; HR 70; Temp 36.6°C; O_2 sat 98% RA

Physical Examination

A&O × 3, NAD, Lungs CTAB, irregularly irregular rhythm, no murmur, rubs, or gallops.

Diagnostic Studies

Given her symptoms and her history, Mrs. Green is sent for an exercise stress test with nuclear imaging. She walks on the treadmill for 4 minutes and 32 seconds. She achieves 85% maximum predicted heart rate for her age. EKG with exercise has 1 to 2 mm downsloping ST depressions in leads V3–V6. Nuclear imaging shows a large, reversible anterior defect. Mrs. Green is referred to a cardiologist. After review of her history, symptoms, and stress test, she is referred for a left heart catheterization in accordance with 2014 guidelines on Diagnosis and Management of patients with SIHD.

In preparation for her LHC, the cardiac catheterization laboratory nurse reviews her chart in advance of her procedure.

- What are some concerns in Mrs. Green's PMH and medication list in relation to a left heart catheterization?
- What assessments should the nurse make when evaluating Mrs. Green's risk for bleeding, stroke off anticoagulation, and contrast-induced nephropathy?
- What interventions should the preprocedure nurse implement to prevent any potential adverse outcomes?

Mrs. Green has an allergy to IV contrast. She will receive IV contrast with her procedure.

Review of the SCAI 2016 Cardiac catheterization best practices consensus statement recommends that Mrs. Green be pretreated with corticosteroids and diphenhydramine (Prednisone 50 mg at 13 hours, 7 hours, and one hour prior to the procedure and diphenhydramine an hour before the procedure). The nurse also notes that Mrs. Green is diabetic and takes metformin. Administration of IV contrast in patients taking metformin can result in lactic acidosis. Current guidelines recommend holding metformin for 48 hours pre- and postcontrast administration. It can be resumed 48 hours postprocedure if renal function is normal. The nurse notes that Mrs. Green's blood sugar is likely to elevate when she takes steroids and will be off her metformin. She notes in the chart to check her blood sugar on arrival.

Mrs. Green is taking warfarin for a history of AF and CVA. The nurse calculates Mrs. Green's CHAD2-VASc score to assess her stroke risk off anticoagulation. Mrs. Green is a female (1 point) who is over 75 years old (2 points), has HTN and DM (1 point each), and had a prior CVA (2 points). Mrs. Green has a CHAD2-VASc score of 7. The nurse knows that any score greater than 5 is considered moderate risk for thromboembolism when not taking anticoagulation according to the 2017 ACC expert consensus decision pathway for periprocedural management of anticoagulation in patients with nonvalvular atrial fibrillation. Additionally, Mrs. Green has a history of prior CVA which also increases her thromboembolism risk. The nurse considers bridging Mrs. Green with LMWH while holding Coumadin to decrease her risk of thromboembolism. Her chart is reviewed in detail and there is no bleeding history.

The nurse remembers that LMWH is renally excreted and should not be given to patients with creatinine clearance <30 mL/min/1.73 m^2. She reviews Mrs. Green's preprocedure labs. Her creatinine is 1.3 mg/dL. Her creatinine clearance calculates to 40 mL/min/1.73 m^2. The nurse discusses all her findings with the physician who agrees with her assessment. Therefore, Mrs. Green will be directed to hold warfarin for 4 days prior to her procedure date. She will start LMWH 2 days prior to her procedure. Her last dose of LMWH will be 24 hours before her procedure.

Given her CKD, the nurse knows Mrs. Green is at increased risk for CIN. She makes a note in the chart to start IV fluids when she arrives and for the duration of her recovery or up to 12 hours postprocedure in accordance with guideline recommendations. The nurse calls Mrs. Green the week before her procedure and reviews directions as described above. Additionally, she tells Mrs. Green that she will need to have nothing by mouth (NPO) after midnight as her procedure is at 7 AM. She should take her aspirin, carvedilol, and amlodipine with a small sip of water. She explains the procedure to Mrs. Green and answers her questions. The nurse advises that she must have someone available to drive her home. They also discuss postprocedure restrictions including no heavy lifting for 2 days. Mrs. Green feels less anxious now that she understands the procedure.

CASE STUDY 2

Patient Profile

Name/Age/Sex: **John Morris, 63-year-old male**

History of Present Illness

Mr. Morris has ischemic cardiomyopathy and has been maintained on maximal medical therapy for heart failure. However, he has noticed increased lower extremity edema despite starting Lasix a few months ago. His weight has slowly increased overtime and he has become SOB when walking on an incline. He has had some subtle, atypical chest pain that occurs intermittently and not necessarily with activity. Recent echocardiogram demonstrated a decrease in his EF from 30% to 20% with global hypokinesis. He has not had repeat angiography since his CABG. Given his new symptoms and reduction in EF, his HF specialist refers him for a right and left heart catheterization in accordance with the 2013 HF Guidelines for Invasive Evaluation. The RHC will provide his physician with hemodynamics and the LHC will image his bypass grafts to determine if ongoing ischemia has impacted his EF.

Past Medical History

CAD s/p CABG × 3 (Left internal mammary artery [LIMA] to LAD, saphenous vein graft [SVG] to OM2, radial to RCA) 10 years ago, peripheral arterial disease (PAD) s/p L SFA PTA/stent 2 years ago, Dyslipidemia, HTN, CKD (creatinine 1.5), LV dysfunction (EF 30%), s/p Implantable cardioverter defibrillator (ICD)

Family History

Brother—MI at age 48, alive at 60, F—HTN, deceased at 70 2/2 aortic dissection, M—dyslipidemia, DM, alive and well at age 88

Social History

Married, disabled after CABG from construction. Tobacco use—2 packs per day × 40 years, quit 10 years ago at time of CABG. ETOH—2–3 beers/day. No other drug use.

Medications

Aspirin 81 mg daily, Clopidogrel 75 mg daily, Metoprolol XL 50 mg daily, Rosuvastatin 40 mg daily, Sacubitril/valsartan 97/103 mg twice daily, Furosemide 40 mg daily

Allergies

NKDA

Patient Examination

Vital Signs

80.9 kg; 177.8 cm; BP 133/78; HR 60; O_2 Sat 99%RA; Temp 36.8°C

Physical Examination

Lungs CTAB, Cardiac rrr, no MRG, DP/PT 1+, A&O × 3, NAD

Diagnostic Studies

Mr. Morris presents on the day of his procedure. He is prepped for right internal jugular vein and left radial artery access. His right radial artery was used for a bypass graft. RIJ access is achieved and the Swan–Ganz catheter is inserted and passed from RA to RV to PA to PCW position while waveform tracings are recorded. These demonstrate volume overload with RA 12 mm Hg, PAP 45/24 mm Hg, PCWP 24 mm Hg. Mixed venous oxygenation is measured at 50%. His arterial oxygen saturation is 96%. Hemoglobin is 12.3 g/dL. His blood pressure is 132/78. Fick cardiac output is calculated at 3.7 L/min. CI is 1.85 L/min/m^2. SVR is calculated at 1816 dynes sec/cm^5. The nurse in the lab discontinues the IVF that is being administered for CIN prevention as the PCWP is elevated and CO is severely reduced. The Swan–Ganz catheter is removed.

The interventionalist attempts to obtain left radial artery access. However, the artery proves to be very tortuous and right femoral access is obtained with some difficulty given his PAD. The native coronary arteries are imaged first. This helps to elucidate what territories are supplied by the native vessels and what territories are missing visible arteries that should be supplied by grafts. The LAD is occluded in the mid portion. The LCX has an 80% stenosis before the OM2. The RCA is also occluded in the proximal segment. The SVG to LCX is imaged and noted to be patent. The radial graft to the RCA is patent as well. Last, the LIMA to the LAD is engaged and also patent. The catheter is removed. It is decided not to use a vascular closure device as Mr. Morris has significant PAD. His sheaths will be removed in the recovery area by the postprocedure nurses. The interventionalist will discuss the results with this HF physician. They will consider intervention of the LCX at a later date as his creatinine is 1.5 and they do not want to increase the amount of contrast that he receives at one time. SCAI 2016 Best Practices notes that the amount of contrast should not exceed 3.7 × GFR. Mr. Morris' GFR is 49 mL/min/1.73 m^2 (3.7 × 49 = 181). Mr. Morris received 100 mL of contrast. Additionally, he is in a low-output state with high SVR and volume overload. He could benefit from increased inotropy and afterload reduction. He will be admitted for medical optimization and diuresis.

Key Questions

What should the postprocedure nurse assess following cardiac catheterization? What complications should the nurse be prepared to identify and treat? What risk factors does Mr. Morris have for bleeding?

Mr. Morris returns to the recovery area. His vital signs are an HR of 80 beats/min (bpm) in sinus rhythm, blood pressure of 130/85 mm Hg, oxygen saturation of 94% on 2 liters nasal canula. The RIJ and RFV catheters are sutured in place. Mr. Morris' vital signs, access sites, and pulses are monitored every 15 minutes for the first 2 hours. The activate clotting time (ACT) is checked to see if his sheaths may be removed. The 2016 SCAI expert consensus document on best practices in the cardiac catheterization laboratory recommends an ACT <180 seconds to safely remove sheaths. Mr. Morris' initial ACT is 210 seconds. After 30 minutes, the ACT is 175 seconds and his nurse prepares to remove his right femoral artery sheath first.

The nurse is prepared for a vagal reaction when pressure is applied to the groin and possible bleeding. Mr. Morris is at increased risk of bleeding based on the HAS-BLED score. His score is 4 (1 point each for HTN, CKD, alcohol use, antiplatelet medication). Scores greater than 3 are highly predictive of bleeding events.

The nurse prepares for possible complications. A liter of normal saline is attached to Mr. Morris' IV. The line is closed but ready if needed. Atropine is removed from the medication cabinet in anticipation of a possible vagal reaction. Another nurse assists Mr. Morris' nurse to monitor HR and blood pressure frequently and to assess for any bleeding or vagal reaction. The nurse removes the right femoral arterial sheath while placing pressure above the arterial puncture site. Hemostasis is achieved initially as there is no external bleeding. Vital signs are stable. The right pedal pulse is occluded initially during maximal pressure. Within a few minutes, Mr. Morris tells the nurse that he does not feel well. He says he feels hot, flushed, and nauseated. The nurse recognizes this as a possible vagal reaction. HR is slowing into the 60s on the monitor. The blood pressure cuff is cycling. The nurses react and open the IV

(*continued*)

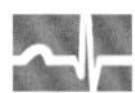

CASE STUDY 2 (*Continued*)

fluid and prepare to administer Atropine. The blood pressure reads 85/40 mm Hg and heart rate is 45 bpm. Atropine 1 mg IV is administered. The HR starts to rise and recycling of the cuff shows a blood pressure of 100/50 mm Hg. Simultaneously, the nurse lessens the pressure on the groin as a nidus for the vagal reaction. Mr. Morris' vital signs remain stable for the remainder of the groin pressure and hemostasis is achieved within 20 minutes. Vital signs continue to be monitored frequently as Mr. Morris has 4 hours of bed rest. His blood pressure returns to his baseline of 130/80. The RIJ sheath is removed without incident and hemostasis is achieved with 5 minutes of pressure.

After 2 hours of bedrest, Mr. Morris complains that he is short of breath. He has increased his work of breathing. Mr. Morris has received a liter of normal saline. The nurse notes his vital signs on the monitor. His HR has climbed to 102 bpm. Oxygen saturation is 85% on 2 liters via nasal cannula and his respiratory rate is 30 breaths/min. Blood pressure cycles to 180/90 mm Hg. The nurse increases the flow of oxygen to 6 liters and calls for another nurse.

They recognize that Mr. Morris has a reduced EF and was volume overloaded with a PCWP of 24 mm Hg before he received additional IV fluid. He has not received any diuretic as yet. With increased blood pressure, Mr. Morris has also increased his vascular resistance. The nurse calls the physician to consider lowering Mr. Morris' blood pressure and prescribing diuretic. He receives a sublingual nitroglycerin and 40 mg IV furosemide. His blood pressure reduces to 160/80 mm Hg. He slowly improves symptomatically as the medications take effect. Within 15 minutes, Mr. Morris has urinated 500 mL and his oxygen is able to be reduced to 2 liters.

Mr. Morris completes his bedrest and ambulates to the bathroom with his nurse. When he returns to his bed, the nurse assesses his right groin. The nurse notes an enlarged area at his access site. The nurse recognizes this as a hematoma. Mr. Morris is assisted to the supine position and the nurse applies manual pressure while asking another nurse for help. Vital signs are taken and his blood pressure is now 100/45. The nurse is concerned that Mr. Morris could be bleeding and hemostasis must be achieved. IV fluids are again connected to help replace lost blood volume and maintain blood pressure and perfusion. The physician is called and simultaneously another nurse draws a complete blood count to check the hemoglobin for significant change from preprocedure. The staff continue to apply pressure to the right groin. The hematoma has decreased in size and blood pressure improves with fluids. The fluids are discontinued given his recent desaturation related to volume overload. The hemoglobin results at 11.7 g/dL from 12.8 g/dL preprocedure. The change can be attributed to dilution with IV fluid administration. After another 20 minutes of pressure, the hematoma has resolved and vital signs are stable. Bedrest resumes. Mr. Morris ambulates after an additional 4 hours. His groin and vital signs remain stable and he is transferred to the cardiac step down unit for ongoing care.

It is the continuous assessment and clinical astuteness of Mr. Morris' nurse that helped to avoid several bad outcomes. Rapidly addressing a vagal reaction prevents cardiovascular collapse. Recognizing acute volume overload and intervening averts possible respiratory decline and intubation. Finally, quick identification and treatment of an expanding hematoma prevented significant hemorrhage and rapid hemodynamic decline.

KEY READINGS

Moscucci M, ed. *Grossman and Baim's Cardiac Catheterization, Angiography, and Interventions*. 8th ed. Philadelphia, PA: Lippincott Williams & Wilkins; 2013.

Naidu SS, Aronow HD, Box LC, et al. SCAI expert consensus statement: 2016 best practices in the cardiac catheterization laboratory: (Endorsed by the Cardiological Society of India, and Sociedad Latino Americana de Cardiologia Intervencionista; Affirmation of value by the Canadian Association of Interventional Cardiology-Association Canadienne de Cardiologie d'intervention). *Catheter Cardiovasc Interv*. 2016;*88*(3):407–423. ISSN 1522–726X. Disponível em: < https://www.ncbi.nlm.nih.gov/pubmed/27137680

Ragosta M. *Textbook of Clinical Hemodynamics*. Philadelphia, PA: Saunders Elsevier; 2008.

Sorajja P, Borlaug BA, Dimas VV, et al. SCAI/HFSA clinical expert consensus document on the use of invasive hemodynamics for the diagnosis and management of cardiovascular disease. *Catheter Cardiovasc Interv*. 2017;*89*(7):E233–E247. ISSN 1522–726X. Disponível em: < https://www.ncbi.nlm.nih.gov/pubmed/28489331

REFERENCES

1. Naidu SS, Aronow HD, Box LC, et al. SCAI expert consensus statement: 2016 best practices in the cardiac catheterization laboratory: (Endorsed by the Cardiological Society of India, and sociedad Latino Americana de Cardiologia intervencionista; Affirmation of value by the Canadian Association of interventional cardiology-Association canadienne de cardiologie d'intervention). *Catheter Cardiovasc Interv*. 2016;88(3): 407–423.
2. Davis J. The society of invasive cardiovascular professionals new 2015 educational guidelines for invasive cardiovascular technology personnel in the cardiovascular catheterization laboratory. *Cath Lab Digest*. 2015; 23(5).
3. Cournand A, Ranges C. Catheterization of the right auricle in man. *Proc Soc Exp Biol Med*. 1941;46:462–470.
4. Cournand A, Riley RL, Breed ES, et al. Measurement of cardiac output in man using the technique of catheterization of the right auricle or ventricle. *J Clin Invest*. 1945;24(1):106–116.
5. Richards D. Cardiac output by catheterization technique in various clinical conditions. *Federal Proceedings*. 1945;4:215–220.
6. Seldinger SI. Catheter replacement of the needle in percutaneous arteriography; a new technique. *Acta Radiol*. 1953;39(5):368–376.
7. Sones FM, Shirey EK. Cine coronary arteriography. *Mod Concepts Cardiovasc Dis*. 1962;31:735–738.
8. Bertrand ME. *The Evolution of Cardiac Catheterization and Interventional Cardiology*. Boxford, MA: Iatric Press and the European Society of Cardiology; 2006.
9. Bourassa MG. The history of cardiac catheterization. *Can J Cardiol*. 2005;21(12):1011–1014.
10. Inoue K, Owaki T, Nakamura T, et al. Clinical application of transvenous mitral commissurotomy by a new balloon catheter. *J Thorac Cardiovasc Surg*. 1984;87(3):394–402.
11. St Goar FG, Fann JI, Komtebedde J, et al. Endovascular edge-to-edge mitral valve repair: short-term results in a porcine model. *Circulation*. 2003;108(16):1990–1993.
12. King TD, Thompson SL, Steiner C, et al. Secundum atrial septal defect. Nonoperative closure during cardiac catheterization. *JAMA*. 1976;235(23):2506–2509.
13. Holzer R, Balzer D, Amin Z, et al. Transcatheter closure of postinfarction ventricular septal defects using the new Amplatzer muscular VSD occluder: Results of a U.S. Registry. *Catheter Cardiovasc Interv*. 2004;61(2):196–201.
14. Reddy VY, Doshi SK, Sievert H, et al. Percutaneous left atrial appendage closure for stroke prophylaxis in patients with atrial fibrillation: 2.3-year

follow-up of the PROTECT AF (Watchman Left Atrial Appendage System for Embolic Protection in Patients with Atrial Fibrillation) Trial. *Circulation*. 2013;127(6):720–729.

15. Leon MB, Smith CR, Mack M, et al. Transcatheter aortic-valve implantation for aortic stenosis in patients who cannot undergo surgery. *N Engl J Med*. 2010;363(17):1597–1607.
16. Heidenreich PA, Trogdon JG, Khavjou OA, et al. Forecasting the future of cardiovascular disease in the United States: A policy statement from the American Heart Association. *Circulation*. 2011;123(8):933–944.
17. Levine GN, Bates ER, Blankenship JC, et al. 2015 ACC/AHA/SCAI Focused Update on Primary Percutaneous Coronary Intervention for Patients With ST-Elevation Myocardial Infarction: An Update of the 2011 ACCF/AHA/SCAI Guideline for Percutaneous Coronary Intervention and the 2013 ACCF/AHA Guideline for the Management of ST-Elevation Myocardial Infarction. *J Am Coll Cardiol*. 2016;67(10):1235–1250.
18. Krumholz HM, Merrill AR, Schone EM, et al. Patterns of hospital performance in acute myocardial infarction and heart failure 30-day mortality and readmission. *Circ Cardiovasc Qual Outcomes*. 2009;2(5):407–413.
19. O'Gara PT, Kushner FG, Ascheim DD, et al. 2013 ACCF/AHA guideline for the management of ST-elevation myocardial infarction: executive summary: a report of the American College of Cardiology Foundation/American Heart Association Task Force on Practice Guidelines: Developed in collaboration with the American College of Emergency Physicians and Society for Cardiovascular Angiography and Interventions. *Catheter Cardiovasc Interv*. 2013;82(1):E1–E27.
20. Duarte AG, Lin YL, Sharma G. Incidence of right heart catheterization in patients initiated on pulmonary arterial hypertension therapies: A population-based study. *J Heart Lung Transplant*. 2017;36(2):220–226.
21. Agarwal M, Patel B, Shah M, et al. Abstract 19490: National trends in diagnostic right heart catheterization in the United States. *Circulation*. 2017;136:A19490.
22. Levine GN, Bates ER, Blankenship JC, et al. 2011 ACCF/AHA/SCAI Guideline for Percutaneous Coronary Intervention. A report of the American College of Cardiology Foundation/American Heart Association Task Force on Practice Guidelines and the Society for Cardiovascular Angiography and Interventions. *J Am Coll Cardiol*. 2011;58(24):e44–122.
23. Sorajja P, Borlaug BA, Dimas VV, et al. SCAI/HFSA clinical expert consensus document on the use of invasive hemodynamics for the diagnosis and management of cardiovascular disease. *Catheter Cardiovasc Interv*. 2017;89(7):E233–E247.
24. Yancy CW, Jessup M, Bozkurt B, et al. 2013 ACCF/AHA guideline for the management of heart failure: A report of the American College of Cardiology Foundation/American Heart Association Task Force on Practice Guidelines. *J Am Coll Cardiol*. 2013;62(16):e147–e239.
25. Fihn SD, Blankenship JC, Alexander KP, et al. 2014 ACC/AHA/AATS/PCNA/SCAI/STS focused update of the guideline for the diagnosis and management of patients with stable ischemic heart disease: a report of the American College of Cardiology/American Heart Association Task Force on Practice Guidelines, and the American Association for Thoracic Surgery, Preventive Cardiovascular Nurses Association, Society for Cardiovascular Angiography and Interventions, and Society of Thoracic Surgeons. *J Am Coll Cardiol*. 2014;64(18):1929–1949.
26. Amsterdam EA, Wenger NK, Brindis RG, et al. 2014 AHA/ACC guideline for the management of patients with non-ST-elevation acute coronary syndromes: executive summary: a report of the American College of Cardiology/American Heart Association Task Force on Practice Guidelines. *Circulation*. 2014;130(25):2354–2394.
27. Patel MR, Calhoon JH, Dehmer GJ, et al. ACC/AATS/AHA/ASE/ASNC/SCAI/SCCT/STS 2017 Appropriate Use Criteria for Coronary Revascularization in patients with stable ischemic heart disease: A Report of the American College of Cardiology Appropriate Use Criteria Task Force, American Association for Thoracic Surgery, American Heart Association, American Society of Echocardiography, American Society of Nuclear Cardiology, Society for Cardiovascular Angiography and Interventions, Society of Cardiovascular Computed Tomography, and Society of Thoracic Surgeons. *J Nucl Cardiol*. 2017;24(5):1759–1792.
28. Grossman W. *Grossman and Baim's Cardiac Catheterization, Angiography, and Interventions*. 8th ed. Philadelphia, PA: Lippincott Williams & Wilkins; 2013.
29. Brockow K, Sánchez-Borges M. Hypersensitivity to contrast media and dyes. *Immunol Allergy Clin North Am*. 2014;34(3):547–564, viii.
30. Pisters R, Lane DA, Nieuwlaat R. A novel user-friendly score (HAS-BLED) to assess 1-year risk of major bleeding in patients with atrial fibrillation: the Euro Heart Survey. *Chest*. 2010;138(5):1093–1100.
31. Doherty JU, Gluckman TJ, Hucker WJ, et al. 2017 ACC Expert consensus decision pathway for periprocedural management of anticoagulation in patients with nonvalvular atrial fibrillation: A report of the American College of cardiology clinical expert consensus document task force. *J Am Coll Cardiol*. 2017;69(7):871–898.
32. Douketis JD, Spyropoulos AC, Kaatz S, et al. Perioperative bridging anticoagulation in patients with atrial fibrillation. *N Engl J Med*. 2015;373(9):823–833.
33. Baron TH, Kamath PS, McBane RD. Management of antithrombotic therapy in patients undergoing invasive procedures. *N Engl J Med*. 2013;368(22):2113–2124.
34. Brockow K, Christiansen C, Kanny G, et al. Management of hypersensitivity reactions to iodinated contrast media. *Allergy*. 2005;60(2):150–158.
35. Schabelman E, Witting M. The relationship of radiocontrast, iodine, and seafood allergies: a medical myth exposed. *J Emerg Med*. 39(5):701–707.
36. Beckett KR, Moriarity AK, Langer JM. Safe use of contrast media: what the radiologist needs to know. *Radiographics*. 2015;35(6):1738–1750.
37. Tsai TT, Patel UD, Chang TI, et al. Validated contemporary risk model of acute kidney injury in patients undergoing percutaneous coronary interventions: insights from the National Cardiovascular Data Registry Cath-PCI Registry. *J Am Heart Assoc*. 2014;3(6):e001380.
38. Tavakol M, Ashraf S, Brener SJ. Risks and complications of coronary angiography: a comprehensive review. *Glob J Health Sci*. 2012;4(1):65–93.
39. Hafiz AM, Jan MF, Mori N, et al. Prevention of contrast-induced acute kidney injury in patients with stable chronic renal disease undergoing elective percutaneous coronary and peripheral interventions: randomized comparison of two preventive strategies. *Catheter Cardiovasc Interv*. 2012;79(6):929–937.
40. Mehran R, Aymong ED, Nikolsky E, et al. A simple risk score for prediction of contrast-induced nephropathy after percutaneous coronary intervention: development and initial validation. *J Am Coll Cardiol*. 2004;44(7):1393–1399.
41. Hirshfeld JW, Ferrari VA, Bengel FM, et al. 2018 ACC/HRS/NASCI/SCAI/SCCT Expert consensus document on optimal use of ionizing radiation in cardiovascular imaging: best practices for safety and effectiveness: A report of the American College of Cardiology Task Force on expert consensus decision pathways. *J Am Coll Cardiol*. 2018;71(24):e283–e351.
42. Barrett BJ, Parfrey PS, Vavasour HM, et al. A comparison of nonionic, low-osmolality radiocontrast agents with ionic, high-osmolality agents during cardiac catheterization. *N Engl J Med*. 1992;326(7):431–436.
43. Hirshfeld JW. Cardiovascular effects of iodinated contrast agents. *Am J Cardiol*. 1990;66(14):9F–17F.
44. Kiemeneij F, Laarman GJ, Odekerken D, et al. A randomized comparison of percutaneous transluminal coronary angioplasty by the radial, brachial and femoral approaches: The access study. *J Am Coll Cardiol*. 1997;29(6):1269–1275.
45. Hamon M, Pristipino C, Di Mario C, et al. Consensus document on the radial approach in percutaneous cardiovascular interventions: Position paper by the European Association of Percutaneous Cardiovascular Interventions and Working Groups on Acute Cardiac Care and Thrombosis of the European Society of Cardiology. *EuroIntervention*. 2013;8(11):1242–1251.
46. Mason PJ, Shah B, Tamis-Holland JE, et al; American Heart Association Interventional Cardiovascular Care Committee of the Council on Clinical Cardiology; Council on Cardiovascular and Stroke Nursing; Council on Peripheral Vascular Disease; and Council on Genomic and Precision Medicine. An update on radial artery access and best practices for transradial coronary angiography and intervention in acute coronary syndrome: a scientific statement from the American Heart Association. *Circ Cardiovasc Interv*. 2018;11(9):e000035.
47. Pancholy SB, Bertrand OF, Patel T. Comparison of a priori versus provisional heparin therapy on radial artery occlusion after transradial coronary angiography and patent hemostasis (from the PHARAOH Study). *Am J Cardiol*. 2012;110(2):173–176.
48. Moscucci M, Hendel R. *Grossman and Baim's Cardiac Catheterization, Angiography, and Interventions*. 8th ed. Philadelphia, PA: Lippincott Williams & Wilkins; 2013.

49. Wilson RF. Assessing the severity of coronary-artery stenoses. *N Engl J Med.* 1996;334(26):1735–1737.
50. Pijls NH, De Bruyne B, Peels K, et al. Measurement of fractional flow reserve to assess the functional severity of coronary-artery stenoses. *N Engl J Med.* 1996;334(26):1703–1708.
51. Lotfi A, Jeremias A, Fearon WF, et al. Expert consensus statement on the use of fractional flow reserve, intravascular ultrasound, and optical coherence tomography: A consensus statement of the Society of Cardiovascular Angiography and Interventions. *Catheter Cardiovasc Interv.* 2014;83(4):509–518.
52. Martinez C, Moscucci M. *Grossman and Baim's Cardiac Catheterization, Angiography, and Interventions.* 8th ed. Philadelphia, PA: Lippincott Williams & Wilkins; 2013.
53. Melikian N, De Bondt P, Tonino P, et al. Fractional flow reserve and myocardial perfusion imaging in patients with angiographic multivessel coronary artery disease. *JACC Cardiovasc Interv.* 2010;3(3):307–314.
54. Fifer MA, Douglas JS. *Measurement of Ventricular Volumes, Ejection Fraction, Mass, Wall Stress, and Regional Wall Motion.* 7th ed. Philadelphia, PA: Lippincott Williams & Wilkins; 2006.
55. Ragosta M. *Textbook of Clinical Hemodynamics.* Philadelphia, PA: Saunders/Elsivier; 2008.
56. Grossman W, Moscucci M. *Grossman and Baim's Cardiac Catheterization, Angiography, and Interventions.* 8th ed. Philadelphia, PA: Lippincott Williams & Wilkins; 2013.
57. Doyle BJ, Ting HH, Bell MR, et al. Major femoral bleeding complications after percutaneous coronary intervention: incidence, predictors, and impact on long-term survival among 17,901 patients treated at the Mayo Clinic from 1994 to 2005. *JACC Cardiovasc Interv.* 2008;1(2): 202–209.
58. Rao SV, Ou FS, Wang TY, et al. Trends in the prevalence and outcomes of radial and femoral approaches to percutaneous coronary intervention: A report from the National Cardiovascular Data Registry. *JACC Cardiovas Interv.* 2008;1(4):379–386.
59. Landau C, Lange RA, Glamann DB, et al. Vasovagal reactions in the cardiac catheterization laboratory. *Am J Cardiol.* 1994;73(1):95–97.
60. Dukkipati S, O'Neill WW, Harjai KJ, et al. Characteristics of cerebrovascular accidents after percutaneous coronary interventions. *J Am Coll Cardiol.* 2004;43(7):1161–1167.
61. Khatri P, Kasner SE. Ischemic strokes after cardiac catheterization: opportune thrombolysis candidates? *Arch Neurol.* 2006;63(6): 817–821.
62. Werner N, Zahn R, Zeymer U. Stroke in patients undergoing coronary angiography and percutaneous coronary intervention: incidence, predictors, outcome and therapeutic options. *Expert Rev Cardiovasc Ther.* 2012;10(10): 1297–1305.
63. Berkhemer OA, Fransen PS, Beumer D, et al. A randomized trial of intraarterial treatment for acute ischemic stroke. *N Engl J Med.* 2015;372(1):11–20.

17 Hemodynamic Monitoring

Tao Zheng

OBJECTIVES

1. Review physiologic concepts, parameters, and technologies of hemodynamic monitoring.
2. Identify elements and rationales of invasive and noninvasive hemodynamic monitoring.
3. Compare different modalities in hemodynamic monitoring across the continuum, the evidence of their use, and how they translate into practice.
4. Examine the most commonly used hemodynamic monitoring technologies, what may be used in the future, and how they could be used in different clinical areas.

KEY QUESTIONS

1. What is new in hemodynamic monitoring technologies?
2. What are the evidences validating the reliability of noninvasive hemodynamic monitoring technologies?
3. What else can you use to evaluate hemodynamic status if you do not have the technologies?
4. How can you use the hemodynamic technologies in clinical practice to optimize patient outcomes?

BACKGROUND

Hemodynamic monitoring provides physiologic indicators of cardiovascular function, including factors that affect cardiac performance: preload, afterload, contractility, heart rate (HR), and the relationship between oxygen supply and demand.[1] Invasive and noninvasive hemodynamic monitoring is used to evaluate cardiovascular performance in critically ill patients. Invasive intravascular catheterization is common in intensive care units (ICUs): Arterial catheterization enables frequent blood sampling and real-time monitoring of blood pressure (BP). A central venous catheter (CVC) can be used to augment hemodynamic monitoring (e.g., determination of central venous oxygenation), administer vasoactive medications, and provide venous access. In the United States, 15 million CVC days occur in the ICUs each year.[2] In an observational cohort study on intravascular catheterization in adult ICUs, Gershengorn et al.[3] found that use of arterial catheterization remained constant and use of CVCs increased. However, less invasive hemodynamic monitoring technology continues to develop and evolve.[4] Hemodynamic monitoring may be utilized across the continuum to guide therapeutic interventions.

This chapter (1) reviews technologies for invasive hemodynamic monitoring, including arterial BP monitoring, central venous pressure (CVP)/pulmonary artery (PA) catheterization, and cardiac output (CO) and mixed venous oxygen (SvO_2) monitoring and (2) discusses the current practice standard and recommendations for the effective use of invasive hemodynamic monitoring and functional hemodynamics. Newer technologies for less invasive hemodynamic evaluation (e.g., bioreactance technology and noninvasive finger cuff), tissue perfusion monitoring, and implantable PA monitoring are also introduced.

PHYSIOLOGIC PRINCIPLES OF HEMODYNAMIC MONITORING

Hemodynamic monitoring includes two major components: the measurement of blood flow and the pressure dynamics based on the cardiac cycle and circulatory physiologic principles. In his publication "de Motu Cordis," English physician William Harvey was the first to describe that the human heart functions as a central pump to circulate blood continuously from arteries and veins.[5]

Cardiac Cycle and Electrocardiogram

Cardiac cycle describes the blood flow through the heart during each cardiac contraction: one complete sequence of cardiac filling, cardiac muscle excitation and contraction with ejection of blood (systole), and then cardiac muscle relaxation (diastole).[6] To understand pressure waveforms of the cardiac cycle, one must know how electrical and mechanical activities of the heart are related. Therefore, it is important to observe the ECG and corresponding hemodynamic pressure tracing.[7,8]

Contraction of the atria follows atrial depolarization, represented by the P wave on the ECG. Atrial contraction results in an increase in pressure within each atrial chamber. On the right side of the heart, the atrial pressure is represented as CVP or right atrial pressure (RAP) waveform. On the left side of the heart, left atrial pressure (LAP) is represented by the pulmonary artery occlusion pressure (PAOP) or pulmonary artery wedge pressure (PAWP) waveforms.[7,8]

The maximum atrial pressure immediately prior to the opening of the atrioventricular (AV) valves generates a rise on atrial pressure waveforms. As the AV valves open, the blood leaves the atria, resulting in a rapid drop in atrial pressure.[7,8]

The isoelectric PR interval on the ECG corresponds to closure of the AV valves (mitral and tricuspid). The AV valve closure signifies the end of diastole, and the blood volume within each ventricle just before the closure of AV valve is known as end-diastolic volume (EDV), or preload.[7,8]

After ventricular depolarization, ventricular systole (QRS complex on the ECG) results in a rise in pressure without a change in the volume within the ventricles, a phase known as isovolumetric contraction. During ventricular systole, blood is ejected at high speed and pressure from the left ventricle (LV) into the aorta, and simultaneously from the right ventricle (RV) into the PA. The outflow of blood from the LV is registered as an arterial pressure (AP) waveform.[7,8]

After ventricular repolarization, ventricular diastole (T wave on the ECG) takes place.[7,8] When ventricular chamber pressure falls below the pressures in greater vessels, the semilunar valves (aortic and pulmonary) are forced to close by backflow of blood into the aorta. Semilunar valve closure is associated with a dicrotic notch (incisura) in the AP and pulmonary artery pressure (PAP) waveforms—graphically a notch on the downward arch of the waveform. The dicrotic notch on the AP waveform signifies the closure of the aortic valve and on the PAP waveform represents the closure of the pulmonic valve.[7,8]

TECHNICAL ASPECTS OF INVASIVE PRESSURE MONITORING

Referencing

There are three components in invasive pressure measurement: dynamic BP, hydrostatic pressure, and static pressure. Having the accurate reference point ensures the accuracy of various pressure readings, which provide clinicians accurate hemodynamic assessment. The reference point for all invasive cardiovascular pressure monitoring is to the level of the heart, rather than the catheter tip or the insertion site.[9–11] The phlebostatic axis/phlebostatic level is the most commonly used as a reference point when taking hemodynamic measurement. The phlebostatic axis is aligned to the level of mid-right atrium (RA) and left atrium (LA). Anatomically, the phlebostatic axis is located at the fourth intercostal space, midpoint of the anterior–posterior diameter. The midaxillary line (MAL) can be used as a valid reference level to the RA and the LA for patients with normal chest wall configuration. Varied chest configuration may result in a pressure difference of up to 6 mm.[1]

Zeroing

Offset can be caused by hydrostatic pressure, pressure transducer, amplifier, oscilloscope, recorder, or digital delay. To compensate these offsets, zeroing must be performed to achieve the goal of calibrating the pressure system to the local atmospheric pressure. To zero the transducer, the hemodynamic system is off to the patient and opened to air, and atmospheric pressure is established as "zero."[1] As the condition of atmospheric pressure fluctuates with weather conditions, using the current atmospheric pressure as the reference point of "zero" for the pressure system provides a standardized baseline to attaining accurate pressure measurement.[12]

Transducer Setup

Transducer setup is required to measure the hemodynamic waveform. One transducer may be used if only AP is obtained. Two additional transducers can be used when measuring both RA and PA waveforms: the proximal port (RA) and distal port (PA) are connected separately to the transducers using saline-flushed, noncompliant tubing. Triple transducer sets can be used if AP, CVP, and PAP are measured. Tubing patency is maintained with a 500-mL normal saline bag enclosed by an inflated pressure bag which delivers approximately 3-mL normal saline per hour. 250- to 300-mm Hg pressure is recommended to ensure pressure measurement accuracy.[13]

Patient Position for Pressure Measurement

Hemodynamic pressures may be accurately obtained with the patient's head of bed elevated up to 60 degrees while patient's legs are parallel to the floor.[1] Other acceptable patient positions while obtaining hemodynamic measurement include the patient in 20-, 30-, or 90-degree lateral position with head of bed at 0 degrees or with the patient prone. Patient's stabilization after position change will ensure accurate measurements: 5 to 15 minutes is recommended, and 30 to 60 minutes with prone.[14] Prone position does not induce any significant clinical differences in measurements of PAP, CVP, or CO when adequate time is allowed for stabilization.[15] In a prospective observational study published in 2015, Jacq et al.[16] evaluated the effects on measured values of various combinations of transducer level, catheter access site, and patient positions. There were statistical and clinically significant overestimations in several modalities used for zeroing and/or transducer leveling in invasive AP measurement. The values obtained when patient's head of bed was elevated to 45 degrees, and the zero-reference point was aligned to the phlebostatic axis, were not significantly different from those taken in supine position and used the same reference point (Fig. 17-1).

Square Wave Test

To ensure that hemodynamic equipment produces an accurate and reliable pressure waveform, a square wave test (also known as a fast flush or dynamic response test) can be performed on initial setup, once at the beginning of the shift or anytime when there is disturbance to the system (e.g., zeroing, a change of fluid in the pressure system, a change of tubing, or obtaining a blood sample).[14] To perform a square wave test, pull and release the pigtail of the pressure system or squeeze the bottom of the flush device. By doing so, the flow through the tubing is increased which creates a sudden rise in the pressure system. The sudden risen pressure in the system produces a square wave on the monitor oscilloscope.[17] Two possible waveforms produced by doing square wave tests will signify inaccurate hemodynamic measurements: one is an underdamped waveform, and the other is an overdamped waveform (Fig. 17-2).

An overdamped waveform is described as sluggish, with an exaggerated or falsely widened and blunt tracing. With an overdamped waveform, the patient's systolic blood pressure (SBP) is recorded falsely low and diastolic blood pressure (DBP) is recorded

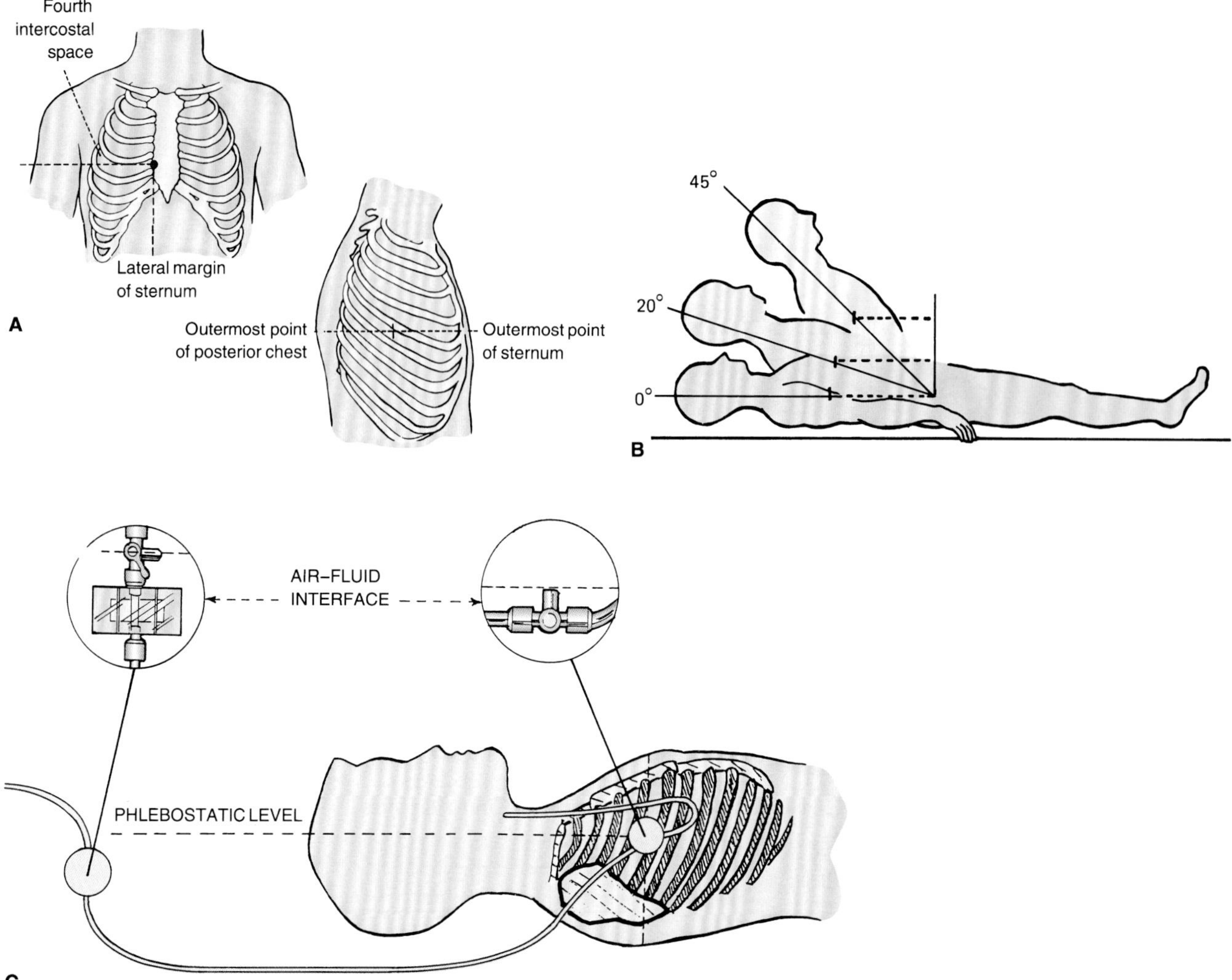

Figure 17-1. The Phlebostatic Axis and the Phlebostatic Level. (**A**) The *phlebostatic axis* is the intersection of two reference lines: first, an imaginary line from the fourth ICS at the point where it joins the sternum, drawn out to the side of the body; second, a line drawn *midway* between the anterior and posterior surfaces of the chest. (**B**) The phlebostatic level is a horizontal line through the phlebostatic axis. The air–fluid interface of the stopcock of the transducer must be level with this axis for accurate measurements. Moving from the flat to erect positions, the patient moves the chest and therefore the reference level; the phlebostatic level stays horizontal through the same reference point. (Adapted from Shinn JA, Woods SL, Huseby JS. Effect of intermittent positive pressure ventilation upon pulmonary capillary wedge pressures in acutely ill patients. *Heart Lung*. 1979;8:324.) (**C**) Two methods for referencing the pressure system to the phlebostatic axis. The system can be referenced by placing the air–fluid interface of either the in-line stopcock or the stopcock on top of the transducer at the phlebostatic level. (From Bridges EJ, Woods SL. Pulmonary artery pressure measurement: state of the art. *Heart Lung*. 1993;22:101.)

falsely high. An underdamped waveform is an overresponded tracing, which can be seen as exaggerated, narrow, artificially peak characteristics. With an underdamped waveform, the patient's SBP is estimated falsely high and DBP is estimated falsely low.[18]

It is essential for clinicians to identify waveform characteristics before taking pressure measurement. In addition, priming the tubing adequately to remove microbubbles during system setup will result in an "adequate" or "optimal" pressure system.[18] It is suggested that using a damping device may improve dynamic response of the system to eliminate the adverse effects from a blood conservation device or a needless access port (Fig. 17-3).[19,20]

Relation of Intracardiac Pressure Measurement to ECG

Intracardiac pressure changes are associated with mechanical events initiated by electronic stimuli during the cardiac cycle. In other words, it is important to observe the ECG when taking hemodynamic measurement. While automated continuous monitoring of CVP and PAP is possible, American Association of Critical Care Nurses (AACN) recommends that the clinician manually measures the parameter by simultaneously capturing the ECG and hemodynamic waveform, as this technique correlates the electrical events with the mechanical events during systole and diastole to allow for accurate

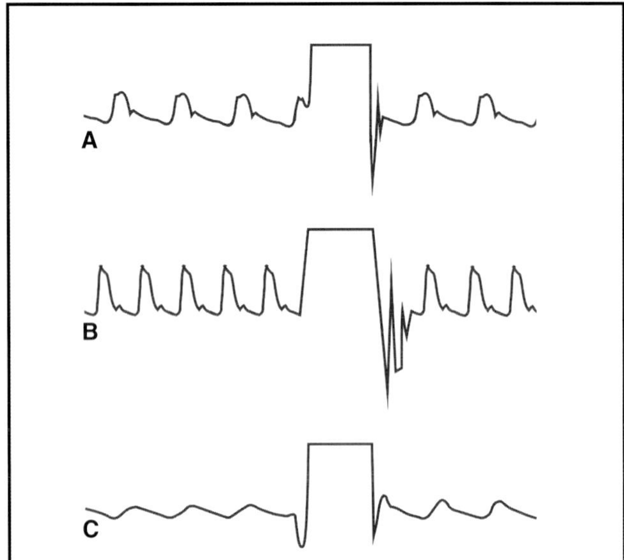

Figure 17-2. Square Wave Test. (**A**) Optimal waveform. (**B**) Underdamped waveform. (**C**) Overdamped waveform. (Created by T. Eric Goffrier.)

measurement.[14] Interpretation of these associations on hemodynamic waveforms will be further discussed later in this chapter.

Blood Sampling and Infection Control

Blood samples such as arterial blood gases, serum electrolytes, and coagulation studies can be drawn from an arterial line. To avoid contamination of the specimen with flushes (such as saline and/or heparin), a blood sample of two times the dead-space volume should be discarded (volume from the catheter tip to the aspiration site).[21] The discard volume includes dead space and the blood diluted by the flush solution (e.g., dead space of 0.5 mL equals to 1 mL discard). For coagulation studies (particularly activated partial thromboplastin time) from a heparinized arterial line, the discard volume should be six times the dead-space volume.[21] If an in-line blood conservation set is used, caution must be exercised to ensure that an adequate discard volume is obtained. If heparin is used in the flush solution and the coagulation results are abnormal, the critical care clinician should consider using a venipuncture specimen to confirm the results.[1]

Blood samples can also be obtained from the CVC hemodynamic monitoring system and PAC. It is important to determine

Decision-Making Algorithm

How to Assess Dynamic Response Characteristics

1. Determine Natural Frequency of System (Fn)
   a. Fast Flush System and Record Strip
   b. Measure period (t) of one cycle
   c. Fn = Paper speed (mm/s)/one cycle (mm)
2. Determine Amplitude Ratio
   Compare the amplitude of two successive peaks (A2/A1)
3. Plot Amplitude Ratio Against Natural Frequency
   -Apply algorithm if system other than OPTIMAL or ADEQUATE

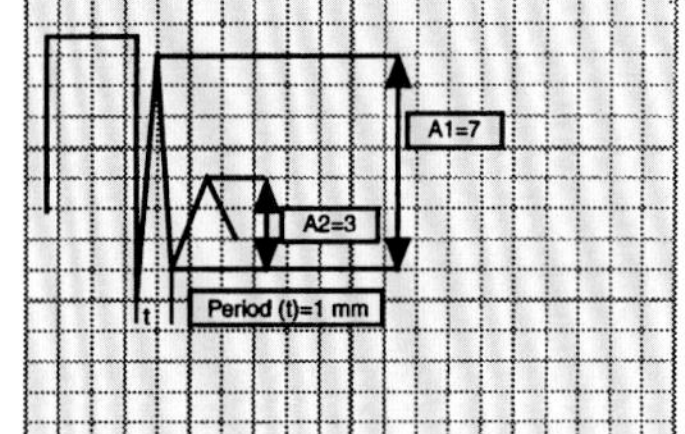

Example:
1) Determine Fn
Paper Speed = 25 mm/s
t = 1 mm
Fn = 25/1 = 25 cycles/s
2) Determine Amplitude
A2/A1 = 3/7 = 0.43
3) Plot on Graph = ADEQUATE

Frequency Versus Amplitude Ratio Plot

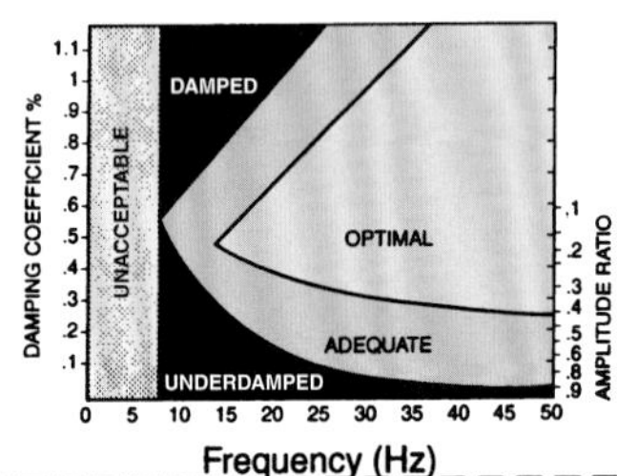

Frequency versus damping coefficient plot that illustrates the five areas into which the catheter, tubing, and transducer systems fall. Systems in the optimal area reproduce even the most demanding (fast heart rate and rapid systolic upstroke) waveforms without distortion. Systems in the adequate area reproduce the most typical waveforms with little or no distortion. All other areas cause serious wave distortion. (Gardner RM, Hollingsworth KW. Optimizing the electrocardiogram and pressure monitoring. *Crit Care Med.* 1986;14:651–658, with permission.)

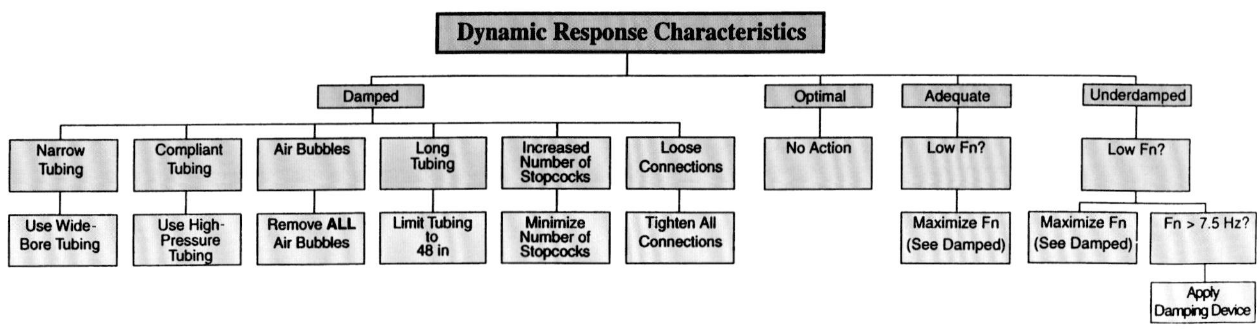

Figure 17-3. Dynamic Response Characteristics. (Adapted with permission from Bridges EJ, Middleton R. Direct arterial vs oscillometric monitoring of blood pressure: stop comparing and pick one [a decision-making algorithm]. *Crit Care Nurse.* 1997;17[3]:58–72.)

whether intravenous solutions or medications are being infused through the CVC, because these solutions and medications must be temporarily paused. Alternative blood access site needs to be considered if critical infusion (i.e., vasoactive mediations) is required for the patient. When using CVC or PAC for blood sampling, the discard volume should include the dead space (from the tip of the distal lumen to the top port of the stopcock) and the blood diluted by the flush solution.[21]

Catheter-related bloodstream infection (CRBSI) and central line–associated bloodstream infection (CLABSI) are often used interchangeably even though the meanings differ. CRBSI requires specific laboratory testing that more thoroughly identifies the catheter as the source of the bloodstream infection (BSI). A CLABSI is a primary BSI in a patient that had a central line within the 48-hour period before the development of the BSI and is not bloodstream related to an infection at another site.[22] CRBSIs independently increase hospital costs and length of stay but have not generally been shown to independently increase mortality. In the United States, a total of 80,000 CRBSIs have been estimated to occur in ICUs each year. Nontunneled CVCs account for the majority of CRBSIs. PACs have similar rates of bloodstream infection as CVCs.[2] Arterial catheter sites are a source of BSIs. It has been estimated that up to 50,000 BSIs per year arise from arterial catheters in the United States alone.[23]

To improve patient outcome and reduce healthcare costs, an effort should be made to reduce the incidence of CRBSI by multidisciplinary team, involving healthcare professionals who order the insertion and removal of CVCs, those personnel who insert and/or maintain intravascular catheters, infection control personnel, healthcare managers including the chief executive officer and those who allocate resources, and patients who are capable of assisting in the care of their catheters.[2] When a CVC is used for pressure measurement, the pressure transducers may become colonized. Septic complications of PACs have been documented in many studies since the early 1970s.[28] In 2011, the Centers for Disease Control and Prevention (CDC) and Healthcare Infection Control Practices Advisory Committee published guidelines for the prevention of intravascular catheter-related infections. These guidelines are intended to provide evidence-based recommendations for healthcare personnel who insert intravascular catheters and for clinicians responsible for surveillance and control of infections in hospital, outpatient, and home healthcare settings.[24] Table 17-1 provides a summary of guidelines on CRBSI prevention for arterial catheterization and CVCs. As these guidelines are often updated and revised, refer to the CDC website for the most current practice recommendations.

INVASIVE BLOOD PRESSURE MONITORING

Indications

With approximately eight million arterial catheters placed yearly in the United States, arterial catheterization is one of the most commonly performed invasive procedures in the ICUs.[25] Arterial catheterization provides vascular access for repetitive blood sampling. In addition, arterial catheterization is the standard for BP monitoring, considered the most accurate measurement of BP compared to other techniques. The primary indication of arterial catheterization is to provide continual, real-time monitoring of the rapidly changing BP and CO in hemodynamic unstable patients.[26] Examples of other clinical indications for direct AP monitoring include hypertensive crisis, hypotension, shock state, frequent drawing of arterial blood samples, monitoring of vasoactive pharmacologic support, and during aggressive respiratory support such as high positive end-expiratory pressure (PEEP).

Arterial Site Selection for Catheter Placement

An arterial catheter can be inserted via a number of arteries, including radial, femoral, axillary, ulnar, brachial, dorsalis pedis, posterior tibial, and temporal arteries.[27] Important considerations in site selection for arterial catheters include patient comfort, ability to secure the catheter, and maintenance of asepsis as well as patient-specific factors (e.g., pre-existing catheters, anatomic deformity, bleeding diathesis), relative risk of mechanical complications (e.g., bleeding, pneumothorax), the availability of bedside ultrasound, the experience of the person inserting the catheter, and the risk for infection. The radial artery has been identified as the most commonly used approach, due to the presence of collateral circulation, which decreases the risk of vascular complications. The second most commonly used arterial site is the femoral artery.[28] Radial and femoral arteries are preferred over others because these two arteries are easily compressible in the case of bleeding complications.[27] Due to a lower infection rate, the radial artery is preferred over the femoral artery.[28] In addition, the ulnar artery provides secondary arterial blood supply to the hand which reduces the risk of ischemia.[12] The femoral artery is often used as an alternative for arterial catheterization. However, an increased risk of infection is associated with the femoral site. The most common complications of radial artery cannulation and femoral artery cannulation are provided in Table 17-2.

The brachial artery is used less frequently due to a lack of good collateral circulation, resulting in an increased risk for diffuse distal ischemia. The axillary artery is a less common insertion site, with complication rates similar to radial and femoral insertions. The dorsalis pedis artery is another option. Complication rates associated with the dorsalis pedis artery are comparable to radial artery insertion. The dorsalis pedis should not be used if the patient has peripheral vascular disease or an absent posterior tibial pulse. In addition, the dorsalis pedis artery pressures are higher than radial pressures, even in the supine position.

Allen Test

The Allen test was first described in 1929 by Dr. Edgar Van Nuys Allen, then modified by Dr. Irving S. Wright in the 1950s. Collateral blood flow to the hand is assessed by using the modified Allen test before an arterial catheter is inserted in the radial artery. The Allen test is most often used clinically to evaluate the baseline of collateral circulation; however, the evidence to support whether this predicts hand ischemia is equivocal.[29] Ruengsakulrach et al.[31] evaluated the sensitivity and specificity of the modified Allen test as compared to Doppler ultrasonography of the thumb artery in 71 patients. Sensitivity and specificity of the modified Allen test were 100% and 97%, respectively. Other studies have provided limited support that the modified Allen test predicts hand ischemia, which is the major argument against its routine use (Fig. 17-4).[29,30]

Complications Related to Arterial Catheterization

The most common complication, temporary occlusion of the artery, occurred 19.7% in radial artery access, and 1.5% in femoral artery access. In comparison, the incidences of

Table 17-1 • CRBSI CONTROL

Category	Recommendations	Level of Evidence
Education, training, and staffing	Educate healthcare personnel regarding the indications for intravascular catheter use, proper procedures for the insertion and maintenance of intravascular catheters, and appropriate infection control measures to prevent intravascular catheter-related infections.	1A
	Periodically assess knowledge of and adherence to guidelines for all personnel involved in the insertion and maintenance of intravascular catheters.	1A
	Designate only trained personnel who demonstrate competence for the insertion and maintenance of peripheral and central intravascular catheters.	1A
	Ensure appropriate nursing staff levels in ICUs. Observational studies suggest that a higher proportion of "pool nurses" or an elevated patient-to-nurse ratio is associated with CRBSI in ICUs where nurses are managing patients with CVCs.	1B
CVC	Weigh the risks and benefits of placing a central venous device at a recommended site to reduce infectious complications against the risk for mechanical complications (e.g., pneumothorax, subclavian artery puncture, subclavian vein laceration, subclavian vein stenosis, hemothorax, thrombosis, air embolism, and catheter misplacement).	1A
	Avoid using the femoral vein for central venous access in adult patients.	1A
	Use a subclavian site, rather than a jugular or a femoral site, in adult patients to minimize infection risk for nontunneled CVC placement.	1B
	Use ultrasound guidance to place central venous catheters (if this technology is available) to reduce the number of cannulation attempts and mechanical complications. Ultrasound guidance should only be used by those fully trained in its technique.	1B
	Use a CVC with the minimum number of ports or lumens essential for the management of the patient.	1B
	Promptly remove any intravascular catheter that is no longer essential.	1A
	When adherence to aseptic technique cannot be ensured (i.e., catheters inserted during a medical emergency), replace the catheter as soon as possible, that is, within 48 hours.	1B
Hand hygiene and aseptic techniques	Perform hand hygiene procedures, either by washing hands with conventional soap and water or with alcohol-based hand rubs (ABHRs). Hand hygiene should be performed before and after palpating catheter insertion sites as well as before and after inserting, replacing, accessing, repairing, or dressing an intravascular catheter. Palpation of the insertion site should not be performed after the application of antiseptic, unless aseptic technique is maintained.	1B
	Maintain aseptic technique for the insertion and care of intravascular catheters.	1B
	Wear clean gloves, rather than sterile gloves, for the insertion of peripheral intravascular catheters, if the access site is not touched after the application of skin antiseptics.	1C
	Sterile gloves should be worn for the insertion of arterial, central, and midline catheters.	1A
	Use new sterile gloves before handling the new catheter when guidewire exchanges are performed.	II
	Wear either clean or sterile gloves when changing the dressing on intravascular catheters.	1C
Maximal sterile barrier precaution	Use maximal sterile barrier precautions, including the use of a cap, mask, sterile gown, sterile gloves, and a sterile full-body drape, for the insertion of CVCs, PICCs, or guidewire exchange.	1B
	Use a sterile sleeve to protect pulmonary artery catheters during insertion.	1B
Skin preparation	Prepare clean skin with an antiseptic (70% alcohol, tincture of iodine, or alcoholic chlorhexidine gluconate solution) before peripheral venous catheter insertion.	1B
	Prepare clean skin with a >0.5% chlorhexidine preparation with alcohol before central venous catheter and peripheral arterial catheter insertion and during dressing changes. If there is a contraindication to chlorhexidine, tincture of iodine, an iodophor, or 70% alcohol can be used as alternatives.	1A
	No comparison has been made between using chlorhexidine preparations with alcohol and povidone-iodine in alcohol to prepare clean skin. Unresolved issue.	
	Antiseptics should be allowed to dry according to the manufacturer's recommendation prior to placing the catheter.	1B
Catheter site dressing regimens	Use either sterile gauze or sterile, transparent, semipermeable dressing to cover the catheter site.	1A
	If the patient is diaphoretic or if the site is bleeding or oozing, use a gauze dressing until this is resolved.	II
	Replace catheter site dressing if the dressing becomes damp, loosened, or visibly soiled.	2B
	Do not use topical antibiotic ointment or creams on insertion sites, except for dialysis catheters, because of their potential to promote fungal infections and antimicrobial resistance.	1B
	Do not submerge the catheter or catheter site in water. Showering should be permitted if precautions can be taken to reduce the likelihood of introducing organisms into the catheter (e.g., if the catheter and connecting device are protected with an impermeable cover during the shower).	1B
	Replace dressings used on short-term CVC sites every 2 days for gauze dressings.	II
	Replace dressings used on short-term CVC sites at least every 7 days for transparent dressings, except in those pediatric patients in which the risk for dislodging the catheter may outweigh the benefit of changing the dressing.	1B
	Ensure that catheter site care is compatible with the catheter material.	1B
	Use a sterile sleeve for all pulmonary artery catheters.	1B
	No recommendation is made for other types of chlorhexidine dressings. Unresolved issue.	
	Monitor the catheter sites visually when changing the dressing or by palpation through an intact dressing on a regular basis, depending on the clinical situation of the individual patient. If patients have tenderness at the insertion site, fever without obvious source, or other manifestations suggesting local or bloodstream infection, the dressing should be removed to allow thorough examination of the site.	1B
	Encourage patients to report any changes in their catheter site or any new discomfort to their provider.	II

Table 17-1 • CRBSI CONTROL (*Continued*)

Category	Recommendations	Level of Evidence
Patient cleaning	Use a 2% chlorhexidine wash for daily skin cleansing to reduce CRBSI.	II
Catheter securement devices	Use a sutureless securement device to reduce the risk of infection for intravascular catheters.	II
Replacement of catheters	Do not routinely replace CVCs or pulmonary artery catheters to prevent catheter-related infections.	1B
	Do not remove CVCs on the basis of fever alone. Use clinical judgment regarding the appropriateness of removing the catheter if infection is evidenced elsewhere or if a noninfectious cause of fever is suspected.	II
	Do not use guidewire exchanges routinely for nontunneled catheters to prevent infection.	1B
	Do not use guidewire exchanges to replace a nontunneled catheter suspected of infection.	1B
	Use a guidewire exchange to replace a malfunctioning nontunneled catheter if no evidence of infection is present.	1B
	Use new sterile gloves before handling the new catheter when guidewire exchanges are performed.	II
Peripheral arterial catheters and pressure monitoring devices	In adults, use of the radial, brachial, or dorsalis pedis sites is preferred over the femoral or axillary sites of insertion to reduce the risk of infection.	1B
	A minimum of a cap, mask, sterile gloves, and a small sterile fenestrated drape should be used during peripheral arterial catheter insertion.	1B
	During axillary or femoral artery catheter insertion, maximal sterile barrier precautions should be used.	II
	Replace arterial catheters only when there is a clinical indication.	II
	Remove the arterial catheter as soon as it is no longer needed.	II
	Use disposable, rather than reusable, transducer assemblies when possible.	IB
	Do not routinely replace arterial catheters to prevent catheter-related infections.	II
	Replace disposable or reusable transducers at 96-hour intervals. Replace other components of the system (including the tubing, continuous-flush device, and flush solution) at the time the transducer is replaced.	IB
	Keep all components of the pressure monitoring system (including calibration devices and flush solution) sterile.	IA
	Minimize the number of manipulations of and entries into the pressure monitoring system. Use a closed flush system (i.e., continuous flush), rather than an open system (i.e., one that requires a syringe and stopcock), to maintain the patency of the pressure monitoring catheters.	II
	When the pressure monitoring system is accessed through a diaphragm, rather than a stopcock, scrub the diaphragm with an appropriate antiseptic before accessing the system.	IA
	Do not administer dextrose-containing solutions or parenteral nutrition fluids through the pressure monitoring circuit.	1A
	Sterilize reusable transducers according to the manufacturers' instructions if the use of disposable transducers is not feasible.	1A
Replacement of administration sets	In patients not receiving blood, blood products, or fat emulsions, replace administration sets that are continuously used, including secondary sets and add-on devices, no more frequently than at 96-hour intervals, but at least every 7 days.	1A
	No recommendation can be made regarding the frequency for replacing intermittently used administration sets. Unresolved issue.	
	No recommendation can be made regarding the frequency for replacing needles to access implantable ports. Unresolved issue.	
	Replace tubing used to administer blood, blood products, or fat emulsions (those combined with amino acids and glucose in a 3-in-1 admixture or infused separately) within 24 hours of initiating the infusion.	1B
	Replace tubing used to administer propofol infusions every 6 or 12 hours, when the vial is changed, per the manufacturer's recommendation.	1A
	No recommendation can be made regarding the length of time a needle used to access implanted ports can remain in place. Unresolved issue.	
Needleless intravascular catheter system	Change the needleless components at least as frequently as the administration set. There is no benefit to changing these more frequently than every 72 hours.	II
	Change needleless connectors no more frequently than every 72 hours or according to manufacturers' recommendations for the purpose of reducing infection rates.	II
	Ensure that all components of the system are compatible to minimize leaks and breaks in the system.	II
	Minimize contamination risk by scrubbing the access port with an appropriate antiseptic (chlorhexidine, povidone-iodine, an iodophor, or 70% alcohol) and accessing the port only with sterile devices.	IA
	Use a needleless system to access IV tubing.	1C
	When needleless systems are used, a split septum valve may be preferred over some mechanical valves due to increased risk of infection with the mechanical valves.	II
Performance improvement	Use hospital-specific or collaborative-based performance improvement initiatives in which multifaceted strategies are "bundled" together to improve compliance with evidence-based recommended practices.	1B

The system for categorizing recommendations in these guidelines is as follows:
Category IA: Strongly recommended for implementation and strongly supported by well-designed experimental, clinical, or epidemiologic studies.
Category IB: Strongly recommended for implementation and supported by some experimental, clinical, or epidemiologic studies and a strong theoretical rationale; or an accepted practice (e.g., aseptic technique) supported by limited evidence.
Category IC: Required by state or federal regulations, rules, or standards.
Category II: Suggested for implementation and supported by suggestive clinical or epidemiologic studies or a theoretical rationale.

Table 17-2 • COMPLICATIONS OF ARTERIAL CANNULATION

Complications	Incidence
Arterial spasm	Radial > femoral
Arterial occlusion	Radial > femoral
Ischemia	Femoral > radial
Internal bleeding	Femoral > radial
Infection	Femoral > radial

Radial artery > femoral artery, more common in a radial artery cannulation.
Femoral artery > radial artery, more common in a femoral artery cannulation.

permanent occlusion of artery are rare (radial 0.09% and femoral 0.18%). Given the associated risks and potentially severe outcomes from arterial occlusion, routine assessment of arterial catheter insertion site is essential to promote early identification of complications. Distal perfusion should be part of the routine assessment, which should include skin color, temperature, and capillary refill, especially after catheter insertion and line manipulation (Table 17-3).

Arterial Pressure Wave

The initial upstroke reflects the increased pressure during the rapid ejection phase of the systole (the LV ejection). The upstroke of the arterial waveform is known as anacrotic limb, which is followed by anacrotic shoulder (a brief, peaked, sustained pressure). During systole, the volume of the blood that enters into the arterial system is greater than the volume that exits through the arterioles, corresponding to the peak pressure (systolic pressure). The dicrotic limb is defined as the downslope of the arterial waveform. At the end of systole, there is decreased pressure in both the aorta and the LV, and the downstroke of the pressure correlates with the decreased aortic pressure, during which there is a decreased ventricular ejection and the continued blood flow to the periphery. The downslope of the arterial waveform is interrupted by a visible sharp dicrotic notch (incisura), which results from an abrupt change of blood flow at the end of systole and right before the aortic valve closes. The downslope of arterial waveform is gradual because the pressure of the aorta continues to decrease until the next ventricular systole. The remainder of the waveform after the dicrotic notch is referred as diastolic run-off throughout the vasculature, which is affected by arterial stiffness and vascular resistance (Fig. 17-5).[12]

Table 17-3 • RISK FACTORS AND ACTIONS TO PREVENT COMPLICATIONS ASSOCIATED WITH ARTERIAL CATHETERIZATION

Risk Factors	Preventive Actions
• Catheter >20 gauge • Catheter in place >3 days • Female • Low CO/hypotension • Peripheral vascular disease • Vasopressor agents • Anticoagulation (↓ risk) • Femoral (↓ risk) • Systemic antithrombotics or anticoagulants (↓ risk) • Insertion site (femoral or axillary) • Insertion site preparation • Catheter in place >5–7 days • Insertion site	• Use of heparinized flush solution to maintain patency is equivocal Consideration should also be given to risk of heparin-induced thrombocytopenia • Aspirate clot or discontinue line if thrombosis is suspected • Perform routine monitoring of distal perfusion (skin color, temperature, and capillary refill) and after line manipulation • No beneficial effect from repeated flushes • No effect from method of blood sampling (waste vs. nonwaste) • Catheter length sheaths/arterial lines (↓ risk) • Maintain system integrity • Monitor waveform for damping (may indicate loose connections)

Direct Arterial Versus Cuff Pressure

There is no basis for the practice of comparing the intra-arterial BP with the auscultatory or oscillometric BP to determine if one system should be followed to guide therapy.

Pressure gradient determines blood flow proportionally between any two areas. The blood flows from areas of higher pressures to those of relatively lower pressure. Inversely, the blood flow is opposed by the resistance of circulatory system.[17] A modification of Ohm's law for the flow of electrons in an electrical circuit can help to demonstrate the relationship between blood flow, resistance, and pressure.[32]

$$\text{Flow (Q)} = \text{Pressure gradient } (\Delta P)/\text{Resistance (R)}$$

where ΔP is the difference in pressure between any two points (proximal and distal) in the system, and R is the hydraulic resistance to blood flow between these two points. The direct AP measurement is based on pressure, while the oscillometric method (noninvasive) is dependent on flow-induced oscillations in the

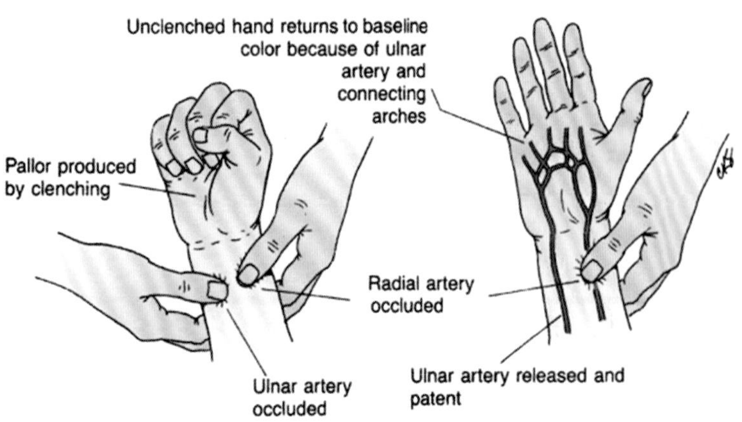

Figure 17-4. Allen Test. To perform the modified Allen test, firm occlusive pressure is applied to both the radial and ulnar arteries. The patient is then instructed to clench his or her hands several times until the color of the palmar skin is blanched. Then the patient is instructed to unclench the hand, the pressure applied to the ulnar artery is released and the occlusion is maintained of the radial artery. The time required for the palmar capillary refill is recorded, and normal hand color should return within 5 to 10 seconds. If it takes longer than 10 seconds, it suggests arterial arch arteries are not intact and arterial catheter should be avoided.[12] (From Diepenbrock, N. H. [2011]. *Quick Reference to Critical Care.* Wolters Kluwer Health.)

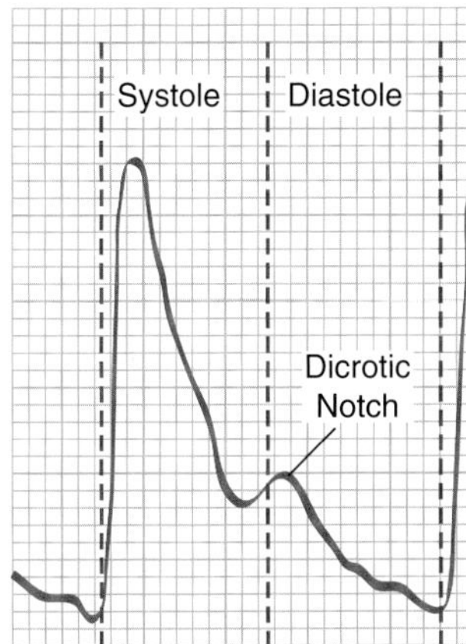

Figure 17-5. Components of Arterial Waveform. The upstroke of the arterial waveform, which begins approximately 0.2 seconds after the onset of the QRS complex, indicates the onset of systole. The dicrotic notch reflects closure of the aortic valve and the onset of diastole.

arterial wall. Based on the above formula, a direct relationship between the flow and the pressure is based on the condition when resistance is constant. In many clinical situations, the resistance is not always constant. Therefore, clinician shall not have the assumption of pressure equals to flow. BP may appear adequate while flow is decreased, or conversely BP may be low although perfusion remains adequate.

Interpretation of Arterial Pressure Data

Evaluation of BP enables identification of abnormalities that would affect hemodynamic status. BP is determined by HR, stroke volume (SV), and size and flexibility of the arteries, known as systemic vascular resistance (SVR). SVR is affected by various factors, including intravascular volume and autonomic nervous system.

Because BP is the product of flow (CO) and resistance (SVR), alterations in BP are reflective of hemodynamic alteration. To understand the changes in BP, one should know the factors that affect SBP, DBP, and mean arterial pressure (MAP). SBP is a measurement taken at the highest point (peak) of the ventricular ejection, which is the indirect reflection of LV contractile force. SBP is affected by left ventricular SV, velocity of LV ejection, systemic arterial resistance, viscosity of the blood, compliance of the aortic and arterial walls, and left ventricular preload. DBP is taken at the lowest point (trough) of the AP, which is primarily affected by arterial peripheral resistance. Other factors that affect DBP include arterial compliance, blood viscosity, SVR, and the length of the cardiac cycle. The difference between the SBP and DBP is called pulse pressure (PP), which is determined by SV, peak rate of ventricular ejection, and arterial wall compliance. An increased PP might be an indication of increased SV or ejection velocity. A narrowed PP can be an indication of cardiac tamponade or ventricular failure.[33]

Both SBP and DBP are clinically significant and important, however neither value is the primary driving pressure of blood flow into organs. The MAP represents the average (mean) of arterial BP over time/through one single cardiac cycle and represents the average driving force in the arterial system through the cardiac cycle. MAP is affected by both CO and SVR as explained using the below formula[32]:

$$\text{MAP} = \text{CO} \times \text{SVR}$$

MAP can be also estimated by using the formulas below[12,34]:

$$\text{MAP} = (1/3 \times \text{SBP}) + (2/3 \times \text{DBP})$$

or

$$\text{MAP} = \text{DBP} + 1/3 \times (\text{SBP} - \text{DBP})$$

These formulas are considering that in normal sinus rhythm, one third of the time in one cardiac cycle is spent in systole, and two thirds is spent in diastole. Therefore, there are limitations with these formulas especially with a faster HR and cardiac arrhythmia. For instance, diastolic filling time is shortened in tachycardia, whereas systolic ejection time remains relatively constant.

Both SBP and DBP may vary in different arterial site, while MAP is unchanged and may be a more consistent value to evaluate and guide therapy. The SBP difference changes with aging, vasoconstriction, vasodilation, and exercise. Both peripheral wave reflection and the end-pressure product, which is the result of the conversion of kinetic energy from flowing blood into pressure as the blood strikes the upstream-looking arterial catheter, cause augmentation of the peripheral SBP. Regardless of the source or site of BP measurement, a key point is that BP and perfusion are not synonymous, and a higher BP does not necessarily translate to higher perfusion.

Noninvasive Blood Pressure Measurement

Most clinical decisions are made based on noninvasive BP measurement due to a lack of availability of invasive BP measurement in all patient care areas. In addition to the physical factors that cause the differences in AP measured in various locations in the body, there are also technical factors that affect measurement accuracy. In addition, the oscillometric system directly measures the mean pressure and extrapolates the systolic and diastolic pressures based on an algorithm which may affect the accuracy of the systolic and diastolic pressure measurements.

For direct and oscillometric BP monitoring, the correct reference is the heart. If the transducer or the arm is positioned above the heart, there will be a decrease in the measured pressure. Conversely, if the transducer/arm is positioned below the heart, there will be an increase in the measured pressure. When the patient is in the sitting position, for oscillometric or auscultated BP measurements, the arm should be supported at the level of the heart (level of the midsternum). If the arm is parallel to the patient or supported on the armrest, the SBP and DBP may be 10 mm Hg higher than if the arm is supported horizontally at heart level (level of the midsternum) and in patients with hypertension, the difference in arm position may cause a 20-mm Hg overestimation of SBP. If the patient is in a lateral recumbent position, the noninvasive BP measurements taken from the "up arm" may be 13 to 17 mm Hg lower than those if the patient is in supine position, and BP measurements from the "down arm" are similar to those taken at supine position or inconsistent. If the "up arm" is used, the measured pressure can be corrected by measuring the distance from the angle-specific phlebostatic axis and correcting the pressure (1 cm equals to 0.73 mm Hg or 1 in equals to 1.8 mm Hg).

Forearm BP measurements may be necessary in cases in which access to the upper arm is not possible or an appropriate cuff is not available (i.e., the existence of morbid obesity or a conical-shaped arm). Two factors need to be considered when comparing the BP from the upper arm and the forearm. First, if the arm is in a dependent position, the hydrostatic pressure increases the BP in the forearm relative to the upper arm. To correct for this hydrostatic effect, the arm should be supported horizontally at heart level. The second factor is that the SBP is normally higher in the periphery (forearm greater than upper arm), although there is limited research comparing noninvasive upper arm and forearm BP in hemodynamically stable patients.

A challenge when performing BP measurements in individuals who are morbidly obese is finding an appropriately sized cuff. For every 5-cm increase in arm circumference (starting at 35 cm), use of a standard cuff leads to an overestimation of SBP by 3 to 5 mm Hg and DBP by 1 to 3 mm Hg compared with an appropriately sized large cuff. To correctly size the cuff, measure the arm circumference half the distance from the elbow to the wrist. Cuff size should be similar to the guidelines for upper arm circumference. The cuff should be centered between the elbow and wrist and the arm should be supported at the level of the heart.

In summary, there is minimal evidence to support the use of direct arterial BP monitoring in the guidance of therapeutic interventions. Despite the potential inaccuracy associated with noninvasive BP measurement with site of measurement, a large amount of observational studies demonstrate the positive association of noninvasive BP measurement and clinical decision making.[35]

VENTRICULAR FUNCTION CURVES

Knowledge of the relationship between preload, afterload, contractility, and SV is essential for effective hemodynamic monitoring and guiding therapeutic interventions that modify these hemodynamic variables. Ventricular function curves demonstrate the interaction between preload, afterload, and contractility and the effects of various disease processes (heart failure [HF], hemorrhage) and therapeutic actions (vasodilator or inotropic drug therapy) on SV and CO. The family of curves varies for each patient but is useful in predicting and evaluating the effects of various therapeutic interventions. The curves are constructed by plotting the PAOP (or some measure of EDV or preload) on the horizontal axis and the CO, CI, or SV on the vertical axis. A key point is that an increase in SV in response to a fluid bolus (change in preload) cannot be reliably predicted on the basis of the standard preload indices (CVP, PAOP) or volumetric indices (RV end-diastolic pressure [RVEDP], global EDV), because the response depends on ventricular function, as indicated by the slope of the ventricular function curve. The traditional preload indices remain useful in the differential diagnosis and determining of a patient's risk for pulmonary edema.

CVP MONITORING

The CVP directly reflects RAP and indirectly reflects the preload of the RV or RVEDP. The CVP is determined by vascular tone, the volume of blood returning to the heart, the pumping ability of the heart, and patient position (supine, standing). The CVP and RAP are generally similar as long as there is no vena caval obstruction. Normally, the CVP ranges from 3 to 8 cm H_2O or 2 to 6 mm Hg (1 mm Hg equals to 1.36 cm H_2O). In the supine/flat position, a CVP of less than 2 mm Hg may indicate hypovolemia, vasodilation, or increased myocardial contractility. An increased CVP may indicate increased circulatory blood volume, vasoconstriction, or decreased myocardial contractility. An increased CVP is also observed in RV failure, tricuspid insufficiency, positive pressure breathing, pericardial tamponade, pulmonary embolus, and obstructive pulmonary disease.

Indications

SV is intrinsically dependent on the preload (the degree to which the ventricles are stretched prior to contracting). An increase in the volume or speed of venous return in the ventricle will increase preload. Through the Frank–Starling law of the heart, an increase in preload will increase SV.[8]

Effect of Catheter Type and Location on CVP

The CVP is measured in the superior vena cava (SVC). Thus, the CVP can be measured from the proximal port of the PA catheter, through a CVC, or the distal port of a multilumen catheter. Very little direct evidence is available to guide the critical clinician to determine which lumen of multilumen CVC provides the most reliable CVP measurement.[36] CVP measurements from the central and peripherally inserted central catheters are considered clinically equivocal.[37]

Limitations

The CVP is not an accurate indicator of LV function or left heart preload. In the presence of normal right heart function, severe deterioration of LV function may not be reflected by a change in CVP. An increased CVP is usually an indication of later stages of LV failure, although the CVP may remain normal even in the presence of high PAP and pulmonary edema.

Complications

Complications associated with CVP monitoring include localized infection, arrhythmias, vessel laceration, RV perforation, thrombophlebitis, hematoma formation at the insertion site, and pneumothorax or a malpositioned catheter. The most common predictor of complications, particularly pneumothorax, is the number of needle insertions required to access the vein. There is an increased risk of arterial puncture, but fewer malpositioned catheters, with the jugular approach. Conversely, there may be a decreased risk of infection with a subclavian versus jugular or femoral insertion.[2]

Interpretation of CVP Waveform

CVP is a key determinant of cardiac function, and one of the determinants of the pressure gradient for organ perfusion (MAP-CVP).[38] Based on the formula for perfusion pressure gradient, an elevated CVP impairs renal perfusion, which is associated with acute kidney injury.[39]

Normal CVP waveform consists of a, c, and v waves and x and y descents, which represent the mechanical components of the CVP tracing. It is important to print a strip with both ECG and CVP tracings and use the correlation of electrical and mechanical events when analyzing the waveform. Both the P wave in the ECG tracing and a wave of the CVP tracing represent the atrial contraction. The a wave is a result of an increased pressure created by atrial contraction, and the a wave follows the P wave on the ECG and generally falls at the beginning of the QRS complex. a wave is not seen in patients with tricuspid stenosis, RV hypertrophy, pulmonary hypertension, pulmonary stenosis, or atrial fibrillation.[17] "Cannon a wave" is defined as a giant a wave which is generated when the RA is attempting to eject blood against a closed tricuspid valve.[40] The next positive deflection

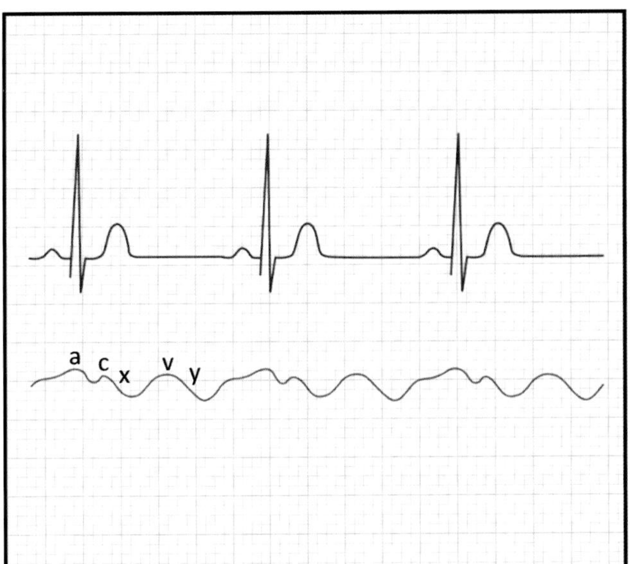

Figure 17-6. CVP With ECG Tracing. (Recreated by T. Eric Goffrier.)

is the c wave (sometimes not seen). The c wave is generated by the bulging of the tricuspid valve into the RA (due to pressure gradient) at the beginning of ventricular systole. Therefore, the c wave represents the closure of tricuspid valve. A large c wave might be present in patients with tricuspid regurgitation.[17] The c wave is followed by the v wave. The v wave represents the filling of the atrium, corresponding to the T wave on the ECG tracing. Acute increase in pressure in the RV might be demonstrated as a giant v wave, which can also be seen in patients with tricuspid regurgitation (Fig. 17-6).

PULMONARY ARTERY CATHETER

History of Pulmonary Artery Catheter

The first human right heart catheterization was performed in 1929. Dr. William Ganz and Dr. HJC Swan then added the flotation device (balloon) and temperature measurement in a pulmonary artery catheter (PAC) for thermodilution CO in 1970. The PAC, also known as the Swan–Ganz catheter, is a flow-directed CVC inserted into a vein (jugular, subclavian, or femoral) to the right side of the heart to obtain direct (RAP, right ventricular pressure [RVP], PAP, PAOP, CO, SvO_2) and indirect/calculated hemodynamic measurements (SV/stroke volume index [SVI], cardiac index [CI], SVR, pulmonary vascular resistance [PVR], delivered oxygen [DO_2]). PAC can be inserted at the bedside sterilely in the critical care units without fluoroscopy guidance if intrajugular vein or subclavian vein is used, or it can be performed in the cardiac catheterization laboratory or operation room. The insertion site may be chosen based on patient preference and provider experience. The jugular vein provides the most direct (shortest and straightest) entry into the heart. Ultrasound may be used to increase success rate.[41]

Indications

The measurements obtained with a PAC may guide clinicians to diagnose critically ill conditions and initiate therapeutic interventions.[13] Although the PAC provides diagnostic and monitoring data that other devices may not provide in the ICUs, debates regarding the risks and benefits of using a PAC have continued for decades with important trials conducted in various patient populations. A Cochrane systematic review in 2013 found that there was no overall benefit or improvement in patient outcomes with the use of the PAC in critically ill adults or high-risk surgical patients.[42] However, there are specific patient populations for whom the PAC may prove useful. In advanced HF patients, particularly in patients with low SBP or are on inotropes, PAC-guided therapy has been found to decrease patient mortality.[43] In trauma populations, the use of PACs appeared to benefit older, more severely injured patients.[44] On the other hand, PAC use is not associated with improved outcomes in patients with severe sepsis and septic shock.[45–47] Taken together, it can be concluded that the PAC is a diagnostic tool; it is not a therapeutic intervention.

There are potential complications of using a PAC, such as central venous puncture, and arrhythmias and pulmonary infarction associated with insertion. Given the decreased utilization of the PAC, adequate, ongoing training is important for critical care clinicians to care for patients with a PAC, manage a PAC adequately to decrease chances of infection, and accurately interpret hemodynamic parameters. It is important to recognize that correct interpretation and application of these measurements by a clinician is required to guide therapy (Display 17-1).

Description

Typically, a 7-french (Fr) introducer catheter is used for insertion of a PAC. A 5-Fr introducer can also be used when a smaller size of PAC is indicated. The PAC is inserted via a port in the introducer catheter, which has a one-way valve. The introducer catheter usually has a side port which can be used as a vascular access for infusion and/or fluid resuscitation.[13]

The length of a PAC is typically 100 to 110 centimeters (cm). There are proximal and distal ports in a PAC. The proximal port (colored blue) is located approximately 30 cm from the tip which lies in the RA and can be used for transducing pressure and infusion. The distal port (colored yellow) is at the tip of the catheter and can be used to measure PAP and PAWP. Because of the location of the distal port, the PA port is not used for any type of infusion but can be used for obtaining a blood sample to measure SvO_2. The balloon is located near the tip of the catheter and can be inflated using the balloon port (colored red) during catheter advancement and while obtaining PAWP. The thermistor of the PAC is used to measure the temperature of the blood. Some PAC has an extra port (colored white), which is called venous infusion port (VIP) and can be used for intravenous therapy. For patients with transvenous pacing needs, a pacing PAC with an extra port can be used (Fig. 17-7).[48]

Insertion of PAC

The catheter is inserted percutaneously. Once the RA is reached, the balloon, located on the distal end of the catheter, is inflated and the catheter is "floated" through the RA and RV and out into the PA, where it occludes a branch of the PA. After the characteristic PAOP tracing has been obtained, the balloon is deflated, allowing the catheter to recoil slightly into the PA. The catheter is left in the balloon-down position to prevent pulmonary infarction.[13] The nursing responsibilities during insertion of the PA catheter are summarized in Display 17-2.

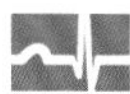

DISPLAY 17-1

Protocol for Obtaining CVP, PAP, and PAOP

1. Explain procedure to patient
2. Position patient in
   a. Supine position with backrest up to 60 degrees
   b. Lateral position at 30 or 90 degrees
   c. CVP and PAP are falsely increased in Trendelenburg and should not be used[10]
3. Allow 5–15 minutes for pressure stabilization after position change depending on the patient's underlying LV function. No specific recommendations are available for required stabilization after prone positioning; measurements have been performed 20–60 minutes after repositioning
4. Reference and zero the pressure-transducer system
   a. Locate the reference point
      Supine: line bisecting fourth ICS at the sternum and one half anteroposterior diameter
      30-degree lateral (right and left): ½ distance from left sternal border to surface of bed
      90-degree lateral (right): fourth ICS at the midsternum
      90-degree lateral (left): fourth ICS left parasternal border
      Prone: line bisecting fourth ICS at the sternum and one half anteroposterior diameter or MAL
   b. Level the air–fluid interface with the reference level (use either the in-line stopcock or the stopcock on the top of the transducer)
   c. Remove the cap from the stopcock using aseptic technique
   d. Turn stopcock "off" to the patient and "open" to air
   e. Activate the "Zero" button on the monitor
   f. Close stopcock and replace cap
   g. Reference and zero the system anytime the patient's position changes
5. Check and troubleshoot the dynamic response characteristics of the system every shift, if the waveform characteristics change, or if the system has been disturbed
6. Confirm zone 3 catheter placement
   a. Review anteroposterior chest radiograph to ensure catheter is below LA (LA is ~3 cm below the carina)
   b. During wedging, the PA waveform should (1) flatten into a characteristic atrial waveform (distinct a and v waves may not be discernible), (2) immediately return to a PA configuration with balloon deflation, and (3) PAOP < mean PA in absence of large V wave
   c. PAEDP-PAOP gradient >4 mm Hg (may indicate zone 1 or 2 placement)
7. Identify end-expiratory waveform
   a. Determine pressures using analog (graphic) tracing
   b. Record end-expiratory pressures
8. If digital data are the only available method, record the PAOP using the following:
   a. Controlled mechanical ventilation: diastolic mode (lowest pressure)
   b. Assisted ventilation: digital mean
   c. Spontaneous ventilation: systolic mode (highest pressure)
9. With active exhalation (suspect if respiratory-induced fluctuation in PAOP is greater than 10–15 mm Hg), read the PAOP at the midpoint between the end-expiratory peak and the end-inspiratory nadir
10. With inverse ratio ventilation, use of the airway pressure waveform may help identify the end-expiratory phase and consideration should be given to correcting for PEEP or auto-PEEP
11. With airway pressure release ventilation (APRV), the PAOP should be measured at the end of the positive pressure plateau, which can be observed on the ventilator and is the point immediately before the release of airway pressure and the initiation of inspiration
12. Evaluate pressures for normal fluctuation and trends
    a. PAS: 4–7 mm Hg
    b. PA mean: 4–5 mm Hg
    c. PAEDP: 4–7 mm Hg
    d. PAOP: 4 mm Hg
13. Improve accuracy of PAOP as an indicator of LAP with high levels of PEEP (>10 cm H_2O)
    a. Position catheter tip dependent to the LA (zone 3—see step 6) or position patient so catheter tip is below LA (e.g., if catheter tip is in right PA, positioning the patient in right lateral position places the tip below the LA). Use an angle-specific reference
    b. Analyze the pulmonary capillary occlusion blood. This confirms correct wedging but does not confirm that PAOP is an accurate indicator of LAP
    c. Estimate effect of increased transmural pressure on PAOP. Subtract ½ applied PEEP (1 cm H_2O = 0.73 mm Hg) from measured PAOP.[13] Example: 15 cm H_2O PEEP; measured PAOP = 18 mm Hg:

       $$15 \text{ cm } H_2O \times 0.73 = 11.1 \text{ mm Hg}$$
       $$18 \text{ mm Hg} - \tfrac{1}{2}(11.1 \text{ mm Hg})$$
       $$\text{Estimated PAOP} = 12.4 \text{ mm Hg}$$

       This is the largest pressure correction possible. Decreased compliance may lessen the effect; for example, with ARDS, only ⅓ of the PEEP may be transmitted to the pleural space.
    d. Suspect nonzone 3 placement if with an increase in PEEP, the PAOP increases greater than ½ the applied PEEP increment (i.e., PEEP increases by 5 cm H_2O (3.7 mm Hg), and PAOP increases greater than 1.8 mm Hg (3.7 mm Hg/2 = 1.8 mm Hg).

Measurement Method

The principle of measuring AP and CVP applies to obtaining measurement using a PAC; the transducer for the PAC needs to be leveled and zeroed to ensure accuracy of hemodynamic measurement (transducer needs to be leveled to phlebostatic axis and head of bed at 0 to 60 degrees with legs parallel to the floor).[14] For consistency, all measurements are preferably obtained with the patient in the same body position.

Right Ventricular Pressure

RVP is not a measurement being monitored continuously in the ICUs, although it is one of the measurements taken during right

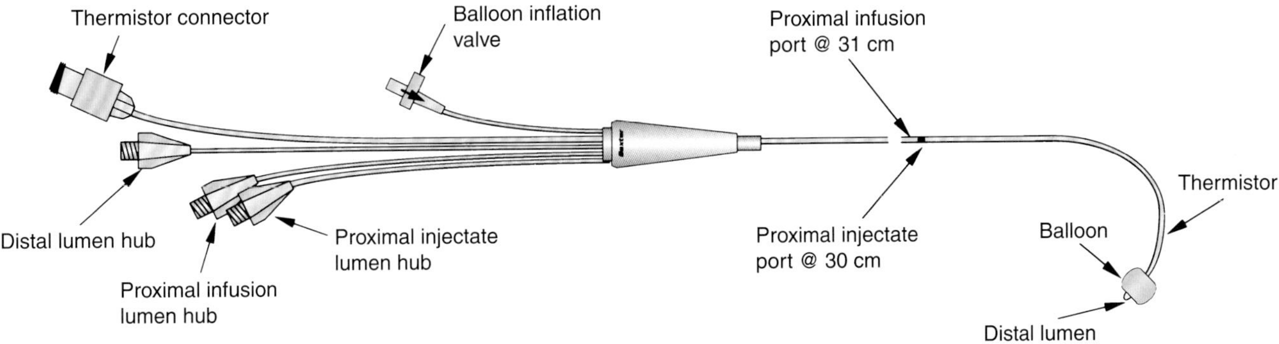

Figure 17-7. Venous Infusion Port PA Catheter. (Courtesy of Baxter Healthcare Corporation, Edwards Critical Care Division, Santa Ana, CA.)

heart catheterization in the cardiac catheterization laboratory. It is important for the critical care clinicians to be able to recognize the distinctive RV waveform shape, as it is an indication that the PAC slips back into the RV. When the tip of the catheter is in the ventricle, there is an increased risk for ventricle irritation that may cause lethal ventricular arrhythmias.[14] Thus, when an RV waveform is noted during routine monitoring, it is required to reposition the PAC immediately (Display 17-3).

PAP and PAWP

The pressure within the PA can be directly measured during right heart catheterization and may be monitored continuously in the intensive care setting using a PAC. Pulmonary artery systolic (PAS), diastolic, and mean pressures are the three pressure measurements obtained. PAS pressure is measured as the blood flow from the RV into the PA. Under the condition of no obstruction of blood flow between the PA and the LV, and the absence of pulmonary vascular disease that increases pulmonary vascular pressure, the PAS is equal to RV systolic pressure; the pulmonary artery end-diastolic pressure (PAEDP) is a reasonable indirect reflection of the LV pressure because there is no valve between the PA and the LA. Left ventricular end-diastolic pressure (LVEDP) can be estimated by using PAWP or LAP. These three pressure measurements are approximately equal with the same above conditions.[49] During diastolic phase of cardiac cycle, the mitral valve opens, and there is a continuous column of blood from the PA to the LA and LV; therefore, the pressures in PA, LA, and LV are approximately equal before the systole (contraction, end diastole) (Fig. 17-8).

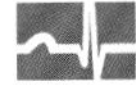 DISPLAY 17-2

Nursing Responsibilities During PA Catheter Insertion

1. Prepare equipment
2. Assist during insertion
   a. Attach pressure tubing to proximal and distal ports and flush system
   b. Determine integrity of balloon (the provider inserting PA catheter will inflate the balloon); the balloon should be symmetric and not cover the catheter tip
   c. Transduce the distal lumen on monitor
   d. Inflate balloon at provider's direction (generally after catheter reaches RA)
   e. Monitor oscilloscope for characteristic waveform changes (see Fig. 17-10A) and ectopy
   f. Record waveforms and pressures as catheter passes from RA to PAOP position
   g. Deflate balloon once PAOP has been obtained, and note return of characteristic PA waveform
   h. Secure catheter and note insertion distance
   i. Apply sterile occlusive dressing (see infection control guidelines—Table 17-1)
   j. Obtain chest radiograph to confirm catheter placement

Measuring PAP

To measure PAP, the ECG and PA pressure waveform must be simultaneously captured. Because the QRS complex in ECG represents the ventricular contraction (systole), a vertical line may be drawn from the end of the QRS complex to the PAP tracing. PAS is measured as the first positive deflection following the QRS complex. The lowest portion of the waveform runoff represents the PA diastolic (PAD) pressure.[13] The rise of systole phase is normally sharp, followed by a downward waveform resulting from a decline in pressure as the blood is ejected out of the PA. A notch is seen during the fall of pressure, known as the dicrotic notch, which is a result of the closure of the pulmonic valve.[13]

1. Increased PVR (Fig. 17-9A)
   a. Pulmonary hypertension
   b. Chronic obstructive pulmonary disease
   c. Acute respiratory distress syndrome (ARDS)
   d. Hypoxia
   e. Pulmonary embolus
2. Increased pulmonary venous pressure
   a. LV failure
   b. Mitral stenosis
3. Increased pulmonary blood flow
   a. Hypervolemia
   b. Atrial and ventricular septal defects
4. Mitral insufficiency (Fig. 17-9B)

Measuring PAOP/PAWP

PAWP is obtained by using a syringe to inflate the balloon at the distal end of the PAC. Balloon inflation allows the tip of the catheter to passively float into the capillary bed, occluding a segment of PA blood flow. Therefore, PAWP is also known as PAOP. The balloon will take up to 1.5 mL of air until the waveform dampens as evidence of the wedge position.[13] Potential risks associated

DISPLAY 17-3

Removal of PAC

1. Verify the order to remove the catheter
2. Assemble necessary equipment
3. Document on the flow sheet the ECG rhythm and vital signs before initiating the procedure
4. Explain the procedure to the patient
5. Transfer IV infusions from PA catheter ports to side port of introducer or discontinue IV solutions if appropriate
6. Ensure that the patient remains in hemodynamically stable condition after transfer of infusions to side port
7. Turn off any remaining infusions to distal and proximal ports
8. Remove syringe from the balloon inflation port. Ensure that the gate valve or stopcock is in the open position by lining up the red lines on the balloon port. This ensures the balloon is deflated passively (level M)[a]
9. Place the patient supine in a slight Trendelenburg position (level E).[b] Turn the patient's head away from the insertion site
10. Open the sterile obturator/introducer cap, ensuring that the sterility of the cap is maintained
11. Put on examination gloves
12. If the catheter dressing is nonocclusive or covers the introducer, after putting on a mask, remove the dressing
13. Instruct the patient to inspire deeply and hold their breath (or apply positive pressure breath on ventilator) during withdrawal of the catheter
14. Unlock the catheter shield from the introducer
15. While securing the introducer with nondominant hand, withdraw the catheter with dominant hand, using a constant steady continuous motion
16. Observe the ECG continuously during withdrawal of the catheter
17. If any resistance is met, do not continue to remove the catheter, and notify the physician immediately
18. Once the PA catheter has been removed, don sterile gloves and insert a sterile adaptor cap into the diaphragm site of the introducer
19. If necessary, reapply a sterile dressing to the catheter site according to policy
20. Elevate head of bed and return patient to position of comfort
21. Examine balloon and catheter to ensure that they are intact. If they are not intact, notify the physician immediately
22. Document on flow sheet the patient's response to procedure, including vital signs and ECG rhythm

[a]**Level M:** Manufacturer's recommendations only.
[b]**Level E:** Multiple case reports, theory-based evidence from expert opinions, or peer-reviewed professional organizational standards without clinical studies to support recommendations.
Zevola DR, Maier B. Improving the care of cardiothoracic surgery patients through advanced nursing skills. *Crit Care Nurse.* 1999;19(1):34–44.

with inflated balloon include PA rupture, pulmonary infarction, pulmonary thrombosis or embolism, and PA hemorrhage. With these potential risks, the duration of balloon inflation should be no more than 8 to 15 seconds (2 to 4 respiratory cycles).[50] Care must be taken to ensure that the balloon is otherwise deflated at all times. Routine PAOP measurement is rarely clinically indicated.

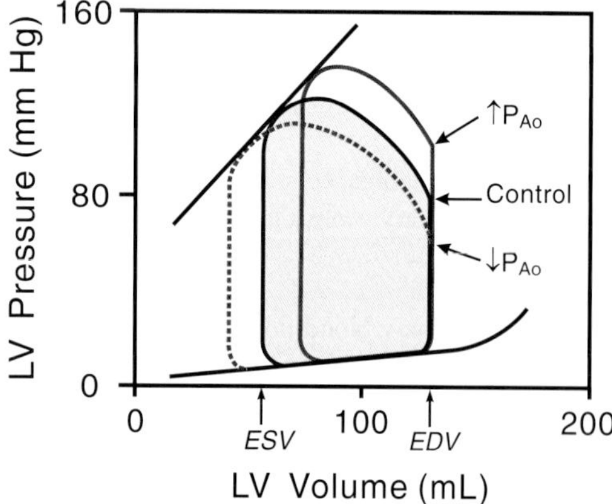

Figure 17-8. Left Ventricular Pressure–Volume Loop. An increase in aortic pressure (*solid red loop*) results in a decrease in stroke volume (width of the loop) and an increase in end-systolic volume (due to less volume pumped out from ventricle). A decrease in aortic pressure (↓PAO *dashed red loop*) results in an increase in stroke volume and a decrease in end-systolic volume). (From Klabunde RE. *Cardiovascular Physiology Concepts*. Baltimore, MD: Wolters Kluwer Health; 2011.)

To measure PAOP, a dual strip of both ECG and PA wedge pressure is obtained (Display 17-4). A vertical line is drawn from the QRS complex to the PAOP tracing, then a and v waves are identified in the PAOP tracing. The wave following the vertical line is a wave, which represents the PAOP at end expiration. The v wave on the other hand represents ventricular systole. The c wave is oftentimes not seen on the PAOP tracing.[13] The v wave of PAOP represents the pressure from the blood retrograde into the LA. A giant v wave indicates an increased retrograded pressure, which can be seen in mitral regurgitation.[51]

Conditions such as chronic obstructive pulmonary disease, ARDS, pulmonary hypertension, and pulmonary embolus impact the pulmonary vasculature while the LV is not affected. Therefore, the PAOP is within normal limits while the PAD is elevated (Fig. 17-10A).[13]

1. Elevated a wave: conditions that increase resistance to LV filling
   a. Mitral stenosis
   b. LV failure (Fig. 17-10B)
   c. Acutely ischemic LV
2. Elevated v wave: conditions that cause increased LA filling during ventricular systole
   a. Acute mitral insufficiency (Fig. 17-10C)
   b. Ventricular septal defect
   c. Aortic regurgitation
3. Elevated a and v waves
   a. Cardiac tamponade
   b. Hypervolemia
   c. Constrictive pericarditis
   d. LV failure (Fig. 17-10B)
   e. Mitral stenosis

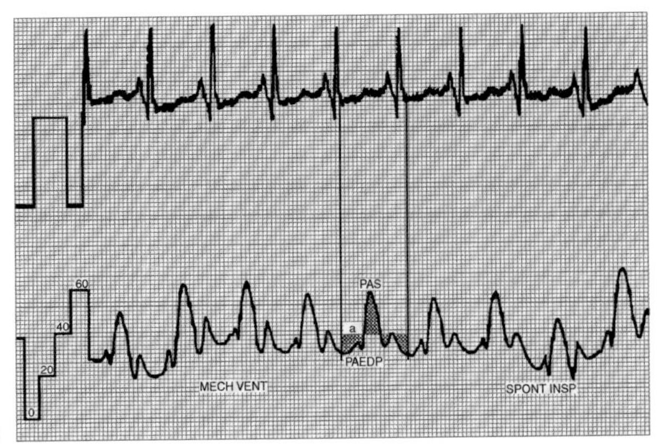

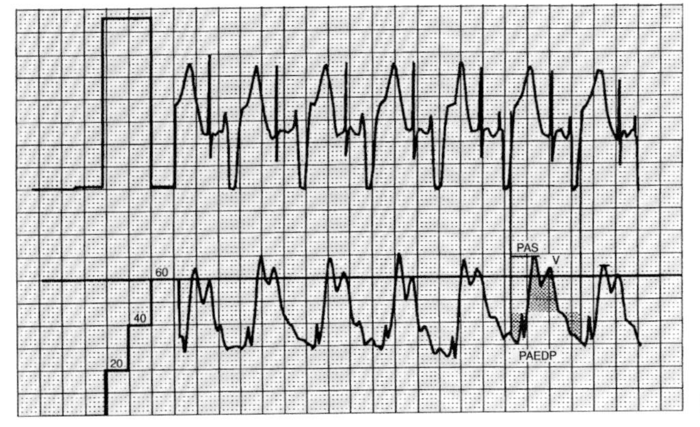

Figure 17-9. (A) Example of the Evaluation of ΔRAP in a Spontaneously Breathing Patient. (B) The CVP (RAP) is read at the base of the a wave or the base of the c wave. The ΔRAP is 1.5 mm Hg, indicating that the patient is likely to respond to a fluid bolus.

Left Ventricular End-Diastolic Pressure

LVEDP is also known as LV preload, which can be visually assessed via left heart catheterization in the cardiac catheterization laboratory setting. In the ICUs, LVEDP can be measured indirectly as PAOP/PAWP. The major function of LV is to pump its content in the end of diastole into the systemic circulation. Therefore, the LV preload is the essential contributor in CO, and it is one of the factors that determine CO.[7] LVEDP can be affected by the presence and timing of atrial kick; conditions such as atrial fibrillation, junction rhythm, and prolonged PR interval (heart block) result in a decrease in LVEDP.[52]

PAEDP and PAWP may be used to estimate LVEDP in the patient with normal cardiac and pulmonary structure and function. PAWP is greater than LVEDP in conditions such as include LA myxoma, mitral valve stenosis, increased pulmonary resistance (such as pulmonary hypertension due to lung disease), and increased intrathoracic pressure with PEEP mechanical ventilation. LVEDP will be higher than PAOP or PAEDP in the presence of aortic regurgitation or aortic insufficiency, noncompliant LV, and pulmonary embolism. Some data suggest that during revascularization procedures, patients with hypovolemia might demonstrate elevated PAOP (Table 17-4) (Display 17-5).[50]

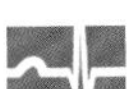 DISPLAY 17-4

Relation of CVP/RAP and PAP to ECG

Pressures/Waveforms	Mechanical Event	ECG Findings	Example
RA Pressure (2–6 mm Hg)			
a wave	RA systole	80–100 milliseconds after P wave	
x descent	RA relaxation	(Downslope of the a wave)	
c wave	Tricuspid valve closure	After the QRS (follows the a wave by a time interval = PR)	**Interpretation:** RAP tracing from patient on mechanical ventilation. The RAP is a mean pressure (bisect an end-expiratory waveform so that the areas above and below are equal or measure at the onset of the c wave). RAP = 15 mm Hg
v wave	RA filling against closed tricuspid valve	Peak of the T wave	
y descent	RA emptying with opening of tricuspid valve (onset of RV diastole)	(Downslope of the v wave)	
PA Pressures Systolic (15–25 mm Hg) Diastolic (8–12 mm Hg) Mean (9–18 mm Hg)	RV ejection of blood into pulmonary vasculature Indirect indicator of LVEDP	T wave (read at peak of waveform 0.08 seconds after onset of QRS; determine by bisecting the wave)	**Interpretation:** PA pressure waveform from spontaneously breathing patient
PAOP (6–12 mm Hg)			
a wave	Left atrial systole	~200–240 milliseconds after P wave	**Interpretation:** PAOP tracing from spontaneously breathing patient. The PAOP is a mean pressure (bisect an end-expiratory waveform so that the areas above and below are equal). PAOP = 6 mm Hg
x descent	Left atrial relaxation	(Downslope of the a wave)	
c wave			
v wave	Left atrial filling against closed mitral valve	TP interval	
y descent	Left atrial emptying associated with opening of mitral valve (onset of LV diastole)	(Downslope of the v wave)	

Bridges EJ. Monitoring pulmonary artery pressures: just the facts. *Crit Care Nurse*. 2000;20(6):59–80.

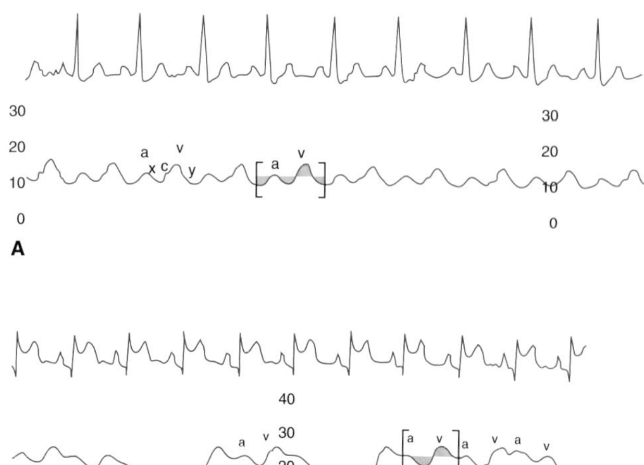

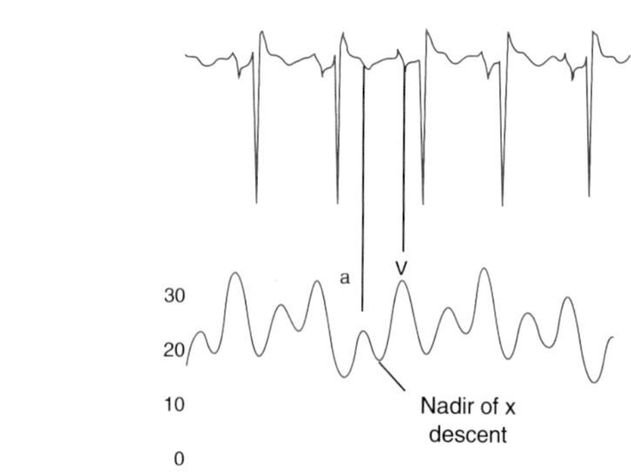

a
V
30
20
10
0
Nadir of x descent
C

Figure 17-10. PAOP Determination. (**A**) Normal PAOP tracing. The mean PAOP is read at end-expiration waveform and is determined by bisecting the a and v waves so there is an equal area above and below the bisection. PAOP = 12 mm Hg. (**B**) Elevated a and v waves. Patient with a history of an inferolateral MI with HF. The increased a and v waves are consistent with LV failure. PAOP = 24 mm Hg. (**C**) PAOP with elevated V wave in a spontaneously breathing patient who was complaining of chest pain. The PAOP is read at the nadir of the *x* descent. Note the relation of the v wave to the TP interval of the electrocardiogram. PAOP = 17 mm Hg.

Respiratory Variations

Understanding the effects of spontaneous breathing and mechanical ventilation on hemodynamic measure will facilitate clinicians to obtain the most accurate reading.[53] Inhalation and exhalation in each breath cycle create cyclic fluctuated pressures within the thoracic cavity, affecting the recording of hemodynamic measurements. Both spontaneous ventilation and mechanical ventilation induce changes in the intrathoracic pressure, and these changes are reflected by corresponding variations in CVP and PA pressures. Pleural pressure is closest to the atmospheric pressure at end expiration when no air flow occurs, and it provides the most accurate distending pressure of cardiac chamber.[54] Thus, it is crucial to measure the hemodynamic values at end expiration.[55] The automatically generated values from the monitoring system are not reliable, because the reading represents the average of what is captured on the monitor without looking at respiration variation in hemodynamic waveform.[56] Additionally, the "stop-cursor" method by freezing the monitor screen is less reliable than the graphic method.[56] It is recommended to identify end-expiratory phase using analysis of graphic recording (see Fig. 17-7).[57]

Spontaneous Ventilation Versus Mechanical Ventilation

In spontaneous breathing, intrathoracic pressure is considered "negative" (decreased) during inspiration due to decreased pleural pressure. During expiration, intrathoracic pressure is considered "positive" (increased). Therefore, in a spontaneously breathing patient, a negative deflection is observed in hemodynamic pressures during inspiration (decreased intrathoracic pressure leads to decreased hemodynamic pressure, e.g., a decreased CVP); thus, all pressure readings derived from the PAC should be measured before the deflection (at end expiration).[57]

Conversely, intrathoracic pressure increases with mechanical ventilation and PEEP due to positive pressure delivered into the patient's thoracic cavity which is above the atmospheric pressure, and the intrathoracic pressure decreases due to passive expiration. PEEP keeps the lung inflated throughout the entire ventilation cycle and increases the intrathoracic pressure. The increased intrathoracic pressure may result in decreased venous return and reduced RV preload.[58] Therefore, when all hemodynamic waveforms from the PAC

Table 17-4 • TROUBLESHOOTING THE PA CATHETER AND MEASUREMENT PROBLEMS

Clinical Problem	Implications	Possible Causes	Interventions
Overdamped pressure tracing	Falsely low systolic readings Falsely increased diastolic readings	Air bubbles in the pressure tubing or transducer More than three stopcocks between catheter and transducer Loose connections Collection of blood in tubing or in and around transducer Catheter kinked internally or at insertion site Catheter wedged against vessel wall Excessive tubing length (>4 ft) Clot or fibrin deposition on catheter tip	Flush all air from system (including microbubbles) Remove excess stopcocks Tighten all connections Flush tubing of all blood (if unable to clear, change transducer-tubing setup) Maintain pressure in infusion bag at 300 mm Hg Aspirate blood from catheter if clot suspected (*do not* flush) If PA catheter kinked, notify MD to reposition If fibrin occluding catheter, catheter may need to be replaced Use noncompliant/wide-bore tubing
Underdamped pressure tracing	Overestimation of systolic pressure Underestimation of diastolic pressure	Air bubbles in tubing, stopcocks, or transducer Excessive tubing length (>4 ft) Excess number of stopcocks	Remove all air bubbles from system Limit tubing to 4 ft maximum Remove unnecessary stopcocks If all attempts to resolve unsuccessful, consider the addition of an in-line damping device

Table 17-4 • TROUBLESHOOTING THE PA CATHETER AND MEASUREMENT PROBLEMS (*Continued*)

Clinical Problem	Implications	Possible Causes	Interventions
Catheter whip (fling) or artifact	Overestimation of systolic pressure Underestimation of diastolic pressure Difficult interpretation of waveform	Location of distal tip of PA catheter near pulmonic valve Hyperdynamic heart Looping of PA catheter in RV External disruption of PA catheter system	Assess dynamic response characteristics (troubleshoot system) Notify MD or qualified RN to reposition PA catheter If fling fails to resolve, use mean pressure
Absence of PA occlusion tracing	Potential for air embolism or blood leaking from balloon port	Balloon rupture Improper positioning of PA catheter	If balloon is inflated without return of air into syringe on passive deflation, assess for signs of air embolism (if present, place in Trendelenburg in left lateral decubitus position, treat symptoms, notify MD) If stable, label balloon port "DO NOT WEDGE." Notify MD of need to replace catheter If balloon is inflated to 1.5 mL, without change in waveform from PA to PA wedge pattern, notify MD or qualified RN of need to reposition catheter Once catheter is repositioned, assess the amount of air required for wedge (ideal volume 1.25–1.5 mL)
Migration of the PA catheter into the RV	Presence of RV arrhythmias Decreased diastolic pressure (equal to RAP)	Accidental or spontaneous withdrawal of catheter into the RV	Inflate the balloon fully to engulf the tip of the catheter and reduce ectopy Notify MD or, if approved for RN, reposition catheter into PA If compromised by arrhythmias, ensure balloon is deflated and withdraw catheter into RA (15–20-cm marking on PA catheter and RAP waveform observed from distal port)
Overwedging	Overwedging (eccentric balloon inflation or inflation in a small vessel) is potential risk for PA perforation and rupture	Catheter migration Balloon position in small pulmonary vessel	Slowly inflate balloon while constantly observing the waveform If overwedge pattern observed, immediately stop inflation and allow balloon to deflate passively Notify MD or, if approved for RN, reposition catheter
Spontaneous wedge	Potential for loss of blood supply to branch of pulmonary vessel and risk of PA infarction	Catheter migration (patient movement, warming up of catheter after placement)	Turn patient to side opposite catheter placement Have patient straighten arm or turn head to dislodge catheter Have patient gently cough Notify MD or RN; reposition catheter

Modified from Gardner PE. Pulmonary artery pressure monitoring. *AACN Clin Issues Crit Care Nurs.* 1993;4:98–119.

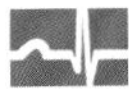 DISPLAY 17-5

PA Thermodilution CO

Factor	Notes	
Catheter position	• Distal port (catheter tip) must be in the PA (confirm by observing PA waveform) • Proximal port should be positioned in RA (verify by observing RA waveform) • Ensure catheter not wedged	
Injection port	• Inject into the proximal port (RA), venous infusion port, or RV port • Injections through side port less accurate than injections through infusion port • Ensure exit of proximal port is outside of introducer sheath	
Calibration constant (CC) (see manufacturer's insert for catheter-specific CC)	• A factor that corrects for the gain of heat from the tubing and thermistor • Specific to (1) catheter type, (2) volume (5 vs. 10 mL), (3) temperature (iced vs. room temperature), (4) solution type (D5W vs. NS)	
Injection technique		
• Injection rate of 4 seconds	• Injection rate demonstrated to produce accurate results with 5–10 mL injectate	
• Avoid handling syringe barrel	• Heat transfer from hands will alter accuracy of measurements	
• Inject at end expiration or throughout respiratory cycle	• Respiratory-induced changes in CO, with up to 30% variability between inspiration/expiration	
• Allow ~60 seconds between measures (monitor will indicate "READY")	• Measurements obtained at end expiration decrease variability in measures (may overestimate CO by 1–1.5 times) • Measurements obtained with random injection throughout respiration increase validity of measures	
• Perform four TDCO measurements (may require more with room temperature injectate or 5 mL vs. 10 mL)	• To determine the CO, average three measurements that are within 10% of median value (e.g., if median value = 5 L/min, include all measures 4.5–5.5 L/min) or average the four measurements to provide 95% confidence that the CO is within 5% of "true" CO	
Injectate temperature/volume Temperature between injectate and blood should be ≥10°C	Iced injectate (0°–5°C) • 5 mL ≅ 10 mL • Low and high CO	Room temperature (19°–25°C) • 10 mL RT ≅ 10 mL IT • CO within normal limits (5 mL IT ≅ 10 mL RT)

(*continued*)

DISPLAY 17-5

PA Thermodilution CO (*Continued*)

Factor	Notes	
There is increased variability in CO measurements between cold and room temperature injectates, particularly in patients with a low EF (<30%)	• Hyperdynamic patients • 10 mL iced is considered the standard[a]	• Normothermia (5 mL if fluid restricted) • Hyperdynamic patients • Hypothermia
Concomitant infusion	• Increased variability with concomitant infusion • Consider discontinuation of infusion if there is no risk to the patient • Avoid performance of TDCO during bolus infusion • Remove all vasoactive medications from proximal port to avoid inadvertent bolus	
Patient position	• Reproducible TDCO measures with backrest up to 20 degrees (Note: CCO reproducible up to 40 degrees backrest elevation) • 250–500-mL/min position-related change in CO in 20-degree side-lying position • Compare side-lying CO to supine CO	
Concurrent use of sequential compression devices (SCDs)	• Note the effect of SCDs on CO measurements—decrease CO an average of 24% during inflation cycle	

[a]It is not necessary to prime the catheter with cold solution before CO measurements.

are measured at end expiration, the values are least affected by air movement in the thoracic cavity. A positive deflection is generated with positive pressure mechanical ventilation (during inspiration); thus, the measurement should be taken just right before the positive deflection (which represents end expiration). Other waveform tracings (such as respiratory tracing from the ECG leads, end-tidal CO_2 [$EtCO_2$] waveform, or continuous airway pressure monitoring) can also be correlated with the PA waveform when available.

For patients with active exhalation or large respiratory excursion, Hoyt and Leatherman[59] recommended using the midpoint of PAP/PAOP (between the peak and the nadir pressure), which should be recorded for clinical use. Boerrigter et al.[60] suggested taking average of PAP/PAOP readings over 2 to 3 ventilatory cycles (Fig. 17-11).

Cardiac Output

Invasive CO may be measured during right heart catheterization and with a PAC in the critical care setting. CO is one of the determining factors of oxygen delivery to the tissue; adequate cardiac function maintains the integrity of tissue perfusion. Maintaining optimal CO has been found to decrease mortality and length of hospital stay.[61]

CO is the measurement of amount of blood moves from the venous to the arterial system per minute, and it is primarily regulated by SV and HR.

$$CO = SV \times HR$$

SV is determined by preload, afterload, and myocardial contractility. Therefore, preload, afterload, HR, and myocardial contractility are the four components that regulate CO (Fig. 17-12).

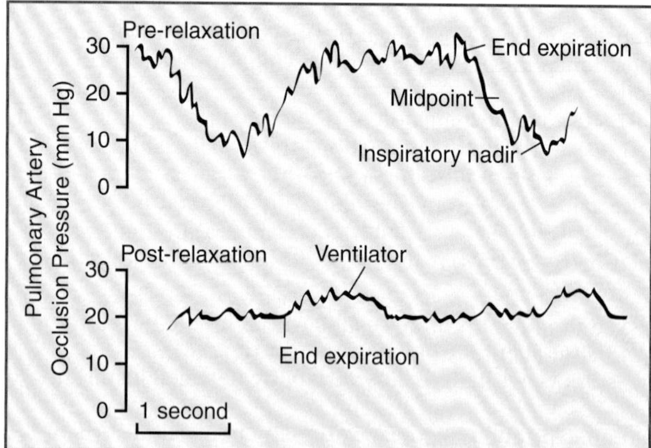

Figure 17-11. PAOP With Respiration Variations. (**Top**) PAOP tracings showing the end-expiratory, end-inspiratory (nadir), and the midpoint values in a patient with marked respiratory variation. (**Bottom**) PAOP in same patient post muscle relaxation with paralytic. (Reprinted with permission from Hoyt JD, Leatherman JW. Interpretation of the pulmonary artery occlusion pressure in mechanically ventilated patients with large respiratory excursion in intrathoracic pressure. *Intensive Care Med.* 1997;23[11]:1126.)

Cardiac Index

CI is a measurement of CO corrected by body size. CI can be calculated using CO divided by body surface area (BSA), which sets a single normal range for patients with varied weight and height.[84]

Preload

Preload reflects the volume of blood in the ventricle being ejected during systole. Any changes in vascular volume and venous return

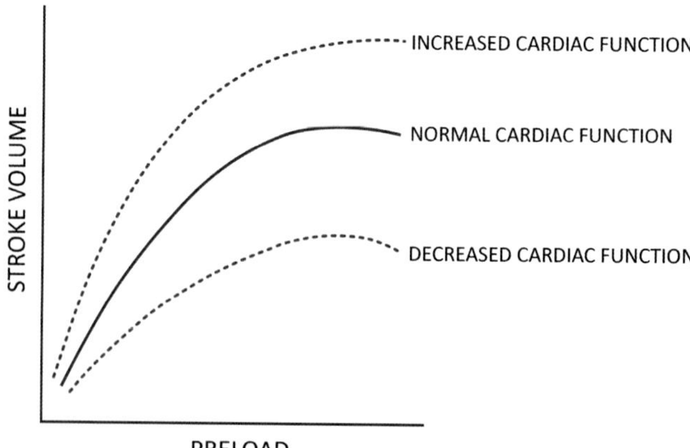

Figure 17-12. Preload and Stroke Volume. With normal ventricular function, an increase in preload results in an increase in stroke volume. With a decreased ventricular function, an increase in preload will not have the same effect in stroke volume. (Created by T. Eric Goffrier.)

affect preload. RV preload can be assessed by obtaining the values of CVP. To evaluate preload of left heart, LVEDP is used as an indirect measurement. In the absence of pulmonary vascular disease, PAWP could be used as an estimate of LVEDP.

Afterload

Afterload is the resistance the ventricles pump against to eject blood, determined primarily by arterial vascular resistance. PVR is the measurement of afterload of right side of the heart and can be calculated using the following formula (MPAP represents mean pulmonary artery pressure):

$$PVR = \frac{(MPAP - PAOP)}{CO} \times 80$$

SVR is used to measure the afterload of left side of the heart and can be calculated using the following formulas:

$$SVR = \frac{CO}{MAP} \text{ or } SVR = \frac{(MAP - CVP)}{co} \times 80$$

The number 80 in these formulas is a constant used to convert resistance into a unit of measurement known as dynes. Because these formulas use CO as a variable other than CI, it is important to take patient body proportion into consideration when evaluating PVR and SVR.

Contractility

Contractility is not directly measured but inferred using the PA catheter. CO is the most common measurement used to evaluate contractility. The calculated SV index may also be used. Based on the Frank–Starling curve, contractility may be affected by preload and afterload. Contractility increases to a point to attempt to overcome resistance created by vessel constriction to maintain SV. Conversely, contractility decreases when the vascular bed dilates and afterload decreases. A low CO may indicate myocardial depression caused by decreased myocardial stretch (preload), myocardial overstretch (high preload), or elevated myocardial resistance (high preload) (Fig. 17-13).

Thermodilution Cardiac Output

Intermittent bolus thermodilution technique to assess CO via the PAC was the clinical standard for decades.[62] The bolus thermodilution technique involves multiple injections (usually 3 to 5

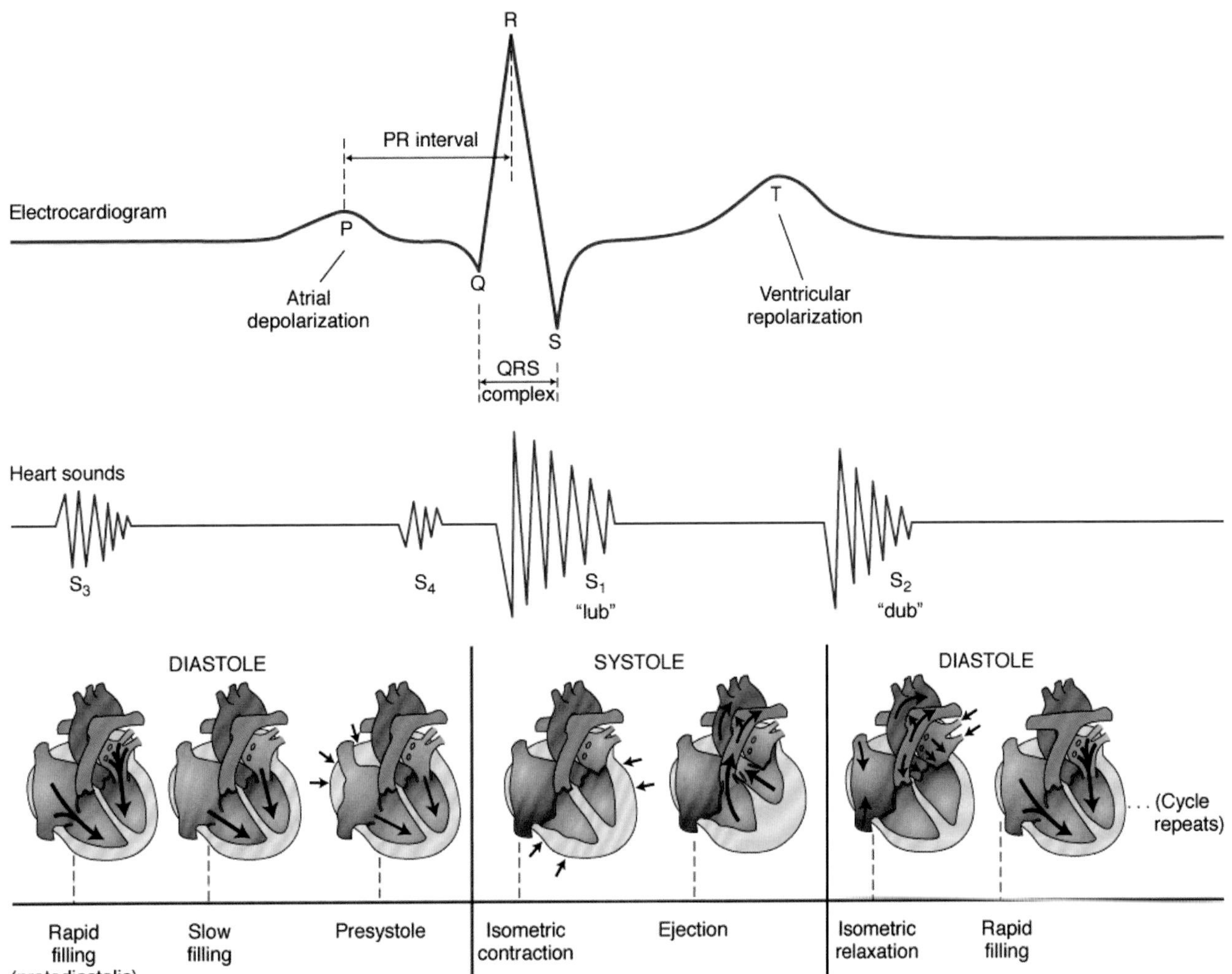

Figure 17-13. Frank–Starling Mechanism. An increase in venous return results in an increase in left ventricular volume, thus increased left ventricular end-diastolic pressure (LVEDP) and stroke volume (from point A to point B). A decrease in venous return decreases the preload and stroke volume (from point A to point C).

injections) of 10 mL of room temperature sterile saline or dextrose into proximal port (into the RA) of the PAC at end expiration. Temperature changes of the blood are sensed by a thermistor on the distal end of the PAC. The Stewart–Hamilton equation is applied to generate the thermodilution curve, which plots the temperature of the PA versus time. The thermodilution curve is viewed on a computer monitor when the bolus of fluid travels from the proximal port to pass the thermistor near the tip of the PAC.

The main limitation of the thermodilution method is inconsistent bolus injection technique. A clinician may generate inconsistent waveforms, resulting in a decreased accuracy of the values obtained. Clinicians may eliminate the outliers and average the remaining measurements.[63] Clinical conditions, such as tricuspid insufficiency and ventricular septal defect, inhibit adequate mixing of the thermal indicator and blood before it is sensed by thermistor, which may cause an underestimation of CO.[64] Significant tricuspid regurgitation is therefore a contraindication for thermodilution CO.

Continuous Cardiac Output

Continuous CO is the most commonly used method for CO measurement. When correctly positioned in the heart, the thermal filament in the PAC is located inside the RV. The thermal filament transmits a heat impulse every 30 to 60 seconds in an on–off fashion. The blood temperature changes are measured. Based on the data transferred to the cardiac monitor, the cardiac monitor displays the average CO obtained over the period of previous 3 to 6 minutes.[1]

Continuous CO monitoring provides the most up-to-date and real-time data, based on which clinicians are able to make appropriate clinical decisions and interventions. Studies have demonstrated that continuous CO monitoring provides accurate and reliable values, and it is easy to use in ICUs.[65,66] It is important to understand that there are conditions that may decrease the accuracy of continuous CO monitoring. For example, a large-volume infusion that changes the blood temperature recorded by the thermodilution filament.[66]

Fick Method

First described by Dr. Adolph Fick in 1870, the Fick method is based on the theory that the blood will absorb the oxygen from the lung entirely; thus, oxygen consumption in the tissue may be determined by evaluating the relationship between the arterial blood and mixed venous blood samples. The Fick method is considered the "gold standard" as it is not affected by tricuspid regurgitation.[13] In addition, the Fick method is the most accurate in low CO states, atrial fibrillation, and ventricular bigeminy.[63] CO can be calculated by knowing three variables: oxygen consumption, hemoglobin concentration, and the difference of oxygen saturation between arterial and mixed venous blood based on the below equation:

$$\text{CO} = \frac{\text{Oxygen consumption}}{(\text{arterial} - \text{venous})\ \text{Oxygen saturation} \times \text{hemoglobin concentration} \times 1.36 \times 10}$$

The constant 1.36 is expressed in mL O_2/g hemoglobin: 1.36 mL represents the amount of oxygen carried by each gram of hemoglobin.[63] 10 is the conversion factor to convert milliliter per deciliter.[13] The method commonly used to determine CO today is called the assumed Fick method. The assumed Fick method uses the formula 125 mL × BSA to calculate the resting oxygen consumption. Direct measurement of oxygen consumption requires use of a tight-fitting gas exchange system, which is a cumbersome and time-consuming process. The assumed Fick method is limited by the large variability in oxygen consumption; thus, assumed values may produce unpredictable errors.[67–69] Other sources of error for determining oxygen consumption can occur, such as oxygen saturation measurement in intracardiac shunts (Table 17-5).

Cardiac Output Measurement in Targeted Temperature Management

Post cardiac arrest hemodynamic profile often suggests myocardial stunning and vasodilation, characterized by impaired vasoregulation, reduced CO, and hypotension, contributing to a decrease in organ perfusion. There is limited research on hemodynamic implication of targeted temperature management (TTM). A randomized study conducted by Bro-Jeppesen et al.[70] suggested that, when compared with a higher actively controlled target temperature (36°C), a lower level of target temperature (33°C) after cardiac arrest was associated with increased systemic vascular tone, decreased CO due to a decrease in HR with unchanged myocardial contractility, and increased levels of lactate. Lower core temperature is also associated with a lower metabolic rate. Bro-Jeppesen et al. concluded that choosing a target temperature regimen with less impact on metabolism and cardiovascular function may be important for balancing the benefits and hazards of TTM in individual patients.[70]

OXYGEN SUPPLY AND DEMAND

The cardiopulmonary system regulates the transport of carbon dioxide (CO_2) and oxygen (O_2) to and from the tissue. The amount of O_2 in the blood and CO determine the oxygen delivery. Tissue oxygenation is not measured by the standard indices of hemodynamic measurement (CVP/RAP, PAP, PAOP, CO/CI) and may be normal in the presence of continued tissue hypoxia. The use of global indices (DO_2, oxygen consumption [VO_2], serum lactate, and SvO_2 or central venous oxygen saturation [$ScvO_2$]) and regional indices (transcutaneous O_2 and CO_2 saturation) offers additional information on oxygen supply and demand and these indices are more sensitive to changes in tissue oxygenation. An understanding of factors that affect DO_2 and VO_2 will help detect potential tissue hypoxia and guide therapeutic interventions (Fig. 17-14).

DO_2 represents oxygen delivery in the body (normal is approximately 1000 mL/min). Oxygen delivery index (Do_2I, or DO_2 corrected to BSA) is the product of CI and arterial oxygen content (CaO_2).[71]

Venous Oxygen Content

Venous oxygen content is the amount of oxygen remaining in the blood after blood passes through the tissue (oxygen consumption in the tissue). The tissue consumes about 25% of the delivered oxygen and leaves about 75% oxygen in the remaining venous blood.[72] Because venous oxygen content represents the oxygen reserve in the body, if there is an increase in demand or a decrease in delivery, the body will extract more oxygen at the cellular level to compensate. The greater the oxygen extraction from the cells,

Table 17-5 • HEMODYNAMIC CHARACTERISTICS OF VARIOUS PATHOLOGIC CONDITIONS

Pathophysiology	Hemodynamic Findings: RAP	PA	PAOP	SV	CO	Additional Findings
Pericardial tamponade	↑	↑	↑	↓	↓	Equalization (within 5 mm Hg) of RAP = PAEDP = PAOP; RAP waveform: prominent *x* descent with attenuated or absent *y* descent (d/t decreased ventricular filling); *pulsus paradoxus* (↓SBP >10 mm Hg and ↓pulse pressure during inspiration; DBP unchanged); *pulsus alternans*; absent S_3 heart sound; cardiac pressures may be normal if the patient is hypovolemic
Pericardial constriction	↑	↑	↑	↓	N/↓	RAP waveform: steep *x* and *y* descent resulting in an "M"- or "W"-shaped waveform; RAP ≅ PAEDP ≅ PAOP (if no tricuspid or mitral regurgitation); decreased respiratory variation in RAP; Kussmaul sign (inspiratory increase in RAP in severe pericardial constriction); *pulsus paradoxus* (approximately 33% of cases). CO maintained by tachycardia
Massive pulmonary embolism	↑	↑	↑/N/↓	↓	↓	Increased RA v wave with steep *y* descent due to tricuspid regurgitation, increased alveolar–arterial oxygen gradient (normal value does not rule out pulmonary embolism), tachypnea, dyspnea, increased pulmonic component of S_2, pleuritic chest pain
Mitral regurgitation			↑			If amplitude of v wave is 10 mm Hg or more than *a* wave amplitude, read PAOP at nadir (base) of the *x* descent; PAOP > PAEDP (regurgitant v wave)
Left ventricular failure	N/↑	↑	↑	↓	↓	Pulmonary congestion or edema, S_3 or S_4, increased *a* wave height (due to decreased ventricular compliance); increased v wave height due to mitral regurgitation, pulsus alternans. Approximately 50% of patients with HF have mild or no impairment in systolic function
RV infarction	↑	↑/↓	↑/↓	N/↓	N/↓	RAP > PAOP or RAP 1–5 mm Hg > PAOP, or RAP >10 mm Hg, RA tracing with prominent *x* and *y* descent (M configuration), increased jugular venous pressure, systemic venous congestion, RV gallop, split S_2, positive hepatojugular reflux, increased RA *a* wave, positive Kussmaul sign (increased RAP with inspiration), RV S_3 or S_4
Acute ventral septal defect	↑	↑	↑	↓	↓	Acute hypotension and pulmonary congestion, systolic thrill, holosystolic murmur, acute right HF with increased jugular venous pressure, late PAOP v wave, oxygen step-up of >10% RA and PA
Hypovolemia	↓	↓	↓	↓	↓/N	Increased SVR (compensatory), decreased $S\bar{v}O_2$
Septic shock (hyperdynamic)	↓	↓	↓/N/↑	N/↑	N/↑	Systemic hypotension, SBP <90 mm Hg, metabolic acidosis with compensatory hyperventilation (respiratory alkalosis), decreased vascular resistance (↓ SVR) and ↑ $S\bar{v}O_2$. This profile may be accompanied by distributive shock
Septic shock (hypodynamic)		↑↓	↑↓	↓	↓	Systemic hypotension, SBP <90 mm Hg, systemic vasoconstriction (increased SVR), decreased $S\bar{v}O_2$. During the early phase of septic shock, this profile may reflect inadequate fluid resuscitation. This profile also reflects cardiogenic shock

N, normal; ↓, decreased; ↑, increased.

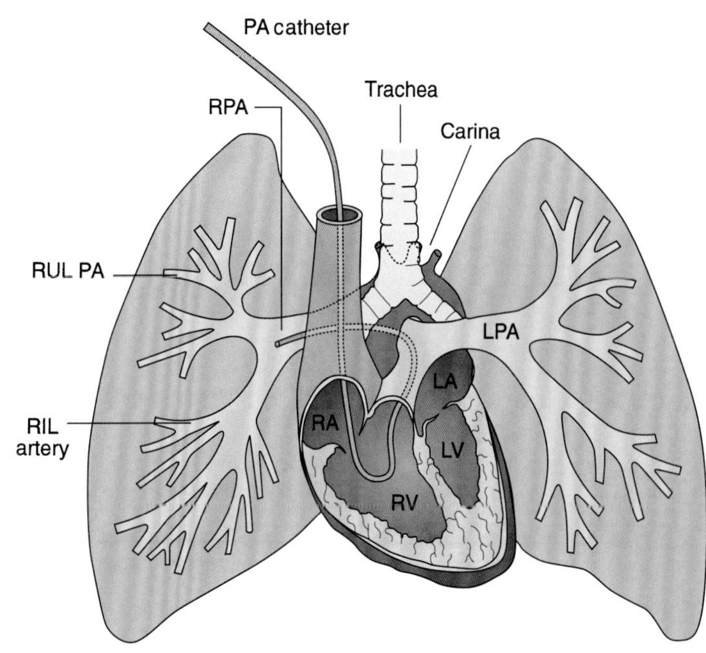

Figure 17-14. Schema of the Cardiopulmonary Structures. Schema of the cardiopulmonary structures demonstrating the relationship between the LA, PA, and pulmonary vasculature, with a correctly positioned PA catheter. RUL PA, right upper lobe PA; RIL, right interlobar PA; RPA, right PA; LPA, left PA; RV, right ventricle.

the less oxygen reserve in the blood (less venous oxygen content). An assessment of venous oxygen content allows the clinician to investigate the relationship between oxygen demand and consumption.[72]

SvO_2

SvO_2 is a measurement taken in the PA, which contains mixed venous blood from organ systems and regions of the body.[72] SvO_2 reflects the average venous saturation of the whole body after tissue extraction of oxygen from the blood, and has been used as a reflection of cardiovascular performance in critically ill patients.[72–74] In addition, SvO_2 was a proposed surrogate of the balance between the systemic oxygen supply (DO_2) and demand (VO_2). Three physiologic components of DO_2 and VO_2 determine SvO_2: the heart, the lung, and the hemoglobin: An adequate CO provided by the heart will supply adequate central venous oxygen. The lung is responsible for converting deoxygenated blood into oxygenated blood. The hemoglobin carries oxygen to the cells and carbon dioxide to the lung.[75,76] SvO_2 is calculated using the following formula (SaO_2 represents arterial oxygen saturation):

$$SvO_2 = SaO_2 - \left(\frac{VO_2}{CO} \times 1.36 \times Hgb\right)$$

When Hgb and SaO_2 are constant, it is assumed that a change in SvO_2 reflects a change in CO. Based on the formula, a decrease in SvO_2 can also be caused by a decrease in arterial oxygen saturation (arterial hypoxemia), an increase in VO_2 (increased O_2 extraction from cell), and a decrease in hemoglobin (e.g., bleeding).[77] To evaluate the clinical significance of changes in hemodynamic status, it is important to examine the relationship of SvO_2 and CO, and the associated trends over the duration of time appropriate for the suspected condition or therapeutic intervention.

SvO_2 can be sampled from a PAC for intermittent monitoring. Blood is drawn from the distal port (PA port) of the PAC. Blood is aspirated slowly to prevent obtaining arterial blood that would overestimate oxygen saturation value. A fiberoptic PAC can be used in the ICUs for continuous SvO_2 monitoring. When the PAC is connected to the SvO_2 monitor, the light source from the optimal module will transmit the light through one of the fiberoptic channels to the tip of the catheter. The oxyhemoglobin absorbs the light and is reflected back through a second fiberoptic channel to a photodetector in the optimal module. The amount of reflected light depends on the amount of saturated hemoglobin. The light source is analyzed by a microprocessor, and a ratio between oxygenated and deoxygenated blood is calculated based on which the SvO_2 is determined.

Normal SvO_2 ranges from 60% to 80%. Anaerobic metabolism occurs when SvO_2 is less than 40%. SvO_2 between 40% and 60% indicates an imbalance of oxygen delivery and oxygen demand; the body compensates by increasing CO to increase O_2 delivery, or increasing O_2 extraction from the blood. SvO_2, a global parameter, does not provide information about oxygen balance in a particular organ or system (Fig. 17-15).

$ScvO_2$

$ScvO_2$ has been used as a surrogate to SvO_2. $ScvO_2$ reflects the venous blood return from the upper body (head, neck, and upper extremities). The $ScvO_2$ is about 2% to 5% higher than SvO_2 in a healthy individual.[78] A blood sample is taken in the SVC right above the RA. Fiberoptic oximetric catheters are used to continuously monitor $ScvO_2$. A blood sample from CVC positioned in the SVC can be drawn to measure $ScvO_2$ intermittently using co-oximetry (Table 17-6).

Serum Lactate

Lactic acid is a by-product of anaerobic metabolism caused by tissue hypoxia; thus, the onset and severity of lactic acidosis reflect oxygen deficiency. Serum lactate became a measurement for shock in the 1960s.[79] Normal serum lactate level is less than 2 mmol/L. In the clinical situation of shock (decreased CO), the lactate level will be greater than 2 mmol/L.

Elevated lactate is associated with increased mortality. Jansen et al.[80] found that correcting a lactate level of more than 3 mmol/L

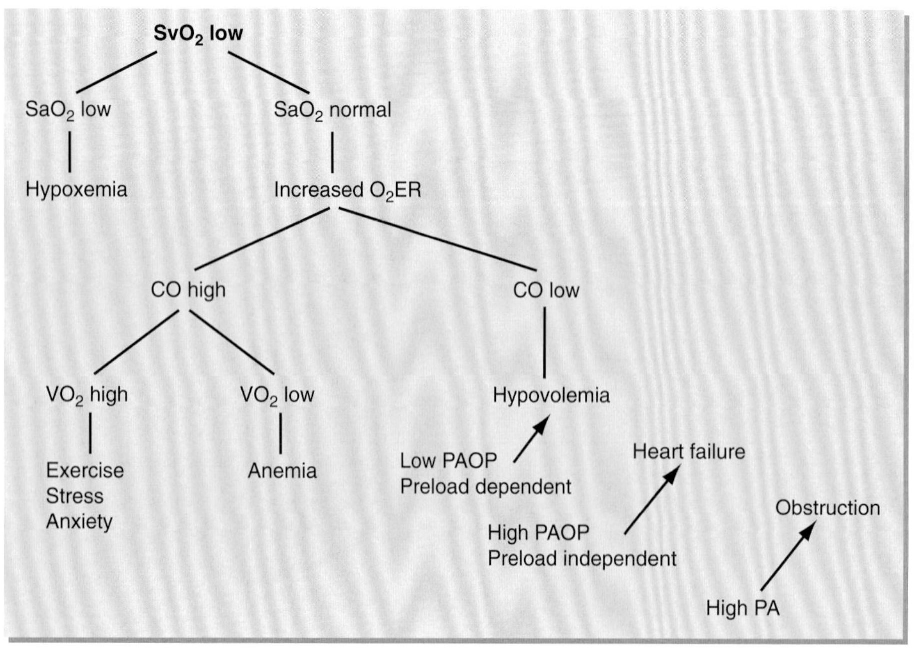

Figure 17-15. Interpretation of Hemodynamic Data Starting With Mixed Venous O_2 Saturation, Svo_2; O_2ER, O_2 Extraction Ratio; Vo_2, O_2 Uptake. (Vincent JL, De Backer D. Cardiac output measurement: is least invasive always the best? *Crit Care Med.* 2002;30[10]:2381.)

Table 17-6 • OXYGEN TRANSPORT EQUATIONS

Variables	Equation/Example	Normal
Arterial oxygen content (Ca_{o2})	(Hgb × 1.36 × Sa_{o2}) + (0.003 × Pa_{o2}) (15 × 1.36 × 0.99) + (0.003 × 100)	20 mL/dL
Venous oxygen content (Cv_{o2})	(Hgb × 1.36 × $S\bar{v}o_2$) + (0.003 × PvO_2) (15 × 1.36 × 0.75) + (0.003 × 40)	15 mL/dL
Oxygen delivery ($\dot{D}O_2$)	CO × Ca_{o2} × 10 5 × (15 × 1.36 × 0.99) × 10	1000 mL/min
Oxygen delivery index ($\dot{D}o_2I$)	CI × Ca_{o2} × 10 3.5 × (15 × 1.36 × 0.99) × 10	600 mL/min/m^2
Oxygen consumption ($\dot{V}o_2$)	CO × 1.36 × Hgb (Sa_{o2} − $S\bar{v}o_2$) 5 × 1.36 × 15 (1.0 − 0.75)	250 mL/min
Oxygen consumption index ($\dot{V}o_2I$)	CI × 1.36 × Hgb (Sa_{o2} − $S\bar{v}o_2$) 3.5 × 1.36 × 15 (1.0 − 0.75)	125 mL/min/m^2
Oxygen extraction ratio (O_2ER)	$\dot{D}o_2/\dot{V}o_2$ (Ca_{o2} × Cv_{o2})/Ca_{o2} [(Hgb × 1.36 × Sa_{o2}) − (Hgb × 1.36 × $S\bar{v}o_2$]/(Hgb × 1.36 × Sa_{o2}) (Sao_2 − $S\bar{v}o_2$)/Sa_{o2}	25%
Cardiac index/oxygen extraction ratio	CI/O_2ER (3.0 ÷ 0.25)	10–12

by 20% over 2 hours is associated with decreased mortality. In septic shock, serum lactate trends are used to guide resuscitation therapy and monitor response.[81]

Increased serum lactate levels may not be due to hypoperfusion. For example, impaired lactate clearance may occur in patients with decreased liver function. It is important to identify the underlying cause of increased serum lactate.

FUNCTIONAL HEMODYNAMICS

One of the most important aspects of caring for the critically ill patient is the evaluation of intravascular volume status. Historically, CVP, PAD, and PAWP have been commonly used to assess for hypo- or hypervolemia and guide subsequent appropriate interventions, namely to determine whether intravenous fluid be administered and the subsequent response to fluid administration.

An observational study showed that static markers of preload (e.g., CVP, PAWP) were still used to predict preload responsiveness in 35.5% (N = 2213) of fluid challenges in ICUs around the world. In addition, CVP was the leading variable used in 89.9% (N = 785) of these cases.[82] In a survey of American and European anesthesiologists, more than 70% of respondents reported that CVP was used to guide fluid management in patients undergoing high-risk surgery.[83] However, numerous studies have indicated that cardiac filling pressures (CVP, PAD, and PAWP) are static markers of preload and have poor sensitivity and specificity for preload responsiveness.[84–87]

The Surviving Sepsis Campaign guidelines and European Society of Intensive Care Medicine have recommended the use of dynamic parameters over static measures to predict fluid responsiveness, because neither standard preload indices (CVP, PAWP) nor volumetric indices (right ventricular diastolic volume, global EDV) can reliably predict an increased SV with a fluid bolus.[88–90]

Fluid (preload) responsiveness is defined as an increased SV and CO with a fluid challenge.[91,92] Assessment is complicated by cardiovascular physiology.[93] Patients may have a significant or negligible increase in SV based on their position in the Frank–Starling curve, which is determined by their ventricular systolic function. An increase in SV by at least 10% after a fluid bolus 30 mL/kg is considered positive fluid responsiveness, and additional fluid may be administered until SV is increased by 10% than what it was with the previous dose. Once the patient reaches the "plateau" phase of the Frank–Starling curve, fluid boluses should be held until volume status is reevaluated.[94]

Functional hemodynamics refers to the dynamic function of the heart, and includes the measurement of systolic pressure variation (SPV), pulse pressure variation (PPV), and stroke volume variation (SVV).[94] SPV, PPV, and SVV are calculated mathematically from AP waveform analysis.[95–97] These variables are more reliable than static pressure measurements for predicting and measuring preload responsiveness.[98–103] Mechanical ventilation induces changes in measurement of BP and SV, which provide the insight of fluid responsiveness of the patient.[104–106] While tidal volume in mechanical ventilation might also affect the accuracy of functional hemodynamics, a meta-analysis demonstrated that, when compared to the traditional static measurements, these dynamic variables were more predictive of preload responsiveness in mechanically ventilated patients (Figs. 17-16 and 17-17).[107,108]

Systolic Pressure Variation

SPV is the difference between inspiration increase and expiration decrease at a given mechanical breath cycle, and it can be calculated using the below equation:

$$SPV = SPV_{max} - SPV_{min}$$

Both mechanical ventilation and spontaneous breathing produce a normal variation in SBP for about 5 to 10 mm Hg.[4] In mechanically ventilated patients, the SBP decreases during expiration and increases during inspiration due to changes in pleural pressure, which is equivalent to pressure outside the heart and the intrathoracic arteries and veins.[108]

A calculated percentage of SPV (SPV%) may be more sensitive and specific at the time of hemodynamic instability.[109] However, Berkenstadt et al.[110] suggested that SPV% might be artificially increased during hypotension.

$$SPV\% = \frac{(SBP_{max} - SBP_{min})}{[(SBP_{max} + SBP_{min})/2]} \times 100$$

SPV and SPV% are directly related to the tidal volume delivered to the patient. SPV greater than 10-mm Hg predicted fluid responsiveness in patients with acute circulatory failure caused by sepsis and who were receiving an 8- to 11-mL/kg tidal volume.[111]

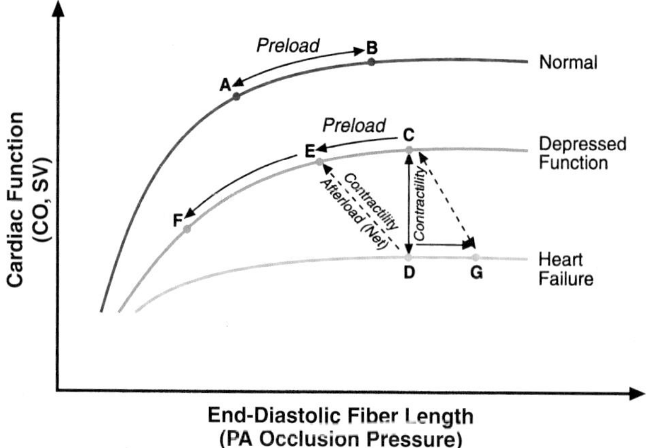

Figure 17-16. End-Diastolic Fiber Length. Family of ventricular function curves representing normal, depressed, and severely depressed function. A change in preload is represented by a move up or down a single curve (Frank–Starling principle). Point A to point B and point B to point A reflect an increase and decrease, respectively, in preload. The response to volume loading is dependent on the position on the ventricular function curve and the shape of the curve. If both ventricles are on the steep portion of the curve, the SV will increase in response to volume (responder). In contrast, if the heart is on the flat portion of the curve, the SV will not increase (nonresponder). A change in afterload results in a shift in the curve that appears similar to that caused by contractility, although the mechanism is different. Point D to E reflects the net effect of a decrease in afterload on a failing heart. This upward and lateral shift is the result of two actions. Point D to C reflects an increase in force of contraction and point C to E a decrease in preload due to increased systolic ejection. A change in contractility is represented by an upward or downward shift of the curve, that is, for any given preload and afterload, the CO is increased or decreased. In a failing heart, an additional effect of decreased contractility is an increase in preload due to decreased systolic ejection; thus, the net effect of a decrease in contractility is to shift the curve down and to the left (point C to point G).

Pulse Pressure Variation

PPV is a calculated percentage that reflects variations in arterial PP between inspiration and expiration.[112,113] PPV can be calculated using the following formula:

$$\text{PPV\%} = \frac{(\text{PP}_{max} - \text{PP}_{min})}{[(\text{PP}_{max} + \text{PP}_{min})/2]} \times 100$$

Left ventricular SV, arterial resistance, and arterial compliance are the three factors that can affect PP. Both arterial resistance and arterial compliance do not change significantly in each breath cycle. Therefore, changes associated in PP from beat to beat reflect changes in left ventricular SV. It is used in advanced hemodynamic monitoring systems to assess fluid volume responsiveness: volume expansion to increase CO.[114–116] PPV is an accurate predictor of fluid responsiveness in critically ill patients who were passively ventilated with tidal volume of greater than 8 mL/kg and without cardiac arrhythmia.[114] Studies have shown that patients with a baseline PPV greater than or equal to 13% were likely to respond positively to a fluid challenge (i.e., increasing their CI by 15% or more).[87,95,96]

Stroke Volume Variation

SV is a measurement for the amount of blood pumped out of the ventricles in one contraction. SV is a calculated percentage over a breath cycle using the below formula:

$$\text{SVV\%} = \frac{(\text{SV}_{max} - \text{SV}_{min})}{[(\text{SV}_{max} + \text{SV}_{min})/2]} \times 100$$

The greater the SVV, the greater the patient's response to fluid, which puts the patient on the steep portion of the Frank–Starling curve.[4] For patients with controlled mechanical ventilation without spontaneous breathing, the normal SVV is from 10% to 15%, and a clinical value at 13% or greater predicted fluid responsiveness (Fig. 17-18).[116]

End-Expiratory Occlusion Test

End-expiratory occlusion (EEO) test is based on the theory that there is a decrease in cardiac preload due to a decrease in venous return with a positive ventilation breath. To perform the test, simply stop the ventilator while measuring both the intrinsic PEEP and the changes in CO. The ventilation pause must be longer than 15 seconds, which is the amount of time required for the preload change to transit through the pulmonary circulation.[38] A PP change of greater than 5% during the end-expiratory occlusion predicted fluid responsiveness with a sensitivity of 87% and a specificity of 100%.[117] The EEO test is valid in ARDS patients when PPV and SSV are not sensitive indicators. Silva et al.[118] concluded that EEO remained valid with PEEP levels of 5 cm H_2O as well as 15 cm H_2O.

Clinical Indications and/or Implications of Functional Hemodynamics

Functional hemodynamic technologies can be used in both ICUs and acute care units. Assessment of the relationship between a

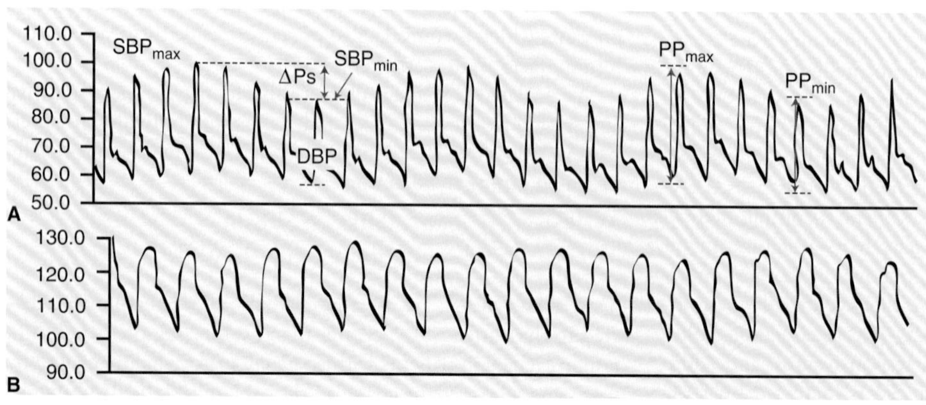

Figure 17-17. Example of SPV and PPV. (**A**) This analog tracing was obtained from the bedside monitor with the paper speed decreased to 6.25 mm/s. In this case, the patient is demonstrating marked variation in their SPV (e.g., SPV = 9 mm Hg) indicating fluid responsiveness. (**B**) In this case, there is minimal variation in the functional indices (e.g., SPV = 4 mm Hg) indicating that the patient would not be fluid responsive and other methods, such as a vasopressor, should be considered to treat the patient's hypoperfusion.

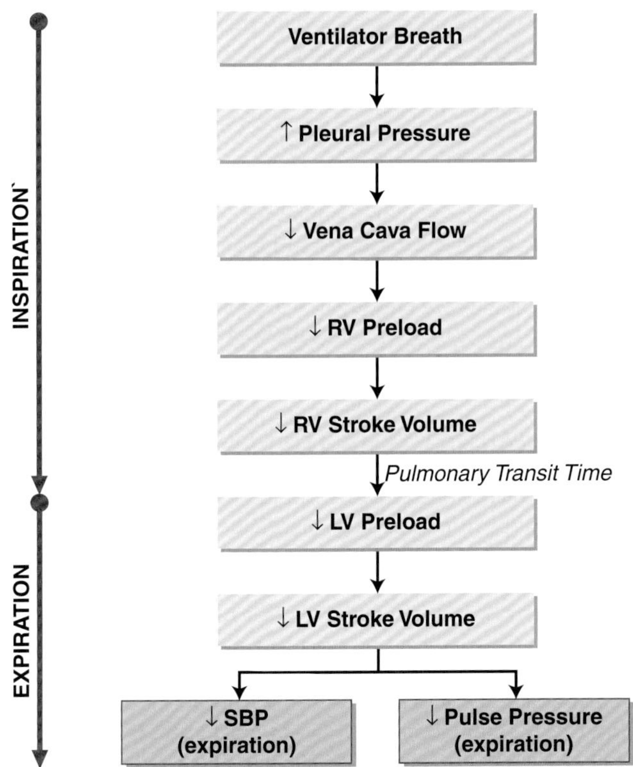

Figure 17-18. Primary Mechanism for Ventilator-Induced Variation in SV, SBP, and Pulse Pressure. The cyclic changes in LV stroke volume are mainly related to the expiratory decrease in LV preload due to the inspiratory decrease in RV filling and output.

fluid challenge and change in SV determines where the patient is on their individual Frank–Starling curve and predicts fluid responsiveness.[119–120] Hypovolemia causes tissue hypoperfusion, tissue hypoxia, and organ failure.[121] Volume expansion can potentially increase CO and oxygen delivery.[122] However, volume overload aggravates the risk of lung and tissue edema and prolongs mechanical ventilation. Hypervolemia also results in organ failure, increased length of ICU stay, and increased mortality.[123a,123b] Fluid overload increases mortality especially in patients with sepsis,[124,125] ARDS,[126,127] intra-abdominal hypertension, and acute kidney injury (see Fig. 17-19).[128]

Marik et al.[129] analyzed the administration of fluids on the first ICU day for patients ($N = 23{,}513$) admitted directly from the emergency department with severe sepsis and septic shock. In

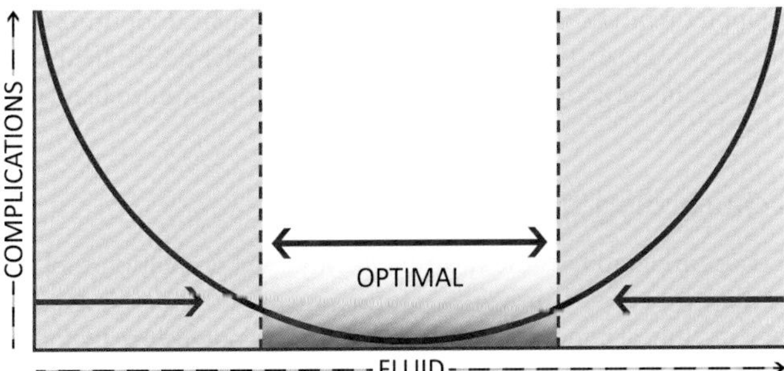

Figure 17-19. Fluid Versus Complication Curve. This curve reflects the balance of fluid resuscitation. Both underresuscitation and overresuscitation can result in complications.
(Created by T. Eric Goffrier.)

patients who received 5 L of fluid or greater, mortality increased by 2.3% for each additional liter. Taken together, both underresuscitation and overresuscitation can have detrimental effects on patient outcomes (Fig. 17-19).[130]

Limitations of Functional Hemodynamics

The primary limitation of these parameters is the impact of conditions associated with varying pleural/intrathoracic or intra-abdominal pressures. PPV and inspiratory changes in RAP failed to predict the response to volume expansion in spontaneously breathing patients.[131] Functional hemodynamic parameters (PPV and SSV) are not recommended for patients with cardiac dysrhythmias. Because under the condition of dysrhythmias, it is impossible to determine whether observed variability in hemodynamic measurement reflects fluid responsiveness or arrhythmia-induced changes in SV.[132]

Low tidal volume and higher PEEP for lung protection are commonly used in ARDS patients. With these ventilation strategies, there is reduced amplitude of change in intrathoracic pressure, altering the magnitude of the ventilator-induced changes in functional dynamic indices.[133–135] Low pulmonary compliance in ARDS reduces the transmission of alveolar pressure to both intravascular and cardiac pressures, which inhibits the use of PPV and SVV.[136] Low lung compliance, rather than low tidal volume, appears to affect accuracy of the diagnostic value of PPV.[136,137] Myatra et al.[138] used a "tidal volume challenge" (transiently increased the tidal volume to 8 mL/kg from 6 mL/kg) in ARDS patients and found that an absolute change of PPV greater than or equal to 3.5% and SVV greater than or equal to 2.5% reliably predicted fluid responsiveness.

About 50% of ICU patients develop intra-abdominal hypertension.[139] The complex relationship of the thoracic and abdominal compartments in intra-abdominal hypertension condition limits the accuracy of PPV and SVV.[140] Respiratory variations of SV are not exclusively related to either normovolemia or hypovolemia, and the threshold values distinguishing responders and nonresponders might be higher than under normal intra-abdominal pressure.[141,142]

There is limited literature in patients with decreased ventricular function. In the condition of right HF, the increase in PVR during mechanical ventilation could induce false positives in PPV or SVV.[38] Further studies might be needed to assess the accuracy of using dynamic indices to predict fluid responsiveness in an open-chest setting during cardiothoracic surgery.[143]

Passive Leg Raising

Passive leg raising (PLR) is a provocative test to assess fluid responsiveness. PLR provides an internal translocation of blood from venous compartment of lower limbs and of the abdominal compartment to increase both right and left cardiac preload.[144,145] One meta-analysis examined almost 1000 adults included in 21 studies, and found PLR predicted fluid responsiveness with 85% pooled sensitivity and 91% specificity.[146]

A number of practical techniques are essential to perform PLR. To induce significant changes in right and left cardiac preload, the patient is positioned on the bed with the head of the bed elevated to 45 degrees, then the position of the bed is changed to flat while both legs are raised off the bed to a 45-degree angle.[147] PLR provides a reversible internal fluid challenge of approximately 300 mL of blood from the legs to the central circulation.[148] With positive fluid responsiveness, increased RV preload will result in an

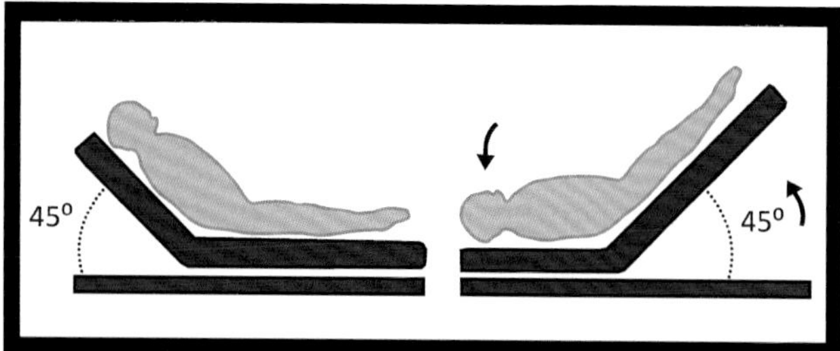

Figure 17-20. Passive Leg Raising. Technique to perform a passive leg raising test. (Created by T. Eric Goffrier.)

increase in LV preload, and if the LV is fluid responsive, SV and CO will increase (Fig. 17-20).

Changes in AP are not reliable assessments of the hemodynamic effects of PLR.[149] The direct measurement of CO is required to assess the effects of PLR.[150] An increase in SV and CO induced by the "internal" preload challenge will occur immediately and reach their maximum within 1 minute after starting the PLR maneuver.[102] The hemodynamic effects will then diminish quickly in some patients, particularly in patients with severe sepsis and capillary leak. An increase of 10% or greater in CO provides the best sensitivity and specificity in assessing fluid responsiveness.[146]

PLR can be repeated as frequently as required without infusing any fluid. Accuracy has been shown in spontaneously breathing patients, and patients with cardiac arrhythmias, low tidal volume ventilation, and low lung compliance.[151,152] In addition, the translocation of blood volume induced by PLR is sufficient to induce a significant increase in perfusion pressure (MAP).[148]

It has been suggested that intra-abdominal hypertension invalidates the PLR test.[153] This is based on the hypothesis that compression of the inferior vena cava (IVC) increases the resistance to venous return; however, only one study has investigated this scenario.[154] Thus, additional studies are required to further investigate this issue.

PLR may be safely performed when a patient's physical condition can tolerate it. In addition, when additional fluid volume may be a concern for patients with certain clinical conditions such as ARDS, PLR does not require fluid administration and is considered a safe maneuver.[155,156]

End-Tidal Carbon Dioxide

Measuring increased end-tidal carbon dioxide ($EtCO_2$) induced by PLR is the original noninvasive method to assess fluid responsiveness.[157–159] Exhaled CO_2 is determined by the production of CO_2 by cell metabolism, the pulmonary flow (venous return, essentially equivalent to CO) that transports CO_2 from periphery to the lungs, and minute ventilation of the pulmonary system to clear the venous blood of CO_2.[160] Based on this reasoning, if cell metabolism is stable and ventilation is unaltered, changes of $EtCO_2$ are only related to changes in CO, and could be used as a noninvasive tool for monitoring CI.

A PLR-induced increase in $EtCO_2$ greater than or equal to 5% and improved SV for more than 15% predicted fluid responsiveness.[156] In addition, in patients with acute circulatory failure on mechanical ventilation, it was found that an increase greater than or equal to 5% in $EtCO_2$ or greater than or equal to 12% in CO during PLR predicted fluid responsiveness with a sensitivity of 90.5%.[158] Xiao-Ting et al.[161] discovered that changes in $EtCO_2$ are not reliable detectors in changes of CO during a mini-fluid challenge with 100 mL of saline, while other studies used 500 mL of fluid as a bolus. Thus, it is important to consider the amount of fluid used in volume expansion, and risk and benefits based on a patient's clinical conditions.

Valsalva Maneuver

Valsalva maneuver is another noninvasive technique that can be performed in spontaneously breathing patients to assess fluid responsiveness. The underlying physiologic concept of maintaining a forced expiratory effort against a closed glottis has been used for decades in assessing volume status in HF patients.[162] Garcia et al.[163] found that a 10-second Valsalva maneuver was a feasible and useful test to predict fluid responsiveness.

Other Tests Using Heart–Lung Interactions

A PEEP challenge (increase PEEP from 5 to 10 cm H_2O within 1 minute) was performed in 52 patients undergoing cardiac surgery based on the theory that PEEP induced changes in pulmonary elimination of carbon dioxide (VCO_2). During the PEEP challenge, a decrease in VCO_2 by 11% predicted fluid responsiveness with a sensitivity of 90% and specificity of 95%.[164]

Respiratory systolic variation test (RSVT) is used to assess fluid responsiveness; its advantage is its independence of tidal volume. RSVT delivers three consecutive mechanical breaths of incremental peak inspiratory pressures of 10, 20, and 30 cm H_2O. The respiratory maneuver produces sequential incremental challenge to LV filling. The lowest values of the systolic AP following these three breaths are measured individually and plotted against their corresponding airway pressures, producing the RSVT slope that is the estimate of the slope of the Frank–Starling curve. An increase of more than 15% in SV is considered fluid responsiveness.[165] Some ventilators are now able to perform the RSVT test automatically.[166]

LESS INVASIVE METHODS FOR HEMODYNAMIC EVALUATION

Esophageal Doppler

Esophageal Doppler is a less invasive option than a PAC. A Doppler probe is placed in the esophagus that intermittently measures the flow in the thoracic aorta. The measurement of aortic blood velocity and aortic root cross-sectional area by echocardiogram yields SV. Other hemodynamic variables, such as CO, preload, afterload, and contractility, can then be calculated by interpreting the esophageal Doppler monitor (EDM) waveform. Esophageal Doppler requires continual esophageal placement to optimize the hands-on signal. The correct position of Doppler probe, held over the root of aorta, requires a skilled operator to minimize bias (Fig. 17-21).[170]

Echocardiography

Echocardiography is the most frequently used evaluation tool for cardiac function. It provides information about underlying etiology of clinical conditions such as low CO, hypotension, hypoperfusion, and lactatemia.[171] In addition, echocardiography provides information about estimate of intracardiac pressures, ventricular systolic and diastolic function, preload, and wall motion abnormalities.[172] There are two principle modes of echocardiography: transthoracic (TTE) and transesophageal echocardiography

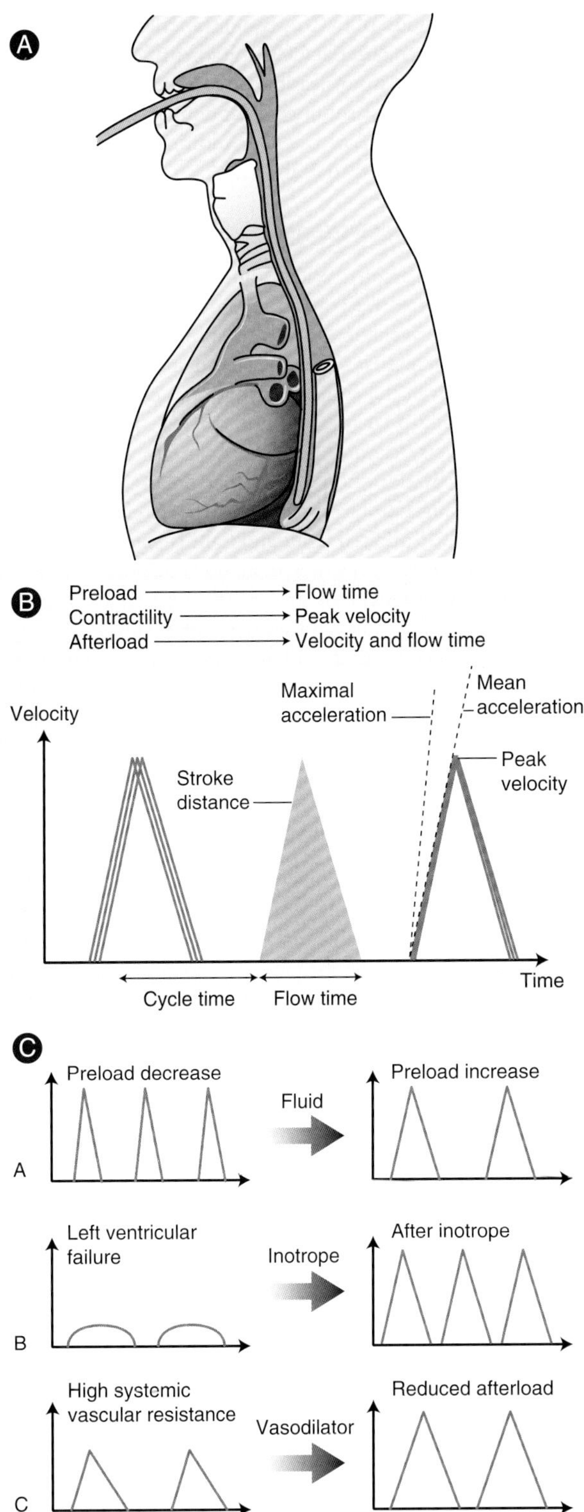

Figure 17-21. (A) Correct Positioning of the Esophageal Doppler Probe. (Reproduced courtesy of Deltex Medical.) (**B**) Doppler flow velocity waveform. (**C**) EDM waveforms. The first graph shows the components of the normal Doppler waveform and the effect of increasing preload, which corresponds to an increased FT_c. The second graph displays poor contractility (decreased PV), which responds to inotropes by increasing PV. The last graph displays increased afterload (decreased FT_c and decreased PV) and the effects of afterload reduction (increased FT_c and increased PV).
(Gan T. The esophageal Doppler as an alternative to the pulmonary artery catheter. *Curr Opin Crit Care.* 2000;6:214–221.)

(TEE). TTE can be challenging when evaluating RV function; the retrosternal position of the RV limits a direct view.[173] While more invasive than TTE, TEE is more accurate than PA catheter–derived diagnosis.[174,175] Expansive discussion on echocardiography may be found elsewhere in this text.

Collapsibility Index

Collapsibility index is a measurement based on the appearance of IVC or SVC. A compliant vessel will respond to a slight increase in CVP by demonstrating a marked increase in IVC diameter.[176] A poor compliant vessel would do the opposite: an increased CVP is unable to dilate the vessel. These two scenarios indicate a patient with a preload reserve versus no preload reserve. Muller et al.[177] found that in spontaneous breathing patients with acute circulatory failure, an IVC collapsibility index of 40% or greater was associated with fluid responsiveness; however, a low value of less than 40% did not exclude volume responsiveness. This finding was in agreement with a previous study conducted by Brennan et al.[178]

Bioreactance Technology

Bioreactance technology is a noninvasive technology to assess fluid responsiveness. The basis of the technology is the use of time delay, also known as phase shift, which occurs when an alternating electrical current passes through the thorax. The phase shift is then used as baseline for SV measurement. To determine fluid responsiveness or volume status, a fluid bolus is given (or using PLR). If the heart is volume responsive, a great outflow will be observed, and it creates a large time delay. Consequently, there is an increased SV.[179] An increase in SV by 10% or greater is considered fluid responsive. This technology has been validated by multiple studies.[180–183] To assess the reliability of bioreactance technology, Marik et al.[181] used PLR which validated the technology with 95% sensitivity and 100% specificity. Rich et al.[184] measured CO using three different methods (Fick, thermodilution, and NICOM™, a bioreactance-based noninvasive CO monitor). In patients undergoing vasodilation challenge, they found bioreactance technology performed with more precision (p <0.001, N = 20). A retrospective cohort study conducted by Latham et al.[185] examined whether SV-guided resuscitation (using bioreactance technology) improved outcomes in patients with severe sepsis and septic shock. The investigators found that SV-guided resuscitation was associated with decreased hypervolemia and improved secondary outcomes.

Noninvasive Finger Cuff

Noninvasive finger cuff technology was first discovered in 1967.[186] The technology provides continuous arterial BP monitoring, and it can be used in all patient care areas. Finger cuff uses infrared photoplethysmography to determine vessel size and blood volume. Depending on the different technologies used, an external measurement as a counterpressure may be required for calibration, and an appropriate algorithm is used to determine SV and CO.[186]

The ClearSight system is a finger cuff developed by Edwards Lifesciences using Nexfin noninvasive technology, which has been validated against other reference standard technologies (thermodilution CO and pulse contour CO).[187] The Nexfin technology is based on two methods: continuous measurement of BP using the volume clamp method, and initial and frequent calibration using the Physiocal method. The volume clamp method involves clamping an artery to a constant volume by dynamically providing equal pressure on either side of the arterial wall.[188] An inflatable bladder built inside the cuff provides a counterpressure to keep arterial volume constant. The blood volume is measured using photoplethysmography. Physiocal method provides automatic and periodic calibration by analyzing the curvature and sharpness of the plethysmogram during short episodes of constant pressure levels. Continuous monitoring using one cuff on one finger is limited to 8 hours. Two cuffs can be used on two different fingers for more than 8 hours of monitoring.[188] In addition to continuous BP monitoring, the ClearSight system provides hemodynamic parameters such as SV, SVV, CO, and SVR.[189,190]

CNAP® (Continuous Noninvasive Arterial Pressure) provides beat-to-beat continuous arterial BP monitoring. CNAP monitor uses an intelligent transfer function to continuously scale the measurements from an upper arm cuff to finger BP to receive absolute values.[191] CNAP® Monitor 500 HD is another model using the same technology which can provide basic CO measurement using pulse contour analysis.[192]

TISSUE PERFUSION MONITORING

Information derived from tissue or peripheral perfusion monitoring devices guides resuscitation to augment hemodynamics and oxygenation. The goal for treating shock or underperfusion is to restore the oxygen delivery to the cells to meet metabolic demand. Under the condition of hypoperfusion and shock, the body will shunt blood away from peripheral and splanchnic tissue (less vital areas) to perfuse vital organs (primarily the brain and heart). In shock, there tends to be a large portion of damage done before it is recognized. It is known that despite normal global oxygen delivery value, regional tissue hypoperfusion still exists.[193,194] Microcirculation dysfunction may lead to multiorgan dysfunction; subsequently, microcirculation hypoperfusion is a major source of pathogenesis in multiorgan dysfunction.[195]

Traditional clinical markers are insensitive in assessing tissue hypoperfusion and have their limitations. The regional markers will reflect the perfusion and oxygenation abnormalities and can be monitored continuously.[196,197] Resuscitation efforts guided by physiologic regional markers help determine the success of therapeutic interventions.[198] Persistent microvascular alterations are associated with increased morbidity and mortality.[199] Vellinga et al.[200] suggested that microcirculation monitoring can potentially be a clinically significant extension to traditional hemodynamic monitoring.

Given the limitations of global hemodynamic parameters for assessment of gastric perfusion or ischemia, CO_2 gastric tonometry emerged to study alteration of gut perfusion by examining the pH of the stomach.[201] The technology was found to be too challenging to perform at the bedside and affected by many factors.[202] The sublingual mucosa was considered as an alternative to assess the adequacy of mucosal blood flow; it was found that PCO_2 (partial pressure of carbon dioxide) gained from the sublingual region and the stomach was interchangeable.[203,204]

Sublingual Capnometry

The sublingual capnometry device uses a fiberoptic probe and a disposable sensor placed in direct contact with sublingual mucosa inside the sublingual pocket. An electronic computer device then analyzes the sublingual CO_2 concentration ($PslCO_2$).[205,206] With tissue hypoperfusion, an increase in venous blood PCO_2 results in a decreased venous pH. Consequently, there is an increase in PCO_2 and the venoarterial PCO_2 gradient.[207,208] Continuous monitoring of $PslCO_2$ is not feasible due to the required position of the probe. Thus, most sublingual capnometry devices provide intermittent measurement of $PslCO_2$. Additionally, some clinical conditions limit the access to oral cavity.[209–211]

Near-Infrared Spectroscopy

Near-infrared spectroscopy (NIS) is one of the noninvasive techniques using spectroscopy measurement and sensor to assess end-organ tissue oxygenation (StO_2). Noninvasive pulse oximetry has been routinely used to measure hemoglobin saturation and assess oxygenation in the clinical setting for decades. Pulse oximetry is traditionally used to assess the oxygen saturation. However, pulse oximetry cannot assess StO_2 due to the attenuation of infrared light by skin, bone, and other organs. NIS is able to measure StO_2 using a probe placed on the thenar eminence or deltoid that emits near-infrared light, and light is passed through the tissue between probes. NIS uses light transmission and absorption to measure hemoglobin and mitochondrial oxygenation. Mitochondrial dysfunction can lead to cellular damage and organ failure.[212,213] Numerous studies demonstrated promising predictability of NIS measurement of StO_2, the accurate relationship to $ScvO_2/SvO_2$, and 28-day mortality. However, NIS remains to be a developing technology, and larger and highly powered studies are needed to examine clinical applications of NIS.

Sidestream Dark Field Imagery

Sidestream dark field (SDF) imagery is another noninvasive technology to measure StO_2 using sublingual photometry. The SDF probe covered with disposable cap is put directly in contact with the tissue surface.[214] The probe emits stroboscopic lights that are absorbed by hemoglobin, allowing visualization of blood vessels and microcirculation. SDF has been studied in patients with hemorrhage shock, septic shock, and postcardiac arrest.[214,215]

IMPLANTABLE PA PRESSURE MONITORING

Implantable PA pressure monitoring devices enable remote PA pressure monitoring, largely used in HF patients. Changes in PA pressure are detected and interventions may be made. Providers may use this advanced technology in conjunction with goal-directed medical therapy to decrease mortality, HF hospitalizations and readmissions, and improve quality of life.[216,217]

CardioMEMS™ HF system is the first and only FDA-approved, fully wireless, implantable HF monitoring device that monitors PAS, PAD, and mean PAP.[218] CardioMEMS HF system uses a sensor that is implanted in the PA to monitor patient's PAP and HR. Daily pressure readings are transmitted wireless to the providers. CardioMEMS will not interfere with a patient's daily activities or other devices such as a pacemaker or defibrillator.[219]

A randomized, controlled, single-blind study conducted by Costanzo et al.[220] included 550 patients with New York Heart Association function class III HF and a history of HF hospitalization in the prior year. This study found that incorporation of a PA pressure–guided treatment algorithm resulted in more frequent adjustment of plan of care for HF patients, particularly in diuretics and vasodilation management. The study showed that CardioMEMS was effective in better managing HF patients with a 33% overall reduction in HF hospitalization, and 50% reduction in hospitalization for HF patients with reserved ejection fraction over an average of 18 months.[221,222]

CONCLUSION

The technologies used in hemodynamic monitoring continue to evolve. Both invasive and less invasive devices provide valuable diagnostic data in managing critically ill patients (Table 17-7). Despite the decreased use of the once ubiquitous PAC, clinician education and training remains paramount to ensure the quality of care and to decrease potential risks and complications. It is expected that future further development of software and refining of the algorithms used will enhance reliability of the different noninvasive systems, particularly in noninvasive continuous arterial BP monitoring. Critical care clinicians should understand that both invasive and less invasive hemodynamic technologies provide diagnostic information but are not therapeutic interventions. Accurate acquisition and interpretation of hemodynamic parameters is key to guiding the initiation of therapeutic interventions and the continuous management of critically ill patients.

Table 17-7 • HEMODYNAMIC INDICES

Indices/Equations	Normal Values	Interpretation
Preload		
RAP or CVP	2–6 mm Hg	RV filling pressure—does not predict fluid responsiveness
PAEDP	8–12 mm Hg	Indirect indicator of LV filling pressure and capillary filling pressure (P_{cap})
PAOP	6–12 mm Hg	Indirect indicator of LV filling pressure and capillary filling pressure (P_{cap})—does not predict fluid responsiveness
Afterload		
SBP	120 mm Hg	Clinical indicator of pressure that must be overcome during ejection phase of cardiac cycle
SVR	800–1200 dynes/s/cm^{-5}	Measure of systemic vascular tone (one factor that affects cardiac afterload, but it is not synonymous with afterload; increased SVR manifested by increased MAP)
SVRI	1900–2400 dynes/s/cm^{-5}/m^2	SVR indexed to BSA
PVR	70–80 dynes/s/cm^{-5} or 1 Wood unit	Measure of resistance to RV ejection
Force of Contraction		
SV	60–180 mL/beat	Amount of blood ejected during each ventricular contraction
Stroke volume index	33–47 mL/beat/m^2	SVR indexed to BSA
RV stroke work index (RVSWI) RVSWI = SVI(MAP – CVP) × 0.0136	5–10 g-m/m^2/beat	Work performed by the RV to eject blood into the pulmonary vasculature. Stroke work determines the energy expenditure (oxygen consumption) of the heart
Left ventricular stroke work index (LVSWI) LVSWI = SVI(MAP – PAOP) × 0.0136	45–65 g · m/m^2/beat	Work performed by the LV to eject blood into the aorta. The factor 0.0136 is used to convert pressure and volume to units of work With high filling pressures or hypotension, this equation may underestimate the amount of work performed
RAP variation (ΔRAP)	ΔRAP >1	Spontaneous inspiratory decrease in RAP >1 mm Hg (on or off the ventilator) predictive of volume response
SPV	≥7–10 mm Hg depending on VT	With VT >8 mL/kg, an SPV >10 mm Hg indicates fluid responsiveness. Unpublished animal research (VT = 8 mL/kg) identified an SPV ≥7 mm Hg as predictive of fluid responsiveness (sensitivity = 0.74, specificity = 0.71, AUC = 0.75).[94] Increased ΔSPV associated with in ΔCI for any given volume infused Patient must be on mechanical ventilation with minimal spontaneous ventilation and stable VT
SPV%	>10% predictive in one study	Unpublished animal research (VT = 8 mL/kg) identified an SPV% >7% as predictive of fluid responsiveness (sensitivity = 0.75, specificity = 0.69, AUC = 0.8) May be artificially increased with severe hypotension Patient must be on mechanical ventilation with minimal spontaneous ventilation and stable VT
PPV%	PPV >12% (VT >8 mL/kg)	Affected only by change in SV (assuming arterial resistance and compliance do not acutely change during a single breath)
	PPV >10% (VT = 8 mL/kg)	May be a more reliable indicator than SPV or SPV% May be artificially increased with severe hypotension
	PPV ≥8% (VT <8 mL/kg	Patient must be on mechanical ventilation with minimal spontaneous ventilation and stable VT
SVV%	>10% (VT = 10 mL/kg)	Requires proprietary technology Patient must be on mechanical ventilation with minimal spontaneous ventilation and stable VT No studies at lower VT
PVI	>14% (VT 8–10 mL/kg)	Only one study describing thresholds. Further research required in unstable patients and patients with changing vascular tone

BSA, body surface area.

CASE STUDY 1

Patient Profile

Mr. Smith is a 48-year-old male under the care of a primary care physician and cardiologist. He was admitted to the Cardiology Medicine Unit after a follow-up appointment for 3 days of increased shortness of breath and notable mild lower extremity edema. Mr. Smith stated that he gained 3 kg (6.6 lb) over 3 days and "slept in my recliner to get better rest."

Current Medical Diagnoses

- Hyperlipidemia
- Hypertension
- Dilated cardiomyopathy
- Chronic Obstructive Pulmonary Disease

Medical History

- Frequent admission to hospital due to decompensated heart failure
- Occasional high dietary sodium intake multiple occasions within the last week
- Recent cardiac catheterization (performed within the last year) demonstrated no evidence of obstructive coronary artery disease

Allergies

- No known allergies

Social History

- Alcohol use: 1–2 glasses of wine every week
- Smoking: never
- Diet: low sodium diet recommended, "But sometimes I cannot help it" per Mr. Smith
- Exercise: basic ADLs
- Occupation: Uber driver

Current Home Medications

- Furosemide 20-mg tablet, 1 tablet by mouth daily
- Lisinopril 10-mg tablet, 1 tablet by mouth daily
- Metoprolol tartrate 100-mg tablet, 1 tablet by mouth daily
- Simvastatin 40-mg tablet, 1 tablet by mouth at night

Physical Examination

Weight: 202 lb

Height: 5 ft 8 in

BP: 140/68 mm Hg

MAP: 92

HR: 110–120 bpm

Respiration: 24 breaths/min

Temperature: 37.5°C

O_2 Sat: 92% on 2 L O_2

Heart sounds revealed audible S_3

Lung sounds revealed bibasilar crackles

Admission Laboratory Data

NA^+: 132 mmol/L

K^+: 4.3 mmol/L

Hgb: 14.5 g/dL

Hct: 46%

Cl^-: 105 mmol/L

BUN: 24 mg/dL

Creatinine: 1.7 mg/dL

Diagnostics

- Admission ECG showed sinus tachycardia. No Q wave, ST segment, or T-wave changes
- Chest x-ray showed mildly increased pulmonary vasculature
- Left ventricular ejection fraction 32% via echocardiogram within the last year

100-mg IV furosemide (Lasix) was ordered STAT. An order for right heart catheterization for potential leave-in PAC was placed to examine hemodynamic parameters.

After receiving 100-mg IV furosemide, Mr. Smith was sent to cardiac catheterization laboratory. Right heart catheterization revealed the following:

CVP: 16 cm H_2O

PAP: 55/22 mm Hg

CO: 4 L/min

CI: 1.9 L/min/m^2

SVR: 2200 dynes/s/cm^{-5}

Svo_2: 58%

Upon transferring to Cardiac Care Unit (CCU) with a "leave-in" PAC, additional 200-mg IV furosemide (Lasix) and dobutamine drip at 2 mcg/kg/min were ordered. After administration of furosemide and dobutamine drip was started, Mr. Smith demonstrated significant improvement in hemodynamic parameters and increased urine output. Mr. Smith stated, "I feel like I am getting more air."

Hemodynamic data revealed the following:

CVP: 10 cm H_2O

PAP: 32/10 mm Hg

CO: 5.5 L/min

CI: 2.62 L/min/m^2

SVR: 1300 dynes/s/com^{-5}

Svo_2: 68%

Take-Home Points

- CVP measures the pressure of the RA and it reflects the pressure of right side of the heart. Right ventricular failure and fluid overload result in an increase in CVP.
- PAP is the pulmonary pressure in the pulmonary bed. The elevated PAP was due to volume overload in the pulmonary system.
- CI is the CO indexed to BSA, which provides realistic indicator of cardiac function.
- SVR measures the afterload of left side of the heart. Mr. Smith's initial elevated SVR was probably due to compensatory mechanism for decreased CO.
- A decreased SvO_2 was due to a decreased CO based on this equation:

$$SvO_2 = SaO_2 - \left(\frac{VO_2}{CO} \times 1.36 \times Hgb\right)$$

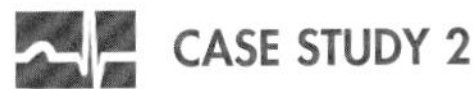

CASE STUDY 2

Patient Profile

Mrs. Burke, a 65-year-old female, came to the emergency room because she had been experiencing some difficulty of breathing since last Thursday. This morning, Mrs. Burke felt her cough was getting worse. She coughed out some sputum several times today which was "more than I have coughed out." Mrs. Burke said that she'd had chest colds in the past, but this time she just cannot seem to be able to "shake this off." Today she was feeling "weaker" and "so cold in the house."

History
- Urinary tract infection 6 months ago

Allergy
- Shellfish

Social History
- Alcohol use: 1 glass of wine every evening with dinner
- Smoking: 1–2 packs of cigarettes a week for 20 years
- Diet: no restriction, tries to eat more lean meat
- Exercise: tries to take a walk 2 or 3 times a week in the evening with husband
- Occupation: retired librarian

Current Medical Diagnoses
- Hyperlipidemia
- Hypertension
- Gastroesophageal reflux disease (GERD)

Current Home Medications
- Lisinopril 10-mg tablet, 1 tablet by mouth daily
- Simvastatin 40-mg tablet, 1 tablet by mouth at night
- Fish oil, 1 tablet by mouth daily
- Multivitamin, 1 tablet by mouth daily

Physical Examination

Weight: 130 lb

Height: 5 ft 2 in

BP: 94/40 mm Hg

MAP: 58

HR: 110 bpm

Respiration: 18 breaths/min

Temperature: 38.8°C

O_2 Sat: 90% placed on 3L O_2

Heart sounds: S_1, S_2

Lung sounds revealed crackles in the lower base with expiratory wheezes.

Mrs. Burke appeared to be very drowsy. Husband said, "That was what she looked like when she had a UTI in January!"

Admission Laboratory Data

NA^+: 138 mmol/L

K^+: 4.0 mmol/L

Hgb: 15.5 g/dL

Hct: 42%

Cl^-: 105 mmol/L

BUN: 22 mg/dL

Creatinine: 1.5 mg/d:

WBC: 22,000/mm^3

Diagnostics
- Chest x-ray showed some consolidation in the right lower lobe

Treatment
- Blood culture was sent
- Broad-spectrum antibiotics was started
- Total of 2 L of lactated Ringer was given

Repeated Vital Signs

BP: 94/46 mm Hg

MAP: 62

HR: 110 bpm

Respiration: 22 breaths/min

O_2 Sat: 85%, now Mrs. Burke was put on 45% oxygen with Venturi mask

Temp: 38.5°C

Mrs. Burke now appeared to be lethargic, and physical stimulation barely kept her awake.

ABG Results

(20 minutes after placement of Venturi mask)

pH: 7.40

PCO_2: 50 mm Hg

PO_2: 57 mm Hg

HCO_3^-: 29 mmol/L

Lactate: 4.5 mmol/L

Repeat Vital Signs

(After another liter of lactated Ringer)

BP: 83/42 mm Hg

MAP: 55

HR: 112 bpm

Respiration: 16 breaths/min

O_2 Sat: 90%

Temp: 38.2°C

Lactate: 3.4 mmol/L

Now the team is debating what the next step is for Mrs. Burke: more IV fluid or start a pressor?

After much discussion, the team decided to use noninvasive hemodynamic system to evaluate Mrs. Burke's SV changes with a passive leg raising test. SV was increased by 12%, which means Mrs. Burke was fluid responsive. Additional 1 L of lactated Ringer was given.

Take-Home Points
- Mrs. Burke demonstrated signs of pneumonia, possibly sepsis. According to Surviving Sepsis Campaign guidelines (2018), fluid and antibiotics are priorities for the plan of care.[82]
- It is important to ask whether fluid or pressor is needed for the patient, due to potential complications associated with volume overload.
- Lactated Ringer is one of the recommended volume expanders, as hyperchloremia with overuse of sodium chloride is associated with decreased renal blood flow and glomerular filtration.[167]
- In sepsis, hyperchloremia is independently associated with all-cause hospital mortality.[168,169]
- Noninvasive hemodynamic technology may provide crucial diagnostic values.

KEY READINGS

Lough ME, ed. *Hemodynamic Monitoring: Evolving Technologies and Clinical Practice.* 1st ed. St. Louis, Missouri: Mosby; 2015.

Marik PE, Linde-Zwirble WT, Bittner EA, et al. Fluid administration in severe sepsis and septic shock, patterns and outcomes: an analysis of a large national database. *Intensive Care Med.* 2017;43(5):625–632.

Stouffer GA, ed. *Cardiovascular Hemodynamics for the Clinician.* 2nd ed. Chichester, West Sussex; Hoboken, NJ: Wiley-Blackwell; 2017.

Truijen J, van Lieshout JJ, Wesselink WA, et al. Noninvasive continuous hemodynamic monitoring. *J Clin Monit Comput.* 2012;26(4): 267–278.

REFERENCES

1. Bridges EJ. Hemodynamic monitoring. In: Woods SL, Froelicher ESS, Motzer SUM, et al., eds. *Cardiac Nursing.* 6th ed. Philadelphia, PA: LWW; 2009:460–492.
2. O'Grady NP, Alexander M, Burns LA, et al. Guidelines for the prevention of intravascular catheter-related infections. *Clin Infect Dis.* 2011;52(9):e162–e193.
3. Gershengorn HB, Garland A, Kramer A, et al. Variation of arterial and central venous catheter use in United States intensive care units. *Anesthesiology.* 2014;120(3):650–664.
4. Headley JM. Arterial waveform and pressure-based hemodynamic monitoring. In: Lough ME, ed. *Hemodynamic Monitoring: Evolving Technologies and Clinical Practice.* 1st ed. St. Louis, Missouri: Mosby; 2015:341–369.
5. Ribatti D. William Harvey and the discovery of the circulation of the blood. *J Angiogenes Res.* 2009;1:3.
6. Mohrman DE, Heller LJ. The heart pump. In: *Cardiovascular Physiology.* 9th ed. United States: McGraw-Hill Education/Medical; 2018.
7. Lough ME. Physiologic principle of hemodynamic monitoring. In: Lough ME, ed. *Hemodynamic Monitoring: Evolving Technologies and Clinical Practice.* 1st ed. St. Louis, Missouri: Mosby; 2015:1–31.
8. Klabunde RE. Cardiac function. In: *Cardiovascular Physiology Concepts.* 2nd ed. Philadelphia, PA: LWW; 2011:60–92.
9. Bridges EM, Middleton R. Direct arterial vs oscillometric monitoring of blood pressure: stop comparing and pick one (a decision-making algorithm). *Crit Care Nurse.* 1997;17(3):58–66, 68–72.
10. Courtois M, Fattal PG, Kovács SJ, et al. Anatomically and physiologically based reference level for measurement of intracardiac pressures. *Circulation.* 1995;92(7):1994–2000.
11. McCann UG, Schiller HJ, Carney DE, et al. Invasive arterial BP monitoring in trauma and critical care. *Chest.* 2001;120(4):1322–1326.
12. Lough ME. Arterial pressure monitoring. In: Lough ME, ed. *Hemodynamic Monitoring: Evolving Technologies and Clinical Practice.* 1st ed. St. Louis, Missouri: Mosby; 2015:55–86.
13. Rosario JJ, Salgado A. Pulmonary artery pressure and thermodilution cardiac output monitoring. In: Lough ME, ed. *Hemodynamic Monitoring: Evolving Technologies and Clinical Practice.* 1st ed. St. Louis, Missouri: Mosby; 2015:115–144.
14. Bridges E. Pulmonary artery/central venous pressure monitoring in adults. *Critical Care Nurse.* 2016;36(4):e12–e18.
15. Hering R, Wrigge H, Vorwerk R, et al. The effects of prone positioning on intraabdominal pressure and cardiovascular and renal function in patients with acute lung injury. *Anesth Analg.* 2001;92(6):1226–1231.
16. Jacq G, Gritti K, Carré C, et al. Modalities of invasive arterial pressure monitoring in critically ill patients. *Medicine (Baltimore).* 2015;94(39):e1557.
17. Zellinger M. Hemodynamic monitoring. In: Hardin SR, Kaplow R, eds. *Cardiac Surgery Essentials for Critical Care Nursing.* 2nd ed. Burlington, MA: Jones & Bartlett Learning; 2015:141–164.
18. Bridges EJ. Pulmonary artery pressure monitoring: when, how, and what else to use. *AACN Advanced Critical Care.* 2006;17(3):286–305.
19. Fujiwara S, Tachihara K, Mori S, et al. Effect of using a PlanectaTM port with a three-way stopcock on the natural frequency of blood pressure transducer kits. *J Clin Monit Comput.* 2016;30(6):925–931.
20. Melamed R, Johnson K, Pothen B, et al. Invasive blood pressure monitoring systems in the ICU: influence of the blood-conserving device on the dynamic response characteristics and agreement with noninvasive measurements. *Blood Press Monit.* 2012;17(5):179–183.
21. Crumlett H, Johnson A. Blood sampling from an arterial catheter. In: Wiegand DL, ed. *AACN Procedure Manual for High Acuity, Progressive, and Critical Care.* 2016:530–539.
22. Centers for Disease Control and Prevention (CDC). *Intravascular Catheter-related Infection (BSI) Guidelines for the Prevention of Intravascular Catheter-Related Infections (2011).* Available at cdc.gov/infectioncontrol/guidelines/bsi/. Accessed April 2, 2019.
23. Gowardman JR, Lipman J, Rickard CM. Assessment of peripheral arterial catheters as a source of sepsis in the critically ill: a narrative review. *J Hosp Infect.* 2010;75(1):12–18.
24. Darovic GO. Pulmonary artery pressure monitoring. In: Darovic GO, ed. *Hemodynamic Monitoring: Invasive and Noninvasive Clinical Application.* 3rd ed. Philadelphia, PA: W.B. Saunders Co.; 2002.
25. Gu WJ, Tie HT, Liu JC, et al. Efficacy of ultrasound-guided radial artery catheterization: a systematic review and meta-analysis of randomized controlled trials. *Crit Care.* 2014;18(3):R93.
26. Hambsch ZJ, Kerfeld MJ, Kirkpatrick DR, et al. Arterial catheterization and infection: toll-like receptors in defense against microorganisms and therapeutic Implications: TLRs in arterial catheterization. *Clin Transl Sci.* 2015;8(6):857–870.
27. Scheer BV, Perel A, Pfeiffer UJ. Clinical review: complications and risk factors of peripheral arterial catheters used for haemodynamic monitoring in anaesthesia and intensive care medicine. *Crit Care.* 2002;6(3):199–204.
28. Brzezinski M, Luisetti T, London MJ. Radial artery cannulation: a comprehensive review of recent anatomic and physiologic investigations. *Anesth Analg.* 2009;109(6):1763–1781.
29. Abu-Omar Y, Mussa S, Anastasiadis K, et al. Duplex ultrasonography predicts safety of radial artery harvest in the presence of an abnormal Allen test. *Ann Thorac Surg.* 2004;77(1):116–119.
30. Asif M, Sarkar PK. Three-digit Allen's test. *Ann Thorac Surg.* 2007;84(2):686–687.
31. Ruengsakulrach P, Brooks M, Hare DL, et al. Preoperative assessment of hand circulation by means of Doppler ultrasonography and the modified Allen test. *J Thorac Cardiovasc Surg.* 2001;121(3):526–531.
32. Klabunde RE. Vascular function. In: Taylor C, ed. *Cardiovascular Physiology Concepts.* 2nd ed. Baltimore, MD: LWW; 2011:93–123.
33. Goda TS, Kaplow R. Postoperative complications of cardiac surgery and nursing interventions. In: Hardin SR, Kaplow R, eds. *Cardiac Surgery Essentials for Critical Care Nursing.* 2nd ed. Burlington, MA: Jones & Bartlett Learning; 2015.
34. Stouffer GA. Arterial pressure. In: Stouffer GA, ed. *Cardiovascular Hemodynamics for the Clinician.* 2nd ed. Chichester, West Sussex; Hoboken, NJ: Wiley-Blackwell; 2017:56–68.
35. Prospective Studies Collaboration. Age-specific relevance of usual blood pressure to vascular mortality: a meta-analysis of individual data for one million adults in 61 prospective studies. *Lancet.* 2002;360(9349):1903–1913.
36. Peterson KJ. Measuring central venous pressure with a triple-lumen catheter. *Critical Care Nurse.* 2012;32(3):62–64.
37. Black IH, Blosser SA, Murray WB. Central venous pressure measurements: peripherally inserted catheters versus centrally inserted catheters. *Crit Care Med.* 2000;28(12):3833–3836.
38. Monnet X, Marik PE, Teboul JL. Prediction of fluid responsiveness: an update. *Ann Intensive Care.* 2016;6:111.
39. Legrand M, Dupuis C, Simon C, et al. Association between systemic hemodynamics and septic acute kidney injury in critically ill patients: a retrospective observational study. *Crit Care.* 2013;17(6):R278.
40. Chen D, Pai PY. Cannon a wave. *Circulation.* 2009;119(13):e381–e383.
41. Keenon A, Crouch ED, Faber JE, et al. Normal hemodynamics. In: Stouffer GA, ed. *Cardiovascular Hemodynamics for the Clinician.* 2nd ed. Hoboken, NJ: Wiley-Blackwell; 2017:37–55.
42. Rajaram SS, Desai NK, Kalra A, et al. Pulmonary artery catheters for adult patients in intensive care. *Cochrane Database Syst Rev.* 2013(2):CD003408.
43. Sotomi Y, Sato N, Kajimoto K, et al. Impact of pulmonary artery catheter on outcome in patients with acute heart failure syndromes with hypotension or receiving inotropes: from the ATTEND Registry. *Int J Cardiol.* 2014;172(1):165–172.
44. Friese RS, Shafi S, Gentilello LM. Pulmonary artery catheter use is associated with reduced mortality in severely injured patients: a national trauma data bank analysis of 53,312 patients: *Crit Care Med.* 2006;34(6):1597–1601.
45. The ProCESS Investigators; Yealy DM, Kellum JA, Huang DT, et al. A randomized trial of protocol-based care for early septic shock. *N Engl J Med.* 2014;370(18):1683–1693.
46. The ARISE Investigators; ANZICS Clinical Trials Group; Peake SL, Delaney A, Bailey M, et al. Goal-directed resuscitation for patients with early septic shock. *N Engl J Med.* 2014;371(16):1496–1506.

47. Mouncey PR, Osborn TM, Power GS, et al. Trial of early, goal-directed resuscitation for septic shock. *N Engl J Med*. 2015;372(14):1301–1311.
48. Vickie S, Stouffer GA. The nuts and bolts of right heart catheterization and PA catheter placement. In: Stouffer GA, ed. *Cardiovascular Hemodynamics for the Clinician*. 2nd ed. Chichester, West Sussex; Hoboken, NJ: Wiley-Blackwell; 2017:17–36.
49. Oakes DF. *Oakes' Hemodynamic Monitoring: A Bedside Reference Manual*. 2010 edition. Orono, ME: Health Educator Publications; 2009.
50. Weinhouse GL. *Pulmonary artery catheterization: Indications, contraindications, and complications in adults*. In: UpToDate. Available at https://www.uptodate.com/contents/pulmonary-artery-catheterization-indications-contraindications-and-complications-in-adults. Accessed June 2, 2018.
51. Hayashi H, Abe Y, Morita Y, et al. The accuracy of a large V wave in the pulmonary capillary wedge pressure waveform for diagnosing current mitral regurgitation. *Cardiology*. 2018;141(1):46–51.
52. Iskandrian AS, Segal BL, Hakki AH. Left ventricular end-diastolic pressure in evaluating left ventricular function. *Clin Cardiol*. 1981;4(1):28–33.
53. Roberson RS. Respiratory variation and cardiopulmonary interactions. *Best Pract Res Clin Anaesthesiol*. 2014;28(4):407–418.
54. Nahouraii RA, Rowell SE. Static measures of preload assessment. *Crit Care Clin*. 2010;26(2):295–305.
55. Johnson MK, Schumann L. Comparison of three methods of measurement of pulmonary artery catheter readings in critically ill patients. *Am J Crit Care*. 1995;4(4):300–307.
56. Ahrens TS, Schallom L. Comparison of pulmonary artery and central venous pressure waveform measurements via digital and graphic measurement methods. *Heart Lung*. 2001;30(1):26–38.
57. Tuggle D. Central venous pressure monitoring. In: Lough ME, ed. *Hemodynamic Monitoring: Evolving Technologies and Clinical Practice*. 1st ed. St. Louis, Missouri: Mosby; 2015:89–111.
58. Magder S. Hemodynamic monitoring in the mechanically ventilated patient. *Curr Opin Crit Care*. 2011;17(1):36–42.
59. Hoyt JD, Leatherman JW. Interpretation of the pulmonary artery occlusion pressure in mechanically ventilated patients with large respiratory excursions in intrathoracic pressure. *Intens Care Med*. 1997;23(11):1125–1131.
60. Boerrigter BG, Waxman AB, Westerhof N, et al. Measuring central pulmonary pressures during exercise in COPD: how to cope with respiratory effects. *Eur Resp J*. 2014;43(5):1316–1325.
61. White MF. Optimizing hemodynamics: strategies for fluid and medication titration in hypoperfusion states. In: Good VS, Kirkwood PL, eds. *Advanced Critical Care Nursing*. 2nd ed. St. Louis, MO: Saunders; 2017:565–587.
62. Phan TD, Kluger R, Wan C, et al. A comparison of three minimally invasive cardiac output devices with thermodilution in elective cardiac surgery. *Anaesth Intens Care*. 2011;39(6):1014–1021.
63. Costello FM, Stouffer GA. Cardiac output. In: Stouffer GA, ed. *Cardiovascular Hemodynamics for the Clinician*. 2nd ed. Chichester, West Sussex; Hoboken, NJ: Wiley-Blackwell; 2017:82–90.
64. Balik M, Pachl J, Hendl J. Effect of the degree of tricuspid regurgitation on cardiac output measurements by thermodilution. *Intensive Care Med*. 2002;28(8):1117–1121.
65. Rocca GD, Costa MG, Pompei L, et al. Continuous and intermittent cardiac output measurement: pulmonary artery catheter versus aortic transpulmonary technique. *Br J Anaesth*. 2002;88(3):350–356.
66. Yelderman ML, Ramsay MA, Quinn MD, et al. Continuous thermodilution cardiac output measurement in intensive care unit patients. *J Cardiothorac Vasc Anesth*. 1992;6(3):270–274.
67. LaFarge CG, Miettinen OS. The estimation of oxygen consumption. *Cardiovasc Res*. 1970;4(1):23–30.
68. Bergstra A, van Dijk RB, Hillege HL, et al. Assumed oxygen consumption based on calculation from dye dilution cardiac output: an improved formula. *Eur Heart J*. 1995;16(5):698–703.
69. Wolf A, Pollman MJ, Trindade PT, et al. Use of assumed versus measured oxygen consumption for the determination of cardiac output using the Fick principle. *Cathet Cardiovasc Diagn*. 1998;43(4):372–380.
70. Bro-Jeppesen J, Hassager C, Wanscher M, et al. Targeted temperature management at 33°C versus 36°C and impact on systemic vascular resistance and myocardial function after out-of-hospital cardiac arrest: a sub-study of the Target Temperature Management Trial. *Circ Cardiovasc Interv*. 2014;7(5):663–672.
71. Ruffolo DC. Shock and end points of resuscitation. In: Good VS, Kirkwood PL, eds. *Advanced Critical Care Nursing*. 2nd ed. St. Louis, MO: Saunders; 2017:545–564.
72. Leeper B. Venous oxygen saturation monitoring. In: Lough ME, ed. *Hemodynamic Monitoring: Evolving Technologies and Clinical Practice*. 1st ed. St. Louis, Missouri: Mosby; 2015:205–229.
73. Hameed SM, Aird WC, Cohn SM. Oxygen delivery. *Critic Care Med*. 2003;31(12):S658–S667.
74. Lee J, Wright F, Barber R, et al. Central venous oxygen saturation in shock: a study in man. *Anesthes*. 1972;36(5):472–478.
75. Krauss XH, Verdouw PD, Hughenholtz PG, et al. On-line monitoring of mixed venous oxygen saturation after cardiothoracic surgery. *Thorax*. 1975;30(6):636–643.
76. Marx G, Reinhart K. Venous oximetry. *Curr Opin Crit Care*. 2006;12(3):263–268.
77. Nichols D, Nielsen ND. Oxygen delivery and consumption: a macrocirculatory perspective. *Crit Care Clin*. 2010;26(2):239–253.
78. Reinhart K, Kuhn HJ, Hartog C, et al. Continuous central venous and pulmonary artery oxygen saturation monitoring in the critically ill. *Intensive Care Med*. 2004;30(8):1572–1578.
79. Weil MH, Tang W. Forty-five-year evolution of stat blood and plasma lactate measurement to guide critical care. *Clin Chem*. 2009;55(11):2053–2054.
80. Jansen TC, van Bommel J, Bakker J. Blood lactate monitoring in critically ill patients: a systematic health technology assessment. *Crit Care Med*. 2009;37(10):2827–2839.
81. Bakker J, Nijsten MW, Jansen TC. Clinical use of lactate monitoring in critically ill patients. *Ann Intensive Care*. 2013;3:12.
82. Cecconi M, Hofer C, Teboul JL, et al. Fluid challenges in intensive care: the FENICE study. *Intensive Care Med*. 2015;41(9):1529–1537.
83. Cannesson M, Pestel G, Ricks C, et al. Hemodynamic monitoring and management in patients undergoing high risk surgery: a survey among North American and European anesthesiologists. *Crit Care*. 2011;15(4):R197.
84. da Silva Ramos FJ, Costa ELV, Amato MBP. Bedside monitoring of heart-lung interactions. In: *Annual Update in Intensive Care and Emergency Medicine 2013*. Annual Update in Intensive Care and Emergency Medicine. Berlin, Heidelberg: Springer; 2013:373–384.
85. Kumar A, Anel R, Bunnell E, et al. Pulmonary artery occlusion pressure and central venous pressure fail to predict ventricular filling volume, cardiac performance, or the response to volume infusion in normal subjects. *Crit Care Med*. 2004;32(3):691–699.
86. Cecconi M, Aya HD. Central venous pressure cannot predict fluid-responsiveness. *Evid Based Med*. 2014;19(2):63.
87. Michard F, Teboul JL. Predicting fluid responsiveness in ICU patients: a critical analysis of the evidence. *Chest*. 2002;121(6):2000–2008.
88. Rhodes A, Evans LE, Alhazzani W, et al. Surviving sepsis campaign: international guidelines for management of sepsis and septic shock: 2016. *Intensive Care Med*. 2017;43(3):304–377.
89. Levy MM, Evans LE, Rhodes A. The surviving sepsis campaign bundle: 2018 update. *Intensive Care Med*. 2018;44(6):925–928.
90. Cecconi M, De Backer D, Antonelli M, et al. Consensus on circulatory shock and hemodynamic monitoring. Task force of the European Society of Intensive Care Medicine. *Intensive Care Med*. 2014;40(12):1795–1815.
91. Raper R, Sibbald WJ. Misled by the wedge? The Swan-Ganz catheter and left ventricular preload. *Chest*. 1986;89(3):427–434.
92. Diebel LN, Wilson RF, Tagett MG, et al. End-diastolic volume: a better indicator of preload in the critically ill. *Arch Surg*. 1992;127(7):817–822.
93. Monnet X, Pinsky MR. Predicting the determinants of volume responsiveness. *Intensive Care Med*. 2015;41(2):354–356.
94. Bridges EJ. Arterial pressure based stroke volume and functional hemodynamic monitoring. *J Cardiovasc Nurs*. 2008;23(2):105–112.
95. Michard F, Boussat S, Chemla D, et al. Relation between respiratory changes in arterial pulse pressure and fluid responsiveness in septic patients with acute circulatory failure. *Am J Respir Crit Care Med*. 2000;162(1):134–138.
96. Michard F, Teboul JL. Respiratory changes in arterial pressure in mechanically ventilated patients. In: *Yearbook of Intensive Care and Emergency Medicine 2000*. Yearbook of Intensive Care and Emergency Medicine. Berlin, Heidelberg: Springer; 2000:696–704.
97. Headley JM. Arterial pressure–based technologies: a new trend in cardiac output monitoring. *Crit Care Nurs Clin North Am*. 2006;18(2):179–187.
98. Osman D, Ridel C, Ray P, et al. Cardiac filling pressures are not appropriate to predict hemodynamic response to volume challenge. *Crit Care Med*. 2007;35(1):64–68.
99. Marik PE, Cavallazzi R. Does the central venous pressure predict fluid responsiveness? An updated meta-analysis and a plea for some common sense. *Crit Care Med*. 2013;41(7):1774–1781.

100. Marik PE, Baram M, Vahid B. Does central venous pressure predict fluid responsiveness? A systematic review of the literature and the tale of seven mares. *Chest.* 2008;134(1):172–178.
101. Perner A, Faber T. Stroke volume variation does not predict fluid responsiveness in patients with septic shock on pressure support ventilation. *Acta Anaesthesiol Scand.* 2006;50(9):1068–1073.
102. Monnet X, Rienzo M, Osman D, et al. Passive leg raising predicts fluid responsiveness in the critically ill. *Crit Care Med.* 2006;34(5):1402–1407.
103. Cavallaro F, Sandroni C, Marano C, et al. Diagnostic accuracy of passive leg raising for prediction of fluid responsiveness in adults: systematic review and meta-analysis of clinical studies. *Intensive Care Med.* 2010;36(9):1475–1483.
104. De Backer D, Pinsky MR. Can one predict fluid responsiveness in spontaneously breathing patients? *Intensive Care Med.* 2007;33(7):1111–1113.
105. Feihl F, Broccard AF. Interactions between respiration and systemic hemodynamics. Part I: basic concepts. *Intensive Care Med.* 2009;35(1):45–54.
106. Feihl F, Broccard AF. Interactions between respiration and systemic hemodynamics. Part II: practical implications in critical care. *Intensive Care Med.* 2009;35(2):198–205.
107. Marik PE, Cavallazzi R, Vasu T, et al. Dynamic changes in arterial waveform derived variables and fluid responsiveness in mechanically ventilated patients: a systematic review of the literature. *Crit Care Med.* 2009;37(9):2642–2647.
108. Kreit JW. Systolic blood pressure variation during mechanical ventilation. *Ann Am Thorac Soc.* 2014;11(3):462–465.
109. Pizov R, Ya'ari Y, Perel A. Systolic blood pressure variation is a sensitive indicator of hypovolemia in ventilated dogs subjected to graded hemorrhage. *Anesth Analg.* 1988;67(2):170–174.
110. Berkenstadt H, Friedman Z, Preisman S, et al. Pulse pressure and stroke volume variations during severe haemorrhage in ventilated dogs. *Br J Anaesth.* 2005;94(6):721–726.
111. Tavernier B, Makhotine O, Lebuffe G, et al. Systolic pressure variation as a guide to fluid therapy in patients with sepsis-induced hypotension. *Anesthes.* 1998;89(6):1313–1321.
112. Colquhoun DA, Forkin KT, Dunn LK, et al. Non-invasive, minute-to-minute estimates of systemic arterial pressure and pulse pressure variation using radial artery tonometry. *J Med Eng Technol.* 2013;37(3):197–202.
113. Lansdorp B, Ouweneel D, de Keijzer A, et al. Non-invasive measurement of pulse pressure variation and systolic pressure variation using a finger cuff corresponds with intra-arterial measurement. *Br J Anaesth.* 2011;107(4):540–545.
114. Yang X, Du B. Does pulse pressure variation predict fluid responsiveness in critically ill patients? A systematic review and meta-analysis. *Crit Care.* 2014;18(6):650.
115. Bentzer P, Griesdale DE, Boyd J, et al. Will this hemodynamically unstable patient respond to a bolus of intravenous fluids? *JAMA.* 2016;316(12):1298–1309.
116. McGee WT. A simple physiologic algorithm for managing hemodynamics using stroke volume and stroke volume variation: physiologic optimization program. *J Intens Care Med.* 2009;24(6):352–360.
117. Monnet X, Osman D, Ridel C, et al. Predicting volume responsiveness by using the end-expiratory occlusion in mechanically ventilated intensive care unit patients. *Crit Care Med.* 2009;37(3):951–956.
118. Silva S, Jozwiak M, Teboul JL, et al. End-expiratory occlusion test predicts preload responsiveness independently of positive end-expiratory pressure during acute respiratory distress syndrome. *Crit Care Med.* 2013;41(7):1692–1701.
119. Ramsingh D, Alexander B, Cannesson M. Clinical review: does it matter which hemodynamic monitoring system is used? *Crit Care.* 2013;17(2):208.
120. Monnet X, Teboul JL. Assessment of volume responsiveness during mechanical ventilation: recent advances. *Crit Care.* 2013;17(2):217.
121. Shoemaker WC, Appel PLM, Kram HB. Tissue oxygen debt as a determinant of lethal and nonlethal postoperative organ failure. *Crit Care Med.* 1988;16(11):1117–1120.
122. Rivers E, Nguyen B, Havstad S, et al. Early goal-directed therapy in the treatment of severe sepsis and septic shock. *N Engl J Med.* 2001;345(19):1368–1377.
123a. Boyd JH, Forbes J, Nakada T, et al. Fluid resuscitation in septic shock: a positive fluid balance and elevated central venous pressure are associated with increased mortality. *Crit Care Med.* 2011;39(2):259–265.
123b. Kelm DJ, Perrin JT, Cartin-Ceba R, et al. Fluid overload in patients with severe sepsis and septic shock treated with early goal-directed therapy is associated with increased acute need for fluid-related medical interventions and hospital death. *Shock.* 2015;43(1):68–73.
124. Micek ST, McEvoy C, McKenzie M, et al. Fluid balance and cardiac function in septic shock as predictors of hospital mortality. *Crit Care.* 2013;17(5):R246.
125. Sirvent JM, Ferri C, Baró A, et al. Fluid balance in sepsis and septic shock as a determining factor of mortality. *Am J Emerg Med.* 2015;33(2):186–189.
126. Rosenberg AL, Dechert RE, Park PK, et al. Review of a large clinical series: association of cumulative fluid balance on outcome in acute lung injury: a retrospective review of the ARDS net tidal volume study cohort. *J Intensive Care Med.* 2009;24(1):35–46.
127. Jozwiak M, Silva S, Persichini R, et al. Extravascular lung water is an independent prognostic factor in patients with acute respiratory distress syndrome. *Crit Care Med.* 2013;41(2):472–480.
128. Kirkpatrick AW, Roberts DJ, Waele JD, et al. Intra-abdominal hypertension and the abdominal compartment syndrome: updated consensus definitions and clinical practice guidelines from the World Society of the Abdominal Compartment Syndrome. *Intensive Care Med.* 2013;39(7):1190–1206.
129. Marik PE, Linde-Zwirble WT, Bittner EA, et al. Fluid administration in severe sepsis and septic shock, patterns and outcomes: an analysis of a large national database. *Intensive Care Med.* 2017;43(5):625–632.
130. Marik PE, Lemson J. Fluid responsiveness: an evolution of our understanding. *Br J Anaesth.* 2014;112(4):617–620.
131. Heenen S, De Backer D, Vincent JL. How can the response to volume expansion in patients with spontaneous respiratory movements be predicted? *Crit Care.* 2006;10(4):R102.
132. Pinsky MR. Functional hemodynamic monitoring. *Crit Care Clin.* 2015;31(1):89–111.
133. Backer DD, Heenen S, Piagnerelli M, et al. Pulse pressure variations to predict fluid responsiveness: influence of tidal volume. *Intensive Care Med.* 2005;31(4):517–523.
134. Kang WS, Kim SH, Kim SY, et al. The influence of positive end-expiratory pressure on stroke volume variation in patients undergoing cardiac surgery: an observational study. *J Thorac Cardiovasc Surg.* 2014;148(6):3139–3145.
135. Kubitz JC, Annecke T, Kemming GI, et al. The influence of positive end-expiratory pressure on stroke volume variation and central blood volume during open and closed chest conditions. *Eur J Cardiothorac Surg.* 2006;30(1):90–95.
136. Monnet X, Bleibtreu A, Ferré A, et al. Passive leg-raising and end-expiratory occlusion tests perform better than pulse pressure variation in patients with low respiratory system compliance. *Crit Care Med.* 2012;40(1):152–157.
137. Liu Y, Wei L, Li G, et al. Pulse pressure variation adjusted by respiratory changes in pleural pressure, rather than by tidal volume, reliably predicts fluid responsiveness in patients with acute respiratory distress syndrome. *Crit Care Med.* 2016;44(2):342–351.
138. Myatra SN, Prabu NR, Divatia JV, et al. The changes in pulse pressure variation or stroke volume variation after a "tidal volume challenge" reliably predict fluid responsiveness during low tidal volume ventilation. *Crit Care Med.* 2017;45(3):415–421.
139. Malbrain ML, Chiumello D, Pelosi P, et al. Prevalence of intra-abdominal hypertension in critically ill patients: a multicentre epidemiological study. *Intensive Care Med.* 2004;30(5):822–829.
140. Díaz F, Erranz B, Donoso A, et al. Influence of tidal volume on pulse pressure variation and stroke volume variation during experimental intra-abdominal hypertension. *BMC Anesthesiol.* 2015;15:127.
141. Duperret S, Lhuillier F, Piriou V, et al. Increased intra-abdominal pressure affects respiratory variations in arterial pressure in normovolaemic and hypovolaemic mechanically ventilated healthy pigs. *Intensive Care Med.* 2007;33(1):163–171.
142. Jacques D, Bendjelid K, Duperret S, et al. Pulse pressure variation and stroke volume variation during increased intra-abdominal pressure: an experimental study. *Crit Care.* 2011;15(1):R33.
143. Piccioni F, Bernasconi F, Tramontano GTA, et al. A systematic review of pulse pressure variation and stroke volume variation to predict fluid responsiveness during cardiac and thoracic surgery. *J Clin Monit Comput.* 2017;31(4):677–684.
144. Rutlen DL, Wackers FJ, Zaret BL. Radionuclide assessment of peripheral intravascular capacity: a technique to measure intravascular volume changes in the capacitance circulation in man. *Circulation.* 1981;64(1):146–152.
145. Jabot J, Teboul JL, Richard C, et al. Passive leg raising for predicting fluid responsiveness: importance of the postural change. *Intensive Care Med.* 2009;35(1):85.

146. Monnet X, Marik P, Teboul JL. Passive leg raising for predicting fluid responsiveness: a systematic review and meta-analysis. *Intensive Care Med.* 2016;42(12):1935–1947.
147. Monnet X, Teboul JL. Passive leg raising: five rules, not a drop of fluid! *Crit Care.* 2015;19(1):18.
148. Guérin L, Teboul JL, Persichini R, et al. Effects of passive leg raising and volume expansion on mean systemic pressure and venous return in shock in humans. *Crit Care.* 2015;19:411.
149. Cherpanath TGV, Hirsch A, Geerts BF, et al. Predicting fluid responsiveness by passive leg raising: a systematic review and meta-analysis of 23 clinical trials. *Crit Care Med.* 2016;44(5):981–991.
150. Monnet X, Teboul JL. Passive leg raising. *Intensive Care Med.* 2008;34(4):659–663.
151. Maizel J, Airapetian N, Lorne E, et al. Diagnosis of central hypovolemia by using passive leg raising. *Intensive Care Med.* 2007;33(7):1133–1138.
152. Teboul JL, Monnet X. Prediction of volume responsiveness in critically ill patients with spontaneous breathing activity. *Curr Opin Crit Care.* 2008;14(3):334–339.
153. Mahjoub Y, Touzeau J, Airapetian N, et al. The passive leg-raising maneuver cannot accurately predict fluid responsiveness in patients with intra-abdominal hypertension. *Crit Care Med.* 2010;38(9):1824–1829.
154. Malbrain ML, Reuter DA. Assessing fluid responsiveness with the passive leg raising maneuver in patients with increased intra-abdominal pressure: be aware that not all blood returns! *Crit Care Med.* 2010;38(9):1912–1915.
155. Benes J, Zatloukal J, Kletecka J, et al. Respiratory induced dynamic variations of stroke volume and its surrogates as predictors of fluid responsiveness: applicability in the early stages of specific critical states. *J Clin Monit Comput.* 2014;28(3):225–231.
156. Biais M, Vidil L, Sarrabay P, et al. Changes in stroke volume induced by passive leg raising in spontaneously breathing patients: comparison between echocardiography and Vigileo™/FloTrac™ device. *Crit Care.* 2009;13(6):R195.
157. Monnet X, Bataille A, Magalhaes E, et al. End-tidal carbon dioxide is better than arterial pressure for predicting volume responsiveness by the passive leg raising test. *Intensive Care Med.* 2013;39(1):93–100.
158. Monge García MI, Gil Cano A, Gracia Romero M, et al. Non-invasive assessment of fluid responsiveness by changes in partial end-tidal CO2 pressure during a passive leg-raising maneuver. *Ann Intens Care.* 2012;2(1):9.
159. Young A, Marik PE, Sibole S, et al. Changes in end-tidal carbon dioxide and volumetric carbon dioxide as predictors of volume responsiveness in hemodynamically unstable patients. *J Cardiothorac Vasc Anesth.* 2013;27(4):681–684.
160. Anderson CT, Breen PH. Carbon dioxide kinetics and capnography during critical care. *Crit Care.* 2000;4(4):207–215.
161. Xiao-ting W, Hua Z, Da-wei L, et al. Changes in end-tidal CO2 could predict fluid responsiveness in the passive leg raising test but not in the mini-fluid challenge test: a prospective and observational study. *J Crit Care.* 2015;30(5):1061–1066.
162. Felker GM, Cuculich PS, Gheorghiade M. The Valsalva maneuver: a bedside "biomarker" for heart failure. *Am J Med.* 2006;119(2):117–122.
163. Monge García MI, Gil Cano A, Díaz Monrové JC. Arterial pressure changes during the Valsalva maneuver to predict fluid responsiveness in spontaneously breathing patients. *Intensive Care Med.* 2009;35(1):77–84.
164. Tusman G, Groisman I, Maidana GA, et al. The sensitivity and specificity of pulmonary carbon dioxide elimination for noninvasive assessment of fluid responsiveness. *Anesth Analg.* 2016;122(5):1404–1411.
165. Preisman S, Kogan S, Berkenstadt H, et al. Predicting fluid responsiveness in patients undergoing cardiac surgery: functional haemodynamic parameters including the respiratory systolic variation test and static preload indicators. *Br J Anaesth.* 2005;95(6):746–755.
166. Trepte CJC, Eichhorn V, Haas SA, et al. Comparison of an automated respiratory systolic variation test with dynamic preload indicators to predict fluid responsiveness after major surgery. *Br J Anaesth.* 2013;111(5):736–742.
167. Karakala N, Raghunathan K, Shaw AD. Intravenous fluids in sepsis: what to use and what to avoid. *Curr Opin Crit Care.* 2013;19(6):537–543.
168. Sen A, Keener CM, Sileanu FE, et al. Chloride content of fluids used for large-volume resuscitation is associated with reduced survival. *Crit Care Med.* 2017;45(2):e146–e153.
169. Yunos NM, Bellomo R, Hegarty C, et al. Association between a chloride-liberal vs chloride-restrictive intravenous fluid administration strategy and kidney injury in critically ill adults. *JAMA.* 2012;308(15):1566–1572.
170. Labovitz AJ, Noble VE, Bierig M, et al. Focused cardiac ultrasound in the emergent setting: a consensus statement of the American Society of Echocardiography and American College of Emergency Physicians. *J Am Soc Echocardiogr.* 2010;23(12):1225–1230.
171. Geisen M, Spray D, Nicholas Fletcher S. Echocardiography-based hemodynamic management in the cardiac surgical intensive care unit. *J Cardiothorac Vasc Anesth.* 2014;28(3):733–744.
172. Ahmed SN, Syed FM, Porembka DTD. Echocardiographic evaluation of hemodynamic parameters. *Crit Care Med.* 2007;35(8):S323–S329.
173. Haddad F, Hunt SA, Rosenthal DN, et al. Right ventricular function in cardiovascular disease, part I: anatomy, physiology, aging, and functional assessment of the right ventricle. *Circulation.* 2008;117(11):1436–1448.
174. Bouchard MJ, Denault A, Couture P, et al. Poor correlation between hemodynamic and echocardiographic indexes of left ventricular performance in the operating room and intensive care unit. *Crit Care Med.* 2004;32(3):644–648.
175. Fontes ML, Bellows W, Ngo L, et al. Assessment of ventricular function in critically ill patients: limitations of pulmonary artery catheterization. *J Cardiothorac Vasc Anesth.* 1999;13(5):521–527.
176. Mohsenin V. Assessment of preload and fluid responsiveness in intensive care unit. How good are we? *J Crit Care.* 2015;30(3):567–573.
177. Muller L, Bobbia X, Toumi M, et al. Respiratory variations of inferior vena cava diameter to predict fluid responsiveness in spontaneously breathing patients with acute circulatory failure: need for a cautious use. *Crit Care.* 2012;16(5):R188.
178. Brennan JM, Blair JE, Goonewardena S, et al. Reappraisal of the use of inferior vena cava for estimating right atrial pressure. *J Am Soc Echocardiogr.* 2007;20(7):857–861.
179. Bioreactance. *Cheetah Medical.* Available at https://www.cheetah-medical.com/how-it-works/bioreactance. Accessed July 23, 2018.
180. Waldron NH, Miller TE, Thacker JK, et al. A prospective comparison of a noninvasive cardiac output monitor versus esophageal Doppler monitor for goal-directed fluid therapy in colorectal surgery patients. *Anesth Analg.* 2014;118(5):966–975.
181. Marik PE, Levitov A, Young A, et al. The use of bioreactance and carotid Doppler to determine volume responsiveness and blood flow redistribution following passive leg raising in hemodynamically unstable patients. *Chest.* 2013;143(2):364–370.
182. Squara P, Rotcajg D, Denjean D, et al. Comparison of monitoring performance of bioreactance vs. pulse contour during lung recruitment maneuvers. *Crit Care.* 2009;13(4):R125.
183. Raval NY, Squara P, Cleman M, et al. Multicenter evaluation of noninvasive cardiac output measurement by bioreactance technique. *J Clin Monit Comput.* 2008;22(2):113–119.
184. Rich JD, Archer SL, Rich S. Noninvasive cardiac output measurements in patients with pulmonary hypertension. *Eur Respir J.* 2013;42(1):125–133.
185. Latham HE, Bengtson CD, Satterwhite L, et al. Stroke volume guided resuscitation in severe sepsis and septic shock improves outcomes. *J Crit Care.* 2017;42:42–46.
186. Truijen J, van Lieshout JJ, Wesselink WA, et al. Noninvasive continuous hemodynamic monitoring. *J Clin Monit Comput.* 2012;26(4):267–278.
187. Ameloot K, Van De Vijver K, Broch O, et al. Nexfin noninvasive continuous hemodynamic monitoring: validation against continuous pulse contour and intermittent transpulmonary thermodilution derived cardiac output in critically ill patients. *ScientificWorldJournal.* 2013:519080.
188. Chen G, Meng L, Alexander B, et al. Comparison of noninvasive cardiac output measurements using the Nexfin monitoring device and the esophageal Doppler. *J Clin Anesth.* 2012;24(4):275–283.
189. Edwards Lifesciences. *ClearSight system.* Available at https://www.edwards.com/gb/devices/Hemodynamic-Monitoring/clearsight. Accessed July 29, 2018.
190. Maguire S, Rinehart J, Vakharia S, et al. Respiratory variation in pulse pressure and plethysmographic waveforms: intraoperative applicability in a North American academic center. *Anesth Analg.* 2011;112(1):94–96.
191. Jeleazcov C, Krajinovic L, Münster T, et al. Precision and accuracy of a new device (CNAPTM) for continuous non-invasive arterial pressure monitoring: assessment during general anaesthesia. *Br J Anaesth.* 2010;105(3):264–272.
192. Wellisch A. *CNAP® blood pressure.* Available at https://www.cnsystems.com/innovation/cnap-technology/cnap-blood-pressure. Accessed July 29, 2018.

193. Verdant CL, De Backer D, Bruhn A, et al. Evaluation of sublingual and gut mucosal microcirculation in sepsis: a quantitative analysis. *Crit Care Med.* 2009;37(11):2875–2881.
194. Lebuffe G, Decoene C, Pol A, et al. Regional capnometry with air-automated tonometry detects circulatory failure earlier than conventional hemodynamics after cardiac surgery. *Anesth Analg.* 1999;89(5):1084–1090.
195. Weil MH, Tang W. Welcoming a new era of hemodynamic monitoring: expanding from the macro to the microcirculation. *Crit Care Med.* 2007;35(4):1204–1205.
196. Wilmot LA. Shock: early recognition and management. *J Emerg Nurs.* 2010;36(2):134–139.
197. Moore K. The physiological response to hemorrhagic shock. *J Emerg Nurs.* 2014;40(6):629–631.
198. Strehlow MC. Early identification of shock in critically ill patients. *Emerg Med Clin North Am.* 2010;28(1):57–66.
199. Sakr Y, Dubois MJ, De Backer D, et al. Persistent microcirculatory alterations are associated with organ failure and death in patients with septic shock. *Crit Care Med.* 2004;32(9):1825–1831.
200. Vellinga NAR, Boerma EC, Koopmans M, et al. International study on microcirculatory shock occurrence in acutely ill patients. *Crit Care Med.* 2015;43(1):48–56.
201. Fiddian-Green RG, Baker SM. Predictive value of the stomach wall pH for complications after cardiac operations: comparison with other monitoring. *Crit Care Med.* 1987;15(2):153–156.
202. Splanchnic hypoperfusion-directed therapies in trauma: a prospective, randomized trial. *Am Surg.* 2005;71(3):252–260.
203. Povoas HP, Weil MH, Tang W, et al. Comparisons between sublingual and gastric tonometry during hemorrhagic shock. *Chest.* 2000;118(4):1127–1132.
204. Creteur J, Backer DD, Sakr Y, et al. Sublingual capnometry tracks microcirculatory changes in septic patients. *Intensive Care Med.* 2006;32(4):516–523.
205. Marik PE. Sublingual capnometry: a non-invasive measure of microcirculatory dysfunction and tissue hypoxia. *Physiol Meas.* 2006;27(7):R37–R47.
206. Creteur J. Gastric and sublingual capnometry. *Curr Opin Crit Care.* 2006;12(3):272–277.
207. Boswell SA, Scalea TM. Sublingual capnometry: an alternative to gastric tonometry for the management of shock resuscitation. *AACN Clin Issues.* 2003;14(2):176–184.
208. Donati A, Tibboel D, Ince C. Towards integrative physiological monitoring of the critically ill: from cardiovascular to microcirculatory and cellular function monitoring at the bedside. *Crit Care.* 2013;17(Suppl 1):S5.
209. Ruffolo DC, Headley JM. Regional carbon dioxide monitoring: a different look at tissue perfusion. *AACN Clin Issues.* 2003;14(2):168–175.
210. Pranskunas A, Koopmans M, Koetsier PM, et al. Microcirculatory blood flow as a tool to select ICU patients eligible for fluid therapy. *Intensive Care Med.* 2013;39(4):612–619.
211. Bezemer R, Bartels SA, Bakker J, et al. Clinical review: clinical imaging of the sublingual microcirculation in the critically ill—where do we stand? *Crit Care.* 2012;16(3):224.
212. van Genderen ME, Lima A, Akkerhuis M, et al. Persistent peripheral and microcirculatory perfusion alterations after out-of-hospital cardiac arrest are associated with poor survival. *Crit Care Med.* 2012;40(8):2287–2294.
213. Abraham WT, Adamson P, Stevenson L, et al. Pulmonary artery pressure management in heart failure patients with reduced ejection fraction significantly reduces heart failure hospitalizations and mortality above and beyond background guideline-directed medical therapy. *J Am Coll Cardiol.* 2015;65(10):A790.
214. Treu CM, Lupi O, Bottino DA, et al. Sidestream dark field imaging: the evolution of real-time visualization of cutaneous microcirculation and its potential application in dermatology. *Arch Dermatol Res.* 2011;303(2):69–78.
215. Spanos A, Jhanji S, Vivian-Smith A, et al. Early microvascular changes in sepsis and severe sepsis. *Shock.* 2010;33(4):387–391.
216. Adamson PB, Abraham WT, Stevenson LW, et al. Pulmonary artery pressure–guided heart failure management reduces 30-day readmissions. *Circ Heart Fail.* 2016;9(6):e002600.
217. Adamson PB, Abraham WT, Bauman J, et al. Abstract 16744: impact of wireless pulmonary artery pressure monitoring on heart failure hospitalizations and all-cause 30-day readmissions in Medicare-eligible patients with NYHA class III heart failure: results from the CHAMPION trial. *Circulation.* 2014;130(Suppl 2):A16744.
218. Adamson PB, Abraham WT, Aaron M, et al. CHAMPION trial rationale and design: the long-term safety and clinical efficacy of a wireless pulmonary artery pressure monitoring system. *J Card Fail.* 2011;17(1):3–10.
219. CardioMEMS™ HF System | Abbott. Available at https://www.sjm.com/en/sjm/cardiomems. Accessed July 23, 2018.
220. Costanzo MR, Stevenson LW, Adamson PB, et al. Interventions linked to decreased heart failure hospitalizations during ambulatory pulmonary artery pressure monitoring. *JACC Heart Fail.* 2016;4(5):333–344.
221. Abraham WT, Stevenson LW, Bourge RC, et al. Sustained efficacy of pulmonary artery pressure to guide adjustment of chronic heart failure therapy: complete follow-up results from the CHAMPION randomized trial. *Lancet.* 2016;387(10017):453–461.
222. Adamson PB, Abraham WT, Bourge RC, et al. Wireless pulmonary artery haemodynamic monitoring in chronic heart failure: a randomized controlled trial. *Circ Heart Fail.* 2014;7(6):935–944.

18 Cardiac Electrophysiology Studies

Monica Knapp

OBJECTIVES

Upon reading this chapter, the reader should be able to:

1. Describe standard catheter positions for performing an electrophysiology (EP) study.
2. Understand how to best prepare patients undergoing EP procedures for their perioperative management.
3. Identify an appropriate patient population suitable for EP testing.
4. Depict appropriate recommendations and associated risks associated with combined EP study and catheter ablation for the management of patients with supraventricular tachycardia (SVT) or atrial fibrillation (AF).
5. Indicate which subset of patients with ventricular arrhythmias should undergo catheter ablation and identify associated risks.

KEY QUESTIONS

1. What are the general principles involved in a basic EP study?
2. How would a provider best prepare a patient undergoing a catheter ablation?
3. Which supraventricular tachycardias (SVTs) are suitable for EP study and catheter ablation? And which have the highest success rate following an ablation?

BACKGROUND

Cardiac electrophysiology (EP) has greatly evolved over the last few decades as a major cardiology subspecialty. Similarly, the scope and technology of cardiac EP continues to expand this evolution. The use of cardiac EP procedures includes diagnostic testing and interventional treatment procedures with the use of catheter ablation. This cardiac subspecialty was reportedly born from ancient Chinese pulse theory which served as the foundation for the study of arrhythmias and clinical EP in the 5th century BC. Much later in 1875, Étienne-Jules Marey born in Beaune, Bourgogne (Côte d'Or), France, discovered the refractory period of heart muscle tissue and recorded the first electrogram in animal hearts using a capillary electrometer in 1876. Eleven years later, Waller recorded the first human electrogram.[1]

Nearly a century later, after the first recording of the His bundle in the 1960s, invasive cardiac catheterization procedures were adapted to allow for simultaneous intracardiac recording and programmed stimulation, thereby giving rise to the EP study. In general, diagnostic EP studies are performed to determine an arrhythmia diagnosis or EP mechanism of a known arrhythmia. Interventional or therapeutic EP studies consist of endocardial catheter ablation of supraventricular and ventricular arrhythmias. Knowledge from EP studies also provided the foundation for antitachycardia pacing, which was incorporated into a key therapy provided by implantable cardioverted defibrillators (ICDs).[2] The placement of ICDs for the management of ventricular tachycardia (VT) and ventricular fibrillation (VF) is also an interventional EP procedure and is discussed in Chapter 36.

The advent of catheter ablation transformed cardiac EP from its status as a marginal subspecialty prior to the late 1980s. Catheter ablation was initially accomplished with the use of high-energy direct current shocks directed at the atrioventricular (AV) junction, but these procedures were limited in terms of utility and safety due to barotrauma.[3] Advances in cardiac EP procedures took a significant leap with the use of radiofrequency (RF) current as the power source for ablation that could target and create ablative lesions by heating the myocardium at the catheter-tissue interface. This power source offered greater safety and control than its predecessor, direct current shocks.[4] The introduction of steerable ablation catheters in the market also advanced EP procedures with their ability to improve intracardiac catheter positioning. Lastly, the birth of EP mapping techniques also allowed for identification of target sites with greater detail and precision. Together, these advances made catheter ablation a successful strategy for treating common supraventricular tachycardias (SVTs) and consequently made arrhythmia surgery obsolete by the early 1990s.[2] Further developments in EP procedures continue to evolve this practice and extend its application to other arrhythmias.

Cardiac EP procedures have grown tremendously in their utility and efficacy since their inception. In the United States, the number of reported ablation procedures has risen from 450 in 1989 to about 15,000 annually. In 1995, Scheinman surveyed 157 laboratories in the United States which demonstrated success rates as follows for AV node ablations, 97%, for accessory pathways in all locations, 90%, for AV node modifications in the treatment of AV nodal reentry tachycardia, 94%, for atrial flutter,

72%, and for atrial tachycardia, 71%.[5] Although complications from such ablation procedures exist and are reviewed later in this chapter, studies have demonstrated clear quality of life improvements in symptomatic patients.[6,7]

Knowledge of electrocardiography, normal cardiac activation, and cardiac activation during arrhythmias is needed to understand EP studies. The foundation for these related subjects is discussed elsewhere in this text.

DIAGNOSTIC EP STUDIES

Before an EP study, a patient needs to be prepared for the procedure. This preparation and the techniques, complications, and indications of EP studies are presented here.

Patient Preparation

Preparation for EP procedures is similar to that for cardiac catheterization as discussed elsewhere in this text. Patients are kept fasting and usually sedated during EP studies. The degree of sedation depends on the type of study being performed and the preferences of the hospital performing the procedures. A peripheral intravenous line is required for administration of medicine. Systemic anticoagulation may be used during EP studies to decrease the incidence of thromboembolic complications.[8] Appropriate emergency and resuscitation equipment is required for all EP procedures.

Nursing Care of the Patient Undergoing EP Procedures

Healthcare professionals caring for arrhythmia patients play a pivotal role for the patient undergoing an EP procedure, catheter ablation procedure, or both. The need for patient education during all phases of the arrhythmia experience has been well documented.[9–11] Teaching before the study must include discussions about the nature of the test, a description of the procedure, procedure length, success rates, and complication rates. Nurses must also include postprocedure instructions and discharge instructions. After the procedure, the patient must keep the affected leg(s) straight for 4 hours to allow the venous puncture site to heal and for 4 to 6 hours if the femoral artery was punctured. The preliminary results of the procedure should be shared immediately with the patient and family. Frequent explanations may be required at first if the patient is recovering from heavy sedation. After a successful ablation, patients have no restrictions and antiarrhythmic medications are usually discontinued.

Most of the intraprocedure and postprocedure nursing care is centered on monitoring the patient for potential complications related to the procedure. In most instances, patients are anxious before and during EP procedures. Adequate sedation to allow for patient comfort should be provided. Oversedation must be prevented. Nurses must be alert for major complications directly related to placement of catheters inside the heart. Bleeding from catheter insertion sites, tamponade from perforation, and tachyarrhythmias and bradyarrhythmias can all occur during and after the EP procedure. Nurses who care for patients with arrhythmias in any setting should be prepared to handle any emergency that may arise. Other potential problems to be monitored include thrombophlebitis, thromboembolism, and infection.

The Heart Rhythm Society (HRS), formerly known as the North American Society of Pacing and Electrophysiology, has developed standards of professional practice for allied professionals (nurses, nurse practitioners, physician assistants, technicians) caring for patients with cardiac rhythm disorders. The standards for EP procedures are threefold and include: (1) the application of scientific principles related to clinical EP to provide technical support and patient care services; (2) the demonstration of technical knowledge and clinical skills to operate laboratory equipment and troubleshoot equipment malfunction; and (3) the integration of cardiovascular and electrical knowledge to effectively monitor the patient throughout the procedure.[12]

Techniques

During invasive EP testing, spontaneous and pacing-induced intracardiac and surface electrical signals are continuously recorded. The normal timing and sequence of electrical activation can be observed and measured during a normal or baseline rhythm. Abnormal timing and electrical activation sequences are recorded and studied during tachyarrhythmias. Programmed electrical stimulation may also be used to induce and analyze paroxysmal arrhythmias that are the same as or similar to a patient's clinical arrhythmia.[13]

Flexible multielectrode catheters, that is, circular or multispline variations, are introduced percutaneously. The catheters are advanced using fluoroscopy into the heart. The right and left femoral, subclavian, and internal jugular veins are the most commonly used venous access sites. One to several catheters may be placed depending on the type of study to be performed (Fig. 18-1). The usual intracardiac recording sites include the high right atrium, right atrial appendage, right ventricular apex, right ventricular outflow tract, coronary sinus, the His bundle region, and occasionally the left atrium. In addition, a roving catheter can be used to map intracardiac electrograms arising from different regions of the heart during tachycardia. Occasionally, the left ventricle is used during a diagnostic study for programmed electrical stimulation if VT cannot be induced from the right ventricle.

After the catheters are in place and connected to the physiologic recording equipment, intervals are measured from both the 12-lead electrocardiogram (ECG) and the intracardiac electrograms in the baseline state (Fig. 18-2). The AH interval is a measurement of conduction time from the low right atrium through the AV node to the His bundle and is an approximation of AV node conduction time. The AH interval can vary a great deal depending on the patient's autonomic state and measures approximately 55 to 120 ms.[13] The HV interval represents conduction time from the onset of His bundle depolarization to the onset of ventricular activity. The normal HV interval measurement is 35 to 55 ms.[14] After baseline recordings, various pacing techniques may be performed to assess the patient's electrical conduction system. Refractory periods for the atrium, AV node, and ventricle are recorded. The presence of retrograde or ventricular–atrial conduction is noted, as is the activation sequence. Attempts to induce and document the arrhythmia using the introduction of extrastimuli in either the atrium or the ventricle are then made. Intravenous isoproterenol or epinephrine may be used to help induce arrhythmias or reveal accessory pathway (AP) or slow pathway conduction.

The patient must be adequately prepared before the study and should understand that arrhythmia induction is often one of the primary goals of the study. The electrophysiologist attempts to gather as much information as possible depending on the type of arrhythmia induced and how well it is hemodynamically tolerated. Special physiologic recording equipment is able to document

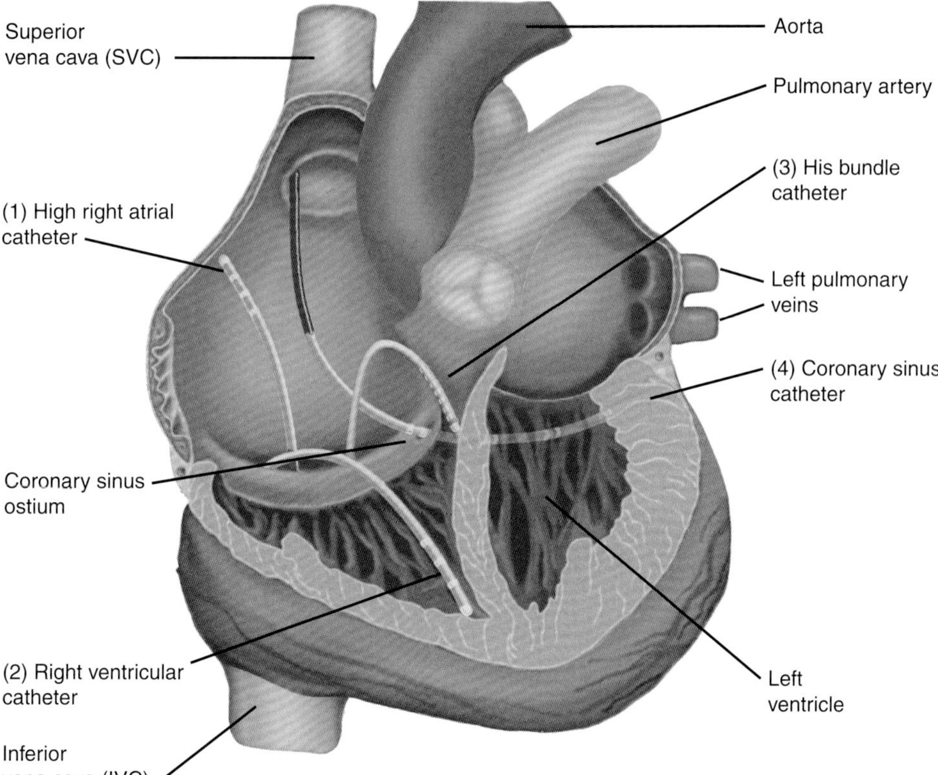

Figure 18-1. Diagram of intracardiac placement of catheters. 1, right atrial recording catheter; 2, right ventricular recording catheter; 3, His recording catheter; 4, coronary sinus catheter.

simultaneously every beat in 12-lead ECG and intracardiac electrogram format. Induced arrhythmias can then be reviewed and analyzed after they are terminated. It is important to note the method of arrhythmia termination. Tachycardias may be self-terminating or require antitachycardia pacing to terminate them. Occasionally, it is necessary to cardiovert or defibrillate the patient to stop the arrhythmia. It is usually necessary to wait until the patient loses consciousness before defibrillation to prevent painful shock in an awake state.

If the patient is hemodynamically stable during a ventricular arrhythmia, attempts to map its origin can be performed, particularly if ablation is planned. Atrial arrhythmias are usually well tolerated and allow for extensive mapping. Recordings are made at various locations in the heart and compared with a reference signal, either a surface ECG lead or a stable intracardiac electrogram. The site of earliest activation is closest to the site where the arrhythmia originates. Occasionally, the clinical arrhythmia cannot be induced or is not sustained long enough for adequate mapping.

Complications

Complications due to programmed electrical stimulation during EP studies are rare and such studies should be performed with a low morbidity.[15] The majority of these complications have been attributed to mechanical aspects of the study, not the EP stimulation protocols. In a large landmark review, Horowitz et al.[8] evaluated the experience of six EP laboratories during a 4-year period: 8545 EP studies were performed on 4015 patients. Five deaths (0.12%) occurred, all caused by intractable VT/VF. The complications that occurred most frequently after EP studies were cardiac perforation (0.5%) and major venous thrombosis (0.5%). Cardiac perforation and pericardial effusion resolved without treatment in most patients; five patients required pericardial drainage or open repair. The femoral catheter site was the location of thrombosis for 20 patients with venous thrombosis (0.5%). Pulmonary emboli followed venous thrombosis in nine of these patients (0.2%).[8] A subsequent frequently cited review (1062 EP studies for 359 patients) by DiMarco et al.[16] reported higher complication rates than Horowitz et al.[8], which may be in part related to a smaller sample and less operator experience at that time: venous thrombosis (1.1%), pulmonary emboli (1.6%), unstable VT requiring countershock for termination (10%), and systemic or catheter site infections (1.7%).

In general, the actual risk of death from electrophysiologic study procedures approaches zero because reentrant VT or fibrillation induced under controlled conditions can be quickly terminated. Furthermore, a more recent study by Josephson et al.[15] demonstrated only a single death and overall complication rate of less than 2% for their reported 12,000 procedures. The prevalence of complications was higher in elderly patients and in those undergoing catheter ablation (2.5%) than in those undergoing diagnostic procedures alone (1%).[15] In contrast, the complication prevalence reported by DiMarco et al. was much higher for diagnostic EP procedures (5.6%).[16]

Major hemorrhage and arterial injury are uncommon complications of EP studies and are substantially less than those with standard cardiac catheterization. Although significant hemorrhage remains uncommon, the prevalence increases in obese patients.[15] Findings from Josephson et al.[15] and Horowitz et al.[8] highlight the overall low rate of thromboembolism (less than 1%) and cardiac perforation of the atrium or ventricle resulting in tamponade (less than 1%). Increased experience and procedural volume may be associated with decreased frequency of adverse events.[15,16,18] Taken as a whole, EP procedures have evolved such that in most cases, they are relatively safe for a wide range of patients.

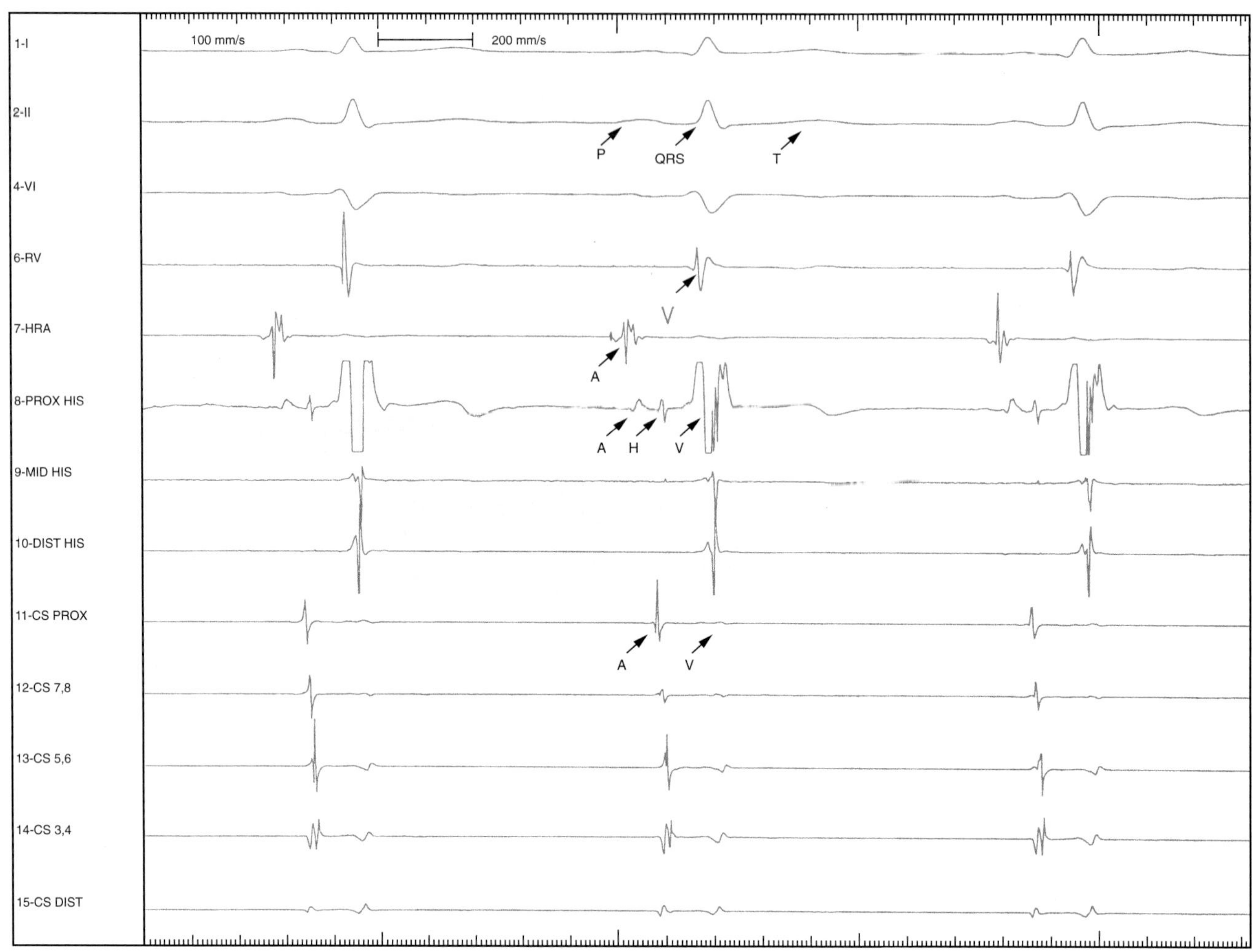

Figure 18-2. Basic intervals. Channel 1-I is lead I; channel 2-II is lead II; channel 4-V1 is lead V_1; channel 6-RV is a right ventricular tracing (*V*); channel 7-RA is a right atrial tracing (*A*); channel 8-HIS PROX is a tracing from the proximal portion of the His bundle; channel 9-HIS MID is a tracing from the middle portion of the His bundle; channel 10-HIS DIST is a tracing from the distal portion of the His bundle. On channel 8-HIS PROX, the first waveform represents atrial depolarization (*A*) and occurs slightly later than the P wave on lead II. The next waveform is the His bundle deflection (*H*). The last waveform represents ventricular depolarization (*V*), corresponding to the QRS complex. Atrial and ventricular tracings are also recorded on channels 11–15-CS and reflect proximal to distal coronary sinus electrograms.

Indications

In general, indications for EP testing include assessing for bradyarrhythmias, reentrant tachyarrhythmias, and focal tachycardias through the use of conduction interval measurements, and the delivery of programmed extrastimuli. Specific clinical indications for both brady- and tachyarrhythmias are discussed in the subsequent sections.

Cardiac Arrest Survivors

People who survive a cardiac arrest not associated with an acute transmural myocardial infarction are at high risk for recurrence. The 2-year recurrence rate has been reported at 47%.[17] VF was the rhythm most commonly found at the time of cardiac arrest.[18,19] VT and VF were induced during EP testing in a baseline, antiarrhythmic, drug-free state in 70% to 80% of patients resuscitated from cardiac arrest.[20,21] A full discussion of sudden cardiac death can be found elsewhere in this text.

Serial, EP-guided, antiarrhythmic drug testing was once common practice in EP laboratories. The goal was to identify a drug that was effective in suppressing inducible VT or VF and subsequent recurrent cardiac arrest. VT or VF suppression with EP-guided antiarrhythmic drug therapy has been reported in 26% to 80% of cardiac arrest survivors.[20,21] Antiarrhythmic medications may also provoke or exacerbate arrhythmias; this situation is referred to as proarrhythmic effect.

In the last couple of decades, several studies have shown ICD therapy as superior to EP-guided antiarrhythmic drugs in reducing all-cause mortality.[22–27] Therefore, ICD therapy is usually recommended as first-line therapy for patients with inducible VT or survivors of cardiac arrest. Specific indications for ICD therapy are discussed elsewhere in this text.

EP testing is often recommended for patients who receive nonpharmacologic drug therapy. Implantation of combination antitachycardia pacemakers and ICDs often requires a baseline EP test and possible further testing after implantation to allow for optimized programming of the device. Knowledge of baseline conduction and the presence of concurrent atrial arrhythmias are also helpful for appropriate device selection as discussed elsewhere in this text. Patients with ischemic or nonischemic cardiomyopathy and reduced left ventricular function may be eligible to undergo prophylactic ICD implantation for primary prevention of cardiac arrest without undergoing prior EP evaluation.[27–29]

Wide-Complex Tachycardias

Wide-complex tachycardias can be caused by VT, SVT with aberration, or pre-excitation syndromes such as antidromic reciprocating tachycardia, in which an accessory bypass tract is the antegrade limb and the AV node is the retrograde limb of the tachycardia. Although guidelines and criteria have been established to help practitioners diagnose wide-complex tachycardias using the 12-lead ECG, necessary criteria may be difficult to identify, and the diagnosis may not be certain, especially in the presence of a rapid ventricular rate response.[30,31] In these cases, EP studies are necessary to confirm or establish a diagnosis so that proper safe treatment can be initiated.[32]

During invasive EP testing for wide-complex arrhythmias, the timing and sequence of atrial activation in relation to ventricular activation are recorded. Although it may be difficult to distinguish the various pre-excitation syndromes from VT, the presence of AV dissociation favors a diagnosis of VT.

Syncope

Syncope is defined as an abrupt, transient loss of consciousness accompanied by loss of postural tone, with spontaneous, rapid recovery. Multiple classifications of syncope exist, but all share a common mechanism of cerebral hypoperfusion as the underlying etiology. Syncope can be broken down to two main subtypes: cardiac and noncardiac syncope. Cardiac syncope is caused by brady- or tachyarrhythmias, or hypotension as seen with decreased cardiac index, obstructed blood flow, vascular dissection, or vasodilatation. Conversely, noncardiac syncope is attributed to other noncardiac etiologies, including volume depletion, reflex syncope, or orthostatic hypotension.[33] These subtypes carry distinct historical characteristics that are associated with increased probability of either cardiac versus noncardiac syncope (Table 18-1).[33] Syncope is a common medical problem that is frequently benign, but has a high rate of mortality in patients with underlying heart disease, transient myocardial ischemia, and other cardiac abnormalities. Data gathered from the history and physical, and laboratory studies are used to assign patients to either a short-term (from presentation and up to 30 days after syncope) or long-term (up to 12 months after syncope) risk group (Table 18-2).[33] The 1-year mortality rate for presumed cardiac causes of syncope has been reported to be 20% to 30%.[34] Therefore, the principal objective when evaluating a patient with syncope is to rule out any life-threatening etiology.

Although patients are routinely referred to EP centers for syncope evaluation, invasive EP testing is not always indicated and plays only a limited role as discussed later in this section. Obtaining a thorough history, physical examination, along with a 12-lead ECG, however, are class I recommendations for the initial evaluation of syncope, and these results can frequently uncover the mechanism and direct treatment.[33] The most common cause of syncope is vasodepressor syncope (otherwise known as neurally mediated syncope (NMS), neurocardiogenic syncope, or vasovagal syncope) followed by primary arrhythmias.

The history, including observers' statements describing the onset and recovery can provide clues for the cause. For example, sudden onset of syncope without any warning signs or symptoms suggests a cardiac arrhythmia. Recovery from syncope caused by a cardiac event is usually rapid, without neurologic sequelae,

Table 18-1 • HISTORICAL CHARACTERISTICS ASSOCIATED WITH INCREASED PROBABILITY OF CARDIAC AND NONCARDIAC CAUSES OF SYNCOPE

More Often Associated With Cardiac Causes of Syncope

- Older age (>60 years)
- Male sex
- Presence of known ischemic heart disease, structural heart disease, previous arrhythmias, or reduced ventricular function
- Brief prodrome, such as palpitations, or sudden loss of consciousness without prodrome
- Syncope during exertion
- Syncope in the supine position
- Low number of syncope episodes (1 or 2)
- Abnormal cardiac examination
- Family history of inheritable conditions or premature SCD (<50 years of age)
- Presence of known congenital heart disease

More Often Associated With Noncardiac Causes of Syncope

- Younger age
- No known cardiac disease
- Syncope only in the standing position
- Positional change from supine or sitting to standing
- Presence of prodrome: nausea, vomiting, feeling warmth
- Presence of specific triggers: dehydration, pain, distressful stimulus, medical environment
- Situational triggers: cough, laugh, micturition, defecation, deglutition
- Frequent recurrence and prolonged history of syncope with similar characteristics

SCD, sudden cardiac death.
Adapted from Shen WK, Sheldon RS, Benditt DG, et al. 2017 ACC/AHA/HRS guideline for the evaluation and management of patients with syncope: a report of the American College of Cardiology/American Heart Association Task Force on clinical practice guidelines and the Heart Rhythm Society. *J Am Coll Cardiol.* 2017;70(5):e39–e110.

Table 18-2 • SHORT- AND LONG-TERM RISK FACTORS OF SYNCOPE

Short-Term Risk Factors (≤30 days)	Long-Term Risk Factors (>30 days)
History: Outpatient clinic or ED evaluation	
Male sex	Male sex
Older age (>60 years)	Older age
No prodrome	Absence of nausea/vomiting preceding syncopal event
Palpitations preceding loss of consciousness	VA
Exertional syncope	Cancer
Structural heart disease	Structural heart disease
HF	HF
Cerebrovascular disease	Cerebrovascular disease
Family history of SCD	Diabetes mellitus
Trauma	High CHADS-2 score
Physical examination or laboratory investigation	
Evidence of bleeding	Abnormal ECG
Persistent abnormal vital signs	Lower GFR
Abnormal ECG	
Positive troponin	

This table includes individual risk predictors from history, physical examination, and laboratory studies associated with adverse outcomes from selected studies.
SCD, sudden cardiac death.
Adapted from Shen WK, Sheldon RS, Benditt DG, et al. 2017 ACC/AHA/HRS guideline for the evaluation and management of patients with syncope: a report of the American College of Cardiology/American Heart Association Task Force on clinical practice guidelines and the Heart Rhythm Society. *J Am Coll Cardiol.* 2017;70(5):e39–e110.

whereas recovery from a seizure is usually associated with a period of drowsiness and confusion. Transient ischemic attacks rarely result in syncope. Syncope precipitated by neck turning may be due to carotid sinus hypersensitivity. Medications taken that may be associated with proarrhythmia or orthostasis should be identified. Finally, a family history of unexpected sudden cardiac death should be ascertained.[35]

The physical examination should include orthostatic vital signs and carotid sinus pressure in patients who do not have cerebrovascular disease or carotid bruits.[36] Orthostatic vital signs can reveal a dehydrated patient. The presence of carotid bruits suggest impaired cerebral blood flow and underlying coronary artery disease. A positive carotid sinus test is documented by recording a pause of 3 seconds or longer or a blood pressure decrease greater than 50 mm Hg without symptoms. A blood pressure decrease of 30 mm Hg with symptoms is also considered an abnormal test result.[37] Reproduction of symptoms may suggest the cause of syncope, especially if other causes are ruled out. Assessment for signs of underlying structural heart disease should be performed, including attention to heart rate and rhythm, or the presence of murmurs, rubs, or gallops. A basic neurologic examination, including assessment for focal deficits such as abnormalities of visual fields, motor strength, sensation, tremor, cognition, and speech, and gait disturbance may point to a neurologic etiology.

Once the practitioner determines that a cardiac cause is most likely, a series of noninvasive tests may be indicated. Noninvasive studies for evaluating syncope are outlined in Table 18-3. The 12-lead ECG should be scrutinized for arrhythmias, long QT syndrome, Brugada syndrome, left ventricular hypertrophy, preexcitation, conduction abnormalities, and ischemia or infarction. An echocardiogram helps to rule out or confirm the presence of structural heart disease, including valvular or obstructive disease and to evaluate left ventricular function. EP study outcomes suggest that an arrhythmia is more likely to be the cause of syncope in patients who have structural heart disease and reduced left ventricular function. Therefore, when ventricular arrhythmias are suspected, hospitalization with immediate EP testing is indicated because these patients are presumed to be at high risk for sudden cardiac death until proven otherwise. Ambulatory monitoring for 24 to 48 hours may be helpful if the patient is having frequent symptoms and is not considered to be at high risk for ventricular arrhythmias. If symptoms are not frequent enough, a patient-activated transtelephonic event recorder, implanted loop recorder system, external loop recorder, mobile cardiac outpatient telemetry, or patch recorder may be helpful in documenting the presence or absence of arrhythmia during symptoms of presyncope or syncope.[33,38,39]

Noninvasive risk stratification tools such as the signal-averaged ECG, T-wave alternans, heart rate variability, and baroreceptor sensitivity may prove helpful in identifying candidates with syncope at risk for VT events or sudden cardiac death. The signal-averaged ECG involves recording, amplifying, and filtering the surface ECG. Low-amplitude, high-frequency signals called late potentials are detected at the terminal portion of the QRS.[40,41] Delayed myocardial activation in areas of scar tissue represented by late potentials is thought to be the cause of ventricular arrhythmias. While the signal-averaged ECG is most accurate in patients with cardiomyopathy or previous myocardial infarction, it is associated with a low positive predictive value.[42] Microvolt T-wave alternans is a test where high-resolution chest electrodes detect tiny beat-to-beat changes in the ECG T-wave morphology during a period of controlled exercise. Spectral analysis, a mathematical method of measuring and comparing time and the electrical signals, is then used to calculate minute voltage changes. The presence of these changes has been associated with an increased risk of ventricular arrhythmias in patients with a history of myocardial infarction or cardiomyopathy. Studies show that the test has good positive and negative predictive accuracy.[43]

There is a growing body of evidence that supports T-wave alternans as the more powerful predictor for future arrhythmic events when compared with the signal-averaged ECG.[43,44] However, to date, no prospective clinical trials have demonstrated enough evidence to support the widespread use of any of these tests for high-risk screening and further research is still needed.[42,45]

The head-upright tilt test is a noninvasive, provocative test used to reproduce and diagnose NMS otherwise known as vasodepressor, neurocardiogenic, or vasovagal syncope. NMS is manifested by a combination of vasodilation and bradycardia, which occurs when the feedback mechanisms between the parasympathetic nervous system and sympathetic nervous system break down. Both systems are thought to activate alternately or simultaneously. Normal circulatory function is interrupted when both systems discharge rapidly. Vagal stimulation becomes exaggerated and causes bradycardia, vasodilation, or both in the presence of sympathetic nervous system stimulation.[46,47] During the head-upright tilt test, the patient is positioned on a tilt table with a footboard. There are various protocols for inducing NMS. Basically, an upright tilt at 60 to 70 degrees for 20 to 45 minutes is performed. If syncope is not induced, adjunctive agents such as with an isoproterenol infusion or sublingual nitrates may be used until a positive result occurs. These agents increase sensitivity but decrease specificity of the test.[48,49] A positive response reproduces the patient's syncope along with documentation of bradycardia, hypotension, or both.[49,51] Indiscriminate use of tilt table testing in patients with clear-cut vasovagal syncope should be avoided as 25% to 30% of these patients will have a "false negative" result, which may confuse the diagnosis. The tilt test is most appropriately used in patients with histories suggestive of vasovagal syncope, but when the diagnosis is uncertain.[35,42]

Invasive EP studies are indicated (class IIa recommendation)[33] when a noninvasive evaluation for syncope is negative and the suspicion for a cardiac cause remains high.[52–54] Sinus node function is evaluated by measuring the sinus node recovery time. Overdrive pacing is performed in the high right atrium for 30 to 60 seconds.[55] A prolonged sinus node recovery time may be an indication of sick sinus syndrome. The His–Purkinje system is evaluated by measuring the HV interval during sinus rhythm, and during incremental atrial pacing and atrial refractory period determinations. A prolonged HV interval is an indication of infra-Hisian disease.[56] AV node function is also evaluated by incremental atrial pacing and refractory period determinations. The Wenckebach point is recorded during incremental pacing, whereas the effective refractory periods of the atrium and AV node are recorded with the introduction of atrial extrastimuli. The atrium is refractory when the atrial extrastimuli fail to capture the atrium. The AV node is refractory when the atrial extrastimuli capture the atrium but fail to result in a His bundle depolarization (AV block). Permanent pacing may be indicated if abnormalities are found. Attempts are also made to induce ventricular and SVT during EP testing for syncope.

In all cases, the findings of the EP study along with reproduction of the patient's symptoms and other findings in the work-up must be evaluated carefully to determine the appropriate course of therapy. The mechanism for syncope remains unexplained in approximately 40% of episodes.[57] The prognosis for this latter group of patients is good.

Table 18-3 • NONINVASIVE STUDIES FOR WORK UP OF SYNCOPE[33]

Study	Description	Indication	Monitoring Period	Patient Considerations
12-lead ECG	Electrodes on the chest skin are connected to a machine that graphically records the electrical activity of the heart.	Multiple indications, including as a baseline and screening test in evaluation of cardiovascular risk and screening for arrhythmias or conduction abnormalities.	One-time real-time "snapshot" of rhythm that can be repeated as needed.	Simplest and fastest test to evaluate the heart rhythm.
Transthoracic echocardiogram	Cardiac imaging modality using sound waves through a device placed on the chest to depict cardiac structure and function.	Useful when there are suspicions about the presence of valvular disease, hypertrophic cardiomyopathy, or left ventricular dysfunction. It helps identify a potential disease substrate related to a patient's prognosis.	An outpatient study that may take around 40 minutes.	A very low risk study. It is not likely to identify the immediate cause of syncope.
Ambulatory monitoring	A test that continuously or intermittently records heart activity by electrocardiography via a small device worn by an ambulatory patient.	To evaluate ambulatory patients with syncope of suspected arrhythmic etiology.	The duration of the monitoring period should be adequate for the likelihood of capturing an event. May be intermittent or continuous, and may last from 24 hours to 3–4 weeks.	The efficacy of any monitoring device for syncope is related to the duration of monitoring, frequency of syncope, duration of prodrome, suddenness of incapacitation, and continuous versus intermittent monitoring.
Patient-activated, transtelephonic monitor (event recorder)	A recording device for electrical heart activity that is triggered by the patient when symptoms occur. The monitor records this data, which is, in turn, transmitted by telephone to an ECG receiving center that evaluates the ECGs.	To evaluate ambulatory patients with frequently recurring syncope or near syncope of suspected arrhythmic etiology.	An outpatient monitoring system that is used over a 2–6 week period.	Limited use in patients who experience sudden incapacitation with syncope. Better for those with frequent symptoms that are likely to recur within 2–6 weeks.
Loop recorder (external or implantable)	A device that continuously records and stores heart rhythm data. Recording ECGs can be patient-activated or auto triggered to record events preceding, during, or after the triggered event. Data is transmitted over a wireless network to a remote monitoring system.	To evaluate ambulatory patients with frequently recurring syncope or near syncope of suspected arrhythmic etiology. The looping memory feature allows it to record a section of the ECG that occurred before and after the patient activated the monitor.	External devices can record data over weeks to months, whereas implantable loop recorders may last up to 3 years.	Better for patients with symptoms that are likely to recur within 2–6 weeks (external loop recorder). Transient, infrequent symptoms can also be captured (implantable loop recorder). Implantable loop recorders require a brief outpatient procedure for implant/explant, but do not require sedation.
Mobile outpatient telemetry	A device that automatically records and wirelessly transmits the patient's ECG data to a central monitoring station which is staffed by trained technicians that can provide immediate and accurate surveillance of the patient's cardiac activity around the clock.	Appropriate for high-risk patients whose rhythm requires real-time, immediate healthcare provider evaluation, or who would be unable to trigger an event recording device in the setting of syncope.	An outpatient monitoring system that is used for a period of up to 30 days.	Appropriate for high-risk patients whose rhythm requires real-time monitoring. No need for triggering monitoring equipment.
Patch recorder	An adhesive patch applied to the chest which continuously records and stores rhythm data. It is auto triggered or patient activated to allow for symptom-rhythm correlation and record events preceding, during and after the triggered event.	Considered as an alternative to external loop recorder.	Various models record heart rhythm from 2 to 14 days.	It can be accurately self-applied since it is leadless and is water resistant. May be more comfortable to wear than an external loop recorder.
Tilt-table test	An orthostatic stress test, which assesses the susceptibility of a vasovagal response to postural change. Patients lie on a table with the head raised to 60 to 80 degrees above the rest of the body for about 40 minutes while the blood pressure and heart rate are monitored. A positive response is when presyncope or syncope is induced and associated with hypotension, with or without bradycardia.	If the diagnosis remains unclear after initial evaluation, this test may be considered for those with suspected vasovagal syncope, orthostatic hypotension, convulsive syncope or psychogenic syncope. Can help distinguish whether syncope is related to abnormal control of heart rate or blood pressure.	This is an outpatient procedure conducted over about 40 minutes, but may require observation in a recovery area for 30–60 minutes afterward.	Exhibiting the patient's usual presyncope or syncope symptoms are to be expected while in a safe, supervised setting by trained providers. Patients should be counseled on being strapped to the table for the duration of this procedure.

INTERVENTIONAL EP AND CATHETER ABLATION

This interventional procedure includes a diagnostic EP study and catheter ablation. The mechanism of the arrhythmia is confirmed during the first part of the procedure, and the ablation takes place during the second part. Most hospitals combine the diagnostic and therapeutic segments of the study into one procedure.[58]

Catheter Ablation

Catheter ablation techniques have been used for more than 20 years. Originally, high-energy, direct current shocks were delivered through catheters, using a standard defibrillator, to the endocardial ablation site.[59,60] The technique was not widely used, however, because of the high complication rate, including cardiac tamponade and late sudden death.[61,62] As a result, efforts to find a safer energy source were pursued. In 1986, RF energy was applied through catheters to create endocardial lesions.[63] RF energy is a form of electrical energy that is produced by high-frequency alternating current. As the current passes through tissue, heat is generated. RF current is used in the operating room to coagulate blood vessels and to ablate abnormal tissue during neurosurgery. RF current used during endocardial catheter ablation is alternating current with a 500,000- to 750,000-Hz frequency range. The current passes from the electrode tip to a large-surface-area skin patch. The current is typically applied for 10 to 60 seconds at a time using higher power (45 to 55 W) for nonirrigated ablation catheters, or lower power (25 to 35 W) for irrigated ablation catheters, depending on the area targeted for ablation. Catheter delivery of RF energy causes tissue heating in a small area around the electrode. The typical lesion is 3 mm × 4 mm × 5 mm.[62]

Although RF energy is the most common source of energy for performing SVT ablations, cryoablation is an effective alternative to RF catheter ablation, which targets a focal site using extremely cold temperatures (−75° to −80°C) to destroy tissue, causing localized scarring. Cryoablation is typically used with ablations for AV nodal reentrant tachycardia (AVNRT), para-Hisian accessory pathways or para-Hisian atrial tachycardias in order to minimize injury to the AV node. A large multicenter prospective randomized trial led by Deisenhofer et al.[64] demonstrated a significantly higher recurrence rate of AVNRT with the cryoablation technique than with the RF ablation technique. However immediate ablation success and risk of AV nodal block did not differ significantly in either group.

Contact force (CF) sensing technology for RF catheter ablation is a newer advancement in the field that possibly allows delivery of better, more durable lesions by measuring the CF between the catheter tip and the myocardium in real time. CF catheters may also improve the safety and efficacy of RF catheter ablation. There is compelling evidence supporting CF sensing technology, but no prospective clinical trial shave demonstrated enough evidence to support this technology as the recommended standard of care for ablations.[65]

Catheter selection and outcomes of ablation depend on operator experience, patient selection, and target area for ablation. Alternate forms of energy for lesion generation are currently under development, including ultrasound, laser, and microwave energy sources.

Techniques

The first part of the procedure, the diagnostic phase, was described previously. After a diagnosis is made, an ablating catheter is positioned at the targeted area. The ablating catheter can be steered and has multiple electrodes, typically 2 to 5 mm apart. The catheter tip is 4 to 8 mm long and serves as the electrode through which RF current is applied. The targeted area is located using fluoroscopy and by observing the electrogram patterns recorded by the distal mapping electrode pair. Recently developed three-dimensional (3D) mapping systems have vastly improved the precision and efficiency of mapping, and also reduced fluoroscopy exposure for the staff and patient.[66] Furthermore, use of these 3D electroanatomic mapping systems has demonstrated success and complication rates for SVT ablation with zero or minimal fluoroscopy that are similar to standard fluoroscopic mapping techniques.[67,68]

Complications

Two of the most common complications associated with catheter ablation are inadvertent complete heart block when ablating in close proximity to the conduction system and cardiac perforation with tamponade when ablating within the atria, coronary sinus, or other cardiac veins, or right ventricle. Fewer than 1% to 2% of the occurrences of these complications have been reported. Rare complications include creating inadvertent arrhythmogenic foci, producing mitral or tricuspid regurgitation when ablating at or near valves, systemic embolization, and stroke (particularly when ablating in the left heart), and the creation of fixed lesions in coronary arteries when RF energy is applied in an adjacent area.[67] Specific complications related to ablation within the left atrium are addressed under the section on atrial fibrillation (AF). Complications rates of SVTs are reviewed in Table 18-4.

Indications

Combination EP study and catheter ablation procedures are a class I indication for patients with SVTs caused by APs, AV nodal reentry tachycardia, intra-atrial tachycardias caused by either automatic or reentrant mechanism, AF, and atrial flutter.[69] These procedures are also indicated for some patients with certain types of VT.

AV Nodal Reentrant Tachycardia

Dual AV nodal pathways are the substrate for AVNRT. This arrhythmia is responsible for 60% to 70% of paroxysmal SVTs.[58] The fast pathway has a longer effective refractory period and the slow pathway has a shorter refractory period. The typical form of AVNRT is initiated when a premature beat from the atrium is blocked in the fast pathway. The early beat conducts down the slow pathway and then reenters back into the atrium through the fast pathway. This impulse continues to conduct down the slow pathway and up the fast pathway, thus perpetuating the reentry circuit and the tachycardia. Uncommon or atypical forms of AVNRT can be found and consist of antegrade fast and retrograde slow pathway conduction, or antegrade and retrograde conduction over multiple slow pathway fibers. Ablation of all forms of AVNRT is generally the same and is accomplished by mapping the slow pathway region, which extends from the posterior/inferior interatrial septum near the coronary sinus ostium up to the anterior/superior interatrial septum. After characteristic electrograms are recorded, RF energy is applied through the distal ablating electrode. An alternative to RF ablation is cryoablation, which has an equivalent acute success rate and lower rate of AV block, but higher recurrence rate of AVNRT in long-term follow-up in recent systematic reviews and randomized trials.[69]

Table 18-4 • PROCEDURAL COMPLICATIONS OF SVT ABLATIONS AT DISCHARGE

	Total	AFIB	AFL	AVNRT	AVRT	Focal AT
Number of procedures, *n*	1256	4672	3755	2919	789	431
Major periprocedural and in-hospital complications, *n* (%)						
Death	4 (<0.1)	2 (<0.1)	1 (<0.1)	1 (<0.1)	0	0
Nonfatal stroke	10 (0.1)	9 (0.2)	1 (<0.1)	0	0	0
Nonfatal MI	3 (<0.1)	2 (<0.1)	1 (<0.1)	0	0	0
MACCE (death, stroke, or MI)	16 (0.1)	13 (0.3)	2 (0.1)	1 (<0.1)	0	0
Hospital stay, median (IQR)	3 (2–5)	3 (2–5)	3 (2–6)	2 (1–3)	2 (1–3)	3 (2–5)
Arrhythmia recurrence, in-hospital	3.3	7.0	1.0	0.5	1.6	4.6
Other arrhythmia, in-hospital	2.6	1.7	4.7	1.6	0.9	3.0

Data are percentages of patients unless stated otherwise. For each variable, data is available in >99.8% of patients.
MACCE, major adverse cardiac and cerebrovascular event; MI, myocardial infarction; AFIB, atrial fibrillation; AFL, atrial flutter and other macro-reentrant atrial tachycardia; AT, atrial tachycardia; AVNRT, atrioventricular nodal reentrant tachycardia; AVRT, atrioventricular reentrant tachycardia including Wolff–Parkinson–White syndrome; $CHADS_2$, risk of stroke ranging from 0 (low) to 6 (high); COPD, chronic obstructive pulmonary disease; IQR, interquartile range; LVEF, left ventricular ejection fraction; SD, standard deviation.
Modified with permission from Brachmann J, Lewalter T, Kuck KH, et al. Long-term symptom improvement and patient satisfaction following catheter ablation of SVT: insights from the German ablation registry. *Eur Heart J.* 2017;38:1317–1326.

Repeat programmed stimulation is performed after the ablation in an attempt to induce the tachycardia. The procedure is considered successful when AVNRT cannot be induced and/or when there is no evidence of slow pathway conduction. Complete heart block is a potentially serious complication because of the close proximity of the slow pathway to the compact AV node and has been reported 1.3% to 3% of the time. The success rate is reported to be greater than 95% in large registry studies.[70,71]

AV Reentrant Tachycardia

Both Wolff–Parkinson–White (WPW) syndrome and concealed AV bypass tracts are responsible for 30% to 40% of paroxysmal SVTs.[72] The anatomy is basically the same. The AP is a small bundle of muscle fibers that crosses the AV groove on either the right or left side of the heart, creating an extra electrical connection that can conduct in one or both directions. When the AP conducts in an anterograde direction, a delta wave can be observed on the ECG and is characteristic of WPW syndrome. Paroxysmal SVT is initiated in the same manner as described for AVNRT. In orthodromic reciprocating tachycardia, the AV node serves as the antegrade limb of the tachycardia and the AP serves as the retrograde limb of the tachycardia. This conduction pattern results in a narrow QRS complex. If conduction travels antegrade over the AP and retrograde up the AV node, then a wide QRS complex is observed and is known as antidromic reciprocating tachycardia. If AF occurs in a patient with WPW syndrome, then a life-threatening situation may develop if conduction over the AP is rapid enough to induce VF. Less common forms of APs are the Mahaim fiber, which slowly conducts only antegrade and is found on the right side of the heart, and the permanent form of junctional reciprocating tachycardia, which slowly conducts only retrograde and is located very near or within the coronary sinus ostium.[73,74]

Catheter ablation of AV bypass tracts on the left side of the heart involves one of two techniques. The mapping and ablating catheter can be advanced from the femoral artery retrograde across the aortic valve. The catheter is then positioned under or on the mitral valve annulus. When the catheter is positioned properly, the AP activation can be recorded and appears as a discrete high-frequency potential (Fig. 18-3).[58,75] RF current is then applied. If the patient has WPW syndrome, the delta wave on the ECG disappears during RF energy application. It is necessary to ablate so that both antegrade and retrograde conduction over the bypass tract are abolished. Testing is performed after ablating to assess for retrograde conduction and to try to induce tachycardia. Another approach to the mitral annulus is by means of transseptal catheterization. In this approach, the ablating and mapping catheter is advanced to the left atrium through the right heart using a special sheath assembly to cross the interatrial septum (Fig. 18-4). Both approaches have an 85% success rate.[76] Catheter ablations of right-sided and septal APs are somewhat more difficult because there is no structure analogous to the coronary sinus to aid in mapping the atrial–ventricular groove. Specialized multielectrode, steerable catheters, and long guiding sheaths have proven useful in providing catheter stability for mapping and ablating on the right side of the heart.

Atrial Flutter

Primary ablation of classic right atrial isthmus–dependent flutter is being performed in most centers and can be offered as a first-line therapy in patients with atrial flutter who are not interested in drug therapy.[77] This procedure involves ablation of a discrete anatomic region in the low right atrium thought to be responsible for the macro-reentrant circuit. Ablation of the right atrial isthmus between the inferior vena cava and tricuspid valve creates a line of block that prevents perpetuation of the arrhythmia (Fig. 18-5). Success rates in an experienced hospital were reported to be 90% ($n = 200$). Although the procedure is safe, with an extremely low complication rate, the recurrence of atrial flutter was 10% to 15%. Repeat ablation was successful in most cases.[78]

Atypical forms of atrial flutter are less common and can arise from the right or left atria. Mapping and ablation of these circuits can be performed but the success rate is lower than that for typical atrial flutter.

Atrial Fibrillation

Classification of AF is a factor of the duration of episodes using the current scheme as depicted in Table 18-4.[79] Outcomes of a given therapy for patients are strongly associated with their classification of AF and thus help guide the selection of the type of therapy being considered as indicated by the top 10 key points made by the 2017 Consensus Statement on Atrial

(*text continues on page 509*)

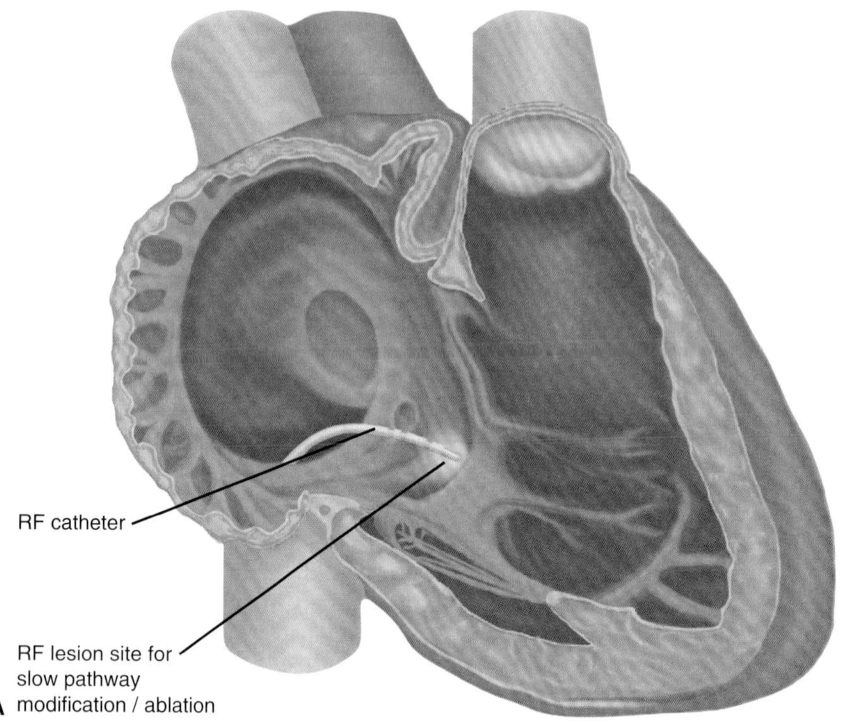

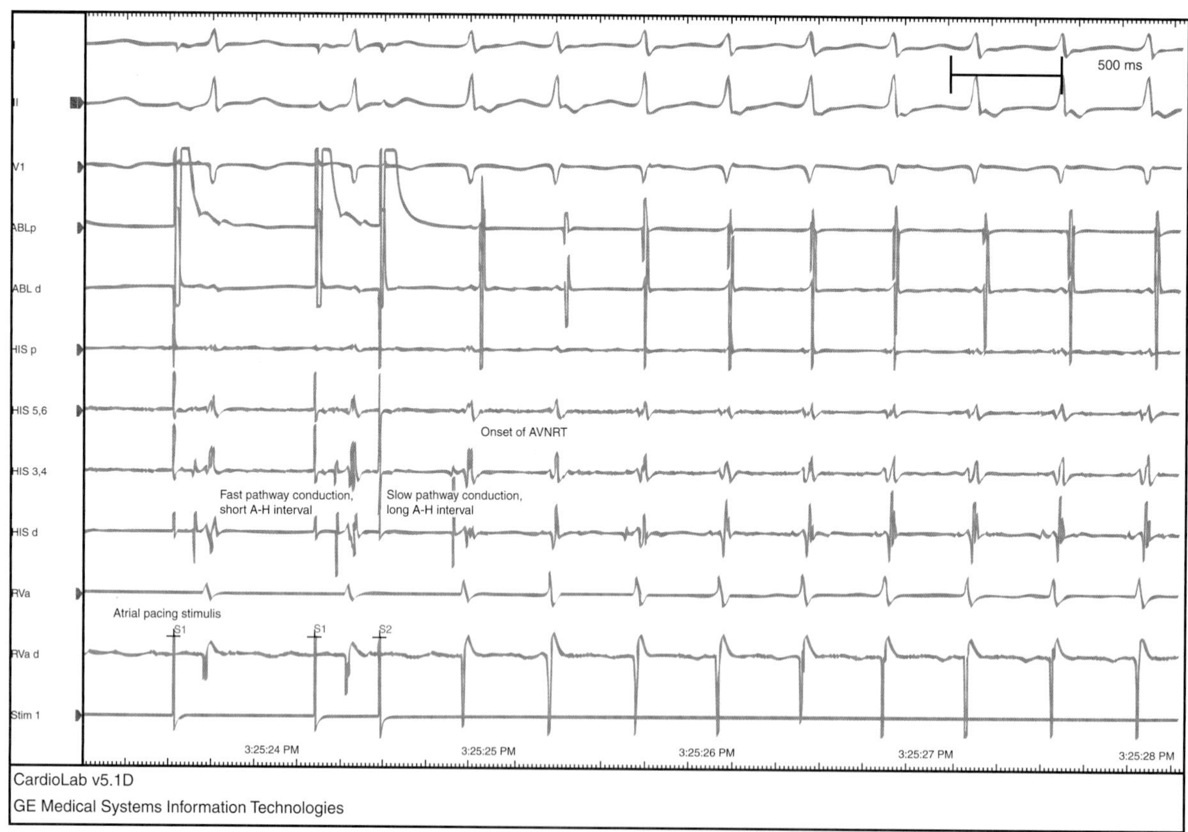

Figure 18-3. A: Diagram of slow pathway catheter ablation for treatment of AVNRT. **B:** Intracardiac electrograms show atrial pacing with AV conduction jumping from fast pathway to slow pathway followed by onset of AVNRT.

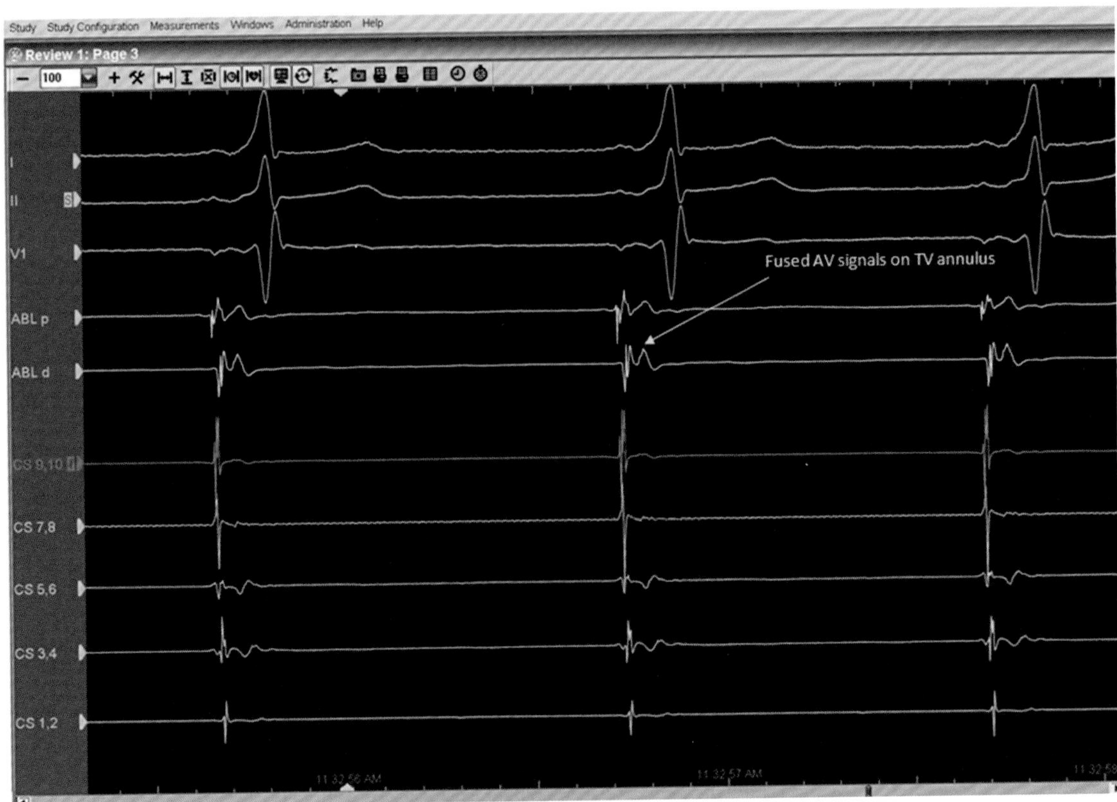

Figure 18-4. High-frequency AP potential noted on distal ablator when it was positioned along the tricuspid annulus at the earliest site mapped. This correlated with a left posteroseptal AP. Note the fused atrial and ventricular electrograms.

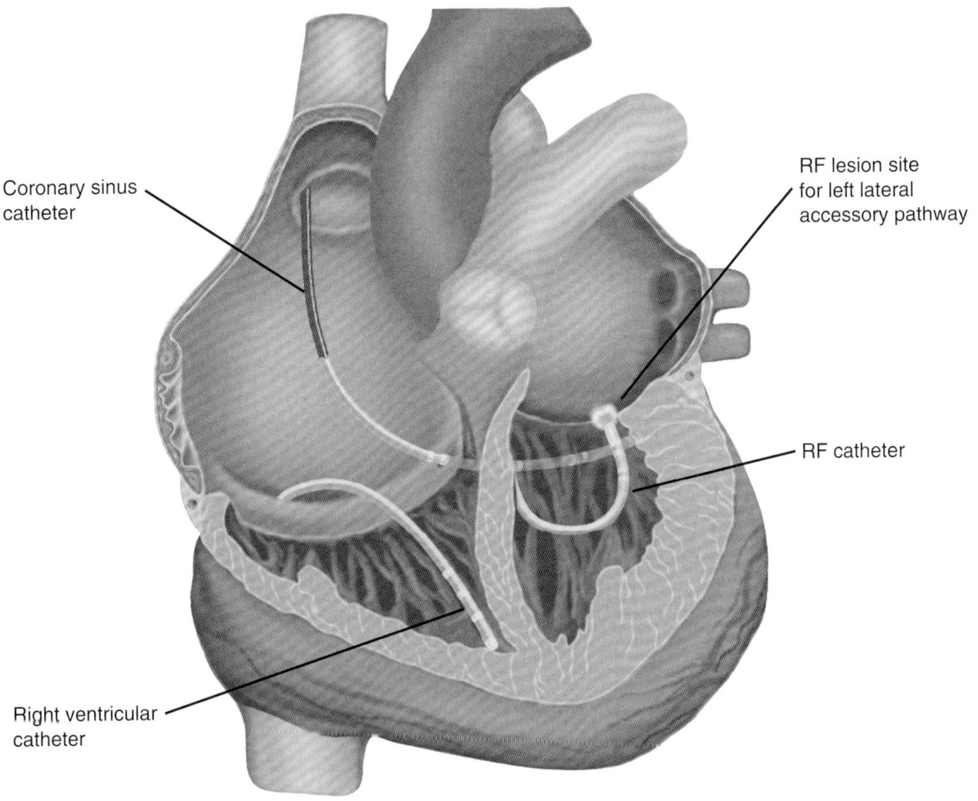

Figure 18-5. Diagram of catheter ablation of **(A)** left lateral AP using aortic approach associated radiograph in the left anterior oblique view and *(continued)*

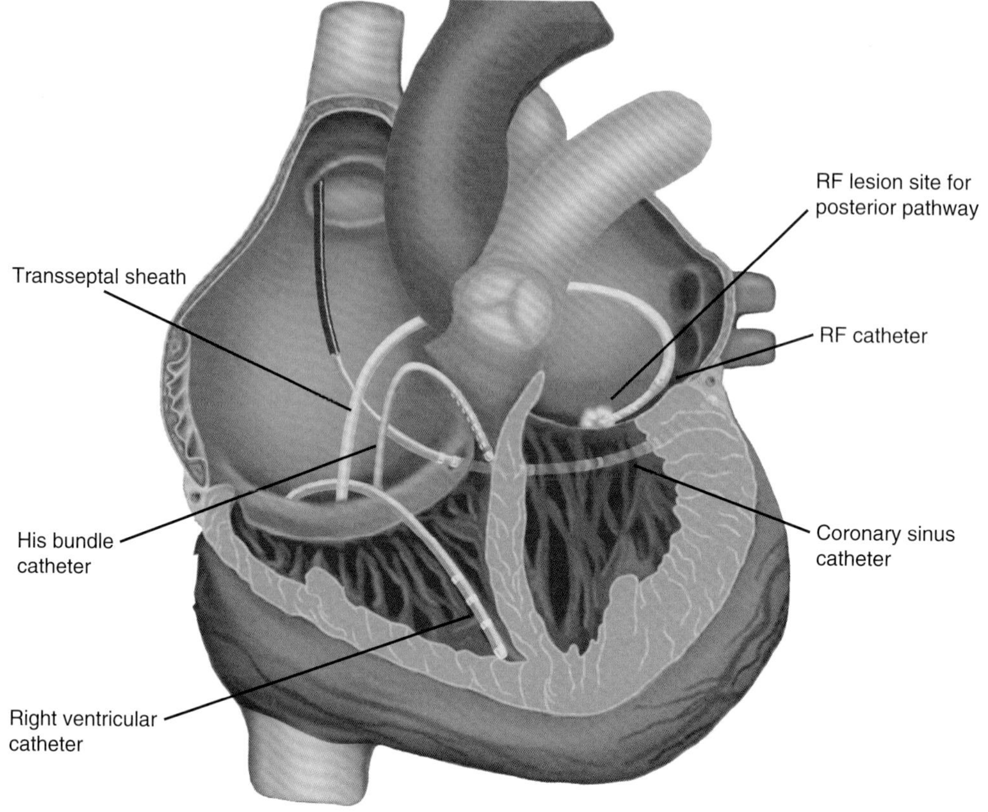

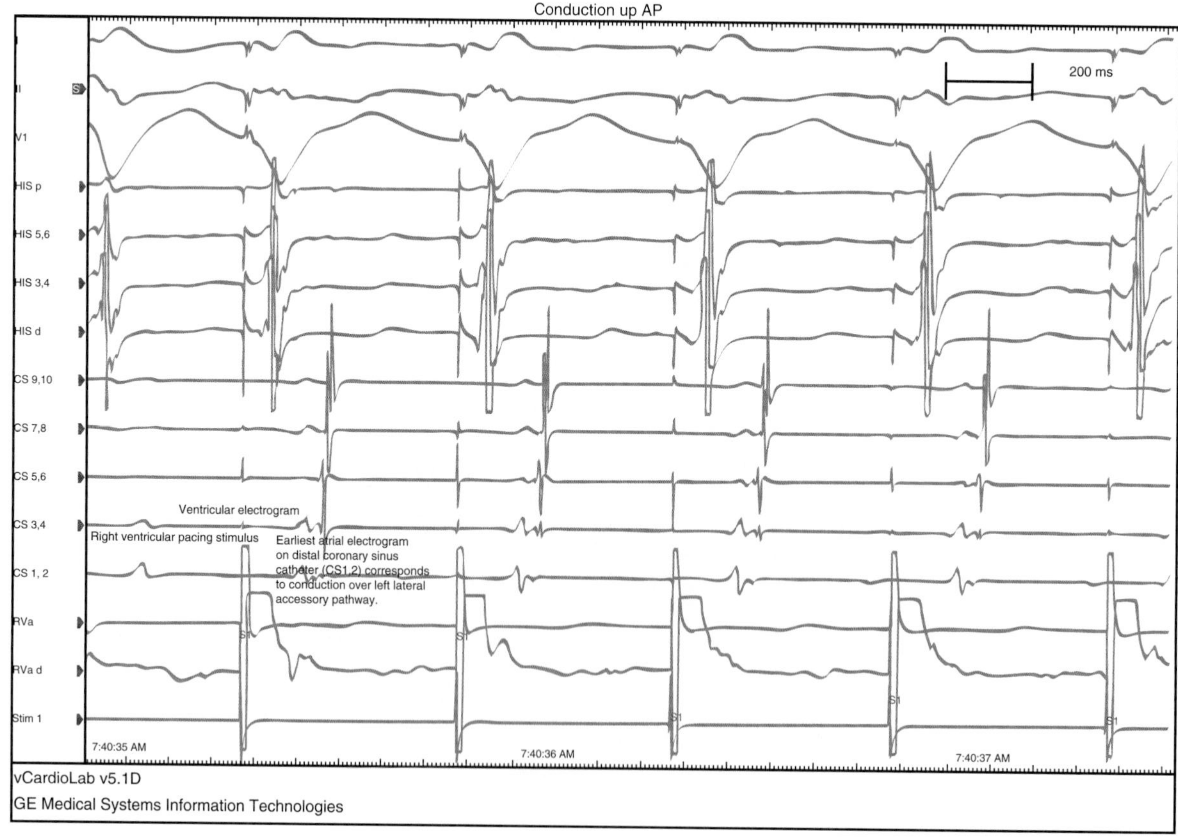

Figure 18-5. (*Continued*) **(B)** left posterior lateral AP using transseptal approach. Intracardiac electrograms show **(C)** retrograde conduction over a left lateral AP during ventricular pacing and

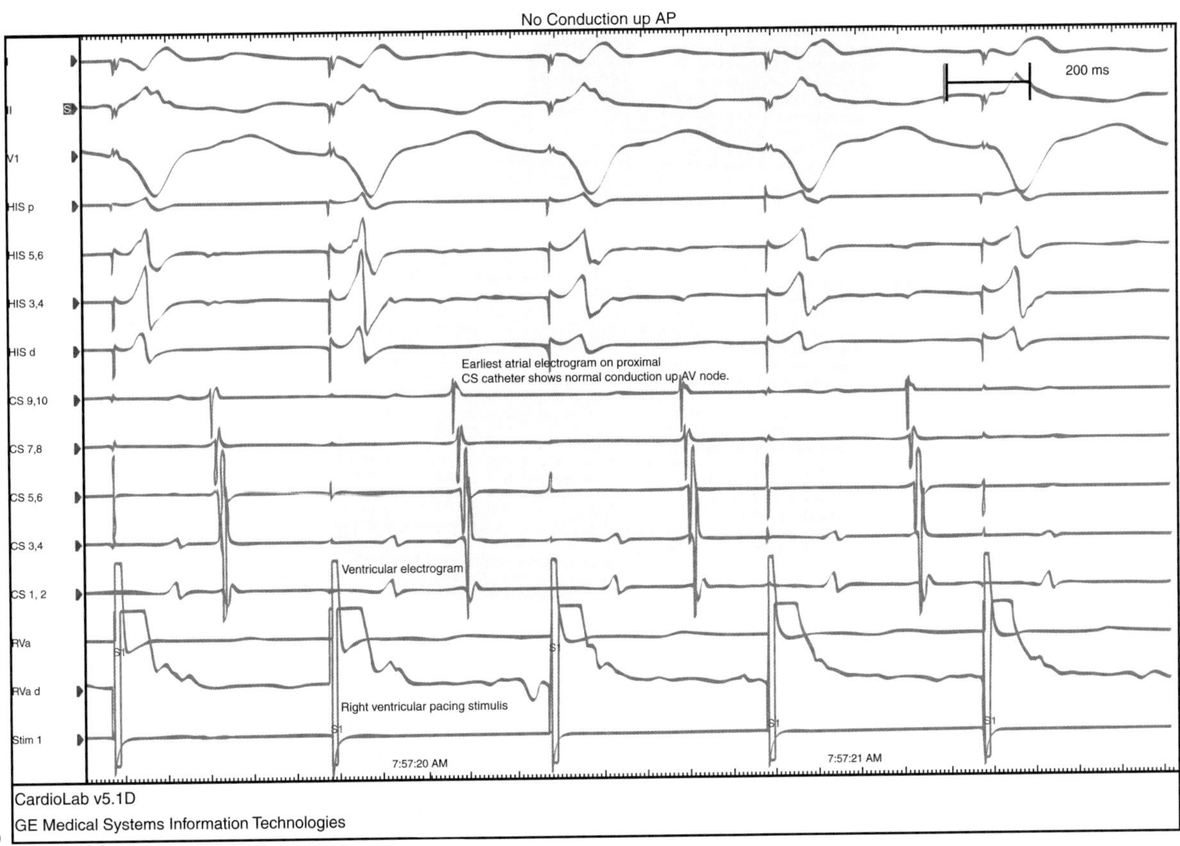

Figure 18-5. (*Continued*) **(D)** retrograde conduction up AV node during ventricular pacing after successful ablation of pathway. Post Ablation: ventricular pacing with retrograde conduction up AV node post successful ablation of left lateral accessory pathway.

Fibrillation Ablation.[80] Indications for ablation of AF are listed in Table 18-5.[81]

Complete AV node ablation is a class IIa indication for patients who have long-standing persistent or paroxysmal AF or flutter with a rapid ventricular response.[79] This procedure should be performed only in patients for whom conventional antiarrhythmic drug therapy has failed or for whom the side effects from effective doses of medication are intolerable. To perform this procedure, the ablating catheter is advanced from the right femoral vein to the area of the AV node (Fig. 18-6). Complete heart block with or without a junctional escape rhythm is the result. Permanent, rate-responsive pacing is indicated after AV node ablation, and the patient may discontinue all antiarrhythmic medications.[63,82] Given the requirement for permanent pacing following an AV node ablation, a permanent pacemaker is implanted prior to the AV node ablation, either the same day, or more often a few weeks prior to the ablation. Following an AV node ablation, continuous anticoagulation is recommended because the underlying arrhythmia is still present. Left ventricular dysfunction caused by chronic, rapid heart rates in AF has been reported to improve after AV node ablation.[83] In addition, more than 80% of the patients report improved quality of life with increased exercise tolerance after this procedure.[84]

FDA approval and use of a percutaneously implanted leadless pacemaker system as an alternative for a single-chamber pacemaker has given rise to the possibility of its utility for patients undergoing the ablate-and-pace technique. Currently, only case reports exist of simultaneous leadless pacemaker implantations combined with an AV node ablation.[85] Prospective, randomized trials are needed to further elucidate the safety and efficacy of this technique, but this strategy may have the potential to alter current common practice with the use of only a single vascular access site.

Recent ablation techniques for AF have focused on the ablation of triggers or ectopic beats that arise from the pulmonary veins (PVs) within the left atrium. In the mid-1990s, Haissaguerre et al. observed that isolated or multiple focal discharges emanated from sleeves of atrial myocardium, which encased the PVs. These discharges often led to the initiation of AF.[86] Catheter ablation

Table 18-5 • DEFINITIONS OF AF: A SIMPLIFIED SCHEME

Term	Definition
Paroxysmal AF	AF that terminates spontaneously within 7 days of onset. Frequency of recurrent episodes may vary.
Persistent AF	Continuous AF that lasts more than 7 days.
Long-standing Persistent AF	Continuous AF that lasts more than 12 months.
Permanent AF	Those with persistent AF where a mutual decision between the patient and clinician has been made to no longer pursue a rhythm control strategy. The acceptance of AF may evolve based on changes in symptoms, therapeutic interventions, and patient/clinician preferences.
Nonvalvular AF	AF in the absence of rheumatic mitral stenosis, a mechanical or bioprosthetic heart valve, or mitral valve repair.

AF, atrial fibrillation.

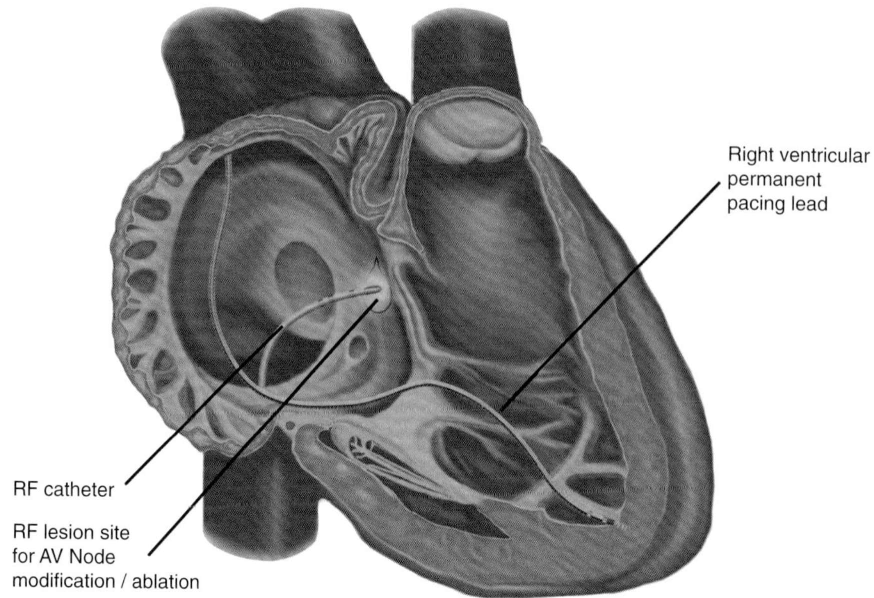

Figure 18-6. Diagram of catheter ablation of AV node and right ventricular pacemaker lead.

of these triggers involves puncture of the intra-atrial septum and placement of the ablation and mapping catheters within the left atrium. The cornerstone of an AF ablation requires PV isolation. Two methods of isolating the PV potentials exist: RF catheter ablation and cryothermal ablation using a balloon catheter (Artic Front©, Medtronic CryoCath LP). PV potentials can be mapped at the ostium of the PVs and focal point-by-point RF current is applied at sites with early potentials (Fig. 18-5). Alternatively, a guidewire is advanced into the PV, over which the cryoballoon is inflated in the left atrium, and then advanced into the PV ostium where it then delivers a cryolesion.

Attaining circumferential tissue contact is the key to delivering an effective cryolesion and lasting PV isolation. The goal of either method is to electrically isolate all four PVs, thereby eliminating the ability for these discharges to enter the left atrium and trigger AF. Another alternative ablation technique involves the creation of linear lesions within the left atrium that encircle the atrial tissue around the outside of the PV ostia. This approach is primarily anatomic, and mapping of electrograms is not necessary. A 3D electroanatomic mapping system is used as a guide.[87] Other lesion sets and ablation techniques for AF may be used depending on the operator's preference and the patient's form of AF (paroxysmal or persistent). Additional techniques include mapping and ablation of complex fractionated atrial electrograms scattered within the left atrium,[88] ablation of ganglionic plexi typically found just outside the PVs,[89] and several other lesion sets currently under development. Generally, persistent AF requires a more aggressive approach and more lesions than does paroxysmal AF to obtain a successful outcome. Potential complications include thromboembolism of air or thrombus, PV stenosis, phrenic nerve injury, atrial–esophageal fistula, pericardial perforation and tamponade, new-onset regular atrial tachycardias, vascular complications, acute coronary artery occlusion, periesophageal vagal injury and gastric hypomotility, prolonged exposure to radiation, and mitral valve trauma due to entrapment with a curvilinear mapping catheter.[90] The risk of major complications appears to be approximately 3% to 6%. Success rates vary with the experience of the centers performing this procedure and range from 70% to 80%, particularly in patients with paroxysmal AF.[87,91,92]

An alternative to endoscopic catheter ablation of AF is surgical ablation. The surgical approach is based on the Maze procedure originally developed by Dr. James Cox in 1987. In this procedure, a series of incisional scars are made across the right and left atrium using a cut-and-sew technique. The intent was to interrupt all macro-reentrant circuits thought to be responsible for AF. Fortuitously, the PVs were also isolated with this process. In addition, the left atrial appendage was amputated. The procedure was highly efficacious in restoring sinus rhythm and AV synchrony, and reducing stroke.[93] Modifications of this approach have resulted in the Cox maze III technique, which uses linear ablation lines in place of the traditional cut-and-sew incisions. In late follow-up, more than 90% of the patients have been free of symptomatic AF using what has become the gold standard for the surgical treatment of AF.[94] Minimally invasive approaches, such as the thoracoscopic AF ablation,[95] are currently under development and could expand the indications for stand-alone AF surgery in the future. Current indications for surgical ablation are listed in Table 18-6.

Atrial Arrhythmias

Arrhythmias that originate in the atria and arise from either reentrant circuits or abnormal foci can often be treated with catheter ablation. Patients who have undergone atrial surgery for congenital heart disease may have fixed anatomic barriers within scar tissue, which facilitate a reentrant tachycardia. Arrhythmias that arise from abnormal atrial foci have increased automaticity as their mechanism and can be found in either the left or right atrium. The effective site for ablation in both cases is determined by methodically mapping the appropriate atrium during tachycardia (Fig. 18-7). Use of a 3D electroanatomic or noncontact mapping system greatly enhances the ability to precisely pinpoint the origin of the tachycardia. The earliest endocardial atrial electrogram marks the origin of the tachycardia.[96]

Ventricular Tachycardia

In past history, catheter ablation of VT was not considered a reasonable therapy for patients who had not previously exhausted

(*text continues on page 515*)

Table 18-6 • INDICATIONS FOR CATHETER AND SURGICAL ABLATION OF ATRIAL FIBRILLATION

	Recommendation	Class	LOE
Indications for catheter ablation of atrial fibrillation			
A. Indications for catheter ablation of atrial fibrillation			
Symptomatic AF refractory or intolerant to at least one class I or III antiarrhythmic medication	Paroxysmal: Catheter ablation is recommended.	I	A
	Persistent: Catheter ablation is reasonable.	IIa	B-NR
	Long-standing persistent: Catheter ablation may be considered.	IIb	C-LD
Symptomatic AF prior to initiation of antiarrhythmic therapy with a class I or III antiarrhythmic medication	Paroxysmal: Catheter ablation is reasonable.	IIa	B-R
	Persistent: Catheter ablation is reasonable.	IIa	C-EO
	Long-standing persistent: Catheter ablation may be considered.	IIb	C-EO
B. Indications for catheter atrial fibrillation ablation in populations of patients not well represented in clinical trials			
Congestive heart failure	It is reasonable to use similar indications for AF ablation in selected patients with heart failure as in patients without heart failure.	IIa	B-R
Older patients (>75 years of age)	It is reasonable to use similar indications for AF ablation in selected older patients with AF as in younger patients.	IIa	B-NR
Hypertrophic cardiomyopathy (HCM)	It is reasonable to use similar indications for AF ablation in selected patients with HCM as in patients without HCM.	IIa	B-NR
Young patients (<45 years of age)	It is reasonable to use similar indications for AF ablation in young patients with AF (<45 years of age) as in older patients.	IIa	B-NR
Tachy–brady syndrome	It is reasonable to offer AF ablation as an alternative to pacemaker implantation in patients with tachy–brady syndrome.	IIa	B-NR
Athletes with AF	It is reasonable to offer high-level athletes AF as first-line therapy due to the negative effects of medications on athletic performance.	IIa	C-LD
Asymptomatic AF[a]	Paroxysmal: Catheter ablation may be considered in select patients[a]	IIb	C-EO
	Persistent: Catheter ablation may be considered in select patients.	IIb	C-EO
Indications for surgical ablation of atrial fibrillation			
C. Indications for concomitant open (such as mitral valve) surgical ablation of atrial fibrillation			
Symptomatic AF refractory or intolerant to at least one class I or III antiarrhythmic medication	Paroxysmal: Surgical ablation is recommended.	I	B-NR
	Persistent: Surgical ablation is recommended.	I	B-NR
	Long-standing persistent: Surgical ablation is recommended.	I	B-NR
Symptomatic AF prior to initiation of antiarrhythmic therapy with a class I or III antiarrhythmic medication	Paroxysmal: Surgical ablation is recommended.	I	B-NR
	Persistent: Surgical ablation is recommended.	I	B-NR
	Long-standing persistent: Surgical ablation is recommended.	I	B-NR
D. Indications for concomitant closed (such as CABG and AVR) surgical ablation of atrial fibrillation			
Symptomatic AF refractory or intolerant to at least one class I or III antiarrhythmic medication	Paroxysmal: Surgical ablation is recommended.	I	B-NR
	Persistent: Surgical ablation is recommended.	I	B-NR
	Long-standing persistent: Surgical ablation is recommended.	I	B-NR
Symptomatic AF prior to initiation of antiarrhythmic therapy with a class I or III antiarrhythmic medication	Paroxysmal: Surgical ablation is reasonable.	IIa	B-NR
	Persistent: Surgical ablation is reasonable.	IIa	B-NR
	Long-standing persistent: Surgical ablation is reasonable.	IIa	B-NR
E. Indications for stand-alone and hybrid surgical ablation of atrial fibrillation			
Symptomatic AF refractory or intolerant to at least one class I or III antiarrhythmic medication	Paroxysmal: Stand-alone surgical ablation can be considered for patients who have failed one or more attempts at catheter ablation and also for those who are intolerant or refractory to antiarrhythmic drug therapy and prefer a surgical approach, after review of the relative safety and efficacy of catheter ablation versus a stand-alone surgical approach.	IIb	B-NR
	Persistent: Stand-alone surgical ablation is reasonable for patients who have failed one or more attempts at catheter ablation and also for those patients who prefer a surgical approach after review of the relative safety and efficacy of catheter ablation versus a stand-alone surgical approach.	IIa	B-NR
	Long-standing persistent: Stand-alone surgical ablation is reasonable for patients who have failed one or more attempts at catheter ablation and also for those patients who prefer a surgical approach after review of the relative safety and efficacy of catheter ablation versus a stand-alone surgical approach.	IIa	B-NR
	It might be reasonable to apply the indications for stand-alone surgical ablation described above to patients being considered for hybrid surgical AF ablation.	IIb	C-EO

[a]A decision to perform AF ablation in an asymptomatic patient requires additional discussion with the patient because the potential benefits of the procedure for the patient without symptoms are uncertain.

AF, atrial fibrillation; LOE, level of evidence; HCM, hypertrophic cardiomyopathy.

Adapted with permission from Calkins H, Hindricks G, Cappato R, et al. 2017 HRS/EHRA/APHRS/SOLAECE expert consensus statement on catheter and surgical ablation of atrial fibrillation. *Heart Rhythm.* 2017;14(10):e275–e444.

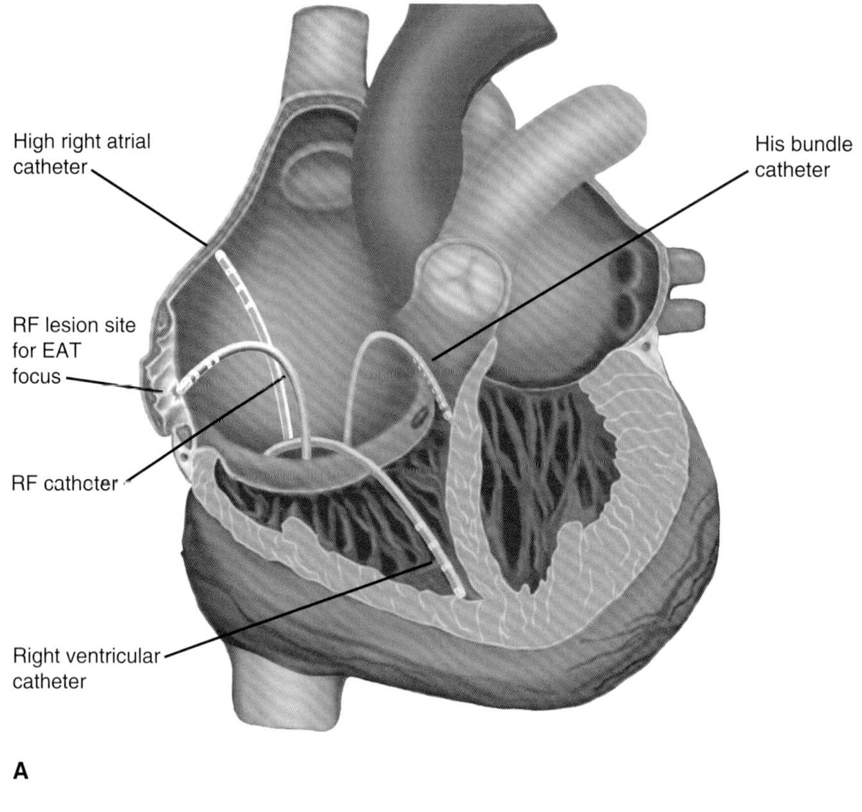

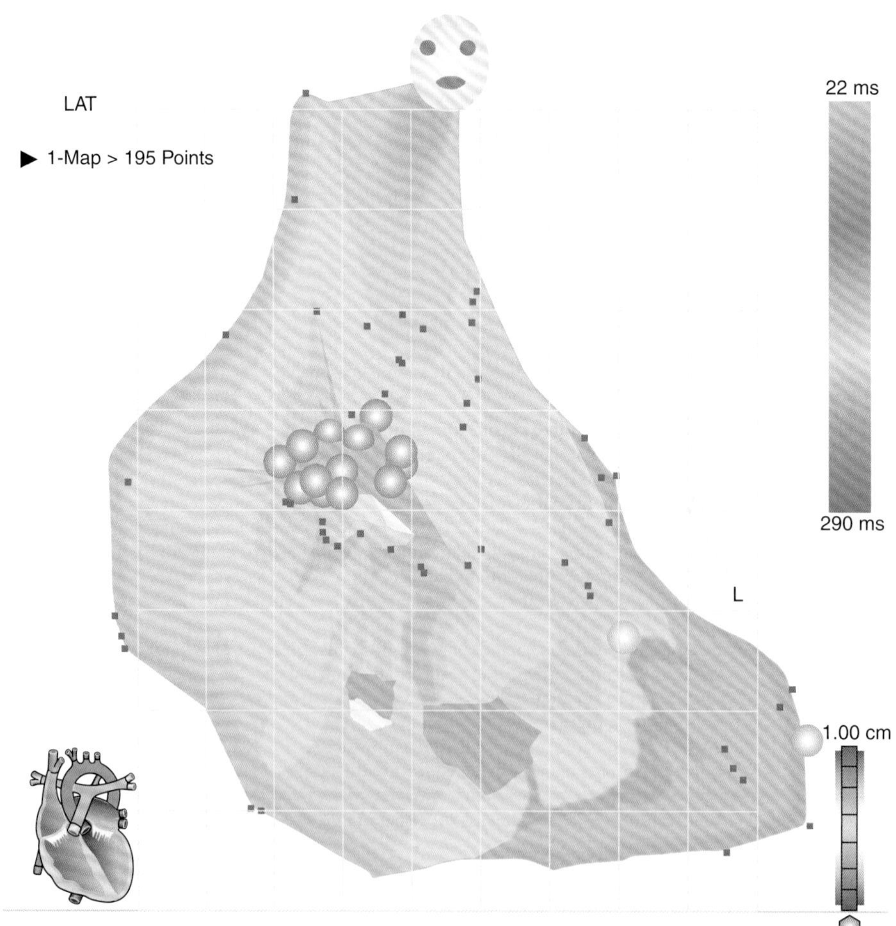

Figure 18-7. Catheter Ablation of Atrial Arrhythmias. **(A)** Diagram of catheter ablation of right atrial ectopic atrial tachycardia. **(B)** Diagram of catheter ablation of ectopic atrial tachycardia with focus on lateral wall of right atrium. Green balls show site of ablation where the atrial tachycardia originates. (2) Image of ectopic atrial focus obtained from 3-D mapping system (Biosense-Webster).

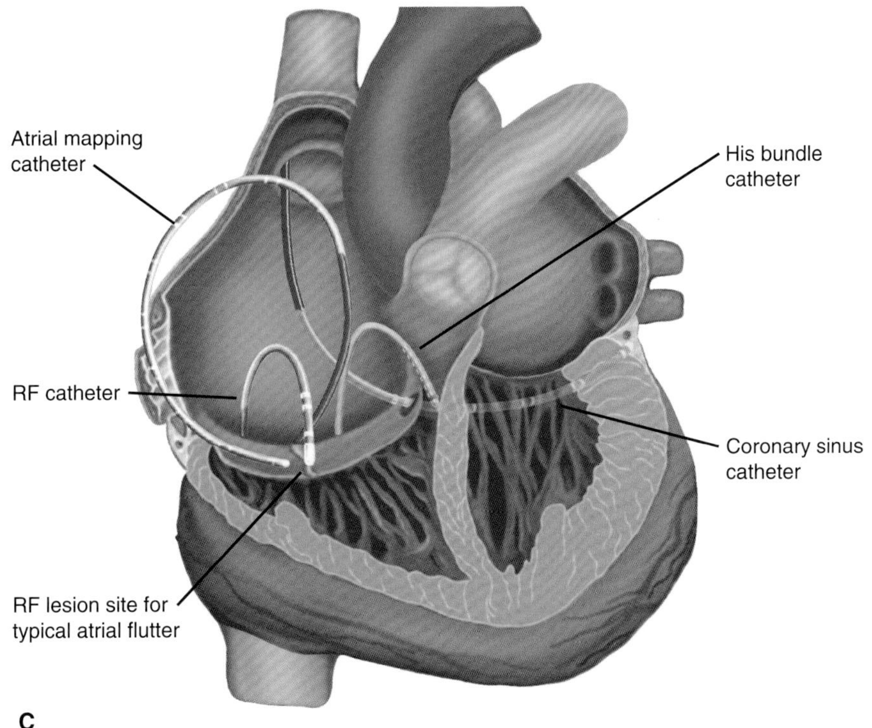

Atrial Flutter Ablation

I
II
V1
ABL p
ABL d
CS 9,10
CS 7,8
CS 5,6
CS 3,4
CS 1,2
Stim 3
P1 ART

500 ms

Ventricular beats

Atrial electrograms in sinus rhythm

Atrial flutter electrograms as seen on coronary sinus catheter

50 mm Hg

11:42:19 AM 11:42:20 AM 11:42:21 AM 11:42:22 AM 11:42:23 AM

CardioLab v5.1D
GE Medical Systems Information Technologies

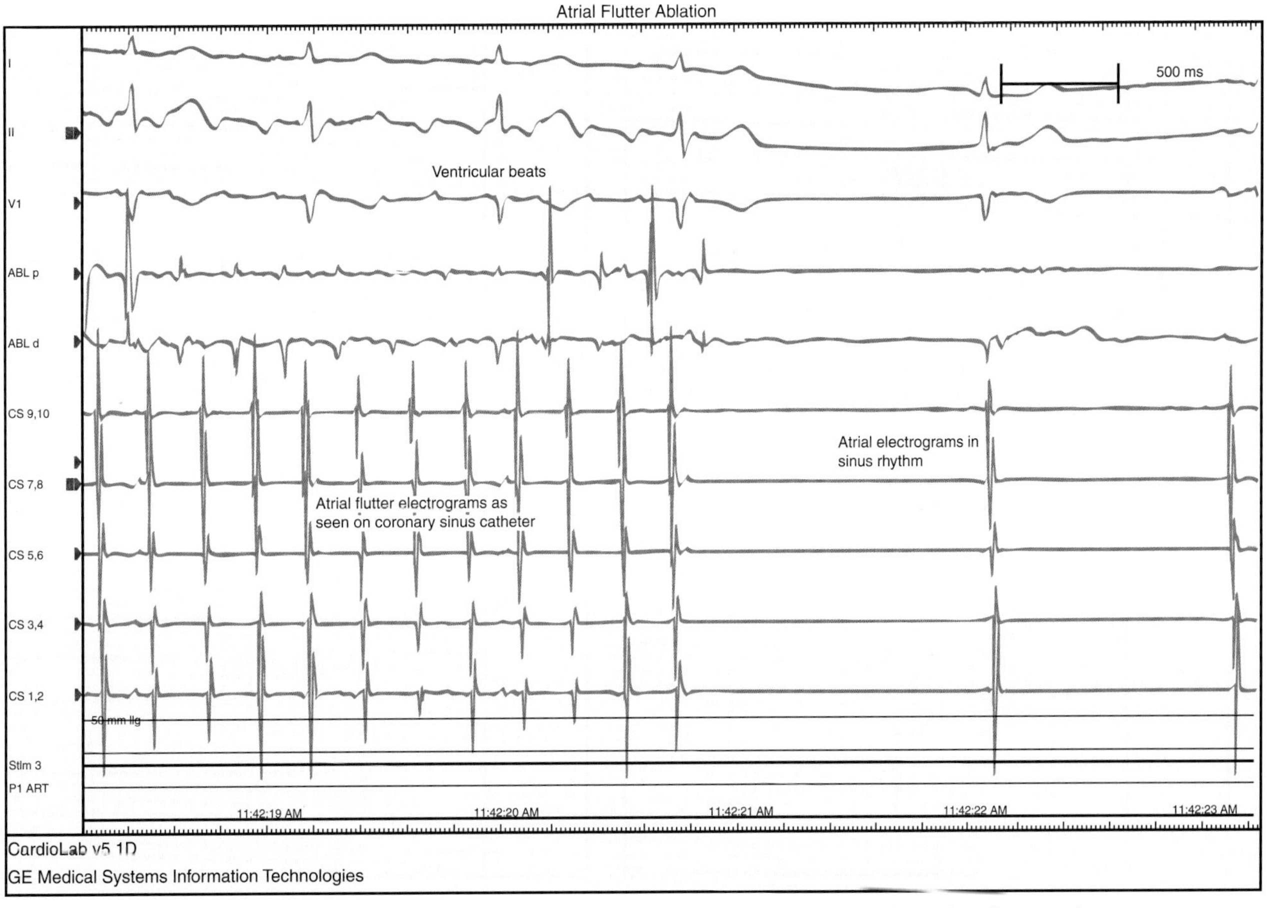

D

Figure 18-7. (*Continued*) **(C)** Diagram of catheter ablation of right atrial isthmus-dependent flutter and **(D)** intracardiac electrograms showing termination of atrial flutter during ablation. (*continued*)

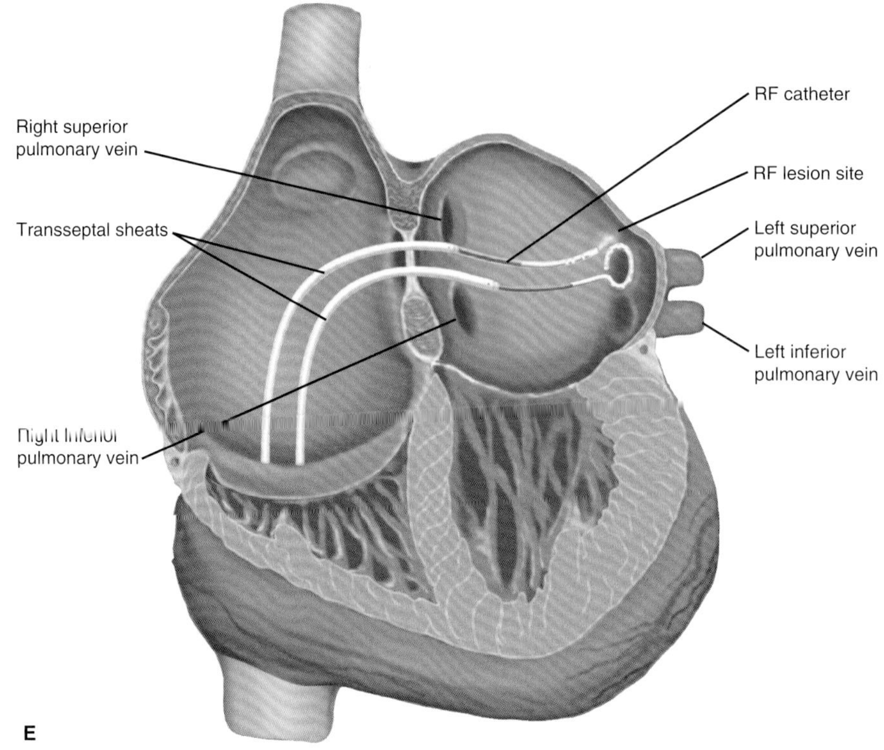

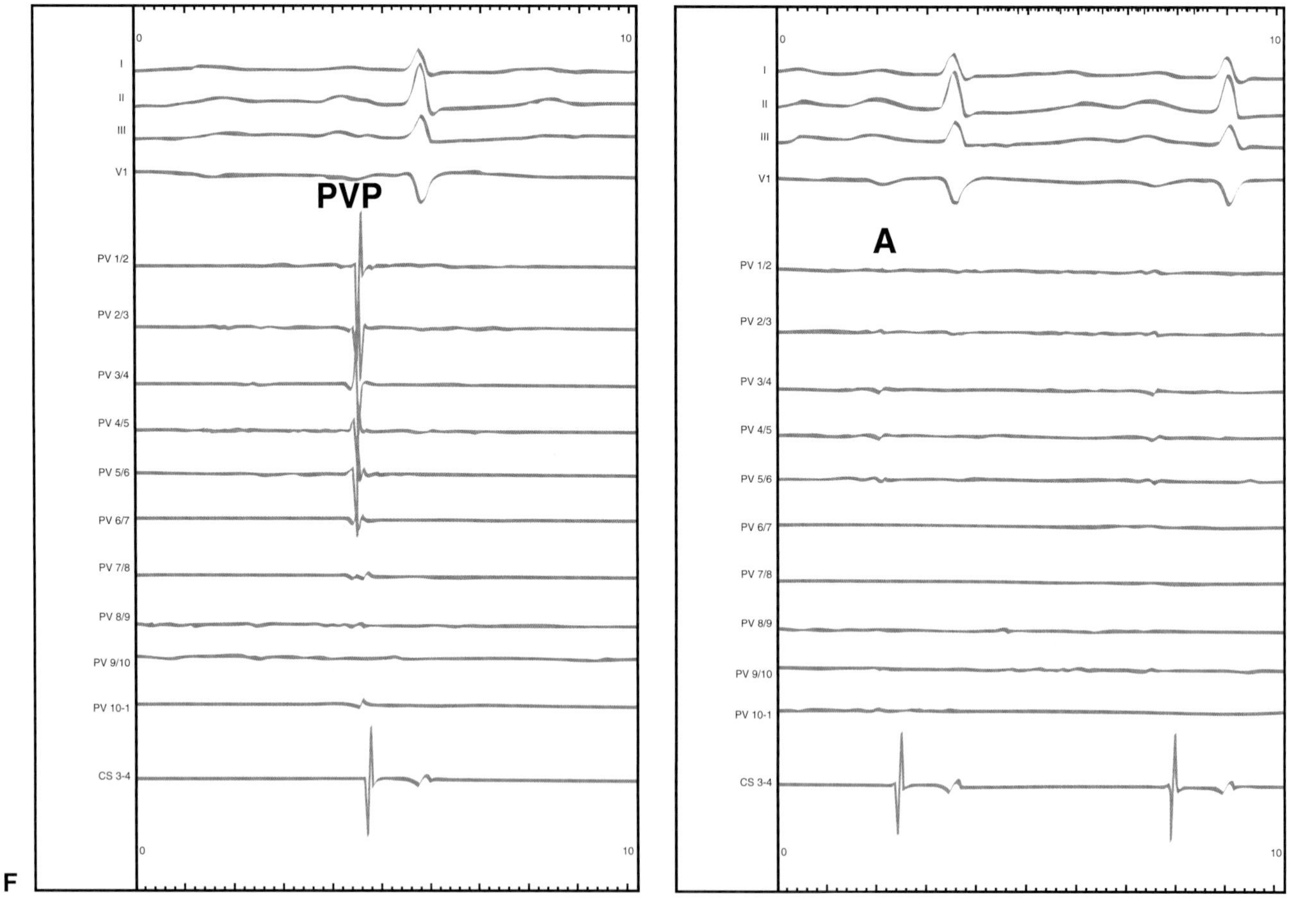

Figure 18-7. (*Continued*) **(E)** Diagram of catheter ablation of atrial fibrillation using a radiofrequency catheter ablation technique and **(F)** Intracardiac electrograms showing pulmonary vein potentials prior to ablation in the left-hand figure and then loss of pulmonary vein potentials (electrical isolation) after ablation in the right-hand figure. A, far field atrial electrogram; EAT, ectopic atrial tachycardia; LAT, left atrial tachycardia; PVP, pulmonary vein potential.

Table 18-7 • INDICATIONS FOR CATHETER ABLATION OF VENTRICULAR TACHYCARDIA

Patients with structural heart disease (including prior MI, dilated cardiomyopathy, ARVC/D) *Catheter ablation of VT is recommended*

1. for symptomatic sustained monomorphic VT (SMVT), including VT terminated by an ICD, that recurs despite antiarrhythmic drug therapy or when antiarrhythmic drugs are not tolerated or not desired[a];
2. for control of incessant SMVT or VT storm that is not due to a transient reversible cause;
3. for patients with frequent PVCs, NSVTs, or VT that is presumed to cause ventricular dysfunction;
4. for bundle branch reentrant or interfascicular VTs;
5. for recurrent sustained polymorphic VT and VF that is refractory to antiarrhythmic therapy when there is a suspected trigger that can be targeted for ablation.

Catheter ablation should be considered

1. in patients who have one or more episodes of SMVT despite therapy with one of more class I or III antiarrhythmic drugs;[a]
2. in patients with recurrent SMVT due to prior MI who have LV ejection fraction >0.30 and expectation for 1 year of survival, and is an acceptable alternative to amiodarone therapy;[a]
3. in patients with hemodynamically tolerated SMVT due to prior MI who have reasonably preserved LV ejection fraction (>0.35) even if they have not failed antiarrhythmic drug therapy.[a]

Patients without structural heart disease

Catheter ablation of VT is recommended for patients with idiopathic VT

1. for monomorphic VT that is causing severe symptoms;
2. for monomorphic VT when antiarrhythmic drugs are not effective, not tolerated, or not desired;
3. for recurrent sustained polymorphic VT and VF (electrical storm) that is refractory to antiarrhythmic therapy when there is a suspected trigger that can be targeted for ablation.

VT catheter ablation is contraindicated

1. in the presence of a mobile ventricular thrombus (epicardial ablation may be considered);
2. for asymptomatic PVCs and/or NSVT that are not suspected of causing or contributing to ventricular dysfunction;
3. for VT due to transient reversible causes, such as acute ischemia, hyperkalemia, or drug-induced torsade de pointes.

[a]This recommendation for ablation stands regardless of whether VT is stable or unstable, or multiple VTs are present.
ARVC/D, arrhythmogenic right ventricular cardiomyopathy/dysplasia; ICD, implantable cardioverter defibrillator; MI, myocardial infarction; NSVT, nonsustained ventricular tachycardia; PVC, premature venticular contraction; VT, ventricular tachycardia; VF, ventricular fibrillation.
Reprinted with permission from Aliot EM, Stevenson WG, Almendral-Garrote JM, et al. EHRA/HRS consensus on catheter ablation of ventricular arrhythmias. *Heart Rhythm*. 2009;6:886–933.

pharmacologic options. However, advances in both understanding of VT substrates and technology for ablation strategies has greatly facilitated VT ablation, making it an acceptable safe and efficacious option in many cases as indicated in Table 18-7.[97] Ablation of paroxysmal VT can be a challenging therapy for patients whose tachycardia is suited to study and ablation. For a VT focus to be effectively ablated, the tachycardia must be inducible, monomorphic, and tolerated for long enough periods to enable accurate mapping. For unstable VT, other interventional modalities, for example, intra-aortic balloon pump, or Impella® (Abiomed), may be used to help facilitate a patient's ability to tolerate the procedure. The advent of electroanatomic and noncontact 3D mapping systems has greatly facilitated mapping and ablation of VT.[98] For a successful ablation, the type of VT must be determined.

Bundle-branch reentrant tachycardia conducts antegrade over the right bundle and retrograde over the left bundle. This type of VT occurs in patients who have severe ischemic or idiopathic cardiomyopathy. The VT is rapid because it uses the His–Purkinje system. Ablation of the right bundle usually abolishes this VT.[99]

Benign monomorphic VT (idiopathic VT) typically occurs in young people with no structural heart disease. The VT most often arises from the right ventricular outflow tract or from the inferior left ventricular septum (fascicular VT). Various EP techniques are used to map the presumed site of origin before ablating. RF ablation is most often successful in this group of patients.

VT associated with coronary heart disease is usually caused by a reentrant mechanism in an area of patchy fibrosis or scar. One of the problems encountered with ablating in this situation is that these patients may have multiple tachycardia circuits.[76] 3D electroanatomic voltage maps can be used to reconstruct the region of scar within the ventricle and identify the critical zones of conduction delay responsible for reentrant VT. This technique is known as "substrate mapping." Ablation is employed to eliminate potential reentrant circuits and can be performed during sinus rhythm. Induction and mapping of the VT is not required prior to ablation. If a single monomorphic VT is identified, the earliest site of activation during VT also can be located and ablated using these mapping systems.[98] Techniques to identify the best ablation strategy for VT are still under development.

CONCLUSIONS

From its conception, cardiac EP has advanced well beyond the scope of its initial pioneers. The introduction of new power sources and mapping catheters, coupled with the development of 3D electroanatomic mapping techniques continue to push the envelope of this field, offering more efficient, safer means of treatment for SVTs and VT to a broader patient population.

Although current ablation techniques for treatment of AF and VT are reasonably effective, future considerations for further research in cardiac EP procedures may include comparing outcomes of PV isolation for treatment of AF using the RF catheter ablation technique to those from using the cryoablation technique as this has been a source of contention in recent literature. New ways to screen for successful patient outcomes are also needed, particularly for patients with AF and VT. Magnetic resonance imaging mapping of scar regions prior to EP ablation procedures as well as intraoperative endocardial mapping assistance with intracardiac echocardiogram imaging may prove to be beneficial for mapping substrate regions of arrhythmias and has the potential to reduce fluoroscopy exposure. Further evidence-based advances in technology and methodology are needed and will hopefully address these shortcomings in the years to come.

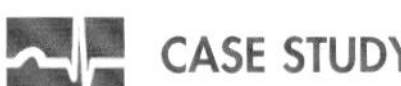

CASE STUDY 1

Patient Profile

History of Present Illness

Mr. Roberts is an 84-year-old male with a history of coronary artery disease status post previous stenting to the right coronary artery in the presence of an acute inferior wall myocardial infarction, hypothyroidism, sleep apnea, and recent episodes of syncope while returning from a cruise to Alaska with reported episodes of prolonged ventricular tachycardia. His left ventricular function is reduced with an LV ejection fraction of 42% and moderate aortic stenosis noted on a transthoracic echocardiogram. He has stable coronary anatomy on a recent heart catheterization.

Family History

No family history of heart disease.

Social History

Retired. Lives with his wife in California and was on a cruise when the syncope event occurred. Nonsmoker. Rare alcohol use.

Medications

Metoprolol XL 25 mg daily, Simvastatin 20 mg daily, Lisinopril 5 mg twice daily, Aspirin 81 mg daily

Allergies

No known allergies

Assessment and Plan

Mr. Roberts is a 64-year-old male with a history of stable coronary artery disease status post remote coronary artery bypass graft surgery who now presents with recurrent syncope due to an unknown etiology. He has known left ventricular dysfunction with a reduced ejection fraction. Shared decision making with Mr. Roberts and the cardiology team determines that he will undergo an EP study to assess for inducibility of VT or other causes of syncope, and furthermore to assess for ability to suppress VT in consideration of an ICD implant (Fig. 18-8).

This patient later underwent an ICD implant during the same hospitalization and 24 hours after this device was implanted, the patient received three ICD shocks. All three shocks were appropriate for rapid VT and delivered despite amiodarone loading.

Key Takeaways

The cardiac nurse must understand that structural heart abnormalities are frequently related to or give rise to electrophysiologic abnormalities. This case highlights the value of an EP study when suspicion of ventricular arrhythmias is high in a patient presenting with syncope and concomitant known structural heart disease with a reduced left ventricular function. The rate of this inducible VT also allowed for successful, individualized ICD tachytherapy programming.

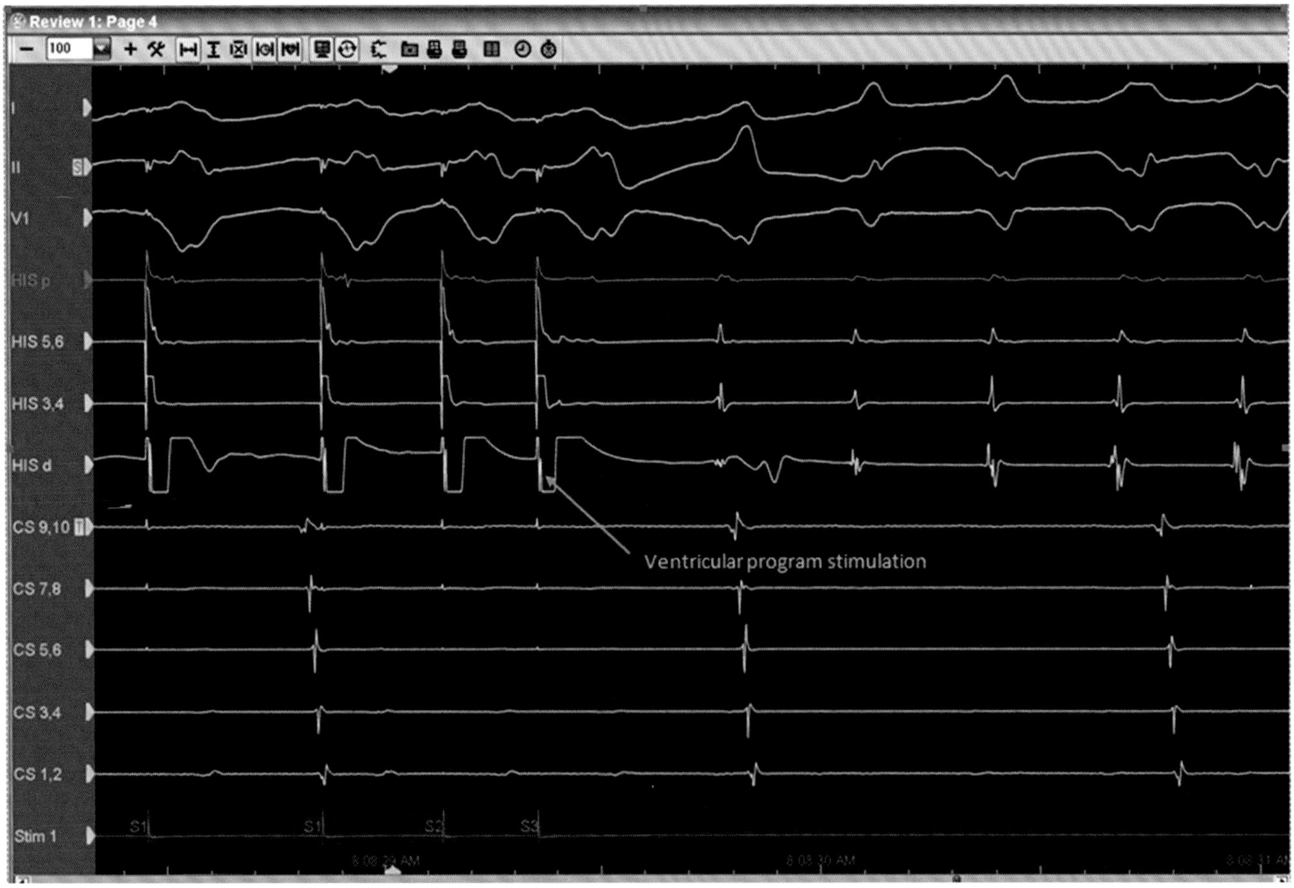

Figure 18-8. Ventricular tachycardia induction with programmed ventricular single extrastimuli pacing. Notable for atrioventricular (AV) dissociation.

CASE STUDY 2

Patient Profile

History of Present Illness

Mr. Barbados is a 24-year-old male with evidence of WPW on a resting ECG as noted during an entrance physical for the officers' training program in the Marine Corps. He has no prior medical history. He is asymptomatic but desires to become a pilot in the Marine Corps and cannot fly with evidence of WPW.

Family History

Parents are alive and well. He is an only child.

Social History

He is in the Marine Corps officers training program. Nonsmoker. Occasionally drinks to excess, drinks about 10 to 12 beers a week.

Medications

None

Allergies

No known allergies

Assessment and Plan

Mr. Barbados is a 24-year-old male who presents with electrocardiographic evidence of WPW. A cardiac EP study confirms the diagnosis of WPW and he is scheduled for an ablation. During the procedure, the following images are obtained (Fig. 18-9).

Key Takeaways

It is important for the nurse to have foundational knowledge of the indications, benefits, risks, and alternatives to any invasive procedures. The cardiac nurse must also understand that the outcome of any cardiovascular diagnostic procedure is impacted by the technology and protocol used. This case highlights the usefulness of the CS catheter in bracketing the position of the AP. A concern for a manifest accessory pathway is the potential for inducibility of ventricular arrhythmias, particularly should the same patient develop atrial fibrillation as this can serve as the trigger for VA in the presence of a bypass tract.

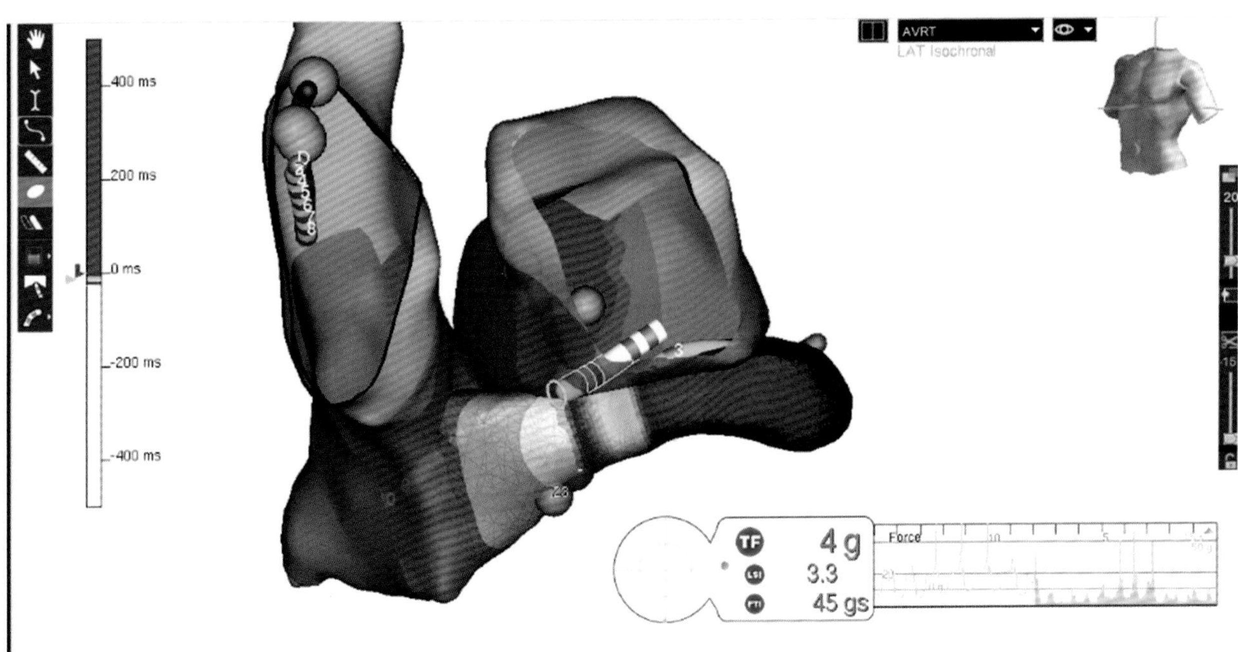

Figure 18-9. **(A)** Electroanatomic map courtesy of Abbott EnSite Velocity depicting earliest site of AP as denoted by red (earliest) and purple (latest) color scheme for activation mapping within the CS. Ablation catheter is positioned in left atrium via transseptal puncture along the mitral valve annulus over the CS 5, 6 position, corresponding to the left posteroseptal position. *(continued)*

CASE STUDY 2 (*Continued*)

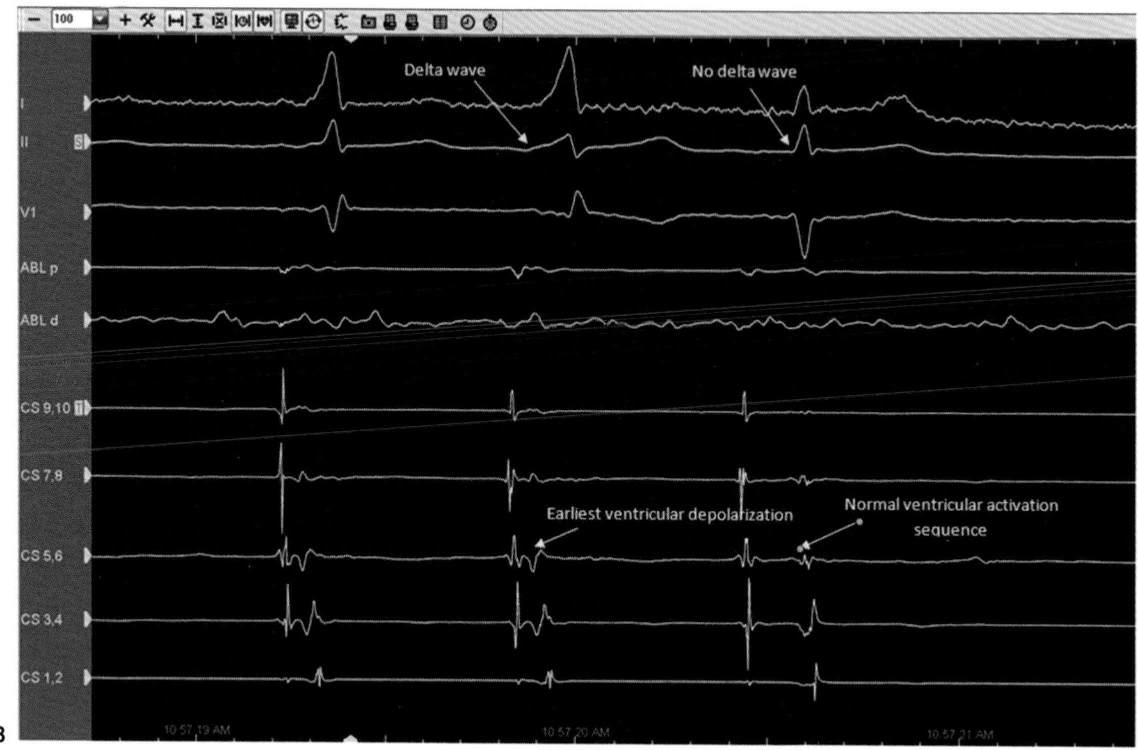

Figure 18-9. (*Continued*) **(B)** Loss of delta wave after onset of RF energy application. Notice that before RF energy is applied, the earliest ventricular depolarization occurs on the CS electrogram labelled CS 5, 6, corresponding to the left posteroseptal position. This location is where the mapping and ablating catheter was positioned under the mitral valve annulus. After RF energy application, the delta wave disappears (leads I, II, V1), and the ventricular activation sequence normalizes on all CS electrograms. (Created by Claude Rickerd of Abbott. St. Jude Medical. Used with permission.)

KEY READINGS

For further enrichment, the following key readings are recommended:

Aliot EM, Stevenson WG, Almendral-Garrote JM, et al. EHRA/HRS consensus on catheter ablation of ventricular arrhythmias. *Heart Rhythm*. 2009;6(6):886–933.

Calkins H, Hindricks G, Cappato R, et al. 2017 HRS/EHRA/APHRS/SOLAECE expert consensus statement on catheter and surgical ablation of atrial fibrillation. *Heart Rhythm*. 2017;14(10):e275–e444.

January CT, Wann LS, Alpert JS, et al. 2014 AHA/ACC/HRS guideline for the management of patients with atrial fibrillation. *J Am Coll Cardiol*. 2014;64(21): e1–e76.

Page RL, Joglar JA, Caldwell MA, et al. 2015 ACC/AHA/HRS guideline for the management of adult patients with supraventricular tachycardia: a report of the American College of Cardiology/American Heart Association Task Force on clinical practice guidelines and the Heart Rhythm Society. *Heart Rhythm*. 2016;13:e136–e221.

REFERENCES

1. Luderitz B. Historical perspectives of cardiac electrophysiology. *Hellenic J Cardiol*. 2009;50:3–16.
2. Bashir Y, Betts TR, Rajappan K. Part I: Essential background information. In: *Cardiac Electrophysiology and Catheter Ablation*. 1st ed. New York: Oxford University Press; 2010:4–6.
3. Scheinman MM, Morady F, Hess DS, et al. Catheter-induced ablation of the atrioventricular junction to control refractory supraventricular arrhythmias. *JAMA*. 1982;248:851–855.
4. Tracy CM, Akhtar M, DiMarco JP, et al. American College of Cardiology/American Heart Association Clinical competence statement on invasive electrophysiology studies, catheter ablation, and cardioversion. A report of the American College of Cardiology/American Heart Association/American College of Physicians-American Society of Internal Medicine task force on clinical competence. *Circulation*. 2000;102:2309–2320.
5. Scheinman MM. NASPE survey on catheter ablation. *Pacing Clin Electrophysiol*. 1995;18:1474–1478.
6. Brachmann J, Lewalter T, Kuck KH, et al. Long-term symptom improvement and patient satisfaction following catheter ablation of SVT: insights from the German ablation registry. *Eur Heart J*. 2017;38:1317–1326.
7. Bathina MN, Mickelsen S, Brooks C, et al. Radiofrequency catheter ablation versus medical therapy for initial treatment of supraventricular tachycardia and its impact on quality of life and healthcare costs. *Am J Cardiol*. 1998;82:589–593.
8. Horowitz LH. Safety of electrophysiologic studies. *Circulation*. 1986;73: II-28–II-30.
9. Berry VA. Wolff-Parkinson-White syndrome and the use of radiofrequency catheter ablation. *Heart Lung*. 1993;22:15–25.
10. Connelly AG. An examination of stressors in the patient undergoing cardiac electrophysiologic studies. *Heart Lung*. 1992;21:335–342.
11. Moulton L, Grant J, Miller B, et al. Radiofrequency catheter ablation for supraventricular tachycardia. *Heart Lung*. 1993;22:3–14.
12. Gure MT, Bubien RS, Belco KM, et al. Policy statement: North American Society of Pacing and Electrophysiology: standards of professional practice for the allied professional in pacing and electrophysiology. *Pacing Clin Electrophysiol*. 2003;26(1):127–131.
13. Josephson ME. Electrophysiologic investigation: general concepts. In: Josephson ME, ed. *Clinical Cardiac Electrophysiology Techniques and Interpretations*. 2nd ed. Philadelphia, PA: Lea & Febiger; 1993:22–70.
14. Hammill SC, Sugrue DD, Gersh BJ, et al. Clinical intracardiac electrophysiologic testing: technique, diagnostic indications, and therapeutic uses. *Mayo Clin Proc*. 1986;61:478–503.

15. Josephson ME. Electrophysiologic investigation: technical aspects. In: *Clinical Cardiac Electrophysiology Techniques and Interpretations*. 3rd ed. Philadelphia, PA: Lippincott Williams & Wilkins; 2002:1–18.
16. DiMarco JP, Garan H, Ruskin JN. Complications in patients undergoing electrophysiologic procedures. *Ann Intern Med*. 1982;97:490–493.
17. Schaffer WA, Cobb LA. Recurrent ventricular fibrillation and modes of death in survivors of out-of-hospital ventricular fibrillation. *N Engl J Med*. 1975;293:259–262.
18. Cobb L, Hallstrom AP. Clinical predictors and characteristics of the sudden cardiac death syndrome. In: *Proceedings USA/USSR First Joint Symposium on Sudden Death. DHEW Publication no. (NIH) 78–1470*. Washington, DC: National Institutes of Health; 1977.
19. Greene HL. Sudden arrhythmic cardiac death: mechanisms, resuscitation, and classification. *Am J Cardiol*. 1990;65:4B–12B.
20. Skale BT, Miles WM, Heger JJ, et al. Survivors of cardiac arrest: prevention of recurrence by drug therapy as predicted by electrophysiologic testing or electrocardiographic monitoring. *Am J Cardiol*. 1986;57:113–119.
21. Wilber DJ, Garan H, Finkelstein D, et al. Use of electrophysiologic testing in the prediction of long-term outcome. *N Engl J Med*. 1988;318:19–24.
22. AVID Investigators. A comparison of antiarrhythmic drug therapy with implantable defibrillators in patients resuscitated from near-fatal ventricular arrhythmias. *N Engl J Med*. 1997;337:1576–1583.
23. Buxton AE, Lee KL, Fisher JD, et al. A randomized study of prevention of sudden death in patients with coronary artery disease. Multicenter Unsustained Tachycardia Trial Investigators. *N Engl J Med*. 1999; 341:1882–1890.
24. Connolly SJ, Gent M, Roberts RS, et al. Canadian implantable defibrillator study (CIDS): a randomized trial of the implantable cardioverter defibrillator against amiodarone. *Circulation*. 2000;101:1297–1302.
25. Kuck K, Cappato R, Siebels J, et al. Randomized comparison of antiarrhythmic drug therapy with implantable defibrillators in patients resuscitated from cardiac arrest: the Cardiac Arrest Study Hamburg (CASH). *Circulation*. 2000;102:748–754.
26. Moss AJ, Hall WJ, Cannom DS, et al. Improved survival with an implantable defibrillator in patients with coronary artery disease at high risk of ventricular arrhythmia. Multicenter Automatic Defibrillator Implantation Trial Investigators. *N Engl J Med*. 1996;335:1933–1940.
27. Moss AJ, Zareba W, Hall J, et al. Prophylactic implantation of a defibrillator in patients with myocardial infarction and reduced ejection fraction. *N Engl J Med*. 2002;346:877–883.
28. Bardy GH, Lee KL, Mark DB, et al. Sudden cardiac death in heart failure trial (SCD-HeFT). *N Engl J Med*. 2005;352:225–237.
29. Al-Khatib SM, Stevenson WG, Ackerman MJ, et al. 2017 AHA/ACC/HRS guideline for management of patients with ventricular arrhythmias and the prevention of sudden cardiac death: a report of the American College of Cardiology/American Heart Association Task Force on clinical practice guidelines and the Heart Rhythm Society. *Circulation*. 2017;138(13):e210–e271.
30. Dongas J, Lehman MH, Mahmud R, et al. Value of preexisting bundle branch block in the ECG differentiation of supraventricular from ventricular origin of wide QRS tachycardia. *Am J Cardiol*. 1985;55:717–721.
31. Wellens HJJ, Brugada P, Heddle WF. The value of the 12 lead ECG in diagnosis type and mechanism of a tachycardia: a survey among 22 cardiologists. *J Am Coll Cardiol*. 1984;4:176–179.
32. Zipes DP, Camm AJ, Borggrefe M. ACC/AHA/ESC 2006 guidelines for the management of patients with ventricular arrhythmias and the prevention of sudden cardiac death: executive summary. *J Am Coll Cardiol*. 2006;9:539–548.
33. Shen WK, Sheldon RS, Benditt DG, et al. 2017 ACC/AHA/HRS guideline for the evaluation and management of patients with syncope: a report of the American College of Cardiology/American Heart Association Task Force on clinical practice guidelines and the Heart Rhythm Society. *J Am Coll Cardiol*. 2017;70(5):e39–e110.
34. Kapoor WN. Syncope. *N Engl J Med*. 2000;343:1856–1862.
35. Strickberger SA, Benson DW, Biaggioni I. AHA/ACCF scientific statement on the evaluation of syncope. *J Am Coll Cardiol*. 2006;47:473–484.
36. Nelson SD, Kou WH, De Buitleir M, et al. Value of programmed ventricular stimulation in presumed carotid sinus syndrome. *Am J Cardiol*. 1987;60:1073–1077.
37. Sugrue DD, Wood DL, McGoon MD. Carotid sinus hypersensitivity and syncope. *Mayo Clin Proc*. 1984;59:637–640.
38. Linzer M, Prystowsky EN, Brunetti LL, et al. Recurrent syncope of unknown origin diagnosed by ambulatory continuous loop ECG recording. *Am Heart J*. 1988;116:1632–1634.
39. Krahn AD, Klein GJ, Norris C, et al. The etiology of syncope in patients with negative tilt table and electrophysiology testing. *Circulation*. 1995;92:1819–1824.
40. Berbari EJ, Lazzara R. An introduction to high resolution ECG recordings of cardiac late potentials. *Arch Intern Med*. 1988;148:1859–1863.
41. Hall PA, Atwood JE, Myers J, et al. The signal averaged surface electrocardiogram and the identification of late potentials. *Prog Cardiovasc Dis*. 1989;31:295–317.
42. Brignole M, Alboni O, Benditt D, et al. Guidelines on management (diagnosis and treatment) of syncope—Updated 2004. *Europace*. 2004; 6(6):467–537.
43. Bloomfield DM, Bigger JT, Steinman RC, et al. Microvolt T-wave alternans and the risk of death or sustained ventricular arrhythmias in patients with left ventricular dysfunction. *J Am Coll Cardiol*. 2006;47(2):456–463.
44. Gold MR, Bloomfield FM, Anderson KP, et al. A comparison of T-wave alternans, signal-averaged electrocardiography and programmed ventricular stimulation for risk stratification. *J Am Coll Cardiol*. 2000;36:2247–2253.
45. Engel G, Beckerman JG, Froelicher VF, et al. Electrocardiographic arrhythmia risk testing. *Curr Probl Cardiol*. 2004;29(7):365–432.
46. Clutter C. Neurally mediated syncope. *J Cardiovasc Nurs*. 1991;5:65–73.
47. Purcell JA. Provoking vasodepressor syncope with head-up tilt-table testing. *Prog Cardiovasc Nurs*. 1992;7:15–18.
48. Morillo CA, Klein GJ, Zandri S, et al. Diagnostic accuracy of a low-dose isoproterenol head-up tilt protocol. *Am Heart J*. 1995;129:901–906.
49. Almquist A, Goldenberg IF, Milstein S, et al. Provocation of bradycardia and hypotension by isoproterenol and upright posture in patients with unexplained syncope. *N Engl J Med*. 1989;320:346–351.
50. Fitzpatrick AP, Theodorakis G, Vardas P, et al. Methodology of head-up tilt testing in patients with unexplained syncope. *J Am Coll Cardiol*. 1991;17:125–130.
51. Sheldon R, Killam S. Methodology of isoproterenol-tilt table testing in patients with syncope. *J Am Coll Cardiol*. 1992;19:773–779.
52. Bass EB, Elson JJ, Fogoros RN, et al. Long-term prognosis of patients undergoing electrophysiology studies for syncope of unknown origin. *Am J Cardiol*. 1988;62:1186–1191.
53. Denes P, Uretz E, Ezri MD, et al. Clinical predictors of electrophysiologic testing in patients with syncope of unknown origin. *Arch Intern Med*. 1988;148:1922–1928.
54. Teichman SL, Felder SD, Matos JA, et al. The value of electrophysiologic studies in syncope of undetermined origin: report of 150 cases. *Am Heart J*. 1985;110:469–479.
55. Yee R, Strauss HC. Electrophysiologic mechanisms: sinus node dysfunction. *Circulation*. 1987;75(suppl 3):12–18.
56. Fogors RN. The electrophysiologic study in the evaluation of the SA node, AV node and His-Purkinje system. In: *Electrophysiology Testing*. 4th ed. Blackwell Publishing; 2006:35–57.
57. Kapoor WN. Current evaluation and management of syncope. *Circulation*. 2002;106:1606–1609.
58. Calkins H, Kim YN, Schmaltz S, et al. Electrogram criteria for identification of appropriate target sites for radiofrequency catheter ablation of accessory connections. *Circulation*. 1992;85:565–573.
59. Gallagher JJ, Svenson RH, Kasell JH, et al. Catheter technique for closed-chest ablation of the atrioventricular conduction system. *N Engl J Med*. 1982;306:194–200.
60. Evans GJ, Scheinman MM, Zipes DP, et al. The percutaneous cardiac mapping and ablation registry: final summary of results. *Pacing Clin Electrophysiol*. 1989;11:1621–1626.
61. Scheinman MM, Morady F, Hess D, et al. Catheter induced ablation of the atrioventricular junction to control refractory supraventricular arrhythmias. *JAMA*. 1982;248:851–855.
62. Hauer R, Straks W, Borst C, et al. Electrical catheter ablation in the left and right ventricular wall in dogs: relation between delivered energy and histopathologic changes. *J Am Coll Cardiol*. 1988;8:637–643.
63. Langberg JJ, Chin MC, Rosenqvist M, et al. Catheter ablation of the atrioventricular junction with radiofrequency energy. *Circulation*. 1989; 80:1527–1535.
64. Deisenhofer I, Zrenner B, Yin Y, et al. Cryoablation versus radiofrequency energy for the ablation of atrioventricular nodal reentrant tachycardia (the CYRANO Study). *Circulation*. 2010;122:2239–2245.
65. Halder S, Wong T. Contact force sensing for atrial fibrillation ablation. *Eur Heart J*. 2013;11(21). Available at https://www.escardio.org/Journals/E-Journal-of-Cardiology-Practice/Volume-11/Contact-force-sensing-for-atrial-fibrillation-ablation. Accessed June 29, 2018.
66. Fisher WG, Swartz JF. Three-dimensional electrogram mapping improves ablation of left sided accessory pathway. *Pacing Clin Electrophysiol*. 1992;15:2344–2356.
67. Razminia M, Manankil MF, Eryazici PLS, et al. Nonfluoroscopic catheter ablation of cardiac arrhythmias in adults: feasibility, safety, and efficacy. *J Cardiovasc Electrophysiol*. 2012;23:1078–1086.

68. Earley MJ, Showkathali R, Alzetani M, et al. Radiofrequency ablation of arrhythmias guided by non-fluoroscopic catheter location: a prospective randomized trial. *Eur Heart J.* 2006;27:1223–1229.
69. Page RL, Joglar JA, Caldwell MA, et al. 2015 ACC/AHA/HRS guideline for the management of adult patients with supraventricular tachycardia: a report of the American College of Cardiology/American Heart Association Task Force on clinical practice guidelines and the Heart Rhythm Society. *Heart Rhythm.* 2016;13:e136–e221.
70. Scheinman MM. Patterns of catheter ablation practice in the United States: results of 1992 NASPE survey. *Pacing Clin Electrophysiol.* 1994;17:873–875.
71. Jackman WM, Beckman KJ, McClelland JH, et al. Treatment of supraventricular tachycardia due to atrioventricular nodal reentry, by radiofrequency catheter ablation of slow-pathway conduction. *N Engl J Med.* 1992;327:313–318.
72. Calkins H, Sousa J, El-Atassi R, et al. Diagnosis and cure of the Wolff-Parkinson-White syndrome or paroxysmal supraventricular tachycardias during a single electrophysiologic test. *N Engl J Med.* 1991;324:1612–1618.
73. McClelland JH, Wang K, Beckman KJ, et al. Radiofrequency catheter ablation of right atriofascicular (Mahaim) accessory pathways guided by accessory pathway activation potentials. *Circulation.* 1994;89:2655–2666.
74. Ticho BS, Saul JP, Hulse JE, et al. Variable location of accessory pathways associated with PJRT and confirmation with radiofrequency ablation. *Am J Cardiol.* 1992;70:1559–1564.
75. Jackman WM, Wang X, Friday KJ, et al. Catheter ablation of atrioventricular pathways (Wolff-Parkinson-White syndrome) by radiofrequency current. *N Engl J Med.* 1991;324:1605–1611.
76. Lesh MD. Interventional electrophysiology: state-of-the-art 1993. *Am Heart J.* 1993;126:686–698.
77. Fuster V, Ryden LE, Cannom DS, et al. ACC/AHA/ESC 2006 guidelines for the management of patients with atrial fibrillation: a report of the American College of Cardiology/American Heart Association Task Force on Practice Guidelines (Writing Committee to Revise the 2001 Guidelines for the Management of Patients with Atrial Fibrillation). *J Am Coll Cardiol.* 2006;48:e149–e246.
78. Fischer B, Jais P, Shah D, et al. Radiofrequency catheter ablation of common atrial flutter in 200 patients. *J Cardiovasc Electrophysiol.* 1996;7:1225.
79. January CT, Wann LS, Alpert JS, et al. 2014 AHA/ACC/HRS guideline for the management of patients with atrial fibrillation. *JACC.* 2014;64(21):e1–e76.
80. Morady F. *2017 consensus statement on atrial fibrillation ablation.* 2017. Available at https://www.acc.org/latest-in-cardiology/ten-points-to-remember/2017/09/26/13/35/2017-hrs-expert-consensus-statement-on-catheter-ablation. Accessed July 13, 2018.
81. Calkins H, Hindricks G, Cappato R, et al. 2017 HRS/EHRA/APHRS/SOLAECE expert consensus statement on catheter and surgical ablation of atrial fibrillation. *Heart Rhythm.* 2017;14(10):e275–e444.
82. Jackman WM, Wang X, Friday KJ, et al. Catheter ablation of atrioventricular junction using radiofrequency current in 17 patients. *Circulation.* 1991;83:1562–1576.
83. Rodriguez LM, Smeets JLRM, Xie B, et al. Improvement of left ventricular function by ablation of atrioventricular nodal conduction in selected patients with lone atrial fibrillation. *Am J Cardiol.* 1993;72:1137–1141.
84. Fitzpatrick AP, Kourouyan HD, Siu A, et al. Quality of life and outcomes after radiofrequency His-bundle ablation and permanent pacemaker implantation: impact of treatment in paroxysmal and established atrial fibrillation. *Am Heart J.* 1996;121:499–507.
85. Ho J, Prutkin JM. Simultaneous atrioventricular node ablation and leadless pacemaker implantation. *Heart Rhythm Case Rep.* 2017;3(3):186–188.
86. Haissaguerre M, Jais P, Shah DC, et al. A focal source of atrial fibrillation by ectopic beats originating in the pulmonary veins. *N Engl J Med.* 1998;339:659–666.
87. Pappone C, Rosanio S, Oreto G, et al. Circumferential radiofrequency ablation of pulmonary vein ostia: a new anatomic approach for curing atrial fibrillation. *Circulation.* 2000;104:2539–2544.
88. Nademanee K, McKenzie J, Kosar E, et al. A new approach for catheter ablation of atrial fibrillation: mapping of the electrophysiologic substrate. *J Am Coll Cardiol.* 2004;43:2044–2053.
89. Scherlag BJ, Nakagawa H, Jackman WM, et al. Electrical stimulation to identify neural elements on the heart: their role in atrial fibrillation. *J Interv Card Electrophysiol.* 2005;13(suppl 1):37–42.
90. Calkins H, Brugada J, Packer F, et al. HRS/EHRA/ECAS expert consensus statement on catheter and surgical ablation of atrial fibrillation: recommendations for personnel, policy, procedures and follow-up. *Heart Rhythm.* 2007;4(6):816–861.
91. Haissaguerre M, Jais P, Shah DC, et al. Electrophysiological end point for catheter ablation of atrial fibrillation initiated from multiple pulmonary venous foci. *Circulation.* 2000;101:1409–1417.
92. Chen SA, Hsieh MH, Tai CT, et al. Initiation of atrial fibrillation by ectopic beats originating from the pulmonary veins: electrophysiological characteristics, pharmacological responses, and effects of radiofrequency ablation. *Circulation.* 1999;100:1879–1886.
93. Schaff HV, Dearani JA, Daly RC, et al. Cox-Maze procedure for atrial fibrillation: Mayo Clinic experience. *Semin Thorac Cardiovasc Surg.* 2000; 12:30–37.
94. Prasad SM, Maniar HS, Camillo CJ, et al. The Cox maze III procedure for atrial fibrillation: long-term efficacy in patients undergoing lone versus concomitant procedures. *J Thorac Cardiovasc Surg.* 2003;126:1822–1828.
95. Koistinen J, Valtonen M, Savola J, et al. Thoracoscopic microwave ablation of atrial fibrillation. *Interact Cardiovasc Thorac Surg.* 2007;6:695–698.
96. Lesh MD, Van Hare GF, Epstein LM, et al. Radiofrequency catheter ablation of atrial arrhythmias results and mechanisms. *Circulation.* 1994;89:1074–1089.
97. Aliot EM, Stevenson WG, Almendral-Garrote JM, et al. EHRA/HRS consensus on catheter ablation of ventricular arrhythmias. *Heart Rhythm.* 2009;6(6):886–933.
98. Kautzner J, Cihak R, Peichl P, et al. Catheter ablation of ventricular tachycardia following MI using 3-dimensional electroanatomic mapping. *Pacing Clin Electrophysiol.* 2003;26(1):342–347.
99. Cohen TJ, Chien WU, Lurie KG, et al. Radiofrequency catheter ablation for treatment of bundle branch reentrant VT: results and long-term follow-up. *J Am Coll Cardiol.* 1991;18:1767–1773.

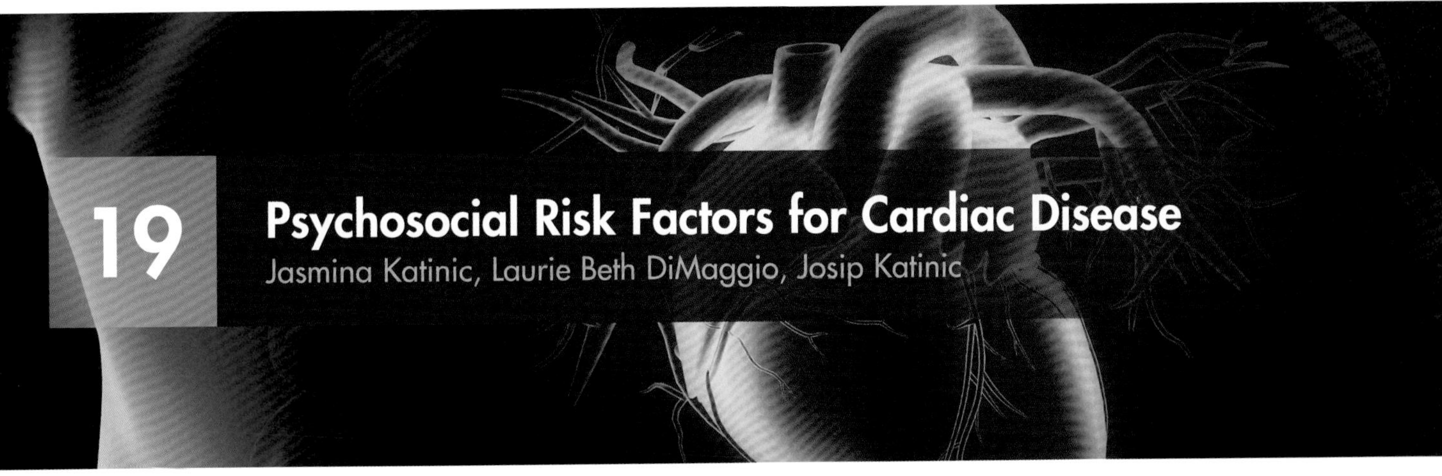

19 Psychosocial Risk Factors for Cardiac Disease

Jasmina Katinic, Laurie Beth DiMaggio, Josip Katinic

OBJECTIVES

1. Verbalize the burden of unrecognized psychosocial impairment within the cardiac population.
2. Describe the psychosocial risk factors that predispose patients to cardiac disease.
3. Demonstrate the impact of undetected psychosocial risk factors on cardiovascular physiology.
4. Utilize the current assessment tools to screen for behavioral cardiopathology.
5. Implement appropriate nursing interventions and knowledge of pharmacologic treatment options.

KEY QUESTIONS

1. What specific emotional, behavioral, and chronic risk factors influence the development of cardiovascular disease?
2. What is the relationship between psychosocial distress and cardiovascular pathology?
3. What are the barriers to effective psychosocial assessment for the cardiac nurse?
4. How does patient perception affect psychosocial outcomes?
5. What are the treatment options for behavioral cardiology patients?

BACKGROUND: PREVALENCE AND EPIDEMIOLOGY

Psychosocial risk factors carry significant cardiovascular implications on patient mortality, morbidity, quality of life, and systematic health care costs. Both self-reported and clinically diagnosed depression have long proven to be significant and independent risk factors for developing cardiovascular disease (CVD).[1] Traditionally, there has been a separation in management of CVD from cardiology and behavioral medicine. The new discipline of behavioral cardiology takes into consideration assessing psychosocial risk factors and unhealthy lifestyles influencing cardiovascular health and treatment modalities.[2]

The symptoms of psychosocial disease and of CVD often overlap, making the complex relationship a difficult problem to describe and assess. Historically, dozens of systematic reviews examining the prevalence of concomitant psychosocial and CVD ranged between 10% and 60%, focusing primarily on depressive symptoms and anxiety.[3] The pervasive influence of psychosocial distress on cardiovascular pathophysiology had previously been not well studied or understood when compared to recent years.[4] Additionally, insight into the efficacy of psychosocial interventions including pharmacotherapy, cognitive-behavioral therapy, and group cardiac rehabilitation has advanced substantially over the past decade.[5]

Currently, an estimated prevalence of psychosocial disease in the general population sits near 5.4%, compared to 45% in patients with coronary artery disease, 77% in patients with heart failure, 36% in patients with persistent atrial fibrillation, and 28% of patients undergoing implantable cardioverter-defibrillator (ICD) placement.[5,6] Moreover, the clinical diagnosis of major depressive disorder demonstrated increased prevalence in the cardiovascular population with 15% to 20% of patients with coronary heart disease, 26% in patients with heart failure, and 15% of chronic atrial fibrillation patients when compared to 2.1% in the general population.[1] These systematic analyses express the likelihood of underdiagnosis for cardiac patients with anxiety and depressive symptoms, estimating failure to diagnose in up to 50% of patients as well as 22% incidence of adequate treatment.[6]

This chapter will address the chronic, recurrent, and progressive nature of psychosocial disease within the cardiovascular population, detailing the risk factors, the physiologic and psychological ramifications, the screening tools for diagnosis, and interventions. Nurses have many opportunities to educate and motivate cardiovascular patients with unfavorable emotional, behavioral, and chronic stressors. Barriers to the proven screening tools will be discussed in order to make the argument that empowered cardiac nurses can improve detection of psychosocial disease within the cardiac population. Equipping the nurse in this crucial role allows for patient care that moves past the stabilization of acute CVD management in favor of treating each patient holistically and effectively.

PSYCHOSOCIAL RISK FACTORS FOR CARDIOVASCULAR DISEASES

Emotional Factors

Depression

Depression is defined as single or multiple episodes of daily mood alterations lasting a minimum of 2 weeks.[7,8] These episodes may be characterized by psychological as well as physiologic symptoms such as apathy, sadness, feelings of shame and guilt, suicidal thoughts, fatigue, sleep disturbance, changes in appetite and weight, trouble concentrating, motor agitation or retardation.[7,9] The diagnostic criteria for major or minor depression is based on assessment of clinical presentation of symptoms, history of duration, and significance of the impairment.[8] In this chapter, the term *depression* will be all-inclusive.

It is not fully understood why the female population is twice as likely to experience depression as males, though a significant element can be attributed to emotional coping strategies and interpersonal-related vulnerability when dealing with stressful events.[10] In an 18-year longitudinal study conducted by the American Heart Association (AHA), depression was largely linked as an independent risk factor for the development of coronary artery disease in women.[11] Unlike women, depressive symptoms in men may be masked by social position, underestimating the relationship between depression and CVD.[10]

Depression is associated with poor compliance in accurately taking medications.[12,13] Affected patients can minimize the significance of cardiac symptoms, therefore delaying seeking medical treatment.[14,15] Besides the individual health consequences of depression in CHD patients, depression increases the systematic impact on the economics of the health care system.[16] The cost of increased hospitalization admissions for recurrent cardiac events and longer hospital stays are also associated with higher emotional distress. The average hospital cost for a depressed cardiac patient is more than four times the cost of a nondepressed patient.[17]

Anxiety

Anxiety itself is characterized by fear, worry, and uncertainty and often unique to individual experience and perception. Anxiety disorder and its influence for developing cardiac events is less studied than depression. One study found a mixed association of anxiety and adverse outcomes in both pre-existing heart conditions and those without.[18] Anxiety disorders account for vast and expensive emergency visits creating a significant economic burden on the health care system. Over a 3-year period studied in Northern Ireland, 58.7% of chest pain presentations were accounted for noncardiac diagnosis.[19]

Hostility and Anger

The research on the relationship between personality and CVD over the years has demonstrated significant impact on morbidity and mortality. Recent studies linked anger and hostility to progression of atherosclerosis and increased risk factor for CVD.[20] In particular, individuals with type A behavior are at increased risk for developing CHD.[21] The cardiac patients suffering from anger and hostility are likely to have poor cardiac prognosis. The acute anger and greater physical activity are associated with increased incidence of ICD discharge in cardiac patients found in the study involving 140 patients 2 months after device implant.[22] The acute anger and increased platelet aggregation have been associated with coronary events.[21]

Behavioral Factors

Sleep is a complex and essential process for normal brain function, mental, and physical health.[23] Heart disease and depression have biologic similarities relevant to the hypothalamic–pituitary–adrenocortical (HPA) and sympathetic adrenal medullary systems, which have overlapping symptoms of sleep disturbance.[24] Poor sleep can be related to both biologic and behavioral mechanisms that cause chronic elevation of inflammatory mediators, and poor sleep hygiene over time is linked to obesity, hypertension, diabetes mellitus, and CVD.[25] In 2015, National Sleep Foundation published new recommendations for sleep time duration for nine age groups: 7 to 9 hours for adults 26 to 64 years of age and 7 to 8 hours for older adults 65 years and older.[26]

Emotional stress such as depression and anxiety can lead to increased appetite and craving of calorie-dense foods.[27] This combination of direct effect of emotional factors on cardiovascular health and indirect factors such as diet and exercise[28] can lead to elevated cortisol levels and activation of endocannabinoid receptors.[27] Due to hormonal alteration and increased appetite, excess calories may be stored in form of intra-abdominal adipose tissue and thus further worsening hormonal imbalance.[27] A 3-month study conducted by Daubenmier et al.[29] evaluated such health behaviors and their effect on cardiovascular health. They examined behavioral factors and their contributions to excess weight, elevated blood pressure, lipids, and hemoglobin A1c and found that improvement in dietary, exercise, and stress management behaviors may lead to reduction in CVD.[29]

In a randomized controlled trial of 134 patients with stable ischemic heart disease, exercise and stress management training reduced emotional distress and improved cardiovascular risk markers as adjunctive to usual medical therapy.[30] Lower baseline exercise tolerance in patients with CHD and hostility demonstrated slower rates in cardiac improvement.[31] Benefit of exercise therapy in patients with depression is likely multifactorial. Factors resulting in better cardiovascular outcomes are related to recognizing depressive behavior, finding the effective method to reduce depressive symptoms, and improving aerobic exercise capacity.[32]

Chronic Psychosocial Stressors

Low Socioeconomic Status

Over 80% of cardiovascular deaths occur in low- and middle-income countries.[33] Health disparities associated with socioeconomic status (SES) can affect cardiovascular health with regard to both poor quality of care and limited access to care.[34] SES is one of the key contributors to CVD due to low income, limited education, and perceived lifestyle stress.[35] Consistent with research in Reasons for Geographic and Racial Differences in Stroke (REGARDS) study and Atherosclerosis Risk in Communities study, low house hold income was associated with higher CVD events and death.[35,36]

Other risk factors that are linked to low SES and negatively affect cardiovascular health include tobacco consumption, high-fat diet, and a sedentary lifestyle.[37] Affordability and easy access to food high in saturated fats contribute to higher obesity rates and increased serum cholesterol levels. Unfortunately, regardless of SES, many patients with high levels of serum cholesterol do not seek preventative care in order to risk stratify for CVD. One of the early preventative assessments is the Framingham Cardiovascular Risk Equation.[38] However, based on data collected from the Atherosclerosis Risk in Communities study, using Framingham risk score alone was not adequate in treatment of high cholesterol levels[36] and it was important to add subjective and objective assessment of individuals of low SES.[38] When SES was included in recommended cholesterol treatment, risk of coronary heart disease was reduced by approximately 50% when compared to Framingham risk score alone.[39] In addition to lifestyle choices within low SES group, the racial and ethnic factors contribute to increased CVD incidence.

Low Social Support and Social Isolation

Social support is the network of family, friends, neighbors, and community members that is accessible to an individual through social ties.[40] Structural support is characterized by social integration and the ability to network and socially participate.[41] Functional support is defined as emotional support and is measured by perception of how much support is received and how much is available.[41] Both structural and functional support influence the outcome of morbidity and mortality related to CVD through emotions and feelings of control.[42] Emotional support has been proven to have cardioprotective properties, whereas low level of emotional support was associated with increased risk in myocardial infarction (MI) and cardiac mortality.[43] In addition to mental health, low social support is associated with multiple physiologic and psychological pathways that foster negative effects on cardiovascular health. Social isolation, as an independent factor, was identified as one of the major risk factors for increased mortality.[41] Loneliness and social isolation describe a strong relationship between social connections and biologic markers of CVD.

Work Stress

Work-related stress is associated with an increased risk for CVD. Numerous studies conducted in Europe, the United States, and Japan support the relationship between work stress and its negative effect on cardiovascular health.[44] Lifestyle behavioral factors like smoking, exercise, and diet exacerbate the adverse effect on work-related stress and CVD. Based on 10-year incidence of CAD in seven cohort studies, individuals with healthy lifestyle had over 50% lower incidence of CAD.[45] There is a higher risk of stroke related to long working hours as well as an increased risk of development of coronary heart disease.[46] Other job factors, like lack of support from coworkers, job insecurity, and juggling family and job demands likely influence a person's perception of employment. However, what one person experiences as stress, another may view as stimulating and exciting. All things considered, clearly substantiated evidence supporting the causal relationship between job stress and CHD is still absent.[47,48]

PATHOPHYSIOLOGIC RELATIONSHIP BETWEEN PSYCHOSOCIAL RISK FACTORS AND CARDIOVASCULAR DISEASE

The physiologic response to chronic psychosocial pathology hinges on the body's adaptability in order to maintain homeostasis.[4] This "stress response" represents the multiorgan mechanism which reacts to the increase in cerebral energy demands and activates the appropriate compensatory response.[49] Though useful and even beneficial for the acute remedy of psychosocial distress, chronic wear and tear on the body, or allostatic load, leads to adverse cardiac outcomes through autonomic, adrenal, endothelial, stress reactivity, and inflammatory pathways.[50]

Autonomic Dysfunction

Depression, anxiety, and stress or perceived stressors stimulate the sympathetic nervous system and catecholamine release of epinephrine and norepinephrine, causing increased heart rate, increased blood pressure, increased myocardial oxygen demand, diaphoresis, and can lead to chest pain.[51] Chronic neurohormonal excitement has been demonstrated to provoke atrial fibrillation, increased risk of stroke due to increased blood pressure, and exacerbate heart failure due to the increase in left ventricular filling pressure.[52] Concomitant impairment of the parasympathetic nervous system response leads to decreased heart rate recovery after exercise, decreased baroreceptor sensitivity, and decreased heart rate variability, which have been studied to carry cyclical increased risk for depression following acute MI.[53]

Adrenal Dysfunction

Psychosocial distress activates the HPA axis, releasing glucocorticoids, increasing hepatic glucose production, and mobilizing energy reserves, impairing the natural circadian rhythm.[49] The resulting chronic cortisol peaks start earlier in the day and do not decrease appropriately in the evening, disrupting the diurnal rhythm of releasing energy stores for performing activities of daily living, and recede to promote sleep.[49] Trying to meet the increased energy demands of the brain under stress, the HPA axis suppresses insulin secretion, potentially decreasing subcutaneous fat stores while increasing circulating blood glucose levels, causing atheroma formation and progression, decreased vascular compliance, and increased risk for impaired glucose metabolism, diabetes mellitus, and dyslipidemia.[54] The associated impairment in serotonin release contributes to a cyclical risk for increased depression and further impairment in adrenal function.[55]

Endothelial Dysfunction

The vascular endothelium separates the lumen from circulation and regulates vascular tone (nitric oxide synthase for potent vasodilation and endothelin-1 for potent vasoconstriction), affecting blood flow, inflammation, and thrombosis.[56] Chronic states of stress affect the ability of the vascular endothelium to mediate homeostasis with inefficient, turbulent arterial blood flow, increasing friction and decreasing bioavailability of nitric oxide and the mechanism for vasodilatory compensation.[50] The resulting vascular remodeling leads to increased uptake of circulating low-density lipoprotein cholesterol (LDL-C) into the endothelium, fostering an environment of oxidation, fibrin proliferation, and atheroma formation, increasing risk of cardiovascular and peripheral arterial disease, dyslipidemia and stroke, and hypertensive heart disease.[57]

Inflammation and Hypercoagulability

The previously mentioned autonomic, adrenal, and endothelial pathophysiologic factors which potentiate atherosclerosis and diminished vagal tone foster a proinflammatory state and ultimately the formation of neurotoxic metabolites instead of neuroprotective metabolites.[58] The inflammatory response to chronic stress includes uninhibited release of macrophages, which increases platelet aggregation and promotes thrombosis, exacerbating plaque instability and potentially leading to rupture. Laboratory markers including C-reactive protein (CRP), tumor necrosis factor (TNF), and interleukin-1B have recently been studied to be the most reliable inflammatory markers in patients with depression.[59] A study comparing these laboratory markers compared with assessed level of depression in patients hospitalized for acute coronary syndrome demonstrated abnormal platelet physiology with higher platelet aggregation, higher CRP, TNF, and interleukin-1B in patients whose depression assessment (by Patient Health Questionnaire [PHQ]-9) was considered at least moderate.[60]

In the setting of acute psychosocial distress, the interaction between autonomic, adrenal, endothelial, inflammatory, and hematologic functions directs energy to the brain, promoting necessary hypervigilance to surmount the activity or incident. Chronic redirection of these compensatory mechanisms increases the risk of coronary, electrophysiologic, hypertensive, vascular, and functional heart disease (see Table 19-1).

ASSESSMENT OF PSYCHOSOCIAL RISK FACTORS IN PATIENTS WITH CARDIOVASCULAR DISEASE

While adequate screening tools have been established and proven to assist in the detection and management of psychosocial diseases in cardiac patients, effective diagnosis and treatment remains low.[6] Barriers to successful assessment and implementation of screening tools for cardiac nurses include lack of standardization in policy, lack of resources or education, lack of homogeneity in screening tools, and lack of sufficient time to perform assessments.[61] The ultimate goal in understanding psychosocial screening tools is to implement changes in order to detect and effectively manage psychosocial risk factors for cardiac patients. Cardiac nurses, equipped with the resources to perform screening instruments, can tailor assessment to institutional policy, allowing for referral to case management and mental health professionals as applicable. The screening tools for depression, anxiety, and low-perceived social support are detailed below.

Depression and Anxiety

The AHA recommends routine implementation of 2- and 9-item PHQs (PHQ-2 and PHQ-9).[1] Developed from the previously recommended Primary Care Evaluation of Mental Disorders (PRIME-MD) (see Table 19-2) 27-question instrument, the PHQ-2 allows for the brevity required to widely implement screening for all patients within inpatient and outpatient settings.[62] The PHQ-2 (see Table 19-3) characterizes the presence and frequency of depressed mood and anhedonia over the past month. The PHQ-9 (see Table 19-4) takes the first two questions from the PHQ-2, then explores the DSM-IV diagnostic criteria for major depressive disorder.[63] According to the AHA recommendation, a positive PHQ-2 should trigger the conducting of PHQ-9.[1] While no study has established that this process improves patient mortality, the screening process when paired with a management protocol has been shown to demonstrate reduced cardiac symptoms and improved blood pressure.[64] These questionnaires are concise and efficient, with favorable negative predictive value of 94% for PHQ-2 and 88% for PHQ-9.[1]

Low-Perceived Social Support

Despite the presence or absence of psychosocial risk factors, the patient perception of psychosocial well-being significantly impacts depressive symptoms and stress, both positively and negatively.[65] The ENRICHD Social Support Instrument (see Table 19-5) was the first screening tool to evaluate emotional, structural, and instrumental support within the patient's living situation.[66] The multicenter, randomized, controlled clinical trial did demonstrate statistically significant improvement in both the detection of social isolation and the patient perception of depressive symptoms.[67] It is a seven-question Likert scale in which the patient rates the availability of social support on a scale from 1 (None of the Time) to 5 (All of the Time). A positive ENRICHD

Table 19-1 • EFFECTS OF PSYCHOSOCIAL RISK FACTORS ON CARDIOVASCULAR PATHOPHYSIOLOGY

Physiologic Pathway	Responsibility in Homeostasis	Pathophysiologic Mechanism Under Chronic Stress	Long-Term Effects of Psychosocial Distress
Sympathetic Nervous System	Catecholamines regulate heart rate, breathing rate, blood pressure, and increased blood flow to brain and musculature	Increased heart rate; increased blood pressure; increased oxygen demand; diaphoresis	Potentiates atrial fibrillation; increased risk of CVA; potentiates diastolic heart failure
Parasympathetic Nervous System	Baroreceptors respond to arterial tension and pulse pressure to vasodilate or reconstrict; acetylcholine is released to slow heart rate following sympathetic nervous system withdrawal	Decreased baroreceptor sensitivity impairs compensatory vasodilation; impaired heart rate recovery following exertion	Chronic hypertension; decreased heart rate variability
Adrenal System	Hypothalamic–pituitary–adrenal (HPA) axis regulates circadian rhythm with hepatic glucose production and mobilization	Increased hepatic glucose production and glucocorticoid release; increased mobilization of stored energy reserves; decreased insulin secretion; decreased serotonin release	Impaired circadian rhythm (daytime fatigue and impaired sleep); increased risk of diabetes mellitus; increased atheroma formation; increased hyperlipidemia; increased depression
Vascular Endothelium	Regulates vascular tone; NOS to decrease blood pressure (vasodilation) and endothelin-1 to increase blood pressure (vasoconstriction)	Increased turbulence of vascular flow; decreased bioavailability of NOS; increased uptake of LDLs into the endothelium; increased oxidation	Chronic hypertension; increased atheroma formation; increased risk of CAD and PAD; increased risk of CVA
Inflammatory Process	Release of prostaglandins, histamine, and bradykinin in response to tissue or vascular injury, increasing the release and recruitment of macrophages	Creation of neurotoxic metabolites and free radicals increases oxidative stress; increased platelet aggregation; increased thrombosis and plaque instability	Increased hyperlipidemia; increased risk of plaque rupture; increased risk of coronary artery disease, peripheral arterial disease, and myocardial infarction

Table 19-2 • PRIME-MD (PRIMARY CARE EVALUATION OF MENTAL DISORDERS), DIAGNOSTIC ASSESSMENT FOR DEPRESSION AND ANXIETY—PATIENT QUESTIONNAIRE

Instructions: This questionnaire will help your health provider better understand problems that you may have.
During the PAST MONTH, have you often been bothered by...

1. Stomach pain
2. Back pain
3. Pain in your arms, legs, or joints (knees, hips, etc.)
4. Menstrual pain or problems
5. Pain or problems during sexual intercourse
6. Headaches
7. Chest pain
8. Dizziness
9. Fainting spells
10. Feeling your heart pound or race
11. Shortness of breath
12. Constipation, loose bowels or diarrhea
13. Nausea, gas, or indigestion
14. Feeling tired or having low energy
15. Trouble sleeping
16. The thought that you have a serious undiagnosed disease
17. Your eating being out of control
18. Little interest or pleasure in doing things
19. Feeling down depressed or hopeless
20. "Nerves" or feeling anxious or on edge
21. Worrying about a lot of different things
22. Have you had an anxiety attack (suddenly feeling fear or panic)
23. Have you thought you should cut down your drinking of alcohol
24. Has anyone complained about your drinking
25. Have you felt guilty or upset about your drinking
26. Was there ever a single day in which you had five or more drinks of beer, wine, or liquor

Overall would you say your health is:
Excellent
Very Good
Good
Fair
Poor

Borrowed with permission from Spitzer RL, Williams JB, Kroenke K, et al. Utility of a new procedure for diagnosing mental disorders in primary care: the PRIME-MD 1000 study. *JAMA.* 1994;272:1749–1756.

Table 19-3 • TWO-ITEM INSTRUMENT—DEPRESSION SCREEN

During the past *month*, have you often been bothered by...		
1. Little interest or pleasure in doing things?	Yes	No
2. Feeling down, depressed, or hopeless?	Yes	No

Adapted from McManus D, Pipkin SS, Whooley MA. Screening for depression in patients with coronary heart disease (data from the Heart and Soul Study). *Am J Cardiol.* 2005;96:1076–1081.

is characterized by a score of less than 18 and should lead to further assessment and intervention for the vulnerable patient.

While beneficial when used in the outpatient setting, the ENRICHD is a critical assessment tool prior to discharge from a cardiac hospitalization.[65] The patient's perception of functional independence (help with chores) along with the emotional isolation (advice, love, affection, support) within the ENRICHD helps identify patients susceptible for negative psychosocial prognosis. Recommendation of consultation with social support services and mental health professionals is always reasonable for the critically thinking cardiac nurse.

NURSING AND PHARMACOLOGIC INTERVENTIONS

Nursing Interventions

Nurses have many opportunities to educate and motivate patients through the implementation of psychosocial interventions. The need for intervention is critical for hospitalized patients, especially after coronary events, life-threatening arrhythmias, and major cardiovascular procedures. Education as a psychosocial support intervention can significantly improve depression and anxiety while encouraging patients to learn and adapt. The psychosocial interventions in this section will target emotional factors, behavioral factors, and chronic stressors (see Fig. 19-1).

Table 19-4 • PATIENT HEALTH QUESTIONNAIRE-9: DEPRESSION MODULE

Over the Past *2 Weeks*, How Often Have You Been Bothered by Any of the Following Problems?	Not at All 0	Several Days 1	More Than Half the Days 2	Nearly Every Day 3
1. Little interest or pleasure in doing things				
2. Feeling down, depressed, or hopeless				
3. Trouble falling or staying asleep, or sleeping too much				
4. Feeling tired or having little energy				
5. Poor appetite or overeating				
6. Feeling bad about yourself—or that you are a failure or have let yourself or your family down				
7. Trouble concentrating on things, such as reading the newspaper or watching television				
8. Moving or speaking so slowly that other people could have noticed; or the opposite—being so fidgety or restless that you have been moving around a lot more than usual				
9. Thoughts that you would be better off dead or hurting yourself in some way				
If you checked off any problems on this questionnaire so far, how difficult have these problems made it for you to complete your work, take care of things at home, or get along with other people?	**Not difficult**	**Somewhat difficult**	**Very difficult**	**Extremely difficult**

Permission obtained from Kroenke K, Spitzer RL, Williams JB. The PHQ-9: validity of a brief depression severity measure. *J Gen Intern Med.* 2001;16:606–613.

Table 19-5 • ESSI: ENRICHD SOCIAL SUPPORT INSTRUMENT

	None of the Time	Little of the Time	Some of the Time	Most of the Time	All of the Time
1. Is there someone available to you whom you can count on to listen to you when you need to talk?	1	2	3	4	5
2. Is there someone available to you to give you advice about a problem?	1	2	3	4	5
3. Is there someone available to you who shows you love and affection?	1	2	3	4	5
4. Is there someone available to you to help you with daily chores?	1	2	3	4	5
5. Can you count on anyone to provide you with emotional support (talking over problems or helping you make a difficult decision)?	1	2	3	4	5
6. Do you have as much contact as you would like with someone you feel close to, in someone you can trust and confide in?	1	2	3	4	5
7. Are you currently married, or living with a partner?	Yes			No	

Adapted from Mitchell PH, Powell L, Blumenthal J, et al. A short social support measure for patients recovering from myocardial infarction: the ENRICHD Social Support Inventory. *J Cardiopulm Rehabil.* 2003;23:398–403.

Emotional Factors

Nursing interventions help improve health outcomes in patients with emotional distress by encouraging patients to engage in positive activities that increase connection with others. Opportunities include attending community lectures, working together on home projects, and other hobbies or activities that impart a sense of accomplishment. Utilizing the cognitive social learning model in stress management training, nurses play a key role in providing adequate education about psychosocial risk factors, emotional stress, and coping skills.[30] These therapeutic techniques may include monitoring irrational thoughts and generating alternative interpretations of situations. Other techniques include progressive muscle relaxation, training in assertiveness, problem solving, and time management. Social support and group interactions have shown great benefit toward improved cardiovascular health and self-esteem.[30] In one study, low levels of emotional support were

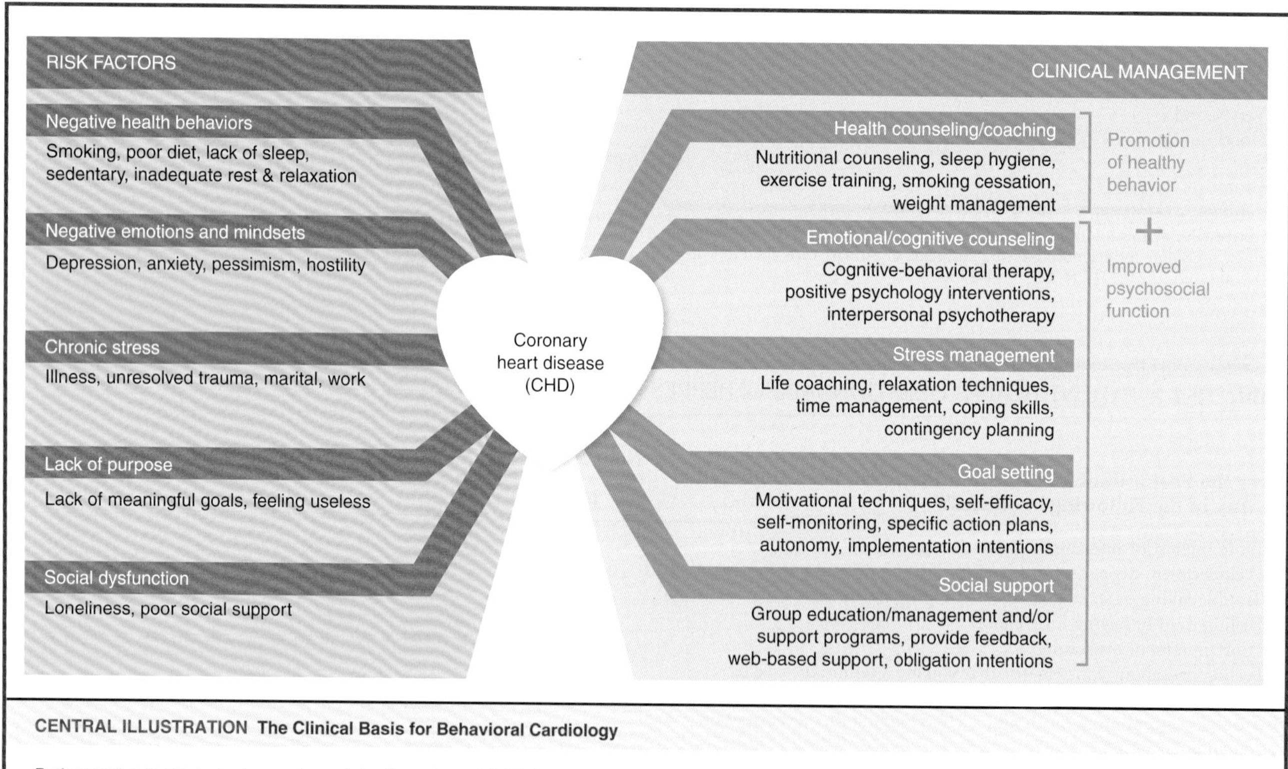

Figure 19-1. The clinical basis for behavioral cardiology. Both negative behaviors and a variety of psychosocial risk factors increase the risk for CHD, often in synergistic fashion. An increasing number of evidence-based techniques have been developed as management strategies for promoting healthy behaviors and the enhancement of psychosocial well-being. CHD, coronary heart disease. (From Rozanski A. Behavioral cardiology: current advances and future directions. *J Am Coll Cardiol.* 2014;64[1]:100–110.)

associated with significant threefold increased risk of incidence of MI and CHD mortality over 6 years of follow-up in a sample of 736 initially healthy individuals.[68]

To further reduce incidence of emotional distress and successfully intervene, nurses may act by implementing effective communications and establishing rapport with hostile and angry patients to decrease angry assumptions, thoughts, and behaviors.[43] Open-ended questions may give insight into patient perception, for example: "What kind of pressure have you been under at home or work, and whom do you turn to for support?"[27] Once psychosocial stress is identified, the nurse may intervene within their scope of practice or refer for psychiatric and/or social service assistance and care.[27]

The hostile and angry patients tend to have unsatisfactory relationships and may have difficulty maintaining relationships. The goal-oriented activities and interventions can nurture and encourage social connectivity thus helping patients learn to (a) recognize their internal reactions in the interpersonal environment, (b) practice expressing their feelings and listening in a reflective and empathetic way, (c) practice assertive skills, like delegation and creating boundaries, and (d) learn the difference between assertive and aggressive responses.[69]

In recent years, the field of behavioral cardiology has sought to manage psychosocial distress, recognizing that emotional factors and chronic life stressors provoke adverse cardiac events and poor clinical outcomes.[70]

Behavioral Factors

There are clear benefits to combined lifestyle interventions like increasing physical activity, exercise, and dietary change to help improve cardiovascular outcomes.[71] The AHA recommends physical activity for at least 150 minutes of moderate-intensity aerobic activity or at least 75 minutes of increased-intensity aerobic activity per week.[72] Adherence to heart-healthy diet and dietary modifications include sodium restriction, Mediterranean diet, Swedish diet, DASH (dietary approaches to stop hypertension) diet, and limited alcohol intake to help reduce the incidence of CVD.[73] There are several different strategies identified to target specific dietary behaviors and other lifestyle changes such as exercise, tobacco use, physical inactivity, and alcohol use. Nutritional resources and educational insight that nurses introduce can motivate patients to change lifestyle.[74] Again, open-ended questions with motivational interviewing techniques, such as "What concerns do you have about your tobacco use?" or "How would you describe your concerns about your sleep habits?" allow for the recruitment of patient buy-in.[70] These intervention strategies for individual behavior change focus on self-monitoring, self-efficacy, and family and peer support.

Another important behavioral factor that plays a key role is exercise. The Novel Technology Strategies, Internet-based programs, and personal tracking devices (i.e., FitBits™, San Francisco, CA) provide affordable solutions to bolster cardiac health.[74] Nurses can educate, motivate, supervise, and encourage patients attending cardiac rehabilitation programs.[70] These group-based interventions may motivate participants to continue with their new strategies of health promotion.[75] Nurses can further enhance those strategies by setting small goals with action plans.

Another important consideration is impaired circadian cycle, which is directly related to increased psychosocial stress. Nurses and other clinicians should educate patients about this significant health risk factor and provide support by promoting rest and relaxation techniques and life coaching.[27] Cost-effective behavioral interventions are emerging in the development of tailored group programs or individual web-based programs to assist patients with practical and useful behavioral strategies regarding sleep hygiene, rest, and stress management.[70]

Chronic Stressors

Chronic stress, poor SES, social isolation, caregiver burden, and job stress have been linked to the development of cardiac disease.[75] The other common psychological disorders leading to chronic stress are depression, anxiety, and posttraumatic stress disorders. Nurses can guide and support patients with goals aimed to lower stress, effectively cope, and improve psychosocial and cardiovascular health outcomes. A nurse can also provide emotional support with empathetic listening, validation, and encouraging social interactions in patients with few social ties or lack of support.[76] In addition to cardiovascular benefit, cardiac rehabilitation programs help with managing psychological disorders in heart disease patients while helping them reduce effects of stress on their minds and bodies.[77] Patients with existing support networks are likely to benefit by having family or significant others involved during the recovery from a cardiac event. Providing information prior to procedures, throughout hospitalization or outpatient treatment process, and during rehabilitation can decrease fears of uncertainty and allow patients to recover more completely. Moreover, educating patients and spouses or significant others about disease processes, courses of treatment, and the recovery process can decrease overprotectiveness and overinvolvement when patients are discharged home from the hospital.[78] For example, treadmill exercise before discharge from the hospital, if observed by the spouse, has shown to enhance patient's self-esteem and to reduce spousal anxiety.[79]

Chronic stress, lack of awareness, social isolation, and lack of support may perpetuate negative heart outcomes. Consider a patient who experiences a cardioverter-defibrillator shock and the worry and anxiety associated with the event. The fear may manifest itself with behavior like avoiding engaging in activities, frequently seeking reassurance, or excessive self-monitoring and overanalyzing. Nurses play a pivotal role in establishing a rapport with patients to gain trust and subsequently intervene by providing support, education, reassurance, and relaxation training exercises.[80] The mainstay of interventional therapy focuses on behavioral strategies to reduce or eliminate posttraumatic stress resulting in improved psychosocial outcomes.[80]

Multiple studies have demonstrated that stress management can decrease psychological distress and thus reduce cardiovascular risk and improve life expectancy.[27] Long working hours and lack of sleep have demonstrated increased risk for developing a cardiac disease. Nurses may effectively contribute to screen such individuals and engage patients in counseling and educate them on lifestyle modification to reduce their risks for CVD. Nurses can set what goals to achieve daily or weekly in order to reduce stress, as individuals who manage their time effectively are experiencing less stress.[81]

Pharmacologic Interventions

The cardiac nurse should be aware of the standard of care for pharmacologic management of psychosocial distress in the cardiac patient population. The most successful combination for moderate to severe depressive disorders within the cardiac population is concomitant pharmacotherapy and psychotherapy.[82] Due to the potential for side effects and drug interactions, as well as the nuances between the drug classes and the effect on the cardiovascular system, collaboration between cardiology and psychiatry is always reasonable in the management of these patients.

Selective serotonin reuptake inhibitors (SSRIs) continue to demonstrate widespread efficacy with fewer drug interactions and side effects when compared to tricyclic antidepressants, selective norepinephrine reuptake inhibitors (SNRIs), monoamine oxidase inhibitors (MAOIs), and atypical antidepressants.[83] Not without side effects, certain SSRIs can cause QT prolongation, decreased bioavailability or variable plasma levels of antiarrhythmic drugs, and potential decreased platelet activity, increasing bleeding risk with warfarin and reducing efficacy of clopidogrel.[84] Specifically, citalopram and escitalopram should be used with caution in electrophysiology and heart failure patients. On the other hand, cardiac patients with inflammatory and endothelial dysfunction have been demonstrated to achieve normalized platelet function, decreased risk of ischemic heart disease, and improved autonomic function.[85]

SNRIs, though demonstrating no QT prolongation when compared to SSRIs, carry risks of hypertension and tachycardia and should be used with caution in patients with heart failure, recent MI or stroke, and uncontrolled hypertension.[86] Tricyclic antidepressants increase risk of orthostatic hypotension and increase heart rate while slowing conduction (PR, QRS, and QT intervals, AV conduction, and ventricular arrhythmias), especially when taken with other antiarrhythmic agents.[82] Tricyclics should not be the first-line choice for patients with cardiac disease and should be considered with extreme caution only in patients refractory to SSRI or SNRI therapy.[84] Monoamine oxidase inhibitor (MAOI) was the original antidepressant therapy to become clinically available. They are largely no longer prescribed due to the risk of hypertensive crisis when taken with tyramine-containing foods, such as cheeses. Hypertensive crisis occurs from the unregulated release of epinephrine, norepinephrine, and dopamine.[82]

As an advocate for each patient, the cardiac nurse should be aware of the basic pharmacologic interventions for cardiac patients with psychosocial concerns and address the potential possibilities with cardiology and psychiatric providers.

Summary

In recent years, the evidence demonstrates the complex state when the two most prevalent diseases, psychosocial and cardiovascular, coexist in a patient. The collaborative approach of both behavioral and cardiology specialties, will further impact comprehensive and efficacious patient-centered care. Assessment and care of patients with emotional, behavioral, and social needs play an important role in the prevention of CVDs. Implementation of the current tools in order to identify patients with these potential risk factors will help nurses tailor their patient care. Despite the advanced understanding of pharmacologic treatment modalities for psychosocial diseases, there is a need for future research on nonpharmacologic guidelines to further advance the assessment and intervention capabilities for cardiac nurses and the treatment options for behavioral cardiology patients.

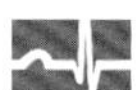

CASE STUDY 1

Patient Profile

Name/Age/Sex: **Linda Taylor, 63-year-old female**

History of Present Illness

Is presented today in a primary care office with complaints of intermittent chest pressure that started 2 weeks ago, occurring several times per day and lasting 10–15 minutes. She rates the pressure 4 on a 10-point scale and denies any associated pain in her back, neck, or arm. She experiences the pressure in her chest when she is climbing stairs. She denies taking any over-the-counter medications to alleviate pain.

She also reports that she feels isolated since her husband died 1 year ago and often feels she has no motivation or energy to do anything alone. She works as a high school teacher for the past 25 years and reports no new or increasing stress related to her work environment. Since her pain started, she feels very fatigued and has not been sleeping well.

Past Medical History

HTN, hyperlipidemia, obesity, and hysterectomy

Family History

Father (Deceased, 86): HTN, CAD
Mother (Deceased, 79): Depression, breast cancer

Social History

Occupation: Chemistry high school teacher for past 25 years
Education: Bachelor's degree in chemistry
Tobacco use: Former smoker 30 pack-year, quit 3 years ago
ETOH: Social, 2–3 glasses of wine/wk
Illicit drugs: None

Medications

Lisinopril 20 mg daily, hydrochlorothiazide 12.5 mg daily, Crestor 20 mg daily, multivitamin 1 tab daily

Allergies

NKDA

Pertinent Findings

Normal ECG
BMI 42 kg/m^2
PHQ-9 score 14

Considerations

Risk for cardiac disease: Recommend continued close follow-up with cardiologist, dietary modification, and increased exercise regimen will help with weight management, depression, and anxiety and thus reduce risk for cardiac disease.

Moderate depression: Patient referred for cognitive and behavioral therapy with positive psychology interventions.

Increased stress: Coping skills and relaxation techniques recommended for stress management including deep diaphragmatic breathing 3–4 times per day, meditation, increased social support, and verbal expression of feelings.

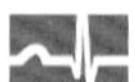

CASE STUDY 2

Patient Profile

Name/Age/Sex: **Mark Byron, 42-year-old male**

History of Present Illness

Presented for his annual general physical examination. He has no current complaints and no changes in his health since last visit. Upon further assessment and evaluation, you discovered that he just recently had a change in employment and that he has been under a lot of financial stress to support his family. His wife is currently unemployed and he is working 2 jobs. Upon further conversation, you also discovered that he has not been eating well and only gets 4 hours of sleep at night.

CASE STUDY 2 (*Continued*)

Past Medical History
None

Family History
Father (76): HTN, hyperlipidemia, CAD, MI
Mother (71): Hypothyroidism, anxiety, depression

Social History
Occupation: Automotive Mechanic
Education: 12 GED, Automotive Technician
Tobacco use: Current smoker, 2 packs/day
ETOH: 1–2 beer/day
Illicit drugs: None
Activity: Does not exercise regularly

Allergies
NKDA

Medications
None

Patient Examination
A&O × 3, NAD
Lungs: CTAB
Cardiac: RRR, no murmur noted
EENT: Sclera white, moist mucous membranes, PERRLA

Diagnostic Testing
Normal ECG
PHQ-9 score 5

Considerations

Risk for cardiac event: Educated on the importance of time management and relaxation techniques to help reduce stress and risk for cardiac disease. Motivational interviewing utilized in order to discuss potential readiness for smoking cessation.

Lack of sleep: Recommended web-based program to assist in useful behavioral strategies to help achieve 7–9 hours of sleep at night, literature provided.

Mild depression: Discussed with patient and mutually agreed upon strategies for the reduction of symptoms of depression with options including a daily exercise routine, meditation, and appropriate social support.

KEY READING

Okereke O, Manson J. Psychosocial factors and cardiovascular disease risk: an opportunity in women's health. *Circ Res.* 2017;120(12):1855–1856.

REFERENCES

1. Huffman JC, Celano CM, Beach SR, et al. Depression and cardiac disease: epidemiology, mechanisms, and diagnosis. *Cardiovasc Psychiatry Neurol.* 2013;2013:695925.
2. Pickering T, Clemow L, Davidson K, et al. Behavioral cardiology—has its time finally arrived? *Mt Sinai J Med.* 2003;70(2):101–112.
3. Shen BJ, Eisenberg SA, Maeda U, et al. Depression and anxiety predict decline in physical health functioning in patients with heart failure. *Ann Behav Med.* 2010;41(3):373–382.
4. Dubois CM, Lopez OV, Beale EE, et al. Relationships between positive psychological constructs and health outcomes in patients with cardiovascular disease: a systematic review. *Int J Cardiol.* 2015;195:265–280.
5. Yohannes AM, Willgoss TG, Baldwin RC, et al. Depression and anxiety in chronic heart failure and chronic obstructive pulmonary disease: prevalence, relevance, clinical implications and management principles. *Int J Geriatr Psychiatry.* 2010;25(12):1209–1221.
6. Zanni GR. Depression: underdiagnosed and undertreated. Pharmacy Times; 2011. Available at https://www.pharmacytimes.com/publications/issue/2011/january2011/counseling-0111. Accessed June 18, 2018.
7. Kasper DL, Fauci AS, Hauser SL, et al. *Harrison's Principles of Internal Medicine.* New York: McGraw-Hill Education; 2015.
8. Diagnostic and Statistical Manual of Mental Disorders (DSM-5). *Mindfulness practices may help treat many mental health conditions.* 2014. Available at https://www.psychiatry.org/psychiatrists/practice/dsm. Accessed July 26, 2018.
9. Ksithija L, Zaved K. Depression—A review. *Res J Recent Sci.* 2012; 1:79–87.
10. Moller-Leimkuhler AM. Gender differences in cardiovascular disease and comorbid depression. *Dialogues Clin Neurosci.* 2007;9(1):71–83.
11. O'Neil A, Fisher AJ, Kibbey KJ, et al. Depression is a risk factor for incident coronary heart disease in women: an 18-year longitudinal study. *J Affect Disord.* 2016;196:117–124.
12. Carney RM, Rich MW, Freedland KE, et al. Major depressive disorder predicts cardiac events in patients with coronary artery disease. *Psychosom Med.* 1988;50(6):627–633.
13. Carney RM, Freedland KE, Rich MW, et al. Depression as a risk factor for cardiac events in established coronary heart disease: a review of possible mechanisms. *Ann Behav Med.* 1995;17(2):142–149.
14. Blumenthal JA, Williams RS. Physiological and psychological variables predict compliance to prescribed exercise therapy in patients recovering from myocardial infarction. *Psychosom Med.* 1982;44:519–527.
15. Finnegan DL, Suler JR. Psychological factors associated with maintenance of improved health behavior in post coronary patients. *J Psychol.* 1985;119:87–94.
16. Davidson KW, Kupfer DJ, Bigger JT, et al. Assessment and treatment of depression in patients with cardiovascular disease: National Health, Lung, and Blood Institute Working Group report. *Psychosom Med.* 2006;68:645–650.
17. Allison TG, Williams DE, Miller TD, et al. Medical and economic costs of psychological distress in patients with coronary artery disease. *Mayo Clin Proc.* 1995;70(8):734–742.
18. Cohen B, Edmondson D, Kronish I. State of the art review: depression, stress, anxiety, and cardiovascular disease. *Am J Hypertens.* 2015;28(11):1295–1302.
19. Mcdevitt-Petrovic O, Kirby K, Shevlin M. The prevalence of non-cardiac chest pain (NCCP) using emergency department (ED) data: a Northern Ireland based study. *BMC Health Serv Res.* 2017;17(1):549.
20. Rozanski A, Blumenthal JA, Davidson KW, et al. The epidemiology, pathophysiology, and management of psychosocial risk factors in cardiac practice. *J Am Coll Cardiol.* 2005;45(5):637–651.
21. Blumenthal JA, Feger BJ, Smith PJ, et al. Treatment of anxiety in patients with coronary heart disease: rationale and design of the UNderstanding the benefits of exercise and escitalopram in anxious patients WIth coroNary heart Disease (UNWIND) randomized clinical trial. *Am Heart J.* 2016;176:53–62.
22. Burg MM, Lampert R, Joska T, et al. Psychological traits and emotion-triggering of ICD shock-terminated arrhythmias. *Psychosom Med.* 2004;66(6):898–902.
23. Pearson QM. Sleep and aging: challenges and recommendations for middle-aged and older adults. *Adultspan Journal.* 2017;16(1):31–46.
24. Norra C, Kummer J, Boecker M, et al. Poor sleep quality is associated with depressive symptoms in patients with heart disease. *Int J Behav Med.* 2011;19(4):526–534.
25. Motivala SJ. Sleep and inflammation: psychoneuroimmunology in the context of cardiovascular disease. *Ann Behav Med.* 2011;42(2):141–152.
26. Hirshkowitz M, Whiton K, Albert SM, et al. National Sleep Foundation's sleep time duration recommendations: methodology and results summary. *Sleep Health.* 2015;1(1):40–43.
27. Das S, O'Keefe JH. Behavioral cardiology: recognizing and addressing the profound impact of psychosocial stress on cardiovascular health. *Curr Hypertens Rep.* 2008;10(5):374–381.
28. Thurston RC, Rewak M, Kubzansky LD. An anxious heart: anxiety and the onset of cardiovascular diseases. *Prog Cardiovasc Dis.* 2013;55(6):524–537.
29. Daubenmier JJ, Weidner G, Sumner MD, et al. The contribution of changes in diet, exercise, and stress management to changes in coronary risk in women and men in the Multisite Cardiac Lifestyle Intervention Program. *Ann Behav Med.* 2007;33(1):57–68.
30. Blumenthal JA, Sherwood A, Babyak MA, et al. Effects of exercise and stress management training on markers of cardiovascular risk in patients with ischemic heart disease. *J Cardiopulm Rehabil.* 2005;25(4):235.

31. Shen BJ, Gau JT. Influence of depression and hostility on exercise tolerance and improvement in patients with coronary heart disease. *Int J Behav Med.* 2016;24(2):312–320.
32. Milani RV, Lavie CJ, Mehra MR, et al. Impact of exercise training and depression on survival in heart failure due to coronary heart disease. *Am J Cardiol.* 2011;107(1):64–68.
33. Camargo KRD. Closing the gap in a generation: health equity through action on the social determinants of health. *Glob Public Health.* 2011; 6(1):102–105.
34. Gallo LC, Matthews KA. Understanding the association between socioeconomic status and physical health: do negative emotions play a role? *Psychol Bull.* 2003;129(1):10–51.
35. Sumner JA, Khodneva Y, Muntner P, et al. Effects of concurrent depressive symptoms and perceived stress on cardiovascular risk in low- and high-income participants: findings from the Reasons for Geographical and Racial Differences in Stroke (REGARDS) Study. *J Am Heart Assoc.* 2016;5(10):e003930.
36. Franks P, Winters PC, Tancredi DJ, et al. Do changes in traditional coronary heart disease risk factors over time explain the association between socio-economic status and coronary heart disease? *BMC Cardiovasc Disord.* 2011;11(1):28.
37. Yusuf S, Reddy S, Ounpuu S, et al. Global burden of cardiovascular diseases: part I: general considerations, the epidemiologic transition, risk factors, and impact of urbanization. *Circulation.* 2001;104(22):2746–2753.
38. Allen JA, McNeely JM, Waldestein SR, et al. Subjective socioeconomic status predicts Framingham cardiovascular disease risk for whites, not blacks. *Ethn Dis.* 2014;24(2):150–154.
39. Franks P, Tancredi DJ, Winters P, et al. Including socioeconomic status in coronary heart disease risk estimation. *Ann Fam Med.* 2010;8(5):447–453.
40. Ozbay F, Johnson DC, Dimoulas E, et al. Social support and resilience to stress: from neurobiology to clinical practice. *Psychiatry (Edgmont).* 2007;4(5):35–40.
41. Reblin M, Uchino BN. Social and emotional support and its implication for health. *Curr Opin Psychiatry.* 2008;21(2):201–205.
42. Uchino BN. Social support and health: a review of physiological processes potentially underlying links to disease outcomes. *J Behav Med.* 2006;29(4):377–387.
43. Everson-Rose SA, Lewis TT. Psychosocial factors and cardiovascular diseases. *Annu Rev Public Health.* 2005;26(1):469–500.
44. Kivimäki M, Kawachi I. Work stress as a risk factor for cardiovascular disease. *Curr Cardiol Rep.* 2015;17(9):74.
45. Kivimaki M, Nyberg ST, Fransson EI, et al. Associations of job strain and lifestyle risk factors with risk of coronary artery disease: a meta-analysis of individual participant data. *Can Med Assoc J.* 2013;185(9):763–769.
46. Virtanen M, Heikkila K, Jokela M, et al. Long working hours and coronary heart disease: a systematic review and meta-analysis. *Am J Epidemiol.* 2012;176(7):586–596.
47. Bunker SJ, Colquhoun DM, Esler MD, et al. Stress and coronary heart disease: psychosocial risk factors. *Med J Aust.* 2003;178:272–276.
48. Smith TW, Ruiz JM. Psychosocial influences on the development and course of coronary heart disease: current status and implications for research and practice. *J Consult Clin Psychol.* 2002;70:548–568.
49. Herman JP, McKlveen JM, Ghosal S, et al. Regulation of the hypothalamic-pituitary-adrenocortical stress response. *Compr Physiol.* 2016;6:603–621.
50. Peters A, McEwen BS. Stress habituation, body shape and cardiovascular mortality. *Neurosci Biobehav Rev.* 2015;56:139–150.
51. Pedersen SS, Kanel R, Tully PJ. Psychosocial perspectives in cardiovascular disease. *Eur J Prev Cardiol.* 2017;24(3):108–111.
52. De Jong MJ, Chung ML, Wu JR, et al. International perspectives on quality of life in cardiopulmonary disorders: linkages between anxiety and outcomes in heart failure. *Heart Lung.* 2011;40(5):393–404.
53. Carney CM, Freedland KE, Veith RC. Depression, the autonomic nervous system, and coronary heart disease. *Psychosom Med.* 2005;67(1):29–33.
54. Hitze B, Hubold H, van Dyken K, et al. How the selfish brain organizes its supply and demand. *Front Neuroenergetics.* 2010;2:7.
55. Nikkheslat N, Zunszain PA, Horowitz MA, et al. Insufficient glucocorticoid signaling and elevated inflammation in coronary heart disease patients with comorbid depression. *Brain Behav Immun.* 2015;48:8–18.
56. Bohm F, Pernow J. The importance of endothelin-1 for vascular dysfunction in cardiovascular disease. *Cardiovasc Res.* 2007;76(1):8–18.
57. Hadi AR, Carr CS, Suwaidi JA. Endothelial dysfunction: cardiovascular risk factors, therapy, and outcome. *Vasc Health Risk Manag.* 2005;1(3):183–198.
58. Halaris A. Inflammation-associated co-morbidity between depression and cardiovascular disease. *Curr Top Behav Neurosci.* 2017;1(31):45–70.
59. Miller AH, Raison CL. The role of inflammation in depression: from evolutionary imperative to modern treatment target. *Nat Rev Immunol.* 2016;16(1):22–34.
60. Williams MS, Rogers HL, Wang NY, et al. Do platelet-derived microparticles play a role in depression, inflammation, and acute coronary syndrome? *Psychosomatics.* 2014;55(3):252–260.
61. Disbrow DK. Barriers cardiac nurses face in addressing psychosocial issues of heart failure patients. Walden University Scholar Works; 2017. Available at https://scholarworks.waldenu.edu/cgi/viewcontent.cgi?article=4773&context=dissertations. Accessed June 24, 2018.
62. Spitzer RL, Kroenke K, Williams JB. Validation and utility of a self-report version of PRIME-MD: the PHQ primary care study. Primary Care Evaluation of Mental Disorders. Patient Health Questionnaire. *JAMA.* 1999;282(18):1737–1744.
63. Kroenke K, Spitzer RL, Williams JB. The Patient Health Questionnaire-2: validity of a two-item depression screener. *Med Care.* 2003;41(11):1284–1292.
64. Katon WJ, Lin EHB, VonKorff M, et al. Collaborative care for patients with depression and chronic illness. *N Engl J Med.* 2011;364(13):1278–1279.
65. Perez GL, Wallston KA, Goggins KM, et al. Effects of stress, health competence, and social support on depressive symptoms after cardiac hospitalization. *J Behav Med.* 2016;39(3):441–452.
66. Mitchell PH, Powell L, Blumenthal J, et al. A short social support measure for patients recovering from myocardial infarction. *J Cardiopulm Rehabil.* 2003;23(6):398–403.
67. Berkman LF, Blumenthal J, Burg M, et al. Effects of treating depression and low perceived social support on clinical events after myocardial infarction: the Enhancing Recovery in Coronary Heart Disease Patients (ENRICHD) Randomized Trial. *JAMA.* 2003;289(23):3106–3116.
68. Orth-Gomér K, Wamala SP, Horsten M, et al. Marital stress worsens prognosis in women with coronary heart disease. *JAMA.* 2000;284(23):3008–3014.
69. Sotile WM. *Psychosocial Interventions for Cardiopulmonary Patients: A Guide for Health Professionals.* Champaign, IL: Human Kinetics; 1996.
70. Rozanski A. Behavioral cardiology. *J Am Coll Cardiol.* 2014;64(1):100–110.
71. Olendzski B, Speed C, Domino FJ. Nutritional assessment and counseling for prevention and treatment of cardiovascular disease. *Am Fam Physician.* 2006;73(2):257–263.
72. American Heart Association Recommendations for Physical Activity in Adults. *How cigarettes damage your body.* 2015. Available at http://www.heart.org/HEARTORG/HealthyLiving/PhysicalActivity/FitnessBasics/American-Heart-Association-Recommendations-for-Physical-Activity-in-Adults_UCM_307976_Article.jsp. Accessed July 28, 2018.
73. Lanier JB, Bury DC, Richardson SW. Diet and physical activity for cardiovascular disease prevention. *Am Fam Physician.* 2016;93(11):919–924.
74. Artinian NT, Fletcher GF, Mozaffarian D, et al. Interventions to promote physical activity and dietary lifestyle changes for cardiovascular risk factor reduction in adults: a scientific statement from the American Heart Association. *Circulation.* 2010;122(4):406–441.
75. Lagraauw HM, Kuiper J, Bot I. Acute and chronic psychological stress as risk factors for cardiovascular disease: insights gained from epidemiological, clinical and experimental studies. *Brain Behav Immun.* 2015;50:18–30.
76. Friedwald VE, Arnold LW, Carney RM, et al. The editor's roundtable: major depression in patients with coronary heart disease. *Am J Cardiol.* 2007;99:519–529.
77. Chauvet-Gelinier JC, Bonin B. Stress, anxiety and depression in heart disease patients: a major challenge for cardiac rehabilitation. *Ann Phys Rehabil Med.* 2017;60(1):6–12.
78. Doerr BC, Jones JW. Effect of family preparation on the state anxiety level of the CCU patient. *Nurs Res.* 1979;28(5):315.
79. Taylor CB, Bandura A, Ewart CK, et al. Exercise testing to enhance wives confidence in their husbands cardiac capability soon after clinically uncomplicated acute myocardial infarction. *Am J Cardiol.* 1985;55(6):635–638.
80. Habibović M, Burg MM, Pedersen SS. Behavioral interventions in patients with an implantable cardioverter defibrillator: lessons learned and where to go from here? *Pacing Clin Electrophysiol.* 2013;36(5):578–590.
81. Papathanasiou IV, Tsaras K, Neroliatsiou A, et al. Stress: concepts, theoretical models and nursing interventions. *Am J Nurs Sci.* 2015;4(2):45–50.
82. Teply RM, Packard KA, White ND, et al. Treatment of depression in patients with concomitant cardiac disease. *Prog Cardiovasc Dis.* 2016;58(5):514–528.
83. Rosse SP. Depression, anxiety, and the cardiovascular system: the psychiatrist's perspective. *J Clin Psychiatry.* 2001;62(8):19–22.
84. Nezafati MH, Vojdanparast M, Nezafati P. Antidepressant and cardiovascular adverse events: a narrative review. *ARYA Atheroscler.* 2015;11(5):295–304.
85. Yekehtaz H, Farokhnia M, Akhondzadeh S. Cardiovascular considerations in antidepressant therapy: an evidence-based review. *J Tehran Heart Cent.* 2013;8(4):169–176.
86. Mavrides N, Nemeroff CB. Treatment of affective disorders in cardiac disease. *Health Commun.* Available at http://europepmc.org/articles/PMC4518697. Accessed July 25, 2018.

20 Obesity: An Overview of Assessment and Treatment

Alison Yam, Anna Dean, Brandy Thomas

OBJECTIVES

1. Define obesity, risk factors, identification, and assessment.
2. Evaluate cardiovascular risk and conditions associated with obesity.
3. Identify potential challenges in prevention of obesity.
4. Recognize weight loss treatment goals and components.
5. Identify current obesity pharmacology, side effects, and treatment duration.
6. Apply knowledge about types of bariatric surgery, benefits, and complications.
7. Differentiate between weight loss and weight loss maintenance strategies.

KEY QUESTIONS

1. What components are assessed in screening for obesity? List associated BMI range.
2. Differentiate between very high absolute risk and high absolute risk for cardiovascular disease. Name three cardiovascular conditions influenced by obesity.
3. Name one short- and one long-term medication for obesity, associated side effect, and range of treatment duration.
4. What is the most common bariatric surgery? What are the associated benefits and complications?
5. Differentiate between strategies for weight loss and weight loss maintenance.

BACKGROUND

Obesity has been on the rise in the United States since 1976. The National Center for Health Statistics (NCHS) reports that from 2015 to 2016, almost 40% of adults in the United States are obese.[1] Should this trend continue, it is projected that 86% of Americans will be either overweight or obese by 2030.[2] Obesity rates have also seen significant increases among children and adolescents. Of particular concern is the increasing number of children who are growing up being either overweight or obese. The 2015–2016 National Health and Nutrition Examination Survey (NHANES) reports that 18.5% of 2 to 19 year olds are obese[3] and other reports show that 35% are overweight.[2] While obesity rates among children have leveled off, extreme obesity (BMI equivalency of greater than or equal to 35 kg/m^2) continues to grow.[3] This is of critical importance as overweight and obese children are more likely to grow up being overweight and obese adults.[2]

Being obese is a risk factor for developing cardiovascular disease (CVD), depression, diabetes, cancer (specifically liver, kidney, breast, endometrial, prostate, and colon), kidney disease, musculoskeletal disorders, and other chronic diseases.[3,4] New research is illuminating how adiposity is perhaps another indicator of overall risk. Tracking adiposity across the life span, researchers are trying to determine what point on the continuum is most critical.[5,6] In this model, adiposity at a young age portends BMI in adulthood. The 2015–2016 NHANES indicates that almost 40% of adults in the United States are obese (BMI greater than or equal to 30 kg/m^2).[3] Prevalence rates may be even higher since the NHANES relies on self-reported survey data. The U.S. Preventive Services Task Force (USPSTF) recommends that individuals 18 years and older be screened for obesity. Screening and interventions are important because being obese is associated with decreased life expectancy by as much as 20 years in obese individuals.[4]

Body mass index (BMI) is the standard measurement used for classifying weight status. Obesity in adults is defined as a BMI of greater than or equal to 30 kg/m^2. BMI alone as a classification of obesity is being challenged as it does not adequately reflect actual body fat composition, or age-related changes in muscle mass versus body fat.[5] Instead, waist circumference is considered more of a true measure of adiposity or body fat. This has important implications for health status as belly fat is metabolically active and contributes to developing CVD. This risk is imparted on individuals with a girth of greater than or equal to 94 cm in men and greater than or equal to 80 in women (Fig. 20-1).[7]

Obesity has been linked to a host of chronic diseases associated with heart disease, including type II diabetes (T2D), dyslipidemia, and hypertension.[2,7] Given the prevalence of obesity in the United States, it is no surprise that T2D is on the rise as well. Among the obese and overweight, 85% have T2D and it is estimated that if trends continue, one in three Americans will be diabetic by 2050.[2,7]

Obesity and diabetes are inextricably linked to CVD and stroke.[2,7] Being obese is associated with deleterious effects on the heart and circulatory system, contributing to an increased risk of arrhythmias, sudden death, heart failure, and ischemic heart disease.[7] Indirectly, obesity contributes to cardiovascular risk as

Body Mass Index Table

	Normal						Overweight					Obese										Extreme Obesity														
BMI	**19**	**20**	**21**	**22**	**23**	**24**	**25**	**26**	**27**	**28**	**29**	**30**	**31**	**32**	**33**	**34**	**35**	**36**	**37**	**38**	**39**	**40**	**41**	**42**	**43**	**44**	**45**	**46**	**47**	**48**	**49**	**50**	**51**	**52**	**53**	**54**
Height (inches)																		**Body Weight (pounds)**																		
58	91	96	100	105	110	115	119	124	129	134	138	143	148	153	158	162	167	172	177	181	186	191	196	201	205	210	215	220	224	229	234	239	244	248	253	258
59	94	99	104	109	114	119	124	128	133	138	143	148	153	158	163	168	173	178	183	188	193	198	203	208	212	217	222	227	232	237	242	247	252	257	262	267
60	97	102	107	112	118	123	128	133	138	143	148	153	158	163	168	174	179	184	189	194	199	204	209	215	220	225	230	235	240	245	250	255	261	266	271	276
61	100	106	111	116	122	127	132	137	143	148	153	158	164	169	174	180	185	190	195	201	206	211	217	222	227	232	238	243	248	254	259	264	269	275	280	285
62	104	109	115	120	126	131	136	142	147	153	158	164	169	175	180	186	191	196	202	207	213	218	224	229	235	240	246	251	256	262	267	273	278	284	289	295
63	107	113	118	124	130	135	141	146	152	158	163	169	175	180	186	191	197	203	208	214	220	225	231	237	242	248	254	259	265	270	278	282	287	293	299	304
64	110	116	122	128	134	140	145	151	157	163	169	174	180	186	192	197	204	209	215	221	227	232	238	244	250	256	262	267	273	279	285	291	296	302	308	314
65	114	120	126	132	138	144	150	156	162	168	174	180	186	192	198	204	210	216	222	228	234	240	246	252	258	264	270	276	282	288	294	300	306	312	318	324
66	118	124	130	136	142	148	155	161	167	173	179	186	192	198	204	210	216	223	229	235	241	247	253	260	266	272	278	284	291	297	303	309	315	322	328	334
67	121	127	134	140	146	153	159	166	172	178	185	191	198	204	211	217	223	230	236	242	249	255	261	268	274	280	287	293	299	306	312	319	325	331	338	344
68	125	131	138	144	151	158	164	171	177	184	190	197	203	210	216	223	230	236	243	249	256	262	269	276	282	289	295	302	308	315	322	328	335	341	348	354
69	128	135	142	149	155	162	169	176	182	189	196	203	209	216	223	230	236	243	250	257	263	270	277	284	291	297	304	311	318	324	331	338	345	351	358	365
70	132	139	146	153	160	167	174	181	188	195	202	209	216	222	229	236	243	250	257	264	271	278	285	292	299	306	313	320	327	334	341	348	355	362	369	376
71	136	143	150	157	165	172	179	186	193	200	208	215	222	229	236	243	250	257	265	272	279	286	293	301	308	315	322	329	338	343	351	358	365	372	379	386
72	140	147	154	162	169	177	184	191	199	206	213	221	228	235	242	250	258	265	272	279	287	294	302	309	316	324	331	338	346	353	361	368	375	383	390	397
73	144	151	159	166	174	182	189	197	204	212	219	227	235	242	250	257	265	272	280	288	295	302	310	318	325	333	340	348	355	363	371	378	386	393	401	408
74	148	155	163	171	179	186	194	202	210	218	225	233	241	249	256	264	272	280	287	295	303	311	319	326	334	342	350	358	365	373	381	389	396	404	412	420
75	152	160	168	176	184	192	200	208	216	224	232	240	248	256	264	272	279	287	295	303	311	319	327	335	343	351	359	367	375	383	391	399	407	415	423	431
76	156	164	172	180	189	197	205	213	221	230	238	246	254	263	271	279	287	295	304	312	320	328	336	344	353	361	369	377	385	394	402	410	418	426	435	443

Source: Adapted from *Clinical Guidelines on the Identification, Evaluation, and Treatment of Overweight and Obesity in Adults: The Evidence Report.*

Figure 20-1. Body mass index table. (Source: National Heart, Lung, and Blood Institute; National Institutes of Health; U.S. Department of Health and Human Services.)

a result of dyslipidemia, hypertension, glucose intolerance, and endothelial dysfunction and inflammation.[2] Obesity is an independent risk factor for CVD, and CVD places individuals with T2D at significant risk for diabetes-related death.[2,7]

In the midst of the mounting evidence demonstrating the deleterious effects of obesity on health in general, and on the cardiovascular system in particular, research has demonstrated that significant benefits to health can be achieved by as little as 5% to 10% reduction in baseline weight.[4,6] This fact highlights the importance of identifying the patient at risk early on and implementing a treatment course that may prevent the development of obesity.

In 1998, the National Heart, Lung, and Blood Institute (NHLBI) issued the *Evidence Report,* which continues to provide evidence-based clinical guidelines for the identification, evaluation, and treatment of adults who are overweight and obese. The USPSTF has also made recommendations regarding screening of all adults over the age of 18 for obesity.[4] This screening should, at a minimum, include weight, BMI, and for those individuals with a BMI of less than 30 kg/m^2, waist circumference measurement.[4,6,8]

Health care professionals play an important role in counseling and educating their patients about maintaining a healthy weight and how to use healthy lifestyle measures to reduce excess weight. The 5As model is a behavior-change approach to counseling and managing patients who are overweight and obese. The components of the 5As are Assess, Advise, Agree, Assist, and Arrange. Providers who use the 5As in their practice show a twofold increase in addressing, managing, and treating obesity.[9]

IDENTIFICATION AND ASSESSMENT OF THE OVERWEIGHT OR OBESE PATIENT

Weight Status

WHO developed the classification of obesity based on BMI. Normal weight is defined as a BMI range of 18.50 to 24.99 kg/m^2, overweight as a BMI of 25.00 to 29.99 kg/m^2, and obese as a BMI of 30 kg/m^2 or more.[2,4,6–8] Asian populations have a higher amount of body fat than Caucasian populations at the same BMI. This suggests that persons of Asian descent may have increasing but tolerable health risks at a BMI range of 18.50 to 23 kg/m^2, an elevated risk with a BMI between 23 and 27.5 kg/m^2, and a high risk at a BMI greater than or equal to 27.5 kg/m^2.[8]

Waist (Abdominal) Circumference

Central or visceral obesity is an excess accumulation of fat in the abdomen that is out of proportion to total body fat.[1,2] Intra-abdominal obesity is considered more sensitive and specific than BMI as a predictor of obesity-related morbidity and mortality.[2] A large waist circumference increases the risk of myocardial infarction, heart failure, and death from all causes in patients with CVD.[2,6,7] Visceral obesity can be measured more accurately by computed tomography or magnetic resonance imaging, but these are expensive and impractical for clinical assessment in a practitioner's office. The NHANES and USPSTF recommend that both waist circumference as well as BMI be evaluated during the clinical assessment.[4,6] In addition, waist circumference can be a valuable marker to monitor weight loss progress.

Gender-specific cutoffs have been established to identify relative risk for development of obesity-associated risks factors. Men with a waistline circumference greater than 40 in (102 cm) and women with a waistline circumference greater than 35 in (88 cm) are at high risk for obesity-related morbidity.[2,8] Variability also exists among certain ethnic groups. In Asians, increased health risk is associated with a smaller waist circumference. South Asian, Chinese, and Japanese individuals have an increased risk at a waist circumference of greater than or equal to 90 cm (35.5 in) for men and greater than or equal to 80 cm (31.5 in) for women.[8]

Patients of normal weight with increased waist circumference measurements may be at increased risk of CVD. Because patients with a BMI of more than 35 kg/m^2 exceed the waist circumference cutoffs, these indicators of relative risk lose their predictive power, making it unnecessary to measure waist circumference in this group.

Assessment of Cardiovascular Disease Risk Factors

Once a patient's relative risk has been established, the absolute risk status specific for CVD should be determined.

Very High Absolute Risk

Patients who are overweight, obese, or have abdominal obesity are considered to be at *very high absolute risk* if they have the following disease conditions: established coronary heart disease (CHD), presence of other atherosclerotic diseases (peripheral arterial disease, abdominal aortic aneurysm, or symptomatic carotid disease), T2D, sleep apnea, or hypertension with evidence of target organ damage. Individuals with any of these conditions require aggressive treatment to mitigate or eliminate their risk for disease progression and exacerbation.

High Absolute Risk

Obese individuals who have three or more risk factors carry a *high absolute risk* for obesity-related comorbid conditions. These risk factors include cigarette smoking; hypertension; low-density lipoprotein (LDL) cholesterol of 160 mg/dL or more; LDL cholesterol of 130 to 159 mg/dL in the presence of two or more other risk factors; high-density lipoprotein (HDL) cholesterol less than 35 mg/dL; impaired fasting glucose; a family history of premature CHD; men aged 45 years or older; and postmenopausal women aged 55 years or older.

Additional Factors That Increase Absolute Risk

The presence of additional risk factors (e.g., physical inactivity and elevated triglycerides) can increase a patient's absolute risk to a level higher than that estimated for very high and high absolute risk.[10] Elevated triglycerides in obesity may be due to a lipoprotein phenotype that includes elevated triglycerides, low HDL levels, and small LDL particles, a pattern considered atherogenic.[2] Excess visceral adiposity, hyperinsulinemia that accompanies insulin resistance, and adipose tissue-released proinflammatory cytokines such as interleukin-1, interleukin-6, tumor necrosis factor-α, resistin, or reduced adiponectin (anti-inflammatory) are also being investigated as contributory risk profiles associate with obesity.[2,7,8]

Cardiovascular-Related Conditions Influenced by Obesity

Increased body weight has a significant deleterious impact on CHD, hypertension, and heart failure requiring additional medical management. It is incumbent on the provider to address these conditions with their patients as cardiovascular health is influenced by weight status.

Undertreated Groups

Individuals older than 65 years are frequently undertreated for weight issues. The elderly are at increased risk for hypertension, diabetes, osteoarthritis (OA), and decreased mobility as a result of being obese. A reason why this is the case is that BMI does not distinguish weight that is a result of fat or muscle. Another reason is that as we age, we lose height and BMI is a calculation of height and weight. So, BMI alone may present an erroneous picture of obesity status in the elderly.[11] Therapeutic goals for treating obesity in this population should include decreasing abdominal fat and preserving muscle mass and strength.[10] Weight reduction improves functional status and reduces concomitant risk factors in the older population in a way similar to that seen in younger adults. The overweight or obese smoker carries excess risk from obesity-associated risk factors. Smoking cessation and weight management should be addressed through lifestyle approaches.[10,12] When attempting to address behavior changes, improved outcomes are more likely with a stepwise approach that focuses on assisting the patient to stop smoking first before initiating weight loss interventions.[10,12]

CLINICAL EVALUATION

Baseline assessment of the cardiac patient should include BMI, waist circumference, and cardiovascular risk profile. Additionally, noncardiovascular conditions such as sleep apnea, OA, gallstones, and gynecologic abnormalities should be part of the assessment. These conditions need to be evaluated so that obesity is treated in the context of the patient's risk profile and comorbid conditions.[2,3,10] Weight loss frequently ameliorates risks by reducing blood pressure and triglycerides, and reducing the impact of other comorbid conditions.[6,10] The NHLBI *Evidence Report*[10] includes an algorithm that is focused on weight-related assessment and treatment, but it does not include evaluation for other disorders for which the patient may be seeing a health care provider. BMI and waist circumference should be evaluated at a minimum of every 2 years even if these are normal at the time of the assessment.[12] For the patient who is of normal weight, brief counseling about prevention of future weight gain should be provided. Knowing that weight gain can be expected from most patients, maintenance of weight is a positive outcome and patients should receive reinforcement for maintaining a healthy weight.

Clinical History

Patient assessment should include a detailed patient history to include identifying problems with controlling or managing weight. If not done so previously, a physical examination should be performed along with blood work to assess lipid profile and glucose level. The provider should identify existing cardiovascular risk factors as well as other risk factors that may pose additional risk to health status.[10]

Eating and Physical Activity Patterns

Assessment of dietary habits, nutritional status, and physical activity provides additional information useful for the treatment plan. The patient should be instructed to complete a food and activity diary over the course of a few days. Included in the food diary should be the type and exact amount of foods eaten, and details from recipes or information from package labels. Information from the food and activity diary will help the provider develop a treatment plan and provide focus for nutrition education.

It is a well-established fact that lack of physical activity leads to obesity.[13] It is important for the provider to ascertain barriers that prevent patients from engaging in some form of physical activity. Not all patients have the financial means to join a gym; however, there are many other options for patients to be active. The provider should help their patients explore these options and advise them on how to get started with an exercise program. One of the best ways for individuals to become more active is by incorporating physical activities into their daily routines.[10,12]

Patient Motivation

A patient's motivation for engaging in weight loss is critical to the success of any weight reduction plan or program. Losing and maintaining weight for good health should be a permanent change. Providers should assess their patient's attitude toward weight loss, prior treatment failures and successes, support systems, comprehension of risk posed by weight status, readiness to initiate lifestyle changes, self-efficacy for achieving weight loss, time commitment, barriers to behavior change, and financial issues especially if the treatment is not covered by insurance.[10,12] Adverse medical events can be a motivating trigger for losing weight. Since these events are associated with a higher success rate for losing and maintaining weight, it has been suggested that health care professionals use these occasions as an opportunity to talk to their patients about weight management.[10,12] Individuals experiencing major life events, such as a relocation, change in marital status, and family illness, may find it better to delay initiating a weight loss program until they can focus on the behavior changes required. Those individuals with significant anxiety, depression, or eating disorders (e.g., binge eating or bulimia) may need to be treated for these conditions before starting a weight loss program. Patients with eating disorders should be referred to a specialist for treatment of the specific eating disorder.[12]

Understanding the risks excess weight has on their health, the benefits of initiating treatment, and what assistance and support will be available to them may sway the unmotivated patient. If the patient remains uninterested in weight loss treatment, the provider should at least address coexisting risk factors and initiate management of these, including prevention strategies to avoid additional weight gain. When the patient is ambivalent about making requisite lifestyle changes or initiating a weight loss program, motivational interviewing (MI), a patient-centered behavior modification strategy, can be used. This strategy has been successful with individuals seeking to lose weight. Once the assessment has been completed, the treatment plan needs to be considered and discussed with the patient.

Environmental Barriers to Weight Loss

Environmental obstacles exist as a result of reduced physical activity and increased access to high-fat, high-calorie convenience food.[2,7,13] Trends also point to the changing food environment as contributing to the obesity problem. Larger portion sizes, high-calorie foods, and access to fast-food restaurants have resulted in Americans consuming on average 570 more calories per day. Those living in food deserts or fast-food rich neighborhoods, also contribute to the increasing rate of obesity. Recent findings revealed that persons who live in areas with a higher number of fast-food restaurants had a higher BMI compared with persons who live in areas with fewer fast-food restaurants (Table 20-1).[2]

Inactivity is also impacted by environmental factors such as air pollution, the availability of green space, recreational facilities, and parks.[13]

WEIGHT LOSS TREATMENT

Treatment Approach

As the global prevalence of overweight and obese patients continues to increase, it is critical for both patients and providers to understand available treatment options.[14] A number of treatment approaches exist for obesity and weight management. These treatment options can be divided into the following three categories: lifestyle changes, pharmacotherapy, and surgical intervention. Health care providers should counsel patients on all three options, but in most cases, the first step for treatment will focus on lifestyle modification. These modifications include diet changes and monitoring, behavioral adjustments, and the implementation of an exercise or increased physical activity program. Lifestyle modifications can be used as an independent treatment, and subsequent pharmacotherapy and/or surgical interventions should occur after or along with lifestyle changes.[15–17] Because obesity markedly increases the risk for comorbidities including diabetes mellitus, hypertension, kidney disease, many types of cancers, stroke, and CVD,[18,19] treatment options must be discussed in depth with the patient and all physical and mental health factors taken into account when formulating a treatment plan.

Goal of Treatment

Because obesity is a patient-centered condition, patients should be assessed for their willingness to participate in a treatment program as well as their understanding of the weight loss plan, prior to its implementation. This includes providing specific information on changing behaviors and habits, safe forms of exercise, and extensive education on nutrition and food portioning. Once the patient is confident and determined with their decision to proceed, it is advisable to start setting goals. Treatment goals will vary greatly across patients, but for patients pursuing weight loss due to medical need, the recommended 6-month treatment target is a 5% to 10% weight reduction.[20] This target equates to a loss estimate of 0.5 to 1 lb/wk for moderate obesity and 1 to 2 lb/wk for more severely obese patients. The Centers for Disease Control and Prevention (CDC) considers a healthy adult BMI, a measure of weight relative to height, to be between 18.5 and 24.9 kg/m^2.[8] This range is primarily used as a screening tool, but it can be used as an overarching baseline treatment goal. However, patient-specific goals, as well as personal goals, should also be considered and implemented. For example, if an overweight or obese patient is suffering from obstructive sleep apnea, a personal goal for that patient may include reversing their sleep apnea diagnosis and no longer requiring a continuous positive airway pressure (CPAP) machine when sleeping.

Table 20-1 • ESTIMATED CALORIE NEEDS PER DAY, BY AGE, SEX, AND PHYSICAL ACTIVITY LEVEL

Males				Females[d]			
Age	Sedentary[a]	Moderately Active[b]	Active[c]	Age	Sedentary[a]	Moderately Active[b]	Active[c]
2	1,000	1,000	1,000	2	1,000	1,000	1,000
3	1,000	1,400	1,400	3	1,000	1,200	1,400
4	1,200	1,400	1,600	4	1,200	1,400	1,400
5	1,200	1,400	1,600	5	1,200	1,400	1,600
6	1,400	1,600	1,800	6	1,200	1,400	1,600
7	1,400	1,600	1,800	7	1,200	1,600	1,800
8	1,400	1,600	2,000	8	1,400	1,600	1,800
9	1,600	1,800	2,000	9	1,400	1,600	1,800
10	1,600	1,800	2,200	10	1,400	1,800	2,000
11	1,800	2,000	2,200	11	1,600	1,800	2,000
12	1,800	2,200	2,400	12	1,600	2,000	2,200
13	2,000	2,200	2,600	13	1,600	2,000	2,200
14	2,000	2,400	2,800	14	1,800	2,000	2,400
15	2,200	2,600	3,000	15	1,800	2,000	2,400
16	2,400	2,800	3,200	16	1,800	2,000	2,400
17	2,400	2,800	3,200	17	1,800	2,000	2,400
18	2,400	2,800	3,200	18	1,800	2,000	2,400
19–20	2,600	2,800	3,000	19–20	2,000	2,200	2,400
21–25	2,400	2,800	3,000	21–25	2,000	2,200	2,400
26–30	2,400	2,600	3,000	26–30	1,800	2,000	2,400
31–35	2,400	2,600	3,000	31–35	1,800	2,000	2,200
36–40	2,400	2,600	2,800	36–40	1,800	2,000	2,200
41–45	2,200	2,600	2,800	41–45	1,800	2,000	2,200
46–50	2,200	2,400	2,800	46–50	1,800	2,000	2,200
51–55	2,200	2,400	2,800	51–55	1,600	1,800	2,200
56–60	2,200	2,400	2,600	56–60	1,600	1,800	2,200
61–65	2,000	2,400	2,600	61–65	1,600	1,800	2,000
66–70	2,000	2,200	2,600	66–70	1,600	1,800	2,000
71–75	2,000	2,200	2,600	71–75	1,600	1,800	2,000
76 and up	2,000	2,200	2,400	76 and up	1,600	1,800	2,000

[a]Sedentary means a lifestyle that includes only the physical activity of independent living.
[b]Moderately active means a lifestyle that includes physical activity equivalent to walking about 1.5 to 3 miles per day at 3 to 4 miles per hour, in addition to the activities of independent living.
[c]Active means a lifestyle that includes physical activity equivalent to walking more than 3 miles per day at 3 to 4 miles per hour, in addition to the activities of independent living.
[d]Estimates for females do not include women who are pregnant or breast-feeding.
Source: Institute of Medicine. *Dietary Reference Intakes for Energy, Carbohydrate, Fiber, Fat, Fatty Acids, Cholesterol, Protein, and Amino Acids*. Washington, DC: The National Academies Press; 2002.

For patients with family histories of obesity-associated comorbidities, goals might focus on preventing that specific disease progression. For instance, a patient with a family history of CVD may work toward reaching a specified waist circumference (less than 40 in for men and less than 35 in for nonpregnant women) used for determining CVD risk.[21,22] Other personal goals may include being able to accomplish previously unattainable physical activities such as running a marathon or rock climbing. Obtaining and maintaining a healthy weight is critical for reducing morbidity, but it is important to discuss and create personal and attainable goals with patients that will provide them with positive outcomes to assist with maintaining their weight loss.

Components of Treatment

Lifestyle Modification

The cornerstone for all weight loss treatments is lifestyle modification that includes the following changes: physical activity, diet, and behaviors. Patients should be thoroughly educated on and should have attempted lifestyle modification before pursuing further weight loss methods such as pharmacotherapy or surgical intervention.[15] It is imperative that patients be provided with in-depth education on all aspects of lifestyle modification in order to be as successful as possible and allow for assessment on further intervention. Before lifestyle modification can be implemented, it is important to understand the different factors that influence food intake and physical activity. Studies show that the human and animal brains regulate food consumption as a behavior. More specifically, the part of the brain known as the hypothalamus contributes to the feeling of hunger by detecting decreased nutrient supply (i.e., food). The brain detects this nutrient deficiency and then elicits ingestive behaviors such as searching for food (i.e., shopping and going to restaurants) and the long-term storage of food (i.e., in cupboards or refrigerator).[23] A proper assessment of behaviors such as these should be completed and discussed in the early stages of lifestyle modification planning.

Dietary Therapy

In order to implement successful dietary therapy, patients and practitioners should familiarize themselves with current dietary guidelines. The American Medical Association (AMA) supports the most recent guidelines put forth by the Dietary Guidelines Advisory Committee[24] which gives extensive, evidence-based recommendations for implementing and maintaining a healthy diet.[25] Although there can be many components involved, weight loss via dietary therapy should primarily focus on reducing total caloric intake.[21] To this end, a general knowledge of how many calories certain foods contain is a good starting point for management. Carbohydrates and proteins contain an average of 4 calories/g, whereas fats contain an average of 9 calories/g and alcohol an average of 7 calories/g. The 2015–2020 Dietary Guidelines for Americans recommends the daily caloric intake from sugars and saturated fats be less than 10% of total calories, less than 2300 mg-daily sodium intake and less than 1 alcoholic drink a day for women or 2 for men.

Patient-specific plans with daily calorie intake goals should take into account the patients' age, height, weight, sex, comorbidities, and exercise capabilities when necessary, but general recommendations include following a healthy eating pattern and should comprise the following: fat-free or decreased fat dairy products, proteins, whole fruits, whole grains, vegetables of all subgroups, and oils. Patients should be made knowledgeable on the recommended serving size of each food group based on their daily calorie goal. For a 2000 calorie-a-day plan, the serving size recommendations are 2.5 cups of vegetables, 2 cups of fruit, 6 oz of grains, 5.5 oz of protein, 5 teaspoons of oils, and 3 cups of dairy for ages 9 years and older regardless of calorie goal.[25]

When practitioners and patients are devising meal plans, they should take into account the patient's taste preferences and ensure understanding that a variety of food types from these groups should be included in meal planning. For example, potatoes should not solely constitute daily vegetable intake. Rather, the patient should alternate between starchy vegetables for some meals and green leafy vegetables for others. Ensuring patients know they can alter recipes by using low-fat and low-sodium substitutes can also aid in their willingness to stick to a diet.[26] Patients can be directed to reputable online resources for easy-to-understand healthy cooking recommendations and how to make healthy choices when grocery shopping. Practitioners should be aware and knowledgeable on current fads, trends, and medications available to patients as over-the-counter treatments. While some of these options are effective, they should be evaluated for safety while taking into consideration the specific needs and history of the patient before implementation.[15] Connecting patients with medical nutrition therapists to assist in finding a diet best suited for their weight and medical needs is also an important option to consider, especially for patients with multiple comorbidities.

Examples of diet plans to consider that are based on specific patient needs are the DASH (dietary approaches to stop hypertension) and the Mediterranean diet. The main focus of the DASH diet is to lower blood pressure by carefully controlling and monitoring what food is consumed. The DASH diet proposes meal planning focused on low sodium, low caffeine, and alcohol consumption and suggests meals primarily be comprised of fruits, vegetables, whole grains, low-fat dairy, and lean meats. Since the DASH diet was created for lowering hypertension and not specifically for weight loss treatment, combining the diet with an exercise or increased physical activity program has shown to yield better weight loss results.[27,28] The DASH diet should be considered in cases where comorbidities are caused secondary to hypertension such as decreased renal function or end-stage renal disease[28] and CVD. The Mediterranean diet has also been found to reduce cardiovascular risk factors and focuses on a diet consisting of plant-based foods, replacing butter with oils, and limiting red meat consumption.[29] Regardless of what diet is chosen, the previously mentioned recommendations regarding calorie decrease[24] should be introduced and included as part of the weight loss plan.[27]

Exercise and Physical Activity

A successful weight loss plan includes a decrease in calories consumed and an increase in energy expenditure due to physical activity and naturally occurring metabolic processes.[15,27,30] Based on guidelines put forth by the Department of Health and Human Services (HHS) for maintaining a healthy physical lifestyle, the CDC recommends all adults should partake in 2.5 hours of moderate aerobic physical activity or 75 minutes a week of vigorous aerobic physical activity and that each instance should be at least 10 minutes in length.[26] By increasing physical activity to 5 hours a week of moderate exercise or 2.5 hours a week of vigorous exercise, more extensive weight loss may be obtained and, most importantly, maintained.[27,31] Barring any medical restrictions, the Academy of Nutrition and Dietetics recommends that patients implement 2.5 to 7 hours or more of physical activity a week for weight loss and 3 to 5 hours or more of a week for weight maintenance into their weight loss management programs.[27] In addition, the CDC recommends that activities involving muscle strengthening be included during physical activity at least 3 days a week.[31]

As with dieting and meal planning, it is important to include the patients' preferences and to assess barriers and factors to make reaching physical activity and exercise goals possible.[27,32] Potential barriers to implementing increased physical activity are emotional or social issues including anxiety of being in a crowd, inability to follow instruction, or dependence on encouragement or support. By contrast, physical limitations can include medical ailments or discomfort.[33] Moreover, environmental barriers such as ability to walk places, residential safety and aesthetics, and the presence of public transportation can positively affect physical activity and exercise adherence.[32,34]

When creating a weight loss program, the above emotional, social, physical, and environmental barriers should be assessed in order to create a physical activity plan that will provide the patient with the highest likelihood for success.[32] For example, if a patient has been resistant to an increase in physical activity because of discomfort caused by OA, options that do not place stress on the joints (e.g., swimming) should be explored. A variety of exercise options should be reviewed before implementation to ensure the best possible outcomes. It is also important to note that sedentary behaviors are more pervasive in contemporary society due to the increase in occupational- and entertainment-related screen use.[25] It is necessary to consider creative options to increase energy expenditure during these activities such as jump roping while watching television or using a bike chair while working at a desk. Providing patients with information regarding other positive aspects of starting and sticking to an exercise program, such as a decrease in symptoms related to depression, stress and anxiety,[35] as well as reduction in the risk of other comorbidities such as CVD and cancer can also be a motivational tool for adherence.[36]

Behavioral Therapy

The third component of lifestyle modification for weight loss is behavioral therapy.[15,27] Behavioral therapy is part of a collaborative weight loss approach that complements nutritional modifications and exercise. The Centers for Medicare and Medicaid Services (CMS) states that "intensive behavioral therapy for obesity" includes the following three aspects: obesity screening, nutritional assessment, and behavioral therapy to achieve a decrease in weight.[37] Behavioral therapy can encompass many types of interventions such as traditional counseling, interviewing, acceptance and commitment training, among others.[27,37] If used correctly, behavioral therapy can assist in an average weight loss of 5% to 8% per year.[38] However, historical compliance with behavioral programs is very low due to time constraints of both the patient and provider that prevent regular meetings and weight loss counseling.[15,38]

Cognitive-behavioral therapy (CBT) is a common approach that focuses on the psychological aspects contributing to poor health outcomes.[39] CBT is not specific to obesity and weight loss and is used to treat other disorders including stress, anxiety, depression, and a variety of personality and mood disorders. Moreover, CBT can be utilized in different ways to fit the patient's specific needs.[40] Although there are many different variations of CBT, some of the most common aspects include self-monitoring, goal setting, stimulus control, cognitive restructuring, problem solving, and relapse prevention.[27,41]

Self-monitoring requires the patient to keep a log or journal on their treatment plan, and is usually comprised of nutritional information such as what foods were consumed and calorie counting or logging fat grams. Self-monitoring can also include logging feelings, moods, and behaviors which can be helpful for identifying trends and barriers while following the weight loss plan.[40] A 2018 study identified that logging or tracking weight loss interventions was a barrier of implementation for many patients,[32] so patients should be made aware of different tracking options such as physically writing in a journal or using a nutrition or fitness tracking application on their phone.

Goal setting, which is identifying the aim or desired end result, is a key element in weight loss and is one of the top three most used techniques according to a recent review of interventions aimed at increasing physical activity.[42] Goal setting can be used in a variety of ways when implementing a weight loss plan. Factors to take into consideration when making goals are timeliness, achievability, measurability, complexity, and individual/personal factors such as age and health status.[43] Goals should be variable in length as meeting short-term goals can provide motivation to stay on track and continue striving to meet long-term goals. Some goals, such as caloric intake or pounds lost, can be numerically tracked. Other goals should be behavior based and may include replacing a high-fat snack with fresh fruit or taking the stairs instead of the elevator. To be most effective, goals should require some difficulty and should be specific. For example, "I will take the stairs every day instead of the elevator when I am at work" rather than "I will try to take the stairs more often" is a specific, daily achievable goal. Feedback on goals should be provided during therapy sessions and all goals and achievements in the journey should be recognized and celebrated.[43,44]

Stimulus control requires behavioral observation to assess what stimulates a particularly unhealthy habit and developing a plan to remove the stimulus and, hence, the unhealthy habit.[41] A common example of stimulus control in a weight loss plan is to replace all unhealthy snacks (the stimulus) in the home or the immediate environment with healthy options, as having the unhealthy snacks readily available contributes to the habit of eating the snacks.[45] Appropriate time should be dedicated to identifying unhealthy behaviors and their stimulants before plans for stimulus control are put into action.

Cognitive restructuring can be described as altering the way you perceive certain things and the value that you apply to it. A large part of implementing cognitive restructuring is balancing an unrealistically positive or laissez-faire attitude with a disproportionately negative response to a given situation. For example, if a patient makes a dietary mistake and eats a large dessert that's not part of their meal plan, they may feel as though the diet as a whole is ruined and they should stop dieting and exercising as they are unable to correctly follow the set meal plan. This is a profoundly negative reaction that can lead to further negative outcomes. Cognitive restructuring for this situation would entail helping the patient to react in a more balanced outlook such that they feel regret while simultaneously recognizing the positive aspects of a given situation. These positive aspects may include the fact that that this was their first slipup in a long time, and if they exercise a little longer today, they can make up for the dessert and be back on track fairly quickly. The overarching goal of cognitive restructuring is based on becoming aware of and pragmatic in how you react to certain situations.

Problem solving is an essential part of CBT and is similar to stimulus control. Patients should spend time identifying the issues that prevent them from being able to meet their goals and make healthier choices and then actively create a plan on how they will tackle that interference the next time it is presented to them. CBT should include evaluation of the person's current problem-solving abilities, communication style, and attitude in order to best coach the patient in different problem-solving techniques.[41]

Relapse prevention is an important CBT topic to discuss before a patient has completed their therapy. Relapsing into unhealthy habits is common, especially during times that evoke strong memories or feelings associated with the habit. For instance, many people experience relapse during holidays, while on vacation, or during times of great stress or depression. Relapse prevention involves identifying these risk factors and developing a strategic plan that can be used for prevention.[46] Some aspects that a relapse prevention plan might include are a list of warning signs that they are falling back into unhealthy patterns, listing the coping tools that have been helpful to them in the past, making a list of family or friends who can be contacted for social support, and identifying certain feelings or actions that necessitate professional help.[41]

Many methods other than CBT can be utilized as behavioral interventions. Such methods include motivational interview and acceptance and commitment therapy, and these can be used independent of or concomitantly with CBT. Regardless of which behavioral techniques are employed, therapy sessions that occur on a regular basis for at least 6 months with face-to-face contact have proven to be more successful than other types of behavioral weight loss programs.[27]

Pharmacotherapy

As obesity continues to become more prevalent and a larger safety concern, more antiobesity drugs have been developed and received Food and Drug Administration (FDA) approval. Historically, antiobesity therapies utilized in the past were associated with significant adverse effects. Phentermine/fenfluramine, phenylpropanolamine, sibutramine, and ephedra caused cardiac valvular abnormalities, stroke, and myocardial infarction, respectively. Rimonabant had limited use in Europe, but was found to increase suicidal risk and FDA approval was withdrawn in 2007.[47] Modern drug therapy for obesity includes a collection of approved antiobesity therapies. Pharmacologic therapy for treatment of obesity is approved with a BMI of greater than or equal to 30 kg/m^2 in the absence of comorbid conditions, or for patients with a BMI of greater than or equal to 27 kg/m^2 with concomitant morbidities such as T2D or hypertension. Individuals who have markedly increased medical risks and who have been unsuccessful with nonpharmacologic therapy could benefit from adjunctive drug therapy.

FDA-approved short-term (approximately 12 weeks) therapy for obesity includes nonadrenergic agents: phentermine, diethylpropion, phendimetrazine, and benzphetamine. These medications reduce appetite by an increase in the activation of dopaminergic and adrenergic receptors. The FDA shortened treatment duration in 1973 because of concerns of long-term efficacy and abuse. Common adverse effects of these agents include insomnia, elevated heart rate, dry mouth, taste alterations, tremors, headache, dizziness, gastrointestinal issues, anxiety, and restlessness. Phentermine is frequently prescribed off-label for longer periods, despite its lack of FDA approval for long-term use. Benzphetamine is the least frequently prescribed, and there is less data from controlled trials to evaluate safety or efficacy.

Current medications approved for long-term drug treatment of obesity work to decrease fat absorption or suppress appetite. Orlistat is the oldest of these medications currently approved, and was FDA approved in 1999. This medication acts peripherally in the gastrointestinal tract to inhibit gastric and pancreatic lipases essential for digestion of fats, thereby decreasing fat absorption by approximately 30%. However, orlistat must be taken three times a day either during meals or up to an hour afterward to achieve these results. This medication is available in both prescription (120 mg) and over-the-counter (60 mg) strengths. Prescription strength orlistat is FDA approved for use by adults and adolescents 12 to 16 years old.[48] When patients continue to consume a diet rich in fat, they will suffer significant gastrointestinal side effects. These include oily or loose stools, and fecal incontinence. Maintaining a low-fat diet can help patients avoid these side effects. Therefore, patient adherence to prescribed diet and medication must be monitored. Another adverse effect of this medication is malabsorption of fat-soluble vitamins and supplementary multivitamins.[49] Orlistat lowers plasma lipids which is beneficial since 60% to 70% of obese patients are also dyslipidemic.[50] This medication also lowers glucose, fatty liver disease, and systemic blood pressure which cause a considerable reduction in cardiovascular risk.[51] Amiodarone, warfarin, levothyroxine, cyclosporine, and some antiepileptic medications should be monitored while taking orlistat.[52]

Lorcaserin (Belviq) was first rejected from the FDA because of concerns of tumor growth in preclinical studies,[51] but it was approved in 2012 for long-term weight management. This medication is a serotonin receptor agonist developed to selectively avoid 5-HT$_{2b}$-mediated valvulopathies which afflicted earlier agent fenfluramine. Lorcaserin stimulates serotonin receptors on anorectic poopiomelanocortin (POMC) neurons to suppress appetite. For those with T2D, a 0.5% reduction in HgA1C was found with this medication during drug trials. These patients should be monitored for hypoglycemia when taking lorcaserin. In addition, there was an average weight loss of 3.0% to 3.6% more than the placebo.[49] Reduction of blood pressure, total cholesterol, LDLs, and triglycerides is another benefit of this medication.[48] This drug is currently not approved for use in Europe due to concerns of valvular abnormalities and psychiatric disorders.[51] Although approved in the United States, it is classified as a schedule IV controlled substance because of incidence of euphoria with use. This medication is contraindicated with pregnancy, creatinine clearance less than 30 mL/min, or severe hepatic deficiency. Common adverse effects with lorcaserin include fatigue, dizziness, dry mouth, headache, and gastrointestinal distress. There is a risk of serotonin syndrome and one should exercise extreme caution if taking other serotonergic agents.[52]

Another medication approved for long-term weight management is phentermine/topiramate. This combination medication is a NE transport inhibitor/GABA agonist thought to work by appetite suppression.[53] This medication was also initially rejected by the FDA, but related to a history of oral cleft in the offspring of women taking topiramate. Qsymia® (phentermine/topiramate) was FDA approved in 2012, but safety precautions were recommended to reduce adverse effects. Women taking this medication must take monthly pregnancy tests. Also, this medication should be avoided in patients with cardiac or cerebrovascular disease secondary to a risk of increased heart rate. Safety concerns about cardiovascular complications of phentermine and risk of depression, anxiety, or cognitive impairment with topiramate have kept this medication off the European market.[51] Patients should be assessed for depression and/or suicidal ideation prior to treatment with this medication. Phentermine/topiramate can increase heart rate, and regular monitoring is critical when starting or increasing the dose. Adverse reactions include insomnia, constipation, dry mouth/impaired taste, paresthesia, and/or dizziness.

Naltrexone/bupropion (Contrave®) is another combination therapy used for long-term weight management, and was FDA approved in 2014. Although the exact mechanism of action is poorly understood, findings suggest that weight loss is secondary to hypothalamic mechanisms and cortical reactivity to food cues, memory, and self-control. There is a black box warning for this medication of increased risk of suicidal ideation, and it is important that patients are assessed prior to placement on this medication.[53] Concerns about cardiovascular safety were the primary reason that the initial application for approval was not accepted in 2010. Prior to treatment with this medication, hypertension should be controlled, and blood pressure monitored for the first 3 months of treatment.[49] Contraindications include uncontrolled hypertension, seizure disorder, eating disorder, end-stage renal failure, pregnancy, and use of monoamine oxidase inhibitor (MAOI) within 14 days. Common adverse effects include nausea, constipation, headache, vomiting, dizziness, insomnia, dry mouth, and diarrhea.

Liraglutide (Saxenda®) is a GLP agonist that stimulates insulin release, delays gastric emptying, controls postprandial glucagon, and decreases food intake.[52] This medication was FDA approved in 2014 for chronic weight management of obesity and overweight adults with at least one weight-related comorbidity (hypertension, diabetes, dyslipidemia, etc.). Saxenda can cause an increase in heart rate, and should be discontinued for a sustained elevated resting heart rate. In addition, there is a boxed warning secondary to thyroid gland tumors found in rodent studies. This medication should be avoided with a personal or family history of thyroid carcinoma or multiple endocrine neoplasia syndrome type II.[53] Most commonly, adverse effects include nausea, diarrhea, constipation, and vomiting.[54] Serious adverse events include acute pancreatitis, chest pain, bronchitis, gallbladder disease, renal impairment, and suicidal thoughts.[52,53]

Numerous drugs are undergoing clinical trial evaluation as potential future obesity pharmacology. These include tesofensine, bupropion/zonisamide, exenatide, metformin, and pramlintide. Each of these drugs has been associated with small weight losses when used in the treatment of disorders for which they are indicated.[48,53]

Lifestyle modifications are always the first intervention in both preventing and treating obesity, but pharmacology can be used adjunctively depending on BMI and/or comorbidities. Sustainable weight loss will likely require long-term use. Medication use needs to be accompanied by a program of behavior modification, a structured eating plan, and increased physical activity. However, for those with a BMI of greater than or equal to 40 kg/m^2 or greater than or equal to 35 kg/m^2 with comorbidities, bariatric surgery should also be considered.[52]

Bariatric Surgery

Morbid obesity (BMI greater than or equal to 40 kg/m^2) and severe morbid obesity (BMI greater than 50 kg/m^2) are major health problems, but surgery is a viable option.[55] Every year there are approximately 280,000 obesity-related deaths in the United States. Surgical treatment can help to reduce this relative risk of death due to significant weight loss.[56] About 15 million Americans have a BMI of at least 40 kg/m^2, but only 1% of the eligible population receives surgical treatment.[52] However, the number of bariatric or metabolic procedures were as many as 579,517 surgical and 14,725 endoluminal procedures performed worldwide in 2014.[57] Economic consequences of obesity are severe, and medical costs are estimated to be as high as 209.7 billion annually in the United States. This accounts for over 20% of all annual health care spending in the United States.[58]

There are numerous bariatric surgical procedures available that include sleeve gastrectomy (SG), Roux-en-Y gastric bypass (RYGB), and adjustable gastric banding (AGB). The IFSO Worldwide Survey of Bariatric surgery and Endoluminal Procedures reports relative percentages of the most common procedures worldwide are SG (45.9%), gastric banding (39.6%), vertical banded gastroplasty (7.4%). Less commonly performed procedures are mini gastric bypass/one anastomosis gastric bypass (1.8%) and biliopancreatic diversion/duodenal switch (1.1%).[57]

SG is bariatric technique that consists of a subtotal vertical gastrectomy that preserves the pylorus to create a duct along the lesser curvature. SG promotes rapid gastric emptying and may trigger hormonal mechanisms with additional benefits. Additional benefits of this procedure include significant weight loss, T2D remission that can occur even prior to weight loss, and an average hypertension remission rate of 69%. SG also has a lower risk of complications such as nutritional deficiencies or dumping syndrome.[58] The Roux-en-Y (RYGB) technique involves the construction of a 30-mL gastric pouch, gastrojejunal anastomosis, attachment of a Roux limb which is 100 to 150 cm in length, and a jejunostomy.[59] Today, more than 90% of the gastric bypass surgeries are performed laparoscopically.[60] The gastric banding procedure is also done laparoscopically and involves placing an adjustable silicone band around the upper part of the stomach approximately 2 cm below the gastroesophageal junction to create a small gastric pouch. The gastric band is then sutured to the stomach to prevent slippage (Fig. 20-2).[61]

In all of these bariatric procedures, postprocedural vomiting is a common difficulty.[56] Staple line leak is the most common complication with SG and occurs with 1% to 2.7% of these procedures.[58] Other complications that can occur include gastric dilation, gastrointestinal reflux disease (GERD), incisional hernias, fistulas, or strictures. Patients undergoing RYGB have an increased risk of experiencing dumping syndrome and nutritional deficiencies (particularly vitamin B_{12}, thiamine, calcium, copper, vitamin D, and iron). They are also at risk for leaks/strictures, ulcers, small bowel obstruction (SBO), and hernias. Rarely, the patient can be at risk for intussusception, a complication of RYGB in which the bowel telescopes and can create ischemia. This typically only occurs after significant weight loss. Gastric banding has the lowest risk perioperative and postoperative mortality rates, but has also

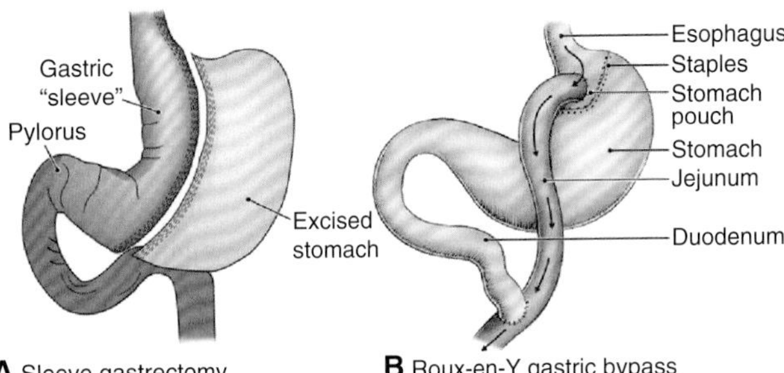

Figure 20-2. Sleeve gastrectomy and Roux-en-Y. (**A**) Sleeve gastrectomy. (**B**) Roux-en-Y gastric bypass. (**A.** Reprinted with permission from Neinstein LS, Katzman DK, Callahan T, et al. *Neinstein's Adolescent and Young Adult Health Care*. 6th ed. Philadelphia, PA: Wolters Kluwer Health; 2016; **B.** *Lippincott's Nursing Advisor 2013*. Philadelphia, PA: Lippincott Williams & Wilkins; 2013.)

resulted in the highest long-term reoperation rate. Reoperation may be necessary if the gastric band is affected by malpositioning, slippage, infection, or erosion. Band slippage can result in the rare complication of gastric volvulus, which twists the proximal stomach around the band. This can result in a closed-loop obstruction causing ischemia, and is a life-threatening complication. Additional complications that may occur include stomal stenosis, gastroesophageal perforation, or pouch dilation.[56,61]

Substantial weight loss can result from these surgical procedures, which can result in a decrease in mortality. The Swedish Obesity Study (SOS), a large prospective controlled trial conducted over a period of 15 years, found a 30.7% higher mortality rate in the control group than the bariatric group.[55] Obesity-associated comorbidities include T2D, hyperlipidemia, CVD, cholelithiasis, gastroesophageal reflux disease, hypertension, obstructive sleep apnea, weight-bearing OA, and back pain, and cancer.[56] Weight loss and maintenance can potentially reverse some of these conditions. Improvements in metabolic risk factors are lost if weight is regained. An increase in weight gain as minimal as 2% to 6% can increase plasma lipids, blood pressure, fasting glucose and insulin levels to baseline or worse.[62]

Maintenance of Weight Loss

Successful long-term weight loss maintenance has been defined as intentionally losing at least 10% of one's initial body weight and maintaining that loss for at least 1 year.[63] Despite the effectiveness of bariatric surgery in achieving weight loss, over 50% of patients return to their previous weight as early as 18 months after surgery.[64] Environmental, behavioral, biologic, and cognitive factors play a role in weight loss maintenance. Lifestyle modification programs that utilize cognitive and behavioral strategies to achieve weight management can improve long-term adherence.[63]

The National Weight Control Registry (NWCR) is an ongoing registry of individuals who have been successful at losing and maintaining a minimum of 13.6 kg for at least 1 year.[65] Behavioral strategies used by these successful individuals include high levels of physical activity (approximately 1 h/day), consuming a low-fat, low-calorie diet, regular self-monitoring of body weight, a consistent eating pattern across weekdays and weekends, and eating breakfast regularly. Another finding from this registry was a correlation between weight maintenance and low levels of depression and disinhibition. QuoVadis (QUality of life in Obesity: eVAluation and DIsease Surveillance), an observational study of 1944 patients with obesity, found differences in the cognitive factors associated with weight loss and weight loss maintenance. Factors correlated with weight lost included increased dietary restraint and reduced disinhibition, whereas, weight loss maintenance was associated with factors such as satisfaction with results achieved and confidence in being able to lose weight without professional help.[63] One randomized controlled trial examining cognitive mechanisms for weight loss and maintenance concluded that both the amount of weight lost and satisfaction with weight loss were associated with weight loss maintenance at 1-year follow-up.[66]

The multidisciplinary team role in long-term weight management is helping facilitate the lifestyle modification program incorporating behavioral and cognitive components that will sustain weight loss. This program should begin with a weight loss phase (approximately 16 to 24 sessions/6 months), followed by a weight maintenance phase (monthly/1 year). Providers should receive training in CBT. Lifestyle counselors or practitioners such as dieticians, physical therapists, or psychologists, must be integrated into the plan for weight loss and maintenance. Providers should routinely assess the effect of treatment on lifestyle and weight, and continue to consider appropriate treatment options for the patient. This may include adding obesity pharmacology to lifestyle approach, rehabilitation treatment, and bariatric surgery in patients that meet criteria.[63]

Summary

Obesity is a chronic medical condition with numerous adverse effects on the cardiovascular system and health-related quality of life. Obesity rates continue to grow, and a number of children are either overweight or obese.[1–3] The goal of treatment varies by patient, but all patients pursuing weight loss reduction for medical reasons should aim for a 5% to 10% reduction over 6 months.[20] Current treatment consists of lifestyle modification interventions with nutrition, exercise, and behavioral therapy.[15,27] Some patients will require addition of pharmacotherapy or bariatric surgery depending on their BMI and comorbidities.[50,52] At least a 10% weight loss at 1 year defines successful weight loss maintenance, and this requires the support of a multidisciplinary team. Key behavioral strategies and frequent follow-up during weight loss and weight loss maintenance phases are essential for the patient's success.[63] Providers can teach patients utilizing CBT, and assess for comorbidities related to obesity. Taking an active role in educating patients about prevention of obesity, nurses can also reduce cardiovascular risks for this increasing patient population. Increased efforts should be focused on obesity prevention and routine screening in order to reduce further progression of this condition.

ACKNOWLEDGMENT

The authors were supported by grants R01 DK58387, R01 DK071817, and F31 NR 009750, National Institutes of Health, National Institute of Diabetes and Digestive and Kidney Diseases, and National Institute of Nursing Research.

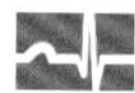

CASE STUDY

Patient Profile

Name/Age/Sex: **John Smith, 50-year-old male**

History of Present Illness

Mr. Smith presents for his annual physical. He has recently started walking twice a week for 30 minutes for exercise. He tries to maintain a healthy diet, but usually binges on sweets on the weekends. He neglects breakfast often. Mr. Smith expresses a desire to lose weight, but feels overwhelmed and "doesn't know how to get on track."

Past Medical History

Coronary artery disease, type II diabetes (T2D), and hyperlipidemia

Surgical History

Tonsillectomy

Family History

Mother, living, htn
Father: Deceased, CAD, DM

Medications

Aspirin 81 mg q daily, metformin 500 mg BID, pravastatin 80 mg q HS

Allergies

NKDA

Patient Examination

Vital Signs

BP 138/74; HR 78; RR 14; Temp 37°C; O_2 Sat 100% RA; BMI 39.2; waist circumference of 45 in, Ht. 5 ft 2 in, and Wt. 215 lb

Physical Examination

Lungs: CTAB
Cardiac: RRR no murmurs noted
Abdomen: soft and tender, BS × 4 quadrants
Skin: Intact, dry
HEENT: PERRLA, sclera white, mucous membranes moist

Key Questions

A. Classify Mr. Smith's BMI (Normal, Overweight, Obese, Morbidly Obese, etc.).
B. How would you classify Mr. Smith's cardiovascular risk? How does this affect his treatment strategy?
C. What exercise and nutrition recommendations would you give Mr. Smith?
D. What options are available to Mr. Smith to assist in weight loss?
E. What strategies are necessary for weight loss maintenance?

Answers

A. Extreme Obesity. Rationale: Normal weight is defined as a BMI range of 18.50 to 24.99 kg/m^2, overweight as a BMI of 25.00 to 29.99 kg/m^2, obese as a BMI of 30 kg/m^2 or more, and extreme obesity BMI greater than or equal to 35 kg/m^2.[2,2–4,6–8] Morbid obesity is a BMI greater than or equal to 40 kg/m^2 and severe morbid obesity is BMI greater than 50 kg/m^2.[55]
B. Mr. Smith's cardiovascular risk is categorized as a *very high absolute risk*. He will require more aggressive treatment because of this classification. *Rationale: Patients who are overweight, obese, or have abdominal obesity are considered to be at very high absolute risk if they have the following disease conditions: established coronary heart disease (CHD), presence of other atherosclerotic diseases (peripheral arterial disease, abdominal aortic aneurysm, or symptomatic carotid disease), T2D, sleep apnea, or hypertension with evidence of target organ damage. Individuals require aggressive treatment to mitigate or eliminate their risk for disease progression and exacerbation.*[10]

CASE STUDY (*Continued*)

C. Encourage Mr. Smith to utilize an activity and food diary, and make him aware he can either physically write in a journal or using a nutrition or use fitness tracking application on his phone. He should also follow up with a nutritionist for dietary recommendations, but can start on a low-fat, low-cholesterol, low-calorie diet. Breakfast should be encouraged, and healthier "sweet" alternatives should be recommended. Mr. Smith should increase amount of exercise to at least 2.5 hours of moderate aerobic physical activity/week. Rationale: A 2018 study identified that logging or tracking weight loss interventions was a barrier of implementation for many patients,[32] so options should be given to the patient. CDC recommends at least 2.5 hours of moderate aerobic physical activity or 75 min/wk of vigorous aerobic physical activity and that each instance should be at least 10 minutes in length.[26]

D. Mr. Smith can start on an antiobesity medication per his current BMI, such as orlistat. Orlistat would also have a beneficial effect on his lipid profile. He is also a surgical candidate for bariatric surgery. Whether considering either or both therapies, it is essential that Mr. Smith also implements recommended exercise and nutrition recommendations. In addition, a low-fat diet will reduce symptoms associated with orlistat. *Rationale: Pharmacologic therapy for treatment of obesity is approved with a BMI of greater than or equal to 30 kg/m² in the absence of comorbid conditions, or for patients with a BMI of greater than or equal to 27 kg/m² with concomitant morbidities such as T2D or hypertension.[50] When patients continue to consume a diet rich in fat, they will suffer significant gastrointestinal side effects from orlistat.[49] Typically, bariatric surgery is reserved for morbidly obese patients, but is also available for those that have a BMI greater than 35 and comorbidities (such as coronary artery disease and T2D).[52]*

E. Frequent follow-up is essential to assist in weight loss maintenance, and providers should be CBT trained. A multidisciplinary team should be utilized for support, but Mr. Smith should be encouraged throughout the process to gain confidence. *Rationale: Weight loss maintenance was associated with factors such as satisfaction with results achieved and confidence in being able to lose weight without professional help.[63]*

KEY READINGS

Gadde K, Martin C, Berthoud H, et al. Obesity. Pathophysiology and management. *J Am Coll Cardiol.* 2018;71(1):69–84.

Lavie CJ, Laddu D, Arena R, et al. Healthy weight and obesity prevention: JACC health promotion series. *J Am Coll Cardio.* 2018;72(13):1506–1531.

REFERENCES

1. Hales CM, Carroll MD, Fryar CD, et al. *Prevalence of obesity among adults and youth: United States, 2015–2016.* U.S. Department of Health and Human Services, NCHS Data Brief. 2017. Available at https://www.cdc.gov/nchs/data/databriefs/db288.pdf
2. Bhupathiraju SN, Hu FB. Epidemiology of obesity and diabetes and their cardiovascular complications. *Circ Res.* 2016;118(11):1723–1735.
3. Parker JD, Talih M, Malec DJ, et al. National Center for Health Statistics data presentation standards for proportions. *Vital Health Stat.* 2017;2(175):2017–1375.
4. Moyer VA. Screening for and management of obesity in adults: U.S. Preventive Services Task Force recommendation statement. *Ann Intern Med.* 2012;157(5):373–378.
5. Song M. Trajectory analysis in obesity epidemiology: a promising life course approach. *Curr Opin Endocr Metab Res.* 2019;4:37–41.
6. Pantalone KM, Hobbs TM, Chagin KM, et al. Prevalence and recognition of obesity and its associated comorbidities: cross-sectional analysis of electronic health record data from large US integrated health system. *BMJ Open.* 2017;7(11):e017583.
7. Hruby A, Hu FB. The epidemiology of obesity: a big picture. *Pharmacoeconomics.* 2015;33(7):673–689.
8. Purnell JQ. Definitions, classification, and epidemiology of obesity. [Updated 2018 Apr 12]. In: Feingold KR, Anawalt B, Boyce A, et al., eds. *Endotext [Internet].* South Dartmouth, MA: MDText.com, Inc; 2000. Available at https://www.ncbi.nlm.nih.gov/books/NBK279167
9. Fitzpatrick SL, Wischenka D, Appelhan BM, et al. An evidence-based guide for obesity treatment in primary care. *Am J Med.* 2016;129(1):115.e1–115.e7.
10. NHLBI Obesity Education Initiative Expert Panel on the Identification, Evaluation, and Treatment of Obesity in Adults (US). *Clinical Guidelines on the Identification, Evaluation, and Treatment of Overweight and Obesity in Adults: The Evidence Report.* Bethesda, MD: National Heart, Lung, and Blood Institute; 1998. Chapter 4, Treatment Guidelines. Available at https://www.ncbi.nlm.nih.gov/books/NBK2004
11. Pietrzykowska NB. Obesity in the elderly. *Obesity Action Coalition.* 2014. Available at https://www.obesityaction.org/community/article-library/obesity-in-the-elderly
12. Uphold CR, Graham MV. Obesity. *Clinical Guidelines in Adult Health.* 3rd ed. Gainesville, FL: Barmarrae Books; 2003.
13. Gray CL, Messer LC, Rappazzo KM, et al. The association between physical inactivity and obesity is modified by five domains of environmental quality in U.S. adults: a cross-sectional study. *PLoS One.* 2018;13(8):e0203301.
14. Roberto CA, Swinburn B, Hawkes C, et al. Patchy progress on obesity prevention: emerging examples, entrenched barriers, and new thinking. *Lancet.* 2015;385:2400–2409.
15. Kushner RF. Weight loss strategies for treatment of obesity: lifestyle management and pharmacotherapy. *Prog Cardiovasc Dis.* 2018;61(2):246–252.
16. Berning J. The role of physicians in promoting weight loss. *Econ Hum Biol.* 2015;17:104–115.
17. Ard J. Obesity in the US: what is the best role for primary care? *BMJ.* 2015;350:g7846.
18. Afshin A, Forouzanfar MH, Reitsma MB, et al. Health effects of overweight and obesity in 195 countries over 25 years. *N Engl J Med.* 2017;377(1):13–27.
19. Centers for Disease Control and Prevention. *Adult obesity facts.* 2018. Available at https://www.cdc.gov/obesity/data/adult.html. Published August 14, 2018. Accessed October 14, 2018.
20. Jensen MD, Ryan DH, Apovian CM, et al. Practice guideline: 2013 AHA/ACC/TOS guideline for the management of overweight and obesity in adults. A report of the American College of Cardiology/American Heart Association Task Force on practice guidelines and the Obesity Society. *J Am Coll Cardiol.* 2014;63(Part B):2985–3023.
21. Centers for Disease Control and Prevention. *Assessing your weight | Healthy weight.* Available at https://www.cdc.gov/healthyweight/assessing/index.html. Accessed October 14, 2018.
22. Gadde KM, Martin CK, Berthoud HR, et al. Obesity: pathophysiology and management. *J Am Coll Cardiol.* 2018;71:69–84.
23. Thomas MA, Xue B. Mechanisms for AgRP neuron-mediated regulation of appetitive behaviors in rodents. *Physiol Behav.* 2018;190:34–42.
24. American Medical Association. *AMA supports newest dietary guidelines to improve public health.* Available at https://www.ama-assn.org/content/ama-supports-newest-dietary-guidelines-americans-improve-public-health. Accessed October 13, 2018.
25. 2015–2020 Dietary Guidelines—health.gov. Available at https://health.gov/dietaryguidelines/2015/guidelines. Accessed October 13, 2018.
26. Centers for Disease Control and Prevention. *Healthy eating for a healthy weight | Healthy weight.* Available at https://www.cdc.gov/healthyweight/healthy_eating/index.html. Accessed October 25, 2018.
27. Raynor HA, Champagne CM. Position of the Academy of Nutrition and Dietetics: interventions for the treatment of overweight and obesity in adults. *J Acad Nutr Diet.* 2016;116(1):129–147.

28. Osté MCJ, Gomes-Neto AW, de Borst MH, et al. Dietary Approach to Stop Hypertension (DASH) diet and risk of renal function decline and all-cause mortality in renal transplant recipients. *Am J Transplant.* 2018;18(10):2523–2533.
29. Greiner BH, Croff J, Wheeler D, et al. Mediterranean diet adherence in cardiac patients: a cross-sectional study. *Am J Health Behav.* 2018;42(6):3–10.
30. Johns DJ, Hartmann-Boyce J, Jebb SA, et al. Diet or exercise interventions vs combined behavioral weight management programs: a systematic review and meta-analysis of direct comparisons. *J Acad Nutr Diet.* 2014;114(10):1557–1568.
31. Centers for Disease Control and Prevention. Physical activity guidelines. 2018. Available at https://www.cdc.gov/cancer/dcpc/prevention/policies_practices/physical_activity/guidelines.htm. Accessed October 27, 2018.
32. McVay MA, Yancy WS Jr, Bennett GG, et al. Perceived barriers and facilitators of initiation of behavioral weight loss interventions among adults with obesity: a qualitative study. *BMC Public Health.* 2018;18(1):854.
33. Franco MR, Tong A, Howard K, et al. Older people's perspectives on participation in physical activity: a systematic review and thematic synthesis of qualitative literature. *Br J Sports Med.* 2015;49(19):1268–1276.
34. Feuillet T, Charreire H, Menai M, et al. Spatial heterogeneity of the relationships between environmental characteristics and active commuting: towards a locally varying social ecological model. *Int J Health Geogr.* 2015;14(1):12.
35. Mikkelsen K, Stojanovska L, Polenakovic M, et al. Exercise and mental health. *Maturitas.* 2017;106:48–56.
36. Apostolopoulos V, Borkoles E, Polman R, et al. Physical and immunological aspects of exercise in chronic diseases. *Immunotherapy.* 2014;6(10):1145–1157.
37. Wadden TA, Butryn ML, Hong PS, et al. Behavioral treatment of obesity in patients encountered in primary care settings: a systematic review. *JAMA.* 2014;312(17):1779–1791.
38. Forman EM, Butryn ML, Manasse SM, et al. Acceptance-based versus standard behavioral treatment for obesity: results from the mind your health randomized controlled trial. *Obesity.* 2016;24(10):2050–2056.
39. Jacob A, Moullec G, Lavoie KL, et al. Impact of cognitive-behavioral interventions on weight loss and psychological outcomes: a meta-analysis. *Health Psychol.* 2018;37(5):417–432.
40. Sears R. *Cognitive Behavioral Therapy & Mindfulness Toolbox: 50 Tips, Tools and Handouts for Anxiety, Stress, Depression, Personality and Mood Disorders.* PESI Publishing & Media; 2017.
41. Wenzel A, Dobson KS, Hays PA. *Cognitive Behavioral Therapy Techniques and Strategies.* Washington, DC: American Psychological Association; 2016.
42. Conn VS, Hafdahl A, Phillips LJ, et al. Impact of physical activity interventions on anthropometric outcomes: systematic review and meta-analysis. *J Prim Prev.* 2014;35(4):203–215.
43. Epton T, Currie S, Armitage CJ. Unique effects of setting goals on behavior change: systematic review and meta-analysis. *J Consult Clin Psychol.* 2017;85(12):1182–1198.
44. Wang L. Abandon your SMART goals: 6 reasons why SMART goal-setting does not work. *Canadian Manager.* 2017;42(2):31–33.
45. Linde JA, Jeffery RW, Crow SJ, et al. The Tracking Study: description of a randomized controlled trial of variations on weight tracking frequency in a behavioral weight loss program. *Contemp Clin Trials.* 2015;40:199–211.
46. Menon J, Kandasamy A. Relapse prevention. *Indian J Psychiatry.* 2018;60:S473–S478.
47. Onakpoya IJ, Heneghan CJ, Aronson JK. Post-marketing withdrawal of anti-obesity medicinal products because of adverse drug reactions: a systematic review. *BMC Med.* 2016;14(191):1–11.
48. Yanovski SZ, Yanovski JA. Long-term drug treatment for obesity: a systematic and clinical review. *JAMA.* 2014;311(1):74–86.
49. Jones BJ, Bloom SR. The new era of drug therapy for obesity: the evidence and the expectations. *Drugs.* 2015;75:935–945.
50. Sahebkar A, Simental-Mendia LE, Reiner Z, et al. Effects of orlistat on plasma lipids and body weight: a systematic review and meta-analysis of 33 randomized controlled clinical trials. *Pharmacol Res.* 2017;122:53–65.
51. Martin KA, Mani MV, Mani A. New targets to treat obesity and metabolic syndrome. *Eur J Pharmacol.* 2015;763:64–74.
52. Bersoux S, Byun TH, Chaliki SS, et al. Pharmacotherapy for obesity: what you need to know. *Cleve Clin J Med.* 2017;84(12):951–958.
53. Narayanaswami V, Dwoskin LP. Obesity: current and potential pharmacotherapeutics and targets. *Pharmacol Ther.* 2016;170:116–147.
54. Nuffer WA, Trujillo JM. Liraglutide: a new option for the treatment of obesity. *Pharmacotherapy.* 2015;35(10):926–934.
55. Abelaal M, Le Roux CW, Docherty CW. Morbidity and mortality associated with obesity. *Ann Transl Med.* 2017;5(7):161.
56. Ma IT, Madura JA. Gastrointestinal complications after bariatric surgery. *Gastroenterol Hepatol.* 2015;11(8):526–535.
57. Angrisani L, Santonicola A, Iovino P, et al. Bariatric surgery and endoluminal procedures: IFSO Worldwide Survey 2014. *Obes Surg.* 2017;27(9):2279–2289.
58. Benaiges D, Más-Lorenzo A, Goday A, et al. Laparoscopic sleeve gastrectomy: more than a restrictive bariatric surgery procedure? *World J Gastroenterol.* 2015;21(41):11804–11814.
59. Alba DL, Wu L, Cawthon PM, et al. Changes in lean mass, absolute and relative muscle strength, and physical performance after gastric bypass surgery. *J Clin Endocrinol.* 2018;104(3):711–720.
60. Seeras K, Prakash S. Laparoscopic gastric bypass. In: *StatPearls [Internet].* Treasure Island, FL: StatPearls Publishing; 2018. Available at https://www.ncbi.nlm.nih.gov/books/NBK518968
61. Levine MS, Carucci LR. Imaging of bariatric surgery: normal anatomy and postoperative complications. *Radiology.* 2014;270(2):327–341.
62. Puhl RM, Quinn DM, Weisz BM, et al. The role of stigma in weight loss maintenance among U. S. adults. *Ann Behav Med.* 2017;51:754–763.
63. Montesi L, El Ghoch M, Brodosi L, et al. Long-term weight loss maintenance for obesity: a multidisciplinary approach. *Diabetes Metab Syndr Obes.* 2016;9:37–46.
64. Masood A, Alsheddi L, Alfayadh L, et al. Dietary and lifestyle factors serve as predictors of successful weight loss maintenance postbariatric surgery. *J Obes.* 2019;2019:7295978.
65. Metzgar CJ, Preston AG, Miller DL, et al. Facilitators and barriers to weight loss and weight loss maintenance: a qualitative exploration. *J Hum Nutr Diet.* 2015;28:593–603.
66. Calugi S, Marchesini G, El Ghoch M, et al. The influence of weight-loss expectations on weight loss and of weight-loss satisfaction on weight maintenance in severe obesity. *J Acad Nutr Diet.* 2016;117(1):32–38.

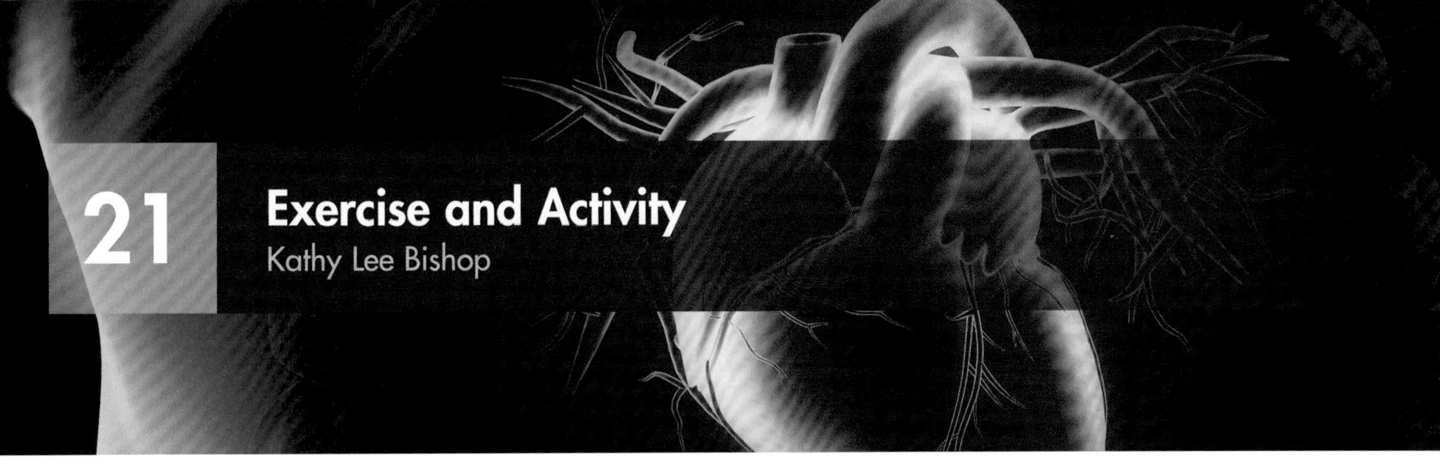

21 Exercise and Activity

Kathy Lee Bishop

OBJECTIVES

At completion of the chapter the reader will be able to:

1. Discuss the benefits of exercise and activity on prevention and health.
2. Understand detrimental effects of bed rest and sedentary lifestyle.
3. Understand the components of an exercise prescription.
4. Develop an exercise prescription for a case.

KEY QUESTIONS

1. What are the physical activity (PA) guidelines for all adults?
2. What are the benefits of PA and exercise?
3. What are the components of an exercise prescription?
4. What are valid tools to measure functional level?

INTRODUCTION

Sedentary lifestyles are associated with increased risk of chronic disease, morbidity, and mortality.[1,2] The fourth leading risk factor for deaths in the world in 2010 was insufficient physical activity (PA).[3] Guidelines were developed by the U.S. Department of Health and Human Services to have all American adults engage in at least 150 minutes of moderate-intensity PA per week.[4] After nearly four decades of recommendations, only 20% of American adults have been found to meet the 2008 guidelines.[4] The concept of PA varies from moderate-intensity walking to dancing, housekeeping, gardening, or mowing the lawn. The premise is to participate in any activity which will raise the heart rate and respiratory rate. Activity does not have to be performed on exercise equipment. Regular exercise or PA can lead to prevention of many diseases (cancer, diabetes, heart disease, mental illness, and mood), weight loss, and improvement in mental health. Regular moderate-to-vigorous PA has been shown to improve sleep, reduce feelings of depression, anxiety, and more importantly improve quality of life.[4] Regularly performed PA also reduces the risk of dementia, falls, and improves overall physical function. Evidence supports that PA can reduce the "risk of bladder, breast, colon, endometrium, esophagus kidney, stomach, and lung cancer."[4] Greater amounts of PA have been shown to reduce risk of mortality from the original cancer (prostrate, colorectal, and women with breast cancer).[4] Table 21-1 represents an overview of health-related benefits for adults and older adults based on the 2018 Physical Activity Guidelines Advisory Committee.

DEFINITIONS

"Physical activity (PA) is bodily movement produced by skeletal muscles that results in energy expenditure."[4] "Exercise is PA that is planned, structured, repetitive, and designed to improve or maintain physical fitness, physical performance, or health."[4] A single metabolic equivalent (MET) is equal to 3.5 mL/kg/min of oxygen consumed. Sedentary behavior is characterized by less than 1.5 METs while sitting, reclining, or lying down. Using METs

Table 21-1 • HEALTH-RELATED BENEFITS OF PHYSICAL ACTIVITY IN ADULTS AND OLDER ADULTS[4]

All-Cause Mortality	Lower Risk
Brain health	Improved cognitive function Improved quality of life Improved sleep Improved cognitive function after aerobic activity Reduced incidence of depression Reduced risk of dementia Reduced feelings of anxiety and depression
Cancer	Lower incidence of various types of cancers
Cardiovascular conditions	Lower incidence of hypertension Lower incidence of Type 2 diabetes Lower incidence and mortality (heart disease/stroke)
Weight status	Weight loss and prevention of weight regain with sufficient dose ratio of moderate-to-vigorous physical activity Reduced risk of excessive weight gain
Falls in older adults	Reduced incidence of falls and fall-related injuries
Physical function in older adults	Improved physical function

Office of Disease Prevention and Health Promotion. https://health.gov/paguidelines/second-edition/report/

Table 21-2 • EXAMPLE OF CATEGORIES OF ENERGY EXPENDITURE[4]

Level of Activity	MET Range	Activity Examples
Vigorous	≥6.0	Brisk walking 4.5–5 mph, shoveling snow, strenuous fitness class, jogging, running
Moderate	3.0–<6.0	Mopping, vacuuming, raking yard, walking 2.5–4 mph, doubles tennis
Light	1.6–3.0	Cooking, leisurely walking pace
Sedentary	1.0–1.5	Standing quietly, sitting, reclining, or lying

Office of Disease Prevention and Health Promotion. https://health.gov/paguidelines/second-edition/report/

is an easy way to compare the demands that specific activities like running, mowing the lawn, doubles tennis, folding laundry, etc. challenge the body. Aerobic PA is simply large muscle groups moved rhythmically over time which requires use of oxygen-supported metabolic energy pathways. Trying to move the "MET" meter to be greater than 1.5 is a starting point. To maintain or improve an individual's cardiorespiratory fitness, an aerobic PA must be intense enough and performed long enough to use the oxygen-supported fuel system. Going out for a comfortable stroll requires only about 2.0 METs. Walking at a pace of 3.0 miles per hour (mph) requires 3.3 METs. The idea is to move more and at a faster pace to achieve the cardiorespiratory benefit (Table 21-2).

Relative intensity can be defined as the "ease or difficulty with which an individual performs any given PA."[4] Two ways to measure relative intensity are percent of aerobic capacity or maximal heart rate. Simple scales of perceived exertion can also be used to guide an appropriate activity level. A scale from 0 to 10 is a simple way to direct a level of intensity for a given PA. The individual "self-perceives" how difficult an activity is to perform. A 0 is essentially sitting at rest and 10 would reflect the greatest effort. Moderate-intensity activities would be about 5 or 6 points (halfway on the scale) and more vigorous would be closer to 7 or 8. A conversation or singing scale can also be used to give the individual immediate feedback. Singing and talking are still achievable during light-intensity activities, but as the intensity increases this becomes more difficult. These scales are simple to use and most individuals can understand these guidelines. If an individual can find their own pulse, a target heart rate range recommended by a healthcare professional would be another option for intensity guidelines. There are a variety of wearable devices that will measure pulse at rest and during exercise. Deciding on the most user-friendly device that fits with the individual's lifestyle is based on multiple factors such as cost, level of training, and desired feedback. If the individual only needs to know a heart rate, a simple, low-cost, reliable device is ideal.

DESIGNING AN EXERCISE PRESCRIPTION

Frequency, intensity, type, time, volume, and progression (FITT-VP) should all be considered when planning to be more physically active.[5] Table 21-3 represents the operational definitions of the FITT-VP model with recommendations for aerobic exercise. Frequency refers to how often the activity or exercise should be done on a weekly basis. The intensity can be measured by the rate of energy expended. For an individual using MET charts (lawn mowing, singles tennis, bowling, hiking, walking a dog), a scale of perceived exertion, ability to sing, carry on a conversation, or target heart rates are all examples of ways to measure intensity.

Another way to measure intensity is related to target heart rate or a percent of oxygen consumption. Setting a target heart rate or a percent of oxygen consumption is typically based on a stress test performed in a clinician's office. A person with no health conditions (comorbidities) who has not had a stress test to provide an individualized target could use a percentage of their age-predicted target range. For example, a healthy 30 year old could use 220 minus their age (30) to get the age-predicted maximum heart rate. This age-predicted maximum heart rate would then be multiplied by a percentage like 70% and 80% to set a target heart rate range. As an individual is just beginning an exercise program, a lower-intensity program is advised to help decrease the incidence of delayed-onset muscle soreness and shortness of breath. If the individual pushes the intensity up too soon, the adverse responses of muscle soreness may cause

Table 21-3 • FITT-VP AEROBIC EXERCISE RECOMMENDATIONS[5]

*F*requency	5 days per week of moderate exercise or ≥3 days per week vigorous exercise, or combination of moderate and vigorous exercise ≥3–5 days per week is recommended.
*I*ntensity	Moderate and/or vigorous intensity is recommended for most adults. Light-to-moderate intensity exercise may be beneficial in deconditioned individuals.
*T*ime	30–60 minutes per day of purposeful moderate exercise, or 20–60 minutes per day of vigorous exercise, or a combination of moderate and vigorous exercise per day is recommended for most adults. <20 minutes' exercise per day can be beneficial, especially in previously sedentary individuals.
*T*ype	Regular, purposeful exercise that involves major muscle groups and is continuous and rhythmic in nature is recommended.
*V*olume	A target volume of ≥500–1000 MET-minutes per week is recommended. Increasing pedometer step counts ≥2000 steps per day to reach ≥7000 steps per day is beneficial. Exercising below these volumes may still be beneficial for individuals unable or unwilling to reach this amount of exercise.
*P*attern	Exercise may be performed in one (continuous) session per day or in multiple sessions of ≥10 minutes to accumulate the desired duration and volume of exercise per day. Exercise bouts of <10 minutes may yield favorable adaptations in very deconditioned individuals.
*P*rogression	A gradual progression of exercise volume by adjusting exercise duration, frequency, and/or intensity is reasonable until the desired exercise goal (maintenance) is attained. This approach may enhance adherence and reduce risks of musculoskeletal injury and adverse cardiac events.

Reprinted with permission from Pescatello LS, Riebe D, Thompson PD, eds. *ACSM's Guidelines for Exercise Testing and Prescription.* 9th ed. Wolters Kluwer Health/Lippincott Williams & Wilkins; 2014.

Table 21-4 • 2018 PHYSICAL ACTIVITY GUIDELINES FOR AMERICANS: RECOMMENDATIONS[6]

Age	Aerobic Activity	Muscle Strengthening
6–17	60 minutes of moderate or vigorous physical activity/day including at least 3 days of vigorous physical activity/wk	3 days/wk and included as part of 60 minutes of daily PA Include weight-bearing activity
18–64	150–300 min of moderate physical activity/wk, 75 min of vigorous physical activity/wk or equivalent combination over week	Muscle strengthening activities at moderate or greater intensity (all major muscle groups) on 2 or more days/week
65 and older	Same as adults, or be as active as health conditions and abilities allow	Same as adults, but include balance training and combination activities (aerobic/strength training together)
All ages	Move more. Sit less. Any and all physical activity counts	

Office of Disease Prevention and Health Promotion. https://health.gov/paguidelines/second-edition/report/

them not to continue. A slow, progressive increase in intensity is a great way to allow the body to accommodate and for instance, lower the risk of musculoskeletal injuries. Making the new exercise program enjoyable and achievable are great goals especially for setting the intensity. If the individual is on medications like a beta blocker, using a rating of perceived exertion scale would be a better way of accessing the level of intensity because the heart rate may not change proportional to the workload. Heart rate should respond in a linear fashion to the intensity of exercise. Beta blockers do not allow for the heart rate to have this same trajectory with a given workload.

Time refers to the length of time the individual is performing the aerobic or moderate to vigorous exercise. Type relates to form of activity to be performed: aerobic, strength training, balance training, or stretching. Volume is the amount of activity accumulated over a specific length of time. Volume is described over a day or a week. This applies to individuals who may not be able to do a 30- to 45-minute bout of exercise, but could accumulate a "volume" of 45 minutes by doing a shorter interval multiple times over the day. Volume is essentially how often the PA is done and for how long while taking into account the MET level achieved. There is evidence to support that total volume of moderate-to-vigorous PA is more important than the number of days per week on which individuals perform the activity.[4] An example of volume would simply be the total amount of minutes walked per week. Steps per day would be another way of using volume/day. If an individual is just starting out with an activity program, walking up to 2000 steps per day may be a good target. As the individual reaches the 2000-step goal then moving up to 5000, 7500, to 10,000 steps may be reasonable over a few months of consistent PA. Starting slowly, avoiding injury by limiting high intensity (running at high speeds for prolonged time, repetitive jumping, etc.), and sticking with the PA is key to success. Table 21-4 represents activity recommendations across the continuum.[6] No matter what the age, trying to get each individual to move more and sit less continues to be an ongoing goal.

CARDIOVASCULAR HEALTH CONDITIONS

Table 21-5 lists the physiologic systems that exhibit benefit from regular exercise.[7] The benefits of exercise are not just for prevention of health conditions, but are also beneficial for individuals that already present with cardiovascular (CV) diagnoses. The next section reviews the benefits of exercise for hypertension, diabetes, heart failure, myocardial ischemia and infarction, peripheral arterial disease (PAD), and rhythm disturbances.

Hypertension

Exercise is recommended for prevention, treatment, and control of hypertension.[8] Hypertension is the most costly, common, and preventable CV risk factor.[2,8] Nearly 40% of adults around the world are impacted by hypertension which is linked to coronary artery disease, heart failure, and stroke.[9] Hypertension is prevalent in greater than 10% of American school-age children.[9] At the other end-of-life spectrum, hypertension has been shown to accelerate brain aging thereby impacting cognitive function such as memory and goal-directed behavior.[10]

Physical exercise is considered a cornerstone of nonpharmacologic therapy for hypertension.[9] A meta-analysis of randomized control trials has concluded that dynamic resistance training can

Table 21-5 • SYSTEM ADAPTATIONS WITH REGULAR EXERCISE[7]

System	Benefit
Cardiovascular	Improves venous return Heart contractility Lowers systolic blood pressure Improves oxygen transport Increases total blood volume Increases red blood cells Lowers heart rate for a given workload Increased cardiac output at rest Improves myocardial contractility Decreases cardiac mortality
Pulmonary	Improved respiratory strength and endurance Desensitization dyspnea and increase overall exercise capacity (chronic obstructive pulmonary disease)
Musculoskeletal	Increases bone density Increases skeletal muscle size Increases metabolism Increases motor recruitment Increases skeletal muscle strength Increases motor control and motor learning Increases number of mitochondria with endurance training
Immune system	Promotes resistance to illness, inflammation, and tumor progression Increased lymphocyte production within 6–24 hours of acute exercise Elevation of number of cytokines and natural killer, B, and T cells Improves immunity by 15–25%
Psychological factors	Improves symptoms of depression Decreases depression associated with cancer, neuromuscular disorders, cardiac conditions, and chronic obstructive lung disease

Adapted from Coglianese D, ed. *Clinical Exercise Pathophysiology for Physical Therapy. Examination, Testing, and Exercise Prescription of Movement-Related Disorders.* Thorofare, NJ: Slack Incorporated; 2015.

lower systolic blood pressure by 2 to 3 mm Hg while aerobic exercise training can lower it by as much as 5 to 7 mm Hg.[8] This change in blood pressure has been shown to lower CV risk by 20% to 30% and parallels first-line antihypertensive modifications. In a recently published review article looking at resistance, aerobic, and combined exercise training, combined training was found to have an impact on arterial stiffness.[11] In the same article, vigorous resistance training was associated with an increase in arterial stiffness. This finding reinforces the importance of designing an individualized exercise program based on type and intensity (FITT-VP). Additional studies are needed to confirm the role that regular physical exercise may have in preventing cognitive impairments related to hypertension.[9]

Diabetes

Diabetes is a major cause of morbidity and mortality related to cardiovascular disease (CVD).[12] The prevalence of type 2 diabetes is increasing globally. Interventions using PA have been shown to reduce the risk by 47% to 58% in groups at high risk for developing type 2 diabetes.[12] The benefits of physical exercise affect metabolic parameters such as blood glucose and lipids levels which in turn have impact on CV risk. There does not seem to be the same glycemic benefit for type 1 diabetes as there is for type 2 diabetes from aerobic and resistance-type exercise.[12] A decrease in blood glucose can be observed with low- and moderate-intensity exercise. Caution is used with higher intensity because a rise in blood glucose can be seen. A thorough medical evaluation is recommended prior to starting a new exercise program to assess any safety concerns. The medical evaluation should include assessment of underlying CVD, autonomic neuropathy, retinopathy, peripheral neuropathy, nephropathy, blood glucose, and risk of ketosis for guidance on program design.[12] A fluctuating blood glucose can pose challenges with initiation of a new exercise program. Glucose monitoring before, during, and after exercise can help guide the use of prepared carbohydrate snacks or even glucose tablets when a severe drop occurs. The individual could expect a fall in the blood glucose levels for upward of 24 to 48 hours after the bout of exercise. As the individual becomes more accustomed to regular exercise, this dramatic drop in blood glucose tends to level off. The blood glucose results should be tracked and shared with their clinician for possible titration of glucose-lowering medication.

Aerobic and resistance exercise are recommended for individuals with type 2 diabetes.[13] Combining an exercise program with both resistance and aerobic components has demonstrated a noticeable improvement in hemoglobin A1c values, but less marked improvement in all CV risk factors. A published meta-analysis and systematic review revealed that a supervised resistance and aerobic program had more of an impact on lipid profiles and decreasing insulin resistance than an unsupervised program.[13] All adults and patients with type 2 diabetes mellitus can benefit from resistance exercise by improving muscle mass, insulin sensitivity, lipid profiles, blood pressure, and physical function. Accessible, cost-effective, medically supervised programs like cardiac rehabilitation may be an ideal way to monitor and progress individuals safely with an exercise program to help manage diabetes and subsequent risk factors for CV events.

Heart Failure

Heart failure is a progressive, chronic disorder that is the fastest-growing CVD.[14] An estimated 5.7 million Americans are affected by heart failure.[15] Exercise has been shown to improve quality of life and survival for heart failure patients.[14] Exercise training is now considered a Class I level recommendation for chronic heart failure.[16]

The most common presentations of exercise intolerance are dyspnea and fatigue.[17] Dyspnea and fatigue can be directly related to cardiac, pulmonary, skeletal muscle, endothelial, and neurohumoral system impairment. Exercise training has been shown to positively improve central hemodynamic function, peripheral vascular and muscle function, autonomic nervous system function, as well as maximal oxygen consumption.[17] The Heart Failure: A Controlled Trial Investigating Outcomes of exercise TraiNing (HF-ACTION) demonstrated the efficacy and benefits of exercise in stable heart failure patients.[17]

An exercise stress test is recommended prior to starting an exercise program to assess patients at high risk for adverse events and to help direct the exercise prescription (FITT-VP).[16] Aerobic exercise is recommended between 3 and 7 MET h/wk. The Borg scale (6–20) can be used to guide perceived exertion between levels of 12 and 14. This equates to having the individual rating the exercise "fairly light" but just below "hard" if the 6–20 scale is used. The target duration should be over 30 minutes per session at least 4 days a week. Resistance training 2 to 3 times per week can be incorporated once tolerance to the aerobic exercise is demonstrated without adverse events. Self-reported quality of life, functional capacity, and symptoms of dyspnea and fatigue have been reported diminished with optimal medical treatment and exercise training.[17] Heart failure patients needing mechanical circulatory assistance from a ventricular assist device (VAD) have also shown improved outcomes in quality of life, improved peak oxygen consumption, and distance walked on a 6-minute walk test with exercise rehabilitation.[14] Most patients with a VAD will not have a palpable pulse. Using the Borg Scale is a great way to help the patient understand intensity. Blood pressures may have to be measured with portable Doppler for auscultation. Each VAD center will have specific parameters for mean arterial pressure and emergency procedures. Cardiac rehabilitation is recommended as a first step for patients with any type of mechanical circulatory support device for medical supervision and safe progression.

Myocardial Ischemia/Myocardial Infarction

CVD is the leading cause of death in the world.[18] The World Health Organization reports that 80% of CVD is related to unhealthy behaviors like alcohol abuse, a diet high in fat, and physical inactivity.[18] A cost-effective intervention is to get more physically active. In a study comparing the incidence of CVD in bus ticket collectors in London who were more active than their bus driver counterparts there was a higher incidence of CVD in those who were sedentary.[19] In another study, a large cohort of over 16,000 college alumni showed PA levels influenced risk of mortality substantially.[19] There is evidence to support that physical exercise may reverse some of the pathologic changes of atherosclerosis.[18]

A systematic review did not conclusively demonstrate the benefit of exercise rehabilitation for patients with stable angina.[20] These studies had small enrollments and demonstrated only low quality of evidence for improvement in exercise capacity compared to usual care. Aerobic exercise may still be a potential countermeasure to protect the myocardium. The benefits can be measured in two phases: an early phase within 30 minutes to a later phase several days post exercise session.[21] The cardioprotective role that physical exercise plays in ischemia and reperfusion injuries needs further study before the recommendation can be supported with a higher quality of evidence.[20,21] On the other hand, there is substantial evidence to support exercise training after myocardial infarction.[22] Prevention of future complications, increased longevity and quality of life, improved exercise tolerance, and decreased cardiac mortality and CV risk have all been demonstrated when exercise training has been adequately prescribed (FITT-VP).

Peripheral Arterial Disease

Lower extremity PAD affects as many as 8.5 million Americans, approximately 5% of the population.[23,24] PAD results from chronic atherosclerosis in which narrowing of the blood vessels results in insufficient blood flow to meet the demands of the lower extremities.[24] A typical clinical symptom is intermittent claudication. Life style modifications are similar to the recommended changes for individuals with CV and cerebrovascular disease. In a recent systematic review and meta-analysis when compared to usual care, an intensive walking program significantly increased pain-free walking distance, and improved the 6-minute walk test distance in patients with PAD.[24] Supervised treadmill exercise has also been shown to significantly improve pain-free and maximal treadmill walking distance.[23] Supervised exercise training for individuals with PAD is now covered by Medicare similar to a cardiac rehabilitation program.

Rhythm Disturbances

The benefits of exercise have been well established for CVD prevention.[25] A reduction of CV mortality by as much as 35% and all-cause mortality by 33% has been demonstrated. Exercise can also trigger life-threatening ventricular arrhythmias and sudden cardiac death in young and older athletes.[25] The American Heart Association has developed a 14-element assessment for CV screening of competitive athletes.[25] Medical history, family history, and physical examination each play a key component to detect or raise suspicion of genetic or congenital CV abnormalities.[25] Once detection and risk for adverse cardiac events has been identified, the athlete should be evaluated by a sports medicine cardiologist who specializes in rhythm disturbances in athletes or specifically an electrophysiologist. One example of preparticipation sports management screening is an athlete with a diagnosis of hypertrophic cardiomyopathy. This athlete should not participate in the majority of competitive sports.[25] Implantation of a defibrillator would make the athlete automatically ineligible for competitive sports.[25] Exercise guidelines and specific parameters should be prescribed even for low level types of sport activities.

The intensity and the duration of the exercise play a role in individuals with CVD or in men with limited PA and in older individuals.[25] There are well-documented benefits of moderate-intensity exercise and the protective role of this extends to individuals with a variety of ventricular and atrial arrhythmias. In the general population, atrial fibrillation (AF) is the most common, sustained arrhythmia.[26] Studies have demonstrated a higher incidence of AF in athletes compared to the rest of the population related to some electrophysiologic and anatomic remodeling.[25] The majority of studies in athletes have looked primarily at men, and not women, at risk for AF. The mechanisms remain unclear, but what can be agreed upon is a dose response of high and sustained levels of exercise has demonstrated an increased risk for AF.[25,26] Exercise intensity is best monitored with a Borg Scale. Having an accurate heart rate parameter as a guide is challenging for the individual in persistent atrial fibrillation (AF). The newer wearable wrist devices that measure heart rate tend to have inconsistent reliability with the rate variability of AF. Using the Borg Scale guide of 11 to 14 allows for an intensity of exercise which is based on the individual's perception of work level.

Exercise also poses risks and benefits for susceptibility to ventricular ectopy (VE).[25] Approximately 1% to 4% of healthy, inactive individuals have premature ventricular beats greater than 60 per hour.[27] Similar to AF, regular physical exercise can either induce or prevent VE depending on dose and intensity. There is evidence to support the benefit of consistent exercise on improved autonomic balance of parasympathetic tone, enhanced myocardial function and perfusion, and resistance of ischemia/reperfusion-induced myocardial injury.[25] The American College of Sports Medicine recommends that men aged 45 and over and women 55 and over should have a symptom-limited exercise test prior to initiating vigorous exercise.[25] For competitive athletes, the American Heart Association recommends CV screening to identify risks related to personal medical history of cardiac-like symptoms, a family cardiac history, and a detailed physical examination.[27] A 12-lead electrocardiogram may be the first indication that there is underlying structural disease in athletes with premature ventricular beats and could help identify which athlete is at high risk for sudden cardiac death.[27] A positive finding in an individual with VE is if the VE occurs at rest, but the VE either decreases or is eliminated during a regular bout of exercise. Sympathetic tone should take over during exercise to have a higher, more consistent inherent pacemaker provide the rhythm during exercise. Further medical evaluation by a cardiologist or electrophysiologist is recommended if there is an increase in VE with exercise or immediately following the bout of exercise. Medical evaluation is also recommended if the individual complains of any type of presyncope, syncope, or dizziness with initiating exercise, increasing intensity of exercise, or immediately following the exercise.

THE CONTINUUM OF CARE: HOSPITAL BASED ACTIVITY TO HOME

Patient care providers should think about the impact of bed rest and how early activity in the hospital could help patients' overall well-being. Table 21-6 represents a system-by-system review of bed rest.[28] If the clock is turned back to the early 1930s, Sir Thomas Lewis stated that "*on the treatment of myocardial infarction: the patient is to be guarded by day and night nursing and helped in every way to avoid voluntary movement and effort.*"[29] Even in the early 1960s bed rest was still being used for immediate treatment of acute myocardial infarction.[30] Prolonged bed rest is associated with increased risk for prolonged ventilation, ventilator-associated pneumonia, increased risk for pressure ulcer development, higher risks for falls, increased workload on the CV system, higher occurrences of delirium, and adverse impact on quality of life post hospital discharge.[31] An uncomplicated cardiac surgical patient could be fast tracked and out of bed to chair and even walking as early as postoperative day 1.[31]

Early progressive mobility in the intensive care unit (ICU) is considered standard of care with reduction in the risk for venous thromboembolism and pulmonary emboli, improvement in airway clearance, decreased length of stay, and reduced need for rehabilitation post discharge.[31] Determining the timing for out-of-bed early mobilization is based on many factors especially if the patient has a complicated CV course. The considerations include hemodynamic status, use of vasoactive medications, cognitive status (Confusion Assessment Method-ICU score), sedation level, and level

Table 21-6 • SYSTEMS IMPACTED BY BED REST[28]

Cardiovascular	↓ Exercise tolerance/↓ maximum oxygen consumption ↓ Cardiac output ↑ Resting heart rate ↓ Resting and maximum stroke volume ↑ Venous compliance ↓ Orthostatic tolerance Venous pooling Reduction in aerobic and muscular power Elevated heart rate with all submaximal workloads Decreased blood volume
Hematologic	↓ Blood volume ↓ Red blood cells ↑ Deep venous thrombosis risk
Metabolic/ endocrine/ electrolytes	↑ Insulin resistance Hypercalcemia/renal stone formation ↑ Urinary excretion of sodium, potassium, calcium, and phosphorus Altered thermoregulatory responses
Musculoskeletal	Muscle atrophy (disuse atrophy) ↓ Mitochondria density/↓ aerobic enzymes Increased bone demineralization/osteopenia/ osteoporosis
Nutrition	Cachexia/malnutrition Obesity
Psychiatric	↑ Agitation ↑ Anxiety ↑ Delirium ↑ Depression
Pulmonary	↓ Lung volumes and capacities ↓ Respiratory muscle strength ↑ Risk for pneumonia/pulmonary emboli Increased risk for pneumonia and atelectasis Dyspnea on exertion Increased desaturation with activity

Reprinted with permission from Malone D, Bishop KL. *Acute Care Physical Therapy: A Clinicians' Guide.* 2nd ed. Thorofare, NJ: Slack Incorporated; 2019.

Table 21-7 • SIMPLE FUNCTIONAL TOOLS[36–42]

6-minute walk test	Measurement of endurance assesses walking distance over 6-minute period Need a stopwatch, instruction sheet, at least a 100 ft to do laps Good test–retest reliability (*ICC* = 0.95) in community-dwelling elderly
Two-minute walk test	Measurement of endurance assesses walking distance over 2-minute period Need a stopwatch, instruction sheet, at least a 100 ft to do laps Normative reference values available for age and gender
Timed up and go test	Assess mobility, balance, walking ability, fall risk Need a stopwatch, instruction sheet, a chair, measure 3 m to turn and walk back to chair Good test–retest reliability (*ICC* = 0.99) in frail elderly
5 times sit to stand	Assesses functional mobility and strength Need a stopwatch, chair, instruction sheet 55% sensitivity, 65% specificity to predict recurrent fallers Inability to rise from a chair 5 times in <13.6 seconds is associated with increased disability and morbidity
AM-PAC® 6-Clicks	System for measuring activity limitations Good validity, interrater reliability, predictive of discharge destination from acute care Scored out of 24; ≥discharge to home; <17 facility
30-second chair stand	Assesses functional leg strength in older adults # of times rising from a chair; scoring available by gender and age Need a stopwatch, instruction sheet, chair 0.95 interrater reliability for community-dwelling elderly

Ahlund K, Back M, Oberg B, et al. Effects of comprehensive geriatric assessment on physical fitness in an acute medical setting for frail elderly. *Clin Interv Aging.* 2017;12:1929–1939; https://www.cdc.gov/steadi/pdf/STEADI-Assessment-30Sec-508.pdf; https://www.sralab.org/rehabilitation-measures/30-second-sit-stand-test; https://www.sralab.org/sites/default/files/2017-06/5x-STS.pdf; https://www.physio-pedia.com/Six_Minute_Walk_Test_/_6_Minute_Walk_Test; Bohannon R. Normative reference values for the two-minute walk test derived by meta-analysis. *J Phys Ther Sci.* 2017;29(12):2224–2227; Jette DU, Stilphen M, Ranganathan VK, et al. Validity of the AM-PAC "6-clicks" inpatient daily activity and basic mobility short forms. *Phys Ther.* 2014;95(3):379–391.

of ventilatory support.[32] An example of how to determine if early mobilization should be restricted is if there have been increases in mechanical ventilation requirements within the previous 12 hours, the fraction of inspired oxygen (F_iO_2) greater than 60%; oxygen saturation less than 90%; and mean arterial pressure less than 65 mm Hg on vasoactive medication.[33–35] Waiting at least 24 hours to mobilize a patient after a fresh tracheostomy is recommended. As well, in-bed activities to facilitate lower extremity activity and airway clearance should be discussed with the Critical Care team following the fresh tracheostomy.

Hospitals should consider adjusting the focus from staying in bed to mobility and early PA so patients do not lose the level of function they had before coming to the hospital. Simple functional tools to assess each patient at time of admission could target high fall risk patients and which patients could remain more mobile during their hospital stay. Table 21-7 lists out a variety of easy tools that could be used to help identify which patients outside of the ICU could get moving sooner rather than waiting for the impact of bed rest to set in.[36–42] The Activity Measure for Post Acute Care (AM-PAC® 6-Clicks) could be done by the patient if able, family members, or caregivers at time of admission.[42] This tool does not need to be done by a professionally trained nurse or rehabilitation specialist. Identifying who needs extra assistance early to better allocate resources (to get out of bed to a chair for meals, to the commode, to the bathroom) during the hospital stay may lessen a host of adverse events. Once the patient is assessed for balance, fall risk, and safety the hospital team could give the patient a daily walking or bedside exercises as part of their care plan. This mindset change that moving early and often while in the hospital has the potential to engage the patient and help them realize the value of PA. Even family members could be educated on the value of "moving more" for a healthier lifestyle. Patients deemed unsafe by screening would be identified as fall risk and would require assistance for out-of-bed activity and a referral for rehabilitation services. Patients deemed safe and not a fall risk should be encouraged to walk in their room, and walk in the hallway to promote a sense of activity leading toward an improvement in overall quality of life and well-being. Hospitals should include improve health and well-being instead of managing health conditions and impairments. Discharge planning could include recommendations for clinician follow-up as well as joining a local gym or activity program to incorporate that value of exercise in the role of patient-centered care. Patients who had impairments and functional limitations at time of discharge would be referred to cardiac rehabilitation, pulmonary rehabilitation, vascular rehabilitation (Supervised Exercise Treatment for Peripheral Arterial Disease), or to specific rehabilitation services (Physical, Occupational, Speech Therapy). The challenge ahead for hospitals is to change the culture to help patients and staff see that moving early and often, whether for rehabilitation or prevention of adverse effects of bed rest, will promote well-being, lifelong healthier habits, and acceptance that *exercise is medicine.*[6]

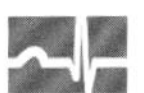 CASE-BASED LEARNING

Patient Profile

Name/Age/Sex: **Ellen Dock, 62-year-old female**

History of Present Illness

Patient came to ED with a chief complaint that "an elephant was sitting on my chest." Initial ER evaluation: troponin of 0.12. ECG NSR with slight ST depression ant/lat leads. CXR negative. Nuclear stress test performed with lateral ischemia. Underwent successful PCI with DES to her LCx. Discharged with prescription for Cardiac Rehab.

Past Medical History

CAD with prior DES × 3 to RCA 2015, MI 2015, HTN, DM, HLD, CVA, OSA

Surgical History

Cholecystectomy, PCI, hysterectomy

Family History

Mother, living, HTN; father, deceased, MVA

Medications

Started on DAPT with ASA/Brilinta. Unable to use Plavix due to previous nonresponder, unable to use Effient given h/o CVA. Reports prior allergy w/ Brilinta (hives/HA). Tolerating Brilinta so far. Will send home on Medrol Dosepak.

Allergies

Brilinta

Vital Signs and Measurements: Temp 36.3°C; BP 139/75 mm Hg; MAP via cuff 92; HR 58 bpm; RR 18 bpm; SpO_2 98% on room air; NSR; no edema; normal peripheral perfusion; S1/S2; Ht. 65 in; Wt. 187 lb

Lab Values

Whole BG POCT 136 mg/dL	WBC 19.8 10^3/mcL
Sodium 134 mmol/L	RBC 4.94 10^3/mcL
Potassium 4.6 mmol/L	Hgb 14.2 gm/dL
Glucose level 201 mg/dL	HCT 40.9%
BUN 15 mg/dL	PLT 433 10^3/mcL
Creatinine 0.69 mg/dL	HgbA1C 6.6
BUN/Creat ratio 22	Troponin 0.12

Diagnostic Evaluations

Nuclear stress test:
HR: 80–136 bpm (85% MPHR)
BP: 147/80 mm Hg–157/81 mm Hg
ECG: SR to ST with septal Q waves
Stress: 1–2 mm inferior horizontal ST depressions, resolved with recovery.
Perfusion: small size, moderate intensity, reversible defect lateral wall

Left heart catheterization:
95% LCx; 60% MLAD at first diagonal; 90% distal first diagonal, patent RCA, and RCA stents
LVEF 60%PCI (DES) of LCx

CXR: negative
ECG: NSR with slight ST depression anterior/lateral leads

Medications

Aspirin 81 mg w breakfast	Insulin glargine 80 units/mL at night
Bacillus coagulans-inulin 1 cap once a day	Insulin lispro 100 units/mL with meals
Carvedilol 6.25 mg w breakfast and dinner	Lisinopril 40 mg
Icosapent (Vascepa) 1 gm BID	Ticagrelor (Brilinta) 90 mg, BID

Family/Social History

Married, lives with spouse; shower chair; four stairs
Physical Therapy Consult: Fall Risk post CVA
6 minute walk test (6 MWT) 11/17 – 1137′, 3.2 ft/s; Berg Balance: 55/56; Five Times Sit To Stand: 17 seconds; Ten Times Sit To Stand: 32 seconds

Exercise Prescriptions: E. Dock
Phase 1. **Hospital (Day 0–Discharge)**
FITT-VP principle: Frequency: 3–5×/day; comfortable pace/conversational without complaint of SOB; Time: 10–15 minutes; Type: Ambulation in halls once cleared by PT; out of bed for meals >30 minutes 3×/day.

Target Heart Range:
Resting HR + 10 bpm
(telemetry monitor)
SR with occasional PVCs

Precautions:
Risk for Falls—consult PT previous CVA
Orthostatic hypotension
Hypoglycemia
DVT prophylaxis
R Groin site
Distal pulses/sensation
R radial site
Distal pulses/sensation

Blunted response:
Hypoglycemia and HR due to DM and beta blocker

BG: >100 mg/dL prior to any type of walking or PT session

Ankle pumps with position change
Diabetes-appropriate snacks between meals as per nutrition consult
PT consult
Social work consult—may need home health evaluation for safety and activity progression

Symptoms:
Watch hypoglycemia
Watch CP and anginal equivalents
Watch HA/cognitive changes

Education:
Weekly weight
Medications
Symptoms: reaction to medications, diabetes, CAD, CVA, PAD
Nutrition plan
Diabetes management
Fall safety

(continued)

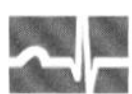 CASE-BASED LEARNING (*Continued*)

Phase 2. **Outpatient Cardiac Rehabilitation (Post discharge day 14–12 weeks)**
FITT-VP principle: Frequency: 3 ×/week; Intensity: Resting HR + 20–30 bpm; Rating of Perceived Exertion: 11–14; Type: Recumbent cycles progressing to treadmill with improved fall risk assessment; Time: 30 minutes continuous (warm up/aerobic/cool down/stretches) exercise progressing to 45 minutes (expand to include light weights with appropriate BG response); Volume: 90 min/wk progressing to 135 min/wk in 6 weeks

Target heart range: Resting HR + 20–30 beats (Telemetry monitor) Rating of perceived exertion: 11–14	BG: pre-exercise: >100 mg/dL; postexercise: >100 mg/dL BP: pre-exercise 200/100 mm Hg (asymptomatic); post exercise 170/90 Heart rhythm: SR to ST with occasional PVCs	Consider a CHO/protein snack prior to exercise Remeasure BG to evaluate drop; prepare BG tablets if drops below 90 BP: resting elevated; review timing of medications and symptoms; have PT track on phone or spreadsheet; report sent to physician for review
Symptoms: Evaluate anginal equivalent, hypoglycemic symptoms, HA, grown and wrist discomfort	**Precautions:** Type/timing of insulin and location of injection Drop in BG with blunted hypoglycemic response (beta blocker) Blunted HR response (beta blocker, possible autonomic neuropathy) Safety/Vision/Balance—recumbent equipment Watch trends in BG—may need medication titrated with increased BG control	**Education:** Daily weight Medications Blood glucose control Symptoms Nutrition plan (CAD, DM) Risk factor reduction Osteoporosis risk Exercise safety

Phase 3. **Home (Discharge from Outpatient Cardiac Rehabilitation—Maintenance)**
FITT-VP principle: Frequency: 5 days/wk; Intensity: Resting HR + 20–30 BPM and/or conversational guidelines; Type: walking in neighborhood, local high school, large box store for environmental controls, walk with a friend/family member; Time: 45 minutes continual pace; Volume: 135 minutes to 300 minutes over 6 months; Progress: Add 2–5 min/wk to 135 minutes—progress from 45 min/wk to 60 min 5×/wk over 6 months

Target heart range: Resting HR + 20–30 beats Patient purchased HR monitor to wear on wrist Patient instructed in conversational intensity guidelines	Continue to measure BG pre- and postexercise Should be >100 prior to start of exercise Track trends and share with physician office Watch for drops in BG not related to exercise Continue to monitor daily BG Continue to monitor symptoms related to medication	Continue to monitor any symptoms: especially HA, change in cognition, angina
Precautions: Balance/cognitive—uneven sidewalks; may want to go to the local high school track or indoors—environmentally controlled at malls or large box stores BG trends—may need medication titrated with increased BG control		**Education:** Participate in free YMCA Diabetes education program Participate in osteoporosis community fall risk program Monitor BG, symptoms Medical contact numbers for follow-up appointments

Abbreviations
ASA, acetyl salicylic acid; BID, twice a day; BP, blood pressure; BG, blood glucose; BUN, blood urea nitrogen; bpm, breaths per minute or beats per minute; CHO, carbohydrate; C, Celsius; CVA, cerebral vascular accident; CXR, chest roentgenogram; CAD, coronary artery disease; dL, deciliter; DVT, deep vein thrombosis; DM, diabetes mellitus; DES, drug-eluding stent; DAPT, dual antiplatelet therapy; ECG, electrocardiogram; ER, emergency room; E, exponent; FITT-VP, frequency, intensity, time, type, volume, progression; gm, gram; HA, headache; HR, heart rate; HCT, hematocrit; Hgb, hemoglobin; h/o, history of; HPI, history of present illness; HLD, hyperlipidemia; HTN, hypertension; LCx, left circumflex; LHC, left heart catheterization; LVEF, left ventricular ejection; lb, pounds; MPHR, maximal predicted heart rate; MAP, mean arterial pressure; mcL, microliter; MLAD, midleft anterior descending; mg, milligrams; mm Hg, millimeters of mercury; mmol/L, millimoles per liter; MVA, motor vehicle accident; MWT, minute walk test; MI, myocardial infarction; NSR, normal sinus rhythm; OSA, obstructive sleep apnea; PCI, percutaneous coronary intervention; PAD, peripheral arterial disease; PT, physical therapy; POCT, point of contact testing; PVC, premature ventricular contraction; RBC, red blood counts; RR, respiratory rate; RCA, right coronary artery; RA, room air; SpO_2, saturation of peripheral oxygen; SOB, shortness of breath; SR, sinus rhythm; ST, sinus tachycardia; T, temperature; WBC, white blood counts; y/o, year old; YMCA, Young Men's Christian Association.

KEY READING

Thomas R, Balady G, Banka G, et al. ACC/AHA clinical performance and quality measures for cardiac rehabilitation. *J Am Coll Cardiol.* 2018;71(16).

REFERENCES

1. Bergeron CD, Tanner AH, Friedman DB, et al. Physical activity communication: a scoping review of the literature. *Health Promot Pract.* 2019;20(3):344–353. https://doi.org/10.1177/1524839919834272
2. Sharman JE, La Gerche A, Coombes JS. Exercise and cardiovascular risk in patients with hypertension. *Am J Hypertens.* 2015;28(2):147–158.
3. Zhang Y, Qi L, Xu L, et al. Effects of exercise modalities on central hemodynamics, arterial stiffness and cardiac function in cardiovascular disease: systematic review and meta-analysis of randomized controlled trials. *PLoS One.* 2018;13(7):e0200829.
4. 2018 Physical Activity Guidelines Advisory Committee. *2018 Physical Activity Guidelines Advisory Committee Scientific Report.* Washington, DC: U.S. Department of Health and Human Services; 2018.
5. American College of Sports Medicine. *ACSM's Guidelines for Exercise Testing and Prescription.* 9th ed. Philadelphia, PA: Wolters Kluwer Health/ Lippincott Williams & Wilkins; 2014.
6. The Miracle Drug. Exercise is Medicine® American College of Sports Medicine®. Available at www.exerciseismedicine.org
7. Coglianese D, ed. *Clinical Exercise Pathophysiology for Physical Therapy. Examination, Testing, and Exercise Prescription of Movement-Related Disorders.* Thorofare, NJ: Slack Incorporated; 2015.
8. Pescatello LS, MacDonald HV, Lamberti L, et al. Exercise for hypertension: a prescription update integrating existing recommendations with emerging research. *Curr Hypertens Rep.* 2015;17(11):87.
9. Rêgo ML, Cabral DA, Costa EC, et al. Physical exercise for individuals with hypertension: it is time to emphasize its benefits on the brain and cognition. *Clin Med Insights Cardiol.* 2019;13:1179546819839411.
10. Lefferts WK, DeBlois JP, White CN, et al. Effects of acute aerobic exercise on cognition and constructs of decision-making in adults with and without hypertension. *Front Aging Neurosci.* 2019;11:41.
11. Li Y, Hanssen H, Cordes M, et al. Aerobic, resistance and combined exercise training on arterial stiffness in normotensive and hypertensive adults: a review. *Eur J Sport Sci.* 2015;15(5):443–457.
12. Lumb A. Diabetes and exercise. *Clin Med (Lond).* 2014;14(6):673–676.
13. Pan B, Ge L, Xun YQ, et al. Exercise training modalities in patients with type 2 diabetes mellitus: a systematic review and network meta-analysis. *Int J Behav Nutr Phys Act.* 2018;15(1):72.
14. Grosman-Rimon L, Lalonde SD, Sieh N, et al. Exercise rehabilitation in ventricular assist device recipients: a meta-analysis of effects on physiological and clinical outcomes. *Heart Fail Rev.* 2019;24:55–67.
15. Scheiderer R, Belden C, Schwab D, et al. Exercise guidelines for inpatients following ventricular assist device placement: a systematic review of the literature. *Cardiopulm Phys Ther J.* 2013;24(2):35–42.
16. Ades PA, Keteyian SJ, Balady GJ, et al. Cardiac rehabilitation exercise and self-care for chronic heart failure. *JACC Heart Fail.* 2013;1(6):540–547.
17. Downing J, Balady GJ. The role of exercise training in heart failure. *J Am Coll Cardiol.* 2011;58(6):561–569.
18. Yang J, Cao RY, Gao R, et al. Physical exercise is a potential "medicine" for atherosclerosis. In: Xiao J, ed. *Exercise for Cardiovascular Disease Prevention and Treatment. Advances in Experimental Medicine and Biology 999.* Singapore: Springer Nature Singapore Pvt. Ltd; 2017:269–285.
19. Adams V, Linke A. Impact of exercise training on cardiovascular disease and risk. *Biochim Biophys Acta Mol Basis Dis.* 2019;1865(4):728–734.
20. Long L, Anderson L, Dewhirst AM, et al. Exercise-based cardiac rehabilitation for adults with stable angina. *Cochrane Database Syst Rev.* 2018;(2):CD012786.
21. Borges JP, da Silva Verdoorn K. Cardiac ischemia/reperfusion injury: the beneficial effects of exercise. In: Xiao J, ed. *Exercise for Cardiovascular Disease Prevention and Treatment. Advances in Experimental Medicine and Biology 999.* Singapore: Springer Nature Singapore Pvt. Ltd; 2017:269–285.
22. Moraes-Silva IC, Rodriques B, Coelho-Junior HJ, et al. Myocardial infarction and exercise training: Evidence from basic science. In: Xiao J, ed. *Exercise for Cardiovascular Disease Prevention and Treatment. Advances in Experimental Medicine and Biology 999.* Singapore: Springer Nature Singapore Pvt. Ltd; 2017:139–153.
23. McDermott MM. Exercise training for intermittent claudication. *J Vasc Surg.* 2017;66(5):1612–1620.
24. Lyu X, Li S, Peng S, et al. Intensive walking exercise for lower extremity peripheral arterial disease: a systematic review and meta-analysis. *J Diabetes.* 2016;8(3):363–377.
25. Manolis AS, Manolis AA. Exercise and arrhythmias: a double-edged sword. *Pacing Clin Electrophysiol.* 2016;39(7):748–762.
26. Flannery MD, Kalman JM, Sanders P, et al. State of the art review: atrial fibrillation in athletes. *Heart, Lung Circ.* 2017;26(9):983–989.
27. Singh TK, Baggish AL. Premature ventricular beats in the athlete: management considerations. *Expert Rev Cardiovasc Ther.* 2018;16(4):277–286.
28. Malone DM, Bishop KL. Acute care physical therapy: a clinician's guide. In: Malone DM, Bishop KL, eds. *Chapter 4. Bed Rest, Deconditioning, and Hospital-Acquired Neuromuscular Disorders.* 2nd ed. Thorofare, NJ: Slack Publishing; 2019:93–110.
29. Magder S. Assessment of myocardial stress from early ambulatory activities following myocardial infarction. *Chest.* 1985;87:442–447.
30. Duke M. Bed rest in acute myocardial infarction a study of physician practices. *Am Heart J.* 1971;82(4):486–491.
31. Freeman R, Maley K. Mobilization of intensive care cardiac surgery patients on mechanical circulatory support. *Crit Care Nurs Q.* 2013;36(1): 73–88.
32. Schweikert WD, Pohlman MC, Pohlman AS, et al. Early physical and occupational therapy in mechanically ventilated, critically ill patients: a randomised controlled trial. *Lancet.* 2009;373(9678):1874–1882.
33. Engel HJ, Tatebe S, Alonzo PB, et al. Physical therapist-established intensive care unit early mobilization program: quality improvement project for critical care at the university of California san Francisco medical center. *Phys Ther.* 2013;93:975–985.
34. Zomorodi M, Topley D, McAnaw M. Developing a mobility protocol for early mobilization of patients in a surgical/trauma ICU. *Crit Care Res Pract.* 2012;2012:964547.
35. Green M, Marzano V, Leditschke IA, et al. Mobilization of intensive care patients: a multidisciplinary practical guide for clinicians. *J Multidiscip Healthc.* 2016;9:247–256.
36. Ahlund K, Back M, Oberg B, et al. Effects of comprehensive geriatric assessment on physical fitness in an acute medical setting for frail elderly. *Clin Interv Aging.* 2017;12:1929–1939.
37. https://www.cdc.gov/steadi/pdf/STEADI-Assessment-30Sec-508.pdf
38. https://www.sralab.org/rehabilitation-measures/30-second-sit-stand-test
39. https://www.sralab.org/sites/default/files/2017-06/5x-STS.pdf
40. https://www.physio-pedia.com/Six_Minute_Walk_Test_/_6_Minute_Walk_Test
41. Bohannon R. Normative reference values for the two-minute walk test derived by meta-analysis. *J Phys Ther Sci.* 2017;29(12):2224–2227.
42. Jette DU, Stilphen M, Ranganathan VK, et al. Validity of the AM-PAC "6-clicks" inpatient daily activity and basic mobility short forms. *Phys Ther.* 2014;95(3):379–391.

22 Smoking Cessation and Effective Treatment

Joelle T. Fathi

OBJECTIVES

1. Describe the neurohormonal mechanism of nicotine addiction.
2. Identify three first-line pharmacologic treatments for nicotine dependence.
3. Recognize nicotine withdrawal and clinical approaches for preventing or alleviating withdrawal symptoms.
4. Assess for signs and symptoms of treatment side effects.
5. Explain approaches for relapse prevention and sustained cessation.

KEY QUESTIONS

1. How does nicotine dependence occur?
2. Why is it so difficult for people to quit smoking cigarettes?
3. How can nurses help people successfully quit smoking?
4. What interventions yield the highest chance that a person will be successful in smoking cessation?
5. Which smoking cessation treatment is the safest in a cardiac patient?

BACKGROUND

Nicotine was introduced to the Europeans in the late 1400s by Christopher Columbus and from there it continued its travels around the world.[1] Jean Nicot, a French diplomat, discovered the plant in Portugal and transported it back to France in 1559, at which time the psychoactive substance of the tobacco plant, "nicotine", was named after Nicot.[2] Although these discoveries are well established, the ancient history and use of nicotine is also deeply rooted with the Native Americans and is archeologically traced to the 16th century through the detection of nicotine in clay pipes, which were notably utilized for ceremonial and ritual purposes.[3]

As a principal alkaloid, nicotine is a potent substance with addictive properties that may be derived from the tobacco leaf.[4–6] Originating in the root of the tobacco plant, nicotine migrates to the leaves of the plant and may be elicited through smoking, chewing, snorting, and even drinking the prepared tobacco leaves[2] with cigarette smoking as the most common method of nicotine delivery worldwide.[7]

Interestingly, smoking-related diseases and evidence of habitual use or nicotine addiction are not historically depicted or documented until the late 1880s. This coincided with the emergence of cigarette manufacturers who forged ahead with mass production and distribution of cigarettes that contained enhanced ingredients with greater addictive properties and toxic additives. Cigarettes were soon sold publicly and disseminated to soldiers at war, in mass quantities. This resulted in a significant rise in consumption of cigarettes in the United States, from "less than 4 billion cigarettes in 1905 to more than 100 billion 20 years later."[8] This access and exposure, as well as public marketing by tobacco companies, in turn, promoted addiction to cigarettes with chronic and habitual use patterns.[2,9,10]

The full impact of routine tobacco smoke exposure on the health of a smoker took many decades to be fully realized but by 1950, researchers were able to demonstrate the ill effects of routine cigarette smoking.[11–13] Following the emergence of scientifically proven risks and a strong causal relationship with smoking and lung disease, lung cancer, and coronary artery disease, the Surgeon General delivered a formal report in 1964 that cautioned the public from use of cigarettes and other tobacco products.[9,14,15]

The prevalence of smoking in the United States has consistently fallen since the Surgeon General's seminal report, when nearly half of all adults in America were smokers.[10,16] Currently, smoking is at an all-time low of 13.7% (approximately 34 million smokers),[17] down from 20.9% in 2005.[18] This downward trajectory of active smokers in the United States is encouraging but the statistical chances for associated morbidity and mortality remain daunting when it is considered that 50% of all smokers today will die of tobacco-related diseases, 10 years before their never-smoking peers. Cigarettes are claiming the lives of 480,000 people each year,[16,19,20] with tobacco smoke being directly associated with 33% of all deaths due to cardiovascular disease and 20% of those related to ischemic heart disease.[21,22]

Populations at Risk for Smoking Afflictions

The burden and disparate patterns of addiction to cigarettes is unfairly weighted in society and leans heavily toward men, people who have a general education development (GED) certificate or less, and live below the poverty level. Additionally, people who belong to diverse populations, suffer from disability or serious mental illness, are uninsured or insured by a Medicaid health plan, and live in the midwest or southern United States are at much higher risk for smoking cigarettes.[16,18,23,24] The burden of addiction to cigarettes is multifactorial and influenced by social, environmental, regional and agricultural factors, as well as state policy.

UNDERSTANDING THE NEUROBIOLOGY AND PATHOPHYSIOLOGY OF NICOTINE ADDICTION

While there are various contributors (pharmacologic, chemical, conditioning, environmental, and social triggers) to addiction, it is critical that nurses first develop foundational knowledge in the neurobiology and pathophysiology of addiction to deliver compassionate and empathetic care to those who are suffering from nicotine addiction. Furthermore, comprehension of such responses to the substance nicotine and subsequent behavioral conditioning clarifies the rationale for effective therapeutic and pharmacologic treatment approaches for successful cessation.

Like other substances that possess addictive properties, neuroreceptors in the brain are stimulated by the substance that elicit expression of neurohormones such as dopamine, GABA, glutamate, and serotonin; these potent neurohormones drive varying levels of euphoria, can elevate mood, stimulate a heightened state of energy, and even improve concentration, and may have a calming effect.[25] Perhaps the most provocative mechanism of addictive substances including nicotine, and what the brain seeks most is the expression and surge of high levels of neurohormones, predominantly dopamine. This high concentration of neurohormones induced by exogenous substances cannot be accomplished by typical triggers and means, like food and sex, in our normal environments.[26] This neurohormonal alteration and the cascading effects that predictably result with a reward effect in the brain are at the core of addiction to tobacco products, including conventional cigarettes and electronic nicotine delivery devices (i.e., electronic cigarettes [e-cigarettes]).

The brain has two types of acetylcholine receptors—muscarinic and nicotinic. These receptors are responsive to certain agonists that when stimulated, initiate a cascade of events. Nicotine has a high affinity for and explicitly influences the nicotinic acetylcholine neuroreceptors (nAChRs) of the brain; these receptors predominantly respond to the presence of nicotine.[27] In the setting of exposure to nicotine, the nAChRs are stimulated by nicotine upon contact which triggers ion channels to open, allowing cations (sodium and calcium) to flow into the neurons and in turn, elicit the expression of neurohormones.[25]

Repetitive exposure to nicotine promotes neuroadaptation wherein tolerance occurs, more binding sites for nicotine open on the nAChRs, dependence/addiction develops, and withdrawal symptoms result in the absence of nicotine.[25]

Recognizing and Understanding Nicotine Cravings and Withdrawal

Recognition of the signs and symptoms of nicotine withdrawal by patients and nurses is very important for the benefit of the patient's overall success in cessation. Nicotine is a potent stimulant that elevates energy, concentration, and mood, but also has a calming effect for many people; these benefits promote nicotine-seeking behaviors and continual use. Once nicotine has metabolized and the systemic nicotine levels drop, the brain sends cues seeking more nicotine and the resulting reward response. These cues are interpreted as cravings for nicotine and the intensity of these cravings is driven by the level of dependence (how much nicotine is regularly consumed), how sharply the nicotine level has dropped, and exposure to environmental triggers and lifestyle rituals that are cognitively associated with smoking. Finally, when nicotine levels decrease without replenishment, the patient experiences a drop in mood, energy, and ability to concentrate, a disruption in sleep patterns, and may even experience anxiety or feel generally ill.

Risk for Nicotine Addiction in Adolescence

Development of lifelong addiction is significantly influenced by the stage of neural development of the brain at time of exposure, the modality by which nicotine is administered, the dose and concentration, and how frequently it is administered.

For all intents and purposes, nicotine addiction can be considered a preventable childhood disease. Extensive research on the brains of adolescent mice provides significant insight into the neurohormonal development of the brain and the irreversible remodeling of the brain, in adolescence, with nicotine exposure. Adolescent nicotine exposure causes irreversible brain cell damage and loss. This exposure, in adolescence, induces a divergent distribution of nAChR receptors and upregulation alteration "in synaptic function in cholinergic and catecholaminergic pathways, characterized by suppressed neural activity and persistent desensitization of cholinergic responses" than when exposure occurs in adulthood.[28]

Furthermore, there is significant evidence demonstrating that structural and neurochemical brain maturation, including the dopaminergic system that drives motivated behaviors and associative learning, is specifically related to continual reorganization of the gray and white matter and neurochemical systems; these changes continue until at least age 25 and even later.[29] This neuroplasticity and evolution of central nervous system development, early in life, are significant drivers in age-specific responses to nicotine with a higher propensity for nicotine addiction and maladaptive, addictive behavioral patterns in adolescence than in adulthood.[29,30] Unfortunately, the adolescent brain is expressly vulnerable and once the neural circuitry has been reorganized under the influence of regular nicotine exposure and use, it never returns to regular neural patterns.[30] Indeed, this science provides a plausible explanation for why the onset of lifelong smoking in 80% of smokers, is before 18 years of age, why the addictive properties of nicotine and contents of cigarettes have such a stronghold on humans, and why cravings may persist long after successful cessation.[31,32]

CARDIOVASCULAR RISK AND SMOKING

Cardiovascular disease is directly correlated with modifiable risk factors including uncontrolled diabetes, cholesterol, hypertension, and tobacco smoke exposure[33,34] either through mainstream smoke (what is inhaled into the smoker's mouth from the tobacco end of the cigarette) or sidestream smoke also known as second-hand exposure.[7,35] Tobacco smoke's deleterious effects on the arterial vessels of the heart result more often in cardiovascular disease than lung cancer and chronic obstructive pulmonary disease.[11]

Smoking cigarettes poses independent cardiovascular risk through mechanisms that raise serum blood sugar levels, suppress protective high-density lipoproteins, raise maleficent low-density lipoproteins, and contribute to hypertension through vasoconstriction.[21] Perhaps even more critical is the exponential rise in risk for cardiovascular heart disease (CHD) when cardiovascular risk factors exist in the setting of cigarette smoking. In the presence of a single cardiovascular risk factor, smoking cigarettes doubles the risk for CHD over that of a never smoker. When a second cardiovascular risk factor is added to smoking, the risk quadruples and when multiple risk factors are present with smoking cigarettes, the risk incrementally skyrockets into the eightfold risk range.[21]

Tobacco Smoke and Atherosclerotic Changes

The composition of cigarettes and combusted tobacco smoke represents "7000 chemicals and 69 carcinogens" with many known to be contributors to systemic disease through their direct effect on human tissues.[12] The primary constituents in tobacco smoke, like N-nitrosamines, polycyclic aromatic hydrocarbons (PAHs), aldehydes, heavy metals, and aromatic and heterocyclic amines are recognized for their volatile and carcinogenic effects.[36,37] The mechanisms by which these and many other chemicals induce endothelial changes at a cellular level, and subsequent atherosclerotic disease, in the setting of tobacco smoke exposure, are complex and multifactorial.[37]

Endothelial damage is directly related to inhalation of the combusted contents of a cigarette, by midstream or sidestream pathways. By its direct effect through oxidative stress and cytotoxic action and proinflammatory processes, inhaled cigarette smoke increases blood pressure, and promotes changes in serum lipids which are all primary contributing factors to CHD.[37] Additionally, the presence of such proinflammatory action stimulates local platelet activation and aggregation, leukocyte recruitment on the endothelial surface, induction of endothelial (structural) damage and dysfunction, necrotic endothelial death, deposition of lipids, and a prothrombotic environment which are all contributors to progressive CHD and increased risk for an acute coronary event.[7,21,35]

Benefits of Quitting Smoking and Cardiac Events

Research demonstrates that cutting back on smoking is not as effective in improving health outcomes or positively impacting all-cause mortality compared to the benefits of sustained abstinence. Quitting smoking is the most effective way to prevent adverse smoking-related health events, slow progression of established disease processes, and improve overall health status.[19] In fact, quitting smoking between the ages of 35 and 44 can greatly reduce the chances of suffering from a smoking-related health event.[20] Given the benefits of quitting smoking at any age, complete cessation should be the end goal for all healthcare providers who are treating patients with tobacco dependence, and patients addicted to cigarettes and other tobacco products.

The drop in energy, change in ability to concentrate, spike in depression and anxiety, constipation, changes in appetite, and disruption of sleep, as discussed earlier, are just a few of the unpleasant symptoms that are experienced in nicotine withdrawal.[19] The physiologic and psychological benefits of nicotine and the drive to avoid these noxious symptoms of withdrawal are potent enough to motivate patients to continue to smoke, even when they know they should quit. Commonly, patients do not recognize these symptoms as those of withdrawal nor do they understand these symptoms can be prevented with proper treatment. Prevention of withdrawal symptoms is central to all smoking cessation treatments which greatly enhance the chances of successful cessation and long-term quit and avoidance of relapse.

The risk of continued smoking and benefits of smoking cessation in cardiac patients, especially those who have suffered an acute cardiac event, is scientifically well established. In a large retrospective population-based study, patients who suffered a recent myocardial infarction and continued smoking demonstrated a 50% increased risk for another cardiac event compared to nonsmoking cardiac patients. Remarkably, for those who quit smoking following an acute cardiac event, an exponential benefit of having quit was realized over time, with the risk for a recurrent cardiac event declining and being that of a nonsmoker by 3 years of cessation.[38] Other researchers have demonstrated similar results with significant risk reduction of recurrent cardiac events with incremental periods of cessation, following the event.[39,40] Helping our patients quit smoking and remain smoke-free are the most effective means for preventing pathogenesis and progression of cardiac disease, and related disability and deaths.

ASSESSING TOBACCO DEPENDENCY

The Fagerström Tolerance Questionnaire (FTQ), a psychometric tool that measures physical dependence to nicotine and assesses behaviors associated with nicotine addiction, was first developed in 1978.[41] Later, a refined version of this widely accepted and utilized tool, the Fagerström Test for Nicotine Dependence (FTND) was created and proved to be a more accurate measurement of heaviness of smoking showing greater consistency with biochemical measurements of nicotine levels (Fig. 22-1).[42,43]

The FTND can be easily administered and is cost-effective compared to biometric testing. Additionally, the patient's score on the FTND may be used to identify patients with higher levels of dependency and potential need for additional services and care by other healthcare professionals, like behavioral therapists, psychotherapists, addiction medicine specialists, or certified tobacco treatment specialists to be successful at quitting.

Approaching the Tobacco Use Conversation With Patients

The 5As (Ask, Advise, Assess, Assist, Arrange) Model for behavior change can be very helpful to nurses when addressing any behavior that impacts a patient's health, including smoking (Table 22-1). Given the chronic nature of nicotine dependence, tobacco use should be addressed, using the 5As, in every patient encounter, to avoid missed opportunities for intervention and cessation.

Table 22-1 • THE "5 AS" MODEL FOR TREATING TOBACCO USE AND DEPENDENCE

Ask	Ask patient about their use
Advise	Advise patient that quitting smoking is recommended
Assess	Assess patient's readiness to quit
Assist	Assist patient in quitting (counseling, pharmacologic treatment, referral)
Arrange	Arrange clinical follow-up for patient

Question	Answers	Points
1. How soon after you wake up do you smoke your first cigarette?	Within 5 minutes	3
	6–30 minutes	2
	31–60 minutes	1
	After 60 minutes	0
2. Do you find it difficult to refrain from smoking in places where it is forbidden (e.g., in church, at the library, in the cinema, etc.)?	Yes	1
	No	0
3. Which cigarette would you hate most to give up?	The first on in the morning	1
	All others	0
4. How many cigarettes/day do you smoke?	10 or less	0
	11–20	1
	21–30	2
	31 or more	3
5. Do you smoke more frequently during the first hours after waking than during the rest of the day?	Yes	1
	No	0
6. Do you smoke if you are so ill that you are in bed most of the day?	Yes	1
	No	0

Figure 22-1. The Fagerstrom tolerance test. (Reprinted with permission from Heatherton T, Kozlowski L, Frecker R, et al. The Fagerstrom test for nicotine dependence: a revision of the Fagerstrom Tolerance Questionnaire. *Br J Addict.* 1991;86:1119–1127.)

This conversation starts with ***Asking*** the patient about and documenting tobacco use in the medical record. Asking patients about their use, improves the likelihood that they will converse about their use, and opens the door for further discussion and next steps. ***Advise*** that quitting smoking is recommended. This should be performed in a clear manner, urging the patient to quit. ***Assess*** the patient's readiness to quit. This can be performed by using the stages of change model (see below) and may facilitate further discussion and determination of next steps. For ex tobacco users and recently quit patients, inquire if there are any challenges to remaining quit. ***Assist*** the patient who is interested in discussing quitting through counseling and provide prompt access to tobacco cessation treatment for those who are ready to make a quit attempt. For patients who are unwilling to consider discussion or a quit attempt at this time, engage motivational interventions to enhance their opportunity to progress in their readiness to quit, and ***Arrange*** for all patients, no matter where they are on the continuum of readiness to quit, to have clinical follow-up soon.[44,45]

Assessing Readiness to Quit

Prochaska and DiClemente designed a theoretical framework, the Transtheoretical Model of Behavior Change (TTM) aka Stages of Change, that can be easily integrated into the ***Assess*** step of the 5As conversation (see above) (Table 22-2). This model may be helpful in determining a patient's readiness to quit, accommodate them based on where they are in their smoking cessation journey, and determining next steps.[46]

Table 22-2 • STAGES OF CHANGE[44]

Precontemplation	Not ready to quit
Contemplation	Considering a quit attempt
Preparation	Actively planning a quit attempt
Action	Actively involved in a quit attempt
Maintenance	Achieved smoking cessation

Motivational Interviewing for Behavior Change

Motivational interviewing (MI) is designed to motivate change in behavior. It is a counseling approach that is empathic and embodies principles of facilitation and guidance, in clinical care conversations, through partnership with patients, acceptance, compassion, and evocation.[47] MI practice is person centered and identifies the patient as an expert, as the clinician elicits change rather than imposing it through "therapeutic alliances"[48] and helps them address and resolve any ambivalence they may have about smoking cessation. This approach guides patients through strategic questions that help them discover their levels of motivation and confidence in quitting smoking, how quitting smoking would make a difference in their lives, and what is to be gained if they quit, or lose if they continue to smoke. This practice also helps patients identify perceived barriers to quitting and can be used in every patient encounter to facilitate moving them through the stages of change and ultimately to quit. A meta-analysis of randomized controlled trials was conducted to evaluate whether there is an association in utilization of MI with higher rates of smoking cessation, compared to usual care or brief advice. This demonstrated clinical correlation with a significant increase in smoking cessation in those who received MI through a general practitioner or trained counselor.[49] Simply put, MI for behavior change works. This communication and counseling technique can be learned by nurses through local or online courses and books that teach MI, implemented in clinical care immediately, and adapted to most health-related behavior change, including smoking cessation efforts.

PHARMACOKINETICS OF NICOTINE IN CIGARETTE SMOKING

Combustion of cigarettes and the resulting gases represent an efficient means for the delivery of nicotine to the brain and other tissues in the human body that are receptive to this substance.

From the time of an inhaled puff on a cigarette to the time nicotine attaches to the α4β2 subunit of the nAChR receptor in the brain is about 20 seconds.[50] This method of transport and the rate of rise of nicotine levels are very efficient as the nicotine-containing gas is inhaled into the lungs, transported across the alveolar membrane into the arterial blood, and swiftly reaches the brain.[50] The α4β2 subunits of the nAChR receptors have a very high affinity for nicotine and instantaneously partner with nicotine upon its arrival. Brody et al. conducted a compelling study that demonstrated the relationship between smoking and occupancy of nicotine at the α4β2*nAChR receptors by utilizing 2-FA PET scanning. This research showed that when smokers took in as little as 0.13 (one to two puffs) of a cigarette, they achieved a 50% occupancy of the α4β2*nAChR receptors for 3.1 hours after smoking. When the study participants smoked a full cigarette (or more) the receptor occupancy reached more than 88% saturation and nicotine cravings were reduced. This research also demonstrates the ability of the smoker to control the dosing effect of nicotine depending on their smoking patterns (how many puffs and intensity of puffing, how often and how much of the cigarette they smoke, and how many cigarettes they smoke over a period).[27]

As a smoker takes in more nicotine and the arterial blood concentration increases, the nicotine not only distributes to the brain, but deposits in the adipose tissues and muscles; over the course of a day of smoking, the concentration of nicotine in the body rises. The CYP2A6 metabolic pathway in the liver is the predominant means for metabolism of nicotine with a half-life that averages about 2 hours, barring any genetic polymorphism (variation) of this liver enzyme. Due to the concentration of chemicals, including nicotine, in the body and rate of metabolism, levels may remain high for the upward of 6 hours, when nicotine has not been replenished. However, it is important to understand that all people metabolize differently and for rapid metabolizers with quicker clearance, there may be a drive to smoke more cigarettes to maintain certain concentrations of nicotine; these people may more commonly experience withdrawal symptoms in between cigarettes. Conversely, slow metabolizers may smoke less cigarettes and suffer less symptoms of withdrawal.[50–52]

The CYP1A2 enzymatic pathway is responsible for metabolism of medications such as some antidepressants, blood thinners, antiplatelet agents, and even substances like caffeine, and directly influences the serum concentration of these medications. This enzymatic pathway is activated by the chemicals in cigarettes, namely PAHs. The implications for CYP1A2 activation can be dramatic, and are dose dependent and correlated with how much someone smokes and inhales. The more cigarettes smoked, the more activated this pathway becomes, in turn causing more efficient and faster clearance of medications that are normally metabolized by the CYP1A2 pathway thus requiring higher doses for therapeutic effect. This can be especially challenging if a patient is taking a medication that has a narrow therapeutic range and is further complicated by changes when a patient is reducing their cigarette intake, abruptly quit in the setting of acute illness and/or hospitalization, or recently quit. These considerations are critical when managing patients and their cessation treatment plan.[50,53]

PHARMACOTHERAPY AND TREATMENT OF TOBACCO DEPENDENCE

In 2015, 68% of adult smokers expressed an interest in quitting smoking and 55.4% reported having attempted to quit in the past year. But only 7.4% were successful in quitting and less than one third of those attempting to quit smoking were engaged in cessation counseling and/or treatment.[22] People are often working on quitting smoking alone, without counseling or treatment and it is largely these same people who are less likely to be successful. However, research clearly demonstrates that being given a chance to help quit with counseling and treatment greatly improves the odds of success in quitting for good.

The seminal work Treating Tobacco Use and Dependence: Clinical Practice Guideline, 2008 Update remains a key resource and is recommended to anyone working in tobacco control and helping people quit smoking.[24] Since the release of this clinical practice guideline, research has continued to demonstrate the effectiveness of tobacco treatment, the safety of current pharmacologic therapies, and how to use them (see Tables 22-1 and 22-2).[24]

All first-line pharmacotherapies for nicotine dependence principally target the α4β2*nAChR receptors and expression of neurohormones with the primary mechanism being prevention of the unpleasant symptoms of nicotine withdrawal that is one of the greatest motivators in continuance of smoking. Partnership with the patient in designing and choosing an effective pharmacotherapy treatment plan is the first monumental step in successful smoking cessation and relapse prevention.

Nicotine Replacement Therapy

Nicotine replacement therapy (NRT) is one of the longest standing, first-line, and most available treatments for smoking cessation and offers a 1.6 to 2.0-fold increased chance of successful cessation compared to placebo.[54,55]

NRT is available in various forms, including long-acting transdermal patch, as well as short-acting delivery systems like gum, nasal spray, inhaler, and lozenges. These can be introduced into any smoking cessation treatment plan and are ideally tailored to the patient's specific preferences and needs.

The mechanism of action of both the long-acting and short-acting delivery systems is replacing the nicotine that the α4β2*nAChR receptors are accustomed to, and if dosed and administered properly, can greatly reduce and ideally prevent nicotine withdrawal and the unpleasant symptoms that accompany this physical phenomenon that often motivates people to reinitiate smoking.

A systematic review of 150 trials of NRT, examining over 50,000 people, illustrates the significant opportunity for successful cessation. All forms of NRT were reported to increase the chances of cessation by as much as 50% to 70% and using a combination of long-acting nicotine transdermal patch with a short-acting nicotine yielded even higher rates of quitting.[56,57]

Nicotine Transdermal Patch as a Long-Acting Delivery System

While outcomes data are favorable, properly dosing NRT is critical in achieving this long-term quit success for patients. It is common for patients to complain that the patch did not work for them, qualifying their reports with evidence that they were still experiencing cravings to smoke, even with the patch in place. These reports are evidence the patient is experiencing withdrawal symptoms and translates to subtherapeutic levels and underdosing of NRT.

The transdermal patch is a long-acting delivery system and should be dosed based on a patient's daily nicotine intake. In the setting of cigarette smoking, each cigarette delivers approximately

1 mg of nicotine. The total number of full cigarettes smoked daily should be accounted for and multiplied by one to determine the necessary dose of the transdermal patch. Ideally, the dosing of the patch will be as closely matched as possible to the daily nicotine intake by cigarettes. This will ensure maintenance of adequate therapeutic levels, allay unnecessary symptoms of nicotine withdrawal, and ease the frequency of breakthrough urges to smoke and dosing requirements of short-acting NRT.

Example calculation: For a patient who smokes one pack per day (20 cigarettes).

$$(20 \text{ cigarettes/day} \times 1 \text{ mg/cigarette} = 20 \text{ mg nicotine needed daily by nicotine patch})$$

The patch is intended to be worn around the clock to deliver a constant and steady dose of nicotine with minimal disruption in serum and tissue concentrations. However, some people complain of feeling too activated at bedtime and may experience insomnia while on the patch. If this is the case, the patient can take the patch off an hour before bedtime and restart a fresh patch as soon as they wake up, with the understanding that the steady state of the nicotine will drop overnight, as the patch has been off, and it takes at least an hour for the nicotine levels to rise to sufficient levels and reduce cravings for smoking.

Sharing this information with patients and educating about cravings in the morning helps them plan for these disruptions. Educating them to treat any cravings, regardless if they wore the patch at night or not, with short-acting nicotine upon waking and until their symptoms abate (i.e., a steady nicotine state is achieved), with the placement of a new patch, will reduce the risk that they will use a cigarette to address their cravings and position them for success.

Patients will ask about cutting their patches in half, when reducing the dose and/or to reduce costs. It is important to preemptively advise patients to never cut the patch. Disruption of the patch through cutting will change the long-acting delivery mechanism of the medication and can be dangerous.

Patients may report that they cannot get the patch to stick to their skin under certain conditions (sweaty and moist skin, hairy areas). They may be counseled that they can place the patch anywhere on their body, including their foot, if necessary. If they have trouble getting the patch to stay on, they may try using a waterproof transparent film dressing over the patch to reinforce adherence to the skin (Table 22-3).

Short-Acting Nicotine Replacement Therapy for Breakthrough Cravings

Whenever patients are experiencing a reduction in their nicotine delivery by cigarettes, whether they are reducing cigarette intake, are embarking upon or are fully engaged in a cessation treatment plan and on any of the treatment modalities that are discussed in this chapter, or working on staying quit, they will experience breakthrough urges or cravings to smoke. Short-acting nicotine replacement is like a rescue medication and referred to as a "reliever" medication. Choosing the best short-acting delivery method, that is a personalized fit for each patient, is a critical step in providing them the backup they need, in case they suffer withdrawal symptoms, nicotine cravings, and cues to smoke a cigarette. Possession of this short-acting nicotine and teaching them to use it, instead of smoking a cigarette when they experience any withdrawal symptoms, will provide them the pharmacologic tools they need, the physiologic and psychological relief from the symptoms they may experience, and the confidence to get smoke-free and ultimately "stay quit" as an ex smoker.

Short-acting NRT is available in a variety of delivery systems and formulas and is used to prevent or treat breakthrough urges to smoke. Understanding the various systems and formulas, the nuances of dosing, and conditions in which these should be prescribed and administered is useful for the nurse to know and facilitate clinical questions, as they review tobacco history, current use, consider appropriate cessation treatment options, discover noncompliance to treatment, and scout for treatment side effects or subtherapeutic dosing with patients.

Table 22-3 • RECOMMENDED INITIAL DOSING OF NICOTINE PATCH THERAPY BASED ON NUMBER OF CIGARETTES SMOKED DAILY

Cigarettes per Day	Patch Dose (mg/day)[a]
<10	7–14
10–20	14–21
21–40	21–42
>40	42+

[a]Nicotine patches are available in the following doses: 7, 14, and 21 mg.
From The ASAM Principles of Addiction Medicine (2014) published by Wolters Kluwer.

Nicotine Gum and Lozenge

Nicotine gum and lozenge are available over the counter in 2-mg and 4-mg doses. Both rely on delivery of nicotine through the mucosal tissue of the mouth.

Due to the mechanism of oral absorption of nicotine by gum or lozenge and metabolism, only 50% of the dose of gum and lozenges is delivered to the brain, even in the most optimal conditions. This means that a 2-mg nicotine gum or lozenge delivers approximately 1 mg of nicotine. Similarly, a 4-mg nicotine gum or lozenge delivers approximately 2 mg of nicotine.

Administration for optimal delivery and therapeutic effects of gum and lozenges is highly dependent on how they are used. Gum is intended to be chewed for a minute (activate and express the nicotine) and tucked in the cheek for 5 minutes (allow absorption of nicotine through direct contact with the mucosal tissue), then chewed for a minute and tucked again for 5 minutes; continuing this cycle for a full 30 minutes. The lozenge is intended to be tucked between only the gum and cheek until fully dissolved, not placed on the tongue or chewed. Some patients experience some burning with the gum and lozenge in which case they can move it side to side in the mouth for relief.

If not administered by the patient as prescribed, nicotine will be swallowed and can lead to nausea, gastrointestinal disturbance, and acid reflux. Furthermore, nicotine will not absorb in an acidic environment or provide therapeutic effect. Acidic beverages and drinking while the gum or lozenge is in the mouth should also be avoided.

Many patients suffer from xerostomia (dry mouth) and some formulations of the lozenge do not dissolve as readily and are reported to take up to several hours to dissolve. This delays the delivery of nicotine and the mediating withdrawal symptoms and is found to be unacceptable for most patients. The over-the-counter, miniature nicotine lozenges dissolve the most readily and are easily snapped in half for half dosing, depending on the intensity of the craving and dosing needs.[8]

Patients who are edentulous (without teeth) or have poor oral health, including missing or broken teeth, or oral sores, will not be able to chew the nicotine gum, therefore nicotine lozenge, inhaler, or nasal spray would be a better choice. It is important to note that no more than 20 lozenges or 24 pieces of gum should be consumed every 24 hours.

Nicotine Inhaler

A nicotine inhaler is NOT an electronic device (e-cigarette, vape, vape pen, Juul, etc.) but available by prescription only. This inhaler is often overlooked as a therapeutic short-acting nicotine delivery system but is covered by many insurers and an effective option for many patients. The inhaler is a small device that has cartridges of dry nicotine (powder). The cartridge is placed in the inhaler and the patient sucks or puffs vigorously to administer the nicotine powder in the mouth with absorption through the mucosal tissue. It is important to let the patient know that they do NOT inhale like smoking a cigarette.

Perhaps the most common error in prescribing and administering this medication is underdosing due to a lack of understanding that each cartridge has approximately 80 puffs of nicotine (i.e., a total of 4 mg of nicotine or the equivalent of 4 cigarettes). It takes 20 puffs to deliver 1 mg of nicotine (equivalent of one cigarette of nicotine). Recommendations for patients would be 20 to 40 puffs every hour as needed for urges to smoke.[58] A patient who normally smokes one pack per day (20 cigarettes) would use five nicotine inhaler cartridges daily. This nicotine replacement option is especially appealing to patients who are attached to the hand-to-mouth rituals of smoking.

There a few key considerations when choosing oral nicotine replacement for patients. Smoking is a significant risk factor for periodontal disease, and it is not uncommon for long-time smokers to have dental decay, broken teeth, and sensitive mouths. Examining patient's mouths and asking them about the comfort with eating, chewing gum, etc. is critical in determining the best option that sets them up for compliance and success.

The gum and inhaler are not good options for patients who wear dentures; the dentures will block the contact of the medication with the mucosal tissue and nicotine will not be absorbed. Nicotine lozenges are the best option for patients who wear dentures.

Nicotine Nasal Spray

Many nurses, healthcare providers, and patients are not familiar with the nicotine nasal spray as a short-acting nicotine delivery system. This is available by prescription and like other intranasal actuation systems is delivered with a spray pump. This medication acts fast and is delivered through the mucosal tissue by spraying in the nostril. One spray delivers 0.5 mg (equivalent of half cigarette) and 2 sprays 1.0 mg (equivalent of one full cigarette) of nicotine. The patient can instill 1 spray in each nostril, up to 10 sprays an hour.[58] It is normal for the spray to burn in the nostril, but patients usually get accustomed to this experience and can tolerate it over time. Educating the patient that they may experience this will prevent any surprise and reassure them that it is normal.

Bupropion

Bupropion has an FDA indication as a first-line treatment for nicotine dependence and increases the chances of quitting smoking by 80% compared to placebo.[59] As an antidepressant, bupropion inhibits dopamine and norepinephrine (neurohormone) reuptake, allowing for higher levels of endogenous neurohormones to circulate. Bupropion also blocks α4β2*nAChR activity and these two mechanisms reduce the cravings for cigarettes while mitigating withdrawal symptoms.

When taking bupropion, side effects most notable in clinical trials are insomnia (30% to 40%), dry mouth (10%), and nausea. These can be largely mitigated if the extended release (SR or XL) formulations are prescribed and when taken with a meal. Bupropion is more activating than sedating and can be too activating for some patients and can even cause anxiety. If this occurs, it can be helpful to lower the dose and sometimes it needs to be stopped, if the symptoms are uncontrollable and/or disruptive.

Seizures are considered a serious adverse event and occur at a rate of 1 in 1000 people who are taking bupropion. Seizure risk is dose dependent (the higher the dose, the higher the risk of seizure) and occurs less frequently in those taking the extended release formulation, excluding participants who have a history of seizure or eating disorder. For this reason, bupropion should be avoided in people with a history of seizures and eating disorders. Furthermore, bupropion is a CYP2D6 inhibitor and caution should be taken especially when prescribing or discontinuing antidepressants, which are commonly inhibitors or inducers of the CYP2D6 pathway.[58,59] It is important to note that it is safe to use both long-acting and short-acting NRT in combination with bupropion.

Varenicline

Varenicline is a partial agonist of the α4β2*nAChR receptors with a 500-fold affinity for these receptors. This medication effectively attaches to and blocks the α4β2*nAChR receptors and the associated nicotine reward, diminishes the chances of nicotine withdrawal, and prevents cravings for nicotine.[60]

The Evaluating Adverse Events in a Global Smoking Cessation Study (EAGLES) trial showed that varenicline is more effective than the other first-line treatments (Bupropion and NRT) and placebo, with sustained smoking cessation at the end of 9 to 12 treatment weeks and 12 to 24 follow-up (nontreatment) weeks.[55] Systematic reviews comparing varenicline to NRT and bupropion demonstrated more than double the chance of smoking cessation on standard doses of varenicline and double the chances of quitting with lower doses of varenicline.[61] Because of the mechanism of action of varenicline and its attachment to the α4β2*nAChR receptors, it directly competes with the presence of nicotine and smoking is not well tolerated when taking varenicline.

Typical dosing of this medication includes a slow increasing taper over 10 days. Patients are generally allowed to smoke during this time, with the intent of reducing cigarette intake and setting a quit date for the day of transition to the full, twice daily, dosing.

There is a 25% prevalence of nausea when taking varenicline.[55] Patients must take this medication with food, and a full glass of water is recommended to avoid nausea. It is possible to flood the α4β2*nAChR receptors if a patient is smoking too much while on varenicline, and this can cause nausea. It is helpful to educate the patients on the mechanism of this medication so as to understand why nausea occurs and most importantly, what they can do to avoid the nausea but to also allow nausea to be a reminder that it is time to reduce the cigarette intake even more, until they have quit. Even when cigarette intake is reduced, or smoking cessation has been achieved, patients may experience nausea. In this case, it is possible to reduce the varenicline dose, still benefit from effect from the medication, and avoid the nausea (or at least reduce it to tolerable levels).

Occupancy of the α4β2*nAChR receptors, whether it be by nicotine or varenicline causes stimulation of the central nervous system. Sometimes varenicline can be too stimulating for patients and can make them feel nervous, jumpy, shaky, or disrupt their sleep patterns. If this occurs, it can be helpful to reduce the dose or take the bedtime dose earlier in the evening (with food). Patients commonly describe active, colorful, and memorable dreaming when they are taking varenicline. This is tolerable for most patients but in the event this activity is disturbing or undesired, reducing the evening dose can mitigate these symptoms.

The protein binding and metabolism of varenicline is minimal (less than 20%) with 92% excreted in the urine. This medication would not be safe for patients with significant kidney impairment and dosing adjustments are indicated if creatinine clearance is less than 30 mL/min. It is safe to prescribe this medication in patients with liver disease; no dose adjustment necessary (Table 22-4).[58]

SAFETY OF PHARMACOTHERAPY IN PSYCHIATRIC DISEASE

For several decades, varenicline and bupropion carried black box warnings with concern that these medications might cause psychiatric side effects. The U.S. Food and Drug Administration (FDA) required the manufacturers of these medications to conduct a randomized trial to study this comprehensively. Referred to previously, the landmark EAGLES trial enrolled over 8000 people and examined the neuropsychiatric safety of varenicline and bupropion compared to NRT and placebo in (1) patients who had documented history of psychiatric disease but were psychiatrically stable at time of enrollment and (2) patients who had no psychiatric history.[55]

This study was a randomized, double-blind, triple-dummy, placebo-controlled, and active-controlled trial where both populations of patients were randomized to treatment with varenicline, bupropion, NRT, or placebo for 12 weeks and 12-week follow-up after treatment. The results of this study did not demonstrate a significant difference in neuropsychiatric adverse events; in fact, the incidence was quite comparable across the two groups.[55] Following the release of these findings, in 2016 the black box warnings for associated neuropsychiatric side effects for varenicline and bupropion were lifted.

Because of the neurohormonal interplay of nicotine and partial-nicotinic acetylcholine receptor blockers, in the setting of smoking cessation and treatment thereof, it is essential to understand that patients can experience disruption of their neurohormones and subsequent symptoms including but not limited to changes in mood, agitation, anxiety, hostility, depression, psychosis, suicidal ideation, or others. Patients should be educated about the neurohormonal changes that occur, how pharmacotherapy for the treatment of nicotine dependence works, and potential symptoms they may experience so they may identify them early and report them as soon as possible.

SAFETY OF PHARMACOTHERAPY IN CARDIOVASCULAR DISEASE

As discussed earlier, patients who are afflicted by addiction to cigarettes carry a significant cardiac risk and an even higher risk if they have had a past cardiac event and continue to smoke; therefore, cessation treatment is a high priority. With the emphasis on addressing and treating tobacco dependence, there has been great interest in studying the potential risk of smoking cessation pharmacologic treatment regimens and the risk of an acute coronary event.

The Canadian health system conducted an interesting observational study in which administrative data was reviewed over a 3.5-year time span, with the purpose of determining, in a real-world setting, if varenicline was associated with a greater risk of acute cardiac events. In this review, 6317 of 56,851 new users of varenicline were hospitalized or admitted to the emergency department for an acute cardiovascular event, demonstrating a 34% higher risk when compared to the control interval.[62]

Table 22-4 • SUGGESTIONS FOR THE CLINICAL USE OF PHARMACOTHERAPIES FOR SMOKING CESSATION[a]

Pharmacotherapy	Adverse Effects	Dosage	Duration
SR bupropion hydrochloride (*Precautions:* history of seizure, history of eating disorders)	Insomnia, dry mouth, seizures	150 mg every morning for 3 days, then 150 mg twice daily (begin treatment 1–2 weeks prequit)	7–12 weeks Maintenance up to 6 months
Nicotine gum	Mouth soreness, dyspepsia	1–24 cigarettes/day: 2 mg gum (up to 24 pieces/day); ≥25 cigarettes/day: 4 mg gum (up to 24 pieces/day)	Up to 12 weeks
Nicotine inhaler	Local irritation of mouth and throat	6–16 cartridges/day	Up to 6 months
Nicotine lozenge	Nausea/heartburn	Time to first cigarette >30 minutes: 2-mg lozenge Time to first cigarette ≤30 minutes: 4-mg lozenge Between 4 and 20 lozenges/day	Up to 12 weeks
Nicotine nasal spray	Nasal irritation	8–40 doses/day	3–6 months
Nicotine patch	Local skin reaction, insomnia	For example, 21 mg/24 h 14 mg/24 h 7 mg/24 h	4 weeks initial dosage 2 weeks decreased dosage 2 weeks decreased dosage OR
		For example, 15 mg/16 h	8 weeks
Varenicline (*Precautions:* significant kidney disease, patients on dialysis	Nausea/trouble sleeping, abnormal or vivid/strange dreams, depressed mood, and other psychiatric symptoms	0.5 mg/day for 3 days 0.5 mg twice/day for 4 days. Then, 1 mg twice/day (begin treatment 1 week prequit)	3–6 months

[a]The information contained in this table is not comprehensive. See package inserts for additional information including safety information.
Reprinted from U.S. Department of Health and Human Services. *Treating Tobacco Use and Dependence: Clinical Practice Guideline, 2008 Update.* Washington, DC: Government Printing Office; 2008.

Conversely, the aforementioned, scrupulously designed EAGLES trial was conducted at 140 multinational centers with 8058 participants. The primary endpoint of this study was time to development of a major adverse cardiovascular event (cardiovascular death, nonfatal myocardial infarction, or nonfatal stroke) during treatment (bupropion, nicotine patch, varenicline, or placebo) and secondary endpoints of this study, during same treatment were new-onset or worsening peripheral vascular disease requiring intervention, coronary revascularization, or hospitalization for unstable angina. The incidence of cardiovascular events during treatment was statistically insignificant for both primary and secondary end points, and was not significantly different across all treatment groups.[63]

This research on cardiac risks of tobacco cessation treatments is mixed with varying outcomes, and may illustrate significant differences due to study design (i.e., observational study versus a high-quality, head-to-head, randomized controlled trial), demographics of study participants, and omissions of independent variables. Regardless, healthcare providers and teams need to evaluate each patient individually, calculate their cardiac risk, share this information with patients, and counsel them about their options, including the potential risks of treatment, and the exponential and temporal risks of no treatment, and the continuance of smoking.

AUGMENTED APPROACHES FOR SUCCESSFUL CESSATION

Reduce-to-Quit Strategies Are Effective in Helping Patients Quit Smoking

For many smokers, it is very difficult to imagine approaching smoking cessation and achieving success in quitting. However, many smokers express interest in quitting, or at least trying to quit, and should be provided the opportunity to take steps toward quitting, rather than assuming an all-or-nothing stance on their cessation options, and risk alienating the patient.

A reduce-to-quit plan can be instrumental in helping smokers try pharmacotherapy and/or reduce their daily cigarette intake, without the fright of committing to a quit date and the risk of failing. Rather, a reduce-to-quit plan provides patients the opportunity to initiate therapy and develop knowledge, experience, and confidence in approaching quitting.

The reduce-to-quit plan on pharmacotherapy is effective. This has been evident in emerging research conducted in patients who were unwilling or unable to commit to a smoking cessation plan, but willing to take medication and reduce cigarette intake. This concept is well illustrated in a randomized-controlled trial that randomly selected participants to either take varenicline or placebo, and all participants were to reduce cigarettes according to a reduction schedule. The varenicline group outperformed placebo with sustained quit rates of 32.1%, compared to 6.9% in the placebo group at 15 through 24 weeks. 37.8% were sustained quit in the varenicline group compared to 12.5% in the placebo group at 21 to 24 weeks, and 27% were sustained quit for the varenicline group compared to 9.9% for the placebo group at 21 through 52 weeks. Comparatively, taking varenicline with a reduce-to-quit cigarette reduction plan triples the chances that a patient will quit smoking.[64] There are many options for patients to approach how to quit smoking, depending on their stages of change and readiness to quit. A reduce-to-quit plan can provide a low-pressure plan that places the patient in control and moves them closer to their goal.

Recognizing and Treating Nicotine Dependence as a Chronic Disease

By all accounts, nicotine dependence is a chronic disease arguably more lethal than many chronic diseases, and should be treated as such. Due to the addictive properties of nicotine, the chronic relapsing nature of nicotine addiction, and the need for ongoing management, like other chronic diseases, it is crucial for nurses to possess foundational knowledge of nicotine dependence, inquire about use of tobacco products, and assess readiness to quit in every patient encounter, including clinical encounters with cardiac patients.

Extended Duration of Nicotine Dependence Treatment

Given the permanent neurohormonal alterations of the brain, accompanying complexities of physiologic dependence, psychological interplay, and behavioral components of nicotine dependence, as discussed earlier in this chapter, some patients will require ongoing treatment to avoid relapse and remain smoke-free.

The current recommendation for a treatment course of NRT is 12 weeks but research has examined the efficacy of longer, treatment courses for better outcomes. Schnoll et al. conducted a parallel randomized, placebo-controlled trial in which 568 adults were randomized to an 8-week treatment with 21-mg nicotine transdermal patch, 16-week with placebo transdermal patch, or an extended 24-week treatment with a 21-mg nicotine transdermal patch. Using biochemical confirmation, this study demonstrated the participants who received the extended therapy with transdermal nicotine were nearly twice as likely to experience successful abstinence at 24 weeks post quit date than those who received standard therapy.[65] Equally important for those on extended therapy with the transdermal nicotine patch, the relapse rates were fewer. Furthermore, for the participants who did relapse, it was later than those who were not on extended therapy and participants who experienced a lapse had a greater chance of recovery.

Like the management of other addictions, and consistent with the chronic disease care model, the option for ongoing pharmacologic treatment and/or behavioral therapy should be considered for highly nicotine-dependent patients, who suffer ongoing cravings or relapse, and are motivated to quit and stay quit. Treating over the continuum and until the patient can confidently get smoke-free and remain so is a much safer option than lifelong smoking.[66]

Behavioral Therapy for Tobacco Dependence

Behavioral therapy includes a broad cadre of interventions and may include individual counseling, group or telephone counseling, text messaging, web-based self-help programs, and smartphone applications. These behavioral interventions are supportive and usually focused on educating patients about withdrawal symptoms, understanding how to identify triggers for smoking and navigating the triggers to avoid smoking, and addressing coping skills as well as stress management strategies.[67]

Treatment for nicotine dependence and smoking with proper management of pharmacotherapy enhances the chances that a patient will be successful in quitting smoking. Combining this treatment with behavioral therapy is also beneficial. Pooled estimates based on 47 randomized and quasirandomized clinical trials demonstrate a 10% to 25% increased chance of successfully quitting smoking when behavioral therapy is provided by phone or in person and in combination with pharmacotherapy.[68] Lancaster et al. conducted a systematic review of high-quality randomized and quasirandomized control trials, examining the relationship between individual in-person counseling compared to minimal behavioral intervention (provision of self-help materials, advice, usual care) and successful smoking cessation. This systematic analysis revealed that when combining individual counseling with or without pharmacotherapy, patients can experience a 40% to 80% increased chance of quitting smoking.[69]

Providing patients with combination behavioral and pharmacotherapy is superior to either intervention as compared to stand-alone interventions. Access to these resources varies and patients may have specific preferences, or hesitancy for certain behavioral interventions. Nurses should be aware of what resources are available so that related discussions with patients may occur and personalized recommendations and referrals may be made with ease.

RELAPSE PREVENTION, SETTING THE STAGE FOR SUCCESSFUL AND SUSTAINED CESSATION

Addiction is a complex and dynamic biopsychosocial and cognitive process that is influenced by physiologic mechanisms that drive the chemical dependence. Addiction is a burden heavily weighted with a psychosocial component that is motivated by learned behaviors and deeply rooted in environmental influences and social exposures. When counseling about cessation, understanding the difference between a "lapse" and a "relapse" and sharing this with patients will assist them in navigating their cessation plan, avoid self-defeat during treatment, and prevent relapse.[70] A *lapse* is defined as a brief disruption in abstinence, and a *relapse* is a break in abstinence with a return to regular patterns of smoking. Lapses in smoking are not uncommon in cessation attempts and often results in relapse.[71]

Relapse rates in smokers are high, especially when they are approaching cessation efforts alone or have a break in their cessation treatment plan.[72,73] Relapse prevention is on the continuum of smoking cessation and once cessation has been achieved, the relapse prevention journey begins. As discussed throughout this chapter, relapse prevention is critically important and begins with behavioral and pharmacologic treatment as the cornerstone for achieving and maintaining successful cessation. Cognitive behavioral processes such as self-efficacy, outcome expectancies, craving, motivation, affective states, coping behaviors, substance use, and perceived effects have all been identified as determinants of relapse and represent the critical and complex constructs of the Cognitive-Behavioral Model of Relapse that assist in understanding the dynamic nature of relapse.[74,75] Integration of relapse models into the implementation of relapse prevention and care of smokers may be useful in helping them understand and address these determinants in order to reduce the risk of lapse and relapse, and succeed in quitting and staying quit.[71] Relapse prevention is a science in and of itself, and worth further inquiry for nurses who are working in smoking cessation. As with all cessation approaches, it is ideal for relapse prevention work to be integrated into a chronic disease care model that includes ongoing behavioral therapy with consideration of extended or intermittent pharmacotherapy, as necessary (Fig. 22-2).

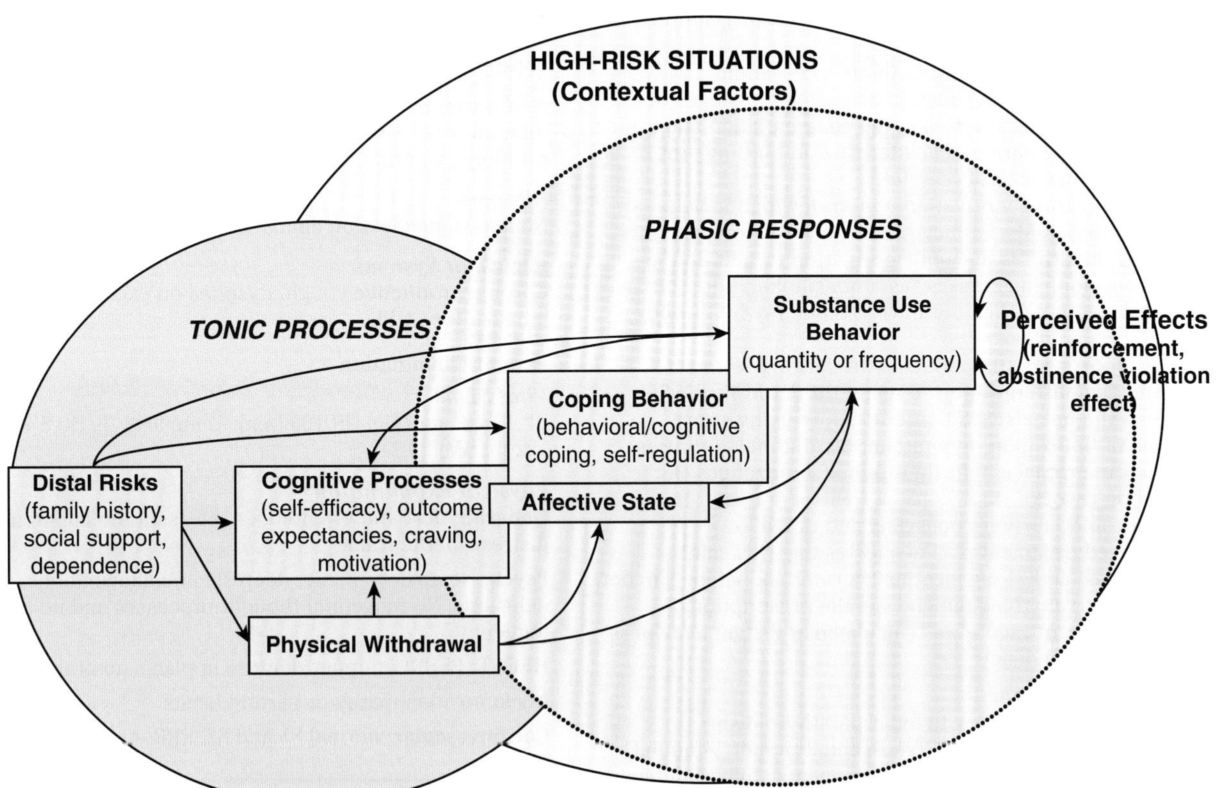

Figure 22-2. Dynamic model of relapse. (From The ASAM Principles of Addiction Medicine [2014] published by Wolters Kluwer.)

Summary

Nurses are instrumental in smoking cessation as front-line members of the healthcare team. They have the unique opportunity to initiate interventions that can be life saving for smokers. By seizing the opportunity to ask key questions and listen to patients to understand their current health state and behaviors, identify tobacco use, assess interest in smoking cessation, and detect the need for medication treatment or adjustments, nurses can initiate effective smoking cessation efforts and literally help save the lives of thousands of smokers in the United States. In the setting of smoking and smoking cessation, the nurse's presence and knowledgeable inquiry can be instrumental in revealing patient misperceptions about treatment, hesitancy, noncompliance with or failure of treatment regimens due to inadequate dosing or side effects, or uncontrolled withdrawal symptoms and breakthrough urges to smoke. All these issues can be addressed by nursing, and greatly influence a patient's trajectory to successful quit.

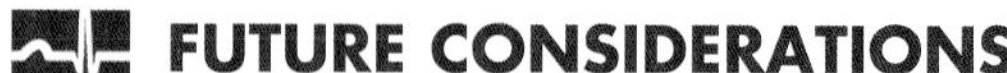

FUTURE CONSIDERATIONS

Although the prevalence of smoking cigarettes is on a continued downward trend in the United States, both the access to and utilization of addictive electronic nicotine delivery systems (e-cigarettes) is on the rise, and global utilization of inhaled tobacco by way of cigarettes, is on a steep upward trajectory with over 900 million people worldwide smoking cigarettes.[7] The contributing factors to this disturbing trend are multifactorial and represent a global epidemic of unnecessary morbidity and mortality from smoking-related cardiovascular disease and other devastating diseases. As the largest healthcare workforce in the world (19.3 million nurses)[76] nurses are perfectly positioned to fight this war on tobacco through proactive patient care and perhaps even more importantly, through their voices and advocacy work to change and implement local, state, and federal health policy, and influence marketing, access to, exposure, and the distribution of tobacco products. Nurses are encouraged to find a way to get involved and strive for meaningful change.

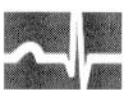

CASE-BASED LEARNING 1

Patient Profile

History of Present Illness

Ms. Quincy is a 73-year-old African American female who presents to the clinic for follow-up medication refill of her cardiac medications. She has an 80 pack-year history of smoking (1.5 packs per day for 53 years), currently smoking 1 to 1.5 packs per day (20 to 30 cigarettes). She starts her day with 2 cigarettes before she sets the coffee; this is followed by 1 to 2 more cigarettes within the first hour of awakening. She reports that it takes her about 7 minutes to smoke a cigarette.

The 5As were engaged to facilitate a cessation conversation with Ms. Quincy. In assessing her stages of change, she identifies herself in the contemplation stage and qualifies this by sharing, "I'm interested in quitting, but I don't think I'll ever be successful."

Upon launching motivational interviewing for behavior change with her, Ms. Quincy reports a 5/10 motivation to quit with "health" as her only motivation to quit and in this discussion, she advises "as a nonsmoker, I don't expect you to understand this, but I LOVE filling my lungs with smoke!".

She reports 6.5/10 confidence in quitting, with one previous 9-month quit period using the "cold turkey" method. She has also had quit attempts using short courses of bupropion, hypnotism, diversional activities, and nicotine replacement therapy (NRT) lozenges but "they didn't work."

SQ accepted further counseling and opted for a personalized treatment plan of short-acting NRT mini-lozenge, 4-mg and 21-mg nicotine transdermal patch. "I'm not committing to anything but give me the prescriptions."

Her Fagerström score was calculated at 8/10 in heaviness of nicotine dependency.

Past Medical History

Hypercalcemia secondary to hyperparathyroidism, pyelonephritis, COPD per PFTs, essential tremor, vitamin D deficiency, osteopenia, urinary incontinence, hyperlipidemia, pulmonary nodule, hyperglycemia, possible TIA, ETOH dependence, subarachnoid hemorrhage secondary to trauma, thyroid nodules, wears glasses and hearing aids.

Past Surgical History

Partial parathyroidectomy

Family History

Father: coronary artery disease (smoker), hyperlipidemia, hypertension
Daughter: morbid obesity, diabetes
Mother: morbid obesity, diabetes, hyperlipidemia

Social History

Widowed × 20 years, born and raised in Washington. Retired data analyst. Writes and reads for fun. Drinks one to two cocktails a night.

Medications

Vitamin B-12, loratadine, atorvastatin, potassium chloride, probiotic, aspirin

Allergies

No known medication allergies

Review of Systems

Chronic productive cough, dyspnea on exertion and on inhalers for COPD

Patient Examination

Vital Signs

BP 138/84 mm Hg; HR 100 bpm; Temp 98.9 °F; Ht. 5′1″; Wt. 122 lb; BMI 23.2

Physical Examination

General: Alert and oriented × 4, pleasant, no apparent distress, petite frame

Psych: No anxiety, panic, depression, hallucinations, or delusions. No tangential thought processes and no suicidal tendency.

HEENT: PERRLA, upper denture in place, no oral lesions

Neck: no adenopathy or carotid bruits

Cardiovascular: normal S1 and S2, RRR, no murmur, gallop, or rub

Pulmonary: Clear to auscultation throughout, no wheezes, rales, or rhonchi

Abdomen: soft, nontender

CASE-BASED LEARNING 1 (*Continued*)

In-Person Smoking Cessation Follow-Up Visit (2 Weeks Later)
Since our last visit, Ms. Quincy filled her prescription for 21-mg nicotine transdermal patches and purchased NRT lozenges. She shares, "I'm not committing to a quit date, but I want to know how to get started." She now identifies herself in the preparation stage of change but demonstrates great hesitancy in starting the replacement therapy. She is counseled on a Reduce-to-Quit plan while integrating NRT lozenges for breakthrough urges to smoke. A follow-up call in a week is scheduled, or sooner as needed.

Telephonic Visit 1 (10 Days Later)
Upon first telephonic follow-up visit, Ms. Quincy shares that she made a chart on her computer to start tracking her daily cigarette intake. Her goal this week was to only smoke 25 cigarettes per day, but she got down to 20 a day. She states: "I can't believe I'm smoking so many less cigarettes! Key is not having the mindless cigarettes. I only did that once. I was at my computer and I had finished one and lit one up without realizing it. Now, I'm using the Nicotine lozenge in my mouth while I'm smoking a cigarette and use it until it's gone; this prevents me from having the urge to smoke a second cigarette."

She denies any symptoms of chemical withdrawal and wants to hold at 20 cigarettes a day for another week. The value of lifestyle ritual and behavior adjustments and journaling was discussed at length. She reports that she has smoked 70 less cigarettes, gained 490 minutes of her life/time not smoking and saved $40! She agrees to a call in a week.

Telephonic Visit 2 (7 Days Later)
Ms. Quincy shares that she was able to maintain her total daily intake at 20 cigs per day using the lozenges (4 mg) about 5 times daily (10 mg total) for breakthrough urges to smoke. She denies withdrawal symptoms and reports that the lozenges are taking a long time to dissolve in her dry mouth. Use of NRT nasal spray for quicker relief of urges to smoke was discussed. She expresses significant interest and prescription sent to pharmacy.

Significant discussion time is spent on behavior modification work, reviewing diversional activities to keep her hands and her mind busy: "My goal is to find things that I can do with my two hands to avoid smoking. I just never thought I could do this and would have never thought of this 'reduce to quit' plan."

Discussion of the nicotine transdermal patch was initiated but she declined to consider this at this time. Introduced the idea of (1) initiating the nicotine transdermal patch (21 mg) when she consistently drops her daily cigarette intake below 20 cigarettes and (2) choosing a quit date. She plans to experiment with the NRT nasal spray for breakthrough urges to smoke and agrees to a follow-up call in 2 weeks.

Telephonic Visit 3 (18 Days Later)
Ms. Quincy reports that she has continued to decrease her daily cigarette intake down and now her rolling daily average cigarette intake is 18! She shares that one day she only had 13 ("I can't believe I did it!") and states "I did have one big fail where I smoked 30 cigarettes and thought I would NEVER do that again!" Discussed what goes well on the days that she only smokes 13 and identified the triggers on the day she smoked 30 cigarettes. She shared that the day she smoked 30 cigarettes, her dog ran away at her apartment complex and she was extremely distressed trying to find the dog on foot due to poor exercise tolerance.

Ms. Quincy reports that she used the nasal spray once for several sprays and got a headache. Discussed that it may have been too much and to only use one spray next time. She purchased the miniature nicotine lozenges, which are more readily dissolving in her mouth; she continues to use the lozenges (4 mg) three to five times daily as needed for urges to smoke, which work to quell the urges. She denies any changes in mood or energy and no thought process changes. She expresses an interest in starting the nicotine transdermal patch but cannot and will not commit to a quit date. She confirmed she has a starter pack and reviewed proper use of the patch, including potential side effects and how to know if she is taking in too little or too much nicotine. She agrees to a follow-up call in a week or sooner as needed.

Telephonic Visit 4 (7 Days Later)
Ms. Quincy reports the rolling average is 16.7 cigs per day: "I know, can you believe it?" She reports using the nasal spray again: one to two sprays upon waking which she's noticed allows her to delay her first cigarette of the day for as much as 2 to 3 hours. She reports needing either the mini-nicotine lozenge (4 mg) or one to two nicotine sprays about 5 times a day. She is averaging one cigarette every hour while awake and now "watching the clock to keep track" of when she can have another cigarette. She shares, "You know, the major change recently is that I don't smoke two cigarettes in a row anymore and that's amazing!" and also reports that she remains reluctant to start the nicotine patch. She is happy with her progress and wants to wait to use it. Current calculated nicotine intake from cigarettes is 16-mg and 10-mg short-acting NRT for a total of 26 mg daily.

Ms. Quincy is in great spirits and focused on goal of getting down to 10 cigs per day by the next call. While she expresses that she is not emotionally ready to choose a quit date, she conveys she is more confident that she may be successful in quitting, in the future.

Telephonic Visit 5 (2 Weeks Later)
Ms. Quincy reports that she has reduced her cigarette intake to 10 cigs per day! She shares, "I have new strategies to reduce. I stopped smoking a cigarette each way to the grocery store every day. This way I could cut another 2 cigarettes a day. I'm keeping myself really busy, and this really helps me avoid smoking."

She reports that she continues the NRT lozenges and spray (one or the other) as needed, average of 4 to 6 times daily. She is experiencing more intense cravings for cigarettes at times. Upon further review and discussion, she realizes that these intense cravings are associated with certain social and environmental triggers like the "after lunch cigarette with my girlfriends or with my cocktail in the evening." Lifestyle ritual and behavior modification were discussed to continue to drive toward cessation. She shares she has employed more strategies to fill her time and avoid smoking by taking more cat naps, making plans out of the house including lunches out and going to the nail salon, and she is reading more books. Current daily nicotine intake calculation is 10 mg from cigarettes smoked and 10 mg from short-acting NRT for a total of 20-mg daily nicotine intake.

When approached about a quit date she shares that she is not ready to choose a quit date but states "I ran out of cigarettes and I didn't buy a carton. I only bought two packs and I don't plan to buy anymore!". Upon further discussion, she agrees to initiate the 21-mg nicotine transdermal patch

(*continued*)

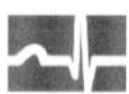

CASE-BASED LEARNING 1 *(Continued)*

and agrees to a follow-up call in a week or sooner as needed.

Telephonic Visit 6 (10 Days Later)

Ms. Quincy instantly shares, "Oh, my GOSH! I went out for the day and forgot to put my cigarettes in my purse, so I didn't smoke all day!" She sees this as "real progress" in her path to getting smoke-free. She had an appointment with her endocrinologist and shares that she got the courage to tell him she is working on quitting. Ms. Quincy relays her annoyance that his reply was, "Well, it just takes will power." She shares, "I thought, 'Well, you know, it does take will power, but it takes a whole lot more than that, including coaching and treatment, to be successful after smoking for 54 years!'". She expressed her gratitude for the calls and guidance. She started the 21-mg nicotine transdermal patch that day and was able to go 20 hours without smoking a cigarette and "didn't go crazy without one". She reports that she has been smoke-free since then with 8 days quit. Cravings are less frequent or intense; she continues to use the short-acting nicotine nasal spray or mini-lozenge just a few times daily with relief.

Ms. Quincy shares, "I walked to the mail box for the first time in many, many years since my husband died. I didn't feel as short of breath and my cough is better. I don't know how in the world I was able to smoke 30 to 40 cigarettes a day!" Positive reinforcement was provided for the progress she is making and ways in which she can continue to identify and avoid triggers to smoke and modify her lifestyle rituals and behaviors to accommodate a smoke-free life.

Telephonic Visit 7 (7 Days Later)

Ms. Quincy finished 2 weeks of the 21-mg nicotine transdermal patch and transitioned to the 14-mg patch a few days ago. She initially noted a surge in breakthrough urges to smoke and was using the short-acting nicotine replacement 5 to 7 times daily (as instructed) but is now only using the NRT spray or mini-lozenge two to three times daily.

She reports that she remains smoke-free! "My strategy is to put all my energy into thinking about NOT smoking. I won't lie; I entertain getting into the car and going to the corner store to buy 'just one more pack'; it is this creeping feeling, like the Devil is on my shoulder, but I won't do it."

Her cessation success was reviewed and strategies discussed to maintain her smoke-free life (cessation maintenance) including the 7-mg nicotine transdermal patch treatment plan. She shares reluctance in stepping down too quickly off the 14-mg patch "because things are going so well, I don't want to fail". She is advised that she can purchase some extra 14-mg patches, if needed and can step down at her own pace. She enthusiastically responds to this plan and displays her comfort in "not feeling rushed." She qualifies this by sharing, "You know, it took me this long to get the courage to quit; I'm going to do it the right way, so it sticks."

Introduced the idea and viable option in long-term use of the short-acting nicotine replacement for any urges or cravings to smoke, after the patch regimen is completed, to optimize chances of long-term quit success. She was receptive to this concept of extended cessation treatment.

Telephonic Visit 8 (3 Weeks Later)

Ms. Quincy shares that she used the 14-mg patch for an additional 7 days then stepped down to the 7-mg patches nearly 2 weeks ago with only three left. She continues to use the short-acting nicotine zero to four times daily with relief and expresses "I am ready to stop the patches when these run out. I'm tired of thinking about them." We engaged in motivational interviewing, reviewed the importance of continued lifestyle ritual and behavior modification to reinforce new life as a nonsmoker, and discussed how to manage lapses and to call ASAP in case of need. A follow-up call is planned for 1 month. She agrees to continue using the short-acting NRT spray or mini-lozenge as needed for any breakthrough urges or cravings to smoke. Tobacco cessation will be addressed at all future healthcare encounters.

Summary

Ms. Quincy continued to track her data throughout the quit process. The following reflect her statistical data from the time she initiated her cessation journey to her quit date.

- 3900 less cigarettes smoked since starting reduce-to-quit plan
- 195 less packs of cigarettes
- Saved $1462 in cigarette purchases
- 455 hours = 27,300 minutes saved in time NOT spent smoking

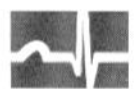

CASE-BASED LEARNING 2

Patient Profile

History of Present Illness

Mrs. Denver is a 60-year-old Caucasian female with a 60 pack-year history of smoking who presents for discussion of new-onset hypertension. She reports an onset of regular smoking at age 14, average one to two packs per day for 41 years, currently smoking one pack per day (20 mg nicotine).

The 5As were engaged to facilitate a cessation conversation. In assessing her stages of change, Mrs. Denver identifies herself as in the contemplation stage and qualifies this by sharing, "I think about quitting smoking all the time, I'm just not sure if I can do it."

She is assessed to have 9/10 motivation to quit. Her motivations are health, cost, and "I'm sick and tired of being controlled by these cigarettes and sometimes it's embarrassing for my kids that I smoke. I want my kids to see that I can quit; I can do it. None of them smoke."

She is rated with 4/10 confidence that she can quit and reports three major attempts to quit in past. Bupropion was discontinued due to anxiety. She used patches when she was in the hospital following a motor vehicle accident (MVA). She was "quit" in hospital but as NRT was not continued upon discharge she resumed smoking. She has used the NRT gum but sticks to her dentures. She has not tried varenicline or combination NRT therapy but is open to any treatment plan.

Her reasons to continue smoking include: "It's my break time when I can get away from everyone. It's me time." She does not live with a smoker but socializes with a group who congregate at the mailboxes in her apartment complex to smoke. She reports having a cigarette within the first 5 minutes upon waking and smokes one half to three

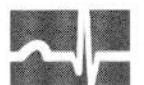

CASE-BASED LEARNING 2 (*Continued*)

quarters of a pack by noon then spreads the remaining 5 to 10 cigarettes out over the balance of the day.

Fagerström score is 8/10 for heaviness of nicotine dependence.

Past Medical History
Bipolar affective disorder, obsessive–compulsive disorder, attention deficit disorder, posttraumatic stress disorder, cervical spine fractures, chronic back pain due to MVA (2000), obesity, hepatitis C, hypothyroidism, obesity, menopause, partial (upper) dentures

Past Surgical History
Spine fusion, appendectomy, two C-sections, left breast biopsy, right knee arthroscopy, left ankle repair, colonoscopy

Family History
Mother: Stroke, myocardial infarction
Father: leukemia
Maternal grandmother: hypothyroid and stroke
Sister: Liver disease

Social History
Mrs. Denver was born and raised in Montana. She is estranged from family and a single mother of four (32-year-old son out of house, 19-year-old daughter cosmetologist and lives at home, 14-year-old twins one of which has special needs and is home schooled). She worked as a retail clerk until she became disabled following the MVA in 2000. She enjoys sewing but has no time to do it.

Medications
Amlodipine 5 mg QD, levothyroxine 25 mcg QD, sertraline 25 mg QD, olanzapine 5 mg QD, lithium carbonate 600 mg QHS, amphetamine-dextroamphetamine 30 mg BID, oxycodone 10 mg QID PRN, ondansetron 4 mg PRN, albuterol multidose inhaler as needed

Allergies
No medication allergies

Review of Systems
No kidney or liver failure. No seizure history. Bipolar disorder has been stable for some time on triple therapy; she is well established with psychiatry with routine follow up. Suffers anxiety intermittently but overall controlled.

Patient Examination

Vital Signs
BP 128/86 mm Hg; HR 85 bpm; SpO_2 98% on room air; Ht. 5′5″; Wt. 90 kg; BMI 38.41

Physical Examination
General: Alert and oriented × 4, calm. No apparent distress. Pleasant.

HEENT: PERRLA, upper denture in place, no oral lesions

Neck: No adenopathy or carotid bruits

Cardiovascular: Normal S1 and S2, RRR; no murmur, gallop, or rub

Pulmonary: Clear to auscultation throughout, no wheezes, rales, or rhonchi

Abdomen: Soft, nontender

Extremities: Upper extremities without edema or clubbing; warm and dry. Lower extremities without edema.

Psych: no anxiety or panic, no evidence for hallucinations, delusions, no tangential thought processes or suicidal tendencies. Positive for pressured speech and high energy but no mania. Humorous.

In-Person Follow-Up Visit (1 Week Later)
Follow-up visit for hypertension and smoking cessation. Mrs. Denver reports that she is still contemplating quitting. She reviewed educational materials and has questions. She was interested in engaging motivational interviewing for behavior change and counseling. She accepted NRT SA nicotine lozenge and was counseled on lozenge use. A reduce-to-quit plan was introduced. She expressed interest in the varenicline and engaged in discussion about this treatment option. By the close of the visit she identified herself in the preparation stage of change and appeared excited to try the NRT. Agreed to a telephonic visit in a few weeks.

Telephonic Visit 1 (14 Days Later)
Mrs. Denver was excited for the call and appreciative for the support. She shared that the lozenges are taking 3 hours to dissolve in her mouth and she feels they are not working. She has a very dry mouth (xerostomia) from psychiatric meds. She expressed frustration but successfully reduced total daily intake of cigarettes by 50% (down to smoking 10 cigarettes a day) and expressed high levels of motivation to continue cessation plan. She accepted NRT nasal spray and engaged in discussion on proper use. A prescription was sent to pharmacy. At the close of the visit, she identified herself in the action phase of change. We discussed the importance of addressing lifestyle and behavior change modification to be successful in quitting. We walked through a typical day and identified areas to start modifying. She agreed to a follow-up call in 1 to 2 weeks and sooner as needed. A clinical note was sent to her psychiatrist and it was requested that she make a follow-up appointment with him soon so he may monitor her psychiatric status and need for any medication adjustments as her cigarette intake is reduced to off.

Telephonic Visit 2 (10 Days Later)
Mrs. Denver shares that she picked up the nasal spray. She was unable to talk due to emergency with son and requested a call back in a week.

Telephonic Visit 3 (7 Days Later)
Mrs. Denver was called for follow-up smoking cessation discussion. She reports not using the nasal spray due to sneezing and burning. She is trying the lozenges but with stress she has relapsed back in her total daily intake to one pack per day. She expressed high motivation to continue cessation efforts and wants to consider varenicline as previously discussed. Given psychiatric history and complex medication regimen, an appointment was made for an in-person visit with the nurse practitioner for further discussion.

In-Person Visit 4 With Nurse Practitioner (7 Days Later)
Mrs. Denver shares that she weaned down to one half pack per day (10 cigarettes) again. She rates her motivation to quit at 10/10 and her confidence in quitting at 6/10 but states "I'm scared to choose a quit date."

Behavioral strategies to accommodate smoke-free living were reviewed. Lifestyle rituals and behaviors that trigger smoking were discussed. She was previously tasked in last telephonic visit to make list of activities she could do instead of smoking and brought in a list of 23 activities, some of which she had adopted with success. She reviewed what is going well and current challenges in quitting. Stress and related anxiety are identified as the major triggers for her to smoke and "that darn brain that just craves smoking."

She denies any depressive/manic swings or suicidal ideation. She is experiencing some anxiety that is controllable. She denies any changes in her psychiatric medications.

(*continued*)

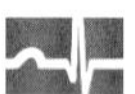

CASE-BASED LEARNING 2 (*Continued*)

Pharmacologic options including varenicline were reviewed. Varenicline starter pack prescribed. She was instructed to continue NRT nasal spray and/or mini-lozenge as needed for cravings and breakthrough urges to smoke. We reviewed side effects and symptoms to report; the majority of time was spent educating on dosing and preventing unpleasant side effects, including taking with food. The visit was closed with motivational interviewing and reinforcement of approaches that support forward progress in her cessation journey. She agreed to telephonic follow-up visit in 2 weeks. Clinical note sent to her psychiatrist.

Telephonic Visit 5 (2 Weeks Later)
Mrs. Denver confirms that she has secured the varenicline. She expressed her gratitude that her insurance company pays for it. She remains unable to choose a quit date but wishes to proceed with a "reduce to quit" plan and has a medication start date in another week.

Varenicline education was provided including avoidance of side effects (take with food and water and pay careful attention to surge in nausea due to concurrent smoking). She voiced a clear understanding of our plan and demonstrated a focused and positive outlook on this plan with humor. Telephonic follow-up in a week is planned, on or around the date of dose increase to twice daily varenicline. She is encouraged to call sooner as needed. The clinic note was sent to her psychiatrist.

Telephonic Visit 6 (1 Week Later)
Today is Mrs. Denver's quit date! She smoked her last cigarette several hours ago and now on the varenicline twice daily, as of today. She has been experiencing intermittent nausea, which she attributes to the varenicline despite taking food, but conveys she was smoking on the medication until today.

She denies any chemical urges to smoke and feels the urges she does experience are all environmental and stress related. She reports she had to stop socializing at the mailboxes with the smokers because "it was a HUGE trigger to smoke".

She denies any neuropsychiatric symptoms, changes in thought processes, or disruption of sleep. She is experiencing anxiety, which remains controllable. A goal was set to start journaling and she identified a sewing project she wants to do to take her mind off smoking. She wants to make pajamas for her kids. Outcome data to track were reviewed including money saved, how much time she's gained in not smoking, and how many less cigarettes she has smoked. A follow-up call later this week is planned, or sooner as needed.

Telephonic Visit 7 (3 Days Later)
Mrs. Denver reports that her last cigarette was 3 days ago! "This is the longest I've never smoked in 40 years! I threw away all the ashtrays yesterday." She shares she is working out each day to some walking tapes and watching movies to stay distracted.

She states, "I am so grateful that you gave me a chance on this medicine and that my insurance company paid for the medication; I want to write them a letter to thank them." She relays she felt more last evening and used an NRT lozenge and went to her room to take a break and calm down, which was effective. She denies any neuropsychiatric symptoms, and continues to sleep well. Mrs. Denver saw her psychiatrist in follow-up last week: "He's so proud of me and I'm proud of myself. I have another appointment with him in a month, but I can call him anytime!" She reports some constipation since quitting smoking. She was reassured that this is normal and was referred to over-the-counter bowel regimens. We reviewed strategies to remain smoke-free and reminded to use the NRT *any* time she experiences anxiety or breakthrough urges to smoke.

Telephonic Visit 8 (2 Weeks Later)
Mrs. Denver has 17 days smoke-free! She reports that the intensity and frequency of the cravings are "Way less! Smoking is not preoccupying my mind." She demonstrates joy and disbelief that she has been successful in quitting smoking.

She shares a stressful social event with her daughter that involved a visit with the police. This would normally "trigger some chain smoking". She went to the store and purchased a pack of cigarettes. But, "even with the chaos, I didn't open the cigarettes, I couldn't do it. I went to the neighbor's and gave the cigs to her."

She did increase the frequency in her use of the NRT nasal spray, which is really helping with cravings and management of anxiety symptoms. She usually starts her day with two to three sprays (1 to 1.5 mg of nicotine).

She further shares "You know, it's working. I'm getting there. This morning I woke up, got my coffee, went to watch the news and after 20 minutes, I realized I hadn't even thought about having a cigarette or using the "snorter" (nasal spray). OH, MY GOLLY, IT'S WORKING!" She is exuberant on the phone, ecstatic about this progress. A clinic note was sent to her psychiatrist.

Telephonic Visit 9 (2 Weeks Later)
Mrs. Denver shares that she's been smoke-free × 31 days now! "I still have urges, like when I finish my chores, or I walk by my balcony where I would normally take a smoke break, so I pulled the drapes and cannot look out there."

Currently using seven to nine NRT (4 to 5 mg nicotine) nasal sprays daily for cravings and anxiety with relief.

"I'm not sure if they are real cravings but the 'snorter' works."

"I'm shocked that I'm smoke-free; I really think the varenicline really, really, works and people should know that!"

"You know, I live in the ghetto, and I have to stay away from the mailbox circle and away from those smokers or I'll cave."

"My daughter bought me a necklace that is a cross with Jesus on it. It commemorates my success in quitting smoking; my kids are watching me closely and they're proud that I quit. I can't let them down."

She was provided positive reinforcement for her success. We discussed continued strategies for medication management and engaged in motivational interviewing for behavior change and reviewed approaches to lifestyle modification to support the behavior changes necessary to stay quit.

Telephonic Visit 10 (1 Month Later)
Mrs. Denver reports that she has been smoke-free for 60 days! She reports, "I cheated once." Her neighbor gave her one and she smoked it and enjoyed it but has not had another and that was 2 weeks ago. She expressed her regret in smoking. "I don't want to go down that road again; it felt awful afterword and wasn't worth it. I've worked too hard to go back now – NO WAY!"

We discussed lapse and relapse and identified this as a lapse. Strategies for these circumstances were reviewed, including how to engage strategies in these risky settings as well as cessation maintenance tools to prevent this from occurring again.

She continues varenicline twice daily. We discussed a plan for a minimum of 3-months' treatment from her quit date. A refill was sent to the pharmacy. She is to continue NRT nasal spray or mini-lozenge, as needed for cravings and anxiety. Cessation maintenance will be addressed at 3-month follow-up hypertension visit or sooner as needed.

CASE-BASED LEARNING CONCLUSIONS

- Nicotine dependence is an addiction and chronic disease and needs to be treated like one.
- Successful smoking cessation requires pharmacologic and behavioral treatment.
- Ongoing quit coaching and counseling is ideal; people are less successful in quitting if they go it alone.
- The cessation journey is highly individual.
- It takes time to quit smoking.
- Do not give up on patients or treatment methods.

Abbreviations: 5As, ask, advise, assist, assess, arrange; COPD, chronic obstructive pulmonary disease; PFTs, pulmonary function tests; TIA, transient ischemic attack; ETOH, alcohol; BP, blood pressure; HR, heart rate; T, temperature; Ht, height; Wt, weight; BMI, body mass index; HEENT, head, eyes, ears, nose, throat; PERRLA, pupils equal round, reactive to light and accommodation; RRR, regular rate and rhythm.

KEY READINGS

Anthenelli RM, Benowitz NL, West R, et al. Neuropsychiatric safety and efficacy of varenicline, bupropion, and nicotine patch in smokers with and without psychiatric disorders (EAGLES): a double-blind, randomised, placebo-controlled clinical trial. *Lancet.* 2016;387(10037):2507–2520.

Barua RS, Rigotti NA, Benowitz NL, et al. 2018 ACC Expert Consensus Decision Pathway on tobacco cessation treatment: a report of the American College of Cardiology Task Force on Clinical Expert Consensus Documents. *J Am Coll Cardiol.* 2018;72(25):3332–3365.

Hurt RD, Ebbert JO, Hays JT, et al. Pharmacologic interventions for tobacco dependence. In: Ries RK, Fiellin DA, Miller SC, et al., eds. *The ASAM Principles of Addiction Medicine.* Philadelphia, PA: Wolters Kluwer; 2014:811–822.

Miller WR, Rollnick S. *Motivational Interviewing: Helping People Change.* 3rd ed. New York: The Guilford Press; 2013.

United States Public Health Service. *Treating Tobacco Use and Dependence: Clinical Practice Guideline 2008 Update.* Rockville, MD: U.S. Dept. of Health and Human Services, Public Health Service; 2008.

REFERENCES

1. Winter JC. *Tobacco Use by Native North Americans: Sacred Smoke and Silent Killer.* Norman, OK: University of Oklahoma Press; 2000.
2. Proctor R. *Golden Holocaust: Origins of the Cigarette Catastrophe and the Case for Abolition.* Berkeley, CA: University of California Press; 2011.
3. Godlaski TM. Holy smoke: tobacco use among Native American tribes in North America. *Subst Use Misuse.* 2013;48(1–2):1–8.
4. La Torre G, Saulle R, Nicolotti N, et al. From nicotine dependence to genetic determinants of smoking. In: La Torre G, ed. *Smoking Prevention and Cessation.* New York: Springer; 2013:1–29.
5. Giardina EG. Cardiovascular effects of nicotine. *Up to Date.* 2017. Availabl at https://www.uptodate.com/contents/cardiovascular-effects-of-nicotine. Accessed June 6, 2018.
6. Stolerman IP, Jarvis MJ. The scientific case that nicotine is addictive. *Psychopharmacology (Berl).* 1995;117(1):2–10; discussion 14–20.
7. Morris PB, Ference BA, Jahangir E, et al. Cardiovascular effects of exposure to cigarette smoke and electronic cigarettes: clinical perspectives from the prevention of cardiovascular disease. *J Am Coll Cardiol.* 2015;66(12):1378–1391.
8. Hurt RD, Ebbert JO, Hays JT, et al. Pharmacologic interventions for tobacco dependence. In: Ries RK, Fiellin DA, Miller SC, et al., eds. *The ASAM Principles of Addiction Medicine.* Philadelphia, PA: Wolters Kluwer; 2014:811–822.
9. Cole HM, Fiore MC. The war against tobacco: 50 years and counting. *JAMA.* 2014;311(2):131–132.
10. Glynn T, Hurt R, Westmaas J. Tobacco. In: Society TAC, ed. *The American Cancer Society's Principles of Oncology: Prevention to Survivorship.* 1st ed. Atlanta, GA: The American Cancer Society; 2018:58–71.
11. Boyle P. *Tobacco and Public Health: Science and Policy.* Oxford, New York: Oxford University Press; 2004.
12. U.S. Department of Health & Human Services. *The Changing Cigarette. How Tobacco Smoke Causes Disease: The Biology and Behavioral Basis for Smoking Attributable Disease.* Rockville, MD: U.S. Department of Health and Human Services; 2010:15–22.
13. Amos A, Mackay J. Tobacco and women. In Boyle P, Gray N, Henningfield J, et al., eds. *Tobacco Science, Policy and Public Health.* New York: Oxford University Press:334.
14. National Institutes of Health, U.S. National Library of Science. *The reports of the surgeon general: The 1964 report on smoking and health.* 2018. Available at https://profiles.nlm.nih.gov/ps/retrieve/Narrative/NN/p-nid/60. Accessed on June 6, 2018.
15. U.S. Department of Health Education and Welfare. *Smoking and Health.* Washington, DC: Report of the Advisory Committee to the Surgeon General of the Public Health Service; 1964:1103.
16. U.S. Department of Health & Human Services. *The Health consequences of smoking—50 years of progress: a report of the Surgeon General 2014. Executive summary.* 2014. Available at https://www.ncbi.nlm.nih.gov/books/NBK179276/pdf/Bookshelf_NBK179276.pdf
17. Department of Health and Human Services. *Smoking Cessation: A Report of the Surgeon General.* Washington (DC): U.S. Department of Health and Human Services, Centers for Disease Control and Prevention, National Center for Chronic Disease Prevention and Health Promotion, Office on Smoking and Health; 2020.
18. Centers for Disease Control and Prevention. Current cigarette smoking among adults—United States, 2016. *MMWR Morb Mortal Wkly Rep.* 2018;67(2):43–59.
19. Rigotti NA. Benefits and risks of smoking cessation. 2018. *Up to Date.* Available at https://www.uptodate.com/contents/benefits-and-risks-of-smoking-cessation. Accessed June 08, 2018.
20. Jha P, Ramasundarahettige C, Landsman V, et al. 21st-century hazards of smoking and benefits of cessation in the United States. *N Engl J Med.* 2013;368(4):341–350.
21. U.S. Department of Health & Human Services. *Cardiovascular Diseases.* Rockville, MD: U.S. Department of Health and Human Services; 2010.
22. Babb S, Malarcher A, Schauer G, et al. Quitting smoking among adults—United States, 2000–2015. *MMWR Morb Mortal Wkly Rep.* 2017;65(52):1457–1464.
23. Centers for Disease Control and Prevention, National Center for Chronic Disease Prevention and Health Promotion, Office on Smoking and Health. *Best Practices for Comprehensive Tobacco Control Programs.* Atlanta, GA: U.S. Department of Health and Human Services; 2014.
24. United States Public Health Service. *Treating Tobacco Use and Dependence: Clinical Practice Guideline 2008 Update.* Rockville, MD: U.S. Department of Health and Human Services, Public Health Service; 2008.
25. Benowitz NL. Nicotine addiction. *N Engl J Med.* 2010;362(24):2295–2303.
26. Volkow ND, Warren KR. Drug addiction: the neurobiology of behavior gone awry. In: Ries RK, Fiellin DA, Miller SC, et al., eds. *The ASAM Principles of Addiction Medicine.* 5th ed. Philadelphia, PA: Wolters Kluwer; 2014:4–7.
27. Brody AL, Mandelkern MA, London ED, et al. Cigarette smoking saturates brain alpha 4 beta 2 nicotinic acetylcholine receptors. *Arch Gen Psychiatry.* 2006;63(8):907–915.
28. Slotkin TA. Nicotine and the adolescent brain: insights from an animal model. *Neurotoxicol Teratol.* 2002;24(3):369–384.
29. Yuan M, Cross SJ, Loughlin SE, et al. Nicotine and the adolescent brain. *J Physiol.* 2015;593(16):3397–3412.
30. Smith RF, McDonald CG, Bergstrom HC, et al. Adolescent nicotine induces persisting changes in development of neural connectivity. *Neurosci Biobehav Rev.* 2015;55:432–443.
31. Green MP, McCausland KL, Xiao H, et al. A closer look at smoking among young adults: where tobacco control should focus its attention. *Am J Public Health.* 2007;97(8):1427–1433.
32. Biener L, Albers AB. Young adults: vulnerable new targets of tobacco marketing. *Am J Public Health.* 2004;94(2):326–330.
33. Jackson E. Cardiovascular risk of smoking and benefits of smoking cessation. *UpToDate.* 2018. Available at https://www.uptodate.com/contents/cardiovascular-risk-of-smoking-and-benefits-of-smoking-cessation. Accessed June 8, 2018.

34. Ebrahim S, Taylor F, Ward K, et al. Multiple risk factor interventions for primary prevention of coronary heart disease. *Cochrane Database Syst Rev.* 2011;(1):CD001561.
35. Ambrose JA, Barua RS. The pathophysiology of cigarette smoking and cardiovascular disease: an update. *J Am Coll Cardiol.* 2004;43(10):1731–1737.
36. Hecht SS, Szabo E. Fifty years of tobacco carcinogenesis research: from mechanisms to early detection and prevention of lung cancer. *Cancer Prev Res (Phila).* 2014;7(1):1–8.
37. U.S. Department of Health & Human Services. *Chemistry and Toxicology of Cigarette Smoke and Biomarkers of Exposure and Harm. How Tobacco Smoke Causes Disease: The Biology and Behavioral Basis for Smoking-Attributable Disease.* Rocksville, MD: U.S. Department of Health and Human Services; 2010:27–80.
38. Rea TD, Heckbert SR, Kaplan RC, et al. Smoking status and risk for recurrent coronary events after myocardial infarction. *Ann Intern Med.* 2002;137(6):494–500.
39. Gordon T, Kannel WB, McGee D, et al. Death and coronary attacks in men after giving up cigarette smoking. A report from the Framingham study. *Lancet.* 1974;2(7893):1345–1348.
40. Dobson AJ, Alexander HM, Heller RF, et al. How soon after quitting smoking does risk of heart attack decline? *J Clin Epidemiol.* 1991; 44(11):1247–1253.
41. Fagerstrom KO. Measuring degree of physical dependence to tobacco smoking with reference to individualization of treatment. *Addict Behav.* 1978;3(3–4):235–241.
42. Heatherton TF, Kozlowski LT, Frecker RC, et al. The Fagerstrom test for nicotine dependence: a revision of the Fagerstrom tolerance questionnaire. *Br J Addict.* 1991;86(9):1119–1127.
43. Pomerleau CS, Carton SM, Lutzke ML, et al. Reliability of the Fagerstrom Tolerance Questionnaire and the Fagerstrom Test for Nicotine Dependence. *Addict Behav.* 1994;19(1):33–39.
44. Rigotti NA. Overview of smoking cessation management in adults. *UpToDate.* 2018. Available at https://www.uptodate.com/contents/overview-of-smoking-cessation-management-in-adults. Accessed July 1, 2018.
45. Agency for Healthcare Research and Quality. *Treating tobacco use and dependence: quick reference guide for clinicians.* Available at https://www.ahrq.gov/professionals/clinicians-providers/guidelines-recommendations/tobacco/clinicians/references/quickref/index.html
46. Prochaska JO, DiClemente CC. Stages and processes of self-change of smoking: toward an integrative model of change. *J Consult Clin Psychol.* 1983;51(3):390–395.
47. Miller WR, Rollnick S. *Motivational Interviewing: Helping People Change.* 3rd ed. New York: The Guilford Press; 2013.
48. Schoo A, Lawn S, Rudnik E, et al. Teaching health science students foundation motivational interviewing skills: use of motivational interviewing treatment integrity and self-reflection to approach transformative learning. *BMC Med Educ.* 2015;15(228):1–10.
49. Lindson-Hawley N, Thompson TP, Bergh R. Motivational interviewing for smoking cessation. *Cochrane Database Syst Rev.* 2015;(3):CD006936.
50. Dani J, Kiosten T, Benowitz N. The pharmacology of nicotine and tobacco. In: Ries RK, Fiellin DA, Miller SC, et al., eds. *The ASAM Principles of Addiction Medicine.* Philadelphia, PA: Wolters Kluwer; 2014:201–216.
51. Benowitz NL. Pharmacokinetic considerations in understanding nicotine dependence. *Ciba Found Symp.* 1990;152:186–200; discussion 200–209.
52. Henningfield J, Benowitz N. Pharmacology of nicotine addiction. In: Boyle P, Gray N, Henningfield J, et al., eds. *Tobacco and Public Health: Science and Policy.* Oxford: Oxford University Press; 2004.
53. Lucas C, Martin J. Smoking and drug interactions. *Aust Prescr.* 2013; 36(3):102–104.
54. Hughes JR. How confident should we be that smoking cessation treatments work? *Addiction.* 2009;104(10):1637–1640.
55. Anthenelli RM, Benowitz NL, West R, et al. Neuropsychiatric safety and efficacy of varenicline, bupropion, and nicotine patch in smokers with and without psychiatric disorders (EAGLES): a double-blind, randomised, placebo-controlled clinical trial. *Lancet.* 2016;387(10037): 2507–2520.
56. Stead LF, Perera R, Bullen C, et al. Nicotine replacement therapy for smoking cessation. *Cochrane Database Syst Rev.* 2012;11:CD000146.
57. Hartmann-Boyce J, Chepkin SC, Ye W, et al. Nicotine replacement therapy versus control for smoking cessation. *Cochrane Database Syst Rev.* 2018;5:CD000146.
58. *Micromedex healthcare series.* Micromedex, Inc. Thomson Reuters; 2018. Available at http://www.micromedex.com/. Accessed July 1, 2018.
59. Cahill K, Stevens S, Perera R, et al. Pharmacological interventions for smoking cessation: an overview and network meta-analysis. *Cochrane Database Syst Rev.* 2013;5:CD009329.
60. Jordan CJ, Xi ZX. Discovery and development of varenicline for smoking cessation. *Expert Opin Drug Discovery.* 2018;13(7):671–683.
61. Cahill K, Lindson-Hawley N, Thomas KH, et al. Nicotine receptor partial agonists for smoking cessation. *Cochrane Database Syst Rev.* 2016;(5):CD006103.
62. Gershon AS, Campitelli MA, Hawken S, et al. Cardiovascular and neuropsychiatric events after varenicline use for smoking cessation. *Am J Respir Crit Care Med.* 2018;197(7):913–922.
63. Benowitz NL, Pipe A, West R, et al. Cardiovascular safety of varenicline, bupropion, and nicotine patch in smokers: a randomized clinical trial. *JAMA Intern Med.* 2018;178(5):622–631.
64. Ebbert JO, Hughes JR, West RJ, et al. Effect of varenicline on smoking cessation through smoking reduction: a randomized clinical trial. *JAMA.* 2015;313(7):687–694.
65. Schnoll RA, Patterson F, Wileyto EP, et al. Efficacy of extended duration transdermal nicotine therapy: a randomized trial. *Ann Intern Med.* 2010;152(3):144–151.
66. Steinberg MB, Schmelzer AC, Richardson DL, et al. The case for treating tobacco dependence as a chronic disease. *Ann Intern Med.* 2008;148(7): 554–556.
67. Park ER. Behavioral approaches to smoking cessation. *UpToDate.* 2018. Available at https://www.uptodate.com/contents/behavioral-approaches-to-smoking-cessation. Accessed June 8, 2018.
68. Stead LF, Koilpillai P, Lancaster T. Additional behavioural support as an adjunct to pharmacotherapy for smoking cessation. *Cochrane Database Syst Rev.* 2015;(10):CD009670.
69. Lancaster T, Stead LF. Individual behavioural counseling for smoking cessation. *Cochrane Database Syst Rev.* 2017;3:CD001292.
70. Collins SE, Witkiewitz K, Kirouac M, et al. Preventing relapse following smoking cessation. *Curr Cardiovasc Risk Rep.* 2010;4(6):421–428.
71. Douaihy A, Daley DC, Marlatt GA, et al. Relapse prevention: clinical models and intervention strategies. In: Ries RK, Fiellin DA, Miller SC, et al., eds. *The ASAM Principles of Addiction Medicine.* 5th ed. Philadelphia, PA: Wolters Kluwer; 2014:991–1007.
72. Witkiewitz K, Marlatt GA. Relapse prevention for alcohol and drug problems: that was Zen, this is Tao. *Am Psychol.* 2004;59(4):224–235.
73. Marlatt GA, Gordon JR. *Relapse Prevention: Maintenance Strategies in the Treatment of Addictive Behaviors.* New York: Guilford Press; 1985.
74. Hunter-Reel D, McCrady B, Hildebrandt T. Emphasizing interpersonal factors: an extension of the Witkiewitz and Marlatt relapse model. *Addiction.* 2009;104(8):1281–1290.
75. Hendershot CS, Witkiewitz K, George WH, et al. Relapse prevention for addictive behaviors. *Subst Abuse Treat Prev Policy.* 2011;6:17.
76. World Health Organization. *World Health Statistics.* 2013. Available at http://www.who.int/gho/publications/world_health_statistics/2013/en/. Accessed July 01, 2018.

23 Hypertension

Yvonne Commodore-Mensah, Binu Koirala, Cheryl R. Dennison Himmelfarb

OBJECTIVES

1. Describe the pathophysiology and epidemiology of hypertension.
2. Discuss clinical manifestations and consequences of uncontrolled hypertension.
3. Define primary hypertension, secondary hypertension, and resistant hypertension.
4. Describe the guideline-based recommendations for diagnosing and staging the severity of high blood pressure and treatment targets for different patient groups.
5. Devise evidence-based treatment plans (incorporating nonpharmacologic and pharmacologic options) for a patient with high blood pressure.

KEY QUESTIONS

1. How is hypertension defined for adults and children based on the current national guidelines?
2. What factors contribute to hypertension?
3. What are the consequences of uncontrolled hypertension?
4. What are the key nonpharmacologic and pharmacologic strategies for managing hypertension?

BACKGROUND

Hypertension (HTN), also known as high blood pressure (BP), is the most common risk factor for cardiovascular disease (CVD) and stroke.[1] In 2010, HTN was the leading cause of death and disability-adjusted life-years worldwide.[2] According to the recent guideline for the Prevention, Detection, Evaluation, and Management of High Blood Pressure in Adults, around 46% of Americans have HTN, and many more individuals have elevated BP, which indicates they are at high risk for developing HTN.[3,4] Since the 1970s, there has been a dramatic decrease in the mortality rate from hypertensive heart disease in Europe and the United States, primarily because of the development of effective antihypertensive drugs in conjunction with increased awareness, treatment, and control of HTN.[5] Despite this progress, worldwide, an estimated 7.6 million premature deaths are caused each year by HTN.[6]

PATHOPHYSIOLOGY

Definitions and BP Classification and Goal

BP has two components, which are continuous variables: systolic BP (SBP) and diastolic BP (DBP). Elevations in either SBP or DBP increase a person's risk for a clinical event. Death from both ischemic heart disease and stroke increases progressively and linearly from levels as low as 115 mm Hg SBP and 75 mm Hg DBP upward among individuals whose ages range from 40 to 89 years.[7] For every 20 mm Hg systolic and 10 mm Hg diastolic increase in BP, there is a doubling of mortality from ischemic heart disease, stroke, and other vascular diseases.[7] Conversely, it is generally true that the lower the pressures, the lower the risk of morbidity and mortality, except in the relatively uncommon situations of sympathetic nervous system dysfunction or hypovolemia.

The word "hypertension" can be confusing to patients, who might believe that they are neither "tense" nor "hyper" and therefore unlikely to have HTN. For this reason, "high blood pressure" may be a better term to use when communicating with the public. HTN can be considered as a sign, a risk factor, and a disease.

Adults

As new research has become available, many countries have established guidelines on the detection, evaluation, and treatment of HTN.[3,8] According to the recent evidence-based American College of Cardiology (ACC) and American Heart Association (AHA) guideline for the Prevention, Detection, Evaluation and Management of High Blood Pressure in Adults, normal blood pressure is below 120/80 (Table 23-1).[3] Blood pressure in the range of systolic 120 to 129 and diastolic less than 80 is classified as elevated blood pressure. This new guideline introduced a new definition of HTN as blood pressure greater than or equal to 130/80. HTN is classified as stage 1 (systolic 130 to 139 or diastolic 80 to 89) or stage 2 (systolic greater than or equal to 140 or diastolic greater than or equal to 90). Blood pressure diagnosis should be based on BP measured in the health care setting an average of greater than or equal to two careful readings on greater than or equal to two occasions. Adults with systolic blood pressure or diastolic blood pressure in two categories should be designated to the higher BP category. Types of HTN are classified as (1) systolic and diastolic HTN (either primary or secondary) and (2) isolated systolic HTN caused

Table 23-1 • BLOOD PRESSURE CLASSIFICATION AND THERAPEUTIC TARGET

Blood Pressure			Blood Pressure Classification	Therapeutic Target (Goal BP)
SBP		DBP		
<120 mm Hg	and	<80 mm Hg	Normal BP	
120–129 mm Hg	and	<80 mm Hg	Elevated BP	
130–139 mm Hg	or	80–89 mm Hg	Stage 1 HTN	<130/80
≥140 mm Hg	or	≥90 mm Hg	Stage 2 HTN	<130/80

BP, blood pressure; HTN, hypertension.
Adapted from Whelton PK, Carey RM, Aronow WS, et al. 2017 ACC/AHA/AAPA/ABC/ACPM/AGS/APhA/ASH/ASPC/NMA/PCNA guideline for the prevention, detection, evaluation, and management of high blood pressure in adults: A report of the American College of Cardiology/American Heart Association Task Force on Clinical Practice Guidelines. *Circulation.* 2018;138(17):e484–e594.

by increased cardiac output or increasing rigidity of the aorta. The incidence of isolated systolic HTN (defined as SBP greater than or equal to 160 mm Hg with normal DBP) increases dramatically with age and thus is of particular concern among older adults.[3]

Children

Criteria used for categorizing BP in adults are not applicable to children. The level of BP, which is considered normal, increases gradually from infancy to adulthood. The definition of HTN in children and adolescents is based on the normative distribution of BP in healthy children.[9] Normal BP is defined as SBP and DBP less than the 90th percentile for gender, age, and height. Preadolescent with 90th to 95th percentile for gender, age, and height is considered to have prehypertension. In adolescents, prehypertension is defined as BP greater than or equal to 120/80 mm Hg to less than 95th percentile or greater than or equal to 90th and less than 95th, whichever is lower.[1] HTN is defined as average SBP or DBP at or greater than 95th percentile for gender, age, and height on at least three separate occasions.[10]

Hemodynamics of HTN

BP is the product of the amount of blood pumped by the heart each minute (cardiac output) and the degree of dilation or constriction of the arterioles (systemic vascular resistance), that is, pressure = flow × resistance. Arterial BP is controlled over short time periods by the arterial baroreceptors that sense changes in pressure within major arteries and then through neurohumoral feedback mechanisms, which modulate heart rate, myocardial contractility, and vascular smooth muscle contraction to maintain BP within normal limits. Over longer time periods (hours to days), neurohumoral and direct renal regulation of vascular volume also play an important role in maintaining normal BP. Baroreceptors in low-pressure components of the cardiovascular system such as the veins, atria, and pulmonary circulation have a role in neurohumoral regulation of vascular volume.

HTN occurs because there is an increase in cardiac output and/or systemic vascular resistance. It may be that either one or both are elevated. Because BP can be measured relatively easily and because it is not easy to measure cardiac output or systemic vascular resistance, we identify dysfunction of these variables as disorders of BP regulation. As discussion in several chapters of this book reveals, each of these variables, cardiac output and systemic vascular resistance, are themselves influenced by many factors. Given all the influencing factors, BP needs to be considered as an extremely complex condition.

Epidemiology

Prevalence of HTN is influenced by the choice of cutpoints used to categorize high BP, methods used for diagnosis, and the population studied. The prevalence of HTN among Americans is substantially increased when HTN is defined as BP greater than or equal to 130/80 mm Hg versus the prior 2003 guideline definition (BP greater than or equal to 140/90 mm Hg), approximately 46% versus 32%.[4] In the U.S. general adult population, HTN awareness, treatment, and control have been steadily improving since the 1960s. Based on data from the National Health and Nutrition Examination Survey (NHANES), conducted between 1999 and 2014, this steady improvement seems to have reached a plateau over the last 10 years (Table 23-2).[5] The most recent estimates indicate that among adults in the United States with HTN, 84% are aware, 75% are in treatment, and 54% had achieved BP control (defined at that time as SBP/DBP less than 140/90 mm Hg).[5] The 54% HTN control rate in 2014 is suboptimal and clearly indicates a need for increased efforts on the part of health systems and health care providers in partnering with patients to better manage HTN.

Risk Factors for Hypertension

Age, Gender, and Weight

SBP and DBP levels correlate with age, height, and weight. Evidence suggests that HTN begins in childhood, perhaps even in

Table 23-2 • TRENDS IN AWARENESS, TREATMENT, AND CONTROL AMONG PARTICIPANTS WITH HYPERTENSION IN THE U.S. POPULATION, 1999–2014

	National Health and Nutrition Examination Survey (%)							
	1999–2000 (n = 4,487)	**2001–2002 (n = 4,945)**	**2003–2004 (n = 4,668)**	**2005–2006 (n = 4,693)**	**2007–2008 (n = 5,615)**	**2009–2010 (n = 5,988)**	**2011–2012 (n = 5,294)**	**2013–2014 (n = 5,641)**
Awareness	70	71	75	78	80	82	82	84
Treatment	59	60	65	68	72	76	75	75
Control[a]	31	35	40	44	48	53	52	54

[a]Among all with hypertension.
From Zhang Y, Moran AE. Trends in the prevalence, awareness, treatment, and control of hypertension among young adults in the United States, 1999–2014. *Hypertension.* 2017;70(4):736–742. Available at http://doi.org/10.1161/HYPERTENSIONAHA.117.09801

utero, although a meta-analysis of 55 studies of birth weight and BP later in life did not support this so-called fetal origins hypothesis.[11] Because HTN in children is defined as a BP greater than the 95th percentile for a child of any given age and height, the initial incidence of HTN in children is automatically 5%. Normally, BP increases in children at a rate between 1 and 4 mm Hg per year for both SBP and DBP and then levels off after age 18 to 20 years. Children whose BP consistently falls above the 95th percentile for height, gender, and age are at risk for sustained HTN and should be evaluated and possibly treated.[10]

In adults, BP tends to increase with age.[12,13] The prevalence of HTN increases with advancing age to the point where more than half of the people aged 60 to 69 years and approximately three fourths of those aged 70 years and older are affected.[14] The age-related rise in SBP, often manifesting as isolated systolic HTN, is primarily responsible for an increase in both incidence and prevalence of HTN with increasing age.[15] Overall, women have lower prevalence of HTN than in men until about 64 years of age, however, is higher after 65 years of age. The age-adjusted prevalence of HTN in adults greater than or equal to 20 years of age for women is 33.4%, and for men, it is 34.5% (Heart disease and stroke statistics 2018 update). Although rates of HTN treatment are higher among women (58%) compared with men (52%), men achieved higher rates of HTN control (66%) than women (63%).[13]

Data from the Framingham and other epidemiologic studies have shown that as body weight increases, so do SBP and DBP in children and adults.[16,17] In the Bogalusa study, children and adolescents who were overweight (body mass index [BMI] greater than 85th percentile) were 2.4 times more likely to have HTN than those with BMI less than the 85th percentile.[18] NHANES III data revealed that the prevalence of HTN in men and women with BMI less than 25 kg/m^2 was 15%, whereas in men and women with a BMI greater than or equal to 30 kg/m^2 prevalence was 42% and 38%, respectively.[19] This relationship between weight and BP is thought to be one of the reasons that BP increases with age. In combined data from four longitudinal studies begun in adolescence with repeat examination in young adulthood to early middle age, being obese continuously or acquiring obesity was associated with a relative risk of 2.7 for developing HTN. Becoming normal weight reduced the risk of developing HTN to a level similar to those who had never been obese.[3]

Family History and Genetic Factors

Family history of HTN has been used as an indicator of genetic influence on HTN. With the progress on the human genome project, it is possible that we may be able to predict risk with more precision; however, expense and issues of privacy must also be considered. Depending on how a positive family history of HTN is defined, a person with a positive history has a relative risk for HTN of between 2.4 and 5.0.[20] The risks are greater when more family members have HTN and if these family members had HTN diagnosed before the age of 55 years. The risk associated with a positive family history is slightly greater for women than for men. The influence of family history is seen in children as well as adults.[20] Genetic studies suggest that rather than a single genetic variant, alleles at many different loci contribute to HTN, with the combinations of causative alleles varying between individuals. Among the most studied genetic markers for the pathogenesis of HTN are the renin–angiotensin system, salt intake, CVD, obesity and insulin resistance, the sympathetic nervous system, and endothelial dysfunction.[21]

Ethnic and Geographic Differences

Geographic differences in the prevalence of HTN have been described for different regions within the United States as well as across the world. The prevalence of HTN is higher in blacks than in whites, Asians, and Hispanic Americans. Based on the BP cutoff of greater than or equal to 130/80 mm Hg for HTN, the prevalence of HTN is highest among non-Hispanic black men (59%) and women (56%) and lowest among non-Hispanic white women (41%) and non-Hispanic Asian women (36%).[3] Within the United States, HTN prevalence, associated stroke mortality, and all-cause mortality vary in geographic patterns and are higher in the Southeast than other regions of the United States. Ten of 11 states in the southeastern United States, the "Stroke Belt," have stroke mortality rates greater than 10% above the national mean. Contributors to this pattern include geographic variations in obesity, physical inactivity, and salt and nutritional intake but not in HTN treatment or control.[22]

The global burden of HTN in regions with the highest estimated prevalence of HTN was roughly twice the rate reported in regions with the lowest estimated prevalence. In men, the highest estimated prevalence was in the Latin America and Caribbean regions, whereas for women the highest estimated prevalence was in the former socialist economies. The lowest estimated prevalence of HTN for both men and women was in the region "other Asian islands" (i.e., Korea, Thailand, and Taiwan). Existing data suggest that the prevalence of HTN has increased in economically developing countries during the past decade.[2,23] Differences in HTN rates across regions may be influenced by differences in BP measurement and treatment, genetics, lifestyle choices, or other confounding variables.

Social Determinants

Social determinants of health are defined by the World Health Organization as the conditions in the social, physical, and economic environment in which people are born, live, work, and age.[24] An inverse relationship between socioeconomic status, including educational level and income, and the prevalence of HTN[25] and risk of CVD[26,27] has been documented. In the Atherosclerosis Risk in Communities (ARIC) study which included 11,441 black and white adults, those with lower income and education level had the greatest risk of cardiovascular events.[28] A meta-analysis of 51 studies has shown an increased risk of HTN among those with the lowest socioeconomic indicators including income, occupation, and education.[29]

It is important to tailor counseling on lifestyle modification to a patient's social and physical environment. Screening for social determinants of health in patients diagnosed with HTN may help identify opportunities for intervention. The Centers for Medicare & Medicaid Services has developed a screening tool[30] to assess five domains of non–health-related measures that impact health outcomes: housing instability, food insecurity, transportation difficulties, utility assistance needs, and interpersonal safety. Community resources such as community health workers may help address social needs of patients diagnosed with HTN.[25,31] Community health workers play a critical role in HTN self-management and their integration into multidisciplinary care teams improves care that is delivered to underserved populations and racial/ethnic minorities.[31]

Causes of HTN

Despite decades of research, the main underlying cause of HTN is unknown. However, HTN has been linked to a family history and other factors, such as obesity, stress, excess sodium dysfunction, and sympathetic nervous dysfunction, which may all contribute to HTN. The interaction of both genetic and environmental factors underpin causal hypotheses for HTN.

Primary HTN

The cause of primary HTN remains in question though it accounts for about 90% of all cases of HTN. BP is a complex variable involving mechanisms that influence cardiac output, systemic vascular resistance, and blood volume. HTN is caused by one or several abnormalities in the function of these mechanisms or the failure of other factors to compensate for these malfunctioning mechanisms. Currently, the genetic basis for rare types of HTN has been identified, and there is hope that soon these discoveries will lead to an understanding of the cause or causes of most HTN.

Genetic factors and the environmental issues of obesity, stress, and excess sodium, as well as sympathetic nervous system dysfunction, may all contribute to HTN. Several hypotheses are linked to understanding the cause of HTN and include the following:

1. Dysfunction of the autonomic nervous system may be a cause due to the inheritance of genes predisposing an individual to increased sympathetic nervous activity.
2. Variations in renal sodium absorption also suggest that genes involved in rare inherited forms of HTN may be related to mutations in several genes that increase one's susceptibility to disorders of renal absorption of sodium, chloride, and water. To date, genes accounting for the vast majority of salt-sensitive HTN have not been identified.[21]
3. Dysfunction of the renin–angiotensin–aldosterone system results in an increase in renin–angiotensin–aldosterone activity resulting in extracellular fluid volume expansion and systemic vascular resistance. Angiotensin II has also been shown to act like a growth factor and a cytokine resulting in growth, differentiation, and apoptosis in vascular tissues. Studies have also identified gene coding for various components of the renin–angiotensin–aldosterone system and their roles in the development of HTN.[21]
4. Impaired vascular responsiveness, that is, impairments in vascular dilation and increased vascular contraction, due to the function of the endothelium, occurs in those individuals with HTN. Oxidative stress is also a critical factor in both HTN and atherogenesis.[32]
5. Insulin resistance may also play a role in the development of HTN. Insulin resistance may be the common factor that links HTN, diabetes, and other metabolic abnormalities. The metabolic syndrome of abdominal obesity, increased BP, dyslipidemia, and insulin resistance with or without impaired glucose tolerance plus prothrombotic and proinflammatory states may place individuals at high cardiovascular risk.

Secondary HTN

Secondary HTN affects 10% of individuals with HTN, and a large number of children younger than 10 years have HTN due to a specific physiologic condition.[5] In children younger than 10 years, the most common causes of persistent HTN are renal disease and vascular problems such as coarctation of the aorta. Common secondary causes of high BP in adults include chronic renal disease, renovascular disease, primary aldosteronism, and, increasingly, sleep apnea. Table 23-3 summarizes the major secondary causes of HTN in both children and adults. Aspects of diagnosis and management of some of the more common conditions are highlighted here.

Table 23-3 • CAUSES OF SECONDARY HYPERTENSION

Renal
Renal parenchymal disease
Renal vascular disease
Renin-producing tumors
Primary sodium retention (Liddle syndrome)
Increased intravascular volume
Endocrine
Acromegaly
Hypothyroidism
Hyperthyroidism
Hyperparathyroidism
Adrenal cortical
Cushing syndrome
Primary aldosteronism
Apparent mineralocorticoid excess
Adrenal medulla
Pheochromocytoma
Carcinoid syndrome
Neurologic
Increase intracranial pressure
Quadriplegia
Guillain–Barré syndrome
Idiopathic, primary, or familial dysautonomia
Other
Diseases of the aorta
Rigidity of the aorta
Coarctation of the aorta
Obstructive sleep apnea
Drugs and exogenous hormones
Pregnancy-induced HTN
Acute stress-related secondary HTN
Isolated systolic HTN due to an incrased cardiac output

Renal Parenchymal Disease. Chronic renal disease causes HTN and, conversely, HTN contributes to the development of 1% to 2% of chronic renal disease.[3] Three factors contribute to the development of HTN in those individuals with renal disease: loss of nephrons leading to retention of sodium, chloride, and water; decreased release of vasodilator substances such as nitric oxide; and activation of the renin–angiotensin system. NHANES III data indicates that 70% of all patients with chronic renal disease have HTN. As aggressive lowering of SBP may slow the progression of kidney disease, health care providers must consider the necessary treatment to reach the BP goal.

Renovascular Disease. Renovascular HTN, found in 5% to 34% of all hypertensives, occurs when one or both of the renal arteries are diseased, leading to decreased perfusion of the kidneys.[3] The most common cause of renal artery stenosis is atherosclerosis, which leads to renal ischemia, release of renin from juxtaglomerular cells of the kidney, and a secondary increase in BP.[33] Diagnosis of renal artery stenosis is made on the basis of difficult-to-control BP or deterioration in renal function or electrolyte imbalance and through identification of an abdominal bruit by physical examination. This is followed by the renal duplex Doppler, ultrasound, magnetic resonance imaging or computed tomography, and a renal angiogram with consideration of medical treatment, angioplasty, or surgery (which is the gold standard for severe renal artery stenosis).[3]

Primary Hyperaldosteronism. Primary aldosteronism is a disease characterized by excess secretion of aldosterone, caused by an adrenocortical adenoma, adrenal hyperplasia, adrenal carcinoma, or the cause may be unknown; in which case it is diagnosed as idiopathic hyperaldosteronism.[33] A common form of primary aldosteronism is a benign aldosterone-producing adenoma. With high levels of aldosterone, there is retention of sodium, chloride, and water resulting in an expanded extracellular fluid volume. This condition is now thought to be the cause of up to 20% of all cases of HTN.[3] Primary hyperaldosteronism may be difficult to diagnose due to low serum potassium; the most common sign is found in only one third of the cases. Currently, the best screening test is the plasma aldosterone to plasma renin activity ratio. Health care providers should look for this condition in those patients younger than 50 years who appear to have resistant HTN or HTN with hypokalemia. Surgical removal of an adenoma reduces BP and if no tumor is present, medical treatment with aldosterone antagonists such as spironolactone is indicated.

Pheochromocytoma. Pheochromocytomas are largely benign neuroendocrine tumors of the adrenal medulla and present in up to 6% of those individuals with HTN. Because excessive amounts of catecholamine occurs with these tumors, individuals may experience chest discomfort, tachycardia and palpitations, panic attack, and headaches.[33] A pheochromocytoma is normally diagnosed by undertaking measurement of urinary and plasma catecholamines, urinary metanephrine, and urinary vanillylmandelic acid. Nuclear imaging may also identify certain extra-adrenal tumors and once detected, surgical intervention is needed.

Obstructive Sleep Apnea. An association between sleep apnea and systemic HTN has been reported since the 1970s. Increasingly, this condition has gained more widespread attention due to the increasing rate of obesity. Obstructive sleep apnea affects 2% to 4% of the general population, and more than 50% of those affected by it have HTN.[33] It is now a significant health problem causing disrupted sleep, memory loss, personality changes, decreased attention span, poor judgment, and frequent episodes of hypopnea (reduced chest movement with 4% or more decrease in oxyhemoglobin) and/or apnea (cessation of airflow for 10 seconds or more). A good medical history about sleep patterns is warranted, and referral to a sleep disorder clinic needed to confirm the diagnosis. Treatment involves not only the use of continuous positive airway pressure, the most common approach to this condition but also weight loss and treatment of concomitant HTN with medicines as needed.[33] Assessment of sleep patterns and snoring is also indicated for those individuals with resistant HTN.

Coarctation of the Aorta. Coarctation or narrowing of the lumen of the aorta is rare in adults but relatively common in children, accounting for 7% of all congenital CVD.[33] The most common narrowing occurs distal to the left subclavian artery. Those individuals with coarctation of the aorta normally have high upper extremity BPs with low pressures in the lower extremities including weak femoral pulses. If this condition is left untreated, it can cause left ventricular hypertrophy (LVH). Bruits may be present on physical findings, and screening tests, which include a transthoracic echocardiogram or contrast computed tomography/magnetic resonance imaging, help to visualize this condition. Treatment includes surgical repair of the lesion or angioplasty. A comparison of the BP and left ventricular mass among patients who had surgical repair of a coarctation and controls found that these patients had significantly higher 24-hour ambulatory SBP and left ventricular mass compared with controls.[34] Thus, follow-up remains important in these patients.

Pregnancy-Induced HTN. HTN occurs in 5.9% of all pregnancies and is classified as preeclampsia–eclampsia, preeclampsia superimposed on chronic HTN, chronic HTN, or gestational HTN.[3] The cause of preeclampsia is not known but it includes proteinuria, renal insufficiency, impaired liver function, and abnormalities including thrombocytopenia, hemolysis, and fetal growth restriction. Early diagnosis is critical and close monitoring of BP essential with treatment being directed at medicines with proven safety for each condition.

As shown in Table 23-3, numerous other causes of secondary HTN are noted. A careful history and physical examination will help reveal many of these secondary causes.

Clinical Manifestations of HTN

Signs and Symptoms

There are few signs and no symptoms of HTN until it becomes very severe and target organ damage (TOD) has occurred. The major sign is the presence of elevated BP based on the criteria for the definition HTN (Table 23-1). Evaluation of hypertensive patients has three objectives: (1) to assess lifestyle and identify other cardiovascular risk factors or concomitant disorders that may affect prognosis and guide treatment (Table 23-4); (2) to reveal identifiable causes of high BP (Table 23-3); and (3) to assess the presence or absence of TOD and CVD (Table 23-4).[3,35,36] Morbidity and mortality associated with HTN are predominately the consequences of damage to a selected set of organs, known as "TOD," which include the blood vessels, heart, brain, kidneys, and eyes. Evidence of TOD is a serious prognostic indicator in a person with HTN. Mechanisms of TOD are described below.

Vascular Changes Associated With HTN

HTN can influence the endothelium, vascular smooth muscle, extracellular matrix, and connective tissue of the arteries.

Table 23-4 • CARDIOVASCULAR RISK FACTORS AND HYPERTENSION-RELATED TARGET ORGAN DAMAGE

Major Risk Factors
Hypertension
Cigarette smoking
Obesity (body mass index ≥30 kg/m^2)
Physical inactivity
Dyslipidemia
Diabetes mellitus
Microalbuminuria or estimated GFR <60 mL/min
Age (older than 55 years for men and 65 years for women)
Family history of premature cardiovascular disease (men younger than 55 years or women younger than 65 years)

Target Organ Damage
Heart
- Left ventricular hypertrophy
- Angina or prior myocardial infarction
- Prior coronary revascularization
- Heart failure

Brain
- Stroke or transient ischemic attack
- Chronic kidney disease

Peripheral arterial disease
Retinopathy

GFR, glomerular filtration rate.

Alterations of vascular structure that occur during chronic HTN may be referred to as remodeling or hypertrophy.[37] Eutrophic inward remodeling, or "remodeling," refers to a decrease in lumen diameter without a change in the thickness of the arterial wall or the characteristic of the material within the vessel wall. In contrast, hypertrophic inward remodeling, or "hypertrophy," is defined as a decrease in lumen diameter associated with an increase in wall thickness and vessel wall material. In either case, narrowing of the vessel lumen is associated with increased vascular resistance.[37] Some of the factors that contribute to the hypertrophy and remodeling processes appear to be different. Mechanisms of hypertrophy may include increased arterial pulse pressure, sympathetic nerve activity, angiotensin II, genetic factors, endothelin-1, nitric oxide, and oxidative stress.[37] Mechanisms of remodeling may include intravascular pressure, angiotensin II, genetic factors, endothelin-1, and αβv3 integrins.[37]

Changes in the Vascular Endothelium. The vascular endothelium is the largest organ in the body. Vascular endothelial cells are extremely active and play a critical role in regulation of blood vessel tone and cellular activity in the vascular wall. Endothelial cells modulate blood vessel tone by secreting a variety of dilator and constrictor substances. In addition to their effect on vascular tone, these substances and other factors produced by the endothelium, may also modify platelet aggregation, thrombogenicity of the blood, vascular inflammation, and oxidative stress and, over the long term, influence cell migration and proliferation with subsequent development and progression of atherosclerosis and its complications.[37]

Impaired endothelial vasodilation has been identified in persons with HTN and even in the normotensive children of hypertensive parents. However, it is not yet clear whether endothelial dysfunction is a precursor of HTN or a sequel. Improved understanding of the molecular basis for endothelial dysfunction in HTN may provide a pathway to developing new therapies to reduce the impact of HTN. Other factors that cause endothelial dysfunction include aging, hyperlipidemia, insulin resistance/diabetes, tobacco use, physical inactivity, and hyperhomocysteinemia.[38]

Atherosclerosis. Atherosclerosis is a complex degenerative condition that is characterized by endothelial dysfunction and lipid accumulation in the endothelium and media, followed by wall thickening and outward remodeling, and later by luminal encroachment, thrombosis, and occlusion.[39] Atherosclerosis manifests as coronary heart disease (CHD), cerebrovascular, and peripheral arterial disease and is a major worldwide source of morbidity and mortality. Atherosclerotic plaque formation involves the interaction of genetic predisposition and environmental risk factors with diffuse vascular injury. Many of these factors are also involved in the pathogenesis of HTN. HTN promotes or accelerates all phases of the development of atherosclerotic lesions, from plaque formation to rupture.[39]

Heart. Parallel structural and functional changes in the large arteries (stiffness), cardiac mass (hypertrophy), and myocardial relaxation and filling (diastolic dysfunction) occur at an accelerated rate with chronic HTN. The pressure overload associated with HTN promotes LVH that leads to left ventricular dysfunction and heart failure (HF). Both HTN and HF advance vascular endothelial and renal dysfunction, which in turn further promotes the progression of each disease state, as well as other conditions. Hypertensive individuals have a two- to fourfold increased risk of CHD and HF and those individuals with prehypertension have a 1.6- to 2.5-fold increased risk of CVD, both compared with those who are normotensive.[37] Aggressive HTN control can prevent the development of LVH and lead to regression of LVH. However, it remains controversial whether there are differential drug effects on reversing LVH related to HTN.

Kidney. HTN is both a cause and consequence of chronic kidney disease (CKD). The incidence and prevalence of CKD and end-stage renal disease, presumed to be secondary to primary HTN, have increased considerably over the past two decades and are particularly high among African Americans. HTN causes renal damage through multiple mechanisms.[40] One mechanism is ischemia with glomerular hypoperfusion causing glomerulosclerosis and subsequently tubulointerstitial fibrosis. Other mechanisms of injury, such as endothelial dysfunction, cholesterol oxidation, cigarette smoking, and proteinuria, act in concert with high systemic and glomerular capillary pressures to accelerate nephrosclerosis. While the presence of macroalbuminuria (proteinuria greater than 300 mg/day) indicates presence of kidney disease, even lower-level microalbuminuria (30 to 300 mg/day) is associated with increased cardiovascular risk.

Antihypertensive drug classes differ in ability to lower proteinuria and slow the progression of CKD. Drugs that block the renin–angiotensin system, that is, angiotensin-converting enzyme inhibitors (ACE-Is) and angiotensin receptor blockers (ARBs), are the most potent antiproteinuric agents and also have been shown to be highly effective in slowing the progression of renal insufficiency.[3]

Eye. HTN has profound effects on the structure and function of the eye. Hypertensive retinopathy refers to a spectrum of microvascular signs in the retina related to HTN.[41] HTN initially causes retinal circulation vasospasm and increased vasomotor tone, which are reflected as the signs of generalized arteriolar narrowing. Persistent HTN leads to arteriosclerotic changes, including intimal thickening, media wall hyperplasia, and hyaline degeneration. This is seen as increasingly severe generalized arteriolar narrowing, arteriolar wall opacification, and focal narrowing. Thickening of the retinal arteriolar wall by these arteriosclerotic processes may compress the venules, resulting in the sign of AV nicking. In the presence of more acute elevations in BP, an exudative stage may occur, manifesting as microaneurysms, hemorrhages, hard exudates, and cotton wool spots. Optic disc swelling and macular edema may occur with severely elevated BP. These processes may not occur in the sequence described above. Numerous studies have confirmed the strong association between the presence of signs of hypertensive retinopathy and elevated BP.[41] The strongest evidence of the usefulness of the evaluation of hypertensive retinopathy for risk stratification is based on its association with stroke as the retinal circulation shares anatomical, physiologic, and embryologic features with the cerebral circulation. A simplified classification of hypertensive retinopathy according to the severity of the retinal signs is presented in Table 23-5.[41]

Brain. HTN has adverse consequences in the brain, including ischemia and hemorrhagic stroke, cognitive impairment/dementia, and encephalopathy. HTN contributes to the development of atherosclerotic plaques in the extracerebral and intracranial vessels as well as the process of microatheroma and hypertensive hyalinosis. Despite the brain's adaptive mechanisms to maintain

Table 23-5 • CLASSIFICATION OF HYPERTENSIVE RETINOPATHY[41]

Retinopathy Grade	Signs	Associations[a]
None	No detectable signs	None
Mild	One or more of the following signs: Generalized arteriolar narrowing, focal arteriolar narrowing, arteriovenous nicking, opacity ("copper wiring")	Modestly associated with risk of clinical and subclinical stroke, coronary heart disease, and mortality
Moderate	Hemorrhage (blot, dot, or flame-shaped), microaneurysm, cotton–wool spot, hard exudate, or a combination of these signs	Strongly associated with risk of clinical and subclinical stroke, cognitive decline, and mortality from cardiovascular causes
Malignant	Signs of moderate retinopathy plus swelling of the optic disc[b]	Strongly associated with mortality

[a]A modest association is defined as an odds ratio of greater than 1 but less than 2. A strong association is defined as an odds ratio of 2 or greater.
[b]Anterior ischemic optic neuropathy, characterized by unilateral swelling of the optic disc, visual loss, and sectorial visual field loss, should be ruled out.
From Wong TY, Mitchell P. Hypertensive retinopathy. *N Engl J Med.* 2004;351(22):2310–2317.

cerebral blood flow, loss or reduction of blood flow results in stroke, producing pathologic changes related to the duration and degree of ischemia. Research has documented the positive relationship between level of BP and stroke and an inverse relationship between HTN control and reduction in stroke.[7,42]

Cognitive impairment spans the spectrum from mild cognitive impairment to dementia. Cerebrovascular damage leading to cognitive impairment can occur not only from atherothrombosis but also through cerebral hemorrhage, hypoperfusion, and other arteriopathies. Longitudinal studies strongly suggest an adverse effect of elevated BP in middle age on cognitive functioning.[43] There is also an adverse effect of low BP in older adults for development of dementia; however, intensive BP lowering has been found to have no impact on cognitive function in high risk subsets, such as older adults with long-standing type 2 diabetes mellitus at high risk for cardiovascular events.[44] Hypertensive encephalopathy is a consequence of accelerated or malignant HTN. Encephalopathy occurs when the BP levels exceed the upper limit of autoregulation so that the cerebral arteries become dilated, disrupting the blood–brain barrier and leading to the formation of cerebral edema; local changes in ion and cytokine concentrations; and/or alteration in neural function.[37]

ASSESSMENT, DIAGNOSIS, AND CLINICAL EVALUATION

Assessment and Diagnosis

HTN is relatively easy to diagnose. However, in part due to the lack of symptoms, an individual may not seek evaluation or treatment of HTN. In fact, though rates of awareness, treatment, and control have improved over the past several decades, nearly 20% of the hypertensive population in the United States are unaware of their condition and about half of those in treatment remain uncontrolled.[5]

BP Measurement

Accurate BP measurement is essential to classify individuals, to ascertain BP-related risk, and to guide HTN management decisions.[45] Proper training of observers, positioning of the patient, and selection of cuff size are all essential (Table 23-6). Because an individual's BP can vary markedly, accurate diagnosis of HTN

Table 23-6 • CHECKLIST FOR ACCURATE MEASUREMENT OF BLOOD PRESSURE

Key Steps for Proper BP Measurements	Specific Instructions
Step 1: Properly prepare the patient	1. Have the patient relax, sitting in a chair (feet on floor, back supported) for >5 minutes. 2. The patient should avoid caffeine, exercise, and smoking for at least 30 minutes before measurement. 3. Ensure patient has emptied his/her bladder. 4. Neither the patient nor the observer should talk during the rest period or during the measurement. 5. Remove all clothing covering the location of cuff placement. 6. Measurements made while the patient is sitting or lying on an examining table do not fulfill these criteria.
Step 2: Use proper technique for BP measurements	1. Use a BP measurement device that has been validated and ensure that the device is calibrated periodically. 2. Support the patient's arm (e.g., resting on a desk). 3. Position the middle of the cuff on the patient's upper arm at the level of the right atrium (the midpoint of the sternum). 4. Use the correct cuff size, such that the bladder encircles 80% of the arm, and note if a larger- or smaller-than-normal cuff size is used. 5. Either the stethoscope diaphragm or bell may be used for auscultatory readings.
Step 3: Take the proper measurements needed for diagnosis and treatment of elevated BP/hypertension	1. At the first visit, record BP in both arms. Use the arm that gives the higher reading for subsequent readings. 2. Separate repeated measurements by 1–2 minutes. 3. For auscultatory determinations, use a palpated estimate of radial pulse obliteration pressure to estimate SBP. Inflate the cuff 20–30 mm Hg above this level for an auscultatory determination of the BP level. 4. For auscultatory readings, deflate the cuff pressure 2 mm Hg/s, and listen for Korotkoff sounds.
Step 4: Properly document accurate BP readings	1. Record SBP and DBP. If using the auscultatory technique, record SBP and DBP as onset of the first Korotkoff sound and disappearance of all Korotkoff sounds, respectively, using the nearest even number. 2. Note the time of most recent BP medication taken before measurements.
Step 5: Average the readings	Use an average of ≥2 readings obtained on ≥2 occasions to estimate the individual's level of BP.
Step 6: Provide BP readings to patient	Provide patients the SBP/DBP readings both verbally and in writing.

requires the documentation of elevated BP (average of two to three BPs) obtained on two to three separate occasions. There is accumulating evidence that suggests that hypertensive patients whose BP remains high at night (nondippers) are at greater risk for cardiovascular morbidity than dippers. Less data are available to define the clinical significance of BP variability, although it has been suggested that it is a risk factor for cardiovascular morbidity.

The recognition of the limitations of the traditional clinic readings has led to two parallel developments: first, increasing use of measurements made out of the clinic, which avoids the unrepresentative nature of the clinic setting and also allows for increased numbers of readings to be taken; and second, the increased use of automated devices, which are being used both in and out of the office setting. It is increasingly recognized that office measurements correlate poorly with BP measured in other settings and that they can be supplemented by self-measured readings taken with validated devices at home. There is increasing evidence that home readings predict cardiovascular events and are particularly useful for monitoring the effects of treatment.

Out-of-Office and Self-Monitoring of BP

Ambulatory BP monitoring (ABPM) is used to obtain out-of-office BP readings at set intervals, usually over a 24-hour period. Self-monitoring, also known as home BP monitoring (HBPM), relies on the patient to record out-of-office BP measurements. Both ABPM and HBPM typically provide BP estimates that are based on multiple measurements. HBPM overcomes many of the limitations of traditional office BP measurement and is both cheaper and easier to perform than ambulatory BP monitoring.[45] Monitors using the oscillometric method are currently available and are accurate, reliable, easy to use, and relatively inexpensive. An increasing number of individuals are using them regularly to check their BP at home. HBPM has been endorsed by national and international guidelines and the AHA recently provided detailed recommendations for their use.[45] HBPM has the potential to improve the quality of care while reducing costs.

White-Coat Hypertension

Approximately 13% to 35% of people with HTN have persistently elevated BP in the presence of a health care worker, particularly a physician. However, when BP is measured elsewhere, including at work, BP is not elevated. When this phenomenon is detected in patients not taking medications, it is referred to as the white-coat HTN. White-coat HTN is usually considered clinically significant when office SBP/DBPs are greater than 20/10 mm Hg higher than home or ambulatory blood pressure monitoring SBP/DBPs. Although it can occur at any age, it is more common in older age, female versus male, and nonsmoking versus current smoking status. Its magnitude can be reduced (but not eliminated) by the use of stationary oscillometric devices that automatically determine and analyze a series of BPs over 15 to 20 minutes with the patient in a quiet environment in the office or clinic. The major clinical relevance of white-coat HTN is that it has typically been associated with a minimal to only slightly increased risk of CVD and all-cause mortality risk.[3]

Masked HTN or Isolated Ambulatory HTN

The converse condition of normal BP in the office and elevated BPs elsewhere, such as at work or at home is somewhat less frequent than white-coat HTN but more problematic to detect.[3] Lifestyle can contribute to this, for example, alcohol, tobacco, and caffeine consumption and physical activity may lead to acute increases in BP away from the clinic or office.

Resistant HTN

Resistant HTN is defined as above-goal elevated BP in a patient despite the concurrent use of three antihypertensive drug classes.[33] These antihypertensive drugs should be administered at maximum or maximally tolerated daily doses. Resistant HTN also includes patients whose BP achieves target values on greater than or equal to 4 antihypertensive medications. The diagnosis of resistant HTN requires assurance of antihypertensive medication adherence and exclusion of the "white-coat HTN" (office BP above goal but out-of-office BP at or below target). The importance of resistant HTN is underscored by the associated risk of adverse outcomes compared with nonresistant HTN.[33]

Clinical Evaluation

The objectives of the medical assessment for HTN are to determine (1) diagnosis and stage of HTN; (2) secondary causes of HTN; (3) presence of TOD; (4) level of global CVD risk; and (5) the plan for individualized monitoring and therapy. The assessment should include a thorough history and physical examination, including orthostatic BP change. Table 23-7 lists many of the important variables to assess during the history and physical examination.[3] It is also important to ask the patient about any nontraditional remedies they may be using including herbs, vitamins, and other supplements. Table 23-8 lists the basic and optional laboratory tests recommended for the assessment of TOD.[3]

Secondary HTN, a potentially curable condition, occurs in an estimated 10% of HTN cases; therefore, health care providers should evaluate for secondary causes (see Table 23-3).[33] Additional evaluation is recommended in patients whose age, severity of HTN, medical history, physical examination, or laboratory findings are suggestive of secondary HTN. Poor response to antihypertensive drug therapy or an accelerated phase of previously well-controlled HTN also indicates a need for further investigation.

Prognosis

HTN cannot be cured but can be managed through lifestyle modification and antihypertensive pharmacologic therapy. The relationship between BP and risk of CVD events is continuous, consistent, and independent of other risk factors. For adults aged 40 to 70 years, each increment of 20 mm Hg in SBP or 10 mm Hg in DBP doubles the risk of CVDs.[3,7] Unlike SBP, which is consistently associated with increased CVD risk after DBP adjustment, DBP is inconsistently associated with CVD risk after SBP adjustment.[46,47] The effectiveness of lifestyle and pharmacologic treatment in reducing BP has been demonstrated and substantial evidence indicates that controlling BP in hypertensive patients significantly lowers risk of CV morbidity and mortality.[48–50] A small reduction in BP markedly reduces the risk of HF, stroke, and myocardial infarction.[48]

PREVENTION AND MANAGEMENT

Prevention

The prevention of HTN is a major public health challenge. In the US, 46% of adults have HTN (defined as BP ≥130/80 mm Hg), and even more adults with elevated BP will develop HTN over their lifetime.[51] There is ample epidemiologic and clinical trial evidence that weight loss, a healthy diet, such as the Dietary

Table 23-7 • IMPORTANT ASPECTS OF THE PATIENT HISTORY

Management of Hypertension
Date of diagnosis
Last known normal BP
Course of BP
Goal BP
Current medications
Prior medications
 types, doses, side effects, intolerances
Intake of agents that may interfere
 Nonsteroidal anti-inflammatory drugs, oral contraceptives, sympathomimetics (including caffeine), adrenal steroids, excessive sodium intake, alcohol (>2 drinks/day), herbal remedies
Dietary history
 weight change, fresh vs. processed foods, sodium intake, saturated fats
Ability to modify lifestyle and maintain therapy
 understanding the nature of HTN and need for regimen; ability to perform physical activity; source of food preparation

Family History
HTN
Premature CVD or CV death
Familial diseases
 congenital heart disease (e.g., coarctation of the aorta); pheochromocytoma; renal disease; diabetes; gout

Social History
Work/profession
Educational level and health literacy (ability to read instructions)
Family structure and support
Social support and resources, including need for care providers
Psychosocial stress
Sexual function

Symptoms of Secondary Causes
Muscle weakness
Spells of tachycardia, sweating, tremor
Thinning of the skin
Flank pain

Symptoms of Target Organ Damage
Headaches
Transient weakness or blindness
Loss of visual acuity
Chest pain
Dyspnea
Edema
Claudication

Presence of Other Risk Factors and Concomitant Diseases
Current or past history of cigarette smoking
Diabetes
Dyslipidemia
Renal disease
Obstructive sleep apnea
 early morning headaches, daytime somnolence, loud snoring, erratic sleep
Physical inactivity

BP, blood pressure; DBP, diastolic blood pressure; SBP, systolic blood pressure. Adapted from Whelton PK, Carey RM, Aronow WS, et al. 2017 ACC/AHA/AAPA/ABC/ACPM/AGS/APhA/ASH/ASPC/NMA/PCNA guideline for the prevention, detection, evaluation, and management of high blood pressure in adults: a report of the American College of Cardiology/American Heart Association Task Force on Clinical Practice Guidelines. *Circulation*. 2018;138(17):e484–e594.

Approaches to Stop Hypertension (DASH) diet which is rich in fruits, vegetables, whole grains, legumes, and fish, reduced dietary sodium, increased dietary potassium intake, increased physical activity, and moderation in alcohol intake are particularly

Table 23-8 • RECOMMENDED AND OPTIONAL LABORATORY TESTS AND DIAGNOSTIC PROCEDURES

Recommended
Fasting blood glucose
Complete blood count
Lipid profile
Serum creatinine with eGFR
Serum sodium, potassium, calcium
Thyroid-stimulating hormone
Urinalysis
Electrocardiogram

Optional
Echocardiogram
Uric acid
Urinary albumin to creatinine ratio

important in the prevention of HTN (Table 23-9).[3] Population health and targeted strategies to prevent HTN should begin during childhood and be maintained throughout life.[10] For those with a normal BP, repeat evaluation every year is reasonable.

Recommendations for Management

Risk-Based Approach to Management

The goal of therapy for patients with HTN is the prevention of morbidity and mortality related to elevated BP, specifically the prevention of TOD and progression of atherosclerotic cardiovascular and renal disease.[3,52] Thresholds for BP-lowering therapy and therapeutic targets are summarized in Table 23-1 and an algorithm on BP thresholds and recommendations for risk-based treatment and follow-up is provided in Figure 23-1.[3] Nonpharmacologic therapy is recommended for all adults with elevated blood pressure and stages 1 and 2 HTN. This recommendation for nonpharmacologic therapy extends to those who are also taking medication to lower their blood pressure. Nonpharmacologic interventions for prevention and treatment of HTN are described in further detail below.

The risk-based approach to treatment involves the calculation of atherosclerotic cardiovascular disease (ASCVD) risk to guide treatment decisions at stage 1 HTN (systolic 130 to 139 mm Hg or diastolic 80 to 89 mm Hg).[35,36] At stage 1, those with low risk (10-year ASCVD risk less than 10%) are recommended nonpharmacologic therapy. Those with higher risk (10-year ASCVD risk greater than or equal to 10%) at stage 1, are recommended blood pressure–lowering medication in addition to nonpharmacologic therapy. Similarly, stage 1 is the threshold for recommending blood pressure–lowering medication in addition to nonpharmacologic therapy for those with comorbid conditions that increase risk such as diabetes, CKD, HF, stable ischemic heart disease, and peripheral arterial disease. At stage 2 (systolic greater than or equal to 140 mm Hg or diastolic greater than or equal to 90 mm Hg), blood pressure–lowering medication in addition to nonpharmacologic therapy is recommended regardless of ASCVD risk. For older adults (greater than or equal to 65 years of age) who are noninstitutionalized and ambulatory with an average systolic blood pressure greater than or equal to 130 mm Hg, blood pressure–lowering medication in addition to nonpharmacologic therapy and a treatment goal of systolic blood pressure less than 130 mm Hg is recommended.

These recommendations encourage aggressive treatment of HTN. However, emphasis is placed on the need to balance using an individualized approach that involves shared decision making through frequent communication to assess patient preferences, goals of care, how they are feeling, and how medications may affect their daily

Table 23-9 • EVIDENCE-BASED NONPHARMACOLOGIC INTERVENTIONS FOR THE PREVENTION AND TREATMENT OF HYPERTENSION[a]

	Nonpharmacologic Intervention	Dose	Approximate Impact on SBP	
			Hypertension	**Normotension**
Weight loss	Weight/body fat	Ideal body weight is best goal but at least 1-kg reduction in body weight for most adults who are overweight. Expect about 1 mm Hg for every 1-kg reduction in body weight.	−5 mm Hg	−2/3 mm Hg
Healthy diet	DASH dietary pattern	Diet rich in fruits, vegetables, whole grains, and low-fat dairy products with reduced content of saturated and trans fat	−11 mm Hg	−3 mm Hg
Reduced intake of dietary sodium	Dietary sodium	<1500 mg/day is optimal but at least 1,000-mg/day reduction in most adults	−5/6 mm Hg	−2/3 mm Hg
Enhanced intake of dietary potassium	Dietary potassium	3500–5000 mg/day, preferably by consumption of a diet rich in potassium	−4/5 mm Hg	−2 mm Hg
Physical activity	Acrobic	• 90–150 min/wk • 65–75% heart rate reserve	−5/8 mm Hg	−2/4 mm Hg
	Dynamic Resistance	• 90–150 min/wk • 50–80% 1 rep maximum • 6 exercises, 3 sets/exercise, 10 rep/set	−4 mm Hg	−2 mm Hg
	Isometric Resistance	• 4 × 2 min (hand grip), 1-minute rest between exercises, 30–40% maximum voluntary contraction, 3 sessions/wk • 8–10 weeks	−5 mm Hg	−4 mm Hg
Moderation in alcohol intake	Alcohol consumption	In individuals who drink alcohol, reduce alcohol† to: • Men: ≤2 drinks daily • Women: ≤1 drink daily	−4 mm Hg	−3 mm Hg

[a]Type, dose, and expected impact on BP in adults with a normal BP and with hypertension.
†In the United States, one "standard" drink contains roughly 14 g of pure alcohol, which is typically found in 12 oz of regular beer (usually about 5% alcohol), 5 oz of wine (usually about 12% alcohol), and 1.5 oz of distilled spirits (usually about 40% alcohol).
Reprinted with permission from Whelton PK, Carey RM, Aronow WS, et al. 2017 ACC/AHA/AAPA/ABC/ACPM/AGS/APhA/ASH/ASPC/NMA/PCNA guideline for the prevention, detection, evaluation, and management of high blood pressure in adults: a report of the American College of Cardiology/American Heart Association Task Force on Clinical Practice Guidelines. *Circulation.* 2018;138(17):e484–e594.

activities. This is of particular importance among older adults with HTN and a high burden of comorbidity and limited life expectancy.

Nonpharmacologic Interventions

Nonpharmacologic interventions alone or in combination with pharmacologic therapy are indispensable in the prevention and management of high BP. Nonpharmacologic therapy alone is effective in preventing HTN in adults with elevated BP, and for the management of those with uncomplicated and milder forms of HTN.[53,54] Evidence-based lifestyle modification strategies that lower BP are described in Table 23-9 and include weight control, a healthy diet, such as the DASH diet which is rich in fruits, vegetables, whole grains, legumes, and fish, reduced dietary sodium, increased dietary potassium intake, increased physical activity, and moderation in alcohol intake. Although other interventions such as stress reduction, guided breathing, fish oil supplementation, low-carbohydrate and vegetarian diet have been reported to lower BP, there is insufficient high-quality data to support wider implementation of these strategies.[3] Also, persons diagnosed with HTN are encouraged to modify other risk factors for CVD such as dyslipidemia and smoking because of their additive impact on the rate of development and progression of atherosclerosis.[3,52]

Weight Control. The relationship between HTN and overweight/obesity is well established. There is also a correlation between the presence of excess abdominal adiposity (defined as an increased waist-to-hip ratio of more than 0.85 in women and 0.95 in men) and the development of HTN, diabetes, dyslipidemia, and increased CHD mortality.[55–57] A number of epidemiologic studies have revealed that overweight people have from two to three times the risk for HTN compared with persons who are not overweight.[58] The influence of weight may be related to alterations in cardiovascular, endocrine, and metabolic factors caused by obesity. These alterations include increased cardiac output, increased blood volume, and sodium retention. Adipose tissue acts as a major endocrine organ, secreting bioactive substances which may induce metabolic disorders, such as hyperinsulinemia, insulin resistance, decreased carbohydrate tolerance, and decreased insulin sensitivity.[59] Alterations in endothelial function have also been demonstrated in persons who are overweight.[60]

Weight loss consistently reduces BP more effectively than any other lifestyle measure.[3] Among adults whose BP was controlled with medications for 5 years, an average weight loss of 10 lb prevented 60% of the overweight participants from having to return to take medications.[61] In addition, weight loss complements pharmacologic management of mild–high BP. In a meta-analysis of 25 randomized control trials, which included trials based on weight reduction through energy restriction, increased physical activity, or both, average reductions of 4.4/3.6 mm Hg for SBP and DBP, respectively were reported for a 5-kg weight loss.[62] A dose–response relationship was observed with greater weight loss, resulting in greater BP reduction.

Counseling an overweight patient with HTN about weight reduction is important, as both a preventive measure as well as an independent or complementary treatment for HTN. A challenge for both health care providers and patients is supporting the maintenance of weight loss, because longitudinal studies have shown that subjects who lose weight initially tend to gain back the weight over time.

Diet High in Fruits and Vegetables. The DASH study examined the effects of an 8-week dietary intervention on BP in normotensive and hypertensive subjects.[77] The DASH diet emphasized fruits, vegetables, and low-fat dairy products; included

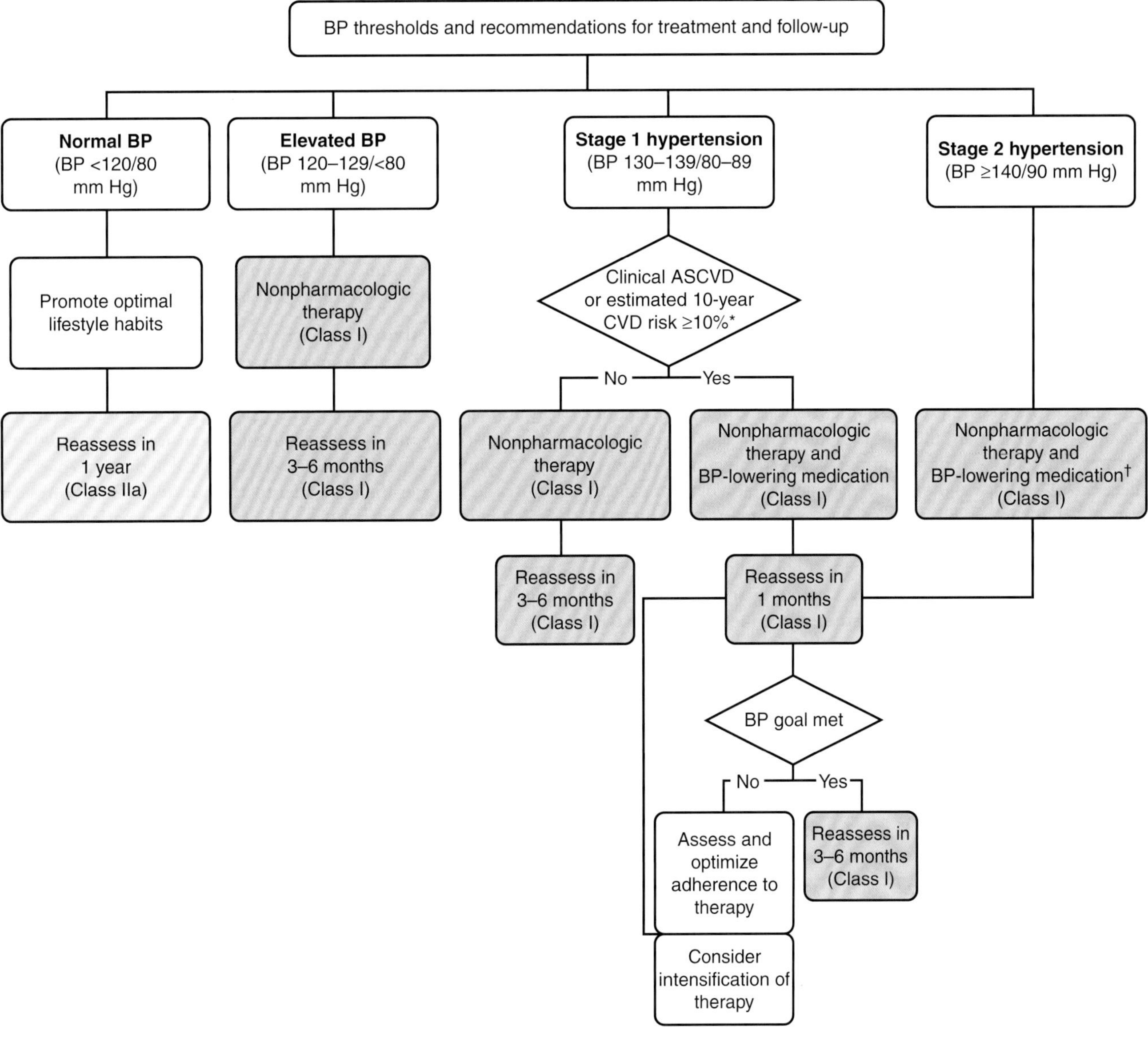

Figure 23-1. Blood pressure thresholds and recommendations for treatment and follow-up. *Using the ACC/AHA Pooled Cohort Equations. Note that patients with DM or CKD are automatically placed in the high-risk category. For initiation of RAS inhibitor or diuretic therapy, assess blood tests for electrolytes and renal function 2 to 4 weeks after initiating therapy. †Consider initiation of pharmacologic therapy for stage 2 hypertension with two antihypertensive agents of different classes. Patients with stage 2 hypertension and BP greater than or equal to 160/100 mm Hg should be promptly treated, carefully monitored, and subject to upward medication dose adjustment as necessary to control BP. Reassessment includes BP measurement, detection of orthostatic hypotension in selected patients (e.g., older or with postural symptoms), identification of white-coat hypertension or a white-coat effect, documentation of adherence, monitoring of the response to therapy, reinforcement of the importance of adherence, reinforcement of the importance of treatment, and assistance with treatment to achieve BP target. ASCVD, atherosclerotic cardiovascular disease; CVD, cardiovascular disease; DM, diabetes mellitus; CKD, chronic kidney disease; RAS, renin-angiotensin system. (Reprinted with permission from Whelton PK, Carey RM, Aronow WS, et al. 2017 ACC/AHA/AAPA/ABC/ACPM/AGS/APhA/ASH/ASPC/NMA/PCNA guideline for the prevention, detection, evaluation, and management of high blood pressure in adults: a report of the American College of Cardiology/American Heart Association Task Force on Clinical Practice Guidelines. *Circulation.* 2018;138[17]:e484–e594.)

whole grains, poultry, fish, and nuts; and was reduced in fats, red meat, sweets, and sugar-containing beverages. Accordingly, it was rich in potassium, magnesium, calcium, and fiber and was reduced in total fat, saturated fat, and cholesterol; it also was slightly increased in protein. In the 133 hypertensive subjects, adherence to a diet rich in fruits, vegetables, and low-fat dairy products and low in saturated and total fat resulted in a marked decline in both SBP and DBP. Compared with normotensive control subjects, subjects with an SBP between 140 and 160 mm Hg and/or a DBP between 90 and 95 mm Hg had decreases in BP of −11.4/−5.5 mm Hg. There was no significant change in weight during the study in any of the study groups. The DASH diet included 8 to 10 servings per day of fruits and vegetables and 2.7 servings of low-fat dairy products. Subsequent clinical trials based on the DASH diets have shown that (1) salt reduction significantly decreases SBP and DBP; and (2) the DASH diet can successfully be combined with other lifestyle modifications specifically limiting alcohol intake to 1 oz or less per day and increasing physical activity to a minimum of 180 minutes (3 hours) each week.[63–65] While the DASH diet is effective, adopting these dietary recommendations presents a great challenge for many individuals.

Sodium Restriction. In general, as the amount of dietary salt (sodium chloride) intake rises, so does BP.[63] The most persuasive evidence about the effects of salt on BP comes from rigorously controlled, dose–response trials.[65] Each of these three trials tested at least three sodium levels, and each documented statistically significant, direct, progressive dose–response relationships. The largest of the dose–response trials, the DASH-Sodium trial, tested the effects of three different levels of sodium intake separately in two distinct diets: the DASH diet and a control diet more typical of what Americans eat. The three sodium levels (lower, intermediate, and higher) provided approximate sodium intakes of 1.5, 2.5, and 3.3 g, respectively. The BP response to sodium reduction, while direct and progressive, was nonlinear. Specifically, decreasing sodium intake by 0.9 g/day (40 mmol/day) caused a greater lowering of BP when the starting sodium intake was 100 mmol/day than when it was above this level. In subgroup analyses of the DASH-Sodium trial, reduced sodium intake significantly lowered BP in each of the major subgroups studied (i.e., men, women, blacks, and non-blacks).[66,67] The effects of sodium reduction on BP tend to be greater in blacks; middle-aged and older persons; and individuals with HTN, diabetes, or CKD.[63] In addition, clinical trials have documented that reduced sodium intake can lower BP in the setting of antihypertensive medication and facilitate HTN control and is associated with a reduced risk of atherosclerotic cardiovascular events and congestive HF.[63]

The 2015–2020 Dietary Guidelines for Americans recommend that adults consume no more than 2300 mg of sodium per day.[68] The 2017 HTN guidelines recommend a goal sodium intake of less than or equal to 100 mmol/day, which is equivalent to approximately 6 g of sodium chloride or 2.4 g of sodium per day.[3] In many of the clinical trials of sodium reduction, the goal levels of sodium intake were even lower than this recommended goal. To reduce salt intake, individuals should choose foods low in salt and limit the amount of salt added to food. However, because greater than 75% of consumed salt comes from processed foods, any meaningful strategy to reduce salt intake must involve the efforts of food manufacturers and restaurants. It may help patients to know that it takes 8 to 12 weeks to adjust one's sense of taste to a lower intake of sodium.

Dietary Potassium Intake. Potassium intake is inversely related to BP and is also inversely related to stroke.[69–71] A higher level of potassium seems to blunt the effect of sodium on BP, with a lower sodium–potassium ratio being associated with a lower level of BP than that noted for corresponding levels of sodium or potassium on their own.[72] Also, a lower sodium–potassium ratio may result in a reduced risk of CVD as compared with the pattern for corresponding levels of either sodium or potassium alone.[73]

Potassium supplementation, preferably in dietary modification, is recommended for adults with elevated BP or HTN, unless contraindicated by the presence of CKD or use of drugs that reduce potassium excretion. Potassium interventions have been effective in lowering BP, especially in adult patients consuming an excess of sodium and in blacks.[74] The typical BP-lowering effect of a 60-mmol (1380-mg) administration of potassium chloride has been about 2 mm Hg and 4 to 5 mm Hg in adults with normotension and HTN, respectively, although the response is up to twice as much in persons consuming a high-sodium diet.[3]

The 2015 Dietary Guidelines for Americans encourage a diet rich in potassium and identify the adequate intake level for adult patients as 4700 mg/day.[68] Good sources of dietary potassium include fruits and vegetables, as well as low-fat dairy products, selected fish and meats, nuts, and soy products. Four to five servings of fruits and vegetables will usually provide 1500 to greater than 3000 mg of potassium. This recommendation can be achieved by a diet, such as the DASH diet, that is high in potassium content.

Physical Activity. A sedentary lifestyle is a risk factor for HTN and contributes to more than 5 million deaths globally.[75] Approximately half of American adults do not meet minimum physical activity guidelines although adults are advised to engage in at least 150 minutes of moderate-intensity physical activity or 75 minutes of vigorous-intensity physical activity per week.[75] Short (i.e., greater than or equal to 10-minute) bouts of physical activity are also as beneficial as longer bouts so patients should be encouraged to focus on the cumulative amount of exercise and reduce sedentary behavior.[75] Those diagnosed with HTN should engage in 30 minutes of moderate-to-vigorous-intensity aerobic activity five times per week. Aerobic exercise has a BP-lowering effect. Specifically, aerobic exercise results in average SBP reduction of approximately 2 to 4 mm Hg and 5 to 8 mm Hg in adults with normal and high blood pressure, respectively.[76] Persons who are physically active experience lower cardiovascular and all-cause mortality rates.

Physical activity is known to have a variety of metabolic and other effects that may partially explain its beneficial effects on BP. These include a reduction in resting cardiac output and peripheral vascular resistance, a humoral mechanism contributing to the reduction of the activity of the renin–angiotensin–aldosterone system and sympathetic nervous system activity, and increase in prostaglandins with vasodilator effect.[76] Importantly, an effect of physical exercise on TOD has also been demonstrated. Two studies of 18 persons with HTN and LVH found that after 24 to 32 weeks of exercising at least three times per week, the participants had significant decreases in indices of LVH suggesting reduction (i.e., improvement) in TOD.[77]

Reduction of Alcohol Intake. Observational studies and clinical trials have documented a direct, dose-dependent relationship between alcohol intake and BP, particularly as the intake of alcohol increases above 2 drinks per day.[63,78] A meta-analysis 15 randomized controlled trials (RCTs) demonstrated that decreased consumption of alcohol (median reduction in self-reported alcohol consumption, 76%; range, 16% to 100%) reduced SBP and DBP by 3.3 and 2.0 mm Hg, respectively.[78] BP reductions were similar in nonhypertensive and hypertensive individuals. Importantly, the relationship between reduction in mean percentage of alcohol and decline in BP was dose dependent though there appears to be a benefit to low–moderate levels of alcohol consumption with a lower incidence of ischemic stroke in persons with an alcohol intake of 1 to 2 drinks per day compared with abstainers.

Alcohol consumption should be limited to less than or equal to 2 alcoholic drinks per day in most men and less than or equal to 1 alcoholic drink per day in women and lighter-weight persons.[3] A standard drink has been defined as approximately 14 g of alcohol, which is the amount contained in 12 oz of beer, 5 oz of wine, or 1.5 oz of distilled liquor such as vodka, gin, or scotch.

Control of Other Risk Factors. Beyond HTN, epidemiologic studies have shown that the other major risk factors such as smoking, dyslipidemia, and diabetes have an additive effect on CVD morbidity and mortality. Therefore, although smoking cessation and improving dyslipidemia will not decrease BP, these interventions will reduce morbidity and mortality from ASCVD.[52]

Pharmacologic Management

Following a diagnosis of HTN, use of BP-lowering medication is recommended (Fig. 23-1) in adults with

1. estimated 10-year ASCVD risk less than 10% and no history of CVD and SBP greater than or equal to 140 mm Hg or DBP greater than or equal to 90 mm Hg for primary prevention of CVD events[7,79,80] and
2. estimated 10-year ASCVD risk greater than or equal to 10% at levels of SBP greater than or equal to 130 mm Hg or DBP greater than or equal to 80 mm Hg for primary prevention of CVD or for secondary prevention of recurrent CVD events.[42,50,79,81–86]

A BP target of less than 130/80 mm Hg is recommended, though this may be individualized based on the health care provider–patient shared decision-making discussion.[42,87–90]

For initiation of antihypertensive pharmacologic therapy, first-line agents include thiazide diuretics, calcium channel blockers (CCBs), and ACE-Is or ARBs.[48,91] Additional classes of antihypertensive medications include (1) adrenergic inhibitors including β-blocking agents, central-acting inhibitors, central α-agonists, α-adrenergic blockers, and combined α-adrenergic and β-adrenergic blockers; (2) vasodilators; and (3) CCBs. Consideration of patient comorbidities, lifestyle, and preferences as well as duration of action may suggest better tolerance or greater effect from one class of medication versus other classes. Multisocietal guidelines should be referenced for detailed recommendations on BP thresholds, BP goals, and pharmacological therapy in patients with HTN and certain clinical conditions.[3,48]

Initiation of antihypertensive pharmacologic therapy with a single antihypertensive drug is reasonable in adults with stage 1 HTN, though the vast majority of persons with BP sufficiently elevated to warrant pharmacologic therapy may be best treated initially with two agents. In fact, initiation of antihypertensive drug therapy with two first-line agents of different classes, either as separate agents or in a fixed-dose combination, is recommended in adults with stage 2 HTN and BP greater than 20/10 mm Hg above their BP target.[48] Evidence favoring this approach comes mostly from studies using fixed-dose combination products showing greater BP lowering with fixed-dose combination agents than with single agents, as well as better adherence to therapy.[91,92]

Combinations of pharmacologic agents that have similar mechanisms of action or clinical effects should be avoided. For example, two drugs from the same class should not be administered together (e.g., two different ACE-Is, or nondihydropyridine CCBs). Likewise, two drugs from classes that target the same BP control system are less effective and potentially harmful when used together (e.g., ACE-Is, ARBs). Exceptions to this rule include concomitant use of a thiazide diuretic, K-sparing diuretic, and/or loop diuretic in various combinations.[3]

Adults initiating a new or adjusted HTN drug regimen should have a follow-up evaluation of adherence and response to treatment at monthly intervals until control is achieved.[3] Follow-up evaluation components include assessment of BP control and evaluation for orthostatic hypotension, adverse effects from medications, adherence to nonpharmacologic and pharmacologic therapy, need for adjustment of medication dosage, laboratory testing (including electrolyte and renal function status), and other assessments of TOD.[3]

Management in Special Populations

Management of HTN is modified on the basis of individual characteristics as well as knowledge of HTN care for specific groups. The following section outlines additional information that guides the management of HTN in several special populations.

HTN in Older Adults

Because of its extremely high prevalence in older adults, HTN is a leading cause of preventable morbidity and mortality and a major contributor to premature disability and institutionalization.[3] Both SBP and DBP increase linearly up to the fifth or sixth decade of life, after which DBP gradually decreases while SBP continues to rise. Thus, isolated systolic HTN is the predominant form of HTN in older persons. RCTs have clearly demonstrated that BP lowering in isolated systolic HTN is effective in reducing the risk of fatal and nonfatal stroke (primary outcome), cardiovascular events, and death.[93–96]

Treatment of HTN in older adults is challenging because of the high degree of variability in comorbidity, polypharmacy, frailty, cognitive impairment, and variable life expectancy. However, over the past 30 years, RCTs of antihypertensive therapy have included large numbers of older persons, and in these trials intensive treatment has safely reduced the risk of CVD for persons over the ages of 65 years.[3,95] Both HYVET (Hypertension in the Very Elderly Trial) and SPRINT (Systolic Blood Pressure Intervention Trial) included those who were frail but still living independently in the community, and both were stopped early for benefit.[95,97] Importantly, BP-lowering therapy is one of the few interventions shown to reduce mortality risk in frail older individuals. RCTs in noninstitutionalized community-dwelling older persons have also demonstrated that improved BP control does not exacerbate orthostatic hypotension and has no adverse impact on risk of injurious falls. It should be noted, that SPRINT excluded those with low (less than 110 mm Hg) standing BP on study entry. Health care providers should educate and routinely evaluate older persons on antihypertensive therapy.

In summary, despite the complexity of management in caring for older persons with HTN, RCTs have demonstrated that in many community-dwelling older adults, even adults greater than 80 years of age, BP-lowering goals during antihypertensive treatment need not differ from those selected for persons less than 65 years of age. Importantly, no randomized trial of BP lowering in persons greater than 65 years of age has ever shown harm or less benefit for older versus younger adults. However, clinicians should implement careful titration of BP lowering and monitoring for orthostatic hypotension in older persons.

HTN in Racial and Ethnic Minorities

It is well established that blacks have higher prevalence of HTN and poorer control rates than whites and other racial and ethnic groups.[3] Furthermore, risk factors, such as obesity, physical inactivity, and poor diet are more prevalent in racial and ethnic minority groups.[1] In addition to behavioral and socioeconomic factors, such as limited health care access, lack of health insurance, and transportation issues, clinical inertia has also been demonstrated to contribute to racial and ethnic disparities in HTN care and control.[98] Non-Hispanic Asian, Hispanic, and non-Hispanic black adults are less likely to have controlled BP than non-Hispanic white adults.[1,5]

Among Hispanic adults in the United States, the lower control rates are attributed to poor awareness and treatment.[99,100] However, among blacks, awareness and treatment are comparable to whites, but HTN is more severe and BP control is poorer in blacks.[100,101]

The 2017 ACC/AHA guidelines have outlined specific recommendations for treating HTN in racial and ethnic minorities. In black adults who are diagnosed with HTN but without a HF or CKD diagnosis, including diabetes, initial antihypertensive drug therapy should include a thiazide-type diuretic or CCB.[3] Furthermore, two or more antihypertensive drugs are recommended to achieve BP control (less than 130/80 mm Hg) in adults diagnosed with HTN and especially blacks. Among blacks who do not achieve BP control with three drugs, resistant HTN should be considered and treated.[3,33]

HTN in Pregnancy

HTN occurs in pregnancy either because of pre-existing chronic HTN or because of the development of pregnancy-induced HTN including gestational HTN, preeclampsia, and eclampsia. HTN that exists prior to pregnancy, develops before the 20th week of pregnancy, or that persists more than 6 weeks after delivery is considered chronic HTN. Gestational HTN is defined as an elevated BP that usually occurs in the third trimester and is not accompanied by other signs and symptoms. In preeclampsia and eclampsia, the elevated BP is considered as one of several signs and symptoms of an underlying disorder of organ perfusion. Edema and proteinuria usually occur with pregnancy-induced HTN. All pregnant women are recommended to be screened for preeclampsia at every prenatal visit.[102]

The 2017 ACC/AHA guidelines recommend that women with HTN who become pregnant, or are planning to become pregnant, should be transitioned to methyldopa, nifedipine, and/or labetalol during pregnancy.[3] ACE-Is, ARBs, or direct renin inhibitors are also contraindicated because of their documented adverse effects on fetal growth and development.[3]

HTN in Patients With Diabetes

HTN prevalence is approximately 80% among adults with diabetes; special consideration must be given to this cohort.[99,103–107] Coexistent HTN and diabetes contribute significantly to the development of CVD, nephropathy, and retinopathy.[108–110] Furthermore, among treated hypertensives, those with diabetes are significantly less likely to have controlled HTN compared to those without diabetes. Most adults with diabetes mellitus have a 10-year ASCVD risk greater than or equal to 10%, requiring initiation of antihypertensive drug therapy at BP greater than or equal to 130/80 mm Hg and a treatment goal of less than 130/80 mm Hg.[111] Meta-analyses of RCTs supported lowering of BP to less than 130/80 mm Hg among those with diabetes mellitus.[50,112] Two meta-analyses addressing target BP in adults with diabetes mellitus restricted the analysis to RCTs that randomized patients to different BP levels.[42,113] Target BP of 133/76 mm Hg provided a significant benefit compared with that of 140/81 mm Hg for major cardiovascular events, MI, stroke, albuminuria, and retinopathy progression.[42]

In the ACCORD (Action to Control Cardiovascular Risk in Diabetes) trial,[99,107] lowering the BP target (SBP less than 120 mm Hg) did not reduce the rate of the composite outcome of fatal and nonfatal major cardiovascular events and was associated with greater risk of adverse events, such as self-reported hypotension and a reduction in estimated glomerular filtration rate. Secondary analyses of the ACCORD trial demonstrated a significant outcome benefit of stroke risk reduction in the intensive BP/standard glycemic group.[114]

Lifestyle interventions are also recommended and include weight control and physical activity, which are keys to BP control in persons with diabetes. The guidelines also recommend the use of all first-line classes of antihypertensive agents (i.e., diuretics, ACE-Is, ARBs, and CCBs) for the treatment of HTN in adults with diabetes.[3] Importantly, ACE-Is and ARBs have beneficial effects in diabetes beyond HTN control, including reducing renal dysfunction, CVD, and stroke.[3]

HTN With Chronic Kidney Disease

Control of HTN is extremely effective in preventing the progression of renal failure in persons with renal disease regardless of etiology. Most patients with CKD have a 10-year ASCVD risk greater than or equal to 10%, requiring initiation of antihypertensive pharmacologic therapy at BP greater than or equal to 130/80 mm Hg with a recommended treatment goal of less than 130/80.[3] Trial data suggests that more intensive BP treatment may further reduce CVD events among patients with CKD. In the Systolic Blood Pressure Intervention trial (SPRINT), those with CKD who were randomized to intensive therapy (SBP target less than 120 mm Hg) had the same beneficial reduction in CVD events and all-cause mortality compared to their counterparts without CKD, with no difference seen in the principal renal outcome.[115] Several meta-analyses support more intensive BP treatment to reduce cardiovascular events but do not demonstrate a reduction in the rate of progression of kidney disease.[42,50,87] It is important to note that more intensive BP treatment may result in a modest reduction in glomerular filtration rate, which is thought to be primarily attributable to a hemodynamic effect and may be reversible. Electrolyte abnormalities are also more likely during intensive BP treatment.

The guidelines recommend the use of ACE-Is and ARBs in treating persons with renal disease based on clinical trials demonstrating their effectiveness.[3] Three or more optimally dosed antihypertensive medications are often needed to achieve the goal BP of less than 130/80 mm Hg. Dietary recommendations for potassium restriction must be considered for patients with more advanced renal disease.

Hypertensive Crisis

Hypertensive emergencies are characterized by severe elevations in BP (greater than 180/120 mm Hg) complicated by evidence of impending or progressive target organ dysfunction.[3] Acute hypertensive crises are rare situations in which patients require immediate intervention to reduce BP. These crises may occur either in persons whose HTN previously was not diagnosed or in persons with known but poorly controlled HTN. Hypertensive crises have been classified into two types: hypertensive emergencies and urgencies. Hypertensive emergency occurs when end-organ damage is acute or imminent and immediate reduction in BP, usually via intravenous medication in an intensive care unit, is required. Hypertensive urgency occurs when the BP is critically high, with signs such as edema of the optic disc, but there is less evidence of TOD, so that BP reduction can occur over a longer period using oral antihypertensive medications. There is a continuum from emergencies to urgencies and excellent assessment and judgment are required. Acute elevations of BP may occur after certain medications such as clonidine are discontinued or the individual either forgets to take or runs out of medication. Adults with hypertensive urgency should be treated immediately with oral combination therapy.[3]

Hypertensive emergencies are defined as severe elevations in BP (greater than 180/120 mm Hg) associated with evidence of new or worsening TOD. In adults with a hypertensive emergency, admission to an intensive care unit is recommended for continuous monitoring of BP and TOD and for parenteral administration of an appropriate agent.[3] In the management of hypertensive emergencies, the goal is to reduce the pressure so that TOD from the HTN is prevented or minimized while preventing the cerebral or myocardial ischemia that could result from too rapid of a reduction in BP. The parenteral drugs that may be used in hypertensive emergencies are detailed in the clinical guideline. After the BP has been brought under control, the patient who has experienced an HTN emergency or urgency will require extended expert outpatient HTN management.

ACHIEVING BP CONTROL

Despite well-established effective lifestyle and pharmacologic treatments for HTN, the rates of HTN awareness, treatment, and control remain low, particularly in racial and ethnic minorities.[3] Several factors contribute to poor HTN control and include patient-, provider-, and system-level factors.[116] Achieving HTN control requires concerted action by patients, providers, and health care organizations. Table 23-10 summarizes strategies to promote HTN control.

Role of Patients

The challenge for patients in achieving HTN control is to modify their lives in ways that support their treatment plan. Deciding to control one's HTN is the critical factor that precedes lifestyle modification and HTN control.[117,118] Each of these HTN care constituents recently identified the key action steps required to substantially improve BP control rates. Patients must take the following actions: (1) take an active and responsible role in personal health management; (2) be appropriately educated; (3) develop skills to monitor and control BP; (4) take a partnership role in treatment; and (5) resolve barriers to BP control.

Role of Health Care Providers

Health care providers in partnership with patients hold the keys to HTN control. Health care providers should: (1) identify, prevent, and correctly treat HTN; (2) promote public and community awareness of HTN; (3) develop communication skills that empower patients; and (4) advocate improved access to health care.[118] The provider's responsibilities range from knowing and using the latest guidelines for HTN control to motivating the patient to follow the treatment plan. At a minimum, the challenges to a provider include correctly diagnosing the patient's condition; communicating

Table 23-10 • STRATEGIES TO PROMOTE BLOOD PRESSURE CONTROL

Identify knowledge, attitudes, beliefs, and experience:
- Assess patient's understanding and acceptance of the diagnosis and expectations of being in care.
- Assess cultural beliefs and practices that may influence care and adherence.
- Discuss patient's concerns and clarify misunderstandings.

Educate about conditions and treatment:
- Inform patient of blood pressure (BP) level.
- Agree with patient on a goal BP.
- Assess patient motivation for change.
- Inform patient about recommended treatment, providing specific oral and written information.
- Elicit concerns and questions and provide opportunities for patient to state specific behaviors to carry out treatment recommendations.
- Emphasize the need to continue treatment, that is an elevated BP is typically undetectable but carries significant consequences, and successful BP control does not mean HTN is cured.
- Teach self-monitoring skills.

Individualize the regimen:
- Actively engage patient in his/her own care by promoting shared decision making, with emphasis on social and cultural factors, including health literacy.
- Include patient in decision making.
- Simplify the regimen.
- Incorporate treatment into patient's daily lifestyle.
- Set, with the patient, realistic short-term objectives for specific components of the treatment plan.
- Encourage discussion of side effects and concerns.
- Encourage self-monitoring of BP.
- Prioritize critical aspects of the regimen.
- Implement treatment plan in steps.
- Modify dosages or change medications to reduce side effects.
- Minimize cost of therapy.
- Indicate you will ask about adherence at next visit.
- When weight loss is established as a treatment goal, discourage quick weight loss regimens, fasting, or unscientific methods, since these are associated with weight cycling which may increase cardiovascular morbidity and mortality.

Provide follow-up and reinforcement:
- Provide feedback regarding BP measurements.
- Ask about behaviors to achieve BP control.
- Give positive feedback for behavioral and BP improvement.
- Hold exit interviews to clarify regimen.
- Make appointment for next visit before patient leaves the office.
- Use appointment reminders and confirm appointments in advance to promote ongoing follow-up.
- For nonadherence, schedule more frequent visits to counsel the patient.
- For missed appointments, contact and follow up with the patient.
- Consider health care provider–patient contracts.
- Consider home visits.
- Establish regular, structured follow-up mechanisms and reminder systems to monitor patient progress both in the office and remotely.
- Provide the most appropriate evidence-based tools and resources designed to maximize self-management (including health behavior change, lifestyle modification, etc.).

Promote social support:
- Educate family members to be part of the BP control process and provide daily reinforcement.
- Suggest small group activities to enhance mutual support and motivation.

Collaborate with other professionals:
- Draw upon complementary skills and knowledge of nurses, pharmacists, community health workers, dietitians, optometrists, dentists, and physician assistants.
- Facilitate communication and care coordination among various team members, patient, family, and caregivers.
- Assure awareness and effective use of evidence-based diagnosis and treatment guidelines by all team members.
- Follow a single, personalized plan of care based on evidence, guidelines, and the individual patient's characteristics and needs.
- Refer and/or obtain consultation for intensive counseling or specialty evaluation as needed.

Adapted from Himmelfarb CR, Commodore-Mensah Y, Hill MN. Expanding the role of nurses to improve hypertension care and control globally. *Ann Glob Health.* 2016;82(2):243–253.

the importance of HTN as a disease and as a risk factor for atherosclerosis; developing an effective treatment plan that fits the patient's lifestyle and economic situation; and evaluating the results of the therapy. To achieve these goals, the provider requires skills in assessment, diagnosis, communication, and behavioral counseling. Table 23-10 lists strategies to promote BP control.

Collaborative Care

The optimal management of HTN requires the collaboration of health care providers.[119,120] HTN care teams are diverse, with the patient as the central figure. Other members may include the nurse, health educator, community health worker, nutritionist, pharmacist, and physician. Nurses have a role in all aspects of HTN management, from measuring BPs to conducting research to setting national policy. The role of the individual nurse depends on his or her preparation and work experience. The successful use of nurses to manage patients with HTN has been reported in the literature since the 1970s.[121–125] The current era of cost containment and the preparation of advanced practice nurses create a receptive climate for further development of the nurses' role in HTN management. Successful HTN teams require expertise in communication, coordination, and an appreciation of the skills of each team member.

Nurses and nurse practitioners play key roles in HTN management including (1) detection, referral, and follow up; (2) diagnostics and medication management; (3) patient education, counseling, and skill building; (4) coordination of care; (5) clinic or office management; (6) population health management; and (7) performance measurement and quality improvement.[126] Furthermore, nurses have expanded their clinical roles to leading community and clinical studies to improve HTN care and address racial and ethnic disparities in HTN outcomes by addressing social determinants of health.[126–131] Strategies to improve BP control are summarized in Table 23-10.

Clinician Inertia

Clinician inertia occurs when health care providers who are treating HTN fail to increase the intensity of drug treatment even though they see the patient regularly and are aware that BP goals have not been achieved.[132,133] The causes of this problem are varied and include a lack of knowledge about the relative risks and benefits of rigorous HTN management and resistance to implementing guidelines.[133–136] Treatment guidelines explicitly indicate that most patients will require two or more antihypertensive agents to achieve HTN control.[7] The intensity of treatment (i.e., dose and/or selection of medication) must be increased until BP is at or below goal, with the requirement that treatment should also remain well tolerated.

Role of Health Care Organizations

Health care systems must be adequately resourced and structured to deliver effective HTN treatment and prevention and to promote public and professional education. Health care organizations can implement specific strategies such as providing education for both providers and patients, setting standards of care, implementing computerized data systems, documenting the impact of care on patient outcomes, and determining which types of care are cost-effective while maintaining quality of life to improve HTN control.[126]

Role of the Community

Communities, including employers, can play an active role in HTN screening and education and promote and support health visits and follow-up care. Community-based interventions in the United States and Europe have demonstrated that community action can reduce the risks of CVD. In a landmark trial of BP reduction in black barbershops in the community,[137] the intervention group which received health promotion by barbers and medication management by specialty-trained pharmacists experienced a 21.6 mm Hg greater reduction in mean SBP than the control group. The FAITH (Faith-Based Approaches in the Treatment of Hypertension) study[138] which consisted of community-based lifestyle intervention plus motivational interviewing delivered in churches resulted in significantly greater reduction in SBP in blacks diagnosed with HTN compared with health education alone. Together, these studies demonstrate the promising role of nontraditional care settings in the community in improving HTN control.

Target:BP™ is a national initiative which is a partnership between the AHA and the American Medical Association (AMA) in response to the rising rates of uncontrolled BP. Target:BP assists organizations in the community to achieve BP control by providing access to an evidence-based quality improvement program to improve BP control and recognizing organizations which meet BP targets.

Summary

In summary, HTN is a common risk factor for cardiovascular, renal, and cerebrovascular disease. HTN often occurs without symptoms and the cause is unclear in most cases. Effective treatment of HTN includes lifestyle modification and pharmacologic treatment. Although evidence-based guidelines for HTN prevention, detection, and treatment have been widely promulgated, HTN control rates remain suboptimal. Achieving further improvements in HTN control will require activated patients, providers, and health care organizations.

CASE STUDY

Patient Profile

A 60-year-old African-American man with prediabetes presents for an annual physical examination. He has no complaints. After measuring his blood pressure twice using proper technique, you obtain an average reading of 143/88 mm Hg. His physical examination is unremarkable except his body mass index is 32 kg/m^2. He has no past history of myocardial infarction, stroke, kidney disease, or heart failure. After the visit, he measures his blood pressure at home and returns 1 month later. The average BP from multiple clinic and home readings is 138/86 mm Hg.

His total cholesterol is 260 mg/dL, HDL cholesterol is 42 mg/dL, and LDL cholesterol is 167 mg/dL. He does not smoke and rarely exercises. His hemoglobin A1C level is 6.1, and he has an estimated GFR of 53 mL/min/1.73 m^2. He has no proteinuria. He has an estimated 10-year ASCVD risk of 10.6%. His ECG is normal.

Considerations

1. How would you classify his blood pressure according to the 2017 ACC/AHA hypertension guidelines?
2. What would be your next step in managing this patient with suspected hypertension?
3. What would be the recommended blood pressure treatment goal for this patient?
4. What self-management strategies will you emphasize when you provide counseling to this patient?

CASE STUDY (*Continued*)

Treatment Plan

With BP exceeding 130/80 mm Hg on at least two separate clinic visits, this patient has stage 1 hypertension according to the 2017 ACC/AHA hypertension guidelines. Since his 10-year risk for ASCVD is greater than 10%, the recommendations suggest that in addition to nonpharmacologic therapy (which is first-line therapy for all with elevated BP or hypertension), he would benefit from a BP-lowering medication.

A shared decision-making discussion, with the patient influenced by health care provider judgment, should drive the ultimate choice of starting first with nonpharmacologic therapy only and initiating BP-lowering medications if BP remains greater than 130/80 mm Hg after 1 month versus immediately starting BP-lowering medications along with recommended lifestyle modification.

This patient would also benefit from setting goals for nonpharmacologic therapy including regular physical activity, a heart-healthy diet such as the DASH (Dietary Approaches to Stop Hypertension) diet, and reducing dietary sodium intake. If he consumes alcohol, he should be instructed to limit his intake to no more than 2 standard drinks a day.

The first-line pharmacologic agents for hypertension include thiazide diuretics, angiotensin-converting enzyme inhibitors (ACE-Is), angiotensin II receptor blockers (ARBs), and calcium channel blockers (CCBs) because these classes of medications reduce the risk of heart attack, stroke, and death. In African Americans, CCBs and thiazide diuretics are more effective for lowering BP and preventing ASCVD compared to ACE-Is or ARBs. Shared decision making which considers his values, preferences, and associated comorbidities should drive the ultimate choice of antihypertensive medication(s). The recommended BP treatment target should be less than 130/80 mm Hg. He should receive counseling on risk factors for hypertension, consequences of uncontrolled hypertension, and effective strategies to lower BP based on his risk factors and clinical profile. He should also be instructed to continue taking prescribed medications once the BP target of less than 130/80 mm Hg is reached. He should be advised to self-monitor his BP at home and report any side effects of the prescribed medications.

After initiating therapy, he should return to the clinic in 1 month to determine his progress in making the recommended lifestyle changes, adherence to drug therapy, and discuss any related side effects. If the BP goal is not met, despite adherence to therapy, treatment intensification should be considered as well as an assessment of barriers to BP control including social determinants of health.

KEY READINGS

Arnett DK, Blumenthal RS, Albert MA, et al. 2019 ACC/AHA guideline on the primary prevention of cardiovascular disease: a report of the American College of Cardiology/American Heart Association Task Force on Clinical Practice Guidelines. *Circulation*. 2019;140(11):e596–e646.

Carey RM, Calhoun DA, Bakris GL, et al. Resistant hypertension: detection, evaluation, and management: a scientific statement from the American Heart Association. *Hypertension*. 2018;72(5):e53–e90.

Himmelfarb CR, Commodore-Mensah Y, Hill MN. Expanding the role of nurses to improve hypertension care and control globally. *Ann Glob Health*. 2016;82(2):243–253.

Whelton PK, Carey RM, Aronow WS, et al. 2017 ACC/AHA/AAPA/ABC/ACPM/AGS/APhA/ASH/ASPC/NMA/PCNA guideline for the prevention, detection, evaluation, and management of high blood pressure in adults: a report of the American College of Cardiology/American Heart Association Task Force on Clinical Practice Guidelines. *Circulation*. 2018;138(17):e484–e594.

REFERENCES

1. Benjamin EJ, Virani SS, Callaway CW, et al. Heart disease and stroke statistics-2018 update: a report from the American Heart Association. *Circulation*. 2018;137(12):e67–e492.
2. Forouzanfar MH, Liu P, Roth GA, et al. Global burden of hypertension and systolic blood pressure of at least 110 to 115 mm Hg, 1990–2015. *JAMA*. 2017;317(2):165–182.
3. Whelton PK, Carey RM, Aronow WS, et al. 2017 ACC/AHA/AAPA/ABC/ACPM/AGS/APhA/ASH/ASPC/NMA/PCNA guideline for the prevention, detection, evaluation, and management of high blood pressure in adults: a report of the American College of Cardiology/American Heart Association Task Force on Clinical Practice Guidelines. *J Am Coll Cardiol*. 2018;71(19):e127–e248.
4. Muntner P, Carey RM, Gidding S, et al. Potential US population impact of the 2017 ACC/AHA high blood pressure guideline. *Circulation*. 2018;137(2):109–118.
5. Zhang Y, Moran AE. Trends in the prevalence, awareness, treatment, and control of hypertension among young adults in the United States, 1999 to 2014. *Hypertension*. 2017;70(4):736–742.
6. Olsen MH, Spencer S. A global perspective on hypertension: a Lancet commission. *Lancet*. 2015;386(9994):637–638.
7. Lewington S, Clarke R, Qizilbash N, et al. Age-specific relevance of usual blood pressure to vascular mortality: a meta-analysis of individual data for one million adults in 61 prospective studies. *Lancet*. 2002;360(9349):1903–1913.
8. Williams B, Mancia G, Spiering W, et al. 2018 ESC/ESH guidelines for the management of arterial hypertension. *Eur Heart J*. 2018;39(33):3021–3104.
9. National High Blood Pressure Education Program Working Group on High Blood Pressure in Children and Adolescents. The fourth report on the diagnosis, evaluation, and treatment of high blood pressure in children and adolescents. *Pediatrics*. 2004;114(2 suppl. 4th Report):555–576.
10. Flynn JT, Kaelber DC, Baker-Smith CM, et al. Clinical practice guideline for screening and management of high blood pressure in children and adolescents. *Pediatrics*. 2017;140(3):e20171904.
11. Law CM, de Swiet M, Osmond C, et al. Initiation of hypertension in utero and its amplification throughout life. *BMJ*. 1993;306(6869):24–27.
12. Hajjar I, Kotchen TA. Trends in prevalence, awareness, treatment, and control of hypertension in the United States, 1988–2000. *JAMA*. 2003;290(2):199–206.
13. Ong KL, Cheung BM, Man YB, et al. Prevalence, awareness, treatment, and control of hypertension among United States adults 1999–2004. *Hypertension*. 2007;49(1):69–75.
14. Burt VL, Whelton P, Roccella EJ, et al. Prevalence of hypertension in the US adult population. Results from the Third National Health and Nutrition Examination Survey, 1988–1991. *Hypertension*. 1995;25(3):305–313.
15. Franklin SS, Jacobs MJ, Wong ND, et al. Predominance of isolated systolic hypertension among middle-aged and elderly US hypertensives: analysis based on National Health and Nutrition Examination Survey (NHANES) III. *Hypertension*. 2001;37(3):869–874.
16. Hubert HB, Feinleib M, McNamara PM, et al. Obesity as an independent risk factor for cardiovascular disease: a 26-year follow-up of participants in the Framingham heart study. *Circulation*. 1983;67(5):968–977.
17. Huang Z, Willett WC, Manson JE, et al. Body weight, weight change, and risk for hypertension in women. *Ann Intern Med*. 1998;128(2):81–88
18. Freedman DS, Dietz WH, Srinivasan SR, et al. The relation of overweight to cardiovascular risk factors among children and adolescents: the Bogalusa Heart Study. *Pediatrics*. 1999;103(6 Pt 1):1175–1182.
19. Brown CD, Higgins M, Donato KA, et al. Body mass index and the prevalence of hypertension and dyslipidemia. *Obes Res*. 2000;8(9):605–619.

20. Hunt SC, Williams RR. Genetics and family history of hypertension. In: Izzo JL Jr, Black HR, eds. *Hypertension Primer. The Essentials of High Blood Pressure. From the Council on High Blood Pressure Research.* American Heart Association; 1999:218–221.
21. Marteau JB, Zaiou M, Siest G, et al. Genetic determinants of blood pressure regulation. *J Hypertens.* 2005;23(12):2127–2143.
22. Howard G, Prineas R, Moy C, et al. Racial and geographic differences in awareness, treatment, and control of hypertension: the REasons for Geographic And Racial Differences in Stroke study. *Stroke.* 2006; 37(5):1171–1178.
23. Mills KT, Bundy JD, Kelly TN, et al. Global disparities of hypertension prevalence and control: a systematic analysis of population-based studies from 90 countries. *Circulation.* 2016;134(6):441–450.
24. Marmot M, Friel S, Bell R, et al. Commission on Social Determinants of Health. Closing the gap in a generation: health equity through action on the social determinants of health. *Lancet.* 2008;372(9650):1661–1669.
25. Havranek EP, Mujahid MS, Barr DA, et al. Social determinants of risk and outcomes for cardiovascular disease: a scientific statement from the American Heart Association. *Circulation.* 2015;132(9):873–898.
26. Schultz WM, Kelli HM, Lisko JC, et al. Socioeconomic status and cardiovascular outcomes: challenges and interventions. *Circulation.* 2018;137(20):2166–2178.
27. Albert MA, Glynn RJ, Buring J, et al. Impact of traditional and novel risk factors on the relationship between socioeconomic status and incident cardiovascular events. *Circulation.* 2006;114(24):2619–2626.
28. Fretz A, Schneider AL, McEvoy JW, et al. The association of socioeconomic status with subclinical myocardial damage, incident cardiovascular events, and mortality in the ARIC study. *Am J Epidemiol.* 2016; 183(5):452–461.
29. Leng B, Jin Y, Li G, et al. Socioeconomic status and hypertension: a meta-analysis. *J Hypertens.* 2015;33(2):221–229.
30. National Academy of Medicine. Standardized screening for health-related social needs in clinical settings: the accountable health communities screening tool. 2017. Available at https://nam.edu/standardized-screening-for-health-related-social-needs-in-clinical-settings-the-accountable-health-communities-screening-tool. Accessed May 5, 2019.
31. Brownstein JN, Bone LR, Dennison CR, et al. Community health workers as interventionists in the prevention and control of heart disease and stroke. *Am J Prev Med.* 2005;29(5 suppl 1):128–133.
32. Oparil S, Zaman MA, Calhoun DA. Pathogenesis of hypertension. *Ann Intern Med.* 2003;139(9):761–776.
33. Carey RM, Calhoun DA, Bakris GL, et al. Resistant hypertension: detection, evaluation, and management: a scientific statement from the American Heart Association. *Hypertension.* 2018;72(5):e53–e90.
34. de Divitiis M, Pilla C, Kattenhorn M, et al. Ambulatory blood pressure, left ventricular mass, and conduit artery function late after successful repair of coarctation of the aorta. *J Am Coll Cardiol.* 2003;41(12): 2259–2265.
35. Goff DC Jr, Lloyd-Jones DM, Bennett G, et al. 2013 ACC/AHA guideline on the assessment of cardiovascular risk: a report of the American College of Cardiology/American Heart Association Task Force on Practice Guidelines. *J Am Coll Cardiol.* 2014;63(25 Pt B):2935–2959.
36. *ASCVD risk estimator.* Available at http://tools.acc.org/ldl/ascvd_risk_estimator/index.html#!/calulate/estimator
37. Baumbach GL. Mechanisms of vascular remodeling. In: Izzo JL, Sica D, Black HR, eds. *Hypertension Primer: The Essentials of High Blood Pressure.* Philadelphia, PA: LWW; 2008.
38. Halcox JPJ, Quyyumi AA. Endothelial function and cardiovascular disease. In: Izzo JL, Sica D, Black HR, eds. *Hypertension Primer: The Essentials of High Blood Pressure.* Philadelphia, PA: LWW; 2008.
39. Giles TD. Atherogenesis and coronary artery disease. In: Izzo JL, Sica D, Black HR,eds. *Hypertension Primer: The Essentials of High Blood Pressure.* Philadelphia, PA: LWW; 2008.
40. Anderson S. Pathogenesis of nephrosclerosis and chronic kidney disease. In: Izzo JL, Sica D, Black HR. *Hypertension Primer: The Essentials of High Blood Pressure.* Philadelphia, PA: LWW; 2008.
41. Wong TY, Mitchell P. Hypertensive retinopathy. *N Engl J Med.* 2004; 351(22):2310–2317.
42. Xie X, Atkins E, Lv J, et al. Effects of intensive blood pressure lowering on cardiovascular and renal outcomes: updated systematic review and meta-analysis. *Lancet.* 2016;387(10017):435–443.
43. Fotherby MD, Eveson DJ, Robinson TG. The brain in hypertension. In: Lip G, Hall JE, eds. *Comprehensive Hypertension.* Amsterdam: Elsevier; 2007:591–605.
44. Williamson JD, Launer LJ, Bryan RN, et al. Cognitive function and brain structure in persons with type 2 diabetes mellitus after intensive lowering of blood pressure and lipid levels: a randomized clinical trial. *JAMA Intern Med.* 2014;174(3):324–333.
45. Muntner P, Shimbo D, Carey RM, et al. Measurement of blood pressure in humans: a scientific statement from the American Heart Association. *Hypertension.* 2019;73(5):e35–e66.
46. Benetos A, Thomas F, Bean K, et al. Prognostic value of systolic and diastolic blood pressure in treated hypertensive men. *Arch Intern Med.* 2002;162(5):577–581.
47. Lindenstrom E, Boysen G, Nyboe J. Influence of systolic and diastolic blood pressure on stroke risk: a prospective observational study. *Am J Epidemiol.* 1995;142(12):1279–1290.
48. Reboussin DM, Allen NB, Griswold ME, et al. Systematic review for the 2017 ACC/AHA/AAPA/ABC/ACPM/AGS/APhA/ASH/ASPC/NMA/PCNA guideline for the prevention, detection, evaluation, and management of high blood pressure in adults: a report of the American College of Cardiology/American Heart Association Task Force on Clinical Practice Guidelines. *Circulation.* 2018;138(17):e595–e616.
49. Dickinson HO, Mason JM, Nicolson DJ, et al. Lifestyle interventions to reduce raised blood pressure: a systematic review of randomized controlled trials. *J Hypertens.* 2006;24(2):215–233.
50. Ettehad D, Emdin CA, Kiran A, et al. Blood pressure lowering for prevention of cardiovascular disease and death: a systematic review and meta-analysis. *Lancet.* 2016;387(10022):957–967.
51. Muntner P, Carey RM, Gidding S, et al. Potential U.S. population impact of the 2017 ACC/AHA High Blood Pressure Guideline. *J Am Coll Cardiol.* 2017;71(2):109–118.
52. Arnett DK, Blumenthal RS, Albert MA, et al. 2019 ACC/AHA guideline on the primary prevention of cardiovascular disease: executive summary: a report of the American College of Cardiology/American Heart Association Task Force on Clinical Practice Guidelines. *J Am Coll Cardiol.* 2019;74(10):1376–1414.
53. Whelton PK, Appel LJ, Espeland MA, et al. Sodium reduction and weight loss in the treatment of hypertension in older persons: a randomized controlled trial of nonpharmacologic interventions in the elderly (TONE). *JAMA.* 1998;279(11):839–846.
54. Appel LJ. Lifestyle modification as a means to prevent and treat high blood pressure. *J Am Soc Nephrol.* 2003;14(7 suppl 2):S99–S102.
55. Blair D, Habicht JP, Sims EA, et al. Evidence for an increased risk for hypertension with centrally located body fat and the effect of race and sex on this risk. *Am J Epidemiol.* 1984;119(4):526–540.
56. Despres JP, Moorjani S, Lupien PJ, et al. Regional distribution of body fat, plasma lipoproteins, and cardiovascular disease. *Arteriosclerosis.* 1990;10(4):497–511.
57. Folsom AR, Prineas RJ, Kaye SA, et al. Incidence of hypertension and stroke in relation to body fat distribution and other risk factors in older women. *Stroke.* 1990;21(5):701–706.
58. Stamler R, Stamler J, Riedlinger WF, et al. Weight and blood pressure. Findings in hypertension screening of 1 million Americans. *JAMA.* 1978;240(15):1607–1610.
59. Katagiri H, Yamada T, Oka Y. Adiposity and cardiovascular disorders: disturbance of the regulatory system consisting of humoral and neuronal signals. *Circ Res.* 2007;101(1):27–39.
60. Yanai H, Tomono Y, Ito K, et al. The underlying mechanisms for development of hypertension in the metabolic syndrome. *Nutr J.* 2008; 7(1):10.
61. Langford HG, Blaufox MD, Oberman A, et al. Dietary therapy slows the return of hypertension after stopping prolonged medication. *JAMA.* 1985;253(5):657–664.
62. Neter JE, Stam BE, Kok FJ, et al. Influence of weight reduction on blood pressure: a meta-analysis of randomized controlled trials. *Hypertension.* 2003;42(5):878–884.
63. Appel LJ, Brands MW, Daniels SR, et al. Dietary approaches to prevent and treat hypertension: a scientific statement from the American Heart Association. *Hypertension.* 2006;47(2):296–308.
64. Appel LJ. Effects of comprehensive lifestyle modification on blood pressure control: main results of the PREMIER clinical trial. *JAMA.* 2003;289(16):2083–2093.
65. Sacks FM, Svetkey LP, Vollmer WM, et al. Effects on blood pressure of reduced dietary sodium and the dietary approaches to stop hypertension (DASH) diet. DASH-Sodium Collaborative Research Group. *N Engl J Med.* 2001;344(1):3–10.
66. Vollmer WM, Sacks FM, Ard J, et al. Effects of diet and sodium intake on blood pressure: subgroup analysis of the DASH-sodium trial. *Ann Intern Med.* 2001;135(12):1019–1028.
67. Bray GA, Vollmer WM, Sacks FM, et al. A further subgroup analysis of the effects of the DASH diet and three dietary sodium levels

on blood pressure: results of the DASH-sodium trial. *Am J Cardiol.* 2004;94(2):222–227.

68. U.S. Department of Health and Human Services and U.S. Department of Agriculture. *2015–2020 Dietary Guidelines for Americans.* 8th ed. December 2015. Available at https://health.gov/dietaryguidelines/2015/guidelines/
69. Mente A, O'Donnell MJ, Rangarajan S, et al. Association of urinary sodium and potassium excretion with blood pressure. *N Engl J Med.* 2014;371(7):601–611.
70. Zhang Z, Cogswell ME, Gillespie C, et al. Association between usual sodium and potassium intake and blood pressure and hypertension among U.S. adults: NHANES 2005–2010. *PLoS One.* 2013;8(10):e75289.
71. Vinceti M, Filippini T, Crippa A, et al. Meta-analysis of potassium intake and the risk of stroke. *J Am Heart Assoc.* 2016;5(10):e004210.
72. Rodrigues SL, Baldo MP, Machado RC, et al. High potassium intake blunts the effect of elevated sodium intake on blood pressure levels. *J Am Soc Hypertens.* 2014;8(4):232–238.
73. Cook NR, Obarzanek E, Cutler JA, et al. Joint effects of sodium and potassium intake on subsequent cardiovascular disease: the trials of hypertension prevention follow-up study. *Arch Intern Med.* 2009;169(1): 32–40.
74. Whelton PK, He J, Cutler JA, et al. Effects of oral potassium on blood pressure: meta-analysis of randomized controlled clinical trials. *J Am Heart Assoc.* 1997;277(20):1624–1632.
75. Piercy KL, Troiano RP, Ballard RM, et al. The physical activity guidelines for Americans. *J Am Heart Assoc.* 2018;320(19):2020–2028.
76. Cornelissen VA, Smart NA. Exercise training for blood pressure: a systematic review and meta-analysis. *J Am Heart Assoc.* 2013;2(1):e004473.
77. Kokkinos PF, Narayan P, Colleran JA, et al. Effects of regular exercise on blood pressure and left ventricular hypertrophy in African-American men with severe hypertension. *N Engl J Med.* 1995;333(22):1462–1467.
78. Xin X, He J, Frontini MG, et al. Effects of alcohol reduction on blood pressure: a meta-analysis of randomized controlled trials. *Hypertension.* 2001;38(5):1112–1117.
79. Blood Pressure Lowering Treatment Trialists' Collaboration. Blood pressure-lowering treatment based on cardiovascular risk: a meta-analysis of individual patient data. *Lancet.* 2014;384(9943):591–598.
80. van Dieren S, Kengne AP, Chalmers J, et al. Effects of blood pressure lowering on cardiovascular outcomes in different cardiovascular risk groups among participants with type 2 diabetes. *Diabetes Res Clin Pract.* 2012;98(1):83–90.
81. Law MR, Morris JK, Wald NJ. Use of blood pressure lowering drugs in the prevention of cardiovascular disease: meta-analysis of 147 randomised trials in the context of expectations from prospective epidemiological studies. *BMJ.* 2009;338:b1665.
82. Thomopoulos C, Parati G, Zanchetti A. Effects of blood pressure lowering on outcome incidence in hypertension: 2. Effects at different baseline and achieved blood pressure levels–overview and meta-analyses of randomized trials. *J Hypertens.* 2014;32(12):2296–2304.
83. Sundstrom J, Arima H, Jackson R, et al. Effects of blood pressure reduction in mild hypertension: a systematic review and meta-analysis. *Ann Intern Med.* 2015;162(3):184–191.
84. Thompson AM, Hu T, Eshelbrenner CL, et al. Antihypertensive treatment and secondary prevention of cardiovascular disease events among persons without hypertension: a meta-analysis. *JAMA.* 2011;305(9): 913–922.
85. Wright JT Jr, Williamson JD, Whelton PK, et al. A randomized trial of intensive versus standard blood-pressure control. *N Engl J Med.* 2015;373(22):2103–2116.
86. Czernichow S, Zanchetti A, Turnbull F, et al. The effects of blood pressure reduction and of different blood pressure-lowering regimens on major cardiovascular events according to baseline blood pressure: meta-analysis of randomized trials. *J Hypertens.* 2011;29(1):4–16.
87. Thomopoulos C, Parati G, Zanchetti A. Effects of blood pressure lowering on outcome incidence in hypertension: 7. Effects of more vs. less intensive blood pressure lowering and different achieved blood pressure levels—updated overview and meta-analyses of randomized trials. *J Hypertens.* 2016;34(4):613–622.
88. Verdecchia P, Angeli F, Gentile G, et al. More versus less intensive blood pressure-lowering strategy: cumulative evidence and trial sequential analysis. *Hypertension.* 2016;68(3):642–653.
89. Bangalore S, Toklu B, Gianos E, et al. Optimal systolic blood pressure target after SPRINT: insights from a network meta-analysis of randomized trials. *Am J Med.* 2017;130(6):707–719.
90. Bundy JD, Li C, Stuchlik P, et al. Systolic blood pressure reduction and risk of cardiovascular disease and mortality: a systematic review and network meta-analysis. *JAMA Cardiol.* 2017;2(7):775–781.
91. Psaty BM, Lumley T, Furberg CD, et al. Health outcomes associated with various antihypertensive therapies used as first-line agents: a network meta-analysis. *JAMA.* 2003;289(19):2534–2544.
92. ALLHAT Officers and Coordinators for the ALLHAT Collaborative Research Group. The Antihypertensive and Lipid-Lowering Treatment to Prevent Heart Attack Trial. Major outcomes in high-risk hypertensive patients randomized to angiotensin-converting enzyme inhibitor or calcium channel blocker vs diuretic: the antihypertensive and lipid-lowering treatment to prevent heart attack trial (ALLHAT). *JAMA.* 2002; 288(23):2981–2997.
93. SHEP Cooperative Research Group. Prevention of stroke by antihypertensive drug treatment in older persons with isolated systolic hypertension. Final results of the Systolic Hypertension in the Elderly Program (SHEP). *JAMA.* 1991;265(24):3255–3264.
94. Beckett NS, Peters R, Fletcher AE, et al. Treatment of hypertension in patients 80 years of age or older. *N Engl J Med.* 2008;358(18):1887–1898.
95. Williamson JD, Supiano MA, Applegate WB, et al. Intensive vs standard blood pressure control and cardiovascular disease outcomes in adults aged ≥75 years: a randomized clinical trial. *JAMA.* 2016;315(24):2673–2682.
96. Duprez DA. Systolic hypertension in the elderly: addressing an unmet need. *Am J Med.* 2008;121(3):179–184.
97. Warwick J, Falaschetti E, Rockwood K, et al. No evidence that frailty modifies the positive impact of antihypertensive treatment in very elderly people: an investigation of the impact of frailty upon treatment effect in the HYpertension in the Very Elderly Trial (HYVET) study, a double-blind, placebo-controlled study of antihypertensives in people with hypertension aged 80 and over. *BMC Med.* 2015;13(1):78.
98. Mueller M, Purnell TS, Mensah GA, et al. Reducing racial and ethnic disparities in hypertension prevention and control: what will it take to translate research into practice and policy? *Am J Hypertens.* 2015; 28(6):699–716.
99. Margolis KL, O'Connor PJ, Morgan TM, et al. Outcomes of combined cardiovascular risk factor management strategies in type 2 diabetes: the ACCORD randomized trial. *Diabetes Care.* 2014;37(6):1721–1728.
100. Cooper-DeHoff RM, Aranda JM Jr, Gaxiola E, et al. Blood pressure control and cardiovascular outcomes in high-risk Hispanic patients–findings from the International Verapamil SR/Trandolapril study (INVEST). *Am Heart J.* 2006;151(5):1072–1079.
101. Margolis KL, Piller LB, Ford CE, et al. Blood pressure control in Hispanics in the antihypertensive and lipid-lowering treatment to prevent heart attack trial. *Hypertension.* 2007;50(5):854–861.
102. Henderson JT, Thompson JH, Burda BU, et al. Preeclampsia screening: evidence report and systematic review for the US Preventive Services Task Force. *JAMA.* 2017;317(16):1668–1683.
103. Emdin CA, Rahimi K, Neal B, et al. Blood pressure lowering in type 2 diabetes: a systematic review and meta-analysis. *JAMA.* 2015;313(6):603–615.
104. Arguedas JA, Leiva V, Wright JM. Blood pressure targets for hypertension in people with diabetes mellitus. *Cochrane Database Syst Rev.* 2013;10:CD008277.
105. Bress AP, Bellows BK, King JB, et al. Cost-effectiveness of intensive versus standard blood-pressure control. *N Engl J Med.* 2017;377(8):745–755.
106. Soliman EZ, Byington RP, Bigger JT, et al. Effect of intensive blood pressure lowering on left ventricular hypertrophy in patients with diabetes mellitus: action to control cardiovascular risk in diabetes blood pressure trial. *Hypertension.* 2015;66(6):1123–1129.
107. ACCORD Study Group; Cushman WC, Evans GW, Byington RP, et al. Effects of intensive blood-pressure control in type 2 diabetes mellitus. *N Engl J Med.* 2010;362(17):1575–1585.
108. Adler AI, Stratton IM, Neil HA, et al. Association of systolic blood pressure with macrovascular and microvascular complications of type 2 diabetes (UKPDS 36): prospective observational study. *BMJ.* 2000;321(7258):412–419.
109. Stamler J, Vaccaro O, Neaton JD, et al. Diabetes, other risk factors, and 12-yr cardiovascular mortality for men screened in the multiple risk factor intervention trial. *Diabetes Care.* 1993;16(2):434–444.
110. Do DV, Wang X, Vedula SS, et al. Blood pressure control for diabetic retinopathy. *Cochrane Database Syst Rev.* 2015;1:CD006127.
111. Reboldi G, Gentile G, Angeli F, et al. Effects of intensive blood pressure reduction on myocardial infarction and stroke in diabetes: a meta-analysis in 73,913 patients. *J Hypertens.* 2011;29(7):1253–1269.
112. Brunström M, Carlberg B. Effect of antihypertensive treatment at different blood pressure levels in patients with diabetes mellitus: systematic review and meta-analyses. *BMJ.* 2016;352:i717.
113. Lv J, Ehteshami P, Sarnak MJ, et al. Effects of intensive blood pressure lowering on the progression of chronic kidney disease: a systematic review and meta-analysis. *Can Med Assoc J.* 2013;185(11):949–957.

114. Action to Control Cardiovascular Risk in Diabetes Study Group; Gerstein HC, Miller ME, Byington RP, et al. Effects of intensive glucose lowering in type 2 diabetes. *N Engl J Med.* 2008;358(24):2545–2559.
115. SPRINT Research Group; Wright JT Jr, Williamson JD, Whelton PK, et al. A randomized trial of intensive versus standard blood-pressure control. *N Engl J Med.* 2015;373(22):2103–2116.
116. Khatib R, Schwalm JD, Yusuf S, et al. Patient and healthcare provider barriers to hypertension awareness, treatment and follow up: a systematic review and meta-analysis of qualitative and quantitative studies. *PLoS One.* 2014;9(1):e84238.
117. Patient behavior for blood pressure control. Guidelines for professionals. *JAMA.* 1979;241(23):2534–2537. doi:10.1001/jama.1979.03290490040024
118. Bakris G, Bohm M, Dagenais G, et al. Cardiovascular protection for all individuals at high risk: evidence-based best practice. *Clin Res Cardiol.*2008;97(10):713–725.
119. Miller NH, Hill M, Kottke T, et al. The multilevel compliance challenge: recommendations for a call to action. A statement for healthcare professionals. *Circulation.* 1997;95(4):1085–1090.
120. Hill MN, Ball J, Williams R, et al. Collaboration in high blood pressure control: among professionals and with the patient. *Ann Intern Med.* 1984;101(3):393–395.
121. Curzio JL, Rubin PC, Kennedy SS, et al. A comparison of the management of hypertensive patients by nurse practitioners compared with conventional hospital care. *J Hum Hypertens.* 1990;4(6):665–670.
122. Logan AG, Milne BJ, Achber C, et al. Work-site treatment of hypertension by specially trained nurses. A controlled trial. *Lancet.* 1979;2(8153):1175–1178.
123. Pheley AM, Terry P, Pietz L, et al. Evaluation of a nurse-based hypertension management program: screening, management, and outcomes. *J Cardiovasc Nurs.* 1995;9(2):54–61.
124. Schultz JF, Sheps SG. Management of patients with hypertension: a hypertension clinic model. *Mayo Clin Proc.* 1994;69(10):997–999.
125. Smith ED, Merritt SL, Patel MK. Church-based education: an outreach program for African Americans with hypertension. *Ethn Health.* 1997;2(3):243–253.
126. Himmelfarb CR, Commodore-Mensah Y, Hill MN. Expanding the role of nurses to improve hypertension care and control globally. *Ann Glob Health.* 2016;82(2):243–253.
127. Hill MN, Bone LR, Kim MT, et al. Barriers to hypertension care and control in young urban black men. *Am J Hypertens.* 1999;12(10 Pt 1): 951–958.
128. Dennison CR, Peer N, Steyn K, et al. Determinants of hypertension care and control among peri-urban black South Africans: the HiHi study. *Ethn Dis.* 2007;17(3):484–491.
129. Commodore-Mensah Y, Hill M, Allen J, et al. Sex differences in cardiovascular disease risk of Ghanaian- and Nigerian-born West African immigrants in the United States: the Afro-Cardiac Study. *J Am Heart Assoc.* 2016;5(2):e002385.
130. Kim MT, Han HR, Hedlin H, et al. Teletransmitted monitoring of blood pressure and bilingual nurse counseling-sustained improvements in blood pressure control during 12 months in hypertensive Korean Americans. *J Clin Hypertens (Greenwich).* 2011;13(8):605–612.
131. Allen JK, Dennison-Himmelfarb CR, Szanton SL, et al. Community outreach and cardiovascular health (COACH) trial: a randomized, controlled trial of nurse practitioner/community health worker cardiovascular disease risk reduction in urban community health centers. *Circ Cardiovasc Qual Outcomes.* 2011,4(6):595–602.
132. Rose AJ, Berlowitz DR, Orner MB, et al. Understanding uncontrolled hypertension: is it the patient or the provider? *J Clin Hypertens (Greenwich).* 2007;9(12):937–943.
133. Rose AJ, Shimada SL, Rothendler JA, et al. The accuracy of clinician perceptions of "usual" blood pressure control. *J Gen Intern Med.* 2008;23(2):180–183.
134. Alderman MH, Furberg CD, Kostis JB, et al. Hypertension guidelines: Criteria that might make them more clinically useful. *Am J Hypertens.* 2002;15(10 Pt 1);917–923.
135. Hyman DJ, Pavlik VN. Characteristics of patients with uncontrolled hypertension in the United States. *N Engl J Med.* 2001;345(7):479–486.
136. Tu K, Mamdani MM, Tu JV. Hypertension guidelines in elderly patients: is anybody listening? *Am J Med.* 2002;113(1):52–58.
137. Victor RG, Lynch K, Li N, et al. A cluster-randomized trial of blood-pressure reduction in black barbershops. *N Engl J Med.* 2018;378(14):1291–1301.
138. Schoenthaler AM, Lancaster KJ, Chaplin W, et al. Cluster randomized clinical trial of FAITH (faith-based approaches in the treatment of hypertension) in blacks. *Circ Cardiovasc Qual Outcomes.* 2018; 11(10):e004691.

24 Lipid Management

Jan L. McAlister

OBJECTIVES

1. To understand the basic pathophysiology of lipid metabolism.
2. To be able to perform risk stratification in order to identify patients for treatment.
3. To improve knowledge of lipid disorders.
4. To identify primary and secondary research studies providing the foundation for lipid management.
5. To identify evidence-based treatment modalities.

KEY QUESTIONS

1. How are lipids metabolized and what are the key organs involved in this process?
2. How is Lp(a) utilized in determining cardiovascular risk?
3. How is familial hyperlipidemia identified and treated?
4. How does the nurse play a role in identifying and understanding treatments for high cholesterol?

BACKGROUND

How did we get to where we are? In 1758, a French physician named François Poulletier de la Salle isolated cholesterol from gallstones.[1] In 1815, a French chemist named Michel Eugène Chevreul isolated and purified sterol from gallstones, naming the substance cholesterol. In 1828, Louis René Le Canu first identified the presence of cholesterol in human blood. Later in 1852, an Irish physician Richard Quain first identified plaque in blood vessels and in 1854, Dr. Rudolf Virchow described this cholesterol deposition as atherosclerosis. In 1913, Nikolai Anitschkow established a link between cholesterol and atherosclerosis by feeding rabbit's purified cholesterol.[2] Then in 1927, Wieland and Adolf Windaus received the Nobel Prize for cholesterol and bile salts, which led to Adolf Windaus clarifying the structure as cholesterol.[1] The first cholesterol blood test was developed in 1934. Biochemists David Rittenberg and Rudolph Schoenheimer studied dietary cholesterol effects in the blood and demonstrated dietary cholesterol had negligible effects on blood cholesterol levels in 1937.

In 1951, Doctors David Barr, Ella M. Russ, and Howard Eder found heart patients had elevated low-density lipoprotein (LDL) cholesterol levels and low high-density lipoprotein (HDL) levels. In 1953, Ancel Keys published controversial Seven Countries Study suggesting an association between fat and mortality, but did not include the data on sugar consumption.[3] In 1955, ultracentrifugation technique for lipid analysis, in which blood is divided into plasma proteins, was discovered by Doctors Richard Havel, Howard Eder, and Joseph Bragdon. This process is still utilized today. Also, in 1955, Canadian physician Rudolf Altschul found high doses of niacin lowered cholesterol levels. Then in 1959, John William Gofman researched the identification, quantification, and clinical implications of lipoproteins. He defined three major classes of lipoproteins in the serum: very–low-density lipoprotein (VLDL), LDL, and HDL and identified that heart attacks correlated with high levels of LDLs.[4–6] In 1963, Doctors Sami Hashim and Theodore Van Itallie found that cholestyramine to lower cholesterol levels in the blood.

In 1964, Dr. Konrad Bloch received the Nobel Prize for explaining cholesterol synthesis establishing hydroxymethylglutaryl coenzyme-A (HMG-CoA) reductase as the enzyme in the synthesis. Cholesterol serves as a precursor for bile acids, sex hormones, and cortisol. Konrad Bloch and Feodor Lynen would receive the Nobel Prize for cholesterol and fatty acid metabolism and cholesterol synthesis with John Cornforth and George Popják.[7–9] In 1967, the classification system of lipoprotein disorders was established by Doctors Donald Fredrickson, Robert Levy, and Robert Lees. In 1969, the Friedewald formula was developed to calculate LDL cholesterol (LDL-C) based on fasting total cholesterol, HDL cholesterol (HDL-C), and triglyceride levels. Later in 1976, Japanese biochemist Akira Endo isolated HMG-CoA reductase inhibitor from the fungal strain *Penicillium citrinum*, which led to the development of statin drugs to reduce cholesterol.[10] In 1987, lovastatin (Mevacor) was the first cholesterol-lowering statin drug approved.[11] Statins are the backbone of our lipid management to this day.

Present

Cardiovascular disease (CVD), the leading cause of death for American women and men, is responsible for approximately 836,546 deaths per year. Approximately, one in every four Americans died from CVD in 2015 with coronary heart disease (CHD) being the most common type of heart disease. From 2005 to 2015, the annual death rate attributable to CHD declined 34.4% and the actual number of deaths declined 17.7%, but the burden and risk factors still remain alarmingly high.[12] A high blood level of LDL-C remains a major risk factor for CVD.[13] Elevated serum cholesterol and, particularly, LDL-C levels are significant modifiable risk factors associated with the development and progression of CVD. More than 123 million Americans have a blood cholesterol higher than the desirable level of 200 mg/dL. Furthermore, of these with cholesterol higher than 200 mg/dL, almost 29 million Americans have a blood cholesterol more than 240 mg/dL.[12] Seven percent of U.S. children and adolescents ages 6 to 19 have high total cholesterol.[14] The good news is, American adults with high total (greater than 240 mg/dL) cholesterol decreased from 18.3% in 1999–2000 down to 11% in 2013–2014.[15] High cholesterol has no symptoms; so many people do not know their cholesterol is too high, unless they have a blood test to check it.

There is a large body of evidence, including animal studies,[16] observational studies,[17] and numerous clinical trials, that consistently point to a relationship between high blood lipids and CVD. An example of this compelling relationship is the INTERHEART study.[18] The INTERHEART study, using data from 52 countries, showed that 90% of population-attributable risk is strongly associated with nine easily measured risk factors.[18] Two thirds (or 66%) of the population-attributable risks are accounted for by abnormal lipids (using the apo B/apo A-I ratio as a marker for abnormal lipids—a surrogate for LDL measure) and by current smoking. This association holds true for both men and women, across different geographic regions, and ethnic groups.[18] Table 24-1 summarizes the results of large randomized lipid-lowering primary and secondary prevention trials.[19–28] Meta-analyses of the cholesterol-lowering clinical trials estimated that a 10-mg/dL reduction in total cholesterol results in a 22% reduction in CVD incidence after 2 years of intervention, and a 25% reduction after 5 years.[29,30] There is some evidence that cholesterol lowering begun at an early age (e.g., age 40 years) may provide greater risk reduction than if started at a later age (e.g., age 70 years).[31] However, recent clinical trials including persons older than 65 years show benefit for CVD risk reduction in older populations.[27,32]

Blood Lipids: Structure and Functions

The complex relationships between genetic and metabolic mechanisms and the molecular interactions within the cell wall help explain the association between lipid abnormalities and CVD. The major lipid particles, cholesterol and triglycerides, both have important functions in the body. Cholesterol is an essential component of cell membranes, functioning to provide stability while permitting membrane transport; it is a precursor to adrenal steroids, sex hormones, and bile and bile acids. Triglycerides are the major source of energy for the body. Both cholesterol and triglycerides are insoluble molecules and must be transported in the circulation as lipoproteins.

Lipoproteins are complexes of nonpolar lipid cores (triglycerides and cholesterol esters) surrounded by a surface coat of polar lipids (phospholipids and free cholesterol) and specific proteins called apoproteins. Total cholesterol, for example, is composed of 18 different lipid and lipoprotein particles.[33] Lipoproteins can be classified according to their density, their migration on an electrophoretic field, or their lipid and apoprotein composition.[34]

During the 1980s, significant advances were made in determining the function of the apoproteins, the lipid-processing enzymes, and lipoprotein receptors. Apoproteins function as more than transport vehicles; they have variant properties that activate enzyme systems or receptor sites to promote the catabolism or removal of lipoproteins from the circulation.[35] The functions of nine apoproteins in the lipid metabolic cascade have been identified: apo A-I, apo A-II, apolipoprotein B-100 (apo B-100), apo B-48, apo C-I, apo C-II, apo C-III, apo E2, apo E3, apo E4, and lipoprotein(a), or Lp(a). In addition, the actions of several lipoprotein-processing enzymes (lipoprotein lipase [LPL], hepatic lipase [HL], lecithin cholesterol acyltransferase, and cholesteryl ester transfer protein [CETP]) and the function of cell receptors, including the LDL and chylomicron remnant receptor, are now established. These advances permit an understanding of lipid metabolism, as well as the abnormalities leading to elevated blood cholesterol. Current data reveals a residual cardiovascular risk in patients despite adequately treating LDL, bringing to question, is there a better target marker for atherogenicity than LDL.[36–38] Apo B represents the total number of circulating atherogenic particles and may serve as a better atherogenic marker.[39] Each VLDL, intermediate-density lipoprotein (IDL), LDL and lipoprotein(a) contains one molecule of apo B-100 and each chylomicron or chylomicron remnant contains one molecule of apo B-48, making apo B a one-to-one relationship.[39,40]

Lipid Metabolism and Transport

The gut and liver are responsible for the production of the six principal lipoproteins. Exogenous lipoproteins are formed in the mucosa of the small intestine after digestion of dietary fats. During the digestive process, hydrolyzed products of ingested fats enter epithelial cells of the small intestine, where they are converted into triglycerides and cholesterol esters. These products are then aggregated into the lipoprotein complexes known as chylomicrons. Chylomicrons pass into small lymph vessels and reach the circulatory system through the thoracic duct. In the peripheral capillaries, chylomicrons are hydrolyzed by the enzyme LPL, located on the capillary endothelium. Free fatty acids and glycerol then enter adipose tissue cells. A cholesterol-rich chylomicron remnant (a second lipoprotein complex) is released into the circulation when lipolysis is nearly complete. Chylomicron remnants are cleared rapidly by the liver (Fig. 24-1).[41,42]

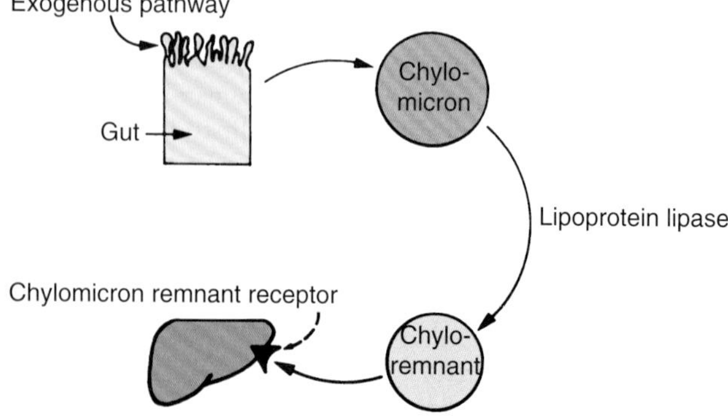

Figure 24-1. The exogenous metabolism of lipoproteins and the transport of chylomicrons to the tissue and chylomicron remnants to the liver.

Table 24-1 • SELECTED, RANDOMIZED, CLINICAL TRIALS USING STATIN THERAPY TO LOWER CHOLESTEROL

Trial	Number of Patients	Age (years)	Lipids (mean, mg/dL)	Average Length of Follow-up	Mean Lipid Reduction	Outcomes
Primary Prevention						
West of Scotland (WOSCOPS)[a]	6595 men	45–64	TC: 272 LDL: 192	4.9 years	TC: ↓20% LDL: ↓26%	Nonfatal MI and CVD death: ↓31%
AFCAPS/TexCAPS[b]	5608 men 997 women		TC: 221 LDL: 150	5.2 years	TC: ↓18% LDL: ↓25%	Major coronary events (MI, unstable angina, or sudden cardiac death: ↓37%)
Primary and Secondary Prevention						
Heart Protection Study[c]	15,454 men 5082 women	40–80 (52% >65)	TC: 228 LDL: 131[j]	5.0 years	LDL: ↓37 mg/dL	All-cause mortality ↓13%, major vascular events ↓24% Coronary death ↓27%, nonfatal/fatal stroke ↓25% Nonfatal MI and coronary death ↓27%
Prospective Study of Pravastatin in the Elderly at Risk[d]	2804 men 3000 women	70–82	TC: 150–350	3.2 years	LDL: ↓34%	Composite of: coronary death, nonfatal MI, fatal or nonfatal stroke ↓24%
Anglo-Scandinavian Cardiac Outcomes Trial–Lipid Lowering Arm[e]	10,350 81% male	40–79	LDL: 132	3.3 (stopped early due to benefit)	LDL ↓29%	Total cardiovascular events ↓21% Total coronary events ↓29% Total fatal and nonfatal stroke ↓7%
Secondary Prevention						
Scandinavian Simvastatin Survival Study (4S)[f]	3617 men 427 women	35–70	TC LDL: 188	5.4 years	TC ↓28% LDL: ↓38%	CHD deaths: ↓42% Nonfatal MI and CVD death ↓37%
CARE[g]	4159	Average 59	LDL: 139	3 years	LDL: ↓27%	Major coronary events ↓25% Coronary mortality ↓24% Total mortality ↓9%
LIPID[h]	9014	31–75	LDL: 150	61 years	LDL: ↓25%	Major coronary events ↓29% Coronary mortality ↓24% Total mortality ↓23%
Pravastatin or Atorvastatin Evaluation and Infection—Thrombolysis in MI[i]	4162	≥18	TC: ≤240 mg/dL Mean LDL: 106	24 months	LDL: ↓22% Pravastatin ↓51% Atorvastatin	Composite death from any cause, MI, hospitalization from unstable angina, revascularization, or stroke ↓16%

TC, total cholesterol; LDL, low-density lipoprotein.

[a]WOSCOPS: Shepherd, J., Cobbe, S. M., Ford, I., et al., for the West of Scotland Coronary Prevention Study Group. (1995). Prevention of coronary heart disease with pravastatin in men with hypercholesterolemia. *New England Journal of Medicine, 333*, 1301–1307.

[b]AFCAPS/TexCAPS: Downs, J. R., Clearfield, M., Weis, S., et al., for the AFCAPS/TexCAPS Research Group. (1998). Primary prevention of acute coronary events with lovastatin in men and women with average cholesterol levels: Results of AFCAPS/TexCAPS. *Journal of the American Medical Association, 279*, 1615–1622.

[c]HPS: Heart Protection Study Collaborative Group. (2002). Heart Protection Study of cholesterol lowering with simvastatin in 20,536 high-risk individuals: A randomised placebo-controlled trial. *Lancet, 360*, 7–22.

[d]Shepherd, J., Blauw, G. J., Murphy, M. B., et al., PROSPER study group. (2002). Pravastatin in elderly individuals at risk of vascular disease (PROSPER): A randomised controlled trial. PROspective Study of Pravastatin in the Elderly at Risk. *Lancet, 360*, 1623–1630.

[e]Sever, P. S., Dahlof, B., Poulter, N. R., et al., ASCOT Investigators. (2003). Prevention of coronary and stroke events with atorvastatin in hypertensive patients who have average or lower-than-average cholesterol concentrations, in the Anglo-Scandinavian Cardiac Outcomes Trial–Lipid Lowering Arm (ASCOT-LLA): A multicentre randomised controlled trial. *Lancet, 361*, 1149–1158.

[f]4S: Scandinavian Simvastatin Survival Study. (1994). Randomised trial of cholesterol lowering in 4444 patients with coronary heart disease: The Scandinavian Simvastatin Survival Study (4S). *Lancet, 344*, 1383–1389.

[g]CARE: Sacks, F. M., Pfeffer, M. A., Moye, L. A., et al., for the Cholesterol and Recurrent Events Trial Investigators. (1996). The effect of pravastatin on coronary events after myocardial infarction in patients with average cholesterol levels. *New England Journal of Medicine, 335*, 1001–1009.

[h]LIPID: Long-Term Intervention with Pravastatin in Ischaemic Disease (LIPID) Study Group. (1998). Prevention of cardiovascular events and death with pravastatin in patients with coronary heart disease and a broad range of initial cholesterol levels. *New England Journal of Medicine, 339*, 1349–1357.

[i]Cannon, C. P., Braunwald, E., McCabe, C. H., et al., for the Pravastatin or Atorvastatin Evaluation and Infection Therapy-Thrombolysis in Myocardial Infarction 22 Investigators. (2004). Intensive versus moderate lipid lowering with statins after acute coronary syndromes. *New England Journal of Medicine, 350*, 1495–1504.

[j]Serum lipids were determined by direct LDL measurement method as baseline samples were nonfasting. If calculated by Friedewald (as in other trials), LDL would be approximately 15% higher.

In the liver, the endogenous lipoprotein cascade begins with the production of VLDLs. Triglycerides are resynthesized from chylomicrons and packaged with specific apoproteins, apo B-100, apo C-I, apo C-II, and apo E, to form VLDL. Once VLDL is released into the circulation, IDLs and VLDL remnants are formed from VLDL lipolysis. This process takes place in the capillary endothelium and is mediated by LPL, the same enzyme responsible for the hydrolysis of chylomicrons. Apo C-II also acts as a cofactor in these processes.[43]

LDL receptors in the liver recognize and bind with apo E on the IDL particle and remove approximately half of the IDL from the circulation. The remainder is converted by HL into smaller cholesterol-rich lipoproteins known as LDL. Apo B-100 is the remaining protein left on the surface coat of LDL particles. The LDL receptors on cells of the liver and other organs that require cholesterol for structural and metabolic functions bind with apo B-100 and facilitate the removal of LDL from the blood. Figure 24-2 illustrates the endogenous pathway. The LDL particle

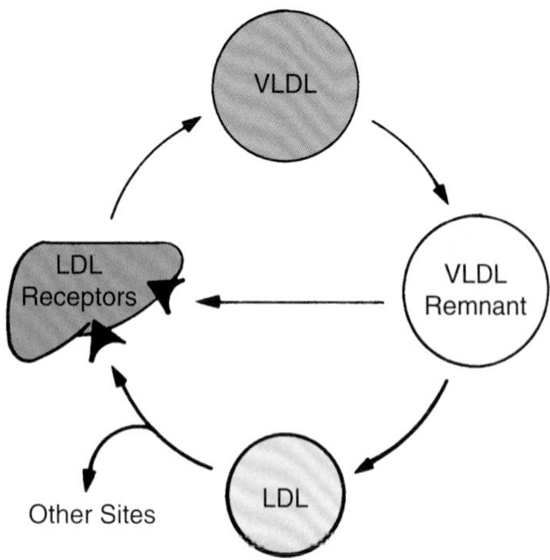

Figure 24-2. The endogenous lipid transport system originates in the liver. LDLs provide essential cholesterol to the tissue cells.

is the major cholesterol-carrying lipoprotein in the blood and, consequently, the most atherogenic lipoprotein.[34] Under normal conditions, more than 93% of the cholesterol in the body is located in the cells, and only 7% circulates in the blood. Two thirds of the blood cholesterol is carried by LDL. Increased cellular uptake of cholesterol through the LDL receptor pathway suppresses the cell's own synthesis of cholesterol by inhibiting the HMG-CoA reductase enzyme. This enzyme determines the rate of cholesterol synthesis. As cellular cholesterol levels increase, the activity of the LDL receptor is downregulated, and synthesis of new LDL receptors is inhibited.[44] These feedback control mechanisms serve as the rationale for determining the treatment of elevated blood cholesterol.

Several metabolic and genetic disorders can be related to elevated LDL-C levels. Habitually high dietary intakes of saturated fats and cholesterol beyond that needed for cell functions result in blood levels of LDL beyond normal and result in inhibited LDL receptor activity. High LDL levels also can result from a decrease in clearance of LDL because of a deficiency in LDL receptors. This deficiency may be caused by genetic abnormalities in the structure of the receptor-binding sites (where apolipoproteins bind) or by a decrease in LDL receptors on the surface of cells. In addition, genetic mutation in apoproteins, particularly apo E and apo B-100, can result in decreased cholesterol clearance. The metabolic consequence is an increased blood level of this atherogenic lipoprotein and the synthesis of cholesterol within cells, a process normally suppressed by LDL uptake.

Reverse Cholesterol Transport

Studies have consistently observed a protective effect of HDL. For example, high levels of HDL have been associated with a reduced risk of CVD.[21,45] It has been suggested that the protective effect of HDL is greater than the atherogenic effect of LDL-C. For men in the Framingham Heart Study, a 50% reduction in coronary risk was found with every 10-mg/dL increment in HDL.[46] Studies have indicated that increased apo A-I levels may also be inversely related to CVD.[47] Early trial data in small clinical trials demonstrated that pharmacologic increases of HDL-C significantly decreased coronary and stroke events among patients with CVD.[48] This data has not been replicated.

At present, the synthesis and metabolism of HDL is not fully elucidated. Over the last couple of decades, research directed at identifying therapeutics to raise HDL levels has led to an increased understanding of the complex mechanisms involved in HDL synthesis and its role in reverse cholesterol transport (the transport of cholesterol from the tissues to the liver resulting in biliary excretion of cholesterol).[49]

HDL particles are composed of proteins approximately 50%, phospholipids approximately 30% and cholesterol approximately 25%, triglycerides approximately 5%, and assorted lipoprotein-processing enzymes.[49] The intestine and liver are responsible for synthesizing the precursors of HDL and its major lipoprotein, apo A-I to form incomplete (or nascent) lipid-poor HDL precursors. These precursors acquire excess cholesterol through a variety of mechanisms outlined below. One early step is the cholesterol efflux from macrophages mediated by the membrane protein, adenosine triphosphate-binding cassette transporter A-1 (ABCA1), one of a family of proteins that transport molecules across cell membranes.[50] It is proposed that ABCA1 allows binding with apo A-I in nascent HDL to form more mature HDL particles.[51] Other steps include the action of the enzyme, lecithin cholesterol acyltransferase, which converts free cholesterol in the tissues into an HDL cholesteryl ester core.[52,53] Apo A-I has been shown to activate lecithin cholesterol acyltransferase and may influence the activity of the CETP. CETP facilitates the exchange of cholesterol esters for the triglycerides in apo B lipoproteins including LDL and VLDL.[54] Apo C-II is a cofactor for LPL. In the presence of circulating triglycerides, apo C-II moves from HDL to the triglyceride particle, activating LPL and promoting the catabolism of VLDL.[55] This mechanism, in part, explains the clinical observation of an inverse association between high triglycerides and low HDL levels. A third apoprotein, apo E, is thought to facilitate direct transfer of cholesterol esters to hepatocyte receptors.[55] Cholesterol esters are then excreted in bile or bile acids.[56]

Although the protective effect of HDL has been linked to its role in the reverse transport of cholesterol, it is clear that other factors, particularly genetic factors, determine coenzyme, apoprotein, and receptor activity. In fact, it is estimated that 50% to 70% of the variation in HDL is genetically determined influencing the receptor and enzyme activity involved in the catabolism of HDL.[57] Deletions or mutations of the apo A-I gene result in very reduced HDL levels (e.g., A-I Milano) and may be associated with increased atherosclerosis. One important recent discovery was that of the ABCA1 genetic defect manifested in Tangier disease as a disorder with extremely low HDL levels and with accelerated cholesterol tissue deposition.[50,58]

Studies have found that plasma HDL levels are regulated by a class of enzymes including LPL, HL, and endothelial lipase (EL).[59] LPL is synthesized by adipose and skeletal muscle cells and acts primarily on the hydrolysis of triglycerides. HL is synthesized in the liver cells and acts on triglyceride and phospholipid catabolism. EL is synthesized in endothelial cells and appears to regulate HDL levels by preventing the transfer of triglycerides and remnant particles to HDL. Evidence includes genetically modified animal models that overexpress EL show a marked decrease in HDL levels.[60] In human studies there have been genetic variants noted to the EL gene in persons with high HDL levels.[57]

While we have gained a greater understanding of the role of HDL in reverse cholesterol transport, studies also suggest that HDL may have both pro- and anti-inflammatory properties and in the face of inflammatory states, HDL may be altered to become proinflammatory.[61,62] This may explain the finding that atherosclerosis (as an inflammatory disease) is observed even in persons with normal to high HDL levels. Studies have also suggested that

HDL may act as an antioxidant, by preventing the oxidation of LDL, thus rendering it less atherogenic,[63,64] or by attenuating the expression of other enzymes and molecules that alter endothelial dilation and chemotactic properties.[65]

At present, there are two major subclasses of HDL based on density and apoprotein composition. HDL3 is richer in apo A-II than HDL2, which has a higher concentration of apo A-I.[47] Production of apo A-I is higher in women than in men and is increased by exercise training, alcohol consumption, and estrogen administration.[34] Premenopausal women have more than three times the concentration of HDL2 than do men. More recent studies[66,67] have increased the controversy surrounding the HDL hypothesis[68] due to multiple reasons: (1.) lack of evidence demonstrating the direct causal role of HDL-C to outcomes through a primary biologic mechanism, (2.) a complex HDL mechanism, which is unlike the apolipoprotein B–containing lipoproteins that generally exhibits dose-depending risk, (3.) mechanisms of action of HDL outside the reverse cholesterol transport and lipid transport, (4.) inability of HDL to accurately reflect reverse cholesterol transport reflux and effect on outcomes. It is suggested that plasma HDL concentration may not replicate the functionality of the HDL in circulation or the effects of a specific HDL-targeted treatment on CVD.[69] Current research is ongoing.

LDL VARIANTS

LDL Particle Size

Mounting evidence suggests that the size of the LDL particle plays an important role in its atherogenicity. Particle size is determined by flotation rates after ultracentrifugation procedures.

LDL can be separated into a small dense LDL particle (phenotype B) and a larger less dense LDL particle (phenotype A).[70] Clinical trial evidence suggests that people with a predominance of small dense LDL particles have a higher incidence of CVD and more accelerated progression of coronary lesions.[71] The exact mechanism of the negative influence of the small dense LDL particle is not completely understood. One possible explanation is that the smaller denser particles have a greater ability to penetrate the endothelial space and participate fully in the subendothelial atherosclerotic process. Small LDL particles also appear to be more susceptible to oxidation than larger LDL particles.[72] In addition, the small dense LDL particle is most commonly found in conjunction with a constellation of other factors, including hypertriglyceridemia, low HDL-C, and insulin resistance.[73]

Research also suggests that it is possible to increase (alter) the size of the LDL particle to the larger (phenotype A) size by reducing triglycerides and normalizing insulin sensitivity. In addition, lipid-lowering drugs such as bile acid–binding resins, niacin, and the fibrates are reported to alter particle size favorably.[70]

Oxidized LDL

The concept that oxidation of LDL and oxidative stress plays a role in atherosclerosis originated over 30 years ago.[74–76] Ongoing research in lipid metabolism continues investigating the issue of oxidation. Molecular biologists have established that modified or oxidized LDL is taken up more rapidly in vitro by monocytes and macrophages than is native LDL.[76] It has also been shown that Lp(a) is a primary carrier of oxidized LDL and accounts for the relationship between elevated Lp(a) and atherosclerosis.[77]

Oxidized LDL has been found to be cytotoxic, and it is postulated that this facilitates endothelial injury, leading to the development of fatty streaks and atherosclerotic lesions.

Oxidative inhibitors can block the modification of LDL to an oxidized form. Studies are ongoing in this area but a clear understanding of oxidized lipids and CVD remains elusive.[78]

The Role of Lp(a)

Lp(a) is a unique and enigmatic lipoprotein particle that is similar to LDL with each particle linked to a molecule of the atherogenic apo B-100 in a 1:1 ratio. There is a covalent association between apo B-100 and lipoprotein(a) (apo[a]), with apo(a) having a unique and similar DNA sequence to plasminogen, a substance that breaks up blood clots.[79–83] Due to the similarity with LDL and the structural homology with plasminogen, Lp(a) plays an atherothrombotic action, therefore, establishing a cardiovascular risk.[82] Recent studies and meta-analysis have found elevated levels of Lp(a) are independent predictors of CVD.[79,84] It is important to note that Lp(a) has also been detected in atherosclerotic plaques.[85] Lp(a) levels vary inversely to the size of the apo(a) protein. Those who are black and South Asian have higher Lp(a) levels compared with those who are Caucasian or from other Asian populations.[86] Circulating levels of Lp(a) above 50 mg/dL but less than 200 mg/dL are found in less than 1% of the general population.[80] Epidemiology studies suggest that Lp(a) levels above 25 to 30 mg/dL constitute CVD risk; further, it is estimated that 37% of those at high risk of CVD have elevated levels of Lp(a).[87] The relationship between Lp(a) concentrations and CVD outcomes,[88–90] as well as cerebrovascular outcomes,[89–91] has been confirmed by at least three meta-analyses for each. Recent data indicates that elevated plasma levels of Lp(a) are also a causal risk factor for aortic valve stenosis.[92,93]

Currently, treatment options are controversial due to the lack evidence-based therapies proving beneficial in high-risk patients. Apheresis is the most effective technique to reduce circulating Lp(a) concentrations up to 75% from baseline and is utilized in very–high-risk patient populations.[94] Lp(a) is refractory to both drug intervention and lifestyle.[80,94] Previous societies had recommended 1- to 3-g nicotinic acid (niacin, B_{12}) daily or extended-release niacin (1 to 2 g) daily as an effective means of lowering Lp(a). In more recent clinical trials, a statin–niacin combination medication was found to be effective in lowering Lp(a), but unfortunately, such reduction was not associated with lower CVD outcomes.[95] Further studies are ongoing to establish effective therapies in management. Like Lp(a), there are a number of emerging lipid risk factors that may further explain the relationship of dyslipidemia to CHD.

Lipoprotein-Associated Phospholipase A_2

The search for biomarkers that identify those at risk for CVD has led to interest in lipoprotein-associated phospholipase A_2 Lp-PLA_2, an enzyme that hydrolyzes lipids and preferentially oxidized LDL.[96] It is produced by inflammatory cells, bound to LDL and other lipoproteins, and once in the arterial wall facilitates hydrolysis of the phospholipids,[97] thereby triggering inflammatory processes. It is known that Lp-PLA_2 is produced by macrophages (prominent in the inflammatory atherosclerotic process) and mainly carried in circulation bound to LDL-C. Several prospective epidemiologic studies have identified Lp-PLA_2 as a significant predictor of CV events and stroke.[98,99] Current lipid-altering medications including statins, fenofibrate, ezetimibe, and prescription omega 3 fatty acids, also including weight loss, have been shown to reduce inflammatory markers, including Lp-PLA_2.[100–104] Despite being shown to be a significant predictor of risk for cardiovascular events, stroke, and mortality in primary and secondary prevention studies, there have been no randomized trials in which the benefits of lowering Lp-PLA_2 with any specific therapies.[105]

Cholesterol and Endothelial Function

Serum cholesterol levels and diets high in saturated fat have been associated with impairments in endothelial functioning. The endothelium acts to regulate vascular tone, platelet adhesion, thrombosis, and growth factors.[106] Studies have demonstrated that elevated cholesterol results in a reduced vasodilation response. Furthermore, when cholesterol is lowered, vasodilation responses improve.[107]

Elevated cholesterol also increases platelet aggregation and monocyte adhesion, factors that lead to thrombus formation and plaque rupture.[108] Continuing research suggests that the lipids influence a variety of endothelial responses that appear to contribute to the atherosclerotic process and continued research may find reliable methods of testing endothelial function.

DYSLIPIDEMIC DISORDERS

Although the metabolic processes related to blood lipids are complex and influenced by both genetic and environmental factors, the management of dyslipidemia has been well characterized. Since 2001, a long history of national recommendations has been developed based on scientific evidence and consideration for the need of both primary and secondary prevention of CVD.[12,19] In general, lipid disorders can be characterized by the specific lipid abnormalities observed (see Table 24-2).

Hypercholesterolemia

Hypercholesterolemia is the most common dyslipidemia and, in most people, decreased LDL clearance is responsible for the observed abnormality. A high intake of dietary cholesterol and saturated fatty acids downregulates LDL receptor activity and receptor synthesis, resulting in decreased LDL clearance.[1]

Familial (Severe) Hypercholesterolemia

Severe hypercholesterolemia is caused most commonly by an autosomal-dominant genetic disorder causing lifelong exposure to elevated LDL levels and is known as familial hypercholesterolemia (FH).[109] There are two types of FH, heterozygous (HeFH) and homozygous (HoFH). If left untreated, patients with HeFH typically develop CHD before age 55 for men and 60 for women.[110] Individuals with HoFH develop CHD before they are 20 years old and as a result, have earlier mortality.[111]

Plasma LDL-C normally binds to cell membrane receptors and is taken into the cell for several biologic functions. In HeFH, there is one normal gene and one abnormal gene for the LDL receptor. Because only half the normal number of LDL receptors is synthesized, LDL is removed from the blood at two thirds the normal rate.[44] The result is a two- to threefold increase in blood

Table 24-2 • LIPID ABNORMALITIES AND ASSOCIATED MECHANISMS

Lipid Abnormality	Mechanisms
Elevated total cholesterol	High dietary intake of saturated fat and cholesterol LDL receptor deficiency and other enzyme/receptor abnormalities
Elevated LDL cholesterol	LDL receptor deficiency Apoprotein B-100 genetic defect, other enzyme/receptor abnormalities High dietary intake of saturated fat and cholesterol
Elevated triglycerides	Deficiency in LPL Obesity, physical inactivity, insulin resistance, glucose intolerance Excessive alcohol intake
Low HDL	Apoprotein A-I deficiency, other enzyme/receptor abnormalities Reduced VLDL clearance Cigarette smoking, physical inactivity Insulin resistance Elevated triglycerides Overweight and obesity Very high carbohydrate (CHO) intake (>60% total calories) Certain drugs (β-blockers, anabolic steroids, progestational agents)
Increased lipoprotein remnants (VLDL is a surrogate marker for lipoprotein remnants when triglyceride (Tg) is >200 mg/dL)	Defective apolipoprotein E seen in familial combined hyperlipidemia
Lp(a)	Level is genetically determined
Lipoprotein phospholipase A^2 ($LpPLA^2$)	An enzyme that hydrolyzes cholesterol and initiates inflammatory processes
Small LDL particles	Particle size is determined by level of triglycerides; LDL particle is denser and more atherogenic at higher levels of TG
HDL subspecies	Low levels of HDL 2 and 3 increase CVD risk? Genetically determined versus lifestyle and other lipid levels
Apolipoprotein B	A potential marker for all atherogenic lipoproteins
Apolipoprotein A-I	Increased CVD risk when apo A-I is low
Combined dyslipidemias small, dense LDL, high triglycerides, low HDL elevated LDL and triglycerides	Defects in VLDL and LDL receptor activities coexisting with environmental influences such as obesity, physical inactivity, diet high in saturated fat, and cigarette smoking

National Cholesterol Education Program (2001).

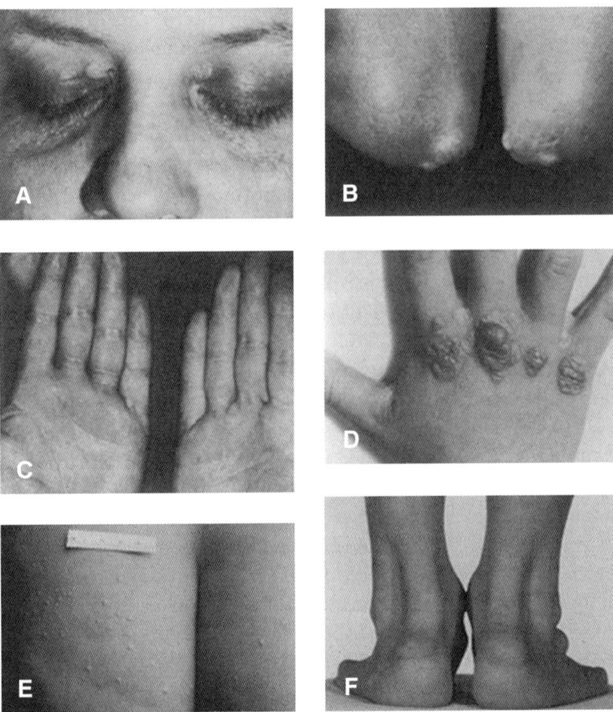

Figure 24-3. Representative xanthomas are illustrated: (**A**) Xanthelasmas (xanthomas of the palpebral fissures). (**B**) Tuberous xanthomas of the elbows. (**C**) Palmar xanthomas. (**D**) Interdigital xanthomas. (**E**) Tuberoeruptive xanthomas of the buttocks. (**F**) Tendon xanthomas of the Achilles tendon. (Reprinted from Fuster V, Ross R, Topol EJ, eds. *Atherosclerosis and Coronary Artery Disease.* 1st ed. Philadelphia, PA: Lippincott-Raven; 1996, with permission.)

LDL levels. Recent studies suggest the prevalence of this genetic disorder is between 1 person in 200 people to 300 people, which results in an increased risk for CHD.[112–114]

The homozygous form of FH develops when two abnormal genes are inherited. These patients may have the same mutation in both alleles of the same gene or they are compound heterozygotes with different mutations in each allele of the same gene or double heterozygotes with mutations in two different genes affecting the low density lipoprotein receptor (LDLR).[115] In recent studies, the prevalence may affect as many as 1 in 160,000 to 300,000 persons.[116] For this patient population, LDL levels are up to six times normal levels and require early initiation of assessment and intervention in order to decrease cardiovascular risks.[115] Individuals with untreated FH often have clinical signs of cholesterol deposits in the tendons and joint called tendon xanthomas, which may lead to tendonitis or corneal arcus when the eyes are examined (Fig. 24-3). Diagnosis of the FH can be made on the basis of genetic or clinical criteria. Cascade screening and family history remain important for the clinician. Genetic testing may provide a definitive diagnosis, however in some patient's genetic confirmation may remain elusive, as additional FH genes cannot be excluded.[116] Early pharmacotherapy should be started as early as possible with target LDL less than 100 mg/dL for those without clinical CVD and less than 70 mg/dL for those with CVD. First-line therapy for FH patients are your traditional lipid lowering therapies, like statin medications, which we will discuss later in the chapter. However, therapies specific to FH, not available to those with regular dyslipidemia include: (1.) lipoprotein apheresis, extracorporeal removal of LDL-C from the plasma[117–120] (2.) lomitapide, oral inhibitor of the microsomal triglyceride transport protein (MTP), which is responsible for transferring triglycerides and phospholipids onto chylomicron and VLDL during assembly in the intestine and liver[121] (3.) mipomersen, an antisense oligonucleotide administered through subcutaneous injection that targets the messenger ribonucleic acid (mRNA) of apo B.[122]

Hypertriglyceridemia

The relationship between triglycerides and CVD remains unclear. Elevated serum triglyceride levels have been associated with CVD. However, the strength of the association is diminished when other CVD risks are accounted for, leading some to suggest that elevated triglycerides are a marker for other atherogenic factors.[123] Chylomicrons and VLDL are lipoprotein carriers of triglyceride and, whereas chylomicrons are not considered to be atherogenic, the remnants of VLDL catabolism are smaller particles that are richer in cholesterol esters.[123] These remnant particles, or IDLs, are considered more atherogenic.[124]

Elevated triglycerides are frequently observed in people who also have low HDL levels (below 40 mg/dL) and small dense size LDL particles. This combination of lipid abnormalities is considered an atherogenic phenotype.[123] In addition, elevated triglyceride levels (and its associated small dense LDL particle size and low HDL-C level) commonly exist with insulin resistance (with or without glucose intolerance), hypertension, obesity (particularly abdominal obesity pattern), and prothrombotic and proinflammatory states. This combination of risk factors is commonly called the metabolic syndrome and is linked to increased CVD risk.[19,29] See Table 24-3 for a summary of the metabolic syndrome characteristics. These associations suggest that elevated triglyceride levels may be a marker for other CVD risk factors. Diabetes also results in increased plasma triglyceride levels because of increased VLDL. LDL-C is more glycated in patients with diabetes compared with nondiabetic subjects. Glycated LDL particles have increased oxidative susceptibility.[123] HDL is often low in patients with diabetes as a result of increased HL triglyceride activity. Additionally, hyperglycemia is associated with significantly increased mortality in patients with acute coronary syndrome. The Heart Protection Study (HPS) further confirmed the importance of lipid management in persons with type 2 diabetes. HPS included 5963 persons with diabetes (ages 40 to 80 years). Those subjects receiving simvastatin 40 mg/day had significant reductions of 25% for major coronary events including stroke and revascularization.[25]

High triglyceride levels are also related to high carbohydrate and alcohol intake. As a marker for CVD risk, the reduction of plasma triglyceride levels to less than 150 mg/dL is a desirable

Table 24-3 • CHARACTERISTICS OF THE METABOLIC SYNDROME

Risk Factor	Comments
Abdominal obesity (waist circumference)	Men: >102 cm (>40 in) Women: >88 cm (>35 in)
Triglycerides	≥150 mg/dL
HDL cholesterol	Men: <40 mg/dL Women: <50 mg/dL
Blood pressure	≥130/≥85 mm Hg
Fasting glucose	≥110–125 mg/dL

Adapted from Expert Panel on Detection, Evaluation, and Treatment of High Blood Cholesterol in Adults. Executive summary of the third report of the National Cholesterol Education Program (NCEP) Expert Panel on detection, evaluation, and treatment of high blood cholesterol in adults (Adult Treatment Panel III). *JAMA.* 2001;285(19):2486–2497.

goal.[19,29] Although not designated as an independent risk predictor by the previous Adult Treatment Panel (ATP) III guidelines, the importance of elevated triglycerides is recognized in a number of ways. In ATP III, triglyceride level is seen as a marker of elevated atherogenic remnant particle level thought to increase risk of coronary artery disease (CAD) and as an indication of lipid and nonlipid risk factors in the metabolic syndrome.[19]

Another target goal in the older ATP III guidelines, utilized for persons with elevated triglycerides is called "non-HDL cholesterol." Non-HDL cholesterol is the total cholesterol minus the HDL cholesterol. This number represents the sum of the LDL and the VLDL cholesterol in determining a treatment goal for LDL-C. If using the ATP III guidelines, the goal for LDL-C is 30 mg/dL higher in persons with triglycerides of 200 mg/dL or more. This is based on a normal VLDL value being 30 mg/dL.[19]

Hypoalphalipoproteinemia

A familial HDL deficiency state, hypoalphalipoproteinemia, has been linked to premature CVD. Although high HDL levels may mobilize cholesterol from arterial luminal surfaces and return it to the liver, low HDL usually reflects an enzymatic or apoprotein abnormality affecting the catabolism of LDL or VLDL (see section titled "Reverse Cholesterol Transport"). Alterations of the human apo A-I gene have been found in those with familial HDL deficiency and premature CVD.[125] This suggests that low HDL may represent a genetic marker for identifying those at risk for CVD. The abnormalities related to VLDL catabolism explain the common coexistence of low HDL with elevated triglycerides. Furthermore, when triglycerides are lowered, increases in HDL are observed. In the absence of a genetic deficiency (i.e., A-I Milano, Tangier disease), lower HDL levels are related to environmental factors such as cigarette smoking and physical inactivity (see Table 24-2 for causes of low HDL-C).

Although raising HDL-C by delaying catabolism (e.g., CETP inhibition) may not enhance reverse cholesterol transport, elevating HDL-C may have other cardioprotective benefits such as antioxidant, anti-inflammatory, and anticoagulant effects that all may improve endothelial function. At present, niacin is the most effective HDL-raising therapy. Although the mechanism by which niacin raises HDL level is not well understood, the predominant hypothesis is that niacin inhibits the holoparticle uptake of HDL, resulting in delayed catabolism.[126] Unfortunately, the most recent clinical trials utilizing prescription strength niacin have failed to show clinical benefit to patients, despite raising HDL.[67,127,128]

Combined Dyslipidemias

Combined dyslipidemias usually represent a combination of genetic lipoprotein or apoprotein defects and environmental effects. The specific lipid abnormalities observed provide clues to the genetic disorders. Table 24-2 summarizes observed lipid abnormalities and associated mechanisms. An understanding of these mechanisms guides the management of lipid abnormalities.

THE MANAGEMENT OF HIGH BLOOD CHOLESTEROL

Since the late 1980s, a large body of evidence has associated elevated blood lipids with CVD. Clinical trials have demonstrated that reducing blood cholesterol is the most effective in preventing CVD for both primary and secondary prevention. The research has prompted groups such as the National Institutes of Health, American Heart Association (AHA), the American College of Cardiology (ACC), and the National Lipid Association to establish health policy guidelines for the detection and treatment of lipid disorders.[19,29,129–131] In 1985, the ATP was set up under the support of the National Cholesterol Education Program (NCEP). Since that time, the NCEP-ATP has been revising and framing guidelines to provide a better treatment structure to cardiovascular patients, as well as to educate the public. As a result, the public has witnessed considerable reduction in cardiovascular-related deaths.[132] All three ATP guidelines, ATP I, ATP II, and ATP III have targeted LDL-C numbers as their primary goal.[133] The first ATP guideline was published in 1988, which outlined the strategy for primary prevention of CHD in individuals with high LDL-C (greater than 160 mg/dL) or with borderline high DL (130 to 159 mg/dL) including two risk factors.[19,134] In 1993, ATP II supported ATP I and added intensive management of LDL-C in patients with established CHD (secondary prevention) and a fixed lower LDL-C goal of less than 100 mg/dL in CHD patients.[135,136] Six years later, in 2001, the ATP III guidelines were developed based on the foundation of the previous ATP guidelines and represented an update on the recommendations for clinical management of high blood cholesterol. The key features in ATP III included: consideration of LDL-C less than 100 mg/dL as optimal level, introduction of the Framingham risk score (10-year CHD risk) to calculate treatment intensity, and therapeutic lifestyle modification (TLC. Secondary targets were introduced such as non-HDL in patients with triglycerides greater than 200 mg/dL and metabolic syndrome (see Table 24-3).[19,29] In 2004, ATP III underwent an update based on clinical trials changing the target LDL-C goal of less than 70 mg/dL as a clinical target for patients at extremely high risk.[29]

Recommendations for the Detection of High Cholesterol

Health policy recommendations for detection of high cholesterol include the measurement of total cholesterol, and HDL-C in all adults aged 20 years and older, with repeat measurement within 5 years based on the ATP III guidelines. Total cholesterol less than 200 mg/dL is considered desirable; levels between 200 and 239 mg/dL are classified as borderline–high, and those more than 240 mg/dL are considered high blood cholesterol.[19] Measures of HDL less than 40 mg/dL are considered low and constitute a risk factor for CVD. HDL more than 60 mg/dL remains a "negative" risk factor and removes one risk factor from the overall risk profile. If total cholesterol is greater than 200 mg/dL or HDL is less than 40 mg/dL, then a full lipoprotein analysis is required and treatment is based on LDL levels.

Other nonlipid factors that contribute to CVD risk status should also be assessed, including cigarette smoking, hypertension, diabetes mellitus, a family history of premature heart disease (age—men younger than 55 years and women younger than 65 years), and the presence of other CVD "risk equivalents" (abdominal aortic aneurysm, peripheral vascular disease, atherosclerotic cardiovascular disease [ASCVD] risk score greater than 7.5%, presence of multiple risk factors).[29]

Evaluation of the Patient With Elevated Cholesterol and Current Guidelines

In 2001, the ATP III was initiated with an update in 2004 guiding health care professionals in assessing risk and promoting therapies for target LDL reduction based on risk.[19,29] In 2013, the ATP IV was convened to establish an updated set of treatment guidelines for adults to reduce ASCVD risk based on randomized controlled trials (RCTs), systematic reviews, and meta-analyses of RCTs, with evidence based on statin therapy. For the ACC/AHA 2013 guidelines, ASCVD includes CHD, stroke, and peripheral arterial disease.[137] The ATP III guidelines continue to be used for the comprehensive approach to the detection and evaluation of lipid disorders (as previously discussed) and the ACC/AHA 2013 guidelines have simplified approach of therapy based on evidence-based trials supporting four treatment groups. Lifestyle modification (adherence to heart-healthy diet, regular exercise, avoiding use of tobacco products, and maintenance of healthy weight) remains a crucial component of health promotion and reducing ASCVD risk.[137]

The Expert Panel did not find evidence to support the use of LDL-C or HDL-C target levels, but instead defined groups indicated for higher-intensity statin medication or moderate-intensity statin medication. The four statin benefit groups defined by the guidelines include: (1) persons with clinical ASCVD (i.e., acute coronary syndrome, myocardial infarction, stable or unstable angina, coronary or other arterial revascularization, stroke, transient ischemic attack, or peripheral arterial disease); (2) persons with primary elevations of LDL-C levels of 190 mg/dL or greater; (3) persons with diabetes mellitus who are 40 to 75 years of age with LDL-C level of 70 to 189 mg/dL, but without clinical ASCVD; and (4) persons without clinical ASCVD or diabetes, who have LDL levels of 70 to 189 mg/dL and an estimated 10-year ASCVD risk (based on the Pooled Cohort Equation) of 7.5% or greater. The guidelines demonstrate an algorithm of statin therapy recommendations based on the four subgroups and their risk (see Fig. 24-4). The Expert Panel found extensive and consistent evidence supporting the use of statins for the prevention of ASCVD in many higher-risk and all secondary prevention individuals. Prior to the 2013 ACC/AHA guidelines, the Framingham Risk Calculator was used to establish a 10-year risk score for primary prevention of CVD to establish risk categories in patients. Since the 2013 ACC/AHA guidelines, a newer pooled cohort equation and a risk calculator were developed to estimate the 10-year risk of developing ASCVD outcomes for the purpose of primary prevention, in order to replace the Framingham Risk Calculator. The ASCVD risk calculator for primary prevention in patients 40–75 age should be performed every 4 to 6 years.[19,29,137] The ASCVD Risk Calculator is derived from several components including age, sex, race, systolic and diastolic blood pressure, total cholesterol, HDL-C, LDL-C, history of statin therapy, history of diabetes, history of smoking, and current therapy for blood pressure. Now, most smartphones or electronic medical records have ASCVD risk score calculator application, making the score easy to assess in clinical practice. Currently, there are multiple national organizations with guideline-directed medical therapy recommendations or consensus statements guiding care based on each patient's individual comorbidities and risk, which are beneficial in evaluating patient risk.[138–140]

At the time of the ACC/AHA guideline's publication, no data supported use of nonstatin therapies for the further reduction in LDL-C. In 2015, IMPROVE-IT was published showing that with the addition of a nonstatin agent, ezetimibe, which reduces the absorption of cholesterol from the gastrointestinal tract, to a statin medication, showed reduction of LDL-C by approximately 24% and demonstrated an improvement in cardiovascular outcomes.[141] Please refer to the most recently published guidelines.

HEART DISEASE IN WOMEN

Since the first women-specific clinical recommendations for the prevention of CVD in women in 1999 by the AHA, enormous progress has been made in the awareness, treatment, and prevention of CVD in women.[142] CVD is the largest killer of women in the United States. Over 500,000 women die of CVD annually.[142] In 2007, CVD still caused approximately 1 death per minute among women in the United States.[143] These represent 421,918 deaths, more women's lives than were claimed by cancer, chronic lower respiratory disease, Alzheimer disease, and accidents combined.[143] Opposing previous trends, CHD death rates in U.S. women 35 to 54 years of age appear to be increasing, likely due to the effects of the obesity epidemic.[144] CVD rates in the United States are significantly higher for black females compared to their white counterparts (286.1/100,000 vs. 205.7/100,000). This disparity substantiates the claims of lower awareness of heart disease and stroke that has been documented among black versus white females.[143,145–147]

The 2011 guideline update introduced an algorithm for risk classification in women based on the absolute 10-year probability of having a coronary event (using the Framingham risk score for women [Table 24-4] and based on clinical diagnosis). Women defined at high risk have a calculated 10-year CHD risk greater than 20% and/or established CHD, other vascular disease, diabetes mellitus, or chronic kidney disease. Women who are at intermediate risk have a 10-year risk of 10% to 20% and may have subclinical CVD (i.e., coronary calcification) metabolic risk factors, markedly elevated levels of one risk factor or a first-degree relative with early CVD. Women at lower risk have a 10-year risk of less than 10% and may have metabolic syndrome or variable numbers of risk factors. Additionally, in the 2011 update, an optimal risk group was defined as women who have desirable levels of risk factors and who have a heart-healthy lifestyle.[148] Also a change in the 2011 guidelines utilizes effectiveness (how interventions and therapies function in a clinical context) as well as evidence on efficacy of interventions (how interventions and therapies function in a clinical research context).

Although previous guidelines briefly discussed the association between pregnancy events and CVD, the updated 2011 guidelines expand upon this association, partly due to adverse pregnancy outcomes that have been proposed as unique risk factors for future CV disease in women. In large epidemiologic studies, preterm birth and small-size-for-gestational age have been associated with future development of maternal CVD.[149,150] Pregnancy complications such as preeclampsia and gestational diabetes are also associated with long-term CVD. The updated guidelines now include a history of preeclampsia, gestational diabetes, and pregnancy-induced hypertension as criteria for at-risk classification for CVD, and recommend that obstetrician-gynecologists refer patients with pregnancy complications to primary care physicians postpartum. All health care providers should feel comfortable and proficient at taking a detailed pregnancy history when seeing new patients later in life in order to assess CVD risk.

Recommendations for women are based on risk category (currently using Framingham risk score for women) and major risk factor interventions targeting hypertension, dyslipidemia, and diabetes.

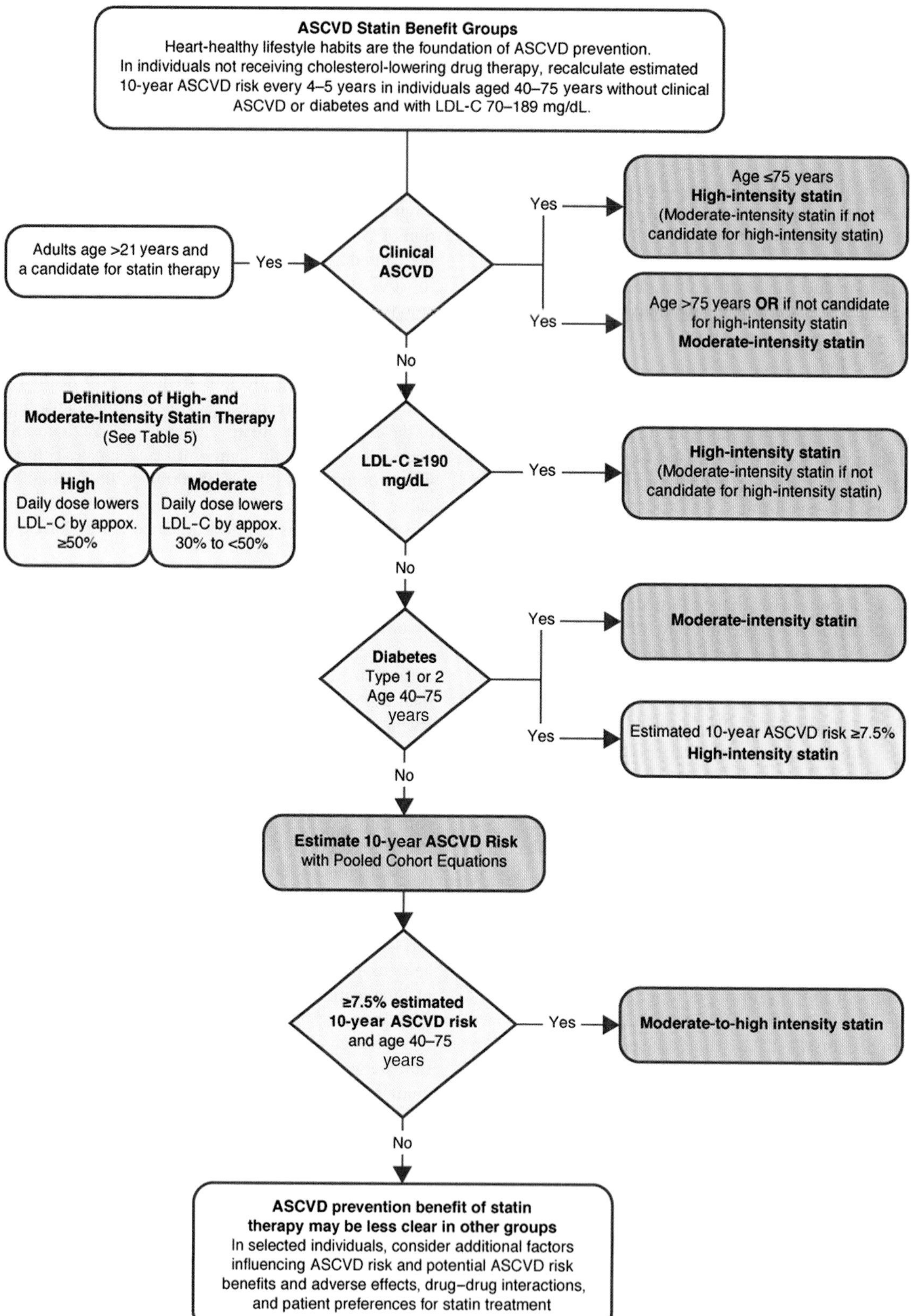

Figure 24-4. ACC/AHA 2013 guideline on the treatment of blood cholesterol to reduce atherosclerotic cardiovascular risk in adults. (From Stone NJ, Robinson J, Lichtenstein AH, et al. 2013 ACC/AHA guideline on the treatment of blood cholesterol to reduce atherosclerotic cardiovascular risk in adults: a report of the American College of Cardiology/American Heart Association Task Force on Practice Guidelines. *Circulation*. 2014;129[25 suppl 2]:S1–S45, with permission.)

Table 24-4 • ESTIMATE OF 10-YEAR CVD RISK FOR WOMEN (FRAMINGHAM POINT SCORES)

Age (years)	Points	HDL (mg/dL)	Points	Systolic BP (mm Hg)	Points: Untreated	Points: Treated
20–34	−7	≥60	−1	<120	0	0
35–39	−3	50–59	0	120–129	0	1
40–44	0	40–49	1	130–139	1	2
45–49	3	<40	2	140–159	1	2
50–54	6			≥160	2	3
55–59	8					
60–64	10					
65–69	12					
70–74	14					
75–79	16					

	Points				
Total Cholesterol (mg/dL)	Age 20–39 Years	Age 40–49 Years	Age 50–59 Years	Age 60–69 Years	Age 70–79 Years
<160	0	0	0	0	0
160–199	4	3	2	1	1
200–239	8	6	4	2	1
240–279	11	8	5	3	2
≥280	13	8	7	4	2
Nonsmoker	0	10	0	0	0
Smoker	9	7	4	2	1

Point Total	10-Year Risk (%)	Point Total	10-Year Risk (%)
<9	<1	17	5
9	1	18	6
10	1	19	8
11	1	20	11
12	1	21	14
13	2	22	17
14	2	23	22
15	3	24	27
16	4	≥25	≥30

Adapted from Expert Panel on Detection, Evaluation, and Treatment of High Blood Cholesterol in Adults. Executive summary of the third report of the National Cholesterol Education Program (NCEP) Expert Panel on detection, evaluation, and treatment of high blood cholesterol in adults (Adult Treatment Panel III). *JAMA*. 2001;285(19):2486–2497.

Recommendations include maintenance of an optimal blood pressure less than 120/80 mm Hg through lifestyle approaches including the dietary approaches to stop hypertension (DASH) eating plan.[151] Pharmacologic intervention is indicated at levels greater than or equal to 140/90 mm Hg or even lower in the setting of blood pressure-related target organ damage. Optimal levels of lipoprotein targets were defined as LDL-C less than 100 mg/dL, triglycerides less than 150 mg/dL, non-HDL less than 130 mg/dL, and HDL-C greater than 50 mg/dL. Women defined as high risk, LDL-C–lowering therapy was recommended with statins preferred to be used in combination with lifestyle therapy. Statin therapy was also recommended for high-risk women with LDL-C less than 100 mg/dL unless contraindicated. For women at intermediate risk, LDL-C lowering with statin therapy was recommended if the LDL-C greater than or equal to 130 mg/dL along with lifestyle modification. Finally, for women at lower risk, LDL-C lowering was recommended if levels were greater than or equal to 190 mg/dL or greater than or equal to 160 mg/dL in the presence of multiple risk factors.[148] At the time of these guidelines, niacin was recommended for women to improve HDL-C, but more recent clinical trials disprove effectiveness on cardiovascular outcomes. Future evidence-based guidelines for CVD prevention in women should reflect the evidence-based data on niacin and fibrates, as well as reflect the new ASCVD risk scoring.

INITIAL EVALUATION OF THE PATIENT WITH ELEVATED CHOLESTEROL

It is appropriate that the patient with high blood cholesterol receives a thorough clinical evaluation in addition to a lipoprotein analysis. Several medical diagnoses have been associated with high cholesterol. Abnormal lipid profiles may be the first clue to undiagnosed endocrine disorders such as hypothyroidism or diabetes. A careful family history is also important. Genetic forms of hypercholesterolemia are relatively common in the general population, for example, FH that we discussed previously. It is therefore advisable that first-degree relatives be screened for lipid disorders. Hyperlipidemia, like hypertension, is a relatively asymptomatic disorder and is usually first recognized by abnormal laboratory findings. Subcutaneous or tendinous lipid deposits, called xanthomas, are the one physical finding that may be prominent in severe lipid disorders (see Fig. 24-3).

Certain types of hyperlipoproteinemia are characterized by abdominal pain. Possible causes for the abdominal pain include pancreatitis and hepatosplenomegaly. Abdominal pain of unknown origin also has been documented as a physical finding. This pain may be associated with ischemic bowel and is related to increased blood viscosity, macrophage ingestion of fat particles, or the effect of the size of the lipid particles on abdominal tissue.[35] Patients with chylomicronemia, or markedly elevated triglycerides levels, have a higher risk for pancreatitis.

Lipoprotein Measurement

The measurement of plasma lipids and lipoproteins is essential for the diagnosis of lipid abnormalities and for the identification of those at risk for CVD. These measurements also provide important feedback to the patient modifying his or her risk profile. The most common lipid analysis includes measurement of total cholesterol, total triglycerides, and HDL-C. This allows calculation of LDL using the following equation: LDL = total cholesterol − (triglycerides ÷ 5) − HDL.[152] This indirect assessment of LDL can be used if triglycerides are less than 400 mg/dL. If triglycerides are more than 400 mg/dL, then LDL must be directly measured using the more complex and costly ultracentrifugation procedure through the laboratory. Included in the calculation methodologies is the non-HDL as measurement of atherogenicity in some of the more current recommendations. The equation is total cholesterol − HDL = non-HDL, which is an apo B surrogate and if high, is a measure of risk.

To interpret the results of lipid measurements, some knowledge of the accuracy and precision of the measure is useful. One of the common scenarios encountered in lipid management is a laboratory report with values extremely different from the previously measured values, and the patient protests, "I have not been doing anything differently." Intraindividual cholesterol measurements have been shown to vary by 4% to 11% over a 1-year period.[153] Although there are several sources for variability or error in cholesterol measures, the most obvious is analytic variability, or laboratory error, which has been estimated to contribute one third to one half of the intraindividual variability. Laboratories must make their standardization criteria available and should strive to achieve less than 3% measurement variability. Biologic and physiologic factors constitute the other major source for measurement variability. To minimize measurement variability, the National Cholesterol Education Laboratory Standardization Panel recommends the following standards of practice[153]:

1. A stable lifestyle, including health status, diet, medication, and activity level, should be followed for at least 2 weeks before measurement.
2. Cholesterol measures should be made no sooner than 8 weeks after MI, surgical procedure, trauma, or an acute bacterial or viral infection.
3. In acute coronary syndrome, it is recommended that a lipid profile be collected at the earliest possible time during hospitalization.[154]
4. Blood collection procedures should include a 12-hour fast (except for water and usual medications) before sampling, if lipid measures other than total cholesterol are to be performed. This is currently being debated in the literature.
5. The patient should sit quietly for 5 minutes before the venipuncture.
6. The sample should be obtained within 1 minute of tourniquet application.
7. Standardized procedures for processing and transporting samples should be followed.

Dietary Management of Hyperlipidemia

A heart-healthy diet remains the cornerstone of CVD prevention and treatment. Initial assessment of a patient's lipid status management should begin with evaluating dietary patterns. As mentioned previously, CVD, diabetes, and obesity have only increased over the years, mostly contributed to our dietary habits. Evidence of the relationship between dietary intake, plasma cholesterol, and CVD has been steadily accumulating. Seminal population studies have shown that countries with the highest incidence of CVD and elevated blood cholesterol levels also have high dietary intakes of saturated fats.[155–158] Developing countries with a mean cholesterol level less than 150 mg/dL have a very low incidence of CVD and also have diets low in total fat, saturated fatty acids, and cholesterol.[156] The target of lifestyle therapies is the level of atherogenic cholesterol, which involves LDL-C and non-HDL levels.

Diet Patterns and Lipid Effects

Current evidence strongly supports the Healthy U.S. Dietary Pattern, the Healthy Mediterranean-Style Dietary Pattern, and the Healthy Vegetarian Dietary Pattern for CVD risk reduction and improvement in CVD risk factors in adults and children 2 years of age or older.[159–163] Epidemiology studies and randomized clinical trials have examined the relationship of dietary patterns including very low fat, reduced saturated fat, vegetarian diets, and the Mediterranean diet with cardiovascular outcomes such as CVD events, mortality, or angiographic disease progression. In general, a benefit was observed if the chosen dietary pattern was continuously maintained.[164] Limited evidence is available from RCT to assess the impacts of lifestyle therapies on CVD risk. In the RCTs, each reduction in 1% of LDL-C or non–HDL-C is associated with a 1% reduction in CHD event risk over a period of approximately 5 years.[29,165] The primary goal of low-fat dietary patterns was to reduce LDL blood concentrations. However, in studies of low-fat dietary plans, researchers have noted detrimental effects on other lipid parameters including reductions in HDL and increases in triglyceride levels leading to a controversy about which diet is best for CVD. The effects of diet on lipid parameters relates to the amount of fat, the type of fat, and whether fat is replaced with protein or carbohydrate. Sacks and Katan[166] have estimated the lipid effects of four common dietary plans: the average Western diet (38% total fat, 17% saturated fat, 42% carbohydrates), a 30% total-fat diet, a 20% total-fat diet, and the Mediterranean diet (a reduced saturated fat diet with increased use of vegetable oils such as olive oil, and increased intake of vegetables, fruits, and fish). Compared with the Western diet, LDL is reduced by 6%, 12%, and 13% in each of the above-mentioned diet patterns, respectively. Conversely, HDL is reduced by 9%, 20%, and 9% in each diet pattern, respectively. The net result is that the cholesterol to HDL ratio increases in both lower-fat diets but is lowest with the Mediterranean diet.[166] Saturated fatty acids, with the exception of stearic acid, raise total and LDL-C probably through a mechanism decreasing LDL receptor synthesis.[167] Studies suggest that diets high in monounsaturated fat relative to saturated fat provide a desirable plasma lipid profile, with lowering of total and LDL cholesterol and no reduction in HDL.[168] The major criticism of these studies has been that the addition of only unsaturated fats to the diet is not practical among free-living individuals. For example, food items high in stearic acid usually contain other highly saturated fatty acids as well. Studies also have found that trans fats (partially hydrogenated unsaturated fats) raise LDL levels but show no effect on HDL levels, resulting in an even higher cholesterol to HDL ratio.[167]

The effect of other dietary additives on plasma lipids has also been studied. Dietary studies on the effect of increased omega-3 fatty acids either by fish intake or supplementation with fish oils have shown an effect on plasma lipids, primarily triglyceride lowering with concomitant increases in HDL.[169,170] The response is dose related and is sufficiently high that it is unlikely to be achieved using food choices only. Omega-3 fatty acids also exert antithrombotic effects through the thromboxane–prostaglandin pathways, resulting in decreases in platelet aggregation and vasoconstriction. Although the safety of consumption of large amounts of fish oils is an issue, most researchers agree that the inclusion of fish several times each week is a safe and prudent alternative. Plant sterols and stanols at doses of 2 g/day or greater can lower LDL-C by 5% to 10% based on recent meta-analyses, and seems to increase LDL-C reduction with increase in dose, but it does plateau in effectiveness.[171–173]

Dietary Recommendations

The goal of diet therapy is to reduce LDL-C to desirable levels predicated by the person's CVD risk status while maintaining a nutritionally sound eating pattern. The most recent dietary recommendations from the AHA/ACC 2013 guideline include both dietary and healthy lifestyle recommendations.[137] The overarching recommendations call for consuming a dietary pattern that emphasizes intake of vegetables, fruits, and whole grains. Included in the dietary plan are low-fat dairy products, poultry, fish legumes, nontropical vegetable oils, and nuts. Emphasis in the new guidelines is placed on limiting intake of sweets, sugar-sweetened beverages, and red meats.[137] The plan of provider is to adopt these recommendations with the appropriate individualized caloric requirements, plus adapt to personal and culture food preferences while considering treatment of other conditions. One should aim to achieve no more than 5% to 6% of total calories derived from saturated fat.[137] An in-depth evaluation of specific components of guideline-directed lifestyle changes is also available through the National Lipid Association's Recommendations for the Patient-Centered Management of Dyslipidemia guidelines.[139] All of these above dietary recommendations are consistent with the DASH and Mediterranean diets (see Table 24-5). The DASH diet is a healthy option that includes limiting sodium for individuals who may have elevated blood pressure.[174] Be aware the responses to dietary intervention is variable and appears related not only to the specific fatty acid composition of the diet but to the level of plasma lipids. Persons with the higher lipid levels usually experience the greatest response to dietary interventions.[175]

Table 24-5 • HEART-HEALTHY DIETARY PLANS[a]

	AHA Healthy Lifestyle[b]	**Mediterranean Diet**[c]	**DASH Diet**[d]
Fats and oils	Two to three servings a day Use vegetable or liquid oils. Examples: 1 tsp of soft margarine or vegetable oil. 2 tbsp mayonnaise. Saturated fat: Less than 7% of daily calories	Olive oil with each meal Used as the principal source of fat ~25–35% of total calories Saturated fat: Less than 7% of daily calories	Two to three servings a day Saturated fat: Less than 6% of daily calories
Trans fat	Less than 1% of daily calories. Minimize use of partially hydrogenated fats.	Very low—likely due to the absence of hydrogenated foods	Not specified
Lean meat, poultry, or fish	Less than 6 oz a day. Examples: grilled or broiled meats, trim fat. Fish intake ~8 oz a week, particularly of oily fish. Do not fry or serve with cream sauces.	Meat: four to five servings a month Poultry: one to three servings a week Fish: four to five servings a week	≤2 servings a day Includes eggs
Whole grains	Six to eight servings a day. Examples: 1 slice of bread, 1 oz dry cereal, ½-cup cooked rice or pasta. At least half of the grains should be whole grains.	Nonrefined whole grains—eight servings a day	Seven to eight servings a day Include at least three servings of whole grains a day
Nuts, seed, legumes	Four to five servings a week. Examples: 2-tbsp peanut butter, or ½ oz of seeds, ½ cup of dried peas or beans.	Greater than four servings a week	Four to five a week
Vegetables	Four to five servings a day. Examples: 1 cup of leafy greens, ½ cup of raw or cooked vegetables	Two to three servings a day. Potatoes four to five servings a week	Four to five servings a day
Fruits	Four to five servings a day. Examples: 1 medium fruit, ¼-cup dried fruit, ½-cup fruit juice	Four to six servings a day.	Four to five a day
Fat-free or low-fat dairy products	Two to three servings a day: Use only low- or nonfat products. Examples: 1 cup of milk, 1 cup of yogurt, 1½ oz of hard cheese.	One to two servings a day White cheese and yogurt intake more common than milk.	Two to three servings a day: Use only low- or nonfat products.
Sweets and sugars	Five or less servings a week. Limit beverages with added sugar. Examples: ½ cup of sorbets or ices, 1 tbsp of jam, 1 tbsp of sugar.	One to three servings a week	Limited
Alcohol	If consumed, use in moderation: 1 drink for women, 2 for men. Examples: 4-oz wine, 12-oz beer, 1½-oz spirits	One to two wine servings a day—accompanying meals	≤1 oz a day men, ≤½ oz women
Dietary cholesterol	<300 mg a day	Not specified	≤150 mg a day

[a]Serving size examples are based on a 2000 daily caloric intake and require adjustment for other calorie intakes.
[b]American Heart Association Nutrition Committee; Lichtenstein, A. H., Appel, L. J., Brands, M., et al. (2006). Diet and lifestyle recommendations revision 2006: A scientific statement from the American Heart Association Nutrition Committee. *Circulation, 114*, 82–96.
[c]Willett, W. C., Sacks, F., Trichopoulou, A., et al. (1995). Mediterranean diet pyramid: A cultural model for healthy eating. *American Journal of Clinical Nutrition, 61*, 1402S–1406S.
[d]Dietary Approaches to Stop Hypertension diet. Retrieved from http://www.nhlbi.nih.gov/health/bublic/heart/hbp/dash/new_dash.pdf

Before initiating dietary change, an assessment of the patient's current dietary pattern and usual eating habits is necessary. Dietary assessments are based on subjective reports and are predisposed to problems of recall accuracy and reliability. Utilizing a dietician to assist in the care of patients is beneficial in obtaining the dietary goals. Several systematic reviews from 1995 to 2014[176,179] and research trials[180–186] support the effectiveness of utilizing dieticians for medical nutrition–guided therapy on ASCVD risk factor modification.

Weight Control and Lipid Management

The prevalence of obesity in the United States has increased since the late 1970s. More than 35% of men and 40% of women in the United States are obese.[187,188] Because both LDL and the incidence of CVD are reduced in people who maintain a normal body weight, the obesity data is alarming. Studies examining weight loss have reported varying effects on lipid profiles. A meta-analysis of 70 studies examining the effect of weight reduction on lipoproteins found that a 1-kg reduction in weight was associated with a 0.05-mmol/L decrease in total cholesterol (1 mmol/L = 38.67 mg/dL).[189] Significant decreases in LDL and triglyceride levels were also found.

The effect of weight loss on HDL varies, generally decreasing during the active weight loss period and increasing after a period of stable reduced weight. Krauss et al. studied the effect of four diet patterns (a 54% carbohydrate, low-saturated fat diet, a 39% carbohydrate, low-saturated fat diet, a 26% carbohydrate, low-saturated fat diet, and a 26% carbohydrate, high-saturated fat diet) consumed during a stable weight period and during a 5-week weight loss period.[190] They observed significant increases in HDL after the weight loss period for all diets combined with the largest decreases in lipid parameters including small dense LDL occurring with the 54% carbohydrate diet as compared to the 26% carbohydrate diet with low-saturated fat content. The diet with the high-saturated fat content showed the smallest decrease in LDL-C level as well as the lowest amount of weight loss,[190] highlighting the importance of dietary restrictions of saturated fat. Of note, the DASH diet reported a 21% increase in HDL among men and a 33% increase among women.[191] The mechanisms postulated to account for these alterations in lipoproteins include decreased HMG-CoA reductase activity and enhanced cholesterol excretion in bile acids. The release of cholesterol from adipose tissues is also thought to inhibit hepatic synthesis of cholesterol.

For all patients with dyslipidemia, the secondary goal of diet intervention is weight reduction. Patients with dyslipidemia should be counseled to expect an initial reduction in HDL during active weight loss. Increasing levels of cardiovascular physical activity may minimize the HDL reduction and facilitate weight loss.[192]

Alcohol and Lipoproteins

Moderate alcohol intake has been reported to be protective for CVD. France, a country with a low rate of CVD, has a markedly higher per capita consumption of alcohol, particularly of wine.[193] One possible mechanism for this protective effect may be related to the increase in HDL observed with alcohol intake. Researchers have established that moderate alcohol intake increases HDL3, apo A-I, and apo A-II.[194,195]

Alcohol may also alter platelet aggregation and lower fibrinogen levels. Alcohol also increases catabolism of VLDL, the triglyceride-carrying lipoprotein. Patients with elevated triglyceride levels may have dramatic improvements in triglyceride levels with cessation of alcohol. Most researchers agree that the inverse association between alcohol intake and CVD risk is a consistent but weak association.[196] Recommendations to consume alcohol must therefore be considered cautiously, given the potential side effects of impaired judgment, decreased motor coordination, and possible addiction associated with alcohol use. The AHA's "scientific advisory" on *Wine and Your Heart* concluded that until randomized clinical trials are undertaken, there is "little justification to recommend alcohol (specifically wine) as a cardioprotective strategy."[197]

Physical Activity and Lipoproteins

There is mounting evidence in population studies linking physical activity and cardiorespiratory fitness with reduction in cardiovascular events. In addition to the effects that physical activity has on lipids and lipoproteins, increasing physical activity in those who were previously sedentary, has been associated with improvements in blood pressure, insulin resistance, and hemostasis.[198–201] The quality of exercise to reduce LDL-C is consistent with the exercise needed for long-term weight control and implementing moderate-intensity physical activity or burning greater than or equal to 2000 kcal/wk, which can be accumulated in repeated 10-minute bouts.[202] Aerobic exercise is the generally preferred method of physical activity recommended in all of the exercise guidelines for weight control and LDL reduction. There is a greater amount of physical activity required to lower LDL-C as suggested in the 2008 Physical Activity Guidelines Advisory Committee. These recommendations include: (1) primary activity—aerobic exercise, (2) intensity—40% to 75% aerobic capacity, (3) frequency—5 or more days a week (4) duration—30 to 60 minutes per session (5) 200 to 300 min/wk of moderate or higher intensity of physical activity (greater than or equal to 2000 kcal/wk).[203]

Hormones and Lipoproteins

In order to understand the present with hormones, specifically hormone replacement therapy (HRT), one needs to evaluate the past to appreciate the present. CHD develops in women almost a decade later in life than in men for reasons not entirely well understood. Several mechanisms have been suggested to account for this beneficial effect. Estrogen therapy can decrease LDL and increase HDL and apo A-I levels.[204] Estrogen use has been associated with lower Lp(a), reduced LDL oxidative susceptibility, and improved endothelial vasodilation responses.[204,205] Large, randomized, placebo-controlled clinical trials have examined the effect of HRT for primary and secondary CAD prevention.

The Heart and Estrogen/Progestin Replacement Study (HERS) evaluated the influence of Premarin plus medroxyprogesterone acetate (MPA) versus placebo in 2763 women with CVD at baseline.[206] After an average follow-up of 4.1 years, no differences were detected in acute MI and coronary death between the two groups. In addition, there was a pattern of early increased risk of CVD and thrombotic events with a pattern of late benefit in the women randomized to HRT. This increased risk seemed to occur primarily in the first year of treatment and there was a suggestion of potential benefit with long-term treatment (i.e., more than 4 years).[206] Because of this interesting potential late benefit, a follow-up study was undertaken. The investigators found that after 6.8 years of follow-up, use of estrogen–progestin did not significantly decrease the risk of primary or secondary CVD events in postmenopausal women with CVD. The effect of other doses and types of estrogen or estrogen only on CVD was not investigated in this trial; therefore, these conclusions can only be applied to women using this specific estrogen–progestin combination.[207]

The Women's Health Initiative (WHI), the largest study of primary and secondary prevention of heart disease in women ever undertaken reported a negative influence of HRT on breast cancer and cardiovascular risk in women. The WHI was a double-blind, randomized, placebo-controlled primary and secondary prevention trial examining the effects of estrogen and estrogen–MPA combination therapy on various cardiovascular, vascular, breast cancer, and other health outcomes. The Data and Safety Monitoring Board stopped the combined estrogen-plus-MPA arm of the trial because the rates of breast cancer in this group were significantly higher compared with placebo. They also found that the overall health risks of the estrogen–MPA combination, including increased risks for acute MI, thromboembolism, and stroke, far exceeded the benefits of the combination therapy.[208] This combined HRT was terminated 3 years earlier than its planned completion date of 2006. The increasing risk of breast cancer was the key factor that led the National Heart, Lung, and Blood Institute (NHLBI) to terminate the combined HRT arm of the study.[209] The breast cancer findings along with the negative CVD outcomes discredit short- or long-term estrogen-plus-progestin use for women with and without CVD.[208,209] Women in the WHI with prior hysterectomy were randomized to the group receiving conjugated equine estrogen only versus the placebo group. After 6.8 years of follow-up, the use of conjugated equine estrogen was found to increase the risk of stroke and did not affect CVD incidence. As a result, conjugated equine estrogen is not recommended for prevention of chronic disease in postmenopausal women.[210] The 2007 AHA guidelines for the primary and secondary prevention of heart disease in women supported these conclusions.[211]

Since the WHI and HERS trials, there has been much controversy in clinically treating women with heart disease risk and who are less than 60 years of age or who are within 10 years of menopause. This controversy led to the 2017 hormone therapy position statement of the North American Menopause Society after establishing an advisory panel of clinicians and researchers evaluating all the current literature and previous comparison of trials. The 2017 position statement reiterates hormone therapy (HT) remains the most effective treatment for vasomotor symptoms (VMS) and the genitourinary syndrome of menopause (GSM) and has been shown to prevent bone loss and fracture. The risks of HT differ depending on type, dose, duration of use, route of administration, timing of initiation, and whether a progestogen is used.

Treatment should be individualized to identify the most appropriate HT type, dose, formulation, route of administration, and duration of use, using the best available evidence to maximize benefits and minimize risks, with periodic evaluation of the benefits and risks of continuing or discontinuing HT.[212]

PHARMACOLOGIC MANAGEMENT OF HYPERLIPIDEMIA

The primary rationale for the treatment of hyperlipidemia is the reduction of CVD morbidity and mortality. Studies using hypolipidemic drug therapy to achieve LDL reductions have demonstrated lower CVD morbidity and mortality and lower overall mortality rates.[21,23] Angiographic studies using lipid-lowering drugs have demonstrated less progression of angiographically determined CVD with reduction of LDL.[213–216] The rate of progression of CVD appears to be a dose-related response, with slower rates of progression associated with greater LDL lowering.

Meta-analytic techniques have been used to analyze lipid-lowering studies and suggest that the decrease in CVD mortality is offset by increased death rates from other causes, particularly cancer deaths and non–illness-related deaths such as injury deaths and suicides.[217–219] These meta-analyses did not include data from the more recent very large clinical trials investigating lipid-lowering drugs.[20,21,23] These studies did not observe any increase in cancer or non–illness-related deaths. Although the explanations for these findings remain controversial, the consensus of experts is that hypolipidemic drug therapy should always be instituted with nonpharmacologic interventions (TLC), including a low-fat, low-cholesterol diet, regular exercise, weight control, smoking cessation, control of hypertension, and control of blood glucose (in patients with diabetes). Hypolipidemic drug therapy requires careful consideration of individual risks as well as the benefits of such drug therapy. There is sufficient evidence that lowering LDL-C, particularly with the use of HMG-CoA reductase inhibitors, in persons with known CAD and with CAD equivalents provides substantial benefit to reduced morbidity and mortality.

Classes of Hypolipidemic Drugs

The major classes of hypolipidemic drugs include the bile acid–binding resins, nicotinic acid, HMG-CoA reductase inhibitors (statins), fibric acid derivatives, and the intestinal absorption blockers. Within the past 5 years, a newer option of therapy for higher-risk individuals has come to the market that dramatically lowers LDL-C called proprotein convertase subtilisin kexin type 9 inhibitors (PCSK9 inhibitors). Individual response to any of these agents is variable, and each of the agents has potential side effects. Nursing can play a major role in the management of patients by assisting the patient to minimize side effects while promoting adherence to the regimen that achieves the desired lipid profile. In this section, the action, indications for use, and specific adherence strategies for each of the classes of hypolipidemic drugs are reviewed, but does not include PCSK9 inhibitors (Table 24-6).

Bile Acid–Binding Resins

Bile acid–binding resins are insoluble in water and are not absorbed from the intestine. These agents bind with bile acids in the intestine, forming an insoluble complex. The enterohepatic circulation of bile acids is interrupted and fecal excretion of bile acids is increased. This results in increased synthesis of bile acids from hepatic cholesterol stores. Reduced hepatic cholesterol stimulates LDL receptor formation and increases HMG-CoA reductase activity, resulting in increased extraction of LDL from the bloodstream and a lower plasma concentration of LDL. Hepatic production of VLDL is also enhanced, resulting in increased triglyceride levels. The expected response to resin therapy is seen in 2 to 4 weeks and may result in a 20% to 25% reduction in LDL.[33]

Strategies for Increased Efficacy and Adherence. The major side effect of the bile acid–binding resins is constipation; the resins can be unpalatable, which may affect compliance. Resins come in both powder and tablet formulations. In powder form, the resins must be mixed with water. Because they are insoluble, they form a gritty solution. It is helpful to demonstrate the mixing process and allow the patient to taste the drug as part of the prescription process. If constipation develops, instruct the patient in the use of fiber, stool softeners, and other hygienic measures, such as increased fluid intake. Bile acid–binding resins should be taken

Table 24-6 • LIPID-LOWERING AGENTS

Drug Class	Average Lipid/Lipoprotein Effects		Side Effects	Contraindications	Clinical Trial Results
HMG-CoA reductase inhibitors (statins)[a]	LDL-C HDL-C TG	↓18–60% ↑5–15% ↓7–37%	Myopathy Increased liver enzymes	Absolute: Active or chronic liver disease Relative: Concomitant use with certain drugs[b]	Reduced major coronary events, CVD deaths, need for coronary procedures, stroke, and total mortality
Bile acid sequestrants[c]	LDL-C HDL-C TG	↓15–30% ↑3–5% No change or an increase	GI distress Constipation Decreased absorption of other drugs	Absolute: Dysbetalipoproteinemia TG >400 mg/dL Relative: TG >200 mg/dL	Reduced major coronary events and CVD deaths
Nicotinic acid[d]	LDL-C HDL-C TG	↓5–25% ↑15–35% ↓20–50%	Flushing Hyperglycemia Hyperuricemia (or gout) Upper GI distress Hepatotoxicity	Absolute: Chronic liver disease Severe gout Relative: Diabetes Hyperuricemia Peptic ulcer disease	Reduced major coronary events
Fibric acid derivatives[e]	LDL-C (May be increased in patients with high TG) HDL-C TG	↓5–20% ↑10–20% ↓20–50%	Dyspepsia Gallstones Myopathy Unexplained non-CVD deaths in WHO study with clofibrate	Absolute: Severe renal disease Severe hepatic disease	Reduced major coronary events
Cholesterol absorption inhibitors[f]	LDL HDL TG	↓18% ↑1% ↑8%	Adverse event profile similar to placebo	Known hypersensitivity to ezetimibe	Studies in progress

[a]Atorvastatin (10 to 80 mg), fluvastatin (20 to 80 mg), lovastatin (20 to 80 mg), pravastatin (20 to 80 mg), simvastatin (20 to 80 mg).
[b]Cyclosporine, macrolide antibiotics, antifungal agents, and cytochrome P450 inhibitors (fibrates and niacin should be used with appropriate caution).
[c]Cholestyramine (4 to 16 g), colestipol (5 to 20 g), colesevelam (2.6 to 3.8 g).
[d]Immediate-release (crystalline) nicotinic acid (1.5 to 3 g), extended-release nicotinic acid (1 to 2 g), and sustained-release nicotinic acid (1 to 2 g).
[e]Gemfibrozil (600 mg BID), fenofibrate (200 mg), clofibrate (1000 mg BID).
[f]Not included in ATP III table of medications; approved for use after the guidelines were released.
Adapted from Expert Panel on Detection, Evaluation, and Treatment of High Blood Cholesterol in Adults. Executive summary of the third report of the National Cholesterol Education Program (NCEP) Expert Panel on detection, evaluation, and treatment of high blood cholesterol in adults (Adult Treatment Panel III). *JAMA*. 2001;285(19):2486–2497, and prescribing information for statins.

with meals, particularly with the largest meal of the day, because intestinal bile acids are greatest during that time. Because these drugs are binding agents, they have the potential to bind and interfere with the absorption of other medications. Consequently, the patient should be instructed to take other medications 1 hour before or 4 hours after taking the resin. Reviewing the mechanism of action with the patient promotes adherence and a better understanding of the rationale for these instructions.

Nicotinic Acid (Niacin)

Nicotinic acid, or niacin, is a vitamin B_3 derivative that in large doses blocks the release of free fatty acids from adipose tissues, resulting in less hepatic conversion of free fatty acids into triglycerides.[220] The hepatic production of VLDL is also decreased. Because VLDL is converted to IDL and LDL, decreased VLDL levels lead to favorable reductions in these lipoproteins as well. Contraindications to use include active liver disease and peptic ulcer disease, and caution should be exercised when it is used in patients with diabetes and atrial arrhythmias.

Strategies for Increased Efficacy and Adherence. The most common side effect of nicotinic acid use is cutaneous flushing caused by a prostaglandin-mediated vasodilation effect on vascular smooth muscle. This effect can be minimized with the use of aspirin taken 30 minutes before the nicotinic acid dose. Other less common side effects include abdominal discomfort; nausea; elevations in glucose, uric acid, and liver enzymes; reversible hepatotoxicity; and potentiation of atrial arrhythmias. Abdominal side effects are reduced if niacin is taken with meals. Niacin use must be monitored by a health professional, with liver enzymes measured before and periodically during therapy. Side effects can be minimized by starting at low doses and increasing the dose gradually. Written instructions, including a suggested dosage schedule, should be provided to the patient. The patient should be informed of the various side effects and instructed to contact a health professional if hepatotoxic side effects, such as flu-like symptoms and malaise, occur.[221]

Due to lack of evidence-based outcomes, niacin has fallen out of favor in daily clinical practice and may be used in very specific circumstances.

CETP Inhibitor

Torcetrapib is a CETP inhibitor that has demonstrated a dose-dependent increase of HDL and, to a lesser extent, apo A-I, resulting in a marked increase in HDL particle size.[222] Unfortunately, torcetrapib results in a 3 to 4 mm Hg increase in blood pressure. In a large outcome trial with torcetrapib in CVD patients, torcetrapib was associated with an increase in total mortality.[223] To date, no CETP inhibitors are commercially available due to the safety issues involving the therapy.

HMG-CoA Reductase Inhibitors (Statins)

The statins inhibit HMG-CoA reductase, the rate-limiting enzyme in cholesterol synthesis. Reduced cholesterol synthesis in the hepatocytes stimulates increased LDL receptor activity, thereby promoting clearance of VLDL and LDL from the bloodstream.[224] Statin medications are your first-line therapy for LDL lowering in patients.

Strategies for Increased Efficacy and Adherence. The statins are well tolerated. Single daily doses may be sufficient to achieve lipid goals. If single-day dosage is used, lipid response has been shown to be greatest with evening use. Side effects of statins include muscle pain, increased risk of diabetes mellitus in those already predisposed, and abnormalities in liver enzyme tests. Liver enzyme elevations occur in 1% to 2% of users and resolve with discontinuation of the drug. Myopathies (muscle aching, soreness, or weakness) associated with elevations in creatine kinase greater than three times the normal occur in 0.5% of users, but the incidence is increased when statins are used in combination with immunosuppressants, gemfibrozil, and niacin.[225] Patients should be instructed to report muscle aches, pain, or weakness. If such symptoms are present, liver aminotransferases and creatine kinase should be measured and the drug stopped. Adjusting dosing options of statin medications or changing types of statins may increase compliance with therapy. Not all statins are the same, so working as a team with the patient to obtain ideal LDL-C levels should be the common goal.

Intestinal Absorption Inhibitors

Intestinal absorption blockers were released by the Food and Drug Administration (FDA) in 2002. The medication (ezetimibe) acts by preventing the absorption of cholesterol at the intestinal brush border. The action of ezetimibe is similar to that of the plant stanols and sterols. This medication appears to be relatively "nonsystemic" in that it works exclusively in the intestine to block the uptake of cholesterol. Through this action, serum cholesterol is lowered, uptake by the liver of LDL is enhanced, and LDL levels decrease. This medication has been shown to lower LDL-C alone or in combination with other cholesterol-lowering medications.[226,227] Ezetimibe is generally well tolerated. The reported side effects include diarrhea, dizziness, abdominal discomfort, and headaches.

Fibric Acid Derivatives

Fibric acid derivatives have been used as hypolipidemic agents. They act primarily to increase LPL activity, which enhances catabolism of VLDL and thereby reduces triglyceride levels.[225] Because of their limited LDL effect, these drugs are not considered first-line therapy for LDL lowering. They are effective in treating hypertriglyceridemia and low HDL-C states. The class of fibric acid derivatives is generally tolerated with side effects including mild stomach upset and myopathies. Because fibrates can increase the cholesterol content of bile, there is an increased risk for gallstones. In research, fibrates reduce nonfatal heart attacks, but do not reduce all-cause mortality.[228,229]

Proprotein Convertase Subtilisin Kexin Type 9 Inhibitors

Human monoclonal antibodies that inhibit PCSK9 comprise a new class of statin combination therapy and have been approved by the FDA for use in addition to diet and maximally tolerated statin therapy in adults with heterozygous FH or with clinical ASCVD, who require additional lowering of LDL-C. PCSK9 has medical importance because it acts in lipoprotein homeostasis. Agents which block PCSK9 can lower LDL particle concentrations. The first two PCSK9 inhibitors, alirocumab and evolocumab, were approved as once every 2-week subcutaneous injections, by the U.S. FDA in 2015 for lowering LDL particle concentrations when statins and other drugs were not sufficiently effective or poorly tolerated. There is also monthly dosing available. The predominant side effects reported include nasopharyngitis, injection site reactions, and general flu-like symptoms. Strategies for compliance include instructing patients on self-injecting and developing a calendar for compliance of injections.

General Adherence Strategies

It is estimated that 50% of patients discontinue drug therapy after 1 year and only one third adhere to dietary interventions beyond 1 year.[230,231] Factors related to nonadherence include lack of knowledge, misconceptions, beliefs and attitudes about the therapy, complexity of the regime, side effects, and the strength of the relationship between the patient and the health care provider.[229] Patient education should include information about the specific drug regime, how the drug works, when and how to use the drug, and how to minimize potential side effects. Barriers to medication adherence include faulty health perceptions. Beliefs and attitudes may interfere with adherence. Social and environmental barriers may include such problems as difficulty taking medication in social settings or restaurants and lack of equipment for mixing medication. It is appropriate to explore common beliefs, attitudes, and difficulties with the patient and develop strategies together to address these issues. Anticipation of potential side effects should also be explored. Studies indicate that adverse side effects and therapeutic ineffectiveness were the major reasons cited for discontinuing lipid-lowering drugs.[231]

Cues to action are important determinants of adherence to medication regimes. Ideal cues are ones that are a part of the patient's habitual routine. Because such cues are habitual, the patient may need assistance in recognizing possible cues. Monitoring and recording medication as it is taken can be useful in identifying potential cues. Feedback is a powerful reinforcer of behavior. Procedures for rapid lipid analysis should be used when possible. Communicating changes in blood lipid response and responding to side effect issues are essential components of lipid management and can often be accomplished by telephone. Consideration should be given to routine telephone contacts to promote adherence and increase the effectiveness of lipid management. Nursing case–managed intervention studies have demonstrated that adherence to lifestyle changes and lipid-lowering drug therapies can be achieved, perhaps caused in part by the strength of the relationship between the nurse and the patient.[214,232]

The nurse is in an excellent position to promote adherence. The focus of the intervention should include the concept of dyslipidemia as a "silent disease," one that is present for life but one for which treatment has been proven effective.

Putting It All Together

Consideration of hypolipidemic drug therapy is divided into primary and secondary prevention. Those individuals with no known existing ASCVD, but may have risk factors are termed primary prevention, while those who have known ASCVD are considered secondary prevention. The 2013 ACC/AHA guidelines[137] define the four statin therapy groups as listed previously (see Fig. 24-4). Based on the four subgroups, one defines the dosage of statin therapy between high, moderate, and low dosing. High-dose statin is defined as atorvastatin 40 to 80 mg and rosuvastatin 20 to 40 mg. Moderate dose statin is defined as atorvastatin 10 to 20 mg, rosuvastatin 5 to 10 mg, pitavastatin 2 to 4 mg, simvastatin

20 to 40 mg, lovastatin 40 to 80 mg, pravastatin 40 to 80 mg, and fluvastatin 80 mg. Low-dose statin is defined as pitavastatin 1 mg, simvastatin 5 to 10 mg, lovastatin 10 to 20 mg, pravastatin 10 to 20 mg, and fluvastatin 20 to 40 mg. The fourth subgroup for treatment in the guidelines is primary prevention and is based on risk factors using the newer pooled cohort equation and a risk calculator to estimate the 10-year risk of developing ASCVD. If the 10-year risk score is greater than 7.5%, then statin therapy is recommended.

However, some clinicians continue to use target goals of LDL-C to dictate therapy based on the ATP III guidelines[19] and more recently the NLA Patient-Centered Management of Dyslipidemia, Part 2[139] defining patients as low risk (0 to 1 ASCVD risk factors), moderate risk (2 major risk factors), high risk (greater than or equal to 3 major ASCVD risk factors, type 1 or 2 diabetes with 0 to 1 other ASCVD risks and no organ damage, chronic kidney disease, LDL greater than or equal to 190, high threshold risk score), and very high risk (known ASCVD and type 1 or 2 diabetes with greater than or equal to 2 other major risk factors or evidence of end-organ damage). Treatment goals are established based on risk of the individual. Those at low, moderate, and high risk have a treatment target of LDL-C less than 100 mg/dL and/or non–HDL-C target of less than 130 mg/dL. Very–high-risk individuals have treatment targets of LDL-C less than 70 mg/dL and/or non-HDL less than 100 mg/dL. Consideration for drug therapy is also dictated by risk. This includes utilizing combination therapy of medications if very–high-risk patients have not achieved target. Consider drug therapy if low-risk patients have LDL-C greater than 160 mg/dL and/or non–HDL-C greater than or equal to 190 mg/dL; moderate-risk patients have LDL-C greater than or equal to 130 mg/dL and/or non–HDL-C greater than or equal to 160 mg/dL; high-risk patients have LDL-C greater than or equal to 100 mg/dL and/or non–HDL-C greater than or equal to 130 mg/dL; and very high risk if LDL-C is greater than or equal to 70 mg/dL and/or non–HDL-C greater than or equal to 100 mg/dL. Either of the treatment guidelines is appropriate to use as long as aggressive treatment for risk is utilized.

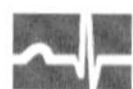

CASE STUDY 1

Patient Profile

Name/Age/Sex: **Jane Greene, 54-year-old female**

History of Present Illness

Mrs. Greene presents to her primary care office for her annual physical. She denies any complaints, other than work-related stress. She states that she has not had any health changes in the past year.

Past Medical History

Hypertension, hyperlipidemia

Surgical History

Hysterectomy 2014

Family History

Father type 2 diabetes and history of stent to LAD at 63; Mother has hyperlipidemia on medication and hypertension controlled with medication.

Social History

Nonsmoker, 2–5 glasses of wine per week, denies illicit drug use. Married for 20 years, works as an attorney for the state.

Medications

Lisinopril 10 mg, refused statin

Allergies

Bee stings

Patient Examination

Vital Signs

BP 152/94; Temp 37.0°C; HR 60; Ht. 168 cm; Wt. 88 kg

Physical Examination

General: Awake, alert, and oriented. No distress noted. Appears younger than stated age.

Skin: Intact, warm, dry. No rashes or lesions are noted.

Cardiac: No murmurs, gallops, or rubs are auscultated. S1 and S2 are heard and are of normal intensity.

Respiratory: Clear to auscultation bilaterally

Abdominal: Abdomen is soft, symmetric, and nontender without distention. No masses, hepatomegaly, or splenomegaly are noted.

Psychiatric: Appropriate mood and affect. Good judgment and insight. No visual or auditory hallucinations. No suicidal or homicidal ideation.

Testing

Total serum cholesterol is 240 mg/dL, LDL-C 150 mg/dL, HDL-C 52 mg/dL, triglycerides 190 mg/dL

Considerations

Key Question

Obtain ASCVD 10-year risk score using the ACC/AHA ASCVD risk calculator:

She is primary prevention (trying to prevent the first vascular event).

Her 10-year risk on the ASCVD risk score is 4.4% if she is Caucasian and 10.4% if she is African American. This shows the difference in risk based on ethnicity.

Evidence

According to the 2013 ACC/AHA Cholesterol Management Guidelines, the two women would be treated differently.

The Caucasian 54-year-old female with a lower 10-year risk score would be treated with behavior modification based on the guideline's behavior management recommendations for diet and physical activity. Blood pressure (BP) management would be increased to two medications from different classes, in order to obtain better BP control. An option to obtain further testing such as coronary calcium scoring or ankle–brachial index, may increase risk potential based on results, which would lead to more aggressive therapy involving statin medication.

The African American 54-year-old female has a higher risk of 10.4%. Based on the 2013 ACC/AHA Cholesterol Management Guidelines, she also benefits from behavior modification, based on the guideline's recommendations for dietary management and physical activity. However, she meets criteria for moderate–high-intensity statin therapy based on her ASCVD risk score being greater than or equal to 7.5%. The guidelines do recommend optimal BP management utilizing two agents from different classes to gain better BP control (see Fig. 24-4).

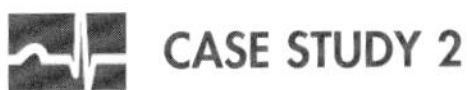

CASE STUDY 2

Patient Profile

Name/Age/Sex: **Philip Blackstone, 60-year-old male**

History of Present Illness

Mr. Blackstone presents to his cardiology office for his annual examination. He states that he has been watching the salt in his diet and walks 1 mile three times a week. He takes medications as directed.

Past Medical History

History of inferior myocardial infarction (MI) at age 30 with coronary artery bypass grafting (CABG) at that time. He had repeat stents later at ages 40 and again at 50.

Surgical History

CABG (1989), PCI × 2 (1999, 2009)

Family History

Father deceased with MI at 69 and brother with CABG in his 40s

Social History

Nonsmoker, 2–5 glasses of wine per week, denies illicit drug use. Married for 20 years, works as an attorney for the state.

Medications

Metoprolol 25 mg daily (beta blocker), amlodipine 5 mg daily (calcium channel blocker), prediabetes (metformin 500 mg daily), and hyperlipidemia (stopped his atorvastatin 40 mg daily due to side effects). Synthroid 0.25

Allergies

ACE-Is (angioedema)

Patient Examination

Vital Signs

BP 118/70; Temp 37.0°C; HR 58; Ht. 178 cm; Wt. 100 kg

Physical Examination

General: Awake, alert, and oriented. No distress noted. Appears younger than stated age.

Skin: Intact, warm, dry. No rashes or lesions are noted.

Cardiac: No murmurs, gallops, or rubs are auscultated. S1 and S2 are heard and are of normal intensity.

Respiratory: Clear to auscultation bilaterally

Abdominal: Abdomen is soft, symmetric, and nontender without distention. No masses, hepatomegaly, or splenomegaly are noted.

Psychiatric: Appropriate mood and affect. Good judgment and insight. No visual or auditory hallucinations. No suicidal or homicidal ideation.

Testing

Total cholesterol is 201 mg/dL, LDL-C 120 mg/dL, HDL-C 45 mg/dL, triglycerides 180 mg/dL

Fasting blood sugar 110; HbA1c 5.8

Considerations

Key Question

Is he primary or secondary prevention?

He is secondary prevention meaning to prevent or reduce the impact of vascular disease after it has already occurred.

Evidence

Based on 2013 ACC/AHA Cholesterol Guidelines, clinical ASCVD is a subcategory in the algorithm recommending if ≤75 years old, patients should be on high-intensity statin medication (atorvastatin 40–80 mg or rosuvastatin 20–40 mg daily). If patient cannot tolerate high-intensity statin medication or if greater than 75 years old, attempt moderate-intensity statin.

Next step would be to initiate the other high-intensity statin medication: rosuvastatin 20 mg for improved management of cholesterol (see Fig. 24-4).

Even though the 2013 ACC/AHA guidelines do not set a target in cholesterol readings, since clinical ASCVD patients are one of the highest-risk categories, lower LDL-C readings are encouraged—preferable goal is below 70. Future guidelines will continue to drive this effort of a lower LDL-C in clinical practice. Continued evaluation and team approach to care is a critical component in secondary prevention in order to improve compliance and outcomes.

Aggressive treatment for all risk factors is encouraged. Smoking cessation, if applicable. Optimal BP control. Optimal blood sugar control. Optimal weight control.

Treatment options should always include 2013 ACC/AHA Cholesterol Guideline recommendations regarding a heart-healthy diet and physical activity recommendation.

KEY READING

Grundy S, Stone N, Bailey A, et al. AHA/ACC/AACVPR/AAPA/ABC/ACPM/ADA/AGS/APhA/ASPC/NLA/PCNA Guideline on the management of blood cholesterol. *J Am Coll Cardiol.* 2019;73(24).

REFERENCES

1. Brown MS, Goldstein JL. A receptor-mediated pathway for cholesterol homeostasis. *Science.* 1986;232:34–37.
2. Anitschkow N. Uber die Veranderungen der Kaninchenaorta bei experimenteller. Cholesterin-steatose. *Beitr Pathol Anat.* 1913;56:379–404.
3. Keys A, Anderson J, Fidanza F, et al. Effects of diet on blood lipids in man, particularly cholesterol and lipoproteins. *Clin Chem.* 1955;1(1):34–52.
4. Gofman JW, Lindgren FT, Elliott H. Ultracentrifugal studies of lipoproteins of human serum. *J Biol Chem.* 1949;179(2):973–979.
5. Gofman J, Lindgren F. The role of lipids and lipoproteins in atherosclerosis. *Science.* 1950;111(2877):166–171.
6. Gofman J. Serum lipoproteins and the evaluation of atherosclerosis. *Ann N Y Acad Sci.* 1956;64(4):590–595.
7. Bloch K. The biological synthesis of cholesterol. *Science.* 1965;150(3692):19–28.
8. Lynen F. The biochemical basis of the biosynthesis of cholesterol and fatty acids. *Wien Klin Wochenschr.* 1966;78(27):489–497.
9. Cornforth J, Popjak G. Biosynthesis of cholesterol. *Br Med Bull.* 1958;14(3):221–226.
10. Kaneko I, Hazama-Shimada Y, Endo A. Inhibitory effects on lipid metabolism in cultured cells of ML-236B, a potent inhibitor of 3-hydroxy-3-methylglutaryl-coenzyme-A reductase. *Eur J Biochem.* 1978;87(2):313–321.
11. Vagelos PR, Galambos L. *Medicine, Science, and Merck.* Cambridge, UK: Cambridge University Press; 2004.
12. Benjamin EJ, Virani SS, Callaway CW, et al. Heart disease and stroke statistics—2018 update: a report from the American Heart Association. *Circulation.* 2018;137:e67–e492.
13. Mozaffarian D, Benjamin EJ, Go AS, et al. Heart disease and stroke statistics—2015 update: a report from the American Heart Association. *Circulation.* 2015;131:e29–e322.
14. Nguyen DR, Bit BK, Carroll MD. Abnormal cholesterol among children and adolescents in the United States, 2011–2014. *NCHS Data Brief.* 2015;(228):1–8.
15. Carroll MD, Fryar CD, Kit BK. Total and high-density lipoprotein cholesterol in adults: United States, 2011–2014. *NCHS Data Brief.* 2015;(226):1–8.
16. Armstrong ML, Warner ED, Connor WE. Regression of coronary atheromatosis in rhesus monkeys. *Circ Res.* 1970;27:59–67.

17. Anderson KM, Castelli WP, Levy D. Cholesterol and mortality: 30 years of follow-up from the Framingham study. *JAMA*. 1987;257:2176–2180.
18. Yusuf S, Hawken S, Ounpuu S, et al. Effect of potentially modifiable risk factors associated with myocardial infarction in 52 countries (the INTERHEART study): case control study. *Lancet*. 2004;364:937–952.
19. Expert Panel on Detection, Evaluation, and Treatment of High Blood Cholesterol in Adults (Adult Treatment Panel III). *National Cholesterol Education Program (NCEP)*. Bethesda, MD: U.S. Department of Health and Human Services; 2001. NIH Publication No. 01–3670.
20. Downs JR, Clearfield M, Weis S, et al. Primary prevention of acute coronary events with lovastatin in men and women with average cholesterol levels: results of AFCAPS/TexCAPS. Air Force/Texas Coronary Atherosclerosis Prevention Study. *JAMA*. 1998;279:1615–1622.
21. Scandinavian Simvastatin Survival Study Group. Randomized trial of cholesterol lowering in 4444 patients with coronary heart disease: the Scandinavian Simvastatin Survival Study (4S). *Lancet*. 1994;344:1383–1389.
22. Sacks FM, Pfeffer MA, Moye LA, et al. The effect of pravastatin on coronary events after myocardial infarction in patients with average cholesterol levels. Cholesterol and Recurrent Events Trial investigators. *N Engl J Med*. 1996;335:1001–1009.
23. Shepherd J, Cobbe SM, Ford I, et al. Prevention of coronary heart disease with pravastatin in men with hypercholesterolemia. West of Scotland Coronary Prevention Study Group. *N Engl J Med*. 1995;333:1301–1307.
24. Long-Term Intervention with Pravastatin in Ischaemic Disease (LIPID) Study Group. Prevention of cardiovascular events and death with pravastatin in patients with coronary heart disease and a broad range of initial cholesterol levels. *N Engl J Med*. 1998;339:1349–1357.
25. Heart Protection Study Collaborative Group. Heart Protection Study of cholesterol lowering with simvastatin in 20,536 high-risk individuals: a randomized placebo-controlled trial. *Lancet*. 2002;360:7–22.
26. Cannon CP, Braunwald E, McCabe CH, et al. Intensive versus moderate lipid lowering with statins after acute coronary syndromes. *N Engl J Med*. 2004;350:1495–1504.
27. Shepherd J, Blauw GJ, Murphy MB, et al. Pravastatin in elderly individuals at risk of vascular disease (PROSPER): a randomized controlled trial. PROspective Study of Pravastatin in the Elderly at Risk. *Lancet*. 2002;360:1623–1630.
28. Sever PS, Dahlof B, Poulter NR, et al. Prevention of coronary and stroke events with atorvastatin in hypertensive patients who have average or lower-than-average cholesterol concentrations, in the Anglo-Scandinavian Cardiac Outcomes Trial–Lipid Lowering Arm (ASCOT-LLA): a multicentre randomized controlled trial. *Lancet*. 2003;361:1149–1158.
29. Grundy SM, Cleeman JI, Bairey Merz CN, et al. Implications of recent clinical trials for the National Cholesterol Education Program Adult Treatment Panel III Guidelines. *Circulation*. 2004;110:227–239.
30. Gould AL, Rossouw JE, Santanello NC, et al. Cholesterol reduction yields clinical benefit: a new look at old data. *Circulation*. 1995;91:2274–2282.
31. Law MR. Lowering heart disease risk with cholesterol reduction: evidence from observational studies and clinical trials. *Eur Heart J*. 1999;1(suppl S):S3–S8.
32. Deedwania P, Stone PH, Bairey Merz CN, et al. Effects of intensive versus moderate lipid-lowering therapy on myocardial ischemia in older patients with coronary heart disease. Results of the Study Assessing Goals in the Elderly (SAGE). *Circulation*. 2007;115:700–707.
33. Castelli WP. Lipids, risk factors and ischaemic heart disease. *Atherosclerosis*. 1996;124(suppl):S1–S9.
34. Schaefer EJ, Levy RI. Pathogenesis and management of lipoprotein disorders. *N Engl J Med*. 1985;312:1300–1320.
35. Gotto AM. High density lipoproteins: biochemical and metabolic factors. *Am J Cardiol*. 1983;54(4):2B–8B.
36. Barter P, Gotto AM, LaRosa JC, et al. HDL cholesterol, very low levels of LDL cholesterol and cardiovascular events. *N Engl J Med*. 2007;357(13):1301–1310.
37. LaRosa JC, Grundy SM, Waters DD, et al. Intensive lipid lowering with atorvastatin in patients with stable coronary disease. *N Engl J Med*. 2005;352(14):1425–1435.
38. Sazonov V, Beetsch J, Phatak H, et al. Association between dyslipidemia and vascular events in patients treated with statins: report from the UK General Practice Research Database. *Atherosclerosis*. 2010;208:210–216.
39. Barter P. Managing diabetic dyslipidaemia—beyond LDL-C: HDL-C and triglycerides. *Atheroscler Suppl*. 2006;7:17–21.
40. Genest J, Libby P, Gotto AM. Lipoprotein disorders and cardiovascular disease. In: Zipes DP, Libby P, Bonow RO, Braunwald E, eds. *Braunwald's Heart Disease: A Textbook of Cardiovascular Medicine*. 7th ed. Philadelphia, PA: Elsevier Saunders; 2005:1013–1034.
41. Grundy SM. Hyperlipoproteinemia: metabolic basis and rationale for therapy. *Am J Cardiol*. 1984;54:20C–26C.
42. Grundy SM. Pathogenesis of hyperlipoproteinemia. *J Lipid Res*. 1984;25:1611–1618.
43. Breslow JL. The genetic basis of lipoprotein disorders: introduction and review. *J Intern Med*. 1992;231:627–631.
44. Goldstein JL, Brown MS. Regulation of low-density lipoprotein receptors: implication for pathogenesis and therapy of hypercholesterolemia and atherosclerosis. *Circulation*. 1987;76:505–507.
45. Gordon DJ, Probstfield JL, Garrison RJ, et al. High density lipoprotein cholesterol and cardiovascular disease: four prospective American studies. *Circulation*. 1989;79:8–15.
46. Kannel WB. High-density lipoproteins: epidemiologic profile and risks of coronary artery disease. *Am J Cardiol*. 1983;52(4):9B–12B.
47. Eisenberg S. High-density lipoprotein metabolism. *J Lipid Res*. 1984;25:1017–1054.
48. Asztalos BF, Schaefer E. HDL in atherosclerosis: actor or bystander? *Atheroscler Suppl*. 2003;4:21–29.
49. Joy T, Hegele RA. Is raising HDL a futile strategy for atheroprotection? *Nat Rev*. 2008;7:143–155.
50. Soumain S, Albrecht C, Davies AH, et al. ABCA1 and atherosclerosis *Vasc Med*. 2005;10:109–119.
51. Curtiss LK, Valenta DT, Hime NJ, et al. What is so special about apolipoprotein A1 in reverse cholesterol transport? *Arterioscler Thromb Vasc Biol*. 2006;26:12–19.
52. Gotto AM. Clinical diagnosis of hyperlipoproteinemia. *Am J Med*. 1983;74(5A):5–9.
53. Tall AR, Small DM. Current concepts: plasma high-density lipoproteins. *N Engl J Med*. 1978;299:1232–1236.
54. Singh IM, Shishehbor MH, Ansell BJ. High-density lipoprotein as a therapeutic target. *JAMA*. 2007;298:786–798.
55. Miller NE. HDL metabolism and its role in lipid transport. *Eur Heart J*. 1990;11:H1–H3.
56. Rifkind BM. *Drug Treatment of Hyperlipidemia*. New York: Marcel Dekker; 1991.
57. de Lemos AS, Wolfe ML, Long CJ, et al. Identification of genetic variants in endothelial lipase in persons with elevated high-density lipoprotein cholesterol. *Circulation*. 2002;106:1321–1326.
58. Rader DJ. Regulation of reverse cholesterol transport and clinical implications. *Am J Cardiol*. 2003;92(suppl):43J–49J.
59. Cohen JC. Endothelial lipase: direct evidence for a role in HDL metabolism. *J Clin Invest*. 2003;111:318–321.
60. Ishida T, Choi S, Kundu RK, et al. Endothelial lipase is a major determinant of HDL level. *J Clin Invest*. 2003;111:347–355.
61. Navab M, Ananthramaiah GM, Reddy ST, et al. The double jeopardy of HDL. *Ann Med*. 2005;37:173–178.
62. Ansell BJ. Targeting the anti-inflammatory effects of high-density lipoprotein. *Am J Cardiol*. 2007;100(suppl):3N–9N.
63. Brown BG, Zhao XQ, Chait A, et al. Lipid altering or antioxidant vitamins for patients with coronary disease and very low HDL cholesterol? The HDL-atherosclerosis treatment study design. *Can J Cardiol*. 1998;14:6A–13A.
64. Tall AR. Overview of reverse cholesterol transport. *Eur Heart J*. 1998;19:A31–A35.
65. Assman G, Gotto AM. HDL cholesterol and protective factors in atherosclerosis. *Circulation*. 2004;109(suppl 3):8–14.
66. Landray MJ, Haynes R, Hopewell JC, et al. Effects of extended-release niacin with laropiprant in high-risk patients. The HPS2-Thrive Collaborative Group. *N Engl J Med*. 2014;371(3):203–212.
67. AIM-HIGH Investigators; Boden WE, Probstfield JL, Anderson T, et al. Niacin in patients with low HDL cholesterol levels receiving intensive statin therapy. *N Engl J Med*. 2011;365:2255–2267.
68. Hafiane A, Genest J. HDL, atherosclerosis, and emerging therapies. *Cholesterol*. 2013;2013:891403.
69. Subedi BH, Joshi P, Jones S, et al. Current guidelines for high density lipoprotein cholesterol in therapy and future directions. *Vasc Health Risk Manag*. 2014;10:205–216.
70. Austin MD, Hokanson JE, Brunzell JD. Characterization of low-density lipoprotein subclasses: methodologic approaches and clinical relevance. *Curr Opin Lipidol*. 1994;5:395–403.
71. Gardner CD, Fortmann SP, Krauss RM. Small low-density lipoprotein particles are associated with the incidence of coronary artery disease in men and women. *JAMA*. 1996;276:875–881.
72. De Graaf J, Hak-Lemmers H, Hector P, et al. Enhanced susceptibility to in vitro oxidation of the low-density lipoprotein subfractions in healthy subjects. *Arterioscler Thromb Vasc Biol*. 1991;11:298–306.
73. Reaven GM, Chen YD, Jeppesen J, et al. Insulin resistance and hyperinsulinemia in individuals with small, dense, low-density lipoprotein particles. *J Clin Invest*. 1993;92:141–146.

74. Steinbrecher UP, Parthasarathy S, Leake DS, et al. Modification of low density lipoprotein by endothelial cells involves lipid peroxidation and degradation of low density lipoprotein phospholipids. *PNAS.* 1984; 81:3883–3887.
75. Quinn MT, Parthasarathy S, Fong LG, et al. Oxidatively modified low density lipoproteins: a potential role in recruitment and retention of monocyte/macrophages during atherogenesis. *PNAS.* 1987;84: 2995–2998.
76. Steinberg D, Parthasarathy S, Carew TE, et al. Beyond cholesterol. Modifications of low-density lipoprotein that increase its atherogenicity. *N Engl J Med.* 1989;320:915–924.
77. Fraley A, Tsimikas S. Clinical applications of circulating oxidized low-density lipoprotein biomarkers in cardiovascular disease. *Curr Opin Lipidol.* 2006;17:502–509.
78. Itabe T. Oxidized low-density lipoproteins: what is understood and what remains to be clarified. *Biological Pharmaceutical Bulletin.* 2003;26:1–9.
79. Kamstrup PR. Lipoprotein (a) and ischemic heart disease—a causal association? A review. *Atherosclerosis.* 2010;211(1):15–23.
80. Nordestgaard BG, Chapman MJ, Ray K, et al. Lipoprotein (a) as a cardiovascular risk factor: current status. *Eur Heart J.* 2010;31:2844–2853.
81. Lippi G, Franchini M, Targher G. Screening and therapeutic management of lipoprotein (a) excess: review of the epidemiological evidence, guidelines and recommendations. *Clin Chim Acta.* 2011;412:797–901.
82. Hoover-Plow J, Huang M. Lipoprotein (a) metabolism: potential sites for therapeutic targets. *Metabolism.* 2013;62:479–491.
83. Boffa MB, Koschinsky ML. Update on lipoprotein (a) as a cardiovascular risk factor and mediator. *Curr Atheroscler Rep.* 2013;15:1–20.
84. Kassner U, Schlabs T, Rosanda A, et al. Lipoprotein(a)—an independent casual risk factor for cardiovascular disease and current therapeutic options. *Atheroscler Suppl.* 2015;18:263–267.
85. Lawn RM. Lipoprotein (a) in heart disease. *Sci Am.* 1992;6:54–60.
86. Berglund L, Raakrishnan R. Lipoprotein(a): an elusive cardiovascular risk factor. *Arterioscler Thromb Vasc Biol.* 2004;24:2219–2226.
87. Koschinsky ML. Novel insights into Lp(a) physiology and pathogenicity: more questions than answers? *Cardiovasc Hematol Disorders Drug Targets.* 2006;6:276–278.
88. Danesh J, Collins R, Peto R. Lipoprotein (a) and cardiovascular disease. Meta-analysis of prospective studies. *Circulation.* 2000;102:1082–1085.
89. Emerging Risk Factors Collaboration; Erqou S, Kaptoge S, Perry PL. Lipoprotein (a) and risk of cardiovascular disease, stroke, and nonvascular mortality. *JAMA.* 2009;302:412–423.
90. Gesner B, Dias KC, Siekmeier R, et al. Lipoprotein (a) and risk of cardiovascular disease—a systematic review and meta-analysis of prospective studies. *Clin Lab.* 2011;57:143–156.
91. Smolders B, Kemmens R, Thijs V. Lipoprotein (a) and stroke: a meta-analysis of observational studies. *Stroke.* 2007;38:1959–1966.
92. Nsaibia MJ, Mahmut A, Boulanger MC, et al. Autotaxin interacts with lipoprotein (a) and oxidized phospholipids in predicting the risk of calcific aortic valve stenosis in patients with coronary artery disease. *J Intern Med.* 2016;280:509–517.
93. Yeang C, Wilkinson MJ, Tsimikas S. Lipoprotein (a) and oxidized phospholipids in calcific aortic valve stenosis. *Curr Opin Cardiol.* 2016;31:440–450.
94. Tziomalos K, Athyros VG, Wierzbicki AS, et al. Lipoprotein a: where are we now? *Curr Opin Cardiol.* 2009;24:351–357.
95. Albers JJ, Slee A, O'Brien KD, et al. Relationship of apolipoproteins A-1 and B, and lipoprotein (a) to cardiovascular outcomes: the AIM-HIGH trial (atherothrombosis intervention in metabolic syndrome with low HDL/high triglyceride and impact on global health outcomes). *J Am Coll Cardiol.* 2013;62:1575–1579.
96. McConnell JP, Hoefner DM. Lipoprotein-associated phospholipase A2. *Clin Lab Med.* 2006;26:679–697.
97. Epps KC, Wilensky RL. Lp-PLA$_2$—a novel risk factor for high-risk coronary and carotid artery disease. *J Intern Med.* 2011;269:94–106.
98. Toth PP, McCullough PA, Wegner MS, et al. Lipoprotein-associated phospholipase A2: role in atherosclerosis and utility as a cardiovascular biomarker. *Expert Rev Cardiovasc Ther.* 2010;8:425–438.
99. Braun LT, Davidson MH. Lp-PLA2: a new target for statin therapy. *Curr Atheroscler Rep.* 2010;12:29–33.
100. Davidson MH. Clinical significance of statin pleiotropic effects: hypotheses versus evidence. *Circulation.* 2005;111:2280–2281.
101. Schaefer EJ, McNamara JR, Asztalos BF, et al. Effects of atorvastatin versus other statins on fasting and postprandial C-reactive protein and lipoprotein-associated phospholipase A2 in patients with coronary heart disease versus control subjects. *Am J Cardiol.* 2005;95:1025–1032.
102. Muhlestein JB, May HT, Jensen JR, et al. The reduction of inflammatory biomarkers by statin, fibrate and combination therapy among diabetic patient with mixed dyslipidemia. The DIACOR (Diabetes and Combined Lipid Therapy Regimen) study. *J Am Coll Cardiol.* 2006; 48:396s–401s.
103. Saiygis VG, Tambaki AP, Kalogirou M, et al. Differential effect of hypolipidemic drugs on lipoprotein-associated phospholipase A2. *Arterioscler Thromb Vasc Biol.* 2007;27:2236–2243.
104. Tzotas T, Filippatos TD, Triantos A, et al. Effects of a low-calorie diet associated with weight loss on lipoprotein-associated phospholipase A2 (Lp-PLA2) activity in healthy obese women. *Nutr Metab Cardiovasc Dis.* 2008;18:477–482.
105. Davidson MH, Ballantyne CM, Jacobson T, et al. Clinical utility of inflammatory markers and advanced lipoprotein testing: advice from an expert panel of lipid specialists. *J Clin Lipidol.* 2011;5:338–367.
106. Fair JM, Berra KA. Endothelial function and coronary risk reduction: mechanisms and influences of nitric oxide. *Cardiovasc Nurs.* 1996; 32:17–22.
107. Treasure CB, Klein JL, Weintraub WS, et al. Beneficial effects of cholesterol-lowering therapy on the coronary endothelium in patients with coronary artery disease. *N Engl J Med.* 1995;332:481–487.
108. Levine GN, Keaney JF, Vita JA. Cholesterol reduction in cardiovascular disease. *N Engl J Med.* 1995;332:512–521.
109. Rader DJ, Cohen J, Hobbs HH. Monogenic hypercholesterolemia: new insights in pathogenesis and treatment. *J Clin Invest.* 2003;111(12): 1795–1803.
110. Knowles JW, O'Brien EC, Greendale K, et al. Reducing the burden of disease and death from familial hypercholesterolemia: a call to action. *Am Heart J.* 2014;168(6):807–811.
111. Cuchel M, Bruckert F, Ginsberg HN, et al. Homozygous familial hypercholesterolaemia: new insights and guidance for clinicians to improve detection and clinical management. A position paper from the Consensus Panel on Familial Hypercholesterolaemia of the European Atherosclerosis Society. *Eur Heart J.* 2014;35(32):2146–2157.
112. Benn M, Watts GF, Tybjaerg-Hansen A, et al. Mutations causative of familial hypercholesterolaemia: screening of 98,098 individuals from the Copenhagen General Population Study estimated a prevalence of 1 in 247. *Eur Heart J.* 2016;37(17):219–223.
113. Besseling J, Kinft I, Hof M, et al. Severe heterozygous familial hypercholesterolemia and risk for cardiovascular disease: a study of a cohort of 14,000 mutation carriers. *Atherosclerosis.* 2014;233(1):219–223.
114. de Ferranti SD, Rodday AM, Mendelson MM, et al. Prevalence of familial hypercholesterolemia in the 1999 to 2012 United States National Health and Nutrition Examination Surveys (NHANES). *Circulation.* 2016;133(11):1067–1072.
115. Migliara G, Baccolini V, Rosso A, et al. Familial hypercholesterolemia: a systematic review of guidelines and genetic testing and patient management. *Front Public Health.* 2017;5(252):1–8.
116. Nordestgaard BG, Chapman MJ, Humphries SE, et al. European Atherosclerosis Society Consensus Panel. Familial hypercholesterolaemia is underdiagnosed and undertreated in the general population: Guidance for clinicians to prevent coronary heart disease: consensus statement of the European Atherosclerosis Society. *Eur Heart J.* 2013;34: 3478–3490.
117. Thompson GR, Barbir M, Davies D, et al. Recommendations for the use of LDL apheresis. *Atherosclerosis.* 2008;98:247–255.
118. Harada-Shiba M, Arai H, Oikawa S, et al. Guidelines for the management of familial hypercholesterolemia. *J Atheroscler Thromb.* 2012; 19:1043–1060.
119. Goldberg AC, Hopkins PN, Toth PP, et al. National Lipid Association Expert Panel on Familial Hypercholesterolemia. Familial hypercholesterolemia: screening, diagnosis and management of pediatric and adult patients: clinical guidelines from the National Lipid Association Expert Panel on Familial Hypercholesterolemia. *J Clin Lipidol.* 2011;5:51–58.
120. Stefanutti C, Julius U. Lipoprotein apheresis: state of the art and novelties. *Atheroscler Suppl.* 2013;14:19–27.
121. Hussain MM, Rava P, Walsh M, et al. Multiple functions of microsomal triglyceride transfer protein. *Nutr Metab.* 2012;9:14.
122. Crooke ST, Geary RS. Clinical pharmacological properties of mipomersen (Kynamro), a second-generation antisense inhibitor of apolipoprotein B. *Br J Clin Pharmacol.* 2013;76:269–276.
123. Grundy SM. Hypertriglyceridemia, atherogenic dyslipidemia, and the metabolic syndrome. *Am J Cardiol.* 1998;91(4A):18B–25B.
124. Krauss RM. Atherogenicity of triglyceride-rich lipoproteins. *Am J Cardiol.* 1998;81(4A):13B–17B.

125. Ordovas JM, Schaefer EJ, Salem D, et al. Apoprotein A-1 gene polymorphism associated with premature coronary artery disease and familial hypoalphalipoproteinemia. *N Engl J Med.* 1986;314:671–677.
126. Zhang LH, Kamanna VS, Zhang MC, et al. Niacin inhibits surface expression of ATP synthase beta chain in HepG2 cells: implications for raising HDL. *J Lipid Res.* 2008;49:1195–1201.
127. HPS-2 Thrive Collaborative Group. HPS2-THRIVE randomized placebo controlled trial in 25,673 high risk patients of ER niacin/laropiprant: trial design, pre-specified muscle and liver outcomes, and reasons for stopping study treatment. *Eur Heart J.* 2013;34:1279–1291.
128. HPS-2 THRIVE Collaborative Group. Effects of extended release niacin with laropiprant in high-risk patients. *N Engl J Med.* 2014;371:203–212.
129. Grundy SM, Balady GJ, Criqui MH, et al. Guide to the primary prevention of cardiovascular diseases. *Circulation.* 1997;95:2329–2331.
130. Smith SC Jr, Blair SN, Criqui SN, et al. Preventing heart attack and death in patients with coronary disease. *Circulation.* 1995;92:2–4.
131. Smith S, Allen J, Blair S, et al. AHA/ACC guidelines for secondary prevention for patients with coronary and other atherosclerotic vascular disease: 2006 update. *Circulation.* 2006;113:2363–2372.
132. Warnick GR, Myers GL, Cooper GR, et al. Impact of the third cholesterol report from the adult treatment pane of the national cholesterol education program on the clinical laboratory. *Clin Chem.* 2002;48:11–17.
133. Talwalkar PG, Sreenivas CG, Gulati A, et al. Journey in guidelines for lipid management: From adult treatment panel (ATP)-I to ATP-III and what to expect in ATP-IV. *Indian J Endocrinol Metab.* 2013;17(4):628–635.
134. Report of the National Cholesterol Education Program Expert Panel on detection, evaluation, and treatment of high cholesterol in adults. The Expert Panel. *Arch Intern Med.* 1988;148:36–69.
135. Summary of the second report of the National Cholesterol Education Program (NCEP) Expert Panel on detection, evaluation, and treatment of high blood cholesterol in adults (Adult Treatment Panel II). *JAMA.* 1993;269:3015–3023.
136. Ansell BJ, Watson KE, Fogelman AM. An evidence-based assessment of the NCEP adult treatment panel II guidelines. National cholesterol education guidelines. *JAMA.* 1999;282:2051–2057.
137. Stone NJ, Robinson JG, Lichtenstein AH, et al. ACC/AHA guideline on the treatment of blood cholesterol to reduce atherosclerotic cardiovascular risk in adults: a report of the American College of Cardiology/American Heart Association Task Force on Practice Guidelines. *J Am Coll Cardiol.* 2014;63:2889–2934.
138. Jacobson TA, Ito MK, Maki KC, et al. National Lipid Association recommendations for patient-centered management of dyslipidemia: part 1—executive summary. *J Clin Lipidol.* 2014;8(5):473–488.
139. Jacobson TA, Maki KC, Orringer C, et al. National Lipid Association recommendations for the patient centered management of dyslipidemia: part 2. *J Clin Lipidol.* 2015;9(6 suppl):S1–S122.e1.
140. Jellinger PC, Handlesman Y, Rosenblit PD, et al. American Association of Clinical Endocrinologists and American College of Endocrinology: guidelines for management of dyslipidemia and prevention of cardiovascular disease. *Endocr Pract.* 2017;23(suppl 2):1–87.
141. Cannon CP, Blazin MA, Giugliano RP, et al. Ezetimibe added to statin therapy after acute coronary syndromes. *N Engl J Med.* 2015;372(25):2387–2397.
142. Mosca L, Grundy SM, Judelson D, et al. Guide to preventative cardiology for women: AHA/ACC Scientific Statement Consensus panel statement. *Circulation.* 1999;99:2480–2484.
143. American Heart Association Statistics Committee and Stroke Statistics Subcommittee; Roger VL, Go AS, Lloyd-Jones DM, et al. Heart disease and stroke statistics—2011 update: a report from the American Heart Association. *Circulation.* 2011;123:e18–e209.
144. Ford ES, Ajani UA, Croft JB, et al. Explaining the decrease in US deaths from coronary disease, 1980–2000. *N Engl J Med.* 2007;356:2388–2398.
145. Mosca L, Mochari-Greenberger H, Dolor RJ, et al. Twelve-year follow-up of American women's awareness of cardiovascular disease risk and barriers to heart health. *Circ Cardiovasc Qual Outcomes.* 2010;3:120–127.
146. Kleindorfer D, Khoury J, Broderick JP, et al. Temporal trends in public awareness of stroke: warning signs, risk factors, and treatment. *Stroke.* 2009;40:2502–2506.
147. American Heart Association: American Stroke Association; Ferris A, Robertson RM, Fabunni R, et al. American Heart Association and American Stroke Association national survey of stroke risk awareness among women. *Circulation.* 2005;111:1321–1326.
148. Mosca L, Benjamin EJ, Berra K, et al. Effectiveness-based guidelines for the prevention of cardiovascular disease in women—2011 update: a guideline from the American Heart Association. *Circulation.* 2011;123(11):1243–1262.
149. Smith GC, Pell JC, Walsh D. Pregnancy complications and maternal risk of ischaemic heart disease: a retrospective cohort study of 129,290 births. *Lancet.* 2001;357(9273):2002–2006.
150. Freibert SM, Mannino DM, Bush H, et al. The association of adverse pregnancy events and cardiovascular disease in women 50 years of age and older. *J Women's Health (Larchmt).* 2011;20(2):287–293.
151. National Heart, Lung, and Blood Institute Joint National Committee on Prevention, Detection, Evaluation, and Treatment of High Blood Pressure; National High Blood Pressure Education Program Coordinating Committee; Chobanian AV, Bakris GI, Black HR, et al. The seventh report of the Joint National Committee on prevention, detection, evaluation and treatment of high blood pressure. The JNC 7 report. *JAMA.* 2003;289:2560–2572.
152. Friedewald WT, Levy RI, Fredrickson DS. Estimation of the concentration of low-density lipoprotein cholesterol in plasma with the use of preparative ultracentrifuge. *Clin Chem.* 1972;18:499–502.
153. Baille EE. *Recommendations from improving cholesterol measurement: A report from the Laboratory Standardization Panel of the Cholesterol Education Program.* Bethesda, MD: U.S. Department of Health and Human Services; 1990.
154. Antman EM, Hand M, Armstrong PW. 2007 Focused update of the ACC/AHA 2004 guidelines for the management of patients with ST-elevation myocardial infarction: a report of the American College of Cardiology/American Heart Association Task Force on Practice Guidelines: Developed in collaboration with the Canadian Cardiovascular Society endorsed by the American Academy of Family Physicians: 2007 Writing group to review new evidence and update the ACC/AHA 2004 guidelines for the management of patients with ST-elevation myocardial infarction, writing on behalf of the 2004 WritingCommittee. *Circulation.* 2008;117:296–329.
155. Arntzenius AC, Kromhout D, Barth JD, et al. Diets, lipoproteins, and the progression coronary atherosclerosis: the leiden intervention trial. *N Engl J Med.* 1985;312:805–811.
156. Keys A. Coronary heart disease in seven countries. *Circulation.* 1979;41(suppl 1):1–211.
157. Kushi LH, Lew RA, Stare FJ, et al. Diet and 20 year mortality from coronary heart disease. *N Engl J Med.* 1985;312:811–818.
158. McGee DL, Reed DM, Yano K, et al. Ten-year incidence of coronary heart disease in the Honolulu Heart Program: relationship to nutrient intake. *Am J Epidemiol.* 1984;119:667–676.
159. Eckel RH, Jakcic JM, Ard JD, et al. 2013 AHA/ACC guideline on lifestyle management to reduce cardiovascular risk: a report of the American College of Cardiology/American Heart Association Task Force on Practice Guidelines. *J Am Coll Cardiol.* 2014;63:2960–2984.
160. U.S. Department of Agriculture and U.S. Department of Health and Human Services. *Dietary Guidelines for Americans.* 7th ed. Washington, DC: U.S. Government Printing Office; 2010.
161. U.S. Department of Agriculture and U.S. Department of Health and Human Services. *Scientific report of the 2015 Dietary Guidelines Advisory Committee. Part A. Executive summary.* Available at http://www.health.gov/dietaryguidelines/2015-scientific-report/02- executive-summary.asp
162. Gidding SS, Lichtenstein AH, Faith MS, et al. Implementing American Heart Association pediatric and adult nutrition guidelines: a scientific statement from the American Heart Association Nutrition Committee of the Council on Nutrition, Physical Activity and Metabolism, Council on Cardiovascular Disease in the Young, Council on Arteriosclerosis, Thrombosis, and Vascular Biology, Council on Cardiovascular Nursing, Council on Epidemiology and Prevention and Council for High Blood Pressure Research. *Circulation.* 2009;119:1161–1175.
163. Expert Panel on Integrated Guidelines for CV Health and Risk Reduction in Children and Adolescents; National Heart, Lung, and Blood Institute. Expert Panel on integrated guidelines for cardiovascular health and risk reduction in children and adolescents: summary report. *Pediatrics.* 2011;128(suppl 5):5213–5256.
164. Zarraga E, Schwarz ER. Impact of dietary patterns and interventions on cardiovascular health. *Circulation.* 2006;114:961–973.
165. Robinson JG, Wang S, Smith BJ, et al. Meta-analysis of the relationship between nonhigh-density lipoprotein cholesterol reduction and coronary heart disease risk. *J Am Coll Cardiol.* 2009;53:316–322.
166. Sacks FM, Katan M. Randomized clinical trial on the effects of dietary fat and carbohydrate on plasma lipoproteins and cardiovascular disease. *Am J Med.* 2002;113(9B):13S–24S.
167. Bonanome A, Grundy SM. Effect of stearic acid on plasma cholesterol and lipoprotein levels. *N Engl J Med.* 1988;318:1244–1248.
168. Grundy SM, Vega GL. Plasma cholesterol responsiveness to saturated fatty acids. *Am J Clin Nutr.* 1983;47:822–824.

169. Connor WE, Connor SL. Diet, atherosclerosis, and fish oil. *Adv Intern Med.* 1990;35:135–172.
170. Leaf A, Weber PC. Cardiovascular effects of n-3 fatty acids. *N Engl J Med.* 1988;318:549–557.
171. Demonty I, Ras RT, van der Knaap HC, et al. Continuous dose-response relationship of the LDL-cholesterol–lowering effect of phytosterol intake. *J Nutr.* 2009;139:271–284.
172. AbuMweis SS, Barake R, Jones PJ. Plant sterols/stanols as cholesterol lowering agents: a meta-analysis of randomized controlled trials. *Food Nutrition Research.* 2008;52. doi:10.3402/fnr.v3452i3400.1811
173. Musa-Veloso K, Poon TH, Elliot JA, et al. A comparison of the LDL-cholesterol lowering efficacy of plant stanols and plant sterols over a continuous dose range: results of a meta-analysis of randomized, placebo-controlled trials. *Prostaglandins Leukot Essent Fatty Acids.* 2011;85:9–28.
174. Obarzanek E, Sacks FM, Vollmer WM, et al. Effects on blood lipids of a blood pressure-lowering diet: the dietary approaches to stop hypertension (DASH) trial. *Am J Clin Nutr.* 2001;74:80–89.
175. Kris-Etherton P, Krummel D, Russell ME, et al. The effect of diet on plasma lipids, lipoproteins, and coronary heart disease. *J Am Diet Assoc.* 1988;88:1373–1400.
176. Lin JS, O'Connor EA, Evans CV, et al. *Behavioral Counseling to Promote a Healthy Lifestyle for Cardiovascular Disease Prevention in Persons with Cardiovascular Risk Factors: An Updated Systematic Evidence Review for the U.S. Preventive Services Task Force.* Rockville, MD: Agency for Healthcare Research and Quality; 2014. PMID: 25232633. Available at http://www.ncbi.nlm.nih.gov/books/NBK241537
177. Aucott L, Gray D, Rothnie H, et al. Effects of lifestyle interventions and long-term weight loss on lipid outcomes—a systematic review. *Obes Rev.* 2011;12:e412–e425.
178. Academy of Nutrition and Dietetics Evidence Analysis Library. *Disorders of lipid metabolism (2007–2011).* 2014. Available from https://www.andeal.org/topic.cfm?menu=5300&cat=4527. Accessed November 24, 2014.
179. McCoin M, Sikand G, Johnson EQ, et al. The effectiveness of medical nutrition therapy delivered by registered dietitians for disorders of lipid metabolism: a call for further research. *J Am Diet Assoc.* 2008;108: 233–239.
180. Daubert H, Ferko-Adams D, Rheinheimer D, et al. Metabolic risk factor reduction through a worksite health campaign: a case study design. *Online J Public Health Inform.* 2012;4(2):ojphi.v4i2.4005.
181. Parker AR, Byham-Gray L, Denmark R, et al. The effect of medical nutrition therapy by a registered dietitian nutritionist in patients with prediabetes participating in a randomized controlled clinical research trial. *J Acad Nutr Diet.* 2014;114:1739–1748.
182. Barakatun Nisak MY, Ruzita AT, Norimah AK, et al. Medical nutrition therapy administered by a dietitian yields favorable diabetes outcomes in individual with type 2 diabetes mellitus. *Med J Malaysia.* 2013;68:18–23.
183. Lim H, Son JY, Choue R. Effects of medical nutrition therapy on body fat and metabolic syndrome components in premenopausal overweight women. *Ann Nutr Metab.* 2012;61:47–56.
184. Adachi M, Yamaoka K, Watanabe M, et al. Effects of lifestyle education program for type 2 diabetes patients in clinics: a cluster randomized controlled trial. *BMC Public Health.* 2013;13:467.
185. Wong VW, Chan RS, Wong GL, et al. Community-based lifestyle modification programme for non-alcoholic fatty liver disease: a randomized controlled trial. *J Hepatol.* 2013;59:536–542.
186. Makrilakis K, Grammatikou S, Liatis S, et al. The effect of a non-intensive community-based lifestyle intervention on the prevalence of metabolic syndrome. The DEPLAN study in Greece. *Hormones (Athens).* 2012;11:316–324.
187. LeBlanc EL, Patnode CD, Webber EM, et al. *Behavioral and Pharmacotherapy Weight Loss Interventions to Prevent Obesity-Related Morbidity and Mortality in Adults: An Updated Systematic Review for the U.S. Preventive Services Task Force Evidence Synthesis No. 168.* Rockville, MD: Agency for Healthcare Research and Quality; 2018. AHRQ Publication 18-05239-EF-1.
188. Ogden CL, Carroll MD, Fryar CD, et al. Prevalence of obesity among adults and youth: United States 2011–2014. *NCHS Data Brief.* 2015;219:1–8.
189. Dattilo AM, Kris-Etherton PM. Effect of weight reduction on blood lipids and lipoproteins: a meta-analysis. *Am J Clin Nutr.* 1992;56:320–328.
190. Krauss RM, Blanche PJ, Raulings RS, et al. Separate effects of reduced carbohydrate intake and weight loss on atherogenic dyslipidemia. *Am J Clin Nutr.* 2006;83:1025–1031.
191. Crawford P, Paden SL. What is the dietary treatment for low HDL cholesterol. *J Fam Pract.* 2006;55:1076–1078.
192. Wood PD, Stefanick ML, Haskell WL. The effect on plasma lipoproteins of a prudent weight reducing diet with and without exercise in overweight men and women. *N Engl J Med.* 1991;325:461–466.
193. Marmot MG. Alcohol and coronary disease. *Int J Epidemiol.* 1984; 13:160–167.
194. Camargo CA Jr, Williams PT, Vranizan KM, et al. The effect of moderate alcohol intake on serum apolipoproteins A-I and A-II. *JAMA.* 1985;253:2854–2857.
195. Haskell WL, Camargo C, Williams PT, et al. The effect of cessation and resumption of moderate alcohol intake on serum high-density lipoprotein subfractions. *N Engl J Med.* 1984;310:805–810.
196. Stampfer MJ, Colditz GA, Willett WC, et al. A prospective study of moderate alcohol consumption and the risk of coronary disease and stroke in women. *N Engl J Med.* 1988;319:267–273.
197. Goldberg IJ, Mosca L, Piano MR, et al. Wine and your heart: a science advisory for healthcare professionals from the Nutrition Committee, Council on Epidemiology and Prevention, and Council on Cardiovascular Nursing of the American Heart Association. *Circulation.* 2001;103:472–475.
198. Whelton SP, Chin A, Xin X, et al. Effect of aerobic exercise on blood pressure: a meta-analysis of randomized controlled trials. *Ann Intern Med.* 2002;136:493–503.
199. Kumar A, Kar S, Fay WP. Thrombosis, physical activity, and acute coronary syndromes. *Journal of Applied Physiology (1985).* 2011;111: 599–605.
200. Mann S, Beedie C, Jimenez A. Differential effects of aerobic exercise, resistance training and combined exercise modalities on cholesterol and the lipid profile: review, synthesis, and recommendations. *Sports Med.* 2014;44:211–221.
201. Mann S, Beedie C, Balducci S, et al. Changes in insulin sensitivity in response to different modalities of exercise: a review of the evidence. *Diabetes Metab Res Rev.* 2014;30:257–268.
202. American College of Sports Medicine. In: Pescatello LS, senior ed. *ACSM's Guidelines for Exercise Testing and Prescription.* 9th ed. Philadelphia, PA: Lippincott Williams & Wilkins; 2014.
203. Haskell WH, Nelson ME. *Physical Activity Guidelines Advisory Committee Report, 2008.* Washington, DC: U.S. Department of Health and Human Services; 2008.
204. Campos H, Wilson PW, Jimenez D, et al. Differences in apolipoproteins and low-density lipoprotein subfractions in postmenopausal women on and off estrogen therapy: results of the Framingham offspring study. *Metabolism.* 1990;39:1033–1038.
205. Sullivan MJ. Estrogen replacement. *Circulation.* 1996;94:2699–2702.
206. Hulley SB, Grady D, Bush T, et al. Randomized trial of estrogen plus progestin for secondary prevention of coronary heart disease in postmenopausal women. *JAMA.* 1998;280:605–613.
207. Grady D, Herrington D, Bittner V, et al. Cardiovascular disease outcomes during 6.8 years of hormone therapy. Heart and Estrogen/progestin Replacement Study follow-up (HERS II). *JAMA.* 2002;288: 49–57.
208. The Writing Group for the Women's Health Initiative Investigators. Risks and benefits of estrogen plus progestin in healthy postmenopausal women. Principal results for the Women's Health Initiative Randomized Trial. *JAMA.* 2002;288:321–333.
209. Fletcher SW, Colditz GA. Failure of estrogen and progestin therapy for prevention. *JAMA.* 2002;288:366–368.
210. The Women's Health Initiative Steering Committee. Effects of conjugated equine estrogen in postmenopausal women with hysterectomy. The Women's Health Initiative Randomized Controlled Trial. *JAMA.* 2004;291:1701–1712.
211. Mosca L, Banka C, Benjamin E, et al. Evidence-based guidelines for cardiovascular prevention in women: 2007 Update. *Circulation.* 2007;115:1481–1501.
212. The NAMS 2017 Hormone Therapy Position Statement Advisory Panel. The 2017 hormone therapy position statement of the North American Menopause Society. *Menopause.* 2017;24(7):728–753.
213. Brown G, Albers JJ, Fisher LD, et al. Regression of coronary artery disease as a result of intensive lipid-lowering therapy in men with high levels of apolipoprotein B. *N Engl J Med.* 1990;323:1289–1298.
214. Haskell WL, Alderman EL, Fair JM, et al. Effects of intensive multiple risk reduction on coronary atherosclerosis and clinical cardiac events in men and women with coronary artery disease. *Circulation.* 1994;89: 975–990.
215. Kane JP, Malloy MJ, Ports TA, et al. Regression of coronary atherosclerosis during treatment of familial hypercholesterolemia with combined drug regimes. *JAMA.* 1990;264:3007–3012.

216. Watts GF, Lewis B, Brunt JN, et al. Effects on coronary artery disease of lipid lowering diet, or diet plus cholestyramine, in the St. Thomas' Arteriosclerosis Regression Study (STARS). *Lancet.* 1992;339:563–569.
217. Hulley SB, Herman TB, Grady D, et al. Should we be measuring blood cholesterol levels in young adults? *JAMA.* 1993;269:1416–1419.
218. Jacobs D, Blackburn H, Higgins M, et al. The conference on low cholesterol: mortality associations. *Circulation.* 1992;86:1046–1060.
219. Muldoon MF, Manuch SB, Matthews KA. Lowering cholesterol concentrations and mortality: a quantitative review of primary prevention trials. *BMJ.* 1990;301:309–314.
220. Schectman G, McKinney, WP, Pleuss J, et al. Dietary intake of Americans reporting adherence to low cholesterol diet (NHANES II). *Am J Public Health.* 1990;80:698–703.
221. Kashyap ML, McGovern ME, Berra K, et al. Long-term safety and efficacy of a once-daily niacin/lovastatin formulation for patients with dyslipidemia. *Am J Cardiol.* 1999;89:672–678.
222. Clark RW, Sutfin TA, Ruggeri RB, et al. Raising high-density lipoprotein in humans through inhibition of cholesteryl ester transfer protein: an initial multidose study of torcetrapib. *Arterioscler Thromb Vasc Biol.* 2004;24:490–497.
223. De Haan W, de Vries-van der Weij J, van der Hoorn JW, et al. Torcetrapib does not reduce atherosclerosis beyond atorvastatin and induces more proinflammatory lesions than atorvastatin. *Circulation.* 2008;117: 2515–2522.
224. Tobert JA. New developments in lipid-lowering therapy: The role of inhibitors of hydroxymethylglutaryl-coenzyme A reductase. *Circulation.* 1987;76:534–538.
225. Gotto AM, Pownall HJ. *Manual of Lipid Disorders.* Baltimore, MD: Williams & Wilkins; 1992.
226. Dujovne CA, Ettinger MP, McNeer JF, et al. Ezetimibe study group efficacy and safety of a potent new selective cholesterol absorption inhibitor, ezetimibe, in patients with primary hypercholesterolemia. *Am J Cardiol.* 2002;90(10):1092–1097.
227. Sudhop T, von Bergmann K. Cholesterol absorption inhibitors for the treatment of hypercholesterolemia. *Drugs.* 2002;62(16):2333–2347.
228. Abourbih S, Filion KB, Joseph L, et al. Effect of fibrates on lipid profiles and cardiovascular outcomes: a systematic review. *Am J Med.* 2009;122(10):962.e1–962.e8.
229. Jun M, Foote C, Lv J, et al. Effects of fibrates on cardiovascular outcomes: a systematic review and meta-analysis. *Lancet.* 2010;375(9729):1875–1884.
230. Miller NH. Compliance with treatment regimens in chronic asymptomatic diseases. *Am J Med.* 1997;102:43–49.
231. Insull W. The problem of compliance to cholesterol altering therapy. *J Intern Med.* 1997;241:317–325.
232. Berra K, Miller N, Fair, JM. Cardiovascular disease prevention and disease management: a critical role for nursing. *J Cardiopulm Rehabil.* 2006;26(4):197–206.

25 Diabetes and Cardiovascular Disease

Laurie Quinn

OBJECTIVES

1. Learn classifications for diabetes and other types of glucose intolerance.
2. Discuss pathophysiology of diabetes.
3. Identify the relationship between diabetes and cardiovascular disease.

KEY QUESTIONS

1. What is the relationship between diabetes and cardiovascular (CVD) disease?
2. What interventions have shown success in reducing CVD in people with diabetes mellitus (DM)?
3. What is the role of nursing helping patients with DM reduce their risk for cardiovascular disease?

There is a global epidemic of diabetes. Currently, there are 425 million people worldwide with diabetes mellitus (DM) and this number is expected to increase to 629 million by 2045.[1] There are 30.3 million people in the United States with diabetes, of which 7.2 million remain undiagnosed. Additionally, there are approximately 84 million people in the United States with prediabetes.

The global rise in diabetes is associated with a corresponding increase in the development of diabetes-related complications. The macrovascular complications of DM include aggressive and extensive coronary heart disease (CHD), stroke, and peripheral vascular disease (PVD). The microvascular complications include end-stage renal disease (ESRD), retinopathy and neuropathy, along with lower extremity amputations (LEAs).[2] There is also growing recognition of diabetes-linked conditions, including cancers, aging-related outcomes (e.g., cognitive dysfunction), infections, and liver disease.[2]

Cardiovascular disease is the leading cause of death for all people with DM.[3] Additionally, metabolic syndrome, a clustering of clinical findings consisting of abdominal obesity, high blood glucose, high triglyceride (TG), low high-density lipoprotein cholesterol (HDL-C) levels, and hypertension (HTN) is associated with increased CVD risk.[4] An estimated 35% of all adults and 50% of those over of 60 years of age have metabolic syndrome.[5]

The objectives of this chapter are (1) to discuss the pathophysiology and diagnostic criteria for T1DM, T2DM, and metabolic syndrome; (2) to describe the relationship between T1DM, T2DM, metabolic syndrome, and CVD; (3) to identify strategies for the prevention of T2DM and metabolic syndrome; (4) to identify the prevention of CVD in T1DM, T2DM, and metabolic syndrome.

CLASSIFICATION OF DIABETES AND OTHER FORMS OF GLUCOSE INTOLERANCE

DM is a group of metabolic disorders characterized by hyperglycemia, resulting from defects in insulin secretion, insulin action, or both. The primary forms of DM are type 1 diabetes mellitus (T1DM) and type 2 diabetes mellitus (T2DM) that account for approximately 5% and 95% of diagnosed diabetes, respectively.[6] There are four clinical classifications of diabetes (DM) and two categories of increased risk for developing DM. The clinical classifications include T1DM, T2DM, other specific types of DM, and gestational diabetes mellitus (GDM). Categories associated with increased risk of DM include impaired fasting glucose (IFG) and impaired glucose tolerance (IGT). IGT and IFG are commonly referred to as prediabetes.

Type 1 diabetes is an autoimmune condition that results in destruction of pancreatic β-cells, which synthesize and secrete insulin. People with T1DM have an absolute insulin deficiency and require pharmacologic insulin therapy for survival. Type 1 diabetes can occur at any age and is frequently diagnosed before 30 years of age; however, there is an adult form of autoimmune T1DM that is termed latent autoimmune of the adult (LADA).[7]

Type 2 diabetes is characterized by hyperglycemia, hyperinsulinemia, insulin resistance, and pancreatic β-cell loss. The organs involved in the development of T2DM include the pancreas, liver, skeletal muscle, kidneys, brain, small intestine, and adipose tissue.[8] The incretin effect, changes in the colon and microbiome, immune dysregulation, and inflammation have emerged as important pathophysiologic factors.[8]

The classification referred to as *Other Types of Diabetes* reflects a variety of causes including monogenic diabetes syndromes, such as neonatal diabetes mellitus (NDM) or maturity-onset diabetes of the young (MODY); diseases of the exocrine pancreas, such as acute pancreatitis; cystic fibrosis; endocrinopathies; drug- or chemical-induced diabetes; infections; rare forms of immune-mediated diabetes; and other genetic syndromes that are associated with diabetes.[9] Monogenic diabetes comprises 1% to 5% of all cases of childhood DM.[10] The monogenic forms of DM mellitus result from a single gene mutation, whereas T1DM and T2DM result from polygenic defects. Neonatal diabetes first occurs in newborns and young infants. MODY usually first occurs in children or adolescents and is characterized by mild hyperglycemia to hyperglycemia requiring insulin therapy.[11]

GDM refers to the onset of DM when first diagnosed during pregnancy. The prevalence of GDM ranges from 2% to 10% of all pregnancies in the United States.[12] Hyperglycemia during pregnancy can result in fetal and maternal complications. GDM resolves after childbirth; however, women with GDM have a 35% to 60% chance of developing DM in the 10 to 20 years following the pregnancy.[13] Individuals who have been diagnosed with GDM need dietary treatment and possibly oral diabetes medications or exogenous insulin to control hyperglycemia. Risk factors for GDM include both modifiable and nonmodifiable factors. The nonmodifiable risk factors include non-white ethnicity; underlying polycystic ovary syndrome (PCOS); previous pregnancies complicated by GDM; family history of T2DM; and maternal age. The modifiable risk factors include pre-gravid obesity or maternal excess adiposity; and dietary factors and physical inactivity in the preconception period.[14]

DIAGNOSIS OF DIABETES AND CATEGORIES OF INCREASED RISK FOR DIABETES

The diagnosis of DM in nonpregnant adults is restricted to those who have one of the following[15]:

- Elevated glycosylated hemoglobin (A1C) greater than or equal to 6.5%.*
- Classic symptoms of DM plus casual plasma glucose concentration greater than or equal to 200 mg/dL (11.1 mmol/L). The classic symptoms of DM include polyuria, polydipsia, and unexplained weight loss. Casual refers to any time of day without regard to time since the last meal.
- Fasting plasma glucose (FPG) greater than or equal to 126 mg/dL (7.0 mmol/L).*
- 2-hour plasma glucose (PG) greater than or equal to 200 mg/dL (11.1 mmol/L) during an oral glucose tolerance test (OGTT). The test should be performed using glucose load containing the equivalent of 75 g of anhydrous glucose dissolved in water.*

*In the absence of unequivocal hyperglycemia with acute metabolic decompensation, these criteria should be confirmed by repeat testing on a different day.

The diagnosis of increased risk for DM (i.e., prediabetes) is based on the following criteria:

- IFG:
  - FPG of 100 to 125 mg/dL (5.6 to 6.9 mmol/L)
- IGT:
  - 2-hour PG during an OGTT of 140 to 199 mg/dL (7.8 to 11.0 mmol/L).
- Elevated A1C:
  - 5.7% to 6.4%

PATHOPHYSIOLOGY OF DIABETES MELLITUS

Normal Physiology and Fuel Metabolism

An understanding of normal physiology and fuel metabolism is needed to understand the pathophysiology of T1DM and T2DM. Glucose is an essential fuel for the brain and central nervous system (CNS). Plasma glucose concentrations are maintained within a narrow range that is achieved by a balance between glucose entry into the circulation from the liver, intestinal absorption, and glucose uptake into the peripheral sites, such as adipose tissue and skeletal muscle. This process is coordinated by hormones, such as insulin, glucagon, catecholamines, cortisol, growth hormone, glucagon-like peptide 1 (GLP-1), and gastric inhibitory polypeptide (GIP), neural signals, and metabolic substrates, such as carbohydrates (CHOs), fats, proteins.

This network of hormones, neural signals and metabolic substrates, is dependent on a number of physiologic processes including *glycolysis, glycogen, glycogenolysis, gluconeogenesis, lipolysis, ketogenesis*, and *insulin resistance*. *Glycolysis* is the process in which glucose is broken down to provide energy in the form of adenosine triphosphate (ATP). *Glycogen* is the storage form of glucose, located primarily in skeletal muscle and the liver. In skeletal muscle, glycogen mostly acts as a fuel reserve for use in the synthesis of ATP during muscle contraction. In the liver, glycogen mostly acts as a fuel reserve used to maintain plasma glucose concentrations, especially during fasting. *Glycogenolysis* is the process through which liver and muscle glycogen are broken down to glucose. *Gluconeogenesis* is the formation of glucose or glycogen from non-CHO sources. The process of *gluconeogenesis* requires a coordinated supply of precursors, such as pyruvate, alanine, glutamine, and other amino acids. These precursors are mobilized from muscle to the liver, where they can be converted to glucose or glycogen through gluconeogenesis.

Fatty acids are stored primarily in the form of triglycerides and serve as the body's main fuel reserve. *Lipolysis* is the process through which triglycerides, composed of a glycerol backbone with three fatty acids attached, are hydrolyzed to fatty acids and glycerol. Triglycerides are stored primarily in adipose tissue and to a smaller extent in muscle. The hydrolysis of triglycerides results in the mobilization of fatty acids and glycerol into the bloodstream. Subsequently, fatty acids can be oxidized for energy; glycerol can be used in the process of glycolysis, gluconeogenesis, and again in the production of triglycerides. *Ketogenesis* is the production of ketones. The two primary ketone bodies are acetoacetate and 3-hydroxybutyrate, which are transported in the blood to peripheral tissues for oxidation by the tricarboxylic acid (TCA) cycle. *Insulin resistance* is defined as the inability of either endogenous or exogenous insulin to achieve its biologic response in its target tissues.

Hormones of the Endocrine Pancreas

The pancreas is divided into the exocrine and endocrine sections, which make up 80% and 20% of the organ, respectively. The exocrine pancreas is primarily composed of small glands called acini; the endocrine pancreas is made up of small cells called islets of Langerhans. These islet cells are distributed throughout the pancreas and are divided into the α-cells which secrete glucagon; β-cells, which secrete insulin; delta cells which secrete somatostatin; and F cells that secrete pancreatic polypeptide.

The primary functions of insulin include the synthesis of glycogen in liver and muscle, protein in liver and muscle, triglycerides in adipose tissue and, to a smaller extent, in muscle. Insulin is necessary for glycolysis and glucose transport into insulin-sensitive tissues, such as muscle. Insulin suppresses gluconeogenesis, glycogenolysis, lipolysis, and ketogenesis. The binding of insulin with its cell membrane receptor results in a series of reactions that enhance glucose transport into insulin-sensitive tissues, including skeletal muscle and adipose tissue.

Collectively, glucagon, cortisol, growth hormone, epinephrine, and norepinephrine are referred to as *counterregulatory hormones*. The primary functions of glucagon, secreted from pancreatic α-cells, include hepatic gluconeogenesis, glycogenolysis, lipolysis, and ketogenesis. Cortisol, secreted by the adrenal cortex, causes protein catabolism, lipolysis and insulin resistance. Growth hormone, secreted by the anterior pituitary, causes lipolysis and insulin resistance. The catecholamines include epinephrine and norepinephrine. Of these, epinephrine has the greatest role in fuel metabolism. This hormone primarily is secreted by the adrenal medulla and is associated with glycogenolysis, gluconeogenesis, lipolysis and insulin resistance.

Normal Fuel Metabolism

Metabolic processes involved in fuel metabolism revolve around absorptive (fed) and postabsorptive (fasted) states. These are described below.

Postabsorptive State

The primary goal of fuel metabolism during the postabsorptive state or fasted state is to provide glucose for the brain and nervous tissue. Glucagon is the predominant hormone during this time. Hepatic glycogenolysis and gluconeogenesis increase plasma glucose levels. Additionally, muscle oxidizes free fatty acids (FFAs), released from adipose tissue lipolysis, that are used as an energy substrate

Absorptive State

Insulin is the primary hormone during the absorptive state. Following ingestion of CHO, insulin levels rise and stimulate glucose uptake into insulin-sensitive tissues, primarily muscle. Glucose is the primary oxidative fuel for all tissues during the absorptive state. Glucose in excess of the oxidative needs of the major tissues is stored as glycogen or lipids.

Starvation

During starvation, insulin remains suppressed, glucagon levels remain elevated, and the principal source of hepatic glucose production is gluconeogenesis. The muscles oxidize FFAs, released from adipose tissue lipolysis, for energy. In addition, the brain begins to oxidize ketones for energy.

Fuel Metabolism in Diabetes Mellitus

A number of metabolic derangements are associated with DM. In T1DM, there is an absolute loss of insulin production. In T2DM, there is decreased insulin production and insulin resistance. The abnormalities of fuel metabolism in DM result from a deficiency in insulin and an increase in plasma glucagon and other counterregulatory hormones. These hormonal abnormalities most profoundly affect the muscle, liver, and adipose tissue. Hyperglycemia results from decreased glucose transport into insulin-sensitive tissues, hepatic gluconeogenesis, and hepatic and muscle glycogenolysis. In T1DM, the increased mobilization of FFAs from adipose tissue leads to increased hepatic synthesis of ketone bodies and can result in an acute complication diabetes, diabetic ketoacidosis (DKA).

TYPE 1 DIABETES MELLITUS

Type 1 diabetes is a chronic disorder resulting from interplay among genetic, autoimmune, and environmental factors, characterized by hyperglycemia secondary to insulin deficiency. There has been a sustained increase in the global incidence of T1DM over the last several decades.[16–20] The current global population of people with T1DM is characterized by diversity in age, race, genetic identity, and phenotype.[21] The pathogenesis can be divided into three stages. These include (1) the appearance of pancreatic β-cell autoimmunity, normal glucose tolerance, and no symptoms; (2) pancreatic β-cell autoimmunity, abnormal glucose tolerance, and no symptoms; and (3) pancreatic β-cell autoimmunity, hyperglycemia, and symptoms of DM.[22]

Genetics: Genetic susceptibility to the development of T1DM is associated with the human leukocyte antigen (HLA) genes that lie in the major histocompatibility complex region on chromosome 6p21.[23] This region accounts for half the genetic risk for T1DM. The HLA-DR3-DQ2 or HLA-DR4-DQ8 haplotypes are most closely associated with the development of T1DM.[23] Against this background of genetic susceptibility, an environmental trigger initiates the development of autoimmunity and progression to overt T1DM.

Autoimmunity: Islet autoimmunity is defined by the persistent presence of autoantibodies to pancreatic islet cell antigens. Type 1 diabetes is associated with circulating autoantibodies (e.g., glutamic acid decarboxylase [GAD] islet antigen-2 [IA-2], insulin and zinc transporter 8 [ZnT8]) to pancreatic β-cell antigens. In general, the development of two or more autoantibodies predicts progression to overt diabetes. The majority of children at risk of T1DM who had multiple islet autoantibody seroconversion progress to diabetes over the next 15 years.[24]

Environmental: There is wide diversity in the incidence of T1DM across geographic areas. The incidence is increasing in countries that previously had low incidences of T1DM, such as China,[25] Brazil,[26] and Kuwait,[27] suggesting socioeconomic factors in the development of T1DM. Several environmental factors have been proposed to explain the progression from autoimmunity to overt T1DM. Environmental triggers include pre- and postnatal infections, diet, and toxins, such as respiratory infections[28]; type of infant formula[29]; and changes in intestinal microbiota induced by C-section and use of antibiotics.[30] The hygiene hypothesis postulates that fewer early childhood infections with less diverse microbiota deviate the immune system toward autoimmunity and atopy. A variant of the hygiene hypothesis blames decreased herd immunity to enterovirus for the rise in T1DM.[30] The accelerator and β-cell hypothesis suggests that several unspecified environmental factors, such as overweight, fast growth, infections, dietary deficiencies, alone or in combination, make the pancreatic β-cells exhausted and eventually fail due to autoimmunity.

TYPE 2 DIABETES MELLITUS

Type 2 diabetes, the most common form of DM, is a heterogeneous polygenic disorder that results from the interaction of genetic susceptibility and environmental factors. This disorder is characterized by insulin resistance in muscle, liver, and peripheral tissues, and reduced insulin secretion from the pancreatic β-cell. Genetic factors can influence both insulin resistance and reduced insulin secretion; however, these processes can be modified by environmental factors such as physical inactivity and high-calorie diets.

Genetic and Environmental Influences: Genes and the environment influence the development of insulin resistance and pancreatic β-cell dysfunction. Changes in the gene pool cannot account for the exponential increase in T2DM over the past two decades.[31] During the past decade, progress in genetic association studies has enabled the identification of at least 75 independent genetic loci for T2DM.[32] These discoveries have increased understanding of the genetic architecture of T2DM, and allow us the ability to examine the interaction between the environment and genetics in explaining the evolution of T2DM.

Individuals at Risk for Type 2 Diabetes: The risk for T2DM is increased in those who (1) are overweight or obese; (2) are age 45 years or older; (3) have a family history of diabetes; (4) are African American, Alaska Native, American Indian, Asian American, Hispanic/Latino, Native Hawaiian, or Pacific Islanders; (5) have high blood pressure (BP); (6) have a low level of HDL cholesterol, or a high level of triglycerides; (7) have a history of gestational diabetes or have given birth to a baby weighing 9 lb or greater; (8) are physically inactive; (9) have a history of heart disease or stroke; (10) have depression; (11) have PCOS; (12) have acanthosis nigricans, which is dark, thick, and velvety skin around the neck or armpits, associated with insulin resistance.[33] Obesity, increased weight gain, and physical inactivity are risks most strongly associated with progression to T2DM.[34]

Pathogenesis of T2DM: In the earliest stage in the development of T2DM, the pancreatic β-cell increases insulin secretion in response to insulin resistance. This compensatory hyperinsulinemia is able to maintain normoglycemia. As insulin resistance increases, this compensatory hyperinsulinemia is insufficient to maintain normoglycemia. With increased insulin resistance, visceral adipose tissue becomes more sensitive to the effects of catecholamines, and lipolysis is enhanced. There is increased FFA production and mobilization, worsening insulin resistance in the liver and muscle. Additionally, insulin-mediated glucose transport into skeletal muscle, the major target for glucose disposal, becomes impaired. FPG levels remain normal, but postprandial plasma glucose levels are elevated.

In the final stage, insulin resistance increases further. The restraining effects of insulin on hepatic glucose production become impaired, and plasma glucose levels increase. In addition, effects of worsening hyperglycemia on the pancreatic β-cell become toxic, and insulin secretion subsequently declines. With increasing insulin resistance, FFA production and mobilization become even greater. The increased FFAs lead to subsequent increases in insulin resistance. Fasting and postprandial hyperglycemia result from increased insulin resistance, unrestrained hepatic glucose production, and glucose toxicity.

METABOLIC SYNDROME

Overview: The metabolic syndrome is a condition characterized by the coexistence of several risk factors for CVD including high BP, hyperglycemia, and dyslipidemia (reduced HDL-C) or elevated triglycerides. Each of these components is related to insulin resistance and appears to be etiologically related to each other. **Definition and Criteria:** The diagnosis of metabolic syndrome has been operationalized through various criteria. The two most common criteria are those developed and updated by the National Cholesterol Education Program (NCEP) Adult Treatment Panel III (ATP III)[35,36] and the International Diabetes Federation (IDF).[37]

The ATP III criteria focus on the risk for CVD and do not require evidence of glucose intolerance. According to the ATP III, adults who are diagnosed with metabolic syndrome must have three or more of the following:

- Abdominal obesity as evidenced by waist circumference greater than 40 in (102 cm) in men and greater than 35 in (88 cm) in women.
- Serum triglycerides greater than or equal to 150 mg/dL (1.7 mmol/L) or pharmacologic treatment for elevated triglycerides
- BP greater than or equal to 130/greater than or equal to 85 mm Hg or pharmacologic treatment for HTN
- Serum HDL-C less than 40 mg/dL (1.03 mmol/L) in men and less than 50 mg/dL (1.3 mmol/L) in women or pharmacologic treatment for low HDL
- FPG greater than or equal to 100 mg/dL (5.6 mmol/L) or pharmacologic treatment for T2DM

Critical to the IDF definition of metabolic syndrome is the presence of abdominal obesity. According to IDF criteria, the diagnosis of metabolic syndrome is based on the following:

- Increased waist circumference with ethnic specific waist circumference cut points PLUS any two of the following:
  - Serum triglycerides greater than or equal to 150 mg/dL (1.7 mmol/L) or pharmacologic treatment for elevated triglycerides
  - Serum HDL-C less than 40 mg/dL (1.03 mmol/L) in men and less than 50 mg/dL (1.3 mmol/L) in women or pharmacologic treatment for low HDL
  - Systolic BP greater than or equal to 130 mm Hg, diastolic BP greater than or equal to 85 mm Hg or treatment for HTN
  - FPG greater than or equal to 100 mg/dL (5.6 mmol/L) or previously diagnosed T2DM; an OGTT is recommended for individuals with an elevated FPG, but is not required

The diagnosis of metabolic syndrome is not without controversy. In a joint statement by the American Diabetes Association (ADA) and the European Association for the Study of Diabetes (EASD), a number of critical issues were explored by an expert panel.[38] In particular, the panel expressed concern as to whether metabolic syndrome was actually a "syndrome," as there was no evidence that the sum of the risk factors conferred risk beyond each original component. Nonetheless, these criteria provide a guideline of individual CVD risk factors that are amenable to pharmacologic and lifestyle treatments. As we proceed through the chapter, the interventions and treatments for metabolic syndrome and T2DM will be similar with the exception of the glucose-lowering medications.

CARDIOVASCULAR DISEASE AND DIABETES

The statistics regarding DM and CVD are striking. Atherosclerotic cardiovascular disease (ASCVD) is the principal cause of death and disability among patients with DM, especially in adults with T2DM, which has been reported to have an equivalent risk to aging 15 years.[39] Approximately two thirds of deaths in people with DM are directly related to CVD. Approximately 40% are from ischemic heart disease, 15% from other forms of heart disease, principally heart failure (HF), and 10% from stroke.[40] Diabetes is considered a CHD risk equivalent.[35]

The development of CVD in diabetes is a highly complex process. The relationship between increased rates of CVD and DM first was reported in the Framingham Study.[41,42] The Diabetes Control and Complications Trial (DCCT)[43] and the United Kingdom Prospective Diabetes Study (UKPDS)[44] identified hyperglycemia as the primary factor in the development of the microvascular complications of DM. The original DCCT results did not demonstrate a protective effect of intensive glucose control on macrovascular disease in T1DM; however, the ongoing follow-up study, Epidemiology of Diabetes Interventions and Complications (EDIC) demonstrated that intensive blood glucose control during the DCCT had a protective effect on the future development of diabetes-related complications including CVD.[45]

The damaging effect of hyperglycemia occurs primarily in capillary endothelial cells in the retina, mesangial cells of the renal glomerulus, and neurons and Schwann cells in the peripheral nerves.[46] These cells become the target of hyperglycemia because they are not able to reduce transport of glucose inside the cell; their internal glucose concentration therefore remains constant. There appear to be four major processes involved including (1) increased flux through the polyol pathway; (2) intracellular production of advanced glycation end product (AGE) precursors; (3) protein kinase C activation; and (4) increased hexosamine pathway activity.[46]

This "glucose hypothesis" in relationship to the development of macrovascular complications in diabetes is not as clear. The primary theory on the pathogenesis of macrovascular suggests that these complications are mediated by both hyperglycemia and insulin resistance. Insulin resistance is associated with increased release of FFAs, which causes an atherogenic lipid and lipoprotein profile. In addition to the lipid and lipoprotein abnormalities, FFA flux increases from adipocytes into arterial endothelial cells. This increased flux results in increased FFA oxidation by the mitochondria and overproduction of reactive oxygen species (ROS). As with hyperglycemia, this FFA-induced increase in ROS causes oxidative stress and activates the same damaging pathways, the polyol pathway, the hexosamine pathway, and PKC and causes increased production of AGE precursors.[46]

AGEs are produced from nonenzymatic glycosylation of lipids, lipoproteins, and amino acids, damaging cells by three different mechanisms. These include (1) alterations of intracellular proteins that are essential in regulation of gene transcription; (2) diffusion of AGE precursors from the cell that modifies the nearby extracellular matrix molecules, altering signaling between the matrix and the cell; and (3) diffusion of AGE precursors from the cell and subsequent alteration of circulating proteins in the blood, such as albumin. These modified circulating proteins bind to AGE receptors and activate them, thereby causing the production of inflammatory cytokines and growth factors, which contribute to CVD and vascular dysfunction.[46] Advanced glycation end products may also directly impact macrophage function, suggesting that part of the accelerated development of CVD in DM is related to altered macrophage function.[47]

Prevention of Type 1 Diabetes

Type 1 diabetes has a preclinical period prior to loss of pancreatic β-cell function. Individuals at risk for developing T1DM can be identified using a combination of autoantibodies, markers of genetic susceptibility, and pancreatic β-cell function.[23] Primary prevention seeks to prevent T1DM in those high-risk individuals that have not developed autoantibodies. Secondary prevention is aimed at preventing T1DM in high-risk individuals that have developed autoantibodies. Theoretically, interventions in those with autoantibodies, such as manipulation of the autoimmune process, can delay or prevent the onset of T1DM. Tertiary prevention refers to using interventions to preserve pancreatic β-cell function shortly following diagnosis. There have been a number of clinical trials testing primary, secondary, and tertiary interventions with limited success.[48] No drug or intervention has provided sufficient preservation of pancreatic β-cell function to warrant use in clinical practice.[49] In a recent phase 2 trial, however, a single course of teplizumab, an anti-CD3 monoclonal antibody, significantly slowed progression to T1DM in high-risk, nondiabetic relatives of patients with T1DM that had at least two autoantibodies and abnormal results of an oral glucose tolerance test at trial entry. The median delay in the diagnosis of T1DM was 2 years. At the conclusion of the trial, the percentages of those without T1DM in the teplizumab and placebo groups were 57% and 28%, respectively.[50] This trial holds promise for future prevention of T1DM.

Prevention of Type 2 Diabetes

Primary prevention is the ultimate goal of global efforts toward reducing the burden of T2DM and complications.

Lifestyle Interventions

There are three major primary prevention intervention studies that have focused on the role of lifestyle changes in preventing T2DM in people at risk for T2DM. These include the Chinese Da Qing Study[51]; the Finnish Diabetes Prevention Study[52]; and the U.S.-based Diabetes Prevention Program (DPP).[53]

Da Qing Study

In the Da Qing Study, 577 adults with IGT were randomly assigned to control, diet, exercise, or diet-plus-exercise groups. The diet and/or exercise interventions led to a significant decrease in the incidence of diabetes over a 6-year period compared to controls among those with IGT. The diet, exercise, and diet-plus-exercise interventions were associated with 31%, 46%, and 42% reductions in risk of developing T2DM, respectively.[51] A 20-year follow-up of this study concluded that group lifestyle interventions over 6 years can prevent or delay diabetes for up to 14 years after the active intervention.[54]

Finnish Diabetes Prevention Study

In the Finnish Diabetes Prevention Study, 522 middle-aged, overweight subjects with IGT were assigned to either an intervention group or control group. Each subject in the intervention group received individualized counseling aimed at reducing weight, total intake of fat, and intake of saturated fat and increasing intake of fiber and physical activity. The risk of T2DM was reduced by 58% in the intervention group during the trial. The reduction in the incidence of T2DM was directly associated with changes in lifestyle. Sustained reductions in the incidence of T2DM by lifestyle intervention were noted during follow-up assessments. Patients who had not developed T2DM at 4 years were followed for an additional 3 years. The reduction in the incidence of T2DM in the original intensive lifestyle group continued, albeit to a lesser degree, with a 36% reduction in risk of developing T2DM. Lifestyle intervention in people at high risk for T2DM resulted in sustained lifestyle changes and a reduction in the incidence of T2DM, which remained after the individual lifestyle counseling was stopped.

Diabetes Prevention Program

In the DPP study, 3234 nondiabetic persons with elevated fasting and postload plasma glucose concentrations were randomized to placebo, metformin (850 mg twice daily), or a lifestyle modification program. The lifestyle intervention reduced the incidence by 58% and metformin by 31% as compared with placebo. Lifestyle changes and treatment with metformin both reduced the incidence of diabetes in persons at high risk; however, the lifestyle intervention was more effective than metformin. During a mean follow-up of 15 years, the incidence of T2DM was reduced by 27% in the lifestyle intervention group and by 18% in the metformin group compared with the placebo.[55]

Pharmacologic Interventions

Pharmacologic agents including metformin,[53] α-glucosidase inhibitors,[56] orlistat,[57] GLP-1 receptor agonists,[58] and thiazolidinediones[59,60] have each been shown to decrease the incidence of T2DM in those with prediabetes. Metformin, however, has the strongest evidence base and demonstrated long-term safety as pharmacologic therapy for diabetes prevention.[61]

TREATMENT OF DIABETES AND PREVENTION OF CARDIOVASCULAR DISEASE

The primary goals of therapy in T1DM and T2DM are optimal glucose control, BP control, and lipid control. These goals primarily are accomplished by pharmacologic treatment, nutrition therapy, and exercise.

Pharmacologic Treatments

Since people with T1DM are unable to produce insulin, they depend on exogenous insulin to sustain life. Pharmacologic treatment of T2DM may include oral antidiabetes medications and/or insulin. The primary goal of these therapies is optimal glucose control. The glycemic goals for nonpregnant adults with diabetes are as follows[62]:

- A1C: less than 7.0% (53 mmol/mol)
- Preprandial capillary plasma glucose: 80 to 130 mg/dL (4.4 to 7.2 mmol/L)
- Peak postprandial capillary plasma glucose less than 180 mg/dL (10.0 mmol/L)

These goals can be more or less stringent for individual patients. Such goals can be individualized based on factors such as duration of diabetes, age and life expectancy, coexisting medical conditions, CVD or advanced microvascular complications, hypoglycemia unawareness, and individual patient considerations. Postprandial glucose measurements, if indicated, should be made 1 to 2 hours after the beginning of the meal.[62]

Insulin preparations are general classified as rapid-acting, short-acting, intermediate-acting, long-acting insulin, ultra–long-acting, and premixed combinations. These are detailed in Table 25-1. The oral classes of medications include biguanides; sulfonylureas; meglitinides; thiazolidinediones; α-glucosidase inhibitors; dipeptidyl peptidase 4 (DPP-4 inhibitors); bile acid sequestrants; dopamine-2 agonists and sodium-glucose cotransporter-2 (SGLT-2 inhibitors). The primary medications in each of these categories are detailed in Table 25-2. Additionally, there are some injectable medications for the treatment of T2DM as detailed in Table 25-3.

Recent clinical trials have provided evidence that specific GLP-1 receptor agonists or SGLT-2 inhibitors improve CVD outcomes in those at high risk for CVD; as well as secondary outcomes such as HF and progression of chronic kidney disease (CKD) in those with established CVD or CKD.[63] In the *Liraglutide Effect and Action in Diabetes Trial* (LEADER), patients with T2DM and high CVD risk were randomly assigned to receive liraglutide, a human analogue of human GLP-1, or placebo. Using a time-event analysis, trial investigators concluded that the first occurrence of death from CVD causes, nonfatal myocardial infarction, or nonfatal stroke was lower with liraglutide than with placebo.[64] In the *Trial to Evaluate Cardiovascular and Other Long-term Outcomes With Semaglutide in Subjects With Type 2 Diabetes* (SUSTAIN® 6), patients with T2DM were randomly assigned to a once-weekly semaglutide, an analogue of human GLP-1 with an extended half-life of approximately 1 week, or placebo. As in the LEADER trial, the investigators concluded that the rate of CVD death, nonfatal myocardial infarction, or nonfatal stroke was significantly lower among patients receiving semaglutide than among those receiving placebo. In the *Exenatide Study of Cardiovascular Event Lowering Trial* (EXSCEL), however, the incidence of major adverse CVD events did not differ significantly between

Table 25-1 • INSULIN FORMULATIONS

Insulin Preparation	Onset of Action (hours)	Peak Action (hours)	Effective Duration of Action (hours)	Maximum Duration (hours)
Rapid-acting analogues				
Insulin lispro (Humalog)	¼–½	½–1½	3–4	4–6
Insulin aspart (NovoLog)	¼–½	½–1¼	3–4	4–6
Insulin glulisine (Apidra)	¼–½	½–1¼	3–4	4–6
Inhaled insulin (Afrezza)	Seconds	12–17 minutes	2–3	2–3
Short-acting				
Regular (soluble)	½–1	2–3	3–6	6–8
Intermediate-acting				
NPH (isophane	2–4	6–10	10–16	14–16
Long-acting analogue				
Insulin glargine (Lantus)	0.5–1.5	8–16	18–20	20–24
Insulin glargine U-300 (Toujeo)	0.5–1.5	None	24	30
Insulin detemir (Levemir)	0.5–1.5	6–8	14	~20
Insulin degludec (Tresiba)	0.5–1.5	None	24	40

Source: The Management of Type 1 Diabetes. © 2000–2019, MDText.com, Inc.

Table 25-2 • ORAL MEDICATIONS FOR TYPE 2 DIABETES

Medication Class	Medication	Mode of Action
Biguanides	Metformin (Glucophage®) Metformin extended release (Glucophage XR®; Glumetza®, Fortamet®)	Reduces hepatic glucose production, gluconeogenesis, and glycogenolysis. Increases insulin-stimulated glucose utilization.
Sulfonylureas	Glimepiride (Amaryl®) Glipizide (Glucotrol®) Glipizide extended release (Glucotrol XL®)	Insulin secretagogues: stimulate insulin secretion from the pancreatic β-cell.
Meglitinides	Nateglinide (Starlix®) Repaglinide (Prandin®)	Nonsulfonylurea insulin secretagogues: stimulate insulin secretion from the pancreatic β-cell.
Thiazolidinedione	Pioglitazone (Actos®)	Promotes glucose uptake into skeletal muscle, adipose tissue, liver.
α-glucosidase inhibitors	Acarbose (Precose®) Miglitol (Glyset®)	Slows intestinal carbohydrate digestion and absorption. Decreases postprandial glucose excursions.
DPP-4 inhibitors	Alogliptin (Nesina®) Linagliptin (Tradjenta®) Saxagliptin (Onglyza®) Sitagliptin (Januvia®) Sitagliptin and metformin (Janumet®) Sitagliptin and metformin extended release (Janumet XR®)	Incretins are released after eating and augment the secretion of insulin released from pancreatic β-cells. DPP-4 increases postprandial incretins: glucagon-like peptide-1 (GLP-1) and gastric inhibitory polypeptide (GIP) concentrations.
Bile acid sequestrants	Colesevelam (Welchol®)	Have demonstrated improved glycemic control through unknown mechanisms. Enhanced reductions may occur when combined with other antidiabetes medications.
Dopamine-2 agonists	Bromocriptine quick release (Cycloset®)	Indicated as an adjunct to diet and exercise to improve glucose control.
SGLT-2 inhibitors	Canagliflozin (Invokana®) Dapagliflozin (Farxiga®) Empagliflozin (Jardiance®) Ertugliflozin (Steglatro®) Ertugliflozin and sitagliptin (Steglujan®) Ertugliflozin and metformin (Segluromet®)	Sodium-glucose cotransporters (SGLTs) are responsible for renal glucose reabsorption from the proximal tubules. These drugs lower glycemia by causing glycosuria.

Adapted from Feingold KR. *Oral and injectable (non-insulin) pharmacological agents for type 2 diabetes*. 2019. Available at www.endotext.org

T2DM patients receiving exenatide, GLP-1 receptor agonist, compared to those receiving placebo.[65] More research is needed to assess whether GLP-1 receptor agonists as a drug class are CVD protective, or if the CVD benefits are related to specific drugs.

In the *Empagliflozin Cardiovascular Outcome Event Trial in Type 2 Diabetes Mellitus Patients* (EMPA-REG OUTCOME), patients with T2DM at high risk for CVD events who received empagliflozin, an SGLT-1 inhibitor, as compared with placebo, had a lower rate of the primary composite CVD outcome (nonfatal myocardial infarction, nonfatal stroke and CVD death) and of death from any cause when the study drug was added to standard care.[66] The CANagliflozin cardioVascular Assessment Study (CANVAS) Program integrated data from two trials (CANVAS and CANVAS-Renal) including participants with T2DM and increased CVD risk. Those treated with canagliflozin, an SGLT-1 inhibitor, had a significantly lower risk of death from CVD causes, nonfatal myocardial infarction, or nonfatal stroke than those who received placebo; however, there was a greater risk of amputation.[67] The EMPA-REG OUTCOME Trial was also associated with reduced mortality and hospitalization for HF.[68] This result was supported by the CANVAS Program.[69]

A consensus report from the *ADA* and the *EASD* concluded:

- Among patients with T2DM who have established CVD, SGLT-2 inhibitors or GLP-1 receptor agonists with proven CVD benefit are recommended as part of glycemic management.[63]
- Among patients with CVD in whom HF coexists or is of special concern, SGLT-2 inhibitors are recommended.[63]

Table 25-3 • INJECTABLE MEDICATIONS FOR TYPE 2 DIABETES

Medication	Type	Primary Action
Amylin	Pramlintide acetate (Symlin®)	Slows gastric emptying, promoting satiety. Inhibits secretion of glucagon.
GLP-1 receptor agonists	Dulaglutide (Trulicity®) Exenatide (Byetta®) Exenatide extended release (Bydureon®, Bydureon BCise®) Liraglutide (Victoza®) Lixisenatide (Adlyxin®) Semaglutide (Ozempic®)	GLP-1 is an incretin secreted by the intestinal mucosa. Stimulation of GLP-1 receptor promotes the release of insulin from the pancreas. GLP-1 receptor agonists also suppress glucagon secretion and slow gastric emptying.
Insulin + GLP-1 receptor agonists	Insulin glargine/ lixisenatide (Soliqua 100/33®) Insulin degludec/ liraglutide (Xultophy® 100/3.6)	Combines effects of specific insulin and GLP agonists.

Adapted from Feingold KR. *Oral and injectable (non-insulin) pharmacological agents for type 2 diabetes*. 2019. Available at www.endotext.org

Medical Nutrition Therapy

The role of medical nutrition therapy (MNT) is to assist people with DM adopt healthy eating habits through education and support. The goals of MNT are to manage blood glucose and reduce CVD risk factors; to reduce risk for diabetes-related complications; and to preserve the pleasure of eating. MNT for people with DM focuses on diet quality and energy restriction. There is no ideal percentage of calories from CHO, protein, and fat for all people with DM. Macronutrient distribution should be based on an individualized assessment of current eating patterns, personal preferences, and metabolic goals.[70] In addition, current medications and comorbidities may influence dietary choices. The *Mediterranean* or *Dietary Approaches to Stop Hypertension* (DASH), low CHO, and low glycemic index are examples of eating patterns that have shown positive results in research.[63,70] Energy-restricted diets are appropriate for overweight and obese people with DM. All overweight and obese people with DM should be encouraged to engage of a program of intensive lifestyle management.[63]

Physical Activity

Physical activity is essential for glycemic management and CVD health. The following strategies, described in the *ADA Standards of Care* can be used to guide people with DM.[70] Children and adolescents with T1DM or T2DM or prediabetes are encouraged to participate in 60 minutes or greater per day of moderate- or vigorous-intensity aerobic activity, with strength-training and bone-strengthening activities at least 3 days/wk. Adults with T1DM or T2DM should engage in 150 minutes or greater of moderate to vigorous intensity aerobic activity each week; this should occur over at least 3 days/wk; there should be no greater than 2 consecutive days without activity. In addition, those with T1DM or T2DM should engage in 2 to 3 sessions/wk of resistance exercise on nonconsecutive days. The amount of time spent in daily sedentary behavior should be decreased with sitting interrupted every 30 minutes. Older adults with DM are encouraged to participate in flexibility training and balance training 2 to 3 times/wk. If an individual chooses, yoga and tai chi may be included in physical activity regimens to increase flexibility, muscular strength, and balance.

Blood Pressure Control

BP control is essential for CVD health. The following general strategies, highlighted in the ADA Standards of Care can be used to guide individuals with DM.[70] Patients with DM should have their BP measured at each routine health care visit. Those patients found to have elevated BP (greater than or equal to 140/90 mm Hg) should have their BP confirmed on another day with several readings to diagnose HTN. In patients with DM and HTN, BP targets should be individualized taking into account risk for CVD, the side effects of antihypertensive medications, and patient preferences. A BP target of less than 130/80 mm Hg may be appropriate for those with DM and HTN at higher CVD risk, while a BP target of less than 140/90 mm Hg may be appropriate for those with DM and HTN at lower risk for CVD disease.

For patients with BP greater than 120/80 mm Hg, lifestyle interventions may include the DASH diet, moderation in alcohol intake, and increased physical activity and weight loss, if appropriate. Patients with confirmed office-based BP greater than or equal to 140/90 mm Hg should be prescribed pharmacologic therapy in addition to lifestyle interventions. Patients with confirmed office-based BP greater than or equal to 160/100 mm Hg should be prescribed two drugs or a single-pill combination of drugs demonstrated to reduce CVD events in addition to lifestyle interventions. Such drugs may include ACE-Is, angiotensin receptor blockers (ARBs), thiazide-like diuretics, or dihydropyridine calcium channel blockers. The recommended first-line treatment for HTN in patients with DM with urinary albumin-to-creatinine ratio greater than or equal to 300 mg/g creatinine or 30 to 299 mg/g creatinine is an ACE-Ir or ARB, at the maximum tolerated dose indicated for BP treatment. Patients with HTN who are not meeting BP targets on three classes of antihypertensive medications should be considered for mineralocorticoid receptor antagonist therapy.

Lipid Management

Management of serum lipids is essential for CVD health. The following general strategies, highlighted in the *ADA Standards of Care* can be used to guide individuals with DM.[70]

Lifestyle modifications including a Mediterranean or DASH diet, reduced intake of saturated and trans fat; increased intake of dietary n-3 fatty acids, viscous fiber, and plant stanols/sterols intake; increased physical activity and weight loss, if appropriate, are recommended. In addition to these lifestyle modifications, optimal glycemic control is necessary for patients with elevated triglyceride levels (greater than or equal to 150 mg/dL [1.7 mmol/L]) and/or low HDL cholesterol (less than 40 mg/dL [1.0 mmol/L] for men, less than 50 mg/dL [1.3 mmol/L] for women).

A high-intensity statin therapy should be added to lifestyle interventions for patients of all ages with DM and CVD or 10-year CVD risk greater than 20%. For patients with DM aged less than 40 years with additional CVD risk factors, a moderate-intensity statin in addition to lifestyle interventions should be considered. For patients with DM aged 40 to 75 years and greater than 75 years without CVD, a moderate-intensity statin can be used in addition to lifestyle therapy. In patients with DM who have multiple CVD risk factors, high-intensity statin therapy might be considered.

For patients with DM and CVD, if LDL cholesterol is greater than or equal to 70 mg/dL on maximally tolerated statin dose, an additional LDL-lowering therapy (e.g., ezetimibe) may be prescribed. Patients with fasting triglyceride levels greater than or equal to 500 mg/dL (5.7 mmol/L) should be evaluated for secondary causes of hypertriglyceridemia and consider medical therapy to reduce the risk of pancreatitis. In adults with moderate hypertriglyceridemia (fasting or nonfasting triglycerides 175 to 499 mg/dL), an evaluation of contributing lifestyle factors, secondary causes of hypertriglyceridemia, and medications that increase serum triglycerides should be explored.

Prothrombotic Factors

Control of prothrombotic factors is essential for CVD health in DM. The following general strategies, highlighted in the *ADA Standards of Care* can be used to guide individuals with DM.[70] Aspirin therapy (75 to 162 mg/day) can be used as a secondary prevention strategy in those with DM and a history of CVD. For those with CVD and DM with a documented aspirin allergy, clopidogrel (75 mg/day) should be used. Dual antiplatelet therapy, consisting of low-dose aspirin and a P2Y12 inhibitor, may be prescribed for a year after an acute coronary syndrome. Aspirin therapy (75 to 162 mg/day) may be considered as a primary prevention strategy in those with DM who are at increased CVD risk, after an assessment of patient benefits versus risks.

NURSING MANAGEMENT OF DIABETES

The above strategies are designed to prevent the development of CVD in people with DM. Central to these strategies is optimal glycemic, BP, lipid control, and a reduction in prothrombotic factors. Optimal metabolic control is necessary to prevent CVD in people with DM. This metabolic control is achieved by lifestyle interventions and pharmacologic treatment. Dodds[71] presents an approach to the management of T2DM. When this approach is modified for CVD prevention in T1DM and T2DM and CVD prevention, the following steps are included: (1) establish the diagnosis of DM; (2) implement insulin management in T1DM; and implement pharmacologic treatment for T2DM, if appropriate; (3) determine individualized glycemic targets; (4) provide DM education; (5) review lipid and BP targets; (6) review and assist with the implementation of lifestyle strategies; and (7) assess for associated comorbidities and treat or refer accordingly. Nurses can play a major role in diabetes education, management, and the prevention of CVD.

Diabetes education is defined as a collaborative process through which individuals who have DM or are at risk for developing DM gain knowledge and skills needed to modify behavior and successfully self-manage the disease and its related conditions.[72] The *American Association of Diabetes Educators* (AADE) has identified seven self-care behaviors that are essential for successful and effective self-management.[72] These behaviors include healthy eating, being active, monitoring, taking medication, problem solving, healthy coping, and reducing risks. The interventions needed to achieve these behaviors are designed to achieve optimal health status, to achieve a better quality of life.

Lifestyle interventions to improve nutrition and physical activity have been described previously. These interventions can be initiated, promoted, and supported by nurses. The pharmacologic therapies have been described above. Nurses can provide support in teaching patients about administering medications, understanding side effects, communicating with health care professionals, and monitoring and supporting adherence to medication regimens. Monitoring of blood glucose levels by fingerstick methods or continuous glucose monitoring (CGM) can help patients with T1DM or T2DM in understanding effects of therapies on blood glucose levels, and provide information needed to adjust medication therapy. Patients with T1DM may use insulin pump therapy with a CGM device that is independent from the pump or communicates with the pump. Nurses are essential in teaching patients about glucose monitoring, examining glucose trends, and correlating medications, insulin, physical activity and diet with these glucose levels. All patients with DM need an understanding of the impact of all therapies on reducing complications. Such an understanding may motivate patients to adhere to such therapies. Also, an understanding of acute risks of hypoglycemia and hyperglycemic emergencies is essential. Nurses can teach patients about such risks and strategies to minimize these acute risks. Living with diabetes is complex, exacting an intense burden on patients and families. Diabetes distress is the negative emotional impact of maintaining multiple treatment regimens; it has clinical importance, and may be associated with suboptimal self-care and glycemic control.[73] Nurses need to be cognizant of the need for support and counseling to address such issues.

Summary

Diabetes is a global epidemic that affects the lives of millions of people, and their families. There is evidence that CVD can be prevented through lifestyle changes and pharmacologic therapy. In addition, aggressive risk factor management, with particular focus on blood glucose, lipid, and BP control can mitigate the complications associated with diabetes, such as CVD. By promoting prevention, early treatment, and risk reduction of diabetes, nurses and health care professionals can improve DM outcomes. Teaching individuals and their families, promoting changes in delivery of care, tracking outcomes, and working within communities to promote access to safe places to exercise and eat healthy foods are all activities that health care professionals can participate in to raise awareness and motivate change. Nurses and health care providers, through advocacy, education, and one-on-one personal care can work to improve patient outcomes. This connection to persons diagnosed with diabetes, as well as their families, impacts patient care and can assist in slowing the pace of this global epidemic.

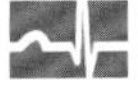

CASE STUDY

Patient Profile

Name/Age/Sex: **Michael Miller, 56-year-old male**

History of Present Illness

Mr. Miller presents for his annual physical. He states that he has been in his usual state of health. No presenting problems. He has been trying to watch his diet, but travels frequently for work and finds it difficult to eat healthy while traveling.

Past Medical History

Hypertension

Surgical History

Tonsillectomy (age 7)

Family History

Mother alive, age 77—HTN; father deceased—colon cancer

Social History

Nonsmoker, social drinker (2–5 drinks/wk), no illicit drug use

Medications

Lisinopril 10 mg PO q daily

Allergies

NKDA

Patient Examination

Vital Signs

BP 142/88; RR 16 breaths per minute; Temp 37.0°C; HR 75 beats per minute; Ht. 175 cm; Wt. 113 kg

Physical Examination

General: Awake, alert, and oriented. No distress noted.

Skin: Warm/dry/intact

Cardiac: No murmurs, gallops, or rubs are auscultated. S1 and S2 are heard and are of normal intensity.

Respiratory: Lung sounds are clear in all fields bilaterally without rales, ronchi, or wheezes.

Abdominal: Abdomen is soft, symmetric, and nontender without distention. No masses, hepatomegaly, or splenomegaly are noted. Obese.

Psychiatric: Appropriate mood and affect. Good judgment and insight. No visual or auditory hallucinations. No suicidal or homicidal ideation.

Testing

Waist circumference 42 in; HDL 36 mg/dL; Fasting glucose 115 mg/dL

Considerations

Key Questions

Patient was diagnosed with metabolic syndrome during his visit. Is there enough data to make this diagnosis? What are potential interventions?

Evidence

There is enough data to make this diagnosis. His waist circumference is above 40 in, in the setting of elevated blood pressure, HDL less than 40, as well as a fasting glucose of 115 mg/dL. At this point, it is recommended for him to start treatments of lifestyle changes as well as metformin. These interventions are based on data from the Da Qing Study, Finnish Diabetes Prevention Study, and the Diabetes prevention program research.

KEY READINGS

Beck J, Greenwood DA, Blanton L, et al. 2017 National standards for diabetes self-management education and support. *Diabetes Educ.* 2018;44(1): 35–50.

Dunlay SM, Givertz MM, Aguilar D, et al. Type 2 diabetes mellitus and heart failure: a scientific statement from the American Heart Association and Heart Failure Society of America. *J Card Fail.* 2019;25(8):584–619.

REFERENCES

1. International Diabetes Federation. *IDF Diabetes Atlas.* 8th ed. 2018. Available at https://www.idf.org/e-library/epidemiology-research/diabetes-atlas/134-idf diabetes-atlas-8th-edition.html. Accessed March 16, 2019.
2. Harding JL, Pavkov MF, Magliano DJ, et al. Global trends in diabetes complications: a review of current evidence. *Diabetologia.* 2019;62(1): 3–16.
3. International Diabetes Federation. *Diabetes and cardiovascular disease.* 2016. Available at http://www.idf.org/cvd. Accessed March 16, 2019.
4. Samson SL, Garber AJ. Metabolic syndrome. *Endocrinol Metab Clin North Am.* 2014;43(1):1–23.
5. Aguilar M, Bhuket T, Torres S, et al. Prevalence of the metabolic syndrome in the United States, 2003–2012. *JAMA.* 2015;313(19):1973–1974.
6. American Diabetes Association. *Statistics about diabetes.* 2018. Available at http://www.diabetes.org/diabetes-basics/statistics. Accessed March 14, 2018.
7. Laugesen E, Ostergaard JA, Leslie RD. Latent autoimmune diabetes of the adult: current knowledge and uncertainty. *Diabet Med.* 2015;32(7): 843–852.
8. Schwartz SS, Epstein S, Corkey BE, et al. The time is right for a new classification system for diabetes: rationale and implications of the beta-cell-centric classification schema. *Diabetes Care.* 2016;39(2):179–186.
9. American Diabetes Association. 2. Classification and diagnosis of diabetes: standards of medical care in diabetes—2018. *Diabetes Care.* 2018; 41(suppl 1):S13–S27.
10. Yang Y, Chan L. Monogenic diabetes: what it teaches us on the common forms of type 1 and type 2 diabetes. *Endocr Rev.* 2016;37(3):190–222.
11. The National Institute of Diabetes and Digestive and Kidney Diseases Health Information Center. *Monogenic diabetes (Neonatal diabetes mellitus & MODY).* 2017. Available at https://www.niddk.nih.gov/health-information/diabetes/overview/what-is-diabetes/monogenic-neonatal-mellitus-mody. Accessed June 16, 2019.
12. Centers for Disease Control and Prevention. Gestational Diabetes. *Gestational diabetes.* 2019. Available at https://www.cdc.gov/diabetes/basics/gestational.html. Accessed June 16, 2019.
13. Centers for Disease Control and Prevention. *National Diabetes Statistics Report, 2017.* Atlanta, GA: Centers for Disease Control and Prevention; 2017.
14. Agha-Jaffar R, Oliver N, Johnston D, et al. Gestational diabetes mellitus: does an effective prevention strategy exist? *Nat Rev Endocrinol.* 2016;12:533–546.
15. American Diabetes Association. 2. Classification and diagnosis of diabetes: standards of medical care in diabetes—2019. *Diabetes Care.* 2019; 42(suppl 1):S13–S28.
16. Dabelea D. The accelerating epidemic of childhood diabetes. *Lancet.* 2009;373(9680):1999–2000.
17. Atkinson MA, Eisenbarth GS, Michels AW. Type 1 diabetes. *Lancet.* 2014;383(9911):69–82.
18. Patterson CC, Harjutsalo V, Rosenbauer J, et al. Trends and cyclical variation in the incidence of childhood type 1 diabetes in 26 European centres in the 25 year period 1989–2013: a multicentre prospective registration study. *Diabetologia.* 2019;62(3):408–417.
19. Harjutsalo V, Sjoberg L, Tuomilehto J. Time trends in the incidence of type 1 diabetes in Finnish children: a cohort study. *Lancet.* 2008; 371(9626):1777–1782.
20. Mayer-Davis EJ, Lawrence JM, Dabelea D, et al. Incidence trends of type 1 and type 2 diabetes among youths, 2002–2012. *N Engl J Med.* 2017;376(15):1419–1429.
21. Snouffer E. An inexplicable upsurge: the rise in type 1 diabetes. *Diabetes Res Clin Pract.* 2018;137:242–244.
22. Pociot F, Lernmark A. Genetic risk factors for type 1 diabetes. *Lancet.* 2016;387(10035):2331–2339.
23. Chetan MR, Thrower SL, Narendran P. What is type 1 diabetes? *Diabetes: Basic Facts.* 2019;47(1):5–9.
24. Ziegler AG, Rewers M, Simell O, et al. Seroconversion to multiple islet autoantibodies and risk of progression to diabetes in children. *JAMA.* 2013;309(23):2473–2479.
25. Wang B, Yuan J, Yao Q, et al. Incidence and temporal trends of type 1 diabetes in China: a systematic review and meta-analysis. *Lancet Diabetes Endocrinol.* 2016;S13.
26. Negrato CA, Lauris JRP, Saggioro IB, et al. Increasing incidence of type 1 diabetes between 1986 and 2015 in Bauru, Brazil. *Diabetes Res Clin Pract.* 2017;127:198–204.
27. Shaltout AA, Wake D, Thanaraj TA, et al. Incidence of type 1 diabetes has doubled in Kuwaiti children 0-14 years over the last 20 years. *Pediatr Diabetes.* 2017;18(8):761–766.
28. Lonnrot M, Lynch KF, Elding Larsson H, et al. Respiratory infections are temporally associated with initiation of type 1 diabetes autoimmunity: the TEDDY study. *Diabetologia.* 2017;60(10):1931–1940.
29. Hummel S, Beyerlein A, Tamura R, et al. First infant formula type and risk of islet autoimmunity in The Environmental Determinants of Diabetes in the Young (TEDDY) study. *Diabetes Care.* 2017;40(3):398–404.
30. Rewers M, Ludvigsson J. Environmental risk factors for type 1 diabetes. *Lancet.* 2016;387(10035):2340–2348.
31. Kahn SE, Cooper ME, Del Prato S. Pathophysiology and treatment of type 2 diabetes: perspectives on the past, present, and future. *Lancet.* 2014; 383(9922):1068–1083.
32. Kwak SH, Park KS. Recent progress in genetic and epigenetic research on type 2 diabetes. *Exp Mol Med.* 2016;48(3):e220.
33. National Institute of Diabetes and Digestive and Kidney Diseases. *Risk factors for type 2 diabetes.* 2016. Available at https://www.niddk.nih.gov/health-information/diabetes/overview/risk-factors-type-2-diabetes. Accessed July 8, 2019.
34. McCulloch DK, Robertson RP. Pathogenesis of type 2 diabetes. In: Nathan DN, ed. *UpToDate 2018.* Available at https://www.uptodate.com/contents/pathogenesis-of-type-2-diabetes-mellitus. Accessed July 8, 2019.
35. National Cholesterol Education Program (NCEP) Expert Panel on Detection, Evaluation, and Treatment of High Blood Cholesterol in Adults (Adult Treatment Panel III). Third report of the National Cholesterol Education Program (NCEP) expert panel on detection, evaluation, and treatment of high blood cholesterol in adults (Adult Treatment Panel III) final report. *Circulation.* 2002;106(25):3143–3421.
36. Grundy SM, Cleeman JI, Daniels SR, et al. Diagnosis and management of the metabolic syndrome: an American Heart Association/National Heart, Lung, and Blood Institute Scientific Statement. *Circulation.* 2005;112(17):2735–2752.
37. Alberti KG, Eckel RH, Grundy SM, et al. Harmonizing the metabolic syndrome: a joint interim statement of the International Diabetes Federation Task Force on Epidemiology and Prevention; National Heart, Lung, and Blood Institute; American Heart Association; World Heart Federation; International Atherosclerosis Society; and International Association for the Study of Obesity. *Circulation.* 2009;120(16):1640–1645.
38. Kahn R, Buse J, Ferrannini E, et al; American Diabetes Association; European Association for the Study of Diabetes. The metabolic syndrome: time for a critical appraisal: joint statement from the American Diabetes Association and the European Association for the Study of Diabetes. *Diabetes Care.* 2005;28(9):2289–2304.
39. Booth GL, Kapral MK, Fung K, et al. Relation between age and cardiovascular disease in men and women with diabetes compared with non-diabetic people: a population-based retrospective cohort study. *Lancet.* 2006;368(9529):29–36.
40. Low Wang CC, Hess CN, Hiatt WR, et al. Clinical update: cardiovascular disease in diabetes mellitus. *Circulation.* 2016;133(24):2459–2502.
41. Kannel WB, McGee DL. Diabetes and glucose tolerance as risk factors for cardiovascular disease: the Framingham study. *Diabetes Care.* 1979;2(2):120–126.
42. Kannel WB, McGee DL. Diabetes and cardiovascular disease. The Framingham study. *JAMA.* 1979;241(19):2035–2038.
43. Diabetes Control and Complications Trial Research Group; Nathan DM, Genuth S, Lachin J, et al. The effect of intensive treatment of diabetes on the development and progression of long-term complications in insulin-dependent diabetes mellitus. *N Engl J Med.* 1993;329(14): 977–986.
44. UK Prospective Diabetes Study (UKPDS) Group. Effect of intensive blood-glucose control with metformin on complications in overweight patients with type 2 diabetes (UKPDS 34). UK Prospective Diabetes Study (UKPDS) Group. *Lancet.* 1998;352(9131):854–865.
45. Nathan DM, Cleary PA, Backlund JY, et al. Intensive diabetes treatment and cardiovascular disease in patients with type 1 diabetes. *N Engl J Med.* 2005;353(25):2643–2653.
46. Brownlee M. The pathobiology of diabetic complications: a unifying mechanism. *Diabetes.* 2005;54(6):1615–1625.

47. Schmidt AM. 22016 ATVB plenary lecture: receptor for advanced glycation endproducts and implications for the pathogenesis and treatment of cardiometabolic disorders: spotlight on the macrophage. *Arterioscler Thromb Vasc Biol.* 2017;37(4):613–621.
48. Wherrett DK. Trials in the prevention of type 1 diabetes: current and future. *Can J Diabetes.* 2014;38(4):279–284.
49. Skyler JS. Prevention and reversal of type 1 diabetes—past challenges and future opportunities. *Diabetes Care.* 2015;38(6):997–1007.
50. Herold KC, Bundy BN, Long SA, et al. An anti-CD3 antibody, teplizumab, in relatives at risk for type 1 diabetes. *N Engl J Med.* 2019;381(7):603–613.
51. Pan XR, Li GW, Hu YH, et al. Effects of diet and exercise in preventing NIDDM in people with impaired glucose tolerance: the Da Qing IGT and Diabetes Study. *Diabetes Care.* 1997;20(4):537–544.
52. Tuomilehto J, Lindström J, Eriksson JG, et al. Prevention of type 2 diabetes mellitus by changes in lifestyle among subjects with impaired glucose tolerance. *N Engl J Med.* 2001;344(18):1343–1350.
53. Knowler WC, Barrett-Connor E, Fowler SE, et al. Reduction in the incidence of type 2 diabetes with lifestyle intervention or metformin. *N Engl J Med.* 2002;346(6):393–403.
54. Li G, Zhang P, Wang J, et al. The long-term effect of lifestyle interventions to prevent diabetes in the China Da Qing Diabetes Prevention Study: a 20-year follow-up study. *Lancet.* 2008;371(9626):1783–1789.
55. Diabetes Prevention Program Research Group. Long-term effects of lifestyle intervention or metformin on diabetes development and microvascular complications over 15-year follow-up: the Diabetes Prevention Program Outcomes Study. *Lancet Diabetes Endocrinol.* 2015;3(11):866–875.
56. Chiasson JL, Josse RG, Gomis R, et al. Acarbose for prevention of type 2 diabetes mellitus: the STOP-NIDDM randomised trial. *Lancet.* 2002;359(9323):2072–2077.
57. Torgerson JS, Hauptman J, Boldrin MN, et al. XENical in the prevention of diabetes in obese subjects (XENDOS) study: a randomized study of orlistat as an adjunct to lifestyle changes for the prevention of type 2 diabetes in obese patients. *Diabetes Care.* 2004;27(1):155–161.
58. le Roux CW, Astrup A, Fujioka K, et al. 3 years of liraglutide versus placebo for type 2 diabetes risk reduction and weight management in individuals with prediabetes: a randomised, double-blind trial. *Lancet.* 2017;389(10077):1399–1409.
59. DeFronzo RA, Tripathy D, Schwenke DC, et al. Pioglitazone for diabetes prevention in impaired glucose tolerance. *N Engl J Med.* 2011;364(12):1104–1115.
60. DREAM (Diabetes REduction Assessment with ramipril and rosiglitazone Medication) Trial Investigators; Gerstein HC, Yusuf S, Bosch J, et al. Effect of rosiglitazone on the frequency of diabetes in patients with impaired glucose tolerance or impaired fasting glucose: a randomised controlled trial. *Lancet.* 2006;368(9541):1096–1105.
61. The Diabetes Prevention Program Research Group. Long-term safety, tolerability, and weight loss associated with metformin in the Diabetes Prevention Program Outcomes Study. *Diabetes Care.* 2012;35(4):731–737.
62. American Diabetes Association. 6. Glycemic targets: standards of medical care in diabetes—2019. *Diabetes Care.* 2019;42(suppl 1):S61–S70.
63. Davies MJ, D'Alessio DA, Fradkin J, et al. Management of hyperglycemia in type 2 diabetes, 2018. A consensus report by the American Diabetes Association (ADA) and the European Association for the Study of Diabetes (EASD). *Diabetes Care.* 2018;41(12):2669–2701.
64. Marso SP, Daniels GH, Brown-Frandsen K, et al. Liraglutide and cardiovascular outcomes in type 2 diabetes. *N Engl J Med.* 2016;375(4):311–322.
65. Holman RR, Bethel MA, Mentz RJ, et al. Effects of once-weekly exenatide on cardiovascular outcomes in type 2 diabetes. *N Engl J Med.* 2017;377(13):1228–1239.
66. Zinman B, Wanner C, Lachin JM, et al. Empagliflozin, cardiovascular outcomes, and mortality in type 2 diabetes. *N Engl J Med.* 2015;373(22):2117–2128.
67. Neal B, Perkovic V, Mahaffey KW, et al. Canagliflozin and cardiovascular and renal events in type 2 diabetes. *N Engl J Med.* 2017;377(7):644–657.
68. Fitchett D, Inzucchi SE, Cannon CP, et al. Empagliflozin reduced mortality and hospitalization for heart failure across the spectrum of cardiovascular risk in the EMPA-REG OUTCOME trial. *Circulation.* 2019;139(11):1384–1395.
69. Radholm K, Figtree G, Perkovic V, et al. Canagliflozin and heart failure in type 2 diabetes mellitus. *Circulation.* 2018;138(5):458–468.
70. American Diabetes Association. Standards of medical care in diabetes—2019 abridged for primary care providers. *Clinical Diabetes.* 2019;37(1):11–34.
71. Dodds S. The how-to for type 2: an overview of diagnosis and management of type 2 diabetes mellitus. *Nurs Clin North Am.* 2017;52(4):513–522.
72. Tomky D, Cypress M, Dang D, et al. AADE position statement; AADE7TM self-care behaviors. *Diabetes Educ.* 2008;34(3):445–450.
73. Dennick K, Sturt J, Speight J. What is diabetes distress and how can we measure it? A narrative review and conceptual model. *J Diabetes Complications.* 2017;31(5):898–911.

26 Cardiovascular Disease in Women

Kristan N.D. Langdon, Stacy Jaskwhich, Rajasree Roy, Divya Gupta, Puja K. Mehta

OBJECTIVES

1. Describe current scope of cardiovascular disease (CVD) in women.
2. Identify unique risk factors that place women at increased risk for development of CVD.
3. Describe sex-specific differences in prevention and pathophysiology of CVD.
4. Demonstrate knowledge of CV conditions common in women.

KEY QUESTIONS

1. When would you suspect a woman is at increased risk of CVD? How would you counsel her on risk factor reduction and management?
2. Women with myocardial infarction often have no obstructive epicardial stenosis. What are possible explanations for this presentation?
3. What is one crucial factor to address with women of childbearing age before being placed on a statin?
4. What is the best way to identify a woman presenting with SCAD? What education would you provide to the patient and her family about treatment?
5. What is a risk factor for development of peripartum cardiomyopathy?
6. What CVD risk factors are unique to women?

INTRODUCTION

Cardiovascular disease (CVD) remains the leading cause of death annually in the United States and is responsible for one in three female deaths.[1] An estimated 44 million women are affected annually by CVD which includes coronary artery disease (CAD) and stroke.[2] Eighty percent of cardiovascular events may be prevented by lifestyle modifications and education.[2] After a decade of aggressive public health awareness campaigns and platforms beginning in the early 1990s, mortality from CVD initially began to decline in women in 2000.[3] Nearly three decades later, in 2013, marked the first time CVD mortality in women dropped below that of men.[3,4] While research and community awareness have increased, "CVD in women continues to be understudied, underdiagnosed, and undertreated."[4] Despite recent overall decline in CVD mortality, there is an uptrend in CVD death in younger women (women between the ages of 35 and 50).[4] In this chapter, we review sex differences in CVD risk factors, presentation, and pathophysiology, and present some clinical cases to highlight CVD in women.

TRADITIONAL RISK FACTORS

Hypertension

Hypertension (HTN) is a major risk factor for both men and women, and is associated with highest CVD mortality risk worldwide.[5,6] Prior to the age of menopause, more men than women have HTN. After menopause, there is a steep incline in the prevalence of HTN in women[7] and more women than men have HTN in their later decades.[5,8] Treatment of HTN in women however remains suboptimal. Women are less likely to be treated to guideline-based target blood pressure goals compared to men.[7,9,81] The greatest risk for HTN is in African-American (AA) women who continue to have the highest prevalence of HTN and increased CVD morbidity and mortality compared to other female and male ethnodemographic groups.[10,11]

Diabetes

Metabolic syndrome, impaired blood glucose regulation, and Diabetes Mellitus type II (DM II) are significant risk factors for CVD and more common in women. Prognostically, diabetes is a stronger predictor of mortality in women compared to men,[12] and women with diabetes have a 40% greater risk of CVD than men.[13] Particularly in young and middle-aged women, who characteristically have lower risk for CVD compared to age-matched males, diabetic comorbidity increases (CAD) risk four- to fivefold.[6,14]

Hyperlipidemia

Presence of hyperlipidemia imparts the highest CV risk for women when adjusted to population-based overall CV risk.[6] During menopause transition, there is a shift in lipid composition with a rise in triglycerides and low-density lipoprotein levels (LDL-C) and a decrease in high-density lipoprotein levels (HDL-C).[6] This shift in lipid distribution is unfavorable. American College of Cardiology and American Heart Association (ACC/AHA) joint lipid guidelines[15] recommend a more intensified approach to statin use based on predicted CVD risk. Updated blood cholesterol guidelines further build on the 2013 ACC/AHA guidelines[16] that were the first to recommend statin therapy based on calculated atherosclerotic cardiovascular disease (ASCVD) risk score alone compared to LDL-C levels. Despite comparable lipid-lowering effect and guideline-based recommendation for statins in men and women, use of statins remains lower in women.[17] Disparity in statin use is not limited only to treatment management in prevention of CVD. Literature indicates that fewer women than men are prescribed a statin post acute myocardial infarction (AMI) despite ACC/AHA AMI guideline recommendations.[6,18]

Familial Hyperlipidemia

Familial hyperlipidemia (FH) is an autosomal dominant inherited disorder that leads to aggressive and premature CVD. In the United States alone, an estimated 1.3 million people live with FH, yet only 10% of them are diagnosed.[19] Men and women are affected equally by FH. If untreated, men have a 50% risk of having a heart attack by age 50, whereas women have a 30% risk by age 60.

Women with FH have additional challenges secondary to changes that occur during pregnancy. Cholesterol increases by about 25% to 50% during pregnancy resulting in extremely high cholesterol levels. Statins are the most effective cholesterol-lowering medications but they are not typically prescribed during pregnancy, which further complicates the treatment of hyperlipidemia. Most recommendations suggest that women should be off statin medications for approximately 3 months before trying to conceive as well as refrain from treatment during breast-feeding.[20] Low-density lipoprotein apheresis and bile acid sequestrants can be helpful during the peripartum and postpartum period with breast-feeding, but are generally not as effective as statin therapy.[20] For women that already have heart disease, it is important to discuss risk prior to conception. There is little data to determine how long it takes for cholesterol levels to return to a safe range after pregnancy.

Tobacco Use

Cigarette smoking is also a potent, yet entirely preventable risk factor for CVD in both men and women. One in four deaths from CVD can be attributed to smoking.[21] Female smokers have a 25% greater risk for CVD and three times the risk for myocardial infarction (MI) compared to male smokers.[6] Smoking cessation can substantially reduce CVD risk in both male and female smokers, and is the single most effective action to reduce CVD risk.[21]

Recently, electronic cigarettes (e-cigarettes) have been marketed and sold as an alternative to tobacco cigarettes. Despite claims of being safer than tobacco cigarettes, health concerns remain about increased lung and CVD health risks with use of e-cigarettes.[22] Nicotine, a powerful chemical of dependence, known to cause vasoconstriction and promote CVD is found in tobacco products, as well in many e-cigarettes. Nicotine, glycerol and its particulates found in e-cigarettes are associated with primary health concern(s).[22]

Physical Inactivity

More women than men in the United States (33.2% vs. 29.9%) are physically inactive.[6] A physically inactive lifestyle is the most prevalent CVD risk factor in women.[6] Physically inactive lifestyle is a term used to describe individuals who have a lifestyle containing insufficient levels of physical activity on a regular basis to meet current health-based activity recommendations. The AHA recommends 30 minutes of moderate physical activity most days of the week. A minimum of 150 minutes of moderate-intensity activity a week or 75 minutes of vigorous activity is recommended by AHA, plus 2 days of moderate–high-intensity muscle-strengthening activity to promote CV health and decrease CVD risk.[23] In order to combat and treat elevated blood pressure levels, cholesterol values, and/or increased body mass index (BMI), more minutes than the minimum 30 minutes most days of the week are needed. The AHA recommends 60 minutes most days of the week to achieve these goals.[23]

Family History

Family history of premature CAD in a first-degree relative, defined as male before the age of 55 years of age or female before 55 years of age, is an independent risk factor for CVD. Many factors contribute to individual and hereditary predisposition to CVD. However, when indicated, report of family history of premature CAD warrants further evaluation and stringent risk management of other potential CVD risk factors to decrease patient's individual risk.

FEMALE-SPECIFIC OR FEMALE PREDOMINATE CARDIOVASCULAR DISEASE RISK FACTORS

In addition to traditional CVD-related risk factors (HTN, diabetes mellitus, smoking, dyslipidemia, sedentary lifestyle, and family history), women have unique risk factors for CVD. Compared to males, women present with CVD with more comorbidities. Both autoimmune disorders and depression are more prevalent in women than men and have been indicated to be risk factors for CVD risk. Careful interviewing and documentation of reproductive history and lifestyle may reveal CVD risks not traditionally screened for and found in women.

Genetic Risk Factors

Lipoprotein(a)

Lipoprotein(a) [Lp(a)] is known to be proinflammatory, proatherogenic, prothrombotic and a strong genetic and independent risk predictor of CVD particularly in women. Even in the absence of other CVD risk factors, elevated Lp(a) alone has demonstrated increased CVD risk.[24] Elevated levels have not only been associated with advanced CAD, but also carotid disease, peripheral arterial disease, and renal artery stenosis.[25] Defined as a level greater than 50 mg/dL, elevated Lp(a) doubles CVD risk in women compared to female population risk with normal Lp(a) levels.[25] At Lp(a) levels greater than 120 mg/dL, a woman has triple the risk for CVD.[25] South Asian and African-American women exhibit the highest CVD risk with presence of elevated Lp(a).[80] In combination with other high-level CVD risk factors, such as diabetes, women with elevated Lp(a) have been associated with a threefold risk of CAD when measured by coronary artery calcium (CAC) scores.[26] There is no recommendation to routinely screen Lp(a) levels in women for primary prevention[27]; however, women at increased risk should be tested for this high marker not only to aid with risk stratification, but also to ensure therapy is optimally managed. It is reasonable to check Lp(a) levels in women with a history of premature CAD, a history of FH, a family history of early-onset CAD, a family history of elevated Lp(a), reoccurrence of CVD despite optimal medical therapy, or in those women with high risk on the 10-year ASCVD global risk score.[25]

Lp(a) levels can increase 8% to 30% as natural estrogen levels decline after menopause.[25] Evidence in the Estrogen/Progestin Replacement Study (HERS) demonstrated lower Lp(a) levels and less cardiovascular events compared to placebo when hormone replacement therapy (HRT) was used in women with known CAD. These results were opposed in the same study in women with low Lp(a), who had higher rates of CAD than the placebo group with HRT. Currently, no guideline recommendation exists for use of HRT in postmenopausal women for cardiovascular benefit.[24,28]

Treatment of Lp(a) remains challenging. The goal is to achieve low LDL levels while modifying all other risk factors. Lifestyle modifications alone through diet and exercise have not shown to improve Lp(a) significantly.[25] Statin drugs increase Lp(a) by potentially as much as 20%.[25] Certain statins, such as rosuvastatin, appear to elevate Lp(a) more frequently compared to other statin drugs. Nonstatin lipid-lowering therapy with nicotinic acid has shown benefit in reducing Lp(a) by 20% to 30%,[25] however has not shown consistent impact on long-term mortality studies.[29] Additionally, there is general consensus that nicotinic acid has a poor compliance rate,[29] possibly secondary to the undesirable side effect(s) of flushing, increased incidence of DM, and adverse events associated with gastrointestinal, musculoskeletal, dermatologic and bleeding complications with nicotinic acid. Some promise of treatment benefit exists with medications such as PCSK9 inhibitors and RNA-targeted therapies.[19] However, currently these medications are more costly and difficult to access.[25]

Autoimmune and Inflammatory Conditions

Inflammation is known to play a crucial role in the atherogenesis process.[30,31] Additionally, evidence shows chronic inflammation has a contributing role in cardiomyopathy.[30] Systemic autoimmune disorders, such as systemic lupus erythematosus (SLE), rheumatoid arthritis, and systemic sclerosis are highly prevalent in women, and are associated with an accelerated atherosclerotic risk.[9] Ischemic heart disease is a leading cause of morbidity and mortality in patients with SLE. Patients with rheumatoid arthritis have a two- to threefold higher risk of MI and increased CVD mortality.[32] Underlying chronic inflammation may contribute to increased risk, beyond the traditional CVD risk factors.[33,34] CAC score may help predict CVD risk in women with SLE and rheumatoid arthritis.[35] Coronary microvascular dysfunction (CMD) in the absence of obstructive CAD contributes to ischemia and chest pain symptoms in patients with autoimmune conditions.[34,36] "Patients with RA have a two to three-fold higher risk of MI and a 50% higher risk of stroke. For SLE, recent case- control series have indicated that the risk of MI is increased between nine to 50-fold over risk in the general population."[37] (p. 7)

Hormone

Oral Contraceptive Pills. Combined oral contraceptive pills (OCPs) can increase blood pressure and thrombotic risk in women but are not associated with increased CVD risk in healthy women without other CVD risk factors. Women who smoke and use OCPs are at significantly greater risk of thrombosis. When combined with use of tobacco cigarettes, OCPs have been associated with a sevenfold risk of CVD in female smokers compared to nonsmokers.[6] It is recommended women 35 years and older who smoke should avoid use of OCPs containing estrogen due to the increased risk of thrombosis. Additionally, in women with a history of venous thromboembolism, stroke, CVD, peripheral vascular disease, or a history of underlying thrombotic disorder, OCPs containing estrogen should be avoided.[38]

Menopause. Estrogen imparts strong anti-inflammatory properties protective against CVD, but because estrogen levels begin to decline in menopause, CVD risk in women increases in the decade after menopause.[39] This timing in increased CVD risk lags behind in men by approximately 10 years. While endogenous estrogen has shown protective effect against CVD, the benefits of HRT use in postmenopausal women are controversial.[28,40] At this time, no indication for use of HRT for primary or secondary prevention of CVD in any population or subpopulation exists.[28]

Pregnancy. Adverse pregnancy outcomes (APOs), such as gestational diabetes mellitus, pregnancy-induced HTN, preeclampsia, low or high birth weight of baby, and preterm delivery are CVD risk factors in women. Health care providers should be aware of these emerging cardiac risk factors in women. A diagnosis of preeclampsia doubles the risk of future diabetes and stroke, and quadruples the risk of HTN later in life.[41] Whether metabolic and physiologic stressors of pregnancy unmask underlying CV risk, or CV risk is exacerbated postpregnancy by APOs, the data demonstrates all women encountering APOs need ongoing monitoring and risk management therapy(ies) postpartum.[4,42] Pregnancy health history helps to identify at-increased risk for developing CVD and need for ongoing surveillance and strict risk factor modification as indicated by risk stratification. A section on pregnancy health history should be included in health history questionnaire(s) to screen for increased CVD risk in women.

Obesity

Obesity in the United States remains at epidemic proportion. Two out of every three adults in the United States are either obese or overweight based on 2013–2014 National Health and Nutrition Examination Survey (NHANES) data.[43] Women are more likely than men (40% vs. 35%) to be obese.[43] Obesity is a primary risk factor for CVD, as well as a risk factor for multiple other CV comorbid risk factors including DM II, HTN, and sleep apnea. Females predominantly develop subcutaneous fat, while men accumulate more visceral fat. Excess visceral fat and pericardial fat are CVD risk factors and nontraditional measures of obesity.[44] Obesity is also linked to heart failure with preserved ejection fraction (HFpEF), which is a heart failure syndrome more common in women.[45]

Psychosocial Factors

Psychological Stress

Psychological stress, including mental stress, appears to contribute to earlier CVD onset, morbidity, and mortality.[46] Young women (defined as women younger than 50 years old) are at particularly disproportionate risk for the adverse effects of mental stress on CVD risk.[47] "Compared to men, women have higher levels of psychological risk factors such as early life adversity, posttraumatic stress disorder, and depression. In addition, women are more prone to develop mental problems as a result of stress."[46] The exact pathways of correlation between increased emotional stress and increased CVD risk are currently unknown. Further research is still needed in this area, particularly in younger women, to better understand the link between emotional stress and CVD risk.

Depression

Depression has been associated with an increased risk of CAD. Women have twofold the rates of depression compared to men. In some studies, depression has been associated as an independent risk factor for CAD, in the absence of other CV risk factors, and poorer prognosis with acute coronary syndromes (ACSs) (unstable angina and MI).[6] Additionally, some studies have found a correlation between the severity of depression and CAD risk.[6] In women less than 55 years of age with CAD, comorbidity with depression has been associated with increased mortality.[6] A 2011 report by ACC/ACCF gave a class IIA rating for depression screening in patients post coronary artery bypass grafting (CABG) or post MI given acknowledged comorbidity between CAD and depression.[48] Treatment of depression was given a class IIb classification in the American College of Cardiology/ American College of Cardiology Foundation (ACC/ACCF) report and considered reasonable to consider given overall clinical benefit when depression was treated, despite no clear correlation between improved CAD outcomes and treatment of depression.[48]

MANAGING ASCVD RISK IN WOMEN

Guidelines for Cardiovascular Disease Risk Assessment in Women

Historically, women have received less preventive treatment and guidance on behavioral and therapeutic risk reduction for CVD compared to men at similar risk.[37] CVD prevention guidelines specifically for women are available and emphasize risk factor identification and treatment as appropriate. Management should include monitoring of efforts toward healthy weight loss and maintenance, optimizing blood pressure and blood glucose control, smoking cessation and avoidance of environmental tobacco exposure, and adequate levels of physical activity.[9]

Pooled Cohort Risk Assessment for ASCVD

The ASCVD risk calculator was developed in 2013 as part of the joint ACC/AHA cholesterol guidelines. A contemporary model to the Framingham and Reynolds Risk Score calculators, it was designed to predict individual 10-year risk for atherosclerotic CVD based on pooled, age-matched cohort population risk taking into account individual's race (which was not incorporated in previous risk calculations).[49] Risk calculation is for individuals between the ages of 20 and 79 years of age. In individuals with 10-year calculated risk greater than 7.5%, initiation of statin therapy is recommended by these cholesterol guidelines.

Advanced Imaging Modalities Used to Identify and Manage CVD Risk

When a patient is at intermediate risk based on ASCVD score, advanced diagnostics such as CAC scoring may be useful to further differentiate risk and help discuss statin initiation.[50,51] According to a study by Shaw et al.,[52] "detectable CAC was associated with 1.3 times higher hazard for CV death among women when compared with men ($P < 0.001$)." Evidence indicates cardiovascular mortality appears to be higher among women with more extensive, numerous, or larger CAC lesions.[52] Evidence of subclinical CAD by CAC can identify a patient's heightened risk. This risk may prompt the health care professional and patient to be more aggressive in treatment than they ordinarily may be based on pooled risk assessment alone.[15]

Aspirin Use in Women

In women younger than 65 years of age, aspirin 81 mg is not indicated for primary prevention of CVD. Earlier use may benefit women with increased risk for stroke, but to date has not been shown to decrease CVD risk.[39]

ATHEROSCLEROTIC CARDIOVASCULAR DISEASE IN WOMEN

Fifty-six percent of women are asymptomatic prior to presenting with MI, and one out of every four women will experience death as the first presenting symptom.[39] Additionally, women have increased in-hospital mortality following MI and tend to do worse overall post MI. Compared to men, more women are likely to have a second CVD event, and higher rates of systolic heart failure following MI.[39]

Nonobstructive CAD in Women

It has become clear over the past several decades that many patients who present with ACS as well as stable ischemic heart disease are found to have no obstructive CAD on further testing. This condition has recently been termed ischemia and no obstructive coronary artery disease (INOCA), and is a growing epidemic associated with an adverse cardiovascular prognosis despite no obstructive epicardial stenosis on angiogram.[17] The finding of INOCA is more common in women compared to men. The Women's Ischemia Syndrome Evaluation (WISE) Study has documented an adverse risk in this population of women which includes MI, stroke, sudden cardiac death, and heart failure, as well as heart failure and angina hospitalization.[53,54] A majority of patients with INOCA have CMD as a cause of their symptoms, and CMD has been liked with adverse CVD risk in both men and women.[55,56] CMD occurs due to endothelium-dependent and endothelium-independent mechanisms that affect myocardial blood flow regulation and contribute to ischemia.[57,58] CMD can occur with or without significant obstructive CAD. If a patient is having persistent angina after coronary stenting, coronary vasospasm related to stent placement and/or CMD may be an explanation of their recurrent symptoms if a cardiac etiology is suspected. CMD also occurs when there is a structural myocardial abnormality, such as in those with hypertrophic cardiomyopathy, left ventricular hypertrophy from HTN, and infiltrative cardiomyopathies such as amyloidosis.

There are structural and functional differences in coronary arteries that contribute to differences in heart disease presentation and pathophysiology. For example, while men most commonly experience myocardial ischemia from obstructive stenosis, women may experience myocardial ischemia and infarction from a wider range etiology including microvascular (small artery) dysfunction, coronary vasospasm, coronary artery dissection, coronary thrombi/emboli, or a combination of these.[59] Additionally, women have

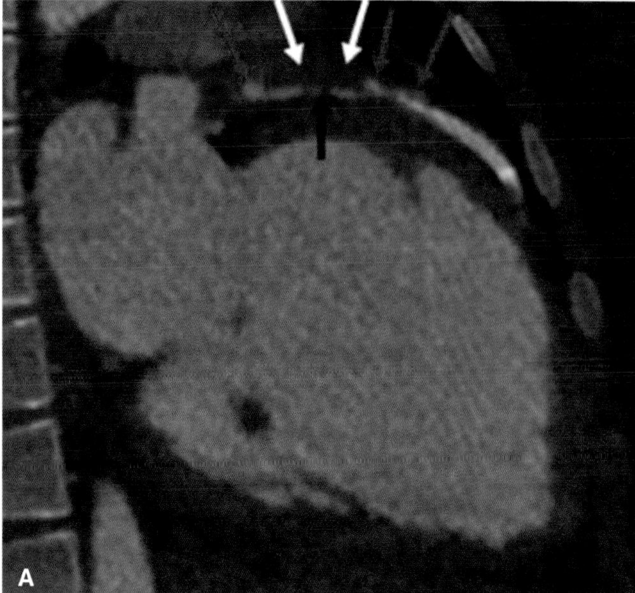

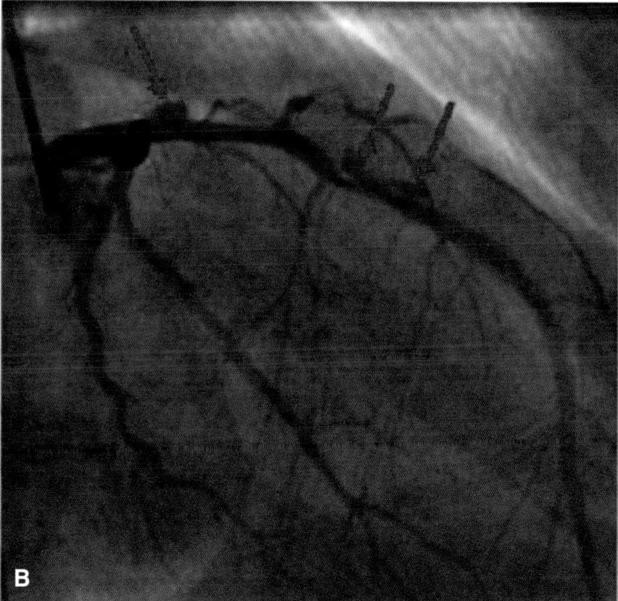

Figure 26-1. Case of a 24-year-old woman with a history of SCAD requiring subsequent coronary stenting. **(A)** Longitudinal image through the proximal LAD shows soft tissue attenuation surrounding the vessel corresponding to the thrombosed false lumen (*white arrows*) which compresses true lumen (*black arrow*). There are a few areas of contrast outpouchings that represent persistent filling of the false lumen (*red arrows*). The left ventricle is severely dilated and the patient's ejection fraction was 31%. **(B)** Right anterior oblique image from a coronary catheterization shows areas of persistent filling of the false lumen (*red arrows*) corresponding to the findings on CTA. (Used with permission from Klein J, Pohl J, Vinson EN, et al., eds. *Brant and Helms' Fundamentals of Diagnostic Radiology.* 5th ed. Philadelphia, PA: Wolters Kluwer Health & Pharma; 2018.)

less collateral coronary circulation growth over time.[39] In women, erosion of arterial intima or vasospasm is the most common etiology for AMI.[39] This is in opposition to plaque rupture, the most common mechanism for AMI in men. Sex-specific differences in CVD arising from differences in gene expression and functioning from the sex chromosomes also have been highlighted as a factor to explain differences between males and females.[37]

NONATHEROSCLEROTIC CARDIOVASCULAR CONDITIONS IN WOMEN

Spontaneous Coronary Artery Dissection

Spontaneous coronary artery dissection (SCAD) occurs with the creation of a false lumen by spontaneous separation within the coronary artery wall. The pressure-driven expansion of the false lumen and compression caused by intramural hematoma can lead to myocardial ischemia and infarction.[60] It is neither iatrogenic nor related to trauma.[61] Nonatherosclerotic SCAD is more common in younger female patients without cardiac risk factors, whereas atherosclerotic SCAD is more prevalent in older male patients with cardiac risk factors.[62,63] Due to underdiagnosis, the prevalence of SCAD in the general population is unknown.[61] Risk factors include hormonal changes during pregnancy or postpartum, fibromuscular dysplasia, stress, connective tissue disorders such as Ehlers–Danlos and Marfan syndromes, and inflammatory conditions such as SLE and ulcerative colitis. SCAD more commonly affects the left anterior descending artery, although other coronary arteries can be involved.[64,65] (p. 20)

Patients presenting with SCAD can have symptoms similar to ACS including chest pain, dyspnea, syncope, diaphoresis, and nausea with troponin elevation. In addition to MI, complications include sudden cardiac death, ventricular arrhythmias, and cardiogenic shock.[61,66] Coronary angiography is the gold standard for diagnosis, although intracoronary imaging with optical coherence tomography and intravascular ultrasound are useful to assess arterial wall integrity.[60,64] Conservative therapy is the preferred initial management, as most dissected segments heal spontaneously. Patients experiencing ongoing ischemia, infarction, hemodynamic instability or left main coronary artery involvement can have percutaneous coronary intervention (PCI) or CABG, with risks associated with both methods of revascularization. Vessel wall fragility often complicates PCI, as instrumentation can further advance the dissection (see Fig. 26-1).[63]

Stress/Takotsubo Cardiomyopathy

Takotsubo cardiomyopathy is a transient left ventricular dysfunction that is often stress induced and without evidence of obstructive CAD. Although there can be several variants, systolic apical ballooning of the left ventricle is the most common form with basal wall hyperkinesis.[67–71] This condition is more common in older women and prevalent in 1% to 2% of patients presenting with symptoms of ACS and troponinemia.[71,72] Although the pathogenesis is not fully understood, catecholamine toxicity, microvascular dysfunction, and coronary artery spasm are implicated.[73–75] While previously thought to be benign, emerging data indicate that it is associated with adverse complications.[76] Familial cases suggest a genetic predisposition,[77] and patients have a higher prevalence of psychiatric and neurologic disorders.[71]

Patients presenting with Takotsubo cardiomyopathy can have symptoms similar to ACS including chest pain, dyspnea, and syncope, frequently but not always triggered by physical or emotional stress.[71,78] Complications can include ventricular arrhythmias, sudden cardiac arrest, and cardiogenic shock.[78] Once pheochromocytoma and myocarditis have been ruled out, diagnostic criteria include transient left ventricular systolic dysfunction and wall motion abnormalities on transthoracic echocardiogram, absence of CAD or acute plaque rupture on angiography in the regions affected, and ECG changes or troponinemia.[79] In patients who are hemodynamically stable and without complications, conservative therapy with alleviating stress factors and treatment with beta blockers, ACE-Is or ARBs, and diuresis is the initial management (see Fig. 26-2).[71]

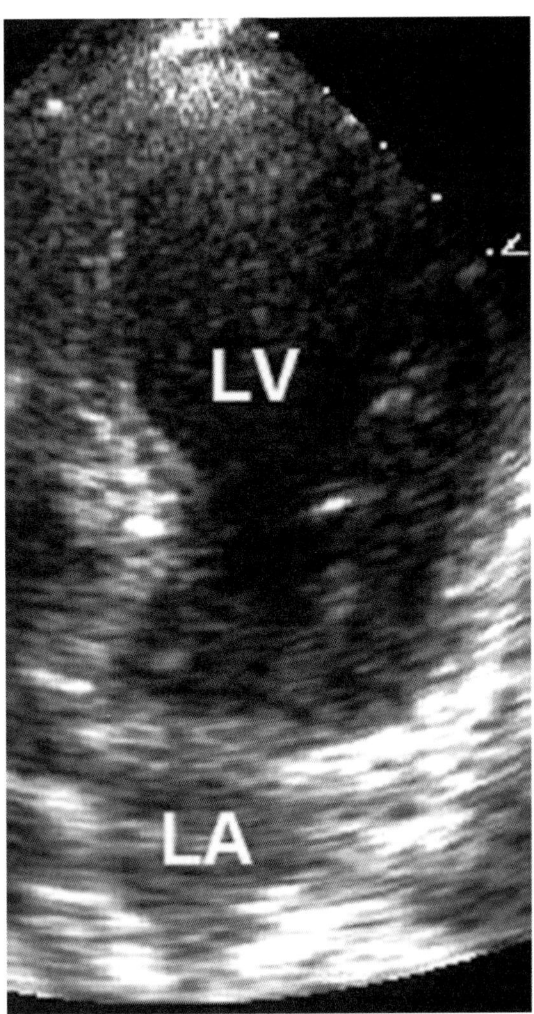

Figure 26-2. Takotsubo cardiomyopathy. LV, left ventricle; LA, left atrium. (Used with permission from Perrino AC, Reeves ST, eds. *Practical Approach to Transesophageal Echocardiography.* 3rd ed. Philadelphia, PA: Wolters Kluwer Health & Pharma; 2013.)

Peripartum Cardiomyopathy

Peripartum Cardiomyopathy occurs in 1/10,000 pregnancies in the United States. In the Southeastern region of the United States, the prevalence of peripartum cardiomyopathy is increased, attributed to the higher percentage of women with HTN, diabetes mellitus, and a larger percentage population of African-American ethnicity. While the entire pathogenic pathway is unknown at this time, several factors contributing to risk for peripartum cardiomyopathy have been proposed, including genetic component, environmental influence, altered physiology, immune factors of mother, and excessive production of prolactin. Sixty-five percent of women with peripartum cardiomyopathy will recover to having a left ventricular ejection fraction (LVEF) greater than 50% at 6 to 12 months post diagnosis. Reported outcomes are best in women with LVEF greater than 50% at the time of diagnosis. African-American women tend to have lower LVEF at the time of diagnosis, and lower recovery rates from peripartum cardiomyopathy. Overall mortality risk from peripartum cardiomyopathy in African-American women is 39%, a 10-fold risk compared to women from other racial groups. Any woman with peripartum cardiomyopathy needs long-term monitoring and informed discussion on increased risk with subsequent pregnancies. Even if LVEF returns to normal range, risk remains heightened. Most women are counseled to avoid subsequent pregnancies secondary to increased mortality risk.

CONCLUSION

CVD remains the leading cause of morbidity and mortality for women in the United States. Comorbidity with other disease states places women at increased risk and needs to be assessed and aggressively managed to decrease risk. Women present with unique risk factors, and prudent awareness of CV presentation differences in men versus women needs to be recognized by astute health care providers. As lifestyle disorders play the largest role in CVD, ongoing education, public awareness campaigns, and appropriate patient management are needed to decrease risk. Providers who care for women should be aware of sex differences in presentation of heart disease and etiologies such as SCAD, CMD, and stress cardiomyopathy. Appropriate risk identification and risk factor management may improve CVD outcomes in women.

FUTURE IMPLICATIONS

While we have made progress in CVD mortality reduction, heart disease remains the leading threat to women. Despite increased knowledge by health professionals and the public, women remain undertreated and understudied for CVD. Ongoing efforts in sex-specific research on women and CV diseases are needed, as well as outcome data to support best practices and patient management. Enhanced collaborative efforts between care providers and specialties will help close the gap when managing women with enhanced CV risk. Encouraging early intervention for primary and secondary prevention of CV-related disorders, and focused efforts at tertiary prevention to support improved patient outcomes and quality in care are still needed.

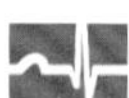

CASE STUDY 1

Patient Profile

Patient is a 45-year-old Caucasian female presenting for initial assessment to a cardiology clinic. She reports being asymptomatic but continues to have concerns about CVD secondary to early-onset CVD in her mother at age 54. She engages in modest exercise several times a week and eats a variety of foods, but a large portion of her diet consists of carbohydrates. She is apprehensive about taking medications and does not want prescription medications.

Medical History
Goiter treated with Synthroid, gestational DM

Family History
Mother had MI age 54; hypothyroidism; father with HTN and DM; both siblings with HTN and dyslipidemia

Lifestyle History
Exercise—45 minutes, 2–3 times/wk—treadmill and tennis; higher carbohydrate diet

Social History
Married, two children, works part time

Patient Examination

Vital Signs
BP 130/82 mm Hg; BMI 23.6; Total cholesterol 204 mg/dL; HDL 45 mg/dL; LDL 130 mg/dL; Triglycerides 145 mg/dL; Lp(a) 88 mg/dL

Workup

- ASCVD risk score 10 year 1.2%, optimal risk 0.4%
- Ordered CAC for further diagnostic evaluation given increased risk with elevated Lp(a), gestational DM, + FH in mother and opposition to medical therapy
- + CAC score 3.18—placing her in the 95th percentile CAD by CAC score

Interventions

What would be your recommendations to patient based on clinical findings during workup?

Recommendations

- Dietary counseling—Mediterranean/DASH diet
  - Low inflammatory diet—low carb/low sugar diet—mostly lean protein (fish, chicken), legumes and nuts, low glycemic fruits and vegetables (berries and greens), limited low-fat dairy, ensure low saturated fat/trans fat/cholesterol; high monounsaturated fats
- Increased soluble fiber
- Avoid processed foods
- Discussed starting Aspirin 81 mg/daily and moderate–high-intensity statin daily for secondary CAD prevention given presence of CAD by CAC scoring on advanced workup
- Increase physical activity to 75 minutes of vigorous intensity, or 150 minutes of moderate intensity per week
- Optimize blood pressure control, SBP less than 120, DBP less than 80 mm Hg
- Monitor HbA1c every 6–12 months over time. Goal less than 5.6

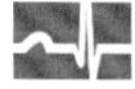

CASE STUDY 2

Patient Profile

A 42-year-old African-American female with no prior cardiac problems presents to hospital with history of fatigue, shortness of breath, and lower extremity edema for the past week, worsening over the past 2 days. Prior to symptoms starting, patient reports being in good health. Hypertension (HTN) has been modestly controlled in the past. Good control during most recent pregnancy. She has uncomplicated vaginal delivery of daughter 4 weeks ago. She is currently breast-feeding.

Medical History
HTN for 15 years. Modest controlled over time. Well-controlled HTN during pregnancy

Family History
Multiple members in immediate family with HTN (mother, father, siblings). Maternal grandmother with DM II

Lifestyle History
No routine exercise but considers self active with children and active job

Social History
Divorced. Has live-in boyfriend for the past 2 years. Three children—12- and 8-year-old sons and 1-month-old daughter; works full time in sales. Currently on maternity leave. Plans to return to work full time in 2 weeks

Patient Examination

Vital Signs
BP 85/60 mm Hg; HR 110 bpm; RR 26 breaths/min; BMI 21; Temp 98.2°F

Workup

- High-speed CT chest with contrast—acute PE found in left upper lobe
- ECHO—biventricular heart failure with LVEF 5–10% and RV and LV thrombi
- ECG—normal sinus rhythm
- BNP—950 pg/mL
- Troponin—0.5 ng/mL

Interventions

- Patient was started on Coumadin for anticoagulation with PE and discharged home on small doses of guideline-driven medical therapy for new-onset systolic heart failure/peripartum cardiomyopathy with ACE-I, B1-selective beta blocker (dose limited secondary to low blood pressure), and as needed, Lasix 20 mg daily. Goal to titrate medical therapy and add aldosterone receptor antagonist and hydralazine/nitrate, as able to complete guideline-driven medical therapy for peripartum cardiomyopathy.
- Started on fluid restriction of less than 2 L of fluid intake daily and less than 1.5-g sodium intake daily.
- Follow-up appointment in outpatient clinic by advanced heart failure team within 7 days postdischarge.
- Daily weight checks on home scale at same time each AM after awakening and using the restroom. Contact provider office for weight gain greater than 2 lb over night, or 4-lb cumulative gain over several days.
- Consider LifeVest application for prevention of sudden cardiac death with low LVEF less than 35%.

CASE STUDY 2 (*Continued*)

Recommendations

- Counseled to stop breast-feeding and to avoid future pregnancies due to enhanced risk with peripartum cardiomyopathy and mortality.
- Close follow-up and management by advanced heart failure team.
- Repeat ECHO and assessment of LVEF within the next 6 months.

Follow-Up

Patient was admitted 2 months after initial presentation with shortness of breath and fluid volume overloaded. Right heart catheterization was performed which revealed a Cardiac Index of 1.3. Patient was evaluated by advanced Heart Failure team and LVAD was placed. She was not a transplant candidate due to high antibody levels.

KEY READINGS

ACC/AHA Blood Cholesterol Guidelines—2018 Update. Rubenfire M. *2018 ACC/AHA multisociety guideline on the management of blood cholesterol.* 2018. Available at https://www.acc.org/latest-in-cardiology/ten-points-to-remember/2018/11/09/14/28/2018-guideline-on-management-of-blood-cholesterol. Accessed November 11, 2018.

Guidelines on Prevention of Cardiovascular Disease in Women—2011 Update. Mosca L, Benjamin EJ, Berra K, et al. Effectiveness-based guidelines for the prevention of cardiovascular disease in women–2011 update: a guideline from the American Heart Association. *Circulation.* 2011; 123:1243–1262.

REFERENCES

1. Centers for Disease Control and Prevention. *Heart disease facts.* 2017. Available at https://www.cdc.gov/heartdisease/facts.htm. Accessed March 3, 2019.
2. American Heart Association. *Heart disease statistics at a glance—Go Red for women.* Available at https://www.goredforwomen.org/about-heart-disease/facts_about_heart_disease_in_women-sub-category/statistics-at-a-glance. Accessed November 12, 2018.
3. Lundberg GP, Mehta LS, Sanghani RM, et al. Heart centers for women. *Circulation.* 2018. Available at https://www.ahajournals.org/doi/abs/10.1161/CIRCULATIONAHA.118.035351
4. Wenger N. *Perspective: a heartfelt plea.* 2017. Available at https://doi.org/10.1038/550S9a
5. Roger VL, Go AS, Lloyd-Jones DM, et al. Heart disease and stroke statistics–2011 update: a report from the American Heart Association. *Circulation.* 2011;123(4):e18–e209.
6. Wenger N. Tailoring cardiovascular risk assessment and prevention for women: one size does not fit all. *Glob Cardiol Sci Pract.* 2017;2017(1):e201701.
7. *Women and hypertension: beyond the 2017 guideline for prevention, detection, evaluation, and management of high blood pressure in adults.* n.d. Available at https://www.acc.org/latest-in-cardiology/articles/2018/07/27/09/02/women-and-hypertension. Accessed November 12, 2018.
8. Gudmundsdottir H, Høieggen A, Stenehjem A, et al. Hypertension in women: latest findings and clinical implications. *Ther Adv Chronic Dis.* 2012;3(3):137–146.
9. Mosca L, Benjamin EJ, Berra K, et al. Effectiveness-based guidelines for the prevention of cardiovascular disease in women–2011 update: a guideline from the American Heart Association. *J Am Coll Cardiol.* 2011; 57(12):1404–1423.
10. American Heart Association. *African Americans and heart disease, stroke.* 2015. Available at https://www.heart.org/en/health-topics/consumer-healthcare/what-is-cardiovascular-disease/african-americans-and-heart-disease-stroke. Accessed April 24, 2019.
11. Jones LM. *Reducing Disparities in Hypertension Among African American Women Through Understanding Information Seeking and Information Use* (Dissertation). Ann Arbor, MI: The University of Michigan; 2014.
12. Golden SH, Brown A, Cauley JA, et al. Health disparities in endocrine disorders: biological, clinical, and nonclinical factors–an Endocrine Society scientific statement. *J Clin Endocrinol Metab.* 2012;97(9):E1579–E1639.
13. Peters SAE, Huxley RR, Woodward M. Diabetes as risk factor for incident coronary heart disease in women compared with men: a systematic review and meta-analysis of 64 cohorts including 858,507 individuals and 28,203 coronary events. *Diabetologia.* 2014;57(8):1542–1551.
14. Kalyani RR, Lazo M, Ouyang P, et al. Sex differences in diabetes and risk of incident coronary artery disease in healthy young and middle-aged adults. *Diabetes Care.* 2014;37(3):830–838.
15. Rubenfire M. *2018 ACC/AHA multisociety guideline on the management of blood cholesterol.* 2018. Available at https://www.acc.org/latest-in-cardiology/ten-points-to-remember/2018/11/09/14/28/2018-guideline-on-management-of-blood-cholesterol. Accessed November 11, 2018.
16. Stone NJ, Robinson JG, Lichtenstein AH, et al. 2013 ACC/AHA guideline on the treatment of blood cholesterol to reduce atherosclerotic cardiovascular risk in adults: a report of the American College of Cardiology/American Heart Association Task Force on Practice Guidelines. *Circulation.* 2014;129(25 suppl 2):S1–S45.
17. Bairey Merz CN, Pepine CJ, Walsh MN, et al. Ischemia and No Obstructive Coronary Artery Disease (INOCA): developing evidence-based therapies and research agenda for the next decade. *Circulation.* 2017;135(11):1075–1092.
18. O'Gara PT, Kushner FG, Ascheim DD, et al. 2013 ACCF/AHA guideline for the management of ST-elevation myocardial infarction. *J Am Coll Cardiol.* 2013;61(4):e78–e140.
19. Familial Hypercholesterolemia Foundation. n.d. *Familial hypercholesterolemia.* Available at https://thefhfoundation.org. Accessed November 11, 2018.
20. Eapen DJ, Valiani K, Reddy S, et al. Management of familial hypercholesterolemia during pregnancy: case series and discussion. *J Clin Lipidol.* 2012;6(1):88–91.
21. Centers for Disease Control and Prevention. *2014 Surgeon General's report: The health consequences of smoking- 50 years of progress.* Available at https://www.cdc.gov/tobacco/data_statistics/sgr/50th-anniversary/index.htm.
22. Morris PB, Ference BA, Jahangir E, et al. Cardiovascular effects of exposure to cigarette smoke and electronic cigarettes: clinical perspectives from the prevention of cardiovascular disease section leadership council and early career councils of the American College of Cardiology. *J Am Coll Cardiol.* 2015;66(12):1378–1391.
23. American Heart Association. *American Heart Association recommendations for physical activity in adults and kids.* n.d. Available at https://www.heart.org/en/healthy-living/fitness/fitness-basics/aha-recs-for-physical-activity-in-adults. Accessed October 30, 2018.
24. Costello BT, Silverman ER, Doukky R, et al. Lipoprotein(a) and increased cardiovascular risk in women. *Clin Cardiol.* 2016;39(2):96–102.
25. Lundberg GP. Lipoprotein(a) and CVD risk in women: Benefit or added cost. *The Heartbeat: A Newsletter for Clinicians.* 2018;1(3):1–3.
26. Verweij SL, de Ronde MWJ, Verbeek R, et al. Elevated lipoprotein(a) levels are associated with coronary artery calcium scores in asymptomatic individuals with a family history of premature atherosclerotic cardiovascular disease. *J Clin Lipidol.* 2018;12(3):597–603.e1.
27. Cook NR, Mora S, Ridker PM. Lipoprotein(a) and cardiovascular risk prediction among women. *J Am Coll Cardiol.* 2018;72(3):287–296.
28. The American College of Obstetricians and Gynecologists (ACOG). *Hormone therapy and heart disease.* 2013. Available at https://www.acog.org/Clinical-Guidance-and-Publications/Committee-Opinions/Committee-on-Gynecologic-Practice/Hormone-Therapy-and-Heart-Disease. Accessed November 7, 2018.
29. The HPS2-THRIVE Collaborative Group. Effects of extended-release niacin with laropiprant in high-risk patients. *N Engl J Med.* 2014;371(3):203–212.
30. Kabbany MT. Cardiovascular diseases in chronic inflammatory disorders. *J Am Coll Cardiol.* 2016. Available at https://www.acc.org/latest-in-cardiology/articles/2016/07/15/10/04/cardiovascular-diseases-in-chronic-inflammatory-disorders. Accessed November 7, 2018.
31. Frostegård J. Atherosclerosis in patients with autoimmune disorders. *Arterioscler Thromb Vasc Biol.* 2005;25(9):1776–1785.
32. Zhang J, Chen L, Delzell E, et al. The association between inflammatory markers, serum lipids and the risk of cardiovascular events in patients with rheumatoid arthritis. *Ann Rheum Dis.* 2014;73(7):1301–1308.

33. Faccini A, Kaski JC, Camici PG. Coronary microvascular dysfunction in chronic inflammatory rheumatoid diseases. *Eur Heart J.* 2016; 37(23):1799–1806.
34. Recio-Mayoral A, Mason JC, Kaski JC, et al. Chronic inflammation and coronary microvascular dysfunction in patients without risk factors for coronary artery disease. *Eur Heart J.* 2009;30(15):1837–1843.
35. Chung CP, Oeser A, Avalos I, et al. Cardiovascular risk scores and the presence of subclinical coronary artery atherosclerosis in women with systemic lupus erythematosus. *Lupus.* 2006;15:562–569.
36. Ishimori ML, Martin R, Berman DS, et al. Myocardial ischemia in the absence of obstructive coronary artery disease in systemic lupus erythematosus. *JACC Cardiovasc Imaging.* 2011;4(1):27–33.
37. Garcia M, Mulvagh SL, Merz CN, et al. Cardiovascular disease in women: clinical perspectives. *Circ Res.* 2016;118(8):1273–1293.
38. Bonnema RA, McNamara MC, Spencer AL. Contraception choices in women with underlying medical conditions. *Am Fam Physician.* 2010;82(6):621–628.
39. Murphy N. *Women & heart disease: An evidence-based update. Webinar presentation by: National Nurse-Led Care Consortium and American Academy of Nurse Practitioners.* 2018.
40. American College of Cardiology. *Hormone replacement therapy associated with lower mortality*, 2017 Available at https://www.acc.org/about-acc/press-releases/2017/03/08/13/09/hormone-replacement-therapy-associated-with-lower-mortality. Accessed November 7, 2018.
41. Carr DB, Newton KM, Utzschneider KM, et al. Preeclampsia and risk of developing subsequent diabetes. *Hypertens Pregnancy.* 2009;28(4):435–447.
42. Mehta PK, Minissian M, Bairey Merz CN. Adverse pregnancy outcomes and cardiovascular risk factor management. *Semin Perinatol.* 2015;39(4):268–275.
43. National Institute of Diabetes and Digestive and Kidney Diseases. n.d. *Overweight & obesity statistics.* Available at https://www.niddk.nih.gov/health-information/health-statistics/overweight-obesity. Accessed October 30, 2018.
44. Mahabadi AA, Massaro JM, Rosito GA, et al. Association of pericardial fat, intrathoracic fat, and visceral abdominal fat with cardiovascular disease burden: the Framingham Heart Study. *Eur Heart J.* 2009;30(7): 850–856.
45. Savji N, Meijers WC, Bartz TM, et al. The association of obesity and cardiometabolic traits with incident HFpEF and HFrEF. *JACC Heart Fail.* 2018;6(8):701–709.
46. National Heart, Lung, and Blood Institute (NHLBI). n.d. *Emotional stress and heart disease in women: An interview with Dr. Viola Vaccarino.* Available at https://www.nhlbi.nih.gov/news/2014/emotional-stress-and-heart-disease-women-interview-dr-viola-vaccarino. Accessed November 10, 2018.
47. Vaccarino V, Wilmot K, Al Mheid I, et al. Sex differences in mental stress-induced myocardial ischemia in patients with coronary heart disease. *J Am Heart Assoc.* 2016;5(9):e003630.
48. Smith SC, Benjamin EJ, Bonow RO, et al. AHA/ACCF secondary prevention and risk reduction therapy for patients with coronary and other atherosclerotic vascular disease: 2011 update. *Circulation.* 2011; 124(22):2458–2473.
49. Preiss D, Kristensen SL. The new pooled cohort equations risk calculator. *Can J Cardiol.* 2015;31(5):613–619.
50. Mitchell JD, Fergestrom N, Gage BF, et al. Impact of statins on cardiovascular outcomes following coronary artery calcium scoring. *J Am Coll Cardiol.* 2018;72(25):3233–3242.
51. Mulders TA, Sivapalaratnam S, Stroes ESG, et al. Asymptomatic individuals with a positive family history for premature coronary artery disease and elevated coronary calcium scores benefit from statin treatment: a post hoc analysis from the St. Francis Heart Study. *JACC Cardiovasc Imaging.* 2012;5(3):252–260.
52. Shaw LJ, Min JK, Nasir K, et al. Sex differences in calcified plaque and long-term cardiovascular mortality: observations from the CAC Consortium. *Eur Heart J.* 2018;39(41):3727–3735.
53. Gulati M, Cooper-DeHoff RM, McClure C, et al. Adverse cardiovascular outcomes in women with nonobstructive coronary artery disease. *Arch Intern Med.* 2009;169(9):843–850.
54. von Mering Gregory O, Arant Christopher B, Wessel Timothy R, et al. Abnormal coronary vasomotion as a prognostic indicator of cardiovascular events in women. *Circulation.* 2004;109(6):722–725.
55. Taqueti VR, Shaw LJ, Cook NR, et al. Excess cardiovascular risk in women relative to men referred for coronary angiography is associated with severely impaired coronary flow reserve, not obstructive disease. *Circulation.* 2017;135(6):566–577.
56. Pepine CJ, Anderson RD, Sharaf BL, et al. Coronary microvascular reactivity to adenosine predicts adverse outcome in women evaluated for suspected ischemia. *J Am Coll Cardiol.* 2010;55(25):2825–2832.
57. Camici PG, d'Amati G, Rimoldi O. Coronary microvascular dysfunction: mechanisms and functional assessment. *Nat Rev Cardiol.* 2015;12(1):48–62.
58. European Society of Cardiology. *Coronary microvascular dysfunction: An update.* 2014. Available at https://www.escardio.org/Journals/E-Journal-of-Cardiology-Practice/Volume-13/Coronary-microvascular-dysfunction-an-update. Accessed November 9, 2018.
59. Pasupathy S, Tavella R, Beltrame JF. Myocardial Infarction With Nonobstructive Coronary Arteries (MINOCA): the past, present, and future management. *Circulation.* 2017;135(16):1490–1493.
60. Alfonso F, Paulo M, Gonzalo N, et al. Diagnosis of spontaneous coronary artery dissection by optical coherence tomography. *J Am Coll Cardiol.* 2012;59(12):1073–1079
61. Saw J, Mancini GBJ, Humphries KH. Contemporary review on spontaneous coronary artery dissection. *J Am Coll Cardiol.* 2016;68(3):297–312.
62. Hayes SN, Kim ESH, Saw J, et al. Spontaneous coronary artery dissection: current state of the science: a scientific statement from the American Heart Association. *Circulation.* 2018;137(19):e523–e557.
63. Nishiguchi T, Tanaka A, Ozaki Y, et al. Prevalence of spontaneous coronary artery dissection in patients with acute coronary syndrome. *Eur Heart J Acute Cardiovasc Care.* 2016;5(3):263–270.
64. Saw J, Aymong E, Sedlak T, et al. Spontaneous coronary artery dissection: association with predisposing arteriopathies and precipitating stressors and cardiovascular outcomes. *Circ Cardiovasc Interv.* 2014;7(5):645–655.
65. Vijayaraghavan R, Verma S, Gupta N, et al. Pregnancy-related spontaneous coronary artery dissection. *Circulation.* 2014;130(21):1915–1920.
66. Tweet MS, Hayes SN, Pitta SR, et al. Clinical features, management, and prognosis of spontaneous coronary artery dissection. *Circulation.* 2012; 126(5):579–588.
67. Akashi YJ, Goldstein DS, Barbaro G, et al. Takotsubo cardiomyopathy. *Circulation.* 2008;118(25):2754–2762.
68. Citro R, Lyon AR, Meimoun P, et al. Standard and advanced echocardiography in Takotsubo (stress) cardiomyopathy: clinical and prognostic implications. *J Am Soc Echocardiogr.* 2015;28(1):57–74.
69. Sato H, Tateishi H, Uchida T, et al. Takotsubo type cardiomyopathy due to multivessel spasm. In: Kodama K, Haze K, Hon M, eds. *Clinical aspect of myocardial injury: from ischemia to heart failure.* Kagaku Hyoronsha, Tokyo: 1990;56–64.
70. Sharkey SW, Maron BJ. Epidemiology and clinical profile of Takotsubo cardiomyopathy. *Circ J.* 2014;78(9):2119–2128.
71. Templin C, Ghadri JR, Diekmann J, et al. Clinical features and outcomes of Takotsubo (stress) cardiomyopathy. *N Engl J Med.* 2015;373(10):929–938.
72. Kurowski V, Kaiser A, von Hof K, et al. Apical and midventricular transient left ventricular dysfunction syndrome (tako-tsubo cardiomyopathy) frequency, mechanisms, and prognosis. *Chest.* 2007;132(3):809–816.
73. Nef HM, Möllmann H, Kostin S, et al. Tako-Tsubo cardiomyopathy: intraindividual structural analysis in the acute phase and after functional recovery. *Eur Heart J.* 2007;28(20):2456–2464.
74. Paur H, Wright PT, Sikkel MB, et al. High levels of circulating epinephrine trigger apical cardiodepression in a β2-adrenergic receptor/Gi-dependent manner: a new model of Takotsubo cardiomyopathy. *Circulation.* 2012;126(6):697–706.
75. Vitale C, Rosano GMC, Kaski JC. Role of coronary microvascular dysfunction in Takotsubo cardiomyopathy. *Circ J.* 2016;80(2):299–305.
76. de Chazal HM, Del Buono MG, Keyser-Marcus L, et al. Stress cardiomyopathy diagnosis and treatment: JACC state-of-the-art review. *J Am Coll Cardiol.* 2018;72(16):1955–1971.
77. Kumar G, Holmes DR, Prasad A. "Familial" apical ballooning syndrome (Takotsubo cardiomyopathy). *Int J Cardiol.* 2010;144(3):444–445.
78. Tsuchihashi K, Ueshima K, Uchida T, et al. Transient left ventricular apical ballooning without coronary artery stenosis: a novel heart syndrome mimicking acute myocardial infarction. *J Am Coll Cardiol.* 2001;38(1):11–18.
79. Scantlebury DC, Prasad A. Diagnosis of Takotsubo cardiomyopathy. *Circ J.* 2014;78(9):2129–2139.
80. Lipoprotein(a) Foundation. n.d. Available at https://www.lipoprotein-afoundation.org/. Accessed November 9, 2018.
81. Sidney S, Rosamond WD, Howard VJ, et al. The "heart disease and stroke statistics—2013 update" and the need for a national cardiovascular surveillance system. *Circulation.* 2013;127(1):21–23.

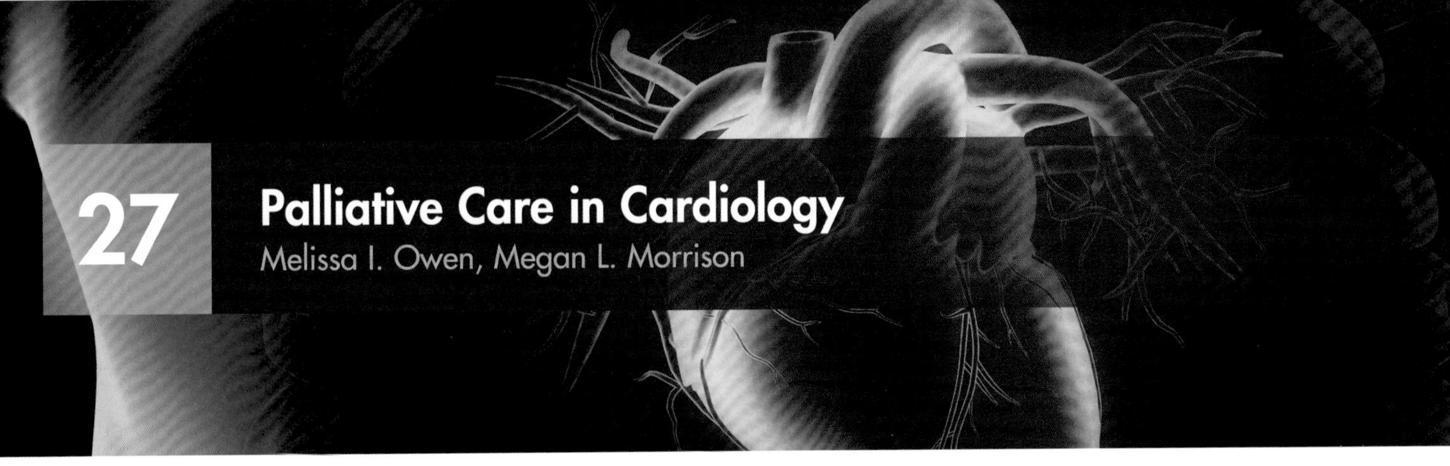

27 Palliative Care in Cardiology

Melissa I. Owen, Megan L. Morrison

OBJECTIVES

1. Describe the scope and implementation of palliative care in cardiology.
2. Differentiate between generalist practice and need for specialty referral.
3. Identify symptom assessment and other palliative care tools appropriate for use in cardiac patients.
4. Describe advance directive use in cardiac patients, including various devices.
5. Describe end-of-life considerations in cardiac disease.

KEY QUESTIONS

1. What is palliative care and how does it differ from hospice?
2. How is palliative care provided to those with cardiac disease?
3. What are important end-of-life considerations for patients with cardiac disease?

BACKGROUND

Historical State and Context

The Hospice and Palliative Care movement is attributed to Dame Cicely Saunders. Saunders was first a nurse in the United Kingdom, and later became a physician. Her focus was on pain and symptom management in the terminally ill. Palliative care was initially developed within the oncology specialty, and focused on creating a better death for those whose cancer was not curable, with the first hospice opening in London, UK in 1967. Over time, the focus of palliative care has shifted from terminal disease and end of life to providing relief of suffering earlier within the course of disease to increase quality of life. It has also expanded to include not only oncology patients, but those patients with any potentially life-limiting illness, including cardiac disease.[1]

SCOPE AND STANDARDS OF PALLIATIVE CARE IN CARDIOLOGY

Overview of Palliative Care

Scope and Standards of Palliative Care in Cardiology Overview of Palliative Care

The World Health Organization (WHO) defines palliative care as "an approach that improves the quality of life of patients and their families facing the problem associated with life-threatening illness, through the prevention and relief of suffering by means of early identification and impeccable assessment and treatment of pain and other problems, physical, psychosocial and spiritual."[2] In 2004, a consortium of the American Academy of Hospice and Palliative Medicine, the center to Advance Palliative Care, Hospice and Palliative Nurses' Association, Last Acts Partnership, and National Hospice and Palliative Care Organization published the first edition of the National Consensus Project (NCP) for Quality Palliative Care: Clinical Practice Guidelines for Quality Palliative Care.[3] The NCP defines palliative care as an interdisciplinary approach to the provision of care designed to reduce suffering and improve quality of life for patients and their families with serious, life-threatening illnesses. Tenets central to this philosophy of care provision include: coordinated services provided by an interdisciplinary team, collaboration and communications among and between patients, families, and nonpalliative care providers, and respect for patient and family hopes and dignity throughout the course of care through death. Most importantly, these services are provided independent of curative or life-prolonging care.[4]

The NCP Clinical Practice Guidelines identify eight domains of care. These include: 1. Structures and Processes of Care, 2. Physical Aspects of Care, 3. Psychological and Psychiatric Aspects of Care, 4. Social Aspects of Care, 5. Spiritual, Religious, and Existential Aspects of Care, 6. Cultural Aspects of Care, 7. Care for the Patient nearing the End of Life, and 8. Ethical and Legal Aspects of Care.[4] Table 27-1 includes brief descriptions of each of these domains. The goal of quality palliative care provision is relief of physical, psychological, emotional, and spiritual suffering and distress of patients and

Table 27-1 • DOMAINS OF PALLIATIVE CARE ACCORDING TO THE NATIONAL CONSENSUS PROJECT

Domain	Description
1. Structures and Processes of Care	Interdisciplinary team collaboration and engagement
2. Physical Aspects of Care	Assessment and treatment of physical symptoms
3. Psychological and Psychiatric Aspects of Care	Assessment, to identify and address mental health aspects of chronic illness
4. Social Aspects of Care	Assessment to identify and address social and family support needs
5. Spiritual, Religious, and Existential Aspects of Care	Assessment of patient and family spiritual concerns and unmet needs
6. Cultural Aspects of Care	Impact of culture on palliative care delivery and patient experience from diagnosis to death and bereavement
7. Care of the Patient Nearing the End of Life	Addresses symptoms and situations common in the last days to weeks of life
8. Ethical and Legal Aspects of Care	Advance care planning and legal considerations in palliative care provision to support patient autonomy

families. Key to this is a comprehensive assessment of needs which includes both the patient's needs as well as the caregiver. Ideally, palliative care is designed to be incorporated across the spectrum of illness, beginning with supportive care at the time of diagnosis of a serious or life-threatening illness and continues throughout the patient's illness trajectory. After the patient's death, care for the family continues through bereavement care. Palliative care was developed from the Hospice model initially used in cancer patients, which have a more predictable clinical course.

The clinical course for patients with noncancer diagnoses is less predictable and nonlinear.[5] Therefore, the model was revised to include an illustration of exacerbations and stabilization, which are relevant in the cardiac patient.

Barriers to Palliative Care Provision

One barrier for the incorporation of palliative care for the cardiac patient is related to poor understanding of the purpose. It is important to note that while end-of-life and hospice care are important palliative care interventions for the patient who meets specific criteria, palliative care is designed to serve a much broader chronically ill or acutely ill population independent of disease prognosis. As noted previously, palliative care evolved from the Hospice model of care. In 1998, the Lasts Acts campaign of the Robert Wood Johnson Foundation released a policy statement which called for an expansion of care to include palliative care as an important treatment modality to be provided in conjunction with curative and life-prolonging therapies.[6] However, confusion surrounding the purpose of palliative care and the association of palliative care with end-of-life care still continues to be identified as a barrier to care provision for patients and healthcare providers.[7] In a 2011 public opinion research survey, 70% of respondents indicated they were "not at all knowledgeable" about palliative care. Furthermore, physician respondents tended to equate palliative care with "comfort care" used at the end of life.[8] Other studies have identified several physician barriers related to incorporation of palliative care in advanced HF patients. These included difficulty in prognostication due to an uncertain disease trajectory, fear of destroying hope in patients if end-of-life discussions are initiated too early, lack of clear referral triggers, and association of palliative care with a specialized team of home care providers.[9–11] In contrast to the healthcare provider perceptions, patients with advanced HF often coped well with this information, although a preconceived equivalence of *palliative care* with *hospice* may make patients less likely to accept these types of services.

Multiple resources exist for provider training in palliative care. One program is the Education in Palliative and End-of-life Care Program (EPEC). This program seeks to educate and enhance healthcare providers on basic skills in palliative care provision including communication, decision making, symptom management, and psychosocial care.[12] Another well-researched program which focuses specifically on care of the dying, is the End-of-Life Nursing Education Consortium (ELNEC) core curriculum. The purpose of this training is to educate nurses and other healthcare providers to improve care. Over 19,500 participants have attended train-the-trainer sessions, and is offered worldwide.[13] Nurses and other healthcare providers can also seek certification through the Hospice and Palliative Credentialing Center.[14]

Cardiac-Specific Guidelines

Several specific cardiac disease management guidelines include indications for palliative care. The American Heart Association/American Stroke Association issued a policy statement in 2016 on the importance of palliative care for patients with advanced cardiovascular disease, and recommendations for consideration.[15] The 2013 *ACCF/AHA Guideline for the Management of Heart Failure* includes palliative care as a recommended care approach for advanced HF. Moreover, this guideline indicates evaluation for cardiac transplantation or VAD placement should include a formal palliative care consult.[16] The Centers for Medicare & Medicaid Services (CMS) requires a tertiary palliative care consult for all patients undergoing evaluation for mechanical circulatory support devices.[17] Finally, palliative care is also recommended for incorporation for those patients with valvular heart disease, especially those patients undergoing transcatheter aortic valve replacement (TAVR). Specific interventions should include advance care planning and goals of care discussions early in the process, including discussion of life expectancy, anticipated improvement postprocedure, and end-of-life planning.[18,19]

Layers of Palliative Care Provision

When considering incorporation of palliative care in the trajectory of chronic illness, it can be provided on three levels—primary, secondary, and tertiary. Primary palliative care involves a holistic approach provided by the patient's primary healthcare provider through mechanisms such as symptom management, psychological and social support, and spiritual care. Primary palliative care is viewed as basic skills that all physicians, nurses, and other team members should possess when caring for patients with life-threatening illnesses. Secondary palliative care includes the addition of an interdisciplinary team with specialized training to support the primary healthcare providers. Tertiary palliative care involves referral to a palliative care specialist for extenuating circumstances such as complex advance care planning or continued symptoms despite prescribed interventions.[20] Provision of primary palliative care requires that healthcare providers are not only aware of patient needs and concerns, but are also willing to provide interventions that address the identified issues, such as symptom management, psychological assessment, and end-of-life discussions as appropriate. Providers need to understand the purpose and intention of palliative care, recognize the appropriate time to initiate a referral, and communicate the purpose of a referral to patients and families. Providers also need to take into consideration patient and family needs and preferences as palliative care interventions are introduced. Referral to a tertiary palliative care team is indicated when a patient's concerns are beyond the scope of the primary practitioner. This can include issues such as refractory symptoms not adequately addressed by conventional therapies, and complex advance care planning needs such as left ventricular device deactivation.

PROVISION OF PRIMARY PALLIATIVE CARE

Symptom Assessment in Cardiology

Healthcare providers who are utilizing primary palliative care with patients should be knowledgeable in assessing symptoms and providing treatment. Symptom assessment in patients with cardiac disease should include a comprehensive approach of both the patient and family/caregiver to inform the development of an individualized care plan. Impact of the symptoms on functional status, quality of life, and patient/family goals are an important consideration when planning intervention to address these needs.[4] Multiple tools are available for use with patients, both generic palliative care tools as well as those that are more specific to cardiac symptoms and are listed in Table 27-2.[21]

An important aspect of symptom assessment for patients and families is to include assessments of both physical and psychological symptoms that affect quality of life and well-being. Common physical symptoms experienced by cardiac patients include generalized pain, chest pain, dyspnea, nausea, constipation, anorexia, and fatigue. Emotional symptoms may include depression and anxiety.[22] The purpose of symptom assessment is to provide timely identification of and reduction in symptoms for patients and families. The National Consensus Guidelines support using standardized and validated measures, when available, for symptom assessment.[4] Moreover, symptoms should be assessed routinely, in addition to after interventions.

The healthcare provider should prescribe interventions in conjunction with the patient and family. The goal of treatment is to reduce the symptoms to an acceptable level for the patient, or the family if the patient is not able to state goals for relief. Treatment options should include both pharmacologic and nonpharmacologic interventions, based upon patient preference.

Presently, there is a crisis in the United States related to the use of opioids, as evidenced by a 200% increase in deaths from opioid overdose since 2000.[23] This has direct impact on patients who require opioids for symptoms relief, as well as challenges and concerns for providers that prescribe opioids. The Centers for Disease Control has issued guidelines related to Opioid prescribing, however it is specified that the guidelines are not intended for use with patients who are in active cancer treatment, palliative care, hospice care.[24] The Hospice and Palliative Nurses Association (HPNA) released a joint statement in 2017 regarding pain management at the end of life, and support the position that nurses have a responsibility to advocate for effective pain and symptom relief receiving end-of-life care without respect to factors including age, disease, or history of substance misuse.[25] Recommendations for healthcare providers who prescribe opioids to patients as part of symptom management include: 1. Screening all patients for pre-existing substance use disorder, 2. Documenting a comprehensive pain and opioid history, 3. Communicating with patients identified as misusing opiates, and 4. Adopting practices such as pain management agreements from substance use disorder treatment programs.[26]

Advance Directives and End-of-Life Planning in Cardiology

Although a fundamental principal of palliative care is that it is interdisciplinary, there has been hesitance within nursing to fully participate in challenging conversations related to disease trajectory and prognosis.[27,28] Some barriers to talking about prognosis and end-of-life care include the uncertainty of survival prognosis, the patient having complex comorbidities, the patient being impaired, fear of taking away hope from the patient, and having inadequate time for communication.[27]

This reluctance to engage in challenging conversations is not limited to nursing. Within physicians and advanced practice providers, often there are perceptions that a *different* physician or provider than themselves should disclose the prognosis in a life-limiting disease. Although the American Heart Association

Table 27-2 • EXAMPLES OF SYMPTOM ASSESSMENT AND QUALITY-OF-LIFE TOOLS

General Symptom Assessment	Heart Failure Specific	Angina Specific
Edmonton Symptom Assessment Scale (ESAS)	ESAS—Heart Failure	Seattle Angina Questionnaire
Memorial Symptom Assessment Scale (MSAS)	MSAS—Heart Failure	MacNew Heart Disease Health Related QoL Questionnaire
Brief Pain inventory	Heart Failure Symptom Survey	Ferrans and Powers QoL Index
Brief Fatigue Inventory	Heart Failure Signs and Symptoms Checklist	Duke Activity Status Index (DASI)
McGill Pain Inventory	Heart Failure Symptoms Checklist	Speak from the Heart Chronic Angina Checklist
Needs at the End of Life Screening Tool (NEST)	MD Anderson Symptom Inventory—Heart Failure	
Palliative Care Outcome Scale	Minnesota Living with Heart Failure Questionnaire	
Short-Form (SF) 8, 12, or 36		
Wong–Baker FACES Pain Rating Scale		

Source: National Palliative Care Research Center, 2018.

recommends annual discussions with patients regarding their prognosis, most of these complex conversations are held at the time of a clinical deterioration.[29] It is generally accepted that high-quality communication and decision making is best not embarked on at the time of a health crisis. A better model is that these conversations about prognosis, expected disease trajectory, goals of care, and decisional support in choosing therapies should begin early in diagnosis, be ongoing, and be integrated into routine cardiac care.[30] Written health directives and planning should represent this ongoing conversation into the values, wishes, and goals of the patient.

Healthcare advance directives (ADs) are a legal document designed with the intent to ensure that one's wishes for their end-of-life care will be followed by their medical care team. In 1967, Luis Kutner, a Chicago lawyer, wrote an article promoting the idea that a person should be able to write an attestation for "permitting death" and he proposed the name, the "living will."[31] By January 1, 1977, California had enacted a law that gave a formal process for a competent person to direct their future care in the case of an incurable disease or injury.[32] Although California was the first, other states would rapidly join creating similar statutory laws. During this incremental progress in advanced directives, there was simultaneous and rapid development in technologies that sustain life.

The growth of ADs coupled with technologic advances revealed many of the inherent deficiencies of ADs, including a narrow scope, inability to adjust as the patient changes their goals and priorities within their care, and poorly defined terms that are notoriously challenging to delineate in bedside care. These challenges in ADs led to the promotion of legal power of attorney for healthcare and proxy decision making. This allowed for a designated agent to make decisions for an individual even after they had lost the capacity to make decisions for themselves.[33] By 1998, all 50 states within the United States had designated laws for power of attorney.

However, there was growing awareness that many people were still having unwanted resuscitative care outside of the hospital, so by 1999 forty-two states had implemented out-of-hospital do not attempt resuscitation protocols for emergency medical system.[34] In the 1990s Oregon piloted a program called, Physician Orders for Life-Sustaining Treatment (POLST). The goal of the POLST is to bridge the gap between high-quality conversations between patients and their healthcare team about their goals for their care and life-sustaining treatments with clear medical orders that follow the patient as they transition throughout the healthcare system and into their homes.

Today, there is form of POLST in 48 states and 23 of those meet the requirements of the National POLST standards. POLST forms are called different names in various states, including Medical Orders for Life-Sustaining Treatment (MOLST), Medical Orders for Scope of Treatment (MOST), Transportable Physician Orders for Patient Preferences (TROPP), and Physician Orders for Scope of Treatment (POST). The forms are different in each state, but they are signed by the provider and, in most states, the patient or possibly the legally recognized decision maker. The POLST does not take the place of the advance directive or the durable power of attorney for healthcare documents. In patients with significant illness or frailty, to whom it would not be surprising if they died within the next year, a patient should be aware of their option to have a POLST in addition to their other advance care planning. Typically the POLST is limited to care for emergency situations, such as whether the patient would want CPR if their heart should stop or mechanical ventilation. If a patient has a POLST, clinicians should be prepared for periodic reviews and updates, including each time a patient makes a transition from one care setting to another.

Within patients with cardiovascular disease, there has been an underutilization of advanced directives found.[35,36] Patients who have completed advanced directives are more likely to be older, be female, identify as Caucasian, not married, have a prior diagnosed malignancy, and have been consulted by palliative or a heart failure specialist.[35–37] Patients with significant cardiac disease who do not already have an AD have been found in studies to be interested in receiving information about ADs.[38] One shortcoming in ADs that is specific to cardiovascular disease, is that completed ADs often fail to mention devices that patients have implanted such as left ventricular assist devices (VADs), implanted pacemakers, and implantable cardioverter defibrillators (ICDs).[36,39,40] This can lead to ethical challenges at the end of life and leave proxy decision makers with added burden.

The use of ADs, durable power of attorney for health, and POLST forms is limited if communication about prognosis, disease trajectory, the values of the patient, and patient-specific guidance is not provided by the healthcare team. This communication should be iterative, multidisciplinary, and ongoing throughout a patient's treatment course. The legal documents cannot replace this communication; in fact, they are a reflection of the high-quality communication and informed decision making that should be transpiring between the patient and their healthcare team.

End-of-Life Considerations

Patients and families with cardiovascular disease need to be prepared with what to expect as they near the end-of-life, which can be difficult to predict with precision in cardiovascular disease. Heart failure is often the end stage of diverse cardiovascular processes such as valvular disease, congenital cardiac conditions, and atherosclerosis. Sudden ischemic events, arrhythmias, or the slower process of pump failure typically classifies death in heart failure. Although in clinical practice, these trajectories can be less distinguishable.

Within heart failure, there are multiple factors that predict increased risk of mortality; increased hospitalizations, increasing age, end-organ dysfunction, elevated natriuretic peptides, declining renal function, decreased exercise capacity, cognitive impairment, and unintentional weight loss.[41–44] The National Hospice and Palliative Care Organization (NHPCO) has identified the criteria for poor prognosis in HF in a patient who has been optimally treated; New York Heart Association Class IV heart failure (symptoms at rest), symptoms such as dyspnea and angina limiting minimal physical activities, nitrate-resistant angina pectoris at rest and not a candidate for any invasive procedures (including by patient choice). NHPCO classifies the following as supporting criteria; ejection fractions of less than 20%, symptomatic ventricular or supraventricular arrhythmias that are treatment resistant, cardiac related syncope, cardiogenic brain embolism, concomitant HIV, and history of cardiac resuscitation.

There are a number of scoring systems available that can be used clinically to estimate survival prognosis; Seattle Heart Failure Model, the Meta-Analysis Global Group in Chronic Heart Failure, Cardio Vascular Medicine Hear Failure Index, the Congestion Score, Heart Failure Survival Score, the Charlson Comorbidity Index, the Organized Program to Initiate Lifesaving Treatment in Hospitalized Patients with Heart Failure, the

Heart Failure Risk Scoring System, and the Acute Decompensated Heart Failure National Registry. The challenge with these prediction tools is that they are accurate at a population level, but are not as reliable at the individual person use. There has been mixed results in the specificity and sensitivity of using the "surprise question" in survival prognostication. The surprise question relies on the clinician's overall gestalt of their patient in response to the question "*would you be surprised if this patient died within the next 12 months.*"[45,46]

Increasing age is associated with increasing incidents of multi-morbidities. Eighty percent of adults over the age of 65 will have two or more chronic conditions and 35% of inpatient hospitals stays are for people with five or more chronic conditions. The number of people living with five or more chronic conditions has increased from 5.1% in 2006 to 8.7% in 2010.[47] Most patients with cardiac disease have at least one comorbidity.[48] In organ failure, it is often a more nuanced cumulative effect of diseases that signals shorter life expectancy. This can be very different than when trying to prognosticate in malignancies.

Hospice is a philosophy of care that falls under the larger umbrella of palliative care. While palliative care is appropriate at any stage of serious illness and in cases where there is not clear expectation of the disease being terminal. In hospice, largely due to insurance and payer regulations, it is restricted to terminal illness with survival prognosis of 6 months or less. As a philosophy of care, hospice care takes place wherever the person considers home. While the care could be provided in a facility, the hospice benefit does not per se provide long-term residential care. Hospice benefits do provide for short-term, nonresidential, inpatient care to manage a symptom that cannot be managed in another setting, this is referred to as general inpatient care (GIP). For most patients receiving hospice care, if they desire or need residential care or paid caregivers in their home, the patient will need insurance or privately pay for this care.

Hospice care that takes place in the home requires caregivers to be present, typically the round-the-clock nature of this care is assumed by family, friends, and paid caregivers. Hospice personnel will typically have episodic contact with the patient and schedule things such as bathing and need nursing care. Patients and families can contact the hospice nurses for pressing needs, but the nurse may provide instructions to them over the phone. Patients and families need anticipatory guidance about the caregiving demands of providing round-the-clock care in end-of-life care and the scope of hospice care. This anticipatory guidance is an essential foundation in helping families gracefully care for their loved one at home and be prepared.

Implantable Cardiac Device Considerations

The number of patients with cardiac assist devices such as pacemakers, cardioverter defibrillators, VADs, and artificial hearts is rising. Anticipatory guidance about what to expect with these devices at the end of life should begin at the time of implantation. Discussions should evolve over time, but basic patient and family education about deactivation of the device to allow for a natural death and simple explanations of what that entails should start prior to implantation. As with all goals of care conversations, clinicians should have ongoing discussions with their patients about their priorities in their care and thoughtful and informed consideration of what the patient would like their end-of-life care to look like, including the management of their implanted cardiac device(s).

There are fundamental ethical principles that clinicians need to be familiar with in considering ethical obligations in deactivating implanted cardiac devices. First, it is ethically permissible for a person to make informed decision to consent and therefore it is also ethical for the person to make the informed decision to refuse. Another important ethical principle is that patients have the right to refuse care that they had prior consented to. An illustration of this is a case where a patient with cancer decides to stop chemotherapy because their cancer has progressed, their quality of life has declined, and the treatment is not benefitting them anymore.

The right to stop or refuse medical treatments includes those that are life sustaining and life prolonging, such as dialysis, mechanical ventilation, and others. The U.S. courts have consistently upheld that patients or their surrogates have the right to stop life-prolonging therapies.[49] An example of this could be the patient with advanced chronic obstructive pulmonary disease in respiratory failure from pneumonia who is willing to have mechanical ventilation temporarily to see if they can recover and resume breathing on their own volition. But this individual could decide that they do not desire to be on long-term or even lifelong mechanical ventilation, and may have mechanical ventilation stopped at a certain point in their course of treatment.

There can sometimes be some confusion about whether stopping or withdrawing life-sustaining care is euthanasia or assisted suicide. It has well established that stopping life-sustaining treatment, of any type, is part of person's right to choose a natural death.[50] Some suggestions for bringing up this topic with a patient is to normalize the topic by saying, "this is something that I bring up with all my patients because it helps me to care for you when I understand what kind of care you would want." Using an *ask-tell-ask* model for communication, the nurse should first elicit what the patient and family understand about their health and their cardiac device. The nurse can than tailor the information to misunderstandings or gaps in knowledge. At the end of life, communication is largely focused on the benefits and burdens of the device. Nurses should enter into these challenging conversations with the mindset that the best outcome is one that represents the values and goals of the patient, and deactivation is not required.

Pacemakers, unless the patient is completely pacemaker dependent, are unlikely to cause immediate death upon deactivation. Typically, pacemakers do not prolong the dying process and may palliate symptoms associated with symptomatic bradycardia. It is important to openly discuss with patients and families that a pacemaker is not a resuscitative device and deactivating a pacemaker will not typically lead to immediate death. With full information on the potential benefits and limitations of a pacemaker at the end of life, a patient or family has the same ethical standing to decide not to implant a device as to deactivate it. An example of this could be deactivating the pacemaker in a patient with advanced dementia who is bed-bound and the family is exercising their loved one's wish to limit medical therapies to only those that provide immediate comfort.

ICDs are intended to provide lifesaving shocks in the case of a potentially lethal arrhythmia. Not all patients have experienced these shocks and other patients are very familiar with the sensation. An ICD can produce a life-preserving electrical impulse to resynchronize the heart. But as disease progresses it is important to remember that the ICD does not treat the underlying physiologic process that is leading to death, such as a failing heart or cancer. Unlike pacemakers, defibrillators can cause physical discomfort if the device detects and appropriately shocks for a rhythm at the end of life. This can lead physical discomfort in an actively dying person and emotional distress for the family and loved ones. It is important to discuss that deactivation of the ICD, like other cardiac devices, does not require surgery and is not invasive. In the case of cardiac resynchronization therapy (CRT), the device can have defibrillation ability or not. In devices with shock therapy, the shock can be deactivated while bradycardia pacing can be maintained in order to avoid things like symptomatic bradycardia.

VAD can be implanted for the purpose of bridging the person to heart transplant, supporting the person to cardiac recovery, or used as destination therapy. These devices assist one or both of the failing ventricles in pumping blood. In destination therapy, the person will live the remainder of their life with their VAD and die with their VAD. VADs are associated with a range of complications such as stoke, gastrointestinal bleeding, and infections. When deactivation prior to death occurs survival is typically short, minutes to an hour. Although this is not always the case with survival exceeding that in some cases to days or greater.[51] Most patients with a VAD will die in the inpatient setting and not on hospice.

CONCLUSIONS

Summary and Implications for Nurses

Palliative care is focused on relieving suffering and improving quality of life in patients with potentially life-limiting disease, including cardiac patients. However, limited provider knowledge of palliative care and confusion between the terms hospice and palliative care, lead to limited incorporation of palliative care in these patients. Heart disease is currently the leading cause of death in the United States, and the population is continuing to age. In order to provide the highest level of care, it is imperative that nurses and other healthcare providers are knowledgeable in palliative care principles.

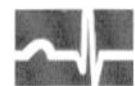

CASE-BASED LEARNING

POLST

Patient Profile

Mrs. Walters is a 91-year-old patient admitted to the telemetry floor for an acute exacerbation of her stage D heart failure. This is her fourth admission in the past 6 months. She resides in a skilled nursing facility and has had a slow loss in her mobility for the past few years, so that now she is wheelchair-dependent. On this admission, Mrs. Walters expressed to her cardiologist and her nurse that she would not want to "go through" CPR or be on a ventilator. Her code status has been *no CPR* and *no intubation* for her entire 6-day hospital stay. She is being discharged back to her rehabilitation facility today. Her nurse notices that there is no POLST in her chart. Mrs. Walter's nurse returns to her room with a blank POLST form and explains the form, including that the form can document the conversations they had in the hospital so the rehabilitation facility will be able to follow the same plan. Mrs. Walters agrees, and the discharging cardiologist completes the form with Mrs. Walters prior to her discharge.

KEY READINGS

Braun LT, Grady KL, Kutner JS, et al. Palliative care and cardiovascular disease and stroke: a policy statement from the American Heart Association/American Stroke Association. *Circulation*. 2016;134(11):e198–e225.

Lampert R, Hayes DL, Annas GJ, et al. HRS expert consensus statement on the management of cardiovascular implantable electronic devices (CIEDs) in patients nearing end of life or requesting withdrawal of therapy. *Heart Rhythm*. 2010;7(7):1008–1026.

National Consensus Project for Quality Palliative Care. *Clinical Practice Guidelines for Quality Palliative Care*. 4th ed. Available at http://www.nationalconsensusproject.org. Updated October 31, 2018. Accessed November 1, 2018.

REFERENCES

1. Clark D. From margins to centre: a review of the history of palliative care in cancer. *Lancet Oncology*. 2007;8(5):430–438.
2. World Health Organization. *Palliative care*. 2018. Available at http://www.who.int/cancer/palliative/definition/en/. Accessed November 1, 2018.
3. American Academy of Hospice and Palliative Medicine, Center to Advance Palliative Care, Hospice and Palliative Nurses Association, Last Acts Partnership, National Hospice and Palliative Care Organization. National consensus project for quality palliative care: clinical practice guidelines for quality palliative care, executive summary. *J Palliat Med*. 2004;7(5):611–627.
4. National Consensus Project for Quality Palliative Care.. *Clinical Practice Guidelines for Quality Palliative Care*. 4th ed. 2014. Available at http://www.nationalconsensusproject.org. Updated October 31, 2018. Accessed November 1, 2018.
5. American Nurses Association and Hospice and Palliative Nurses Association. Scope and standards of practice. *Palliative Nursing: An Essential Resource for Hospice and Palliative Nurses*. Silver Spring, MD: American Nurses Association; 2014.
6. Task Force on Palliative Care, Last Acts Campaign, Robert Wood Johnson Foundation. Precepts of palliative care. *J Palliat Med*. 1998;1(2):109–112.
7. McKenna M, Clark SC. Palliative care in cardiopulmonary transplantation. *BMJ Support Palliat Care*. 2015;5(4):427–434.
8. Center to Advance Palliative Care. *2011 public opinion research on palliative care: a report based on research by public opinion strategies*. 2011 Available at https://media.capc.org/filer_public/18/ab/18ab708c-f835-4380-921d-fbf729702e36/2011- public-opinion-research-on-palliative-care.pdf. Updated June 1, 2011. Accessed November 1, 2018.
9. Boyd KJ, Worth A, Kendall M, et al. Making sure services deliver for people with advanced heart failure: a longitudinal qualitative study of patients, family carers, and health professionals. *Palliat Med*. 2009;23(8):767–776.
10. Brannstrom M, Forssell A, Pettersson B. Physicians' experiences of palliative care for heart failure patients. *Eur J Cardiovasc Nurs*. 2011;10(1):64–69.
11. Kavalieratos D, Mitchell EM, Carey TS, et al. "Not the 'grim reaper service'": an assessment of provider knowledge, attitudes, and perceptions regarding palliative care referral barriers in heart failure. *J Am Heart Assoc*. 2014;3(1):e000544.
12. Hauser JM, Preodor M, Roman E, et al. The evolution and dissemination of the education in palliative and end-of-life care program. *J Palliat Med*. 2015;18(9):765–770.
13. Ferrell B, Malloy P, Virani R. The end of life nursing education nursing consortium project. *Ann Palliat Med*. 2015;4(2):61–69.
14. Hospice and Palliative Credentialing Center. *Certification*. 2018. Available at https://advancingexpertcare.org/HPNA/HPCC/CertificationWeb/Certification.aspx. Accessed November 1, 2018.
15. Braun LT, Grady KL, Kutner JS, et al. Palliative care and cardiovascular disease and association. *Circulation*. 2016;134(11):e198–e225.
16. Yancy CW, Jessup M, Bozkurt B, et al. 2013 ACCF/AHA guideline for the management of heart failure: a report of the American College of Cardiology Foundation/American Heart Association Task Force on practice guidelines. *Circulation*. 2013;128(16):e240–e327.
17. Centers for Medicare & Medicaid Services. *Decision memo for ventricular assist devices and for bridge to transplant and destination therapy*. 2013. Available at https://www.cms.gov/medicare-coverage-database/details/nca-decision-memo.aspx?NCAId = 268. Updated October 30, 2013. Accessed November 1, 2018.
18. Otto CM, Kumbhani DJ, Alexander KP, et al. 2017 ACC expert consensus decision pathway for transcatheter aortic valve replacement in the management of adults with aortic stenosis: a report of the American College of Cardiology Task Force on clinical expert consensus documents. *J Am Coll Cardiol*. 2017;69(10):1313–1346.
19. Steiner JM, Cooper S, Kirkpatrick JN. Palliative care in end-stage valvular heart disease. *Heart*. 2017;103(16):1233–1237.
20. Bakitas M, Bishop MF, Caron PA. Hospital-based palliative care. In: Ferrell BR, Coyle N, eds. *Oxford Textbook of Palliative Nursing*. 3rd ed. New York: Oxford University Press; 2010:53–86.

21. National Palliative Care Research Center. *Measurement and evaluation tools*. 2013. Available at http://www.npcrc.org/content/25/Measurement-and-Evaluation-Tools.aspx. Accessed November 1, 2018.
22. Alpert CM, Smith MA, Hummel SL, et al. Symptom burden in heart failure: assessment, impact on outcomes, and management. *Heart Fail Rev*. 2017;22(1):25–39.
23. Rudd RA, Seth P, David F, et al. Increases in drug and opioid-involved overdose deaths—United States, 2010–2015. *MMWR Morb Mortal Wkly Rep*. 2016;65(50–51):1445–1452.
24. Centers for Disease Control and Prevention Public Health Service U. S. Department Of Health And Human Services. Guideline for prescribing opioids for chronic pain. *J Pain Palliat Care Pharmacother*. 2016;30(2):138–140.
25. Hospice and Palliative Nurses Association and American Society for Pain Management Nursing. *Position statement: pain management at the end of life*. 2017. Available at https://advancingexpertcare.org/position-statements/. Accessed November 1, 2018.
26. Gabbard J, Jordan A, Mitchell J, et al. Dying on hospice in the midst of an opioid crisis: what should we do now? *Am J Hosp Palliat Care*. 2019;36(4):273–281.
27. Hjelmfors L, Stromberg A, Friedrichsen M, et al. Communicating prognosis and end-of-life care to heart failure patients: a survey of heart failure nurses' perspectives. *Eur J Cardiovasc Nurs*. 2014;13(2):152–161.
28. Newman AR. Nurses' perceptions of diagnosis and prognosis-related communication: an integrative review. *Cancer Nurs*. 2016;39(5):E48–E60.
29. Dunlay SM, Foxen JL, Cole T, et al. A survey of clinician attitudes and self-reported practices regarding end-of-life care in heart failure. *Palliat Med*. 2015;29(3):260–267.
30. Whellan DJ, Goodlin SJ, Dickinson MG, et al. End-of-life care in patients with heart failure. *J Card Fail*. 2014;20(2):121–134.
31. Kutner L. Euthanasia: due process for death with dignity; the living will. *Indiana Law J*. 1979;54(2):201–228.
32. Jonsen AR. Dying right in California—the natural death act. *Clin Toxicol*. 1978;13(4):513–522.
33. Sabatino CP. The evolution of health care advance planning law and policy. *Milbank Q*. 2010;88(2):211–239.
34. Sabatino CP. Survey of state EMS-DNR laws and protocols. *J Law Med Ethics*. 1999;27(4):297–315, 294.
35. Butler J, Binney Z, Kalogeropoulos A, et al. Advance directives among hospitalized patients with heart failure. *JACC Heart Fail*. 2015;3(2):112–121.
36. Dunlay SM, Swetz KM, Mueller PS, et al. Advance directives in community patients with heart failure. *Circ Cardiovasc Qual Outcomes*. 2012;5(3):283–289.
37. Portanova J, Ailshire J, Perez C, et al. Ethnic differences in advance directive completion and care preferences: what has changed in a decade? *J Am Geriatr Soc*. 2017;65(6):1352–1357.
38. Kirkpatrick JN, Guger CJ, Arnsdorf MF, et al. Advance directives in the cardiac care unit. *Am Heart J*. 2007;154(3):477–481.
39. Pasalic D, Tajouri TH, Ottenberg AL, et al. The prevalence and contents of advance directives in patients with pacemakers. *Pacing Clin Electrophysiol*. 2014;37(4):473–480.
40. Tajouri TH, Ottenberg AL, Hayes DL, et al. The use of advance directives among patients with implantable cardioverter defibrillators. *Pacing Clin Electrophysiol*. 2012;35(5):567–573.
41. Solomon SD, Dobson J, Pocock S, et al. Influence of nonfatal hospitalization for heart failure on subsequent mortality in patients with chronic heart failure. *Circulation*. 2007;116(13):1482–1487.
42. Lee DS, Gona P, Albano I, et al. A systematic assessment of causes of death after heart failure onset in the community: impact of age at death, time period, and left ventricular systolic dysfunction. *Circ Heart Fail*. 2011;4(1):36–43.
43. O'Connor CM, Hasselblad V, Mehta RH, et al. Triage after hospitalization with advanced heart failure: the ESCAPE (evaluation study of congestive heart failure and pulmonary artery catheterization effectiveness) risk model and discharge score. *J Am Coll Cardiol*. 2010;55(9):872–878.
44. Adejumo OL, Koelling TM, Hummel SL. Nutritional risk index predicts mortality in hospitalized advanced heart failure patients. *J Heart Lung Transplant*. 2015;34(11):1385–1389.
45. Johnson M, Nunn A, Hawkes T, et al. Planning for end-of-life care in heart failure: experience of two integrated cardiology-palliative care teams. *Br J Cardiol*. 2012;19(2):152–161.
46. Treece J, Chemchirian H, Hamilton N, et al. A review of prognostic tools in heart failure. *Am J Hosp Palliat Care*. 2018;35(3):514–522.
47. Gerteis J, Izrael D, Deitz D, et al. *Multiple Chronic Conditions Chartbook. AHRQ Publications No. Q14-0038*. Rockville, MD: Agency for Healthcare Research and Quality; 2014.
48. Tran J, Norton R, Conrad N, et al. Patterns and temporal trends of comorbidity among adult patients with incident cardiovascular disease in the UK between 2000 and 2014: a population-based cohort study. *PLoS Med*. 2018;15(3):e1002513.
49. Lampert R, Hayes DL, Annas GJ, et al. HRS expert consensus statement on the management of cardiovascular implantable electronic devices (CIEDs) in patients nearing end of life or requesting withdrawal of therapy. *Heart Rhythm*. 2010;7(7):1008–1026.
50. Mueller PS, Jenkins SM, Bramstedt KA, et al. Deactivating implanted cardiac devices in terminally ill patients: practices and attitudes. *Pacing Clin Electrophysiol*. 2008;31(5):560–568.
51. Dunlay SM, Strand JJ, Wordingham SE, et al. Dying with a left ventricular assist device as destination therapy. *Circ Heart Fail*. 2016;9(10):e003096.

28 Medical, Surgical, and Catheter-Based Therapy for Cardiovascular Disease

Sarah E. Clarke, Amanda M. Kirby

OBJECTIVES

1. Identify methods for treatment for coronary, valvular, and structural heart disease.
2. Define cardiac conditions that may benefit from medical, surgical, or percutaneous treatment.
3. Analyze current versus future therapies for valvular heart disease.

KEY QUESTIONS

1. Name potential treatments for coronary artery disease (CAD) to include medical versus intervention.
2. How does treatment for mitral regurgitation (MR) differ depending on causation?
3. When is it indicated to consider PFO closure?

Decision-making regarding treatment options for patients with cardiovascular disease is becoming increasingly thought-provoking with the advent of alternative treatment options, technologic advancements, and patients' ability to educate themselves regarding available options for treatment. This age of innovation offers patients a great deal of opportunity to individually develop their treatment plan and discuss this with a team of experts. Many cardiac disease processes that were previously treated with medical management due to lack of available options are now at the forefront of technologic advancement. Healthcare providers now have the ability to offer patients alternatives that were previously not available. In an age of technology and improved opportunity for our patients to receive multiple treatment options, understanding the strength and limitations of these treatments is imperative to guiding therapy.

INTRODUCTION

Treatment of patients with cardiovascular disease has changed greatly over the last decade. Advancements in how we care for patients and how decisions are made regarding the care and treatment that is provided have invigorated new discussions. There is a focus on the team approach to care, commonly referred to as a multidisciplinary approach or heart team approach to care. The necessity of this practice has become increasingly important as the complexity of patient treatment options continues to evolve.[1] The multidisciplinary heart team approach is utilized differently in each of the specialities of cardiovascular care, however the goal of keeping the patient at the center of the care is paramount. Providing a multifaceted approach to, not only evaluate, but also optimize treatment planning is a significant advancement for patients. The topics discussed throughout this chapter will each have multidisciplinary team approach criteria/recommendations to aid in continued adoption of this important topic.

BACKGROUND

Cardiovascular surgery developed rapidly in the mid-late 20th century as a result of technologic advances in intracardiac repair, cardiopulmonary bypass (CPB), revascularization techniques, and valve replacement techniques and technology. In the early 2000s the focus turned to minimally invasive cardiovascular surgery (MICS) in response to innovations in percutaneous coronary interventions (PCIs), developing endoscopic technology, and cost-containment efforts.

Historical Evolution of Cardiovascular Technology

Patient preference was integral to the growth in MICS. Patients, and some doctors, held the perception that a smaller incision is associated with a lower risk of morbidity and mortality. In some cases, the evidence does not support this perception. In a review published by Doenst et al., 10 prospective randomized controlled trials (RCTs) (7 aortic valve replacement and 3 mitral valve replacement trials) were analyzed and none of the studies found a difference in perioperative mortality.[2] There were some benefits noted. In the aortic trials, the benefits trended toward fewer blood transfusions, decreased pain, and early mobilization. In the mitral valve surgery trials, the results were neutral except for the smaller incision and longer periods on the heart–lung machine for the minimally invasive group. The appeal of minimal interventional trauma and a decrease in postoperative pain required reconciliation with the prolonged procedure times and limited visibility associated with minimally invasive procedures. Despite equivocal results, patients are increasingly requesting an approach that leaves the sternum intact

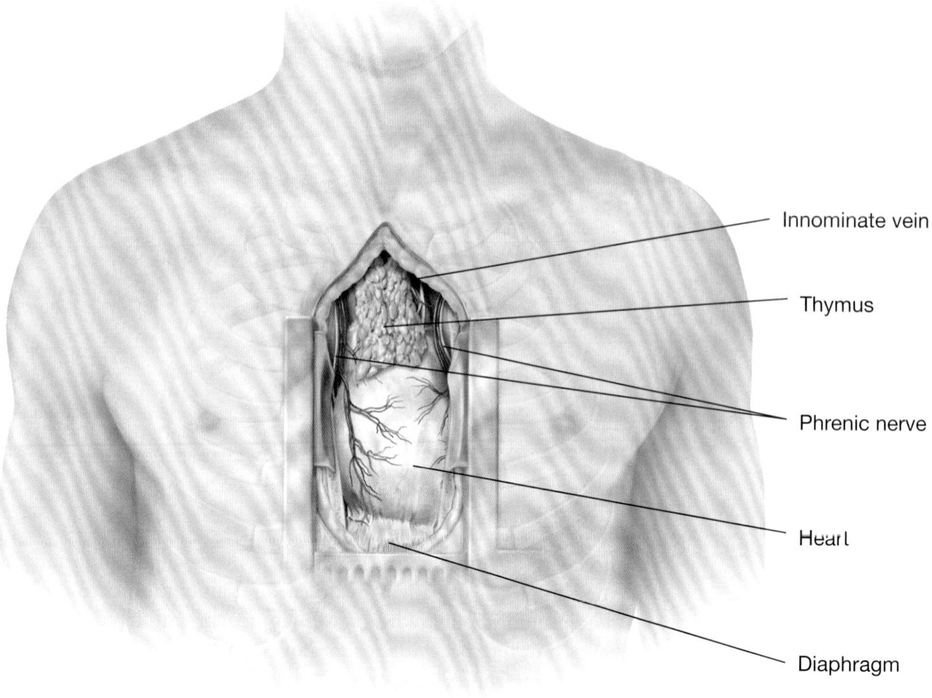

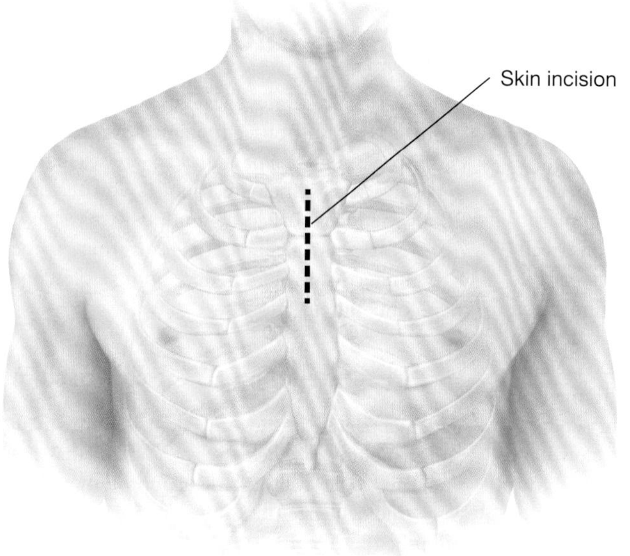

Figure 28-1. **(A, B)** Traditional versus minimal sternotomy. (Used with permission from Mulholland MW, Albo D, Dalman R, et al. *Operative Techniques in Surgery (2 Volume Set)*. Philadelphia, PA: Wolters Kluwer; 2014.)

and meeting these expectations using minimal incisions in cardiac surgery requires advanced technical skills (Fig. 28-1).[2–4]

The growing use of less invasive methods has shifted the focus away from open surgery toward catheter-based interventional techniques. In fact, September 2017 marked the 40-year anniversary of the first human PCI, which changed the course of contemporary cardiovascular care. PCI is now the most frequently performed coronary revascularization procedure. This success is due in part to:

- Collaboration with industry to develop technology and approaches
- Safety and effectiveness assessment with comparison to traditional therapies with the completion of RCTs
- Development of evidence-based recommendations based on substantial mass of data
- Dissemination of these findings and recommendations at an international, national, regional, and local level

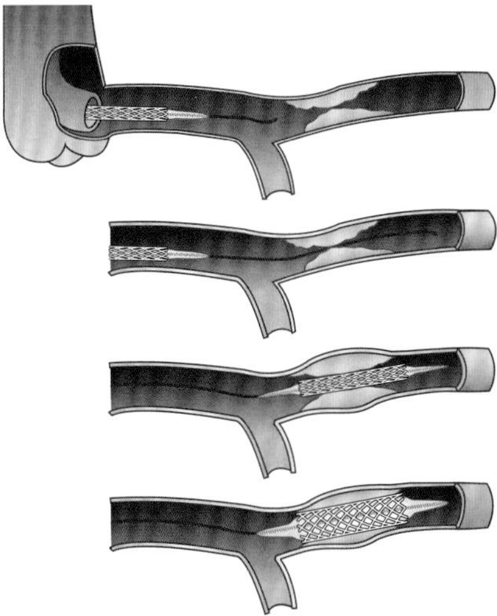

Figure 28-2. Coronary stent. (Used with permission from Norris TL. *Porth's Essentials of Pathophysiology*. 5th ed. Philadelphia, PA: Wolters Kluwer; 2019.)

- Creation of educational programs to share data and experiences utilizing innovative models such as simulation, 3D printing, and transmitted live cases

Continuation in the use of these methods is paramount as new technologies are discovered, studied, and indicated in the treatment of patients with cardiovascular disease (Fig. 28-2).[5]

Minimally Invasive Circulatory Support

Innovation in perfusion techniques is one of the reasons cardiac surgery has been able to progress to less invasive approaches. The initial goals for developments in CPB are decreased invasiveness, blood product conservation, and improved management of anticoagulation. Minimizing invasiveness is critical to curtail systemic inflammation after a surgical procedure involving CPB. Balancing systemic anticoagulation and clotting can be a challenge. Technologic advances in maintaining a closed loop circuit, monitoring and handling air in the system, biocompatibility, and oxygenation have been evaluated and considered safe.[3,6]

Percutaneous Mechanical Circulatory Support

Currently, there are three types of percutaneous mechanical circulatory support devices available: the intra-aortic balloon pump (IABP), percutaneous ventricular assist devices (pVAD), and extracorporeal membrane oxygenation (ECMO). IABPs provide less hemodynamic support compared to the pVAD and ECMO devices. The two pVAD systems available for use in the United States are Impella (Abiomed, Danvers, MA) and TandemHeart (TandemLife, Pittsburgh, PA).

Intra-Aortic Balloon Pump

The IABP assists the heart indirectly by decreasing the afterload and increases diastolic aortic pressure with subsequent improvement in diastolic blood flow resulting in better perfusion of the peripheral organ as well as a potential improvement in the coronary blood flow. The IABP inflates during diastole at the same time as the aortic valve closes. This results in the displacement of blood from the thoracic aorta into the peripheral circulation that is followed by rapid deflation of the balloon before the onset of systole phase of the cardiac cycle. Essentially, this results in improved diastolic pressure and reduced systolic aortic pressure by reducing the afterload. This results in decreased left ventricle wall stress reducing the myocardial oxygen demand. These hemodynamic changes improve the cardiac output by increasing stroke volume.[7]

Indications for use of an IABP include the following:

- acute heart failure with hypotension
- prophylaxis during a high-risk PCI
- post myocardial infarction with decreased left ventricular function causing hypotension
- myocardial infarction with complications of cardiogenic shock
- low cardiac output post coronary artery bypass graft (CABG)
- bridge to treatment in patients with intractable angina, myocardial ischemia, refractory heart failure, or intractable ventricular arrhythmias

Contraindications for use include uncontrolled sepsis, uncontrolled bleeding, moderate to severe aortic regurgitation (AR), aortic aneurysm, aortic dissection, or severe peripheral artery disease not pretreated with stenting.[7]

Percutaneous Ventricular Assist Devices

U.S. Food and Drug Administration (FDA) has approved pVAD for treatment of cardiogenic shock in specific instances. These instances include alternative to extracorporeal membrane oxygenation (ECMO) or optimal medical management and conventional treatments have failed to produce sufficient improvements or patient is suspected to have a reversible cardiac injury.[8]

pVADs are also available for use during PCI to support patients with severe coronary artery disease (CAD), complex anatomy, or extensive comorbidities. Clinical guidelines from the American College of Cardiology (ACC), Heart Failure Society of America (HFSA), Society for Cardiovascular Angiography and Interventions (SCAI), Society of Thoracic Surgeons (STS) consensus document support the use of Impella in patients with severe CAD, in the presence of normal or decreased left ventricular function, of anticipated technically challenging or prolonged PCI patients.[9]

Extracorporeal Membrane Oxygenation

ECMO is a form of temporary life support, to aid respiratory and/or cardiac function. It is the early 1970s and is based on CPB technology and diverts venous blood through an extracorporeal circuit and returns it to the body after gas exchange through a semipermeable membrane. ECMO can be used for oxygenation, carbon dioxide removal, and hemodynamic support. Additional components allow thermoregulation and hemofiltration. The two most common forms of ECMO are venovenous (VV) and venoarterial (VA). In VV-ECMO, used to support gas exchange, oxygenated blood is returned to a central vein. In VA-ECMO, used in cases of cardiac or cardiorespiratory failure, oxygenated blood is returned to the systemic arterial circulation, bypassing both the heart and lungs (Fig. 28-3).[10]

CORONARY ARTERY DISEASE

Medical Management for Coronary Artery Disease

Medical management of CAD is multifactorial. Medications, lifestyle modifications, as well as assessment of nonmodifiable risk

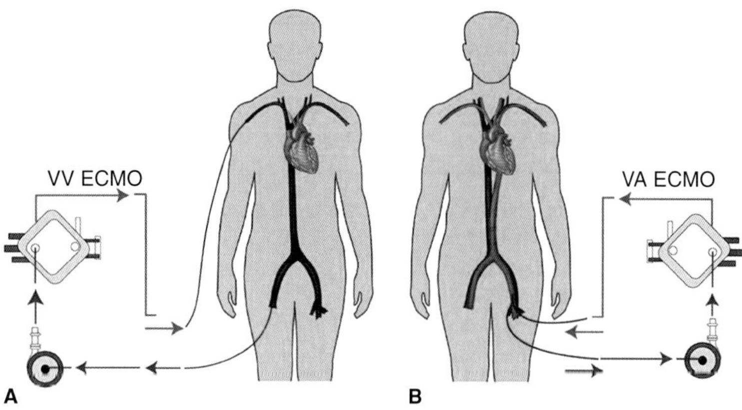

Figure 28-3. Extracorporeal membrane oxygenation. (Used with permission from Griffin BP. *Manual of Cardiovascular Medicine*. 5th ed. Philadelphia, PA: Wolters Kluwer; 2018.)

factors are components of management. Treatment is aimed at controlling symptoms as well as slowing the progression of disease. Patient symptoms, physical examination findings, as well as diagnostic testing determine treatment.

Risk factors may be modifiable or nonmodifiable. Nonmodifiable risk factors include male gender, advanced age, as well as family history of heart disease (especially if developed before age 50). Modifiable risk factors include smoking and tobacco use, hyperlipidemia, hypertension, control of diabetes, sedentary lifestyle, being overweight or obese, stress, as well as a high fat diet. Attention should be given to patient education for lifestyle modification.

Medications for CAD typically include lipid-lowering agents, antihypertensives, and antiplatelet agents. They may also include antianginals. Goal of medications is aimed at modifiable risk factor control as well as hastening the development of disease.

Diagnostic testing includes invasive and noninvasive testing. Noninvasive testing include electrocardiograph testing (ECG), exercise stress tests, as well as laboratory testing. Invasive testing includes cardiac catheterization. Other testing may include nuclear imaging, echocardiography, computerized tomography, magnetic resonance imaging, or positron emission tomography.

Catheter-Based Management of Coronary Disease

In the United States, less than 30% of coronary revascularizations are surgical and greater than 70% are done by interventional cardiologists inserting coronary stents.[11] Advances in stent technology and improved outcomes likely drive this evolution after PCI. A recent individual patient-data pooled analysis of 11 randomized clinical trials comparing CABG with PCI using stents demonstrated significantly lower 5-year stroke rates after PCI compared with CABG.[12] A significant financial investment has been made in the development of coronary stents with novel vascular skeletons and different eluted drugs.

Stents

A stent is a device, which is inserted into a blood vessel, or other internal duct. It is used to expand the vessel to prevent or relieve a blockage. Traditionally, stents are manufactured from metal mesh and can be removed in some instances. However, in cardiac cases they are permanent. There are three types of stents that are available for use during PCI: bare metal stents (BMSs), drug-eluting stents (DESs), and bioresorbable stents (BRSs). Each stent has potential benefits and risks and should be considered dependent on patient characteristics and condition.

Bare Metal Stents

Current BMS are comprised of stainless steel, cobalt chromium, or platinum chromium. Use of BMS reduced the incidence of abrupt vessel closure and restenosis over the use of plain old balloon angioplasty (POBA). Stent endothelialization takes approximately 12 weeks. Restenosis can develop in approximately 20% to 30% of lesions. Current indications for use of a BMS is patients likely to be nonadherent to oral antithrombotic and patients scheduled for procedures requiring the patient to cease use of antithrombotic post 6 weeks of their procedure.[13]

Drug-Eluting Stents

DESs are metal stents that are coated with a pharmacologic agent known to suppress restenosis. Patient who may benefit from a DES include those who can take an antithrombotic for at least 1 year. The size of the coronary lesion can also make a difference. Lesions that are in smaller vessels or longer in length may benefit from a DES. DES is contraindicated in those who cannot take antithrombotics or have a known allergy to the components of the stent.[13]

Bioresorbable Stent Technology

Interest in BRSs was fueled by drawbacks in use of metal DESs. These stents can have late stent thrombosis, vessel remodeling, hinder future surgical revascularization, as well as impair the ability to perform imaging due to artifact.[14]

Interest in developing BRS technology was soaring for a couple years until September 2017. In the last year, BRS platforms with thinner struts (comparable in strut size to the leading metallic DES) have been tested and been submitted for European CE mark. This indicates the product has been assessed to meet high safety, health, and environmental protection requirements to be used commercially in Europe.

Robotic PCI

Patient access to timely, definitive care is impacted by geographic barriers, socioeconomic status, and a decreasing number of specialists.[15] These issues are of more concern in emergent medical events where patient outcomes are improved when patients receive treatment in a timely basis. Access to technologically advanced centers and approaches will continue to offer challenges for these advanced techniques, like robotic PCI. Two robotic PCI systems are currently approved for use in the United States. The robotic system consists of a bedside robotic arm containing a drive unit and a mobile interventional cockpit. The drive unit is controlled by buttons and two joysticks contained within the cockpit. These controls allow precise movements of guidewires, balloons, and stents. The lead-lined cockpit has monitors that display real-time fluoroscopy and cineangiography images, as well as hemodynamic and ECG information. Robotic PCI (R-PCI) is an emerging technology with the potential for transforming PCI. The interventional cardiologist is subjected to less radiation exposure and potentially less orthopedic injuries. Currently there are some limitations to its use. Incompatibility with some devices as well as lacking the ability to manipulate multiple devices simultaneously limits its use in complex cases.[13] One benefit of R-PCI is the ability to perform this procedure remotely therefore increasing access to care.

In addition to patient access benefits, there are also significant benefits to operators as this decreases the level of radiation exposure, which has been linked to cancers, orthopedic issues, and cataracts. In addition, musculoskeletal stress associated with performing long procedures in heavy lead vests that must be worn to comply with radiation exposure protocols. These robotic technologies offer improved procedural control and precision. Robotic devices also make available sub-millimeter device positioning, allowing for optimal stent delivery. Additional studies are required to determine if future advancements in robotics will facilitate improved access to care, procedural success, and patient outcomes (Fig. 28-4).

Surgical Management of Coronary Artery Disease

Surgical management of CAD includes coronary artery bypass grafting (CABG), robotic-assisted CABG, as well as hybrid revascularization. Determination of surgical versus percutaneous approach is dependent on location of lesion, comorbid conditions, as well as acuity.[16]

CABG bypasses the diseased coronary arteries utilizing a graft that is made from the saphenous vein or the internal mammary. The procedure is completed under general anesthesia and a central sternotomy. The patient is placed on CPB during the procedure.

Robotic-assisted CABG can be used in patients who only require a single bypass. The cardiothoracic surgeon makes a small incision and is able to do the procedure with robotic assistance. Four to five small incisions are made in the chest without a central

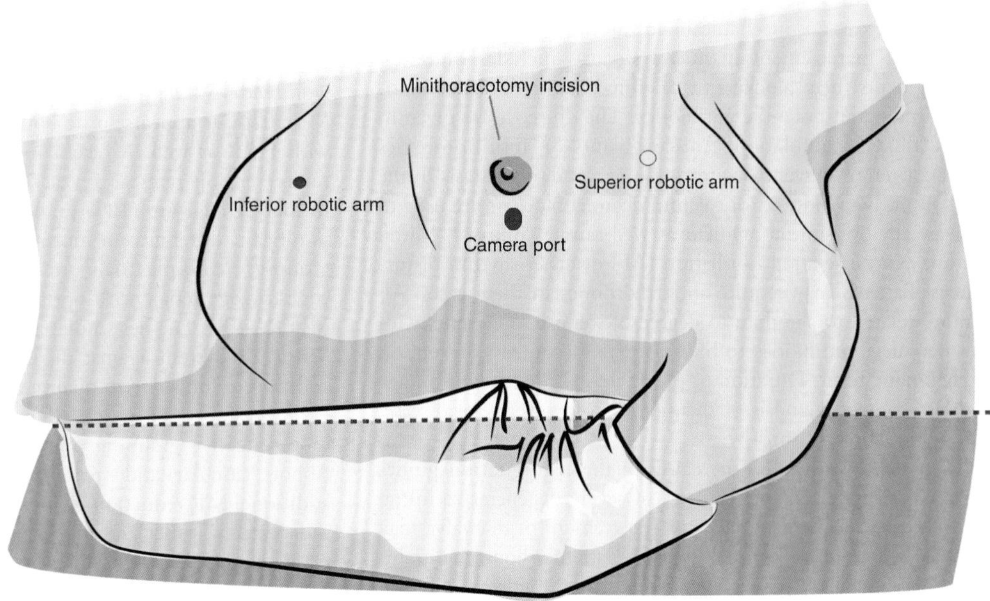

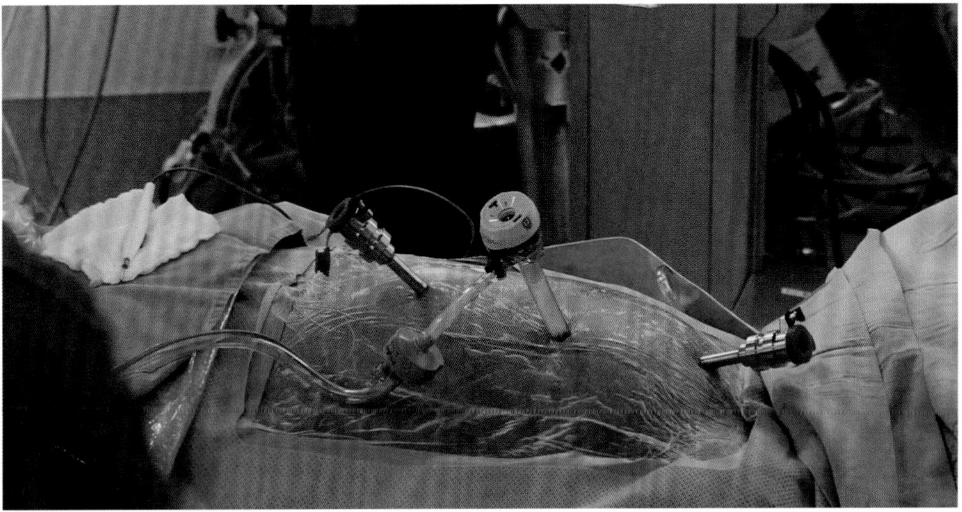

Figure 28-4. Robotic surgery. (Used with permission from Grover F, Mack MJ. *Cardiac Surgery*. Philadelphia, PA: Wolters Kluwer; 2016.)

sternotomy. The procedure does not require CPB. Hospital stay and recovery is typically less time than that of traditional CABG.

In patients diagnosed with a blockage of the left anterior descending coronary artery hybrid revascularization may be an option for treatment. Hybrid revascularization involves a combination of robotic-assisted bypass surgery as well as PCI.

VALVULAR HEART DISEASE

Management of valvular heart disease has dramatically changed in the past 10 years. With the advent of transcatheter therapies, options to treat certain valvular conditions have created an option for treatment in those who may not have had options otherwise. This section will explore transcatheter treatment methodologies.

Mitral Valve Disease

Medical Management of Mitral Disease

Medical management of mitral valve disease is dependent on the cause of valvular heart disease. The treatment is different if the cause is stenosis, functional MR (FMR), or degenerative MR (DMR). In some cases medical management may not be an option if the cause is mechanical and causing symptoms.

Medical management in mitral stenosis includes diuretics, anticoagulants, beta blockers or calcium channel blockers, antiarrhythmics, and potential antibiotics. The diuretics are given to reduce fluid accumulation. Anticoagulants or antithrombotics may be given to prevent clot formation secondary to stasis in the left atrium. Beta blockers or calcium channel blockers are used to decrease the transmitral gradient as well as rate control.[17] Mitral stenosis can cause atrial fibrillation (AF) or other rhythm disturbances. Patients may require antiarrhythmics in these cases. AF is more related to age than to degree of stenosis.[18] Patients with MS may need antibiotics to be treated for secondary prevention of rheumatic fever. Duration of prophylaxis is dependent on age and last known diagnosis of rheumatic fever, severity of disease, and potential reexposure.

In patients with MR, the cause of the regurgitation guides the medical management. In cases of severe degenerative mitral valve disease, mechanical repair or replacement of the valve may be indicated. In cases of function MR patients should be evaluated for heart failure management inclusive of guideline-directed medical therapy (GDMT), device therapy, and or surgical repair/replacement.

Guideline-Directed Medical Therapy

Various medications have been proven to improve morbidity and mortality in patients with heart failure with reduced ejection fraction (HFrEF) and severe MR.[19] GDMT medications include beta blockers, angiotensin receptor/neprilysin inhibitors (ARNIs), diuretics, nitrates, Angiotensin-converting enzyme inhibitors (ACE-Is) or angiotensin receptor blockers (ARBs), as well as aldosterone antagonists. Medications should be uptitrated as conditions allow.[19]

Device Therapy

Cardiac resynchronization therapy (CRT) for patients with heart failure, depressed left ventricle ejection fraction, and intraventricular conduction delays have shown therapeutic benefits.[19] CRT has shown to reduce morbidity and mortality rates as well as improvement in symptoms and quality of life.[19] Typically there are three leads placed, one in the right atrium, one in the right ventricle, and one in the left ventricle. The purpose of the CRT is to have simultaneous biventricular stimulation to delay the electrical impulse improving the overall contraction increasing the left ventricle efficiency.[20]

Mitral Transcatheter Therapies

MR is one of the most prevalent valvular heart diseases.[21] There are two types of MR, degenerative and functional. DMR is caused by structural disease of the mitral leaflets or subvalvular apparatus. FMR results from dilation and dysfunction of the left atrium, ventricle, and mitral annulus. The treatment results are often dependent on the type of mitral disease. Advances in mitral technologies are sluggish in part due to the complexities of the mitral valve anatomy and thus, surgical mitral valve repair or replacement remains the current gold standard. However, surgical treatment options are often not suitable for patients at prohibitive surgical risk. The development of transcatheter technologies are already established or under development to mimic surgical repair (TMVr) and replacement strategies (TMVR). The following will outline some of the recent technologic advancements to treat MR without surgery.

Repair: Edge-to-Edge

Edge-to-edge repair with the MitraClip technology (Abbott Vascular) has drastically changed the landscape for symptomatic severe MR patients with more than 60,000 procedures performed worldwide. While the DMR etiology may be considered ideal for MitraClip, it appears to be both safe and efficacious in patients with FMR as well. A recent meta-analysis demonstrated higher reintervention rates at 1 year in the DMR group as compared to the FMR group (10% vs. 4%, respectively; $p = 0.04$) but no significant difference in mortality between the FMR and DMR groups.[22] Multiple trials are ongoing comparing percutaneous edge-to-edge repair with optimal medical therapy (COAPT and MITRA-FR). Further studies are needed to carefully evaluate the MitraClip system against medical management and surgery, in addition to longer-term quality-of-life outcomes.

Newer/next-generation edge-to-edge devices are designed for more effective grabbing of the leaflets (MitraClip NTR/XTR, Abbott Vascular) and streamlined steering within the left atrium, additional MR reduction by incorporation of a central spacer, and independent leaflet grasping (PASCAL transcatheter mitral valve repair system, Edwards Lifesciences Corp). The first-in-human study of the PASCAL device showed procedural success and residual MR ≤2+ in 96% of patients.[23] The CLASP Study to assess the safety and efficacy of the Edwards PASCAL is ongoing.

Repair: Annuloplasty

The durability of transcatheter edge-to-edge FMR repair is unclear due to its narrow approach by targeting the valve leaflets only. Interventional therapies mimicking annular dimension reduction, the surgical gold standard for FMR, are also being investigated. These devices are delivered via transseptal atrial access and the ring is implanted directly to the atrial side of the mitral annulus. The band can be tensioned to reduce the annular circumference and reduce the degree of MR. In the United States, there are a number of RCT currently enrolling patients to evaluate the efficacy of percutaneous annuloplasty.

Replacement

To date, there have been early cases of catheter-based mitral valve replacements (TMVR), with the majority of these early cases being performed in patients with a previous surgical bioprosthetic valve utilizing a valve-in-valve (ViV) or ring, valve-in-ring (ViR) using an inverted balloon expandable valve. Fewer cases of TMVR in severe mitral annular calcification (ViMAC) have been reported. Because of the early success, ViV in failed surgical mitral valve is considered a viable and approved treatment option with inverted balloon expandable valve.[24] Conversely, ViR and ViMAC are associated with increased adverse events and high 30-day and 1-year mortality.[24,25] Research is ongoing in this area.

Transcatheter mitral valve replacement technologies are under development specifically for treatment of MR. Currently, there are a number of RCTs studying the use of transcatheter mitral valve replacements. The initial data from these trials appear to be favorable, however, more research needs to be done. Limitations to the current TMVR therapies are the anchoring of the device within the mitral valve, left ventricular outflow tract obstruction, and the need for a transapical access.[26]

Surgical Therapies for Mitral Valve Disease

Mitral valve surgery is indicated for severe valvular disease, usually symptomatic, although surgery is also indicated in selected asymptomatic cases. Valvular heart disease severity is typically determined by echocardiographic criteria. The most common indication for MV surgery is severe DMR with an LVEF of >30%.[27] Mitral valve repair is the preferred surgery, however replacement can be considered if the likelihood of success is low in repair.[27] Asymptomatic patients appropriate for surgery include those with LV dysfunction, preserved LV ejection fraction, and AF secondary to the MR or pulmonary hypertension.[27] In patients with ischemic MR, surgery is more limited. If the patient is undergoing concomitant CABG, surgery on the mitral valve is indicated in this patient population.

Mitral valve surgery is only indicated for severe mitral stenosis in patients not judged suitable for mitral balloon valvuloplasty (MBV) by the Heart Team secondary to unfavorable characteristics or contraindications valvuloplasty. Contraindications include severe pulmonary hypertension, AF, left atrial appendage (LAA) thrombus, previous commissurotomy, high echocardiographic anatomic scores (Wilkins, Cormier), and concomitant aortic or tricuspid valvular disease or significant CAD.[27]

Tricuspid Valve

Severe tricuspid regurgitation (TR) affects approximately 1.6 million Americans. The majority (85%) of TR is functional in nature. Untreated TR is associated with progressive right-sided heart failure, and carries a poor prognosis causing high morbidity and mortality. Surgical repair is still the gold standard for TR, but only a small proportion of patients undergo surgical repair leaving a high clinical demand for alternatives to conventional surgery. There are anatomical challenges when performing a percutaneous transcatheter procedure compared to a surgical annuloplasty. Noted challenges are approach, access, landing zone, proximal structures, and visibility.[28]

Recently, promising transcatheter tricuspid technologies, along with a growing body of knowledge, has ignited inquiry within the interventional and surgical communities. Transcatheter tricuspid valve repair (TTVr) devices are currently under preclinical or early clinical trials. Primarily, there are two approaches with different subgroups that exist for percutaneous TR treatment—repair (leaflet coaptation or annuloplasty) and replacement.

Medical Management

Heart failure is a main cause of TR. Diseases of the left side of the heart lead to chronic pressure overload of the right ventricle. This leads to right ventricle dilation, causing functional TR.[29] In these patients, medical therapy typically includes diuretics and heart failure medication is commonly ineffective.[29] Severe TR secondary to RV failure is considered a high risk for cardiac surgery and carries a poor prognosis.

Another culprit of TR is pulmonary disease. Treatment should be aimed at the underlying condition rather than heart failure focused.[29] Increases in right atrial pressure is transmitted to the central and hepatic veins leading to portal hypertension and subsequent ascites. Ascites is present in 90% of those with severe TR.[29]

Primary TR occurs less frequently than functional TR. Primary TR is seen when there is damage to the structure of the tricuspid valve (leaflets, chordae, papillary muscles, or the annulus). This occurs independently of the right ventricle. Primary TR can be seen in endocarditis, congenital disease, rheumatic fever, carcinoid disease, as well as other conditions.[29] Diagnosis of TR is made using echocardiography.

Surgical Approach

Diagnoses where surgical annuloplasty or valve replacement is considered include structural deformity (e.g., Ebstein anomaly), bacterial endocarditis, or ventricular dilation uncontrolled by medical therapy. Significant mortality is associated with surgery for the tricuspid valve. Surgery is considered in severe primary TR, even if the patient is asymptomatic or if the patient is undergoing a left-sided heart surgery.[29] In contrast, patients with secondary severe TR are only considered for surgery if they are undergoing a left-sided heart surgery.

Surgical interventions for TR focus on restoring valvular function by reducing annular size. Annular size reduction is achieved by use of annular ring or partial purse string technique (DeVega technique).[29] Rigid rings are associated with lower incidence of recurrent TR than flexible rings or DeVega technique. Valve replacement should be considered in cases where the valve is structurally compromised as in cases of endocarditis or carcinoid disease.[30] Patients in need of valve replacement should be considered for both bioprosthetic and mechanical valves. Age, pathology, and comorbid conditions will help determine valve choice. It is important to note that the right side of the heart has lower pressure and consideration should be given to anticoagulation.[30] Another important consideration is mechanical valves may limit future pacemaker implantation.

Percutaneous Approach

Repair: Edge-to-edge. The use of one or more of the MitraClip device (Abbott Vascular, Santa Clara, California), albeit off-label use, in the tricuspid position has become a popular approach for high-risk patients with functional TR. This is likely due in part to global accessibility and operator familiarity.[31] Worldwide, roughly 1,000 cases have been performed and patients receiving this therapy represent the majority of patients included in the international registry assessing different available transcatheter TR devices.[32,33] Registry results indicate 1+ grade reduction in 91% of patients and is often accompanied by symptom and functional class improvements.[34]

A modified version of the MitraClip (Abbott Vascular) to address the tricuspid valve is currently under investigation (TRILUMINATE). Trials are also underway studying technologies focused on coaptation using the Pascal Device (Edwards Lifescience). There are a number of other devices being studied in early feasibility in the United States as well as in other parts of the world.

Repair: Annuloplasty. Surgical repair in functional TR is typically performed using either suture annuloplasty or ring annuloplasty. Current percutaneous annuloplasty systems either obtain a direct or an indirect annuloplasty. Both direct and indirect percutaneous annuloplasties are modeled after surgical procedures. Percutaneous annuloplasty systems are designed to address functional TR. Caution must be used not to interfere with the right coronary artery secondary to its proximity to the tricuspid valve. The wall of the right ventricle is very thin and not ideal for a transapical approach. Another limitation is the unfavorable angle between the tricuspid annulus and the inferior vena cava.[35]

There are two types of annuloplasty devices, complete or incomplete. Complete devices include Cardioband (Edwards Lifesciences, Irvine, CA), IRIS (Millipede, Santa Rosa, CA), Minimally Invasive Annuloplasty (MIA) (Micro Interevntional Devices, Inc., Newtown, PA), and Transatrial Intrapericardial Annuloplasty (TRAIPTA). Incomplete devices include TriCIncy (4Tech, Galway, Ireland) and Trialign (Mitralign, Tewksbury, Massachusetts).[35]

Replacement

While many companies are working on percutaneous tricuspid valve replacement devices, currently only a few have been successfully implanted in humans and there are a number of devices in development. The tricuspid valve has some challenges when it comes to percutaneous replacement. The annulus is less fibrous than the mitral valve and the RCA surrounds the parietal attachment of the valve. The shape of the valve changes throughout the cardiac cycle.[36]

Access is a concern when it comes to replacement of the tricuspid valve. The dimensions of the valve are dynamic and the TV annulus is larger than that of the mitral. Current delivery systems are up to 45 French making access assessments critical. Percutaneous accesses include transjugular, femoral vein, or transapical. The femoral vein is considered the safest access point.[36]

In addition to access determination other aspects of replacement require a through assessment. Valve anchoring, conduction disturbances, durability, residual regurgitation, and acute increases in right ventricle afterload are areas that continue to need addressing for percutaneous TVR to be successful. The tricuspid valve, due to the low-flow nature of the right side of the heart will likely require life-long anticoagulation.[36] This will need to be discussed with the patient for shared decision making.

Patients currently undergoing transcatheter tricuspid valve therapy are predominantly high risk, with a functional etiology. Early results reveal potential feasibility, however clinical efficacy requires further investigation.[32] Several devices implementing more complex multi-stage approaches to treat TR are under development or investigation.

Aortic Valve Procedures

Increasing accessibility to transcatheter aortic valve replacement (TAVR) has solidified its use as a viable alternative to traditional surgical aortic valve replacement (SAVR). While TAVR use is continuing to increase, there remains a need for open surgical valve replacement in patients who may have concomitant valvular heart disease, anatomical considerations, or CAD. Due to this need, the surgical aortic valve market continues to advance their technology to make surgical time and CPB time as short as possible. Due to this more sutureless valves are being utilized. These valves utilize a balloon cuff for more rapid deployment and only three sutures to minimize the time needed to suture in place. When compared to a traditional surgical aortic valves which require 12 to 15 sutures to secure.

RCTs proved the superiority of TAVR over medical therapy and over SAVR in patients having prohibitive or high surgical risk.[37–39] Evidence supporting the use of TAVR in intermediate-risk patients has also been published.[40,41] Most recently, data supporting the use of TAVR in low-risk patients have been established.[42,43] The FDA has approved TAVR for use in all surgical risk categories. To improve access to care and provide flexibility for starting and maintaining TAVR programs, the Centers for Medicare and Medicaid Services have approved new guidelines that will expand the use of TAVR procedures to additional hospitals.[44]

Aortic Insufficiency

Currently, SAVR is the preferred therapeutic option for a patient with severe AR. Almost 8% of these patients are not eligible for surgical intervention due to increased age or presence of comorbid conditions.[45,46] TAVR for pure AR of the native valve is being explored as off-label treatment alternative to surgery, however due to the lack of calcium the predictability is lacking. Causes of AR vary and can include inflammatory, infectious, degenerative, and genetic processes leading to structural leaflet dysfunction or aortopathy. Absence of valve calcification and aortic root dilation can compromise device success and decrease procedural safety. Despite these challenges, several reports proved the feasibility of the procedure in high-risk patients with favorable impact on clinical outcomes.[47] The J-Valve system (JC Medical) is intended for the treatment of patients who suffer from AR. First in human studies began in 2018.

Bicuspid Aortic Valve

As bicuspid aortic valves are more prevalent in younger AS patients, the feasibility of TAVR in bicuspid AS is of particular importance. Bicuspid aortic valves tend to be eccentric and heavily calcified. This anatomy has typically been treated with surgery due to the predictability of TAVR and the potential for aortopathy in this patient population. Complication rates are reported to decrease with the introduction of newer devices.[48] TAVR RCTs have systematically excluded patients with a bicuspid aortic valve anatomy due to the presence of a noncircular annulus and concerns for increased perivalvular leaks and presence of severe calcification which was worrisome for increased risk of rupture or periprocedural strokes. Additionally, patients with bicuspid aortic valve anatomy often require treatment at a young age and may have an associated ascending aortic aneurysm.[48,49] TAVR for bicuspid aortic stenosis is under investigation.

Valve-in-Valve

ViV procedures have been successful in treating degenerated aortic bioprostheses and implanting transcatheter valves into surgical mitral annuloplasty rings.[50] However, implanting a second valve within the previous valve or ring can create a smaller orifice. Thus, ViV procedures have the potential for increased postprocedural gradients and prosthesis–patient mismatch (PPM) which adversely affect long-term durability.[51] This deleterious outcome can be more pronounced in younger patients[52] and create a vicious circle of increased gradients, PPM, rapid prosthesis degeneration, and reinterventions. The problem of bioprosthesis failure in younger patients warrants further investigation.

These next-generation TAVR devices demonstrate improved safety and efficacy with various features that can accommodate different clinical and anatomical situations, thus treating an increasing number of patients. Long-term follow-up in patients can provide definitive guidance on the optimal treatment strategy in younger, low-risk patients.

Development and improvement of catheter-based structural heart interventions have enabled more patients to receive minimally invasive heart valve interventions. Increasingly, these procedures are improving survival and/or quality of life for many patients who, previously, were considered unsuitable for surgery. Continued technical and device advances and amassed evidence will expand the future of structural heart disease interventions. The role of professional societies and the Heart Team will be even more prominent in the future while translating trial results into everyday clinical practice (Table 28-1).

Other Structural Interventions

Left Atrial Appendage Occlusion

An estimated 7.2 million Americans ≥20 years of age self-report having had a stroke. It is forecasted by 2030, an additional 3.4 million adults in the United States representing will have had a stroke, reflecting a 20% increase from 2012.[11] Over 85% of all strokes are ischemic. AF is an independent risk factor for ischemic stroke severity, recurrence, and mortality.[53,54] Oral Anticoagulants (OACs) and Direct Oral Anticoagulants (DOACs) are currently the first line of treatment for the prevention of thromboembolism in AF. Unfortunately, anticoagulation under utilization continues to be a global issue[11] and there are several limitations associated with their use, including the risk of bleeding.

In patients with AF who have been diagnosed with thrombus or emboli, the LAA is the site of thrombus formation more than 90% of the time.[54] Over time, AF leads to a loss of contractile function of the LAA, which promotes stasis and thrombus formation that may be the source of the emboli. LAA closure is a promising alternative for reducing systemic thromboembolic events in these patients without increasing the risk of bleeding.[54] This proves beneficial for patients who have not tolerated anticoagulation due to gastrointestinal and other bleeding.

Devices are available for LAA occlusion in the management of stroke and systemic thromboembolism. Endocardial transcatheter closure is the most widely used and tested method for the closure of LAAs. The WATCHMAN™ (Boston Scientific) is the first percutaneous LAA occlusive device approved by the FDA for the prevention of thromboembolism by addressing the LAA in patients with nonvalvular AF.[55,56] The AMPLATZER™ Amulet™ (Abbott Vascular) is a second-generation device with a longer lobe and waist than the AMPLATZER™ Cardiac Plug (Abbott Vascular) is currently being evaluated in an RCT.[57]

The LARIAT® device (SentreHeart Inc.) is a suture-based device and the procedure incorporates a combined endo–epicardial

Table 28-1 • NURSING INTERVENTIONS

	Surgical Treatment	Percutaneous Treatment	Medical Treatment
Shared Decision Making	• Goals of care • Values and preferences • Patient desires • Understanding of indications, alternatives, and personalized risks and benefits for medical, surgical, and percutaneous treatment options • Advanced directive		
Anatomical Concerns	• Porcelain aorta • Previous surgery • Cardiac structures proximal to the sternum prohibiting sternotomy (patent LIMA) • History of radiation to the chest • Pectus deformities	• Vascular disease • Endocarditis • Atheromas	• None
Physiologic Concerns	• Cognitive impairment • Comorbid conditions (COPD, DM, CKD, prior CVA) • Functional impairment (ADLs, IADLs, gait) • Nutritional impairment	• Comorbid conditions (CKD-limiting contrast administration) • Cognitive impairment	• Tolerance of medications and side effects • Interactions of medications, especially with polypharmacy
Social Concerns	• Social support pre/peri/postprocedure • Ability to afford medications • Driver to return for visits	• Social support pre/peri/postprocedure • Ability to afford medications	• Social support to care for patient as illness progresses • Ability to afford medications
Educational Needs	• Procedural expectations • Postprocedural care • Importance of medications • Diet and exercise instructions • Importance of cardiac rehabilitation	• Procedural expectations • Postprocedural care • Importance of medications • Diet and exercise instructions • Importance of cardiac rehabilitation	• Prognosis and course of disease • Routine monitoring (follow-up visits, laboratory studies) • When to call provider • Instructions for activity (limitations) • Diet education
Patient Preparation	• Chest scrub • Dental care • Preoperative testing • Medications	• Groin care • Preprocedure testing • Medications	• Medication awareness • List of providers

Courtesy of Keegan P, Perpetua E.

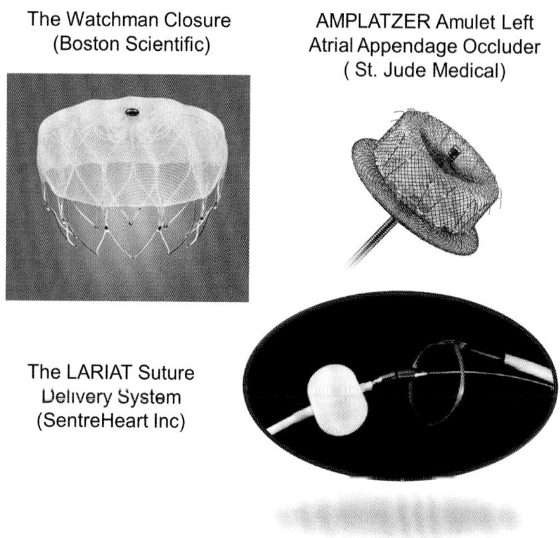

Figure 28-5. Left atrial appendage occuluder. (Used with permission from Herzog E. *Herzog's CCU Book*. Philadelphia, PA: Wolters Kluwer; 2017.)

ligation of the LAA. This procedure may be considered if the LAA is too large for one of the occlude devices but does not have an FDA indication specifically for LAA closure. Other epicardial approaches involve the placement, during open cardiac surgery, of an epicardial clip, such as the ATRICLIP® device (AtriCure), at the base of the LAA which has demonstrated favorable safety and efficacy.[58] Other LAAO devices are in various stages of development and/or clinical trials.

The advantage of LAA closure in reducing the incidence of stroke in patients with nonvalvular AF is promising but further evaluation of its efficacy will be understood over longer treatment duration. Improvements in safety and decreased procedural times are the focus of newer devices and techniques. Further studies are also necessary to determine anticoagulation or antiplatelet regimen and duration post LAAO (Fig. 28-5).

Atrial Septal Defect and Patent Foramen Ovale

An atrial septal defect (**ASD**) is a type of congenital **heart** defect in which there is an abnormal opening in the septum of the heart between the atria. A **patent foramen ovale** (**PFO**) is a hole in the **heart** that did not close the way it should after birth. During fetal development, a small flap-like opening, the foramen ovale, is normally present in the atrial septum.

The causal relationship between PFO and cryptogenic stroke has historically been controversial. Although the prevalence of PFO is significantly higher in patients with cryptogenic stroke, a PFO has not been shown to increase the risk of ischemic stroke.[59] Additionally, roughly 40% adults with an idiopathic ischemic stroke have a PFO.[60] Thus, transient embolism across a PFO may be associated with cryptogenic strokes.

Currently, there are two devices commercially available for ASD and PFO closures in the United States although several are available worldwide. The Amplatzer PFO Occluder (Abbott Vascular) was the first device to be FDA approved in the United States for PFO closure. The device has two self-expanding discs composed of nickel titanium designed to conform to either side of the septum. The discs are connected by a thin neck, which spans the atrial connection. The Gore Cardioform Septal Occluder® (W.L. Gore and Assoc) is currently FDA approved for both ASD and PFO closure and is also comprised of two platinum-filled Nitinol discs covered by a thrombo-resistant polyetrafluoroethylene (PTFE) material.[61]

A single device might not be suitable for optimal treatment of all PFOs due to highly variable anatomical morphology of the PFO. Devices uniquely suited to specific anatomical variants will minimize complications as well as residual shunts and improve the overall success rate of the procedure. In addition, the residual PFO closure device makes future access to the left atrium challenging. With the growth of left-sided procedures, including percutaneous mitral valve interventions, LAA closure, and left-sided ablations, access to the left atrium through the IAS is becoming increasingly important. This has ignited interest in developing a bioresorbable PFO device. Early iterations demonstrated a positive safety profile, however residual shunting at follow-up tempered enthusiasm (Fig. 28-6).

Summary

With the plethora of technologic advancements on the horizon, the concept of the multidisciplinary heart team will continue to be a mainstay in decision making for patient treatment options.[1] The landscape of treatment options for cardiovascular and structural disease is continuing to develop. The nurse will need to stay abreast of these innovations as well as implications for care and patient educational needs.

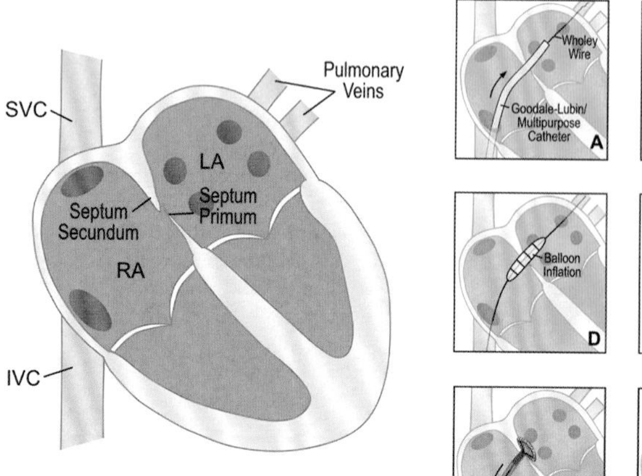

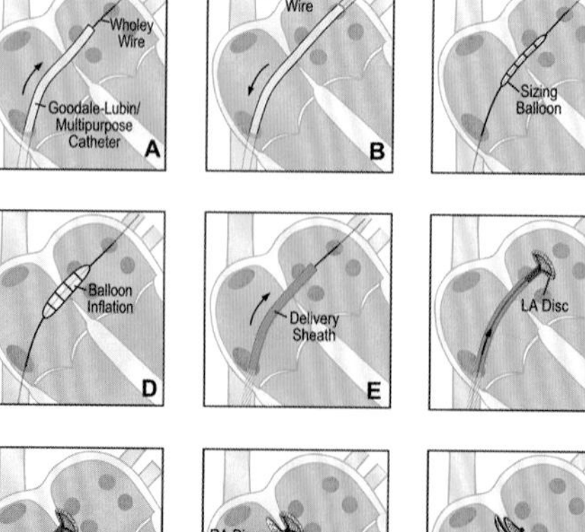

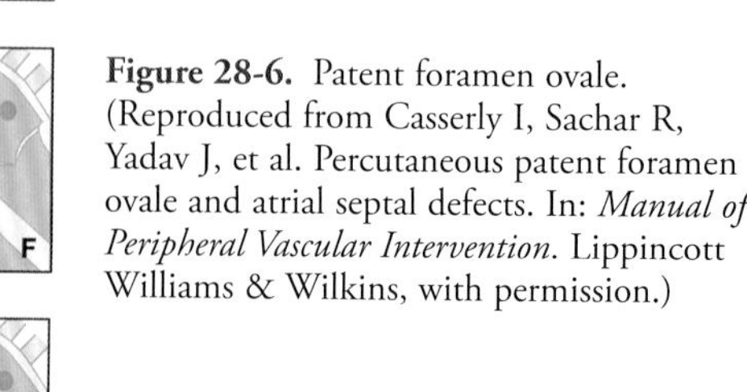

Figure 28-6. Patent foramen ovale. (Reproduced from Casserly I, Sachar R, Yadav J, et al. Percutaneous patent foramen ovale and atrial septal defects. In: *Manual of Peripheral Vascular Intervention*. Lippincott Williams & Wilkins, with permission.)

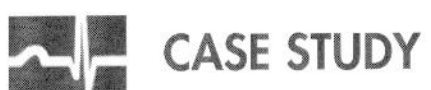

CASE STUDY

Patient Profile
Name/Age/Sex: **Janet Jones, 44-year-old female**

History of Present Illness
Ms. Jones was referred to the structural heart program for evaluation of her PFO. She recently had a stroke and upon workup for causes was found to have a PFO. She denies any other history.

Past Medical History
Stroke 6 months ago

Surgical History
Cholecystectomy, tonsillectomy, appendectomy

Family History
Mother bladder cancer, father diabetes

Social History
Denies alcohol, tobacco, or illicit drug use

Medications
Rosuvastatin 20 mg, aspirin 325 mg (placed on after her stroke)

Allergies
NKDA

Patient Examination

Vital Signs
BP 114/68; Resp 16; Temp 37°C; HR 75; Ht. 160 cm; Wt. 68 kg

Physical Examination
General: Awake, alert and oriented. No distress noted.

Skin: Clean, dry, intact.

Cardiac: No murmurs, gallops, or rubs are auscultated. S1 and S2 are heard and are of normal intensity.

Respiratory: Lung sounds are clear in all lobes bilaterally without rales, ronchi, or wheezes.

Abdominal: Abdomen is soft, symmetric, and nontender without distention. No masses, hepatomegaly, or splenomegaly are noted.

Psychiatric: Appropriate mood and affect. Good judgment and insight. No visual or auditory hallucinations. No suicidal or homicidal ideation.

Testing: Echo with bubble study confirming PFO with left-to-right shunting

Considerations

Key Questions
Should PFO be closed?

Evidence
PFO is associated with strokes of unclear etiology. Even though PFO is present in approximately 20% of the population, it is present in 40% of those with cryptogenic stroke. Three clinical trials, CLOSURE, PC trial, and RESPECT short term did not show a clear benefit for percutaneous closure. However, in 2016, the meta-analysis of CLOSURE I, PC, and RESPECT showed percutaneous PFO closure was superior to medical therapy for the prevention of recurrent stroke. Two other trials, CLOSE and REDUCE, showed benefit to PFO closure. Of note, percutaneous PFO closure patients had a higher risk of development of AF and should be closely monitored.[62]

KEY READINGS

Arnett DK, Goodman RA, Halperin JL, et al. Citation tools. AHA/ACC/HHS strategies to enhance application of clinical practice guidelines in patients with cardiovascular disease and comorbid conditions: from the American Heart Association, American College of Cardiology, and U.S. Department of Health and Human Services. *J Am Coll Cardiol.* 2014;64(17):1851–1856.

Levine GN, O'Gara PT, Beckman JA, et al. Recent innovations, modifications, and evolution of ACC/AHA clinical practice guidelines: an update for our constituencies: a report of the American College of Cardiology/American Heart Association Task Force on clinical practice guidelines. *J Am Coll Cardiol.* 2019;73(15):1990–1998.

Nishimura RA, Otto CM, Bonow RO, et al. 2014 AHA/ACC guideline for the management of patients with valvular heart disease: a report of the American College of Cardiology/American Heart Association Task Force on Practice Guidelines. *J Am Coll Cardiol.* 2014;63(22):e57–e185.

REFERENCES

1. Holmes DR, Rich JB, Zoghbi WA, et al. The heart team of cardiovascular care. *J Am Coll Cardiol.* 2013;61(9):903–907.
2. Doenst T, Diab M, Sponholz C, et al. The opportunities and limitations of minimally invasive cardiac surgery. *Dtsch Arztebl Int.* 2017;114(46):777–784.
3. Cooley DA, Frazier OH. The past 50 years of cardiovascular surgery. *Circulation.* 2000;102(20 Suppl 4):IV87–IV93.
4. Iribarne A, Easterwood R, Chan EYH, et al. The golden age of minimally invasive cardiothoracic surgery: current and future perspectives. *Future Cardiol.* 2011;7(3):333–346.
5. Holmes DR Jr, Williams DO. Catheter-based treatment of coronary artery disease: past, present, and future. *Circ Cardiovasc Interv.* 2008;1(1):60–73.
6. Fromes Y, Bical OM. MIECT: how did it start? *J Thorac Dis.* 2019;11(Suppl 10):S1492–S1497. Available at https://www.researchgate.net/profile/Yves_Fromes/publication/331982461_MIECT_How_did_it_start/links/5c98da62299bf111694696f2/MIECT-How-did-it-start.pdf
7. Khan TM, Siddiqui AH. Intra-aortic balloon pump (IABP). (Updated September 10, 2019). In: *StatPearls [Internet].* Treasure Island (FL): StatPearls Publishing; 2019. Available at https://www.ncbi.nlm.nih.gov/books/NBK542233
8. Ergle K, Parto P, Krim SR. Percutaneous ventricular assist devices: a novel approach in the management of patients with acute cardiogenic shock. *Ochsner J.* 2016;16(3):243–249.
9. Rihal CS, Naidu SS, Givertz MM, et al. 2015 SCAI/ACC/HFSA/STS Clinical Expert Consensus Statement on the use of percutaneous mechanical circulatory support devices in cardiovascular care (Endorsed by the American Heart Association, the Cardiological Society of India, and Sociedad Latino Americana de Cardiologia Intervencion; Affirmation of Value by the Canadian Association of Interventional Cardiology-Association Canadienne de Cardiologie d'intervention). *J Card Fail.* 2015;21(6):499–518.
10. Ali J, Vuylsteke A. Extracorporeal membrane oxygenation: indications, technique and contemporary outcomes. *Heart.* 2019;105:1437–1443.
11. Benjamin EJ, Virani SS, Callaway CW, et al. Heart disease and stroke statistics-2018 update: a report from the American Heart Association. *Circulation.* 2018;137(12):e67–e492.
12. Head SJ, Milojevic M, Daemen J, et al. Stroke rates following surgical versus percutaneous coronary revascularization. *J Am Coll Cardiol.* 2018;72(4):386–398.
13. Chakravartti J, Rao SV. Robotic assisted percutaneous coronary intervention: hype or hope? *J Am Heart Assoc.* 2019;8(13):e012743.
14. Serruys, PW, Ormiston JA, Onuma Y, et al. A bioabsorbable everolimus-eluting coronary stent system (ABSORB): 2-year outcomes and results from multiple imaging methods. *Lancet.* 2019;373(9667):897–910.

15. National Research Council (US); Institute of Medicine (US); Woolf SH, Aron L, eds. *U.S. Health in International Perspective: Shorter Lives, Poorer Health*. Washington, DC: National Academies Press (US); 2013. 4, Public Health and Medical Care Systems. Available at https://www.ncbi.nlm.nih.gov/books/NBK154484/
16. Spadaccio C, Benedetto U. Coronary artery bypass grafting (CABG) *vs*. percutaneous coronary intervention (PCI) in the treatment of multivessel coronary disease: quo vadis? a review of the evidences on coronary artery disease. *Ann Cardiothorac Surg*. 2018;7(4):506–515.
17. Tyagi G, Pasca I, Dang P, et al. Rates and correlates of progression of degenerative mitral stenosis: potential beneficial effect of beta blockers. *J Am Coll Cardiol*. 2012;59(13 suppl):E2033.
18. Lung B, Leenhardt A, Extramiana F. Management of atrial fibrillation in patients with rheumatic mitral stenosis. *Heart*. 2018;104:1062–1068.
19. Yancy C. Jessup M, Bozkurt B, et al. 2017 ACC/AHA/HFSA focused update of the 2013 ACCF/AHA guideline for the management of heart failure: A Report of the American College of Cardiology/American Heart Association Task Force on Clinical Practice Guidelines and the Heart Failure Society of America. *J Am Coll Cardiol*. 2107;70(6):776–803.
20. Yanez I, Egea-Serrano P, Nicolas-Franco S. The use of cardiac resyn chronization to manage mitral regurgitation. *Eur Soc Cardiol*. 2016;(14):28.
21. Obadia JF, Armoiry X, Iung B, et al. The MITRA-FR study: design and rationale of a randomised study of percutaneous mitral valve repair compared with optimal medical management alone for severe secondary mitral regurgitation. *EuroIntervention*. 2015;10(11):1354–1360.
22. Chiarito M, Pagnesi M, Martino EA, et al. Outcome after percutaneous edge-to-edge mitral repair for functional and degenerative mitral regurgitation: a systematic review and meta-analysis. *Heart*. 2018;104(4):306–312.
23. Praz F, Spargias K, Chrissoheris M, et al. Compassionate use of the PASCAL transcatheter mitral valve repair system for patients with severe mitral regurgitation: a multicentre, prospective, observational, first-in-man study. *Lancet*. 2017;390(10096):773–780.
24. Yoon SH, Whisenant BK, Bleiziffer S, et al. Outcomes of transcatheter mitral valve replacement for degenerated bioprostheses, failed annuloplasty rings, and mitral annular calcification. *Eur Heart J*. 2019;40(5):441–451.
25. Guerrero M, Urena M, Himbert D, et al. 1-year outcomes of transcatheter mitral valve replacement in patients with severe mitral annular calcification. *J Am Coll Cardiol*. 2018;71(17):1841–1853.
26. Bapat V, Rajagopal V, Meduri C, et al. Early experience with new transcatheter mitral valve replacement. *J Am Coll Cardiol*. 2018;71(1): 12–21.
27. Sayeed R. Mitral valve disease: when should we call the cardiac surgeon. *Eur Soc Cardiol*. 2018;16:28.
28. Donatelle M, Lim DS. Percutaneous tricuspid annuloplasty. *Minerva Cardioangiol*. 2018;66(6):713–717.
29. Beckhoff F, Alushi B, Jung C, et al. Tricuspid regurgitation – medical management and evolving interventional concepts. *Front Cardiovasc Med*. 2018;5:49.
30. Belluschi I, Del Forno B, Lapenna E, et al. Surgical techniques for tricuspid valve disease. *Front Cardiovasc Med*. 2018;5:118.
31. Asmarats L, Puri R, Latib A, et al. Transcatheter tricuspid valve interventions: landscape, challenges, and future directions. *J Am Coll Cardiol*. 2018;71(25):2935–2956.
32. Taramasso M, Hahn RT, Alessandrini H, et al. The international multicenter trivalve registry: which patients are undergoing transcatheter tricuspid repair? *JACC Cardiovasc Interv*. 2017;10(19):1982–1990.
33. Curio J, Demir OM, Pagnesi M, et al. Update on the current landscape of transcatheter options for tricuspid regurgitation treatment. *Interv Cardiol*. 2019;14(2):54–61.
34. Nickenig G, Kowalski M, Hausleiter J, et al. Transcatheter treatment of severe tricuspid regurgitation with the edge-to-edge mitraclip technique. *Circulation*. 2017;135(19):1802–1814.
35. Mangieri A, Lim S, Rogers J, et al. Percutaneous tricuspid annuloplasty. *Interv Cardiol Clin*. 2018;7(1):31–36.
36. Demir OM, Regazzoli D, Mangieri A, et al. Transcatheter tricuspid valve replacement: principles and design. *Front Cardiovasc Med*. 2018;5:129.
37. Leon MB, Smith CR, Mack M, et al. Transcatheter aortic-valve implantation for aortic stenosis in patients who cannot undergo surgery. *N Engl J Med*. 2010;363(17):1597–1607.
38. Popma JJ, Adams DH, Reardon MJ, et al. Transcatheter aortic valve replacement using a self-expanding bioprosthesis in patients with severe aortic stenosis at extreme risk for surgery. *J Am Coll Cardiol*. 2014;63(19):1972–1981.
39. Adams DH, Popma JJ, Reardon MJ, et al. Transcatheter aortic-valve replacement with a self-expanding prosthesis. *N Engl J Med*. 2014;370(19):1790–1798.
40. Leon MB, Smith CR, Mack MJ, et al. Transcatheter or surgical aortic-valve replacement in intermediate-risk patients. *N Engl J Med*. 2016;374(17):1609–1620.
41. Reardon MJ, Van Mieghem NM, Popma JJ, et al. Surgical or transcatheter aortic-valve replacement in intermediate-risk patients. *N Engl J Med*. 2017;376(14):1321–1331.
42. Mack MJ, Leon MB, Thourani VH, et al. Transcatheter aortic-valve replacement with a balloon-expandable valve in low-risk patients. *N Engl J Med*. 2019;380(18):1695–1705.
43. Popma JJ, Deeb GM, Yakubov SJ, et al. Transcatheter aortic-valve replacement with a self-expanding valve in low-risk patients. *N Engl J Med*. 2019;380(18):1706–1715.
44. CMS Finalizes Updates to Coverage Policy for Transcatheter Aortic Valve Replacement (TAVR) | CMS. Available at https://www.cms.gov/newsroom/press-releases/cms-finalizes-updates-coverage-policy-transcatheter-aortic-valve-replacement-tavr. Accessed July 28, 2019.
45. Iung B, Baron G, Butchart EG, et al. A prospective survey of patients with valvular heart disease in Europe: The Euro Heart Survey on Valvular Heart Disease. *Eur Heart J*. 2003;24(13):1231–1243.
46. Franzone A, Pilgrim T, Stortecky S, et al. Evolving indications for transcatheter aortic valve interventions. *Curr Cardiol Rep*. 2017;19(11):107.
47. Testa L, Latib A, Rossi ML, et al. CoreValve implantation for severe aortic regurgitation: a multicentre registry. *EuroIntervention*. 2014;10(6): 739-745.
48. Yoon SH, Bleiziffer S, De Backer O, et al. Outcomes in transcatheter aortic valve replacement for bicuspid versus tricuspid aortic valve stenosis. *J Am Coll Cardiol*. 2017;69(21):2579–2589.
49. TAVR for Bicuspid Aortic Valves: Is Surgery Still the Gold Standard?—American College of Cardiology. American College of Cardiology. Available at https://www.acc.org/latest-in-cardiology/articles/2019/04/17/07/14/tavr-for-bicuspid-aortic-valves. Accessed August 4, 2019.
50. Webb JG, Mack MJ, White JM, et al. Transcatheter aortic valve implantation within degenerated aortic surgical bioprostheses: PARTNER 2 valve-in-valve registry. *J Am Coll Cardiol*. 2017;69(18):2253–2262.
51. Del Trigo M, Muñoz-Garcia AJ, Wijeysundera HC, et al. Incidence, timing, and predictors of valve hemodynamic deterioration after transcatheter aortic valve replacement: multicenter registry. *J Am Coll Cardiol*. 2016;67(6):644–655.
52. Johnston DR, Soltesz EG, Vakil N, et al. Long-term durability of bioprosthetic aortic valves: implications from 12,569 implants. *Ann Thorac Surg*. 2015;99(4):1239–1247.
53. Lin HJ, Wolf PA, Kelly-Hayes M, et al. Stroke severity in atrial fibrillation. The Framingham Study. *Stroke*. 1996;27(10):1760–1764.
54. Chava R, Turagam M, Lakkireddy D. Left atrial appendage occlusion: what are the options and where is the evidence? *J Innov Cardiac Rhythm Manage*. 2018;9(4):3095–3106.
55. Reddy VY, Holmes D, Doshi SK, et al. Safety of percutaneous left atrial appendage closure: results from the Watchman Left Atrial Appendage System for Embolic Protection in Patients with AF (PROTECT AF) clinical trial and the Continued Access Registry. *Circulation*. 2011;123(4):417–424.
56. Reddy VY, Doshi S, Sievert H, et al. Long term results of PROTECT AF: The mortality effects of left atrial appendage closure versus warfarin for stroke prophylaxis in AF. *Heart Rhythm*. 2013;10:1411–1415.
57. Landmesser U, Schmidt B, Nielsen-Kudsk JE, et al. Left atrial appendage occlusion with the AMPLATZER Amulet device: periprocedural and early clinical/echocardiographic data from a global prospective observational study. *EuroIntervention*. 2017;13(7):867–876.
58. Ailawadi G, Gerdisch MW, Harvey RL, et al. Exclusion of the left atrial appendage with a novel device: early results of a multicenter trial. *J Thorac Cardiovasc Surg*. 2011;142(5):1002–1009, 1009.e1.
59. Hagen PT, Scholz DG, Edwards WD. Incidence and size of patent foramen ovale during the first 10 decades of life: an autopsy study of 965 normal hearts. *Mayo Clin Proc*. 1984;59(1):17–20.
60. Lechat P, Mas JL, Lascault G, et al. Prevalence of patent foramen ovale in patients with stroke. *N Engl J Med*. 1988;318(18):1148–1152.
61. Collado FMS, Poulin MF, Murphy JJ, et al. Patent foramen ovale closure for stroke prevention and other disorders. *J Am Heart Assoc*. 2018;7(12):e007146.
62. Mojadidi M, Zaman M, Elgendy I, et al. Cryptogenic stroke and patent foramen ovale. *J Am Coll Cardiol*. 2018;71(9):1035–1043.

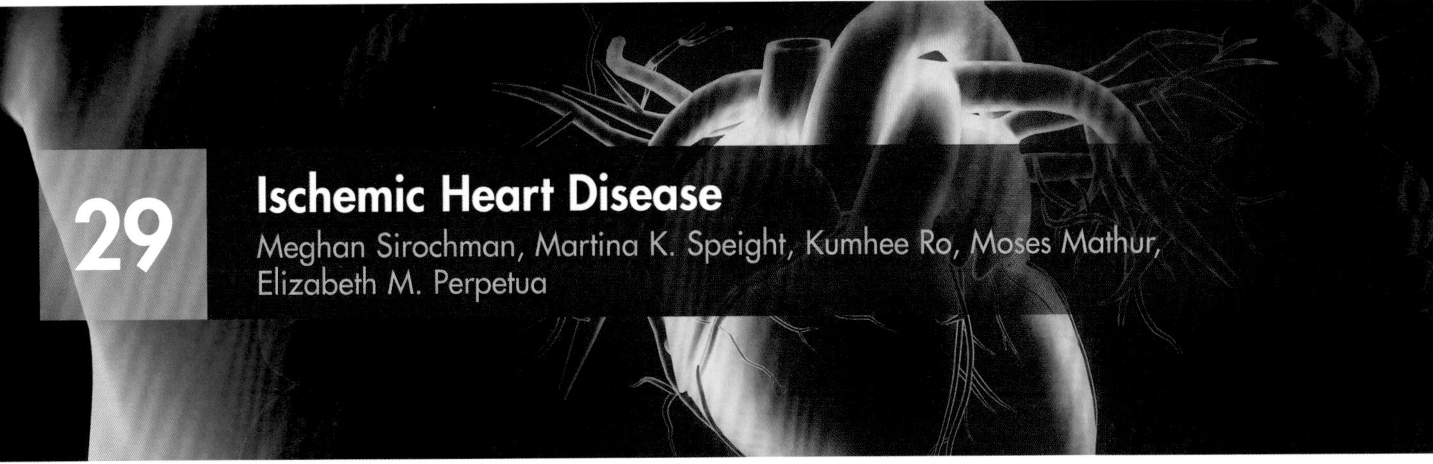

29 Ischemic Heart Disease

Meghan Sirochman, Martina K. Speight, Kumhee Ro, Moses Mathur, Elizabeth M. Perpetua

OBJECTIVES

1. Understand the pathogenesis of atherosclerosis and inflammation.
2. Describe the etiology, diagnosis and management of acute coronary syndrome (ACS), including acute myocardial infarction (AMI), ST-elevation myocardial infarction (STEMI), non–ST-elevation MI (NSTEMI) and other etiologies of MI in nonobstructive coronary artery disease (MINOCA).
3. Describe the etiology, diagnosis, and management of chronic stable ischemic heart disease (SIHD).
4. Compare and contrast the management of ACS versus chronic SIHD.
5. Review nursing care of the patient undergoing coronary revascularization via a catheter-based approach (percutaneous coronary intervention [PCI]) or a surgical approach (coronary artery bypass graft [CABG] surgery).

KEY QUESTIONS

1. What are the pathophysiologic processes responsible for coronary artery disease (CAD) and its consequences?
2. What defines and characterizes ACS and SIHD? How do these diagnoses and their management differ?
3. What is the role of the cardiac nurse in caring for these patients?

BACKGROUND

Most if not all nurses will care for a patient with a history of ischemic heart disease (IHD) also known as coronary artery disease (CAD) or coronary heart disease (CHD). The term IHD and its continuum (Fig. 29-1) includes patients who are asymptomatic, stable, and acutely symptomatic and encompasses the diagnoses of stable angina or low-risk unstable angina (UA); acute coronary syndromes (ACS) including UA/non–ST-elevation MI (NSTEMI), ST-elevation MI (STEMI); sudden cardiac death (SCD); and treatments such as percutaneous coronary intervention (PCI) and coronary artery bypass graft (CABG) surgery.[1]

The spectrum of IHD remains the number one cause of death in the world, attributable to nearly 9 million deaths globally.[2] An estimated 18 million Americans aged 20 years and older have CHD, an overall prevalence of 7%, which is higher in males than females and increases with age.[2] Further, the American Heart Association (AHA) estimates that every 40 seconds an American has a myocardial infarction (MI).[2] In 2019, it was estimated that 720,000 Americans will have a new coronary event (a first hospitalized MI or CHD death) and 335,000 will have a recurrent event.[3] Some of these events are the primary reason for a hospitalization; however, many of these events may occur during hospitalizations for other illnesses.[4] Finally, approximately 35% of people who have a coronary event will not survive.[2] Understanding the various presentations of IHD and how to care for these patients across the continuum are therefore important competencies not only relevant to the cardiac nurse, but all nurses. This chapter describes the pathogenesis, diagnosis, and management of ACS and chronic SIHD. The implications for patient care and the role of the cardiac nurse are discussed.

PATHOGENESIS

Atherosclerosis

The leading cause of myocardial ischemia is atherosclerotic plaque or atheroma disease.[5] Atherosclerosis is a disease of the large and medium arteries, especially the aorta and arteries supplying the heart, brain, kidneys, and lower extremities. The intima or innermost arterial layer is thickened by the development of fibrous tissue and the accumulation of lipid-forming atheromatous plaques (Fig. 29-2). These plaques or atheromas continue to develop and grow over the years, resulting in a narrowed arterial lumen. Occlusion of arterial blood flow can lead to angina, MI, or stroke (Fig. 29-3).

Atherosclerosis is a slow progressive disease that may start in childhood. In some persons, this condition may progress rapidly to cause symptoms in their third decade, whereas in others it does not become clinically significant until the fifth or sixth decades.[6] Atherosclerosis evolves from deposits of lipids, cellular debris, calcium, and fibrin (a clotting agent) that accumulate in the lining of large arteries, all of which initiates and is compounded

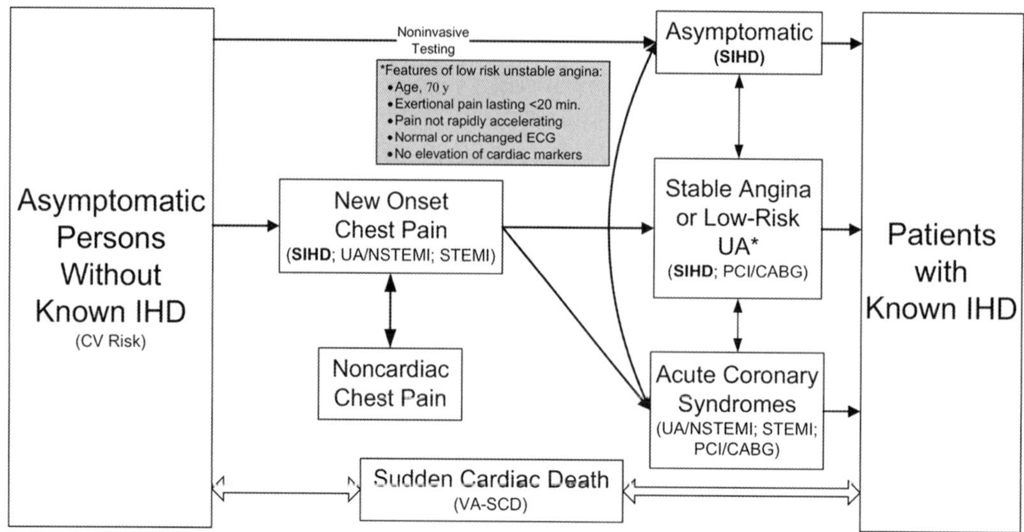

Figure 29-1. Spectrum of IHD. *Guidelines relevant to the spectrum of IHD are in parentheses. CABG, coronary artery bypass graft; CV, cardiovascular; ECG, electrocardiogram; IHD, ischemic heart disease; PCI, percutaneous coronary intervention; SCD, sudden cardiac death; SIHD, stable ischemic heart disease; STEMI, ST-elevation myocardial infarction; UA, unstable angina; UA/NSTEMI, unstable angina/non–ST-elevation myocardial infarction; VA, ventricular arrhythmia. (Adapted from Fihn SD, Gardin JM, Abrams J, et al. 2012 ACCF/AHA/ACP/AATS/PCNA/SCAI/STS Guideline for the diagnosis and management of patients with stable ischemic heart disease: executive summary. *Circulation.* 2012;126[25]:3097–3137.)

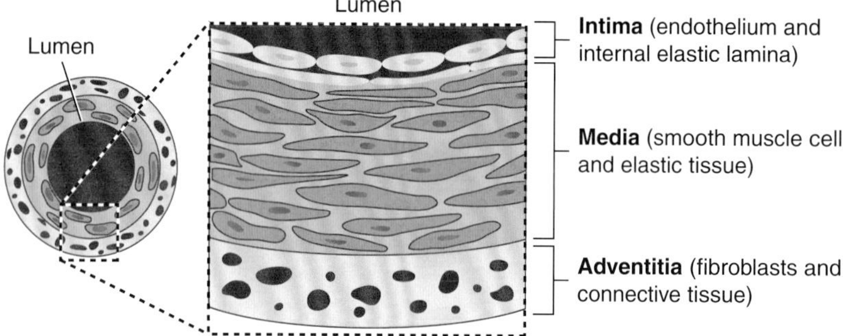

Figure 29-2. Schematic representation of normal coronary artery wall **(top)** and development of atheroma **(bottom).** (Modified from Grech ED. ABC of interventional cardiology: pathophysiology and investigation of coronary artery disease. *BMJ.* 2003;326[7397]:1027–1030.)

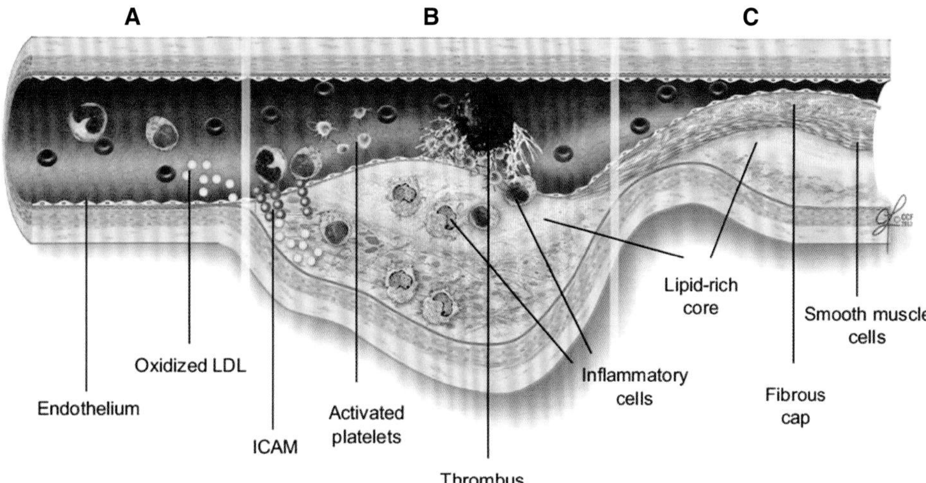

Figure 29-3. Pathophysiology of coronary artery disease **(A)** the "silent period" of atherosclerosis. Asymptomatic endothelial dysfunction predominates during this period which last for decades. Key events include the decreased production of endothelium-derived nitric oxide resulting in local vasoconstriction, the attraction of inflammatory cells to the subendocardial space, the development and destruction of lipid-laden macrophages, increased matrix metalloproteinase activity, and apoptosis. **B:** The vulnerable plaque. Some plaques develop large lipid-laden cores beneath the endothelium. These pockets contain large numbers of inflammatory cells and debris and are covered by a thin layer of smooth muscle cells and fibrous tissue. These thin caps are prone to rupture, exposing blood to the toxic and thrombogenic material in the plaque. This results in platelet activation and thrombosis with abrupt narrowing of the coronary lumen, manifesting as an acute coronary syndrome (unstable angina, myocardial infarction). **C:** The stable plaque. Some plaques develop thick fibrous caps and a dense layer of subendothelial smooth muscle cells that separate the blood from the contents of the plaque. These plaques are much less likely to rupture and gradually encroach upon the coronary lumen, manifesting as stable angina. ICAM, intracellular adhesion molecule; LDL, low-density lipoprotein. (Reprinted with permission from Cleveland Clinic Center for Medical Art & Photography © 2013. All Rights Reserved.)

by a progressive inflammatory component.[7] The later stages of these lesions are termed plaques. Plaques can enlarge to partially or completely impede blood flow through an artery. From the fourth decade, some plaques may hemorrhage within the plaque or rupture, initiating thrombus formation at the site with possible embolic consequences (Fig. 29-4).

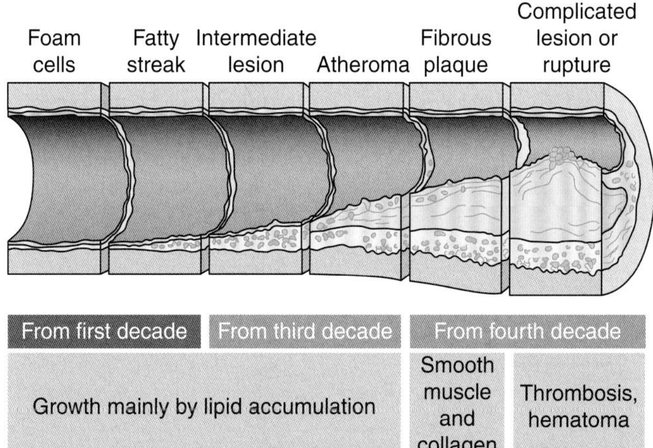

Figure 29-4. Progression of atheromatous plaque from initial lesion to complex and ruptured plaque. (Modified from Grech ED. ABC of interventional cardiology: pathophysiology and investigation of coronary artery disease. *BMJ*. 2003;326[7397]:1027–1030.)

AHA Lesion Classification System

Coronary artery lesions can be grouped into seven major types (Table 29-1). Consistent morphologic data would seem to indicate that each lesion type is relatively stable and will not progress to the next lesion type without additional factors or pressures (Fig. 29-5). While the advanced lesions (types IV to VII) can manifest clinically, the early lesions (types I to III) are clinically silent and can be organized temporally.[6]

Types I and II are generally found in children, whereas type III tends to occur later and bridges early and advanced lesions. Lipid-laden macrophages (termed "foam cells") are the predominant cellular components of type I lesions. Clearly, individuals with greater plasma concentrations of atherogenic lipoproteins will provide the opportunity for accelerated influx and early accumulation of lipid in the lesion-prone areas. In individuals with very high plasma levels of atherogenic lipoproteins, such as those with familial hypercholesterolemia, type II lesions rapidly evolve into advanced lesions, even in arterial locations outside the progression-prone zones. It is noteworthy that by middle age, the development of advanced lesions outside the progression-prone areas occurs even in the absence of high plasma cholesterol (i.e., even in individuals free of premature risk factors). Perhaps the most important observation is that the clinically silent lesions (types I to III) have been shown capable of regression in animal models.[8]

Advanced lesions are generally disorganized and lead to thickening and eventual compromise of the vessel wall. In types II and III lesions, intimal smooth muscle cells dominate, with minimal

Table 29-1 • TERMS USED TO DESIGNATE DIFFERENT TYPES OF HUMAN ATHEROSCLEROTIC LESIONS IN PATHOLOGY

Terms for Atherosclerotic Lesions in Histologic Classification			**Other Terms for the Same Lesions Often Based on Appearance With the Unaided Eye**	
Type lesion	I	Initial lesion	Fatty dot or streak	Early lesions
Type lesion	IIa	Progression-prone type II lesion		
	IIb	Progression-resistant type II		
Type lesion	III	Intermediate lesion (preatheroma)		
Type lesion	IV	Atheroma	Atheromatous plaque, fibrolipid plaque, fibrous plaque	
Type lesion	Va	Fibroatheroma (type V lesion)		Advanced lesions, raised lesions
	Vb	Calcific lesion (type VII lesion)	Calcified plaque	
	Vc	Fibrotic lesion (type VIII lesion)	Fibrous plaque	
Type lesion	VI	Lesion with surface defect, and/or hematoma-hemorrhage, and/or thrombotic deposit	Complicated lesion, complicated plaque	

Reproduced from Stary HC, Chandler AB, Dinsmore RE, et al. A report from the committee on vascular lesions of the council on arteriosclerosis, American Heart Association. *Arterioscler Thromb Vasc Biol.* 1995;15:1512–1531.

involvement of lymphocytes, plasma cells, and mast cells in the pathologic processes. This group of inflammatory cells becomes quite active in advanced (types IV and V) lesions. This lesion, referred to as atheroma, is the first "advanced" lesion of atherosclerosis, characterized histologically by a lipid core, intimal disorganization, and arterial deformity, which predispose this lesion type to sudden progression that may precipitate clinical symptoms. Macrophages within the lesions are primed for immune and/or inflammatory responses, expressing major histocompatibility complex receptors, and a variety of cytokines and growth regulatory molecules. Lesion types V and VI may undergo disruption of the lesion surface or develop hematoma, hemorrhage, or thrombotic deposits. They account for the majority of atherosclerotic morbidity and mortality. Any one of these complications is sufficient to recategorize type IV or V lesions as type VI lesions; they are also referred to as complicated lesions.

Clinical assessment of atherosclerotic lesions was once confined to advanced, gross vascular abnormalities, including aneurysms and vascular stenosis. Integration of imaging modalities, paired with new and emerging technologies, has permitted more accurate depiction of lesion morphology, which in turn, informs more specific interventions. These are listed in

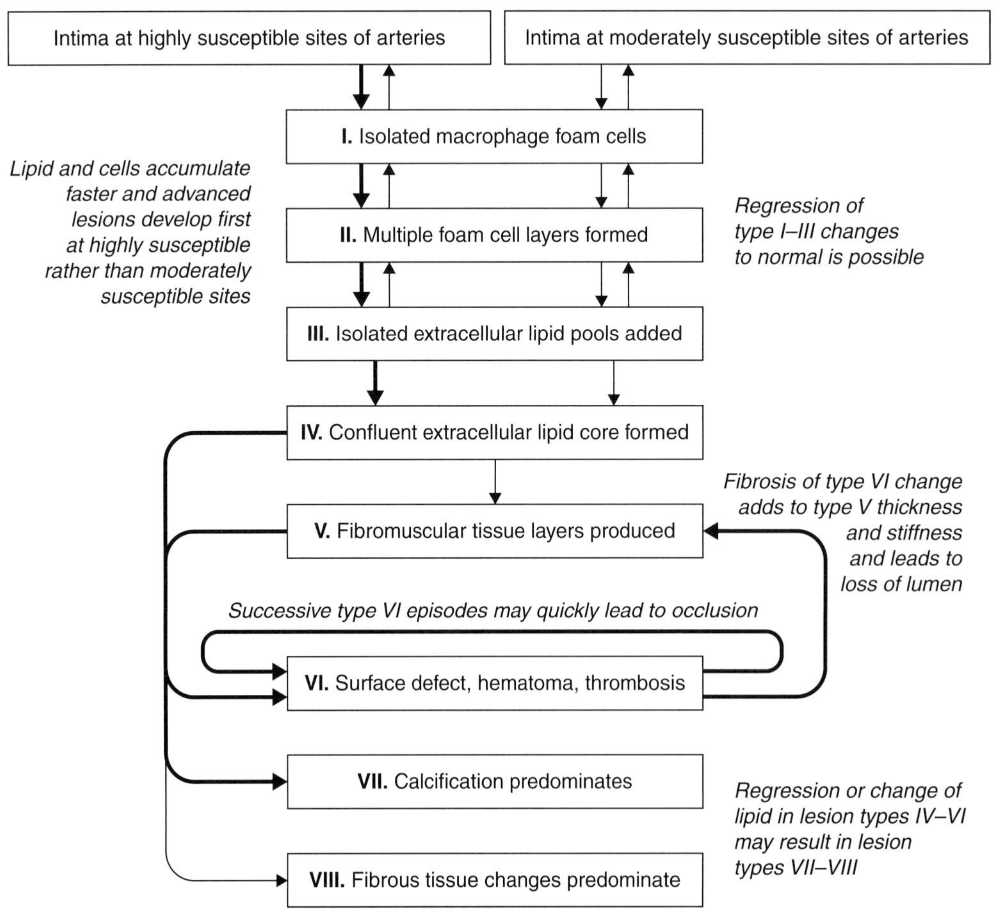

Figure 29-5. The sequence in the evolution of atherosclerotic lesions from type I to type IV and the various possible subsequent pathways of progression to lesion types beyond type IV. (Used with permission from the Natural History and Histological Classification of Atherosclerotic Lesions.)

Table 29-2 • TECHNOLOGIES PERMITTING EARLIER DETECTION AND ESTIMATION OF LESION VOLUME

Method	Features Detected
B-mode ultrasonography and Doppler flow	Permits measurement of the severity of stenosis in peripheral arteries
Intravascular ultrasound	Produces cross-sectional images of the vascular wall, revealing lesion composition and lumen contour
Magnetic resonance angiography	A noninvasive alternative to angiography, permitting study of major vessels (the aorta and carotid arteries and coronary arteries)
Angioscopy	Direct vascular vascularization detects specific morphologic features such as thrombus
Ultrafast computed tomography	A noninvasive method detecting coronary artery calcium

Table 29-2 and described in detail in earlier chapters on cardiac imaging.

Targeting treatment has been honed further by the growing understanding of the pathophysiology of lesion progression and associated clinical events. This has permitted clinicians to move beyond simple diagnosis to proactive prevention of complicated lesions through detection of earlier lesions and more accurate lesion characterization. Morphologic, immunohistochemical, and epidemiologic data have supported the construction of a lesion classification system, which has helped clinical decision making and research into the underlying pathophysiology and potential therapeutic interventions. These diagnoses and their interventions are generally categorized by presentation and acuity: ACS or chronic/stable IHD (SIHD). The cardiac nurse with knowledge of the stages, progression, and clinical manifestations of atherosclerosis is better positioned to anticipate the treatment plan. As a clinician, educator, and patient educator, it is critical that the cardiac nurse understand the rationale for each patient's plan of care, as well as the risks, benefits, and alternatives.

Vascular Surface Defects and Hematomas

The degree of luminal narrowing by an atheroma has little relation to whether thrombosis will occur. MIs of most patients often result from atheromas of less than 50% luminal narrowing or occlusion. Fissuring and disruption of atherosclerotic plaque can occur at any time during this chronic process. The ability of the plaque to disrupt is a major factor in future ischemic events. Plaque composition, rather than the amount of narrowing, is a major determinant of the vulnerability of the plaque formation. Both mechanical and inflammatory changes affect the vulnerability of the plaque and propensity for thrombosis. Superimposed thrombosis on the ruptured, ulcerated plaque can impede blood flow and the delivery of nutrients to the myocardium.

As lesions progress, disruptions of the lesion surface may present as fissures or even ulcerations and are highly variable in their severity and scope. Fissures of the lesion surface vary in length and depth and most likely reseal, leading to lesion progression by incorporating hematoma and thrombus.[9] Ulcerations can range from minor focal loss of a microscopic portion of the endothelial cell layer to deep ulcerations that can expose lipid cores and release lipid and other components that activate the coagulation cascade. Atheromatous lesions (types IV and V) are particularly prone to intimal disruptions and ultimately thrombosis.[9] This susceptibility is caused in part by the presence of activated inflammatory cells within the lesions, the release of proteolytic enzymes by macrophages within the lesions, coronary spasm, structural weakness related to lesion composition, the release of toxic factors from cell death (necrosis), and shear stress. Intimal hematoma from lesion surface tearing and hemorrhage may begin.

Atherothrombosis

Although plaque disruption and thrombosis can be separate processes, they appear to be interrelated. Thrombosis formation may be exacerbated by changes in the endothelium. Contractility, secretory, and mitogenic activities of the vessel wall all are factors that affect ischemia.[10] A dysfunctional endothelium leads to the potential for thrombosis and the development of atherosclerotic lesions. Platelets migrate quickly to the site of plaque rupture and adhere. Platelet aggregation releases metabolic substances that cause vasoconstriction. Thrombin formation is activated by factor XII, and the coagulation pathway results in the formation of fibrin.[11] A fibrin mesh binds with the platelets and leads to formation of a clot or thrombus.[12]

Advanced atherosclerotic lesions containing thrombi or their remnants become common by the fourth decade of life, ranging in size from microscopic to grossly visible deposits, with some consisting of stratified layers of lesions of different ages.[13] Incorporation of recurrent hematomas and thrombi over time (months to years) results in the progressive narrowing of the arterial lumen. Thrombus remnants contain increasing numbers of smooth muscle cells derived by ingrowth from the intima. These smooth muscle cells synthesize collagen, providing the stratum for overgrowth of endothelial cells at the lumen. Ultimately, thrombi may continue to enlarge, with the potential to rapidly occlude the lumen of a medium-sized artery (within days or even hours). This pathophysiologic process results in ACS (Fig. 29-6).

The degree of luminal narrowing by an atheroma has little relation to whether thrombosis will occur. Several mechanisms can influence the location, frequency, concentration, and size of thrombi. Shear stress participates in lesion progression, with thrombotic occlusions being common at vessel bifurcations and locations of arterial angulation.[14] Increased levels of low-density lipoproteins (LDLs), nutrition, tobacco smoke, and elevated lipoprotein(a) levels have been associated with greater risk for clinical CAD. Taken together, systemic factors play a significant role in modulating the development of thrombi.

Atherosclerotic Aneurysms

A common sequela of advanced lesions (types IV, V, and VI) is the development of distensions in the entire vascular wall. These aneurysms are usually associated with type VI lesions, when the intimal surface is eroded. Both old and new mural thrombi permeate atherosclerotic aneurysms, and the thrombi become layered in older aneurysms. Whereas the thrombi can form large masses that can fill an aneurysm, the underlying lumen remains generally well preserved and approximates the dimensions of the original vessel. The evolution of atherosclerotic aneurysms is preceded by a series of changes in the locale of the lesion. Matrix fibers are continuously degraded and resynthesized, causing a progressive decay of matrix architecture that results in dilation and potentially rupture.[15] Susceptibility to atherosclerotic aneurysm is modulated by secondary risk factors resulting in increased hemodynamic and/or tensile stress (e.g., hypertension) and by genetic variation. While atherosclerotic aneurysms can form in all parts of the body, they are most commonly found in the abdominal aorta and iliac arteries.

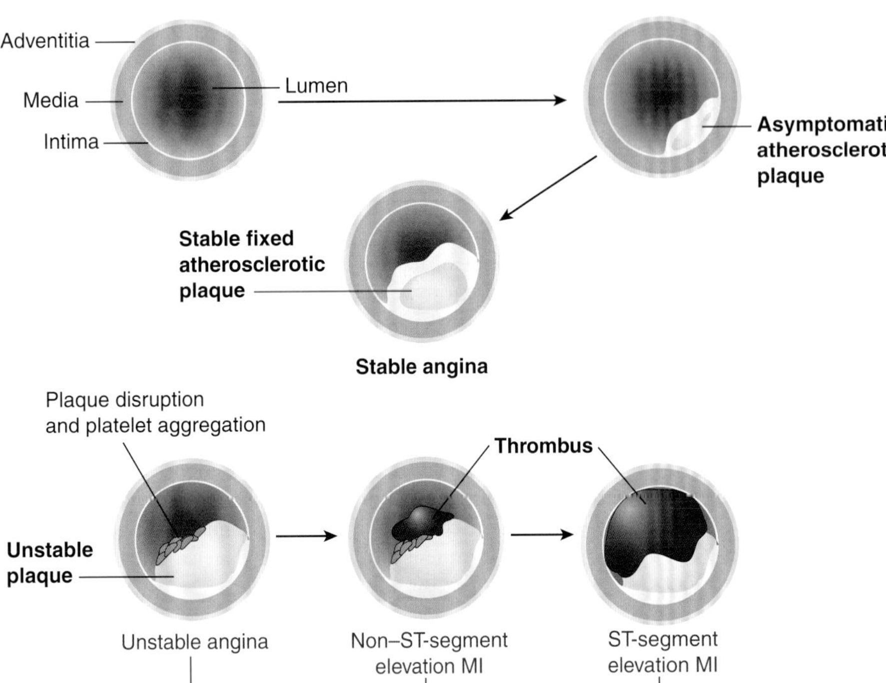

Figure 29-6. Atherosclerotic plaque: stable fixed atherosclerotic plaque in stable angina and unstable plaque with plaque disruption and platelet aggregation in the acute coronary syndromes. (Used with permission from Norris TL, Lalchandani L. *Porth's Pathophysiology*. Philadelphia, PA: Wolters Kluwer; 2018.)

Severity of Stenosis

The severity of lesion stenosis modulates the degree of impaired blood flow. The degree of stenosis is estimated by the ratio of the maximum diameter of a stenosed artery in comparison to an adjacent normal arterial diameter. Coronary artery blood flow begins to decrease to a clinically significant degree with 50% stenosis and blood flow decreases rapidly when stenosis exceeds 70%, and the determination of stenosis is of particular clinical benefit above and below these cutoffs. This decrease in blood flow (physiologic marker) cannot be assessed angiographically and assessment may fail to account for certain factors (e.g., rate of lesion growth and lesion length and/or geometry). In the last decade, the guideline-directed standard for physiologic lesion assessment is invasive fractional flow reserve (FFR) (e.g., pressure wire assessment with maximal hyperemia using intravenous nitroglycerin [NTG] or adenosine) for lesions of indeterminate severity.[16] Quantification of the stenosis severity (%) is a clinically useful starting parameter, which in certain situations (e.g., 50% to 69% stenosis, long lesions) should be coupled with direct physiologic FFR assessment of the decrease in blood flow.[16]

Cells and Extracellular Matrix of Lesions

A host of changes exist in the cellular compartment and extracellular matrix composition of lesions. Interaction of the apolipoprotein B on LDL with cell surface glycosaminoglycans appears to be a mechanism for trapping LDL in the arterial intima. Moreover, production of glycosaminoglycans increases during the early stages of atherosclerosis, which contribute to more avid cellular lipoprotein recruitment. Dermatan sulfate proteoglycans are another surface moiety hypothesized to increase the rate of progression of atherosclerosis. This class of molecules also binds plasma LDL under physiologic conditions with increased affinity in comparison with other molecules of this class. Macrophages contribute to atherogenesis by secretion of a range of factors modulating the formation and modeling of advanced lesions, including monocyte chemotactic protein-1 and tumor necrosis factor (TNF). Enzymatic digestion of the chondroitin sulfate proteoglycan, versican, leads to progression of the lesion because of its role in maintaining the viscoelasticity and the integrity of the vessel wall against the passage of plasma materials.

Lipid and Lipoprotein in the Extracellular Matrix

While the transfer of lipoproteins from the plasma into the intima is a physiologic process, the concentrations of these particles are particularly elevated in advanced lesions. Definitive identification of the types and amounts of extracellular lipid are difficult and depend largely on methods of tissue preparation and study. More extracellular lipid is observed in lesion types III, IV, Va, and VI. In addition, extracellular lipid accumulates and pools, forming "lipid cores," in lesion types IV, Va, and VI. Lesions contain many lipid-laden cells that die or can be found in various stages of disintegration, evidence that much of the extracellular lipid is derived from cells and lipoproteins originally internalized by cells.

Fibrinogen

The degree and extent to which fibrinogen accumulates in advanced lesions or parts of advanced lesions varies. Immunohistochemical techniques show that the cores of advanced lesions stain for fibrinogen more than any other part of advanced lesions, except superimposed thrombi. Immunohistochemical staining alone cannot distinguish thrombus-associated fibrinogen from physiologic infiltration of fibrinogen from the plasma. However, it is generally accepted that intensely fibrinogen-positive bands found in the majority of advanced lesions constitute evidence of incorporated past thrombi. Fibrinogen contributes directly and indirectly (by promoting smooth muscle cell growth) to the volume of most advanced lesions.

Calcium

Mineralization of atherosclerotic lesions is a well-substantiated phenomenon. Accumulation of calcium in the arterial wall in the course of the atherogenic process is considered to be a manifestation of advanced atherosclerosis. Factors controlling the quantity of calcium in the lesions are complex and not necessarily caused by dietary intake. Deposition of lipids, platelets, cellular debris, and calcium stimulate cells in the locale of the damaged artery wall to produce still other substances that contribute further to the atherosclerotic process. This results in recruitment of immune cells into the lesion as well as proliferation of arterial smooth muscle cells in an attempt to "heal" the lesion. As a result, the innermost layer of the artery, the intima, thickens, enlarges, and eventually encroaches on the vessel lumen, progressively restricting the flow of blood (and thus oxygen) to the vascular bed.

Inflammation and Biomarkers

Inflammation has been expressed as a key feature of all stages of atherothrombogenesis. Its effects are detrimental in plaque rupture, occlusive thrombosis, and consequent tissue hypoxia.[17] Furthermore, the presence of inflammatory cytokines in patients with heart failure sparked interest in the role that these molecules play in regulating cardiac structure and function, particularly with respect to their potential role in the progression of heart failure. When expressed in the circulation at sufficiently high concentrations, cytokines are potent enough to duplicate many facets of heart failure, including progressive left ventricular (LV) dysfunction and remodeling, pulmonary edema, and cardiomyopathy.[18] Heart failure progresses in part as a result of the deleterious effects of cytokines in the heart and peripheral circulation, thus exacerbating heart failure.[19] Inflammation indicated by inflammatory markers such as high-sensitivity C-reactive protein, fibrinogen, homocysteine, and serum amyloid A is known to be associated with CVD risk however serial monitoring and management guided by these laboratory studies is not as well understood.[20] Risk factors for CVD and laboratory studies are discussed at length in their respective chapters in this text.

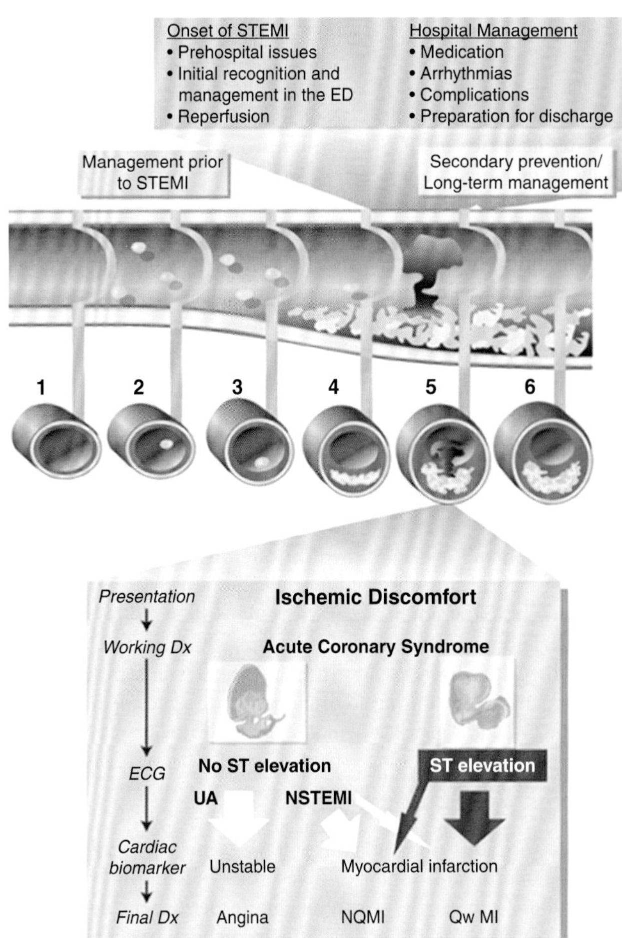

Figure 29-7. Spectrum of pathologic and clinical ST-segment elevation and NSTEMI acute coronary syndromes. (Used with permission from Woods SL, Sivarajan Froelicher E. S., Adams (Underhill) Motzer S, Bridges EJ. *Cardiac Nursing*. Philadelphia, PA: Wolters Kluwer; 2009.)

ACUTE CORONARY SYNDROME

ACS encompasses the clinical diagnoses of acute myocardial ischemia and infarction and their respective events and terminology. For descriptive purposes, myocardial ischemia put simply is an imbalance of the supply of blood flow and oxygen given the demand on the myocardium; MI is necrosis or cell death of the myocardium due to prolonged ischemia. These definitions have advanced from epidemiologic and electrocardiographic classifications to a universal system informed by the acuity of the patient's presentation and the underlying pathophysiologic events (Fig. 29-7).

Definitions

An acute MI is defined as myocardial injury evidenced by an elevation of cardiac troponin with at least one value above the 99th percentile of the upper reference limit with necrosis and a clinical setting with myocardial ischemia.[21] AMI is then characterized based on symptoms (angina or other symptoms of ischemia) as ACS and electrocardiogram (ECG) findings as STEMI or NSTEMI. The nomenclature may appear as STEMI-ACS, NSTEMI-ACS, and the less used unstable angina UA-ACS, which direct treatment strategies.

AMI are further classified into a number of different types, the majority falling into types 1 and 2. Type 1 MI criteria include evidence of acute coronary atherothrombosis and new ischemic ECG changes (majority are STEMI vs. NSTEMI) or development of pathologic Q waves. Type 2 MI criteria include evidence of an imbalance of myocardial supply and demand without acute coronary atherothrombosis and new ischemic ECG changes, or imaging evidence of myocardial loss or ischemic pattern, or development of pathologic Q waves.[21] A newer category of AMI/type 2 MI is MI with nonobstructive coronary arteries (MINOCA). While MINOCA is a newer term in ACS, related conditions are well known: coronary emboli, coronary artery spasm, and spontaneous coronary artery dissection (SCAD).[22] Other working diagnoses of MINOCA include Takotsubo cardiomyopathy, which is also classified as a type 2 MI, and the patient with cardiac involvement of systemic acute respiratory syndrome novel coronavirus (SARS-CoV) or COVID19, which may also present as ACS. This section will review the epidemiology, pathophysiology, presentation, diagnosis and medical management of ACS.

Epidemiology

In the United States, the prevalence and incidence of ACS has declined since the 1970s, primarily due to advances in health systems and aggressive cardiovascular risk factor managements annually. However ACS is still one of the leading causes of morbidity and mortality for both women and men. Of the 7.6 million people that present to the ED with the chest pain annually,[23] 13% to 25% lead to a final diagnosis of ACS.[24]

The incidence of ACS in the United States exceeds 780,000 annually of which approximately 60% have UA and 40% have MI.[25] The distribution of STEMI and NSTEMI patients is roughly 1/3 and 2/3, respectively, of which the latter have more comorbidities, both cardiac and noncardiac.[26] Moreover, greater than 50% of NSTEMI admissions proceed to invasive management with revascularization. Early postprocedure mortality may be higher after STEMI but survival after 6 months has been found to be worse after NSTEMI, possibly due to the presence of chronic conditions.[27]

Health disparities exist across ethnic groups, genders, and ages. Black and Hispanic patients presenting with ACS are more likely to have comorbidities, experience longer delays before treatment, and suffer worse outcomes when compared with non-Hispanic White patients.[28] Access to medical care often is delayed after a coronary event. Morbidity and mortality appear to be particularly worrisome in older adults, men with AMI (threefold higher than women), and women who experience procedural complications.[29] These disparities have been attributed to delays in symptom recognition and underutilization of guideline-directed medical therapy (GDMT) and invasive management.

Etiology and Pathogenesis

Many factors affect the pathophysiologic events that lead to ischemia, infarction, and injury of myocardial muscle. Injury to the myocardium can range from reversible to permanent damage of cellular components in localized tissue. Ischemia occurs from a transient imbalance of blood supply to an area of tissue, with the chief result being tissue hypoxia. Ischemia can be a sudden event or a gradual occurrence from a partial or totally occluded coronary vessel or vessels. The burden of the ischemic event depends on the sensitivity of the tissue to hypoxia, the degree and duration of ischemia, and the ability of the tissue to recover when conditions improve.[30,31]

The coronary arteries supply blood flow to meet the specific demands of the myocardium under varying workloads such as stress, sleep, or exercise. If oxygen needs are not met, then normal coronary arteries dilate to increase delivery of oxygenated blood to the myocardium.[5] Various pathologic states can affect the endothelium of the epicardial arteries impairing and impacting the normal vasomotor response of vasodilatation when myocardial demand increases. Atherosclerotic plaques are the primary cause of endothelial injury and dysfunction, interfering with normal vasomotor response causing a paradoxical response of vasoconstriction.[10–15] Low blood pressure causing decreased blood return can lead to imbalances of oxygen supply and demand. Examples are hypotension or hypovolemia. Increased oxygen demand is caused by conditions such as hyperthyroidism, anemia, or hyperviscosity of the blood.

The usual initiating mechanism for AMI is rupture or erosion of a vulnerable, lipid-laden atherosclerotic coronary plaque, resulting in exposure of circulating blood to highly thrombogenic plaque core and matrix materials. In the statin era, this epidemiology is shifting toward erosion as an increasingly common cause. Platelets adhere, become activated, and aggregate. Thrombin is generated, accelerating platelet activation, and fibrin formed, trapping red blood cells, and forming a thrombus. A totally occluding thrombus typically leads to STEMI. Partial occlusion, or occlusion in the presence of collateral circulation, results in NSTEMI often with ST depression. Ischemia resulting from reduced coronary flow leads to myocardial cell injury or death, ventricular dysfunction, and cardiac arrhythmias. Myocardial necrosis begins after as little as 20 minutes of coronary occlusion. The occurrence of AMI in the absence of critical epicardial coronary disease accounts for ~10% of AMI and is believed to be varied in its mechanism(s) though primarily due to microvascular disease and endothelial dysfunction. An additional mechanism in NSTEMI is spontaneous lysis of thrombus on an eroded but nonobstructive plaque; this mechanism is increasingly relevant in the setting of prompt administration of anticoagulation and antiplatelet therapy to patients on arrival at the emergency department prior to angiography.

MI in nonobstructive coronary artery disease (MINOCA) may have several etiologies as described earlier in this chapter. A clinical algorithm for the diagnosis of MINOCA (e.g., coronary artery vasospasm or SCAD is presented in Figure 29-8. Dynamic obstruction may be triggered by spasms of coronary arteries as seen with Prinzmetal angina induced by cocaine or methamphetamine. Plaque disruption and microvascular disease may also result in MINOCA. Additional assessment is indicated for these clinical scenarios.

Demand versus Supply Ischemia

Myocardial ischemia can occur as a result of increased metabolic *demand* to meet tissue needs or reduced oxygen and nutrient *supply.* The demand or supply mismatch is coupled with the inadequate removal of metabolites because of reduced perfusion to the heart muscle (Fig. 29-9). Pure anoxia or hypoxia, without metabolic clearance, can occur in patients with congenital heart disease, severe anemia, asphyxiation, carbon monoxide poisoning, or cor pulmonale.[32]

In the presence of CAD, acute occlusion of blood flow differentiates supply versus demand ischemia. Acute coronary artery occlusion results in *supply ischemia* and results from an abrupt increase in coronary vascular tone, such as coronary vasospasm, or more commonly from atherothrombi or platelet aggregation secondary to ruptured plaque. *Supply ischemia* is seen in patients with UA or MI. In contrast, an increase in oxygen demand requirements from exercise or emotional stress can cause a transitory imbalance known as *demand ischemia.*

Principles of Diagnosis and Treatment

The cardiac nurse caring for the patient with ACS must keep in mind the time-old adage "time is muscle": A delay to treatment leads to myocardial necrosis. The goal is to rapidly identify the likely diagnosis and by whom, where, and when patients will be evaluated and treated. The faster adequate blood supply can be restored, the better the survival and quality of life via reducing the effects of end organ tissue damage and dysfunction.

The cardiac nurse will be tasked to provide evidence-based care for patients with IHD. In the United States, practice guidelines pertaining to IHD are put forth by several specialties: cardiology (American College of Cardiology Foundation and American Heart Association Task Force on Practice Guidelines), interventional cardiology (Society for Cardiovascular Angiography and Interventions), cardiothoracic surgery (American Association for Thoracic Surgery and Society of Thoracic Surgeons), and cardiovascular nursing (Preventative Cardiovascular Nurses Association). Clinical studies and national guidelines are periodically reviewed and updated in a standardized fashion via an exhaustive evidence review.

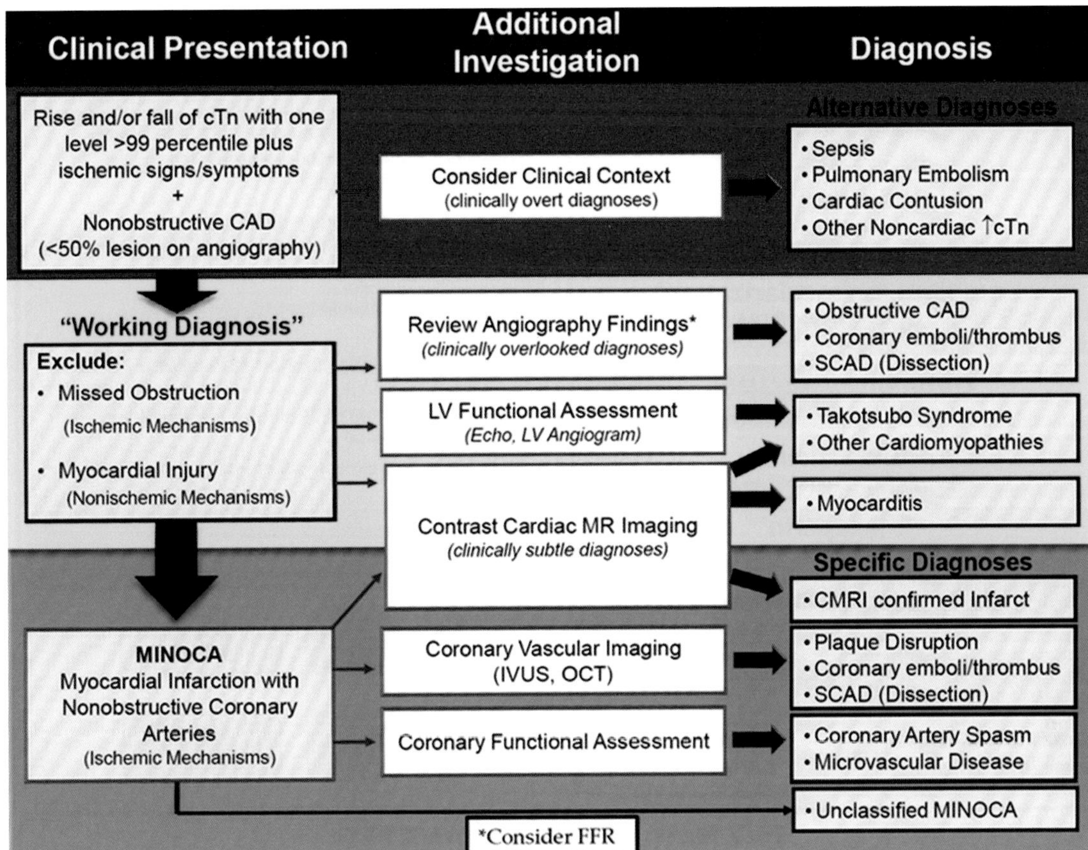

Figure 29-8. Clinical algorithm for the diagnosis of MINOCA. CAD, coronary artery disease; CMRI, cardiac magnetic resonance imaging; cTn, cardiac troponin; FFR, fractional flow reserve; IVUS, intravascular ultrasound; LV, left ventricular; MINOCA, myocardial infarction in the absence of obstructive coronary artery disease; MR, magnetic resonance; OCT, optical coherence tomography; SCAD, spontaneous coronary artery dissection.*Consider FFR.

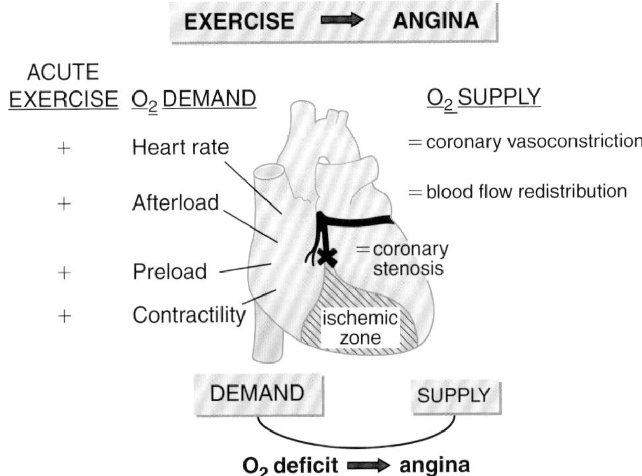

Figure 29-9. Myocardial oxygen balance. The major determinants in the normal heart are heart rate, afterload, preload, and contractility. When the myocardial oxygen demand increases and blood flow is not concomitantly increased or even reduced, as in exercising patients with coronary stenosis, the result is the chest pain called angina pectoris. Clinically, the heart rate increase during exercise is one of the major determinants of myocardial oxygen uptake. (From Opie LH. *Heart Physiology: From Cell to Circulation.* 4th ed. New York: Lippincott Williams & Wilkins; 2004:526.)

Nurses caring for patients with IHD are expected to have knowledge of the latest guidelines for practice updates, institutional policies, credible sources (e.g., peer-reviewed journals; credible clinical/educator experts such as clinical nurse specialists, nurse practitioners, physicians; hospital practice councils, journal clubs, or educational offerings including grand rounds) for high-quality evidence; and literature reviews (e.g., UpToDate). At the time of this publication the most recent U.S. guidelines for STEMI were published in 2013[33] and for NSTEMI in 2014.[34]

Reflective of more recent evidence, the European Society of Cardiology (ESC) ACS-STEMI guidelines were published in 2017.[35] Figure 29-10 depicts the ESC summary synthesis of recommendations, evidence, and landmark clinical trials. The intuitive color scheme facilitates clinician understanding and decision making. For example, the cardiac nurse reviewing this figure may readily conclude that ESC strongly recommends PCI via radial access based on the results of the MATRIX study, and may use this guideline to advocate for a patient in a relevant scenario.

Diagnosis

Physical Assessment

Criteria. Defining criteria for the diagnosis of AMI and the subtypes have become clear and prescriptive.[21] For the diagnosis of ACS, the criteria may remain somewhat challenging as the

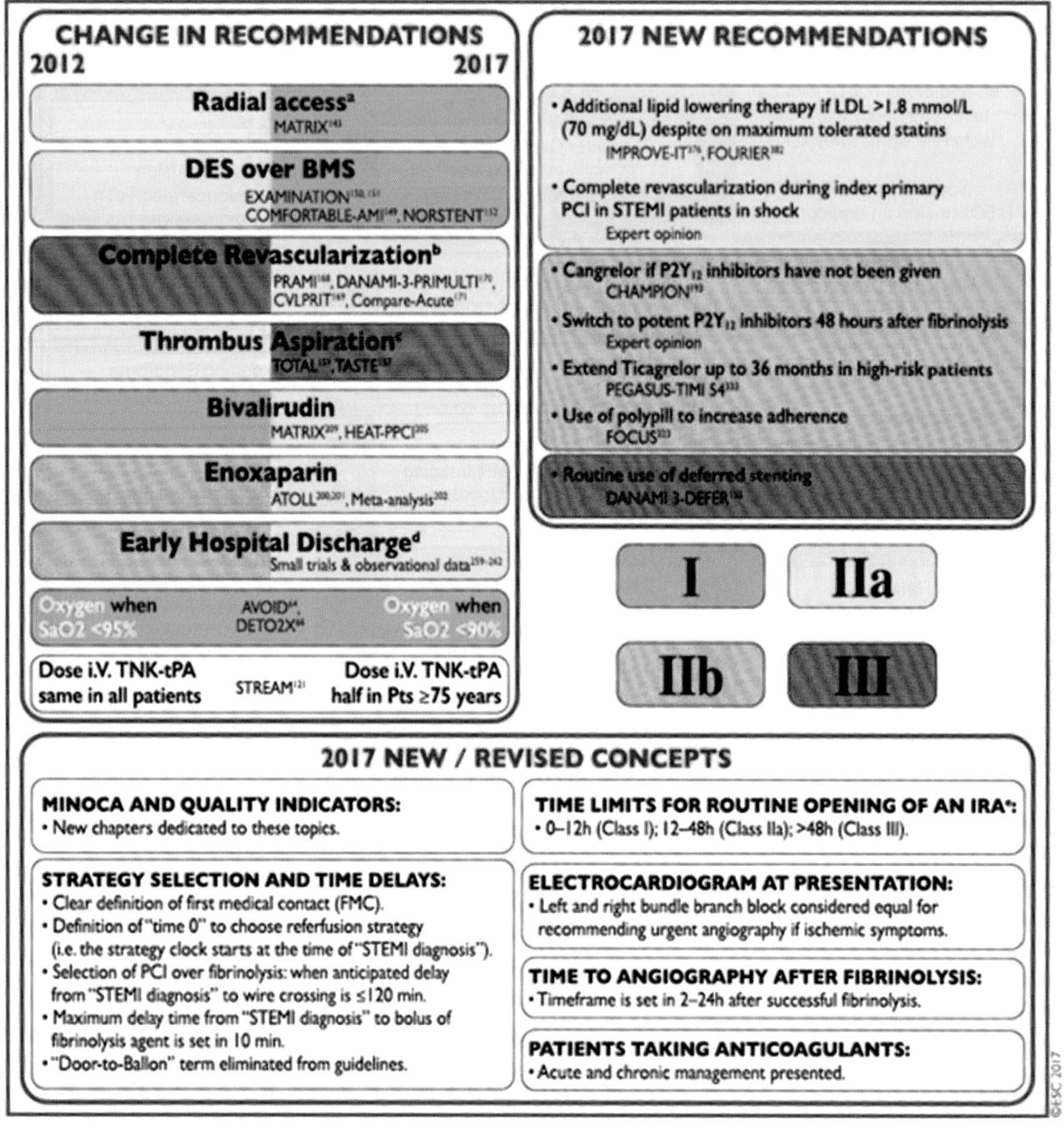

Figure 29-10. European Society of Cardiology What is New in 2017 STEMI Guidelines. BMS, bare metal stent; DES, drug eluting stent; IRA, infarct related artery; i.v., intravenous; LDL, low-density lipoprotein; PCI, percutaneous coronary intervention; SaO_2, arterial oxygen saturation; STEMI, ST-elevation myocardial infarction; TNK-tPA, Tenecteplase tissue plasminogen activator.
[a]Only for experienced radial operators.
[b]Before hospital discharge (either immediate or staged).
[c]Routine thrombus aspiration (bailout in certain cases may be considered).
[d]In 2012 early discharge was considered after 72h, in 2017 early discharge is 48–72h.
[e]If symptoms or hemodynamic instability IRA should be opened regardless time from symptoms onset.
(Used with permission from Ibanez B, James S, Agewall S, et al. 2017 ESC Guidelines for the management of acute myocardial infarction in patients presenting with ST-segment elevation: The Task Force for the management of acute myocardial infarction in patients presenting with ST-segment elevation of the European Society of Cardiology (ESC). *Eur Heart J.* 2017;39[2]:119–177.)

more subjective components such as history, presentation, and chest pain do not reliably exclude ACS. It is important that cardiac nurses are vigilant and know how to synthesize this information to identify patients at risk for ACS.

Systematic Acquisition of the History of Present Illness. ACS may be difficult to distinguish on clinical presentation. A systematic assessment as described in the earlier chapter on history and physical examination will provide an excellent foundation. An acronym such as OLDCART: Onset, location, duration, characteristics, associated/aggravating factors, relieving factors, and treatments attempted may be helpful to guide patient inquiry. Highly predictive symptoms, signs, and risk scores for myocardial ischemia including exertional chest discomfort, Levine sign, and the TIMI risk score are also recommended for diagnostic assessment.

Angina. *Angina pectoris* is chest pain or discomfort that results from myocardial ischemia.[36] UA in general is not relieved with rest. Several presentations of UA may be recognized: resting, new-onset, crescendo, variant angina (Fig. 29-11). First, resting angina pectoris, as the name implies, occurs during a period of nonexertion and lasts longer than 20 minutes. Second,

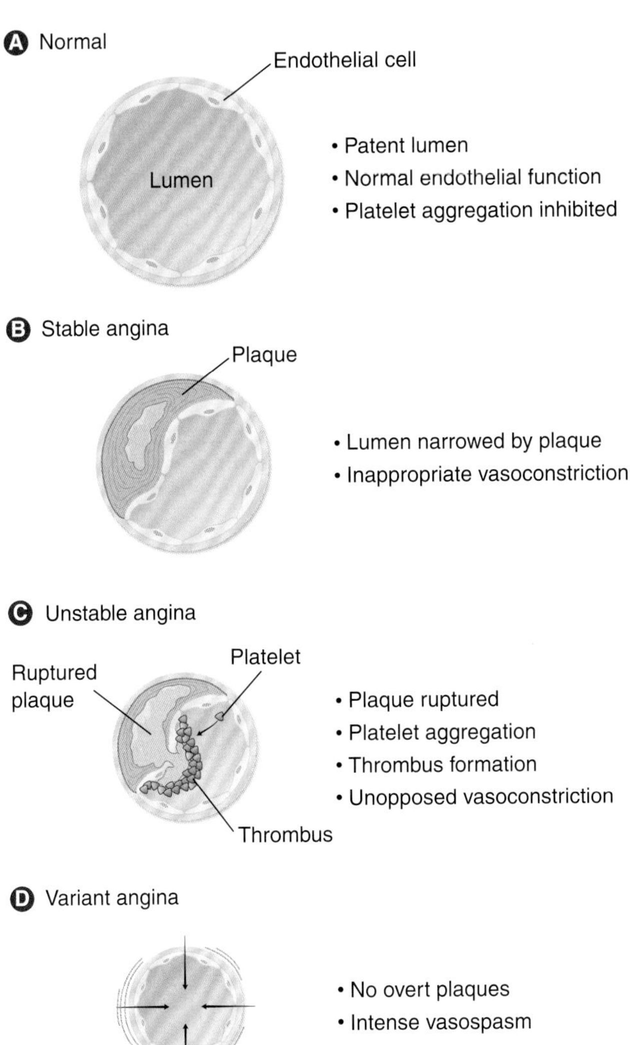

Figure 29-11. Pathophysiology of angina syndromes. **A:** Normal coronary arteries are widely patent, the endothelium functions normally, and platelet aggregation is inhibited. **B:** In stable angina, atherosclerotic plaque and inappropriate vasoconstriction (caused by endothelial damage) reduce the vessel lumen diameter and hence decrease coronary blood flow. **C:** In unstable angina, rupture of the plaque triggers platelet aggregation, thrombus formation, and vasoconstriction. Depending on the anatomic site of plaque rupture, this process can progress to non–Q wave (non–ST-elevation) or Q wave (ST-elevation) myocardial infarction. **D:** In variant angina, atherosclerotic plaques are absent, and ischemia is caused by intense vasospasm. (Used with permission from McCabe JM, Armstrong EJ. Integrative cardiovascular pharmacology: hypertension, ischemic heart disease, and heart failure. In: Golan DE, Armstrong EJ, Armstrong AW, eds. *Principles of Pharmacology: The Pathophysiologic Basis of Drug Therapy*. 4th ed. Philadelphia, PA: Wolters-Kluwer Health; 2017:480.)

new-onset angina presents within the past 2 months without rest pain. Thirdly, *crescendo angina* is a worsening chest pain that may lead to MI or preinfarct angina. Crescendo angina occurs with less exertion than previous angina; an increase in pain may reflect intensity, duration, and/or frequency of ischemic symptoms and warrants urgency. In contrast, patients with *chronic stable angina* experience demand ischemia when they exert themselves yet obtain relief with rest. *Variant (Prinzmetal) angina* is an unusual form of UA that occurs spontaneously and frequently is not related to exertion. Discomfort tends to be prolonged and severe. This spasm of the epicardial coronary artery/arteries is classically characterized by transient ST-segment elevation and resolved with NTG use. Variant angina usually does not progress to MI. Uncommonly, prolonged vasospasm can result in MI, atrioventricular block, ventricular tachycardia, or sudden death. Attacks can be precipitated by emotional stress, hyperventilation, exercise, or exposure to cold. These anginal attacks tend to occur more in the morning. Patients with variant angina tend to be younger with fewer coronary risk factors. This type of angina is usually responsive to NTG, long-acting nitrates, and calcium antagonists, all of which are first-line therapies.

Atypical Chest Pain. While chest pain is not required for the diagnosis of ACS, reported symptoms will frequently include midsternal or substernal compression or crushing chest discomfort. Often patients will report chest discomfort as opposed to actual chest pain. Characteristics of chest pain such as duration, frequency, intensity, previous episodes, and past history of coronary disease risk factors may influence the cardiac nurses consider the presence of ACS. It is important to understand whether the discomfort occurs with exertion, defined as routine activities, exercise, emotional exertion, and/or stress. The patient may describe the chest pain as a cramping, burning, or an aching sensation in the midsternal area. The discomfort may also be described as pressure, tightness, or heaviness in the chest. Unexplained indigestion or belching with or without epigastric pain is also a common subjective complaint. The pain may radiate to the neck, jaw, shoulders, back, or one or both arms. Sometimes patient may report low-grade fever due to inflammatory response within the myocardium. Women more often present with atypical chest pain. Patients with diabetes also may present atypically due to diabetes-associated autonomic dysfunction. Up to 25% of acute MIs are silent and cause only vague symptoms.[37] Older adults may present with stroke, syncope, a change in mental status, and/or generalized weakness.

Physical Examination

A physical examination has limited usefulness in recognizing the patients with ACS. However, a focused physical examination by cardiac nurses should include assessment of vital signs, hemodynamic status, and an assessment of neurologic examination as thrombolysis may be a potential therapy. The physical examination will likely be normal, although findings suggestive of a high-risk situation include: dyskinetic apex, elevated JVP, presence of S3 or S4 murmur, new apical systolic murmur, presence of rales and crackles, or hypotension.[38]

Potential precipitating factors of myocardial ischemia, such as uncontrolled hypertension, thyrotoxicosis, or gastrointestinal (GI) bleeding, are identified on physical examination. Identification of any comorbid conditions, such as pulmonary disease or malignancy, is critical because both therapeutic risk and clinical decision making could be altered. Immediate evaluation is important to rule out alternative diagnoses of noncardiac chest pain, including aortic dissection (suggestive with findings of unequal pulses, blood pressures, or a loud new aortic murmur), acute pericarditis (presents with pleuritic chest pain and/or the presence of a friction rub), pulmonary embolism, tension pneumothorax, myocarditis, perforating peptic ulcer, and esophageal rupture.[38] The physical examination will also give indications as to the hemodynamic effect of the myocardial ischemia, such as hypotension and organ hypoperfusion seen in cardiogenic shock, which is a medical emergency.

Diagnostic Testing

Refer to earlier chapters in the text for a complete discussion of the cardiovascular history and physical examination, laboratory studies, and electrocardiographic findings for MI, and diagnostic imaging studies for MI. Previously in this chapter, the diagnostic criteria were reviewed and depicted in Figure 29-7.

Electrocardiogram. ECG is the single most important test and should be obtained in all patients with suspected ACS within 10 min of arrival to the emergency department. However, the initial ECG with normal tracing does not exclude the presence of ACS. The ECG should be repeated at 15- to 30-minute intervals if the initial study is not diagnostic but the patient remains symptomatic and high clinical suspicion for ACS persists.[38] Serial ECGs increase diagnostic sensitivity and are recommended because ST-segment elevation on the 12-lead ECG is the principal criterion for reperfusion therapy. For STEMI, initial ECG is usually diagnostic, showing ST-segment elevation greater than or equal to 1 mm in two or more contiguous leads subtending the damaged area. STEMI exists when the ECG of the patient presenting with acute chest pain shows (1) greater than or equal to 1-mm ST-segment elevation in at least two anatomically contiguous limb leads (aVL to III, including aVR), (2) greater than or equal to 1-mm ST-segment elevation in a precordial lead V4 through V6, (3) greater than or equal to 2-mm ST-segment elevation in V1 through V3, or (4) a new left bundle branch block.[19] As a subset of ACS, UA/NSTEMI is defined by electrocardiographic ST-segment depression or prominent T-wave inversion. Inverted T waves, particularly if greater than or equal to 2 mm, can also be indicative of UA/NSTEMI. ST-segment elevations and new pathologic Q waves are absent in both UA/NSTEMI.[38]

Table 29-3 • EARLY HOSPITAL CARE FOR NSTEMI

Recommendations	Class of Recommendation	Level of Evidence
Oxygen		
Administer supplemental oxygen only with oxygen saturation <90%, respiratory distress, or other high-risk features for hyponatremia	I	C
Nitrates		
Administer sublingual nitroglycerin (NTG) every 5 min × 3 for continuing ischemic pain and then assess need for intravenous (IV) NTG	I	C
Administer IV NTG for persistent ischemia, heart failure (HF), or hypertension	I	B
Nitrates are contraindicated with recent use of a phosphodiesterase inhibitor	III: Harm	B
Analgesic Therapy		
IV morphine sulfate may be reasonable for continued ischemic chest pain despite maximally tolerated anti-ischemic medications	IIb	B
NSAIDs (except aspirin) should not be initiated and should be discontinued during hospitalization for NSTE-ACS because of the increased risk of major adverse cardiac events (MACE) associated with their use	III	B
Beta-Adrenergic Blockers		
Initiate oral beta blockers within the first 24 h in the absence of heart failure, low output state, risk for cardiogenic shock, or other contraindications to beta blockade	I	A
Use of sustained-release metoprolol succinate, carvedilol, or bisoprolol is recommended for beta-blocker therapy with concomitant NSTE-ACS, stabilized heart failure, and reduced systolic function	I	C
Reevaluate to determine subsequent eligibility in patients with initial contraindications to beta blockers	I	C
It is reasonable to continue beta-blocker therapy in patients with normal LV function and NSTE-ACS	IIa	C
IV beta blockers are potentially harmful when risk factors for shock are present	III: Harm	B
Calcium Channel Blockers (CCBs)		
Administer initial therapy with nondihydropyridine CCBs with recurrent ischemia and contraindications to beta blockers in the absence of LV dysfunction, increased risk for cardiogenic shock, PR interval >0.24 s, or second- or third-degree atrioventricular (AV) block without a cardiac pacemaker	I	B
Administer oral nondihydropyridine calcium agonists with recurrent ischemia after use of beta blockers and nitrates in the absence of contraindications	I	C
CCBs are recommended for ischemic symptoms when beta blockers are not successful, are contraindicated, or cause unacceptable side effects	I	C
Long-acting CCBs and nitrates are recommended for patients with coronary artery spasm	I	C
Immediate-release nifedipine is contraindicated in the absence of a beta blocker	III: Harm	B
Cholesterol Management		
Initiate or continue high-intensity statin therapy in patients with no contraindications	I	A
Obtain a fasting lipid profile, ideally within 24 h	IIa	C

Note: Short-acting dihydropyridine antagonists should be avoided.
NSTE-ACS, non-ST elevation acute coronary syndrome.
Used with permission from O'Gara PT, Kushner FG, Ascheim DD, et al. 2013 ACCF/AHA Guideline for the management of ST-elevation myocardial infarction. A Report of the American College of Cardiology Foundation/American Heart Association Task Force on Practice Guidelines. *Circulation*. 2013;61(4):e78–e140.

Laboratory Studies. Elevation of cardiac biomarker troponin-I or -T is characteristic of diagnosis in UA/NSTEMI and should be obtained in all patients who presents with chest discomfort suggestive of ACS. NSTEMI is distinguished from UA by the presence of an elevated troponin, a biomarker of myocardial necrosis. That said, UA/NSTEMI can be challenging to distinguish at initial presentation, since an elevation in serum cardiac biomarker concentration rises 3 to 6 hours after onset of ischemic symptoms and at least 8 to 12 hours are required to detect elevations in all patients.[38]

MEDICAL MANAGEMENT

Nurses are advised to directly review the literature and hospital protocols due to emerging evidence and focused guidelines updates in this arena. The treatment algorithms for guideline-directed core medical management in the setting of early hospital care are described. Plans for anticoagulation and antiplatelet therapy, as well as for PCI, are also reviewed.

Early Hospital Care

The early management of ACS involves the achievement of multiple concurrent goals. The cardiac nurse endeavors not only to relieve patient discomfort but to implement a care plan initiating therapies that have immediate short-term benefits as well as well as those that improve long-term prognosis. Table 29-3 reviews the early hospital medical management for NSTEMI. It is critical that patients should be assessed for any contraindications to these therapies, including the recent use of phosphodiesterase-5 inhibitors (e.g., sildenafil) before the administration of nitrates. Careful monitoring of hemodynamics and cardiac rhythm is important given the risk of disturbance in the early stages of presentation and treatment.

Initial Antiplatelet/Anticoagulation Strategy

For patients with ACS (STEMI and UA/NSTEMI), antiplatelet and anticoagulant therapy should be initiated at the time of presentation to prevent thrombus-related events (Tables 29-4 and 29-5).[39] Nurses are often the first interaction with patients as they

Table 29-4 • INITIAL ANTIPLATELET AND ANTICOAGULATION STRATEGY FOR NSTEMI

Recommendations	Dosing and Special Considerations	Class of Recommendation	Level of Evidence
Aspirin			
Nonenteric-coated aspirin to all patients promptly after presentation	162–325 mg	I	A
Aspirin maintenance dose continued indefinitely	81–325 mg/day	I	A
$P2Y_{12}$ inhibitors			
Clopidogrel loading dose followed by daily maintenance dose in patients unable to take aspirin	75 mg	I	B
$P2Y_{12}$ inhibitor, in addition to aspirin, for up to 12 mo for patients treated initially with either an early invasive or initial ischemia-guided strategy:			
Clopidogrel	300 or 600 mg loading dose, then 75 mg/day	I	B
Ticagrelor[a]	180 mg loading dose, then 90 mg BID	I	B
Glycoprotein (GP) IIb/IIIa Inhibitors			
GP IIb/IIIa inhibitor in patients treated with an early invasive strategy and DAPT with intermediate/high-risk features (e.g., positive troponin)	Preferred options are eptifibatide or tirofiban	IIb	B
Parenteral Anticoagulant and Fibrinolytic Therapy			
Subcutaneous enoxaparin for duration of hospitalization or until PCI is performed	1 mg/kg subcutaneously every 12 h (reduce dose to 1 mg/kg/day in patients with creatinine clearance <30 mL/min) Initial 30 mg IV loading dose in selected patients	I	A
Bivalirudin until diagnostic angiography or PCI is performed in patients with early invasive strategy only	Loading dose 0.10 mg/g loading dose followed by 0.25 mg/kg/h Only provisional use of GP IIb/IIIa inhibitor in patients also treated with DAPT	I	B
Subcutaneous fondaparinux for the duration of hospitalization or until PCI is performed	2.5 mg subcutaneously per day	I	B
Administer additional anticoagulant with anti-IIa activity, if PCI is performed while on fondaparinux	NA	I	B
IV UFH for 48 h or until PCI is performed	Initial loading dose 60 IU/kg (max 4000 IU) with initial infusion 12 IU/kg/h (max 1000 IIU/hour) Adjusted to therapeutic aPTT range	I	B
IV fibrinolytic treatment not recommended in patients with NSTE-ACS	NA	III: Harm	A

[a]Note that the recommended dose of aspirin is 81 mg daily, if used in combination with ticagrelor.
DAPT, dual antiplatelet therapy; NSTE-ACS, non-ST elevation acute coronary syndromes; PCI, percutaneous coronary intervention; UFH, unfractionated heparin; aPTT, activated partial thromboplastin time.
Used with permission from O'Gara PT, Kushner FG, Ascheim DD, et al. 2013 ACCF/AHA Guideline for the management of ST-elevation myocardial infarction. A Report of the American College of Cardiology Foundation/American Heart Association Task Force on Practice Guidelines. *Circulation.* 2013;61(4):e78–e140.

Table 29-5 • ANTICOAGULANT THERAPY IN ACUTE CORONARY SYNDROME: STEMI AND NSTEMI

Class	Drug Names[a]	Clinical Pearl
Unfractionated heparin (UFH)	Heparin (UFH)[a] Enoxaparin (LMWH)	Heparin is the most common and well-studied anticoagulant used for STEMI PCI.[25]
Low-molecular weight heparin (LMWH)	Enoxaparin[b] Dalteparin	Enoxaparin is effective than UFH in patients who underwent fibrinolytic therapy prior to PCI.[35]
Direct thrombin inhibitors	Bivalirudin[b] Hirudin Argatroban Dabigatran	Bivalrudin has a short half-life (25 min) and therefore may have a lower risk of bleeding than other anticoagulants however it is costly. European guidelines suggest only using in patients with highest bleeding risk.[36]
Factor Xa inhibitor	Fondaparinux[b] Apixaban Endoxaban Rivaroxaban	Fondaparinux is a synthetic pentasaccharide anticoaguant or "tiny" heparin and does not induce HIT.[37]

[a]Note this list is not exhaustive and not all drugs are routinely used or recommended for treatment of STEMI/NSTEMI, however nurses should be familiar with the names of the drugs in their respective class when caring for patients before and after ACS. For example, a patient taking Apixaban for atrial fibrillation would not be a good candidate to be given Fondaparinux during ACS.
[b]Notes most commonly used in its class.

enter the health system and play an important role in facilitating door-to-intervention times for STEMI and UA/NSTEMI patients. Nursing assessment should include screen for risks and contraindications of anticoagulation like recent or prior stroke, heparin-induced thrombocytopenia (HIT), active or history of bleeding, and allergies. Furthermore, it is important for the nurse caring for post-STEMI/NSTEMI to know what anticoagulant the patient received and monitor for signs and symptoms of bleeding, especially at arterial access points from the angiographic procedure.

Comprehensive Plan of Care

Early hospital care, antiplatelet/anticoagulation strategy, and the determination for invasive intervention are part of a comprehensive plan of care that encompasses the patient's multisystem, psychosocial, spiritual, immediate care, and long-term follow-up needs. Table 29-6 shows the depth and breadth of the scope of the guideline-directed patient care relevant for cardiac nurses in all settings.

Fibrinolysis With Invasive Intervention

If a patient with STEMI is at a facility or location where the first-medical-contact (FMC) to PCI-capable hospital time is greater than 120 minutes, administration of a fibrinolytic agent is advised, albeit with caution. Fibrinolytic agents dissolve fibrin, the molecule that binds clots together work by catalyzing the conversion of plasminogen to plasmin. Refer to Table 29-7 for a list of fibrinolytic agents and Table 29-8 to better understand the contraindications, and cautions for fibrinolysis use in STEMI.

INVASIVE INTERVENTION

Percutaneous Revascularization

Revascularization with PCI is the primary goal for patients who present with STEMI. This strategy is reflective of the underlying pathophysiology (thrombus) and principle of treatment (time is muscle). This section provides an overview of PCI and focuses on strategies for revascularization in STEMI and NSTEMI.

Percutaneous Coronary Intervention

Interventional cardiology has drastically evolved and improved techniques and procedures for percutaneous treatment of CHD. Interventional coronary devices used to restore or enhance myocardial blood flow include angioplasty balloons, atherectomy devices, and intracoronary stents. Pharmacologic therapies have been an important partner in the development of device technology. The term *PCI* refers to the collective group of interventional procedures performed through a percutaneous approach in the coronary arteries. PCI was initially limited to percutaneous transluminal coronary angioplasty (PTCA, or balloon angioplasty) (Fig. 29-12) but has long encompassed other procedures using atherectomy devices, thrombectomy devices, and various stents including bare metal stents (BMS) and drug-eluting stents (DES). More recent developments that would be more appropriate in the elective PCI setting include robotic PCI in which the operator is not in the procedure room but in the control room, unexposed to lead or fluoroscopy; bifurcation stenting; bioabsorbable stenting; drug-coated balloons; and many techniques and devices to recanalize chronic totally occluded coronary arteries. Factors that have improved the overall success and complication rates include operator experience, modifications in procedural instruments, newer interventional devices, and advances in adjunctive pharmacologic therapy. These improvements have led to the expansion of interventional cardiology treatment to higher-risk patients with more complex coronary lesions and comorbidities. These improvements have influenced the short- and long-term success of PCI.[40]

Intracoronary stents provide structural support to an artery thereby opposing elastic recoil, preventing vasoconstriction, and preventing or treating dissections of the arterial wall seen with other coronary devices. There are a variety of different types of intracoronary stents, categorized by mechanism of deployment, structure, metals, sizes, and stent coating (including bare metal, drug eluting, and covered). Stents are deployed using balloon-expandable or self-expandable mechanisms. BMS dramatically decreased acute and threatened closure with PTCA but did not eliminate the significant problem of restenosis.[41] DES are coated with a medication to prevent neointimal hyperplasia, the thickening of arterial walls and decreased arterial space, and allow normal development of endothelial lining on the stent struts.

Endothelialization is important for preventing direct contact between bare metal and circulating blood, a circumstance that can lead to clot formation and stent thrombosis. The DES platform is coated with a polymer that allows the intended antiproliferative drug to adhere to the stent struts and allow local delivery. In essence it slows down the body's ability to grow endothelial cells in the location of the stent and therefore slows down the progression and possibility of endothelial cells occluding the stent (restenosis).

Dual antiplatelet therapy (DAPT) aims to prevent stent thrombosis that may occur with endothelialization. With BMS

Table 29-6 • PLAN OF CARE FOR PATIENTS WITH NSTEMI-ACS

Plan of Care	Resources
Medications	
Antithrombotic therapies	• 2013 NSTEMI CPG
Beta blockers	• 2013 NSTEMI CPG
ACE inhibitors/ARBs/ aldosterone antagonists	• 2013 NSTEMI CPG
CCBs	• 2013 NSTEMI CPG
Statins	• 2013 Blood cholesterol CPG
Discontinuation of antithrombotic therapies for elective surgical and medical procedures with increased risk of bleeding	• 2014 SIHD focused update • 2012 SIHD CPG • 2012 Management of AMI in patients with persistent STEMI CPG • 2011 Secondary prevention CPG • 2007 Science Advisory on the prevention of premature discontinuation of DAPT in patients with coronary artery stents
Inappropriate use of analgesics (NSAIDs)	• 2010 Expert consensus document on PPIs and thienopyridines
Use of PPIs	• 2011 PCI CPG
Risk factor modification/lifestyle interventions and physical activity/ cardiac rehabilitation	
Smoking cessation	• Tobacco cessation toolkit
Diet nutrition	• 2013 Lifestyle CPG
Physical activity	• 2013 Lifestyle CPG • 2011 Secondary prevention CPG
Cardiorespiratory fitness (MET capacity)	• 2011 Secondary prevention CPG • 2010 Performance measures on cardiac rehabilitation • 2012 Scientific statement on sexual activity and cardiovascular disease
Management of comorbidities	
Overweight/obesity	• 2013 Obesity CPG • 2011 Secondary prevention CPG
Statins	• 2013 Lifestyle CPG • 2013 Blood cholesterol CPG
Hypertension	• 2014 Report on high BP • 2013 Science advisory on high BP control
Diabetes mellitus	• 2013 Position statement on standards of medical care in diabetes
HF	• 2013 HF CPG
Arrhythmia/arrhythmia risk	• 2012 Focused update incorporated into the 2008 DBT CPG • 2014 AF CPG
Psychosocial factors	
Sexual activity	• 2012 Scientific statement on sexual activity and cardiovascular disease • 2013 Consensus document on sexual counseling for individuals with cardiovascular disease and their partners
Gender-specific issues	• 2007 Cardiovascular disease prevention in women CPG
Depression, stress, and anxiety	• 2008 Science advisory on depression and coronary heart disease
Alcohol use	• 2011 Secondary prevention CPG
Culturally sensitive issues	• 2009 Consensus report on a comprehensive framework and preferred practices for measuring and reporting cultural competency
Return to work schedule	
Clinician follow-up	
Cardiologist	• 2011 Secondary prevention CPG • 2013 Hospital to Home Quality Initiative
Primary care clinician	
Advanced practice nurse/ physician assistant	
Pharmacists	• 2013 Discharge counseling for patients with HF or MI
Other relevant medical specialists	
Electronic personal health records	
Influenza vaccination	• 2005 Recommendations for prevention and control of influenza
Patient/family education	
Plan of care for AMI	• 2010 CPG for cardiopulmonary resuscitation and emergency cardiovascular care–part 9: postcardiac arrest care • 2013 STEMI CPG
Recognizing symptoms of MI	
Activating EMS, signs and symptoms for urgent versus emergency evaluations	
CPR training for family members	
Risk assessment and prognosis	
Advanced directives	
Social networks/social isolation	
Socioeconomic factors	
Access to health insurance coverage	
Access to clinicians	• Effective communication and care coordination
Disability	• Cardiovascular disability: updating Social Security listings
Social services	
Community services	

ACE, angiotensin-converting enzyme; AF, atrial fibrillation; AMI, acute myocardial infarction; ARB, angiotensin receptor blocker; BP, blood pressure; CCB, calcium channel blocker; CPG, clinical practice guideline; CPR, cardiopulmonary resuscitation; DAPT, dual antiplatelet therapy; DBT, device-based therapy; EMS, emergency medical services; HF, heart failure; MET, metabolic equivalent; MI, myocardial infarction; NSAID, nonsteroidal anti-inflammatory drug; PCI, percutaneous coronary intervention; PPI, protein pump inhibitor; SIHD, stable ischemic heart disease; and STEMI, ST-elevation myocardial infarction. Please note that there may be updated versions of these CPGs; this is table is reproduced here to demonstrate the scope of patient care and education involved for this diagnosis. (Used with permission from O'Gara PT, Kushner FG, Ascheim DD, et al. 2013 ACCF/AHA Guideline for the Management of ST-Elevation Myocardial Infarction. *A Report of the American College of Cardiology Foundation/American Heart Association Task Force on Practice Guidelines*. 2013;61(4):e78–e140.)

Table 29-7 • FIBRINOLYTIC AGENTS

	Streptokinase (SK)	Alteplase (t-PA)	Reteplase (r-PA)	Tenecteplase (TNK-tPA)
Generation	First	Second	Third	Forth
Half-life (min)	23	<5	13–16	20[a]
Fibrin specific	–	++	+	+++
Hypotension	Yes	No	No	No

[a]The terminal phase half-life 90 to 130 min.[34,35]

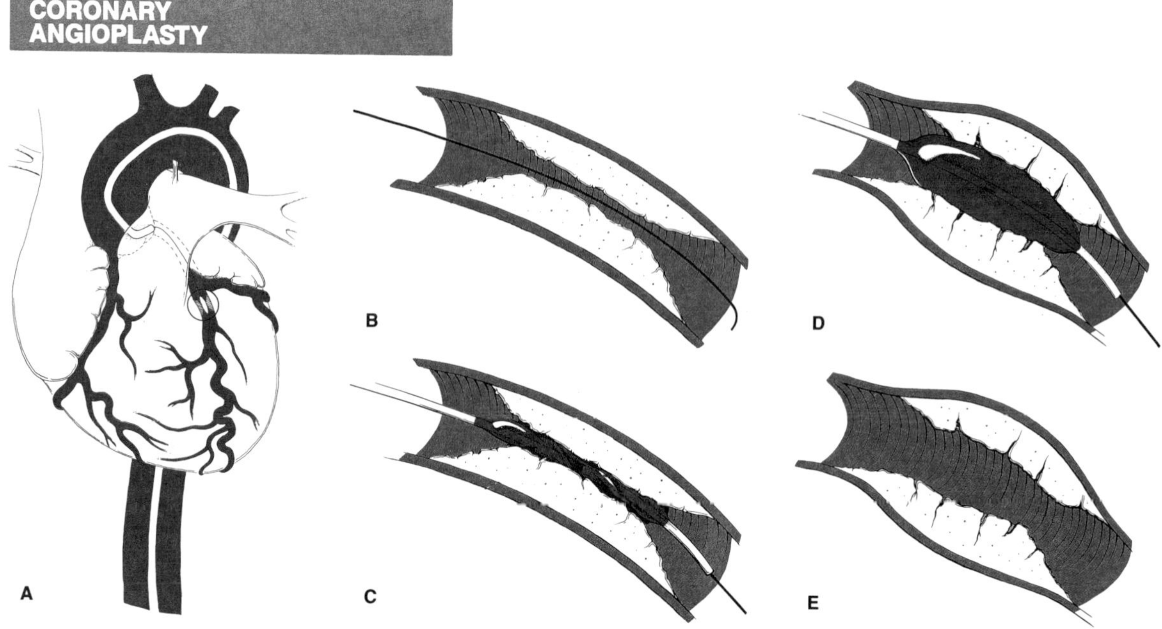

Figure 29-12. Mechanism of intracoronary balloon angioplasty. **A:** A balloon catheter is introduced into the coronary artery through a guide catheter in the aorta. **B:** A guidewire is advanced across the area of narrowing. **C:** The balloon catheter is advanced over the wire across the lesion. **D:** The balloon is inflated. **E:** Coronary artery after PTCA. (Courtesy of Boston Scientific Corporation, Maple Grove, MN.)

Table 29-8 • CONTRAINDICATIONS AND CAUTIONS FOR FIBRINOLYSIS USE IN STEMI

Absolute Contraindications[a]

- Any prior intracranial hemorrhage
- Known structural cerebral vascular lesion (e.g., AVM)
- Known malignant intracranial neoplasm (primary or metastatic)
- Ischemic stroke within 3 mo EXCEPT acute ischemic stroke within 3 hr
- Suspected aortic dissection
- Active bleeding or bleeding diathesis (excluding menses)
- Significant closed head or facial trauma within 3 mo

Relative Contraindications[a]

- History of chronic severe, poorly controlled hypertension
- Severe uncontrolled hypertension on presentation (SBP >180 mm Hg or DBP >110 mm Hg)[b]
- History of prior ischemic stroke greater than 3 mo, dementia, or known intracranial pathology not covered in contraindications
- Traumatic or prolonged (greater than 10 min) CPR or major surgery (less than 3 wk)
- Recent (within 2 to 4 wk) internal bleeding
- Noncompressible vascular punctures
- For streptokinase/anistreplase: prior exposure (more than 5 days ago) or prior allergic reaction to these agents
- Pregnancy
- Active peptic ulcer
- Current use of anticoagulants: the higher the INR, the higher the risk of bleeding

[a]Viewed as advisory for clinical decision making and may not be all-inclusive or definitive.
[b]Could be an absolute contraindication in low-risk patients with STEMI.
AVM, arteriovenous malformation; SBP, systolic BP; DBP, diastolic BP; CPR, cardiopulmonary resuscitation; INR, international normalized ratio.
Adapted from O'Gara PT, Kushner FG, Ascheim DD, et al. 2013 ACCF/AHA Guideline for the Management of ST-elevation myocardial infarction. A Report of the American College of Cardiology Foundation/American Heart Association Task Force on Practice Guidelines. *J Am Coll Cardiol.* 2013;61(4):e78–e140.

Table 29-9 • CONSIDERATIONS FOR DURATION OF DUAL ANTIPLATELET THERAPY AFTER PERCUTANEOUS CORONARY INTERVENTION

Favor Increased DAPT Duration

Factors associated with increased risk of ischemia

- Advanced age
- ACS presentation
- Multiple prior MIs
- Extensive CAD
- Diabetes mellitus
- Chronic kidney disease

Factors associated with increased risk of stent thrombosis

- ACS presentation
- Diabetes mellitus
- LVEF <40%
- First generation
- Stent undersizing
- Stent underdeployment
- Small stent diameter
- Greater stent length
- Bifurcation stents
- In-stent restenosis

Favor Decreased DAPT Duration

Factors associated with increased bleeding risk

- History of prior bleeding
- Oral anticoagulant therapy
- Female sex
- Advanced age
- Diabetes mellitus
- Chronic kidney disease
- Anemia
- Chronic steroid or NSAID therapy

DAPT, dual antiplatelet therapy; ACS, acute coronary syndrome; MI, myocardial infarction; CAD, coronary artery disease; LVEF, left ventricular ejection fraction.
Adapted from Levine GN, Bates ER, Bittl JA, et al. 2016 ACC/AHA guideline focused update on duration of dual antiplatelet therapy in patients with coronary artery disease. A Report of the American College of Cardiology/American Heart Association Task Force on Clinical Practice Guidelines. *J Am Coll Cardiol.* 2016;68(10):1082–1115.

the risk of clot formation is lower and DAPT duration is usually 1 month. With DES the metal of the stent will be exposed longer as a result of the slowing of endothelialization, patients will be required to stay on DAPT for a longer period of time until endothelialization of the stent eventually occurs. Typically, patients are prescribed DAPT for 12 months after DES placement, but this treatment is tailored to patient-specific risks and comorbid conditions (e.g., GI bleeding or current anticoagulation therapy) per the latest guideline recommendations. Some of these are considerations are listed in Table 29-9.

Percutaneous Intervention for ACS

A revascularization strategy is pursued for ACS based upon the diagnosis of STEMI or NSTEMI. The algorithms depicted in Figures 29-13 and 29-14 outline the decision making for STEMI and NSTEMI, respectively. For STEMI, the drivers of the revascularization strategy are patient eligibility for PCI, and access to a PCI-capable hospital. While rapid and safe treatment of the STEMI culprit lesion(s) takes priority, patient eligibility considerations for PCI may include other comorbid conditions (e.g., diabetes, cancer, or diagnoses for which other treatments or procedures may be planned or warranted), absolute and relative contraindications for antiplatelet therapy, or lifestyle considerations. A door-to-balloon (DTB) time is specified and includes time to transport to a PCI-capable hospital if needed. DTB time is a quality measure defined as the time interval that begins with the patient's initial presentation to the hospital and ends with the time of intra-arterial coronary balloon inflation to restore intraluminal flow.[33]

For NSTEMI, patients are initiated on antiplatelet/anticoagulation therapy and undergo cardiac catheterization with coronary angiography. The timing of invasive management with PCI (or CABG) is determined based on symptoms, hemodynamic stability, biomarkers, and risk factors. Immediate invasive management (within 2 hours) is warranted for patients with recurrent/refractory angina or angina at rest, heart failure or mitral regurgitation, sustained ventricular tachycardia, and hemodynamic instability.

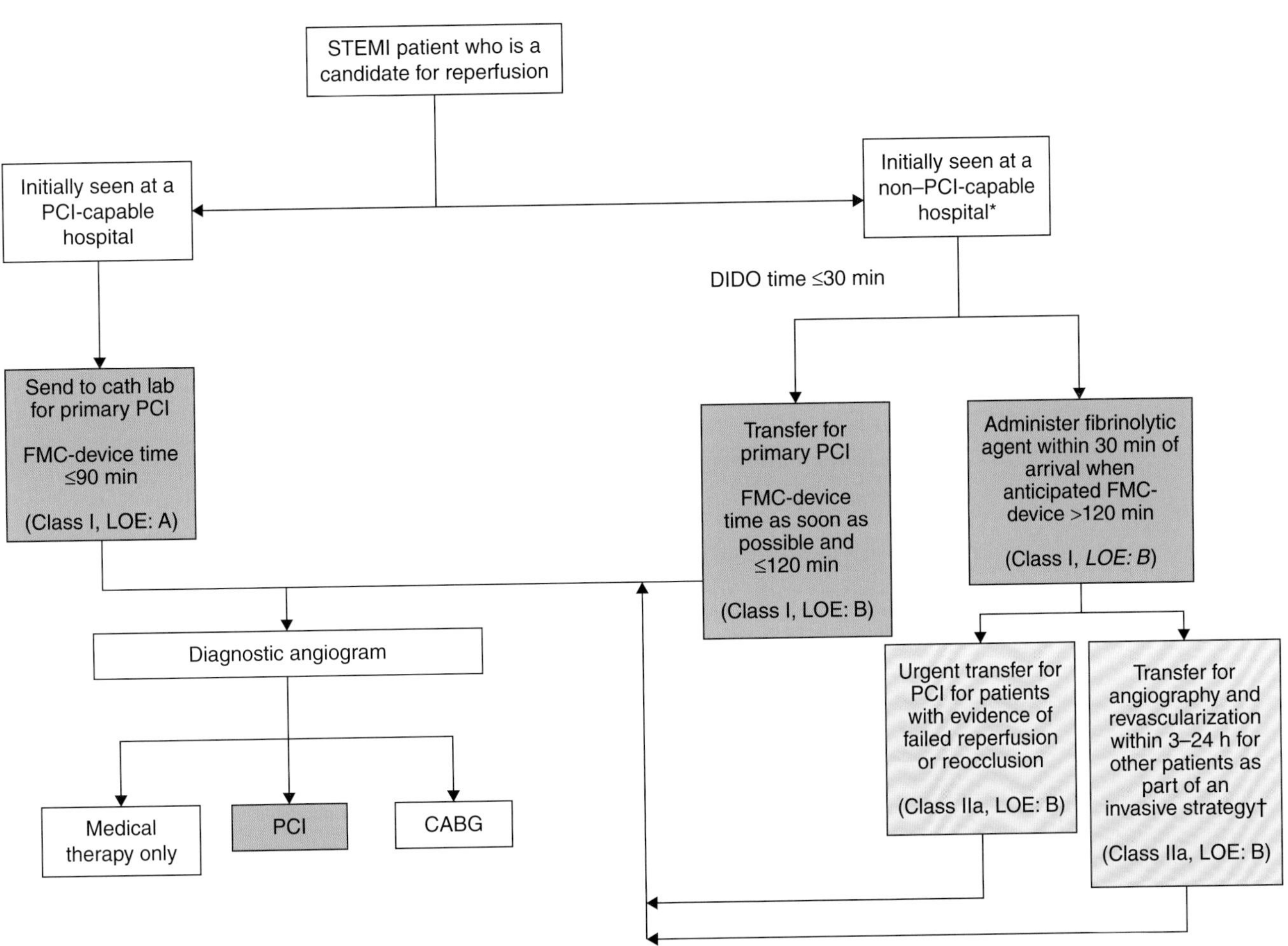

Figure 29-13. Reperfusion therapy for patients with STEMI. The *bold arrows* and *boxes* are the preferred strategies. Performance of PCI is dictated by an anatomically appropriate culprit stenosis. *Patients with cardiogenic shock or severe heart failure initially seen at a non–PCI-capable hospital should be transferred for cardiac catheterization and revascularization as soon as possible, irrespective of time delay from MI onset (Class I, LOE: B). †Angiography and revascularization should not be performed within the first 2 to 3 hours after administration of fibrinolytic therapy. CABG, coronary artery bypass graft; DIDO, door-in–door-out; FMC, first medical contact; LOE, level of evidence; MI, myocardial infarction; PCI, percutaneous coronary intervention; STEMI, ST-elevation myocardial infarction. (Used with permission from O'Gara PT, Kushner FG, Ascheim DD, et al. 2013 ACCF/AHA Guideline for the Management of ST-Elevation Myocardial Infarction. *A Report of the American College of Cardiology Foundation/American Heart Association Task Force on Practice Guidelines.* 2013;61(4):e78–e140).

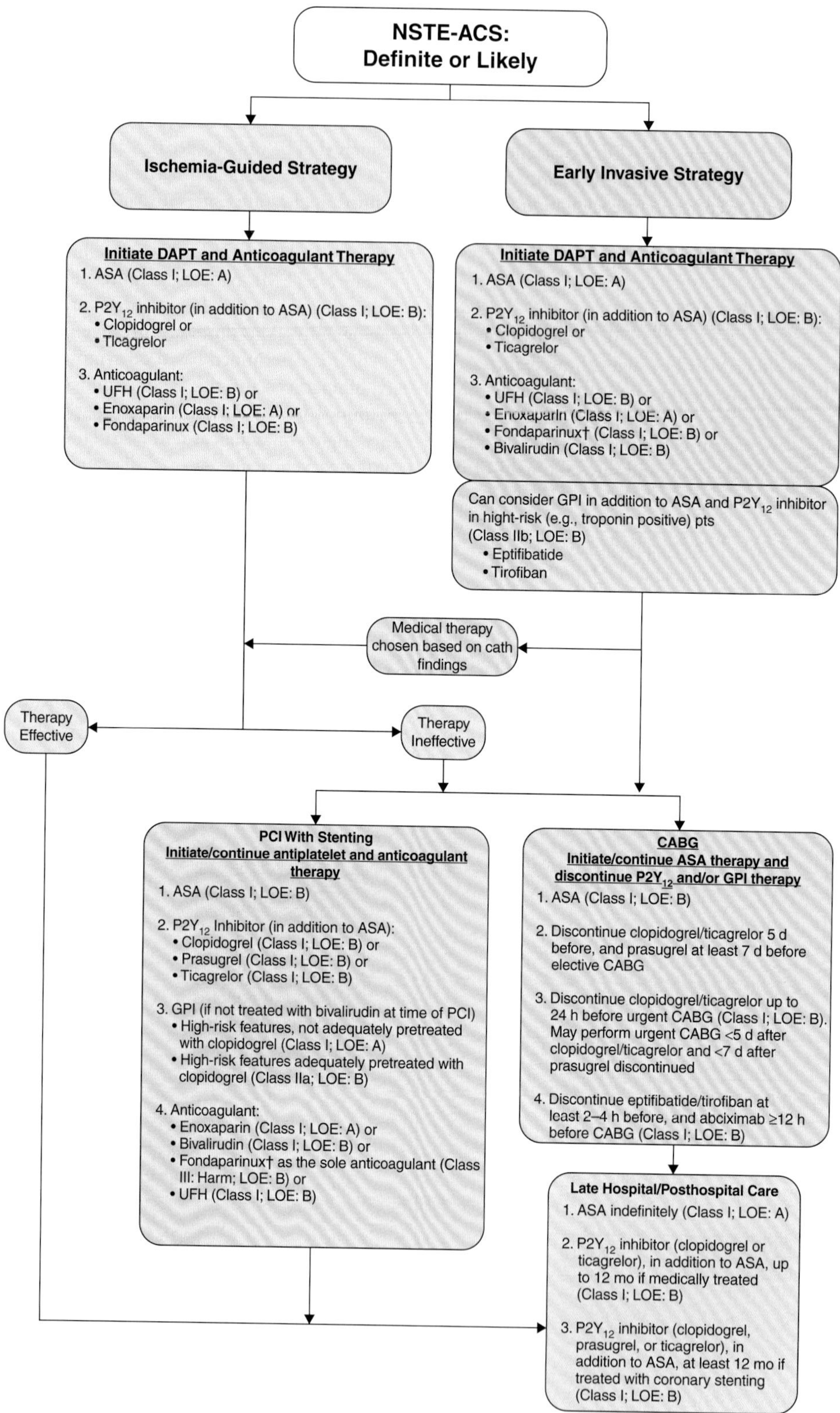

Figure 29-14. Algorithm for management of patients with definite or likely NSTE-ACS. †In patients who have been treated with fondaparinux (as upfront therapy) who are undergoing PCI, an additional anticoagulant with anti-IIa activity should be administered at the time of PCI because of the risk of catheter thrombosis. ASA, aspirin; CABG, coronary artery bypass graft; cath, catheter; COR, class of recommendation; DAPT, dual antiplatelet therapy; GPI, glycoprotein IIb/IIIa inhibitor; LOE, level of evidence; NSTE-ACS, non–ST-elevation acute coronary syndrome; PCI, percutaneous coronary intervention; pts, patients; UFH, unfractionated heparin. (Used with permission from Amsterdam EA, Wenger NK, Brindis RG, et al. 2014 AHA/ACC guideline for the management of patients with non–ST-elevation acute coronary syndromes. A Report of the American College of Cardiology/American Heart Association Task Force on Practice Guidelines. *J Am Coll Cardiol.* 2014;64[24]:e139–e228.)

Other criteria guide the timing for an early (within 24 hours) or delayed (25- to 72-hour) invasive strategy.[38] The treatment algorithm for DAPT and anticoagulation in ACS versus stable IHD is depicted in Figure 29-15.

Surgical Revascularization

In the patient with STEMI, surgical revascularization with CABG may be indicated if the patient does not have favorable anatomy for PCI and has ongoing or recurrent ischemia, cardiogenic shock, severe heart failure, or other high risk features.[33] Specifically, CABG has been found to significantly reduce rates of death, MI, and stroke compared to PCI in patients ($N = 1900$) with diabetes and multivessel CAD.[42]

CABG surgery especially when urgently or emergently performed is accomplished via a median sternotomy incision and cardiopulmonary bypass (CPB) (Fig. 29-16). During the CABG procedure, coronary artery revascularization is accomplished by the surgeon sewing a graft vessel that "bypasses" the coronary blockage. Blood flow is rerouted around the blockage via the new bypass graft. While the saphenous vein is easier to harvest and served as the first bypass conduit, the internal mammary artery

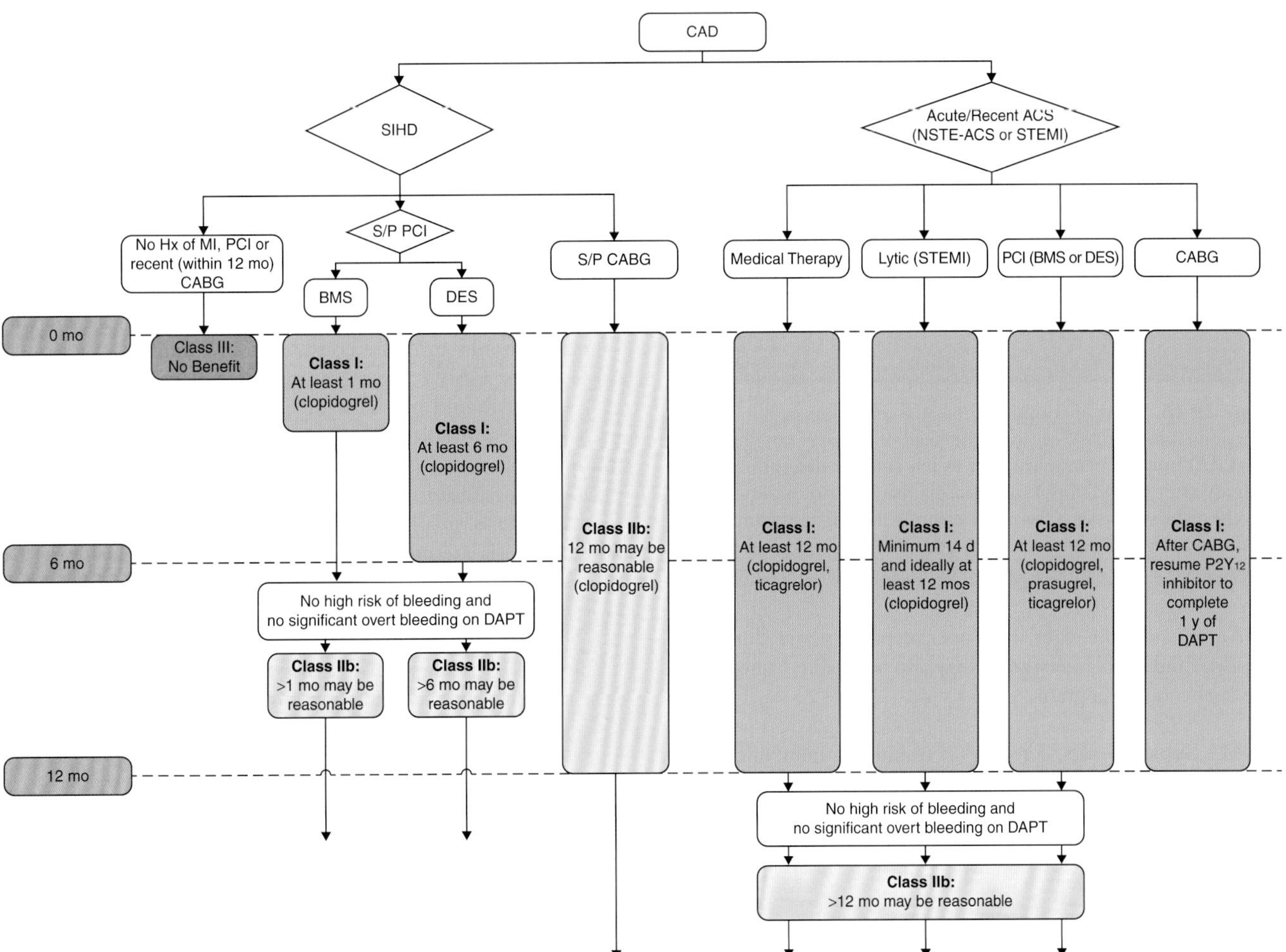

Figure 29-15. Master treatment algorithm for duration of $P2Y_{12}$ inhibitor therapy in patients with CAD treated with DAPT colors correspond to class of recommendation per ACCF/AHA. Clopidogrel is the only currently used $P2Y_{12}$ inhibitor studied in patients with SIHD undergoing PCI. Aspirin therapy is almost always continued indefinitely in patients with CAD. Patients with a history of ACS >1 year prior who have since remained free of recurrent ACS are considered to have transitioned to SIHD. In patients treated with DAPT after DES implantation who develop a high risk of bleeding (e.g., treatment with oral anticoagulant therapy), are at high risk of severe bleeding complication (e.g., major intracranial surgery), or develop significant overt bleeding, discontinuation of $P2Y_{12}$ inhibitor therapy after 3 months for SIHD or after 6 months for ACS may be reasonable. *Arrows* at the bottom of the figure denote that the optimal duration of prolonged DAPT is not established. ACS, acute coronary syndrome; BMS, bare metal stent; CABG, coronary artery bypass graft surgery; CAD, coronary artery disease; DAPT, dual antiplatelet therapy; DES, drug-eluting stent; Hx, history; lytic, fibrinolytic therapy; NSTE-ACS, non–ST-elevation acute coronary syndrome; PCI, percutaneous coronary intervention; SIHD, stable ischemic heart disease; S/P, status post; and STEMI, ST-elevation myocardial infarction. (Used with permission from Levine GN, Bates ER, Bittl JA, et al. 2016 ACC/AHA guideline focused update on duration of dual antiplatelet therapy in patients with coronary artery disease. A Report of the American College of Cardiology/American Heart Association Task Force on Clinical Practice Guidelines. *J Am Coll Cardiol.* 2016;68[10]:1082–1115.)

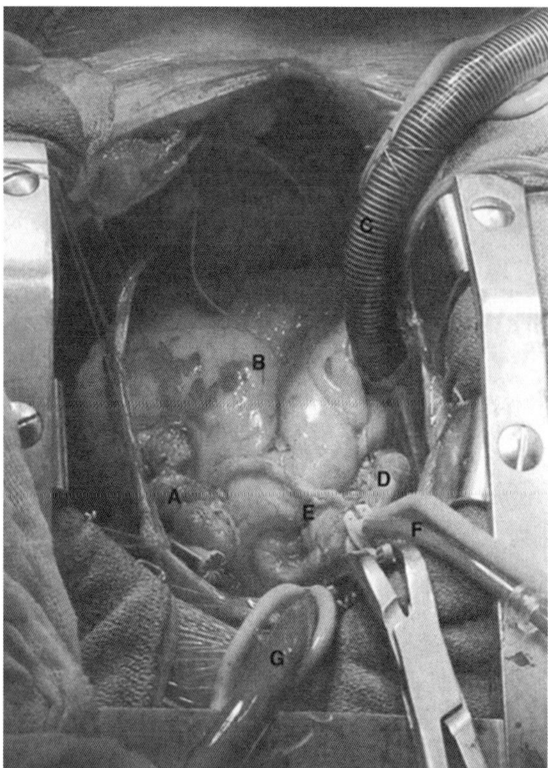

Figure 29-16. View of completed internal mammary and saphenous vein grafts. View from the head of the operating table shows: **(A)** internal mammary graft to left anterior descending coronary artery; **(B)** temporary epicardial pacing wires inserted into the right ventricle; **(C)** venous cannula into right atrium; **(D)** ascending aorta; **(E)** saphenous vein graft; **(F)** cardioplegia delivery catheter; **(G)** aortic cannula. (Photo by D. LeDoux, 2003.)

(IMA), left over the right, has superior patency and durability. The IMA and radial artery grafts may also be used in combination with saphenous vein grafts.

IMA Bypass Grafts. The IMA is technically more difficult to harvest than the saphenous vein graft. After the sternum is cut open, the IMA is dissected away from the chest wall. A special retractor is used to expose the IMA in the retrosternal bed. A 2-cm-wide pedicle strip is removed from the chest wall muscle, fat, and pleura that surround the IMA. The pedicle strip, with the IMA lying in the center, is exposed from the IMA origin at the subclavian artery down to the level of the fourth to sixth intercostal space. The branches of the IMA are exposed, divided, and ligated. An incision is made into the coronary artery to be bypassed (usually the left anterior descending [LAD]) and the distal end of the IMA is sutured into place. The IMA can be used as a free graft rather than a pedicle graft if it is not long enough to reach the target.

Saphenous Vein Bypass Grafts. While the sternal incision is made and the patient is readied for CPB, the saphenous vein is prepared. The saphenous vein can be harvested using endoscopic techniques and small incisions at the same time that the IMA graft is taken down from the retrosternal bed. A long segment of vein is carefully exposed, the branches are ligated and divided, and the vein is removed. The vein is flushed with a cold heparinized solution and checked for leaks. One side of the untwisted vein is marked with a surgical pencil, and the vein is filled with and stored in a cold solution. CPB is instituted, a clamp is placed across the distal aorta, and cold cardioplegia is injected into the aortic root. Portions of saphenous vein are sutured to coronary arteries beyond the arterial stenoses. Distal anastomoses to the LAD artery are usually made first, followed by distal anastomoses to the coronary arteries located on the back of the heart. After all distal anastomoses are completed, the aortic cross-clamp is removed and patient warming is begun. Small openings in the ascending aorta are made with a punch, and the proximal end of the saphenous vein is anastomosed to the aorta. After the proximal anastomoses are completed, CPB is discontinued and the chest is closed.

Radial Artery Bypass Grafts. The radial artery graft is used for bypass conduit only after collateral circulation of the ulnar artery has been assessed by vascular ultrasound or Allen test. Although both radial arteries can be used, the radial artery from the patient's nondominant hand is the usual choice and can be harvested before the chest is opened. The radial graft is a desirable conduit because of its length and ability to reach most distal targets. Postoperative nursing care includes evaluation of ulnar pulse and distal circulation.

In some cases, other minimal incision types can be accomplished such as thoracotomy but is dependent on the bypassed lesions and patient anatomy. Anticoagulant and antiplatelet therapies should carefully considered in regard to the timing of an urgent CABG due to the risk of patient bleeding, however aspirin should not be withheld.[33] Conditions that greatly increase the mortality risk during surgery and anatomic limitations are relative contraindications to CABG surgery. Lack of adequate conduit to create bypass, coronary arteries distal to the stenosis smaller than 1 to 1.5 mm, and severe aortic atherosclerosis are anatomic abnormalities that may limit the success of the revascularization for technical reasons. Severe LV failure and coexisting pulmonary, renal, carotid, and peripheral vascular disease may significantly increase the risk of surgery by predisposing to complications during the perioperative period. Patients with low ejection fraction are sicker at baseline and more than four times the mortality than patients with high ejection fraction.[43]

NURSING CONSIDERATIONS

Nurses play a very important role in identifying patients through careful history taking and identifying early signs and symptoms of ischemia. Early intervention of establishing and restoring coronary blood flow will salvage myocardium and save the patient short-term and long-term postinfarction complications. This section covers the nursing considerations for PCI, CABG, and complications of MI.

Percutaneous Coronary Intervention

Preprocedural Management

Preparation for PCI requires informed consent after physician discussion of risks and benefits, provisional consent for emergency CABG surgery, and patient education. Patient education includes expectations during the procedure and postprocedural care using visual, written, and verbal information. The nursing history (including all current medications and herbal supplements) and physical examination are documented, with abnormalities reported to the physician and catheterization laboratory staff prior to the PCI.

The potential risks and benefits should be discussed in detail with the patient and family and be weighed against timing of therapy or alternative therapies. Patients should understand the possible complications associated with the procedure, the possibility of restenosis, stent thrombosis (see complications) post-procedure, and the potential for incomplete revascularization in patients with diffuse CAD. The clinical and angiographic variables associated with increased mortality include advanced age, female sex, diabetes mellitus, prior MI, multivessel disease, left main disease or equivalent (severe stenosis of the LAD artery and circumflex arteries proximal to any major branch), a large area of myocardium at risk, pre-existing impairment of LV function or renal function, and collateral vessels supplying significant areas of myocardium that originate distal to the segment to be treated.

Most preprocedural nursing assessment and intervention pertain to known or likely risks for complications due to comorbidities, medications, and possible interactions or contra-indications with likely pharmacologic therapy or contrast. For diabetic patients, oral hypoglycemic agents are usually held prior to the PCI. The combination of contrast medium and metformin should be completely avoided in patients with renal dysfunction, hepatic dysfunction, alcohol abuse, or severe congestive heart failure because all these conditions limit metformin excretion and can increase lactate production, possibly leading to fatal lactic acidosis and worsening end organ damage (e.g., acute renal injury).

Isosmolar contrast agents used to opacify the coronary arteries during PCI may result in contrast-induced nephropathy (CIN). CIN occurs in 2% of patients with normal renal function and up to 20% to 30% in patients with a baseline of creatinine of 2 mg/dL.[44] In patients with renal insufficiency and diabetes, creatinine clearance and maximal contrast doses should be estimated by the cardiac nurse and procedural team. The most important intervention to prevent CIN is adequate hydration before and after the procedure. Other strategies such as N-acetylcysteine and/or sodium bicarbonate infusion before and after contrast administration have not been recommended.[39]

Intraprocedure Management

Patient preparation is similar to the patient having a diagnostic cardiac catheterization. Conscious sedation is given at the discretion of the cardiologist and the patient monitored by the catheterization laboratory staff as per protocol. A sheath is placed in the radial or femoral artery. A bolus of heparin is given to maintain an activated clotting time (ACT) of 250 to 300 seconds. ACT below 250 seconds has been associated with thrombotic complications during PCI with multiple catheters, wires, or devices being placed in the aorta and coronary arteries. Use of low–molecular-weight heparin (LMWH) or direct thrombin inhibitors can be used as an alternative to heparin (see anticoagulation options for PCI). Baseline angiographic views are obtained of the coronary artery to be treated using the standard diagnostic catheter or the guiding catheter. Coronary injections may be repeated after administration of intracoronary NTG to exclude spasm as a significant component of the target stenosis and to minimize the occurrence of coronary spasm during the PCI. The appropriate guiding catheter is positioned in the coronary ostium and a guidewire is directed across the stenotic lesion. After the wire tip is confirmed to be in the distal portion of the coronary artery to be treated, the angioplasty balloon or other device is selected. The patient is monitored for hemodynamic stability and electrocardiographic changes during the procedure. During the procedure additional heparin or a direct thrombin inhibitor is given by the cardiologist to maintain an adequate ACT and anticoagulation status. A glycoprotein (GP) IIb/IIIa receptor inhibitor infusion is selected for patients with ACS or angiographic thrombus.

After the procedure is complete, the patient is prepared for transfer to the postinterventional ward. Vital signs are monitored and patient placed on a portable monitor for transfer. The arterial access site is assessed for bleeding or hematoma prior to transfer. Report is called to the receiving staff, including type of procedure performed, specific artery treated, vital signs, status of the arterial sheath, and other pertinent information. (See vascular sheath removal under postprocedure management.)

Postprocedure Management

The patient with ACS status post-PCI is monitored for manifestations of myocardial ischemia, such as chest pain, ECG changes, arrhythmias, or hemodynamic instability. A 12-lead ECG is obtained postprocedure to establish a baseline for comparison. Laboratory tests are drawn and should minimally include hematocrit, platelet count, blood urea nitrogen, and creatinine. All patients who have UA, MI, or a complicated procedure should have cardiac enzymes CK-MB and troponin measured. Patients may be relatively extracellular fluid (ECF) depleted after PCI because of nothing-by-mouth status and radiographic contrast-induced diuresis. Hydration is maintained by normal or half-normal saline until oral intake is sufficient to meet patient requirements. Anticoagulants, antithrombin agents, or GP IIb/IIIa receptor inhibitors infusions are continued as per institutional protocol or physician orders.

Vascular Sheath Removal

Vascular sheath removal, mobilization, and ambulation protocols vary according to the device protocol and hospital policies. In general, the sheaths are removed 4 to 6 hours after the procedure, when the ACT falls below 180 seconds, by either the patient care unit nursing staff or catheterization technician. Vascular sheaths are removed by manual pressure and either an adjunctive compression device or a vascular closure device. Manual pressure is applied for at least 20 minutes or longer, as warranted, to provide homeostasis with strict attention to the arterial site and distal circulation. Recognition and treatment of complications are essential to prevent peripheral vascular injuries.

Access Site Management

The vascular site is monitored for bleeding, hematoma formation, distal circulation, and sensation, initially every 15 minutes and advancing to every hour until stable. Manual compression remains the standard method for femoral sheath removal worldwide, however arterial closure devices are commonly used and do require special training for the physician and staff. Frequently used closure devices with active hemostasis components include collagen plugs (Angio-Seal, St. Jude Medical, St. Paul, MN), suture devices (Perclose, Abbott Vascular, Redwood City, CA), and surgical staples/clips (StarClose, Abbott Vascular, Redwood City, CA). Pressure dressings and sand bags to groin sites are uncomfortable and ineffective in controlling recurrent or persistent bleeding. A specialty compression band (Terumo TR Band, Terumo Interventional Systems, Somerset, NJ) used after radial artery access however has been found quite comfortable and effective for hemostasis without resulting in radial artery occlusion.[45] Minor or tract oozing after a compression or a vascular closure device can be managed with light manual pressure, injection of xylocaine with epinephrine, or light pressure dressing.

Prevention and early recognition of access site complications is essential to avoid peripheral vascular injury. Many of these complications may be averted through frequent and systematic nursing assessment of the vascular access site for bleeding and hematoma formation, and distal circulation, sensation, and intact movement of the associated limb per protocol. Risk factors for vascular complications are also assessed, including difficulty maintaining hemostasis due to anticoagulants or antiplatelet therapy, or increased blood pressure in the setting of pain, anxiety, or discontinuation of antihypertensive therapy. In contrast, a hypotensive response may suggest hypovolemia or even retroperitoneal bleeding. Back pain, groin pain, or pain with knee-to-chest flexion to assess psoas muscle irritation may suggest a retroperitoneal bleed and warrant an imaging study such as a CT scan. Pain, hematoma, and bruit over the access site may indicate pseudoaneurysm formation necessitating Doppler vascular ultrasound study. Vasovagal reactions can occur at the time of sheath insertion or removal. This syndrome is triggered by pain and anxiety, particularly in the setting of ECF deficit, and can result in difficulty maintaining hemostasis as well as hemodynamic instability. Common symptoms associated with a vasovagal reaction include hypotension, nausea, vomiting, yawning, and diaphoresis. Treatment includes cessation of painful stimuli, rapid volume administration with normal saline, and atropine intravenously. If hypotension persists, additional hemodynamic support with intravenous vasopressor agents may be needed.

CABG Surgery

Preoperative Assessment and Preparation

The patient with acute CHD may be hospitalized for only hours or days before surgery. A MI may have occurred, or the patient may be experiencing UA. Before cardiac surgery, patients complete a cardiac work-up. For the patient urgently or emergently referred for CABG surgery, the evaluation at a minimum may include cardiac catheterization to define coronary artery anatomy and target vessels for revascularization and echocardiography to delineate valvular lesions, ventricular function, and focal wall-motion abnormalities. The patient should have a complete physical examination with special attention given to the cardiovascular examination. A new history and physical examination, chest radiograph, ECG, complete blood count, serum electrolytes, coagulation screen, and typing and cross-matching of blood are performed. These data provide information about other disease conditions and cardiac problems. The goal is to optimize the evaluation and intervention timing to preserve myocardium and prevent complications.

Due to the risks involved with blood loss, hemodynamic instability, CPB and its related metabolic derangements, additional diagnostic testing is performed for risk stratification and anticipatory care management. Patients with symptomatic carotid bruits undergo carotid duplex to assess for carotid stenosis as patients with pre-existing cerebrovascular disease are at increased risk for neurologic complications. Patients with chronic lung disease undergo pulmonary function testing and arterial blood gas testing to evaluate difficulty weaning from the ventilator.

Patients are maintained on antianginal, antihypertensive, and heart failure medications until surgery. Antiplatelet medications are usually discontinued before surgery: aspirin, clopidogrel, and nonsteroidal anti-inflammatory agents should be stopped before surgery to prevent perioperative bleeding however intravenous anticoagulation is used in the setting of ACS. Patients on warfarin usually have their dose withheld 3 to 5 days preoperatively. Patients on warfarin for previous mechanical valve replacements may be admitted 1 to 2 days before surgery for intravenous heparin. Heparin is withheld 1 to 2 hours before surgery, whereas enoxaparin is usually stopped 12 hours beforehand.

The preoperative nursing assessment should be thorough and well documented because this serves as a primary source of baseline data for postoperative comparison. The history should include a social assessment of family roles and support systems, and a description of the patient's usual functional level and typical activities. Elderly patients or those with limited social and emotional support may need additional assistance from social service for effective discharge and rehabilitation planning.

Intraprocedural Management

Cardiopulmonary Bypass

In standard CABG surgery, the heart is accessed through a median sternotomy then arrested. Circulation is maintained by placing the patient on CPB. CPB comprises an extracorporeal circuit that circulates systemic throughout the body during periods of time the heart and lungs are not functioning during cardiac surgical procedures. CPB has been the standard method used during cardiac surgery for diverting blood from the heart and lungs to provide a stationary, bloodless surgical field and to promote preservation of optimal organ function. The aorta is "cross-clamped" at this time. Heparin is used for anticoagulation during CPB to prevent clotting in the CPB circuit. ACT is monitored a minimum of every 30 minutes during CPB.

Once CPB is completed, heparin is reversed using protamine sulfate. Care is taken to administer protamine slowly and watch for a possible protamine reaction, which may vary from mild hypotension to full-blown anaphylaxis. Patients at greater risk for protamine reaction include those with insulin-dependent diabetes and those with an allergy to fish. While the patient is connected to the CPB machine, the surgeon, anesthetist, and CPB perfusionists control many physiologic variables. Hemodilution with crystalloid solutions is used to reduce hematocrit and the blood's viscosity. CPB flow rates are controlled to maintain a cardiac index of 2.2 L/min/m^2 and a mean arterial pressure around 60 mm Hg. Blood may be cooled to reduce metabolic demands or warmed to normothermia toward the end of the procedure.

CPB produces a systemic inflammatory response that releases biologically active substances that impair coagulation and the immune response. Proinflammatory cytokines contribute to neutrophil adhesion.[9] In response to the vascular permeability changes that occur with CPB and to the decrease in plasma oncotic pressure that occurs with hemodilution, large amounts of fluid move from intravascular to interstitial spaces. Movement of fluid into interstitial spaces causes postoperative edema. This generalized edema that occurs after CPB resolves after the first few days postoperative or fluid mobilization may be facilitated with the use of diuretics. The longer the CPB time, the more severe the physiologic derangements during the postoperative recovery.

Systemic warming is started approximately 30 minutes before the anticipated time of discontinuing CPB. If the left atrium, left ventricle, or aorta has been entered, air must be evacuated before aortic cross-clamp removal to prevent air embolism. The heart is warmed and resumes spontaneous rhythm or is paced with epicardial wires. Ventricular fibrillation may occur and is converted with internal defibrillation. Under the direction of the surgeon and anesthesiologist, CPB weaning begins by ventilation of the lungs. CPB is gradually weaned by decreasing the amount of blood diverted through the CPB circuit. When the heart is functioning normally with adequate blood pressure and adequate cardiac index, CPB is discontinued, heparin is reversed, and cannulae are removed. If the heart cannot support an adequate cardiac index and mean arterial pressure after weaning from CPB, the patient may have to be placed back on CPB to rest the heart, and other measures for heart failure may need to be instituted, such as inotropic treatment or intra-aortic balloon pump. In patients who continue to have severe hemodynamic compromise, ventricular assist devices may be used.

Myocardial Protection

Myocardial protection refers to the intraoperative techniques intended to protect the myocardium from damage resultant from the ischemic state that occurs with CPB. In cardiac surgical procedure requiring CPB, cross-clamping of the aorta without the use of myocardial protection would result in anaerobic metabolism and depletion of myocardial energy stores. Cross-clamping the aorta without protection for more than 15 to 20 minutes would result in profound myocardial dysfunction. Cardioplegia is infused to arrest the heart and provide a bloodless, motionless operative field as well as protect the heart during cardiac surgery. Cardioplegic solution is infused into the aorta or coronary sinus or into the coronary arteries themselves to cause cardiac arrest.

Hearts with LV hypertrophy may receive incomplete delivery to the subendocardium. In patients with aortic insufficiency, the left ventricle may become distended because of the retrograde flow of cardioplegia across the valve. Although cardioplegia can be delivered through saphenous vein grafts, it cannot be delivered through IMA grafts. Insufficient delivery of cardioplegia results in poor myocardial protection, which results in postoperative myocardial damage and dysfunction.

Postoperative Management

The extremes of this intraoperative milieu result in severe derangements in temperature, hemodynamic, coagulation, and inflammation. After CABG surgery, the patient is admitted to an intensive care unit for close monitoring for 6 to 24 hours after surgery. Report from the operative team should include the type of surgery, vessels grafted and their conduits, total number of minutes of aortic cross-clamp time, number, type and location of invasive lines and vascular access, vasoactive infusions, ventilator settings, chest tube numbers and locations, incisions, and complications.

On arrival in the intensive care unit, the critical care nurse performs a number of rapid assessments to ensure patient stability. Routine care includes continuous ECG monitoring, measurement of blood pressure by arterial line, pulse oximetry, pulmonary artery pressures, and body temperature measurement. Intermittent parameters may include cardiac output measurement as well as calculation of derived hemodynamic parameters, such as afterload, cardiac index, and contractility indices. Specialty pulmonary artery catheters, such as the continuous cardiac output pulmonary artery catheter, may be used to evaluate minute-to-minute changes in cardiac output. Oximetry pulmonary artery catheters may be used continuously to monitor mixed venous oxygen concentration, and values can be used to calculate oxygen consumption and delivery parameters during periods of critical illness.

Sinus bradycardia or other hemodynamically significant bradycardic dysrhythmias such as accelerated junctional rhythm can occur postoperatively and may be treated with an atrial or atrioventricular pacemaker set at a rate of 70 or 100 beats/min. Heart block may occur after valve repair or replacement because of edema and trauma at the suture lines close to the conduction system. Hypertension may be treated with either intravenous nitrates or sodium nitroprusside. Hypotension occurs often during the first 12 hours after surgery as the patient warms and as systemic vascular resistance decreases to normal levels. Hypovolemia (right or left atrial or pulmonary artery wedge pressure of less than 8 to 10 mm Hg) may be present because of the fluid volume alterations that occur with CPB or if diuretic was administration at the end of CPB. Hypovolemia may be treated with crystalloid or colloid volume expanders such as 5% albumin or hetastarch, or with crystalloid. If the patient's hemoglobin is less than 8 g/dL, packed red blood cells or whole blood may be administered. Blood may be recovered through the chest tubes for autotransfusion during the first 4 to 12 hours after surgery. If patients are normovolemic, they are usually placed on a salt and free-water restriction. Potassium replacement is often necessary. Patients are usually maintained on a respirator for the first 1 or 2 hours after surgery, until the effects of anesthesia have reversed. Patients are on prophylactic antibiotics, usually a second-generation cephalosporin, to prevent wound infection for 48 hours or less.

Stable, uncomplicated patients are earmarked to "fast track" by extubating early and minimizing their intensive care unit and hospital stay. Patient care is directed by an established care map or "roadmap." When the patient is hemodynamically stable and pain and bleeding are controlled, the patient can be extubated. As a result, cardiac surgery patients may stay in the intensive care unit as little as 8 to 12 hours, thus freeing up critical care beds and reducing costs to the patient. Patients who are "fast tracked" in rapid recovery programs are discharged 3 to 5 days after surgery. Nurse practitioners or physician assistants in collaboration may manage cardiac surgery patients with the physician.

Complications range from common to uncommon, and may occur early or late in the postoperative course. Atrial arrhythmias and pulmonary complications are the most common variances that keep patients in hospital longer than planned by the care map. Other less common but notable early complications include bleeding, cardiac tamponade, perioperative MI, renal failure, and postcardiotomy delirium. Late complications are also uncommon and encompass postpericardiotomy syndrome with pleural inflammation and pleural and/or pericardial effusions, late cardiac tamponade which may or may not be related to post pericardiotomy syndrome, and lastly wound infections. Staphylococcus is the most common culprit genus. Superficial wounds are treated with antibiotics and local drainage. Deep sternal wounds and mediastinitis are treated with surgical débridement and closure or plastic surgical closure with muscle flap. Although rare, postoperative management of these complications may expand discharge into the outpatient clinic.

COMPLICATIONS OF MI

The nurse must monitor for complications of MI, which usually occur within 24 hours of an acute MI. Complications of MI are best mitigated through early presentation to emergency services for evaluation and treatment however mechanical complications may occur in the first week after acute MI, even after PCI. Mechanical complications include LV septal rupture, LV free wall rupture, LV aneurysm, and mitral regurgitation. The patient may present with symptoms and signs of acute decompensated heart failure including dyspnea, orthopnea, flash pulmonary edema, a cardiac murmur. Complications are further described in Table 29-9.

MANAGEMENT OF THE WORKING DIAGNOSIS OF MINOCA

Etiologies and an algorithm for the diagnosis of MI due to nonobstructive coronary arteries are presented earlier in this chapter. The management of patients with a differential and/or working diagnosis of MINOCA is presented in Table 29-10. Two specific conditions are further described in this section: SCAD and SARS-CoV or COVID19 (Table 29-11).

Spontaneous Coronary Artery Dissection

First described in 1931,[46] SCAD is the dissection of an epicardial coronary artery that cannot be attributed to atherosclerosis, trauma, or an iatrogenic cause. SCAD may be the etiology of up to 4% of ACS cases and commonly occurs in patients with minimal to no conventional cardiovascular risk factors.[47] Women appear to be overwhelmingly predisposed to SCAD, which may be responsible for up to 35% of MIs in women aged 50 and older, and is the most common cause of pregnancy associated MI.[47] Coronary artery obstruction is caused by an intramural hematoma or intimal disruption of the coronary artery due to dissection. The LAD coronary artery is typically the most often affected.

The clinical presentation of SCAD is that of ACS: chest pain and ST-T wave changes on ECG consistent with STEMI. This ACS presentation, combined with a patient profile suspicious for SCAD, prompts invasive coronary angiography. Initial management involves intracoronary nitrates along with intracoronary imaging if safe and feasible. A conservative approach with medical management or an early invasive strategy with stenting, particularly if there is ongoing pain or ischemia, may be pursued.[48]

The duration of hospitalization depends upon the management strategy but typically lasts 48 hours to monitor symptoms, medications, and effort tolerance prior to discharge. Longer hospitalizations or repeated coronary angiography may be warranted if there is concern for early hazard detection or ongoing dissection.[49]

Increased attention has been paid to the recognition and management of SCAD. This diagnosis however may go overlooked, particularly in the patient that does not present with overt or typical pain. In addition, the cardiac nurse should note that depression and anxiety are highly reported in these patients and

Table 29-10 • COMPLICATIONS OF MYOCARDIAL ISCHEMIA

Complication	Characteristics and Management
Ventricular free wall rupture	• Occurs in 10% of acute MI-associated mortality • Presents within first week of MI • Risk factors are large Q-wave infarct and increased age • High mortality
Ventricular septal rupture	• Occurs in 1–3% of acute MI • Presents 3–7 days post-MI • Presents with new loud holosystolic murmur and systemic hypoperfusion due to left-to-right shunting • Emergent treatment for repair • Greater than 20% mortality
Mitral regurgitation	• May occurs due to ischemic mitral valve apparatus (papillary muscles) or ventricle) • New or worsening systolic murmur • Most frequently occurs in inferior MI or non–Q-wave MI • Pulmonary congestion may be intermittent or persistent • Treatment may include percutaneous or surgical revascularization
Arrhythmias	• Can occur at any time in the course of MI • Due to electrophysiologic alterations in ischemic myocardium, pharmacotherapeutic interventions, electrolyte imbalances, or endogenous catecholamine release • Treatment depends upon the type of arrhythmia
Pericarditis/ Dressler Syndrome	• Most commonly occurs several weeks post-MI • Results of localized inflammatory response in the pericardium adjacent to the infarcted area • Patients describe sharp, substernal, severe chest pain, it can radiate to the neck shoulders, or back • Pericardial friction rub may be auscultated • Classic multilead ST-segment elevation is present with diffuse pericarditis, but not present if the pericarditis is localized to the infarct region
Heart failure and cardiogenic shock	• Complication of approximately 5–8% of acute MI[38] • Characterized by systemic hypoperfusion due to low cardiac output despite high filling pressures (i.e., confirmed absence of intravascular hypovolemia) • Risk factors are increased age, female sex, prior MI or diagnosis of heart failure, hypertension, diabetes mellitus, anterior ST-elevated MI, and complete heart block • Commonly a result of left ventricular failure • Advanced hemodynamic monitoring, mechanical circulatory assist devices, and revascularization may improve survival • Associated with high mortality

are highest in the setting of peripartum SCAD.[50] As an advocate and educator, it is most important for the cardiac nurse to recall the patient profile among a working diagnosis of MINOCA and unique considerations for patients ultimately diagnosed with SCAD.

Systemic Acute Respiratory Syndrome Coronavirus (SARS-CoV or COVID19)

A contemporary working diagnosis for MINOCA includes cardiovascular involvement of SARS-CoV or COVID19. This

Table 29-11 • MANAGEMENT OF PATIENTS WITH A WORKING DIAGNOSIS OF MYOCARDIAL INFARCTION DUE TO NONOBSTRUCTIVE CORONARY ARTERIES (MINOCA)

Underlying Mechanism/Clinical Disorder	Selected Diagnostic Investigations	Selective/Empirical Therapies
Ischemic presentation (MINOCA)		
Plaque disruption	Angiographic review Intravascular imaging (IVUS or OCT)	Aspirin, high-intensity statin β-Blockers, in presence of left ventricular dysfunction, and possibly with preserved ejection fraction ACE inhibitors/ARBs in presence of left ventricular dysfunction, and possibly with preserved ejection fraction Consider clopidogrel/ticagrelor
Coronary artery spasm	Resolution with coronary vasodilators (e.g., intracoronary nitroglycerin) Provocative spasm testing Blood toxicology testing (e.g., cocaine, methamphetamines) Review of medication and nonprescription drug use (e.g., migraine medications, cocaine)	Calcium channel blockers Other antispastic agents (nitrates, nicorandil, cilostazol) Consider statin
Coronary microvascular dysfunction	Angiographic review Coronary microvascular functional testing	Conventional antianginal therapies (e.g., calcium channel blocker, β-blocker) Unconventional antianginal therapies (e.g., L-arginine, ranolazine, dipyridamole, aminophylline, imipramine, α-blockers)
Coronary embolism/thrombus	Angiographic review Intravascular imaging (IVUS or OCT) Thrombophilia screen	Antiplatelet or anticoagulant therapy Other targeted therapies for hypercoagulable condition
Spontaneous coronary artery dissection	Angiographic review Intravascular imaging (IVUS or OCT)	Aspirin, β-blocker Consider clopidogrel
Supply–demand mismatch	Review history for potential stressors	Treatment for underlying condition
Presentations mimicking MINOCA (ischemic or nonischemic)		
Branch "flush occlusion" or severe branch stenosis (from coronary embolism/thrombus or ruptured plaque)	Angiographic review Consider intracoronary imaging to identify plaque rupture or dissection, or echocardiography review for a new source of thrombus (screen valves for endocarditis; left atrium and left ventricle for thrombus source and tumor; the possibility of a patent foramen ovale should also be evaluated)	Antiplatelet or anticoagulant if ischemic, statin, β-blockers ACE inhibitors/ARBs in presence of left ventricular dysfunction, and possibly with preserved ejection fraction
Spontaneous coronary artery dissection	Angiographic review	Aspirin, β-blocker Consider clopidogrel
Takotsubo syndrome	Left ventricular angiogram Contrast CMRI	ACE inhibitors Medical or device therapies for heart failure/left ventricular dysfunction Consider β-blockers
Cardiomyopathies	Contrast CMRI	Medical or device therapies for heart failure/left ventricular dysfunction
Myocarditis	Contrast CMRI	Medical or device therapies for heart failure/left ventricular dysfunction. Consider immunomodulatory and immunosuppressive therapies

IVUS, intravascular ultrasound; OCT, optical coherence tomography; CMRI, contrast magnetic resonance imaging; ACE-I, angiotensin-converting enzyme inhibitor; ARB, angiotensin receptor blocker.
Adapted from Tamis-Holland JE, Jneid H, Reynolds HR, et al. Contemporary diagnosis and management of patients with myocardial infarction in the absence of obstructive coronary artery disease: a scientific statement from the American Heart Association. *Circulation.* 2019;139(18):e891–e908.

condition may present with ECG findings resembling ACS, however cardiac catheterization reveals angiographically normal coronary arteries.

An observational study in 2020 by Lala et al.[51] revealed that myocardial injury is prevalent among hospitalized patients with COVID19 infections. Troponin elevations in COVID19 patients may represent acute myocardial injury but not necessarily ACS. Mechanisms by which the virus causes myocardial injury are not fully understood but may be a result of a noncoronary mechanism. Those with existing cardiovascular disease are more likely to have elevated troponins associated with their COVID19 infection. Elevated troponin levels in the setting of COVID19 may be associated with poorer outcomes and therefore may provide better prognostic and risk stratification information.[51] For these patients, responsibilities of the cardiac nurse may include screening for COVID19, appraisal of emerging high-quality evidence, and adherence to hospital-specific policies to improve outcomes and decrease the risk of transmission.

STABLE ISCHEMIC HEART DISEASE

Definition

SIHD as described in multisocietal guidelines encompasses a heterogeneous group of patients, including those with new-onset low-risk chest pain or UA and stable chronic pain syndromes which may present as ischemic equivalents (e.g., dyspnea or exertional arm pain). Guidelines for SIHD also apply to patients who are asymptomatic or pursuing symptom management with appropriate GDMT and/or revascularization such as PCI or CABG surgery.

Diagnostic Evaluation

Clinical presentation, electrocardiographic, and physiologic biomarkers guide the distinction between ACS/UA/NSTEMI and SIHD. If the patient is deemed stable and at low risk for an acute ischemic event, GDMT is initiated and invasive coronary angiography may be pursued to define the coronary anatomy.

Guideline-Directed Medical Therapy

The foundation of management for SIHD is GDMT, which includes therapeutic lifestyle management as tertiary prevention and pharmacologic therapy. The first landmark trial to support this was the Clinical Outcomes Using Revascularization and Aggressive Drug Evaluation (COURAGE) trial[52] (*N* = 2287) which randomized patients with stable CAD to optimal medical therapy versus optimal medical therapy and PCI. While angina improved in patients in both groups, most importantly it was found that PCI did not decrease major adverse cardiac events.[52] This finding was attributed to the efficacy of GDMT, and aligned with the Class I recommendations for antiplatelet, beta-blocker, and statin therapy, as well as angiotensin converting enzyme inhibitor and angiotensin receptor blocker (ACE-I/ARB) therapy in the setting of diabetes or LV dysfunction. In the setting of anginal symptoms, first-line therapy includes sublingual NTG, beta-blockers, and calcium channel blockers (Class I recommendation). Ranolazine may also be added.[1,8] Intolerances to these medications should be assessed and noted. The algorithm for GDMT is detailed in Figure 29-17.

The International Study of Comparative Health Effectiveness of Medical and Invasive Approaches (ISCHEMIA) trial[53] was conducted to evaluate optimal medical therapy versus optimal medical therapy and PCI in patients with moderate to severe ischemia on noninvasive stress testing, a criterion that was not specified—and thus a criticism—of the COURAGE trial. Again, PCI did not decrease major adverse cardiac events, all-cause mortality, or cardiovascular mortality or MI. Routine PCI was associated with early harm (i.e., increased periprocedural MI) and late benefit (i.e., decreased spontaneous MI). Heart Teams considering revascularization in patients with SIHD however must recall that these findings do not generalize to patients with ACS or recent MI, greater than or equal to 50% left main stenosis, LVEF less than 35%, or NYHA Class III–IV (i.e., exclusion criteria for ISCHEMIA trial).

Heart Team decision making on invasive intervention for SIHD must be a patient-centered process that incorporates patient goals, angina burden, GDMT, and likelihood of optimal coronary revascularization. While GDMT remains the cornerstone of treatment, the patient with SIHD and ongoing anginal symptoms may be evaluated for possible revascularization.

Invasive Intervention

The strategy for invasive intervention for the patient with SIHD is based upon several key clinical trials and Heart Team decision for revascularization. The multidisciplinary Heart Team is comprised of cardiologists, interventional cardiologists, cardiothoracic surgeons, imaging specialists, and nursing and allied health professionals involved in the care of the patient with SIHD. Guidelines[1,8,40,54] and prescriptive directions, or appropriate use criteria (AUC),[55] are used to guide the Heart Team approach to intervention. Risk stratification scores incorporated into the decision-making process are the Society for Thoracic Surgeons (STS) predicted risk score of mortality and morbidity for the appropriate operation (STS Adult Cardiac Surgery Data Risk Calculator http://riskcalc.sts.org/stswebriskcalc/calculate) and SYNTAX score[56] of the angiographic complexity of coronary artery lesions (http://www.syntaxscore.com/calculator/start.htm). These guidelines for revascularization are summarized in Table 29-12 and Figure 29-18.

Underpinning the decision-making algorithm for invasive intervention of SIHD is important evidence, particularly for the revascularization of left main and multivessel CAD and chronic totally occluded coronary arteries. Particular attention is paid to the evidence and revascularization strategy of these anatomies.

Left Main and Multivessel CAD

Left main CAD (LMCAD) is prevalent in approximately 5% of patients undergoing coronary angiography but is more likely to be associated with multivessel or concomitant coronary disease.[57] Untreated LMCAD (greater than or equal to 50% stenosis) may yield a poorer prognosis, given the large myocardial territory supplied, and therefore revascularization is recommended.[58] CABG is a long-standing safe treatment for LMCAD with effective outcomes. PCI is also feasible and historically had been applied to nonsurgical candidates only. However, many randomized clinical trials have compared these two forms of revascularization in patients deemed to be surgical candidates: Synergy between Percutaneous Coronary Intervention with Taxus and Cardiac Surgery (SYNTAX) Trial[56]; Evaluation of XIENCE versus Coronary Artery Bypass Surgery for Effectiveness of Left Main Revascularization (EXCEL) trial[59]; and Nordic-Baltic-British Left Main (NOBLE) Revascularisation Study.[60]

The SYNTAX Trial (*N* = 1800) randomized patients with multivessel and/or LMCAD to either PCI (with a paclitaxel-eluting stent) or CABG. The trial favored surgery over PCI, especially for those with complex disease resulting in intermediate to high SYNTAX scores. PCI was considered to be an acceptable alternative in those with less complex lesions, or those with lower SYNTAX scores.[56]

The EXCEL trial (*N* = 1905) randomly assigned and compared patients with unprotected LMCAD considered to be a low or intermediate risk to treatment with either PCI with everolimus-eluting stents or CABG. PCI was found to be noninferior to CABG with no significant difference between the groups at 3 and 5 years. However, the rate of ischemia-driven revascularization was higher in the PCI group at both intervals.[59] Similarly, the NOBLE trial (*N* = 1201) randomly assigned patients with LMCAD to PCI with biolimus-eluting stent or CABG. PCI

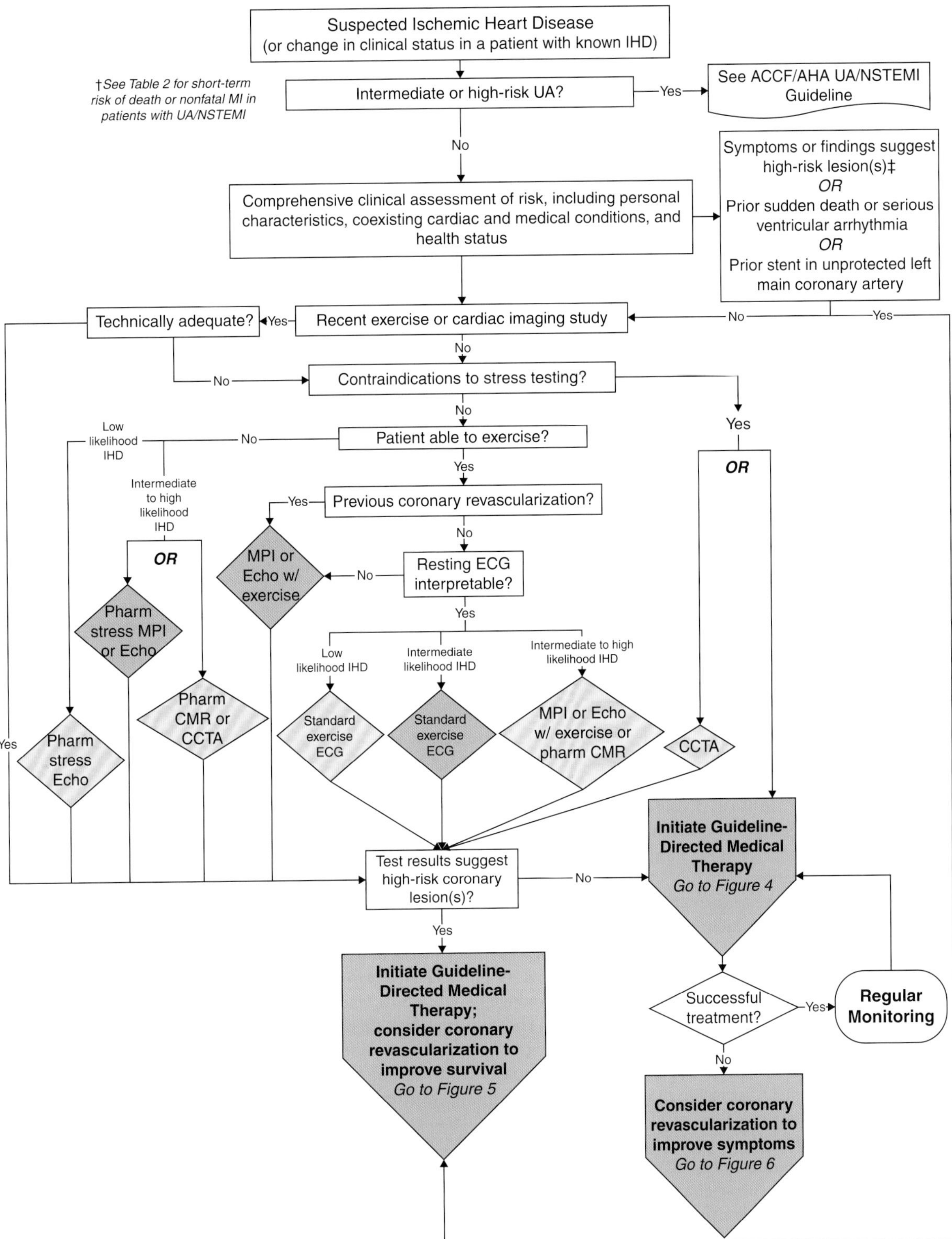

Figure 29-17. Diagnosis of patients with suspected IHD. This image is displayed here to demonstrate the full breadth and depth of the guideline-directed diagnosis and management of suspected IHD. Colors correspond to the class of recommendations per ACCF/AHA. The algorithms do not represent a comprehensive list of recommendations (see full guideline text[2] for all recommendations). ‡CCTA is reasonable only for patients with intermediate probability of IHD. CCTA, computed coronary tomography angiography; CMR, cardiac magnetic resonance; ECG, electrocardiogram; echo, echocardiography; IHD, ischemic heart disease; MI, myocardial infarction; MPI, myocardial perfusion imaging; pharm, pharmacologic; UA, unstable angina; and UA/NSTEMI, unstable angina/non–ST-elevation myocardial infarction. (Used with permission from Fihn SD, Gardin JM, Abrams J, et al. 2012 ACCF/AHA/ACP/AATS/PCNA/SCAI/STS guideline for the diagnosis and management of patients with stable ischemic heart disease: executive summary. *Circulation.* 2012;126[25]:3097–3137.)

Table 29-12 • REVASCULARIZATION STRATEGY FOR STABLE ISCHEMIC HEART DISEASE

Heart Team Approach	Class of Recommendation	Level of Evidence
Heart Team approach is recommended for revascularization of unprotected left main and complex multivessel CAD	I	B
Heart Team approach is recommended for revascularization in patients with diabetes and complex multivessel CAD	I	B
CABG		
CABG is recommended for unprotected LM disease	I	A
CABG is generally recommended in preference to PCI to improve survival in patients with DM and multivessel CAD for which revascularization is likely to improve survival (3-vessel CAD or complex 2-vessel CAD involving the proximal LAD) particularly if a LIMA graft can be anastamosed to the LAD artery, provided the patient is a good candidate for surgery	I	B
CABG is not recommended and deemed to cause harm in 1-vessel CAD without proximal LAD involvement	III: Harm	B
CABG is recommended for survivors of sudden cardiac death with ischemia-mediated ventricular tachycardia	I	B
PCI		
PCI is recommended for unprotected LM when both of the following are present: • Anatomic conditions associated with a low risk of PCI procedural complications and a high likelihood of good long-term outcome (e.g., low SYNTAX score of ≤22, ostial or trunk LM CAD) • Clinical characteristics that predict a significantly increased risk of adverse surgical outcomes (e.g., STS PROM ≥ 5%)	IIa	B
PCI is recommended for unprotected LM when BOTH of the following are present: • Anatomic conditions associated with a low to intermediate risk of PCI procedural complication and an intermediate to high likelihood of good long-term outcome (e.g., low–intermediate SYNTAX score <33, bifurcation LM CAD) • Clinical characteristics that predict an increased risk of adverse surgical outcomes (e.g., moderate to severe COPD, disability from prior stroke, or prior cardiac surgery, STS PROM >2%)	IIb	B
PCI is of uncertain benefit for 3-vessel disease with or without proximal LAD involvement	IIb	B
PCI is of uncertain benefit for 2-vessel disease with or without proximal LAD involvement	IIb	B
PCI is not recommended and deemed to cause harm in patients who have unfavorable anatomy for PCI and who are good candidates for CABG	III: Harm	B
PCI is recommended for survivors of sudden cardiac death with ischemia-mediated ventricular tachycardia	I	C

CAD, coronary artery disease; CABG, coronary artery bypass graft; LM, left main; PCI, percutaneous coronary intervention; LIMA, left internal mammary graft; LAD, left anterior descending; STS, society for Thoracic Surgeons; PROM, predicted risk of mortality.
Adapted from Hillis LD, Smith PK, Anderson JL, et al. 2011 ACCF/AHA Guideline for coronary artery bypass graft surgery. *Circulation.* 2011;124(23):e652–e735.

was found to be inferior to CABG at 5 years. Mortality between the two groups was not significantly different; however, patients treated with PCI had higher rates of nonprocedural MI and required repeat revascularization.[60]

In December 2019, controversy surrounded the EXCEL trial[59] due to questions about trial conduction and data interpretation of the 5-year follow-up results.[61] Consequently, the European Association for Cardio-Thoracic Surgery (EACTS) withdrew its endorsement of the 2018 ESC clinical guidelines section covering the management of LMCAD. The American Association of Thoracic Surgeons (AATS) issued a statement acknowledging the possibility of misrepresented treatment guidelines. The EXCEL trial investigators issued a statement, rebutting the accusation of concealed data. A subsequent meta-analysis of PCI versus CABG in LMCAD ($N = 4612$, including SYNTAX, EXCEL, and NOBLE trials) found no significant differences in major cardiovascular outcomes between the two treatment groups, however unplanned revascularization was found to be less frequent in the patients who underwent CABG (Fig. 29-19).[62]

Chronic Totally Occluded Arteries

Up to 20% of patients with CAD are known to have chronic total occlusions (CTOs).[63] These lesions are commonly ischemic; collateral circulation does not equate normal coronary flow. Presence of a CTO has been found to be associated with worse morbidity and mortality.[64]

Even when patients meet the indications (symptomatic despite optimal medical therapy and ischemic in the territory of the CTO), revascularization may not be offered or pursued. In fact, a CTO was the most common reason for incomplete revascularization in the SYNTAX trial.[56] The technical challenges of CTO PCI have been addressed with advanced technologies, education, and algorithms, which have improved the rate of procedural success (86%) and decreased the rate of complications (7% major adverse cardiac and cerebrovascular events [MACCE]) and death (0.9%).[65] A successful CTO PCI has been associated with improved LVEF, decreased arrhythmogenicity, decreased angina and heart failure symptoms, and improved quality of life.[65] Randomized clinical trial data are needed; however, there remain overall few sites and operators skilled in CTO PCI of these complex procedures thus introducing bias into these studies.

Current multisocietal guidelines[1,8] and AUC[55] for SIHD revascularization do not take into account whether a lesion is a CTO. The 2011 ACC/AHA/SCAI Guideline for PCI do however recommend CTO PCI in patients with favorable anatomy, clinical indication for PCI, and access to operators with the necessary expertise (Class IIa, LOE B).[40]

Nursing Considerations

The equivocal, controversial, and emerging clinical trial results emphasize the importance of multidisciplinary evaluation to offer the safest and most appropriate treatment plan. Consideration of the patient's preference and expectations should be considered and discussed. The cardiac nurse has an important role in advocacy, education, and adherence to optimal GDMT and tertiary preventative measures. A primer of nursing considerations for the patient with SIHD is itemized in Table 29-13.

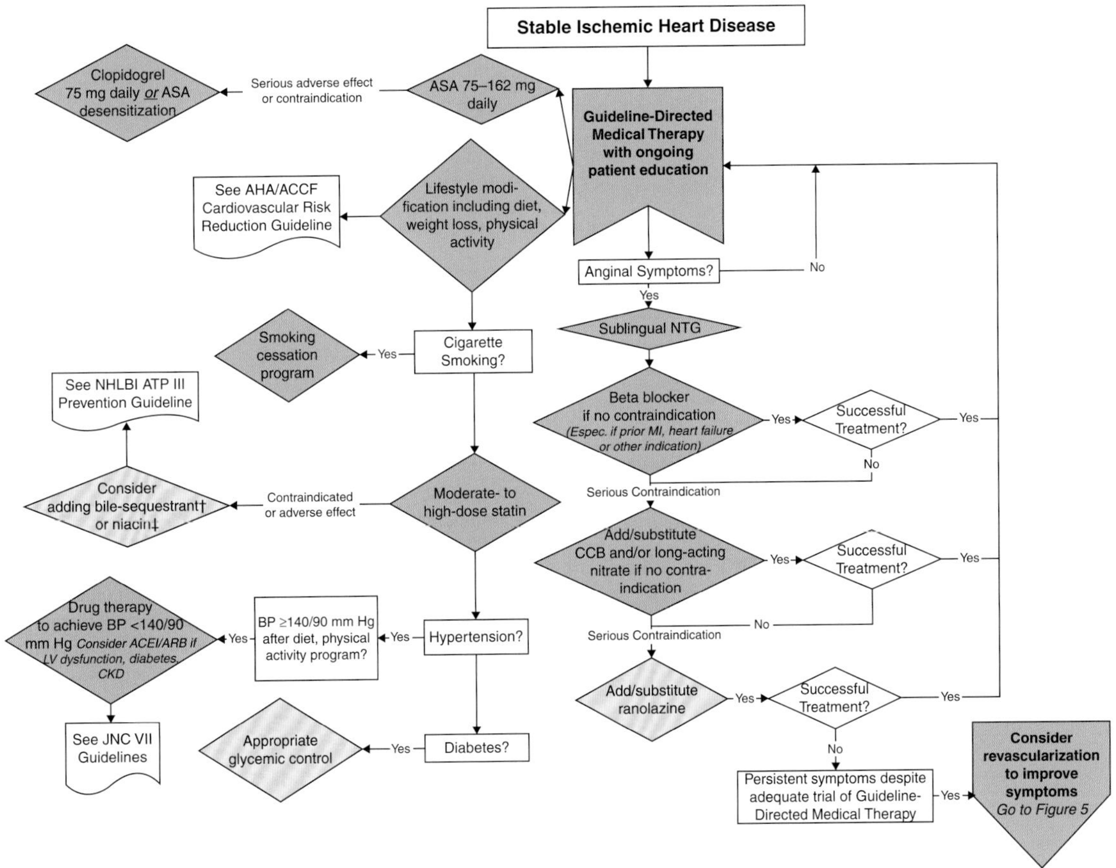

Figure 29-18. Algorithm for guideline-directed medical therapy for patients with SIHD. Colors correspond to the class of recommendations per ACCF/AHA. The algorithms do not represent a comprehensive list of recommendations (see the text and the guidelines for all recommendations). †The use of bile acid sequestrant is relatively contraindicated when triglycerides are ≥200 mg/dL and is contraindicated when triglycerides are ≥500 mg/dL. ‡Dietary supplement niacin must not be used as a substitute for prescription niacin. ACCF, American College of Cardiology Foundation; ACE-I, angiotensin-converting enzyme inhibitor; AHA, American Heart Association; ARB, angiotensin-receptor blocker; ASA, aspirin, ATP III, adult treatment panel 3; BP, blood pressure; CCB, calcium channel blocker; CKD, chronic kidney disease; HDL-C, high-density lipoprotein cholesterol; JNC VII, Seventh Report of the Joint National Committee on Prevention, Detection, Evaluation, and Treatment of High Blood Pressure; LDL-C, low-density lipoprotein cholesterol; LV, left ventricular; MI, myocardial infarction; NHLBI, National Heart, Lung, and Blood Institute; NTG, nitroglycerin. Note: Current hypertension guidelines are JNC VIII, Eighth Report. (Used with permission from Fihn SD, Gardin JM, Abrams J, et al. 2012 ACCF/AHA/ACP/AATS/PCNA/SCAI/STS Guideline for the diagnosis and management of patients with stable ischemic heart disease: executive summary. *Circulation*. 2012;126[25]:3097–3137.)

Table 29-13 • CONSIDERATIONS OF THE CARDIAC NURSE CARING FOR THE PATIENT WITH STABLE ISCHEMIC HEART DISEASE

1. What is the patient's goal?
2. Is the patient on optimal guideline-directed medical therapy for stable ischemic heart disease? If not, why not? Have issues with medical therapy been well assessed and documented in the medical record?
3. Does the patient have angina? Has the patient's angina/anginal equivalent(s) been well assessed and documented in the medical record?
4. Does that patient have evidence of ischemia? Has there been an imaging study that has demonstrated myocardial viability of this territory?
   - Recent hospitalization for chest pain with equivocal cardiac enzymes
   - Echocardiogram with transient regional wall motion abnormalities
   - Myocardial perfusion imaging study with ischemic territories
   - Positron emission tomography (PET) myocardial viability study
5. Does the patient have coronary artery lesions (location; angiographic and physiologic severity) that are concordant with the territory of ischemia?
6. Are the lesions suitable for revascularization?
7. What is the optimal strategy for revascularization: percutaneous (PCI), surgical (CABG), or hybrid?
8. Is the patient goal consistent with the evaluation findings and the treatment options?
9. What is the optimal PCI strategy? Where is the best treatment center and team, given the complexity of the intervention?
10. Has a patient-centered, Heart Team approach to shared decision making occurred to determine the best treatment plan for this individual patient, considering the patient goals, preferences and specific risks, benefits, and considerations for medical management, percutaneous or surgical coronary (PCI or CABG), or a hybrid approach?

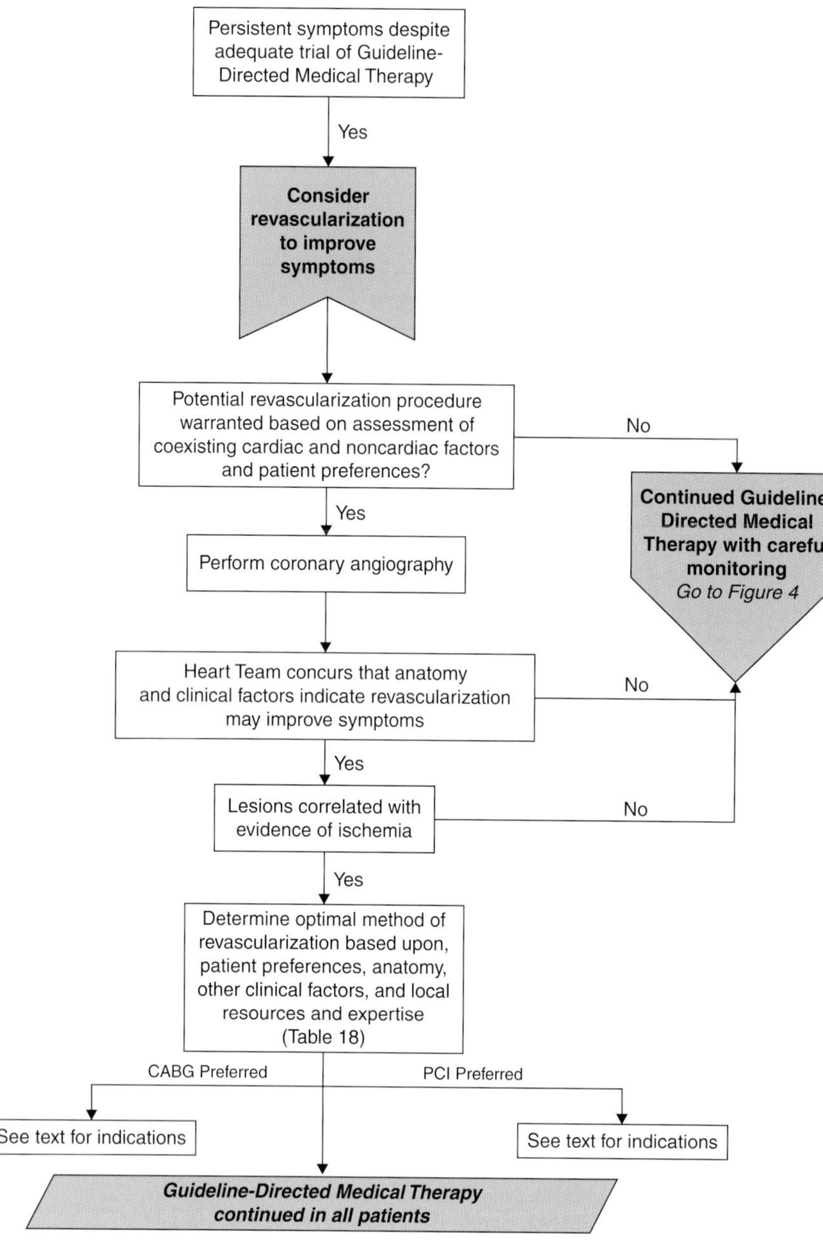

Figure 29-19. Algorithm for revascularization to improve symptoms of patients with SIHD. Colors correspond to the class of recommendations per ACCF/AHA. The algorithms do not represent a comprehensive list of recommendations (see text and guidelines for all recommendations). CABG, coronary artery bypass graft; PCI, percutaneous coronary intervention. (Used with permission from Fihn SD, Gardin JM, Abrams J, et al. 2012 ACCF/AHA/ACP/AATS/PCNA/SCAI/STS guideline for the diagnosis and management of patients with stable ischemic heart disease: executive summary. *Circulation.* 2012;126[25]: 3097–3137.)

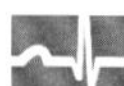 CASE-BASED LEARNING 1

Acute Coronary Syndrome

Patient Profile

Lawrence Zimmer, a 61-yr-old male, is brought to the emergency department (ED) by an ambulance. He appears to be in distress, pale and diaphoretic. The paramedics indicate that his wife called 911 and reported anterior mid sternal chest pain that radiated to his bilateral shoulders. This lasted for 20 minutes. He describes the pain as severe, squeezing, and uncomfortable pressure, "like a giant elephant is sitting on my chest. Feels worse than past chest pain" Mr. Lawrence states that he took his own "baby aspirin" when his symptoms occurred. Sublingual nitroglycerin tablets were taken two times without relief. Arrival to the ED occurs at 45 minutes into this episode of chest pain. IV access and supplemental oxygen for S_aO_2 at 93% were already placed by the paramedics. Labs were drawn and 12-lead ECG was also repeated in the ED.

Past Medical History/Problem List

Hypercholesterolemia
Type II diabetes mellitus
Essential hypertension
Mild aortic stenosis (LVEF [left ventricular ejection fraction] 65%)

Family History

Father—Hx of MI at age 58 (deceased), mother—HTN, died at age 85 from stroke

Social History

Married for 35 yr. Works as a post office worker for almost 30 yr. Sedentary lifestyle with no regular exercises. Smoked

CASE-BASED LEARNING 1 *(Continued)*

for almost 20 yr but quit about 5 yr ago. Recreational drug use when teenager only. Occasional alcohol intake. Three grown children all in good health.

Medications

Atorvastatin 20 mg daily, Metformin 1000 mg twice daily, Aspirin 81 mg daily, Norvasc 5 mg daily, Nitroglycerin 0.4 mg po as needed

Allergies

Sulfa

Clinical Considerations

1. **Repeated 12-lead ECG in the ED noted inferior MI with ST elevation in ECG leads II, III and aVF with reciprocal ST depression in lead aVL. Given his history and presentation, what are the nursing implications for Mr. Lawrence?**

   It is important for cardiac nurses to be familiar with inferior wall MIs, as they are estimated to be about 40–50% of all MIs. Inferior wall myocardial infarction (IWMI) occurs when the tissue supplied by right coronary artery (RCA) is occluded, with decreased perfusion to the inferior region of the myocardium. Due to this etiology, right ventricular (RV) infarct should be suspected in all patients who present with an acute IWMI.

   Approximately 30–50% of patients with IWMI will also involve RV infarction. Because the standard 12-lead electrocardiogram is insufficient for the assessment of RV involvement, right-sided precordial leads should always be included. The addition of right-sided ECGs leads is the most sensitive and specific, especially ST elevation V4R >1.0 mm. This finding has 100% sensitivity and 87% specificity. It can aid in the diagnosis of RV infarction with RCA occlusion. ST elevation greater in lead III than lead II is also suggestive of RV involvement. Due to less myocardium than the LV, RV is dependent on adequate preload to assure adequate cardiac function.

   If there is evidence of RV infarction involvement that is very preload dependent, cardiac nurses should avoid administering nitrates such as nitroglycerin or diuretics, beta blockers, calcium channel blockers, and phosphodiesterase inhibitors as that may precipitate significant hypotension and can cause hemodynamic instability in 10–15% of patients. In this case, Mr. Lawrence has taken his nitroglycerin prior to his ED presentation. His hemodynamic status should be monitored closely and if notes hypotension, fluid resuscitation should be administered to maintain an adequate preload. Additionally, Mr. Lawrence should also be given three more doses of 81 mg of chewable aspirin (total to 324 mg) as he has only taken a baby aspirin of 81 mg at home. The evidence-based guideline states that a loading dose of nonenteric-coated aspirin is 162–325 mg at initial antiplatelet therapy.

2. **Given Mr. Lawrence's inferior MI with right ventricle infarct, what might you expect to find on his physical examination?**

   Although hemodynamically unstable RV infarction occurs in less than 10% of the patients, it is important for cardiac nurses to know the classic clinical triad of RV infarction. These include elevated jugular vein pressure, clear lung fields, and hypotension. These findings are significantly different in patients who may present with left ventricular infarction where pulmonary congestion, third or fourth heart sounds, and a new mitral valve murmur can occur.

   The primary effects of RV infarction result from decreased RV contractility. This leads to a reduction in blood flow from the venous system to the lungs, and finally to the left side of the heart. Additionally, patients with RVMI may exhibit rhythm abnormalities. The heart rate in patients with RVMI may range from bradycardia to complete heart block more frequently than those with predominant left ventricular MI. As these findings may not be present at the admission and do not occur until certain medications such as diuretics or nitrates are administrated, cardiac nurses should be aware of these possible clinical manifestations.

3. **What initial lab work-up and diagnostic might you expect to be ordered for Mr. Lawrence prior to undergoing emergent PCI?**

   The following initial lab work-up will be ordered for Mr. Lawrence in the ED before he undergoes emergent PCI.

   - Complete Blood Count—other conditions may be found to be contributing to infarction (e.g., anemia) and abnormal platelet count may alter management (e.g., severe thrombocytopenia)
   - Comprehensive Metabolic Panel and Magnesium Level—will evaluate electrolyte abnormality including liver function (e.g., hyperkalemia may explain the ECG changes or hypokalemia may contribute to low conduction) and abnormal kidney function will be important to know for medication adjustments.
   - Troponin T or I—these assays are highly specific and sensitive markers of myocardial necrosis.
   - B-type natriuretic peptide (BNP) should be checked, as an elevated level is associated with higher mortality.
   - Prothrombin time with INR and PTT—coagulation studies will be ordered as Mr. Lawrence will receive anticoagulation treatment.
   - XR Chest 1 view—a chest x-ray will show the heart size and the size of the mediastinum.

   Additional labs and diagnostic imaging will be ordered by the inpatient cardiologist and hospitalist.

4. **What is the rationale for administration of dual antiplatelets and anticoagulants before percutaneous intervention? What are the nursing implications for these medications?**

   Dual antiplatelet therapy (DAPT), use of two antiplatelet agents, plus anticoagulant has been referred to as "triple oral antithrombotic therapy" or "triple therapy." Mr. Lawrence needs two antiplatelet agents which include aspirin 325 mg chewable and one of the $P2Y_{12}$ inhibitors mentioned in this chapter. The studies noted administration of clopidogrel or ticagrelor with aspirin was superior to administration of aspirin alone in patients undergoing PCI as it improves ischemic outcomes.

   The cornerstone of antithrombotic therapy is antiplatelet therapy. Platelets play a key role in mediating stent thrombosis, the major cause of ischemic events following percutaneous coronary intervention (PCI). For this reason, antiplatelet therapy is started at the time of PCI and continued for at least 30 days afterward. Aspirin protects the endothelium and reduces platelet activity and aggregation undergoing PCI.

   Nursing implications include assessing patients who are contraindicated to take Aspirin which may be due to active bleeding or has severe allergies to non-steroidal anti-inflammatory drugs (NSAIDs) or Aspirin. $P2Y_{12}$ inhibits platelet aggregation by blocking the adenosine diphosphate $P2Y_{12}$ receptor. This group of drugs include: prasugrel, ticagrelor, and clopidogrel. Mr. Lawrence is given ticagrelor in this case prior to PCI because clopidogrel requires conversion into active metabolites from prodrug agents whereas ticagrelor does not require the biotransformation pathway of platelet aggregation. Ticagrelor reversibly binds

(continued)

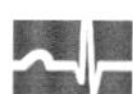

CASE-BASED LEARNING 1 (*Continued*)

$P2Y_{12}$ inhibitor, have onsets of action considerably faster than that of clopidogrel, and is more potent. Therefore, unless it is contraindicated, ticagrelor is recommended with Aspirin per guideline. Prasugrel is not recommended for "upfront" therapy at this time.

Mr. Lawrence is also given an anticoagulant, unfractionated heparin (UFH). Anticoagulation in addition to DAPT is recommended prior to undergoing PCI. Guideline recommendation is 60 IU/kg bolus with maximum dose at 4000 IU/kg. UFH prevents the growth and propagation of a formed thrombus to allow the body's thrombolytic system to degrade the clot. If Mr. Lawrence has a history of heparin-induced thrombocytopenia (HIT) this medication would be contraindicated and other anticoagulation such as bivalirudin can be used instead. While the use of triple oral antithrombotic therapy is necessary to reduce the rate of cardiac ischemic events after PCI, cardiac nurses need to understand when these medications are contraindicated and may not be appropriate to administer.

Patient Examination

Vital Signs

Ht. 180 cm; Wt. 80 kg; BMI 26 kg/m^2; BP 100/50 mm Hg; HR 60; RR 16; SaO_2 93% on 2 L; Temp 37°C

Physical Examination

- General: alert, diaphoretic, pale, in great distress
- HENT—normocephalic, atraumatic
- Eyes—no xanthomas, normal conjunctiva
- Cardiovascular: regular rate and rhythm, no murmur, rub or gallop, pulses 2+ intact and symmetric, no clubbing, cyanosis or lower-extremity edema, jugular venous distention (JVD) is normal
- Respiratory: clear to auscultation bilaterally without crackles or wheezes, normal respiratory effort
- GI—normal bowel sounds, abdomen soft, nondistended, nontender to palpation, no rebound or guarding, no masses or organomegaly appreciated
- Neurologic: no focal deficits, alert and oriented to person, place, time, and event
- Musculoskeletal: no gross deformities appreciated
- Skin: cool skin, pallor
- Psych: appropriate mood and affect given his history and situation

Diagnostic Studies

XR Chest 1 View

Heart size is normal. Basilar opacities likely represent atelectasis. No consolidation to suggest infection. No pulmonary edema, effusion or pneumothorax

Select Labs

Sodium 138 meq/dL
Potassium 3.6 meq/dL
Glucose 115 mg/dL
Blood urea nitrogen 15 mg/dL
Creatinine 0.74 mg/dL
Magnesium 1.8 meq/dL
Hemoglobin 14.5%
Hematocrit 42%
Platelet 191 billion/L
Prothrombin time INR 10.0
Partial thromboplastin time 27
Troponin I 0.1 ng/mL

ED Clinical Course

Mr. Lawrence, a 61-yr-old male, with multiple comorbidities is diagnosed with inferior MI. In the Emergency Department, Mr. Lawrence was resuscitated with fluids and has been hemodynamically stable. Mr. Lawrence was given additional doses of chewable aspirin. Cardiology team was consulted for emergent PCI.

Assessment and Plan

STEMI. Plan for emergent revascularization with PCI, the cornerstone of STEMI management. In consultation with cardiology team, Mr. Lawrence was transferred to cardiac catheterization lab for PCI in satisfactory condition.

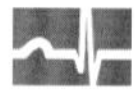

CASE-BASED LEARNING 2

Stable Ischemic Heart Disease

Patient Profile

History of Present Illness

Mr. Chinook is a 62 year old male who presents to the emergency department (ED) in Juneau Alaska with complaints of band-like pressure around his chest and shortness of breath with exertion. However, his wife reports she has noticed him becoming short of breath with regular walks to the mailbox for the past 6 weeks. He reports that chest pressure has been intermittent for the past day and goes way with rest. Pain reminds him of the discomfort he had when he had his heart attack. He had a prescription for nitroglycerin but has not refilled it since his CABG surgery 8 years ago. He remains relatively active working in his wood shop at home, hunting, and fishing.

Medical History

Hypertension, type II diabetes, obesity (BMI 33), 22-pack-yr history of smoking (quit 8 yr ago after his CABG), hyperlipidemia, mild chronic obstructive pulmonary disease (COPD), motor vehicle accident (MVA)

Surgical History

CABG × 3

- LIMA to the left anterior descending (LAD) artery
- SVG to unknown target vessels

Left knee arthroplasty s/p MVA, required left knee replacement

Allergies

Bees (anaphylaxis)
Shellfish (itching)
Statins (muscle aches)

Medications

Aspirin 81 mg daily, metformin 1000 mg BID, lisinopril 10 mg daily, atenolol 50 mg twice daily, CoQ 10, biotin, turmeric, cinnamon, krill oil, and coconut oil capsules

Physical Examination

Vital Signs

Temp 98.2 F; HR 82; BP 145/72; RR 20

Diagnostic Studies

- ECG: sinus rhythm with right bundle branch block (RBBB), HR 82

CASE-BASED LEARNING 2 (*Continued*)

PR 240, QRS 120 ms, no R wave in lead V1
RBBB as noted and unchanged from ECG 2 years ago
Mild ST depression (V1-3) and T-wave inversion

- Labs: complete blood count

Considerations

1. What are your thoughts on this patient's clinical presentation? Does this seem consistent with typical angina (i.e., ischemic chest pain)? Do you suspect this discomfort to be acute or chronic and stable?
2. What medications is this patient on for coronary artery disease? What medications are warranted based on the current guidelines for stable ischemic heart disease? What questions might you ask him to understand what medications or treatments have been effective?
3. Based on current guidelines, what options would you anticipate for diagnostic evaluation or treatment?

Assessment/Plan

Mr. Chinook is a 62-yr-old male with a history of CAD status post CABG ×3 with no recent risk stratification or evaluation of the patency of his bypass grafts or LV function. As this patient is 8 years status post CABG, it is likely that the SVGs to unknown target vessels are no longer patent. He presents today with typical angina reminiscent of his index symptoms at the time of MI and CABG. This presentation is also worrisome as he states he had been quite active until recently.

Based on the diagnostic studies reported in the chart, it appears he has a first degree AV block and a right bundle branch block versus a bifascicular block. There is no change between this ECG and a previous ECG on record from two years ago. It is unclear how well his comorbidities (HTN, DM, dyslipidemia, COPD) have been managed. He is on appropriate guideline-directed medical therapy, including aspirin, beta-blocker, ACE-inhibitor for CAD but no statin due to intolerance. BP is presently above goal. He is on metformin for diabetes with no recent hemoglobin A1C (HA1C) test available.

1. Continue current medical therapy.
2. Refill SLNTG.
3. Risk stratification to include:
   a. Echocardiography to evaluate for a structurally and functionally normal heart, specifically rapid and targeted assessment of LV dysfunction and regional/segmental wall motional abnormalities suggestive of ischemia or infarct
   b. Myocardial perfusion scan with pharmacologic stress
   c. HA1C.
4. Arrange for local stay and coordination with provisional dates to complete diagnostic studies and likely coronary angiography.

KEY READINGS

Maron DJ, Hochman JS, Reynolds HR, et al. Initial invasive or conservative strategy for stable coronary disease. *N England J Med.* 2020;382(15):1395–1407.

Patel MR, Calhoon JH, Dehmer GJ, et al. ACC/AATS/AHA/ASE/ASNC/SCAI/SCCT/STS 2017 appropriate use criteria for coronary revascularization in patients with stable ischemic heart disease. A Report of the American College of Cardiology Appropriate Use Criteria Task Force, American Association for Thoracic Surgery, American Heart Association, American Society of Echocardiography, American Society of Nuclear Cardiology, Society for Cardiovascular Angiography and Interventions, Society of Cardiovascular Computed Tomography, and Society of Thoracic Surgeons. *J Am Coll Cardiol.* 2017;69(17):2212–2241.

Tamis-Holland JE, Jneid H, Reynolds HR, et al. Contemporary diagnosis and management of patients with myocardial infarction in the absence of obstructive coronary artery disease: a scientific statement from the American Heart Association. *Circulation.* 2019;139(18):e891–e908.

Thygesen K, Alpert JS, Jaffe AS, et al. Fourth universal definition of myocardial infarction (2018). *J Am Coll Cardiol.* 2018;72(18):2231–2264.

REFERENCES

1. Fihn SD, Gardin JM, Abrams J, et al. 2012 ACCF/AHA/ACP/AATS/PCNA/SCAI/STS guideline for the diagnosis and management of patients with stable ischemic heart disease: executive summary: a Report of the American College of Cardiology Foundation/American Heart Association Task Force on Practice Guidelines, and the American College of Physicians, American Association for Thoracic Surgery, Preventive Cardiovascular Nurses Association, Society for Cardiovascular Angiography and Interventions, and Society of Thoracic Surgeons. *Circulation.* 2012;126(25):3097–3137.
2. World Health Organization. *Global Health Estimates 2016: Deaths by cause, age, sex, by country and by region. 2000–2016.* Geneva: World Health Organization; 2016.
3. Atherosclerosis Risk in Communities Study. ARIC Study. 2005–2014; http://www.cscc.unc.edu/aric/displaydata.php?pg_id=37. Accessed February 17, 2020.
4. Levitan EB, Olubowale OT, Gamboa CM, et al. Characteristics and prognosis of acute myocardial infarction by discharge diagnosis: the reasons for geographic and racial differences in stroke study. *Ann Epidemiol.* 2015;25(7):499–504.e491.
5. Hackam DG, Anand SS. Emerging risk factors for atherosclerotic vascular disease: a critical review of the evidence. *JAMA.* 2003;290(7):932–940.
6. Stary HC. Natural history and histological classification of atherosclerotic lesions: an update. *Arterioscler Thromb Vasc Biol.* 2000;20(5):1177–1178.
7. Grech ED. Pathophysiology and investigation of coronary artery disease. *BMJ.* 2003;326(7397):1027–1030.
8. Fihn SD, Blankenship JC, Alexander KP, et al. 2014 ACC/AHA/AATS/PCNA/SCAI/STS focused update of the guideline for the diagnosis and management of patients with stable ischemic heart disease. A Report of the American College of Cardiology/American Heart Association Task Force on Practice Guidelines, and the American Association for Thoracic Surgery, Preventive Cardiovascular Nurses Association, Society for Cardiovascular Angiography and Interventions, and Society of Thoracic Surgeons. *J Am Coll Cardiol.* 2014;64(18):1929–1949.
9. Falk E, Shah PK, Fuster V. Coronary plaque disruption. *Circulation.* 1995;92(3):657–671.
10. Corti R, Fuster V, Badimon JJ. Pathogenetic concepts of acute coronary syndromes. *J Am Coll Cardiol.* 2003;41(4 Suppl):S7–S14.
11. Kullo IJ, Edwards WD, Schwartz RS. Vulnerable plaque: pathobiology and clinical implications. *Ann Internal Med.* 1998;129(12):1050–1060.
12. Davies MJ, Thomas A. Thrombosis and acute coronary-artery lesions in sudden cardiac ischemic death. *N Engl J Med.* 1984;310(18):1137–1140.
13. Bini A, Fenoglio JJ, Mesa-Tejada R, et al. Identification and distribution of fibrinogen, fibrin, and fibrin(ogen) degradation products in atherosclerosis. Use of monoclonal antibodies. *Arteriosclerosis.* 1989;9(1):109–121.
14. Taeymans Y, Théroux P, Lespérance J, et al. Quantitative angiographic morphology of the coronary artery lesions at risk of thrombotic occlusion. *Circulation.* 1992;85(1):78–85.
15. Langille BL, O'Donnell F. Reductions in arterial diameter produced by chronic decreases in blood flow are endothelium-dependent. *Science.* 1986;231(4736):405–407.
16. Patel MR, Calhoon JH, Dehmer GJ, et al. ACC/AATS/AHA/ASE/ASNC/SCAI/SCCT/STS 2016 Appropriate use criteria for coronary revascularization in patients with acute coronary syndromes. A Report of the American College of Cardiology Appropriate Use Criteria Task Force, American Association for Thoracic Surgery, American Heart Association, American Society of Echocardiography, American Society of Nuclear Cardiology, Society for Cardiovascular Angiography and Interventions, Society of Cardiovascular Computed Tomography, and the Society of Thoracic Surgeons. *J Am Coll Cardiol.* 2011;69(5):570–591.
17. Libby P, Ridker PM, Hansson GK. Progress and challenges in translating the biology of atherosclerosis. *Nature.* 2011;473(7347):317–325.

18. Bozkurt B, Kribbs SB, Clubb FJ, et al. Pathophysiologically relevant concentrations of tumor necrosis factor-alpha promote progressive left ventricular dysfunction and remodeling in rats. *Circulation.* 1998;97(14):1382–1391.
19. Seta Y, Shan K, Bozkurt B, et al. Basic mechanisms in heart failure: the cytokine hypothesis. *J Cardiac Failure.* 1996;2(3):243–249.
20. Cozlea DL, Farcas DM, Nagy A, et al. The impact of C reactive protein on global cardiovascular risk on patients with coronary artery disease. *Curr Health Sci J.* 2013;39(4):225–231.
21. Thygesen K, Alpert JS, Jaffe AS, et al. Fourth universal definition of myocardial infarction (2018). *J Am Coll Cardiol.* 2018;72(18):2231–2264.
22. Tamis-Holland JE, Jneid H, Reynolds HR, et al. Contemporary diagnosis and management of patients with myocardial infarction in the absence of obstructive coronary artery disease: a scientific statement from the American Heart Association. *Circulation.* 2019;139(18):e891–e908.
23. Rui P, Kang K. National hospital ambulatory medical care survey: 2017 emergency department summary tables. National Center for Health Statistics 2017; https://www.cdc.gov/nchs/data/nhamcs/web_tables/2017_ed_web_tables-508.pdf. May 2, 2020.
24. Bhuiya FA PS, McCaig LF. Emergency department visits for chest pain and abdominal pain: United States 1999–2008. *NCHS Data Brief.* 2010;43:1–8.
25. Ward MJ, Kripalani S, Zhu Y, et al. Incidence of emergency department visits for ST elevation myocardial infarction in a recent 6 year period in the United States. *Am J Cardiol.* 2015,115(2):167–170.
26. Benjamin EJ, Muntner P, Alonso A, et al. Heart disease and stroke statistics—2019 Update: a Report from the American Heart Association. *Circulation.* 2019;139(10):e56–e528.
27. Rosell-Ortiz F, Mellado-Vergel FJ, Fernández-Valle P, et al. Initial complications and factors related to prehospital mortality in acute myocardial infarction with ST segment elevation. *Emerg Med J.* 2015;32(7):559–563.
28. Graham G. Disparities in cardiovascular disease risk in the United States. *Curr Cardiol Rev.* 2015;11(3):238–245.
29. Yusuf S, Hawken S, Ôunpuu S, et al. Effect of potentially modifiable risk factors associated with myocardial infarction in 52 countries (the INTERHEART study): case-control study. *Lancet.* 2004;364(9438):937–952.
30. Virchow R. *Cellular Pathology*. London: John Churchill; 1858.
31. Anderson JL, Morrow DA. Acute myocardial infarction. *N Engl J Med.* 2017;376(21):2053–2064.
32. Scheuer J. Myocardial metabolism in cardiac hypoxia. *Am J Cardiol.* 1967;19(3):385–392.
33. O'Gara PT, Kushner FG, Ascheim DD, et al. 2013 ACCF/AHA guideline for the management of ST-elevation myocardial infarction. A Report of the American College of Cardiology Foundation/American Heart Association Task Force on Practice Guidelines. *J Am Coll Cardiol.* 2013;61(4):e78–e140.
34. Amsterdam EA, Wenger NK, Brindis RG, et al. 2014 AHA/ACC guideline for the management of patients with non-ST-elevation acute coronary syndromes. *Circulation.* 2014;130(25):e344–e426.
35. Ibanez B, James S, Agewall S, et al. 2017 ESC Guidelines for the management of acute myocardial infarction in patients presenting with ST-segment elevation: The Task Force for the management of acute myocardial infarction in patients presenting with ST-segment elevation of the European Society of Cardiology (ESC). *Eur Heart J.* 2017;39(2):119–177.
36. Keefer C, Resnik W. Angina pectoris: a syndrome caused by anoxemia of the myocardium. *Arch Int Med.* 1928;41:769.
37. Braunwald E, Morrow DA. Unstable angina. Is it time for a requiem? *Circulation.* 2013;127:2452–2457.
38. Amsterdam EA, Wenger NK, Brindis RG, et al. 2014 AHA/ACC guideline for the management of patients with non–ST-elevation acute coronary syndromes. A Report of the American College of Cardiology/American Heart Association Task Force on Practice Guidelines. *J Am Coll Cardiol.* 2014;64(24):e139–e228.
39. ACC/AHA Guidelines for the management of patients with ST-elevation myocardial infarction. *Circulation.* 2004;110(9):e82–e292.
40. Levine GN, Bates ER, Blankenship JC, et al. 2011 ACCF/AHA/SCAI guideline for percutaneous coronary intervention. A Report of the American College of Cardiology Foundation/American Heart Association Task Force on Practice Guidelines and the Society for Cardiovascular Angiography and Interventions. *J Am Coll Cardiol.* 2011;58(24):e44–e122.
41. Schmidt T, Abbott JD. Coronary stents: history, design, and construction. *J Clin Med.* 2018;7(6):126.
42. Farkouh ME, Domanski M, Sleeper LA, et al. Strategies for multivessel revascularization in patients with diabetes. *N Engl J Med.* 2012;367(25):2375–2384.
43. Hillis GS, Zehr KJ, Williams AW, et al. Outcome of patients with low ejection fraction undergoing coronary artery bypass grafting. *Circulation.* 2006;114(1 Suppl):I-414–I-419.
44. McCullough PA, Wolyn R, Rocher LL, et al. Acute renal failure after coronary intervention: incidence, risk factors, and relationship to mortality. *Am J Med.* 1997;103(5):368–375.
45. Pancholy SB, Bernat I, Bertrand OF, et al. Prevention of radial artery occlusion after transradial catheterization: the PROPHET-II randomized trial. *JACC Cardiovasc Interv.* 2016;9(19):1992–1999.
46. Pretty H. Dissecting aneurysm of coronary artery in a woman aged 42. *Br Med J.* 1931;1:667.
47. Tweet MS, Hayes SN, Pitta SR, et al. Clinical features, management, and prognosis of spontaneous coronary artery dissection. *Circulation.* 2012;126(5):579–588.
48. Saw J, Mancini GB, Humphries K, et al. Angiographic appearance of spontaneous coronary artery dissection with intramural hematoma proven on intracoronary imaging. *Catheter Cardiovasc Interv.* 2016;87(2):E54–E61.
49. Hayes SN, Kim ESH, Saw J, et al. Spontaneous coronary artery dissection: current state of the science: a scientific statement from the American Heart Association. *Circulation.* 2018;137(19):e523–e557.
50. Liang JJ, Tweet MS, Hayes SE, et al. Prevalence and predictors of depression and anxiety among survivors of myocardial infarction due to spontaneous coronary artery dissection. *J Cardiopulm Rehabil Prev.* 2014;34(2):138–142.
51. Lala A, Johnson KW, Januzzi JL, et al. Prevalence and impact of myocardial injury in patients hospitalized with COVID-19 infection. *J Am Coll Cardiol.* 2020:533–546.
52. Boden WE, O'Rourke RA, Teo KK, et al. Optimal medical therapy with or without PCI for stable coronary disease. *N Engl J Med.* 2007;356(15):1503–1516.
53. Maron DJ, Hochman JS, Reynolds HR, et al. Initial invasive or conservative strategy for stable coronary disease. *N Engl J Med.* 2020;382(15):1395–1407.
54. Hillis LD, Smith PK, Anderson JL, et al. 2011 ACCF/AHA guideline for coronary artery bypass graft surgery. *Circulation.* 2011;124(23):e652–e735.
55. Patel MR, Calhoon JH, Dehmer GJ, et al. ACC/AATS/AHA/ASE/ASNC/SCAI/SCCT/STS 2017 Appropriate Use Criteria for Coronary Revascularization in Patients With Stable Ischemic Heart Disease. A Report of the American College of Cardiology Appropriate Use Criteria Task Force, American Association for Thoracic Surgery, American Heart Association, American Society of Echocardiography, American Society of Nuclear Cardiology, Society for Cardiovascular Angiography and Interventions, Society of Cardiovascular Computed Tomography, and Society of Thoracic Surgeons. *J Am Coll Cardiol.* 2017;69(17):2212–2241.
56. Serruys PW, Morice MC, Kappetein AP, et al. Percutaneous coronary intervention versus coronary-artery bypass grafting for severe coronary artery disease. *N Engl J Med.* 2009;360(10):961–972.
57. Ragosta M, Dee S, Sarembock IJ, et al. Prevalence of unfavorable angiographic characteristics for percutaneous intervention in patients with unprotected left main coronary artery disease. *Catheter Cardiovasc Interv.* 2006;68(3):357–362.
58. Conley MJ, Ely RL, Kisslo J, et al. The prognostic spectrum of left main stenosis. *Circulation.* 1978;57(5):947–952.
59. Stone GW, Kappetein AP, Sabik JF, et al. Five-year outcomes after PCI or CABG for left main coronary disease. *N Engl J Med.* 2019;381(19):1820–1830.
60. Holm NR, Mäkikallio T, Lindsay MM, et al. Percutaneous coronary angioplasty versus coronary artery bypass grafting in the treatment of unprotected left main stenosis: updated 5-year outcomes from the randomised, non-inferiority NOBLE trial. *Lancet.* 2020;395(10219):191–199.
61. Riordan M. EACTS pulls out of left main guidelines after BBC bombshell alleging EXCEL trial cover. 2019. https://www.tctmd.com/news/eacts-pulls-out-left-main-guidelines-after-bbc-bombshell-alleging-excel-trial-cover. Accessed June 2, 2020.
62. Ahmad Y, Howard JP, Arnold AD, et al. Mortality after drug-eluting stents vs. coronary artery bypass grafting for left main coronary artery disease: a meta-analysis of randomized controlled trials. *Eur Heart J.* 2020; ehaa135.
63. Azzalini L, Jolicoeur EM, Pighi M, et al. Epidemiology, management strategies, and outcomes of patients with chronic total coronary occlusion. *Am J Cardiol.* 2016;118(8):1128–1135.
64. Claessen BE, Dangas GD, Weisz G, et al. Prognostic impact of a chronic total occlusion in a non-infarct-related artery in patients with ST-segment elevation myocardial infarction: 3-year results from the HORIZONS-AMI trial. *Eur Heart J.* 2012;33(6):768–775.
65. Sapontis J, Salisbury AC, Yeh RW, et al. Early procedural and health status outcomes after chronic total occlusion angioplasty: a report from the OPEN-CTO Registry (Outcomes, patient health status, and efficiency in chronic total occlusion hybrid procedures). *JACC: Cardiovasc Interv.* 2017;10(15):1523–1534.

30 Peripheral Arterial Disease

Julie Bumgardner

OBJECTIVES

1. Describe the prevalence of PAD.
2. Identify the risk factors for PAD.
3. Describe the pathophysiology process of PAD.
4. Recognize signs and symptoms of PAD.
5. Appropriate diagnostic testing to diagnose PAD.
6. Choose treatment plan for patients.

KEY QUESTIONS

1. Who is at risk for PAD?
2. What is the number one preventable risk factor contributing to PAD?
3. Why is PAD underdiagnosed?
4. What are the common diagnostic tools utilized in diagnosing PAD?
5. When is medical management versus surgical intervention recommended for lower extremity PAD?

INTRODUCTION

The vascular system, also called **the circulatory system**, is made up of the vessels that carry blood and lymph through the body (Fig. 30-1).

Peripheral arterial disease (PAD) is a circulatory problem, defined as diseased arteries outside the heart or brain that effects circulation and decreases blood flow to end targets. PAD is primarily caused by atherosclerosis and associated thrombus that narrows the arteries and slows down blood flow. The more plaque that builds up inside the blood vessel walls, the more the arteries loose flexibility, narrow or occlude. While PAD is common, it is estimated the majority of patients with PAD are undiagnosed and undertreated.[1] Awareness of PAD with both men and women are low. Symptoms can be vague, episodic, and often misconstrued as other medical conditions. PAD is a chronic disease with varied presentations. The medical management of PAD aims to decrease the risk of cardiovascular and cerebrovascular mortality. In addition to medical management, surgical intervention is warranted in advanced PAD to prevent critical ischemia that can lead to stroke, limb loss, end-organ damage, or death. PAD can occur in any blood vessel, but most commonly seen in the aorta, carotid, renal, mesenteric, and lower extremity arteries.

Risk factors of PAD include: smoking, hypertension, diabetes, high cholesterol, advanced age, diet high in saturated fats, obesity, lack of exercise, and genetics. PAD effects greater than 200 million people worldwide, with a prevalence of 8.5 million persons in the United States. The prevalence rises with age and effects 12% to 20% of patients greater than age of 60. People with PAD have a higher risk for coronary disease and stroke.[2] The disease does not improve on its own, gradually becomes worse if untreated, and requires management by a vascular specialist or vascular surgeon. Treatment depends on the symptoms and the severity of the disease. Management includes modifying risk factors, medication, endovascular intervention, or open surgery.

Pathogenesis

Atherosclerosis (see Fig. 30-2) is often referred to as "hardening of the arteries." It has been recognized in humans for thousands of years. First identified as early as the 15th century BC in Egyptian mummies with pictographs referring to heat and redness as concomitants of disease. Cellular research developed over the years, and by the mid-19th century, Rudolf Virchow proposed that some form of injury to the artery wall associated with an inflammatory response, resulted in degenerative atherosclerotic lesions. Nikolay Anichkov expanded this idea to include the role of platelets and thrombogenesis. Modern views of atherogenesis stemmed from the work of John French, who believed alterations in the structural integrity of the endothelial lining of an artery precedes a sequence of events that leads to the various lesions and atherosclerosis.[3]

The process of atherosclerosis is a chronic fibro proliferative disease of arteries fueled by inflammation and lipids. This physiologic process occurs at the cellular and molecular levels. The basic steps in the formation of an intraluminal narrowing are as follows. First, low-density lipoprotein (LDL) cholesterol in the blood passes through the dysfunctional endothelial cells and oxidizes in the intima media. Second, monocytes sense the local inflammation and migrate to the arterial wall. Third, monocytes absorb the oxidized LDL and become foam cells, appearing as a fatty streak. As the foam cells die, the lipid content is released, creating a lipid core. Fourth, smooth muscle cells proliferate, forming a

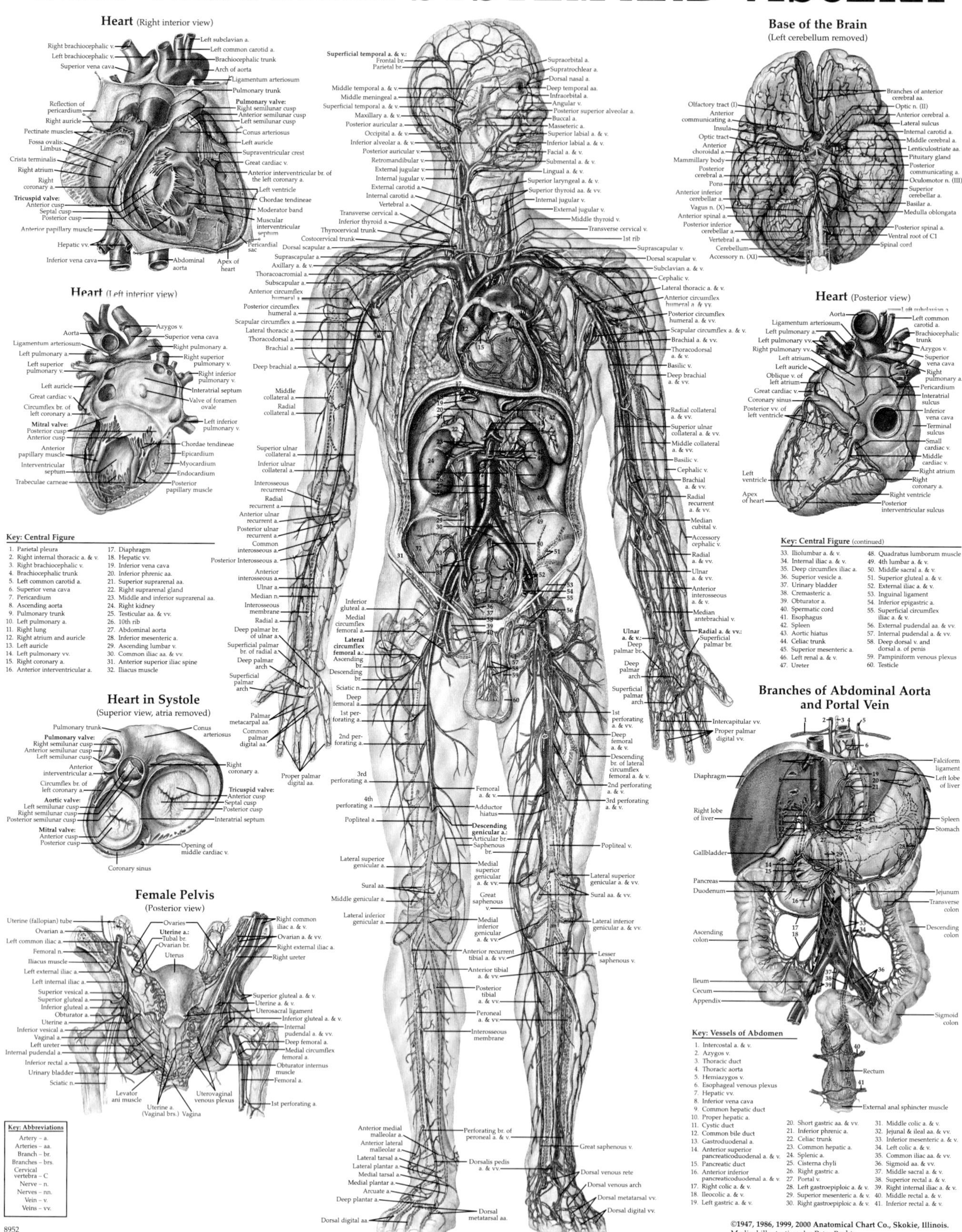

Figure 30-1. Vascular system labeled.

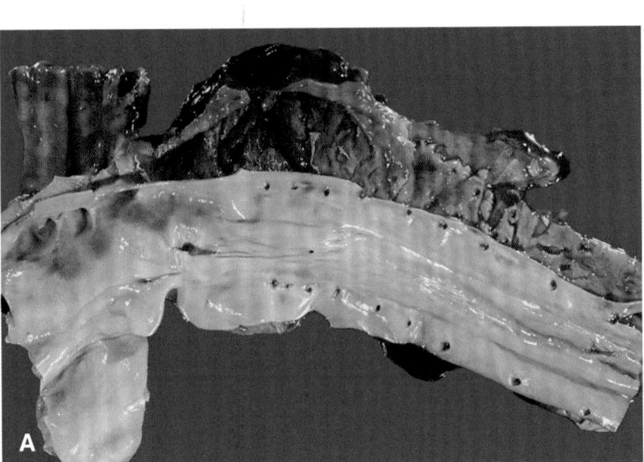

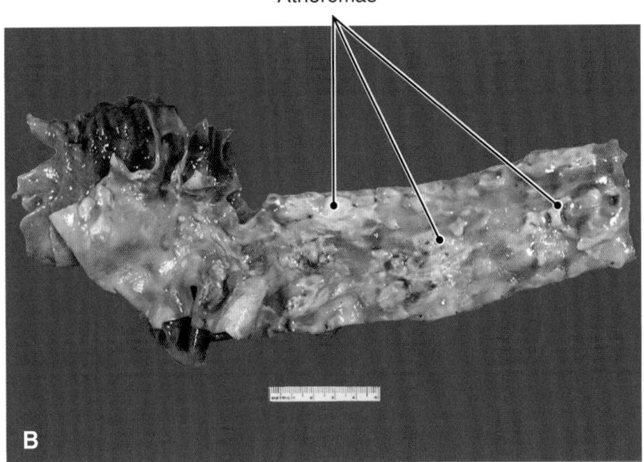

Figure 30-2. Atherosclerosis of the aorta. **A:** The normal aorta. **B:** Severe atherosclerosis. (From McConnell TH. *Nature of Disease*. 2nd ed. Wolters Kluwer Health and Pharma; 2013.)

fibrinous cap over the lipid core. Fifth, as more LDL accumulates, the external elastic membrane expands outward in an effort to maintain blood flow. Eventually the vessel cannot compensate and the plaque will protrude into the lumen, leading to resistance, stiffness, and narrowing of the arteries. The end result is reduced perfusion to distal targets.[4]

Carotid Artery Disease

Extracranial carotid artery disease occurs as a result of luminal narrowing of the neck arteries responsible for the majority of brain perfusion. The most common cause is atherosclerosis, but inflammation, dissection, or abnormal cellular growth such as fibromuscular dysplasia can also cause carotid stenosis.[5] The carotid bifurcation where the common carotid artery divides into the internal and external carotid arteries is a common location for plaque accumulation (Fig. 30-3). Rupture of the plaque can cause a piece to break off and travel to the brain, resulting in ischemia, death of brain tissue, and/or stroke. Transient ischemic attack (TIA) or "mini-strokes" are temporary interruptions of blood flow to the brain, producing transient neurologic symptoms, but do not cause a significant infarction. They are warning signs of a possible future stroke. About one in three patients that have a TIA will eventually have a stroke.[6] Even if the plaque does not cause symptoms, patients with carotid stenosis remain at higher risk of a stroke than the general population.

Stroke is the third leading cause mortality, and the most common cause of long-term disability. Carotid stenosis accounts for 20% to 25% of all ischemic strokes.[7] The prevalence of significant carotid artery disease is 7% in women and 9% in men. Up to 3% of individuals older than 65 have carotid artery disease, with a heightened risk in patients who smoke, have high blood pressure, high cholesterol, diabetes, or heart disease.[8] Physical exam, including detailed neurologic evaluation along with risk assessment and diagnostic imaging will determine patient management.

Patient Presentation

- Unilateral numbness or weakness
- Facial drooping
- Visual disturbances in one eye
- Sudden loss of balance or dizziness
- Slurred speech or difficulty communicating
- Confusion
- Loss of consciousness
- Carotid bruit

Evaluation

- Carotid Doppler
- Computed tomography angiography (CTA)
- Magnetic resonance angiography (MRA)
- Carotid angiogram

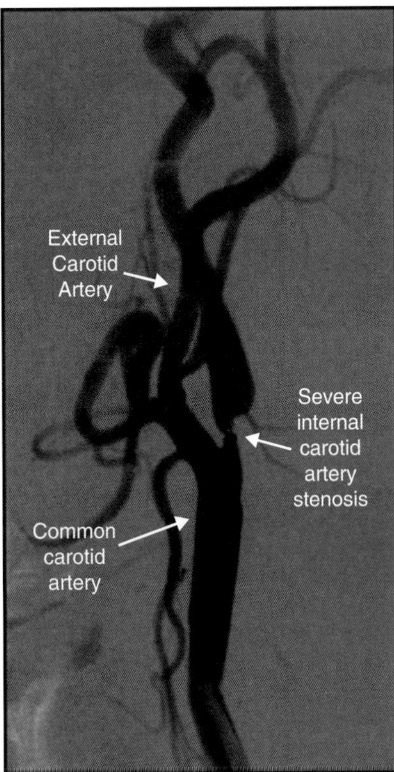

Figure 30-3. Common carotid artery angiography. High magnification view shows the distal bifurcation of the common carotid artery into the external and internal carotid arteries. A severe stenosis is noted in the proximal internal carotid artery. (Garcia MJ. *Noninvasive Cardiovascular Imaging: A Multimodality Approach*. Wolters Kluwer Health and Pharma; 2011.)

Carotid Doppler should be considered for the initial screening. It is an ultrasound imaging test that uses sound waves to produce pictures of the arteries in the neck. It is a low cost, noninvasive test that can also measure blood flow velocities and patterns through the carotid arteries. It provides a range of stenosis that is useful in determining percentage of carotid stenosis. CTA and MRA are often confirmatory studies, allowing for detailed assessment of the carotid arteries, aortic arch, and intracranial parts. Evaluation is done in multiple views, with reconstructions that allow for plaque evaluation. Stenosis measurement is based on North American Symptomatic Carotid Endarterectomy Trial (NASCET) criteria that determine an exact stenosis rather than a range. CTA is less expensive and more readily available than an MRA, but requires iodine contrast medium and radiation. An MRA may be recommended in patients with renal dysfunction or significant dye allergies. Conventional angiography is usually reserved for patients with discordant results from noninvasive imaging studies or in combination with a planned endovascular intervention.[9]

Treatment and Management

Management depends on the severity of disease, assessment of comorbid conditions, life expectancy, and symptoms. Significant disease is defined as any stenosis with greater than 50% stenosis. There has been some controversy over the management of carotid artery disease and what treatment provides the best clinical outcomes. Medical management includes lipid lowering therapy, optimal glycemic control, smoking cessation, antiplatelet, and antihypertensive medication.[10]

Surgical management for carotid disease includes carotid endarterectomy (CEA) or carotid artery stent (CAS). Acute stroke patients, referred within 30 days, with significant carotid stenosis has been studied in two large randomized clinical trials and determined patients will benefit from carotid intervention to prevent further ischemic events. CEA and CAS may be recommended for symptomatic patients who have greater than 50% stenosis or asymptomatic patients with greater than 70% stenosis. CEA is the standard treatment, however patients with significant comorbidities or difficult anatomy may be considered for CAS.[7]

There have been many randomized clinical trials comparing CEA and CAS. One of the largest clinical trial today is the carotid revascularization endarterectomy versus stenting trial (CREST). This trial included over 2000 patients from multidisciplinary centers across North America with symptomatic and asymptomatic disease assigned to CAS or CEA. Their analysis concluded that compared with CEA, CAS was associated with reduced risk of perioperative MI, but an increased risk of periprocedural stroke. The CREST results confirm that CEA and CAS can be done with relatively low complication rates in asymptomatic patients when performed with very experienced practitioners who use their clinical expertise in choosing the most appropriate patients.[11]

Meta-analysis of randomized trials seems to support the superiority of CEA over CAS with regard to stroke or death rate within 30 days, however long-term results are inconclusive. CAS continues to evolve with advanced devices, technology, and training. The management of carotid stenosis is complicated. Stroke prevention without complications remains the goal of treatment.[7]

Operative Management

CAS is an endovascular procedure using a catheter that is placed in another artery, threaded into the carotid artery where a balloon is used to expand the artery and a stent placed to keep the artery open. Indications for carotid stenting include history of prior vocal cord damage, previous neck surgery or radiation, inability to tolerate general anesthesia or surgically "inaccessible" lesions.[12]

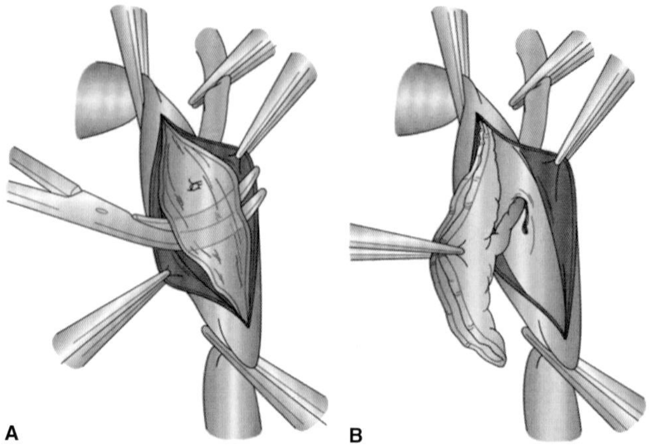

Figure 30-4. A: During carotid endarterectomy, vascular clamps are applied to the common carotid, external carotid, and internal carotid arteries. Carotid plaque is elevated from the carotid lumen. **B:** Carotid plaque is removed and the arteriotomy is closed either primarily or with a patch angioplasty. (Mulholland MW. *Greenfield's Surgery.* 6th ed. Wolters Kluwer Health and Pharma; 2016.)

CEA remains the gold standard in treating severe carotid disease (Fig. 30-4). The common and internal carotid arteries are the arteries of concern because they supply blood to the brain. An incision is made on the side of the neck with the patient under local or general anesthesia. The plaque that forms in the inner layer of the artery, or endothelium is removed, hence the name of the procedure "endarterectomy" which simply means removal of the endothelium of the artery. Patients usually stay 1 or 2 nights in the hospital. Most common risks to the procedure include stroke in 2% to 3% of the patients with no preprocedural symptoms and 5% to 7% with preprocedural symptoms.[13]

Patients should be monitored for any neurologic changes following a carotid intervention, including visual disturbances, slurred speech, dysphagia, facial drooping, and unilateral weakness. A postoperative Doppler is recommended at 2 to 6 weeks after intervention, again at 6 months, 1 year, and then annually.[10]

Renal Artery Stenosis

Renal artery stenosis (RAS) is the narrowing of one or both renal arteries (Fig. 30-5). About 90% of RAS is caused by atherosclerosis. Most other cases are caused by fibromuscular dysplasia, a noninflammatory disease that causes abnormal growth within the artery wall making the vessel appear like a "string of beads." Other less common causes include thromboembolic disease, arterial dissection, aortic aneurysm, and vasculitis. RAS is a common cause of secondary hypertension and is found between 0.5% and 5% of all hypertensive patients. The incidence of atherosclerotic RAS has been increasing and was found in 6.8% of all individuals over 65 years and older on one U.S. study.[14]

Patient Presentation

- Young onset hypertension with negative family history
- Onset of severe hypertension after the age of 55

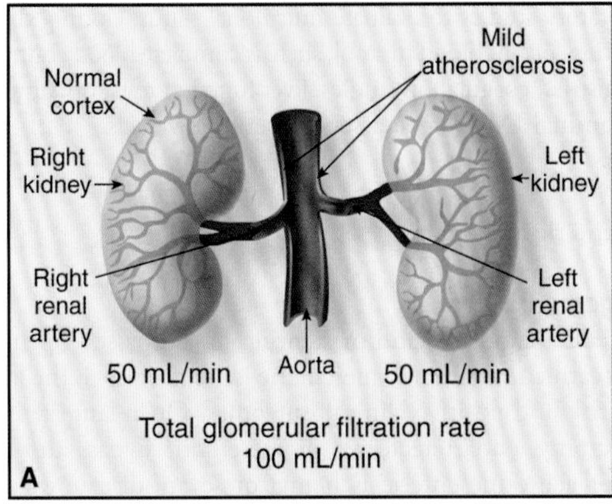

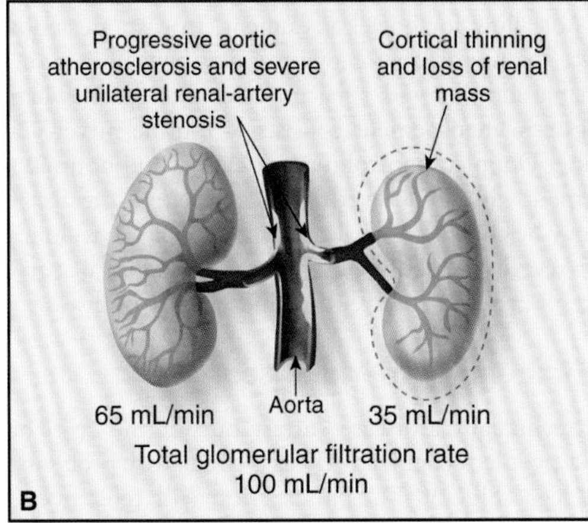

Figure 30-5. Progressive atherosclerosis, renal-artery stenosis, and ischemic nephropathy. In the early phase (**A**), there is mild atherosclerosis of the perirenal abdominal aorta and normal renal function. Renal blood flow, renal mass, and the serum creatinine concentration are normal. The dimensions of the kidneys are normal, and there is no cortical atrophy. The total glomerular filtration rate (100 mL/min) and the glomerular filtration rate in each kidney (50 mL/min) are normal. As the disease progresses (**B**), there is progressive aortic atherosclerosis and severe unilateral renal-artery stenosis. The left kidney is smaller than the right kidney, and there may be cortical thinning and asymmetry in renal blood flow. The serum creatinine concentration remains normal as long as the right kidney is normal, despite the loss of renal mass. The total glomerular filtration rate may be normal (100 mL/min) or only slightly depressed owing to compensatory changes in the right kidney, but renal blood flow is decreased in the left kidney (35 mL/min). (From Safian RD,Textor SC. Renal-artery stenosis. *New England Journal of Medicine* 2001;344:431–442.)

- Accelerated hypertension (sudden and persistent worsening of previously controlled hypertension)
- Resistant hypertension or malignant hypertension (failure of blood pressure control despite full doses of appropriate 3 drug regime including a diuretic)
- Unexplained atrophic kidney or size discrepancy of greater than 1.5 cm between the kidneys
- Unexplained renal failure
- Flash pulmonary edema
- Abdominal or flank bruit
- Lack of evidence supporting an alternative cause, for instance and abnormal urinalysis, proteinuria, or nephrotoxic drug[15]

Evaluation

- Laboratory studies including serum creatinine
- GFR and 24-hour urine analysis to accurately assess the level of renal dysfunction and measuring the degree of proteinuria
- Serologic tests for systemic causes like systemic lupus erythematous or vasculitis
- Renal ultrasound
- CTA
- MRA
- Renal angiogram[15]

Treatment and Management

Treatment depends on symptoms and severity of stenosis. The Society for cardiovascular angiography and interventions categories stenosis severity as follows: Mild less than 50% blockage, moderate 50% to 70% blockage, severe greater than 70% blockage. Intervention can be considered in moderate to severe stenosis, in the setting of malignant hypertension or declining renal function.[16] The degree of RAS that would justify any intervention attempt is greater than 80% blockage with bilateral stenosis or solitary kidney, regardless of the presence of renal insufficiency.[15]

Surgical intervention includes renal artery angioplasty, renal artery stent, or renal artery bypass. An endovascular procedure using angioplasty or stent is generally preferred to limit hospitalization, avoid general anesthesia, and minimize open operative risks. A randomized study by van de Ven compared angioplasty or angioplasty with stent and showed a higher vessel patency with stenting. The primary success rate was 57% for angioplasty alone compared to 88% for angioplasty with concomitant stenting. Restenosis was decreased by 34% with stenting.[16]

Open surgical bypass includes endarterectomy or renal bypass, commonly aortorenal, with either autologous veins or prosthetic material. Open surgery may be considered for extensive blockages, arteries with small caliber, or restenosis from prior endovascular repair. Unfortunately, revascularization may not always result in restoration of renal function because of intrinsic damage sustained to the kidney during the period of reduced blood flow. However, it may be necessary to preserve blood supply to the kidney and avoid further decline in renal function.[17]

Long-term management consists of routine surveillance with laboratory studies, blood pressure control, lipid, antiplatelet therapy, and renal Doppler to monitor kidney size and renal artery blood flow. CTA or MRA may be considered if renal Doppler studies are technically difficult or reveals restrictive blood flow.

Mesenteric Ischemia

Mesenteric ischemia occurs when there is inadequate blood flow through the mesenteric vessels that results in organ ischemia (Fig. 30-6). The mesenteric circulation is complex, connecting collateral networks between visceral and nonvisceral vessels. The primary vessels involved include the celiac, superior mesenteric artery (SMA), and inferior mesenteric artery (IMA). The celiac is the first major branch of the abdominal aorta, around T12. It supplies blood to the liver, stomach, abdominal esophagus, spleen, duodenum, and the pancreas. The SMA arises below the celiac around L1 and supplies blood to the lower part of the duodenum, the transverse colon, and the pancreas. The IMA arises at level L3 and supplies blood to the descending colon, sigmoid colon, and part of the rectum. Severity of ischemia depends on

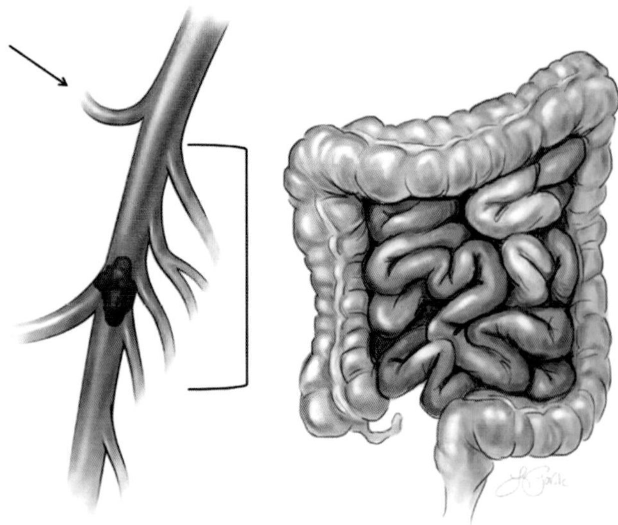

Figure 30-6. Pattern of embolic mesenteric ischemia—SMA emboli typically spare the middle colic artery (*arrow*) and proximal jejunal branches (*bracket*) resulting in an ischemic pattern that spares the jejunum and distal transverse colon. (Mulholland MW. *Greenfield's Surgery.* 6th ed. Wolters Kluwer Health and Pharma; 2016.)

the vessel involved and the extent of collateral blood flow. It is one of the least common causes of abdominal pain, accounting for 1 of every 1000 hospital admissions, however, is a potentially life-threatening condition.[18] Mesenteric venous thrombosis is the least common of the ischemias. It is often related to trauma, thrombophilia, or inflammatory disorders that are often managed with anticoagulation.[19]

Mesenteric ischemia can be acute or chronic. Acute mesenteric ischemia is typically related to embolic phenomena or arterial thrombosis. Less common causes include: isolated dissection, vasculitis, or obstruction, that is, tumor. Acute mesenteric ischemia is a surgical emergency and focuses of restoring mesenteric blood flow, assessing bowel viability, and resecting nonviable bowel if needed. Mortality is as high as 90% once bowel-wall infarction occurs.[20]

Chronic mesenteric ischemia, sometimes referred to intestinal angina, refers to episodic or persistent hypoperfusion of the bowel. The majority of cases are caused by atherosclerotic disease that produces multivessel narrowing. More than one primary mesenteric vessel is usually effected to produce symptoms because of the extensive network of collateral bowel circulation.[20] Conservative management consisting of smoking cessation, antiplatelet medications, and statin therapy may be initiated with asymptomatic patients. Symptomatic patients with abdominal pain, weight loss, and/or bowel changes typically benefit from intervention.

Patient Presentation

- Postprandial pain, generally epigastric or periumbilical
- Fear of eating
- Nausea/vomiting
- Diarrhea/constipation
- Flatulence
- Signs of malnutrition
- Abdominal bruit
- History of vascular disease[19,21]

Evaluation

- Laboratory studies to evaluate nutritional status, clotting disorders, infection, occult blood in stool, such as complete blood count, blood chemistries, coagulation studies, liver function tests, urinalysis
- Abdominal Doppler to assess mesenteric vessels
- CTA
- MRA
- Mesenteric angiogram[19,21]

Management

Mesenteric angioplasty and/or stenting has surpassed open bypass in the treatment of chronic mesenteric ischemia due to the low procedure risk and positive clinical outcomes. Open surgery includes embolectomy, endarterectomy, or mesenteric bypass and is indicated for acute mesenteric ischemia or severe disease that is not accessible with an endovascular approach. Endovascular treatments are generally not applied to acute mesenteric ischemia because it does not allow for bowel assessment. In cases of endovascular approach, the use of laparoscopy to assess bowel function may be a reasonable addition with subacute cases and high-risk patients.[17]

Long-term management consists of routine surveillance with abdominal Doppler, controlling risk factors and optimal medical management with lipid lowering and antiplatelet therapy. CTA or MRA may be considered if abdominal Doppler is technically difficult or reveals restrictive blood flow. Frequency of surveillance depends on previous intervention and severity of disease.

Lower Extremity Arterial Disease

PAD is technically a diseased artery outside the heart or brain, but most people recognize PAD as a circulatory problem involving the legs (Fig. 30-7). This section will reference PAD as

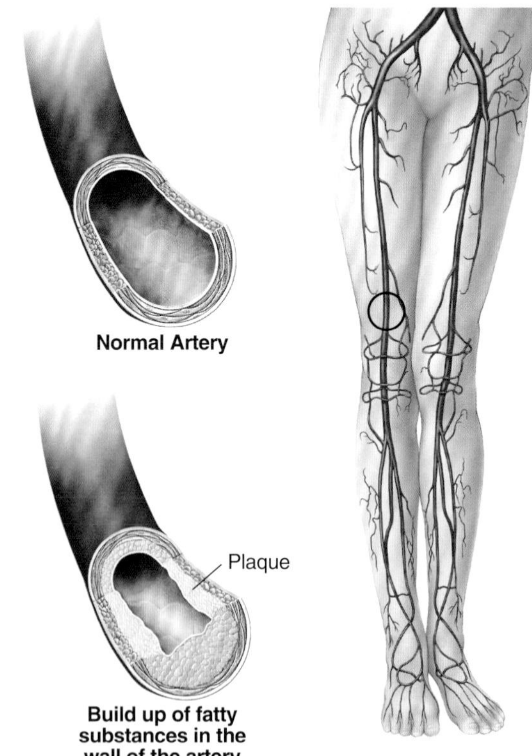

Figure 30-7. Rebar C, Heimgartner N, Gersch C. Peripheral Arterial Disease. (*Pathophysiology Made Incredibly Visual.* 3rd ed. Wolters Kluwer Health and Pharma; 2016.)

diseased arteries in the lower limbs that causes narrowing and reduces blood flow. The most common cause of blocked or narrowed leg arteries is from atherosclerosis, but thromboembolism and rare disorders such as Buerger disease, popliteal entrapment, and Raynaud phenomena can also cause lower extremity ischemia. Worldwide prevalence of lower extremity arterial disease is between 3% and 12%, more common in low to mid income countries. It is estimated that approximately 50% of patients with lower extremity arterial disease present concomitantly with coronary artery disease.[22]

PAD affects about 13% of the Western population in patients over 50 years old. Almost two thirds of patients with mild PAD are asymptomatic, therefore many patients remain undiagnosed. Risk factors include: diabetes, hypertension, high cholesterol, renal disease, inflammatory disorders, genetics, with smoking being the biggest risk factor. A systemic review suggests that half of all PAD can be attributed to heavy smoking. The course of asymptomatic PAD is relatively benign, however patients with diabetes or patients who continue to smoke, the clinical manifestations can be both rapid and unpredictable.[23]

Rutherford classification of PAD includes six stages:

- Stage 0 if the patient is asymptomatic.
- Stage 1 if mild intermittent claudication is present.
- Stage 2 if moderate intermittent claudication is present.
- Stage 3 if severe intermittent claudication is present.
- Stage 4 if ischemic rest pain is present.
- Stage 5 if patient has minor tissue loss.
- Stage 6 if the patient has ulceration or gangrene[17]

Claudication is identified as a cramping, numbness, or weakness in the legs with ambulation which is relieved by rest. It does not occur with sitting, standing, or changing positions. Mild PAD may go undiagnosed because persons may not be able to walk far or fast enough due to other comorbidities to elicit symptoms. Patients may have no problems ambulating at a slow steady pace, but become symptomatic with fast pace walking or up an incline. Location of symptoms correlates with level of disease. For example, aorta iliac disease manifests as pain in the hip or buttocks, femoral popliteal manifests as pain in calf. Collateral circulation may develop with chronic PAD, reducing symptoms to intermittent claudication and gradual decline.[24]

Some of the highest-risk groups have diabetes and/or end-stage renal disease. Complex microvascular changes and increased arterial calcifications combined with neuropathy are often seen with more accelerated disease. They are one of the highest-risk groups for both ulceration and amputation.[25] Acute lower extremity arterial disease is caused by embolism, trauma, or dissection. These conditions can cause abrupt obliteration of blood vessels and require emergent care. Delayed restoration of blood flow, beyond 6 hours, can lead to permanent nerve damage, limb loss, or death (Fig. 30-8).

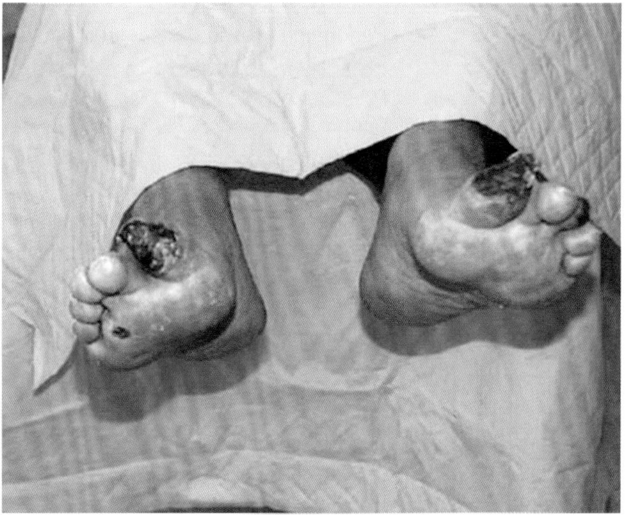

Figure 30-8. Patient with diabetes mellitus, dense peripheral sensory neuropathy, and advanced peripheral arterial disease with critical limb ischemia. (Topol EJ, Califf RM, Prystowsky EN, et al. *Topol Solution.* Wolters Kluwer Health and Pharma; 2006.)

Patient Presentation

- "Five P's" pulselessness, paralysis, paresthesia, pain, and pallor.[25]
- Claudication
- Pulse examination, including femoral, popliteal, DP, and PT pulses
- Arterial bruits
- Color, temperature, and integrity of the skin including capillary refill
- Dependent rubor
- Hair loss or hypertrophic nails
- Tissue loss or nonhealing ulceration
- Gangrene[26]

Evaluation

Ankle–brachial indices (ABIs) are frequently used for initial PAD screening due to low cost and availability (Fig. 30-9). The noninvasive measurement of blood flow using ankle and brachial systolic blood pressure can be assessed at the bedside or vascular lab. Ultrasonography is more accurate because it provides characterization of velocity wave forms and digit pressures, useful in patients with calcified vessels. Patients with diabetes or renal failure have noncompressible arteries, leading to a falsely elevated ABI. An ABI of 1.4 or higher indicates a falsely elevated level from noncompressible vessels and is associated with cardiovascular events and lower quality of life. The lower the ABI, the more restrictive the arterial blood flow, with mild claudication presenting with a range of 0.7 to 0.8.[26]

ANKLE–BRACHIAL INDEX RANGES

ABI 0.9–1.2	Normal
ABI 0.6–0.9	Mild
ABI 0.4–0.6	Moderate
ABI < 0.4	Severe

- Exercise ABI. Recommended for patients with normal resting ABI and a strong suspicion of claudication symptoms to differentiate between diminished arterial supply versus nerve or musculoskeletal disorders. A drop of 20% or greater is indicative of PAD.[27]
- Pulse volume recording (PVR) is a record of brachial and arterial waveforms with velocities at different levels in the legs, including the high thigh, low thigh, calf, ankle, and foot. Segmental pressures and waveforms are analyzed to identify the level and severity of disease.[28]
- CTA
- MRA
- Angiogram

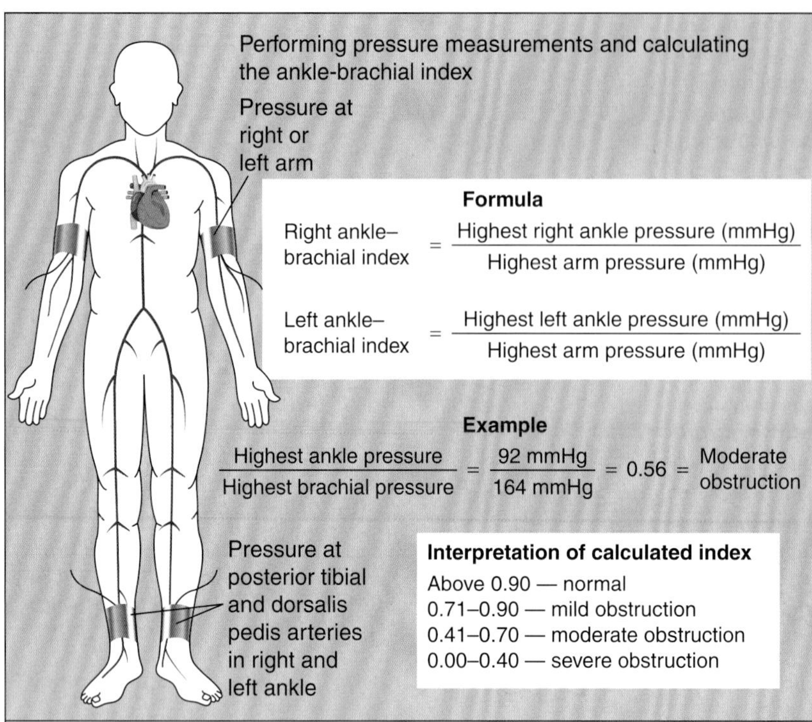

To calculate the ankle-brachial index, systolic pressures are determined in both arms and both ankles with the use of a hand-held Doppler instrument. The highest readings for the dorsalis pedis and posterior tibial arteries are used to calculate the index.

Figure 30-9. Performing pressure measurements and calculating the ankle-brachial index. (From White C. Intermittent claudication. *N Engl J Med.* 2007;356:1241–1250, with permission.)

Management

Conservative management with risk factor modification and medications should be the primary therapy in patients with mild PAD. Smoking is the most important controllable risk factor, followed by uncontrolled diabetes, renal disease, sedentary lifestyle, and diets high in saturated fat. A simple goal of any lower extremity exercise, such as walking 30 minutes a day, three to four times a week can improve quality of life.[29] Cilostazol (Pletal) and pentoxifylline (Trental) are the two medications used to treat claudication. They work by dilating the arteries and preventing platelet aggregation. Cilostazol is noted to be superior to pentoxifylline in meta-analysis studies, increasing walking distance in approximately 75% of patients after 12 weeks of treatment.[30]

Guidelines for initial mild PAD management are as follows:

- Refer to smoking cessation program
- Treatment of hypertension with blood pressure reduced to less than 140/90 mm Hg
- Control diabetes mellitus with the hemoglobin A_{1c} level reduced to less than 7.0%
- Treat dyslipidemia and reduce serum low-density lipoprotein cholesterol to less than 70 mg/dL
- Antiplatelet drug therapy with aspirin or clopidogrel
- Treatment with an angiotensin-converting enzyme inhibitor (ACE-I)
- Treatment with β-blockers in patients with coronary artery disease in the absence of contraindications to these drugs
- Use of statins
- Treatment with cilostazol in patients with intermittent claudication
- Exercise rehabilitation program
- Foot care to monitor for nonhealing wounds and or skin perfusion
- Low saturated fat diet

Indications for lower extremity percutaneous transluminal angioplasty or bypass surgery include:

1. Incapacitating claudication in persons interfering with work or lifestyle
2. Limb salvage in persons with limb-threatening ischemia as manifested by rest pain, nonhealing ulcers, and/or infection or gangrene
3. Vasculogenic impotence

Amputation of lower extremities should be performed for tissue loss that has progressed beyond the point of salvage, intractable pain, low life expectancy, or if surgery is too risky or functional limitations diminish the benefit of limb salvage.[26]

Surgical Management

Revascularization is considered for three main clinical presentations: claudication, critical limb ischemia, and acute limb ischemia. Patients with claudication that fail to risk modification, exercise, and medical therapy typically will benefit from endovascular procedures. Historically, endovascular therapy is preferred for focal lesions, whereas more extensive or long disease segments require open repair. However, technologic advances in equipment have increased options for more complex disease. A combination of techniques can be used for lesions, including atherectomy, balloon angioplasty, and/or stent. Atherectomy is indicated for crossing chronic total occlusions or debulking plaque and is typically used in combination with angioplasty or stenting. Certain regions or lesions dictate preferred treatment techniques. Regions that may increase stent fracture or have repeated compression such as the common femoral or popliteal arteries are not typically treated with a stent. The aortic bifurcation is a common area for atherosclerosis and can be treated with endostents for nonocclusive or less complex disease, especially patients at high risk for open repair.[31] Atherosclerosis involving the anterior tibial, posterior tibial, and peroneal arteries, otherwise known as infrapopliteal disease, has a higher incidence of restenosis and occlusion with stents.[32] Stents are commonly utilized to treat focal and nonocclusive iliac and superficial femoral arterial segments. Initial success of endovascular procedures is lower with occlusions and longer lesions and is more consistently associated with restenosis.[32] An endovascular-first approach for complex disease has gained popularity over the last decade. An important limitation of balloon angioplasty or stenting remains the occurrence of restenosis. Drug-coated balloons and stents have emerged as a new technology to address restenosis. These devices are coated with paclitaxel, a chemotherapy agent that inhibits neointimal growth of vascular smooth muscle cells, potentially limiting restenosis. Current evidence suggests these devices are safe and efficient in increasing patency rates. However, it remains unknown whether these improved results can translate into long-term beneficial clinical outcomes.[33]

Open Repair

Aortobifemoral bypass (ABF) is the most common open surgical procedure to treat aortoiliac disease. It is a durable, but major abdominal surgery that uses a prosthetic graft to connect the aorta to the femoral arteries to increase blood flow to the legs. Preoperative assessment includes cardiac evaluation and/or pulmonary function tests for lung disease. Surgical risks include: bleeding, infection, respiratory failure, heart attack, stroke, renal failure, and/or death. It requires postoperative intensive care, approximately a week hospital stay and 2 to 3 months for full recovery. This surgery is reserved for patients with debilitating claudication or critical lower extremity ischemia.[34]

Axillobifemoral bypass or less common thoracofemoral bypasses are anatomic bypasses that treat aortoiliac disease. They are less invasive and require a small clavicle incision and groin incision. A graft is connected from the axillary artery to the femoral arteries, and is an alternative for patients that are too high risk for an ABF. Surgical risks are lower and recovery is much quicker, but they are less durable, with a higher incidence of graft thrombosis and infection compared to an ABF.[35]

Leg bypass is an open arterial reconstruction that bypasses blockages in the leg. A leg bypass may be recommended for patients with lifestyle-limiting claudication or critical limb ischemia that are not candidates for endovascular techniques. The principles of surgical revascularization are based on inflow, outflow, and conduit. The goal is to provide in-line flow to target vessels. Arterial supply such as the common femoral, deep femoral, profunda, or popliteal are common inflow sites. Inflow vessels (the artery from which the bypass will originate) must have adequate flow, pressure, and allow for suturing. Significant atherosclerotic disease of inflow arteries may require adjunctive procedures such as endarterectomies to ensure adequate blood supply to the bypass. Distal target vessels (outflow) may include any artery that is distal to the blockages, but commonly include the popliteal, posterior tibial, anterior tibial, or peroneal.[36] The outflow vessel should be the least diseased artery with dominant blood supply to the foot.

The autologous vein remains the preferred conduit for surgical revascularization. Doppler studies with vein mapping of the great and small saphenous veins, sometimes cephalic veins, will determine if patients have an acceptable vein. The ipsilateral vein is preferred and should be noncalcified, nonsclerotic, and 2.5 mm or greater in diameter. Prosthetic grafts, such as polytetrafluorethylene (PTFE) may be used if there are no acceptable veins available. Patency rates vary depending on level of disease, length of bypass, conduit, and risk factors.[37] Many studies have attempted to determine the best techniques for lower extremity bypasses. Data obtained from multiple sources revealed 77% of femoral to above-knee popliteal bypasses with vein were patent at 5 years compared to 50% with prosthetic graft. These patency rates drop with femoral to infrapopliteal bypasses: vein 74% and 18% with prosthetic conduit at 5 years.[38]

Lower extremity bypass requires an average hospital stay of 3 to 5 days and fully recovered in 4 to 8 weeks. Like most invasive surgical procedures, risks include heart attack, infection, bleeding, respiratory failure, or death. Extremities should be monitored for nonhealing wounds, temperature, color, sensation changes, loss of pulses, or any evidence of incisional infection. Some postoperative pain and swelling is expected, particularly pedal edema that gradually improves over a few weeks following bypass.

Long-term management for any lower extremity revascularization includes optimal medical management and modifying risk factors. Medications should include lipid lowering and antiplatelet therapy. Other medications, such as cilostazol may be added for patients with persistent claudication. Controlling hypertension and diabetes along with an exercise program is recommended. Smoking cessation remains the most crucial factor, increasing the chance of graft failure threefold compared to patients who quit smoking.[39] Routine follow-up with Doppler studies is recommended. Arterial imaging including graft surveillance and ABI monitors patency of stents, grafts, and blood vessels. Abnormal velocities can detect failing grafts or stents, allowing for early intervention and prevent occlusions.[40]

Determining an optimal revascularization strategy for patients with symptomatic lower extremity PAD requires integration of surgeon and patient preferences, available resources, patient comorbidity, and relevant anatomy. Given availability of both endovascular and open revascularization options, we show that an endovascular approach is associated with improved long-term amputation free survival. There is initially an increased risk of subsequent intervention after an endovascular procedure; however, this risk is modest and confined to the first 30 days after primary intervention. As always, the selection of interventions cannot be generalized and should be individualized for each patient based upon multiple factors and local expertise.[41]

CONCLUSION

PAD is a distinct subtype of atherosclerotic disease that is associated with considerable morbidity, frailty, poor quality of life, and high medical costs. It is a disease that often goes unrecognized due to lack of awareness and gradually deteriorating symptoms that are often contributed to other causes or old age. As our population ages, so will the incidence of PAD. Early detection, controlling risk factors, and optimizing medical management will continue to be mainstay of treatment. The management of PAD continues to change on the basis of current trials and advanced diagnostic and treatment strategies. Advancing technologies are rapidly evolving and outcomes are steadily improving. The complexity and chronicity of PAD will continue to require a multidisciplinary approach, but with proper diagnosis and treatment, patients can still enjoy a quality life.

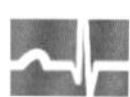

CASE STUDY 1

Patient Profile

Name/Age/Sex: **Matthew Sample, 62-year-old male**

History of Present Illness

Mr. Sample was referred to vascular surgery for left-sided neck bruit on routine physical exam. He is a current smoker and admits to a sedentary lifestyle. He does not follow any types of diet and eats a wide variety of food. He feels stressed at work daily. Review of systems the patient denies any evidence of amaurosis fugax, difficulty with speech, or unilateral weakness. He has no prior history of stroke or TIA.

Past Medical History

Kidney stones, CAD with MI and PTCA 2014, HTN, HLD, Obesity, borderline DM HgB A1C 5.8

Surgical History

PTCA 2014

Family History

Father died age 72 with ruptured aneurysm, CAD with CABG. Mother has HLD, osteoporosis. Brother HLD and COPD

Social History

1 PPD smoker (44 Pack-Year History), no EtOH, no illicit drug use. Married, 2 grown children. Eats fast food for lunch every workday.

Medications

Metoprolol 50 MG QD, Lipitor 20 mg QD, and aspirin.

Allergies

None

Patient Examination

Vital Signs

BP 148/88; BMI 32.6

Physical Examination

General: Awake, alert, and oriented. No distress noted. Appears younger than stated age. No neurologic deficits

Skin: Intact, warm, dry. No rashes or lesions are noted.

Cardiac: No murmurs, gallops, or rubs are auscultated. S1 and S2 are heard and are of normal intensity. +R carotid bruit, Pulse exam within normal limits. +2 radial, +2 DP, and +2 PT pulses bilaterally. Aorta prominent and pulsatile.

Respiratory: Clear to auscultation bilaterally.

Abdominal: Abdomen is soft, symmetric, and nontender without distention. No masses, hepatomegaly, or splenomegaly are noted.

Psychiatric: Appropriate mood and affect. Good judgment and insight.

Testing

Total cholesterol 220; HDL 35; LDL 145; Triglycerides 155
Carotid Doppler revealed: Right peak systolic velocity of internal carotid artery/end diastolic 312/110 cm/s; ICA/CCA ratio 4.74 80–99% stenosis
Left peak systolic velocity of internal carotid artery/end diastolic 88/22 cm/s; ICA/CCA ratio 1.2 less than 39% stenosis
CTA carotids revealed: High-grade 88% stenosis of proximal right internal carotid artery. Left internal carotid artery 30% stenosis.

Considerations

Key Questions

What would your recommendations be to the patient based on family history and clinical findings during his workup?

Evidence

Per the 2016 AHA/ACC Guideline on the Management of Patients With Lower Extremity Peripheral Artery Disease
Right carotid endarterectomy can be considered as well as the following

Recommendations

Abdominal Doppler screening for abdominal aortic aneurysm
Dietary counseling/Mediterranean DASH diet
Avoid fast foods and processed foods
Increase physical activity walk briskly around job site instead of driving cart. Exercise 5× week at least 15 minutes to target HR.
Weight loss BMI less than 24.9
Optimize blood pressure less than 130 systolic less than 70 diastolic, add ACE-I
Lipid management with statin, increase dose
Smoking cessation and counseling

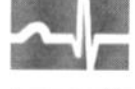

CASE STUDY 2

Patient Profile

Name/Age/Sex: **Judy Applebaum, 70-year-old female**

History of Present Illness

Ms. Applebaum, a 70-year-old female was referred to vascular surgery for leg pain and lower extremity diminished pulses. She reports leg fatigue and calf cramping after 15 minutes of walking, right leg worse than left × 1 year. Her right leg symptoms have gotten worse in the last month, right foot leg feels weak after 5 minutes of walking associated with foot numbness. She wears warm socks to bed because her feet get cold, but she is able to sleep through the night without any leg pain. She has a history of heavy smoking 2 packs × 10 years in her 20 years, then ¼ pack per day × 30 years with brief intermittent periods of cessation. She cleans her house, does yard work, but has never exercised. In general, she doesn't have a lot of stamina, gets short of breath, she contributes this to getting older. Avoids going the doctor, unless she has too.

Past Medical History

Hyperlipidemia, depression, osteoarthritis

Surgical History

Breast mass with surgical excision, benign. Hysterectomy for uterine fibroids

Family History

Father died of MI age 68, Mother still living in fair health, had breast cancer. Younger brother has CAD, s/p CABG.

Social History

Divorced. No alcohol. Current smoker. Retired clerk. Cooks for herself occasionally, but eats a lot of frozen dinners.

Medications

Crestor 10 mg QD, Lexapro 10 mg QD

Allergies

None

CASE STUDY 2 (*Continued*)

Patient Examination

Vital Signs

BP 132/76; BMI 22

Physical Examination

General: Awake, alert, and oriented. No distress noted. Appears younger than stated age. No neurologic deficits.

Skin: Intact, warm, dry. No rashes or lesions are noted

Cardiac: No murmurs, gallops, or rubs are auscultated. S1 and S2 are heard and are of normal intensity +2 femoral pulses bilaterally, nonpalpable right DP and PT pulses, L +1 DP +1 PT pulses. Feet are warm to touch with delayed R capillary refill, no wounds. L less than 3 seconds capillary refill.

Respiratory: Clear to auscultation bilaterally

Abdominal: Abdomen is soft, symmetric, and nontender without distention. No masses, hepatomegaly, or splenomegaly is noted.

Psychiatric: Appropriate mood and affect. Good judgment and insight.

Testing

Total cholesterol 188; HDL 45; LDL 126; Triglycerides 190
ABI's Right 0.48; TBI 0.22; Left 0.75; TBI 0.54
CTA abdomen with runoff revealed: Moderate aorto iliac disease without significant stenosis.
Right: Patent common femoral with severe stenosis. R superficial femoral artery occlusion. Patent popliteal with mild to moderate stenosis. Anterior tibial occlusion. 2 vessel runoff via peroneal and posterior tibial runoff.
Left: Patent common femoral with mild stenosis. Left superficial femoral artery occlusion. Patent popliteal with mild stenosis. Peroneal occlusion. 2 vessel runoff via anterior tibial and posterior tibial.

Considerations

Key Questions

What would your recommendations be to the patient based on family history and clinical findings during his workup?

Evidence

Per the 2016 AHA/ACC Guideline on the Management of Patients With Lower Extremity Peripheral Artery Disease

Treatment

Right common femoral endarterectomy and right superficial femoral artery stent. Left superficial femoral artery stent vs. optimal medical management and observation after right leg intervention.

Recommendations

Exercise program 5× week, walking or physical activity of choice at least 15 minutes a day, working up to 30 minutes per day.
Dietary counseling/Mediterranean DASH diet.
Avoid processed foods, eat more fresh fruits, vegetables, and lean proteins.
Cardiac stress test, considering significant family history, risk factors, and recent diagnosis of peripheral arterial disease.
Smoking cessation and counseling.
Add Plavix and aspirin therapy.

KEY READINGS

Aboyans V, Sevestre MA, Desormais I, et al. Epidemiology of lower extremity arterial disease. *Presse Med.* 2018;47(1):38–46. Available at https://www.ncbi.nlm.nih.gov/pubmed/29449058

Eslami MH, Pounds LC. Carotid artery disease. *Soc Vasc Surg.* Available at https://vascular.org/patient-resources/vascular-conditions/carotid-artery-disease

Society for Vascular Surgery Lower Extremity Guidelines Writing Group; Conte MS, Pomposelli FB, Clair DG, et al. Society for Vascular Surgery practice guidelines for atherosclerotic occlusive disease of the lower extremities: management of asymptomatic disease and claudication. *J Vasc Surg.* 2015;61(3):2S–41S.

REFERENCES

1. Hardman RL, Jazaeri O, Yi J, et al. Overview of classification of symptoms of peripheral arterial disease. *Semin Intervent Radiol.* 2014;31(4):378–388.
2. Centers for Disease Control and Prevention. *Peripheral Arterial Disease.* Updated December 19, 2019. Available at https://www.cdc.gov/dhdsp/data_statistics/fact_sheets/fs_pad.htm. Accessed December 20, 2019.
3. Wilson S, Veith F, Hobson R, et al. Vascular surgery. *Princ Pract.* 1987;2:12–13.
4. Singh RB, Mengi SA, Xu YJ, et al. Pathogenesis of atherosclerosis: a mutifactorial process. *Exp Clin Cardiol.* 2002;7(1):40–53.
5. Zohrabian D, Brenner BE. *Carotid artery dissection.* 2017. Available at https://emedicine.medscape.com/article/757906-overview
6. Mozzafarian D, Benjamin EJ, Go AS, et al; on behalf of the American Heart Association Statistics Committee and Stroke Statistics Subcommittee. Heart disease and stroke statistics—2016 update: a report from the American Heart Association. *Circulation.* 2016;133(4):e38–360.
7. Noiphithak R, Liengudom A. Recent update on carotid endarterectomy versus carotid stenting. *Cerebrovasc Dis.* 2017;43(1–2):68–75.
8. Prasad K. Pathophysiology and medical treatment of carotid stenosis. *Inte J Angiol.* 2015;24(3):158–172.
9. Adla T, Adlova R. Multimodality imaging of carotid stenosis. *Int J Angiol.* 2015;24(3):179–184.
10. Haggani O, Rowe VL. *Carotid endarterectomy.* 2018. Available at https://emedicine.medscape.com/article/1895291-overview
11. Ricotta JJ, AbuRahma A, Ascher E. Updated Society for Vascular Surgery guidelines for management of extracranial carotid disease. *J Vasc Surg.* 2011;54(3):e1–e31.
12. Aziz F. *Carotid artery stenting.* 2018. Available at https://emedicine.medscape.com/article/1839544-overview#a3
13. Pounds L. Carotid endarterectomy. *Soc Vasc Surg.* Available at https://vascular.org/patient-resources/vascular-treatments/carotid-endarterectomy
14. The National Institute of Diabetes and Digestive and Kidney Diseases Health Information Center. *Renal artery stenosis.* Available at https://www.niddk.nih.gov/health-information/kidney-disease/renal-artery-stenosis
15. Bokhari MR, Bokhari RA. *Renal artery stenosis.* 2018. Available at https://www.ncbi.nlm.nih.gov/books/NBK430718/
16. Spinowitz BS, Batuman V. *Renal artery stenosis* guidelines. 2018. Available at https://emedicine.medscape.com/article/245023-guidelines.
17. Cronenwett JL, Johnston KW. *Rutherfords Vascular Surgery.* Vol 2. 7th ed. Philadelphia, PA: Saunders-Elsevier; 2010:2196–2198.
18. Clair DG, Beach JM. Mesenteric ischemia. *N Engl J Med.* 2016;374:959–968.
19. Dang CV, Geibel J. *Acute mesenteric ischemia.* 2018. Available at https://emedicine.medscape.com/article/189146-overview#a7
20. Tendler DA, Lamont JT. Chronic mesenteric ischemia. *UpToDate.* 2017. Available at https://www.uptodate.com/contents/chronic-mesenteric-ischemia
21. Alrayes A, Cagir B. *Chronic mesenteric ischemia workup.* 2017. Available at https://emedicine.medscape.com/article/183683-workup#c6
22. Harris L, Dryjski M. *Epidemiology, risk factors, and natural history of peripheral arterial disease.* 2018. Available at https://www.uptodate.com/contents/epidemiology-risk-factors-and-natural-history-of-peripheral-artery-disease
23. Morley RL, Sharma A, Horsch A. Peripheral arterial disease. *BMJ.* 2018;360. doi:https://doi.org/10.1136/bmj.j5842. Accessed February 1, 2018.
24. Stephens E. *Peripheral vascular disease clinical presentation.* 2017. Available at https://emedicine.medscape.com/article/761556-clinical

25. Lepäntalo M, Fiengo L, Biancari F. Peripheral arterial disease in diabetic patients with renal insufficiency: a review. *Diabetes Metab Res Rev.* 2012;28:40–45.
26. Aronow WS. *Peripheral arterial disease of the lower extremities.* 2012. Available at https://www.ncbi.nlm.nih.gov/pmc/articles/PMC3361053/
27. Hammand TA, Hiatt WR, Gornik HL, et al. Prognostic value of an increase in post-exercise ankle–brachial index. *Vasc Med.* 2017;22(3): 204–209.
28. Gerhard-Herman M, Beckman JA, Creager MA. *Vascular laboratory testing.* 2017. Available at https://www.sciencedirect.com/sdfe/pdf/download/eid/3-s2.0-B9781437729306000124/first-page-pdf
29. Barnes G. *Society for vascular surgery guidelines for peripheral artery disease management | Ten points to remember.* American College of Cardiology. 2015. Available at https://www.acc.org/latest-in-cardiology/ten-points-to-remember/2015/03/20/00/48/society-for-vascular-surgery-practice-guidelines-for-atherosclerotic
30. Chi YW, Lavie CJ, Milani RV, et al. Safety and efficacy of cilostazol in the management of intermittent claudication. *Vasc Health Risk Manag.* 2008;4(6):1197–1203.
31. Nagarsheth KH, Rowe VL. Area occlusive disease treatment and management. *Medscape.* 2017. Available at https://emedicine.medscape.com/article/461285-treatment#d10
32. Thukkani AK, Kinlay S. Endovascular intervention for peripheral arterial disease. *Circ Res.* 2015;116(9):1599–1613.
33. Barkat M, Torella F, Antoniou GA. Drug eluting balloon catheters for lower extremity peripheral arterial disease: the evidence up to date. *Vascu Health Risk Manag.* 2016;12:199–208.
34. Shabir B, Rowe VL. *Aortobifemoral bypass technique.* 2018. Available at https://emedicine.medscape.com/article/1830241-technique
35. Mishall PL, Matakas JD, English K, et al. Axillobifemoral bypass: a brief surgical and historical review. *Einstein J Biol Med.* 2016;31(1–2): 6–10.
36. Lee CJ. *Infrapopliteal disease.* 2017. Available at https://emedicine.medscape.com/article/1895511-overview#a4
37. Park KM, Kim YW, Yang SS, et al. Comparison between prosthetic vascular graft and saphenous vein graft in above-knee popliteal bypass. *Ann Surg Treat Res.* 2014;87(1):35–40.
38. Shishehbor MH, White CJ, Gray BH. Critical limb ischemia: an expert statement. *J Am Cardiol.* 2016;68(18):2002–2015.
39. Willigendael EM, Teijink JAW, Bartelink ML. Smoking and the patency of lower extremity bypass grafts: a meta-analysis. *J Vasc Surg.* 2005;42(1): 67–74.
40. Park KM, Park YJ, Shin-Seok Y, et al. Treatment of failing vein grafts in patients who underwent lower extremity bypass. *J Korean Surg Soc.* 2012; 83(5):307–315.
41. Wiseman JT, Fernandes-Taylor S, Saha S, et al. Endovascular versus open revascularization for peripheral arterial disease. *Ann Surg.* 2017;265(2): 424–430.

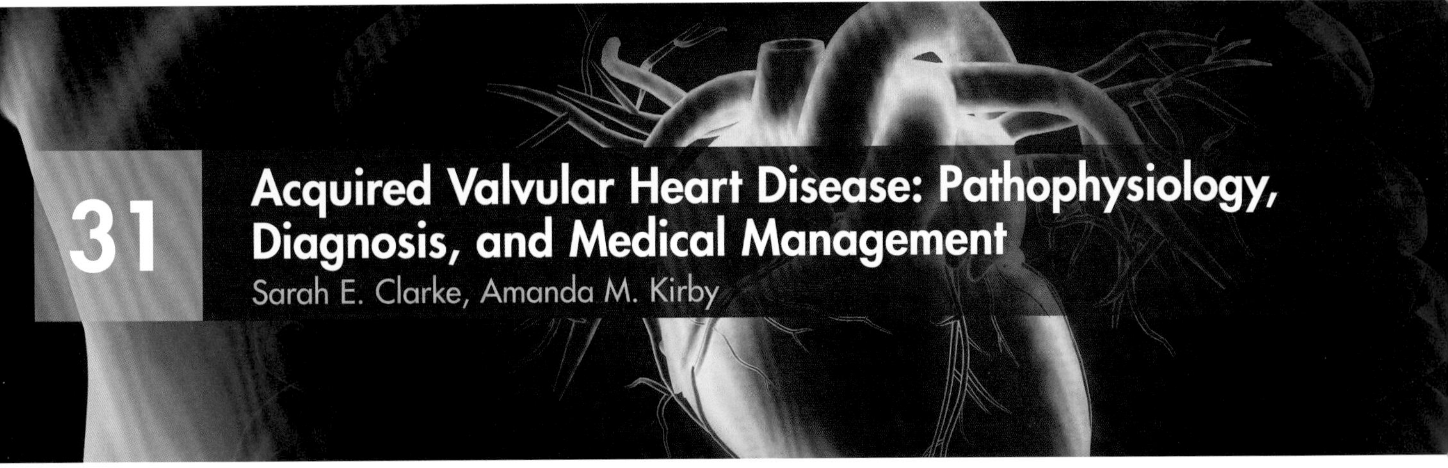

31 Acquired Valvular Heart Disease: Pathophysiology, Diagnosis, and Medical Management

Sarah E. Clarke, Amanda M. Kirby

OBJECTIVES

1. Define the normal function, pathology, and assessment of the aortic, mitral, and tricuspid valves.
2. Describe the appropriate evaluation techniques and rationale for testing each valvular dysfunction.
3. Understand the current evidence-based practices for diagnosis and treatment for valvular heart disease (VHD).

KEY QUESTIONS

1. What are the typical clinical manifestations for patients with VHD?
2. Which diagnostic tests can be helpful in assessing patients with VHD?
3. Which document would you reference to investigate the stages of VHD?

GENERAL PRINCIPLES

Valvular heart disease (VHD) continues to be a common source of cardiac dysfunction and mortality. In fact, the number of patients with VHD in developed countries is growing due to the aging population, enhanced awareness of various treatments, as well as improved noninvasive imaging tests. Timely referrals and development of a treatment strategy provides an opportunity for improved outcomes and preservation of cardiac function. Some treatment recommendations are straightforward; however, certain disease processes and select patient populations require more thoughtful decision-making processes. Guidelines support the management of such patients and/or complex severe VHD is best achieved by an interdisciplinary Heart Team.[1]

Mechanisms of Dysfunction

Competent cardiac valves maintain unidirectional flow of blood through the heart as well as to the pulmonary and systemic circulations. Diseased cardiac valves that restrict the forward flow of blood because they are unable to open fully are referred to as *stenotic*. Stenotic valves elevate afterload and cause hypertrophy of the atria or ventricles pumping against the increased pressure. Cardiac valves that close incompetently and permit the backward flow of blood are referred to as *regurgitant, incompetent,* or *insufficient.* Regurgitant valves cause an elevated volume load and dilation of the cardiac chambers receiving the blood reflux. Valvular dysfunction may be primarily stenotic or regurgitant, or may be "mixed," which refers to a valve that neither opens nor closes adequately.

Duration and Severity of Dysfunction

VHD is usually described by the duration of the dysfunction (acute vs. chronic), the valves involved, and the nature of the valvular dysfunction (stenosis, insufficiency, or a combination of stenosis and insufficiency). The degree of cardiac dysfunction is defined by the New York Heart Association's (NYHA) Functional and Therapeutic Classification. This chapter focuses on the mitral, aortic valves, and tricuspid valve disease. Pulmonic disease is primarily congenital; therefore, it is described in Chapter 33.

Patient Education

Patient education is an essential health intervention to promote self-care or change health behaviors, but assessing patient understanding and effectiveness of the intervention can be challenging. Patient education formats vary depending on the degree of standardization versus individualization. The mode of information transfer has evolved and can include but not be limited to verbal instructions, written communication, videos, podcasts, websites, games, applications, and even social media. Patient education is critical to facilitate shared decision making. The goal(s) of patient education are vast and typically include: to inform the patient about their disease process, diagnostic tests that are relevant to assess the disease process, risk and benefits of the treatment options, expectation for progression or recovery, monitoring of signs and symptoms readmission avoidance, performance of specific health behaviors, and post hospital discharge recovery period and follow-up.

Shared Decision Making

Due to the increasing complexity of VHD management strategies and therapies, there is an increased interest by clinicians in shared decision making between patient and healthcare providers.

In parallel, hospitals are being challenged to make high-quality and safe services more transparent and efficient and this need requires new models and ways of thinking about how health services are delivered. Lastly, clinical guidelines are evolving from verbiage that supports informed patient preferences[2] to choice of valve prosthetics should be a "shared decision process."[1] In current clinical practice, patients who require valve replacement often experience decisional conflict and suboptimal involvement.[3] The majority of patients want to be involved in prosthetic valve selection, while significantly fewer patients actually feel involved. There is a discernible need for improved information conveyance on treatment options and their associated risks and benefits.[4,5] Nurses are key patient advisors and counselors in practice settings where shared decision making is an increasing expectation.

CAUSES OF ACQUIRED VHD

Rheumatic Heart Disease

Rheumatic fever is an acute autoimmune disorder that results as a complication of streptococcal upper respiratory tract infections. Tissues involved in rheumatic fever include the lining and valves of the heart, skin, and connective tissue (Fig. 31-1). The group A β-hemolytic streptococcal organism is responsible for initial and recurrent attacks of rheumatic fever. Lymphatic channels from the tonsils are thought to transmit group A streptococci to the heart.

The incidence of rheumatic fever has declined to less than 1/100,000 in industrialized nations but remains higher than 100/100,000 in endemic, less-developed countries. Reasons for the decline in rheumatic fever include the use of antibiotics to treat and prevent streptococcal infections, as well as improved social conditions such as decreased crowding, better housing and sanitation, and access to health care. Rheumatic fever persists in underdeveloped countries in which socioeconomic conditions enable the spread of streptococcal bacteria and limit access to adequate health care.[6] Acute rheumatic fever involves diffuse

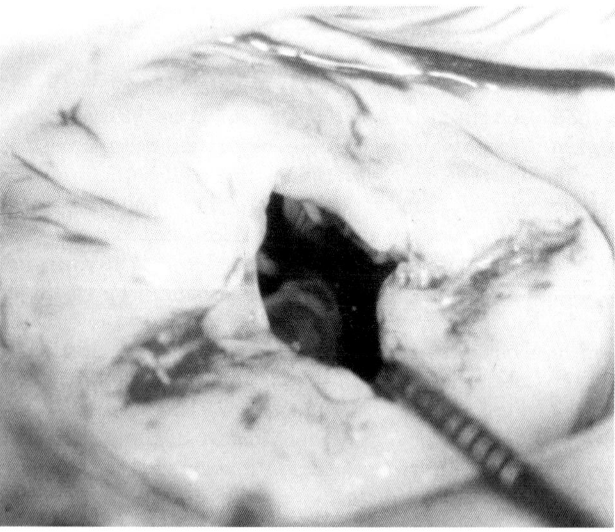

Figure 31-1. Rheumatic mitral valve with leaflet thickening and commissural fusion. (From Alpert JS, Sabick J, Cosgrove DM. Mitral valve disease. In: Topol EJ, Califf RM, Isner JM, et al., eds. *Textbook of Cardiovascular Medicine*. Philadelphia, PA: Lippincott-Raven; 1998:511.)

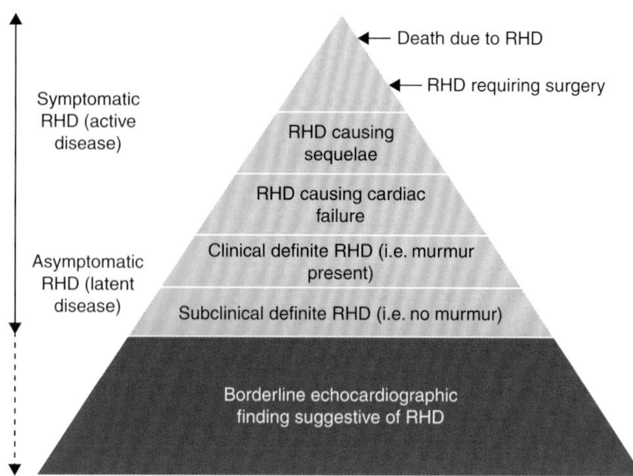

Figure 31-2. Asymptomatic and symptomatic rheumatic heart disease. (Adapted from Beaton A, Engelman D, Mirabel M. *Acute Rheumatic Fever and Rheumatic Heart Disease*. Philadelphia, PA: Elsevier; 2021.)

exudative and proliferative inflammatory reactions in the heart, joints, and skin. There are obvious distinctions between asymptomatic and symptomatic rheumatic heart disease, which can be reviewed in Figure 31-2.[6] Active disease begins with increasing symptoms including cardiac failure and ultimately leads to surgery and in some patients potential for recurrence of rheumatic fever.

Jones criteria, based on expert opinion rather than clinical trials, were introduced in 1944 for the diagnosis of rheumatic fever. Major diagnostic criteria include carditis, polyarthritis, chorea, erythema marginatum (pink skin rash), and subcutaneous nodules. Minor criteria include arthralgia, fever, and elevated C-reactive protein. Figure 31-3 outlines the current Jones criteria for rheumatic heart disease.[7]

Auscultatory signs of aortic and mitral insufficiency are frequently apparent. In more than 90% of patients with carditis, the mitral valve is affected. When the mitral valve is affected, there may be a high-pitched, blowing, pansystolic murmur. A Carey Coombs murmur, a low-pitched, mid-diastolic murmur of short duration, may be noted at the apex. The Carey Coombs murmur may be attributed to swelling and stiffening of mitral valve leaflets, increased flow across the valve, and alteration in left ventricular compliance.

Infective Endocarditis

Infective endocarditis is an endovascular infection that supports continuous bacteremia from the source of the infection, usually a vegetation, on a heart valve. While endocarditis is uncommon, affecting only 10,000 to 20,000 people in the United States each year, it may result in serious complications such as stroke, need for surgery, and death.[1] Although incidence of infective endocarditis is low, between 1.5 and 6 cases per 100 cases per year, morbidity and mortality are high. There is also an inhospital mortality of 15% to 20% and 1-year mortality of as much as 40%.[8] Rheumatic heart disease, calcific aortic stenosis, hypertrophic cardiomyopathy, congenital heart disease, and the presence of prosthetic heart valves predispose to endocarditis. Intravenous drug abusers are at risk for infective endocarditis caused by recurrent bacteremias related to injection from contaminated needles and localized infections at injection sites. Patients with long-term intravenous

A. For all patient populations with evidence of preceding GAS infection	
Diagnosis: initial ARF	2 Major manifestations or 1 major plus 2 minor manifestations
Diagnosis: recurrent ARF	2 Major or 1 major and 2 minor or 3 minor
B. Major criteria	
Low-risk populations*	Moderate- and high-risk populations
Carditis† • Clinical and/or subclinical	Carditis • Clinical and/or subclinical
Arthritis • Polyarthritis only	Arthritis • Monoarthritis or polyarthritis • Polyarthralgia‡
Chorea	Chorea
Erythema marginatum	Erythema marginatum
Subcutaneous nodules	Subcutaneous nodules
C. Minor criteria	
Low-risk populations*	Moderate- and high-risk populations
Polyarthralgia	Monoarthralgia
Fever (≥38.5°C)	Fever (≥38°C)
ESR ≥60 mm in the first hour and/or CRP ≥3.0 mg/dL§	ESR ≥30 mm/h and/or CRP ≥3.0 mg/dL§
Prolonged PR interval, after accounting for age variability (unless carditis is a major criterion)	Prolonged PR interval, after accounting for age variability (unless carditis is a major criterion)

ARF indicates acute rheumatic fever; CRP, C-reactive protein; ESR, erythrocyte sedimentation rate; and GAS, group A streptococcal infection.

*Low-risk populations are those with ARF incidence ≤2 per 100000 school-aged children or all-age rheumatic heart disease prevalence of ≤1 per 1000 population per year.

†Subclinical carditis indicates echocardiographic valvulitis as defined in Table 3.

‡See section on polyarthralgia, which should only be considered as a major manifestation in moderate- to high-risk populations after exclusion of other causes. As in past versions of the criteria, erythema marginatum and subcutaneous nodules are rarely "stand-alone" major criteria. Additionally, joint manifestations can only be considered in either the major or minor categories but not both in the same patient.

§CRP value must be greater than upper limit of normal for laboratory. Also, because ESR may evolve during the course of ARF, peak ESR values should be used.

Figure 31-3. Jones criteria for rheumatic heart disease. (Reprinted with permission from Kumar D, Bhutia E, Kumar P, et al. Evaluation of the American Heart Association 2015 revised Jones criteria versus existing guidelines. *Heart Asia.* 2016;8[1]:30–35.)

lines or dialysis catheters are also at increased risk. Acute endocarditis can also occur in normal heart valves from infection somewhere else in the body. In patients with community-acquired, native valve endocarditis, *Staphylococcus aureus* is the most common causative pathogen.[9] Pathogens that are most commonly responsible for subacute endocarditis include streptococci, enterococci, coagulase-negative staphylococci, and the HACEK group of organisms (*Haemophilus* species, *Actinobacillus actinomycetemcomitans*, *Cardiobacterium hominis*, *Eikenella* species, and *Kingella kingae*). Clinical presentations of endocarditis range from fever and malaise to symptoms related to systemic emboli (Table 31-1).

Diagnosis is made based on the widely accepted and utilized Modified Duke criteria seen in Figure 31-4.[9]

Blood cultures are an essential diagnostic tool in infective endocarditis. Three separate sets of blood cultures drawn from different venipuncture sites, obtained over 24 hours, usually identify the organism. Patients with infective endocarditis whose cultures remain negative may have fastidious organisms or may have received intravenous antibiotics before blood samples were drawn. In acute endocarditis, antibiotic therapy should be started after blood cultures have been obtained using strict aseptic technique and optimal skin preparation.[9] The clinical approach in acute endocarditis includes appropriate antibiotics and monitoring for complications (Display 31-1). The usual course is 6 full weeks of intravenous antibiotics. Patients who do not respond well to standard antibiotic therapy may be referred for surgical valve replacement (Display 31-2).

Table 31-1 • CLINICAL MANIFESTATIONS OF INFECTIVE ENDOCARDITIS

Symptoms	Physical Examination Findings
Fever	Fever
Chills and sweats	Changing or new heart murmur
Malaise	Evidence of systemic emboli
Weight loss	Splenomegaly
Anorexia Stroke symptoms	Janeway lesions (small hemorrhages on palms or soles of feet)
Myalgias Arthralgias	Splinter hemorrhages (hemorrhagic streaks at finger nail tips)
Confusion CHF	Osler nodules (small, tender nodules on finger or toe pads)

Definition of IE According to the Modified Duke Criteria*
Definite IE
Pathological criteria
Microorganisms demonstrated by culture or histological examination of a vegetation, a vegetation that has embolized, or an intracardiac abscess specimen; or pathological lesions; vegetation or intracardiac abscess confirmed by histological examination showing active endocarditis
Clinical criteria
2 Major criteria, 1 major criterion and 3 minor criteria, or 5 minor criteria
Possible IE
1 Major criterion and 1 minor criterion, or 3 minor criteria
Rejected
Firm alternative diagnosis explaining evidence of IE; or resolution of IE syndrome with antibiotic therapy for ≤4 d; or no pathological evidence of IE at surgery or autopsy with antibiotic therapy for ≤4 d; or does not meet criteria for possible IE as above

IE indicates infective endocarditis.

Modifications appear in boldface.

*These criteria have been universally accepted and are in current use.

Reprinted from Li et al[24] by permission of the Infectious Diseases Society of America. Copyright © 2000, the Infectious Diseases Society of America.

Figure 31-4. Definition of IE according to the modified Duke criteria. (Baddour LM, Wilson WR, Bayer AS, et al. Infective endocarditis in adults: diagnosis, antimicrobial therapy, and management of complications. *Circulation*. 2015;132[15]:1435–1486.)

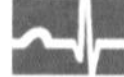 DISPLAY 31-1

Clinical Approach to Endocarditis

Establish diagnosis
- Blood cultures
- Physical examination findings
- Echocardiography
- Establish source that seeded endocarditis

Start appropriate antibiotics based on blood cultures
Monitor telemetry for conduction defects
Treat valvular regurgitation with afterload reduction agents
Repeat blood cultures 3 days after antibiotics started to ensure response
Insert long-term intravenous access for antibiotics
Monitor drug levels when appropriate
Monitor for systemic emboli

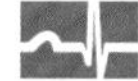 DISPLAY 31-2

Indications for Cardiac Surgery in Infective Endocarditis

Heart failure with hemodynamic instability
Persistent bacteremia and fever despite optimal antibiotic therapy
Paravalvular abscess or fistula
Recurrence of endocarditis after full course of antibiotics
Systemic emboli
Heart failure due to prosthetic valvular dysfunction
Valve dehiscence (in prosthetic valvular endocarditis)
New conduction system defects
Fungal endocarditis

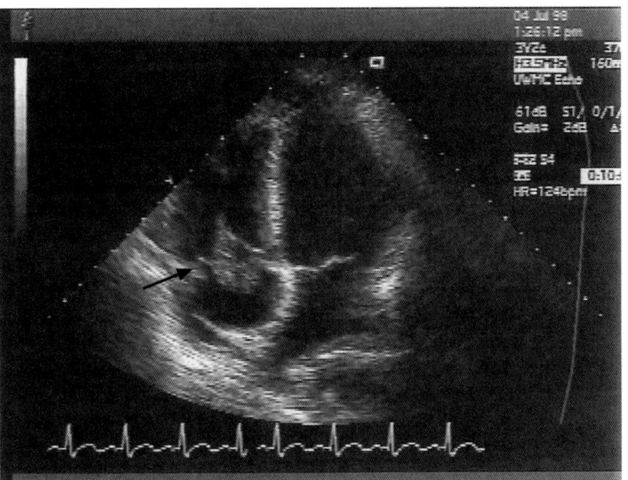

Figure 31-5. Transesophageal echocardiography (TEE). Two-dimensional echocardiogram view of vegetation on tricuspid valve in 27-year-old woman with endocarditis (*arrow*).

Echocardiography is frequently used to verify the presence of vegetations on the valves (Fig. 31-5). A transesophageal echocardiogram (TEE) provides better resolution and can identify smaller vegetations than a transthoracic echocardiogram (TTE). TEE is also useful to identify paravalvular leaks and annular abscesses seen in prosthetic valve endocarditis.[1] Echocardiographic evidence of endocarditis is confirmatory for diagnosis when large vegetations exist (Fig. 31-6).

The American College of Cardiology/American Heart Association (ACC/AHA) guidelines now recommend antibiotic prophylaxis for patients with prosthetic cardiac valves or rings; previous endocarditis; unrepaired cyanotic congenital heart disease; repaired congenital heart disease with prosthetic material or residual defects adjacent to prosthetic device or patch; and cardiac transplant recipients.[1]

MITRAL STENOSIS

Cause

The predominant cause of mitral stenosis is rheumatic fever. The mitral valve is the valve most often damaged by rheumatic carditis.[10] Rheumatic fever causes thickening and decreased mobility of the mitral valve leaflets associated with fusion of the commissures and destruction of normal leaflet structure. In addition to rheumatic disease, degenerative mitral stenosis is increasingly prominent and is related to atherosclerotic heart disease, advanced age, and uncontrolled hypertension.[10]

Pathology

The rheumatic process causes the mitral valve to become fibrinous, resulting in leaflet thickening, commissural or chordal fusion, and calcification. As a result, the mitral valve apparatus becomes funnel shaped with a narrowed orifice. Fusion of the mitral valve commissures results in narrowing of the principal orifice, whereas interchordal fusion obliterates the secondary orifices.

Pathophysiology

The normal mitral valve area is 4 to 6 cm^2. Once the cross-sectional area of the mitral valve is reduced to 2 cm^2 or less, a pressure gradient between the left atrium and left ventricle (LV) occurs. The reduced orifice impedes left atrial emptying. Increased left atrial pressure and dilation occurs along with left atrial hypertrophy in an attempt to maintain normal diastolic flow into the LV. Increased left atrial pressure is transmitted to the pulmonary circuit, resulting in pulmonary hypertension and pulmonary congestion.[10] Women have mitral stenosis more frequently than men.

Clinical Manifestations

Mild dyspnea on exertion occurs as the most common symptom of mild mitral stenosis (valve area of 1.6 to 2.0 cm^2). As mitral

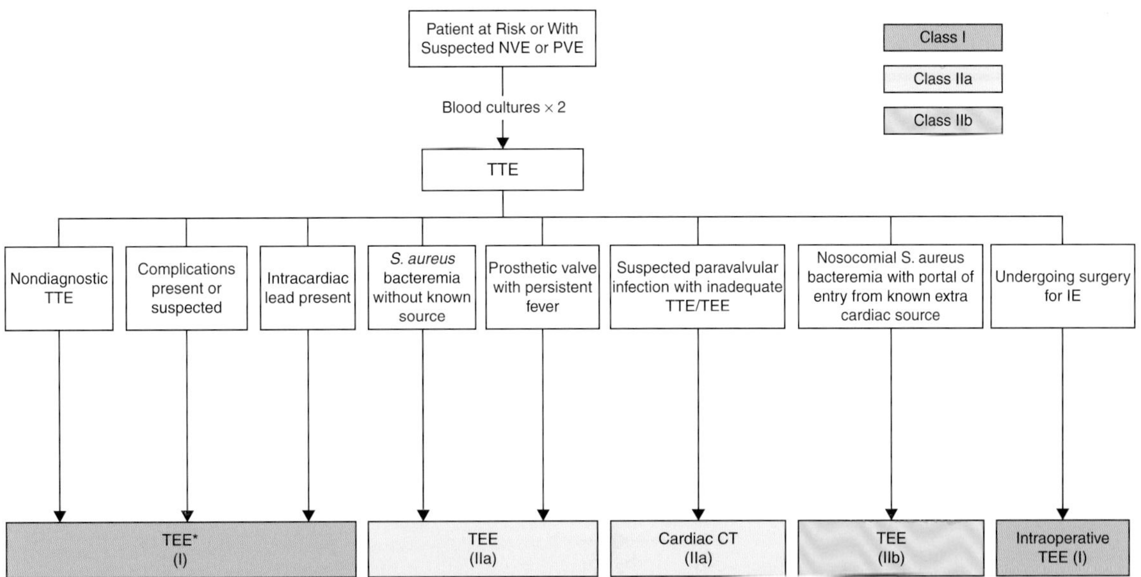

Figure 31-6. Transesophageal echocardiography in native valve and prosthetic valve endocarditis. (Used with permission from Nishimura RA, Otto CM, Bonow RO, et al. 2014 AHA/ACC guideline for the management of patients with valvular heart disease: a Report of the American College of Cardiology/American Heart Association Task Force on practice guidelines. *J Am Coll Cardiol.* 2014;63[22]:e57–e185.)

Stage	Definition	Valve Anatomy	Valve Hemodynamics	Hemodynamic Consequences	Symptoms
A	At risk of MS	• Mild valve doming during diastole	• Normal transmitral flow velocity	• None	• None
B	Progressive MS	• Rheumatic valve changes with commissural fusion and diastolic doming of the mitral valve leaflets • Planimetered MVA >1.5 cm^2	• Increased transmitral flow velocities • MVA >1.5 cm^2 • Diastolic pressure half-time <150 ms	• Mild-to-moderate LA enlargement • Normal pulmonary pressure at rest	• None
C	Asymptomatic severe MS	• Rheumatic valve changes with commissural fusion and diastolic doming of the mitral valve leaflets • Planimetered MVA ≤1.5 cm^2 • (MVA ≤1.0 cm^2 with very severe MS)	• MVA ≤1.5 cm^2 • (MVA ≤1.0 cm^2 with very severe MS) • Diastolic pressure half-time ≥150 ms • (Diastolic pressure half-time ≥220 ms with very severe MS)	• Severe LA enlargement • Elevated PASP >30 mm Hg	• None
D	Symptomatic severe MS	• Rheumatic valve changes with commissural fusion and diastolic doming of the mitral valve leaflets • Planimetered MVA ≤1.5 cm^2	• MVA ≤1.5 cm^2 • (MVA ≤1.0 cm^2 with very severe MS) • Diastolic pressure half-time ≥150 ms • (Diastolic pressure half-time ≥220 ms with very severe MS)	• Severe LA enlargement • Elevated PASP >30 mm Hg	• Decreased exercise tolerance • Exertional dyspnea

The transmitral mean pressure gradient should be obtained to further determine the hemodynamic effect of the MS and is usually >5 mm Hg to 10 mm Hg in severe MS; however, due to the variability of the mean pressure gradient with heart rate and forward flow, it has not been included in the criteria for severity.

LA indicates left atrial; LV, left ventricular; MS, mitral stenosis; MVA, mitral valve area; and PASP, pulmonary artery systolic pressure.

Figure 31-7. Stages of mitral stenosis. (Used with permission from Nishimura RA, Otto CM, Bonow RO, et al. 2014 AHA/ACC guideline for the management of patients with valvular heart disease: a Report of the American College of Cardiology/American Heart Association Task Force on practice guidelines. *J Am Coll Cardiol.* 2014;63[22]:e57–e185.)

stenosis becomes more severe (valve area of 1 to 1.5 cm^2), dyspnea, fatigue, paroxysmal nocturnal dyspnea, and atrial fibrillation may occur. When mitral stenosis becomes severe (valve area of 1 cm^2 or less), symptoms include fatigue and dyspnea with mild exertion and heart failure presentation. With advanced mitral stenosis, pulmonary hypertension and symptoms of right-sided heart failure occur (i.e., edema, hepatomegaly, ascites, elevated jugular venous pressure). Increased left atrial pressure, atrial fibrillation, and stagnation of left atrial blood flow can result in the formation of mural thrombi, with resultant embolic events, including cerebrovascular accidents.[11] Women who had previously been asymptomatic with mitral stenosis may become symptomatic and even experience severe hemodynamic decompensation during pregnancy due to increased cardiac output and increased heart rate. A summary of stage, anatomy, hemodynamic considerations and symptoms can be found in Figure 31-7.[1]

Physical Assessment

In severe mitral stenosis, on auscultation, there are four typical findings including (1) an accentuated S_1; (2) an opening diastolic snap; (3) a mid-diastolic rumble noted best at the apex (in sinus rhythm), followed by presystolic accentuation; and (4) an increased pulmonic S_2 intensity associated with pulmonary hypertension (Table 31-2).

Table 31-2 • DIASTOLIC MURMURS IN ACQUIRED VALVULAR HEART DISEASE

Origin of Murmur	Auscultatory Location and Radiation	Configuration	Quality and Frequency	Maneuvers That Alter Intensity
Aortic insufficiency	Third and fourth left intercostal spaces	Decrescendo S_1 S_2 S_1	Blowing High pitched	Increases with isometric exercise and squatting Decreases with amyl nitrate and Valsalva maneuver
Mitral stenosis	Apex	Decrescendo Opening snap OS S_1 S_2 S_1	Rumbling Low pitched	Increases with expiration, squatting, amyl nitrate, and isometric exercise Decreases with Valsalva maneuver
Pulmonic insufficiency	Second left intercostal space	Crescendo-decrescendo S_1 S_2 S_1	Blowing High pitched	Increases with inspiration and amyl nitrate Decreases with Valsalva maneuver
Tricuspid stenosis	Parasternal at left fourth and fifth intercostal spaces	Decrescendo S_1 S_2 S_1	Rumbling Low pitched	Increases with inspiration, squatting, and amyl nitrate Decreases with Valsalva maneuver

Table 31-3 • DIAGNOSTIC TESTING FOR MITRAL STENOSIS

Diagnostic Test	Rationale/Considerations
Echocardiogram	• Quantify the valve area and gradient • Quantify the degree of mitral insufficiency; • Define the degree of left atrial enlargement; • Assess mitral annular calcification; • Assess pulmonary artery pressures and degree of pulmonary hypertension; • Evaluate right- and left-sided ventricular function.
Cardiac Catheterization	• Define and delineate coronary anatomy • Right heart catheterization can evaluate right heart and pulmonary artery pressures.
Electrocardiogram	• Electrocardiogram is nonspecific and does not indicate the severity of mitral stenosis. If the patient remains in sinus rhythm and left atrial enlargement has occurred, characteristic P mitrale (broad, bifid P waves in leads II and V_1) may be identified. Right axis deviation and right ventricular hypertrophy may be noted in severe mitral stenosis. Atrial fibrillation is common in patients with long-standing mitral stenosis and is usually coarse in appearance.
Chest radiography	• Correlates with the degree of mitral stenosis. As mitral stenosis becomes more severe, the chest radiograph demonstrates straightening of the left heart border caused by left atrial enlargement, elevation of the left mainstem bronchus caused by distention of the left atrium, and distribution of blood flow from the lower to upper lobes. • Although heart size remains normal, central pulmonary arteries become prominent. Kerley B lines and interstitial edema are often present.

Patients with mitral stenosis may exhibit malar blush (pink discoloration of the cheeks). Patients with severe mitral stenosis may have weak pulses secondary to reduced cardiac output. The apical pulse is tapping in quality and is nondisplaced. A lower left parasternal lift or heave caused by right ventricular hypertrophy may be present. Cardiac rhythm is often irregularly irregular, indicating atrial fibrillation. Diagnostic evaluation and criteria for mitral stenosis are detailed in Table 31-3.

Medical Management

Medical therapy for mitral stenosis is aimed at managing symptoms of shortness of breath and heart failure as well as preventing the complications of systemic embolization and atrial fibrillation in the event that it occurs.[11] Medical management is aimed at symptom management, however conservative management incurred a significantly higher mortality and heart failure rate as illustrated in Figure 31-8.[11]

MITRAL INSUFFICIENCY

Cause

Mitral insufficiency (also termed *regurgitation*) may be either chronic or acute (Table 31-4). Primary (degenerative) mitral regurgitation is defined as involvement of the leaflets and chordae tendinae as the cause of the insufficiency. Myxomatous disease, mitral valve prolapse, and endocarditis can cause primary mitral valve regurgitation. Secondary (functional) mitral regurgitation is caused by changes to the left ventricular function or changes to

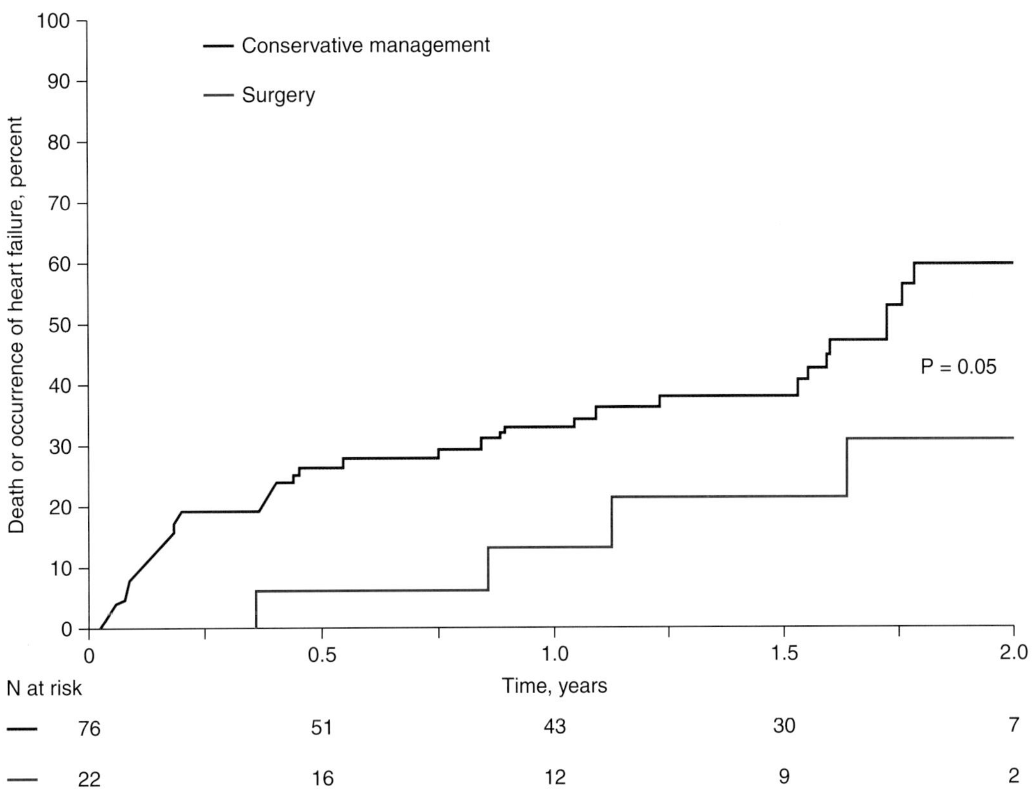

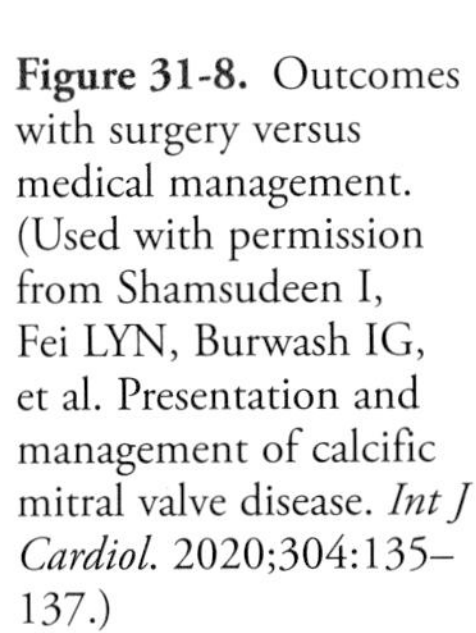
Figure 31-8. Outcomes with surgery versus medical management. (Used with permission from Shamsudeen I, Fei LYN, Burwash IG, et al. Presentation and management of calcific mitral valve disease. *Int J Cardiol.* 2020;304:135–137.)

Table 31-4 • ETIOLOGIES OF MITRAL REGURGITATION

Chronic Mitral Regurgitation	Acute Mitral Regurgitation
Rheumatic heart disease	Myocardial infarction causing:
Ischemia to subvalvular apparatus	Papillary muscle rupture or dysfunction
Infective endocarditis	Rupture of chordae
Myxomatous degeneration	Infective endocarditis
Hypertrophic cardiomyopathy	Trauma
Left ventricular dilation	Myxomatous degeneration with chordal rupture
Systemic lupus erythematosus	
Marfan syndrome	
Calcification of annulus	
Ankylosing spondylitis	
Scleroderma	
Ehlers–Danlos syndrome	
Prosthetic paravalvular leak	
Deterioration of prosthetic mitral valve	

the size and shape of the ventricle. This may or may not include dilatation of the mitral valve annulus. Ischemic cardiomyopathy is the most common cause of secondary mitral regurgitation.[12] Mixed mitral regurgitation is the third type of mitral regurgitation and is caused by a component of both primary and secondary mitral regurgitation, as the name describes.[12]

Pathology

Primary mitral regurgitation occurs when the mitral valve annulus, leaflets, chordae, or papillary muscles are affected by ischemia, collagen disease, infection, calcification, trauma, or degenerative changes, causing incompetent coaptation of the mitral leaflets. Secondary mitral regurgitation occurs with ventricular dilation when ventricular geometry is changed, causing malalignment of the papillary muscles.[12] Echocardiogram in Figure 31-9 depicts anatomy of the prolapsed mitral valve.

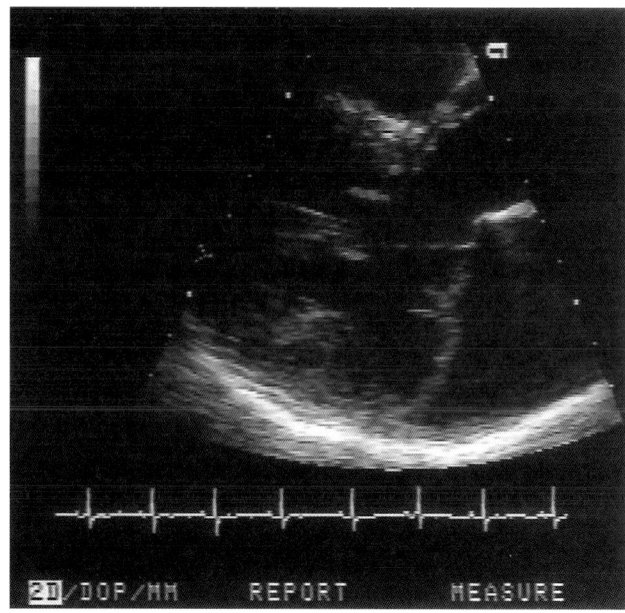

A

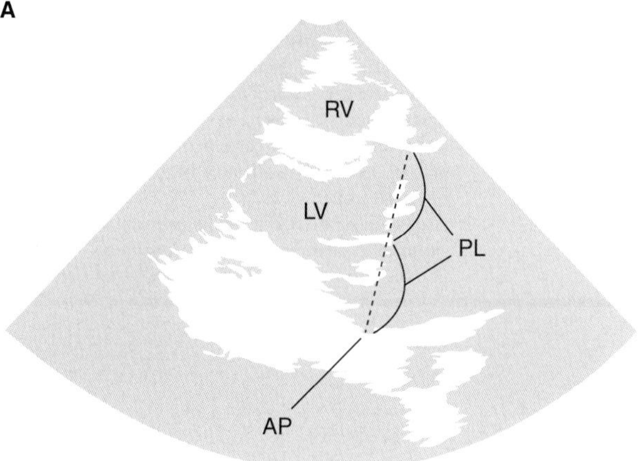

B

Figure 31-9. **A:** Long-axis echocardiographic view of mitral valve with bileaflet prolapse above the annular plane into the left atrium. **B:** Illustration corresponding to echocardiogram. RV, right ventricle; LV, left ventricle; AP, annular plane; PL, prolapsing leaflet.

Pathophysiology

Mitral regurgitation occurs as the result of inadequate closure of the mitral valve, allowing regurgitant flow back into the left atrium during each left ventricular systole. Its severity depends on the volume of regurgitant flow. Regurgitant flow also increases left atrial pressure, causing left atrial dilation and pulmonary congestion. During diastole, the regurgitant volume returns to the LV and increases its volume load. In chronic mitral regurgitation, persistent volume overload results in progressive ventricular dilation and mild hypertrophy. Over time, chronic volume overload will result in systolic heart failure. In acute mitral regurgitation, neither the left atrium nor the ventricle has had sufficient time to adjust to the increased volume load. Left atrial pressure rises quickly, resulting in pulmonary congestion and edema.[13] These clinical, echocardiographic, and hemodynamic findings are classified into stages of MR severity (Figs. 31-10 and 31-11).[1]

Clinical Manifestations

Patients with acute versus chronic mitral regurgitation will vary in their clinical presentation and physical examination. The acute and chronic phases can occur with both primary and secondary causes of mitral regurgitation.[12] In acute mitral regurgitation, symptoms progress rapidly. Symptoms are typically those of left ventricular failure. The patient is usually tachycardiac to compensate for the reduced forward stroke volume. Patients are dyspneic secondary to pulmonary congestion and edema; they are often orthopneic and have paroxysmal nocturnal dyspnea and poor exercise tolerance. Patients may also have signs of biventricular failure because right-sided failure may occur secondary to pulmonary hypertension. Patients with acute mitral regurgitation often present to the emergency department with reports of sudden inability to breathe. New-onset atrial fibrillation can occur. Patients with ischemic mitral insufficiency or papillary muscle rupture may also report chest pain.[12] Determination of whether the patient has primary or secondary mitral regurgitation will aid in the determination of sequelae and treatment options.

Physical Assessment

On examination, the most easily noted characteristic of either chronic or acute mitral regurgitation is the holosystolic murmur, which is heard best at the apex and radiates to the axilla (see Table 31-5). The murmur of mitral regurgitation may vary

Grade	Definition	Valve Anatomy	Valve Hemodynamics*	Hemodynamic Consequences	Symptoms
A	At risk of MR	• Mild mitral valve prolapse with normal coaptation • Mild valve thickening and leaflet restriction	• No MR jet or small central jet area <20% LA on Doppler • Small vena contracta <0.3 cm	• None	• None
B	Progressive MR	• Severe mitral valve prolapse with normal coaptation • Rheumatic valve changes with leaflet restriction and loss of central coaptation • Prior IE	• Central jet MR 20%–40% LA or late systolic eccentric jet MR • Vena contracta <0.7 cm • Regurgitant volume <60 mL • Regurgitant fraction <50% • ERO <0.40 cm^2 • Angiographic grade 1–2+	• Mild LA enlargement • No LV enlargement • Normal pulmonary pressure	• None
C	Asymptomatic severe MR	• Severe mitral valve prolapse with loss of coaptation or flail leaflet • Rheumatic valve changes with leaflet restriction and loss of central coaptation • Prior IE • Thickening of leaflets with radiation heart disease	• Central jet MR >40% LA or holosystolic eccentric jet MR • Vena contracta ≥0.7 cm • Regurgitant volume ≥60 mL • Regurgitant fraction ≥50% • ERO ≥0.40 cm^2 • Angiographic grade 3–4+	• Moderate or severe LA enlargement • LV enlargement • Pulmonary hypertension may be present at rest or with exercise • C1: LVEF >60% and LVESD <40 mm • C2: LVEF ≤60% and LVESD ≥40 mm	• None
D	Symptomatic severe MR	• Severe mitral valve prolapse with loss of coaptation or flail leaflet • Rheumatic valve changes with leaflet restriction and loss of central coaptation • Prior IE • Thickening of leaflets with radiation heart disease	• Central jet MR >40% LA or holosystolic eccentric jet MR • Vena contracta ≥0.7 cm • Regurgitant volume ≥60 mL • Regurgitant fraction ≥50% • ERO ≥0.40 cm^2 • Angiographic grade 3–4+	• Moderate or severe LA enlargement • LV enlargement • Pulmonary hypertension present	• Decreased exercise tolerance • Exertional dyspnea

*Several valve hemodynamic criteria are provided for assessment of MR severity, but not all criteria for each category will be present in each patient. Categorization of MR severity as mild, moderate, or severe depends on data quality and integration of these parameters in conjunction with other clinical evidence.

ERO indicates effective regurgitant orifice; IE, infective endocarditis; LA, left atrium/atrial; LV, left ventricular; LVEF, left ventricular ejection fraction; LVESD; left ventricular end-systolic dimension; and MR, mitral regurgitation.

Figure 31-10. Stages of chronic primary mitral regurgitation. (Used with permission from Nishimura RA, Otto CM, Bonow RO, et al. 2014 AHA/ACC guideline for the management of patients with valvular heart disease: a Report of the American College of Cardiology/American Heart Association Task Force on practice guidelines. *J Am Coll Cardiol.* 2014;63[22]:e57–e185.)

Grade	Definition	Valve Anatomy	Valve Hemodynamics*	Associated Cardiac Findings	Symptoms
A	At risk of MR	• Normal valve leaflets, chords, and annulus in a patient with coronary disease or cardiomyopathy	• No MR jet or small central jet area <20% LA on Doppler • Small vena contracta <0.30 cm	• Normal or mildly dilated LV size with fixed (infarction) or inducible (ischemia) regional wall motion abnormalities • Primary myocardial disease with LV dilation and systolic dysfunction	• Symptoms due to coronary ischemia or HF may be present that respond to revascularization and appropriate medical therapy
B	Progressive MR	• Regional wall motion abnormalities with mild tethering of mitral leaflet • Annular dilation with mild loss of central coaptation of the mitral leaflets	• ERO <0.20 cm^2† • Regurgitant volume <30 mL • Regurgitant fraction <50%	• Regional wall motion abnormalities with reduced LV systolic function • LV dilation and systolic dysfunction due to primary myocardial d isease	• Symptoms due to coronary ischemia or HF may be present that respond to revascularization and appropriate medical therapy
C	Asymptomatic severe MR	• Regional wall motion abnormalities and/or LV dilation with severe tethering of mitral leaflet • Annular dilation with severe loss of central coaptation of the mitral leaflets	• ERO ≥0.20 cm^2† • Regurgitant volume ≥30 mL • Regurgitant fraction ≥50%	• Regional wall motion abnormalities with reduced LV systolic function • LV dilation and systolic dysfunction due to primary myocardial disease	• Symptoms due to coronary ischemia or HF may be present that respond to revascularization and appropriate medical therapy
D	Symptomatic severe MR	• Regional wall motion abnormalities and/ or LV dilation with severe tethering of mitral leaflet • Annular dilation with severe loss of central coaptation of the mitral leaflets	• ERO ≥0.20 cm^2† • Regurgitant volume ≥30 mL • Regurgitant fraction ≥50%	• Regional wall motion abnormalities with reduced LV systolic function • LV dilation and systolic dysfunction due to primary myocardial disease	• HF symptoms due to MR persist even after revascularization and optimization of medical therapy • Decreased exercise tolerance • Exertional dyspnea

*Several valve hemodynamic criteria are provided for assessment of MR severity, but not all criteria for each category will be present in each patient. Categorization of MR severity as mild, moderate, or severe depends on data quality and integration of these parameters in conjunction with other clinical evidence.

†The measurement of the proximal isovelocity surface area by 2D TTE in patients with secondary MR underestimates the true ERO due to the crescentic shape of the proximal convergence.

2D indicates 2-dimensional; ERO, effective regurgitant orifice; HF, heart failure; LA, left atrium; LV, left ventricular; MR, mitral regurgitation; and TTE, transthoracic echocardiogram.

Figure 31-11. Stages of chronic secondary mitral regurgitation. (Used with permission from Nishimura RA, Otto CM, Bonow RO, et al. 2014 AHA/ACC guideline for the management of patients with valvular heart disease: a Report of the American College of Cardiology/American Heart Association Task Force on practice guidelines. *J Am Coll Cardiol.* 2014;63[22]:e57–e185.)

Table 31-5 • SYSTOLIC MURMURS RELATED TO ACQUIRED VALVULAR HEART DISEASE

Origin of Murmur	Auscultatory Location and Radiation	Configuration	Quality and Frequency	Maneuvers That Alter Intensity
Aortic stenosis	Right second intercostal space Radiates to carotid arteries and apex	Crescendo-decrescendo "Diamond shaped" S_1 S_2	Harsh High pitched	Increases with squatting, amyl nitrate Decreases with standing, Valsalva maneuver, and isometric exercise
Mitral regurgitation	Apex Radiates to axilla and back	Holosystolic S_1 S_2	Harsh or blowing High pitched	Increases with expiration, squatting, and isometric exercise Decreases with Valsalva maneuver, standing, and amyl nitrate
Mitral valve prolapse	Apex Radiates to axilla and back	Mid- to late systolic, with systolic click S_1 Click S_2	Harsh High pitched	Increases with Valsalva maneuver, amyl nitrate, and inspiration Decreases with squatting, standing, and isometric exercise
Tricuspid regurgitation	Fourth and fifth left intercostal spaces Radiates to right parasternal border	Holosystolic S_1 S_2	Harsh High pitched	Increases with amyl nitrate and inspiration Decreases with Valsalva maneuver and standing
Pulmonic stenosis	Second left intercostal space Radiates to back	Crescendo-decrescendo "Diamond shaped" S_1 S_2	Harsh High pitched	Increases with amyl nitrate, squatting, and inspiration Decreases with Valsalva maneuver and standing

Table 31-6 • DIAGNOSTIC TESTING FOR MITRAL REGURGITATION

Diagnostic Test	Rationale/Considerations
Echocardiogram	• Assess structural cause of the mitral regurgitation. • Assess left atrial size, left ventricular dimensions and performance, pulmonary artery pressures, and right heart function. • Color flow Doppler allows for the assessment of severity of regurgitation.
Transesophageal echocardiogram	• Superior to transthoracic echocardiography for evaluating mitral valve anatomy/pathoanatomy and the mechanism of mitral regurgitation, especially for prosthetic valve dysfunction or failure and paravalvular dysfunction or leak.
Cardiac catheterization	• Identify coexisting coronary artery disease. • Grade the severity of mitral regurgitation. • Left ventriculography can assess left ventricular function and distinguish any wall motion abnormalities. • Right heart catheterization quantifies pulmonary artery pressures and allows for evaluation of the large V waves in the pulmonary artery wedge tracing. • Direct left atrial pressure indicates the left ventricular filling pressure in patients who have systolic or diastolic left ventricular dysfunction or valvular heart disease.
Electrocardiogram	• Electrocardiography in chronic mitral regurgitation may demonstrate left ventricular hypertrophy and left atrial enlargement or P mitrale (characterized by M-shaped P waves). • Atrial fibrillation may occur with acute and chronic mitral regurgitation. • Patients with ischemic papillary muscle dysfunction may demonstrate ischemic changes, and patients with papillary muscle rupture can show acute inferior, posterior, or anterior myocardial infarction.
Chest radiography	• Chronic mitral regurgitation shows left ventricular hypertrophy and left atrial enlargement. • Calcification of the mitral valve annulus and apparatus may also be seen. • In acute or decompensated chronic mitral regurgitation, pulmonary vascular redistribution and pulmonary edema can be observed. • If the heart is of normal size, the degree of mitral regurgitation is so mild or so acute that eccentric left ventricular hypertrophy has not had time to develop.

somewhat depending on the underlying cause. Patients may have an S_3 gallop in moderate to severe regurgitation caused by high diastolic flow into the ventricle. An S_4 gallop is uncommon in chronic mitral regurgitation. However, in acute mitral regurgitation, an S_4 gallop is common because the left atrium and ventricle are noncompliant. The patient with rheumatic heart disease may also have a diastolic murmur related to coexisting mitral stenosis.

Because of left ventricular dilation, patients with chronic mitral regurgitation have an easily palpated, left laterally displaced point of maximal impulse. Patients with a markedly enlarged left atrium may have a left parasternal lift because of anterior displacement of the apex. Jugular venous pressure can be normal or elevated in the patient with right-sided heart failure. Breath sounds can range from basilar crackles to dullness secondary to pleural effusion. In addition, hepatosplenomegaly, hepatojugular reflux, peripheral edema, and ascites may be present in the patient with right-sided heart failure. Bonow et al. describe the complexity of the evaluation and referral pathway for patients with mitral regurgitation (Table 31-6).[12]

Medical Management

Medical therapy for mitral regurgitation is geared toward afterload reduction to promote forward flow and minimize regurgitation into the left atrium and pulmonary vasculature. In patients with acute or decompensated chronic mitral regurgitation, intravenous vasodilators such as nitroprusside can reduce filling pressures and ventricular cavity size and promote forward flow with afterload reduction. Intravenous diuretics are used to reduce volume overload. In acutely ill patients refractory to medications, intra-aortic balloon counterpulsation can be used further to reduce afterload while maintaining coronary perfusion with diastolic augmentation.

Symptom management is most important in patients with secondary (functional) mitral regurgitation. Optimal medical therapy showed to decrease LV damage in 40% of patients on guideline directed therapy.[14] Diuretics can treat chronic and acute volume overload. The patient should be carefully monitored and referred for mitral valve repair or replacement before significant left ventricular dysfunction or pulmonary hypertension occurs. Treatment considerations are based largely on the type and severity of the mitral regurgitation in the setting of failed maximized medical therapy.

TRICUSPID VALVE DISEASE

The tricuspid valve has been referred to as the "forgotten valve" and management of tricuspid disorders have historically been overshadowed by left-sided VHD. Of late, a growing understanding of the long-term adverse consequences of tricuspid valve disease, and in particular of severe tricuspid regurgitation, coupled with continued advances in surgical and percutaneous transcatheter techniques, has led to more aggressive treatment recommendations. Although, tricuspid stenosis is rare, tricuspid regurgitation is more common. Only 5% of the approximately 1.6 million patients in the United States with moderate to severe tricuspid regurgitation undergo tricuspid surgery annually resulting in an extremely large number of untreated patients with secondary tricuspid regurgitation.[15]

Cause

Roughly 80% of significant cases of tricuspid regurgitation are functional (secondary) as a result of dilation of the right ventricle and the annulus of the tricuspid valve in the setting of right ventricular (RV) remodeling due to pressure and/or volume overload. The causes of primary and secondary tricuspid regurgitation are summarized in Table 31-7.[16] Understanding the differences between primary and secondary tricuspid regurgitation is crucial for clinical decision making and treatment recommendations.

Table 31-7 • ETIOLOGIES OF TRICUSPID REGURGITATION

Primary TR
Congenital
Ebstein anomaly
Tricuspid valve tethering associated with ventricular septal aneurysm or defect
Tricuspid valve dysplasia, hypoplasia, or cleft
Tricuspid valve with two openings
Massive right atrium
Acquired
Myxomatous degeneration (Barlow disease) tricuspid valve prolapse, flail
Endocarditis
Carcinoid syndrome
Rheumatic disease
Trauma (chest wall trauma or tricuspid valve trauma following a cardiac procedure)
Pacemaker or device related
Secondary TR: Underlying disease

Adapted from Dahou A, Levin D, Reisman M, et al. Anatomy and physiology of the tricuspid valve. *JACC Cardiovasc Imaging*. 2019;12(3):458–468.

Pathophysiology

Disruption of these interactions through annular dilatation and apical displacement of the papillary muscles results in secondary tricuspid regurgitation. Secondary tricuspid regurgitation is classified by the underlying pathoanatomy (see Figs. 31-12 and 31-13): (1) tethering or tenting of the tricuspid leaflets, (2) displacement of the papillary muscles, (3) RV dysfunction, and (4) dilation of the annulus and/or right atrium.[16]

History and Physical Examination

Functional tricuspid regurgitation usually accompanies mitral stenosis and pulmonary hypertension because of the increased pressure and volume load on the right ventricle. Symptoms include signs of right-sided heart failure, large V waves in their right atrial or central venous pressure trace, and pulsatile neck veins. Other causes of tricuspid regurgitation include trauma, infective endocarditis, right atrial tumor, and tricuspid valve prolapse. The murmur of tricuspid regurgitation is a holosystolic murmur heard along the left sternal border and may extend over the precordium, sounding like the murmurs of mitral regurgitation and ventricular septal defect (see Table 31-5). Patients with mild tricuspid regurgitation normally do not require treatment. There is increasing evidence that functional tricuspid regurgitation is prognostically significant and may warrant intervention. Appropriate patient selection for and timing of intervention are important clinical tasks that require a comprehensive understanding of the pathophysiology and natural history of functional tricuspid regurgitation (Table 31-8).

Medical Management

Patients with severe tricuspid regurgitation (TR) usually present with signs or symptoms of right-sided HF, including peripheral

Stage	Definition	Valve Anatomy	Valve Hemodynamics*	Hemodynamic Consequences	Symptoms
A	At risk of TR	Primary • Mild rheumatic change • Mild prolapse • Other (eg, IE with vegetation, early carcinoid deposition, radiation) • Intra-annular RV pacemaker or ICD lead • Postcardiac transplant (biopsy related) Functional • Normal • Early annular dilation	• No or trace TR	• None	• None or in relation to other left heart or pulmonary/pulmonary vascular disease
B	Progressive TR	Primary • Progressive leaflet deterioration/ destruction • Moderate-to-severe prolapse, limited chordal rupture Functional • Early annular dilation • Moderate leaflet tethering	Mild TR • Central jet area <5.0 cm² • Vena contracta width not defined • CW jet density and contour: soft and parabolic • Hepatic vein flow: systolic dominance Moderate TR • Central jet area 5–10 cm² • Vena contracta width not defined but <0.70 cm • CW jet density and contour: dense, variable contour • Hepatic vein flow: systolic blunting	Mild TR • RV/RA/IVC size normal Moderate TR • No RV enlargement • No or mild RA enlargement • No or mild IVC enlargement with normal respirophasic variation • Normal RA pressure	• None or in relation to other left heart or pulmonary/pulmonary vascular disease
C	Asymptomatic severe TR	Primary • Flail or grossly distorted leaflets Functional • Severe annular dilation (>40 mm or 21 mm/m²) • Marked leaflet tethering	• Central jet area >10.0 cm² • Vena contracta width >0.7 cm • CW jet density and contour: dense, triangular with early peak • Hepatic vein flow: systolic reversal	• RV/RA/IVC dilated with decreased IVC respirophasicvariation • Elevated RA pressure with "c-V" wave • Diastolic interventricular septal flattening may be present	• None, or in relation to other left heart or pulmonary/pulmonary vascular disease
D	Symptomatic severe TR	Primary • Flail or grossly distorted leaflets Functional • Severe annular dilation (>40 mm or >21 mm/m²) • Marked leaflet tethering	• Central jet area >10.0 cm² • Vena contracta width >0.70 cm • CW jet density and contour: dense, triangular with early peak • Hepatic vein flow: systolic reversal	• RV/RA/IVC dilated with decreased IVC respirophasicvariation • Elevated RA pressure with "c-V" wave • Diastolic interventricular septal flattening • Reduced RV systolic function in late phase	• Fatigue, palpitations, dyspnea, abdominal bloating, anorexia, edema

CW indicates continuous wave; ICD, implantable cardioverter-defibrillator; IE, infective endocarditis; IVC, inferior vena cava; RA, right atrium; RV, right ventricle; and TR, tricuspid regurgitation.

*Several valve hemodynamic criteria are provided for assessment of severity of TR, but not all criteria for each category will necessarily be present in every patient. Categorization of severity of TR as mild, moderate, or severe also depends on image quality and integration of these parameters with clinical findings.

Figure 31-12. Stages of tricuspid regurgitation. Demonstrates stages (A through D) of primary and functional tricuspid regurgitation. Severe TR (stages C and D) is associated with poor prognosis and patients with signs or symptoms of right-sided HF are considered to fit stage D category irrespective of other criteria. (Used with permission from Nishimura RA, Otto CM, Bonow RO, et al. 2014 AHA/ACC guideline for the management of patients with valvular heart disease: a Report of the American College of Cardiology/American Heart Association task force on practice guidelines. *J Am Coll Cardiol.* 2014;63[22]:e57–e185.)

edema and ascites. Diuretics can be used to decrease volume overload in these patients. Loop diuretics are typically provided and may relieve systemic congestion, but their use can be limited. Recent guidelines also support aldosterone antagonists' use in the setting of hepatic congestion, which may promote secondary hyperaldosteronism.[1]

Attention should be focused on the causative factor(s) in patients with functional TR. Medical treatment is limited and is aimed at reducing pulmonary artery pressures and right heart afterload in patients with severe TR. Reduction of pulmonary artery pressures and pulmonary vascular resistance with specific pulmonary vasodilators may be helpful to reduce RV afterload and functional TR in selected patients with pulmonary hypertension who demonstrate acute responsiveness during invasive testing. Medical treatment of conditions that elevate left-sided filling pressures, such as systemic hypertension, should be optimized. If tricuspid regurgitation is severe and symptomatic, tricuspid valve repair may be performed. Tricuspid valve replacement is uncommon and is done only if a satisfactory tricuspid repair cannot be accomplished.

Table 31-8 • DIAGNOSTIC TESTING FOR TRICUSPID REGURGITATION

Diagnostic Test	Considerations
Transthoracic echocardiogram	• Primary assessment modality
Transesophageal echocardiogram	• Utilized in situations where further detailed evaluation is necessary
Cardiac catheterization	• Assess coronary anatomy

Tricuspid Stenosis

The causes of native valve tricuspid stenosis are limited to rheumatic heart disease, congenital defects, and obstructing masses, such as prolapsing myxoma. Rheumatic tricuspid stenosis, the most common type of tricuspid stenosis, is often accompanied by tricuspid regurgitation and left sided VHD.[1,17] Tricuspid stenosis has a pathologic process similar to that of mitral stenosis.

The murmur of tricuspid stenosis is comparable to the murmur of mitral stenosis, including an opening snap followed by a diastolic rumble. The murmur of tricuspid stenosis is a diastolic decrescendo murmur along the left sternal border (see Table 31-2). Common symptoms of tricuspid stenosis include fatigue, minimal orthopnea, paroxysmal nocturnal dyspnea, hepatomegaly, and anasarca (Table 31-9).

Table 31-9 • DIAGNOSTIC TESTING FOR TRICUSPID STENOSIS

Diagnostic Test	Rationale/Considerations
Transthoracic echocardiogram	Evaluation of function • Reveal chordal thickening and calcification • Elevated mean pressure gradient • Pressure half-time greater than or equal to 190 ms • Valve area less than or equal to 1.0 cm^2 • Right atrial and inferior vena cava enlargement[1,22]
Cardiac catheterization	Assess coronary anatomy

Stage	Definition	Valve Anatomy	Valve Hemodynamics	Hemodynamic Consequences	Symptoms
A	At risk of AS	• Bicuspid aortic valve (or other congenital valve anomaly) • Aortic valve sclerosis	• Aortic V_{max} <2 m/s	• None	• None
B	Progressive AS	• Mild-to-moderate leaflet calcification of a bicuspid or trileaflet valve with some reduction in systolic motion or • Rheumatic valve changes with commissural fusion	• Mild AS: Aortic V_{max} 2.0–2.9 m/s or mean ΔP <20 mm Hg • Moderate AS: Aortic V_{max} 3.0–3.9 m/s or mean ΔP 20–39 mm Hg	• Early LV diastolic dysfunction may be present • Normal LVEF	• None
C: Asymptomatic severe AS					
C1	Asymptomatic severe AS	• Severe leaflet calcification or congenital stenosis with severely reduced leaflet opening	• Aortic V_{max} ≥4 m/s or • mean ΔP ≥40 mm Hg • AVA typically is ≤1.0 cm^2 (or AVAi ≤0.6 cm^2/m^2) • Very severe AS is an aortic V_{max} ≥5 m/s or mean ΔP ≥60 mm Hg	• LV diastolic dysfunction • Mild LV hypertrophy • Normal LVEF	• None: Exercise testing is reasonable to confirm symptom status
C2	Asymptomatic severe AS with LV dysfunction	• Severe leaflet calcification or congenital stenosis with severely reduced leaflet opening	• Aortic V_{max} ≥4 m/s or mean ΔP ≥40 mm Hg • AVA typically ≤1.0 cm^2 (or AVAi ≤0.6 cm^2/m^2)	• LVEF <50%	• None
D: Symptomatic severe AS					
D1	Symptomatic severe high-gradient AS	• Severe leaflet calcification or congenital stenosis with severely reduced leaflet opening	• Aortic V_{max} ≥4 m/s or • mean ΔP ≥40 mm Hg • AVA typically ≤1.0 cm^2 (or AVAi ≤0.6 cm^2/m^2) but may be larger with mixed AS/AR	• LV diastolic dysfunction • LV hypertrophy • Pulmonary hypertension may be present	• Exertional dyspnea or decreased exercise tolerance • Exertional angina • Exertional syncope or presyncope
D2	Symptomatic severe low-flow/low-gradient AS with reduced LVEF	• Severe leaflet calcification with severely reduced leaflet motion	• AVA ≤1.0 cm^2 with resting aortic V_{max} <4 m/s or mean ΔP <40 mm Hg • Dobutamine stress echocardiography shows AVA ≤1.0 cm^2 with V_{max} ≥4 m/s at any flow rate	• LV diastolic dysfunction • LV hypertrophy • LVEF <50%	• HF • Angina • Syncope or presyncope
D3	Symptomatic severe low-gradient AS with normal LVEF or paradoxical low-flow severe AS	• Severe leaflet calcification with severely reduced leaflet motion	• AVA ≤1.0 cm^2 with aortic V_{max} <4 m/s or mean ΔP <40 mm Hg • Indexed AVA ≤0.6 cm^2/m^2 and • Stroke volume index <35 mL/m^2 • Measured when patient is normotensive (systolic BP <140 mm Hg)	• Increased LV relative wall thickness • Small LV chamber with low stroke volume • Restrictive diastolic filling • LVEF ≥50%	• HF • Angina • Syncope or presyncope

AR indicates aortic regurgitation; AS, aortic stenosis; AVA, aortic valve area; AVAi, aortic valve area indexed to body surface area; BP, blood pressure; HF, heart failure; LV, left ventricular; LVEF, left ventricular ejection fraction; ΔP, pressure gradient; and V_{max}, maximum aortic velocity.

Figure 31-13. Stages of valvular aortic stenosis. (Used with permission from Nishimura RA, Otto CM, Bonow RO, et al. 2014 AHA/ACC guideline for the management of patients with valvular heart disease: a Report of the American College of Cardiology/American Heart Association Task Force on practice guidelines. *J Am Coll Cardiol.* 2014;63[22]:e57–e185.)

Medical management is similar to that of TR with special attention to left-sided valve disease and atrial fibrillation. Loop diuretics may be useful to relieve systemic and hepatic congestion in patients with severe, symptomatic TS.

AORTIC STENOSIS

Cause

Disease processes that result in aortic valve stenosis can be classified as congenital or acquired. The acquired group largely consists of calcific (formerly "degenerative") and postinflammatory (or rheumatic) disease. Aortic stenosis is one of the most common valve diseases and is expected to increase in prevalence due to aging of the world population. Aortic stenosis is a gradually progressive disease that may have a long asymptomatic phase often lasting for decades that is then followed by a much shorter symptomatic phase with severe narrowing of the aortic valve orifice (Fig. 31-13). The age at which aortic stenosis becomes symptomatic is determined by the underlying cause. Aortic stenosis occurring from 1 to 30 years of age usually represents congenital aortic stenosis. Aortic stenosis presenting at the ages of 40 to 60 years is primarily rheumatic in origin or secondary to calcific aortic stenosis in a congenitally bicuspid aortic valve. In patients past the age of 60 to 70 years, calcific degenerative stenosis is the most prevalent cause.

Pathology

Aortic stenosis is characterized by a fibrocalcific transformation of the valve leaflets, resulting in progressive narrowing of the aortic valve opening. Often, it is accompanied by a hypertrophic response of the LV, which may result in dyspnea, heart failure, syncope, angina, and ultimately death.

Pathophysiology

Over the past decade, evidence has emerged suggesting that the pathophysiology of aortic stenosis occurs in two phases. The initiation phase is characterized by endothelial damage, lipid infiltration, and inflammation mimicking atherosclerosis. The propagation phase is next, in which valve fibrosis and calcification (similar to skeletal bone) occurs in a proliferative cycle Valve injury appears to be the central driver of cyclical calcium formation and disease progression.[18,19] As the valve cusps become less mobile, the valve orifice decreases in size, resulting in an increasingly higher left ventricular systolic pressure necessary to eject blood across the stenosed valve. Increased left ventricular afterload results first in compensatory concentric left ventricular hypertrophy. Onset of severe symptoms of aortic stenosis—angina, syncope, and heart failure (Fig. 31-14)—remains the major demarcation point in the disease's course.[20] Even with severe obstruction, asymptomatic patient's survival is minimally impacted whereas an individual with symptoms has a mortality rate of about 25% per year.[20]

Although initially adaptive in aortic stenosis and helps to preserve ejection performance, left ventricular hypertrophy impairs coronary blood-flow reserve, reduces diastolic function, and is associated with increased mortality. With higher pressure gradients, blood from the LV is ejected back into the left atrium worsening underlying mitral regurgitation process. Even moderate AS adds a hemodynamic burden on the LV. Patients with heart failure with reduced EF (HFrEF) have significant myocardial dysfunction and LV performance is more sensitive to changes in afterload conditions than in patients with normal EF.[21] As aortic stenosis becomes severe, left ventricular systolic function may also decline, resulting in congestive heart failure (CHF).

The heart is unique in that coronary perfusion occurs primarily during diastole. Additionally, oxygen extraction is always close to maximum. Subsequently, the only way in which the myocardium can meet an increased oxygen demand is by increasing coronary blood flow. Myocardial oxygen demand is increased secondary to increased left ventricular wall stress and muscle mass. Myocardial oxygen delivery is reduced as a result of decreased coronary perfusion pressure. Angina may result even in the absence of CHD because of an imbalance in myocardial oxygen supply and demand.

Another ominous symptom of aortic stenosis is syncope. The exact mechanism of syncope in aortic stenosis remains unclear but is probably unrelated to the presence of hypertrophy. In patients with aortic stenosis, syncope is usually exercise induced. Syncope or near syncope may be secondary to reduced cerebral perfusion pressure, inappropriate left ventricular baroreceptor response, or arrhythmia. Orthostatic blood pressure changes may occur during exertion when arterial pressure drops because of systemic vasodilation in the setting of a fixed cardiac output. Increased left ventricular pressure may result in inappropriate baroreceptor response. Finally, arrhythmias potentiated by exercise-induced ischemia might also produce syncope. Patients at risk for recurrence of arrhythmias should be considered for further electrophysiologic testing.

History and Physical Findings

Aortic stenosis is most readily detected by auscultation of its classic mid-systolic (systolic ejection) murmur (see Table 31-10). In

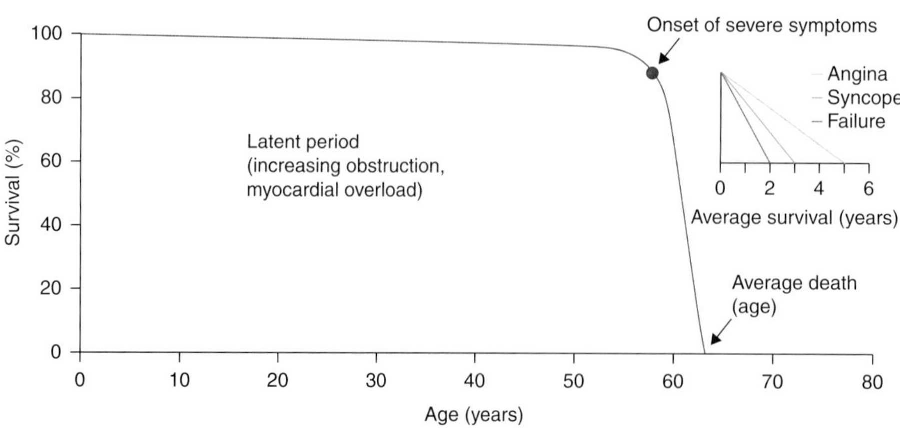

Figure 31-14. Survival of aortic stenosis. (Adapted from Ross J Jr, Braunwald E. Aortic stenosis. *Circulation*. 1968;38 (1 Suppl):61–67.)

Table 31-10 • DIAGNOSTIC TESTING FOR AORTIC STENOSIS

Diagnostic Test	Rationale/Considerations
Echocardiogram	• Quantify the valve area, peak velocity and mean gradient. • Evaluate for any aortic insufficiency. • Define the degree of left atrial enlargement. • Evaluate right- and left-sided ventricular function. • For asymptomatic patients, repeat transthoracic echocardiography is recommended to assess the inevitable progression of obstruction. – Patients with mild AS should undergo repeat TTE approximately every 3–5 yr. – Patients with moderate AS approximately every 1–2 yr. – Patients with severe AS approximately every 6–12 mo. – Earlier imaging is warranted for a change in symptoms or clinical condition.
Cardiac catheterization	• Performed in patients with aortic stenosis primarily to rule out concomitant coronary heart disease. • A full hemodynamic study and crossing of the aortic valve is no longer recommended if noninvasive assessment of the valve is adequate to assess valve function. • Invasive hemodynamic study should be considered when a patient's history, physical examination, and echocardiographic measurements are inconsistent and leave doubt about stenosis severity. • Left ventriculography can quantify the left ventricular ejection fraction and the transvalvular gradient can be established by direct pressure measurement. • Right heart catheterization to quantify pulmonary artery pressures and cardiac output.
Electrocardiogram	• Nondiagnostic • May show – Left ventricular hypertrophy pattern. – Left atrial abnormalities. – Nonspecific ST and T-wave changes. – QRS voltage changes in the precordial leads correlates poorly with the severity of obstruction in aortic stenosis in adults.
Chest radiography	• Nonspecific and may be negative even in advanced disease. • Heart size may be normal or only minimally enlarged. The left ventricular border and apex may be rounded, demonstrating a boot-shaped silhouette. • Calcification of the aortic valve and aorta may be present. • Left atrial enlargement and congestive heart failure may be noted in advanced stages. • Poststenotic dilation of the proximal ascending aorta may be noted along the right heart border. 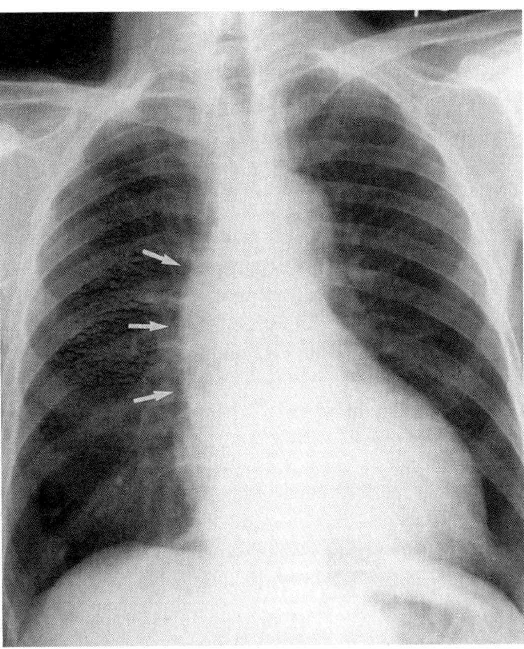 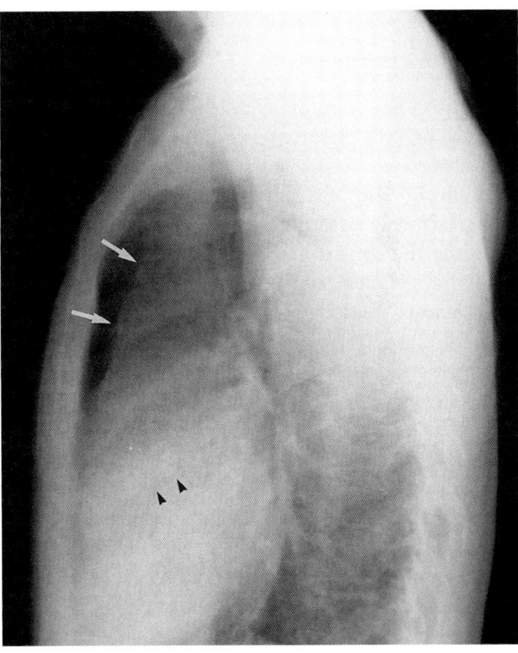 A B **A:** Posteroanterior chest radiograph showing rounded border of left ventricle (*arrows*). **B:** Lateral chest radiograph showing calcified aortic valve (*arrowheads*) and filling of the retrosternal airspace with dilated ascending aorta (*arrows*). (From Boxt LM. [1998]. Plain film examination of the chest. In Topol EJ, Califf RM, Isner JM, et al., eds. *Textbook of cardiovascular medicine*. Philadelphia, PA: Lippincott-Raven; 1988:511.)
Gated blood pool radionuclide scans	• Provides information regarding ventricular function similar to echocardiography and left ventriculography. • Gated pool scans may be useful in patients in whom left ventriculography cannot be performed (i.e., patients with elevated creatinine), or those in whom the left ventricle cannot be clearly imaged with echocardiography.
Exercise testing	• In patients with mild to moderate aortic stenosis with equivocal symptoms may be accomplished with caution in the hands of a cardiologist and can provide relevant information regarding exercise tolerance. • Contraindicated in patients with known severe aortic stenosis and classic symptoms such as syncope, dyspnea, and chest pain, exercise testing due to increased risk of ventricular tachyarrhythmias/fibrillation.

mild disease, the murmur peaks early in systole, S_2 is physiologically split, and carotid upstrokes are normal. As aortic stenosis progresses, the murmur becomes louder and peaks progressively later. As the stenosis becomes critical, the murmur intensity can decrease as stroke volume becomes reduced. The murmur often radiates to one or both carotids. The murmur may be diminished at the base of the heart and radiate to the apex. An S_4 gallop is usually present in patients in sinus rhythm. The point of maximal intensity is sustained but may not be displaced. Blood pressure is normal to hypertensive until advanced aortic stenosis. Jugular venous pressure is normal in most patients except in patients with severe aortic stenosis associated with heart failure. Reduction in stroke volume and cardiac output may cause diminished carotid upstrokes and late systolic peak (tardus) in severe or critical aortic stenosis. The course of aortic stenosis varies in its progression; therefore, patients should be followed up carefully by their healthcare providers with serial physical examinations and periodic echocardiography. Patients should be taught to recognize the symptoms of worsening aortic stenosis, such as dyspnea, chest pain, and near syncope or syncope.

The diagnosis of aortic stenosis is usually made when the routine physical examination reveals a systolic murmur. In patients with a single second heart sound, a history of bicuspid aortic valve, or symptoms that may be due to aortic stenosis, a transthoracic echocardiogram (TTE) is recommended in patients with an unexplained systolic murmur. The diagnosis of AS is based on the presence of a *structurally* abnormal valve (thickened and/or calcified or congenitally abnormal) with restricted motion and Doppler evidence of hemodynamic obstruction.

Medical Management

Although AS is a common condition, medical therapies are still lacking to prevent the progression. Insights in the pathophysiology of aortic stenosis progression have resulted in the identification of fibrosis and calcification pathways. However, clinical trials for treatments targeting these pathways are in their infancy.[19]

Despite the similarities between aortic stenosis and atherosclerosis progression, statin trial results are mixed in reducing aortic stenosis disease progression.[23–26] Emerging evidence has supported that elevated Lp(a) levels exacerbate valve calcification and are associated with increased incidence and progression of aortic stenosis which may suggest that an Lp(a) reduction may be an effective treatment option in patients with aortic stenosis.[27,28] Although niacin is able to reduce Lp(a) plasma levels, it has failed to reduce cardiovascular events in randomized trials. PCSK9 inhibitors lower both LDL cholesterol and Lp(a). Clinical trials are in the early phases however, the findings from one recent study demonstrated that PCSK9 inhibitor use is also associated with reduced risk of aortic valve stenosis.[29]

Given the similarities between cardiovascular calcification and bone metabolism, some have suggested that drugs targeting osteoporosis may be effective in treating aortic stenosis. Although observational studies have suggested that bisphosphonate use is associated with reduced cardiovascular calcification and slowed progression of aortic stenosis, data are inconsistent.[30–33] The data on medications to slow the progression of aortic stenosis are equivocal and thus, often the goal of medical management in patients with aortic stenosis is directed at minimizing the gradients and improving cardiac output.

Aortic stenosis typically arises in elderly patients. As such, stiffening of the vasculature typically leads to systemic hypertension and, in the presence of outflow obstruction, further increases the workload on the LV. Diuretics, used alone, often do not offer full BP control. Beta-blockers reduce inotropy, which can be deleterious in an already strained ventricle. Vasodilators—typically angiotensin-converting-enzyme inhibitors (ACE-I) may be initiated at a low dose then cautiously titrated upward. Initially, maximizing preload can be beneficial to augment the Frank–Starling curve. However, as the disease progresses, avoidance of HF is paramount. In the long run, medical management is not effective and requires interventional and/or surgical treatment.

The role of percutaneous balloon valvuloplasty (BAV) has evolved. In the 1980s, it was thought to be curative. However, BAV did not emerge as a definitive treatment due to high restenosis rates and procedural complications. In patients for whom the risk-to-benefit ratio of a valve replacement is unclear, a BAV may be used to evaluate the clinical response or as a bridge to transcatheter or surgical aortic valve replacement. A BAV may also be used as a palliative treatment in patients that are not candidates for definitive therapy. In daily clinical practice, a successful BAV is usually characterized as a reduction in mean gradient after the procedure, increase in the aortic valve area, and improvement in symptoms.

AORTIC REGURGITATION

Causes

Aortic regurgitation is the diastolic reversal of blood from the aorta into the ventricle. It may be caused by either intrinsic abnormalities of the aortic valve leaflets or disease of the perivalvular structures. Aortic regurgitation may occur acutely or as a chronic valvular disease and typical causes are included in Table 31-11. Both presentations are unique with different etiologies, clinical manifestations (Table 31-12), and management strategies.

Pathology

Rheumatic fever leads to fibrinous infiltrates on the valve cusps, causing them to contract and become maligned and incompetent. Patients with rheumatic disease may have a "mixed lesion" that includes both aortic regurgitation and aortic stenosis. In acute or subacute infective endocarditis of the aortic valve, tissue destruction of the leaflets causes cusp perforation or prolapse. Vegetations adherent to the aortic valve may also interfere with valve closure, causing incompetence. In patients with aortic root dilation or ascending aortic dissection, the aortic annulus becomes

Table 31-11 • ETIOLOGIES OF AORTIC REGURGITATION

Leaflet/Cusp Abnormalities	Disease of Perivalvular Structures
Infectious: rheumatic fever, endocarditis	Systemic hypertension
Inflammatory: systemic lupus erythematosus, rheumatoid arthritis	Aortic root dilation: Marfan syndrome, syphilis, aortitis, ankylosing spondylitis, Ehlers–Danlos syndrome
Congenital: bicuspid aortic valve; Marfan Syndrome	Loss of commissural support: ventricular septal defect, aortic dissection, trauma
Trauma	
Drug-induced valvulopathy	

greatly enlarged, the aortic leaflets separate, and aortic incompetence follows.

Pathophysiology

Acute volume overload occurs secondary to regurgitant volume reentering the LV from the aorta through the incompetent aortic valve. In response to the left ventricular volume overload associated with acute regurgitation, progressive left ventricular dilation occurs. This results in increased wall stress, which leads to LVH that normalizes wall stress. Patients with severe aortic regurgitation may have elevated end-diastolic *volumes*, however, their end-diastolic *pressures* are not uniformly elevated. Consistent with the Frank–Starling mechanism, the stroke volume is also increased. Therefore, despite the presence of regurgitation, a normal cardiac output can be maintained and continue for many years.

Conversely, in patients with acute aortic regurgitation, the LV has not had time to compensate with either concentric or eccentric hypertrophy and cannot accommodate the large volume caused by acute aortic regurgitation. As a result, left ventricular and left atrial pressures rise sharply, causing acute CHF and pulmonary edema. Patients with acute aortic regurgitation usually require surgical intervention.

Stages of Chronic AR

The management of patients with aortic regurgitation hinges upon accurate diagnosis of the cause and stage of the disease process. Figure 31-15 shows the stages of aortic regurgitation and range from patient at risk (stage A) or patients with progressive mild to moderate aortic regurgitation (stage B) to patients with severe asymptomatic (stage C) and symptomatic aortic regurgitation (stage D). This classification tool incorporates the valve

Stage	Definition	Valve Anatomy	Valve Hemodynamics	Hemodynamic Consequences	Symptoms
A	At risk of AR	• Bicuspid aortic valve (or other congenital valve anomaly) • Aortic valve sclerosis • Diseases of the aortic sinuses or ascending aorta • History of rheumatic fever or known rheumatic heart disease • IE	• AR severity: none or trace	• None	• None
B	Progressive AR	• Mild-to-moderate calcification of a trileaflet valve bicuspid aortic valve (or other congenital valve anomaly) • Dilated aortic sinuses • Rheumatic valve changes • Previous IE	• Mild AR: o Jet width <25% of LVOT; o Vena contracta <0.3 cm; o RVol <30 mL/beat; o RF <30%; o ERO <0.10 cm²; o Angiography grade 1+ • Moderate AR: o Jet width 25%–64% of LVOT; o Vena contracta.03–0.6 cm; o RVol 30–59 mL/beat; o RF 30%–49%; o ERO.010–0.29 cm²; o Angiography grade 2+	• Normal LV systolic function • Normal LV volume or mild LV dilation	• None
C	Asymptomatic severe AR	• Calcific aortic valve disease • Bicuspid valve (or other congenital abnormality) • Dilated aortic sinuses or ascending aorta • Rheumatic valve changes • IE with abnormal leaflet closure or perforation	• Severe AR: o Jet width ≥65% of LVOT; o Vena contracta >0.6 cm; o Holodiastolic flow reversal in the proximal abdominal aorta o RVol ≥60 mL/beat; o RF ≥50%; o ERO ≥0.3 cm²; o Angiography grade 3+ to 4+; o In addition, diagnosis of chronic severe AR requires evidence of LV dilation	C1: Normal LVEF (≥50%) and mild-to-moderate LV dilation (LVESD ≤50 mm) C2: Abnormal LV systolic function with depressed LVEF (<50%) or severe LV dilatation (LVESD >50 mm or indexed LVESD >25 mm/m²)	• None; exercise testing is reasonable to confirm symptom status
D	Symptomatic severe AR	• Calcific valve disease • Bicuspid valve (or other congenital abnormality) • Dilated aortic sinuses or ascending aorta • Rheumatic valve changes • Previous IE with abnormal leaflet closure or perforation	• Severe AR: o Doppler jet width ≥65% of LVOT; o Vena contracta >0.6 cm; o Holodiastolic flow reversal in the proximal abdominal aorta; o RVol ≥60 mL/beat; o RF ≥50%; o ERO ≥0.3 cm²; o Angiography grade 3+ to 4+; o In addition, diagnosis of chronic severe AR requires evidence of LV dilation	• Symptomatic severe AR may occur with normal systolic function (LVEF ≥50%), mild-to-moderate LV dysfunction (LVEF 40%–50%), or severe LV dysfunction (LVEF <40%); • Moderate-to-severe LV dilation is present	• Exertional dyspnea or angina or more severe HF symptoms

AR indicates aortic regurgitation; ERO, effective regurgitant orifice; HF, heart failure; IE, infective endocarditis; LV, left ventricular; LVEF, left ventricular ejection fraction; LVESD, left ventricular end-systolic dimension; LVOT, left ventricular outflow tract; RF, regurgitant fraction; and RVol, regurgitant volume.

Figure 31-15. Stages of aortic regurgitation. (Used with permission from Nishimura RA, Otto CM, Bonow RO, et al. 2014 AHA/ACC guideline for the management of patients with valvular heart disease: a Report of the American College of Cardiology/American Heart Association Task Force on practice guidelines. *J Am Coll Cardiol.* 2014;63[22]:e57–e185.)

anatomy (such as congenital abnormalities, diseases of the aortic sinuses and ascending aorta, valve leaflet abnormalities, and prior history of rheumatic fever), valve hemodynamics (i.e., jet width, regurgitant volume and fraction, effective regurgitant orifice area, and angiographic grade), hemodynamic consequences (i.e., LV systolic function and size), and patient symptoms in the overall assessment.[1]

Clinical Manifestations

Chronic

Patients with chronic aortic regurgitation are often asymptomatic for many years. Common symptoms of aortic regurgitation include fatigue and exertional dyspnea. Patients may report palpitations, dizziness, and the sensation of a forceful heartbeat, especially when lying on their left side. Angina may also be noted, but it occurs less frequently in aortic regurgitation than in aortic stenosis. As HF ensues, patients experience orthopnea, paroxysmal nocturnal dyspnea, and cough related to left-sided failure.

Acute

Severe acute aortic regurgitation is usually a hemodynamic emergency. It results in acute volume overload of a normal sized LV that cannot rapidly adapt to the sudden increase in volume from the combined aortic regurgitant flow combined with the normal left atrial inflow. This causes a sudden increase in LV end-diastolic (LVEDP) and filling pressures. When LVEDP exceeds the left atrial pressure premature closure of the mitral valve during diastole can occur leading to further decompensation. Elevated LVEDP leads to mitral regurgitation and increased pulmonary venous pressure. Symptoms of pulmonary edema and left-sided HF develop rapidly. Cardiac output falls due to the inability of the LV to rapidly adapt to the increased volume. Compensatory tachycardia may occur and initially obviate the symptoms related to decline in forward flow. The combination of elevated LVEDP and shortened diastole from tachycardia decreases coronary blood flow dynamics resulting in myocardial ischemia. Profound hypotension and cardiogenic shock ensues in the absence of acute intervention.[34]

Physical Assessment

Chronic

The typical murmur of aortic regurgitation is a high-pitched, early diastolic decrescendo murmur with a blowing quality (see Table 31-2). Patients also may have a physiologic murmur of mitral stenosis caused by the regurgitant aortic jet, which partially prevents mitral valve closure (Austin Flint murmur). As the severity of aortic regurgitation increases, the murmur becomes louder and longer. In chronic aortic regurgitation, the point of maximal impulse is displaced laterally. Systolic hypertension and decreased diastolic pressure create a widened pulse pressure. Patients with chronic aortic regurgitation may have a host of other physical findings that may not be present in acute aortic regurgitation (Table 31-13 and 31-14).

Acute

Acute severe aortic regurgitation typically present with sudden onset dyspnea and rapidly progressing hemodynamic collapse. Hypotension, tachycardia, and pulmonary congestion are commonly seen in addition to severe peripheral vasoconstriction. Acute aortic dissection should be considered in a patient that presents with a significant difference in blood pressure obtained between bilateral extremities. Unlike chronic aortic regurgitation, one would expect a normal or only slightly widened pulse pressure. S_1 may be diminished as a result of the mitral valve prematurely closing. S_3 and S_4 may be present. A short and low-pitched diastolic murmur is heard, but may be difficult to auscultate see Table 31-2.

Table 31-12 • SPECIFIC PHYSICAL EXAMINATION FINDINGS IN AORTIC REGURGITATION

Sign	Physical Description
Quincke sign	Pulsatile flushing/blanching of nail bed with application of gentle pressure
de Musset sign	Bobbing of head with each pulse
Corrigan pulse (water hammer)	Sharp systolic upstroke and diastolic collapse of pulse
Müller sign	Bobbing of uvula with each pulse
Traube sign	"Pistol shot" sound auscultated over the femoral arteries
Duroziez sign	Biphasic femoral bruit auscultated with mild pressure
Hill sign	Blood pressure higher in arms than legs

Medical Management

In symptomatic patients who are candidates for surgery, medical therapy is not a viable alternative to surgery. Medical management does not prevent disease progression but may be useful in alleviating symptoms in patients in patients deemed inoperable. The 2014 AHA/ACC guideline for the management of patients with VHD describes criteria for the use of specific medications. The use of vasodilators such as dihydropyridine calcium channel blockers, ACE-Is, or angiotensin II receptor blockers (ARB) reduces systolic pressure in chronic AR and improves forward flow (especially in chronic aortic regurgitation stage B and C).[34] Beta blocker use is controversial in chronic aortic regurgitation stage B and C for blood pressure control due to the negative chronotropic effect resulting in larger stroke volume and higher systolic pressure.[1] The guidelines recommend the routine use of vasodilator therapy for afterload reduction in patients with chronic asymptomatic mild, moderate, or severe aortic regurgitation and normal LV systolic function however, randomized clinical trial results are not conclusive. Diltiazem and verapamil are contraindicated in aortic regurgitation because they have a more potent negative inotropic effect and may produce bradycardia, which may worsen HF. In addition to long-acting nifedipine and felodipine, ACE-Is may be used to reduce afterload. Sodium nitroprusside reduces preload and afterload and can be used to stabilize patients with acute aortic regurgitation before surgery.

CONCLUSION

VHD is complex. Understanding the etiology and pathology of valve dysfunction is paramount for evaluation, diagnosis, and setting expectation through the process. Nurses are at the forefront of patient advocacy and can be key contributors in helping the patient to get appropriate evaluation at the appropriate time. While medical management strategies are available for each of the valvular pathologies, it is important to understand that surgical intervention and definitive treatment, described in Chapter 32, will decrease long-term complications and preserve outcomes.

Table 31-13 • DIAGNOSTIC TESTING FOR CHRONIC AORTIC REGURGITATION

Diagnostic Test	Rationale/Considerations
Echocardiogram	• First-line imaging modality in the evaluation, accurate diagnosis, and assessment of chronic AR. • Evaluation of regurgitant jet severity, LV size, and systolic function. • Hallmark findings associated with congenital, rheumatic, and infectious etiologies of AR may be detected. • Leaflet perforation, flail leaflet, and fibrosis. • TTE may be used to visualize the surrounding structures including the ascending aorta, although a TEE will provide more details. • TTE can be useful to provide guidance on the timing of valve intervention.
Cardiac catheterization	• Indicated when cardiac MR is not available or there are contraindications for CMR. • In symptomatic patients, cardiac catheterization is useful to assess hemodynamics, coronary artery anatomy, and severity of AR. • Coronary angiography should be completed in patients with known or suspected coronary heart disease. • In patients with aortic root dilation, aortic root angiography may be performed concurrently with coronary angiography.[1]
Electrocardiogram	• May be normal. • Patients with moderate to severe chronic regurgitation may have left-axis deviation and a pattern of left ventricular strain (Q waves in leads I, aVL, and V_3 to V_6, with small R wave in V_1). • Intraventricular conduction defects may occur with left ventricular dysfunction or annular abscess.
Chest radiography	• Congestive heart failure, if present.
Cardiac MR	• Provides accurate assessments of aortic morphology, LV volume, and LV systolic function in addition to regurgitant volume and regurgitant fraction. • Provides clarity in patients with suboptimal echocardiographic data as well in patients whose clinical assessment is not consistent with the severity of AR by echocardiography. • CMR measurement of regurgitant severity is more consistent than echocardiographic measurement.

AR, aortic regurgitation; TTE, transthoracic echocardiogram; TEE, transesophageal echocardiogram; CMR, cardiac magnetic resonance; LV, left ventricle.

Table 31-14 • DIAGNOSTIC TESTING FOR ACUTE AORTIC REGURGITATION

Diagnostic Test	Rationale/Considerations
Transthoracic echocardiogram	• Preferred modality for detecting the cause and estimating the severity of AR.[35] • TTE reveals an equilibration of aortic and LV diastolic pressures along with an elevated LVEDP. • There may be a premature opening of the aortic valve in addition to a delayed opening of the mitral valve. AR regurgitant jet(s) are present. • LV size and ejection fraction may be normal.
Transesophageal echocardiogram	• May be performed to diagnose valvular vegetation or abscess in endocarditis, aortic dissection, or congenital abnormalities
Cardiac catheterization	• In patients with suspected coronary artery disease, especially coronary artery bypass grafting, angiography may be considered only if noninvasive imaging is nondiagnostic.
Computed tomography of chest	• Computed tomography provides rapid and accurate diagnosis of aortic dissection if suspected as a cause of acute AR.
Electrocardiogram	• The electrocardiogram in acute AR is nondiagnostic and may show nonspecific ST-T wave changes and/or LVH.
Chest radiography	• May show pulmonary edema. • Widened mediastinum if aortic dissection is present, with a normal cardiac silhouette.
Cardiac MR	• CMR use is limited in these patients due to hemodynamic instability.

AR, aortic regurgitation; TTE, transthoracic echocardiogram; TEE, transesophageal echocardiogram; CMR, cardiac magnetic resonance; LV, left ventricle; LVH, left ventricular hypertrophy; LVEDP, left ventricular end diastolic pressure.

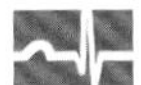

CASE STUDY

Patient Profile

Name/Age/Sex: **Minnie Petersen, 52-year-old female**

History of Present Illness

Mrs. Minnie Petersen is a 52-year-old female who presents to the emergency department for shortness of breath. Her history is notable for breast cancer now in remission, 20 pack-year history of smoking, and recent admission for bacterial endocarditis for which intravenous (IV) antibiotics were initiated per infectious disease. She was discharged 2 weeks ago and continued IV antibiotics via home infusion, administered via peripherally inserted central catheter (PICC) line. She reports worsening shortness of breath over the last week with difficultly climbing stairs or doing inclines. She has avoided walking to the mailbox. Tonight she woke up from sleep extremely short of breath and could not lie flat or catch her breath. Mrs. Petersen is now in the ED triage room.

Medical History

Breast cancer status post bilateral mastectomy 2018, radiation and chemotherapy, in remission
Smoking, 20 pack-year history, quit in 2010
Bacterial endocarditis as described

Allergies

None

Medications

Unsure what antibiotic she is taking
Medication list unavailable

Patient Examination

Vital Signs

Temp 99.9°F; BP 108/48 mmHg; HR 130 bpm; RR 24 breaths/min; SaO_2 92% on 4 L
Cardiac telemetry shows rapid atrial fibrillation at a rate of 130 bpm.

(continued)

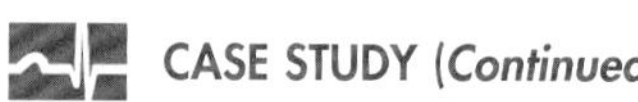

CASE STUDY (*Continued*)

Targeted Physical Examination for Triage
Cardiac: Irregularly irregular. Holosystolic murmur @ LLSB with radiation to the apex and posteriorly. PMI nondisplaced.

Chest: Pectus excavatum. Dull to percussion 1/2 up the left posteriorly and 1/3 up the right.

Respiratory: Shallow, distressed, tachypneic, and labored.

What is the most likely working diagnosis for this patient? What diagnostic tests will be ordered?
Mrs. Petersen's history and physical examination is consistent with acute systolic heart failure and pleural effusions/pulmonary edema secondary to what is likely acute mitral regurgitation. The mechanism is likely degenerative related to endocarditis. Cardiac telemetry and physical exam are consistent with atrial fibrillation which appears to be new. An electrocardiogram, full panel of laboratory studies, chest x-ray and possible pleurocentesis, diuretic, anticoagulation, rate control for atrial fibrillation, transthoracic echocardiogram (and likely transesophageal echocardiogram once stable) are anticipated. The cardiac nurse provides education to the patient and family regarding the working diagnosis, rationale for diagnostic testing, and next steps in the care plan.

KEY READINGS

American Heart Association. *Heart Valve Toolkit for Health Care Professionals.* 2020. Available at https://www.heart.org/en/health-topics/heart-valve-problems-and-disease/heart-valve-disease-resources/heart-valve-toolkit

Maheshwari V, Barr B, Srivastava M. Acute valvular heart disease. *Cardiol Clin.* 2018;36(1):115–127.

Nishimura RA, Otto CM, Bonow RO, et al. 2017 AHA/ACC focused update of the 2014 AHA/ACC guideline for the management of patients with valvular heart disease: a Report of the American College of Cardiology/American Heart Association Task Force on clinical practice guidelines. *Circulation.* 2017;135:e1159–e1195.

REFERENCES

1. Nishimura RA, Otto CM, Bonow RO, et al. 2014 AHA/ACC guideline for the management of patients with valvular heart disease: a Report of the American College of Cardiology/American Heart Association Task Force on practice guidelines. *J Am Coll Cardiol.* 2014;63(22):e57–e185.
2. Joint Task Force on the Management of Valvular Heart Disease of the European Society of Cardiology (ESC); European Association for Cardio-Thoracic Surgery (EACTS), Vahanian A, et al. Guidelines on the management of valvular heart disease (version 2012). *Eur Heart J.* 2012;33(19):2451–2496.
3. Korteland NM, Bras FJ, van Hout FMA, et al. Prosthetic aortic valve selection: current patient experience, preferences and knowledge. *Open Heart.* 2015;2(1):e000237.
4. Hess EP, Coylewright M, Frosch DL, et al. Implementation of shared decision making in cardiovascular care: past, present, and future. *Circ Cardiovasc Qual Outcomes.* 2014;7(5):797–803.
5. Lindman BR, Perpetua E. Incorporating the patient voice into shared decision-making for the treatment of aortic stenosis. *JAMA Cardiol.* 2020;5(4):380–381.
6. Beaton A, Engelman D, Mirabel M. *Acute Rheumatic Fever and Rheumatic Heart Disease.* Philadelphia, PA: Elsevier; 2020.
7. Kumar D, Bhutia E, Kumar P, et al. Evaluation of the American Heart Association 2015 revised Jones criteria versus existing guidelines. *Heart Asia.* 2016;8(1):30–35.
8. Pettersson GB, Hussain ST. Current AATS guidelines on surgical treatment of infective endocarditis. *Ann Cardiothorac Surg.* 2019;8(6):630–644.
9. Baddour Larry M, Wilson Walter R, Bayer Arnold S, et al. Infective endocarditis in adults: diagnosis, antimicrobial therapy, and management of complications. *Circulation.* 2015;132(15):1435–1486.
10. Ranjan R, Pressman GS. Aetiology and epidemiology of mitral stenosis. Available at https://www.escardio.org/Journals/E-Journal-of-Cardiology-Practice/Volume-16/Aetiology-and-epidemiology-of-mitral-stenosis. Accessed May 16, 2020.
11. Shamsudeen I, Fei LYN, Burwash IG, et al. Presentation and management of calcific mitral valve disease. *Int J Cardiol.* 2020;304:135–137.
12. Bonow RO, O'Gara PT, Adams DH, et al. 2020 Focused Update of the 2017 ACC Expert Consensus Decision Pathway on the Management of Mitral Regurgitation: a report of the American College of Cardiology Solution Set Oversight Committee. *J Am Coll Cardiol.* 2020;75(17):2236–2270.
13. Torii S, Romero ME, Mori H, et al. The spectrum of mitral valve pathologies: relevance for surgical and structural interventions. *Expert Rev Cardiovasc Ther.* 2017;15(7):525–535.
14. Nasser R, Van Assche L, Vorlat A, et al. Evolution of functional mitral regurgitation and prognosis in medically managed heart failure patients with reduced ejection fraction. *JACC Heart Fail.* 2017;5(9):652–659.
15. Taramasso M, Vanermen H, Maisano F, et al. The growing clinical importance of secondary tricuspid regurgitation. *J Am Coll Cardiol.* 2012;59(8):703–710.
16. Dahou A, Levin D, Reisman M, et al. Anatomy and physiology of the tricuspid valve. *JACC Cardiovasc Imaging.* 2019;12(3):458–468.
17. Rodés-Cabau J, Taramasso M, O'Gara PT. Diagnosis and treatment of tricuspid valve disease: current and future perspectives. *Lancet.* 2016;388(10058):2431–2442.
18. Pawade TA, Newby DE, Dweck MR. Calcification in aortic stenosis: the skeleton key. *J Am Coll Cardiol.* 2015;66(5):561–577.
19. Zheng KH, Tzolos E, Dweck MR. Pathophysiology of aortic stenosis and future perspectives for medical therapy. *Cardiol Clin.* 2020;38(1):1–12.
20. Ross J Jr, Braunwald E. Aortic stenosis. *Circulation.* 1968;38(1 Suppl):61–67.
21. Harris AW, Pibarot P, Otto CM. Aortic stenosis: guidelines and evidence gaps. *Cardiol Clin.* 2020;38(1):55–63.
22. Baumgartner H, Hung J, Bermejo J, et al. Echocardiographic assessment of valve stenosis: EAE/ASE recommendations for clinical practice. *Eur J Echocardiogr.* 2009;10(1):1–25.
23. Cowell SJ, Newby DE, Prescott RJ, et al. A randomized trial of intensive lipid-lowering therapy in calcific aortic stenosis. *N Engl J Med.* 2005;352(23):2389–2397.
24. Rajamannan NM, Otto CM. Targeted therapy to prevent progression of calcific aortic stenosis. *Circulation.* 2004;110(10):1180–1182.
25. Novaro GM, Tiong IY, Pearce GL, et al. Effect of hydroxymethylglutaryl coenzyme a reductase inhibitors on the progression of calcific aortic stenosis. *Circulation.* 2001;104(18):2205–2209.
26. Moura LM, Ramos SF, Zamorano JL, et al. Rosuvastatin affecting aortic valve endothelium to slow the progression of aortic stenosis. *J Am Coll Cardiol.* 2007;49(5):554–561.
27. Zheng KH, Tsimikas S, Pawade T, et al. Lipoprotein(a) and oxidized phospholipids promote valve calcification in patients with aortic stenosis. *J Am Coll Cardiol.* 2019;73(17):2150–2162.
28. Capoulade R, Chan KL, Yeang C, et al. Oxidized Phospholipids, lipoprotein(a), and progression of calcific aortic valve stenosis. *J Am Coll Cardiol.* 2015;66(11):1236–1246.
29. Langsted A, Nordestgaard BG, Benn M, et al. PCSK9 R46L loss-of-function mutation reduces lipoprotein(a), LDL cholesterol, and risk of aortic valve stenosis. *J Clin Endocrinol Metab.* 2016;101(9):3281–3287.
30. Aksoy O, Cam A, Goel SS, et al. Do bisphosphonates slow the progression of aortic stenosis? *J Am Coll Cardiol.* 2012;59(16):1452–1459.
31. Elmariah S, Delaney JAC, O'Brien KD, et al. Bisphosphonate use and prevalence of valvular and vascular calcification in women MESA (the multi-ethnic study of atherosclerosis). *J Am Coll Cardiol.* 2010;56(21):1752–1759.
32. Innasimuthu AL, Katz WE. Effect of bisphosphonates on the progression of degenerative aortic stenosis. *Echocardiography.* 2011;28(1):1–7.
33. Skolnick AH, Osranek M, Formica P, et al. Osteoporosis treatment and progression of aortic stenosis. *Am J Cardiol.* 2009;104(1):122–124.
34. Akinseye OA, Pathak A, Ibebuogu UN. Aortic valve regurgitation: a comprehensive review. *Curr Probl Cardiol.* 2018;43(8):315–334.
35. Griffin BP. *Manual of Cardiovascular Medicine.* Lippincott Williams & Wilkins; 2018.

32 Therapeutic Intervention for Acquired Valvular Heart Disease: Surgical and Catheter-Based Approaches

Marian Hawkey, Sandra Lauck

OBJECTIVES

1. Describe surgical treatment options for acquired valvular heart disease.
2. Describe FDA-approved transcatheter treatment options for acquired valvular heart disease.

KEY QUESTIONS

1. What are the current treatment options for acquired valvular heart disease?
2. Which patients may be best suited for transcatheter valve therapies?
3. How do priorities for care differ for patients undergoing surgical versus transcatheter procedures?

BACKGROUND

Valvular heart disease remains highly prevalent and, for some patients, challenging to manage and treat definitively. Surgery for heart valve repair and replacement has developed over the past several decades and has been the gold standard of life-saving treatment for countless numbers of patients. However, not all are appropriate candidates for surgical valve repair or replacement because of comorbid burden, frailty, or prohibitive anatomic features.

Transcatheter valve therapy has evolved over the past two decades with the early feasibility procedures of pulmonary and aortic valve implantation and mitral valve repair procedures. Transcatheter aortic valve replacement (TAVR) is currently approved by the Food and Drug Administration (FDA) for patients with symptomatic severe, calcific aortic stenosis at intermediate or higher risk for traditional surgery using the Sapien 3 valve (Edwards, Irvine, CA) and CoreValve (Medtronic, Minneapolis, MN, USA) systems. Transcatheter mitral valve repair (TMVr) using the MitraClip system (Abbott, Abbott Park, IL, USA) is FDA approved for patients with moderate to severe or severe primary (degenerative) mitral regurgitation at prohibitive risk for traditional open-heart surgery, and patients with secondary mitral regurgitation with heart failure symptoms despite optimal medical therapy. Clinical trials are ongoing for a variety of additional transcatheter aortic valve systems and indications, as well as for mitral and tricuspid indications.

The availability and ongoing evaluation of less invasive treatment strategies for valvular heart disease provide options for an increasing number of people for whom traditional open-heart surgery may pose a significant or prohibitive risk. Additionally, an important consequence of developing transcatheter valve programs has been the emergence of the Heart Team as a central force to direct clinical care pathways. The Heart Team includes multidisciplinary healthcare professionals such as surgeons, interventionalists, imaging experts, cardiologists, anesthesiologists, other physician subspecialists (as indicated) and many non-physician caregivers who help to evaluate the patients and coordinate the clinical care before, during, and after transcatheter valve procedures. The collective expertise of these experts transcends the skills of the individual team member and helps to provide an environment for collaborative, optimized clinical decision making.

SURGICAL APPROACHES

Overview

Prosthetic cardiac valves have been used since the mid-1960s to treat acquired valvular heart disease. Because no "perfect" prosthetic valve exists, the patient with valvular heart disease is managed medically as long as it is safely feasible. Timing of valve replacement depends on the patient's functional status, ventricular dysfunction, and the natural course of the lesion.

Before a decision is made to use a particular valve, factors in valve design, specifically durability, thrombogenic potential, and hemodynamic properties, are weighed against annulus size and certain clinical conditions such as the desirability of long-term anticoagulation. Table 32-1 summarizes the characteristics considered in selection of prosthetic valves. Because of their proven durability, mechanical valves are most often chosen for patients younger than 65 to 70 years unless contraindicated (e.g., previous bleeding problems, desire to become pregnant, or poor compliance with medication and follow-up). Prosthetic heart valves differ in design, echocardiography image, and radiologic appearance (Fig. 32-1).

Table 32-1 • SELECTION OF TYPE OF PROSTHETIC VALVE BASED ON PATIENT CHARACTERISTICS

Biologic Valve	Mechanical Valve
History of bleeding	Age <65 years
Inability to take warfarin	Already on anticoagulation
Desire to become pregnant	History of embolic cerebral vascular accident
History of thrombosis with mechanical valve	
History of atrial fibrillation	
Age >65 years	

Mechanical Valves

Mechanical (nonbiologic) valves have excellent durability but are usually thrombogenic. Bileaflet and tilting-disk valves are the mechanical valves in common use today. Caged-ball valves are used less frequently in the United States but may be used in other areas of the world. In patients with aneurysm or dissection of the ascending aorta, composite grafts of conduit and mechanical valves may be used.

Bileaflet valves, such as St. Jude, ATS (advancing the standard), and the CarboMedic are low-profile valves that have centrally mounted leaflets attached to the seating ring with butterfly hinges. These hinges allow the leaflets to open to 85 degrees, making these valves the least obstructive of the mechanical valves. These valves are composed of pyrolytic carbon. With adequate anticoagulation, thromboembolic risk is low with bileaflet valves.

The tilting-disk valve is a low-profile valve consisting of a disk that sits in a seating ring; the flat or convexo–concave disk tilts in response to pressure changes. The Medtronic Hall valve is a tilting-disk valve commonly used today. Tilting-disk valves open to an angle of 60 to 75 degrees in relation to the seating ring. When open, tilting-disk valves produce a minor and major orifice for blood to pass through. Tilting disks have more central flow, but usually more turbulence, than caged-ball valves. Tilting disks close with an audible click. The technology for production of tilting-disk valves has evolved so that a single piece of metal is used to avoid welded struts.

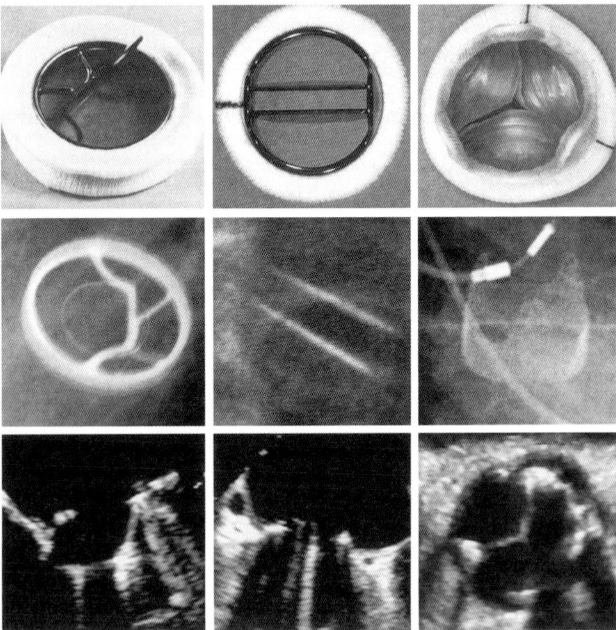

Figure 32-1. Photographic (*top row*), radiographic (*middle row*), and echocardiographic (*bottom row*) appearance of prosthetic valves. From left to right: Bjork–Shiley single tilting disk, St. Jude's Medical bileaflet mechanical valve, and Carpentier–Edwards xenograft (radiographs courtesy of Dr. Carolyn van Dyke). (Adapted from Garcia ML. Prosthetic valve disease. In: Topol EJ, Califf RM, Isner JM, et al., eds. *Textbook of Cardiovascular Medicine.* Philadelphia, PA: Lippincott-Raven; 1998:580.)

Caged-ball valves have been used since the 1960s and have an excellent durability record. Changes in pressure cause the ball to move forward and back within its caged structure. Flow is directed laterally through the valve rather than centrally. Because of its high profile, the caged-ball valve prosthesis can become obstructive, especially when used in patients with small aortic roots or small left ventricles. The Starr–Edwards and the Sutter were two of the most commonly used caged-ball valves. Caged-ball prostheses have been largely abandoned in favor of lower-profile bileaflet valves.

Tissue Valves

Tissue (biologic) valves are characterized by having low rates of thrombotic episodes associated with their use. Porcine or bovine tissue is strengthened and made nonviable by treatment with glutaraldehyde. Homografts are tissue valves from cadavers. They are preserved cryogenically, but are difficult to procure, and their longevity has not been well proven. The main advantages of tissue valves are the associated low rates of thromboembolism and the subsequent decrease in patient morbidity when anticoagulant therapy is not required. Nonthrombogenicity is particularly important for those patients in whom long-term anticoagulation should be avoided, such as children, young adult women, those older than 70 years, or those with a history of bleeding.

The Hancock porcine valve, the Medtronic Mosaic porcine bioprosthesis (treated with α-oleic acid to retard calcification), and the Carpentier–Edwards porcine valve are xenografts using porcine aortic valves preserved with glutaraldehyde under pressure, mounted on a stent.[1] The Carpentier–Edwards pericardial bioprosthesis is made of leaflets fashioned from bovine pericardium fixed without pressure in glutaraldehyde.

Stentless bioprosthetic porcine xenograft valves such as the St. Jude Medical-Toronto, the Medtronic Freestyle Stentless, and the Edwards Prima Plus porcine bioprosthesis have been developed to improve the durability and enhance the hemodynamic performance of porcine aortic valves. Stentless aortic biologic valves were developed secondary to the recognition that conventional bioprosthesis have limitations of long-term durability and residual obstruction that may impede left ventricular mass regression.[2] Use of the stentless aortic bioprosthesis has resulted in enhanced survival and hemodynamic superiority.[3] It is expected that reducing mechanical stress on valve leaflets, and the associated degeneration of the bioprosthesis, may be slowed.

Homografts or allografts from human cadavers are virtually free of any associated thrombosis. They are especially useful in patients with small aortic roots or in patients with active endocarditis. Earlier homografts were preserved with glutaraldehyde and demonstrated early failure. Homografts are now stored "fresh" after harvesting in an antibiotic solution and are then cryopreserved, increasing their longevity to at least 10 years. Valve failure is uncommon and usually the result of progressive valve incompetence. Aortic allografts have demonstrated excellent freedom from thromboembolism, endocarditis, and progressive valve incompetence.[4] Because of lack of availability, use of homografts has been limited.

In the Ross procedure (also known as pulmonary autograft), the aortic valve is replaced with a pulmonary autograft, and the native

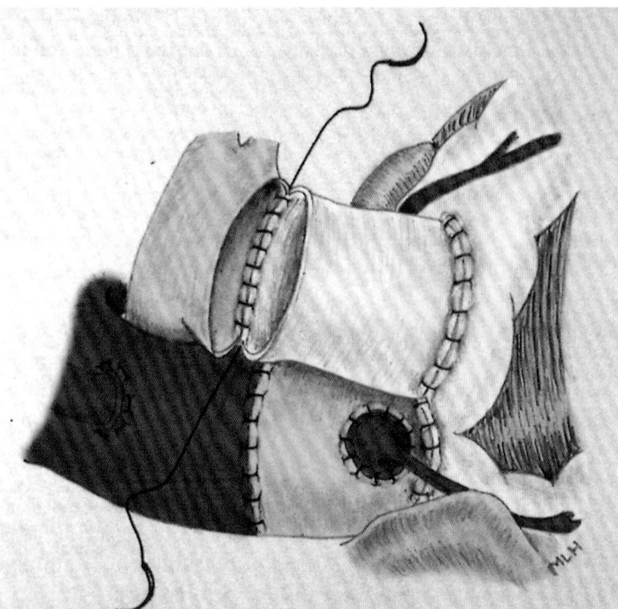

Figure 32-2. Illustration of Ross procedure. Suture line of pulmonary homograft is shown. (From Elkins RC. Valve repair and valve replacement in children, including the Ross procedure. In: Kaiser LR, Kron IL, Spray TL, eds. *Mastery of Cardiothoracic Surgery.* Philadelphia, PA: Lippincott-Raven; 1998:947.)

pulmonary valve is replaced with a pulmonic allograft. Although this procedure introduced by Donald Ross in 1967 was originally developed for pediatric application, it has been expanded to adult surgery as well.[5] In patients undergoing the Ross procedure, the native pulmonary valve is excised and then implanted in the aortic position (autograft); a pulmonary homograft (allograft) is implanted into the pulmonic position (Fig. 32-2). The pulmonary autograft has been shown to be resistant to degeneration and calcification. The actuarial freedom from pulmonary autograft valve replacement is 90% ± 3% at 13 years. The Ross procedure cannot be performed in patients with bicuspid aortic valves or dilated aortic roots.[6] Although the Ross procedure has limited acceptance due to the complexity of the surgery and the replacement of both the aortic and pulmonic valves, in young adults who wish to avoid anticoagulation, it offers an alternative with favorable midterm results.[7]

Minimally Invasive Valve Surgery

Minimally invasive valve surgery is now used for both aortic valve replacement and mitral valve repair and replacement. Minimally invasive surgical approaches are possible because a wide assortment of technologic advances, such as endoscopic and surgical equipment, have been developed to evolve toward more complex, video- and robot-assisted procedures.[8] Although patients undergoing minimally invasive valve surgery still require cardiopulmonary bypass, classic median sternotomy may be avoided, thus reducing pain, improving cosmetic results, and expediting recovery. Endoscopic mitral and tricuspid repair is feasible even after previous cardiac surgery.[9] As minimally invasive valve surgery continues to evolve, it will likely become a mainstay in the treatment of valvular heart surgery.

Aortic valve replacement can be performed through an upper "T" ministernotomy without intraoperative difficulties. Postoperative pain is reduced and recovery is expedited, with patients discharged to home as early as postoperative day (POD) 3.[10] Compared with patients with median sternotomy, patients undergoing mitral valve replacement through the right parasternal approach had a shortened length of stay and reduced direct hospital costs.[11] Most clinical series demonstrates that minimally invasive port-access approach to mitral valve surgery has low morbidity and mortality, with echocardiographic outcomes equivalent to conventional mitral valve surgery.[12] More recently, minimally invasive mitral valve surgery has evolved to include computer-assisted robotic techniques in current clinical trials. The da Vinci Surgical System allows the surgeon to operate from a console through an end-affecter using microwrist instruments, which are mounted on robotic arms, inserted through the chest wall.

Complications of Prosthetic Valves

Thromboembolism remains the most common complication of patients with prosthetic valves. Anticoagulant therapy with warfarin is begun in all patients 48 hours after surgery. All patients with mechanical valves require life-long anticoagulation because of the risk of thrombosis and embolization. The highest thromboembolic risk for mechanical and biologic valves occurs in the first few days to months after implantation, before the valve is fully endothelialized. The American Heart Association and the American College of Cardiology recommend international normalized ratio of 2.0 to 3.0 for mechanical aortic valves and international normalized ratio of 2.5 to 3.5 for mechanical mitral valves.[13] Tissue valves other than homografts also usually require anticoagulation for 6 to 12 weeks after surgery, after which patients have their therapy converted to aspirin. Homografts or the Ross procedure requires no anticoagulation.

Prosthetic valvular thrombosis is a serious complication and can result in severe hemodynamic compromise. In patients with prosthetic valves who are not anticoagulated into a therapeutic range, thrombosis of the prosthetic valve can occur. Thrombus or pannus formation on the valve may occlude the orifice or entrap the pivoting mechanisms, causing acute stenosis or regurgitation. Symptoms of valve thrombosis include embolic events and CHF. If there are large thrombi or valve dysfunction, urgent or emergency valve replacement is usually indicated. Fibrinolytic therapy may be used for right-sided valve thrombosis or left-sided thrombosis with a small clot burden.[6]

Although symptoms of prosthetic valve endocarditis are similar to those of native valve endocarditis, the infection may be difficult to control with antibiotics alone because of the prosthetic material involved. Early prosthetic valve endocarditis (within the first 60 days) carries a high mortality rate. Early prosthetic valve endocarditis occurs in less than 1% of patients who have had valve replacements and frequently requires the patient to undergo additional operations.[14] The most common organism in early prosthetic valve endocarditis is *Staphylococcus epidermidis*. Fever, heart failure, new murmur, and embolic events are common manifestations. Late prosthetic valve endocarditis (more than 60 days after surgery) occurs most commonly in patients with bioprosthetic valves in the aortic position. The incidence is less than 1% per year and is generally caused by the same bacterial species that cause subacute bacterial endocarditis.[14]

Prosthesis malfunction is uncommon for the first 10 years after artificial valve implantation. The best-known problems with mechanical failures were those affecting the Bjork–Shiley convexo–concave tilting-disk valves first manufactured in 1978, with the peak incidence of valve failure in the 1981–1982 models. Subsequent modifications improved the valve area but also increased stress forces. Although these valves have been withdrawn from the market, approximately 40,000 had been implanted worldwide. Because acute valve strut fracture can be fatal, patients with these valves should be evaluated for partial strut fracture using high-resolution cineradiography. Valve degeneration is the primary complication of patients with tissue prostheses. Degeneration of biologic prostheses can occur as lipid or calcium deposits cause valve cusps to stiffen and become stenotic. Failure of tissue valves often occurs slowly over months to years and presents as progressive heart failure. Prosthetic valve degeneration and failure are most easily diagnosed with echocardiography.

Paravalvular leaks between the prosthetic ring and the annulus occur because of tearing of the suture line, spontaneously or after infection. Presence of a new murmur and signs of heart failure alert the clinician to paravalvular leaks. The patient's clinical course should be followed; when the leak becomes significant, surgical repair or replacement is indicated. Hemolysis may also accompany paravalvular leaks.

Hemolytic anemia is a consequence of shortened red cell survival time in all patients with prosthetic valves. Movement of the valve ball or disk causes varying degrees of destruction of the red blood cells. Hemolysis may also occur with paravalvular leak.

Commonly, hemolysis is mild and the patient can compensate by increasing red blood cell production. Rarely, hemolytic anemia occurs. Chronic intravascular hemolysis results in loss of iron in the urine; iron deficiency anemia may result after several years.

Aortic Stenosis

Aortic valve replacement should be considered the treatment of choice for severe aortic stenosis in spite of age.[15] Aortic valve replacement for mechanical relief of obstruction to flow is the only effective treatment.[16] The natural history of aortic stenosis is used as a guide to determine the timing of aortic valve replacement surgery. Patients with asymptomatic aortic stenosis have nearly the same survival rate as the age-matched general population. Once the patient experiences symptoms of angina, syncope, or heart failure, there is an abrupt decline in survival rate. In patients presenting with CHF, only 50% survive 2 years. For patients who present with syncope, the 3-year survival rate is only 50% without aortic valve replacement. The average life expectancy of patients with apnea is only 5 years without aortic valve replacement.[17] Aortic valve replacement is recommended in all patients with severe, symptomatic aortic stenosis. Selection of aortic valve prostheses is discussed earlier in this chapter.

Aortic Regurgitation

Acute aortic regurgitation requires urgent aortic valve replacement. Without adequate time for compensatory mechanisms to develop, aortic regurgitation triggers rapid onset of CHF, tachycardia, and diminished cardiac output. It is desirable to treat patients with acute aortic regurgitation secondary to infective endocarditis with a minimum of 48 hours of appropriate intravenous antibiotics before implanting a prosthetic valve. In patients with active endocarditis who are hemodynamically unstable, use of cadaveric human aortic homografts may minimize the risk of prosthetic valve endocarditis. Patients who have aortic regurgitation caused by ascending aortic dissection or dilation require replacement of the ascending aorta as well.

In chronic aortic regurgitation, the aortic valve must be replaced before irreversible left ventricular dysfunction develops. In asymptomatic patients, it is usually recommended that the aortic valve be replaced when left ventricular function begins to deteriorate. Aortic valve replacement is recommended for the symptomatic patient when left ventricular ejection fraction drops to 0.50 or less, left ventricular systolic dimension is 55 mm or more, and left ventricular diastolic dimension is 75 mm or more.[6]

Mitral Stenosis

Surgical replacement of the mitral valve is required when there is severe mitral regurgitation coexisting with mitral stenosis or if the mitral stenosis is not amenable to percutaneous balloon valvuloplasty. Although some valves with mitral stenosis may be repaired by open commissurotomy and reconstruction, heavily calcified rheumatic mitral valves are often beyond the point of repair. For patients with coexistent tricuspid regurgitation, combined mitral valve surgery with tricuspid repair is related to better clinical outcomes than mitral balloon valvuloplasty alone.[18] A mechanical prosthesis is frequently chosen for patients with mitral stenosis as many already require anticoagulation for existing atrial fibrillation or have a high likelihood of developing atrial fibrillation.[19] For young women who wish to become pregnant, a bioprosthesis may be recommended.

Mitral Regurgitation

Two surgical approaches are used to treat mitral regurgitation. Mitral valve repair uses reconstructive techniques as well as a rigid prosthetic ring to repair the mitral valve apparatus, thus sparing the valve and avoiding the consequences of valve replacement. Mitral valve replacement involves implantation of a prosthetic valve, either mechanical or bioprosthetic. The mitral valve apparatus is preserved whenever possible as it contributes to the preservation of left ventricular function (Fig. 32-3). In patients with chronic mitral regurgitation, mitral replacement should occur

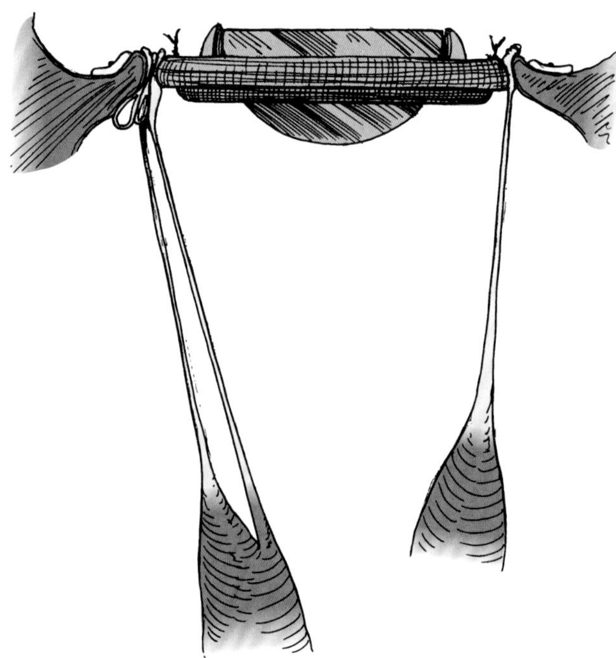

Figure 32-3. Valve replacement with chordal preservation. (From Chitwood WR. Mitral valve repair: ischemic. In: Kaiser LR, Kron IL, Spray TL, eds. *Mastery of Cardiothoracic Surgery.* Philadelphia, PA: Lippincott-Raven; 1998:321.)

Table 32-2 • PRIORITIES FOR CARE FOLLOWING SURGICAL HEART VALVE REPLACEMENT

1. Ventilation	• Maintain proper positioning of endotracheal tube • Collect arterial blood gas samples and manage ventilator settings according to institutional protocol • Wean from ventilator according to institutional protocol
2. Hemodynamic stability	• Achieve return to normothermia according to institutional protocol • Maintain hemodynamics according to prescribed parameters • Verify proper positioning of invasive monitoring lines • Observe for alterations in cardiac rhythm and initiation of treatment, i.e., pacing as indicated • Wean from vasoactive infusions according to institutional protocol • Assess peripheral perfusion
3. Bleeding surveillance	• Maintain sump tube patency and measure output according to institutional protocol • Observe for change/increase in incisional bleeding • Monitor serial CBC results • Initiate anticoagulation therapy according to institutional protocol and monitor for adverse effects
4. Neurologic function	• Administer sedation and analgesia according to institutional protocol • Perform neurologic assessments at prescribed intervals • Report alterations in neurologic status promptly
5. Prevention of infection	• Administer postoperative antibiotics according to institutional protocol • Remove indwelling lines, pacing wires and catheters as soon as appropriate
6. Multi-system function	• Monitor creatinine level and urine output • Assess for bowel sounds and changes in abdominal exam • Monitor lab results for significant changes • Repletion of electrolytes according to institutional standards
7. Return to independent function	• Advance diet according to institutional protocol • Advance activity according to institutional protocol • Initiate postoperative teaching according to institutional protocol

before the patient has had irreversible left ventricular dysfunction. Mitral valve replacement or repair can preserve left ventricular function and ejection fraction. Patients with NYHA class II symptoms should be considered for surgery.

In most patients, mitral valve repair may be undertaken for patients with mitral insufficiency as an alternative to replacement. Surgical techniques involve reconstructing the leaflets and annulus in such a way as to narrow the orifice. These procedures consist of direct suture of the valve cusps, repair of the elongated or ruptured chordae tendineae (chordoplasty), or repair of the valve annulus (annuloplasty). With an annuloplasty, the incompetent valve is remodeled using a ring prosthesis that is attached to the leaflets and the annulus. Mitral valve repair has demonstrated excellent short- and long-term results with low perioperative mortality rate (not greater than 2% in most reported series). In patients with acute mitral regurgitation secondary to myocardial infarction, coronary angiography should be performed to define coronary anatomy for concomitant coronary bypass surgery at the time of mitral valve repair or replacement.

Mitral Valve Prolapse

Mitral valve prolapse is the most common cause of chronic primary MR in developed countries. Outcomes are determined by both lesion severity as well as the presence of negative prognostic features such as symptoms, LV dysfunction, and pulmonary hypertension. Such features are usually present only in the setting of severe MR.

Patients with MVP and severe mitral regurgitation or flail leaflets should be evaluated for surgery. They often can undergo repair rather than replacement. For discussion of surgical options, refer to the section on surgical intervention for mitral regurgitation.

Tricuspid Regurgitation

If tricuspid regurgitation is severe and symptomatic, tricuspid valve repair may be performed, most commonly using an annuloplasty ring. Tricuspid valve replacement is uncommon and is done only if a satisfactory tricuspid repair cannot be accomplished. Surgical correction of tricuspid regurgitation is most often considered at the time of aortic or mitral valve surgery.

Priorities for Care

Patient acuity is high in the immediate postoperative period following heart valve replacement and vigilant clinical management is essential. The trajectory to recovery is usually quite rapid and is facilitated by careful attention to priorities for care (Table 32-2). The operative course including cardiopulmonary bypass and aortic cross-clamp times must be taken into account as well as medical history and comorbid conditions.

There are usually well-defined institutional protocols and processes of care for postoperative cardiac surgery patients which guide clinician practice and help to ensure optimal surveillance and management.

TRANSCATHETER HEART VALVE INTERVENTIONS

The emergence of safe, reproducible, minimally invasive catheter-based interventions has become a game changer in the management of valvular heart disease. The first reports emerged in the early years of our century, describing the feasibility of using a percutaneous approach, and stent and catheter technology to deliver a device in the aortic position.[20–22] Although significant barriers and challenges surfaced in the early development phase, an intense era of early clinical trials contributed to a paradigm shift in treatment options and patient care.[23–25] Innovations are ongoing, and evidence continues to emerge to guide case selection, procedural approaches, and the continuum of care in people with varying heart valve diseases and clinical presentation.

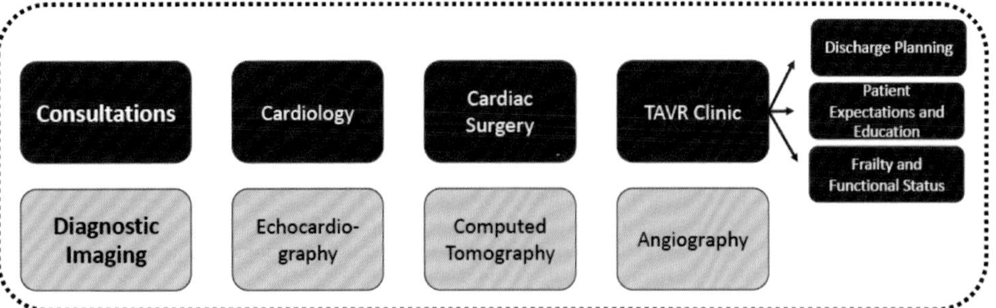

Figure 32-4. Consultations and diagnostic imaging required in patients considered for transcatheter aortic valve replacement.

Overview

Transcatheter interventions are established or emerging for the management of stenosis or regurgitation in all diseased valves. These treatment options share the common principles of percutaneous or minimally invasive surgical vascular access and closure, use of a catheter-based system to deliver an expandable prosthesis that is placed in the diseased native annulus or failed bioprosthetic valve, and opportunities to avoid conventional surgical practices (sternotomy, cardiopulmonary bypass, general anesthesia, use of invasive monitoring devices, and vasoactive medication support), facilitate shorter length of stay and rapid recovery. Although early efforts focused on children with congenital pulmonary valve disease, conclusive advances were made in the development of TAVR (also known as TAVI—implantation). More recently, transcatheter mitral valve repair (TMVr) and replacement (TMVR) options have become available, while innovative approaches continue to be explored to treat the diseased tricuspid valve. Together, these rapidly evolving options offer new opportunities for patients while challenging clinicians to adapt to the continuous emergence of evidence to guide practice. In this context, we focus our discussion on case selection, procedural approaches and nursing care for the most established interventions available to patients with valvular heart disease.

AORTIC STENOSIS

Transcatheter Aortic Valve Replacement

Over the rapid span of the past decade, TAVR has become the established and recommended treatment options for patients who present with higher surgical risk profiles (including intermediate, high, and prohibitive operative risks). As recent clinical trials in lower surgical risk patients have found TAVR to be superior or equal to surgical aortic-valve replacement (SAVR), TAVR is positioned to become the standard of care for most people with aortic stenosis. Given current indications, it is estimated that over 170,000 potential patients are eligible for TAVR annually in North America and Europe.[26] Indications are evolving in international guidelines while policy makers and funders are challenges to facilitate patient access to care and monitor quality of health services. There is sustained consensus that careful case selection, a procedure matched to patient and procedural needs, and standardized postprocedure protocols are essential to program and procedural success.[27]

Case Selection

Heart Team Approach. A central component of case selection rests on the foundational importance of a multidisciplinary team approach to case selection and procedure planning. The Heart Team model of consensus treatment decision is a Class I recommendation in the U.S. and European guidelines.[28] The goal is to leverage the expertise and skillset of cardiologists, cardiac surgeons, nursing and other disciplines to optimize quality of patients care and safety. At the time of case selection, the primary activities of the Heart Team include the review of patients' medical condition and valve disease, the consensus recommendation of indicated, technically feasible, and reasonable interventions, and the inclusion of patients and family in treatment decision.[13] Although significant challenges to implementing and sustaining an effective and well-functioning Heart Team approach have been identified.[29] Patient and program benefits continue to drive the mandated or strong recommendation to maintain a multidisciplinary approach. The role of Valve Program Clinician (VPC) has emerged as centrally important to foster patient-centered coordination of care, program leadership, and multidisciplinary communication and engagement.[30]

Evaluation Pathway. Patients referred for TAVR must undergo a comprehensive evaluation to determine their eligibility for treatment (Fig. 32-4). A careful medical history inclusive of symptoms and comorbidities is essential to assess physical status and risk profile. The advanced age of most patients with severe aortic stenosis warrants the systematic and rigorous assessment of frailty to further inform the determination of risk and the likelihood to derive mortality, morbidity, and quality-of-life benefit.[31] Cardiac nurses' leadership and clinical expertise in promoting the inclusion of measurement of frailty, functional status, and disabilities has been instrumental in setting the standard of care.[32] High-quality multimodality imaging diagnostic testing further augments the essential components of the evaluation pathway. Echocardiography remains the gateway diagnostic to determine severity of disease, valve anatomy, concomitant valvular lesions, cardiac functions (left ventricular ejection fraction), and wall motion abnormalities. Limited cusp motion, decrease in maximal cusp separation, and the presence of left ventricular hypertrophy confirm the presence of aortic stenosis, while mean hemodynamic gradient, maximum jet velocity across the valve orifice, stroke volume, and aortic valve area are pivotal findings that determine the need for valve replacement. Multidetector computed tomography (MDCT) is increasingly used to inform procedure planning. Imaging of the aortic root, aorta, aortic valve, and peripheral vascular systems enables the selection of optimal procedural approach, device, and implantation strategy. Cardiac catheterization and coronary angiography are performed to obtain an assessment of the coronary system, determine the need for revascularization, and provide information about eligibility for a transfemoral approach. Although inaccurate at predicting outcomes after TAVR, surgical risk assessments remain in use across most regions. The U.S. Society of Thoracic Surgeons (STS) Predicted Risk of Mortality and the EuroSCORE employ models based on cardiac surgery

Table 32-3 • RISK ASSESSMENT COMBINING STS RISK ESTIMATE, FRAILTY, MAJOR ORGAN SYSTEM DYSFUNCTION, AND PROCEDURE-SPECIFIC IMPEDIMENTS

	Low Risk (Must Meet ALL Criteria in This Column)	Intermediate Risk (Any 1 Criterion in This Column)	High Risk (Any 1 Criterion in This Column)	Prohibitive Risk (Any 1 Criterion in This Column)
STS PROM	<4% AND	<4–8% OR	>8% OR	Predicted risk with surgery of death or major morbidity (all-cause) >50% at 1 year
Frailty	None AND	1 Index (mild) OR	≥2 Indices (moderate to severe) OR	OR
Major organ system compromise not to be improved postoperatively	None AND	1 Organ system OR	No more than 2 organ systems OR	≥3 Organ systems OR
Procedure-specific impediment	None	Possible procedure-specific impediment	Possible procedure-specific impediment	Severe procedure-specific impediment

Nishimura RA, Otto CM, Bonow RO, et al. 2014 AHA/ACC guideline for the management of patients with valvular heart disease: executive summary: a report of the American College of Cardiology/American Heart Association Task Force on Practice Guidelines. *J Am Coll Cardiol.* 2014;63(22):2438–2488.

variables to derive a predictor score of operative mortality and other adverse events. The American College of Cardiology/American Heart Association (ACC/AHA) recommend using the STS score in conjunction with measurement of frailty, major organ system compromise, and procedure-specific impediment to guide TAVR risk assessment.[13,33]

Importantly, there is not a single score or variable that determines suitability and eligibility for TAVR. Together, these consultations and diagnostic imaging tests constitute the core information that clinicians need to provide a treatment recommendation to guide shared decision making with patients with complex aortic stenosis (Table 32-3).

Patient Education. As the boundaries between risk-based indications continue to evolve and possibly blur, the importance of embedding a shared decision-making process in patient and family education and developing robust patient decision aids is rising.[34,35] Shared decision making is a component of patient-centered care, and refers to a deliberate joint and meaningful communication process between patients and clinicians to achieve the best possible account for the patient. In this exchange, clinicians are accountable for providing and explaining treatment options (including doing nothing) based on the best available evidence including the risks and benefits of each option, and verifying patients' understanding. Patients are responsible for sharing their preferences and values for the outcomes of each option. The goal is to achieve a concordance between values and choices, and a treatment decision that matches what is most desirable for the patient.[36] A patient decision-aid is a carefully developed, evidence-based, and user-tested valid and reliable tool that is used to supplement and help guide shared decision making. They do not replace the face-to-face discussion but rather help guide the discussion. The objectives of a patient decision-aid are to (1) explicitly state the treatment choices that are under consideration, (2) provide evidence-based information about these options, including the potential benefits and harms, and (3) help patients and their family members recognize the sensitivity to their values and priorities that are inherent to their appraisal of treatment options and their ultimate decision.[37] The American College of Cardiology has led the development of impactful resources focused on making the decision between TAVR and SAVR in patients who present with intermediate, high, or prohibitive surgical risks.[38] Such initiatives are gaining momentum to ensure that patients remain at the center of treatment decision.

Periprocedure Approach

Vascular Access. The selection of vascular access approach is driven by femoral artery anatomy, especially arterial size and tortuosity, atherosclerotic burden and location, and the presence of thrombus. Transfemoral access is the least invasive and the preferred procedural approach. Over 90% of procedures are now performed transfemorally as the minimally iliofemoral artery diameter can be as small at 5 mm to be suitable for safe percutaneous access and closure (Fig. 32-5).[39] In the presence of small diameter vessels, excessive calcification or tortuosity, alternative access routes may be considered, including transapical, transaortic, and transsubclavian among others. Regardless of vascular access approach, the main components of the procedure include establishing vascular access for the delivery system and cardiac catheterization, use of angiography augmented by echocardiography as required, catheter-based device delivery, and vascular access closure. Continuous hemodynamic monitoring is essential to guide the procedure. Transvenous right ventricular rapid pacing is often used to temporarily decrease stroke volume at the time of device deployment and helps maintain stability for optimal placement.[40]

TAVR Devices. The main determinants of device selection are valve anatomy and size. There are currently two devices approved by the U.S. FDA while a larger number have received European approval (CE Mark). The primary mechanisms of deployment include balloon-expandable (e.g., the Edwards SAPIEN3 device uses the rapid inflation of a valvuloplasty-type balloon) and self-expanding (e.g., the Medtronic EVOLUT TAVR System uses a catheter pull back technique).

Procedure Room Nursing. The skillset and competencies of cardiac nurses who support TAVR patients in the periprocedure phase must match the unique needs of the procedural approach. Depending on the region and the procedural approach (transfemoral vs. alternative surgical approach), the procedural setting for TAVR may be a conventional or hybrid cardiac catheterization laboratory or operating room with high fidelity imaging and hemodynamic monitoring capability. In the United States, centers report using a hybrid procedure rooms whereas European centers are more likely to use a conventional cardiac catheterization laboratory. In all cases, international societies recommend adherence to high standards of sterility and air circulation.[40] Therefore, cardiac nurses working in this field are challenged to acquire and maintain a "hybrid" skillset

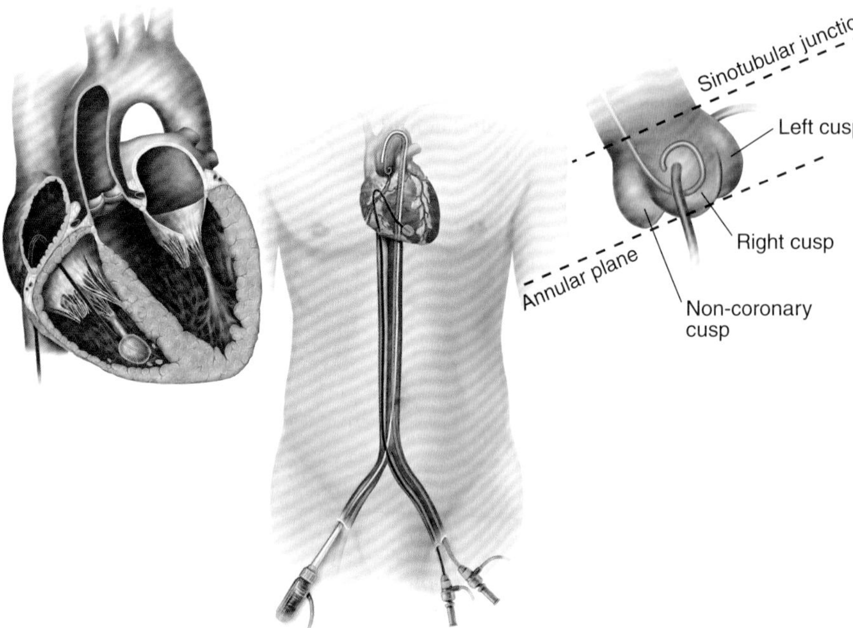

Figure 32-5. Transfemoral approach for transcatheter aortic valve replacement. Setup depicting typical access for transfemoral transcatheter aortic valve replacement with delivery and nondelivery sides. *Insets* depict balloon-tipped pacing catheter in right ventricle and coplanar alignment of aortic cusps ("deployment angle") with an angled pigtail. (Reprinted with permission from Grover FL, Mack MJ, eds. *Cardiac Surgery.* Philadelphia, PA: Wolters Kluwer; 2017.)

that includes components of interventional cardiology nursing (e.g., competency in catheter-based intervention, interpretation of invasive hemodynamic monitoring data) and cardiac surgery nursing (e.g., asepsis, support for various anesthesia strategies). To this end, there is increasing interest in enabling cardiac nurses to become proficient in the specialized field of periprocedure TAVR, or opting for a mixed staffing model of interventional cardiology and surgical nurses who develop similar competencies while contributing their unique skillsets to optimize patient safety (Fig. 32-6).

Anesthesia Strategies and Periprocedure Monitoring. The maturation of TAVR has been associated with a decrease in the intensity of anesthesia. Although general anesthesia and the use of transoesophageal echocardiography became rapidly established as the standard of care in the early years, there is increasing interest in the transition to the use of local anesthesia or monitored anesthesia care, combined with postprocedure transoesophageal echocardiography to ascertain valve function and patient safety.[41] Potential benefits of local anesthesia with minimal sedation include hemodynamic stability, improved ability to detect early warnings of complications (e.g., vascular injury), reduced risk/elimination of postprocedure delirium, accelerated mobilization and reconditioning, shorter procedure time, and decreased costs.[42] Importantly, patient safety remains central to the selection of the optimal

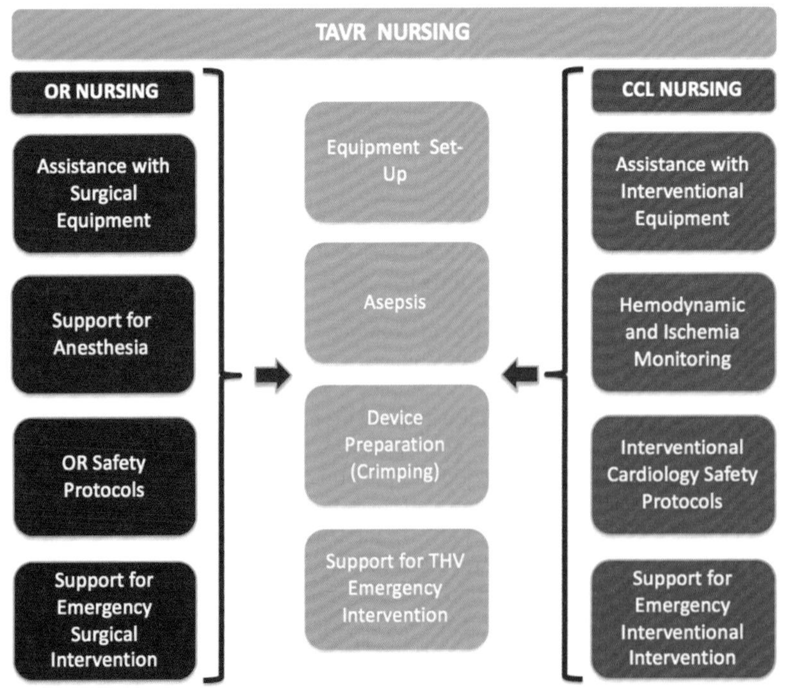

Figure 32-6. Periprocedural nursing responsibilities for transcatheter aortic valve replacement.

anesthesia strategy to consistently achieve excellent outcomes as evidence continue to emerge to guide practice. Similarly, the historical practice of the insertion of multiple invasive lines, including pulmonary artery, central venous, and/or urinary catheters is under review and practices are shifting rapidly.[42] Combined, these strategies pave the way for the transformation of the way TAVR is performed to continue to improve outcomes and reduce costs.

MITRAL STENOSIS

Percutaneous Mitral Catheter Balloon Valvuloplasty

Percutaneous mitral catheter balloon valvuloplasty is an alternative, less invasive procedure than surgical treatment for mitral stenosis. Balloon valvuloplasty is performed in the cardiac catheterization laboratory by a cardiologist experienced with invasive techniques. A small balloon valvuloplasty catheter is introduced percutaneously at the femoral vein and passed into the right atrium. The catheter is then directed transseptally and positioned across the mitral valve. Mitral balloon valvuloplasty is recommended in patients with moderate to severe mitral stenosis that is symptomatic with favorable valve morphology.[6]

Inflation of either one large balloon (23 to 25 mm) or two smaller balloons (12 to 18 mm) stretches the valve leaflets (Fig. 32-7). Inflation of the balloon separates the fused commissures thus improving valve mobility. The best results from this technique to date have been in patients with rheumatic mitral stenosis with commissural fusion. An echocardiographic scoring system rates leaflet thickening, leaflet mobility, calcification, and subvalvular deformity, with a maximum score of 4 in each division. Patients with a total echo score of less than or equal to 8 respond most favorably.[43] Balloon valvuloplasty has been associated with complications including systemic embolization (1% to 3%), severe mitral regurgitation (3% to 5%), and death (0% to 1%).[44] An atrial septal defect also may occur in as many as 10% of patients undergoing balloon valvuloplasty as a result of the transseptal approach, but the defect closes or decreases in most patients.[45] Results have been promising, with the average gradient reduction being approximately 18 to 6 mm Hg and, on the average, an increase in calculated valve area of 50% to 100%. Mitral balloon valvuloplasty is reserved for patients who continue to be symptomatic despite adequate medical therapy. Mitral balloon valvuloplasty may be used in women who experience hemodynamic decompensation during pregnancy due to mitral stenosis as it offers less risk to the fetus than mitral valve replacement and cardiopulmonary bypass.

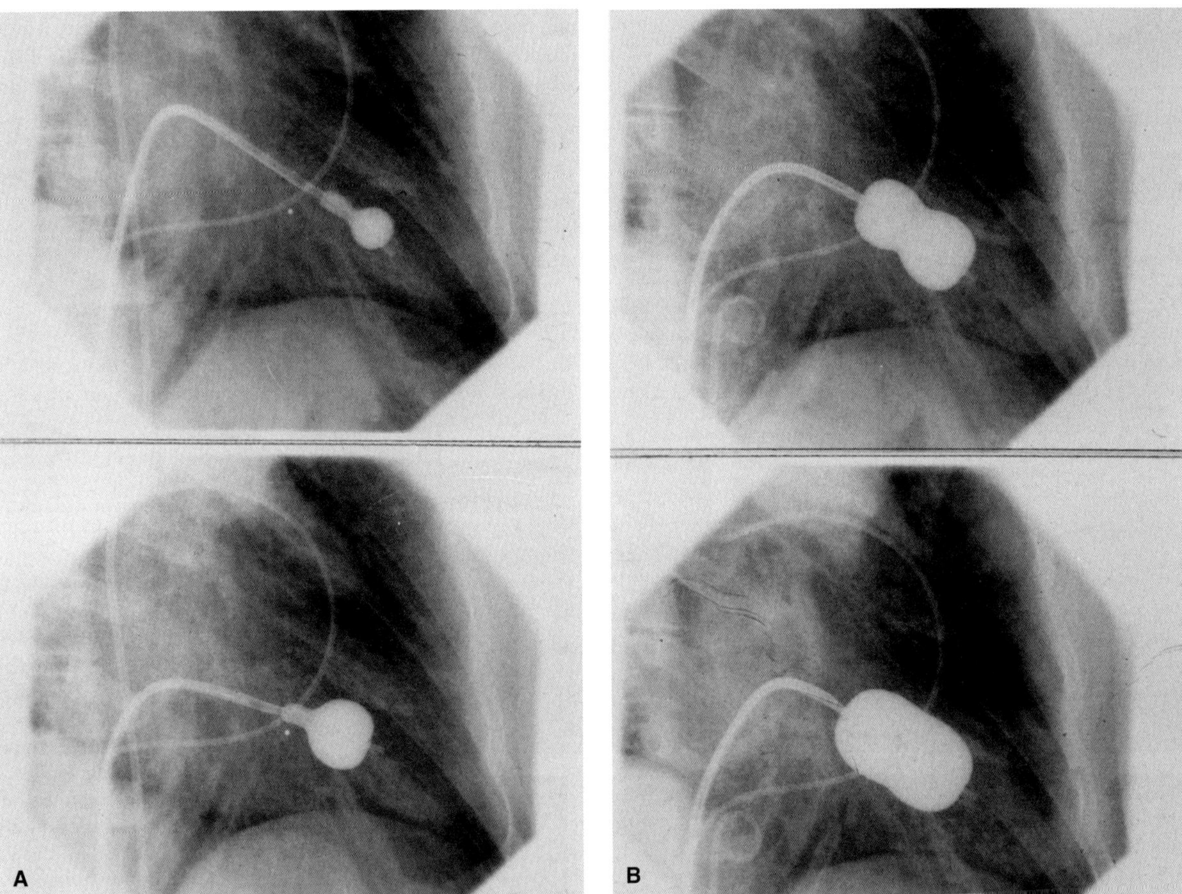

Figure 32-7. Mitral valvuloplasty: Inoue's technique. **(A)** Inflation of distal portion of balloon, which is then pulled back and anchored at the mitral valve. **(B)** Inflation of proximal and middle portions of balloon. At full inflation, the narrowed "waist" of the balloon has disappeared. (From Vahanian AS. Valvuloplasty. In: Topol EJ, Califf RM, Isner JM, et al., eds. *Textbook of Cardiovascular Medicine.* Philadelphia, PA: Lippincott-Raven; 1998:2157.)

MITRAL REGURGITATION

Transcatheter Mitral Valve Repair

Catheter-based approaches for the treatment of mitral regurgitation remain available largely in clinical trials. The sole exception is the MitraClip system (Abbott, IL, USA), approved by the FDA in 2013, as a mitral valve repair option for patients with severe symptomatic primary (degenerative) mitral regurgitation who are determined to be at prohibitive risk for traditional surgery.[46] The randomized clinical trials which preceded FDA approval of the MitraClip demonstrated reduction of severity of mitral regurgitation, improvement in heart failure symptoms and reverse remodeling of the left ventricle.[47]

The 2014 AHA/ACC Valvular Heart Disease Guidelines indicate that percutaneous mitral valve repair should be utilized only for patients with chronic primary mitral regurgitation who are severely symptomatic (NYHA III-IV) despite optimal medical therapy and who are considered to be inoperable.[13] Determination of inoperability should be made by a multidisciplinary Heart Team experienced in the treatment of patients with mitral valve disease. In 2019, the FDA expanded the approved indication for percutaneous mitral valve repair with the MitraClip to include patients with secondary mitral regurgitation and heart failure symptoms despite optimal medical therapy. In the United States, the Centers for Medicare & Medicaid Services further delineates the conditions which must be met in order for a provider to proceed with an FDA-approved TMVr procedure.[48]

The MitraClip delivery system is introduced via the femoral vein and advanced to the left side of the heart by transeptal puncture. The device is positioned over the mitral valve and the clip is deployed when positioning is deemed optimal. In some cases, a second MitraClip may be deployed if further reduction in the degree of mitral regurgitation is desired (Fig. 32-8).

PRIORITIES FOR CARE

The strongest evidence available to guide cardiac nurses' priorities for care of patients undergoing transcatheter heart valve procedures focuses on the development of postprocedure protocols for TAVR patients. The lessons learned in the past decade have contributed to improving outcomes and informing best practices for all present and future transcatheter heart valve therapies. Length of stay across most programs has decreased significantly, with many centers achieving routine discharge on PODs 1 or 2 without negatively impacting early or late readmission rates.[42,49] This is the cumulative result of multiple quality improvement initiatives, often led by cardiac nurses, that have contributed to the development of priorities of care matched to contemporary TAVR.

Close Monitoring of Potential Complications

The incidence of vascular injury, bleeding, stroke, new conduction delay, acute kidney injury, and other complications continues to decrease.[50,51] Nevertheless, close monitoring of TAVR patients in the early recovery period requires a unique nursing skillset. The expertise required to ensure vascular access hemostasis remains central to the care of TAVR patients. The insertion of multiple sheaths can compound the challenge of vascular access management. Although the use of closure devices is associated with prompt hemostasis,[52] nursing expertise in managing minor, major, and life-threatening bleeding is an essential competency of TAVR care.

The management of the onset of new conduction delay can augment the complexity and uncertainty of postprocedure management due to the close proximity and mechanical interaction between the newly implanted device and conduction tissue. The risks of conduction disturbances (i.e., high-degree atrioventricular block requiring permanent pacemaker implantation and new-onset left bundle branch block) warrant significant vigilance. Risk factors of conduction include the presence of baseline right bundle branch block, the use of some self-expanding valve systems, and the depth of prosthesis implantation within the left ventricular outflow tract.[53] Serial electrocardiography and continuous telemetry are essential tools for cardiac nurses to ensure patient safety. If indicated, the implantation of a new permanent pacemaker may be warranted if the conduction delay does not resolve spontaneously in the early phase of recovery.[54]

Early Mobilization and Reconditioning

In the absence of significant vascular complications and hemodynamic instability, a strategy of early mobilization after 4 hours

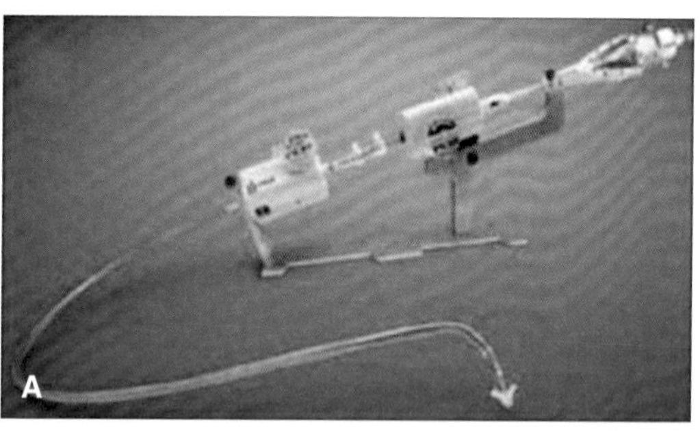

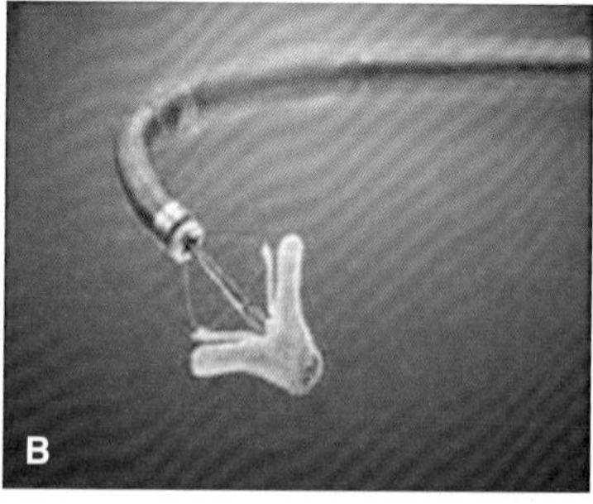

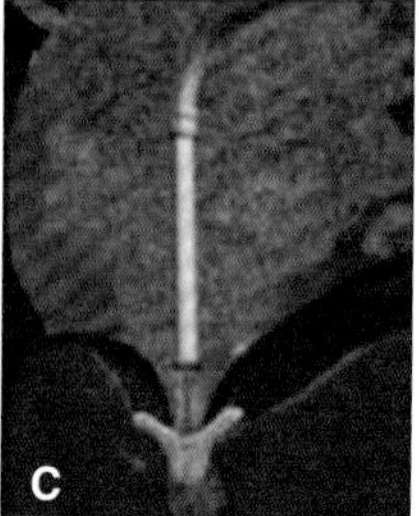

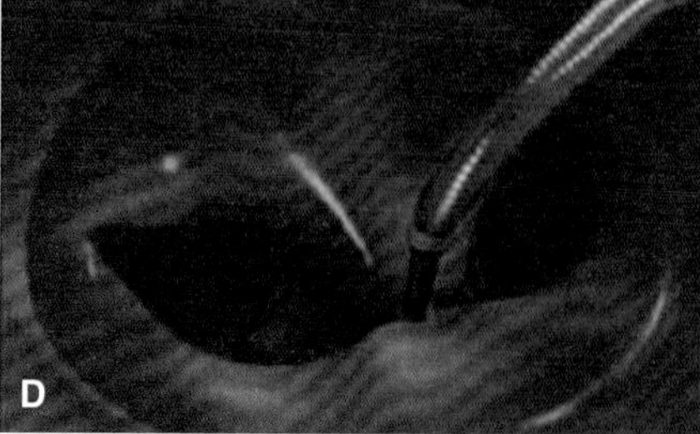

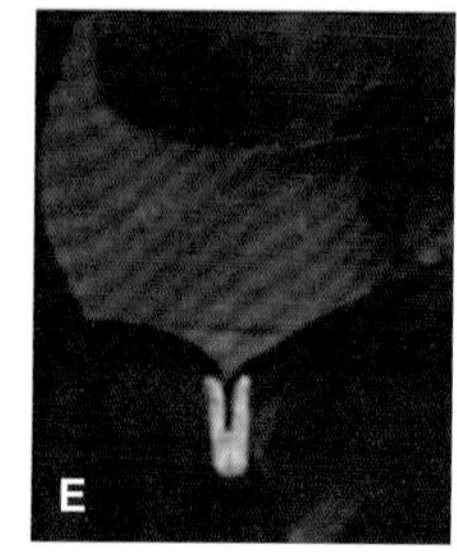

Figure 32-8. MitraClip system. (**A**) The MitraClip system with the steerable guide catheter, the clip delivery system, and the MitraClip positioned in the stabilizer. (**B**) The MitraClip is attached to the delivery system. The two arms are open, and the grippers are almost touching the arms. (**C**) The MitraClip is being positioned directly below the mitral valve with each leaflet on one side between the clip arms and the grippers in the region of mitral regurgitation. (**D**) Surgical view from the left atrium onto the valve: the grippers fix the leaflets to the clip arms, and the clip arms are closed, resulting in a dual orifice during diastole. The clip is still attached to the delivery system. (**E**) The clip is released from the delivery system after grasping the anterior and posterior mitral leaflet. (Pictures and graphics courtesy of Abbott Structural Heart.)

of bedrest is associated with safe outcomes and the avoidance of physical deconditioning.[42] Deconditioning refers to the decrease in muscle mass and other physiologic changes that result from aging and immobility, and contribute to overall weakness. Days of bedrest, rather than days of hospitalization, is a strong predictor of functional dependency and cognitive decline in the elderly.[55] Low mobilization is a major cause of preventable iatrogenic disability in the elderly, and is associated with longer length of stay and higher odds of needing care after discharge.[56] Similarly, rapid rehydration and nutrition, and the avoidance of urinary catheterization are important interventions to facilitate a rapid return to baseline function and mitigate the risks associated with the rapid onset of the "geriatric giants" of immobility, instability, incontinence, and delirium.[57] The priorities for care after TAVR are summarized in Table 32-4.

Table 32-4 • PRIORITIES FOR CARE FOLLOWING TRANSCATHETER AORTIC VALVE REPLACEMENT

Process	Activity/Assessment
Monitoring	
Focused assessment/monitoring	Vital signs Neurologic vital signs Vascular access site and extremities (color, warmth, movement, sensitivity) Cardiac rhythm Pain and discomfort
Laboratory and other diagnostics	Hemoglobin, complete blood count, renal function 12-lead electrocardiogram Transthoracic echocardiogram if required
Rapid removal of invasive lines	If present: Non-TAVR side sheaths Radial arterial line Central venous line
Rapid Reconditioning	
Mobilization	Bedrest × 4–6 hours Nurse-led mobilization at least every 4–6 hours/daytime
Elimination	Avoid urinary catheterization Mobilize to toilet
Hydration and nutrition	Oral fluids as soon as safe Resume regular meal(s) as soon as safe Mobilize to chair for meals
Discharge Planning	
Discharge plan	Confirm discharge plan developed preprocedure Confirm discharge date and time Complete discharge teaching Confirm follow-up plan

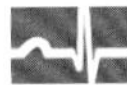

CONCLUSION

In the era of transcatheter valve therapies there are increased options for the management of acquired valvular heart disease with FDA-approved indications for the transcatheter treatment of aortic stenosis and mitral regurgitation. Ongoing clinical trials are evaluating new generation devices for aortic, mitral and tricuspid repair or replacement, as well as indications for new patient sub-sets.

This expanding array of therapies provides definitive treatment options for a broader population of patients and further enables practitioners to tailor treatment to the needs of the individual patient.

CASE STUDY 1

Transcatheter Aortic Valve Replacement

Patient Profile

History of Present Illness

Mr. Kruger is an 80-year-old male who presented to his family physician with increasing shortness of breath on exertion and one episode of syncope that resulted in a large lower upper limb hematoma. Transthoracic echocardiography confirmed severe aortic stenosis.

Past Medical History

Severe symptomatic aortic stenosis (aortic valve area: 0.8 cm^2; transvalvular pressure gradient: 42 mm Hg)
NYHA Class III
Syncope
Moderate chronic lung disease (FEV_1 65% predicted)
Diabetes
Chronic atrial fibrillation
Previous percutaneous coronary intervention (proximal LAD 80% stenosis)
Moderate frailty

Family History

Noncontributory

Social History

Widowed
Lives alone with support of adult son
Performs all activities of daily living
Assistance with instrumental activities of daily living (managing finances, shopping)
Housekeeper weekly

Medications

ACE-I
Beta blocker
Diuretic
Novel oral anticoagulant (NOAC)
Bronchodilator
Insulin

Considerations

- Given advanced age, frailty, and comorbidities, the patient was referred to TAVR center for evaluation of eligibility. He underwent a coronary angiogram that showed a patent proximal LAD stent and diffuse mild to moderate disease. Multidetector computed tomography was completed to assess his femoral vasculature and cardiac anatomy.
- The patient was seen by the team of TAVR cardiologist and surgeon. Cardiac nursing assessment confirmed moderate frailty but high function with completion of all activities of daily living and self-care. Patient reported that his goals of treatment were to feel less fatigued and short of breath, to be able to attend a weekly event at the local community center, and spend time with his family.

(continued)

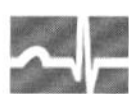
CASE STUDY 1 (*Continued*)

Transcatheter Aortic Valve Replacement

Assessment and Plan

Mr. Kruger is an 80-year-old male with symptomatic severe aortic stenosis who has completed a full evaluation to consider his goals and treatment options. When all findings were discussed at the weekly TAVR multidisciplinary team meeting, the consensus treatment recommendation was to offer transfemoral TAVR. The patient agreed to proceed with the proposed treatment plan.

Interval Course

- Mr. Kruger was admitted on the morning of his procedure. He had his procedure in the hybrid cardiac catheterization laboratory under local anesthesia with minimal sedation using percutaneous access and closure. A focused transthoracic echocardiogram performed at the end of the procedure confirmed absence of paravalvular leak, well-seated device, and 5 mm Hg transvalvular valve gradient.
- He was recovered in the cardiac short stay unit adjacent to the cardiac catheterization laboratory for 2 hours and transferred to the telemetry cardiac unit for overnight monitoring. After 4 hours of bedrest, he mobilized twice with nursing assistance on the evening of his procedure, and sat in a chair for dinner.

Conclusion

Mr. Kruger was discharged the following day in the care of his son who stayed with him overnight. The housekeeper was scheduled to be in the house on postoperative day 2. The TAVR center contacted the patient 2 and 7 days after the procedure to confirm his clinical status. The patient returned to the TAVR center for his 30-day follow-up inclusive of transthoracic echocardiography and clinical consultations.

Key Takeaways

1. Comprehensive physical examination and diagnostic assessment are essential to formulation of an appropriate treatment plan.
2. Patient goals of care must be taken into account when deciding on a treatment plan.
3. The postprocedure care pathway should include careful monitoring for potential complications while concurrently facilitating independent function.[58,59]

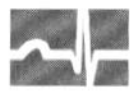
CASE STUDY 2

Transcatheter Mitral Valve Repair

Patient Profile

History of Present Illness

Mrs. Webber is an 86-year-old retired RN admitted to the intensive care unit for acute decompensated heart failure. She suffered a mechanical fall 1 week prior to admission; she was seen then in local ED and discharged. She reported feeling progressively weak with poor intake and some alteration in mental status; returned to ED, normal CXR and head CT, given IV hydration and discharged. The following day Mrs. Webber returned to the ED with worsening weakness, dyspnea and tachypnea, intubated and admitted. Patchy pulmonary edema and effusions on chest CT, diuresis, and antibiotics were initiated. Hypotension required initiation of vasopressors. Transthoracic echocardiogram revealed severe MR, TEE revealed MVP and flail P2 leaflet, torrential MR. Intra-aortic balloon counterpulsation was initiated.

Past Medical History

Chronic MR (mitral valve prolapse), asymptomatic
Declined surgery 15 years ago
Hypertension
History of bowel resection after appendix perforation with subsequent malabsorption

Family History

Noncontributory

Social History

Retired RN
Lives with son, daughter-in-law and granddaughters
Fully ambulatory with self-described excellent quality of life at baseline; cognitively intact
Former smoker

Medications

Lisinopril
Metoprolol
Imodium
Fluoxetine

Assessment and Plan

Mrs. Webber is an 86-year-old female with acute decompensated heart failure due to severe degenerative mitral regurgitation/mitral valve prolapse. She will be transferred to a center with capability for transcatheter mitral valve repair.

Interval Course

Treatment continued as above and remained fully alert and oriented. Deemed to be high risk for surgery because of age and frailty (STS-PROM 39.7%).

- Following complete evaluation and consultation including shared decision making with the patient and Heart Team, Mrs. Webber underwent a successful MitraClip procedure (2 MitraClips placed) with reduction in mitral regurgitation from severe to mild.
- She was extubated on postprocedure day 1. The postprocedure transthoracic echocardiogram demonstrated 2 well-seated MitraClips with mild MR and no significant gradient across the mitral valve (mean diastolic pressure gradient 4 mm Hg).
- Mrs. Webber discharged to an inpatient rehabilitation facility on postprocedure day 3. She returned home from rehab after 2 weeks with ongoing follow-up with local cardiologist.

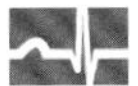

CASE STUDY 2 (*Continued*)

Transcatheter Mitral Valve Repair

Key Takeaways

1. Patients with asymptomatic valvular heart disease should be under surveillance by their health care provider at prescribed intervals to detect changes in presence of symptoms and lesion severity.
2. Transcatheter therapies are viable, and in some cases preferred, treatment options for patients with valvular heart disease.
3. Discharge to a rehab facility can facilitate return to independence as a bridge from hospital to home.

KEY READINGS

Hawkey MC, Lauck SB, Perpetua EM, et al. Transcatheter aortic valve replacement program development: recommendations for best practice. *Catheter Cardiovasc Interv.* 2014;84(6):859–867.

Hawkey MC, Lauck SB, Perpetua E, et al., eds. *Transcatheter Aortic Valve Replacement Program Development: A Guide for the Heart Team.* New York: Wolters Kluwer; 2019.

Lauck SB, Wood DA, Baumbusch J, et al. Vancouver transcatheter aortic valve replacement clinical pathway: minimalist approach, standardized care, and discharge criteria to reduce length of stay. *Circ Cardiovasc Qual Outcomes.* 2016;9(3):312–321.

REFERENCES

1. Jamieson WRE. Update on new tissue valves. In: Franco KL, Verrier ED, eds. *Advanced Therapy in Cardiac Surgery.* Hamilton, Ontario, Canada: BC Decker; 2003:177–195.
2. Goldman BS, Mallidi H. Update on stentless valves. In: Franco KL, Verrier ED, eds. *Advanced Therapy in Cardiac Surgery.* Hamilton, Ontario, Canada: BC Decker; 2003:196–203.
3. David TE, Puschmann R, Ivanov J, et al. Aortic valve replacement with stentless and stented porcine valves: a case-match study. *J Thorac Cardiovasc Surg.* 1998;116(2):236–241.
4. Doty JR, Salazar JD, Liddicoat JR, et al. Aortic valve replacement with cryopreserved aortic allograft: ten-year experience. *J Thorac Cardiovasc Surg.* 1998;115(2):371–379; discussion 379–380.
5. Elkins RC. Pulmonary autograft. In: Franco KL, Verrier ED, eds. *Advanced Therapy in Cardiac Surgery.* Hamilton, Ontario, Canada: BC Decker; 2003:156–167.
6. Otto CM, Bonow RO. Valvular heart disease. In: Libby P, Bonow RO, Mann DL, et al., eds. *Braunwald's Heart Disease.* 8th ed. Philadelphia, PA: Saunders Elsevier; 2008:1625–1712.
7. Sievers HH, Hanke T, Stierle U, et al. A critical reappraisal of the Ross operation: renaissance of the subcoronary implantation technique? *Circulation.* 2006;114(1 suppl):I504–I511.
8. Chitwood WR, Rodriguez E. Minimally invasive and robotic mitral valve surgery. In: Cohn LH, ed. *Cardiac Surgery in the Adult.* New York: McGraw-Hill; 2008:1079–1100.
9. Casselman FP, La Meir M, Jeanmart H, et al. Endoscopic mitral and tricuspid valve surgery after previous cardiac surgery. *Circulation.* 2007;116(11 suppl):I270–I275.
10. Izzat MB, Yim AP, El-Zufari MH, et al. Upper T mini-sternotomy for aortic valve operations. *Chest.* 1998;114(1):291–294.
11. Cosgrove DM 3rd, Sabik JF, Navia JL. Minimally invasive valve operations. *Ann Thorac Surg.* 1998;65(6):1535–1538; discussion 1538–1539.
12. Sharony R, Grossi EA, Ribakove GH, et al. Minimally invasive cardiac valve surgery. In: Franco KL, Verrier ED, eds. *Advanced Therapy in Cardiac Surgery.* Hamilton, Ontario, Canada: BC Decker; 2003:147–155.
13. Nishimura RA, Otto CM, Bonow RO, et al. 2014 AHA/ACC guideline for the management of patients with valvular heart disease: executive summary: a report of the American College of Cardiology/American Heart Association Task Force on Practice Guidelines. *J Am Coll Cardiol.* 2014;63(22):2438–2488.
14. Crawford MH, Durack DT. Clinical presentation of infective endocarditis. *Cardiol Clin.* 2003;21(2):159–166, v.
15. Hara H, Pedersen WR, Ladich E, et al. Percutaneous balloon aortic valvuloplasty revisited: time for a renaissance? *Circulation.* 2007;115(12): e334–e338.
16. Carabello BA. Aortic stenosis: two steps forward, one step back. *Circulation.* 2007;115(22):2799–2800.
17. Ross J Jr, Braunwald E. Aortic stenosis. *Circulation.* 1968;38(1 suppl):61–67.
18. Song H, Kang DH, Kim JH, et al. Percutaneous mitral valvuloplasty versus surgical treatment in mitral stenosis with severe tricuspid regurgitation. *Circulation.* 2007;116(11 suppl):I246–I250.
19. Bloomfield P. Choice of heart valve prosthesis. *Heart.* 2002;87(6):583–589.
20. Cribier A, Eltchaninoff H, Bash A, et al. Percutaneous transcatheter implantation of an aortic valve prosthesis for calcific aortic stenosis: first human case description. *Circulation.* 2002;106(24):3006–3008.
21. Webb JG, Chandavimol M, Thompson CR, et al. Percutaneous aortic valve implantation retrograde from the femoral artery. *Circulation.* 2006;113(6):842–850.
22. Lichtenstein SV, Cheung A, Ye J, et al. Transapical transcatheter aortic valve implantation in humans: initial clinical experience. *Circulation.* 2006;114(6):591–596.
23. Leon MB, Smith CR, Mack M, et al. Transcatheter aortic-valve implantation for aortic stenosis in patients who cannot undergo surgery. *N Engl J Med.* 2010;363(17):1597–1607.
24. Smith CR, Leon MB, Mack MJ, et al. Transcatheter versus surgical aortic-valve replacement in high-risk patients. *N Engl J Med.* 2011;364(23):2187–2198.
25. Adams DH, Popma JJ, Reardon MJ. Transcatheter aortic-valve replacement with a self-expanding prosthesis. *N Engl J Med.* 2014;371(10):967–968.
26. Mack MJ, Leon MB, Thourani VH, et al. Transcatheter aortic-valve replacement with a balloon-expandable valve in low-risk patients. *N Engl J Med.* 2019;380(18):1695–1705.
27. Popma JJ, Deeb GM, Yakubov SJ, et al. Transcatheter aortic-valve replacement with a self-expanding valve in low-risk patients. *N Engl J Med.* 2019;380(18):1706–1715.
28. Durko AP, Osnabrugge RL, Van Mieghem NM, et al. Annual number of candidates for transcatheter aortic valve implantation per country: current estimates and future projections. *Eur Heart J.* 2018;39(28):2635–2642.
29. Otto CM, Kumbhani DJ, Alexander KP, et al. 2017 ACC expert consensus decision pathway for transcatheter aortic valve replacement in the management of adults with aortic stenosis: a report of the American College of Cardiology Task Force on Clinical Expert Consensus Documents. *J Am Coll Cardiol.* 2016;69(10):1313–1346.
30. Bonow RO, Brown AS, Gillam LD, et al. ACC/AATS/AHA/ASE/EACTS/HVS/SCA/SCAI/SCCT/SCMR/STS 2017 appropriate use criteria for the treatment of patients with severe aortic stenosis: a report of the American College of Cardiology Appropriate Use Criteria Task Force, American Association for Thoracic Surgery, American Heart Association, American Society of Echocardiography, European Association for Cardio-Thoracic Surgery, Heart Valve Society, Society of Cardiovascular Anesthesiologists, Society for Cardiovascular Angiography and Interventions, Society of Cardiovascular Computed Tomography, Society for Cardiovascular Magnetic Resonance, and Society of Thoracic Surgeons. *J Am Soc Echocardiogr.* 2018;31(2):117–147.
31. Coylewright M, Mack MJ, Holmes DR Jr, et al. A call for an evidence-based approach to the Heart Team for patients with severe aortic stenosis. *J Am Coll Cardiol.* 2015;65(14):1472–1480.
32. Hawkey MC, Lauck SB, Perpetua EM, et al. Transcatheter aortic valve replacement program development: recommendations for best practice. *Catheter Cardiovasc Interv.* 2014;84(6):859–867.
33. Afilalo J, Lauck S, Kim DH, et al. Frailty in older adults undergoing aortic valve replacement: the FRAILTY-AVR study. *J Am Coll Cardiol.* 2017;70(6):689–700.

34. Lauck SBN, Norekvål TM. Frailty, quality of life, and palliative approach. In: Hawkey MC, Lauck SB, Perpetua E, et al., eds. *Transcatheter Aortic Valve Replacement: A Guide for the Heart Team*. New York: Wolters Kluwer; 2019.
35. Keegan PA, Achtem L. From referral to procedure: clinic evaluation pathway. In: Hawkey MC, Lauck SB, Perpetua E, et al., eds. *Transcatheter Aortic Valve Replacement: A Guide for the Heart Team*. New York: Wolters Kluwer; 2019.
36. Coylewright M, Palmer R, O'Neill ES, et al. Patient-defined goals for the treatment of severe aortic stenosis: a qualitative analysis. *Health Expect.* 2016;19(5):1036–1043.
37. Coulter A, Stilwell D, Kryworuchko J, et al. A systematic development process for patient decision aids. *BMC Med Inf Decis Making.* 2013;13(suppl 2):S2.
38. Lewis KB, Carroll SL, Birnie D, et al. Incorporating patients' preference diagnosis in implantable cardioverter defibrillator decision-making: a review of recent literature. *Curr Opin Cardiol.* 2018;33(1):42–49.
39. Stacey D, Legare F, Lewis K, et al. Decision aids for people facing health treatment or screening decisions. *Cochrane Database Syst Rev.* 2017;4:CD001431.
40. American College of Cardiology. *Aortic stenosis: TAVR/SAVR*. 2018. Available at https://www.cardiosmart.org/SDM/Decision-Aids/Find-Decision-Aids/Aortic-Stenosis. Accessed November 4, 2018.
41. Grover FL, Vemulapalli S, Carroll JD, et al. 2016 Annual Report of The Society of Thoracic Surgeons/American College of Cardiology Transcatheter Valve Therapy Registry. *J Am Coll Cardiol.* 2017;69(10):1215–1230.
42. Wyman JF. The right care in the right place: a United States perspective on procedure planning. In: Hawkey MC, Lauck SB, Perpetua E, et al., eds. *Transcatheter Aortic Valve Replacement: A Guide for the Heart Team*. New York: Wolters Kluwer; 2019.
43. Hyman MC, Vemulapalli S, Szeto WY, et al. Conscious sedation versus general anesthesia for transcatheter aortic valve replacement: insights from the National Cardiovascular Data Registry Society of Thoracic Surgeons/American College of Cardiology Transcatheter Valve Therapy Registry. *Circulation.* 2017;136(22):2132–2140.
44. Lauck SB, Wood DA, Baumbusch J, et al. Vancouver transcatheter aortic valve replacement clinical pathway: minimalist approach, standardized care, and discharge criteria to reduce length of stay. *Circ Cardiovasc Qual Outcomes.* 2016;9(3):312–321.
45. Palacios IF, Sanchez PL, Harrell LC, et al. Which patients benefit from percutaneous mitral balloon valvuloplasty? Prevalvuloplasty and postvalvuloplasty variables that predict long-term outcome. *Circulation.* 2002;105(12):1465–1471.
46. Mayes CE, Cigarroa JE, Lange RA, et al. Percutaneous mitral balloon valvuloplasty. *Clin Cardiol.* 1999;22(8):501–503.
47. Mazur W, Parilak LD, Kaluza G, et al. Balloon valvuloplasty for mitral stenosis. *Curr Opin Cardiol.* 1999;14(2):95–103.
48. U.S. Food & Drug Administration. *Premarket approval*. 2013. Available at https://www.accessdata.fda.gov/scripts/cdrh/cfdocs/cfpma/pma.cfm?id=P100009
49. Feldman T, Foster E, Glower DD, et al. Percutaneous repair or surgery for mitral regurgitation. *N Engl J Med.* 2011;364(15):1395–1406.
50. Centers for Medicare & Medicaid Services. *Decision memo for transcatheter mitral valve repair (TMVR)*. Available at https://www.cms.gov/medicare-coverage-database/details/nca-decision-memo.aspx?NCAId=273. Accessed November 4, 2018.
51. Sud M, Qui F, Austin PC, et al. Short length of stay after elective transfemoral transcatheter aortic valve replacement is not associated with increased early or late readmission risk. *J Am Heart Assoc.* 2017;6(4):e005460.
52. Sorajja P, Kodali S, Reardon MJ, et al. Outcomes for the commercial use of self-expanding prostheses in transcatheter aortic valve replacement: a report from the STS/ACC TVT registry *JACC Cardiovasc Interv.* 2017;10(20):2090–2098.
53. Carroll JD, Vemulapalli S, Dai D, et al. Procedural experience for transcatheter aortic valve replacement and relation to outcomes: the STS/ACC TVT registry. *J Am Coll Cardiol.* 2017;70(1):29–41.
54. Dencker D, Taudorf M, Luk NH, et al. Frequency and effect of access-related vascular injury and subsequent vascular intervention after transcatheter aortic valve replacement. *Am J Cardiol.* 2016;118(8):1244–1250.
55. Auffret V, Puri R, Urena M, et al. Conduction disturbances after transcatheter aortic valve replacement: current status and future perspectives. *Circulation.* 2017;136(11):1049–1069.
56. Fadahunsi OO, Olowoyeye A, Ukaigwe A, et al. Incidence, predictors, and outcomes of permanent pacemaker implantation following transcatheter aortic valve replacement: analysis from the U.S. Society of Thoracic Surgeons/American College of Cardiology TVT Registry. *JACC Cardiovasc Interv.* 2016;9(21):2189–2199.
57. Calero-Garcia MJ, Ortega AR, Navarro E, et al. Relationship between hospitalization and functional and cognitive impairment in hospitalized older adults patients. *Aging Ment Health.* 2017;21(11):1164–1170.
58. Lafont C, Gerard S, Voisin T, et al. Reducing "iatrogenic disability" in the hospitalized frail elderly. *J Nutr Health Aging.* 2011;15(8):645–660.
59. Lauck SB, Kwon JY, Wood DA, et al. Avoidance of urinary catheterization to minimize in-hospital complications after transcatheter aortic valve implantation: an observational study. *Eur J Cardiovasc Nurs.* 2018; 17(1):66–74.

33 Adult Congenital Heart Disease

Christine Peverini

OBJECTIVES

1. You will be able to identify common congenital cardiac diagnoses and understand their unique physiology.
2. You will be able to apply your understanding of congenital cardiac anatomy to guide physical exam findings.
3. You will recognize common long-term implications associated with congenital heart disease.
4. You will identify special management issues that may arise when caring for an adult with congenital heart disease.

KEY QUESTIONS

1. Describe the implications family planning has in relation to the adult with congenital heart disease?
2. How does cyanotic heart disease impact care?
3. What risk factors are associated with prior cardiac surgeries?
4. Which patients should be followed by a specialist in adult congenital cardiology?

BACKGROUND

Congenital heart disease (CHD) encompasses structural abnormalities of the heart or great vessels present at birth associated with actual or potential functional consequences.[1] CHD is the most common birth defect.[2] Severity depends on native anatomy, surgical repair, and current physiology.[3] Advances in medical and surgical techniques have resulted in improved survival of adults with congenital heart disease (ACHD).[4] Current wisdom appreciates that CHD is not "cured" after treatment in childhood. In fact, majority of ACHD patients have long-term consequences of either their native CHD or its surgical repair.[3] Expert care in ACHD centers is needed across the lifespan to optimize outcomes.[3,5]

HISTORICAL STATE AND CONTEXT

Innovations in pediatric cardiology have led to improved survival for individuals with CHD.[1] Thanks to advances in diagnostic techniques, intensive care and surgical procedures, a large number of those with disorders previously fatal in childhood survive to adulthood. In the 1960s 35% of children born with CHD died by age 18 and in 2010 this was reduced to less than 5%. Despite improved life expectancy most ACHD survivors are rarely "cured" of their disease. For some patients with the most severe defects, palliative repairs which modify native anatomy create potential for entirely new problems.[2]

EPIDEMIOLOGY

The prevalence of CHD has generally been estimated to be 4 per 1000 adults[6] and has steadily increased with most recent estimates at 6.12 per 1000 adults.[7,8] CHD has increased by 5% per year and now there are over 1.4 million adults with CHD.[4] In fact, the number of adults with CHD outnumbers children living with CHD.[9] Utilizing a more conservative estimated prevalence of 4 per 1000 adults to a world population of 7.2 billion yields an estimated 34 million adults with CHD worldwide.[9] There is similar prevalence of CHD between males and females. However, in adults, a higher prevalence of CHD has been reported in women.[9] Mortality rates, when adjusted for heart defect and age, remained higher for males (4%) than females (3%).[9] These numbers demonstrate the increasing number of ACHD patients that will be presenting for care in the adult setting.

CURRENT STATE AND CONTEXT

There are two groups of adults with CHD: those operated in infancy or childhood and those reaching adulthood without diagnosis or surgical treatment.[10] Those who underwent repairs in childhood continue to require follow-up in centers with CHD expertise due to the complexity of their heart defects. Those left untreated were often undiagnosed due to lack of symptoms or with such mild symptoms that may have been overlooked.[10] Common sequelae encountered in the ACHD patient include arrhythmias, heart failure and pulmonary vascular disease, and multiorgan dysfunction.[3] ACHD patients demonstrate higher rates of healthcare utilization than their age-matched counterparts.[3]

A detailed review of all congenital heart defects is beyond the scope of this chapter; therefore, those defects most commonly encountered in the ACHD will be discussed here.

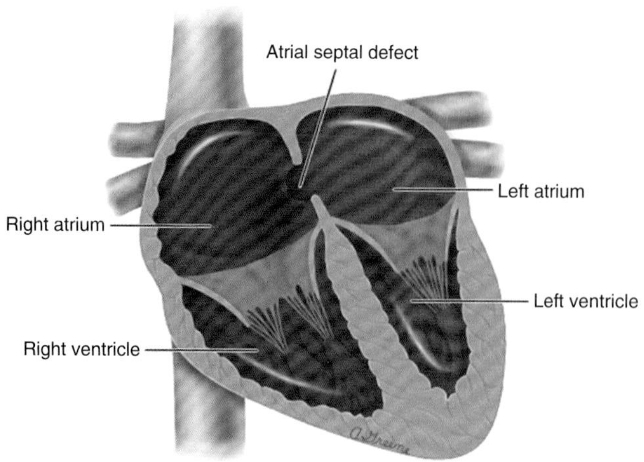

Figure 33-1. Atrial septal defect. The heart has four sections, or "chambers." The upper chambers are called "atria" and the lower chambers are called "ventricles." When the heart is working normally, blood comes in from the body through the right atrium and into the right ventricle. From there it goes to the lungs, where it picks up oxygen. Then the blood comes back through the left atrium, into the left ventricle, and back out to the body. A person with an atrial septal defect (ASD) has a hole between the right atrium and the left atrium. This can change the way blood flows through the heart.

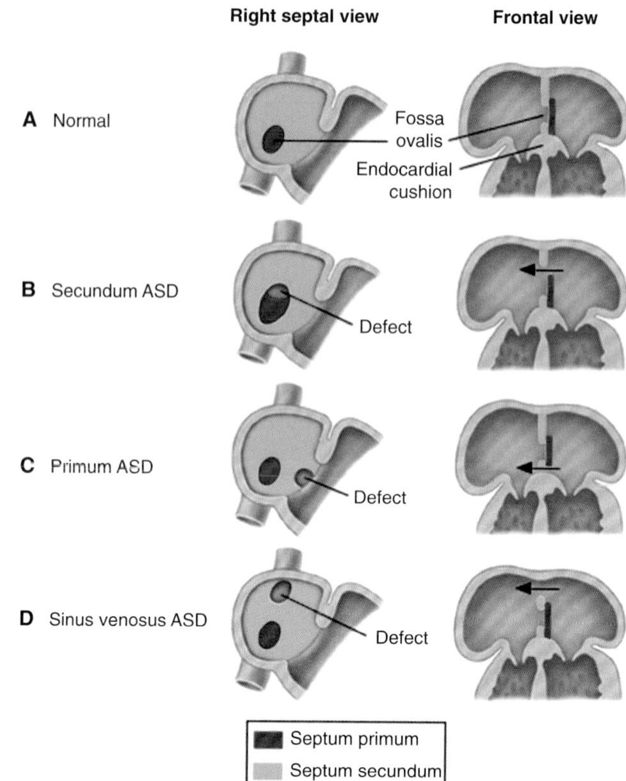

Figure 33-2. Types of atrial septal defects. Panel **A:** The normal atrial septum as well as various types of ASD are shown. Panel **B:** Secundum ASD is formed by the poor growth of the septum secundum or excessive absorption of the septum primum. Panel **C:** Primum ASD is formed by the failure of the septum primum to fuse with the endocardial cushions. The fossa ovalis is normal. The frontal view of the primum ASD shows the caudal location of the ASD just above the endocardial cushion. Panel **D:** Sinus venosus ASD is caused by the malposition of the insertion of the superior or inferior vena cava and is outside the area of the fossa ovalis.

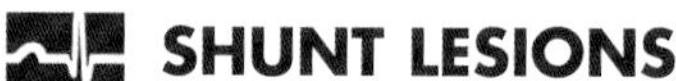

SHUNT LESIONS

This group of heart defects is characterized by a continuous flow of oxygen-saturated blood from the left heart circulation to the right side of the heart. This left-to-right shunting is associated with an increased pulmonary blood flow.

Atrial Septal Defects

Description

Atrial septal defects (ASDs) are abnormal communications between the left and right atria (Fig. 33-1). They constitute 10% of all congenital heart anomalies and may occur as a result of different anatomic defects.[5] There is a female predominance.[1] In addition, 25% of adults have persistence of the foramen ovale (PFO), which is a normal interatrial communication in fetal life.[3] ASDs are differentiated by their occurrence within the septum. *Ostium secundum* ASD, the most common type, usually represents a defect(s) in the septum primum.[3] *Ostium primum* ASD, which occurs low in the atrial septum, has an associated cleft anterior mitral valve leaflet with varying degree of mitral insufficiency. *Sinus venosus* ASDs are commonly located at the posterior aspect of the junction of the right atrium and superior vena cava[3] and may be associated with the partial anomalous right pulmonary venous connection (Fig. 33-2). Owing to the trivial or absent physical signs, ASD may go undetected until the fourth or fifth decade.

Pathophysiology

The hemodynamic consequences of ASD are dependent on (1) the magnitude and direction of the shunt[3]; (2) the compliance of the left and right ventricles[3]; and (3) the responsive behavior of the pulmonary vascular bed. In infancy, the persistence of increased pulmonary vascular resistance and the relatively equally compliant left and right ventricles limit the amount of left-to-right shunting. With increasing age, pulmonary vascular resistance decreases, and the right ventricle becomes thinner, offering less resistance to filling than the left. Consequently, the conditions are appropriate for left-to-right flow across the defect. Individuals with moderate or large defects will have left-to-right shunting even though left atrial pressure is only slightly higher than right atrial pressure.[3] This leads to volume overload of the right side of the heart, enlargement of the right atrium and ventricle as well as a substantial increase in pulmonary blood flow.[3]

Major problems of adults with unrepaired ASD include the development of congestive heart failure, pulmonary hypertension, and atrial arrhythmias, which increase in frequency with age.[11] A persistent rise in pulmonary vascular resistance leading eventually to shunt reversal and cyanosis, or Eisenmenger syndrome. The latter is usually the result of associated diseases affecting left ventricular function, such as systemic hypertension[3] or ischemic heart disease. Left ventricular failure reduces the distensibility of the left ventricle, increasing the volume of left atrial blood being shunted across the defect, thus adding to the burden of an already volume-overloaded right ventricle.

Clinical Manifestations

Many patients with ASDs are asymptomatic.[3,11] Individuals with large left-to-right shunts may have exertional dyspnea or exercise intolerance.[3] A transient ischemic attack or embolic cerebrovascular accident may present as the first symptom of an ASD or patent foramen ovale (PFO).[3] Characteristic of the increased pulmonary flow across the pulmonic valves is a grade 2 to 3 systolic ejection murmur at the left upper sternal border. Increased flow across the tricuspid valve may cause a soft mid-diastolic murmur at the left lower sternal border. A fixed-split second heart sound is often heard at the left upper sternal border. The presence of a systolic thrill reflects a large shunt or coexisting pulmonic stenosis. In ostium primum defect, there is the additional murmur of mitral regurgitation at the apex.

Management

Closure of ASD is recommended if the pulmonary-to-systemic blood flow ratio (Q_p/Q_s) is greater than or equal to 1.5:1.[3] However, severe pulmonary arterial hypertension (PAH) is a contraindication to closure and must be excluded prior to proceeding with closure. Most surgical repairs are performed in infancy by simple suture closure; in larger defects a pericardial or prosthetic patch may be required to close the defect. For *Ostium primum* defects, repair of the mitral valve cleft is also undertaken. Patients are followed longitudinally to determine need for further valve repair or replacement.

Today, transcatheter closure of ASD is the preferred method of closure for patients with secundum ASD with success rates of greater than 95% being reported.[5,12,13] While occurring infrequently, several concerns for these devices include incomplete closure of the shunt, acute embolization of the devices, and the potential for thromboembolic complications.

Adults with simple ASD repaired in infancy and no residual effects may be followed at the community level. Patients with residual lesions or patients in whom the ASD is diagnosed in adulthood should be evaluated at a regional ACHD center. Indications for specialty care include pre- or postoperative arrhythmias, valvular and/or ventricular dysfunction, and elevated pulmonary pressures. Endocarditis prophylaxis is only indicated within the first 6 months after percutaneous closure with a device or surgical closure using prosthetic material.[5]

Ventricular Septal Defects

Description

Ventricular septal defect (VSD) is a defect or opening of the ventricular septum which results in shunting of blood between right and left ventricles (Fig. 33-3). VSDs are the most common heart defects, representing about 37% of all congenital cardiac anomalies.[14] There are three main categories of VSD, each classified according to its location: perimembranous VSD, muscular VSD, and subarterial VSD (Fig. 33-4). Perimembranous defects are the most common type of defect accounting for 75% to 80% of all VSDs and occur in the membranous part of the ventricular septum and the surrounding muscular septum.[3,14] A muscular VSD occurs in the muscular portion of the septum and accounts for approximately 5% to 20%.[3,14] Subarterial VSDs occur in only 6% of cases and are located directly below the semilunar valves. VSDs are further categorized as either restrictive or unrestrictive. Restrictive VSDs are small defects resulting in a high-pressure gradient between right and left ventricles, while nonrestrictive VSDs are larger defects in which the pressure between right and left ventricles is equalized. Unrestricted defects are typically repaired in childhood, but restrictive VSDs account for 7% of congenital heart defects found in adults. Isolated VSDs occur with equal frequency in men and women. The 25-year follow-up indicates that the majority of patients managed medically or surgically, who do not develop Eisenmenger syndrome will fare well.[14,15]

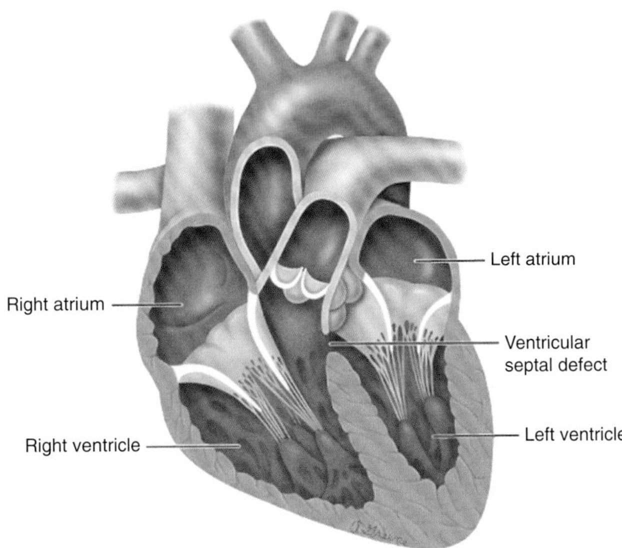

Figure 33-3. Ventricular septal defect. The heart has four chambers: right atrium, left atrium, right ventricle, and left ventricle. A person with a ventricular septal defect (VSD) has a hole between the right and left ventricles.

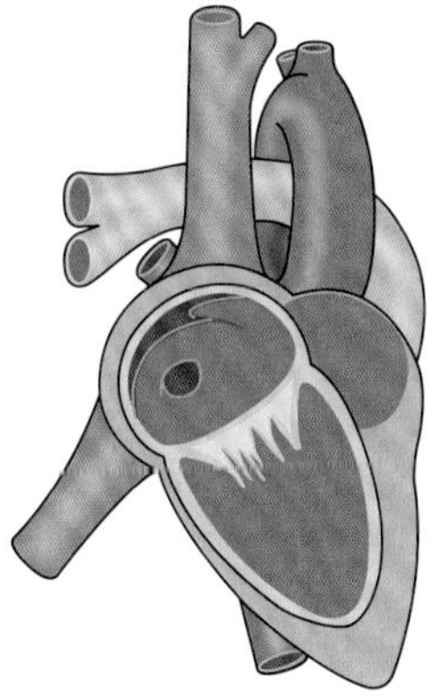

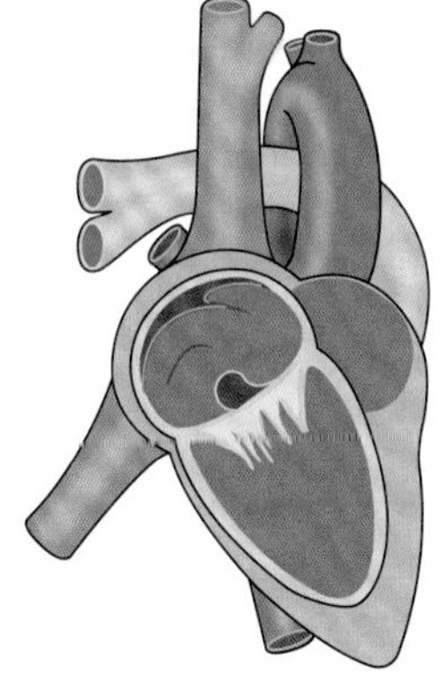

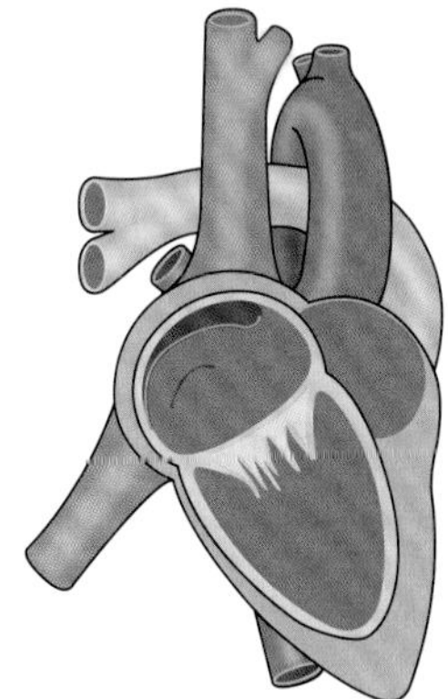

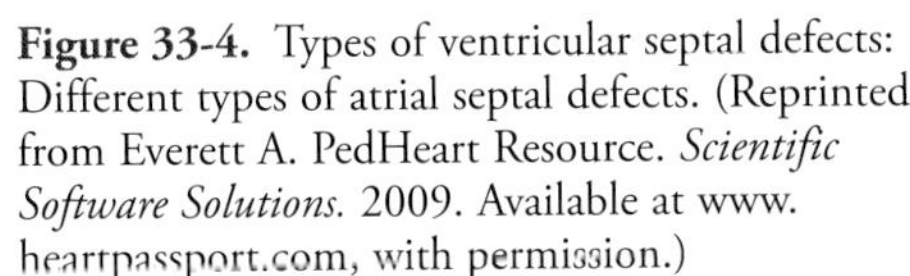

Figure 33-4. Types of ventricular septal defects: Different types of atrial septal defects. (Reprinted from Everett A. PedHeart Resource. *Scientific Software Solutions*. 2009. Available at www.heartpassport.com, with permission.)

Pathophysiology

Defects may be single or multiple, with the degree of shunting dependent on the size of the defect rather than the anatomic location. Defects vary in size from a millimeter or two in diameter to large openings with little or no septal wall, which behave physiologically like a single ventricle. Small isolated VSDs (less than 7 mm in diameter) produce minimal shunting. Those with moderate-sized defects (7 mm to 1.25 cm) will have shunting from the left-to-right ventricle during systole. Both have minimal hemodynamic changes and produce little or no symptomatology. If the defect is large (1.5 to 3 cm), systemic pressure in the right ventricle is equal or slightly lower than the left ventricle creating a left-to-right shunt and increased pulmonary blood flow (unrestricted VSD). This increase in blood flow is returned to the left heart, creating volume overload of the left atrium and ventricle.[3] In addition, increased pulmonary blood flow may eventually result in pulmonary hypertension. Because of the open communication between the two ventricles, there is equalization of pressures. Flow across the defect is determined by relative resistance across the systemic vascular and pulmonary vascular beds.[3] If the pulmonary artery pressure continues to increase and pulmonary vascular resistance approaches or exceeds systemic pressure, shunt reversal (right to left) occurs, rendering the patient cyanotic and no longer a candidate for surgical correction. This condition is referred to as Eisenmenger syndrome.[3]

Clinical Manifestations

Clinical features depend on the volume of pulmonary blood flow, which in turn depends on the size of the defect and the pulmonary vascular resistance. A harsh holosystolic murmur and palpable thrill along the lower left sternal border may be the only findings of a small or moderate defect. A normal splitting second sound indicates the pulmonary arterial pressure is below systemic pressure. In large shunts, the murmur is lower in intensity, a mid-diastolic rumble may be heard at the apex and the second heart sound will be accentuated due to the excess pulmonary flow.[3]

Management

Patients with small VSD (less than 7 mm in diameter) have minimal hemodynamic changes and produce little or no symptoms. While medical interventions are not necessary, they still require follow-up for potential consequences such as aortic valve prolapse or double-chamber right ventricle.[3] In the absence of high or fixed pulmonary vascular obstructive disease, surgical correction is indicated in patients with moderate to large left-to-right shunt. VSD closure will be considered if the Q_p/Q_s is higher than 1.5:1 if the PA systolic pressure is less than 50% systemic and PVR is less than 1/3 systemic.[5] According to the 2018 guidelines, endocarditis prophylaxis is no longer indicated, except for patients with prosthetic material (e.g., patch for VSD closure) with residual defect or within the first 6 months after an operation in which prosthetic material is placed.[5]

Patients with isolated, small VSDs or those with successful surgical repair require periodic follow-up visits every 3 years[5] and may be cared for in general medical community. On the other hand, patients with residual defects or those who develop clinical sequelae such as right or left ventricular outflow tract obstruction, atrial or ventricular arrhythmias, or aortic regurgitation, annual cardiac evaluation is recommended. Patients who had late repairs of moderate-sized or large defects should have follow-up every 1 to 2 years to assess for left ventricular dysfunction and elevated pulmonary pressures.[5] Endocarditis prophylaxis in VSD is only indicated within the first 6 months after percutaneous closure with a device or surgical closure using prosthetic material.[5]

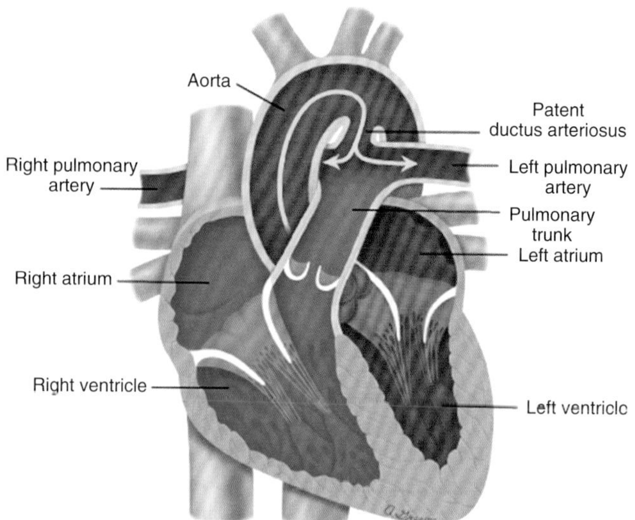

Figure 33-5. Patent ductus arteriosus.

Patent Ductus Arteriosus

Description

The ductus arteriosus is a vascular connection, which during fetal life directs blood flow from the pulmonary artery to the aorta, bypassing the lungs (Fig. 33-5). Functional closure of the ductus occurs within hours or days after birth, in some cases taking 6 months to several years to close. If the ductus remains patent, the direction of blood flow is reversed to left-to-right, because of high systemic pressure in the aorta. A patent ductus arteriosus (PDA), which can escape recognition until adulthood, accounts for 5% to 10% of all cases of CHD and predominates in women (2:1).[11,16] The incidence of PDA is higher at high altitude than at sea level. It is reported that the risk for PDA may be increased at high altitudes. This increased risk is due to a postnatal persistence of pulmonary hypertension. There is reversal of pulmonary hypertension after prolonged residence at sea level.[17]

The hemodynamic changes and clinical manifestations depend on the magnitude of the pulmonary blood flow. The amount of left-to-right shunt is related to the length of the PDA and the size of the ductal lumen as well as the resistance in the pulmonary vascular bed. When the ductus is small, the pulmonary artery pressure remains normal; when larger, aortic pressure is transmitted to the pulmonary artery.

Pathophysiology

A PDA connects the pulmonary artery to the aorta. Blood flows from left to right through the PDA and reenters the pulmonary circulation, increasing the work of the left ventricle. The major complications are left ventricular volume overload leading to congestive heart failure and pulmonary over circulation leading to increased pulmonary vascular resistance. PDA size may be characterized as small (Q_p:Q_s less than 1.5:1), moderate (Q_p:Q_s between 1.5 and 2.2:1), or large (Q_p:Q_s greater than 2.2:1). Adults with small left-to-right shunts from a persistent ductus have no symptoms and life expectancy is normal. Patients with larger shunts and prolonged exposure to increased pulmonary blood flow may lead to increased pulmonary vascular resistance, pulmonary hypertension, and right ventricular hypertrophy.[11] Once pulmonary resistance exceeds systemic pressure, flow reverses to a right-to-left shunt and over time these patients develop cyanotic heart disease[16] (Eisenmenger syndrome) at which point they are rendered inoperable.

Clinical Manifestations

The clinical appearance characterizing a moderate or large PDA with normal pulmonary arterial pressure includes bounding peripheral pulses, a widened pulse pressure, with diastolic pressures as low as 30 to 50 mm Hg. The left ventricular impulse is hyperdynamic, and, if present, a systolic thrill may be palpated over the suprasternal notch area. A continuous loud murmur may be heard in the left infraclavicular region, S1 is normal and S2 may be split with an accentuated P2 component. In the setting of increased pulmonary vascular resistance, the diastolic component of the murmur disappears, leaving only the systolic component. There may be differential cyanosis with cyanosis and clubbing of the toes but not the fingers. This occurs if the defect is large and pulmonary pressures are suprasystemic. The high pulmonary pressures lead to a reversal of flow from right to left, causing deoxygenated blood to flow through the PDA and to the aorta, distal to the subclavian arteries.

Patients with a moderate shunt may have no symptoms during infancy but may begin to develop fatigue, dyspnea, or palpitations during childhood or adulthood. Antibiotic prophylaxis is not recommended in patients with unrepaired PDA unless they have developed Eisenmenger syndrome.[16]

Management

In the absence of pulmonary vascular disease, it is recommended that all PDAs be closed either by surgical ligation or by interventional catheterization using percutaneous closure devices. Patients with moderate- to large-sized PDAs who go unrepaired are at risk for endocarditis, heart failure, and pulmonary hypertension. Once closed, periodic long-term surveillance is recommended because residual problems such as pulmonary hypertension and atrial arrhythmias may develop, particularly in those repaired later in life. Endocarditis prophylaxis is required after surgical or device closure until endothelialization occurs by 6 months, unless a residual shunt persists.[5]

LEFT-SIDED LESIONS

This category of heart defects is characterized by obstructed outflow of the left heart.

Congenital Aortic Stenosis

Description

Left ventricular outflow obstructions (LVOTs) account for 5% to 10% of all congenital heart defects.[18] Congenital aortic stenosis (AS) is characterized by an obstruction to left ventricular outflow and can occur at three levels: valvular, supravalvular, or subvalvular (Fig. 33-6). The majority of adults with congenital AS have "valvar" AS in the form of a bicuspid aortic valve. Congenital AS occurs more frequently in men than in women (4:1).[19] In about 20% of the cases, valvular AS may be associated with coarctation of the aorta (CoA) or PDA.[3] Obstructions to aortic outflow are not only congenital defects but are considered genetic disorders of cardiac and aortic development.[19] Aortopathy associated with bicuspid valve disease likely results from the combination of inherited genetic structural abnormalities of the aortic wall, post-valve

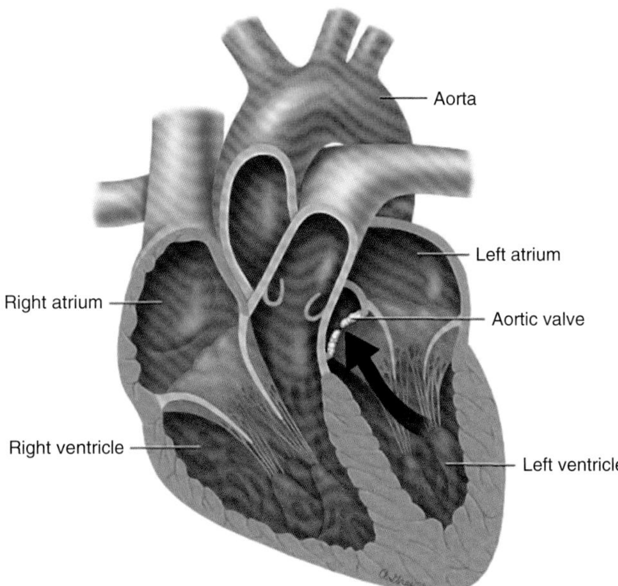

Figure 33-6. Aortic stenosis. When people have aortic stenosis, the aortic valve does not open fully. This prevents blood from flowing normally from the left ventricle, through the aortic valve, and to the aorta. The direction of blood flow is shown by the *black arrow*. The aorta is a big blood vessel that carries blood to the rest of the body.

hemodynamics and traditional cardiac risk factors. The prevalence of aortic dilation with bicuspid aortic valve ranges from 35% to 80% depending on which criteria and screening method are used.[18] Autosomal dominant transmission with variable penetrance is suggested in the literature[5,19] and the 8% to 10% prevalence rate of bicuspid valves in asymptomatic first-degree relatives supports the American College of Cardiology/American Heart Association recommendation for echocardiogram screening.[5,18] Women with Turner syndrome are also at considerable risk of bicuspid valve, coarctation and aortic dilation resulting in increased morbidity and mortality if left untreated.[5] Therefore, screening is recommended for all women with Turner syndrome. Congenital valvular AS is usually a progressive disorder. Up to 20% of patients with gradients less than 25 mm Hg will end up requiring intervention during their lifetime.[3] Complications include aortic regurgitation, infective endocarditis, and aortic aneurysm and dissection.

Pathophysiology

AS is characterized by thickening and rigidity of the valve tissue with a varying degree of commissure fusion in childhood and adolescence. Worsening of the obstruction results from increased cardiac output that occurs during growth along with decrease in the effective valve orifice.[3] Calcification of the aortic valve in adults requires that most individuals who need intervention will include an aortic valve replacement.[5] However, young patients with relatively little calcification may be candidates for balloon valvuloplasty.[5] The adaptation response to chronic AS is left ventricular hypertrophy, which can sustain large pressure gradients across the aortic valve without a drop in cardiac output, left ventricle dilatation, or development of symptoms.[19] Mean systolic pressure gradients with a normal cardiac output reflect the severity of the obstruction. Mild obstruction produces a mean pressure gradient of less than 20 mm Hg, a moderate obstruction produces a mean gradient of 20 to 39 mm Hg; severe stenosis produces mean gradients greater than 40 mm Hg (an aortic valve area indexed to body surface area [AVA*i*] of

$0.6\ cm^2/m^2$); reflecting severe obstruction to left ventricular outflow. While resting cardiac output and stroke volume are generally within normal limits, the cardiac output increases with exercise. The gradient across the area of obstruction also increases with exercise, causing the obstruction to become more severe.

In severe AS, the hemodynamic abnormalities produced by the obstruction to the left ventricle outflow increase myocardial oxygen demand, decreased diastolic coronary perfusion time and coronary flow reserve contribute to ischemia in patients with severe AS without obstructive CAD,[3] thereby interfering with coronary blood flow. As a result, significant stenosis may result in reduced subendocardial perfusion, particularly during exercise, leading to ischemia. Subendocardial ischemia plays a key role in the angina, syncope, ventricular arrhythmias, and sudden death reported in patients with AS.[3] Exertional syncope, which can occur in patients with gradients exceeding 50 mm Hg, is related to the inability of the left ventricle to increase its output and to maintain cerebral flow during exercise. The onset of clinical symptoms in adults may not occur until the fourth or fifth decade and is usually the result of aortic valve regurgitation and/or calcification.[5]

Clinical Manifestations

The symptoms of valvular AS may be inconspicuous. When they occur, those most noted are fatigue, exertional dyspnea, angina, heart failure, and syncope.[18] Classically, a loud (grade 4/6), late peaking systolic murmur which radiates to the carotids is appreciated. A systolic ejection click may be heard after the first heart sound with bicuspid valve. However, this sound decreases as the cusps stiffen due to progressive calcification. With significant stenosis, diminished carotid upstroke with and a left ventricle lift are common. A precordial systolic thrill is palpated over the base of the heart and is transmitted to the suprasternal notch and over both carotid arteries.[18]

Management

Therapeutic decisions are guided by the presence or absence of symptoms. The development of symptoms characterizes a critical point in the natural progression of AS, after which there is a dramatic increase in morbidity and mortality.[18] Asymptomatic patients with mild AS and peak-to-peak gradients less than 25 mm Hg may be treated medically. With higher peak-to-peak gradients greater than 50 mm Hg and no more than mild aortic insufficiency, balloon valvuloplasty may be successfully performed resulting in at least a 50% reduction in the transvalvar gradient.[3] However, balloon valvuloplasty is utilized less often in adults due to calcification of the valves.[3] Case reports demonstrate the successful use of balloon aortic valvuloplasty as a bridge to delivery in pregnancy.[18] The preferred treatment in adults is surgical aortic valve replacement, especially if more than mild aortic regurgitation is present.[3] For patients with a narrowed left ventricle outflow tract and small aortic valve annulus, the Ross–Konno surgical procedure may be performed to relieve left ventricular obstruction to outflow.

Patients with mild AS should be followed in an adult congenital heart center every 3 to 5 and those with moderate AS every 1 to 2 years.[5] Prophylaxis against endocarditis is not required, unless prosthetic cardiac valves have been placed.[5,20]

Coarctation of the Aorta

Description

CoA is a common defect accounting for 5% to 9% of CHD with male predominance of 2:1.[3,18] CoA often presents as a discrete narrowing just opposite of the ductus arteriosus near the left subclavian artery (Fig. 33-7).[3,5] Occasionally, the coarctation occurs above the origin of the right subclavian. It is strongly associated with bicuspid aortic valve, VSD, PDA, and left-sided (aortic and/or mitral) valve abnormalities.[3,5] There is also associated abnormalities in the tissue of the aortic wall which predisposes the ascending aorta to dissection and rupture. A noncardiac anomaly associated with CoA is a saccular aneurysm of the circle of Willis (berry aneurysm) seen in approximately 10% of those with CoA.[5,18] For this reason, it is recommended that every patient with coarctation have at least one CT or MRI to evaluate the intracranial vessels.[5]

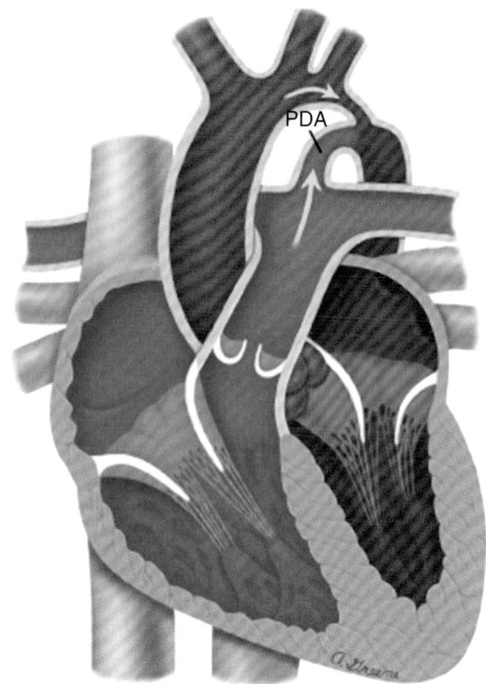

Figure 33-7. Coarctation of the aorta. Coarctation of the aorta is a narrowing of the descending aorta. The narrowing typically is at the isthmus, the segment just distal to the left subclavian artery. In critical coarctation, the narrowing is severe and blood flow to the descending aorta is dependent on a patent ductus arteriosus (PDA). When the PDA closes, neonates with critical coarctation develop heart failure and/or shock. On physical exam, femoral pulses are weak or absent.

Pathophysiology

The physiologic consequences of coarctation stem primarily from systemic hypertension, whether repaired or unrepaired. The increased resistance produced by aortic narrowing results in increased pressure in the aorta proximal to the coarctation and decreased pressure distal to the narrowing. Because renal artery blood flow is decreased, plasma renin release is stimulated, contributing further to the upregulation of systemic arterial pressure. Complications include dissection and rupture of the aorta, seen more commonly in the second and third decades; early atherosclerotic heart disease, stroke, myocardial infarction, endocarditis; heart failure, which increases in incidence after the fourth decade; and cerebral hemorrhage due to rupture of an aneurysm of the circle of Willis.

Clinical Manifestations

Cardinal features of CoA include upper body hypertension; weak or absent femoral pulses, radial–femoral delay (delay between the radial and femoral pulses); a drop in blood pressure between upper and lower extremities and palpable collateral arteries over the scapula, intercostal and lateral chest walls.[18] As the patient grows older, systolic pressures rise more than diastolic, resulting in a widened pulse pressure. Arterial pressures may also vary between right and left arms depending on the zone of coarctation relative to the subclavian artery. In the presence of an anomalous right subclavian artery, the blood pressure in the right arm is lower than the left. When the coarctation involves the origin of the left subclavian artery, the blood pressure in the left arm is lower than the right. Differences between arm and leg blood pressure are accentuated further by exercise, with the brachial blood pressure rising, whereas the femoral pressure remains unchanged or may decrease. Patients may present with exertional headaches, nosebleeds, tinnitus, dizziness, abdominal angina, claudication, and intracranial hemorrhage.[18] Additional physical findings include a thrill palpated at the suprasternal notch or carotids and a left ventricular heave. Continuous murmurs may be heard in the left parascapular region if collaterals are present. A systolic crescendo–decrescendo murmur associated with LVOT obstruction may be heard. An early diastolic murmur, suggestive of aortic regurgitation and an aortic ejection sound may be heard, particularly with a bicuspid aortic valve.[18]

Management

Patients with mild coarctation pressure gradients (less than 20 mm Hg in the absence of significant collateral flow) may be treated medically with β-blockers or angiotensin-receptor blockers, but should be followed carefully to monitor for an increase in the gradient. In patients with higher-pressure gradients, surgical resection of the coarctation has been the treatment of choice for several decades. However, since the 1990s, balloon angioplasty and stenting are commonly utilized for treatment of discrete native recurrent coarctation.[18] Choice of percutaneous versus surgical intervention should be determined in consultation with congenitally trained cardiologist, interventionalist, and surgeons at a CHD center.[5,18]

Patients with CoA are prone to arterial hypertension and coronary heart disease, due to arterial wall stiffness and alterations in vascular reactivity.[3,18] The presence of traditional cardiac risk factors (hypertension, dyslipidemia, diabetes, male sex, and age) in patients with CoA highlights the usefulness of screening for and treating associated CV conditions.[21] Aggressive risk factor management for prevention of general acquired heart disease should be undertaken. ACE-Is, ARBs, and β-blockers are particularly useful in the management of these patients.[3,5,18] Other long-term residual effects include re-coarctation of the previously treated area and aneurysms of the ascending aorta.

Follow-up for patients with CoA is required to monitor for late complications such as hypertension and restenosis. Such follow-up and subsequent treatment should be scheduled every 1 to 2 years in an ACHD center.[5] According to the 2007 guidelines on the prevention of infective endocarditis, antibiotic prophylaxis is only required within the first 6 months after placement of prosthetic material, or when residual defects occur at the site or adjacent to the site of prosthetic material.[5,20]

RIGHT-SIDED LESIONS

These defects are characterized by a right ventricular outflow tract (RVOT) obstruction. The most commonly occurring heart defect in this category is a pulmonic valve stenosis.

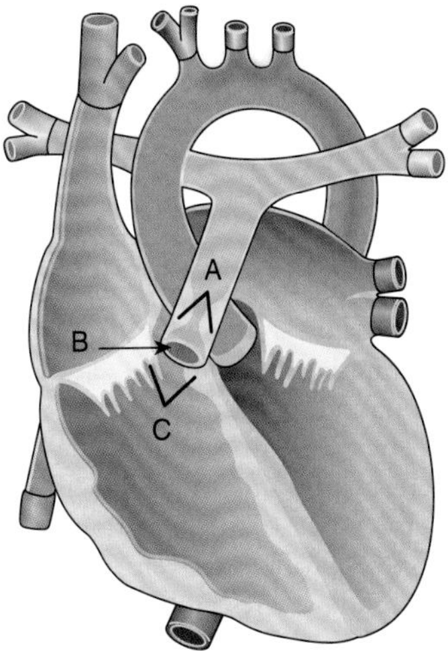

Figure 33-8. Pulmonic stenosis. **A:** Supravalvular pulmonic stenosis. **B:** Valvular pulmonic stenosis. **C:** Infundibular stenosis. (Reprinted from Everett A. PedHeart Resource. *Scientific Software Solutions.* 2009. Available at www.heartpassport.com, with permission.)

Pulmonic Valve Stenosis

Description

Pulmonary valve stenosis (PS) is often an isolated lesion that occurs in 7% to 12% of patients with CHD.[18] The result of PS is obstruction of the ejection of blood from the right ventricle leading to an increase in right ventricular pressure. PS can occur at the valvular, subvalvar (infundibular or subinfundibular), or supravalvular level (stenosis of the pulmonary artery and its branches) (Fig. 33-8). It may occur as an isolated defect or in combination with other congenital cardiac defects, including VSD or ASD.[5,18] Life expectancy depends on the severity of the stenosis. Patients with mild pulmonary stenosis or patients who have undergone balloon valvuloplasty have an excellent survival.[18] They must, however, be periodically evaluated for recurrent pulmonary stenosis, or for pulmonary regurgitation which can occur as a result of valvuloplasty. Long-term follow-up of these patients shows a survival rate similar to that of the general population; morbidity is infrequent, and risk of endocarditis is rare.[5,18]

Pathophysiology

The clinical course of pure, isolated pulmonic valve stenosis is dependent on the degree of right ventricular obstruction. Common findings associated with valvar PS include poststenotic dilation of the main pulmonary artery and dysplastic valve cusps.[5] Most patients with mild PS (peak gradient across the valve less than 36 mm Hg) are asymptomatic and intervention is not usually necessary.[5] However, those with moderate PS (when the gradient is 36 to 64 mm Hg) have a more variable course and may present with exercise intolerance. The functional consequences of pulmonic valve stenosis are related to the degree of stenosis and the adaptive response of the right ventricle. The right ventricle hypertrophies in proportion to the degree of stenosis. Over time, changes in the right ventricle, such as myocardial fibrosis, infundibular stenosis, and subvalvar muscular hypertrophy, can lead to alterations in right ventricle function, which contributes further to the obstruction to the right ventricle outflow. Furthermore, with advancing age, a congenitally deformed pulmonic valve can become thickened, fibrotic, and even calcified, thus reducing valve mobility and increasing the degree of obstruction. In more severe cases, right atrial hypertrophy must be present and be of sufficient degree to open a previously closed foramen ovale leading to right-to-left shunting. Severe pulmonic valve stenosis (peak grading greater than 64 mm Hg) eventually leads to tricuspid regurgitation and clear right ventricular failure.

Clinical Manifestations

Physical findings in mild–moderate PS include normal jugular venous pulse, no RV lift, and a pulmonary ejection sound that decreases with inspiration. A pulmonic ejection click which is louder during expiration may be heard at the left upper sternal border (produced by sudden opening of the pulmonary valve). In severe PS, one typically finds a prominent jugular waveform (due to the forceful right atrial contraction, required to fill the hypertrophied noncompliant right ventricle), an RV lift, and a harsh systolic crescendo–decrescendo murmur heard along the left upper sternal border. The ejection sound is no longer heard but wide splitting of the pulmonic component of the second heart (S2) sound may be present. A right-sided S4 may also be heard.

Management

Patients with mild pulmonic stenosis should be followed at a congenital center every 3 to 5 years,[18] but have no restrictions. Patients with moderate gradients (36 to 64 mm Hg) or severe gradient (greater than 64 mm Hg) are usually managed with balloon valvuloplasty.[5,18] Restenosis is observed in 6.5% of the patients who underwent balloon dilatation.[18] Surgical valvotomy is indicated when the pulmonary valve is dysplastic rendering balloon valvuloplasty less effective. Valve replacement in the presence of significant obstruction with calcification of the pulmonic valve is seen in older adults. Prophylaxis against endocarditis is not required in patients with pulmonic valve stenosis, unless prosthetic cardiac valves have been placed.[20]

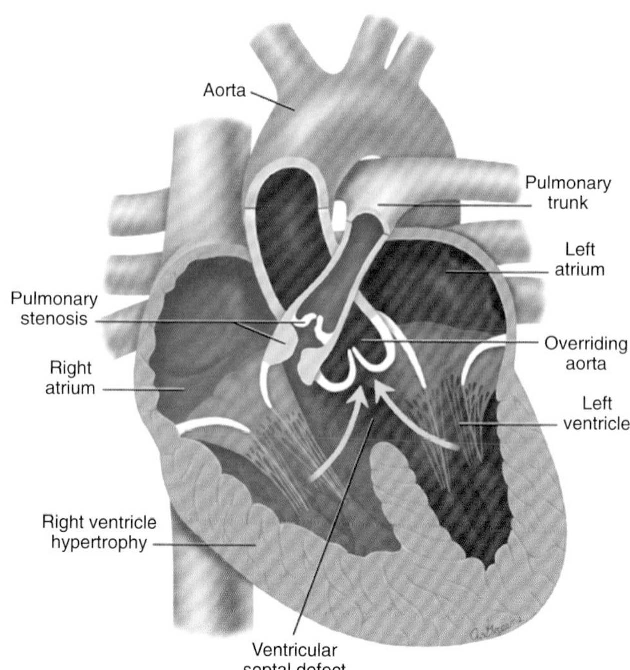

Figure 33-9. Tetralogy of Fallot. Tetralogy of Fallot is characterized by a large ventricular septal defect (VSD), an aorta that overrides the left and right ventricles, obstruction of the right ventricular outflow tract, and right ventricular hypertrophy. As a result of the substantial obstruction of the right ventricular outflow tract, there is right-to-left shunting through the VSD resulting in cyanosis.

Tetralogy of Fallot

Description

Tetralogy of Fallot (TOF) is the most common form of cyanotic heart defects and accounts for 10% of all CHDs.[18] There is a slight predominance of male sex distribution.[18] Up to 15% of patients with TOF have deletion of chromosome 22q11 (DiGeorge syndrome).[18] While a wide anatomic and clinical spectrum exists, the classic cyanotic tetrad includes a nonrestrictive VSD, severe pulmonic stenosis causing obstruction to pulmonary blood flow, right ventricular hypertrophy, and various degrees of overriding aorta which is displaced over the VSD, rather than over the left ventricle (Fig. 33-9). Today, surgical repair is undertaken in early childhood; however, natural survival of an unoperated adult is possible if RVOT obstruction is mild. Morbidity and mortality in adults with unrepaired TOF is high and is related to cyanosis, exercise intolerance, arrhythmia, tendency to thrombosis and cerebral abscess. Those who survive until their 40s or 50s mortality occurs due to heart failure caused by long-standing right ventricular hypertension or suddenly presumably to arrhythmia.[18]

Pathophysiology

The physiologic consequences of TOF depend on the degree of right ventricular outflow obstruction. Since the VSD is usually nonrestrictive, the pressure in the ventricles equalize and the direction of blood flow across the VSD follows the path of least resistance. The pulmonary stenosis is usually infundibular but may occur at the valvular level or in the pulmonary trunk and its branches. When the stenosis is mild, the shunt remains left-to-right with no cyanosis and is referred to as "acyanotic" or "pink" TOF. As pulmonic obstruction increases, the shunt reverses to right to left. Right ventricular hypertrophy develops due to resistance to the outflow. When total obstruction to pulmonary flow exists, and the pulmonary trunk and its branches are present, blood flow to the lung is mainly through enlarged bronchial arteries and, at times, also through a PDA. This severe form of TOF is referred to as pulmonary atresia.

Clinical Manifestations

Invariably, the patients with TOF present with cyanosis. The hypercyanotic episodes ("tet spells") associated with TOF are virtually absent in the adult. If the patient has only mild cyanosis, development is normal. A loud (3–5/6) systolic murmur is heard over the left upper and middle sternal border with a thrill is characteristic; however, with severe right ventricular outflow obstruction (such as during a "tet" spell) the murmur will become softer due to the right-to-left shunting across the VSD. This is due to the absence of turbulent blood flow between the two high-pressure ventricles. When total obstruction (pulmonary atresia) is present, the murmur of the pulmonic stenosis vanishes and is replaced by a soft mid-systolic murmur. Continuous murmurs, an auscultatory sign of pulmonary atresia, indicate collateral circulation by way of bronchial arteries or presence of a PDA.

Management

The majority of patients born with TOF have survived as a result of having undergone a series of surgical procedures. During infancy, a palliative systemic to pulmonary arterial shunt procedure would have been undertaken to permit pulmonary arterial blood flow and increase oxygen saturation. Later in childhood, patients underwent repair that included closure of the VSD and relief of the right ventricle outflow obstruction. Today, while palliative shunt procedures are still performed in selected cases, the majority of patients born with TOF undergo reparative surgery in infancy.[18] The most commonly observed sequelae to repaired TOF is pulmonary valve insufficiency.

Survival at 32 to 36 years after repair is excellent and has been reported at 86% and 85%, respectively.[18] However, a number of late effects resulting from prior surgeries must be monitored on a regular basis, including degree of pulmonary regurgitation, right ventricular enlargement, residual RVOT obstruction, aortic root and valve dilation, atrial and ventricular arrhythmias, and sudden cardiac death.[5,18] A small number of patients with TOF remain cyanotic. These are usually patients who have developed irreversible PAH and are no longer surgical candidates and are managed symptomatically.[20]

Patients with TOF should have follow-up visits with a congenitally trained cardiologist at least annually.[5] Endocarditis prophylaxis indicated for 6 months following a repair when prosthetic materials are used (e.g., for VSD patch closure) or when residual shunts are present.[20]

Ebstein Anomaly

Description

Ebstein anomaly is a rare heart defect involving the tricuspid valve and right ventricle. It is characterized by a downward displacement of portions of the tricuspid valve into the right ventricle (Fig. 33-10). The portion of the normal right ventricle that underlies the tricuspid valve becomes mechanically a part of the right atrium (atrialized right ventricle). As a result, the right atrium is exceptionally large, the right ventricle is small, and the tricuspid valve is incompetent. Ebstein anomaly occurs in less than 1% of all congenital heart defects and affects men and women equally.[20]

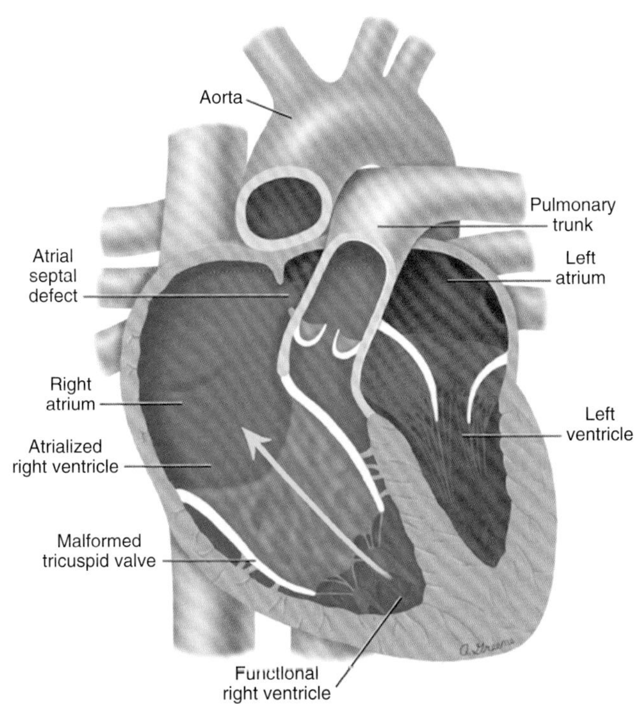

Figure 33-10. Ebstein anomaly. Pathophysiology of Ebstein anomaly.

In patients with Ebstein anomaly, 75% to 95% have either an ASD or PFO, often resulting in a right-to-left shunt.[18] In the presence of an atrial communication, central cyanosis may be present. The presence of shunt places patients at risk of CVA due to risk of paradoxical embolization. In addition, 10% to 45% of patients have one or more accessory pathways (Wolff–Parkinson–White). In fact, arrhythmia including atrial fibrillation, flutter or ectopic atrial tachycardia is commonly the presenting symptom occurring in 40% of patients.[18]

There is significant variation in presentation of Ebstein's patients. Age at presentation depends on the anatomic (displacement of the TV) and functional severity of the anomaly as well as presence of any associated lesions. Report of surgical repair at some stage was seen in 39% of patients.[22] Unoperated patients presenting late have decreased survival due to biventricular heart failure.[18] Sudden cardiac death presumably due to ventricular arrhythmias is well documented.

Pathophysiology

Hemodynamically abnormal function of the right heart is related to three problems: a malformed tricuspid valve, the atrialized portion of the right ventricle, and the reduced size of the pumping portion of the right ventricle. Ineffective emptying of the right atrium may result in an increase in right atrial volume and a right-to-left shunt through a PFO or ASD. Tricuspid regurgitation caused by malformed leaflets adds to the hemodynamic burden. Important complications associated with Ebstein anomaly include supraventricular tachycardia resulting from Wolff–Parkinson–White pre-excitation or other accessory conduction pathways.[18]

Clinical Manifestations

Cardiac exam may reveal a soft parasternal heave. Jugular distention is uncommon despite severe tricuspid regurgitation. This is related to the high compliance of the atrialized right ventricle. The systolic murmur of tricuspid regurgitation may be heard at the left lower sternal border. Intensity will depend on degree of severity and RV function. Splitting of the first and second heart sounds is common. An S3 is common due to abnormal filling characteristics of the functional right ventricle. In addition, an S_4 may be present, producing a quadruple gallop. Lower extremity edema may be present with advanced heart failure. Digital clubbing may be seen when cyanosis is significant if a shunt is present. Clinically, patients commonly present with exercise intolerance due to dyspnea or fatigability.

Management

Medical management of patients with Ebstein anomaly is directed toward the prevention of complications and to the treatment of symptoms as they present themselves. Those patients with supraventricular tachycardia, or persistent atrial fibrillation or flutter may be treated with appropriate catheter-based ablation. If percutaneous ablation is not possible, mapping may be done to augment operative therapies.[18] Surgical repair of the tricuspid valve and closure of the ASD are recommended in symptomatic patients. Valve repair using annuloplasty ring is preferred to replacement, which is reserved for nonreparable valves. When required, a bioprosthetic valve is preferred to mechanical prosthesis.[18]

Patients with Ebstein anomaly should have follow-up visits with an ACHD cardiologist every 1 or 2 years.[18] Endocarditis prophylaxis is needed in cyanotic patients or those with a prosthetic tricuspid valve. It is not indicated for acyanotic unoperated patients.[20]

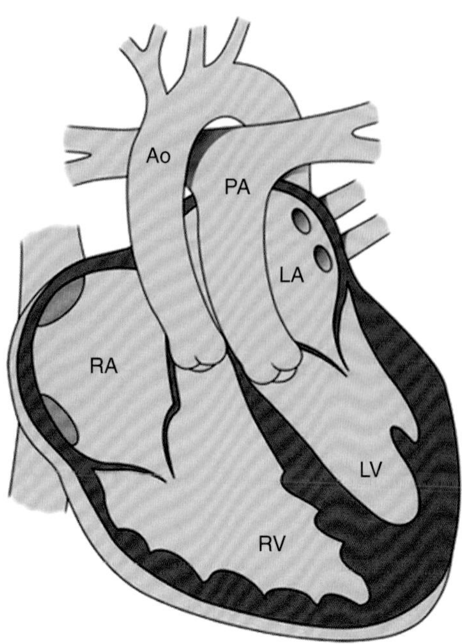

Figure 33-11. Complete transposition of the great arteries (d-TGA). Diagram of the dextro type of transposition of the great arteries showing the abnormal position of the aorta (Ao) and the pulmonary artery (PA).

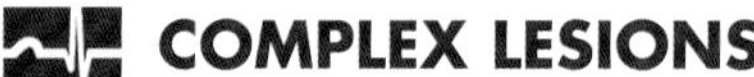

COMPLEX LESIONS

Complete Transposition of the Great Arteries (TGA)

Description

There is only one heart defect that can be firmly classified under cyanotic heart defects with an increased pulmonary blood flow: a *complete* TGA. Complete transposition of the great arteries describes the anatomical arrangement where the aorta arises from the right ventricle (anterior to the pulmonary artery) and the pulmonary artery arises from the left ventricle (Fig. 33-11). Blood circulates in two separate parallel circuits. Blood returning to the heart from the systemic circulation leaves the right ventricle and goes to the aorta, sending deoxygenated blood back into systemic circulation. Mixing of blood is required to supply oxygenated blood to vital organs. This may take place through a PFO and/or via a PDA. When TGA is suspected, therapy is directed at maintaining or restoring patency of the ductus to allow mixing. Complete TGA, also referred to as *d-transposition of great arteries*, occurs in 5% to 7% of all CHDs.[18] There is a male predominance of 2:1 in patients with transposition of the great arteries.[18] Natural survival is extremely rare, and survival into adulthood is dependent on the early use of palliative shunting procedures (atrioseptectomy, atrioseptostomy), pulmonary artery banding to regulate pulmonary flow, and, later, the atrial switch techniques known as the Mustard or Senning operation. Both procedures form a baffle within the atria to "switch" the flow of blood leading to return of normal flow of blood in the heart. However, the LV remains the subpulmonary ventricle and the RV the systemic ventricle.[18]

In the Mustard procedure, venous blood is diverted to the mitral valve by means of an atrial baffle created from the pericardium or other synthetic material. In the Senning procedure, a tunnel is created within the right atrial wall with no synthetic material. While mid-term survival rates associated with the atrial switch procedures have been relatively good, commonly occurring complications include arrhythmias, baffle obstruction, and progressive failure of the systemic right ventricle.[23] This led surgeons to replace the Mustard and Senning procedures with an arterial switch operation.[18] Carried out in an infant's first few weeks of life, the arterial switch procedure, pioneered by Adib Jatene, involves surgically detaching the origin of the coronary arteries from the aorta, then separating the aorta and pulmonary arteries above the semilunar valves. The aorta is then reimplanted to the stump of the pulmonary trunk, and the pulmonary artery is reimplanted to the stump of the aortic root. The coronary arteries are then attached to the "new" or neoaorta. Though complex, the arterial switch operation (ASO) has become the standard of care for those with d-TGA without significant LVOT. The overall perioperative mortality is less than 4%.[24] The quality of life and health status of children ages 11 to 15 after ASO were similar to norms and better than those who had undergone the atrial switch operation.[25]

Pathophysiology

Systemic right ventricular failure and sudden cardiac death are the primary morbidity and mortality for individuals who underwent Mustard or Senning repairs. Sudden death has been found to occur in 7% to 15% of patients after atrial baffle repair. In addition individuals are at risk for both bradyarrhythmias from sinus node dysfunction and atrial reentry tachycardias resulting from the multiple suture lines.[18] The long-term outlook for patients following baffle repair is mainly concerned with the function of the systemic right ventricle. While the right ventricle can endure functioning at the systemic level in the short to medium term, it may fail when required to serve in this capacity indefinitely. Additional long-term complications that increase demand on the right ventricle include tricuspid regurgitation, sinus node dysfunction, atrial re-entrant tachycardia, pulmonary hypertension, and baffle obstruction or leaks. In a 20-year postoperative course, up to 50% of the patients experience at least one form of arrhythmias.[18,23] After arterial switch operation, the majority of patients are asymptomatic, ventricular function is good, and rhythm disturbances are infrequent. The major concern in the long-term survival of these patients is the status of coronary arteries. Survival rates without coronary events were 92.7%, 91%, and 88.2% at 1, 10, and 15 years, respectively.[26]

Clinical Manifestations

Following an atrial switch operation, the second heart sound is usually single, due to the anterior position of the aortic valve. Splitting of the second heart sound may signify the development of pulmonary hypertension. In the absence of an associated defect, there may be no murmurs. In the presence of tricuspid insufficiency, a systolic murmur is audible, and if due to the presence of a VSD, a pansystolic murmur is audible along the left sternal border. A harsh systolic ejection murmur along the left midsternal border will be heard in the setting of valvar or subvalvar pulmonary stenosis.

Management

All patients who have had surgical repair for TGA should be followed at a regional ACHD center at least every 12 months.[5] In addition to an echocardiogram, a cardiac MRI for more detailed assessment of right ventricular function is recommended at least every 2 to 3 years.[5]

Medical management is directed to maintain right ventricle function or to support a failing systemic right ventricle as well as control and/or treat development of complications. Arrhythmias are mainly treated using antiarrhythmic drugs, catheter ablation or implantable cardiac defibrillators. In patients who develop poor chronotropic response to exercise, permanent pacemaker may be indicated.

In Mustard and Senning patients, reoperation is most frequently performed in the setting of baffle obstruction or leaks that result in shunting. The latter is more often observed in patients after the Mustard operation than after the Senning operation. Following the arterial switch operation, patients are monitored for right and left ventricle outflow tract obstructions in the supravalvular areas, due to suture line stenosis. If an outflow tract obstruction occurs, balloon angioplasty or surgical intervention with patch augmentation is the treatment of choice. Endocarditis prophylaxis is indicated for the following circumstances: following valve replacements, prior episode of endocarditis, unrepaired or palliated cyanotic heart disease, repaired disease with residual shunt that inhibits endothelialization.[20]

Congenitally Corrected Transposition of the Great Arteries

Description

CCTGA occurs only less than 1% of all cardiac anomalies.[18] CCTGA is also referred to as *L-transposition of the great arteries.* In CCTGA, the great arteries are reversed, whereby the aorta arises from the right ventricle and the pulmonary trunk from the left ventricle. In addition the ventricles are inverted where the right ventricle occupies the left side of the heart, and the left ventricle is on the right (Fig. 33-12). This is a case where two "wrongs" make a right in that physiologic blood flow is physiologically maintained. However, the morphologic right ventricle functions as the systemic ventricle. Since the atrioventricular valves follow the ventricles, the left-sided atrioventricular valve is the anatomical tricuspid valve, whereas the right-sided valve is the anatomical mitral valve. The coronary arteries and ventricles are morphologically concordant meaning a morphologic right ventricle would still be supplied by the right coronary artery.

CCTGA is frequently associated with VSD (70% to 88%),[18] pulmonic valve stenosis (50% to 70%),[18] and tricuspid valve regurgitation due to an Ebsteinoid configuration (29% to 70%).[18] If a right-lo-left shunt is present, the patient is classified as cyanotic. Surgical intervention is dictated by symptoms and the presence of associated lesions such as VSD or pulmonary stenosis. While most cases are detected in childhood, many go undetected until clinical signs and symptoms appear. Patients with corrected transposition without associated anomalies may reach adulthood, leading normal lives. In general, 20-year survival rate after conventional repair is between 48% and 80%.[18]

Pathophysiology

The most common clinical sequelae and/or complications with CCTGA include right ventricular dysfunction, tricuspid regurgitation, residual left ventricle outflow obstruction, and cardiac conduction abnormalities. Progressive right ventricle dysfunction leading to heart failure is associated with advanced age, typically in the fifth decade, as the morphologic right ventricle begins to fail as the systemic ventricle.[20,27] Complete heart block, if not present at birth, is likely to develop at a rate of 2% per year, due to the displacement of the atrioventricular node in the right atrium.[18] In patients without associated lesions, it is expected that up to 27% will need a pacemaker. This percentage increased up to 45% in patients with associated heart defects.[27]

Clinical Manifestations

Many adults with CCTGA present as one of two groups: (1) those diagnosed and repaired in infancy and now presenting with residual defects associated with a VSD or pulmonic stenosis, or (2) those with no associated lesions who have essentially remained asymptomatic but have developed symptoms related to progressive right ventricle dysfunction or to systemic atrioventricular valve regurgitation. The latter group of patients may have been referred to evaluate pulmonary congestion, a systolic murmur at the apex of the heart, or because of ECG abnormalities, including atrial tachycardias or

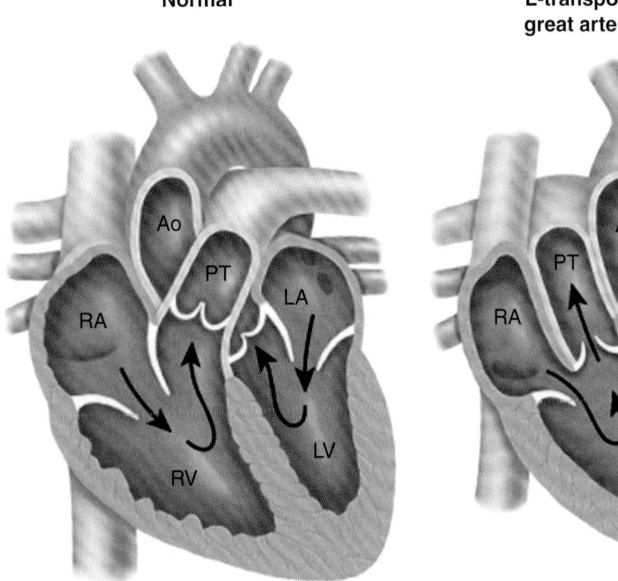

Figure 33-12. Congenitally corrected transposition of the great arteries. RA, right atrium; RV, right ventricle; Ao, aorta; LV, left ventricle; LA, left atrium; PT, pulmonary trunk.

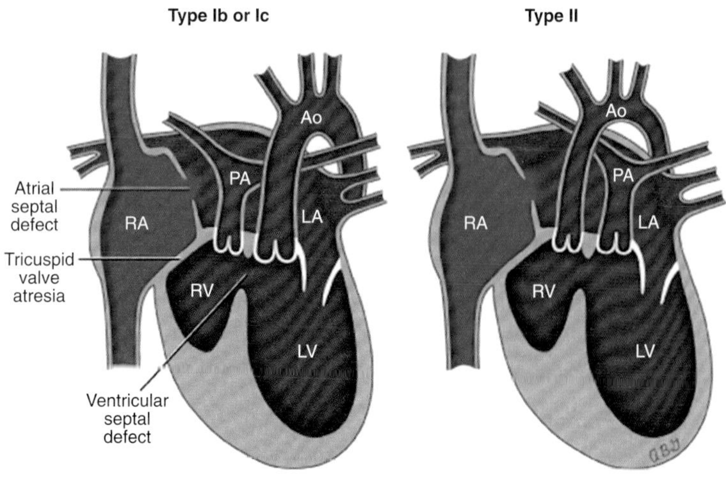

Figure 33-13. Tricuspid atresia. Schematic diagram demonstrating the anatomical and physiologic features of TV atresia type Ib or Ic (normally related great arteries and VSD), and TV atresia type IIc (d-loop transposition of the great arteries with no pulmonary stenosis). TV atresia with normally related great arteries and no VSD is classified as type Ia. In all types of TV atresia, the obligate atrial level shunt results in mixing of systemic and pulmonary venous blood in the left atrium. In types Ib and Ic, there is a left-to-right shunting at the level of the VSD, which serves as the source of pulmonary blood. In type II, the VSD is critical for systemic output, as the right ventricle, which provides the systemic circulation through the aorta, is dependent on blood flowing from the left ventricle through the VSD. In TV atresia type II, blood flow to the pulmonary artery is derived directly from the left ventricle. TV, tricuspid valve; VSD, ventricular septal defect; RA, right atrium; RV, right ventricle; LA, left atrium; LV, left ventricle; PA, pulmonary artery; Ao, aorta.

heart block. On examination, a right ventricular parasternal lift is common, along with the holosystolic murmur of tricuspid regurgitation heard best at the apex and a single second heart sound. In patients with residual pulmonary stenosis, a systolic ejection murmur may be heard at the upper left sternal border.

Management

The goal of treatment for both operated and unoperated patients is preservation of the systemic right ventricle by avoiding dilatation and failure. Tricuspid valve replacement is recommended to avoid morphologic right ventricle volume overload and deterioration of systemic right ventricle function. Ideally, the valve replacement should be performed before the ejection fraction deteriorates to less than 45%.[5] Periodic Holter monitoring to assess the status of AV conduction is recommended and may be useful to clarify relationship between symptoms and arrhythmias.[27]

The complex double-switch procedure is less commonly utilized to convert the morphologic LV into the systemic pumping chamber. This operation combines the atrial (Mustard or Senning) and the arterial switch procedures (Jatene) (see section "Complete Transposition of the Great Arteries"), or alternatively combines the atrial switch procedure and Rastelli operation. This long and extensive surgical operation with higher perioperative mortality, and significant risk of developing complications inherent to both atrial and arterial switch.[18]

Patients with CCTGA should be followed at least annually in a regional ACHD center. The frequency is dependent upon the presence or absence of associated cardiac abnormalities as well as degree of ventricular dysfunction or tricuspid regurgitation. For those who remain asymptomatic, an annual evaluation that includes ECG and echocardiography is recommended.[5,18] Endocarditis prophylaxis is not required in the unrepaired patient, but is recommended in repaired patients with prosthetic material or artificial valves.[20]

Tricuspid Atresia and Single Ventricle

Description

There are multiple heart abnormalities that are not amenable to a two ventricle repair.[20] These include tricuspid atresia, mitral atresia, double-inlet left ventricle, single ventricle, hypoplastic right ventricle or left ventricle, and heterotaxy syndromes.[20] Tricuspid atresia is the most common type of univentricular physiology and the third most common cyanotic heart defect.[18,28] The prevalence is reported to be 0.5 to 1.2 per 10,000 live-births and accounts for 1% to 3% of all congenital heart defects.[28,29] The male-to-female ratio is 1.45:1.[18] The heart with tricuspid atresia (TA) has absence (atresia) of the tricuspid valve. The only remaining valve is connected to the dominant ventricle. Systemic venous blood returns to the right atrium and can only exit via an ASD into the left atrium (Fig. 33-13). This results in a total right-to-left shunt at the atrial level. Blood then enters the left ventricle via the remaining (mitral) valve. There is usually an associated VSD which leads to a rudimentary right ventricular chamber. Whereas all types of tricuspid atresia have in common the absence of the tricuspid valve, various forms exist. The 20-year survival rate in patients with tricuspid atresia is about 60%.[30] Survival is determined by the adequacy of pulmonary blood flow and the pressure in the pulmonary vascular bed, and the 10-year unoperated survival rate is only 46%.[18]

Pathophysiology

In 70% of cases tricuspid atresia, great arteries are normally related.[18] Because of the atretic tricuspid valve, systemic venous blood crosses from the right atrium to the left atrium via an ASD. Oxygenated and deoxygenated blood mix and continue to the left ventricle, where blood is then ejected into the aorta, with some blood reaching the pulmonary circulation by way of the VSD. In most cases, pulmonary blood flow is restricted due to subvalvar or valvular pulmonary stenosis. As a result of the mixing of systemic and pulmonary venous blood in the left atrium, these patients are hypoxic and cyanotic.[18,31]

Less often, patients with transposition of the great arteries have the pulmonary artery coming off the dominant left ventricle and they present with excessive pulmonary blood flow (overcirculation) resulting in marked ventricular volume overload, breathlessness, and minimal cyanosis. The overload caused by the increased pulmonary blood flow often leads to congestive heart failure.[18]

Clinical Manifestations

Clinically, the patient with tricuspid atresia is characterized by cyanosis and clubbing. There is a dominant left ventricle impulse, and a noticeably absent right ventricle impulse. The second heart sound is usually single. In the majority of patients (those with normally related great arteries), a loud pulmonary ejection murmur is heard and may have an associated thrill.

Management

All surgical options are staged and considered palliative as two-ventricle repair is not possible. However, shunts such as a modified Blalock–Taussig (BT) shunt (a synthetic graft connecting the innominate artery to the pulmonary artery) is performed in infancy to ensure a reliable source of pulmonary blood flow. Management aims to complete Fontan circulation which utilizes passive blood flow from the inferior vena cava to the pulmonary artery, and bidirectional Glenn (connection of the superior vena cava to the pulmonary artery and removal of the BT shunt). The end result is passive deoxygenated blood flow to the lungs which returns oxygenated blood to the (common) left atrium to the systemic left ventricle where it is pumped to the body. Normal Fontan physiology requires an elevated central venous pressure and a preload dependent state as there is no subpulmonary ventricle. For patients who underwent a Fontan operation and survived the perioperative period, the 20-year survival rate was more than 80%.[32] However, the long-term concerns associated following Fontan operation include the physiologic effects of persistent low cardiac output, preload starvation, and elevated systemic venous pressure on end organs. Vigilance is needed to detect problems with stenosis or obstruction of the various conduits. Patients with failing Fontan circulation often present with symptoms of right heart failure. Hepatic fibrosus related to chronic hepatic congestion is universal. Chronic hepatic congestion leads to fibrotic changes in the liver and in a small number of cases may lead to hepatocellular carcinoma. Chronic lymphatic congestion may lead to protein-losing enteropathy (PLE).

Patients with tricuspid atresia require continuous long-term care in regional ACHD centers with providers trained in surveillance of potential complications.[18] In the setting of a Fontan physiology, endocarditis prophylaxis is imperative.[20]

Truncus Arteriosus

Description

Truncus arteriosus is an uncommon congenital anomaly which occurs in 1% to 4% of all CHDs.[18] In truncus, the primitive trunk fails to divide into two great arteries (Fig. 33-14). Thus, a large single great vessel emerges from the base of the heart through a single semilunar valve (truncal valve), straddling both ventricles over a large VSD. The truncus, which is the aorta, receives blood from both ventricles and gives rise to both pulmonary and systemic circulations, as well as coronary arteries. The second semilunar valve is absent but a short pulmonary trunk without a valve may emerge from the left side of the truncus and give rise to the right and left pulmonary arteries (type I), or both pulmonary arteries may arise closely spaced but separately from the posterior or lateral walls of the truncus (type II).[33] Pulmonary blood flow then arises entirely by way of collaterals from bronchial arteries or a PDA. A large, nonrestrictive VSD is usually present.[18]

Unoperated mortality rates are dismal at 70% to 90% by 1 year, usually from heart failure. Given the poor natural history, early operation is the mainstay for truncus. Initial surgery consists of banding one or both pulmonary arteries. However, there were many untoward effects from this which led to complete repair as a neonate or early infancy being preferred. Complete repair includes dividing the right and left pulmonary arteries from the common trunk, patch closure of the VSD, and placement of a right ventricular to pulmonary artery (RV-PA) valved conduit.[18]

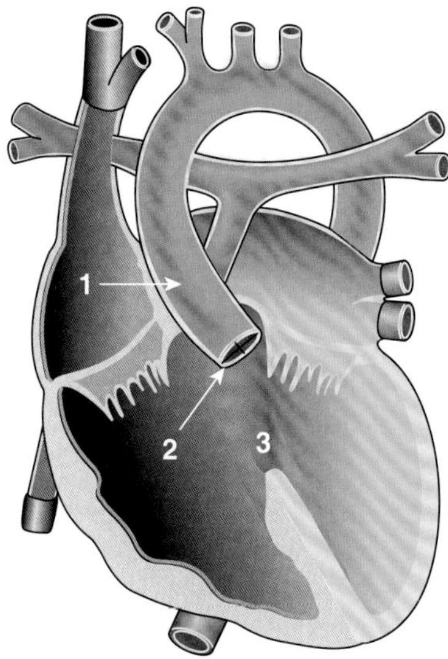

Figure 33-14. Truncus arteriosus. 1, common trunk; 2, truncal valve; 3, VSD. (Reprinted from Everett A. PedHeart Resource. *Scientific Software Solutions.* 2009. Available at www.heartpassport.com, with permission.)

Pathophysiology

The hemodynamic consequences of truncus arteriosus depend on the magnitude of pulmonary blood flow, which reflects the presence and the size of the pulmonary arteries and the resistance to flow through the lungs. In the types with large unobstructed pulmonary arteries arising from the arterial trunk, pulmonary blood flow is greatly increased, clinically resembling patients with large VSD with left-to-right shunts.

Clinical Manifestations

Early presentation consists of heart failure with pulmonary and hepatic congestion. Mixing of systemic and pulmonary blood at the heart and great vessels, may result in mild or moderate cyanosis. Right ventricle pressure is equal to systemic pressure because both ventricles eject directly into the single trunk. The patient with mild cyanosis and a large pulmonary blood flow has a loud systolic murmur along the lower left sternal border. The second heart sound is single and loud. Diastolic flow murmurs may be present if truncal valve regurgitation results from truncal dilatation. Variations may be caused by the resistance to flow into the pulmonary circuit (i.e., a higher resistance leads to shortening and softening of the murmur). There is excellent long-term survival reported after repair with 15-year survival at 83%.[34]

Management

Palliative procedures such as a bilateral pulmonary artery banding to restrict pulmonary blood flow have been performed with limited success in the past. Today, however, the majority of infants will undergo primary surgical repair which includes closure of the VSD, committing the truncus valve to the left ventricle, and thus serving as an aortic valve. In the right ventricle, a homograft or conduit is constructed connecting the right ventricle to the pulmonary artery. Replacement of the right ventricle–pulmonary artery conduit is often required as the conduits are subject to calcification or valve degeneration. Multiple catheter-based interventions are common.[34]

Patients require regular follow-up in a specialized adult congenital heart disease center,[5,18,20] with focus on any evidence of conduit stenosis or regurgitation, aortic root dilatation, branch pulmonary artery stenosis, residual VSD, ventricular dysfunction, truncal valve stenosis or regurgitation, arrhythmias, or pulmonary hypertension and right heart failure.[18] Both repaired and unrepaired patients are considered to have the highest risk of adverse outcome from endocarditis.[20] Therefore, antibiotic prophylaxis is recommended in all patients with truncus arteriosus.

Eisenmenger Syndrome

Description

Eisenmenger syndrome occurs as a result of increased pulmonary vascular resistance and reversed or bidirectional shunts at the aortopulmonary, ventricular, or atrial levels. Pulmonary vascular endothelial proliferation occurs in response to chronic exposure to high pressures (Fig. 33-15). It is associated with decreased oxygen saturation in the systemic circulation, cyanosis and multi-organ involement.[20] The term Eisenmenger syndrome applies to a number of shunting defects that are hemodynamically similar because of the presence of PAH and an associated right-to-left shunt. World Health Organization (WHO) group 1 (PAH) is defined as mean pulmonary artery pressure greater than 25 mm Hg at rest and pulmonary capillary wedge pressure less than or equal to 15 mm Hg with pulmonary vascular resistance 3 WU/m^2 (or a transpulmonary gradient of 6 mm Hg for cavopulmonary shunts).[10] Eisenmenger syndrome is the extreme end of the spectrum of PAH and occurs when the pulmonary artery pressure equals or exceeds the systemic pressure and shunt reversal occurs.[20] It may be a consequence of delayed surgical repair and may go undetected until adolescence or adulthood when operation is no longer possible.

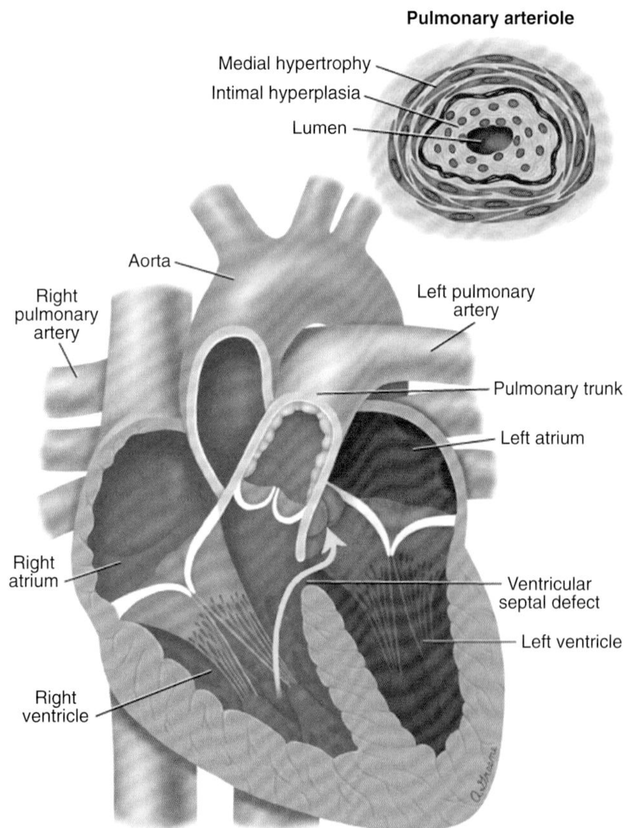

Figure 33-15. Eisenmenger physiology. Eisenmenger syndrome is the triad of systemic-to-pulmonary cardiovascular communication, pulmonary arterial disease, and cyanosis. Pulmonary arterial disease develops as a consequence of increased pulmonary blood flow.

It is estimated that more than 50% of the patients with Eisenmenger syndrome reach the fifth decade of life,[35] and, although rare, patients living into the seventh decade have been reported.[36] While rates of survival are better than previously reported, prognosis appears to be dependent on the age at diagnosis. When diagnosis is made during adulthood, the estimated 10-year survival rate of patients is 58%.[37] Predictors of mortality include functional class, heart failure, history of arrhythmias, early age at presentation, QRS duration, and QTc interval.[35] Progressive subpulmonary ventricular failure and premature death are the outcome in Eisenmenger syndrome.[20] Other causes of death include massive hemoptysis due to bronchial artery rupture, pulmonary infarction from arterial thrombosis, cerebrovascular events including thrombotic stroke, cerebral abscesses, systemic paradoxical embolization.[18,20] The chronic hypoxemia associated with Eisenmenger reaction results in erythrocytosis, an adaptive increase in red blood cell production. Patients may have a "normal" hemoglobin and hematocrit but have a relative anemia due to their increased needs. Iron stores are quickly depleted and iron deficiency has been reported in up to 56% of patients with Eisenmenger syndrome.[38] Because of the viscous effects of excessive red cell volume, a minor increase in hematocrit above 65% to 75% may produce marked increase in whole blood viscosity which can lead to a number of symptoms including headache, lightheadedness, myalgias, and visual disturbances. Therapeutic phlebotomy is avoided in stable "compensated" patients, but may be indicated in symptomatic patients with unstable hematocrits of 65% to 70%. When indicated, phlebotomy must be accompanied by replacement of volume, usually with isotonic saline.[40] Hyperuricemia is proportional to hemodynamic severity and is independently associated with long-term mortality.[40]

Clinical Manifestations

Typical presentation is dyspnea on exertion followed by palpitations, edema, hemoptysis, syncope, and worsening cyanosis.[20] Eventually, overt right heart failure occurs with symptoms of syncope, peripheral edema, ascites, and pleural effusion.[20] A loud second heart sound is the result of increased intensity of closure of the pulmonic valve. As the right ventricle hypertrophies, a prominent A wave may be seen in the jugular pulse. The holosystolic murmur of tricuspid regurgitation may be heard on auscultation. However, loud murmurs may not be present if the RV pressure is similar to the LV pressure.[20]

Management

Supportive therapy includes routine follow-up by trained PAH-CHD physicians, avoidance of pregnancy/adequate contraception, regular immunization against influenza and pneumococcal infections, symptom-limited exercise, treatment of iron deficiency/relative anemia, relief of hyperviscosity syndrome.[20] Patient teaching is imperative and should include education on avoidance of dehydration, extreme fatigue, high-altitude exposure, and cigarette smoke.[20] Increased morbidity and mortality is associated with noncardiac surgical procedures and should be approached by a team which includes CHD-trained physicians and cardiac anesthesia familiar with management of this population.[20] While traditional medical management has had little to offer these patients, recent attention has been given to the use of selective pulmonary vasodilators in improving hemodynamics and exercise capacity in patients with pulmonary hypertension.[41,42] A number of approved and investigational therapies are now available, offering the potential for improved survival for these patients.[41]

CONCLUSIONS

The wide heterogenicity of congenital heart defects presents many challenges to developing evidence-based guidelines for this population. However, the constant innovations in medicine and surgery point toward exponential growth as these patients are now reaching adulthood. Patients with CHD are rarely cured. Late complications include dysrhythmias, need for future cardiac surgeries or catheter-based interventions, heart failure, and multi-system disease.

Summary

There is a high proportion of fear and anxiety in ACHD. Many times, those with long-term chronic health concerns ask questions which may be perceived as provider distrust. This is usually best addressed early by establishing a rapport and building trust. ACHD patients need to stay in care for life, live a healthy lifestyle, and consult with an ACHD center for family planning.

FUTURE CONSIDERATIONS/ IMPLICATIONS FOR PRACTICE

Improved infrastructure to track prevalence and outcomes is needed in this population. Comprehensive care centers are being credentialed and urged to develop multicenter population registries which are needed in order to have adequate numbers for drawing statistical conclusions to address clinical questions. How do we safeguard children from being lost to follow-up as they transition to adult centers? How do providers ensure ACHD patients receive accurate heart transplantation listing priority? How will changes in the Affordable Care Act impact healthcare coverage for this population?

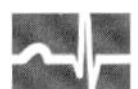

CASE STUDY 1

Patient Profile

Name/Age/Sex: **Alexandra Schwartz, 34-year-old female**

Past Medical History/Problem List

Tetralogy of Fallot s/p classic left Blalock–Taussig shunt in infancy followed by complete repair at age 5. Small residual VSD noted by echocardiogram with left-to-right shunt.
s/p pulmonary valve replacement at age 28
History of *Streptococcus viridans* bioprosthetic pulmonary valve endocarditis treated with 6 weeks antibiotics
History of AV nodal re-entry tachycardia s/p ablation
Genetic syndrome: 22q11 deletion syndrome (DiGeorge syndrome)
Obesity
Hypertension
Diabetes mellitus

Family History

55 y/o mother with hypothyroidism and diabetes mellitus, 56 y/o father with history of hypertension and atherosclerotic heart disease, 28 y/o sister in good health.

Social History

Recently married, works full time as a kindergarten teacher. Lifelong nonsmoker, EtOH 1–2 per month, no illicit drug use.

Medications/Allergies

NKDA
Lisinopril 20 mg po daily
Metformin 500 mg po bid
ASA 81 mg po daily

Case Scenario

- Mrs. Schwartz presents to a local OB/GYN clinic for contraception counseling as she is recently married. Her BP in her left arm is 90/50 mm Hg and 160/90 in her right arm, pulse is 78 and regular, respirations 16. *Why is there a discrepancy in the blood pressure readings? (Answer: in a classis BT shunt, the left subclavian artery is attached to the pulmonary artery. The blood is then supplied to the left arm by collateral circulation) Which reading is useful? (The higher BP is used when making treatment decisions) Why is family planning important and what are considerations for this patient? (History of valve replacement and prior endocarditis both have implications as to the use of antibiotics prior to delivery. DiGeorge syndrome (22Q11 deletion) is a genetic syndrome with an autosomal dominant inheritance pattern. Pre-pregnancy meeting with a genetic counselor is recommended. There is a 50% chance of passing the deletion to their children therefore, fetal screening is recommended).*
- Prior to prescribing contraception a pregnancy test is performed and indicates that she is currently pregnant. Her provider informs her and instructs her to stop her Lisinopril and contact her cardiologist and start prenatal vitamins. On arrival to her congenital cardiology appointment her right arm BP is 220/110 mm Hg, HR 100, RR 20. She is having chest tightness and shortness of breath. Labetalol 20 mg IVP is ordered. *Given her history, what is important to remember prior to giving her IV medication? (She has a residual VSD and as a precaution air filters should be used on her IV to reduce the risk of paradoxical embolization)* She is started on labetalol 100 mg po bid at discharge.
- She continues to follow each trimester for the remainder of her pregnancy with her cardiologist and her high-risk OB team. What is she at risk for in the peripartum period? (Arrhythmias, heart failure, thrombus formation, premature delivery) Given her history of endocarditis and valve replacement—are there any precautions recommended during delivery? (Current recommendations include the use of antibiotics for endocarditis prophylaxis.[1,2,43,44])

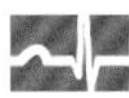

CASE STUDY 2

Patient Profile

Name/Age/Sex: **Daphne Harris, 24-year-old female**

Past Medical History/Problem List

Hypoplastic left heart syndrome s/p Norwood palliation, bidirectional Glenn and eventual lateral tunnel Fontan
Baseline SpO_2 89%
Hepatocellular carcinoma (HCC) s/p radiofrequency ablation in May 2014
Idiopathic thrombocyoptenic purpura (ITP)
Atrial tachycardia previously cardioverted with adenosine; not on anticoagulation d/t ITP
h/o large subdural hematoma related to ITP

Family History

Father with hypothyroidism, mother in good health, paternal GF deceased (h/o MI), paternal GM in good health, maternal GF deceased, maternal GF deceased (renal cancer)

Social History

Recently married, works full time in marketing. Lifelong nonsmoker, EtOH 1–2 per month, no illicit drug use.

Medications/Allergies

Contrast reaction (renal failure)
Carvedilol 25 mg po bid
Digoxin 250 mcg po qday
Enalapril 10 mg po qday
Eplerenone 100 mg po qday
Torsemide 20 mg po qday

History of Present Illness

- Ms. Harris presents to the emergency room July 5th with complaints of palpitations. She reports they started at 3 in the afternoon. She took an extra digoxin (as instructed by her electrophysiologist). However, her heart rate did not return to baseline and so her husband brought her in for treatment. BP is 122/74 mm Hg right arm, 126/80 left arm, HR is 156 bpm, RR 20, oxygen saturation is 88% on room air. While you are discussing her history you learn that she went to the lake with her family for the 4th of July celebration. She admits it was hot and she did not stay hydrated. She also reports she got sick after eating and threw up several times after lunch. She took all her medications. *Why is avoidance of dehydration important for someone with Fontan circulation? (Fontan circulation is preload dependent since there is no subpulmonary ventricle. Blood flow through the pulmonary circulation is the difference between the central venous pressure and atrial pressure. Dehydration is poorly tolerated as cardiac output is dependent on pulmonary blood flow)*
- An IV lock was started—her congenital team has recommended an air filter be attached to her lock prior to starting IV fluids. *Why? (There is risk for paradoxical embolism. This type of embolism crosses from venous to arterial circulation.)*
- The electrophysiology team has recommended adenosine IV rapid push. Ms. Harris successfully returns back to a normal sinus rhythm. *Why are dysrhythmias poorly tolerated in the single ventricle population? (Tachycardia can result in hemodynamic compromise due to the loss of cardiac output. Also, prolonged duration of arrhythmia can lead to clot formation due to sluggish blood flow)*
- Ms. Harris had a liver ultrasound while she was in the ER which revealed a nodular liver and evidence of chronic congestion. Why does normal Fontan physiology lead to chronic hepatic congestion? (There is no subpulmonary ventricle to pump blood through the lungs. So blood that exits from hepatic circulation to the IVC is sluggish and leads to chronic congestion).

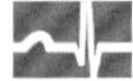

CASE STUDY 3

Patient Profile

Name/Age/Sex: **Matthew Agasu, 47-year-old male**

Past Medical History/Problem List

Unrepaired secundum ASD
Pulmonary arterial hypertension
Cyanosis (baseline oxygen saturation is 82%)

Family History

Maternal and paternal osteoarthritis, paternal HTN, grandmother with hypothyroidism.

Social History

Married, works full time as an accountant. Lifelong nonsmoker, EtOH 1–2 per month, no illicit drug use.

Medications/Allergies

NKA
ASA 81 mg daily
Sildenafil 20 mg po tid
Bosentan 125 mg po bid

History of Present Illness

- Mr. Agasu presents for annual follow-up at his primary care office. BP is 130/88 mm Hg in the right arm and 134/86 in the left arm. HR is 76 and SpO_2 is 82% on room air. He is bothered by tooth pain and wants to know if he *needs antibiotics prior to going to the dentist?*
  - Endocarditis prophylaxis recommended for those at the highest risk of adverse outcomes from endocarditis—which includes those with unrepaired cyanotic heart defects
- He reports erectile dysfunction and asks for a prescription of Viagra. *Why is this contraindicated?*
  - He is on sildenafil which is the generic version of Viagra
- Annual labs are completed and the lab calls in critical values on his hemoglobin at 19 and hematocrit of 62%. Why are his blood counts so high and what risks are associated with this?
  - The increase in RBCs is compensatory to improve oxygen transport in cyanotic patients. The increase may result in increased blood viscosity (hyperviscosity). Routine therapeutic phlebotomy should be avoided unless symptoms of hyperviscosity are present. Symptoms include: headache, dizziness/lightheadedness, slow mentation/impaired alertness, irritability, sense of dissociation/distance; visual disturbances (blurred/double); paresthesia of fingers or toes; tinnitus; fatigue/lethargy; myalgias/muscle weakness/anorexia; restless legs

KEY READINGS

Gatzoulis M, Webb G, Daubeney P. *Diagnosis and Management of Adult Congenital Heart Disease.* 3rd ed. Philadelphia, PA: Elsevier; 2017.

Stout K, Daniels C, Aboulhosn J, et al. 2018 AHA/ACC guideline for the management of adults with congenital *heart disease. J Am Colleg Cardiol.* 2019;139(14).

REFERENCES

1. Egbe A, Uppu S, Lee S, et al. Temporal variation of birth prevalence of congenital heart disease in the United States. *Congenit Heart Dis.* 2014; 10(1):43–50.
2. Orwat MI, Kempny A, Bauer U, et al. The importance of national and international collaboration in adult congenital heart disease: a network analysis of research output. *Int J Cardiol.* 2015;195:155–162.
3. Correa-Villaseñor A, Graham T, Wyszynski D. *Congenital Heart Defects.* Oxford: Oxford University Press; 2010.
4. van der Linde D, Konings E, Slager M, et al. Birth prevalence of congenital heart disease worldwide. *J Am Coll Cardiol.* 2011;58(21): 2241–2247.
5. Stout K, Daniels C, Aboulhosn J, et al. 2018 AHA/ACC guideline for the management of adults with congenital heart disease: a report of the American college of cardiology/American heart association task force on clinical practice guidelines. *J Am Coll Cardiol.* 2018;73(12):e81–e192.
6. Diller G, Kempny A, Alonso-Gonzalez R, et al. Survival prospects and circumstances of death in contemporary adult congenital heart disease patients under follow-up at a large tertiary centre. *Circulation.* 2015; 132(22):2118–2125.
7. van der Bom T, Bouma B, Meijboom F, et al. The prevalence of adult congenital heart disease, results from a systematic review and evidence based calculation. *Am Heart J.* 2012;164(4):568–575.
8. Kaouache M, Ionescu-Ittu R, Mackie A, et al. Lifetime prevalence of congenital heart disease in the general population in 2010. *J Am Coll Cardiol.* 2013;61(10):E505.
9. Webb G, Mulder B, Aboulhosn J, et al. The care of adults with congenital heart disease across the globe: current assessment and future perspective. *Int J Cardiol.* 2015;195:326–333.
10. Cayre R, Milei J. *Congenital Heart Diseases.* Nova Science Publishers, Inc; 2014:137–164.
11. Kenner C, Lott JW. *Neonatal Nursing Care Handbook: An Evidence-Based Approach to Conditions and Procedures.* New York: Springer Publishing Company; 2016.
12. Wilson N, Smith J, Prommete B, et al. Transcatheter closure of secundum atrial septal defects with the amplatzer septal occluder in adults and children—follow-up closure rates, degree of mitral regurgitation and evolution of arrhythmias. *Heart Lung Circ.* 2008;17(4):318–324.
13. Egred M, Andron M, Albouaini K, et al. Percutaneous closure of patent foramen ovale and atrial septal defect: procedure outcome and medium-term follow-up. *J Interv Cardiol.* 2007;20(5):395–401.
14. Dakkak W, Oliver T. *Ventricular Septal Defect.* 2019.Available at https://www.ncbi.nlm.nih.gov/books/NBK470330/. Accessed March 26, 2019.
15. Rooshesselink J. Outcome of patients after surgical closure of ventricular septal defect at young age: longitudinal follow-up of 22–34 years. *Eur Heart J.* 2004;25(12):1057–1062.
16. Doyle T, Kavanaugh-McHugh A. *UpToDate.* Uptodate.com. 2019. Available at https://www.uptodate.com/contents/clinical-manifestations-and-diagnosis-of-patent-ductus-arteriosus-in-term-infants-children-and-adults. Accessed March 27, 2019.
17. Penaloza D, Arias-Stella J. The heart and pulmonary circulation at high altitudes. *Circulation.* 2007;115(9):1132–1146.
18. Gatzoulis M, Webb G, Daubeney P. *Diagnosis and Management of Adult Congenital Heart Disease.* 3rd ed. Philadelphia, PA: Elsevier; 2018.
19. Jashari H, Rydberg A, Ibrahimi P, et al. Left ventricular response to pressure afterload in children: aortic stenosis and coarctation. *Int J Cardiol.* 2015;178:203–209.
20. Warnes C, Williams R, Bashore T, et al. ACC/AHA 2008 guidelines for the management of adults with congenital heart disease: a report of the American College of Cardiology/American Heart Association Task Force on Practice Guidelines (writing committee to develop guidelines on the management of adults with congenital heart disease). *Circulation.* 2008;118(23): e714–e833.
21. Roifman I, Therrien J, Ionescu-Ittu R, et al. Coarctation of the aorta and coronary artery disease. *Circulation.* 2012;126(1):16–21.
22. Celermajer D, Bull C, Till J, et al. Ebstein's anomaly: presentation and outcome from fetus to adult. *J Am Coll Cardiol.* 1994;23(1):170–176.
23. Dennis M, Kotchetkova I, Cordina R, et al. Long-term follow-up of adults following the atrial switch operation for transposition of the great arteries—a contemporary cohort. *Heart Lung Circ.* 2018;27(8):1011–1017.
24. Hutter P, Kreb D, Mantel S, et al. Twenty-five years' experience with the arterial switch operation. *J Thorac Cardiovasc Surg.* 2002;124(4):790–797.
25. Culbert E, Ashburn D, Cullen-Dean G, et al. Quality of life of children after repair of transposition of the great arteries. *Circulation.* 2003; 108(7):857–862.
26. Legendre A. Coronary events after arterial switch operation for transposition of the great arteries. *Circulation.* 2003;108(suppl 1):II186–II190.
27. Graham T, Bernard Y, Mellen B, et al. Long-term outcome in congenitally corrected transposition of the great arteries. *J Am Coll Cardiol.* 2000;36(1):255–261.
28. Rao P. Tricuspid atresia. *Curr Treat Options Cardiovasc Med.* 2000;2(6): 507–520.
29. Stockman J. Prevalence of congenital heart defects in metropolitan Atlanta, 1998–2005. *Yearbook of Pediatrics.* 2010;167–170. doi:10.1016/s0084-3954(09)79390-x
30. Sittiwangkul R, Azakie A, Van Arsdell G, et al. Outcomes of tricuspid atresia in the Fontan era. *Ann Thorac Surg.* 2004;77(3):889–894.
31. Balasubramanian S, Tacy T. Tricuspid valve atresia. Uptodate.com. Available at https://www.uptodate.com/contents/tricuspid-valve-tv-atresia?search=tricuspid%20atresia&source=search_result&selectedTitle=1~24&usage_type=default&display_rank=1. 2019. Accessed March 29, 2019.
32. Khairy P, Fernandes S, Mayer J, et al. Long-term survival, modes of death, and predictors of mortality in patients with Fontan surgery. *Circulation.* 2008;117(1):85–92.
33. Kirby M. Pulmonary atresia or persistent truncus arteriosus. *Circ Res.* 2008;103(4):337–339.
34. Rajasinghe H, McElhinney D, Reddy V, et al. Long-term follow-up of truncus arteriosus repaired in infancy: a twenty-year experience. *J Thorac Cardiovasc Surg.* 1997;113(5):869–879.
35. Diller G. Presentation, survival prospects, and predictors of death in Eisenmenger syndrome: a combined retrospective and case-control study. *Eur Heart J.* 2006;27(14):1737–1742.
36. Su-Mei A, Ju-Le T. Large unrepaired aortopulmonary window? Survival into the seventh decade. *Echocardiography.* 2007;24(1):71–73.
37. Oya H, Nagaya N, Uematsu M, et al. Poor prognosis and related factors in adults with Eisenmenger syndrome. *Am Heart J.* 2002;143(4): 739–744.
38. Galiè N, Humbert M, Vachiery J, et al. 2015 ESC/ERS guidelines for the diagnosis and treatment of pulmonary hypertension. *Eur Heart J.* 2015;37(1):67–119.
39. Oechslin E. Hematological management of the cyanotic adult with congenital heart disease. *Int J Cardiol.* 2004;97:109–115.
40. Oechslin E, Mebus S, Schulze-Neick I, et al. The adult patient with Eisenmenger syndrome: a medical update after Dana Point Part III: specific management and surgical aspects. *Curr Cardiol Rev.* 2010;6(4): 363–372.
41. D'Alto M, Diller G. Pulmonary hypertension in adults with congenital heart disease and Eisenmenger syndrome: current advanced management strategies. *Heart.* 2014;100(17):1322–1328.
42. Archer S, Michelakis E. An evidence-based approach to the management of pulmonary arterial hypertension. *Curr Opin Cardiol.* 2006;21(5): 526–527.
43. Wilson W, Taubert KA, Gewitz M, et al. Prevention of infective endocarditis: guidelines from the American Heart Association—a guideline from the American Heart Association Rheumatic Fever, Endocarditis, and Kawasaki Disease Committee, Council on Cardiovascular Disease in the Young, and the Council on Clinical Cardiology, Council on Cardiovascular Surgery and Anesthesia, and the Quality of Care and Outcomes Research Interdisciplinary Working Group. *Circulation.* 2007;116:1736–1754.
44. The American College of Obstetrics and Gynecologists, Women's Health Care Physicians. *Use of prophylactic antibiotics in labor and delivery.* June, 2011. Practice Bulletin number 120.

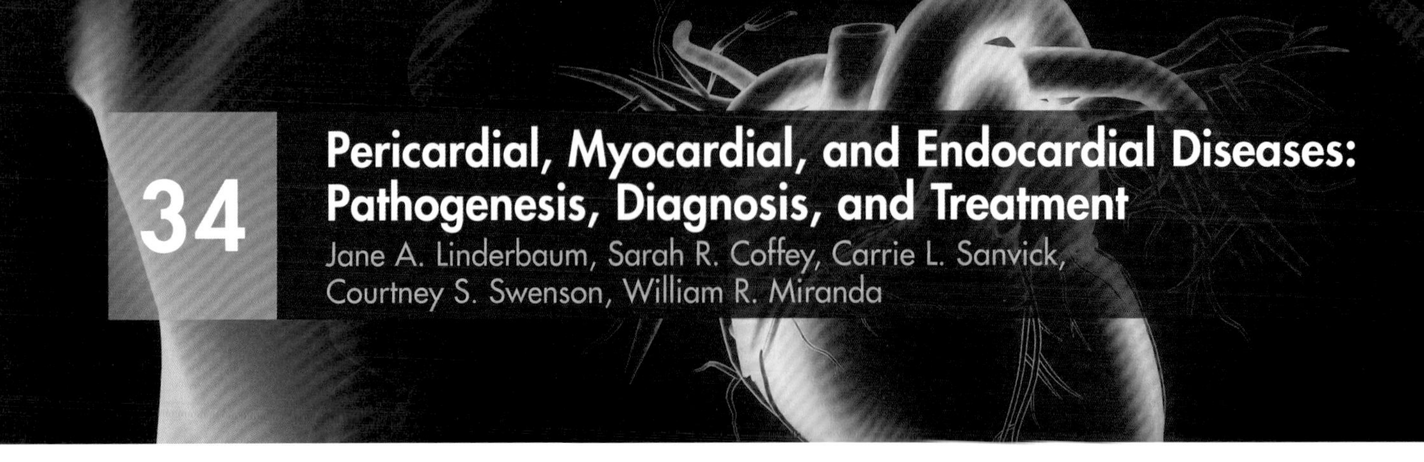

34 Pericardial, Myocardial, and Endocardial Diseases: Pathogenesis, Diagnosis, and Treatment

Jane A. Linderbaum, Sarah R. Coffey, Carrie L. Sanvick, Courtney S. Swenson, William R. Miranda

OBJECTIVES

1. Describe the current scope of pericardial, myocardial, and endocardial diseases.
2. Identify risk factors including comorbid conditions that may be clues to optimal diagnosis and early treatment for patients presenting with pericardial, myocardial, or endocardial conditions.
3. Describe common clinical presentations requiring urgent or emergent treatment and/or specialty referral.
4. Identify patient-centric education principles and priorities to optimize treatment adherence and patient outcomes for patients with pericardial, myocardial, and endocardial conditions.

KEY QUESTIONS

1. What testing is indicated based on best available evidence to guide treatment, and education plans for pericardial, myocardial, and endocardial conditions?
2. Why is patient-centric education important for treatment adherence in pericardial, myocardial, and endocardial disease treatment plans?
3. When should patients with pericardial, myocardial, and endocardial diseases be referred for specialty management?

BACKGROUND

Pericardial, myocardial, and endocardial diseases impact the health of populations across the world, and can ultimately impact cardiac function and quality of life. These diseases contribute to a tremendous economic health care burden; thus, it is imperative to optimize efficient assessment, accurate diagnosis, and appropriate and timely referrals for patients with urgent and emergent clinical findings. Prompt and accurate assessment, diagnosis, and treatment of patients with pericardial, myocardial, and endocardial disorders will optimize patient outcomes and minimize long-term cardiac sequela.

This chapter will provide a practical overview to these conditions with clues to clinical assessment and diagnosis followed by general treatment strategies for busy clinicians. Key learning points and references are provided for additional reading and complex case guidance.

PERICARDIAL DISEASE

The pericardium is a double-layered fibroserous sac that surrounds the heart, covering almost the entire surface and part of the great vessels.[1] The pericardium is composed of two layers, the *serosa* and the *fibrosa,* which contain nerves, blood vessels, and lymphatics. The fibrous outer layer, also called the *parietal pericardium*, is attached to the sternum, great vessels, and diaphragm. The phrenic nerves innervate the majority of the parietal pericardium. A serosal layer of cuboidal cells one cell-layer thick lines the pericardium. The monocellular serosa covers the myocardial surface and is also known as the *visceral pericardium* or the *epicardium*. The pericardial space, which lies between the pericardial layers, contains normally between 15 to 50 mL of serous pericardial fluid. The pericardium is relatively inelastic, and acts as a barrier to inflammation as it exerts a powerful restraining effect on the size of the heart in situations of acute volume overload.[2–4] The pericardium also exerts a mechanical effect that enhances normal ventricular interactions that contribute to the balance of right and left cardiac outputs.[5] The pericardial fluid reduces friction over the surface of the myocardium. Pericarditis may be suspected when the pericardium becomes inflamed or irritated, most commonly of idiopathic origin. This diagnosis is most often made on clinical examination and electrocardiogram findings. Treatment of many types of pericarditis is usually self-limiting and symptoms typically improve within 48 to 72 hours. However, sometimes symptoms can become more bothersome and be associated with patient discomfort and hemodynamic instability. Some of the more common etiologies of pericardial diseases include:

- Idiopathic postviral, following upper respiratory infection or virus, post chest surgery such as in Dressler syndrome
- Infectious—mycobacterial, fungal, protozoal, AIDS associated
- Neoplastic—primary or secondary malignancies (e.g., breast, lung, lymphoma, leukemia, melanoma)
- Connective tissue or autoimmune conditions—examples include rheumatoid arthritis, lupus, scleroderma, or mixed connective tissue diseases

- Others—including uremic/metabolic—for example, renal failure, myxedema, amyloidosis
- Iatrogenic—related to a procedure such as catheter ablation, device placement, or cardiac surgery, medication side effects, or postcardiopulmonary resuscitation

Pericarditis, when complicated with a pericardial effusion, and/or cardiac tamponade are important acute clinical presentations requiring urgent or emergent identification, treatment and surveillance, and will be summarized in this chapter.

Pericarditis

Pericarditis is the inflammation or irritation of the pericardium. The acute inflammatory process can produce either serous or purulent fluid, or a dense fibrinous material.[6] The possible sequelae of pericarditis include cardiac tamponade, recurrent pericarditis, and pericardial constriction.[7]

The most common presentation of pericarditis is idiopathic inflammation and without associated symptom causing effusion. This most common presentation, inflammatory pericarditis, usually lasts 1 to 3 weeks and does not lead to further problems. Treatment with nonsteroidal anti-inflammatories typically results in continuous gradual improvement of symptoms.

Etiology

Pericarditis may be caused by many different conditions. The more common etiologic classifications of pericardial diseases are summarized below. The large majority of these cases resolve without complication within several weeks.

Fortunately, there has been significant decline in infectious pericarditis in the last two decades with improved antiviral and antibacterial regimens, such as in immunocompromised individuals, and significant advances in treatments for acquired immunodeficiency syndrome (AIDS), and the near irradiation of tuberculosis in the United States. Viruses associated with pericarditis include influenza, coxsackie A or B, varicella, mumps, hepatitis B, mononucleosis, and human immunodeficiency virus (HIV).[8] Idiopathic pericarditis is thought often to be the result of previously undetected viral or bacterial etiology. Bacterial infections, such as tuberculosis, *Staphylococcus*, *Pneumococcus*, and *Streptococcus* species and *aspergillosis* and *histoplasmosis* are among the fungal infections that sometimes are identified in pericarditis.

A thorough and complete physical examination and patient history may identify a viral infection preceding the onset of the clinical presentation. Pericarditis and associated symptoms may be the initial presenting symptoms of an infection, or a systemic disease, such as systemic lupus erythematosus or a malignancy.

In viral pericarditis, the pericardial fluid is most commonly serous, of low volume, and resolves spontaneously.[5] Exudative, hemorrhagic, and leukocyte-filled large effusions may be associated with neoplastic, tuberculosis, and purulent pericarditis.[8]

Symptoms

The onset of symptoms can be acute, as is commonly seen in idiopathic or viral pericarditis, or insidious, as seen in uremic pericarditis. Commonly, acute viral pericarditis is nearly always preceded by a recent respiratory, gastrointestinal, or "flu-like" illness. A prodrome of fever, malaise, and myalgia is common in younger patients with acute pericarditis, and older patients may or may not experience fever in their presenting symptomatology. Common presenting symptoms may include any of the following:

- Chest pain, which may be prolonged in the retrosternal or left precordial region.
- Radiation and/or associated shoulder discomfort may be present.
- Pain often may be localized and worsened with supine position.
- Pain may be lessened or resolved with sitting up or leaning forward.

A major symptom of pericarditis is chest pain that is retrosternal or left precordial, radiating to the trapezius ridge and varying with posture. The pain is often transmitted through the phrenic nerves, and usually occurs on the left side. Shoulder pain should be distinguished from trapezius ridge pain by having the patient physically point to the specific site of pain. Clinical examination findings often found in pericarditis may include:

- Shallow respirations, during pain, and the patient may be tachypneic.
- Splinting may be present, and/or the patient may prefer the forward leaning, sitting position. The pain is generally worse when lying supine and is relieved by sitting.
- A pericardial friction rub may be present (may be best heard with the stethoscope diaphragm, at the left lower sternal border [LLSB] and present throughout the cardiac cycle). Presence of a friction rub may be best heard sitting forward and is characterized as "raspy, crunchy" or synonymous to the sound made while walking on fresh snow. A pericardial friction rub is pathognomonic for pericarditis, but is frequently not present, and when present may be intermittent, and variable in quality and intensity. A pericardial friction rub may be best heard at end expiration while the patient is leaning forward; the sound is classically a rasping or creaking with a triple cadence, but can also be bi- or monophasic.[1]
- Pulsus paradoxus may be present. Frequently the chest pain caused by pericarditis induces shallow tachypnea as patients attempt to splint their chest movement.[2]

TESTING

Importantly, the initial diagnosis and treatment of pericardial disease is based on symptomatology, clinical examination, and electrocardiogram. Testing should be considered following a comprehensive history and physical examination. Initial testing includes an electrocardiogram and additional tests as clinically indicated based on the current symptoms and coexisting clinical conditions (e.g., infections, known viral illness, recent cardiac surgery).

- Electrocardiography (ECG) and history and clinical examination
- Inflammatory markers (e.g., sedimentation rate, C-reactive protein)
- CBC with differential
- Troponin-T

Additional consults/testing as clinically indicated may include:

- Cardiology collaboration for expert management guidance and testing interpretation.
- Echocardiography is not necessary for diagnosis but warranted to evaluate for the presence of pericardial effusion or hemodynamic compromise when the clinical situation suggests low cardiac output (hypotension, dyspnea, elevated jugular venous pressure, or edema).

Table 34-1 • FEATURES THAT DIFFERENTIATE PERICARDITIS FROM MYOCARDIAL ISCHEMIA OR INFARCTION AND PULMONARY EMBOLISM[9]

Symptom and Clinical Finding	Myocardial Ischemia or Infarction	Pericarditis	Pulmonary Embolism
Chest pain			
Location	Retrosternal	Retrosternal	Anterior, posterior, or lateral
Onset	Sudden, often waxing and waning	Sudden	Sudden
Character	Pressure-like, heavy, squeezing	Sharp, stabbing, occasionally dull	Sharp, stabbing
Change with respiration	No	Worsened with inspiration	In phase with respiration (absent when the patient is apneic)
Change with position	No	Worse when patient is supine; improved when sitting up or leaning forward	No
Radiation	Jaw, neck, shoulder, one or both arms	Jaw, neck, shoulder, one or both arms, trapezius ridge	Shoulder
Duration	Minutes (ischemia); hours (infarction)	Hours to days	Hours to days
Response to nitroglycerin	Improved	No change	No change
Physical examination			
Friction rub	Absent (unless pericarditis is present)	Present (in 85% of patients)	Rare; a pleural friction rub is present in 3% of patients
S_3 sound, pulmonary congestion	May be present	Absent	Absent
Electrocardiogram			
ST segment elevation	Convex and localized	Concave and widespread	Limited to lead III, aVF, and V_1
PR segment depression	Rare	Frequent	None
Q waves	May be present	Absent	May be present in lead III or aVF or both
T waves	Inverted when ST segments are still elevated	Inverted after ST segments have normalized	Inverted in lead II, aVF, or V_1–V_4 while ST segments are elevated
Atrioventricular block, ventricular arrhythmias	Common	Absent	Absent
Atrial fibrillation	May be present	May be present	May be present

- Cardiac MRI or CT typically reserved for difficult or recalcitrant cases or in individuals not improving with treatment, or when diagnosis is uncertain.
- Rheumatology and/or Cardio-Rheumatology consultation may be helpful in recalcitrant cases.

A diagnosis of **acute pericarditis** is made if the patient has a pericardial friction rub or chest pain, and widespread ST segment elevation on electrocardiography.[6] It is important to differentiate pericarditis from myocardial infarction (MI) and pulmonary embolism. Table 34-1 describes the different features differentiating these conditions.[9]

The electrocardiogram changes in acute pericarditis (typically widespread ST segment elevation, often in 9 of the 12 ECG leads that may be seen in pericarditis) are a result of inflammation of the myocardium below the pericardium. The ECG of a patient with pericarditis may be normal, atypically abnormal with nonspecific changes, or have a four-stage sequence that is diagnostic. Figure 34-1 shows the electrocardiographic manifestations of pericarditis.

In stage I, there are ST segment deviations, primarily due to inflammation on the ventricular surfaces. PR segment deviations are also usually present. Stage I is characteristic of acute pericarditis when it involves all or almost all leads (e.g., 9/12 leads in a standard 12-lead ECG) with early ST junction elevations that produce an appearance of upsloping T waves on the QRS interval, but that are otherwise normal.[2] The ST segment is nearly always depressed in aVR.[3]

In early stage II, the ST segments return to baseline, and PR segments may now be depressed. In late stage II, the T waves flatten and then become inverted. In stage III, the ECG is characteristic of diffuse myocardial injury. In stage IV, the ECG evolves back to the pre-pericarditis state.[2] Stage IV may last days or months.[3]

The changes seen in the ECG of a patient with pericarditis can occur over hours to weeks, particularly from stages I to II, or can take place over days or weeks, most often as stage III evolves to stage IV. Prompt and early diagnosis and intervention may impact the identification of all stages, and thereby impact the characteristic staging in some cases. The ST elevation seen in pericarditis is usually distinguished from that of acute MI by the absence of Q waves, upward ST segments, and the absence of associated T-wave inversion.[10]

Common laboratory findings:

- Elevated erythrocyte sedimentation rate (marker of inflammation).
- Leukocytosis, and/or lymphocytosis.
- Serum cardiac enzymes typically normal, but may be increased when the myocardium is involved.
- Troponin I elevation may or may not be present, but typically does not increase as rapidly as in acute coronary syndromes.

Medical Management

Treatment goals of acute pericarditis include symptom control, identification of the underlying etiology, and prevention of complications.

Initial treatment considerations of acute pericarditis in an adult patient are as follows:

- Colchicine (adult dosing: 1 to 2 mg the first day followed by 0.6 mg once daily for 3 to 6 months)

PLUS (one of the following)

- Aspirin (adult dosing: 650 mg every 6 to 8 hours) for 1 to 2 weeks followed by a taper over 4 to 6 weeks **OR**

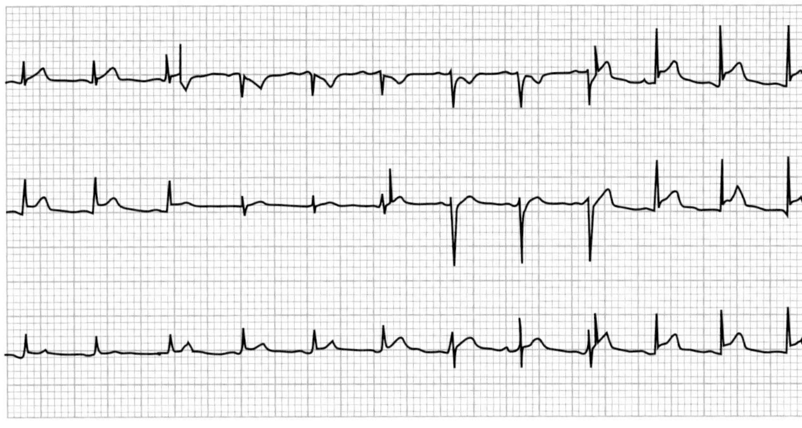

A

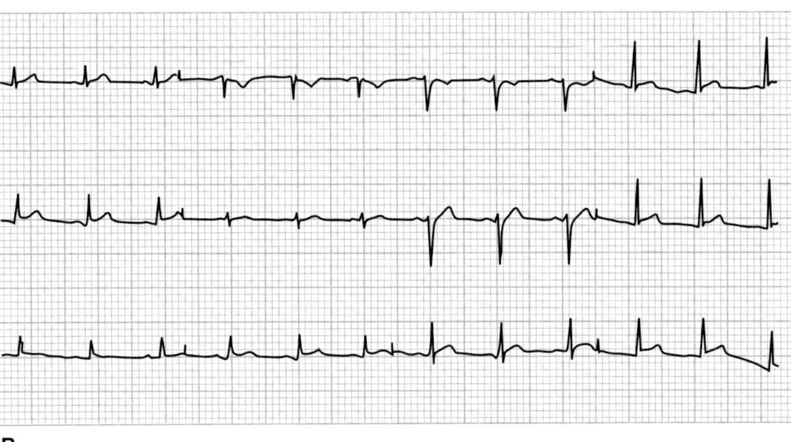

B

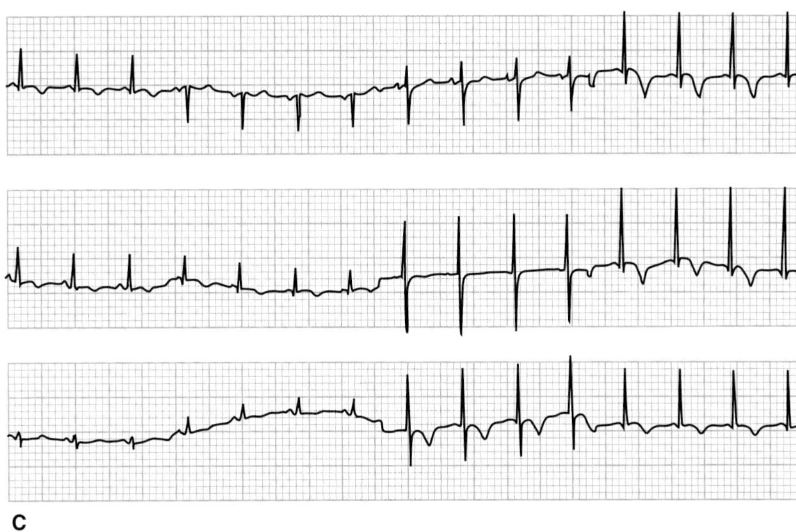

C

Figure 34-1. ECG manifestations of pericarditis. (**A**) Typical, quasi-diagnostic stage I ECG: J (ST) elevated in all leads except aVL, depressed aVR, and V_1. PR segment deviated except in aVL where P is small. (**B**) Early stage II. J (ST) returning to baseline. (**C**) Stage III. T waves inverted in most leads and typically upright in aVR and V_1. (From Spodick DH. Electrocardiographic abnormalities in pericardial disease. In: Spodick DH, ed. *The Pericardium: A Comprehensive Textbook.* New York: Marcel Dekker; 1997:40–64.)

- Ibuprofen (adult dosing: 400 to 800 mg every 6 to 8 hours) for 1 to 2 weeks followed by a taper over 4 to 6 weeks **OR**
- Indomethacin (adult dosing: 50 mg 3 times daily for 1 to 2 weeks followed by a taper over 4 to 6 weeks)

Providers should use with caution in renal disease; dose reduction may be required. Concomitant GI protection with a proton pump inhibitor (PPI) should be considered in most patients on extended use of NSAIDs. Postprocedural or post-MI pericarditis treatment and duration may differ depending on the individual clinical situation and examination findings.

Lack of response to initial treatment or presence of complications (e.g., cardiac tamponade, constriction) warrants further evaluation to an expert for evaluation and consideration of other treatment options.

Important Caveat

Due to the adverse effects of oral corticosteroids (including relapsing pericarditis) and the risk of inducing steroid dependency, oral corticosteroids should not be used routinely for acute pericarditis. In select circumstances, typically after expert advisement, a short-term course of oral corticosteroids may be useful in select circumstances, such as in the presence of postoperative effusive constrictive pericarditis or in the context of some systemic inflammatory disease (e.g., connective tissue disease). The duration of therapy varies depending on the underlying cause and should be managed collaboratively with ongoing surveillance expert involvement when indicated. Symptomatic improvement should be noted with a few days, however complete symptom resolution may take weeks to months. Thus, clinical reassessment and symptom management and reassurance are essential.

Advanced therapies for chronic, recalcitrant pericarditis:

- Alternative immunosuppressant agents may be considered in consultation with a cardiologist and/or rheumatologist.
- Although pericardiectomy is rarely needed, it may be considered for documented recurrent bouts of acute pericarditis (especially when medical treatment proves ineffective, and/or the pericardium remains thickened and/or calcified).
- Advanced hemodynamic catheterization may be indicated for diagnostic purposes in prolonged or recalcitrant cases of pericardial disease.

Complications of Pericardial Disease

Constrictive Pericarditis. Constrictive pericarditis results from a fibrotic, thickened, or calcified pericardium that limits diastolic (relaxation) and ventricular filling.[9] Tuberculosis is responsible for most cases of constrictive pericarditis in Africa and Asia.[11] Other causes of constrictive pericarditis are idiopathic, postradiation, and postsurgical.[12,13] In constrictive pericarditis, the sometimes thickened, adherent pericardium restricts ventricular filling and limits chamber expansion and maximal diastolic volumes.

Physical examination findings in constriction may include:

Kussmaul sign, inspiratory jugular venous distention, replaces the normal inspiratory venous "collapse" that reflects a normal inspiratory decrease of 3 to 7 mm Hg in right atrial pressure. This sign is a hallmark of constrictive pericarditis.[2] Heart failure signs and symptoms may be present, but typically present without clinical evidence of pulmonary congestion and/or edema.

Testing considerations for suspected constrictive pericarditis:

- Chest radiograph: may reveal a calcified pericardium.
- Echocardiogram is indicated, and may be consistent with findings associated with constrictive pericarditis, such as premature opening of the pulmonic valve and rapid posterior motion of the left ventricular posterior wall in early diastole, with little or no posterior motion during the rest of diastole. However, these findings are not specific for constrictive pericarditis and can be caused by other conditions such as restrictive cardiomyopathy (RCM).[14,15]
- Advanced hemodynamic cardiac catheterization may be indicated to confirm the diagnosis and differential diagnosis of constriction from restriction.
- Based on expert guidance and availability, CT, MRI, and echocardiography are diagnostic tests used in collaboration with a comprehensive history and physical examination to diagnose restrictive and constrictive pathologies.

Treatment for constrictive pericarditis may include a pericardiectomy, which involves surgical removal of the pericardium, and remains the mainstay of treatment for confirmed, symptomatic constrictive pericarditis.[16] This surgical procedure may be either a total or a partial pericardiectomy, and should be done at a high-volume center by an experienced cardiothoracic surgical team.

Recurrent or Relapsing Pericarditis. Recurrent pericarditis is a complication of acute pericarditis. Recurrence is diagnosed by recurrent pain and one or more of the following signs: fever, pericardial friction rub, ECG changes, effusion on echocardiography, and elevation of white blood count, C-reactive protein level, or the erythrocyte sedimentation rate.[12] The rate of recurrence is reported to vary from 15% to 50%, and considered an autoimmune phenomenon.[12] Recurrent pericarditis is increased when corticosteroids are used during treatment of the initial presenting episode of pericarditis. Risk factors for recurrence include previous corticosteroid use, female gender, and previous episodes of recurrent pericarditis.[15] Recurrence rate is decreased with the systematic use of colchicine partnered with NSAIDs during a first episode of pericarditis and managed with clinical surveillance and conservative tapering of therapies when improvement in noted sometimes over months to years.

Early Acute Post-MI Pericarditis. In the immediate period after MI, an early pericardial syndrome may develop and then resolve over the following 7 to 10 days. Pericardial involvement following MI can be related to infarct size, patient comorbidities, and clinical course. Post-MI pericarditis is illustrated by the clinical (e.g., evidence of a pericardial friction rub and positions chest discomfort) as well as the ECG characteristic of pericarditis.

The course is most often self-limiting and treatment involves aspirin and NSAIDs. Dressler syndrome occurs in less than 3% of patients following myocardial infarct and typically presents in the 1 to 8 weeks following MI and may present with any of the following: chest pain, pleurisy, pericarditis with friction rub, severe malaise, moderate fever, and leukocytosis. The underlying pathologic process is unknown, but it is thought to reflect a late autoimmune reaction mediated by antibodies to circulating antigens.[16] In contrast to early post-MI pericarditis, inflammation in Dressler syndrome is more diffuse, not localized to the myocardial injury site, and treatment is similar to postinfarction pericardial pain as outlined above.

Pericardial Effusion

Pericardial effusion is an increased amount of fluid within the pericardial space. This involves more than the physiologic amount of pericardial fluid, typically more than 50 cc.

Etiology

Many conditions cause acute pericarditis and pericardial effusions, including uremia, tuberculosis, neoplasms, and connective tissue diseases. Effusions may also be associated with acute idiopathic pericarditis. Benign pericardial effusions occur with heart failure and LVH, and are also common after cardiac surgery, and most often resolve spontaneously without requiring intervention. Other, more malignant pericardial effusions include neoplastic conditions, such as metastatic processes, and can sometimes be the first clinical manifestation of an existing malignancy. Renal failure and hypothyroidism are conditions that may precede uremic pericardial effusions. Tuberculosis remains a more common cause of pericardial effusions in developing countries.

Pathophysiology

The normal pericardium has a reserve capacity of 150 to 250 mL. An increase of volume of this amount in the pericardial space will not result in a major increase in intrapericardial pressure. Intrapericardial pressure will increase once this reserve volume

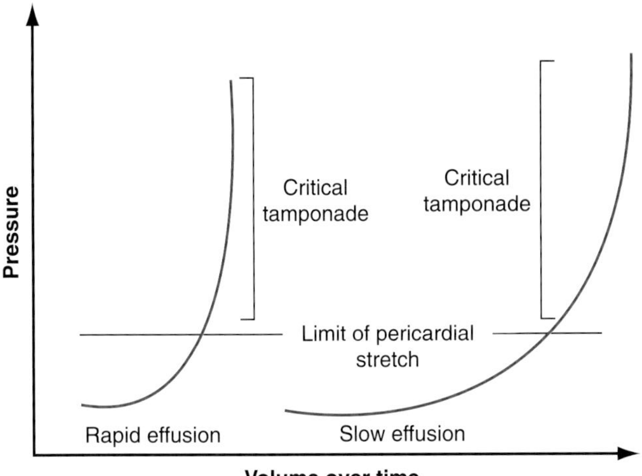

Figure 34-2. Cardiac tamponade. Pericardial pressure–volume (or strain–stress) curves are shown in which the volume increases slowly or rapidly over time. In the left-hand panel, rapidly increasing pericardial fluid first reaches the limit of the pericardial reserve volume (the initial flat segment) and then quickly exceeds the limit of parietal pericardial stretch, causing a steep rise in pressure, which becomes even steeper as smaller increments in fluid cause a disproportionate increase in the pericardial pressure. In the right-hand panel, a slower rate of pericardial filling takes longer to exceed the limit of pericardial stretch, because there is more time for the pericardium to stretch and for compensatory mechanisms to become activated.

is exceeded, and is also a function of how quickly the volume in the pericardial space accumulates. If fluid accumulates slowly, the normally stiff pericardium will stretch. However, if there are increased stiffness of the pericardium, as seen in constrictive pericarditis, small amounts of fluid will result in increased pericardial pressure. Once the intrapericardial pressure is elevated, the filling of the cardiac chambers becomes limited due to compression, resulting in hemodynamic effects.[4] Figure 34-2 shows the difference in effects of rapid versus slow effusion accumulation.

Assessment Findings

Echocardiography is the gold standard for clinical evaluation of pericardial effusion. Pericardial effusions are classified according to the distance between the left ventricular posterior wall and pericardium. Echocardiography can classify mild (less than 10 mm), moderate (10 to 20 mm), and severe (greater than 20 mm) effusions.[11] "Noncompressing" effusions do not produce changes in CO or pulsus paradoxus. If the effusions are caused by a systemic disease, then the symptoms are related to that disease. A pericardial rub may or may not be appreciated. The ECG may reveal reduced voltage, and these changes are nonspecific and unreliable for diagnosis. Cardiomegaly on chest x-ray film may be observed if effusion is present. If the effusion is visible on radiography, then most clinicians would estimate 300 mL of effusion is present in the pericardial space.

Medical Management

Pericardial effusion can be treated medically, with pericardiocentesis or with surgery.[9] Patients presenting for the first time with pericardial effusion are typically treated in the acute setting to define the underlying etiology, treatment plan, and ongoing evaluation for hemodynamic consequences such as cardiac tamponade. Management involves treatment of the pericarditis as discussed above with NSAIDs. Conservative treatment with clinical and echocardiographic monitoring is usually the approach for small or moderate effusions.[3] Uremic pericardial effusions are often treated with aggressive hemodialysis.[9]

Pericardiocentesis is typically conducted with ultrasound guidance in the echocardiography laboratory. Pericardiocentesis is generally indicated in the presence of hemodynamic compromise as in cardiac tamponade, or for diagnostic purposes when malignancies or infectious processes, such as tuberculosis are suspected. Most often, a pericardial tap, or indwelling catheter drainage (pericardial pigtail) is the procedure to treat pericardial effusions. This can be done at the bedside with echo guidance by an experienced echocardiographer ideally in a high-volume center. Small or posteriorly located effusions are more challenging, and require expert referral and may require surgical support for complex cases.

Cardiac Tamponade

Cardiac tamponade is a life-threatening hemodynamic condition resulting from a pericardial effusion that has compressed the cardiac silhouette and impeded cardiac filling. This restriction decreases cardiac output and may cause signs and symptoms of heart failure. Cardiac tamponade can be caused by varying amounts of fluid. The speed of fluid accumulation typically affects the severity of symptoms. Previous scarring, calcification, or pericardial thickening may decrease the flexibility and compensation of the pericardium to pericardial fluid accumulation, thus the importance of rapid identification, diagnosis, and treatment.

Etiology

The most common causes of cardiac tamponade include:

- Procedure complications, such as catheter- or pacemaker-induced perforation of the right heart, coronary vessel perforation during percutaneous interventions, and cardiac surgery
- Acute MI, resulting in pericarditis and/or cardiac rupture
- Pericardial effusions secondary to neoplasm
- Idiopathic pericarditis
- Trauma, cardiac contusions

Cardiac tamponade results from a pericardial effusion that increases **intrapericardial** pressure, compresses the heart, leading to diminished filling volumes and heart failure. If the effusion accumulates rapidly, as seen in trauma, then tamponade can occur with smaller volumes of 300 mL. Rapid accumulation does not allow time for the stiff pericardium to stretch. But an effusion that accumulates slowly, as seen in neoplasm, can be up to 1000 mL, with modest hemodynamic effect. Slowly developing pericardial effusions allow the pericardium to accommodate the effusion with modest hemodynamic compromise in spite of presence of a large effusion.

Pericardial pressure decreases cardiac volume and capacity. In any cardiac condition, the measured filling pressure only reflects true preload in the setting of normal chamber compliance, normal pericardial space, and normal pericardial layers.[4] The decreased stroke volume results in neurohormonal compensatory responses to maintain organ perfusion. Increased sympathetic stimulation results in catecholamine release and increased contractility, tachycardia, and vasoconstriction. Sinus tachycardia reflects exhaustion of compensatory mechanisms and signals—not only the presence of a hemodynamically important effusion, but may be indicative of impending hemodynamic collapse.[4]

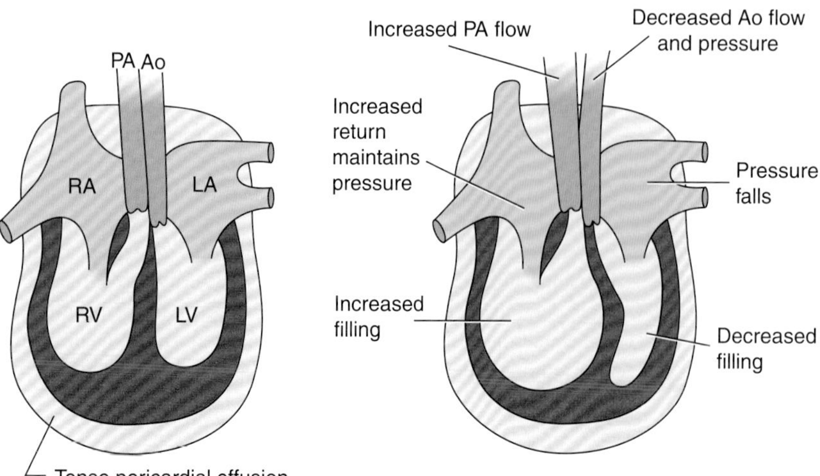

Figure 34-3. Mechanism of pulsus paradoxus.

Clinical Assessment in Cardiac Tamponade

A hemodynamically significant effusion may result in the symptoms of dyspnea, right heart failure, sinus tachycardia, and hypotension. Cardiac tamponade can be a life-threatening condition diagnosed by clinical examination including elevated jugular venous pressure, hypotension, and pulsus paradoxus in the presence of a pericardial effusion. Although cardiac tamponade increases filling pressures, cardiac volumes are reduced. Right and left heart filling pressures are increased and equalized, but the volume in the pulmonary veins may be modest. Therefore, there may be persistence of dyspnea, fatigue, and heart failure in the presence of clear lung fields.

Pulsus paradoxus is defined as an inspiratory decrease in systolic blood pressure greater than 10 mm Hg.[4] Figure 34-3 illustrates the mechanism of pulsus paradoxus in pericardial tamponade.[4]

To measure pulsus paradoxus:

1. Measure the blood pressure change using a blood pressure cuff; inflate the cuff to 15 mm Hg above the highest systolic reading.
2. Slowly deflate the cuff until the first Korotkoff sounds are heard. The sounds are heard only with some heartbeats; these are the ones occurring during expiration.
3. Slowly deflate the cuff until all of the Korotkoff sounds can be heard. The difference between these two readings gives the size of the pulsus paradoxus.

Medical Management of Cardiac Tamponade

The treatment of pericardial tamponade is pericardiocentesis, drainage of the accumulated pericardial fluid by pericardiocentesis. This is typically completed with the use of echocardiographic imaging or fluoroscopy. Hemodynamic monitoring throughout the acute pericardiocentesis and recovery is important and necessary. In the event that the fluid accumulated rapidly and/or is thought to recur, a pericardial pigtail catheter can be placed for prolonged, intermittent drainage, until diagnostic management is defined, symptoms improve, and accumulation ceases.

Pericardial Disease Management Summary

In summary, the priority of management in pericardial disease is the recognition of patient stability, thorough and thoughtful clinical evaluation and treatment planning, while maintaining an adequate cardiac output for optimal organ perfusion in acute patient presentations.

Treatments need to be individualized and always begin with a thorough history and clinical examination and thoughtful consideration of comorbid medical and surgical conditions. Management thereafter may include oxygen, cardiac monitoring, anti-inflammatories, vasoactive mediations, fluid volume management, pain control, and patient education. The cardiac team evaluates the patient's hemodynamic state, evaluating vital signs, symptoms, presence of pulsus paradoxus, and jugular venous distention. Acute decompensations, including cardiac tamponade, should be identified and treated to prevent hemodynamic collapse.

Ongoing and interval comprehensive evaluation includes a comprehensive history, a thorough physical examination, laboratory results, ECGs, and vital signs. Additional stepwise testing is indicated based on the individual patient stability and clinician insight. Stabilization of symptoms and proactive pain control and intervention remain important clinical considerations. Definitive diagnosis should guide optimal treatment.

Differential diagnosis of chest pain and definitive diagnosis of pericarditis and other causes of chest pain, such as MI, pulmonary embolus, and aortic dissection remain important cardiac differential diagnoses. The characteristics of pericardial pain, including intermittent pain presence, location, quality, presence of a pericardial friction rub, and the impact of positional changes, are hallmark signs and symptoms of pericardial etiology (see Table 34-1).

Patient Education for Pericardial Disease. Team-based care and management goals include pain control, definitive diagnosis, and stepwise treatment planning with ongoing management and surveillance. Details such as establishing patient expectations, clinical follow-up and medication titration, and anticipated treatment duration remain important. Discussion and prevention of complications, resumption of activity, and prevention of recurrent symptoms are important patient considerations. Symptoms and pain control, including use of both narcotics and NSAIDs, positioning, diversion, and bed rest or limitation of activities, are indicated. Patients should be counseled on a progressive activity program based on symptoms, and advised to avoid strenuous activity during acute exacerbations of pericardial pain. Patients require reassurance and support in partnership with adherence to medication regimens, sometimes lengthy titration schedules, and lifestyle and activity alterations.

CARDIOMYOPATHIES

The World Health Organization (WHO) defines cardiomyopathies as diseases of the myocardium associated with cardiac dysfunction. The WHO classification of cardiomyopathies includes dilated, hypertrophic, restrictive, and arrhythmogenic right ventricular cardiomyopathies, and unclassified cardiomyopathies.

Dilated Cardiomyopathy

Dilated Cardiomyopathy (DCM) is characterized by dilation and impaired contraction of the left or both ventricles.[17] The dilation often becomes severe and is invariably accompanied by an increase in total cardiac mass. The diagnosis of DCM is made after exclusion of known, specific causes of heart failure.[18] DCM causes considerable morbidity and mortality, and it is one of the major causes of sudden cardiac death. DCM is responsible for approximately 10,000 deaths and 46,000 hospitalizations each year in the United States.[19] Idiopathic DCM is the most common reason for cardiac transplantation.[19]

Etiology

DCM can by caused by a variety of disorders. Causes of DCM include stress-induced, infectious, toxic, genetic, peripartum, tachycardia-mediated, sarcoidosis, end-stage renal disease, autoimmune disease, endocrine dysfunction, and nutritional deficiencies. Frequently, definitive etiology cannot be determined, and the cardiomyopathy is deemed idiopathic. It is estimated that 50% of patients diagnosed with idiopathic cardiomyopathy have a familial DCM.[20] Multiple genes have been identified to be associated with DCM. These genes appear to encode two major subgroups of proteins: cytoskeletal and sarcomeric proteins.[21] The diagnosis of familial DCM is made when DCM is present in the setting of positive family history.

Pathophysiology

DCM is characterized by an increase in myocardial mass and a reduction in ventricular wall thickness. The heart assumes a globular shape and there is pronounced ventricular chamber dilation, diffuse endocardial thickening, and atrial enlargement often with thrombi in the appendages.[22] The histologic changes seen in DCM are nonspecific.[17] Familial DCM is caused by mutations in structural proteins comprising the myocyte cytoskeleton or sarcolemma.[22] Intraventricular conduction delay and left bundle branch block (LBBB) commonly occur in patients with idiopathic DCM. When cardiomyopathy causes left ventricular failure, conduction abnormalities add further to left ventricular (LV) dysfunction by compounding dyssynchrony in the contractile motion of the LV wall.[23]

Assessment Findings

Presentation of DCM is usually with heart failure, which is often progressive. The most typical symptoms include progressive dyspnea with exertion, impaired exercise capacity, orthopnea, paroxysmal nocturnal dyspnea, and peripheral edema. Arrhythmias, thromboembolism, and sudden death are common, and may occur at any stage during the disease.[17] Complaints of abdominal discomfort or anorexia are frequent in late stages of the disease and suggest hepatomegaly or bowel edema, respectively. Other common late complications include thromboembolic events, which may be systemic, originating from the left atria and ventricle, or pulmonary thrombi from the lower extremities.[24] Mitral regurgitation is common in DCM, as are ventricular arrhythmias, particularly ventricular tachycardia, torsade de pointes, and ventricular fibrillation.[25]

Echocardiography is a cornerstone in the evaluation and management of patients with DCM. Two-dimensional echocardiography and Doppler echocardiography can, in most cases, define the anatomic and functional characteristics of the heart that are diagnostic of dilated, hypertrophic, arrhythmogenic right ventricular, or RCM. Doppler echocardiography allows the evaluation of valvular regurgitation or stenosis, and the quantification of cardiac output.[24] This important information regarding the patient's condition helps guide therapy. Cardiac MRI or Cardiac CT may be useful in some patients to further make diagnosis.

Cardiac catheterization usually reveals increased left ventricular end-diastolic pressures and pulmonary artery wedge pressures. Pulmonary hypertension may range from mild to severe. The right ventricle is frequently involved and enlarged, manifested with increased right ventricular end-diastolic pressures, right atrial pressures, and central venous pressures.[24]

Medical Management

The initial evaluation of patients presenting with DCM should focus on identifying reversible and secondary causes.[24] Medical management focuses on optimizing cardiac function. Treatment with neurohormonal antagonists to prevent disease progression and the use of diuretics to maintain the volume balance are the therapeutic cornerstones for the management of patients with DCM.[26] Medications identified through clinical trials as providing beneficial effects for patients with DCM include diuretics, angiotensin-converting enzyme inhibitors (ACE-Is) or angiotensin receptor blockers (ARBs) if ACE intolerant, and β-blockers.[26] β-blocker therapy induces significant reductions in intraventricular dyssynchrony and improved contractility in DCM patients with heart failure.

Successful treatment of the patient with alcoholic cardiomyopathy must include cessation of alcohol consumption, which can have significant benefits in improving symptoms of heart failure. Ongoing alcohol consumption significantly worsens the patient's prognosis. Additional therapy includes a regimen of neurohormonal blockers. Administration of thiamine is also indicated in the possibility that malnutrition may play a role in the presentation. Anticoagulation should only be considered in the presence of a clear-cut and pressing indication because of the increased risk of trauma, catastrophic bleeding, and increased anticoagulation caused by hepatic dysfunction related to alcohol abuse.[24]

In research on patients with severe, nonischemic DCM who were treated with ACE-Is and β-blockers, the implantation of a cardioverter-defibrillator significantly reduced the risk of sudden death from arrhythmia.[27] This intervention has become an important mainstay of treatment. Cardiac resynchronization therapy (CRT) with biventricular pacing is used for patients with medically refractory heart failure.[28] CRT corrects dyssynchrony by synchronous pacing from transvenous pacing catheters implanted in the right atrium and right ventricle. The CRT device usually includes an implantable defibrillator.[23]

Patients with valvular heart disease, pericardial disease, or congenital heart defects should be considered for surgical correction.

Left ventricular assist devices provide aggressive mechanical support to patients with advanced decompensated heart failure.[26]

DCM is a leading reason for cardiac transplantation.[29] Cardiac transplantation becomes a possible treatment option when all medical therapies have been maximized, and no other surgical procedures will correct the underlying disease process.[30]

HYPERTROPHIC CARDIOMYOPATHY

Hypertrophic cardiomyopathy (HCM) is a familial cardiac disorder characterized by unexplained LV hypertrophy, associated with nondilated ventricular chambers in the absence of another cardiac or systemic disease that itself would be capable of producing that degree of hypertrophy.[31] The manifestations of HCM are complex and may include dynamic left ventricular outflow tract obstruction (LVOTO), mitral regurgitation, diastolic dysfunction, myocardial ischemia, and cardiac arrhythmias. HCM is the most common cause of heart-related sudden death in competitive athletes and people age less than 30 years of age. In patients with HCM, the sudden cardiac death mortality rate is 1% per year.[32]

Etiology

HCM is a familial disease with an autosomal dominant inheritance. This disorder affects 1:500 in the general population.[22] Mutations in sarcomeric contractile protein genes cause disease.[17,33] Most common mutations are in the cardiac myosin-binding protein C gene and β-myosin heavy chain.[31] Mechanisms thought to lead to septal hypertrophy include reduced contractile dysfunction leading to compensatory hypertrophy of cardiac myocytes, insufficient levels of muscle ATP resulting in deranged sarcomere function, and the induction of growth factors that stimulate hypertrophy and fibrosis.[34]

Pathophysiology

In HCM, the left ventricular volume is typically normal or reduced, and systolic gradients are common. LVOTO causes an increase in left ventricular systolic pressure, which leads to prolonged ventricular relaxation, increased left ventricular diastolic pressure, myocardial ischemia, and decreased cardiac output. The obstruction can be dependent on changes in preload, afterload, and contractility, so anything that influences these factors can affect the LVOTO.[33] Mitral valve regurgitation is due to systolic anterior motion of the mitral valve.[35] Typical morphologic changes include myocyte hypertrophy and disarray surrounding areas of increased loose connective tissue.

Assessment Findings

HCM is diagnosed by echocardiography in the presence of left ventricular hypertrophy in the absence of other mechanical, metabolic, or genetic causes.[33,36] MRI can also aid in diagnosis.[36] Peak instantaneous LV outflow pressure gradients greater or equal 50 mm Hg either at rest or with provocation represent the conventional threshold for intervention with either myectomy or ablation if symptoms are not controlled with medications. There can often be variation in the severity of the gradient during day-to-day activities. Exacerbation of symptoms during the postprandial period is common.[31] The preferred method of eliciting presence of latent gradients during and/or immediately following exercise is treadmill or bicycle exercise testing along with Doppler echocardiography.

Classic findings in HCM include a systolic ejection murmur that becomes increasingly loud during maneuvers that decrease preload, such as standing from a squatting position or Valsalva maneuver.[33] Systolic pressure gradients in the left ventricular outflow tract during resting conditions are only found in approximately one fourth of patients.[37,38] A mitral regurgitation murmur can be heard because the mitral leaflet is open as it is pulled into the left ventricular outflow tract during systole.[34]

The majority of patients are asymptomatic throughout life. However, some will present with severe symptoms of dyspnea, angina, and syncope.[33] The ECG will display signs of left ventricular hypertrophy. Ventricular arrhythmias and premature sudden death are common and appear to be genetically linked.[17,33,39] Atrial fibrillation is also commonly seen and thought to be due to atrial enlargement.[35]

Medical Management

Treatment strategies in HCM are directed toward prevention of sudden cardiac death and symptom relief.[40] An ICD and amiodarone are used to prevent sudden cardiac death in patients at high risk.[35] Risk factors for sudden cardiac death include sudden cardiac death in first-degree family members, unexplained syncope, abnormal blood pressure response to exercise, resting left ventricular outflow gradient greater than 30 mm Hg, ventricular ectopy, and massive LVH.[39,41]

Pharmacologic therapy is designed to increase diastolic filling, decrease LVOTO, and decrease myocardial oxygen demand. β-Blockers are recommended for the treatment of symptoms in adult patients with nonobstructive or obstructive HCM. Verapamil therapy is recommended for treatment of symptoms in patients who do not respond or cannot take β-blockers. Disopyramide can also be added to β-blockers and verapamil if symptoms persist.[31]

The goal of surgical intervention is to reduce permanently the LVOTO and gradient, thereby decreasing symptoms and improving quality of life. The size of the ventricular septum, and therefore the LVOTO, can be reduced through surgical myectomy or alcohol septal ablation.[35] Successful surgical myectomy results in marked improvement of symptoms. Percutaneous alcohol septal ablation involves the introduction of alcohol into a target septal perforator branch of the left anterior descending coronary artery to induce an MI within the proximal ventricular septum. This treatment results in a decrease in septal thickness. Patients are at risk for conduction problems so a temporary pacemaker is placed prior to the ablation. Some patients may require a permanent pacemaker.[39] There are no randomized clinical trials comparing surgery to ablation; therefore, long-term outcomes for these strategies are unknown.[39,42]

Because of the genetic nature of HCM, annual clinical screening of adolescent relatives aged 12 to 18 years, consisting of a history and physical examination, 12-lead ECG, 24-hour Holter monitor, and two-dimensional echocardiography is indicated. Because some individuals do not manifest HCM until adulthood, screening beyond adolescence is recommended every 5 years.[36]

Restrictive Cardiomyopathy

RCM is characterized by restrictive filling and reduced diastolic volume of either or both ventricles with normal or near-normal systolic function and wall thickness.[17] It is an uncommon type of cardiomyopathy in countries like the United States.[43]

Etiology

RCM may be idiopathic, or associated with other diseases, such as amyloidosis and endomyocardial fibrosis.[17,43,44]

Pathophysiology

The pathophysiologic feature that defines RCM is an increase in stiffness of the ventricular walls, which causes impaired diastolic filling of the ventricle and heart failure. In RCM, interstitial fibrosis may be present.[17] In the early stages of RCM, systolic function may be normal, although deterioration in systolic function is usually observed as the disease progresses.[24]

Assessment Findings

Clinically, RCM mimics constrictive pericarditis. RCM typically presents with heart failure and is frequently associated with pulmonary hypertension and atrial arrhythmias. Patients with RCM frequently present with exercise intolerance because of an impaired ability to augment cardiac output during increasing heart rate because of the restriction of diastolic filling. With advanced disease, profound edema occurs that includes peripheral edema, hepatomegaly, ascites, and anasarca.[24] Physical examination reveals an elevated jugular venous pulse, often with the Kussmaul sign, and an increasing jugular pressure during inspiration due to the restriction to filling. Both S_3 and S_4 heart sounds are common. Classic imaging features of idiopathic RCM include normal ejection fraction, biatrial enlargement, grades 3 to 4 diastolic dysfunction, and nondilated and nonhypertrophied left ventricle.[38] Patients with RCM may present with, or develop, atrial fibrillation. CT and MRI as well as advanced hemodynamic catheterization are valuable for differentiating constrictive and restrictive disease.

Medical Management

There are no proven medical therapies for treatment of idiopathic RCM. Treatment depends on etiology and manifestations.[45] RCM patients require higher pulmonary artery wedge pressures to maintain stroke volume; therefore, diuretics should be used cautiously to treat volume overload. Since cardiac output is dependent on heart rate, bradycardia should be avoided in these patients. Cardiac transplant evaluation may be necessary.

Arrhythmogenic Right Ventricular Cardiomyopathy

Arrhythmogenic right ventricular cardiomyopathy (ARVC) is also known as arrhythmic right ventricular dysplasia. ARVC is characterized by replacement of the ventricular myocardium with fatty and fibrous tissue that most commonly affects the right ventricle, but involvement of the ventricular septum and left ventricle has been reported.[46]

Etiology

Familial disease is common in ARVC, typically with autosomal dominant inheritance and incomplete penetrance. Familial occurrence of arrhythmogenic right ventricular dysplasia is present in approximately 50% of cases.[47]

Pathophysiology

The myocardium of the right ventricular free wall and frequently the left ventricle is replaced by fibrous and/or fibrofatty tissue. The mechanism of this disease leads to the progressive loss of myocytes.[22] Structural and functional abnormalities of the right ventricle lead to arrhythmias and progressive right ventricular failure.[48]

Assessment Findings

Presenting features of ARVC may include palpitations, presyncope, syncope, right ventricular failure, ventricular arrhythmias, or sudden cardiac death. ARVC should always be suspected when sudden cardiac death occurs in a young adult.[47]

Medical Management

The diagnostic criteria for ARVC involve features obtained from ECG, Holter monitor, echocardiography, cardiac MRI, Cardiac CT with IV contrast, as well as genetic testing.[47]

Patients diagnosed with ARVC should be educated to avoid participation in sports, with the exception of low-intensity exercise. β-Blockers are recommended. Class 3 antiarrhythmic therapy with amiodarone or sotalol may decrease ventricular arrhythmia burden, but have not been shown to protect against sudden death. ARVC may warrant implantation of implantable cardioverter-defibrillator especially when there is a personal or family history of presyncope, syncope, or sudden cardiac death. Standard medical therapy with ACE-Is or ARBs, and/or diuretic should be used when heart failure is present.[47] Consideration of heart transplantation is indicated for patients with overt cardiac failure.[26] Screening is recommended for all first- or second-degree relatives.[47]

Unclassified Cardiomyopathies

Unclassified cardiomyopathy was added to the classification system to describe disorders that do not fit into any of the phenotypic categories. Examples of these would include LV noncompaction and stress-induced takotsubo cardiomyopathy. Left ventricular noncompaction is an inherited form of cardiomyopathy characterized by increased left ventricular trabeculations resulting in thickened myocardium with two layers consisting of noncompacted myocardium and a thin compacted layer of myocardium.[49]

Stress-induced cardiomyopathy, also referred to as apical ballooning syndrome, broken heart syndrome, or takotsubo cardiomyopathy, most commonly occurs in postmenopausal women[50] and is characterized by transient regional systolic dysfunction of the left ventricle, mimicking MI, in the absence of angiographic evidence of obstructive coronary artery disease or acute plaque rupture.

Etiology

Apical ballooning syndrome is most often triggered by emotional or physical stressors. The recurrence rate is approximately 1% to 2% per year.[50]

Pathophysiology

Pathophysiology of apical ballooning syndrome is not yet well understood. Hypothesized mechanisms include microvascular dysfunction, catecholamine excess, and coronary artery spasm.[51,52] Left ventricular noncompaction may be caused by intrauterine arrest of compaction of the loose interwoven meshwork that makes up the fetal myocardial primordium.[53]

Assessment Findings

Presenting symptoms of apical ballooning syndrome may include chest pain and dyspnea. Testing may include ECG, troponin levels, echocardiography, or left ventriculography on cardiac catheterization. ECG may show diffuse ST segment change or elevation. Diagnostic criteria include transient hypokinesis, dyskinesis, or akinesis of the left ventricular segments with or without apical involvement with absence of obstructive coronary artery disease or angiographic evidence of plaque rupture.[54,55] Left ventricular noncompaction is typically diagnosed with echocardiography, cardiac MRI, or cardiac CT. Complications of LV noncompaction may include heart failure, tachyarrhythmias, or thromboembolic events.[49]

Medical Management

There are no data regarding effectiveness of any therapies for ventricular noncompaction. Anticoagulation should be considered. Standard heart failure medications are generally used to treat an associated reduction in left ventricular ejection fraction. Implantable cardioverter-defibrillator therapy should be considered in high-risk patients. Echocardiographic screening is indicated for all first-degree relatives of patients who have ventricular noncompaction.[49]

Apical ballooning syndrome is most often treated with supportive measures such as β-blocker therapy and ACE-Is or ARB therapy. Optimal duration of these therapies remains to be established at this time, but should continue at least until there is complete recovery of ventricular systolic function.[50]

Myocarditis

Myocarditis is an inflammatory disease of the myocardium. Myocarditis can be categorized as acute or chronic, and can lead to the development of DCM.[36] Myocarditis may be idiopathic, infectious, or autoimmune.[18] Primary or postviral myocarditis can be categorized by its clinical pathologic manifestations. This includes fulminant, chronic active, eosinophilic, and giant-cell myocarditis.[36] In some cases, myocarditis spontaneously resolves without ongoing complications; although severe myocarditis may result in DCM, or increased risk of MI, stroke, or sudden death usually from ventricular arrhythmias.

Etiology

There are many etiologies of myocarditis. The cause may be viral, bacterial, fungal, protozoal, and parasitic. Toxins, hypersensitivity to medications, and immunologic syndromes can also cause myocarditis.[56] Viruses are considered the predominant cause. Age-related and regional differences may be important when looking at the viral etiology of myocarditis.[56]

Pathophysiology

Myocarditis is the result of both myocardial infections and autoimmunity that results in active inflammatory destruction of myocytes. Inflammation of the myocardium affects its function, and heart failure can result.

Assessment Findings

The clinical appearance of myocarditis is varied; the features range from systemic symptoms of fever, myalgias, palpitations, and dyspnea, to arrhythmia, syncope, sudden death, acute right or left ventricular failure, cardiogenic shock, or DCM.[18,56] Myocarditis may resolve, or result in relapse, DCM requiring heart transplantation, or death.

Imaging used to evaluate myocarditis may include cardiac MRI, echocardiography, and positron emission tomography scan to help diagnose suspected cardiac sarcoidosis.[57] Endomyocardial biopsy can be performed if clinically indicated.

ECG and measurement of serum troponin are additional required tests when myocarditis is suspected.[56] In myocarditis, the ECG may show low-voltage QRS complexes, ST segment elevation, or heart block. Nonsustained atrial or ventricular arrhythmias are common. An S_4 and systolic ejection murmurs may be present on auscultation.

Medical Management

Supportive care is the first line of treatment in myocarditis. Management includes treatment of heart failure, with the goal of improving symptoms and hemodynamic status.[56] Patients may require cardiac device placement in the presence of ventricular arrhythmias, conduction system disease, or when there is increased risk of sudden cardiac death.

Patient Education

Education needs to be individualized based on the type and cause of cardiomyopathy. Patient education includes understanding the disease process, prognosis, diet, activity level, medications, indications for genetic testing, and treatment options for symptom management, screening and surveillance, and finally prevention of disease progression. Following a heart-healthy lifestyle, daily weight monitoring, and when to call a provider are further educational priorities for patients with cardiomyopathy.

ENDOCARDIAL DISEASE

Infective Endocarditis

Infective endocarditis (IE) is a disease in which infective organisms invade the endothelial lining of the heart, usually involving one or more valves, or an intracardiac device. The endocardium covers the valves and surrounds the chordae tendineae. The infection that forms, an irregularly shaped echogenic mass adherent to the endothelial cardiac surface, often on the valve of the heart, is called a vegetation.[58] Destruction, ulceration, or abscess formation can also occur. Approximately 10,000 to 15,000 new cases of IE are diagnosed in the United States each year.[59] IE is considered an uncommon infectious disease but it continues to be characterized by increased morbidity and mortality. IE is now considered one of the top five most common life-threatening infections.[59]

Types of IE

- Native Valve
  - Occurs in patients when their natural heart valves are infected.
- Prosthetic Valve
  - Can arise early or late after surgery. Tends to occur in 1% to 6% of patients and is associated with high morbidity and mortality.[60] The greatest risk tends to occur initially 3 months after surgery but remains high through a 6-month period and then falls gradually each year thereafter.
- Injection Drug Users
  - Involves the right side of the heart and tricuspid valve. Pneumonia and septic pulmonary emboli are also common. Often associated with coinfections with HIV, hepatitis B, or hepatitis C which may alter their clinical presentation, complications, or outcomes.
- Intracardiac Devices

- Complete cardiac implantable electronic device removal is warranted when transesophageal echocardiogram demonstrates a vegetation on the device, positive blood cultures, other high-grade bacteremia without alternative source, or an implanted cardiac device pocket infection.

A variety of microorganisms can cause IE. The three most common causes worldwide are staphylococci, structural cocci, and enterococci. In the United States and most developed countries, *Staphylococcus aureus* is the most common cause.[61] Staphylococci infections account for the majority of cases of health care–associated IE, while streptococci are the most prominent community acquired.[62,63] Gram-negative bacteria such as *Escherichia coli* and *Klebsiella pneumoniae* tend to adhere last readily to heart valves than the previously discussed gram-positive organisms. Fungal IE is fairly rare.

Clinical Findings

Features of IE are nonspecific and are highly variable. Symptoms may include unexplained fever, new-onset heart murmur, heart valve dysfunction, night sweats, weight loss, new-onset heart block, bacteremia, peripheral embolic lesions, central nervous system emboli, stroke, pulmonary emboli, malaise, headache, myalgias, arthralgias, abdominal pain, dyspnea, cough, or pleuritic pain. Cardiac murmurs are observed in approximately 85% of patients.[64] Most often, clinical manifestations reflecting complications of IE may be present initially or develop subsequently. Common complications include but are not limited to valvular insufficiency, heart failure, stroke, septic emboli of internal organs, and metastatic infections.

Risk Factors

IE may be acquired within the community or in the context of a health care exposure. Patient risk factors for developing IE include complex congenital heart disease, pre-existing cardiac valvular abnormalities including prosthetic heart valves, long-term indwelling vascular catheters, intravenous drug use, previous history of endocarditis, age greater than 60 years, and poor dentition or dental infection. Males tend to have a higher incidence of IE as well.[65–70]

Diagnostic Testing

Testing for patients who are suspected to have IE could include:

- Blood cultures (ideally three separate cultures from different venipuncture sites with the first and last samples drawn at least 1 hour apart)
- Transthoracic and transesophageal echocardiography
- Electrocardiography
- CT scan
- Chest x-ray
- MRI
- Dental examination

The modified Duke criteria help stratify patient in the three different categories: definite IE, possible IE, and rejected IE. The Duke criteria should be used as a diagnostic guide together with clinical judgment.[71] Definitive IE is established in the presence two major clinical criteria, one major and three minor clinical criteria, or five minor clinical criteria. Possible IE is defined as the presence of one major clinical criterion and one minor clinical criterion for the presence of three minor clinical criteria. The diagnosis of IE can be rejected if any of the following are present: A firm alternative diagnosis is made, resolution of clinical manifestation occurs less than 3 days after antibiotic therapy, no pathologic evidence is found at surgery or autopsy, or clinical criteria for possible or definitive endocarditis are not met.[72]

Major criteria include:

- Positive blood cultures with typical microorganisms
- Persistently positive blood cultures
- Echocardiogram positive for vegetation, abscess, or partial dehiscence of prosthetic valve
- New valvular regurgitation

Minor criteria include:

- Temperature greater than 38.0°C
  - Predisposition: intravenous drug use or presence of a predisposing heart condition
  - Vascular phenomena: major arterial emboli, septic pulmonary infarcts, intracranial hemorrhage, conjunctival hemorrhages
  - Immunologic phenomena: glomerulonephritis
  - Microbiologic evidence: positive blood cultures that do not meet major criteria[72]

Referrals are based on the patient's symptoms and complications which arise from IE. These could include but are not limited to cardiology, infectious disease, cardiovascular surgeon, neurology, and pulmonary medicine.[73]

Management of patients with IE should be considered multidisciplinary. The cornerstone of treatment of IE is early recognition and elimination of the infecting organism. Antibiotic therapy is most often indicated and patients are usually on this long term. Specific antibiotic therapy is based on the infecting organism. The most frequent complication of IE is congestive heart failure. Continuous close monitoring for symptoms of hemodynamic decompensation and heart failure is vital when caring for these patients. Quite often, these patients require surgical interventions because of compilations that arise from IE. Cardiac conduction issues can also develop secondary to IE or because of surgery, making continuous cardiac monitoring of these patients essential. When caring for these patients, it is essential to be vigilant in monitoring for other complications that could include but are not limited to stroke, pulmonary embolism, and renal dysfunction. Hospital stay for patients who have IE tends to be lengthy. Patients may also require oxygen therapy, medication management and titration, physical and occupational therapy, and discharge education depending on their hospital course.

Prophylaxis

The American Heart Association states that the practice of routinely giving antibiotics to patients at risk for endocarditis prior to a dental procedure is not recommended except for patients with the highest risk of adverse outcomes resulting from IE.[74] Patients who may benefit from prophylaxis include:

- Prosthetic cardiac valves, including transcatheter-implanted prostheses and homografts
- Prosthetic material used for cardiac valve repair such as annuloplasty rings and chords
- Previous endocarditis

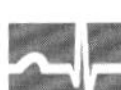 CASE-BASED LEARNING 1

Patient Profile

A 59-year-old Caucasian woman presents with concerns regarding 12 hours of intermittent chest pain. She relates the onset associated with heavy lifting while doing housekeeping, and does describe some relief of her discomfort when sitting down. The pain has been intermittently present over the past few days and associated with a cough. She does describe improvement of the pain when leaning forward, and relates that she has been sleeping in her recliner.

She has no known history of coronary artery disease, however is a current smoker, and has been told she has borderline hypertension. Renal function is normal. Lipid status is unknown. She is on no medications.

Physical examination: On cardiac examination, she has a normal S_1, S_2 without any murmurs, heaves, or rubs. Her lungs are clear. Pulses are intact and she has no edema. The rest of the examination is noncontributory.

Testing: Electrocardiogram reveals sinus rhythm with a 3 mm of upsloping ST segment elevation in leads I, II, III, AVF, V_4, V_5, and V_6. There are inverted T-waves present in AVF and aVL. Laboratories: Reveal a normal CBC, electrolyte panel, negative troponin, and a slightly increased sedimentation rate. Your next best step in clinical management includes:

1. Transfer to local emergency room for further evaluation and treatment.
2. Treat as an acute ST-elevation myocardial infarction.
3. Consider proceeding with an echocardiogram in the evaluation of possible pericarditis.
4. Treat patient with ibuprofen and send patient home with instructions to return if symptoms persist in 1 week.

The 59-year-old Caucasian woman with 12 hours of intermittent chest pain, With a history of exacerbation when leaning back and improvement in discomfort with leaning forward should be considered for pericarditis. She reports a history of cough and on further questioning, you learn she has had a recent upper respiratory infection. This patient should be considered for idiopathic pericarditis. In the setting of a normal CBC, electrolyte, and slightly elevated sedimentation rate, an echocardiogram would be indicated to assess any evidence of pericardial effusion.

Treatment should include a loading dose of colchicine followed by maintenance colchicine of 0.6 mg daily and the addition of a nonsteroidal agent such as aspirin, ibuprofen, or indomethacin in the doses outlined above. The patient should be counseled on reducing activity, telling his symptoms improved, and reporting any increased symptoms, breathlessness, fever, and chills. Finally, the patient should be counseled that it may take weeks to months for her symptoms to completely resolve but in the setting of idiopathic pericarditis, likely related to her recent upper respiratory infection, she can expect initial improvement in the first 48 to 72 hours with the medical program described above. Surveillance and follow-up is important, awaiting complete resolution of symptoms at which time the nonsteroid can be tapered, and the colchicine could be stopped.

- Cardiac transplantation recipients with valve regurgitation due to a structurally abnormal valve
- Specific cases with patients with congenital heart disease[74]

Patient Education

Patient Education. Patients should be educated on the importance of infectious endocarditis prevention, as well as their individualized risk for recurrence. Education should be provided specifically including types of procedures requiring prophylaxis as well as their personal indication for prophylaxis. Prevention starts with routine professional dental care, twice annually, and good daily oral hygiene including both brushing and flossing. Prevention of superficial infection including care for minor cuts and abrasions is imperative. Patients should be instructed to notify a health care provider urgently in the setting of infection, including fever, fatigue, weight loss, or night sweats.

Prevention. High-risk patients can obtain and should carry a wallet card from the American Heart Association. This card delineates the high-risk condition and recommendations for prophylactic antibiotic treatment for specific medical procedures. Patient education for hospitalized patients with IE includes medical and nursing management, treatment options and plan of care, including treatment and prophylaxis prior to surgery when medically indicated.[75]

Summary

Pericardial, myocardial, and endocardial diseases impact global health. These diseases contribute to the economic health burden necessitating rapid, safe, and efficient treatment. Prompt assessment and treatment can benefit patient outcomes and minimize long-term complications.

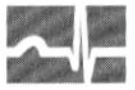 CASE-BASED LEARNING 2

Patient Profile

A 68-year-old female presents to the ER with midsternal chest pain that developed 24 hours after a family emergency. Patient noted she had been under a tremendous amount of stress with recent family emergency. ECG upon arrival to ER showed diffuse ST segment changes. Slight increase in troponins noted on laboratory data. Patient was taken to the coronary catheterization laboratory to rule out acute coronary syndrome. Coronary angiogram showed normal coronary arteries. Left ventriculography on cardiac catheterization shows regional wall-motion abnormalities involving the mid and apical segments. Patient was diagnosed with apical ballooning syndrome or stress-induced cardiomyopathy. Patient initiated on β-blocker and ACE-I prior to discharge from hospital. Patient returned in 3 months for follow-up with normalization of systolic function.

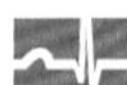 CASE-BASED LEARNING 3

Patient Profile

M. Hill is a 54-year-old male who presents to his primary care provider with a history of generalized malaise, night sweats, and weight loss over the last 2 weeks. He has noticed a slight decrease in his physical activities. His vital signs include temperature of 38.8, pulse rate of 92, respiratory rate of 20, and blood pressure of 105/60. He has no other significant medical history.

CASE-BASED LEARNING 3 (*Continued*)

Once examined, M. Hill was noted to have a 3/6 systolic murmur at the apex. His provider ordered a complete metabolic panel, CBC, blood cultures, and transthoracic echocardiogram. The transthoracic echocardiogram demonstrated severe mitral regurgitation, but no visible vegetations could be noted on the valve. Before his blood cultures came back, M. Hill reported to his local ER for increased dyspnea on exertion. Cardiology was consulted and he was admitted to the hospital for further workup which included transesophageal echocardiogram. His blood cultures came back positive for *Staphylococcus aureus*. His transesophageal echocardiogram again demonstrated severe mitral regurgitation with a 6-mm vegetation noted on the posterior leaflet of the mitral valve. Infectious disease service and cardiovascular surgery.

M. Hill was placed on IV antibiotic therapy for approximately 6 weeks. CV surgery wished to hold off with surgical intervention until it was completed. A repeat TEE showed resolution of the vegetation and only mild mitral regurgitation. M. Hill's symptoms had improved significantly after the 6 weeks and a follow-up in 6 months was recommended with his cardiologist.

KEY READINGS

Adler Y, Charron P, Imazio M; ESC Scientific Document Group. 2015 ESC guidelines for the diagnosis and management of pericardial diseases: The Task Force for the Diagnosis and Management of Pericardial Diseases of the European Society of Cardiology (ESC) Endorsed by: The European Association for Cardio-Thoracic Surgery (EACTS). *Eur Heart J.* 2015;36(42):2921–2964.

Baddour LM, Wilson WR, Bayer AS, et al. Infective endocarditis in adults: diagnosis, antimicrobial therapy, and management of complications: a scientific statement for healthcare professionals from the American Heart Association. *Circulation.* 2015;132:1435–1486.

Cahill TJ, Prendergast BD. Infective endocarditis. *Lancet.* 2016;387:882–893.

Chatterjee K, Anderson M, Heistad D, et al. Pericardial disease. Chapter 86. In: Khandaker MH, Nishimura RA, eds. *Cardiology: An Illustrated Textbook.* New Dehli, India: Jaypee Brothers Medical Publishers; 2017: 1489–1504.

Gersh BJ, Maron BJ, Bonow RO. 2011 ACCF/AHA guideline for the diagnosis and treatment of hypertrophic cardiomyopathy: a report of the American College of Cardiology Foundation/American Heart Association Task Force on Practice Guidelines. *Circulation.* 2011;124:e783–e831.

Habib G, Lancellotti P, Antunes MJ, et al. 2015 ESC guidelines for the management of infective endocarditis: the Task Force for the management of infective endocarditis of the European Society of Cardiology (ESC). Endorsed by: European Association for Cardio-Thoracic Surgery (ACTS), the European Association of Nuclear Medicine (EANM). *Eur Heart J.* 2015;36:3075–3128.

Khandaker MH, Espinosa RE, Nishimura RA, et al. Pericardial disease: diagnosis and management. *Mayo Clin Proc.* 2010;85(6):572–593.

Nishimura RA, Ottow CM, Bonow RO, et al. 2014 AHA/ACC guideline for the management of patients with valvular heart disease: a report of the American College of Cardiology/American Heart Association Task Force on Practice Guidelines. *J Am Coll Cardiol.* 2014;63:e57–e185.

REFERENCES

1. Imazio M. Contemporary management of pericardial diseases. *Curr Opin Cardiol.* 2012;27:308–317.
2. Spodick DH. Acute cardiac tamponade. *N Engl J Med.* 2003;349: 684–690.
3. Kytö V, Sipilä J, Rautava P. Clinical profile and influences on outcomes in patients hospitalized for acute pericarditis. *Circulation.* 2014;130: 1601–1606.
4. Imazio M, Cecchi E, Demichelis B, et al. Myopericarditis versus viral or idiopathic acute pericarditis. *Heart.* 2008;94:498–501.
5. Imazio M, Gaita F, LeWinter M. Evaluation and treatment of pericarditis: a systematic review. *JAMA.* 2015;314:1498–1506.
6. Permanyer-Miralda G, Sagristá-Sauleda J, Soler-Soler J. Primary acute pericardial disease: a prospective series of 231 consecutive patients. *Am J Cardiol.* 1985;56:623–630.
7. Imazio M, Demichelis B, Cecchi E, et al. Cardiac troponin I in acute pericarditis. *J Am Coll Cardiol.* 2003;42:2144–2148.
8. Imazio M, Cecchi E, Demichelis B, et al. Indicators of poor prognosis of acute pericarditis. *Circulation.* 2007;115:2739–2744.
9. Imazio M, Bobbio M, Cecchi E, et al. Colchicine in addition to conventional therapy for acute pericarditis: results of the COlchicine for acute PEricarditis (COPE) trial. *Circulation.* 2005;112:2012–2016.
10. Imazio M, Demichelis B, Parrini I, et al. Day-hospital treatment of acute pericarditis: a management program for outpatient therapy. *J Am Coll Cardiol.* 2004;43:1042–1046.
11. Klein AL, Abbara S, Agler DA, et al. American Society of Echocardiography clinical recommendations for multimodality cardiovascular imaging of patients with pericardial disease: endorsed by the Society for Cardiovascular Magnetic Resonance and Society of Cardiovascular Computed Tomography. *J Am Soc Echocardiogr.* 2013;26:965–1012.e15.
12. Imazio M, Spodick DH, Brucato A, et al. Controversial issues in the management of pericardial diseases. *Circulation.* 2010;121:916–928.
13. Maisch B, Ristić AD. The classification of pericardial disease in the age of modern medicine. *Curr Cardiol Rep.* 2002;4:13–21.
14. Adler Y, Charron P, Imazio M, et al. 2015 ESC guidelines for the diagnosis and management of pericardial diseases: the Task Force for the diagnosis and management of pericardial diseases of the European Society of Cardiology (ESC). Endorsed by: the European Association for Cardio-Thoracic Surgery (EACTS). *Eur Heart J.* 2015;36:2921–2964.
15. Imazio M, Demichelis B, Parrini I, et al. Recurrent pain without objective evidence of disease in patients with previous idiopathic or viral acute pericarditis. *Am J Cardiol.* 2004;94:973–975.
16. Hoit BD. Diseases of the pericardium. In: Fuster V, Alexander RW, O'Rourke RA, eds. *Hurst's the Heart.* 11th ed. New York: McGraw-Hill; 2004:2061–2085.
17. Richardson P, McKenna W, Bristow M, et al. Report of the 1995 World Health Organization/International Society and Federation of Cardiology Task Force on the definition and classification of cardiomyopathies. *Circulation.* 1996;93(5):841–842.
18. Caforio AL, Daliento L, Angelini A, et al. Autoimmune myocarditis and dilated cardiomyopathy: focus on cardiac autoantibodies. *Lupus.* 2005;14(9):652–655.
19. Manolio TA, Baughman KL, Rodeheffer R, et al. Prevalence and etiology of idiopathic dilated cardiomyopathy. *Am J Cardiol.* 1992;69:1458.
20. Karkkainen S, Peuhkurinen K. Genetics of dilated cardiomyopathy. *Ann Med.* 2007;39(2):91–107.
21. Towbin JA, Bowles NE. Dilated cardiomyopathy: a tale of cytoskeletal proteins and beyond. *J Cardiovasc Electrophysiol.* 2006;17(8):919–926.
22. Hughes SE, McKenna WJ. New insights into the pathology of inherited cardiomyopathy. *Heart.* 2005;91(2):257–264.
23. Friedewald VE Jr, Boehmer JP, Kowal RC. The editor's roundtable: cardiac resynchronization therapy. *Am J Cardiol.* 2007;100(7):1145–1152.
24. Hare JM. The dilated, restrictive, and infiltrative cardiomyopathies. In: Libby P, Bonow RO, Mann DL, et al., eds. *Braunwald's Heart Disease: A Textbook of Cardiovascular Medicine.* 8th ed. Philadelphia, PA: Saunders Elsevier; 2007.
25. Ivens EL, Munt BI, Moss RR. Pericardial disease: what the general cardiologist needs to know. *Heart.* 2007;93(8):993–1000.
26. Hunt S, Abraham W, Chin M. ACC/AHA 2005 guideline update for the diagnosis and management of chronic heart failure in the adult. *Circulation.* 2005;112:e154–e235.
27. Kadish A, Dyer A, Daubert JP, et al. Prophylactic defibrillator implantation in patients with nonischemic dilated cardiomyopathy. *N Engl J Med.* 2004;350(21):2151–2158.
28. Takemoto Y, Hozumi T, Sugioka K, et al. Beta-blocker therapy induces ventricular resynchronization in dilated cardiomyopathy with narrow QRS complex. *J Am Coll Cardiol.* 2007;49(7):778–783.
29. Bruce J. Getting to the heart of cardiomyopathies. *Nursing.* 2005;35(8): 44–47.
30. Robert Wood Johnson University Hospital. *Advanced heart failure and transplant cardiology program.* 2008. Available at http://www.rwjuh.edu/medical_services/heart_failure_transplant.html. Accessed January 30, 2008.
31. Gersh BJ, Maron BJ, Bonow RO, et al. 2011 ACCF/AHA Guideline for the Diagnosis and Treatment of Hypertrophic Cardiomyopathy: a report of the American College of Cardiology Foundation/American Heart

Association Task Force on Practice Guidelines. Developed in collaboration with the American Association for Thoracic Surgery, American Society of Echocardiography, American Society of Nuclear Cardiology, Heart Failure Society of America, Heart Rhythm Society, Society for Cardiovascular Angiography and Interventions, and Society of Thoracic Surgeons. *J Am Coll Cardiol.* 2011;58(25):e212–e260. Available at https://www.ncbi.nlm.nih.gov/pubmed/22075469

32. Ommen SR, Linderbaum JA, Rhodes DJ. *Ask Mayo expert. Hypertrophic cardiomyopathy*. 2018. Available at http://www.askmayo expert.mayoclinic.org
33. Nishimura RA, Holmes DR Jr. Clinical practice. Hypertrophic obstructive cardiomyopathy. *N Engl J Med.* 2004;350(13):1320–1327.
34. Elliott P, McKenna WJ. Hypertrophic cardiomyopathy. *Lancet.* 2004; 363(9424):1881–1891.
35. Jurynec J. Hypertrophic cardiomyopathy: a review of etiology and treatment. *J Cardiovasc Nurs.* 2007;22(1):65–73.
36. Maron BJ, Ackerman MJ, Nishimura RA, et al. Task Force 4: HCM and other cardiomyopathies, mitral valve prolapse, myocarditis, and Marfan syndrome. *J Am Coll Cardiol.* 2005;45(8):1340–1345.
37. Hanson E, Jakobs P, Keegan H, et al. Cardiac troponin T lysine 210 deletion in a family with dilated cardiomyopathy. *J Card Fail.* 2002;8: 28–32.
38. Li D, Czernuszewicz GZ, Gonazalez O, et al. Novel cardiac troponin T mutation as a cause of familial dilated cardiomyopathy. *Circulation.* 2001;104:2188–2193.
39. Frenneaux MP. Assessing the risk of sudden cardiac death in a patient with hypertrophic cardiomyopathy. *Heart.* 2004;90(5):570–575.
40. Sherrid MV. Pathophysiology and treatment of hypertrophic cardiomyopathy. *Prog Cardiovasc Dis.* 2006;49(2):123–151.
41. Ho CY, Seidman CE. A contemporary approach to hypertrophic cardiomyopathy. *Circulation.* 2006;113:e858–e862.
42. Olivotto I, Ommen SR, Maron MS, et al. Surgical myectomy versus alcohol septal ablation for obstructive hypertrophic cardiomyopathy. Will there ever be a randomized trial? *J Am Coll Cardiol.* 2007;50(9): 831–834.
43. Seth S, Thatai D, Sharma S, et al. Clinico-pathological evaluation of restrictive cardiomyopathy (endomyocardial fibrosis and idiopathic restrictive cardiomyopathy) in India. *Eur J Heart Fail.* 2004;6(6):723–729.
44. Hassam W, Fawzy M, Helaly S, et al. Pitfalls in diagnosis and clinical, echocardiographic, and hemodynamic findings in endomyocardial fibrosis. *Chest.* 2005;128(6):3985–3992.
45. Goldstein JA. Cardiac tamponade, constrictive pericarditis, and restrictive cardiomyopathy. *Curr Probl Cardiol.* 2004;29(9):503–567.
46. Ask Mayo Expert. *Idiopathic restrictive cardiomyopathy*. 2019. Available at http://www.askmayo expert.mayoclinic.org
47. Ask Mayo Expert. *Arrhythmogenic right ventricular cardiomyopathy*. 2018. Available at http://www.askmayo expert.mayoclinic.org
48. Tandri H, Saranathan M, Rodriguez ER, et al. Noninvasive detection of myocardial fibrosis in arrhythmogenic right ventricular cardiomyopathy using delayed-enhancement magnetic resonance imaging. *J Am Coll Cardiol.* 2005;45(1):98–103.
49. Ask Mayo Expert. *Left ventricular noncompaction*. 2018. Available at http://www.askmayo expert.mayoclinic.org
50. Ask Mayo Expert. *Apical ballooning syndrome*. 2018. Available at http://www.askmayo expert.mayoclinic.org
51. Paur H, Wright PT, Sikkel MB, et al. High levels of circulating epinephrine trigger apical cardiodepression in a β2-adrengeric receptor/Gi-dependent manner: a new model of Takotsubo cardiomyopathy. *Circulation.* 2012;126:697–706.
52. Wittstein IS, Thiemann DR, Lima JA, et al. Neurohormonal features of myocardial stunning due to sudden emotional stress. *N Engl J Med.* 2005;352:539–548.
53. Chen H, Zhang W, Li D, et al. Analysis of ventricular hypertrabeculation and noncompaction using genetically engineered mouse models. *Paediatr Cardiol.* 2009;30:626–634.
54. Bybee KA, Kara T, Prasad A, et al. Systemic reviews: transient left ventricular apical ballooning: a syndrome that mimics ST-segment elevation myocardial infarction. *Intern Med.* 2004;141:858.
55. Prasad A, Lerman A, Rihal CS. Apical ballooning syndrome: a mimic of acute myocardial infarction. *Am Heart J.* 2008;155:408–417.
56. Magnani JW, Dec GW. Myocarditis: current trends in diagnosis and treatment. *Circulation.* 2006;113(6):876–890.
57. Ask Mayo Expert. *Mayocarditis*. 2018. Available at http://www.askmayo expert.mayoclinic.org
58. Bashore T, Cabell CH, Fowler V. Update on infective endocarditis. *Curr Probl Cardiol.* 2006;31:274–352.
59. Baddour LM, Wilson WR, Bayer AS, et al. Infective endocarditis in adults: diagnosis, antimicrobial therapy, and management of complications: a scientific statement for healthcare professionals from the American Heart Association. *Circulation.* 2015;132:1435–1486.
60. Habib G, Lancellotti P, Antunes MJ, et al. 2015 ESC guidelines for the management of infective endocarditis: the Task Force for the management of infective endocarditis of the European Society of Cardiology (ESC). Endorsed by: European Association for Cardio-Thoracic Surgery (ACTS), the European Association of Nuclear Medicine (EANM). *Eur Heart J.* 2015;36:3075–3128.
61. Tleyjeh IM, Abdel-Latif A, Rahbi H, et al. A systematic review of population-based studies of infective endocarditis. *Chest.* 2007;132:1025.
62. Fowler VG Jr, Miro JM, Hoen B, et al. Staphylococcus aureus endocarditis: a consequence of medical progress. *JAMA.* 2005;293:3012–3021.
63. Selton-Suty C, Célard M, Le Moing V, et al. Preeminence of Staphylococcus aureus in infective endocarditis: a 1-year population-based survey. *Clin Infect Dis.* 2012;54:1230–1239.
64. Cahill TJ, Prendergast BD. Infective endocarditis. *Lancet.* 2016;387: 882–893.
65. Hill EE, Herijgers P, Claus P, et al. Infective endocarditis: changing epidemiology and predictors of 6-month mortality: a prospective cohort study. *Eur Heart J.* 2007;28:196–203.
66. Cantrell M, Yoshikawa TT. Infective endocarditis in the aging patient. *Gerontology.* 1984;30:316–326.
67. Durante-Mangoni E, Bradley S, Selton-Suty C, et al. Current features of infective endocarditis in elderly patients: results of the International Collaboration on Endocarditis Prospective Cohort Study. *Arch Intern Med.* 2008;168:2095–2103.
68. Castillo FJ, Anguita M, Castillo JC, et al. Changes in clinical profile, epidemiology and prognosis of left-sided native-valve infective endocarditis without predisposing heart conditions. *Rev Esp Cardiol (Engl Ed).* 2015;68:445–448.
69. Lerner PI, Weinstein L. Infective endocarditis in the antibiotic era. *N Engl J Med.* 1966;274:199–206.
70. Watanakunakorn C. Changing epidemiology and newer aspects of infective endocarditis. *Adv Intern Med.* 1977;22:21–47.
71. Durack DT, Lukes AS, Bright DK. New criteria for diagnosis of infective endocarditis: utilization of specific echocardiographic findings. Duke Endocarditis Service. *Am J Med.* 1994;96:200–209.
72. Prendergast BD. Diagnostic criteria and problems in infective endocarditis. *Heart.* 2004;90:611–613.
73. Ask Mayo Expert. *Infective endocarditis*. 2018. Available at https://askmayoexpert.mayoclinic.org/topic/clinical-answers/gnt-20152237/sec-20137142
74. Nishimura RA, Ottow CM, Bonow RO, et al. 2014 AHA/ACC guideline for the management of patients with valvular heart disease: a report of the American College of Cardiology/American Heart Association Task Force on Practice Guidelines. *J Am Coll Cardiol.* 2014;63:E57–E185.
75. Adler Y, Charron P, Imazio M; ESC Scientific Document Group. 2015 ESC Guidelines for the diagnosis and management of pericardial diseases: The Task Force for the Diagnosis and Management of Pericardial Diseases of the European Society of Cardiology (ESC) Endorsed by: The European Association for Cardio-Thoracic Surgery (EACTS). *Eur Heart J.* 2015;36(42):2921–2964.

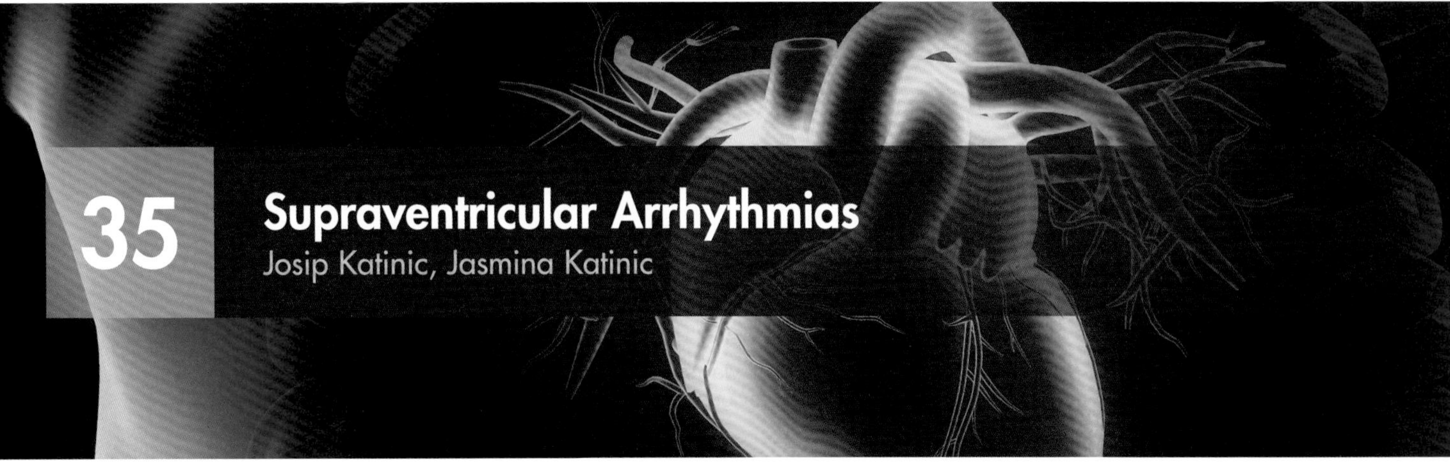

35 Supraventricular Arrhythmias

Josip Katinic, Jasmina Katinic

OBJECTIVES

1. Understand the mechanism of normal impulse initiation.
2. Describe the difference in mechanism of supraventricular arrhythmias.
3. Describe the diagnosis and medical management of supraventricular arrhythmias.
4. Utilize the current guidelines for management of supraventricular arrhythmias.

KEY QUESTIONS

1. What cardiac rhythms are classified as supraventricular arrhythmias?
2. What are the most common symptoms associated with supraventricular tachycardia (SVT) and how is it diagnosed?
3. What are the three types of reentrant tachycardias and how do they differ in pathogenesis?
4. What is the difference between atrial flutter and atrial fibrillation (AF)?
5. What is the role of the cardiac nurse in the care of patients with these arrhythmias?

BACKGROUND

The field of cardiac electrophysiology changed significantly with the development of the electrocardiogram (ECG) in the beginning of the 20th century. Development of intracavitary recording and ability to record bundle of His ECGs with program stimulation of the heart in late 1960s has marked the beginning of the modern clinical electrophysiology. Over the last three decades, the development of intracardiac mapping, programmed stimulation, and radiofrequency catheter-ablation techniques have enabled interventional cardiac electrophysiologists to treat variety of arrhythmias.[1] The supraventricular tachycardia (SVT) is a general term for group of arrhythmias, which arise from or involve at least some part in atria or atrioventricular (AV) junction.[2] The SVTs are a common form of arrhythmias frequently seen in emergency departments. In the United States, the most common subtypes of SVTs are atrial fibrillation (AF) and atrial flutter affecting well over two million patients. These numbers have incrementally risen higher in recent years. Most recent surveys suggest that an estimated 2.7 to 6.1 million of people in the United States are suffering from AF.[3] The incidence of SVT is estimated at 35 cases per 100,000 patient.[2] The other subtypes of SVT (e.g., atrioventricular nodal reentrant tachycardia [AVRNT]) account for approximately 60%, and the other two subtypes of SVT, atrioventricular reentrant tachycardia (AVRT) and atrial tachycardia (AT), account for approximately 30% and 10%, respectively.[2] The other uncommon mechanisms of SVT include sinus node reentry, junctional ectopic tachycardia, intrahisian reentry, and nodoventricular or nodal fascicular reentrant tachycardias.[4] This chapter aims to review the pathophysiology, types, diagnosis, and management of supraventricular arrhythmias.

PATHOPHYSIOLOGY

Cardiac arrhythmias result from abnormalities of electrical impulses due to degeneration, abnormalities of conduction, or both.[1] The most common mechanism responsible for majority of SVTs is *reentry*. This mechanism requires two distinct pathways with two different speeds of conduction (slow and fast) and varying refractory times and it may be based on anatomic, functional, or a combination of both abnormalities, which is required for sustained reentry. Oftentimes early or extra beats such as premature atrial or ventricular contractions (PACs or PVCs), may fail to conduct down the normal pathway (fast to conduct and slow to recover), although they can travel down the fast recovering and slow conducting pathway.[5] Because the slow pathway has a longer conduction time, and by the time the depolarization travels to the slow pathway and arrives at the compact AV junction, the fast pathway may have recovered excitability, so that depolarization travels in a retrograde manner through the fast pathway and back down to the slow pathway (see Fig. 35-1). If this reentry process continues, a sustained tachycardia occurs.[4] The enhanced impulse formation may be due to the enhanced phase 4 automaticity in normal or abnormal cells (abnormal automaticity) or due to the triggered activity. Tachycardias that are due to enhanced automaticity, either normal or abnormal, can neither predictively be initiated nor terminated by electrical stimulation.[6]

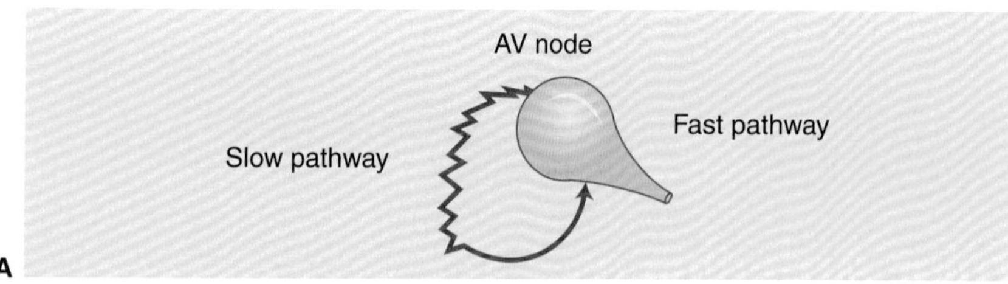

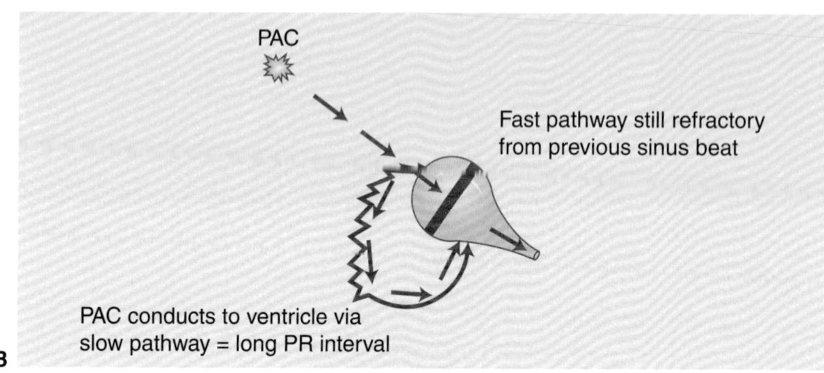

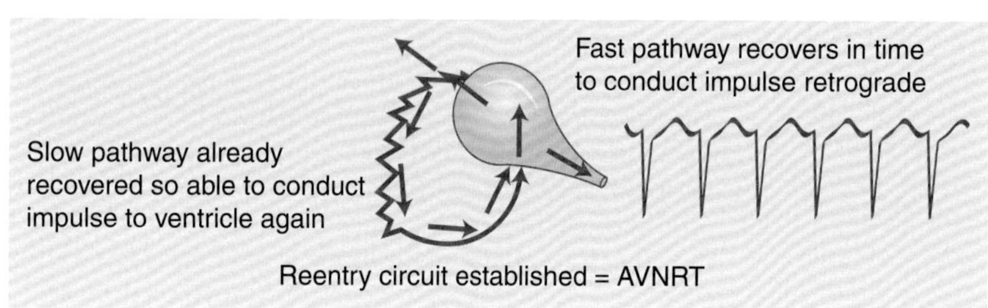

Figure 35-1. Mechanism of AVNRT. **A:** The dual AV nodal pathways responsible for AVNRT. The normal AV node is the fast conducting pathway with a long refractory period; the slow conducting pathway lies outside the AV node and has a shorter refractory period. **B:** A PAC finds the fast pathway still refractory but is able to conduct through the slow pathway. **C:** When the impulse arrives at the end of the slow pathway it finds the AV node recovered and ready to conduct retrograde to the atria. The slow pathway has already recovered due to its short refractory period and is able to conduct the same impulse back into the ventricle. This sets up the reentry circuit and causes AVNRT.

Mechanism of Normal Impulse Initiation

Automaticity is the ability of certain cardiac cells to spontaneously depolarize and initiate an electrical impulse without external stimulation. Knowledge of normal anatomy and physiology of the cardiac conduction system is critical to understanding normal automaticity before considering other mechanisms.

The impulse is transmitted slowly through nodal tissue to the anatomically complex atria where it is then conducted more rapidly to the atrioventricular node (AVN), inscribed on the ECG as the P wave. After a perceptible delay in conduction through the AVN the time needed for activation of the atria and the AVN delay is represented as the PR interval on the ECG. The electrical impulse that emerges from the AVN is transmitted to the His–Purkinje system and more specifically the common bundle of His, then the left and right bundle branches, and finally to the Purkinje network facilitating activation of ventricular muscle. The ventricles are activated rapidly in well-defined fashion as determined by the course of the Purkinje network, representing the QRS complex on the ECG. The recovery of electrical excitability occurs more slowly and it is dependent upon the time of activation and duration of regional action potential. The duration of epicardial extra potentials in the ventricle result in repolarization that occurs first on the epicardial surface and then proceeds to the endocardium which inscribes the T wave on the ECG. The duration of activation recovery, however, is determined by the action potential duration, and represented on the ECG as the QT interval.[1]

The sinoatrial (SA) node, located at the junction of right atrium and superior vena cava, is normally the site of impulse generation. The large P cells are thought to be origin of the electrical impulses in the SA node, which is surrounded by transitional cells and fiber tract extending through the perinodal area into the right atrium proper. Other cells in the heart also have the property of automaticity, including cells in several areas of the atria, coronary sinus, pulmonary veins, AV junction, AV valves, and Purkinje system. The rates of these other pacemakers are slower than the rate of the SA node; therefore, they are suppressed by the SA node under normal conditions, a phenomenon known as overdrive suppression. The site of fastest impulse initiation is commonly referred to the dominant pacemaker, whereas sites of impulse formation that are suppressed by the dominant site are subsidiary or latent pacemakers.

Alteration of Normal Impulse Initiation

Abnormal impulse initiation can be due to enhanced normal automaticity, abnormal automaticity, or afterdepolarizations. Atrial and ventricular myocardial cells that do not normally have automaticity can develop abnormal automaticity when their transient receptor potential (TRP) is reduced and is referred to as depolarization-induced automaticity.[6] Subsidiary pacemakers like those in the Purkinje system that are normally overdrive suppressed by the faster SA node can also develop abnormal automaticity when their TRP is reduced. This abnormal automaticity is thought to be mediated by the slow inward current carried mainly by calcium (slow channels) because the normal fast sodium channels are inactivated at reduced membrane potentials.[7,8] However, both sodium and calcium channels play a role in the development of abnormal automaticity. Abnormal automaticity that develops at more negative diastolic potentials, between −70 and −50 mV, can be suppressed by sodium channel blockers, indicating that a sodium current is involved, whereas automaticity that develops at less negative diastolic potentials, from −50 to −30 mV, can be suppressed by calcium channel blockers.[9]

The resting potential of a cell can be reduced (e.g., from −90 to −70 mV) and the cell partially depolarized by anything that increases the extracellular potassium concentration, decreases the intracellular potassium concentration, increases the permeability of the membrane to sodium, or decreases the membrane permeability to potassium.[7–9] Ischemia, hypoxia, acidosis, hyperkalemia, digitalis toxicity, chamber enlargement or dilation, stretch, and other metabolic abnormalities or drugs can reduce the resting potential and result in abnormal automaticity. Hypoxia and ischemia affect the TRP by decreasing the amount of oxygen available to supply adenosine triphosphate in amounts sufficient to operate the sodium–potassium pump efficiently. Anything that interferes with proper operation of this pump, such as digitalis, reduces normal resting ionic gradients across the cell membrane and results in reduction of the resting potential. When the TRP is reduced at rest, the cell is partially depolarized and the time required for spontaneous diastolic depolarization to reach threshold is reduced, thus increasing pacemaker activity. For the same reason, automaticity is increased when the threshold potential is reduced (e.g., from −40 to −50 mV) by ischemia or drug effects because less time is required for phase 4 depolarization to reach the lower threshold. The rate of phase 4 depolarization can be increased by several factors, including local norepinephrine release at ischemic sites, systemic catecholamine release, reduced vagal tone, and drugs.

Triggered Activity due to the Afterdepolarization

Triggered automaticity or activity refers to impulses' initiation that is dependent on afterdepolarization. Afterdepolarizations are membrane voltage oscillation that occur during (early afterdepolarization, EAD), or after (delayed afterdepolarization, DAD) an action potential.

EADs occur during the action potential and interrupt the orderly repolarization off the myocyte. It was once though that EADs arise from action potential prolongation and reactivation of the depolarizing current, but more recent experimental evidence suggested previously unappreciated interrelationship between intracellular calcium loading and EADs. Cytosolic calcium may increase when action potentials are prolonged, and in turn appears to enhance L-type calcium current thus further prolonging action potential duration. Intracellular calcium loading by action potential prolongation may also enhance the likelihood of DADs.[7–9]

EAD-triggered arrhythmias exhibit rate dependence and in general the amplitude of an EADs is augmented at slow rates when action potentials are longer thereby a fundamental condition that underlies development of the EADs is action potential and QT prolongation. The EADs are often caused by conditions that delay repolarization of the action potential and frequently occur in the presence of hypokalemia, hypomagnesemia, hypothermia, bradycardia catecholamines, and many drugs. Gene mutations that alter sodium and potassium ion channel activity and result in prolonged action potential duration have been identified and shown to cause EADs. The antiarrhythmics medicine class IA and III produce action potential and QT prolongation but also frequently causing arrhythmias. Other noncardiac medicines such as nonsedating antihistamines, certain antibiotics, and phenothiazines may also prolong action potential duration and predispose to EAD-mediated trigger arrhythmias.[7–9]

The presence of increase calcium load in the cytosol and sarcoplasmic reticulum is a common cellular feature inducing a DAD. The DAD begins during late phase 4 and beginning of phase 4, after the membrane has repolarized to its original level after an action potential but before the next propagated impulse. Subthreshold afterdepolarizations do not result in triggered activity, although if the DAD is large enough to reach threshold, a triggered impulse arises, which may also be followed by its own afterdepolarization, thus leading to triggered beats. This mechanism of DAD is poorly understood however factors that could increase DAD amplitude and contribute to triggered arrhythmias include high concentrations of catecholamines, digitalis toxicity, and hypokalemia.[7–9] The triggered impulse can lead to series of rapid depolarizations and subsequently development of the accelerated junctional rhythm, atrial tachyarrhythmia, idiopathic VT originating in the right ventricular outflow tract (RVOT), accelerated idioventricular rhythm after MI, and tachycardias originating in the coronary sinus.

Mechanism of Reentry Tachycardias

The most common arrhythmia mechanism is reentry and defined as circulation of an activation wave around the inexcitable obstacle. This mechanism is also the most important because reentrant tachyarrhythmias are common cause of death in thousands of people every year. Classification as a reentrant mechanism requires that two of the following criteria are met: (1) An anatomic circuit must be present in which two portions of the circuit (pathways) have electrophysiologic properties that differ from one another in critical way and (2) an area of unidirectional block is necessary to allow an impulse to conduct in one direction and to provide a return pathway by which the original stimulus can reenter a previously depolarized area.[10] Conduction velocity in the normal unblocked pathway must be slow enough relative to the refractory period of blocked pathway to allow recovery of the stimulated area to recover its ability to conduct in a retrograde direction. Previously blocked pathway must be slow enough and conducted in retrograde fashion to allow normal pathway to recover and again be capable being excited.[10]

Reentrant tachycardias can be divided in two different forms, anatomic or functional, based upon type of anatomical substrate used for the development of the arrhythmia. Anatomic reentry requires anatomic obstacle such as area of fibrosis in which the circulating wave of depolarization can travel. A tachycardia is initiated when depolarization wave splits into two limbs after going around obstacle creating the circus movement.[11] The common examples of anatomic reentry are SVT (associated with accessory pathway pre-excitation syndrome), AVNRT, and typical right atrial flutter, ventricular tachycardia originating within His–Purkinje system or around an area of infarcted tissue (scar-mediated arrhythmia).

Functional reentry does not require an anatomical obstacle but it depends upon intrinsic factors of electrophysiology properties of cardiac muscle fibers such as dispersion of excitability or refractoriness to allow for functional circuits. The atypical atrial flutter in some cases of AF and VT in structurally normal heart, are examples of functional reentry.[11] Leading circle concept of functional reentry involves the propagation of impulse around the functionally determined region of unexcitable tissue or refractory core.

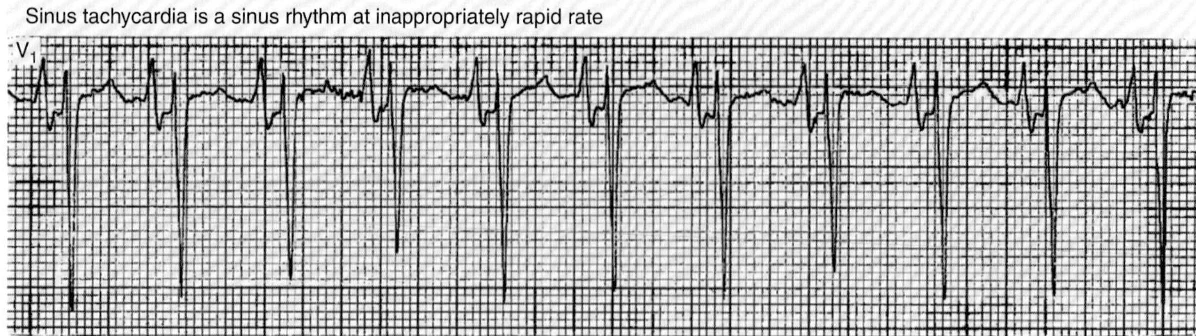

Figure 35-2. Sinus tachycardia.

TYPES OF SUPRAVENTRICULAR ARRHYTHMIA

There are several types of supraventricular arrhythmia. The term paroxysmal supraventricular tachycardia (PSVT) is applied to subset of narrow QRS complex tachycardias. In contrast to PSVTs, AF, atrial flutter, and multifocal atrial tachycardia (MAT) have an irregular ventricular response and they are distinctly different. Examples of ECGs and cardiac rhythm recordings (i.e., "strips") may be referenced in the titular chapter.

Sinus Tachycardia

Sinus tachycardia is a rhythm in which the rate of impulses arising from SA node is elevated. Historically heart rate 60 to 100 beats per minute (bpm) is considered normal sinus rhythm and rates exceeding 100 bpm is defined as sinus tachycardia. The ECG demonstrates a normal-appearing P-wave axis, however occurring at rates greater than 100 bpm. It is important to distinguish sinus tachycardia from other forms of SVT. The P wave is upright in leads II, III and aVF and negative in lead aVR (see Fig. 35-2). Sinus tachycardia can be normal or appropriate response to physiologic stress, anxiety, or fever. Some pathologic conditions such as anemia, hypotension, and thyrotoxicosis could produce sinus tachycardia. The treatment is directed toward underlying condition and pharmacologic therapy with beta-blocker medicine is often used to help minimize the symptoms.[1]

Inappropriate Sinus Tachycardia

Inappropriate sinus tachycardia represents an uncommon medical condition in which heart rate increases spontaneously. It is defined with a resting heart rate greater than 100 bpm. Also called chronic nonparoxysmal sinus tachycardia, it often occurs in an individual without heart disease or secondary causes. The range of observed symptoms often includes dizziness, near syncope, palpitations, chest pain, headaches, and gastrointestinal upset. The features of the P-wave axis and morphology on the ECG are identical to sinus rhythm/sinus tachycardia. The pathophysiology is poorly understood, although the history and physical examination, ECG, and Holter monitor study are helpful in patient evaluation.

Atrial Tachycardia

AT is a less frequently seen type of SVT, comprising a group of atrial arrhythmias including microreentrant AT, right AT, and left AT.[2] Its mechanism may be due to abnormal automaticity, triggered activity, or reentry particularly in patients with scarred atrial myocardium.[4] The AT typically originates in the right atrium along the Crista terminalis or in left atrium.[4] This is a rapid atrial rhythm occurring at a rate of 100 to 250 bpm often arising from a single site within the right or left atrium. This rhythm may be due to rapid firing of an ectopic atrial focus (automaticity), an atrial microreentry circuit that allows an impulse to travel rapidly and repeatedly around a pathway in the atria, or to afterdepolarizations resulting in a triggered AT (see Fig. 35-3).[12–15] Incessant AT is less common and typically lasts for more than half a day, sometimes being present more than 90% of the time.[15] AT has been associated with caffeine, tobacco, alcohol, mitral valve disease, rheumatic heart disease, chronic obstructive pulmonary disease (COPD), acute MI, theophylline administration, electrolyte disturbance, and digitalis toxicity.

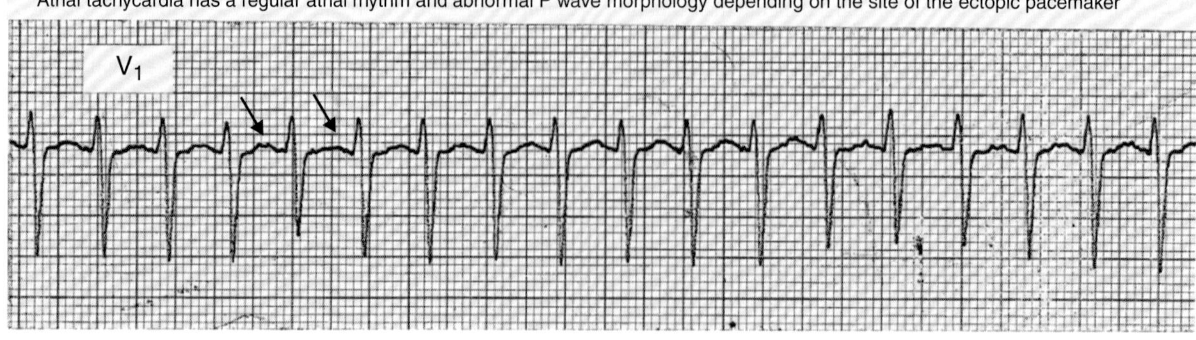

Figure 35-3. Atrial tachycardia.

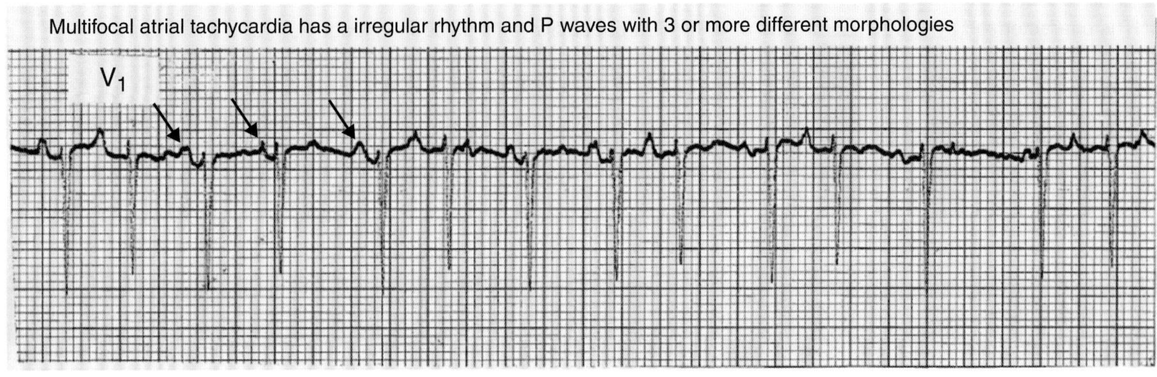

Figure 35-4. Multifocal atrial tachycardia.

Multifocal Atrial Tachycardia

MAT is type of cardiac arrhythmia that often occurs in patients in chronic pulmonary disease and elderly patients. This rhythm is characterized by at least three morphologically distinct P waves and at least three different PR intervals. The atrial and ventricular rates both are typically ranging from 100 to 150 bpm (see Fig. 35-4). The mechanism of MAT is not well understood; however, electrolyte imbalance and DAD leading to the triggered automaticity could result in development of arrhythmia. As previously mentioned a wide range of underlying diseases are associated with development of MAT such as COPD, heart disease, diabetes, hypomagnesemia, sepsis, hypokalemia, and methylxanthine toxicity. The common symptoms may include shortness of breath, light-headedness, dizziness, chest pain, syncope, and palpitations. Physical examination, electrocardiography, laboratory studies (e.g., chemistry panel, arterial blood gases), and chest x-ray are helpful in the evaluation of underlying medical conditions that contribute to the development of this arrhythmia. Acute treatment is directed toward the underlying cardiopulmonary process. Pharmacologic choices of treatment include calcium channel blockers such as diltiazem or verapamil, and beta blockers such as metoprolol and esmolol. Antiarrhythmic agents such as amiodarone or flecainide may be used. Before considering antiarrhythmic medications, patients should be screened for significant ventricular dysfunction or coronary artery disease. The prevention of MAT consists of monitoring electrolyte disturbances, and preventing respiratory failure.[16]

Sinoatrial Nodal Reentrant Tachycardia

Sinoatrial nodal reentrant tachycardia (SANRT) is a form of AT. Its activation sequence is similar to that of normal sinus rhythm and P waves on ECG appears to be normal (see Fig. 35-5). The exact mechanism of SANRT is unknown although it may involve reentry occurring within the SA node and perinodal tissue. This type of arrhythmia is uncommon, primarily seen in adults and children with structural heart disease. Atrial premature beats and atrial pacing are also known to initiate SANRT. Patients are largely asymptomatic although common symptoms range from palpitation to light-headedness and in rare cases syncope. Physical examination reveals the presence of a regular but rapid pulse. ECG will show P wave with rates between 100 and 150 bpm. This type of arrhythmia is commonly misdiagnosed with inappropriate sinus tachycardia and the surface ECG alone is not reliable in distinguishing this type of arrhythmia from other types of SVT. The electrophysiology study can be performed to confirm the diagnosis. Vagal maneuver are generally considered helpful and often result in termination of arrhythmia. Treatment is directed toward symptom relief and prevention of long-term sequelae such as tachycardia-mediated cardiomyopathy. Chronic suppressive therapy with pharmacologic agents (e.g., verapamil, amiodarone) had had some success although catheter ablation has been treatment of choice for chronic management.[17]

Atrioventricular Nodal Reentrant Tachycardia

AVNRT is most commonly seen in women, with a female-to-male gender ratio of 2:1. This subtype of PSVT may occur at any age however most commonly manifests itself during the fourth and fifth decades of life. This rhythm is caused by the reentrant mechanism (fast and slow) risk previously described.[4] On examination, neck pulsations are usually felt because of the simultaneous atrial and ventricular contraction. A "frog sign" (characteristic flapping or bulging appearance of the neck vein) may be identified. Because the fast pathway has a rapid conduction velocity, ventricular atrial conduction time during typical AVRNT is very short. Thus, on the ECG retrograde P waves may be buried within the QRS complexes and not visible or only partially visible at the end of the QRS complex. P waves are typically inverted in the inferior leads (II, III, aVF) and may manifest as pseudo-S waves upright in V1 thus leading to the pseudo-R appearance (see Fig. 35-6). In contrary, in atypical form of AVRNT the fast pathways is utilized as antegrade limb and the slow pathway as the retrograde limb of the reentrant circuit thus

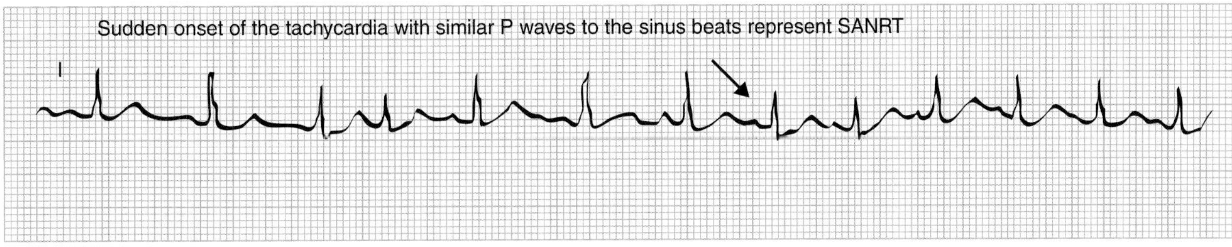

Figure 35-5. Sinoatrial nodal reentrant tachycardia.

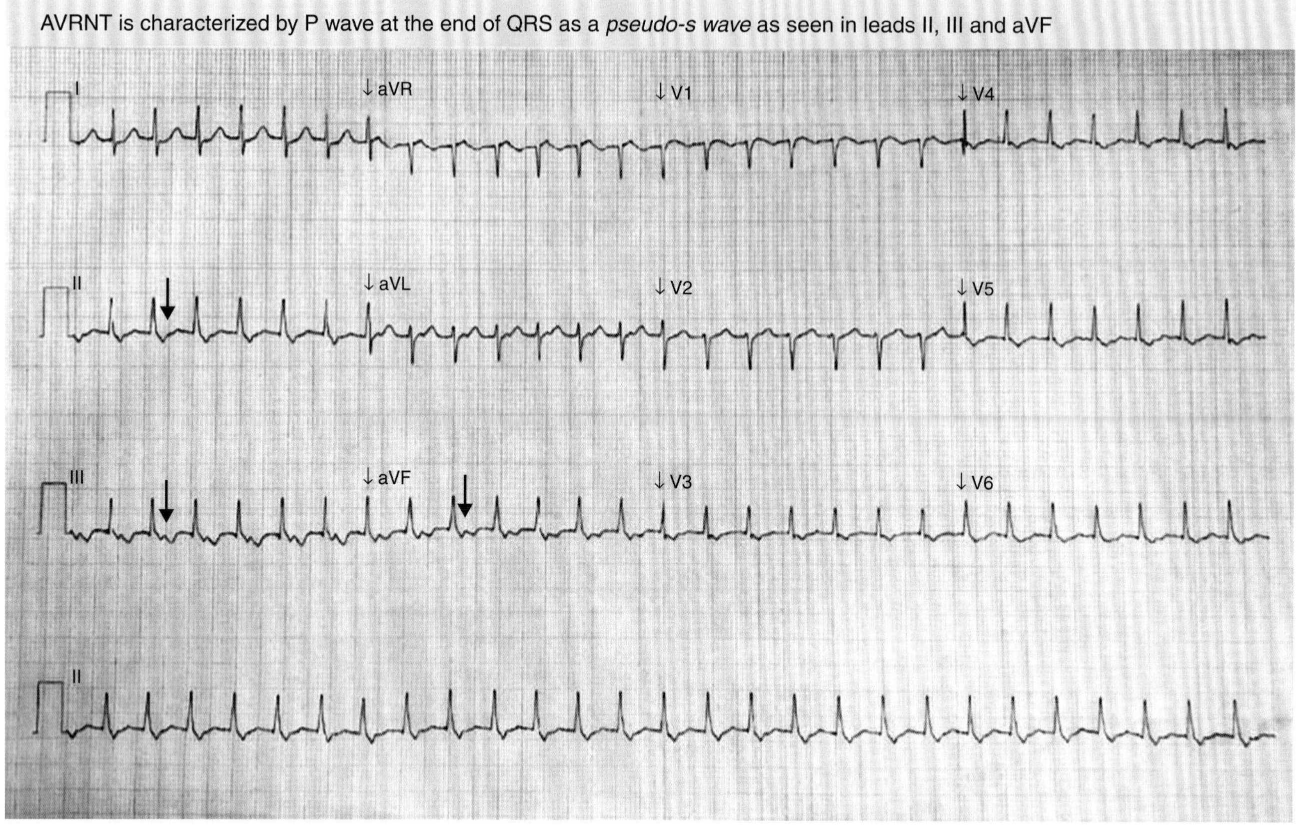

Figure 35-6. 12-lead ECG of AVRNT.

the ventriculoatrial conduction time is prolonged. The surface ECG demonstrates P waves in inferior leads and a long RP interval.[4]

Atrioventricular Reentrant Tachycardia

AVRT is a reentrant arrhythmia with two subcategories of orthodromic and antidromic variance. In orthodromic tachycardia, the antegrade limb is AV node (AVN)–His–Purkinje system and the retrograde limb is the accessory pathway. This subtype of tachycardia consists of 95% of spontaneously- and laboratory-induced AVRT.[5] The conducted impulses reach the ventricular insertion site of the accessory pathway, which may have regained excitability and may conduct in retrograde manner, thus initiating tachycardia.[4] In antidromic reciprocating tachycardia, it is a type of reentry circuit in which an accessory pathway is utilized as the antegrade limb and AVN–His–Purkinje system is utilized as the retrograde limb.[4]

AVRT and Wolff–Parkinson–White (WPW) syndrome have gained more interest in recent years because of their significant increase of morbidity and mortality. Patients with WPW pattern have a short PR interval and slurred upstroke of the QRS complex, better known as a delta wave (Fig. 35-7).[5] Accessory pathways that only conduct in the retrograde direction are called concealed accessory pathways, because no delta waves are present on ECG, whereas antegrade conduction over an accessory pathway leads to ventricular pre-excitation, with typical ECG manifestation of a short PR interval and delta waves (WPW pattern).[4]

Permanent Junctional Reciprocating Tachycardia

Permanent junctional reciprocating tachycardia (PJRT) is a type of orthodromic AVRT that mostly occurs in childhood but may also be seen in older adults. The typical heart rates ranges from 120 to 200 bpm with normal QRS duration. The ECG is characterized by long RP interval and negative P waves in leads II, III, and aVF. This rhythm is caused by an AV reentry using the AVN as antegrade limb and a slowly conducting accessory pathway as the retrograde limb. This arrhythmia commonly originates close to ostium of the coronary sinus.[18] Since this arrhythmia predominantly occurs in childhood, the definitive treatment of choice is radiofrequency catheter ablation of the accessory pathway.[19] Radiofrequency catheter ablation is also a first choice of treatment in adults, as the procedure is highly successful and rate of complications are low.[20]

Atrial Flutter

The macroreentrant arrhythmias involving atrial myocardium are collectively referred to as atrial flutter. The most common atrial flutter circuit rotates in a clockwise and counter-clockwise direction in the right atrium, in the periphery of the tricuspid valve annulus. The counter-clockwise right atrial flutter represents approximately 80% of all atrial flutter. The typical atrial flutter involves a microreentrant circuit of the cavotricuspid isthmus (CTI), a region of right atrial tissue between the orifice of inferior vena cava and tricuspid valve annulus. This type of atrial flutter is also called CTI-dependent atrial flutter and usually has counter-clockwise rotation. The right atrial or classic atrial flutter has a typical atrial rate of 260 to 300 bpm with 2:1 AV conduction at rate of 120 to 150 bpm. The ECG demonstrates sawtooth appearance of P wave in leads II, III, aVF, whereas clockwise atrial flutter produces positive P wave in II, III and aVF leads (Fig. 35-8).

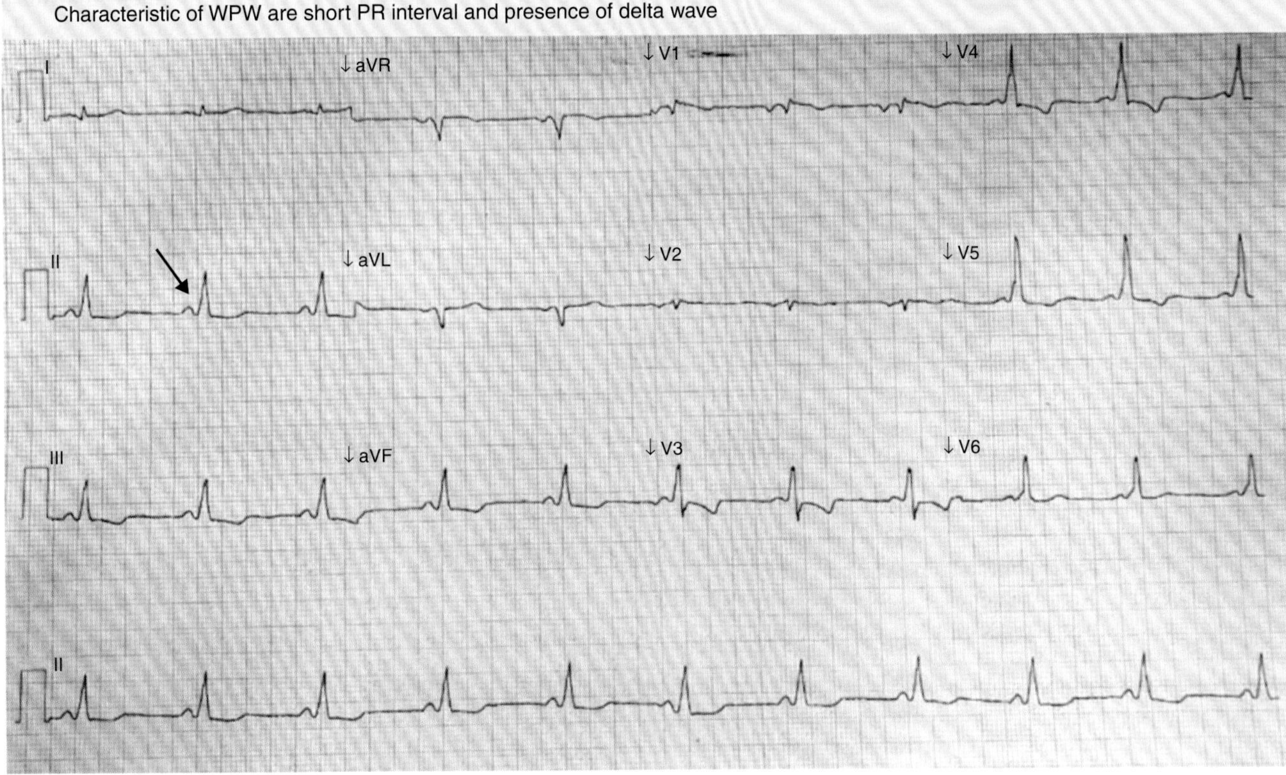

Figure 35-7. 12-lead ECG, Wolff–Parkinson–White.

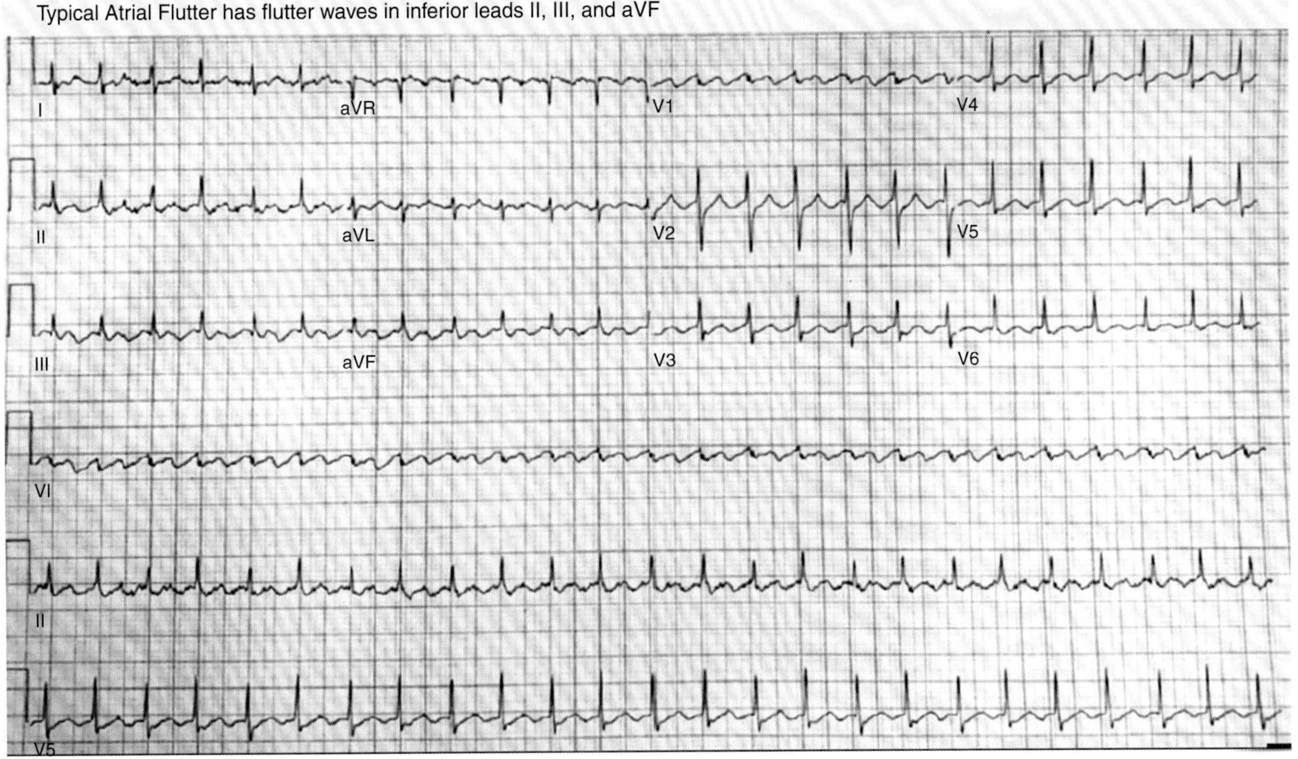

Figure 35-8. 12-lead atrial flutter, typical.

Atypical atrial flutter may evolve from regions of the right or left atria or scar tissue (e.g., status post ablation, Maze procedure, or surgical repair for congenital heart disease). This type of atrial flutter is often dependent on septal macroreentrant loops manifested by prominent voltage in lead V1 and the flat voltage in limb leads. It is important to understand that in patients who underwent a surgical or transcatheter procedures the surface ECG may be different from the typical findings seen in CTI-dependent atrial flutter (see Fig. 35-9).[21]

Atrial Fibrillation

AF is the most common sustained cardiac arrhythmia affecting estimated 2.7 to well over 6 million people in the United States and its prevalence increases with age. In general, the pathophysiology AF can be divided in three categories: triggers, substrate, and sustaining mechanisms.[22] The presence of underlying cardiac diseases such as structural heart disease underlies most cases of the AF. Recent genetic testing suggests that the region of chromosome 10 (10q22-q24) contains a gene responsible for AF in families in which arrhythmia is isolated as an autosomal dominant trait.[23] This is a disorganized, rapid, irregular atrial arrhythmia. It is known that foci of rapid ectopic activity are located in the left atrium, and pulmonary veins also play a role in the initiation of AF. The ventricular response is irregular with typical rates above 100 to 160 bpm and sometimes greater than 200 bpm in some patients (see Fig. 35-10). In contrast, in patients with heightened vagal tone or intrinsic AV nodal conduction defects, the rate may be less than 100 bpm and even profoundly slow.[1] The symptoms vary greatly among individual patients, however, most common include shortness of breath, palpitations, chest pain, syncope, dizziness, dyspnea, and profound fatigue. The mechanism of AF initiation is rather complex and includes drivers responsible for the initiation of AF and the complex anatomical substrate that promotes maintenance of multiple wavelets of (micro)reentry.[1]

DIAGNOSIS AND MANAGEMENT

Supraventricular Tachyarrhythmias

The SVTs can cause a plethora of symptoms ranging from palpitations, pulsation in the neck, chest pain, fatigue, light-headedness, dizziness, and dyspnea. Typically, SVTs have an abrupt onset and termination; however, its duration and symptoms depend on the mechanisms of the tachycardia and presence of underlying structural heart disease. In some patients paroxysmal supraventricular arrhythmias present with presyncope and syncope. The patient's symptoms may vary; thus, patient history is important to aid in uncovering the diagnosis, whereas the physical examination may not be as helpful.[24] A surface 12-lead ECG may be helpful in determining the mechanism of PSVT. The surface ECG shows heart rate greater than 100 bpm and narrow QRS complexes that are less than 120 milliseconds in duration. Approximately 20% of the cases mechanism of PSVT cannot be determined from surface ECG therefore an event recorder may be helpful to determine if SVTs are cause of patient's symptoms. The event recorder may range from 24 hours (i.e., a typical

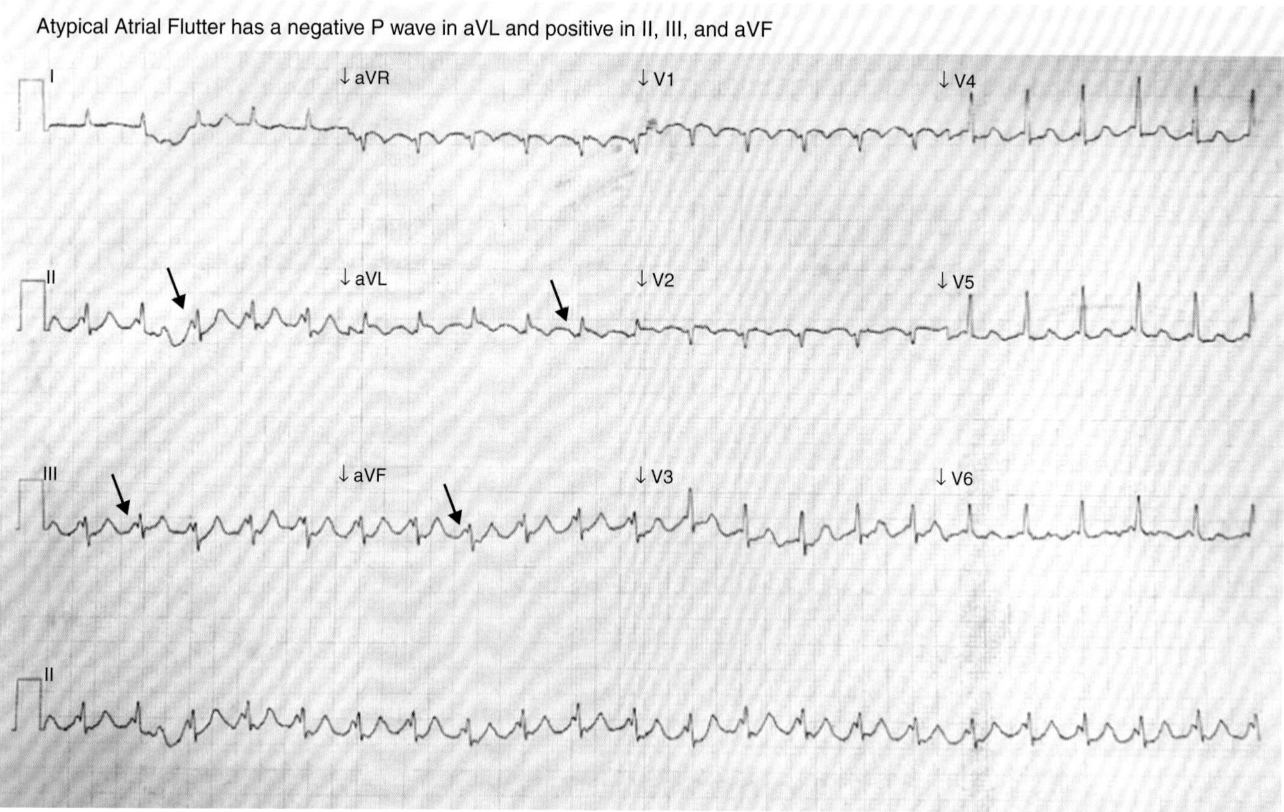

Figure 35-9. 12-lead ECG atrial flutter, atypical.

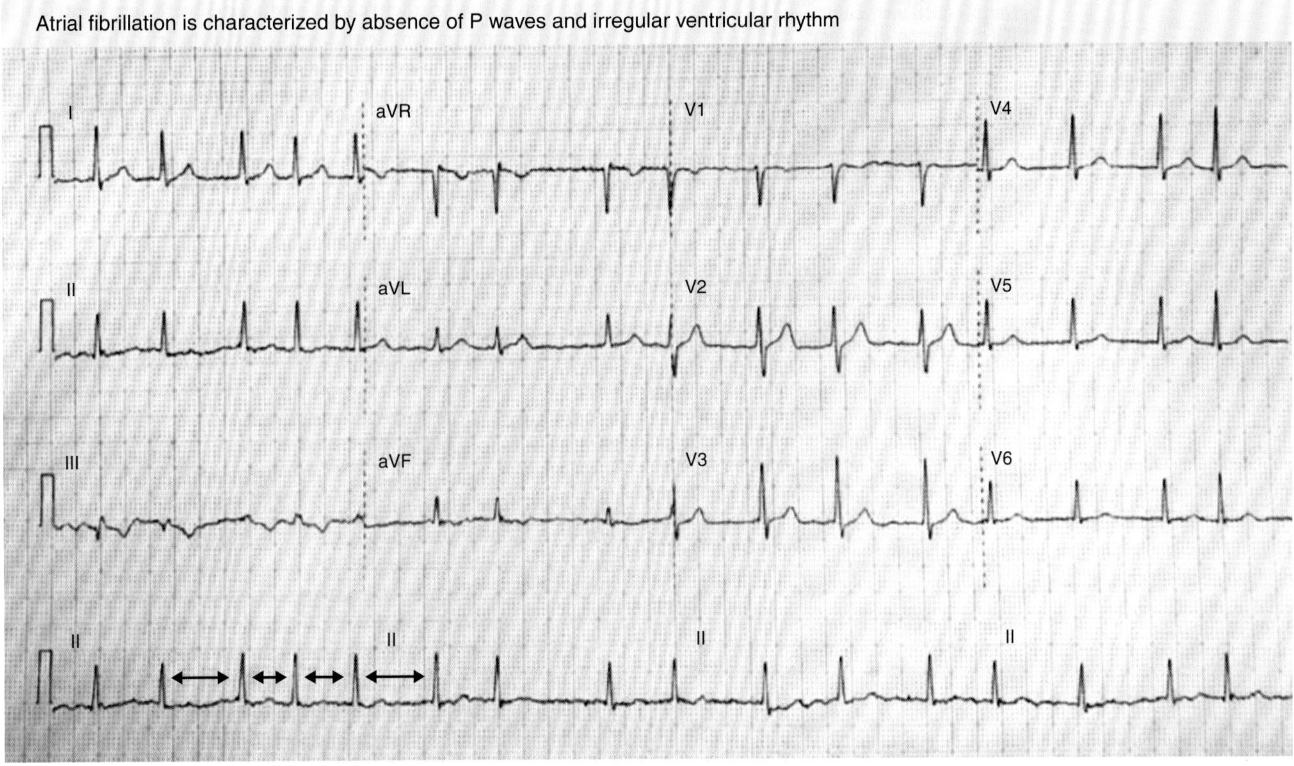

Figure 35-10. Atrial fibrillation.

Holter monitor) to up to 30 days. More recently implementing a minimally invasive procedure such as implanting a loop recorder device may be helpful. An invasive electrophysiology study remains a gold standard for determining mechanism of SVTs. Once the mechanism of SVT and diagnoses of the patient clinical arrhythmia is confirmed a radiofrequency catheter ablation can be performed.[4]

A 12-lead ECG obtained on a patient presenting with SVT may potentially identify the arrhythmia mechanism. If presenting tachycardia has a narrow QRS and has a regular rate, this may represent AT with 1:1 conduction or an SVT that involves AVN. In SVTs that involve the AVN such as AVRNT and AVRT, the retrograde conducted P wave may be difficult to detect. For patients presenting with narrow complex QRS tachycardia, differential diagnoses may be established by potentially identifying the arrhythmia mechanism (Fig. 35-11).[25]

The primary goal of treatment for any SVT is termination of arrhythmia especially in hemodynamically unstable patients who cannot tolerate prolonged tachyarrhythmia. The treatment is further subcategorized in two categories short-term or urgent management and long-term management. The short-term management can be further sub catheterized in two separate categories pharmacologic and nonpharmacologic strategies.[26] Acute treatment is directed toward altering conduction within the AVN. For acute conversion of SVTs carotid sinus massage (after absence of bruit has been confirmed by auscultation), vagal and Valsalva maneuvers can be performed quickly and should be first-line intervention to terminate SVTs.[27]

A pharmacologic strategy for acute management includes intravenous adenosine treatment 6 to 12 mg intravenously. Other intravenous medicine such as beta blockers and calcium channel blockers are considered a second-line treatment. The patients who are hemodynamically unstable with AVNRT and have failed both adenosine and vagal maneuvers may undergo synchronized electrical cardioversion using 100 to 200 J to terminate the arrhythmia. The goal of therapy is to promptly restore sinus rhythm in those patients who are hemodynamically unstable. In hemodynamically stable patients the pharmacologic treatment includes use of beta blockers and calcium channel blockers.[24] The long-term management of SVT is based on SVT type, frequency, and intensity of episode as well as overall impact of quality of life of the patient. The prophylactic pharmacologic therapy may include use of beta blockers (metoprolol, atenolol), calcium channel blockers (verapamil, diltiazem), and digoxin. These pharmacologic agents may be used as "pill in the pocket" strategy to help terminate the arrhythmia. A prophylactic phamacologic strategy may also be considered, including the use of class 1C or III antiarrhythmic agents (Table 35-1).[25] The further treatment considerations are based on significance of symptoms such as development of pre-excitation, syncope, or high-risk occupation and failed pharmacologic therapy. In those patients with recurrence of SVT electrophysiology testing with subsequent catheter ablation if indicated is recommended.

Atrial Flutter

Evaluation of atrial flutter typically involves performing a careful history and physical, ECG, and echocardiogram, and may include other studies such as an exercise stress test and a Holter monitor. In general, the diagnosis of atrial flutter is usually confirmed by observation characteristic patterns on the surface ECG. Most commonly reported symptoms may include dizziness, syncope, palpitations, fatigue, and dyspnea.

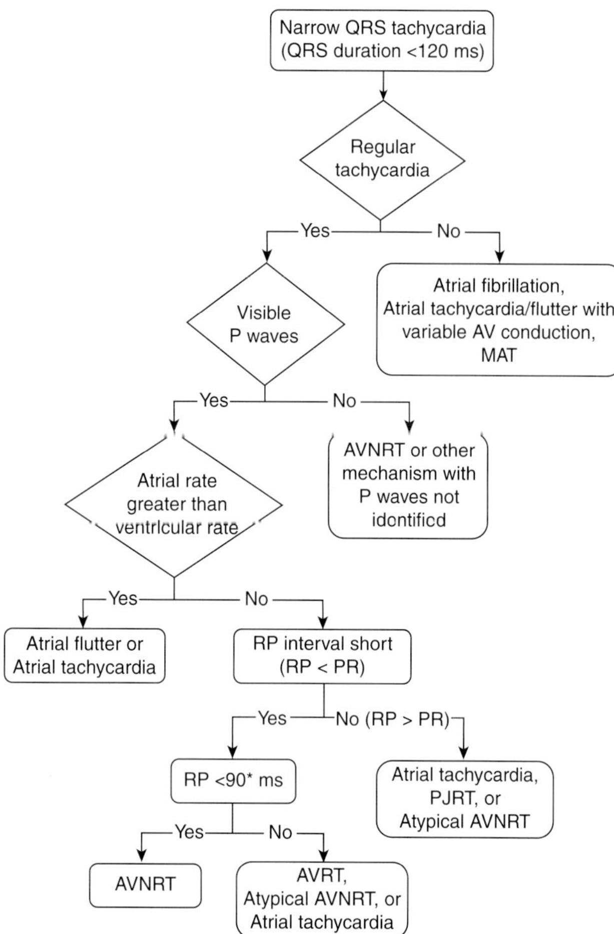

Figure 35-11. Differential diagnosis for adult narrow QRS tachycardia. Patients with junctional tachycardia may mimic the pattern of slow-fast AVNRT and may show AV dissociation and/or marked irregularity in the junctional rate. *RP refers to the interval from the onset of surface QRS to the onset of visible P wave. AV, atrioventricular; AVNRT, atrioventricular nodal reentrant tachycardia; AVRT, atrioventricular reentrant tachycardia; ECG, electrocardiogram; MAT, multifocal atrial tachycardia; PJRT, permanent form of junctional reentrant tachycardia.[27] (Adapted from Page RL, Joglar JA, Caldwell MA, et al. Correction to: 2015 ACC/AHA/HRS guideline for the management of adult patients with supraventricular tachycardia: executive summary: a Report of the American College of Cardiology/American Heart Association Task Force on clinical practice guidelines and the Heart Rhythm Society. *Circulation.* 2016;134[11]:e232–e233, used with permission from Elsevier, STM Signatory Guidelines http://www.stm-assoc.org/permissions-guidelines/)

The treatment of atrial flutter will depend on the symptoms and may involve a rate control strategy, pharmacologic therapy, anticoagulation therapy, electrical cardioversion, and catheter ablation. The rate control strategy may consist of a calcium channel blocker such as diltiazem or verapamil; beta blockers and/or digoxin may also be attempted. The risk of thromboembolic event is high; thereby anticoagulation is recommended (see Table 35-2 for summary of anticoagulation medications). If pharmacologic therapies are the only option in patients unsuitable for catheter ablation, the following antiarrhythmic agents may be used: ibutilide, sotalol, amiodarone, and procainamide. Patients with atrial flutter may develop tachycardia-induced severe left ventricular dysfunction and present with symptoms of heart failure. Antiarrhythmic agents such as ibutilide and sotalol carry the risk of QT prolongation and Torsades de Pointes. The definitive treatment option is catheter ablation.

Atrial Fibrillation

Diagnosis of AF involves a multimodality evaluation. A systematic review concluded that although pulse rate is 94% sensitive and 72% specific for diagnosis, AF is best confirmed by surface 12-lead ECG.[28] Alternatively, if clinical suspicion of AF exists, a Holter monitor or event monitor up to 30 days may be considered. The history and physical examination should assess for conditions and precipitating factors for AF: comorbidities (e.g., COPD, HTN); cardiac and noncardiac etiologies; thyroid disease; sleep apnea; acute illnesses; and substances (e.g., alcohol, diet pills, and illicit drugs). Further diagnostic studies may include blood tests (e.g., complete blood count, chemistries, and thyroid hormone levels); chest radiograph especially if the presentation is acute; transthoracic echocardiogram to evaluate for structural abnormalities; and stress echocardiography. Additional testing may be required if patient history and risk factors such as coronary artery disease exists in which case a myocardial nuclear perfusion stress test or cardiac catheterization may be warranted to evaluate for ischemia.

The treatment considerations for AF depend on acuity of the presentation. In hemodynamically unstable patients, immediate evaluation and treatment including electrical emergent cardioversion is recommended. In the hemodynamically stable patients, the treatment depends on duration of AF and presence of underlying cardiac disease and other comorbidities. As AF is associated with five-fold increased risk for stroke, anticoagulation must be considered. The decision to anticoagulate is based on assessment and risks for stroke assessed with CHA_2DS_2-VASc score (congestive heart failure, hypertension, age 65 to 74, 75 or older doubled risks, diabetes mellitus, stroke, transient ischemic attack, thromboembolism, vascular disease, sex female more risks) (see Table 35-3) and HAS-BLED scoring system (hypertension, abnormal liver and renal function, stroke, bleeding, labile international normalized ratio, elderly [greater than 65 years of age], drugs and alcohol) (see Table 35-4).[28,29]

If the patient is at increased risk for bleeding events with anticoagulation, then determination of alternative, nonpharmacologic strategies to prevent stroke such as left atrial appendage occlusion may be considered. A summary of the most recent AF guideline update incorporated the newer classes of anticoagulants and their considerations (Fig. 35-12).[29]

Possible treatment to control the arrhythmia may employ a rhythm or rate control strategy and includes pharmacologic therapy and invasive procedures such as ablation or surgery. The goals of therapy depend on whether AF is paroxysmal, persistent, or permanent. The most common medicines used to achieve rate control include beta blockers (metoprolol, esmolol) and nondihydropyridine calcium channel blockers (diltiazem, verapamil). Therapy with digoxin may also be considered. Electrical cardioversion is successful short term when combined with pharmacologic conversion, or pharmacologic cardioversion could be attempted alone with antiarrhythmic medications (sotalol, propafenone, flecainide, dofetalide, or amiodarone). Maintaining sinus rhythm is challenging due to limited

(*text continues on page 780*)

Table 35-1 • ONGOING DRUG THERAPY FOR SVT, ORAL ADMINISTRATION

Drug	Initial Daily Dose(s)	Maximum Total Daily Maintenance Dose	Potential Adverse Effects	Precautions (Exclude or Use With Caution) and Interactions
Beta Blockers				
Atenolol	25–50 mg QD	100 mg QD (reduced dosing in patients with severe renal dysfunction)	Hypotension, bronchospasm, bradycardia	• AV block greater than first degree or SA node dysfunction (in absence of pacemaker) • Decompensated systolic HF • Hypotension • Reactive airway disease • Severe renal dysfunction • Drugs with SA and/or AV nodal–blocking properties
Metoprolol tartrate	25 mg BID	200 mg BID	Hypotension, bronchospasm, bradycardia	• AV block greater than first degree or SA node dysfunction (in absence of pacemaker) • Decompensated systolic HF • Hypotension • Reactive airway disease • Drugs with SA and/or AV nodal–blocking properties
Metoprolol succinate (long acting)	50 mg QD	400 mg QD	Hypotension, bronchospasm, bradycardia	• AV block greater than first degree or SA node dysfunction (in absence of pacemaker) • Decompensated systolic HF • Hypotension • Reactive airway disease • Drugs with SA and/or AV nodal–blocking properties
Nadolol	40 mg QD	320 mg QD (reduced dosage with renal impairment)	Hypotension, bronchospasm, bradycardia	• AV block greater than first degree or SA node dysfunction (in absence of pacemaker) • Reactive airway disease • Cardiogenic shock • Decompensated HF • Hypotension • Renal dysfunction • Drugs with SA and/or AV nodal–blocking properties
Propranolol	30–60 mg in divided or single dose with long-acting formulations	40–160 mg in divided or single dose with long-acting formulations	Hypotension, worsening HF, bronchospasm, bradycardia	• AV block greater than first degree or SA node dysfunction (in absence of pacemaker) • Reactive airway disease • Decompensated systolic HF • Hypotension • Drugs with SA and/or AV nodal–blocking properties
Nondihydropyridine Calcium Channel Antagonists				
Diltiazem	120 mg daily in divided or single dose with long-acting formulations	360 mg daily in divided or single dose with long-acting formulations	Hypotension, worsening HF in patients with pre-existing ventricular dysfunction, bradycardia, abnormal liver function studies, acute hepatic injury (rare)	• AV block greater than first degree or SA node dysfunction (in absence of pacemaker) • Hypotension • Decompensated systolic HF/severe LV dysfunction • WPW with AF/atrial flutter • Drugs with SA and/or AV nodal–blocking properties • Diltiazem is a substrate of CYP3A4 (major) and a moderate CYP3A4 inhibitor • Apixaban, itraconazole, bosutinib, ceritinib, cilostazol, cyclosporine, everolimus, ibrutinib, idelalisib, ivabradine, lomitapide, olaparib, ranolazine, rifampin, simeprevir
Verapamil	120 mg daily in divided or single dose with long-acting formulations	480 mg daily in divided or single dose with long-acting formulations	Hypotension, worsening HF in patients with pre-existing ventricular dysfunction, pulmonary edema in patients with hypertrophic cardiomyopathy, bradycardia, abnormal liver function studies	• AV block greater than first degree or SA node dysfunction (in absence of pacemaker) • Decompensated systolic HF/severe LV dysfunction • Hypotension • WPW with AF/atrial flutter • Verapamil is a moderate CYP3A4 inhibitor and also inhibits P-glycoprotein • Contraindicated with dofetilide • Itraconazole, bosutinib, ceritinib, cilostazol, colchicine, cyclosporine, everolimus, dabigatran, edoxaban, flecainide, ibrutinib, ivabradine, olaparib, ranolazine, rivaroxaban, rifampin, silodosin, simeprevir, rivaroxaban, rifampin, simvastatin, topotecan, trabectedin, vincristine, grapefruit juice

(continued)

Table 35-1 • ONGOING DRUG THERAPY FOR SVT, ORAL ADMINISTRATION (*Continued*)

Drug	Initial Daily Dose(s)	Maximum Total Daily Maintenance Dose	Potential Adverse Effects	Precautions (Exclude or Use With Caution) and Interactions
Cardiac Glycosides				
Digoxin	Loading: 0.5 mg, with additional 0.125- to 0.25-mg doses administered at 6–8-h intervals until evidence of adequate effect (maximum dose 8–12 mcg/kg over 24 h)	0.25 mg QD maintenance: 0.125–0.25 mg QD, with dosing based on patient's age, lean body weight, and renal function and drug interactions; occasionally down to 0.0625 mg in cases of renal impairment (trough serum digoxin level 0.5–1 ng/mL)	Bradycardia, heart block, anorexia, nausea, vomiting, visual changes, and cardiac arrhythmias in cases of digoxin toxicity (associated with levels >2 ng/mL, although symptoms may also occur at lower levels)	• Renal dysfunction • WPW with AF/atrial flutter • AV block greater than first degree or SA node dysfunction (in absence of pacemaker) • Drugs with SA and/or AV nodal–blocking properties • Reduce dose by 30–50% when administering with amiodarone and by 50% when administering with dronedarone • Monitor digoxin concentrations with verapamil, clarithromycin, erythromycin, itraconazole, cyclosporine, propafenone, flecainide
Class Ic Antiarrhythmic Agents				
Flecainide	50 mg every 12 h	150 mg every 12 h (PR and QRS intervals should be monitored. May consider monitoring flecainide plasma levels, keeping trough plasma levels below 0.7–1.0 mcg/mL)	Atrial flutter with 1:1 AV conduction, QT prolongation, torsades de pointes, worsening HF, bradycardia	• Sinus or AV conduction disease (in absence of pacemaker) • Cardiogenic shock • Avoid in structural heart disease (including ischemic heart disease) • Atrial flutter (unless concomitant AV nodal therapy to avoid 1:1 conduction) • Brugada syndrome • Renal dysfunction • Hepatic dysfunction • QT-prolonging drugs • Amiodarone, digoxin, ritonavir, saquinavir, tipranavir
Propafenone	150 mg every 8 h (immediate release); 225 mg every 12 h (extended release)	300 mg every 8 h (immediate release); 425 mg every 12 h (extended release) (PR and QRS interval should be monitored. Consider dosage reduction with hepatic impairment)	Atrial flutter with 1:1 AV conduction, QT prolongation, torsades de pointes, bradycardia, bronchospasm	• Sinus or AV conduction disease (in absence of pacemaker) • Cardiogenic shock • Hypotension • Reactive airway disease Avoid in structural heart disease (including ischemic heart disease) • Atrial flutter (unless concomitant AV nodal therapy to avoid 1:1 conduction) • Brugada syndrome • Hepatic dysfunction • QT-prolonging drugs • Drugs with SA and/or AV nodal–blocking properties • Amiodarone, ritonavir, saquinavir, tipranavir
Class III Antiarrhythmic Agents				
Amiodarone	400–600 mg QD in divided doses for 2–4 wk (loading dose); followed by 100–200 mg QD (maintenance dose)	Up to 1,200 mg QD may be considered in an inpatient monitoring setting (loading dose); up to 200 mg QD maintenance (to minimize long-term adverse effects)	Bradycardia, QT prolongation, torsades de pointes (rare), gastrointestinal upset, constipation, hypothyroidism, hyperthyroidism, pulmonary fibrosis, hepatic toxicity, corneal deposits, optic neuritis, peripheral neuropathy, photosensitivity, adult respiratory distress syndrome after cardiac or noncardiac surgery (rare)	• Sinus or AV conduction disease (in absence of pacemaker) • Inflammatory lung disease • Hepatic dysfunction • Hypothyroidism, hyperthyroidism • Peripheral neuropathy • Abnormal gait/ataxia • Optic neuritis • Drugs with SA and/or AV nodal–blocking properties • Amiodarone is a substrate of and inhibits • P-glycoprotein and CYP2C9 (moderate), CYP2D6 (moderate), and CYP3A4 (weak); amiodarone is a substrate for CYP3A4 (major) and CYP2C8 (major); amiodarone is an inhibitor of OCT2 • Reduce warfarin dose by 50%, and reduce digoxin dose by 30–50% • Agalsidase alfa, agalsidase beta, azithromycin, bosutinib, ceritinib, colchicine, dabigatran, edoxaban, flecainide, ivabradine, ledipasvir/sofosbuvir, lopinavir, lopinavir/ ritonavir, lovastatin, nelfinavir, pazopanib, propafenone, simvastatin, ritonavir, rivaroxaban, saquinavir, sofosbuvir, topotecan, vincristine, grapefruit juice

Table 35-1 • ONGOING DRUG THERAPY FOR SVT, ORAL ADMINISTRATION (*Continued*)

Drug	Initial Daily Dose(s)	Maximum Total Daily Maintenance Dose	Potential Adverse Effects	Precautions (Exclude or Use With Caution) and Interactions
Dofetilide	500 mcg every 12 h (if CrCl >60 mL/min) 250 mcg every 12 h (if CrCl 40–60 mL/min) 125 mcg every 12 h (if CrCl 20 to <40 mL/min) Not recommended if CrCl <20 mL/min Adjust dose for renal function, body size, and age Initiate for minimum of 3 d in a facility that can provide continuous ECG monitoring and cardiac resuscitation Contraindicated if the baseline QTc interval or QTc >440 ms or 500 ms in patients with ventricular conduction abnormalities	Repeat ECG 2–3 h after administering the first dose to determine QTc; if the QTc increased by >15% compared with baseline or if QTc is >500 ms (550 ms in patients with ventricular conduction abnormalities), subsequent dosing should be down titrated by 50%; at 2–3 h after each subsequent dose, determine QTc (for 2nd, 3rd, 4th and 5th in-hospital doses); if at any time after the second dose the QTc is >500 ms (550 ms in patients with ventricular conduction abnormalities), dofetilide should be discontinued	QT prolongation, torsades de pointes	• Severe renal dysfunction (contraindicated if CrCl <20 mL/min) • Prolonged QT • History of torsades de pointes • Concomitant use of hydrochlorothiazide, cimetidine, dolutegravir, itraconazole, ketoconazole, megestrol, trimethoprim, prochlorperazine trimethoprim/ sulfamethoxazole or verapamil, contraindicated • Avoid other QT-prolonging drugs
Sotalol	40–80 mg every 12 h (Patients initiated or reinitiated on sotalol should be placed in a facility that can provide cardiac resuscitation and continuous electrocardiographic monitoring for a minimum of 3 d). Contraindicated if the QTc interval is >450 ms. CrCl should be calculated before dosing. If CrCl >60 mL/min, then dosing frequency is twice daily. If CrCl 40–60 mL/min, dosing interval is every 24 h. If CrCl <40 mL/min, should not be used.)	160 mg every 12 h (during initiation and titration, the QT interval should be monitored 2–4 h after each dose. If the QT interval prolongs to ≥500 ms, the dose must be reduced or the drug discontinued.)	QT prolongation, torsades de pointes, bradycardia, bronchospasm	• Prolonged QT • Renal dysfunction • Hypokalemia • Diuretic therapy • Avoid other QT-prolonging drugs • Sinus or AV nodal dysfunction (in absence of pacemaker) • Decompensated systolic HF • Cardiogenic shock • Reactive airway disease • Drugs with SA and/or AV–nodal blocking properties
Miscellaneous				
Ivabradine	5 mg BID	7.5 mg BID	Phosphenes, AF	• Concomitant drugs that can exacerbate bradycardia • Contraindicated in decompensated HF • Contraindicated if BP <90/50 mm Hg • Contraindicated in severe hepatic impairment • Hypertension • Ivabradine is a substrate of CYP3A4 (major) • Avoid use with concomitant strong CYP3A4 inhibitors (boceprevir, clarithromycin, indinavir, itraconazole, lopinavir/ritonavir, nelfinavir, ritonavir, saquinavir, telaprevir, posaconazole, voriconazole) • Avoid use with strong CYP3A4 inducers (carbamazepine, phenytoin, rifampin, St. John wort) • Avoid use with diltiazem, verapamil, grapefruit juice

Adapted from Page RL, Joglar JA, Caldwell MA, et al. Correction to: 2015 ACC/AHA/HRS guideline for the management of adult patients with supraventricular tachycardia: executive summary: a Report of the American College of Cardiology/American Heart Association Task Force on clinical practice guidelines and the Heart Rhythm Society. *Circulation.* 2016;134(11):e232–e233.

Table 35-2 • ORAL ANTICOAGULANTS FOR AF

	Warfarin	Dabigatran	Rivaroxaban	Apixaban	Edoxaban
Dose	Variable od	150 or 110 bd 75 mg bd if CrCl 15–30 mL/min	20 mg od 15 mg od if CrCl 15–30 ml/min	2.5–5 mg bd 2.5 mg bd if Cr ≥1.5 mg/dl, ≥80 yrs of age, body weight ≤60 kg	30–60 mg od (no data in renal impairment)
Target	Vitamin K-dependent factors	Thrombin (factor II)	Factor Xa	Factor Xa	Factor Xa
Half-Life	40 h	12–14 h	9–13 h	8–11 h	8–10 h
Renal Clearance	0	80%	60%	25%	40%
Onset of Action Inhibition	3–5 h	2 h	2.5–4.0 h	3 h	1–5 h
Anticoagulation Monitoring	INR 2–3	Not required	Not required	Not required	Not required
Interactions	Multiple	P-gp	P-gp; CYP3A4	P-gp; CYP3A4	P-gp; CYP3A4
Antidote	Vitamin K	3- and 4-factor prothrombin complex concentrates idarucizumab	4-factor prothrombin complex concentrates andexanet alfa, aripazine	4-factor prothrombin complex concentrates andexanet alfa, aripazine	4-factor prothrombin complex concentrates andexanet alfa, aripazine

P-gp, P-glycoprotein.
Adapted from Katritsis DG, Gersh BJ, Camm AJ. Anticoagulation in atrial fibrillation—current concepts. *Arrhythm Electrophysiol Rev.* 2015;04(2):100–107.[30]

Table 35-3 • CHA_2DS_2-VASC SCORE

Age	<65 0	65–74 +1	≥75 +2
Sex	Female +1	Male 0	
CHF History	No 0	Yes +1	
Hypertension History	No 0	Yes +1	
Stroke/TIA/Thromboembolism History	No 0	Yes +2	
Vascular Disease History	No 0	Yes +1	
Diabetes History	No 0	Yes +1	

CHA_2DS_2-VASc Score	Risk of Ischemic Stroke	Risk of Stroke/TIA/ Systemic Embolism
0	0.2%	0.3%
1	0.6%	0.9%
2	2.2%	2.9%
3	3.2%	4.6%
4	4.8%	6.7%
5	7.2%	10.0%
6	9.7%	13.6%
7	11.2%	15.7%
8	10.8%	15.2%
9	12.2%	17.4%

Adapted from MDCalc, available http://www.mdcalc.com.

Table 35-4 • HAS-BLED SCORE

Hypertension Uncontrolled, >160 mm Hg systolic	No 0	Yes +1
Renal Disease Dialysis, transplant, Cr >2.26 mg/dL or >200 µmol/L	No 0	Yes +1
Liver Disease Cirrhosis or bilirubin >2× normal with AST/ALT/AP >3× normal	No 0	Yes +1
Stroke History	No 0	Yes +1
Prior Major Bleeding or Predisposition to Bleeding	No 0	Yes +1
Labile INR Unstable/high INRs, time in therapeutic range <60%	No 0	Yes +1
Age >65	No 0	Yes +1
Medication usage predisposing to bleeding Aspirin, clopidogrel, NSAIDs	No 0	Yes +1
Alcohol Use ≥8 drinks/wk	No 0	Yes +1

HAS-BLED Score	Risk Group	Risk of Major Bleeding[b]	Bleeds Per 100 Patient-Years[c]	Recommendation
0	Relatively low	0.9%	1.13	Anticoagulation should be considered
1		3.4%	1.02	
2	Moderate	4.1%	1.88	Anticoagulation can be considered
3	High	5.8%	3.72	Alternatives to anticoagulation should be considered
4		8.9%	8.70	
5		9.1%	12.50	
>5[a]	Very high	–	–	

Adapted from MDCalc, available http://www.mdcalc.com. [a]Scores greater than 5 were too rare to determine risk, but are likely over 10%. [b]Lip GY. Implications of the CHA(2)DS(2)-VASc and HAS-BLED Scores for thromboprophylaxis in atrial fibrillation. *Am J Med.* 2011;124(2):111-114. doi:10.1016/j.amjmed.2010.05.007. [c]Pisters R, Lane DA, Nieuwlaat R, de Vos CB, Crijns HJ, Lip GY. A novel user-friendly score (HAS-BLED) to assess 1-year risk of major bleeding in patients with atrial fibrillation: the Euro Heart Survey. *Chest.* 2010;138(5):1093-1100. doi:10.1378/chest.10-0134.

Key Distinctions: 2014 Atrial Fibrillation (AF) Guideline - 2019 AF Focused Update		
	2014 AF Guideline	2019 AF Focused Update
NOACs approved for stroke prevention	Dabigatran, Rlovaroxaban, Apixaban (Class I)	Dabigatran, Rlovaroxaban, Apixaban, and Edoxaban (Class I)
Oral anticoagulants recommended for eligible patients	Warfarin or NOACs (Class I)	NOACs recommended over Warfarin (Class I)
Oral anticoagulants recommended for patients with end-stage renal disease or on dialysis	Warfarin (Class IIa)	Warfarin or Apixaban (Class IIb)
FDA-approved reversal agent for Dabigatran	N/A	Idarucizumab (Class I)
FDA-approved reversal agent for Rivaroxaban and Apixaban	N/A	Andexanet Alfa (Class IIa)
Left atrial appendage occlusion	N/A	May be considered for patients with contraindications to long-term anticoagulation (Class IIb)
AF catheter ablation	N/A	May be reasonable in symptomatic patients with HF and a reduced EF to reduce mortality and HF hospitalizations. (Class IIb)
Anticoagulation for AF after percutaneous coronary Intervention (PCI) with stent placement	N/A	If triple therapy (oral anticoagulant, aspirin, and $P2Y_{12}$ inhibitor) is prescribed, it is reasonable to choose Clopidogrel in preference to Prasurgrel. (Class IIa) If triple therapy is prescribed: a transtion to double therapy (oral anticoagulant and $P2Y_{12}$ inhibitor) at 4-6 weeks may be considered. (Class IIa) Double therapy [$P2Y_{12}$ inhibitor (Clopidogrel or Ticagrelor) and dose-adjusted vitamin K antagonist] is reasonable to reduce the risk of bleeding as compared with triple therapy. (Class IIa) Double therapy with $P2Y_{12}$ inhibitor (Clopidogrel) and low-dose Rivaroxaban (15 mg daily) is reasonable to reduce the risk of bleeding as compared with triple therapy. (Class IIa) Double therapy with $P2Y_{12}$ inhibitor (Clopidogrel) and Dabigatran 150 mg twice daily is reasonable to reduce the risk of bleeding as compared with triple therapy. (Class IIa)
Device detection of AF and atrial flutter	N/A	In patients with cryptogenic stroke in whom extemal ambulatory monitoring is inconclusive, implantation of a cardiac loop monitor is reasonable. (Class IIa)
Weight loss	N/A	For overweight and obese patients with AF, weight loss, combined with risk factor modification, is recommended. (Class I)

Figure 35-12. Summary of 2019 guideline updates for the management of atrial fibrillation. (From January CT, Wann LS, Calkins H, et al. AHA/ACC/HRS Focused Update of the 2014 AHA/ACC/HRS guideline for the management of patients with atrial fibrillation: a report of the American College of Cardiology/American Heart Association Task Force on clinical practice guidelines and the Heart Rhythm Society. *J Am Coll Cardiol.* 2019;74[1]:104–132, used with permission from Elsevier, STM Signatory Guidelines http://www.stm-assoc.org/permissions-guidelines/). DOI: 10.1016/j.jacc.2019.01.011

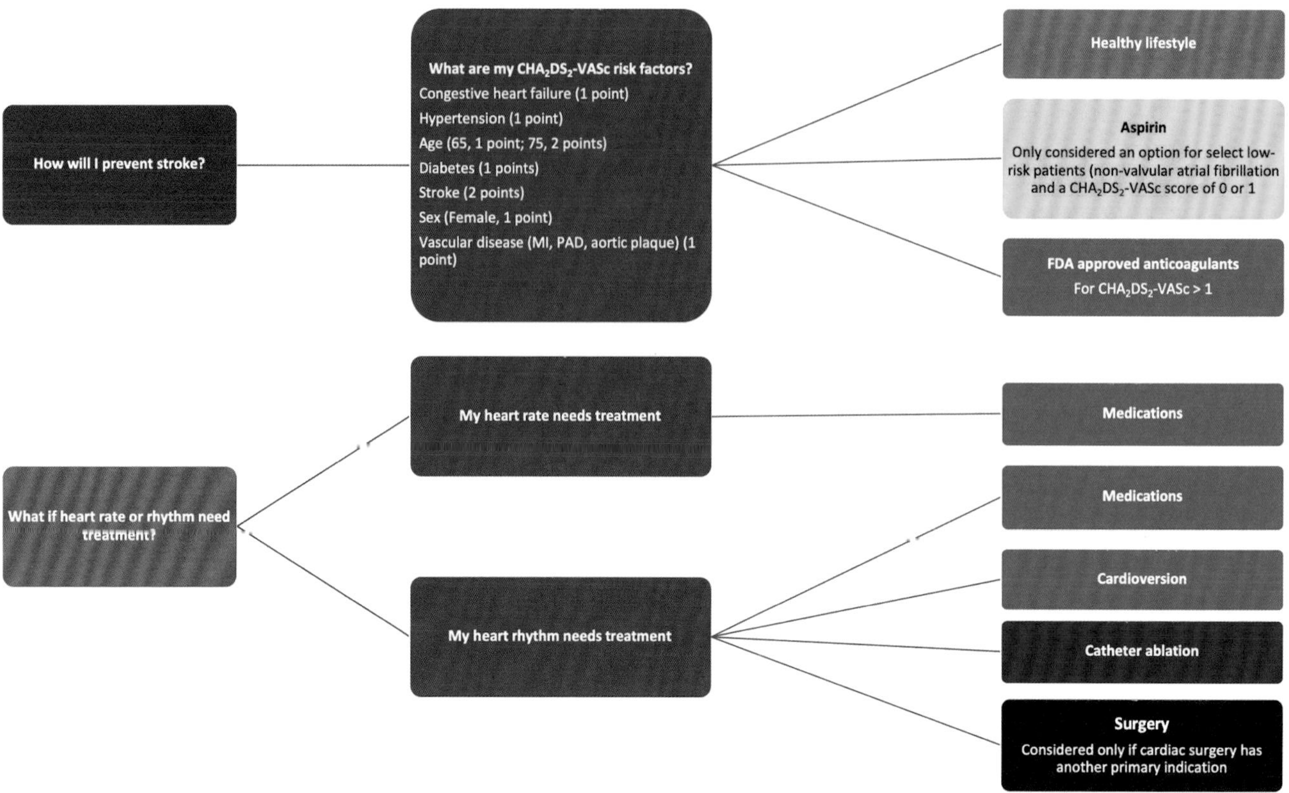

Figure 35-13. Patient education and decision-making aid for treatment of atrial fibrillation. (Adapted from American Heart Association. *My AFib Experience, Simplified Guidelines.* 2016. https://myafibexperience.org/media/38145/7ca93e05039d26fde39d965b41ba4ede-vp_simplified_guidelines_mae-v7.pdf)

long-term effectiveness of pharmacologic agents and the side effects associated with aforementioned medicines.[28]

Catheter ablation such as cryoablation with a cryoballoon and radiofrequency catheter ablation is reasonable treatment option based on the symptomology or, if intolerant to pharmacologic therapy, in younger patients with no structural heart disease. In general, optimal treatment in patients with persistent AF remains controversial and should be individualized.

The Role of the Cardiac Nurse in Management of Supraventricular Arrhythmias

Given the prevalence of these arrhythmias, the cardiac nurse will care for patients with these diagnoses and must understand the evidence and guidelines for evaluation and treatment. As patient education and advocacy are key competencies of the nurse, it is paramount to have current, high-quality information to assist patients to understand their arrhythmia and the decision-making touchpoints for its management. Professional societies such as the American Heart Association and American Stroke Association have developed patient-centered tools that may be used by the cardiac nurse and cardiology care teams for this purpose. An example is provided for the management of AF (Fig. 35-13).

Summary

Supraventricular arrhythmias are the most common arrhythmias requiring medical evaluation and intervention. Treatment options with catheter ablation continue to gain higher degree of success and lower complications rate, whereas pharmacologic interventions carry ongoing concern about potential adverse effects. An area of continued need for research is first-line intervention with vagal maneuvers and which maneuver represents best technique without variation in which it has been administered. The goal of all treatment options is to improve quality of life. A shared decision-making process between a patient and the care team should be utilized to ensure patient-centered care reflective of current evidence and all available options and their short- and long-term considerations. The cardiac nurse provides important patient care, education, and advocacy in the evaluation and management of supraventricular arrhythmias.

CASE STUDY 1

Patient Profile

History of Present Illness

Ms. Blumenthal, a 29 year-old female, presents to emergency room with complaint of palpitations 3 weeks in duration, light-headedness, and dizziness. She carries long-standing history of palpitations however, she never had formal cardiac evaluation and instead she was diagnosed with anxiety. Differential diagnoses considered by the care team are sinus tachycardia and panic attack.

Past Medical History

Anxiety

Family Medical History

No cardiac disease or sudden cardiac death

Social History

Nonsmoker, no alcohol or drug abuse

Allergies

NKDA

Home Medications

None

Patient Examination

Physical Examination

General appearance—alert, diaphoretic
Neck—no JVD distention
Respiratory—no adventitious lung sounds
Cardiovascular—regular rhythm rapid heart rate, no murmurs
Peripheral pulses—regular pulses
Extremities—normothermic, no edema, no pallor

Diagnostic Studies

Surface 12-Lead ECG was performed with following findings:

- Suspicious for SVT, (Fig. 35-14)
- Rate—166 bpm
- Rhythm—regular, rapid
- P waves hidden (pseudo R wave sometimes seen in V1 lead)
- Narrow QRS complex
- No evidence of infarcts/ischemia (Q waves, ST elevation, ST depression, T-wave inversion)

ECG Findings

ECG represents SVT regular, narrow complex tachycardia with reentry, more specific AVRNT.

Echocardiography showed no evidence of structural heart disease and preserved left ventricular function.
Laboratory tests (electrolytes and TSH) within normal limits.

Assessment and Plan

A 29-year-old female with symptomatic AVNRT in the absence of structural or functional cardiac abnormalities.

1. Valsalva maneuver was attempted twice (bear down) prior to arrival in emergency room without relief of symptoms.
2. In the emergency room, adenosine 6 mg was administered which successfully terminated arrhythmia.
3. Low-dose beta blocker was added to reduce symptoms and maintain normal sinus rhythm.
4. Patient was scheduled for follow up with cardiac electrophysiology for possible electrophysiology study and catheter ablation.

Key Takcaways

- Valsalva maneuver is a first-line strategy and can be initiated by the patient with instruction from the nurse to "bear down" as one would when having a bowel movement. Alternatively, the nurse can instruct the patient to engage in moderately forceful attempted exhalation against a closed airway, otherwise known as "popping the ears" as one would on an airplane when trying to balance air pressure in the ears.
- Intravenous (IV) adenosine is a first-line drug for the patient with symptomatic or hemodynamically unstable SVT. Because adenosine is rapidly metabolized, in order to reach the heart adenosine must be administered rapidly over 1 to 3 seconds followed by a 20-mL bolus of normal saline. The first dose of adenosine is 6 mg IV. If the patient does not convert within 1 to 2 minutes, a second dose of 12 mg IV may be administered in the same fashion as the first.
- An oral medication such as metoprolol is also administered following successful restoration of sinus rhythm to decrease the likelihood of SVT recurrence.
- To prevent future episodes of SVT, patient should be educated to avoid use of alcohol, illicit drug use, over-the-counter medication containing stimulants, smoking cessation, and reducing stress.

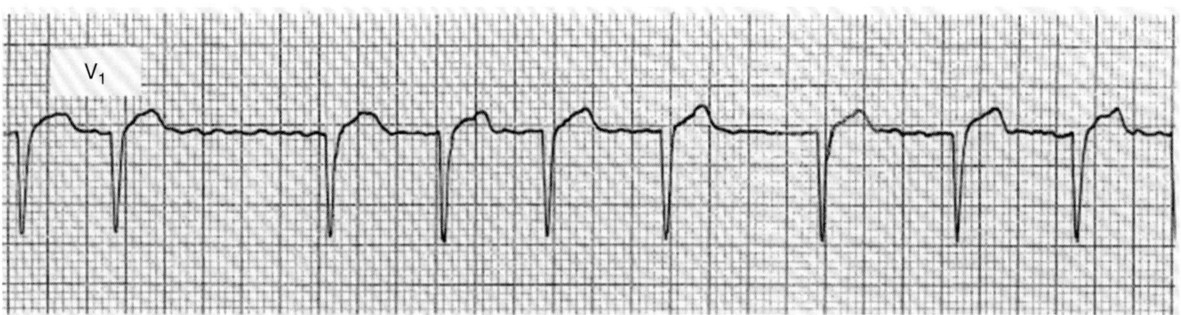

Figure 35-14. Case Study 1, cardiac rhythm telemetry strip.

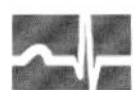

CASE STUDY 2

Patient Profile

History of Present Illness

Mr. Thompson is a 70-year-old male patient with a history of paroxysmal atrial fibrillation, coronary artery disease, hypertension, and aortic stenosis who underwent a CABG in 2002. This hospitalization he underwent a redo-CABG with, aortic valve replacement, mitral valve replacement, LAA ligation, and complex MAZE procedure. He is postoperative day 3 and complains of shortness of breath, dizziness, and palpitations. Initial ECG confirmed atrial fibrillation with rapid ventricular response of 152 bpm and he was given a single dose of 5 mg metoprolol IV, which helped slow his heart rate down.

Patient Examination

Physical Examination

Vital Signs: 158/72 mm Hg, respiration 26.

General appearance—alert, diaphoretic
Neck—no JVD distention
Respiratory—no adventitious lung sounds
Cardiovascular—irregularly irregular rhythm with normal rate, no murmurs
Peripheral pulses-regular pulses
Extremities-normothermic, no edema, no pallor

Diagnostic Studies

ECG (see Fig. 35-15)

- AF with ventricular rate of 96 bpm
- Rate—96 bpm
- Rhythm—irregularly irregular
- No P waves
- QRS complex 88 ms
- Inferior nonspecific ST–T-wave changes

Assessment and Plan

A 70-year-old male status post redo-CABG with AVR, MVR, LAA ligation, and MAZE procedure who presents with new-onset symptomatic atrial fibrillation with rapid ventricular response, improved after administration of IV metoprolol.

1. IV amiodarone bolus with subsequent continuous infusion.
2. Transition to oral amiodarone after IV bolus and restoration of sinus rhythm.
3. Schedule outpatient follow-up appointments with cardiothoracic surgery and electrophysiology upon discharge.

Key Takeaways

- Some patients could experience atrial fibrillation immediately after surgery, within a few weeks or months after maze surgery due to swelling and inflammation of atrial tissue. Patients who have atrial fibrillation after maze procedure will continue to use anticoagulants and antiarrhythmic medications for a few months.
- Amiodarone lowers the incidence of postoperative atrial fibrillation recurrence. Nurse should inform patient about possible side effects associated with this medication such as increased liver enzymes, renal impairment, thyroid disease, visual disturbance, and long-term use may cause pulmonary fibrosis. Periodic monitoring of liver, kidney, and thyroid studies are necessary to avoid unwanted side effects. In addition, yearly chest x-ray and eye examination are recommended.
- Beta blockers may be used to optimize blood pressure and rate control in atrial fibrillation patients. This is very important in postoperative period to prevent adrenergic stimulation by catecholamines such as epinephrine and norepinephrine.

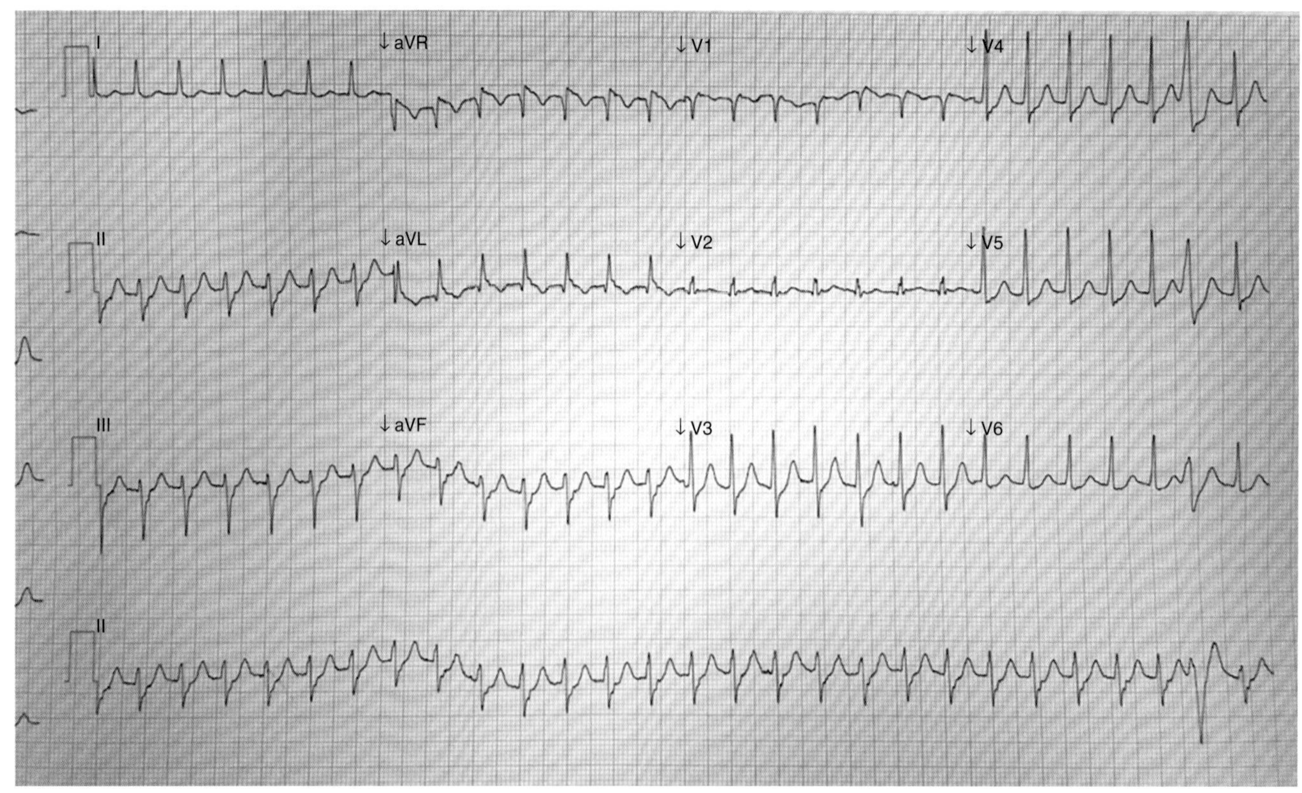

Figure 35-15. Case Study 2, 12 lead ECG.

KEY READINGS

American College of Cardiology. CardioSmart (patient engagement program including tools, decision aids).

a. Atrial Fibrillation https://www.cardiosmart.org/topics/atrial-fibrillation/

b. Supraventricular Tachycardia https://www.cardiosmart.org/topics/supraventricular-tachycardia

January CT, Wann LS, Calkins H, et al. 2019 AHA/ACC/HRS Focused Update of the 2014 AHA/ACC/HRS Guideline for the Management of Patients With Atrial Fibrillation: A Report of the American College of Cardiology/American Heart Association Task Force on Clinical Practice Guidelines and the Heart Rhythm Society in Collaboration With the Society of Thoracic Surgeons. *Circulation.* 2019;140(2):e125–e151.

Page RL, Joglar JA, Caldwell MA, et al. 2015 ACC/AHA/HRS Guideline for the Management of Adult Patients With Supraventricular Tachycardia. *Circulation.* 2016;133(14):e506–e574.

REFERENCES

1. Kasper DL, Fauci AS, Hauser SL, et al. *Harrisons Principles of Internal Medicine.* New York: McGraw-Hill Education; 2015.
2. Sohinki D, Obel OA. Current trends in supraventricular tachycardia management. *Ochsner J.* Winter 2014;14(4):586–595.
3. Atrial fibrillation fact sheet|data & statistics|DHDSP|CDC. Centers for Disease Control and Prevention. https://www.cdc.gov/dhdsp/data_statistics/fact_sheets/fs_atrial_fibrillation.htm. Published August 8, 2017. Accessed July 14, 2019.
4. Eagle KA, Baliga RR. *Practical Cardiology: Evaluation and Treatment of Common Cardiovascular Disorders.* LWW; 2013.
5. Steinberg JS. *Electrophysiology: The Basics.* Philadelphia, PA: Wolters Kluwer; 2017.
6. Josephson ME, Seides Stuart F. *Clinical Cardiac Electrophysiology: Techniques and Interpretations.* Philadelphia, PA: Lea and Febiger; 1979.
7. Antzelevitch C, Burashnikov A. Overview of basic mechanisms of cardiac arrhythmia. *Card Electrophysiol Clin.* 2011;3(1):23–45.
8. Bonow RO, Braunwald E, Libby P, et al. *Braunwalds Heart Disease: A Textbook of Cardiovascular Medicine.* Philadelphia, PA: Elsevier/Saunders; 2019.
9. Issa ZF, Miller JM, Zipes DP. *Clinical Arrhythmology and Electrophysiology: A Companion to Braunwalds Heart Disease.* Philadelphia, PA: Elsevier; 2019.
10. Ferguson JD, DiMarco JP. Contemporary management of paroxysmal supraventricular tachycardia. *AHA Journal.* 2003;107(8):1096–1099.
11. Podrid PJ, Kowey PR. *Cardiac Arrhythmia: Mechanisms, Diagnosis, and Management.* Philadelphia, PA: Lippincott William & Wilkins; 2001.
12. Goldberger JJ, Kadish AH. In: Podrid PJ, Kowey PR. *Cardiac Arrhythmia: Mechanisms, Diagnosis, and Management.* Philadelphia, PA: Lippincott William & Wilkins; 2001.
13. Prystowsky EN, Waldo AL. Atrial fibrillation, atrial flutter, and atrial tachycardia. In: Fuster V, Harrington RA, Narula J, et al., eds. *Hurst's the Heart.* New York: McGraw-Hill Education; 2017.
14. Olgin JE, Zipes DP. Specific arrhythmias: Diagnosis and treatment. In: Bonow RO, Braunwald E, Libby P, et al. *Braunwalds Heart Disease: A Textbook of Cardiovascular Medicine.* Philadelphia, PA: Elsevier/Saunders; 2019.
15. Wyndham CR, Arnsdorf MF, Levitsky S, et al. Successful surgical excision of focal paroxysmal atrial tachycardia. Observations in vivo and in vitro. *Circulation.* 1980;62(6):1365–1372.
16. Tandon N. Multifocal atrial tachycardia: overview of multifocal atrial tachycardia. https://emedicine.medscape.com/article/155825-overview. Published February 1, 2019. Accessed February 25, 2019.
17. Homoud MK, Levy S, Downey BC. Sinoatrial nodal reentrant tachycardia. UpToDate. https://www.uptodate.com/contents/sinoatrial-nodal-reentrant-tachycardia-sanrt. Published September 14, 2017. Accessed January 25, 2019.
18. Meiltz A, Weber R, Halimi F, et al. Permanent form of junctional reciprocating tachycardia in adults: peculiar features and results of radiofrequency catheter ablation. *EP Europace.* 2006;8(1):21–28.
19. Dorostkar PC. Persistent junctional reciprocating tachycardia. In: Macdonald II D, ed. *Clinical Cardiac Electrophysiology in the Young.* 2nd ed. New York: Springer, 2015; 83–89.
20. Dorostkar PC, Silka MJ, Macdonald D, et al. Clinical course of persistent junctional reciprocating tachycardia. *J Am Coll Cardiol.* 1999;33(2):366–375.
21. Garan H. Atypical atrial flutter – heart rhythm. https://www.heartrhythmjournal.com/article/S1547-5271(07)01086-7/fulltext. Published April 2008. Accessed February 3, 2019.
22. Cantillon DJ, Amuthan R. Atrial fibrillation. http://www.clevelandclinicmeded.com/medicalpubs/diseasemanagement/cardiology/atrial-fibrillation/. Published August 2018. Accessed January 14, 2019.
23. Markides V. Atrial fibrillation: classification, pathophysiology, mechanisms and drug treatment. *Heart.* 2003;89(8):939–943.
24. Colluci RA, Silver MJ, Shebrook J. Common types of supraventricular tachycardia: diagnosis and management. *Am Fam Physician.* 2010;82(8):942–952. https://www.aafp.org/afp/2010/1015/p942.html. Accessed January 13, 2019.
25. Page RL, Joglar JA, Caldwell MA, et al. Correction to: 2015 ACC/AHA/HRS guideline for the management of adult patients with supraventricular tachycardia: executive summary: a Report of the American College of Cardiology/American Heart Association Task Force on clinical practice guidelines and the Heart Rhythm Society. *Circulation.* 2016;134(11):e232–e233.
26. Krul SP, Driessen AH, Zwinderman AH, et al. Navigating the mini-maze: systematic review of the first results and progress of minimally-invasive surgery in the treatment of atrial fibrillation. *Int J Cardiol.* 2013;166(1):132–140.
27. Page RL, Joglar JA, Caldwell MA, et al. 2015 ACC/AHA/HRS guideline for the management of adult patients with supraventricular tachycardia: a Report of the American College of Cardiology/American Heart Association Task Force on clinical practice guidelines and the Heart Rhythm Society. *J Am Coll Cardiol.* 2016;67(13):e27–e115.
28. Gutierrez C, Blanchard DG. Diagnosis and treatment of atrial fibrillation. American family physician. https://www.aafp.org/afp/2016/0915/p442.html. Published September 15, 2016. Accessed January 12, 2019.
29. January CT, Wann LS, Calkins H, et al. 2019 AHA/ACC/HRS focused update of the 2014 AHA/ACC/HRS guideline for the management of patients with atrial fibrillation: a Report of the American College of Cardiology/American Heart Association Task Force on clinical practice guidelines and the Heart Rhythm Society. *J Am Coll Cardiol.* 2019;74(1):104–132.
30. Katritsis DG, Gersh BJ, Camm AJ. Anticoagulation in atrial fibrillation—current concepts. *Arrhythm Electrophysiol Rev.* 2015;04(2):100–107.

36 Ventricular Arrhythmias, Cardiac Arrest, and Sudden Cardiac Death

Josip Katinic, Jasmina Katinic

OBJECTIVES

1. Verbalize the difference in pathophysiology of ventricular arrhythmias.
2. Describe medical management and treatment of ventricular arrhythmias.
3. Utilize the current algorithms for management of ventricular arrhythmias and cardiac arrest.
4. Implement appropriate nursing interventions and knowledge in management of ventricular arrhythmias and cardiac arrest patients.

KEY QUESTIONS

1. What causes ventricular tachycardia and what are the treatment options?
2. What types of arrhythmias require immediate defibrillation and how is it performed?
3. What are the causes of cardiac arrest and which adult cardiac life support (ACLS) algorithms are initiated in the emergency response?
4. Which interventions define high-quality cardiopulmonary resuscitation (CPR)?
5. What is the nursing role in managing patients after cardiac arrest?

VENTRICULAR ARRHYTHMIAS

Background

Ventricular arrhythmias are a major cause of morbidity and mortality and subsequent cause of sudden cardiac deaths (SCDs).[1] The ventricular arrhythmias include premature ventricular complex (PVC), accelerated idioventricular rhythm, ventricular tachycardia (VT), ventricular flutter, and ventricular asystole.

There are many etiologies of ventricular arrhythmias. VT usually occurs in patients with underlying structural heart disease. Myocardial disease and scarring cause abnormal cardiac impulse formation and propagation, which ultimately leads to VT.[2] Nonischemic conditions associated with VT, ventricular fibrillation (VF), and SCD include genetic conditions, cardiomyopathies, and idiopathic ventricular tachyarrhythmia in structurally normal hearts.[3] The likelihood of developing VT is proportionate to the degree of ventricular dysfunction. Arrhythmogenic right ventricular dysplasia is infiltrative disorder predominantly over the right ventricle that is characterized by fatty infiltration and fibrosis and may be a cause of cardiac arrest in apparently healthy individuals.[2]

Sustained VT and ventricular fibrillation have adverse effect on long-term prognosis and high mortality despite treatment. Asymptomatic nonsustained VT also demonstrates higher long-term mortality if programmed stimulation induces sustained VT. Development of VT or VF in 48 hours of an acute myocardial infarction (MI) significantly increases in-hospital mortality.[3] Evidence of a ventricular tachyarrhythmia and/or ventricular fibrillation following cardiac surgery increases both in-hospital mortality as well as poor long-term prognosis. The ventricular tachyarrhythmia is frequently observed in men because of ischemic heart disease.[4] Ventricular arrhythmias originate in the ventricular muscle or Purkinje system and are considered to be more dangerous than other arrhythmias because of their potential to severely limit cardiac output. As with any arrhythmia, ventricular rate is a key determinant of how well a patient can tolerate a ventricular rhythm. The sudden cardiac event is a significant cause of long-term mortality in ischemic heart disease accounting for approximately 22% of all causes of death.

This chapter reviews (1) the types of ventricular arrhythmias and their diagnosis and management, (2) cardiac arrest and SCD, and (3) nursing management of these conditions.

Types of Ventricular Arrhythmias

Premature Ventricular Complexes

PVCs are caused by premature depolarization of cells in the ventricular myocardium or Purkinje system due to enhanced normal automaticity or abnormal automaticity, reentry in the ventricles, or afterdepolarizations.[5,6] PVCs can be caused by hypoxia, myocardial ischemia, hypokalemia, acidosis, exercise, increased levels of circulating catecholamines, digitalis toxicity, caffeine, alcohol, and other causes. PVCs increase with aging and are more common in people with coronary heart disease, valve disease, hypertension, cardiomyopathy, and other forms of heart disease. Generally, PVCs are not dangerous in people with structurally normal hearts but are associated with higher mortality rates in patients with structural heart disease or acute MI, especially if left ventricular function is

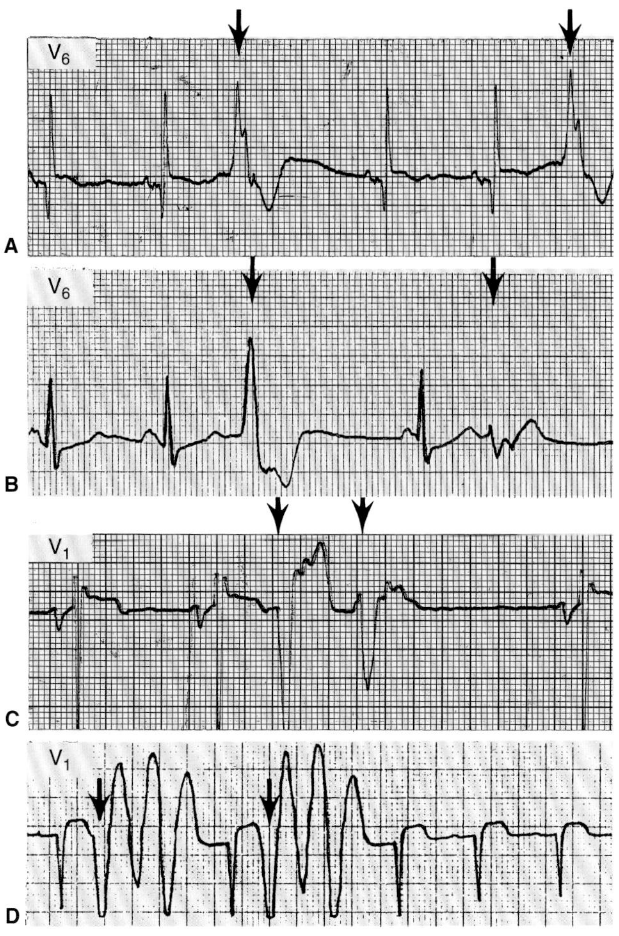

Figure 36-1. Examples of PVCs. Cardiac rhythm recording strips. (**A**) Normal sinus rhythm with unifocal PVCs. (**B**) Sinus rhythm with multifocal PVC. (**C**) Paired PVC. (**D**) R-on-T PVC, resulting in short runs of VT.

reduced. PVCs are considered potentially malignant when they occur more frequently than 10 per hour or are repetitive (i.e., occur in pairs, triplets, or more than three in a row) in patients with coronary disease, previous MI, cardiomyopathy, and with reduced ejection fraction.[7,8]

PVCs have the following ECG characteristics (Fig. 36-1):

Rate: 60 to 100 beats per minute or the rate of the basic rhythm

Rhythm: Irregular because of the early beats

P waves: Not related to the PVC. Sinus rhythm is often not interrupted, so sinus P waves can frequently be seen occurring regularly throughout the rhythm. P waves may follow a PVC because of retrograde conduction from the ventricle backward through the atria; these P waves are inverted in the inferior leads (II, III, aVF).

PR interval: Not present before most PVC. If a P wave happens, by coincidence, to precede a PVC, the PR interval is short.

QRS complex: Wide and bizarre, usually greater than 0.12 second in duration. May vary in morphology if PVCs originate from more than one focus in the ventricles. T waves are usually in the opposite direction from the QRS complex.

Conduction: Impulses originating in the ventricles conduct through the ventricular myocardium from muscle cell to muscle cell rather than through Purkinje fibers, resulting in wide QRS complexes. Some PVCs may conduct retrograde into the atria, resulting in inverted P waves that follow the PVC. When the sinus rhythm is undisturbed by PVCs, the atria depolarize normally.

The significance of PVCs depends on the clinical setting in which they occur. Many people have chronic PVCs that do not need to be treated, and most of these people are asymptomatic. There is no evidence that suppression of PVCs reduces mortality, especially in patients with no structural heart disease. If PVCs cause bothersome palpitations, patients should be instructed to avoid caffeine, tobacco, other stimulants, and try stress reduction techniques. Low-dose β-blockers may reduce PVC frequency and the perception of palpitations and can be used for symptom relief. In the setting of an acute MI or myocardial ischemia, PVCs may be precursors of more dangerous ventricular arrhythmias, especially when they occur near the apex of the T wave (R-on-T PVC). Prophylactic treatment of asymptomatic nonsustained ventricular arrhythmias is not recommended.[9]

Accelerated Idioventricular Rhythm

Accelerated idioventricular rhythm occurs when an ectopic focus in the ventricles fires at a rate of 50 to 100 beats per minute. Accelerated idioventricular rhythm commonly occurs in the presence of inferior MI and during reperfusion with thrombolytic therapy, when the rate of the SA node slows below the rate of the latent ventricular pacemaker.

The ECG characteristics of accelerated ventricular rhythm include the following (Fig. 36-2):

Rate: 50 to 100 beats per minute

Rhythm: Usually regular

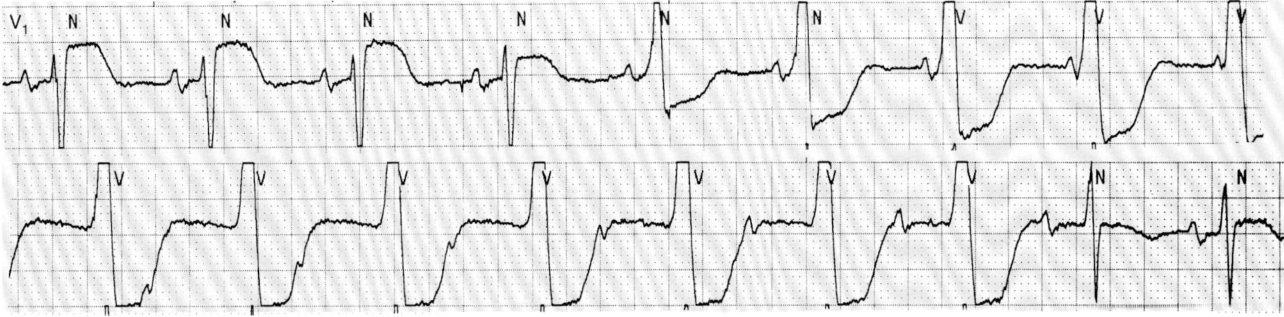

Figure 36-2. Example of accelerated idioventricular rhythm. Cardiac rhythm recording strip demonstrates sinus rhythm with accelerated ventricular rhythm at a rate of 70 beats per minute. Note sinus P waves that continue uninterrupted during the period of accelerated ventricular rhythm (an example of AV dissociation). *N* = arrhythmia computer's interpretation of normal beat, *V* = computer's interpretation of ventricular beat.

P waves: May be seen but are dissociated from the QRS. If retrograde conduction from the ventricle to the atria occurs, P waves follow the QRS complex.

PR interval: Not present

QRS complex: Wide and bizarre

Conduction: If sinus rhythm is the basic rhythm, atrial conduction is normal. Impulses originating in the ventricles conduct through the ventricular myocardium by cell-to-cell conduction, resulting in the wide QRS complex.

The treatment of accelerated ventricular rhythm depends on its cause and how well it is tolerated. This arrhythmia alone is usually not harmful because the ventricular rate is within normal limits and usually adequate to maintain cardiac output. If the patient is symptomatic because of the loss of atrial kick during long episodes of AV dissociation, atropine can be used to increase the rate of the SA node and overdrive the ventricular rhythm. Suppressive therapy is rarely used because abolishing the ventricular rhythm may leave an even less desirable heart rate. Usually, accelerated ventricular rhythm is transient and benign and does not require treatment.

Ventricular Tachycardia

VT is a rapid ventricular rhythm most likely due to reentry in the ventricles, although automaticity of an ectopic focus and afterdepolarizations may also be mechanisms of VT.[5,10] VT can be classified according to (1) duration—nonsustained (lasts less than 30 seconds), sustained (lasts greater than 30 seconds), incessant (VT present most of the time); (2) morphology (ECG appearance of QRS complexes)—monomorphic (QRS complexes have the same shape during tachycardia), polymorphic (QRS complexes vary randomly in shape), bidirectional (alternating upright and negative QRS complexes during tachycardia). The terms salvos and bursts are often used to describe short runs of VT (i.e., 5 to 10 or more beats in a row).

The VT is caused by electrical reentry or abnormal automaticity. Myocardial scarring increases the likelihood of electrical reentrant circuits. Most common cause of sustained monomorphic VT is ventricular scar formation from prior MI.[4] More than 170 mutations of genes have been identified as cause of congenital long QT syndrome (LQTS), potassium channel genes, and sodium channel genes. Polymorphic VT occurs in patients as a result of early afterdepolarization. The Brugada syndrome is caused by sodium channel defect and incomplete right bundle branch block with ST-segment elevation in leads V1 to V3 and can lead to ventricular fibrillation.[2] Nonsustained ventricular tachycardia (NSVT) is defined by 3 sometimes 5 or more consecutive beats in arising the low atrioventricular node with an RR interval of less than 600 milliseconds, more than 100 per and lasting less than 30 seconds. There are no strictly defined diagnostic criteria and this definition is not universal.[11]

During the VT cardiac output is reduced as a consequence of decreased ventricular filling from the rapid heart rate and lack of properly timed or coordinated atrial contraction. Ischemia in mitral insufficiency may also contribute to decreased ventricular stroke volume, hemodynamic intolerance, and collapse.[4] The underlying left ventricular dysfunction leads to diminished cardiac output, which ultimately results in diminished myocardial perfusion thus worsening the inotropic response and degeneration to ventricular fibrillation resulting in sudden death.[4] The monomorphic episodes of NSVT are often due to the idiopathic ventricular outflow arrhythmias, which usually present in the form of repetitive uniform premature ventricular contractions (PVCs)

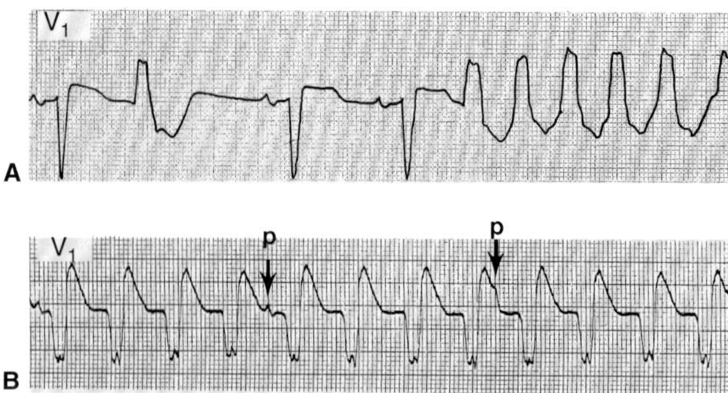

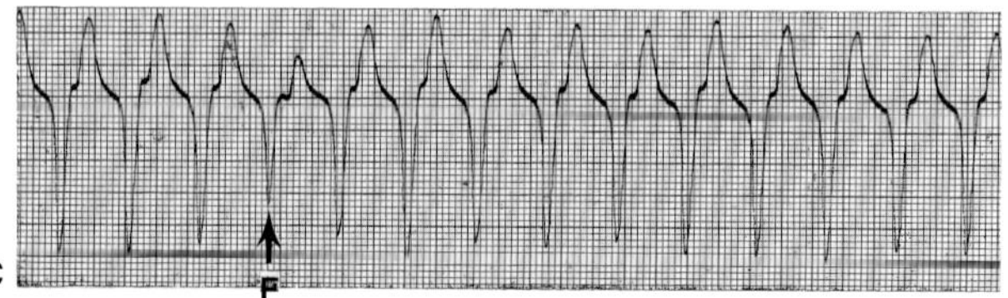

Figure 36-3. Examples of ventricular tachycardia. Cardiac rhythm recording strip demonstrates (**A**) Sinus rhythm with a PVC and a run of monomorphic VT. (**B**) AV dissociation is evidenced by independently occurring P waves. (**C**) VT with a fusion beat (fourth complex).

and paroxysmal-sustained monomorphic VT that is usually exercise provoked.[11] In asymptomatic healthy persons runs of nonsustained ventricular tachyarrhythmia could be recorded at rest although frequent ventricular ectopy during recovery and after exercise poses increased risk for death.[11] The most common anatomic substrate for sustained monomorphic VT is chronic coronary artery disease (CAD) with the vast majority of ventricular arrhythmias in ischemic heart disease originating the left ventricle or interventricular septum. Each area of infarction is associated with characteristic VT morphology.[12] Idiopathic VT is VT that occurs in patients with no known structural heart disease.[8,10,13]

ECG characteristics of monomorphic VT include the following (see Fig. 36-3):

Rate: Ventricular rate is usually 100 to 220 beats per minute

Rhythm: Usually regular but may be slightly irregular

P waves: Often dissociated from QRS complexes. If sinus rhythm is the underlying basic rhythm, regular P waves may be seen but are not related to QRS complexes. P waves are often buried in QRS complexes or T waves. VT may conduct retrograde to the atria with P waves visible after each QRS.

PR interval: Not measurable because of dissociation of P waves from QRS complexes

QRS complex: Wide and bizarre, greater than 0.12 second in duration

Conduction: Impulse originates in one ventricle and spreads by muscle cell-to-cell conduction through both ventricles. There may be retrograde conduction through the atria, but often the SA node continues to fire regularly and depolarizes the atria normally. Rarely, one of these sinus impulses may conduct normally through the AV node and into the ventricle before the next ectopic ventricular impulse fires, resulting in a normal QRS complex, called a capture beat. Occasionally, a fusion beat may occur as the ventricles are depolarized by a descending sinus impulse and the ventricular ectopic impulse simultaneously, resulting in a QRS complex that looks different from both the normal beats and the ventricular beats.

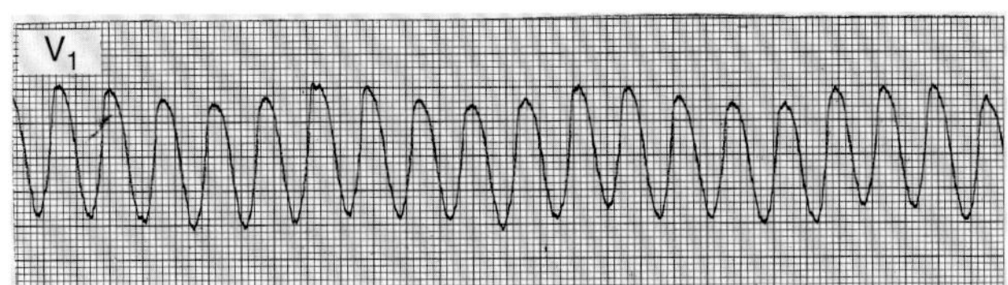

Figure 36-4. Example of ventricular flutter. Cardiac rhythm recording strip demonstrates regular, large oscillations with a loss of organized electrical activity.

The two main determinants of patient tolerance of any tachycardia are ventricular rate and underlying left ventricular function. VT can be an emergency if cardiac output is severely decreased because of a very rapid rate or poor left ventricular function. Defibrillation is the immediate treatment of pulseless VT. Synchronized electrical cardioversion is the immediate treatment for hemodynamically unstable VT with a pulse present. The American College of Cardiology (ACC)/AHA/ESC practice guidelines for managing ventricular arrhythmias recommend procainamide as initial drug treatment of stable sustained VT, and amiodarone for hemodynamically unstable VT or VT that is refractory to cardioversion or recurrent despite procainamide.[9]

Long-term drug therapy for ventricular arrhythmias includes β-blockers because they are effective in suppressing ventricular arrhythmias and reducing SCD in patients post-MI, those with HF, and cardiomyopathy. Amiodarone and sotalol are effective in suppressing ventricular arrhythmias but most studies show no long-term survival benefit. Nonpharmacologic therapy for recurrent VT includes radiofrequency catheter ablation and the implantable cardioverter defibrillator (ICD).

Ventricular Flutter

Ventricular flutter is similar to VT, but the rate is faster. Hemodynamically, ventricular flutter is more dangerous because there is virtually no cardiac output.

ECG characteristics of ventricular flutter are as follows (Fig. 36-4):

Rate: Ventricular rate is usually 220 to 400 beats per minute
Rhythm: Usually regular
P waves: None seen
PR interval: None measurable
QRS complex: Very wide, regular, sine-wave type of pattern
Conduction: Originates in the ventricle and spreads through muscle cell-to-cell conduction, resulting in very wide, bizarre complexes

Ventricular flutter is fatal unless treated immediately by defibrillation. If a defibrillator is not immediately available, cardiopulmonary resuscitation (CPR) should be started. After the rhythm is converted, antiarrhythmic drug therapy should be initiated to prevent recurrence. Drug therapy is similar to that used for VT.

Ventricular Fibrillation

VF is rapid, ineffective quivering of the ventricles; is fatal without immediate treatment; and is the most frequent cause of SCD. Electrical activity originates in the ventricles and spreads in a chaotic, irregular pattern throughout both ventricles. There is no cardiac output or palpable pulse with VF.

ECG characteristics of VF include the following (Fig. 36-5):

Rate: Rapid, uncoordinated, ineffective
Rhythm: Chaotic, irregular
P waves: None seen
PR interval: None
QRS complex: No formed QRS complexes seen; rapid, irregular undulations without any specific pattern. This erratic electrical activity can be coarse or fine.
Conduction: Random electrical activity in ventricles depolarizes them irregularly and without any organized pattern. There is no organized conduction and the ventricles do not contract.

VF requires immediate defibrillation. Synchronized cardioversion is not possible because there are no formed QRS complexes on which to synchronize the shock. CPR must be performed if a defibrillator is not immediately available. The American Heart Association (AHA) guidelines for VF and pulseless VT call for CPR until a defibrillator is available, then immediate defibrillation using and automatic external defibrillator; or manual defibrillation with 360 J if using a monophasic defibrillator or device-specific energy recommendation (200 J if this is not known) if using a biphasic defibrillator.[14] Immediate CPR for 2 minutes is recommended following the first shock.

Amiodarone and lidocaine are the drugs recommended for antiarrhythmic therapy in VF following defibrillation. Drugs have not been shown to improve survival in patients with recurrent hemodynamically unstable ventricular arrhythmias; even amiodarone, which is the most effective antiarrhythmic, is inferior to ICD in reducing the incidence of SCD. However, amiodarone and β-blockers, often in combination, are used in patients with recurrent ventricular arrhythmias who are not eligible for ICD implantation or in those who have an ICD but have recurrent ventricular arrhythmias that cause frequent ICD shocks. Sotalol is also effective in suppressing ventricular arrhythmias in many patients.

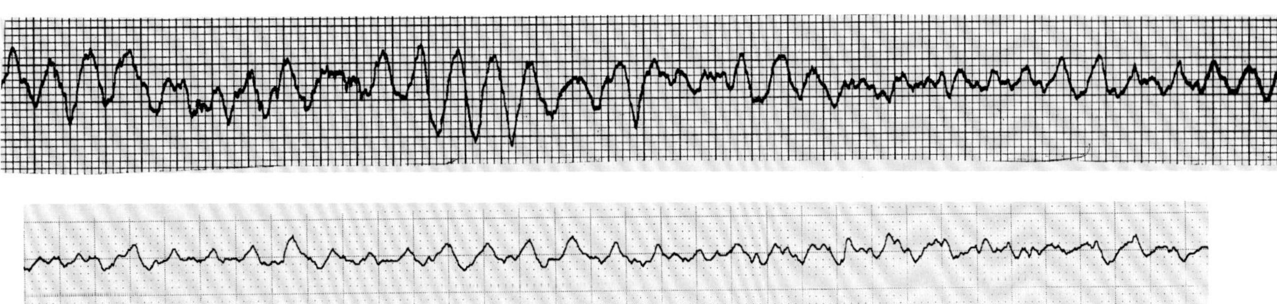

Figure 36-5. Examples of ventricular fibrillation. Cardiac rhythm recording strips demonstrate electrical activation in the ventricles is fractionated, resulting in an ECG of irregular undulations without recognizable ventricular complexes.

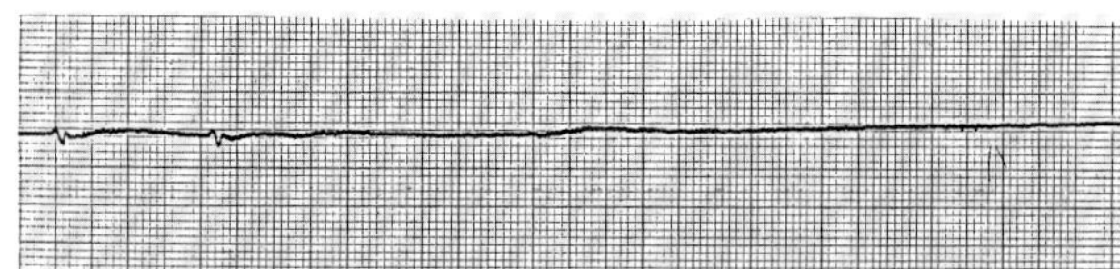

Figure 36-6. Example of ventricular asystole. Cardiac rhythm recording strip demonstrates two P waves are seen at the beginning of the strip followed by absence of electrical activity.

Ventricular Asystole

Ventricular asystole is the absence of any ventricular rhythm; there is no QRS complex, no pulse, and no cardiac output. The term "ventricular standstill" is sometimes used when atrial activity is still present but no ventricular activity occurs. Both situations are fatal unless treated immediately.

Ventricular asystole has the following characteristics (Fig. 36-6):

Rate: None

Rhythm: None

P waves: May be present if the SA node is functioning

PR interval: None

QRS complex: None

Conduction: Atrial conduction may be normal if the SA node is functioning. There is no conduction into the ventricles.

CPR must be initiated immediately if the patient is to survive. IV epinephrine and atropine may be given in an effort to stimulate a rhythm; vasopressin can be used instead of epinephrine as a vasopressor. Asystole has a very poor prognosis despite the best resuscitation efforts because it usually represents extensive myocardial ischemia or severe underlying metabolic problems.

Diagnosis of Ventricular Tachycardia

Patients who develop VT can be asymptomatic although often times, the symptoms are associated with other causes such as acute MI.[4] Most common presenting symptoms are palpitations, lightheadedness, and syncope. The patient having sustained VT may be pulseless on examination, may experience loss of consciousness, pulmonary edema or signs of shock (for detailed assessment and presenting symptoms, see Table 36-1).[2] In patients with suspected VT rapid but accurate recognition of arrhythmia is imperative by performing surface 12-lead electrocardiogram, which must be systematically analyzed to reach the correct diagnosis.[3]

The Kindwall criteria format morphologic differences to four specific criteria for VT with a left bundle branch block; an R wave in V1 or V2 greater than 30 ms in duration; any Q wave in V6; a duration of greater than 60 ms from the onset of the QRS to the nadir of the S wave in V1 or V2; and notching on the down stroke of the S wave in V1 or V2.[12] The QRS complexes can be classified as a monomorphic (constant in form) or polymorphic (variable form). The monomorphic VT tends to be reproducible recurrent phenomena and may be initiated with pacing. In contrary polymorphic VT is more dynamic and unstable process by its very nature thus less reproducible.[15] Sustained polymorphic VT, ventricular flutter and ventricular fibrillation all lead to immediate hemodynamic collapse thereby emergency asynchronous defibrillation is therefore required.[15] Patients with sustained VT or ventricular fibrillation must undergo careful physical examination, review of medication, and measurement of electrolyte and cardiac enzymes. Most patients should undergo coronary angiography and left ventriculography to gain more clinical data.[2] In those patients who have significant ventricular dysfunction or are at increased risk of dying suddenly further evaluation by performing electrophysiology testing is recommended. Patients with sustained VT reproduced during programmed electrostimulation are at higher risk for cardiac arrest and those patients may benefit from implantation of cardiac defibrillator to prevent SCD.[3] Other noninvasive helpful tests used to risk stratify patient with nonsustained VT include signal-averaged electrocardiography, measurement of heart rate variability, and assessment of T-wave alternans, however their clinical use appears to be limited.[2]

Table 36-1 • EVALUATION OF PATIENTS WITH KNOWN OR SUSPECTED VENTRICULAR ARRHYTHMIA AND SUDDEN CARDIAC DEATH

Component	Assessment and Findings Relevant for VA and/or SCD Risk
Presenting symptoms	• Symptoms/events related to arrhythmia: Palpitations, lightheadedness, syncope, dyspnea, chest pain, cardiac arrest • Symptoms related to underlying heart disease: Dyspnea at rest or on exertion, orthopnea, paroxysmal nocturnal dyspnea, chest pain, edema • Precipitating factors: Exercise, emotional stress
Risk factors	• Known heart disease: Coronary, valvular (e.g., mitral valve prolapse), congenital heart disease, other • Risk factors for heart disease: Hypertension, diabetes mellitus, hyperlipidemia, and smoking
Medications	• Antiarrhythmic medications • Other medications with potential for QT prolongation and torsades de pointes • Medications with potential to provoke or aggravate VA (stimulants including cocaine and amphetamines, supplements including anabolic steroids) • Medication interactions that could cause QT prolongation and torsades de pointes
Past medical history	• Thyroid disease • Acute kidney injury, chronic kidney disease, or electrolyte abnormalities • Stroke or embolic events • Lung disease • Epilepsy (arrhythmic syncope can be misdiagnosed as epilepsy) • Alcohol or illicit drug use • Use of over-the-counter medications that could cause QT prolongation and torsades de pointes • Unexplained motor vehicle crashes

Family history	• SCD, SCA, or unexplained drowning in a first-degree relative
	• SIDS or repetitive spontaneous pregnancy losses given their potential association with cardiac channelopathies
	• Heart disease
	  • IHD
	  • Cardiomyopathy: Hypertrophic, dilated, ARVC
	  • Congenital heart disease
	  • Cardiac channelopathies: Long QT, Brugada's, short QT, CPVT
	  • Arrhythmias
	  • Conduction disorders, pacemakers/ICDs
	• Neuromuscular disease associated with cardiomyopathies
	  • Muscular dystrophy
	• Epilepsy

Examination	• Heart rate and regularity, blood pressure • Jugular venous pressure • Murmurs • Pulses and bruits • Edema • Sternotomy scars

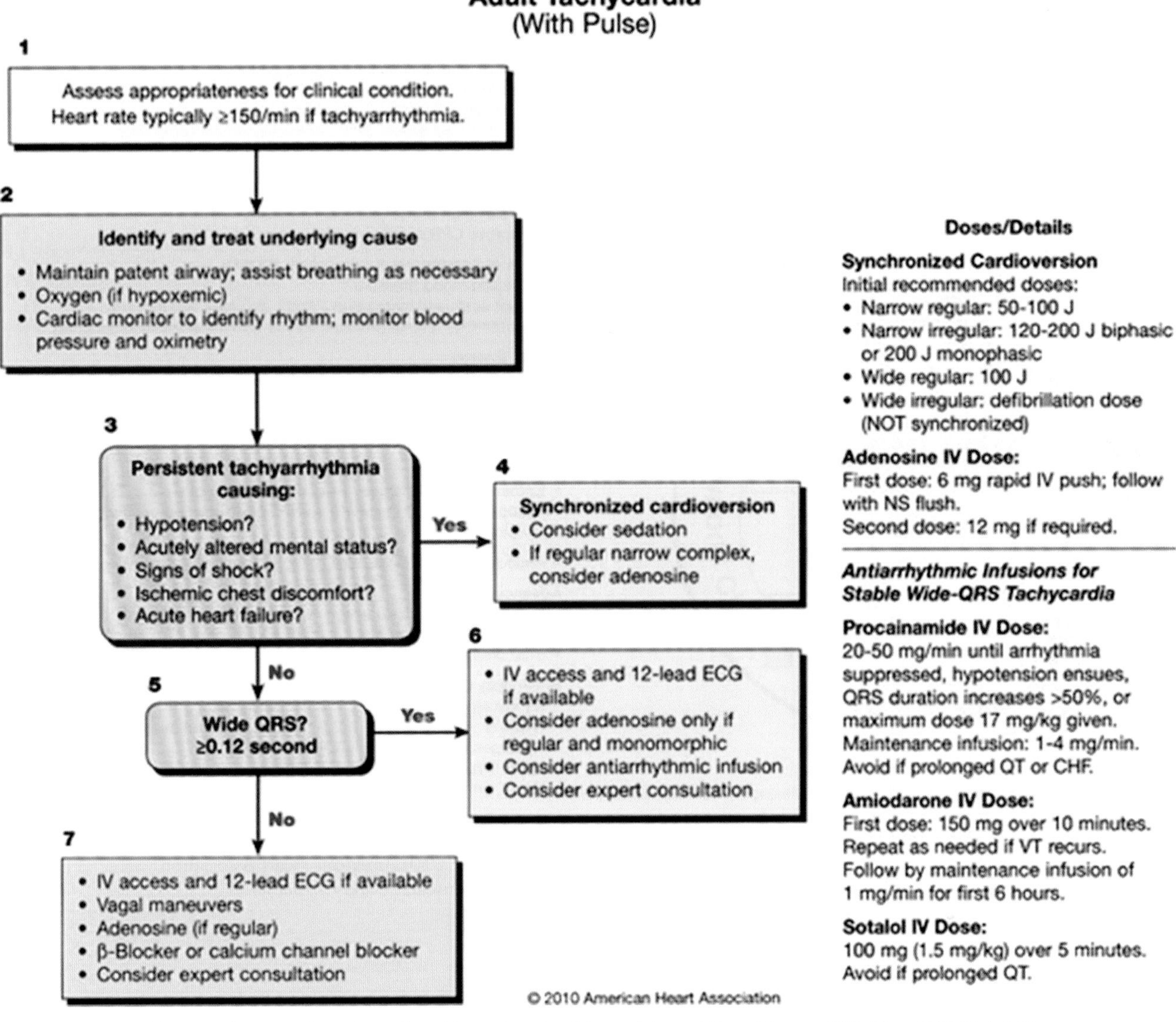

Figure 36-7. Adult tachycardia with a pulse algorithm. (Adapted from Neumar RW, Otto CW, Link MS, et al. Part 8: Adult advanced cardiovascular life support: 2010 American Heart Association Guidelines for Cardiopulmonary Resuscitation and Emergency Cardiovascular Care. *Circulation*. 2010;122(Suppl 3):S729–S767.)

Medical Management and Treatment of Ventricular Tachycardia

Acute management of patients with ventricular tachyarrhythmia should follow advanced cardiovascular life support (ACLS) guidelines (Figs. 36-7 and 36-8). Most effective method for restoring sinus rhythm is a synchronized direct current electrical shock. Patients with ventricular fibrillation or pulseless VT should undergo basic CPR followed by three attempts of defibrillation until sinus rhythm is restored. The recommended energy levels using a biphasic defibrillator are 120 J, followed by 200 J or the maximum possible joules, and monophasic 360 J. If these measures are ineffective drugs should be administered in stepwise manner followed by repeat attempts at defibrillation.[2] The intravenous antiarrhythmic medicine often used for ventricular arrhythmias include lidocaine, procainamide, and amiodarone. Procainamide is preferred for pharmacologic cardioversion of stable VT in patients with normal systolic function, whereas lidocaine is useful for VT during acute ischemia.[3] The amiodarone is the most effective antiarrhythmic medicine for ventricular tachyarrhythmia although requires loading time. Patients who have experienced episodes of sustained VT or ventricular fibrillation are at risk of having recurrence unless there is evidence of correctable cause. Long-term management of patients with ventricular arrhythmias can be divided into drug therapy, device therapy, and catheter ablation. Most recent guidelines for management of ventricular arrhythmias and prevention of SCD published by AHA/ACC/Heart rhythm Society published in 2017 recommend treatment modalities (Figs. 36-9 to 36-12) including pharmacologic therapy, catheter ablation, and implantation of cardiac defibrillator.[16]

Pharmacologic Therapies for Ventricular Arrhythmia and Sudden Cardiac Death

The antiarrhythmic medication therapy except β-blocker therapy (metoprolol, carvedilol) has not shown any evidence in randomized clinical trials to improve survival in ventricular arrhythmias when given for primary or secondary prevention of SCD. The antiarrhythmic medication however remains essential

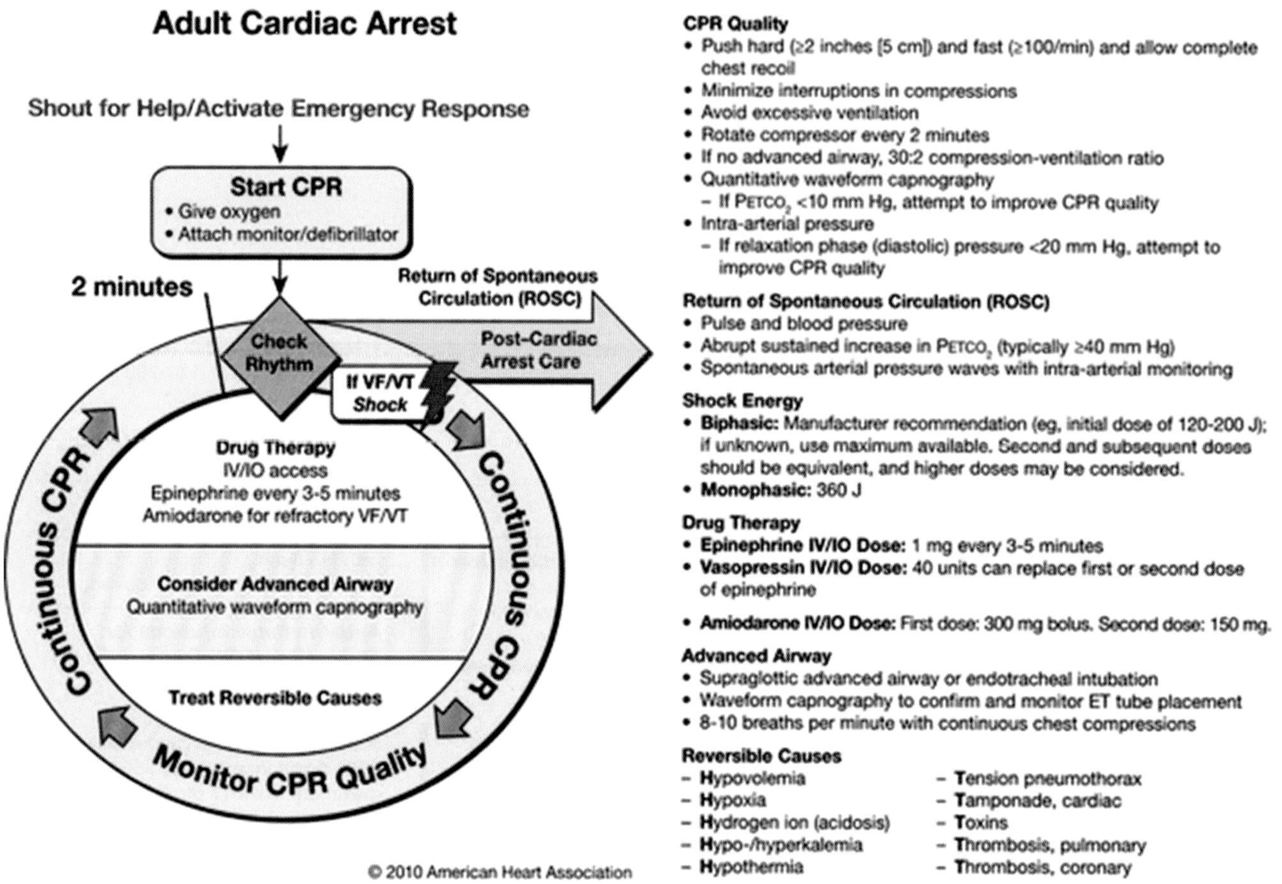

Adult Cardiac Arrest

Shout for Help/Activate Emergency Response

Start CPR
- Give oxygen
- Attach monitor/defibrillator

2 minutes

Check Rhythm

Return of Spontaneous Circulation (ROSC)

Post-Cardiac Arrest Care

If VF/VT Shock

Drug Therapy
IV/IO access
Epinephrine every 3-5 minutes
Amiodarone for refractory VF/VT

Consider Advanced Airway
Quantitative waveform capnography

Treat Reversible Causes

Continuous CPR

Continuous CPR

Monitor CPR Quality

© 2010 American Heart Association

CPR Quality
- Push hard (≥2 inches [5 cm]) and fast (≥100/min) and allow complete chest recoil
- Minimize interruptions in compressions
- Avoid excessive ventilation
- Rotate compressor every 2 minutes
- If no advanced airway, 30:2 compression-ventilation ratio
- Quantitative waveform capnography
  - If P_{ETCO_2} <10 mm Hg, attempt to improve CPR quality
- Intra-arterial pressure
  - If relaxation phase (diastolic) pressure <20 mm Hg, attempt to improve CPR quality

Return of Spontaneous Circulation (ROSC)
- Pulse and blood pressure
- Abrupt sustained increase in P_{ETCO_2} (typically ≥40 mm Hg)
- Spontaneous arterial pressure waves with intra-arterial monitoring

Shock Energy
- **Biphasic:** Manufacturer recommendation (eg, initial dose of 120-200 J); if unknown, use maximum available. Second and subsequent doses should be equivalent, and higher doses may be considered.
- **Monophasic:** 360 J

Drug Therapy
- **Epinephrine IV/IO Dose:** 1 mg every 3-5 minutes
- **Vasopressin IV/IO Dose:** 40 units can replace first or second dose of epinephrine
- **Amiodarone IV/IO Dose:** First dose: 300 mg bolus. Second dose: 150 mg.

Advanced Airway
- Supraglottic advanced airway or endotracheal intubation
- Waveform capnography to confirm and monitor ET tube placement
- 8-10 breaths per minute with continuous chest compressions

Reversible Causes
- Hypovolemia
- Hypoxia
- Hydrogen ion (acidosis)
- Hypo-/hyperkalemia
- Hypothermia
- Tension pneumothorax
- Tamponade, cardiac
- Toxins
- Thrombosis, pulmonary
- Thrombosis, coronary

Figure 36-8. Adult cardiac arrest circular algorithm—2018 update. (Adapted from Neumar RW, Otto CW, Link MS, et al. Part 8: Adult advanced cardiovascular life support: 2010 American Heart Association Guidelines for Cardiopulmonary Resuscitation and Emergency Cardiovascular Care. *Circulation.* 2010;122(Suppl 3):S729–S767.)

to control arrhythmia and improve symptoms. These medicines are divided in four categories by Vaughan Williams class I through IV (Table 36-2).[16]

- Class I (sodium channel blockers) but also further subdivided in a, b, c subclass have a limited role in VT/SCD based on lack of survival benefit and increased mortality observed during chronic therapy.
- Class II (β-blockers) have an excellent safety profile, effective in treating VA and preventing VT. In addition, they reduce all-cause mortality and SCD in patients with heart failure (HF), and reduced ejection fraction (EF).
- Class III (potassium channel blockers) the overall long-term effects on survival remain controversial, however some studies showed a reduction in SCD in primary prevention using amiodarone. In contrary, for secondary prevention of SCD using amiodarone showed neither risk nor benefit.
- Class IV (nondihydropyridine calcium channel blockers) for treatment of VA have not shown any benefit, in fact a calcium channel blockers should be not given to patients with VT in the setting of HF and reduced EF.[16]

In patients with heart failure and reduced EF (LVEF less than 40%) randomized controlled trials have demonstrated that chronic therapy with β-blockers reduces all-cause mortality, VA, and SCD.[17–19] In addition, mineralocorticoid receptors antagonists, ACE (angiotensin-converting enzyme), an angiotensin-receptor blocker, or angiotensin receptor-neprilysin inhibitor is recommended to reduce an SCD and all-cause mortality.[20–22] Three β-blockers (carvedilol, bisoprolol, and metoprolol succinate) have particularly proven to reduce mortality in patients with current or prior symptoms of heart failure and reduced ejection fraction.[16] Mineralocorticoid receptor antagonist such as spironolactone and eplerenone also demonstrated reduction seen both all-cause mortality an SCD.[16] More recently angiotensin receptor-neprilysin (sacubitril/valsartan) demonstrated reduction in ICD and cardiac mortality.[23]

CARDIAC ARREST AND SUDDEN CARDIAC DEATH

Background

Cardiac arrest is defined as cardiac mechanical and circulatory cessation. It is predominantly related to cardiac diseases unless

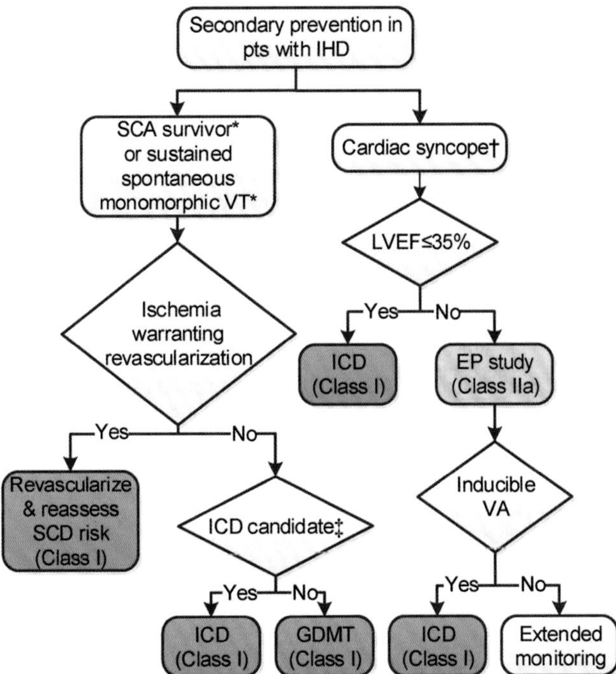

Figure 36-9. Secondary prevention of ventricular arrhythmias and sudden cardiac death in patients with ischemic heart disease. (Adapted from Al-Khatib SM, Stevenson WG, Ackerman MJ, et al. 2017 AHA/ACC/HRS guideline for management of patients with ventricular arrhythmias and the prevention of sudden cardiac death: Executive Summary. A Report of the American College of Cardiology/American Heart Association Task Force on Clinical Practice Guidelines and the Heart Rhythm Society. *J Am Coll Cardiol.* 2018;72(14):1677–1749.)

it is known or likely to be caused by trauma, drug overdose, or other noncardiac-related causes as determined by first responders. According to AHA, approximately 350,000 people annually experienced out-of-hospital cardiac arrests in the United States. Despite being a leading cause of SCD, there are currently no nationwide standards for surveillance to monitor the incidence and outcome.[24]

SCD is a major clinical and public health problem in the United States and the overall incidence has remained unchanged as our population ages. It is defined as an unexpected death caused by cardiac causes that occurs within 1 hour of symptom onset. The person may or may not have had pre-existing heart disease. Cardiac arrest, usually caused by cardiac arrhythmias, is the term used to describe the sudden collapse, loss of consciousness, and loss of effective circulation that precedes biologic death.[25,26] A subclassification of sudden death uses the term instantaneous death, a death with immediate collapse without preceding symptoms. Other causes of death may also be instantaneous, such as stroke, massive pulmonary embolism, or rupture of an aortic aneurysm. It is also important to note that not all arrhythmic deaths are sudden. A patient may be successfully resuscitated from a cardiac arrest but may die days later from complications.[27]

Pathogenesis

The epidemiology of SCD tends to follow that of CAD. The incidence of SCD increases with the aging population in both men and women, whites and nonwhites, just as ischemic heart disease increases. Hypertension, left ventricular hypertrophy (LVH), intraventricular conduction defect, hypercholesterolemia, vital capacity, smoking, relative weight, and heart rate were all noted as risk factors per the 26-year follow-up of the Framingham

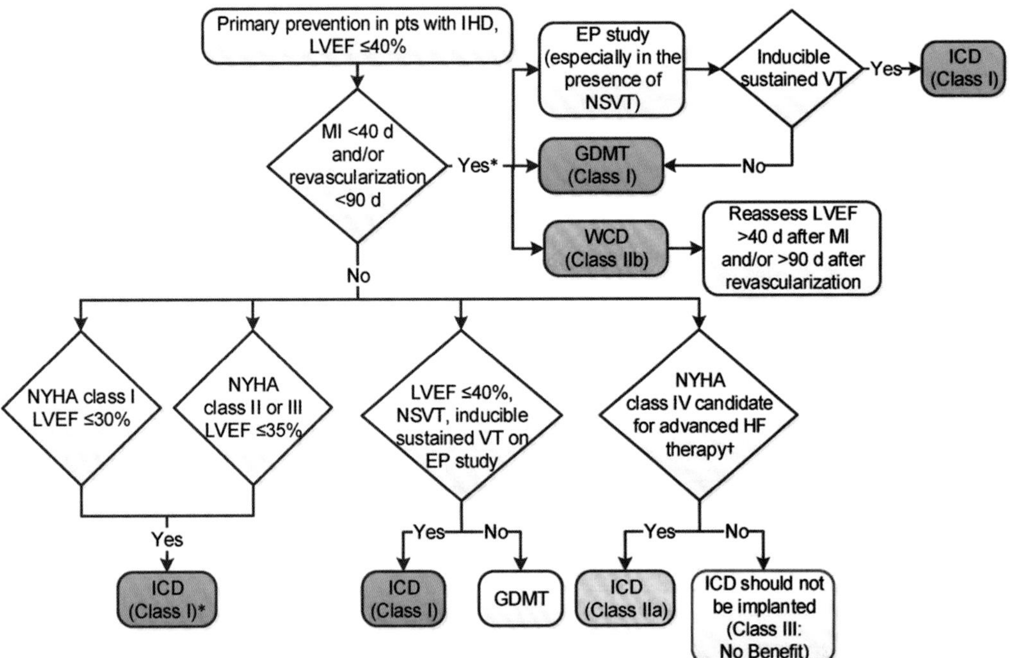

Figure 36-10. Primary prevention of ventricular arrhythmias and sudden cardiac death in patients with ischemic heart disease and left ventricular dysfunction. (Adapted from Al-Khatib SM, Stevenson WG, Ackerman MJ, et al. 2017 AHA/ACC/HRS guideline for management of patients with ventricular arrhythmias and the prevention of sudden cardiac death: Executive Summary. A Report of the American College of Cardiology/American Heart Association Task Force on Clinical Practice Guidelines and the Heart Rhythm Society. *J Am Coll Cardiol.* 2018;72(14):1677–1749.)

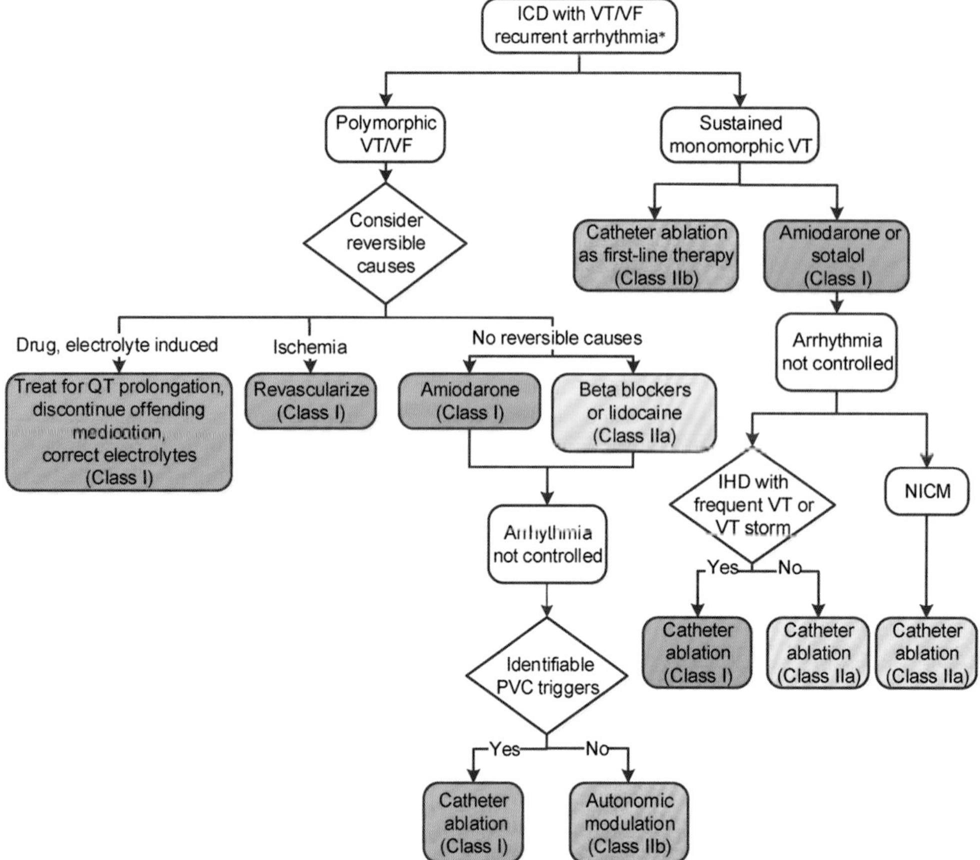

Figure 36-11. Ventricular arrhythmias and sudden cardiac death in patients with implantable cardioverter defibrillator and recurrent ventricular tachycardia/ ventricular fibrillation. (Adapted from Al-Khatib SM, Stevenson WG, Ackerman MJ, et al. 2017 AHA/ACC/HRS guideline for management of patients with ventricular arrhythmias and the prevention of sudden cardiac death: Executive Summary. A Report of the American College of Cardiology/ American Heart Association Task Force on Clinical Practice Guidelines and the Heart Rhythm Society. *J Am Coll Cardiol.* 2018;72(14):1677–1749.)

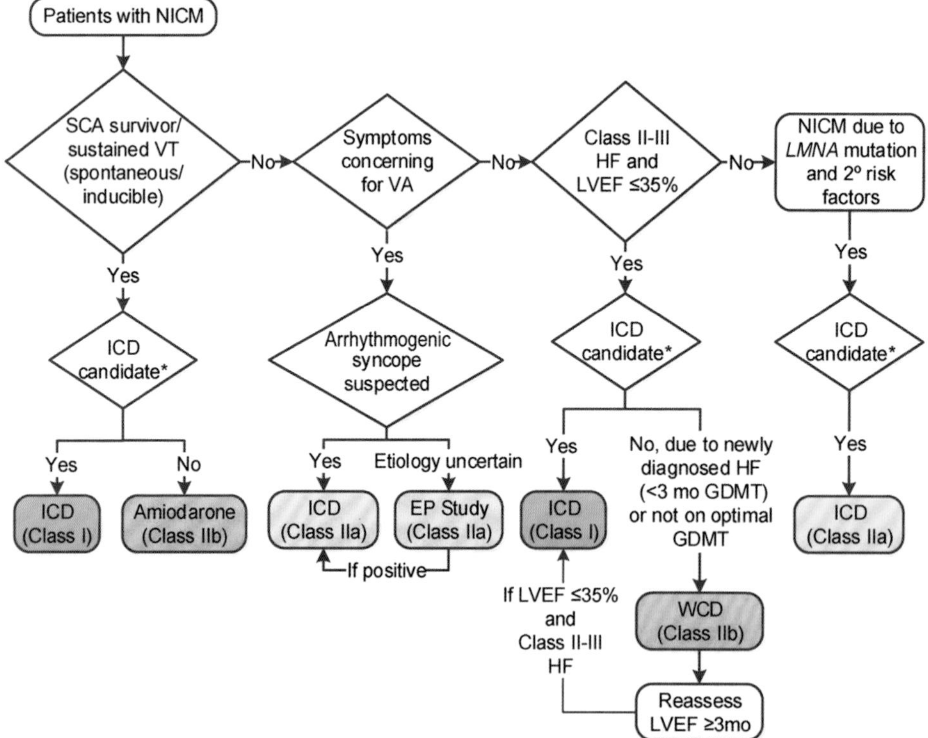

Figure 36-12. Secondary prevention of ventricular arrhythmias and sudden cardiac death in patients with nonischemic cardiomyopathy. (Adapted from Al-Khatib SM, Stevenson WG, Ackerman MJ, et al. 2017 AHA/ACC/HRS guideline for management of patients with ventricular arrhythmias and the prevention of sudden cardiac death: Executive Summary. A Report of the American College of Cardiology/American Heart Association Task Force on Clinical Practice Guidelines and the Heart Rhythm Society. *J Am Coll Cardiol.* 2018;72(14):1677–1749.)

Table 36-2 • ANTIARRHYTHMIC MEDICATIONS FOR TREATING VENTRICULAR ARRHYTHMIAS

Antiarrhythmic Medication (Class) and Dose	Uses in VA/SCA	Electrophysiologic Effects	Common Adverse Effects
Acebutolol PO 200–1200 mg daily or up to 600 mg bid	VT, PVCs	Sinus rate slowed AV nodal refractoriness increased	Cardiac: Bradycardia, hypotension, HF, AVB Other: Dizziness, fatigue, anxiety, impotence, hyper-/hypoesthesia
Amiodarone (III) IV: 300 mg bolus for VF/pulseless VT arrest; 150-mg bolus for stable VT; 1 mg/min × 6 h, then 0.5 mg/min × 18 h PO: 400 mg q 8–12 h for 1–2 wk, then 300–400 mg daily; reduce dose to 200 mg daily if possible	VT, VF, PVC,	Sinus rate slowed QRS prolonged QTc prolonged AV nodal refractoriness increased; increased DFT	Cardiac: Hypotension, bradycardia, AVB, TdP, slows VT below programmed ICD detection rate, increases defibrillation threshold Other: Corneal microdeposits, thyroid abnormalities, ataxia, nausea, emesis, constipation, photosensitivity, skin discoloration, ataxia, dizziness, peripheral neuropathy, tremor, hepatitis, cirrhosis, pulmonary fibrosis, or pneumonitis
Atenolol (II) PO: 25–100 mg qd or bid	VT, PVC, ARVC, LQTS	Sinus rate slowed AV nodal refractoriness increased	Cardiac: Bradycardia, hypotension, HF, AVB Other: Dizziness, fatigue, depression, impotence
Bisoprolol (II) PO: 2.5–10 mg once daily	VT, PVC	Sinus rate slowed AV nodal refractoriness increased	Cardiac: Chest pain, bradycardia, AVB Other: Fatigue, insomnia, diarrhea
Carvedilol (II) PO: 3.125–25 mg q 12 h	VT, PVC	Sinus rate slowed AV nodal refractoriness increased	Cardiac: Bradycardia, hypotension, AVB, edema, syncope Other: Hyperglycemia, dizziness, fatigue, diarrhea
Diltiazem (IV) IV: 5–10 mg qd: 15–30 min Extended release: PO: 120–360 mg/day	VT specifically RVOT, idiopathic LVT	Sinus rate slowed PR prolonged AV nodal conduction slowed	Cardiac: Hypotension, edema, HF, AVB, bradycardia, exacerbation of HF*r*EF Other: Headache, rash, constipation
Esmolol (II) IV: 0.5 mg/kg bolus, 0.05 mg/kg/min	VT	Sinus rate slowed AV nodal refractoriness increased	Cardiac: Bradycardia, hypotension, HF, AVB Other: Dizziness, nausea
Flecainide (IC) PO: 50–200 mg q 12 h	VT, PVC (in the absence of structural heart disease). Has a role in treating patients with CPVT	PR prolonged QRS prolonged; increased DFT	Cardiac: Sinus node dysfunction, AVB, drug-induced Brugada syndrome, monomorphic VT in patients with a myocardial scar, exacerbation of HF*r*EF Other: Dizziness, tremor, vision disturbance, dyspnea, nausea
Lidocaine (IB) IV: 1 mg/kg bolus, 1–3 mg/min 1–1.5 mg/kg. Repeat 0.5–0.75 mg/kg bolus every 5–10 min (max cumulative dose 3 mg/kg). Maintenance infusion is 1–4 mg/min although one could start at 0.5 mg/min	VT, VF	No marked effect on most intervals; QTc can slightly shorten	Cardiac: Bradycardia, hemodynamic collapse, AVB, sinus arrest Other: Delirium, psychosis, seizure, nausea, tinnitus, dyspnea, bronchospasm
Metoprolol (II) IV: 5 mg q 5 min up to 3 doses PO: 25–100 mg Extended release qd or q 12 h	VT, PVC	Sinus rate slowed AV nodal refractoriness increased	Cardiac: Bradycardia, hypotension, AVB Other: Dizziness, fatigue, diarrhea, depression, dyspnea
Mexiletine (IB) PO: 150–300 mg q 8 h or q 12 h	T, VF, PVC, has a role in patients with LQT3	No marked effect on most intervals; QTc can slightly shorten	Cardiac: HF, AVB Other: Lightheaded, tremor, ataxia, paresthesias, nausea, blood dyscrasias
Nadolol (II) PO: 40–320 mg daily	VT, PVC, LQTS, CPVT	Sinus rate slowed AV nodal refractoriness increased	Cardiac: Bradycardia, hypotension, HF, AVB Other: Edema, dizziness, cold extremities, bronchospasm
Procainamide (IA) IV: loading dose 10–17 mg/kg at 20–50 mg/ min Maintenance dose: 1–4 mg/min PO (SR preparation): 500–1,250 mg q 6 h	VT	QRS prolonged QTc prolonged; increased DFT	Cardiac: TdP; AVB, hypotension and exacerbation of HF*r*EF Other: Lupus symptoms, diarrhea, nausea, blood dyscrasias
Propafenone (IC) PO: Immediate release 150–300 mg q 8 h Extended release 225–425 mg q 12 h	VT, PVC (in the absence of structural heart disease)	PR prolonged QRS prolonged; increased DFT	Cardiac: HF, AVB, drug-induced Brugada syndrome Other: Dizziness, fatigue, nausea, diarrhea, xerostomia, tremor, blurred vision
Propranolol (II) IV: 1–3 mg q 5 min to a total of 5 mg PO: Immediate release 10–40 mg q 6 h; extended release 60–160 mg q 12 h	VT, PVC, LQTS	Sinus rate slowed AV nodal refractoriness increased	Cardiac: Bradycardia, hypotension, HF, AVB Other: Sleep disorder, dizziness, nightmares, hyperglycemia, diarrhea, bronchospasm

(continued)

Table 36-2 • ANTIARRHYTHMIC MEDICATIONS FOR TREATING VENTRICULAR ARRHYTHMIAS (*Continued*)

Antiarrhythmic Medication (Class) and Dose	Uses in VA/SCA	Electrophysiologic Effects	Common Adverse Effects
Quinidine (IA) PO: sulfate salt 200–600 mg q 6 h–q 12 h gluconate salt 324–648 mg q 8 h–q 12 h IV: loading dose: 800 mg in 50 mL infused at 50 mg/min	T, VF, (including short QT syndrome, Brugada's)	QRS prolonged QTc prolonged; increased DFT	Cardiac: Syncope, TdP, AVB Other: Dizziness, diarrhea, nausea, esophagitis, emesis, tinnitus, blurred vision, rash, weakness, tremor; blood dyscrasias
Ranolazine (not classified) PO: 500–1000 mg q 12 h	VT	Sinus rate slowed Tc prolonged	Cardiac: Bradycardia, hypotension Other: Headache, dizziness, syncope, nausea, dyspnea
Sotalol (III) IV: 75 mg q 12 h PO: 80–120 mg q 12 h, may increase dose every 3 d; max 320 mg/d	VT, VF, PVC	Sinus rate slowed QTc prolonged AV nodal refractoriness increased; decreased DFT	Cardiac: Bradycardia, hypotension, HF, syncope, TdP Other: Fatigue, dizziness, weakness, dyspnea, bronchitis, depression, nausea, diarrhea
Verapamil (IV) IV: 2.5–5 mg q 15–30 min Sustained release PO: 240–480 mg/d	VT (specifically RVOT, verapamil-sensitive idiopathic LVT)	Sinus rate slowed PR prolonged AV nodal conduction slowed	Cardiac: Hypotension, edema, HF, AVB, bradycardia, exacerbation of HFrEF Other: Headache, rash, gingival hyperplasia, constipation, dyspepsia

Study.[28] There is gender disparity; SCD occurs 75% more often in men. However, SCD does appear to be increasing in women. From 1989 to 1999, SCD increased by 21% among women aged 35 to 44 years in the United States. During this same time frame there was a 2.8% decline among men of the same age group.[29] Risk profiling for CAD is useful for identifying populations and individuals at risk, but does not identify an individual patient at risk for SCD. The inability to identify individuals is a major reason why SCD remains an important public health problem.[30]

There are several different arrhythmia mechanisms responsible for SCD. The most common arrhythmia leading to SCD appears to be VT accelerating into ventricular fibrillation (VF), often followed by asystole or pulseless electrical activity (PEA). Acquired structural and functional changes that occur in a diseased heart, and genetic factors may contribute to sudden death. However, the mechanism that produces the potentially fatal arrhythmia among patients with CAD is difficult to define.[31,32]

The episode could be caused from pure ischemic injury because of occlusion of a major artery in a patient with a normal ventricle in whom VF develops in the first minutes of an acute infarction. The other type of mechanism is one in which a patient with a previous MI has postinfarction scarring that provides the anatomic substrate for VT that leads to hemodynamic collapse and SCD. Patients could also have complex substrates consisting of dense scar tissue with aneurysms or other areas where disorganized arrhythmias predominate. This complex interaction and multiplicity of influences that occur in a cardiac arrest episode differ for all patients.[32]

The incidence of sudden cardiac arrest increases with age in both men and women, white and nonwhite, because of the prevalence of ischemic heart disease increases with age. Data suggest that sudden cardiac arrest has a much higher incidence in men than women (approximately 75% vs. 25%). The peaks in incidence of sudden cardiac that occur between birth and 6 months of age because of the sudden infant death syndrome, and then again between ages 45 and 75 because of CAD. The impact of activity on SCD is widely argued and controversial. Impact of physical activity is somewhat controversial. Although vigorous exercise can trigger SCD and acute MI, in part possibly by increasing platelet adhesiveness and aggregability, moderate physical activity may be beneficial by decreasing platelet adhesiveness and aggregability.[28] During stress testing cardiac arrest occurs at rate of 1 per 2000 and in the rehabilitation programs cardiac arrest occurs at a rate of 1 in 12,000 to 15,000.[28]

In the U.S. there are 100 to 150 sudden cardiac deaths (SCD) during competitive sports each year. In Europe, particularly Northern Italy, arrhythmogenic right ventricular dysplasia/cardiomyopathy, is the predominant anatomic finding with SCD.[28] Another uncommon finding related to the concussion of the heart from nonpenetrating blunt trauma to the anterior chest known as Commotio Cordis can lead to fatal cardiac arrest due to either myocardial trauma or mechanoelectrical triggering of ventricular tachyarrhythmia during the vulnerable period of T-wave.[28]

Other risk factors such as age, hypertension, LVH, intraventricular conduction block, elevated serum cholesterol, glucose intolerance, decreased vital capacity, smoking, relative weight, and heart rate identify individuals at risk for SCD.[28] Smoking is identified as a particularly important risk factor as described in the Framingham study. The incidence of SCD in smokers is 1.3%. For people who smoke more than one pack per day, the incidence of SCD is nearly 2.5 times greater. Emotional stress, especially depression, can also be an important trigger for SCD after MI and a significant predictor of the 18-month post-MI cardiac mortality. After MI, SCD increases threefold in men, related to socioeconomic factors such as low levels of education and complex ventricular ectopy.[28]

Sudden Cardiac Death With Structural Heart Disease

Coronary Artery Disease

CAD is the major structural abnormality found in most sudden cardiac arrest (SCA) victims. In 80% of patients who have had an SCA, CAD is present. SCA is often the first manifestation of CAD.[30,33] Pathology studies of SCD patients have shown that coronary atherosclerosis is the major predisposing cause. Plaque rupture and plaque erosion are the underlying pathologies in the majority of cases of SCD. Evidence shows a difference in the mechanism of MI and death between men and woman. Men tend to have coronary plaque rupture, while women tend to have plaque erosion.[34] Data from the Nurses' Health Study of 121,701 women have shown that 94% of women who had SCD had one risk factor for heart disease.[29] The evolution and clinical manifestation of CAD leading to SCA has been identified as four separate stages. The first stage is atherogenesis, which is the beginning of plaque formation and occurs over a long period of time. This stage should be thought of as the stage that determines risks for CAD. The second stage is the transitional stage where changes in plaque anatomy and pathophysiology are taking place. During this stage, the disease has moved from quiet to active. The third level of the process is the acute coronary syndrome phase when the acute ischemic event may be triggered by plaque disruption and the onset of the thrombotic process. The time to a fatal arrhythmia is close, leaving less time for preventative actions. The final phase is the arrhythmogenesis, when an interaction is occurring between the active ischemic process and the onset of cardiac arrhythmias.[35]

Changes in coronary artery blood flow from other causes such as coronary vasospasms or nonatherosclerotic coronary artery abnormalities can also provoke ischemia and create myocardial electrical disturbances and the development of VF. Structural coronary artery abnormalities without atherosclerosis are rare and include congenital lesions, coronary artery emboli from aortic valve endocarditis, or from thrombotic material released from prosthetic aortic or mitral valve.[36]

Cardiomyopathy

The second largest group of patients who experience SCD includes patients with cardiomyopathy. Severely depressed left ventricular function is an independent predictor of SCD in patients with ischemic and nonischemic cardiomyopathy. An ejection fraction equal to or less than 35% is considered the most powerful predictor of SCD. Improved treatment options for patients with heart failure provide them with better long-term survival. However, there is an increasing proportion of patients with heart failure who die suddenly.[36] Three primary prevention studies have shown reduction in total mortality for ischemic and nonischemic cardiomyopathy patients. The Multicenter Automatic Defibrillator Implantation Trial (MADIT II) has shown that the ICD will reduce total mortality in patients with ischemic cardiomyopathy with ejection fractions less than 30%. The Sudden Cardiac Death in Heart Failure Trial (SCD-HeFT) enrolled patients with either ischemic or nonischemic cardiomyopathy with ejection fractions less than 35%, and NYHA classes II and III heart failure. The results confirmed reduced mortality in the ischemic patients, but also in the nonischemic cardiomyopathy patients. The Defibrillators in Nonischemic Cardiomyopathy Treatment Evaluation (DEFINITE) trial also showed reduction in death from arrhythmias with ICD therapy.[37–39]

A highly prognostic independent risk factor for SCD is LVH. ECG changes consistent with LVH and echocardiographic evidence of LVH have both been associated with sudden and unexpected cardiac death.[9,28] The underlying causes for myocardial hypertrophy include hypertensive or valvular heart disease, obstructive and nonobstructive hypertrophic cardiomyopathy (HCM), and right ventricular hypertrophy secondary to pulmonary hypertension or congenital heart disease. All of these conditions are associated with increased risk of SCD, but it has been suggested that people with severely hypertrophic ventricles are especially susceptible to SCD.[36]

HCM is a familial cardiac disease that occurs in 1 out of 500 people. HCM is the most common cause of sudden death in people under 30 years of age, and it often goes undiagnosed.[40,41] Sudden death often occurs with vigorous exercise in this group of patients. Various risk factors for SCD with HCM include family history of sudden death, documented nonsustained VT, recurrent and unexplained syncope, and extreme thickness of 30 mm or more of the left ventricle. Polymorphic VT and VF are thought to be the initial rhythm for patients with HCM who experience SCD.[36,42] Genetic studies of HCM have confirmed autosomal dominate inheritance patterns. Typically HCM is caused by mutations in any one of 10 genes that encode proteins of the cardiac sarcomere. DNA testing can identify patients with HCM at an early onset, helping to modify medical therapy and recommendations for placement of an implantable defibrillator, or withdrawing from intense physical activities and competitive sports.[41] For the list of other causes of SCD, see Display 36-1.

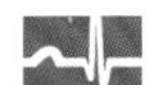
DISPLAY 36-1

Causes of Sudden Death

Cardiac Causes

Acute myocarditis
Aortic or ventricular aneurysm with dissection or rupture
Aortic stenosis
Cardiomyopathies
- Ischemic cardiomyopathy
- Nonischemic dilated cardiomyopathy
- Hypertrophic cardiomyopathy
- Alcoholic cardiomyopathy

Chagas disease
Congenital heart disease
Coronary artery abnormalities
- Myocardial infarction
- Coronary artery spasm
- Coronary artery embolism

Endocarditis
Electrophysiologic abnormalities
- Brugada syndrome
- Complete AV block
- Wolff–Parkinson–White
- Long QT syndrome—congenital and acquired
- Catecholaminergic polymorphic ventricular tachycardia

Prolapsed mitral valve syndrome
- Prosthetic aortic or mitral valves

Right ventricular dysplasia
Sarcoidosis

Noncardiac Causes

Cerebral or subarachnoid hemorrhage
Choking
Dissecting aneurysm of the aorta
Electrolyte abnormalities
Metabolic disturbances
Pulmonary hypertension (primary, particularly during pregnancy)
Pulmonary embolism
Sudden infant death syndrome (should at least in part be included in cardiac causes)

Valvular Heart Disease

The risk of sudden death in patients with valve disease is low but present. After prosthetic or heterograft aortic valve replacements, patients are at risk for SCD caused by arrhythmias, prosthetic valve dysfunction, or existing CHD. The risk of SCD after surgery peaks at 3 weeks and plateaus after 8 weeks. Sudden death can also occur with exertion in young adults with congenital aortic stenosis. The mechanism is uncertain but thought to be from sudden changes in ventricular filling or aortic obstruction with secondary arrhythmias.[42] Mitral valve prolapse is associated with a high incidence of symptomatic atrial and ventricular arrhythmias; however, whether it causes SCD is unresolved.[36]

Rare reports of sudden death have been reported from coronary embolism due to valvular vegetations, which trigger a fatal ischemic arrhythmia. Endocarditis of the aortic or mitral valve may cause deterioration of the valvular apparatus, and abscesses of the valvular rings or septum leading to sudden death.[36]

Sudden Cardiac Death Without Structural Heart Disease

A reported 5% to 10% of those patients who experience SCD have no apparent structural heart disease.[9] There are many potential causes of SCD in this small percentage of patients. The most common of these are electrophysiologic abnormalities including LQTS, short QT syndrome (SQTS), Brugada syndrome, and catecholaminergic polymorphic ventricular tachycardia (CPVT). LQTS is either congenital or acquired by use of drugs, such as antiarrhythmic and psychotropic drugs, or with electrolyte imbalances. The list of drugs that are generally accepted to have an increased risk of torsades de pointes is ever expanding, and can be found at online sites such as www.qtdrugs.org. Torsades de pointes is a type of polymorphic VT, which leads to syncope or SCD. SQTS is relatively newly defined syndrome, with short refractory periods both in the atria and the ventricles. Brugada syndrome is a genetic disease characterized by a right ventricular conduction delay. CPVT is characterized by ventricular arrhythmias that develop during physical activity in the presence of a normal resting ECG.[9,43]

Patients with the classic long QT intervals corrected for heart rate (QTc interval) are at increased risk for torsades de pointes.[9,43,44] Congenital long QT (LQT) is hereditary; mutations in eight genes have been identified. The most common mutations are LQT1 (42%), LQT2 (45%), and LQT3 (8%). Most mutations affect the cardiac potassium-channel genes KCNQ1 and KCNH2 and cause the most frequent forms of long QT. An impaired sodium channel gene, SCN5A, is the cause for LQT3. However, the mutation LQT4 has been identified as a mutation from a membrane adaptor protein, and not an ion channel.[32,43] QT interval duration was identified as the strongest predictor of SCD, even before genetic mutation identification. A QTc greater than 500 ms in a patient identified with an affected gene carries the highest risk of syncope or SCD by the age of 40.[9] Two patterns of long QT have been reported: the Romano Ward syndrome, which is an autosomal dominant syndrome, and the Jervell and Lange-Nielsen syndrome. The latter is autosomal recessive, more severe, and often associated with congenital deafness.[9,45]

In individuals with long QT, ventricular arrhythmias often occur in the setting of stress and activity, but also can occur during rest and sleep. Exercise, particularly swimming, is often a trigger for arrhythmias in the LQT1 patients. LQT2 patients have arrhythmias that are triggered during both rest and emotion, often associated with acoustic stimuli. The LQT3 patients are more prone to having arrhythmias at rest and during sleep.[9,46] Avoidance of competitive sports is recommended for LQT1 and LQT2 patients, but not for LQT3 patients.[41]

Brugada syndrome is an inherited disease that is associated with a high incidence of sudden death. A mutation of cardiac sodium-channel gene SCN5A, has been identified in about 20% of persons with the syndrome, and occurs more often in men. Brugada syndrome is confirmed with ST-segment elevation in the precordial leads, right bundle branch block conduction pattern, and history of SCD. The ECG changes may be present all the time or elicited when antiarrhythmic drugs are given that block sodium channels. Fever has been reported to unmask ECG changes of Brugada syndrome and elicit an electrical VT storm.

Wolff–Parkinson–White (WPW) is associated with an accessory pathway that allows for conduction between the atria and ventricles. Normally, WPW is associated with nonlethal arrhythmias. However, if atrial fibrillation develops and conduction is rapid over the accessory pathway, the ventricular rate can become so fast that the rhythm degenerates into VF. SCD in the setting of WPW is quite low, and has been reported at 0.39% per year.[43,47]

CPVT is a catecholamine-dependent arrhythmia that occurs in the absence of a long QT interval. The arrhythmia often occurs during physical activity or emotional distress; therefore, β-adrenoceptor–blocking agents can be helpful in treating this condition. The first episode often occurs during childhood. The arrhythmia is characterized by bidirectional and polymorphic VT. The condition is rare, and is related to a genetic disorder. CPVT is caused by mutations involving the cardiac ryanodine receptor, and calsequestrin, a calcium-buffering protein.[9,43,48]

Medical Management and Treatment of Cardiac Arrest and Sudden Cardiac Death

The outcome of cardiac arrest is determined by how promptly treatment is initiated with advanced cardiac life support (ACLS). To improve outcome from SCA, the following must occur as rapidly as possible: (1) early recognition of warning signs, (2) early activation of the emergency medical system, (3) early basic CPR, (4) early defibrillation, and (5) early ACLS. These events have been described as "links in a chain of survival," because they are all connected and indispensable to the overall success of emergency cardiac care (see Fig. 36-8).

Although this section summarizes ACLS recommendations for the adult patient, it is not a complete reference. For the cardiac nurse, participation in an ACLS provider course by the AHA is strongly recommended.

Adult Advanced Cardiac Life Support

ACLS teaches the appropriate skills and knowledge, as determined by leaders in emergency cardiovascular care (ECC), to improve survival from SCA and acute life-threatening cardiopulmonary events. In 2018, the AHA updated the guidelines for CPR and ECC (Fig. 36-13). ACLS includes early recognition of prearrest, basic life support (BLS), the use of airway and circulation adjuncts, cardiac monitoring, and defibrillation and other arrhythmia control techniques. ACLS also includes establishment of intravenous access, drug therapy, and postresuscitation care.

Electrical Therapy of Malignant Arrhythmias

Defibrillation and cardioversion are a delivery of electrical energy that totally depolarizes and stuns the myocardium, which allows the sinus node to resume its function as the pacemaker for the heart. Defibrillation is, by definition, the therapy for VF. Cardioversion, which is a synchronized shock, is the electrical therapy

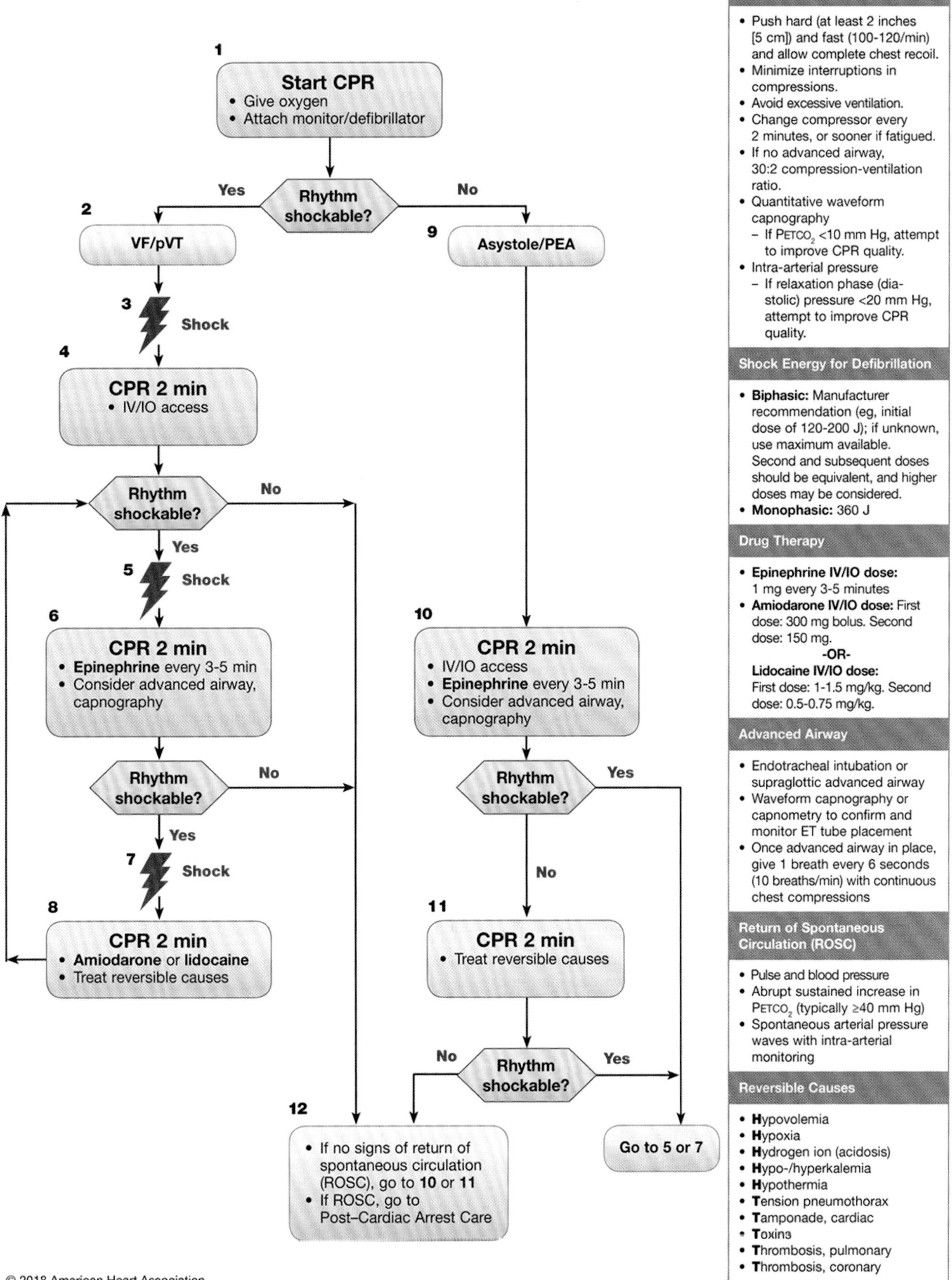

Figure 36-13. Adult cardiac arrest algorithm—2018 update. (Adapted from American Heart Association. Link MS, Berkow LC, Kudenchuk PJ, et al. Part 7: Adult advanced cardiovascular life support. *Circulation.* 2015;132[18 suppl 2]:S444–S464.)

for all other tachyarrhythmias. Transcutaneous and transvenous pacing are additional types of electrical therapy used in ACLS for patients with hemodynamically compromised bradycardias.

VT and VF are the most common arrhythmias during cardiac arrest. Defibrillation is the definitive therapy for cardiac arrest caused by VF. Rapid, early defibrillation is a key step and the most important intervention likely to save lives. Survival rates are best when immediate bystander CPR is provided and defibrillation occurs within 3 to 5 minutes. A major obstacle to rapid, early defibrillation is that most cardiac arrests occur outside of the hospital, indicating a need for public health initiatives to improve early recognition of heart attack signs and symptoms.[24] The widespread use of automated external defibrillators (AEDs) assists in making early defibrillation a reality by expanding the number of rescuers available to treat SCD. The AHA integrates the use of AEDs with BLS skills because VF is the most common rhythm found in adults with witnessed, nontraumatic SCA.[49]

Defibrillators

Defibrillators are the power source used to deliver the electrical therapy. Defibrillators typically include a capacitor charger, a capacitor to store energy, a charge switch, and discharge switch to complete the circuit from the capacitor to the electrodes. The capacitor charger converts power from a low-voltage source, such as direct current, to a voltage level sufficient for a shock. Portable defibrillators derive their power from a battery, which must be kept charged. Electrical output of defibrillators is quantified in terms of Joules (J), or watt-seconds, of energy.

Defibrillators deliver energy to the electrode in either a biphasic or a monophasic waveform. Biphasic waveforms deliver current in a positive direction for a specific duration, and then reverse the current to a negative direction for the remaining discharge. A monophasic waveform delivers the current in one polarity or direction. Studies show that biphasic waveforms achieve shock success rates at lower energies, 150 J compared to 200 J, and produce less ST-segment change than shocks delivered with monophasic waveforms.[38,50,51] Lower-energy requirements reduce the size and weight of the defibrillator, which in turn increases public access to AEDs because they are easier to handle, less expensive, and more convenient.

Rapid defibrillation can be performed with manual, automatic, or semiautomatic external defibrillators. Well-trained personnel, often ACLS responders, who are able to interpret cardiac rhythms on a rhythm strip or monitor, must operate manual defibrillators. Automatic advisory or semiautomatic external defibrillators have been developed for use by first responders. AEDs are accurate and easy to use and, unlike standard defibrillators, have detection systems that analyze the rhythm and advise the operator to shock when VF/VT characteristics are determined. Thus, successful defibrillation can be achieved without requiring the operator to have rhythm recognition skills. AEDs are attached to the patient with the use of adhesive sternal and apex pads that are connected to a cable, allowing for "hands-free defibrillation." AEDs were shown to help emergency personnel deliver the first shock on an average of 1 minute sooner than personnel using conventional defibrillators.[52] Early defibrillation with an AED has been shown to significantly increase survival in both out-of-hospital and in-hospital cardiopulmonary arrests.[49,53]

Transthoracic Impedance

The ability to defibrillate requires the passage of sufficient electric current through the heart. Current flow is determined by transthoracic impedance (TTI), or resistance to current flow, and the selected energy (Joules). If TTI is high, a low-energy shock may fail to produce sufficient current to defibrillate. The factors that determine TTI include energy setting, electrode size and composition, electrode–skin interface, number of and time between previous electrical discharges, electrode pressure, ventilation phase, and electrode placement.[54,55]

Resistance between the electrode and the chest wall must be minimized. Bare electrodes produce high resistance to electrical flow. Defibrillation electrode gel or paste, made specifically for defibrillation, will help to decrease impedance. Self-adhesive monitor or defibrillator pads are also available and effective. The adhesive defibrillator pads are thought to be more convenient and safer, as they reduce the possibility of electrical arcing. AHA recommends the use of adhesive pads. The pads can be placed as the patient's condition deteriorates, allowing for monitoring of the patients heart rhythm and providing the ability to deliver a shock rapidly if necessary.[49]

Elevated TTI reduces the chance of successful defibrillation. Common causes of increased TTI include chest hair, which can increase impedance by 35%, and improper paddle position.[55] The optimal paddle size for adults in hand-held and self-adhesive pads is 8.5 to 12 cm in diameter, although defibrillation success may be higher with the electrodes that are 12 cm in diameter.[52]

Energy Requirements

The type of waveform the defibrillator delivers determines the amount of energy required to convert VF or pulseless VT. Defibrillators available today deliver either a monophasic waveform or one of two types of biphasic waveforms. A single immediate defibrillation must be performed followed by CPR, instead of the previously recommended three-stacked shocks. Both low-energy and high-energy biphasic waveform shocks are effective. There is no evidence to support that escalating energy or nonescalating energy is more effective.[49] AHA stresses that the most important factor in surviving an adult VF arrest is rapid defibrillation by either a monophasic or biphasic defibrillator.

Biphasic defibrillators use either a biphasic truncated exponential waveform that delivers an effective shock of 150 to 200 J, or a rectilinear biphasic waveform that is effective with a 120-J shock. AHA recommends that subsequent shocks remain the same, but can also be increased if the defibrillator is capable of delivering higher-energy shocks. If a manual biphasic defibrillator is in use and the rescuer does not know the effective shock range for that particular defibrillator, the first shock should be 120 to 200 J. If an older model monophasic defibrillator is used, the rescuer should always select 360 J for all shocks. All defibrillators should be clearly labeled, so that the rescuer knows the starting effective energy level. All healthcare providers should be familiar with all models of defibrillators in their facility as there are many different models available. Rescuers who perform defibrillation must announce that they are about to deliver a shock. They must then check that all personnel are clear of the patient and stretcher before defibrillating. If the first shock successfully terminates VF but the patient subsequently goes back into VF, the energy should be kept at the last successful level rather than increasing the energy level.[49]

Electrode Position

Electrode placement is critical in ensuring that a critical mass of myocardium is depolarized. Any of three electrode positions may

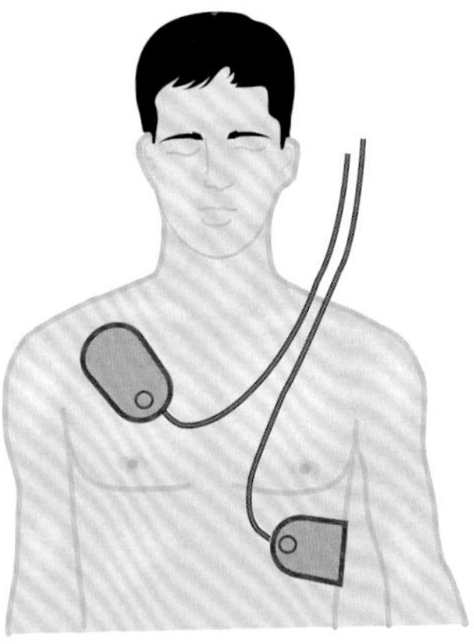
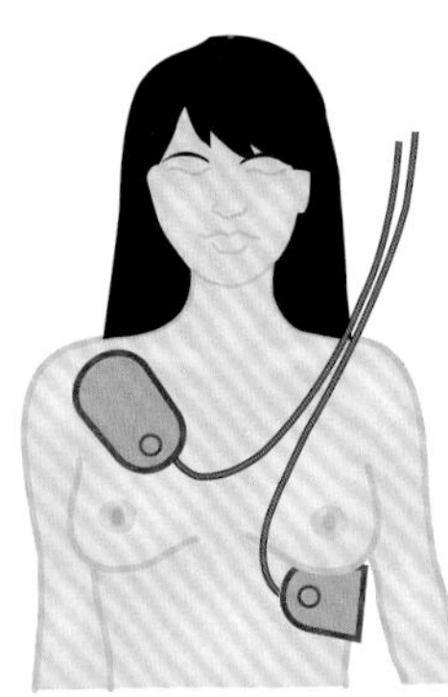

Figure 36-14. Standard positioning of defibrillator pads.

be used. Standard or anterolateral electrode placement involves one electrode being placed to the right of the upper sternum just below the right clavicle. The other electrode is placed on the left chest, lateral to the left breast in the mid-axillary line (Fig. 36-14). Two other patch positions are listed as class IIa recommendations in the updated AHA guidelines[49]: patches on the lateral chest wall on the right and left sides (biaxillary); or one patch in the standard left apical position and the other pad on the right or left upper back. In patients with permanent pacemakers, electrode placement should be as far as possible from the pacemaker pulse generator, and when possible an anterior–posterior position should be considered.

Defibrillation Procedure

Identify the rhythm as VF. If the rhythm appears to be asystole, check the rhythm in another lead to confirm that the rhythm is not fine VF.

- Turn on the defibrillator.
- Apply the adhesive pads in proper electrode position. The chest may need to be shaved, as hair will increase impedance. If electrode paddles are used, apply conductive materials.
- Set energy level to 120 to 200 J for biphasic defibrillator (device specific) and 360 J for monophasic defibrillator.
- Charge capacitors. Charging may take several seconds. Many defibrillators emit a sound or light signal, or both, to indicate that the unit has charged.
- Ensure proper electrode placement on chest.
- If using paddles, apply pressure of 25 lb per paddle. Do not lean forward because of the danger of the paddles slipping.
- Scan the area to ensure that no personnel are in contact directly or indirectly with the patient. Make sure there is no flowing oxygen source in electrical field.
- State firmly, "all clear" or other warning chant.
- Check rhythm—if patient remains in VF, deliver shock by depressing both buttons simultaneously on the paddles or discharge button on defibrillator.
- Start CPR immediately, beginning with compressions and resume for 2 minutes.
- Repeat assessment procedure. Continue with either same or higher energy shock for biphasic defibrillator. (If biphasic defibrillator has ability to increase energy level a higher dose can be selected.) Continue with 360 J for monophasic defibrillator. Scan for personnel in contact with the patient, giving a warning signal prior to delivering shock.

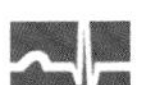
DISPLAY 36-2

The Crucial Links in the Adult Out-of-Hospital Chain of Survival

Rapid identification of potential cardiac arrest by dispatchers, with immediate provision of CPR instructions to the caller
Presence of mobile phones that can allow the rescuer to activate emergency response system without leaving the victim's side
High-quality CPR (see Table 36-3)
Simultaneous, choreographed approach to performance of chest compressions, airway management, rescue breathing, rhythm detection, and shocks by an integrated team of trained rescuers

Adapted from Kleinman ME, Brennan EE, Goldberger ZD, et al. Part 5: Adult basic life support and cardiopulmonary resuscitation quality: 2015 American Heart Association guidelines update for cardiopulmonary resuscitation and emergency cardiovascular care. *Circulation*. 2015;132(18 suppl 2): S414–S435.

- Resume CPR immediately beginning with compressions. If VF continues, refer to management of pulseless arrest algorithm (see Fig. 36-3).

Management of Cardiac Arrest—ACLS Algorithms

A general framework for the crucial links in the adult out-of-hospital chain of survival is outlined in Display 36-2. The initial approach to the management of cardiac arrest is outlined in the ACLS pulseless arrest algorithm. ACLS providers must always start with this algorithm by activating the emergency medical system and beginning BLS. The foundation of good ACLS is good BLS (Table 36-3).[56] The basics of circulation, airway, and breathing remain important during the entire resuscitation continuum. Once the patient is attached to a monitor, determine the rhythm and potential cause for the arrest. If VF or pulseless VT is present, the left side of the

Table 36-3 • BASIC LIFE SUPPORT, ADULT HIGH-QUALITY CARDIOPULMONARY RESUSCITATION

Rescuers Should	Rescuers Should Not
Perform chest compression at a rate of 100–120/min	Compress at a rate slower than 100/min or faster than 120/min
Compress to a depth of at least 2 in (5 cm)	Compress to a depth of less than 2 in (5 cm) or greater than 2.4 in (6 cm)
Allow full recoil after each compression	Lean on the chest between compressions
Minimize pauses in compressions	Interrupt compressions for greater than 10 seconds
Ventilate adequately (2 breaths after 30 compressions, each breath delivered over 1 second, each causing chest rise)	Provide excessive ventilation (i.e., too many breaths or breaths with excessive force)

Adapted from Kleinman ME, Brennan EE, Goldberger ZD, et al. Part 5: Adult basic life support and cardiopulmonary resuscitation quality: 2015 American Heart Association guidelines update for cardiopulmonary resuscitation and emergency cardiovascular care. *Circulation*. 2015;132 (18 suppl 2):S414–S435.

algorithm should be followed. If electrical activity is present without a pulse, or asystole is present then the right side of the algorithm should be followed.

The AHA guidelines use algorithms as an educational tool. They are an illustrative method to summarize information. Providers of emergency care should view algorithms as a summary and a memory aid. They provide ways to treat a broad range of patients. Algorithms by nature oversimplify. The effective teacher and care provider use them wisely, not blindly. Some patients may require care not specified in the algorithms. When clinically appropriate, flexibility is accepted and encouraged. Many interventions and actions are listed as "considerations" to help providers think. These lists should not be considered endorsements or requirements or "standard of care" in a legal sense. Algorithms do not replace clinical understanding. Although the algorithms provide a good "cookbook," the patient always requires a "thinking cook."

Post–Cardiac Arrest Care

Management of the post–cardiac arrest patient is complex and requires performance of both diagnostic and therapeutic interventions to achieve best outcomes of the survivors. It involves determining and treatment of the causes of cardiac arrest, minimizing brain injury, managing cardiovascular dysfunction, and managing problems that may arise from global ischemia and reperfusion injury. Focused review of patient's history, examination, and review of diagnostic studies completed will aid in identification of the probable cause and ongoing medical management.[57]

Methodic sequence of interventions will focus on adequate ventilation, neurologic evaluation, completion of cardiac studies, hemodynamic stability, and reperfusion therapy (see Table 36-4).[57]

NURSING CARE OF CARDIAC ARREST AND SUDDEN CARDIAC DEATH SURVIVORS

Background

The survivors of SCA and their families have physiologic, psychological, and educational needs based on the underlying cause of SCA. The nursing diagnosis of Knowledge Deficit describes an individual's lack of information regarding his or her healthcare. In addition to comprehensive, holistic nursing cardiovascular assessment a more focused assessment, designed to identify a particular learning needs must be employed.

Physiologic Nursing Management

Following the cardiac arrest, patients are admitted in the intensive care unit and in typical sequence they are aggressively treated for acute ischemia. During hospitalization, several treatment options are proposed that require a patient and family to make choices (such as medications or ICD). Continuous cardiac rhythm or ECG monitoring is required until an ICD is implanted. In cases of transient-reduced EF due to cardiac ischemia and increased risk for recurrent ventricular fibrillation or VT, patients will be placed and discharged home on wearable lightweight vest equipped with external cardioverter defibrillator during first 90 days following the heart attack.[58] Patients and families need to be educated about the importance of wearing the vest at all times and risks associated during times when vest is temporarily removed, for example, showering.

Emotional Support

Emotional support is one of the primary roles of the continuous nursing care. Patients and families face an emotionally challenging situation with prognostic uncertainty. Reassurance, effective communication and support through those challenging times are critical to ensure appropriate decision making regarding risk management, discharge planning, and prevention of complications.[59] A common scenario requiring emotional support is the patient with a fear of transferring out of intensive care unit, which can lead to a physical complaint, and increased levels of anxiety thus negatively influence clinical progress.[60] The effect that SCD survival has on quality of life and anxiety is not well defined. After discharge and patients who return home hesitate to call their physician, however the reassurance that they can call a nurse may help alleviate anxiety. By addressing the major issues and consistently educate patient and family about disease process, treatment and recovery will ease the process and decrease anxiety. The nurses certainly play a major therapeutic role in the managing SCA survivors and their families.[27]

Patient and Family Education

The cardiac nurse plays an important role to deliver care focused on individual needs but also in developing a specific education intervention for SCA survivors. As a part of the interdisciplinary team, nurses have a significant impact on preventing or at least minimizing consequences of SCA. The hypoxia that frequently occurs due to cardiac arrest leads to both diffuse brain injury and injury of focal memory regions of the brain. Patient education is increasingly difficult in the presence of compromised memory; therefore family members will need to be involved early in the process to help with ongoing patient education recovery.[61,62] According to Dougherty et al.[63] interviewed partners of SCA survivors who received an ICD during first year or recovery had eight major concerns: physical care, emotional care, memory, ICD, financial impact, uncertain future, healthcare providers, and family. Nurses must assess and incorporate these factors when providing education and support. Given the overwhelming amount of information and concerns, it is almost impossible for patient and families to remember all the information given. This is particularly true of those patients who have repeated episodes, recurrent ICD shocks, and elderly patients with multiple comorbidities. The use of teaching aids such as educational booklets, video resources, images, online resources, and support groups have shown to be effective in educating survivors of SCA. Many excellent examples of such tools and decision aids are available through CardioSmart (http://www.cardiosmart.org), a patient education and empowerment initiative of the ACC.

Nurses often coordinate and provide care related to the ICD, as well as for end-of-life issues. The cardiac nurse has an essential role in education and support for patients and their families, often facilitating discussion, encouraging questions, and documenting accordingly. Unfortunately, information regarding the impact of specific education intervention for SCA survivors is limited and mostly focused on patients with an ICD thus more training and nursing research is needed to enhance intervention and education.[64,65]

Table 36-4 • POST–CARDIAC ARREST CARE

Multiple System Approach to Post–Cardiac Arrest Care				
Ventilation	**Hemodynamics**	**Cardiovascular**	**Neurologic**	**Metabolic**

• Capnography
  • Rationale: Confirm secure airway and titrate ventilation
  • Endotracheal tube when possible for comatose patients
  • $Petco_2$ ~35–40 mm Hg
  • $Paco_2$ ~40–45 mm Hg
	• Frequent blood pressure monitoring/arterial line
	  • Rationale: Maintain perfusion and prevent recurrent hypotension
	  • Mean arterial pressure ≥65 mm Hg or systolic blood pressure ≥90 mm Hg
		• Continuous cardiac monitoring
		  • Rationale: Detect recurrent arrhythmia
		  • No prophylactic antiarrhythmics
		  • Treat arrhythmias as required
		  • Remove reversible causes
			• Serial neurologic exam
			  • Rationale: Serial examinations define coma, brain injury, and prognosis
			  • Response to verbal commands or physical stimulation
			  • Pupillary light and corneal reflex, spontaneous eye movement
			  • Gag, cough, spontaneous breaths
				• Serial lactate
				  • Rationale: Confirm adequate perfusion

• Chest x-ray
  • Rationale: Confirm secure airway and detect causes or complications of arrest: pneumonitis, pneumonia, pulmonary edema
	• Treat hypotension
	  • Rationale: Maintain perfusion
	  • Fluid bolus if tolerated
	  • Dopamine 5–10 mcg/kg per min
	  • Norepinephrine 0.1–0.5 mcg/kg per min
	  • Epinephrine 0.1–0.5 mcg/kg per min
		• 12-lead ECG/Troponin
		  • Rationale: Detect Acute Coronary Syndrome/ST-Elevation Myocardial Infarction; Assess QT interval
			• EEG Monitoring if comatose
			  • Rationale: Exclude seizures
			  • Anticonvulsants if seizing
				• Serum potassium
				  • Rationale: Avoid hypokalemia which promotes arrhythmias
				  • Replace to maintain K >3.5 mEq/L

• Pulse oximetry/ABG
  • Rationale: Maintain adequate oxygenation and minimize Fio_2
  • Spo_2 ≥94%
  • Pao_2 ~100 mm Hg
  • Reduce Fio_2 as tolerated
  • Pao_2/Fio_2 ratio to follow acute lung injury
	...	• Treat acute coronary syndrome
		  • Aspirin/heparin
		  • Transfer to acute coronary treatment center
		  • Consider emergent PCI or fibrinolysis
			• Core temperature measurement if comatose
			  • Rationale: Minimize brain injury and improve outcome
			  • Prevent hyperpyrexia >37.7°C
			  • Induce therapeutic hypothermia if no contraindications
			  • Cold IV fluid bolus 30 mL/kg if no contraindication
			  • Surface or endovascular cooling for 32–34°C × 24 hours
			  • After 24 hours, slow rewarming 0.25°C/hr
				• Urine output, serum creatinine
				  • Rationale: Detect acute kidney injury
				  • Maintain euvolemia
				  • Renal replacement therapy if indicated

• Mechanical ventilation
  • Rationale: Minimize acute lung injury, potential oxygen toxicity
  • Tidal Volume 6–8 mL/kg
  • Titrate minute ventilation to $Petco_2$ ~35–40 mm Hg $Paco_2$ ~40–45 mm Hg
  • Reduce Fio_2 as tolerated to keep Spo_2 or Sao_2 ≥94%
	...	• Echocardiogram
		  • Rationale: Detect global stunning, wall-motion abnormalities, structural problems or cardiomyopathy
			• Consider nonenhanced CT scan
			  • Rationale: Exclude primary intracranial process
				• Serum glucose
				  • Rationale: Detect hyperglycemia and hypoglycemia
				  • Treat hypoglycemia (<80 mg/dL) with dextrose
				  • Treat hyperglycemia to target glucose 144–180 mg/dL
				  • Local insulin protocols

	...	• Treat myocardial stunning
		  • Fluids to optimize volume status (requires clinical judgment)
		  • Dobutamine 5–10 mcg/kg per min
		  • Mechanical augmentation (IABP)
			• Sedation/Muscle relaxation
			  • Rationale: To control shivering, agitation, or ventilator desynchrony as needed
				• Avoid hypotonic fluids
				  • Rationale: May increase edema, including cerebral edema

Adapted from Callaway CW, Donnino MW, Fink EL, et al. Part 8: Post–cardiac arrest care: 2015 American Heart Association guidelines update for cardiopulmonary resuscitation and emergency cardiovascular care. *Circulation.* 2015;132(18 suppl 2):S465–S482.

Summary

SCA remains the primary cause of cardiac death in the United States despite the current therapies and advances in technology. Unfortunately, the overall out-of-hospital survival for SCA remains low and estimated at 6%.[66] Largely the pathophysiology of SCD remains poorly understood. The advances in genetic testing helped to correlate LQTS patients and other inherited diseases linking genetic substrate as an important marker for SCD. In general, to reduce risks for SCD, healthcare workers are focusing on education of training to prevent SCD and identification of individuals at risk for ischemic heart disease and ventricular arrhythmias. The SCD continues to be a major challenge and continued improvements in out-of-hospital resuscitation and the widespread availability of defibrillation devices aims to increase survival cardiac arrest. The cardiac nurse has an important role in these efforts and in the care, education, and advocacy of these patients.

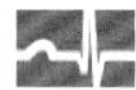

CASE STUDY 1

Patient Profile

History of Present Illness

Mr. Bertolli, a 51-year-old male, presents to the emergency room (ER) with weakness and fatigue. He reports that he was lightheaded and dizzy prior to coming to the ER; emergency medical services witnessed a near syncopal event. In the ER, he was found to have wide complex ventricular tachycardia at 218 bpm confirmed by 12-lead ECG. His prior medical history includes hypertension and premature ventricular contractions treated with low-dose β-blocker.

Clinical Course

The initial basic metabolic panel showed normal potassium, magnesium, sodium, BUN, and creatinine. Subsequently he was cardioverted and given bolus of IV amiodarone. Cardiac catheterization was performed which showed no evidence of coronary artery disease and preserved normal left ventricular systolic function. Transthoracic echocardiography revealed no evidence of structural heart disease with left ventricular ejection fraction estimated at 55%. His ECG after cardioversion demonstrated normal sinus rhythm with normal PR, QRS, and QTc interval.

The possible diagnosis of idiopathic VT was made, as he presented with hemodynamically unstable monomorphic VT. Treatment options were discussed in length and included an electrophysiology study for inducibility of ventricular tachyarrhythmia, catheter ablation if indicated, antiarrhythmic medication, and the option of implantation of ICD for VT protection. After careful consideration patient underwent an ICD implant. After ICD implantation, β-blocker therapy and an angiotensin II receptor blocker medicine for hypertension was resumed. He declined treatment with antiarrhythmic medication. In addition, he was provided with teaching that his ICD will record recurrent ventricular tachycardia and option with ablative therapy could be considered at later date.

Key Takeaways

- Antiarrhythmic therapy is indicated to treat symptomatic and recurrent VT episodes, to reduce incidence of ICD shocks, and to potentially improve quality of life and reduce hospitalizations related to cardiac arrhythmia.
- ICD implantation is often performed by the electrophysiologist, cardiologist, or cardiac surgeon. Primary care advanced patient providers will continue to provide general patient care, but electrophysiologist and electrophysiology nurse practitioner will closely monitor patients for shocks and arrhythmias.
- Routine technical follow-up visits in ICD clinics are scheduled every 3 months due to safety concerns. Remote monitoring systems now available will enable wireless data transmission without the patient's active assistance. Transmission includes all data within the device memory, including device parameters, diagnostics, and stored arrhythmic events.

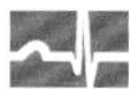

CASE STUDY 2

Patient Profile

Mr. Patel, a 69-year-old man, presented to the ER complaining of intermittent dizziness, which started 2 days ago and progressively became worse. Approximately 1 week prior, he began noticing a shortness of breath on exertion and mild chest pressure. Patient had a recent myocardial perfusion stress test (nuclear imaging study) revealing inferior wall scarring. On presentation, patient's vital signs were stable with normal CBC, normal chemistry, and mildly elevated troponin. The patient's past medical history is significant for hyperlipidemia, hypertension, and tobacco use. His surgical history included cataract surgery and benign abdominal cyst removal. There are no known allergies to the medicine or food. He reported that his father died at age 46 of sudden cardiac death.

Clinical Course

In the emergency department the ECG performed revealed a sustained monomorphic ventricular tachycardia (Fig. 36-15), wide-complex tachycardia.

Intravenous lidocaine was initiated at 2 mg/min resulting in subsequent termination of arrhythmia and conversion to sinus rhythm. Patient hemodynamics remained stable but he continued to complain of chest pressure despite use of sublingual nitroglycerin. Based on the previous myocardial perfusion study, a decision was made to proceed with

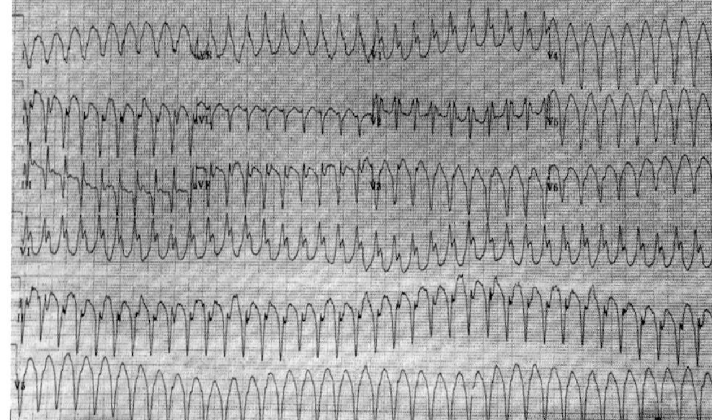

Figure 36-15. ECG, Case study. 12-lead ECG.

CASE STUDY 2 (*Continued*)

cardiac catheterization with possible percutaneous coronary intervention. Lidocaine was discontinued in preparation for cardiac catheterization. Cardiac catheterization revealed no evidence of obstructive coronary artery disease and preserved left ventricular function estimated at 55%. Following the procedure, the patient was transferred to intensive care unit for further observation. Overnight, the nursing staff observed frequent episodes of nonsustained ventricular tachycardia. The cardiac electrophysiologist was consulted. Patient received a low dose of metoprolol tartrate. After receiving the medicine patient had no further arrhythmias overnight and it was recommended he undergo an electrophysiology study with implantation of ICD if indicated. An electrophysiology was performed revealing no evidence of conduction abnormality despite multiple attempts to induce ventricular tachycardia. Since no further arrhythmia could be induced after procedure he was continued on metoprolol. In event of arrhythmia recurrence, repeat electrophysiology study was recommended. He had no further chest pressure, dizziness, or shortness of breath.

Throughout the hospitalization nurses played vital role in patient care but and teaching both patient and family about the disease process, medications, emergency management, and follow-up care. In addition, nurses provided an educational booklet on ventricular dysrhythmias and other written and online resources.

Key Takeways

- A family history of premature cardiac disease is a known risk factor for development of cardiovascular events. Initial assessment should include Framingham risk score which includes information of family history of premature CHD. In addition, coronary artery calcium score is an alternative test for early screening of coronary atherosclerotic plaque in selected patients and it is a good predictor for CHD.
- Lidocaine may be considered as an alternative to amiodarone during cardiac arrest related to VF and VT. In patients with myocardial infarction and VT, initiation of lidocaine was associated with possible higher risk of mortality due to increased risk of asystole and bradyarrhythmias.
- Patients who develop myocardial scaring are at risk for developing VT. The scar is not a homogeneous tissue and some areas of surviving fibers have a higher voltage, thus these areas are corridors of slow conduction that can form part of reentrant circuits of VT. Contrast-enhanced magnetic resonance imaging of a scar heterogeneity is a possible predictor of appropriate ICD therapy.

KEY READINGS

American Heart Association. Watch, Learn and Live—American Heart Association's interactive cardiovascular library. https://watchlearnlive.heart.org/?moduleSelect=arrhyt

CardioSmart. The patient education initiative of the American College of Cardiology. https://www.cardiosmart.org/SuddenCardiacArrest

Knight BP. Up to Date. Patient Education: Implantable cardioverter-defibrillators (Beyond the Basics). 2019. https://www.uptodate.com/contents/implantable-cardioverter-defibrillators-beyond-the-basics

REFERENCES

1. Steinberg JS, Mittal S. *Electrophysiology: The Basics: A Companion Guide for the Cardiology Fellow During the EP Rotation*. Philadelphia, PA: Wolters Kluwer; 2010.
2. Eagle KA, Baliga RR. *Practical Cardiology: Evaluation and Treatment of Common Cardiovascular Disorders*. Place of publication not identified: LWW; 2013.
3. Schleifer WJ, Srivathsan K. Ventricular arrhythmias state of the art. *Clin Cardiol.* 2013;31:595–605.
4. Compton SJ, Rottman JN. Ventricular tachycardia clinical presentation. *Medscape.* 2017:1–48.
5. Conover MB. *Understanding Electrocardiography*. St. Louis, MO: Mosby; 2003.
6. Buxton AE, Duc J, Berger EE, et al. Nonsustained ventricular tachycardia. *Cardiol Clin.* 2000;18(2):327–336.
7. Bigger J. Definition of benign versus malignant ventricular arrhythmias: targets for treatment. *Am J Cardiol.* 1983;52(6):47C–54C.
8. Valentin F. *Hurst's the Heart*. New York: McGraw-Hill; 2008.
9. Zipes DP, Camm AJ, Borggrefe M, et al. ACC/AHA/ESC 2006 guidelines for management of patients with ventricular arrhythmias and the prevention of sudden cardiac death. *Circulation.* 2006;114(10):e385–e484.
10. Olgin JE, Zipes DP. Specific arrhythmias: diagnosis and treatment. In: Bonow RO, Braunwald E, Libby P, et al., eds. *Braunwalds Heart Disease: A Textbook of Cardiovascular Medicine*. Philadelphia, PA: Elsevier/Saunders; 2008.
11. Karritsis DG, Zareba W, Camm J. Nonsustained ventricular tachycardia. *J Am Coll Cardiol.* 2012;60(20):1993–2004.
12. Pellegrini CN, Scheinman MM. Clinical management of ventricular tachycardia. *Curr Probl Cardiol.* 2010;35(9):453–504.
13. Lerman BB, Stein KM, Markowitz SM, et al. Ventricular tachycardia in patients with structurally normal hearts. *Card Electrophysiol.* 2004:668–682. doi:10.1016/b0-7216-0323-8/50075-0.
14. Field JM. *ACLS Resource Text: For Instructors and Experienced Providers.* Dallas, TX: American Heart Association; 2008.
15. Kasper DL, Fauci AS, Hauser SL, et al. *Harrisons Principles of Internal Medicine*. New York: McGraw-Hill Education; 2015.
16. Al-Khatib SL, Page RL. 2017 guideline for management of ventricular arrhythmias and prevention of SCD. *Am Coll Cardiol.* 2017;72(14). doi:10.1016/j.jacc.2017.10.054.
17. Packer M, Bristow MR, Cohn JN, et al. The effect of carvedilol on morbidity and mortality in patients with chronic heart failure. *N Engl J Med.* 1996;334(21):1349–1355.
18. Dargie HJ. Effect of carvedilol on outcome after myocardial infarction in patients with left-ventricular dysfunction: the CAPRICORN randomised trial. *Lancet North Am Ed.* 2001;357(9266):1385–1390.
19. Hjalmarson Å, Goldstein S, Fagerberg B, et al. Effects of controlled-release metoprolol on total mortality, hospitalizations, and well-being in patients with heart failure. *JAMA.* 2000;283(10):1295–1302.
20. Pitt B, Remme W, Zannad F, et al. Eplerenone, a selective aldosterone blocker, in patients with left ventricular dysfunction after myocardial infarction. *N Engl J Med.* 2003;348(14):1309–1321.
21. Pitt B, Zannad F, Remme WJ, et al. The effect of spironolactone on morbidity and mortality in patients with severe heart failure. *N Engl J Med.* 1999;341(10):709–717.
22. Zannad F, Mcmurray JJ, Krum H, et al. Eplerenone in patients with systolic heart failure and mild symptoms. *N Engl J Med.* 2011;364(1):11–21.
23. Desai AS, Mcmurray JJ, Packer M, et al. Effect of the angiotensin-receptor-neprilysin inhibitor LCZ696 compared with enalapril on mode of death in heart failure patients. *Eur Heart J.* 2015;36(30):1990–1997.
24. Zheng ZJ, Croft JB, Giles WH, et al. Sudden cardiac death in the United States, 1989 to 1998. *Circulation.* 2001;104(18):2158–2163.
25. Callans DJ. Management of the patient who has been resuscitated from sudden cardiac death. *Circulation.* 2002;105(23):2704–2707.
26. Prystowsky EN. Primary and secondary prevention of sudden cardiac death: the role of the implantable cardioverter defibrillator. *Rev Cardiovasc Med.* 2001;2(4):197–205.
27. Ali B, Zafari AM. Narrative review: cardiopulmonary resuscitation and emergency cardiovascular care: review of the current guidelines. *Ann Intern Med.* 2007;147(3):171–179.
28. Zipes DP, Wellens HJ. Sudden cardiac death. *Circulation.* 1998;98:2334–2351.

29. Albert CM, Chae CU, Grodstein F, et al. Prospective study of sudden cardiac death among women in the United States. *Circulation.* 2003;107(16):2096–2101.
30. Myerburg RJ, Castellanos A. Emerging paradigms of the epidemiology and demographics of sudden cardiac arrest. *Heart Rhythm.* 2006;3(2): 235–239.
31. Lopshire JC, Zipes DP. Sudden cardiac death. *Circulation.* 2006; 114(11):1134–1136.
32. Rubart M. Mechanisms of sudden cardiac death. *J Clin Invest.* 2005; 115(9):2305–2315.
33. Eisenberg MS, Mengert TJ. Cardiac resuscitation. *N Engl J Med.* 2001; 344(17):1304–1313.
34. Burke AP, Farb A, Malcom GT, et al. Effect of risk factors on the mechanism of acute thrombosis and sudden coronary death in women. *Circulation.* 1998;97(21):2110–2116.
35. Myerburg RJ. Scientific gaps in the prediction and prevention of sudden cardiac death. *J Cardiovasc Electrophysiol.* 2002;13(7):709–723.
36. Myerburg RJ, Junttila MJ. Sudden cardiac death caused by coronary heart disease. *Circulation.* 2012;125(8):1043–1052.
37. Moss AJ, Zareba W, Hall WJ, et al. Prophylactic implantation of a defibrillator in patients with myocardial infarction and reduced ejection fraction. *N Engl J Med.* 2002;346(12):877–883.
38. Bardy G, Lee K, Mark D. Amiodarone or an implantable cardioverter-defibrillator for congestive heart failure. *ACC Curr J Rev.* 2005; 14(4):44.
39. Kadish A, Dyer A, Daubert JP, et al. Prophylactic defibrillator implantation in patients with nonischemic dilated cardiomyopathy. *N Engl J Med.* 2004;350(21):2151–2158.
40. Maron BJ. Hypertrophic cardiomyopathy. *Circulation.* 2002;106(19): 2419–2421.
41. Maron BJ, Seidman J, Seidman CE. Proposal for contemporary screening strategies in families with hypertrophic cardiomyopathy. *J Am Coll Cardiol.* 2004;44(11):2125–2132.
42. Dimarco JP. Sudden cardiac death. In: Crawford MH, ed. *Current Diagnosis & Treatment Cardiology.* New York: McGraw-Hill Medical; 2014.
43. Turakhia M, Tseng ZH. Sudden cardiac death: epidemiology, mechanisms, and therapy. *Curr Probl Cardiol.* 2007;32(9):501–546.
44. Imboden M, Swan H, Denjoy I, et al. Female predominance and transmission distortion in the long-QT syndrome. *N Engl J Med.* 2006; 355(26):2744–2751.
45. Napolitano C, Priori SG, Schwartz PJ, et al. Genetic testing in the long QT syndrome. *JAMA.* 2005;294(23):2975–2980.
46. Moss AJ, Robinson JL, Gessman L, et al. Comparison of clinical and genetic variables of cardiac events associated with loud noise versus swimming among subjects with the long QT syndrome. *Am J Cardiol.* 1999; 84(8):876–879.
47. Pappone C, Santinelli V, Rosanio S, et al. Usefulness of invasive electrophysiologic testing to stratify the risk of arrhythmic events in asymptomatic patients with Wolff-Parkinson-White pattern. *J Am Coll Cardiol.* 2003;41(2):239–244.
48. Priori SG, Napolitano C. Intracellular calcium handling dysfunction and arrhythmogenesis. *Circ Res.* 2005;97(11):1077–1079.
49. Link MS, Berkow LC, Kudenchuk PJ, et al. Part 7: Adult advanced cardiovascular life support. *Circulation.* 2015;132(18 suppl 2):S444–S464.
50. Morrison LJ, Dorian P, Long J, et al. Out-of-hospital cardiac arrest rectilinear biphasic to monophasic damped sine defibrillation waveforms with advanced life support intervention trial (ORBIT). *Resuscitation.* 2005;66(2):149–157.
51. Schneider T, Martens PR, Paschen H, et al. Multicenter, randomized, controlled trial of 150-J biphasic shocks compared with 200- to 360-J monophasic shocks in the resuscitation of out-of-hospital cardiac arrest victims. Optimized Response to Cardiac Arrest (ORCA) Investigators. *Circulation.* 2000;102:1780–1787.
52. Stults KR, Brown DD, Kerber RE. Efficacy of an automated external defibrillator in the management of out-of-hospital cardiac arrest: validation of the diagnostic algorithm and initial clinical experience in a rural environment. *Circulation.* 1986;73(4):701–709.
53. Zafari A, Zarter SK, Heggen V, et al. A program encouraging early defibrillation results in improved in-hospital resuscitation efficacy. *J Am Coll Cardiol.* 2004;44(4):846–852.
54. Kerber RE, Kouba C, Martins J, et al. Advance prediction of transthoracic impedance in human defibrillation and cardioversion: importance of impedance in determining the success of low-energy shocks. *Circulation.* 1984;70(2):303–308.
55. Sado DM, Deakin CD. How good is your defibrillation technique? *J R Soc Med.* 2005;98(1):3–6.
56. Kleinman ME, Brennan EE, Goldberger ZD, et al. Part 5: Adult basic life support and cardiopulmonary resuscitation quality: 2015 American Heart Association guidelines update for cardiopulmonary resuscitation and emergency cardiovascular care. *Circulation.* 2015;132(18 suppl 2):S414–S435.
57. Callaway CW, Donnino MW, Fink EL, et al. Part 8: Post–cardiac arrest care: 2015 American Heart Association guidelines update for cardiopulmonary resuscitation and emergency cardiovascular care. *Circulation.* 2015;132(18 suppl 2):S465–S482.
58. Francis J, Reek S. Wearable cardioverter defibrillator: a life vest till the life boat (ICD) arrives. *Indian Heart J.* 2014;66(1):68–72.
59. Norekvål TM, Kirchhof P, Fitzsimons D. Patient-centred care of patients with ventricular arrhythmias and risk of sudden cardiac death: what do the 2015 European Society of Cardiology guidelines add? *Eur J Cardiovasc Nurs.* 2017;16(7):558–564.
60. Tel H, Tel H. The effect of individualized education on the transfer anxiety of patients with myocardial infarction and their families. *Heart Lung.* 2006;35(2):101–107.
61. Bunch TJ, Hammill SC, White RD. Outcomes after ventricular fibrillation out-of-hospital cardiac arrest: expanding the chain of survival. *Mayo Clin Proc.* 2005;80(6):774–782.
62. Bunch T, White RD, Smith GE, et al. Long-term subjective memory function in ventricular fibrillation out-of-hospital cardiac arrest survivors resuscitated by early defibrillation. *Resuscitation.* 2004;60(2):189–195.
63. Dougherty CM, Pyper GP, Benoliel JQ. Domains of concern of intimate partners of sudden cardiac arrest survivors after ICD implantation. *J Cardiovasc Nurs.* 2004;19(1):21–31.
64. Dickerson SS, Posluszny M, Kennedy MC. Help seeking in a support group for recipients of implantable cardioverter defibrillators and their support persons. *Heart Lung.* 2000;29(2):87–96.
65. Shea JB. Quality of life issues in patients with implantable cardioverter defibrillators. *AACN Clin Issues.* 2004;15(3):478–489.
66. Berger S. Survival from out-of-hospital cardiac arrest: are we beginning to see progress? *J Am Heart Assoc.* 2017;6(9):e007469.

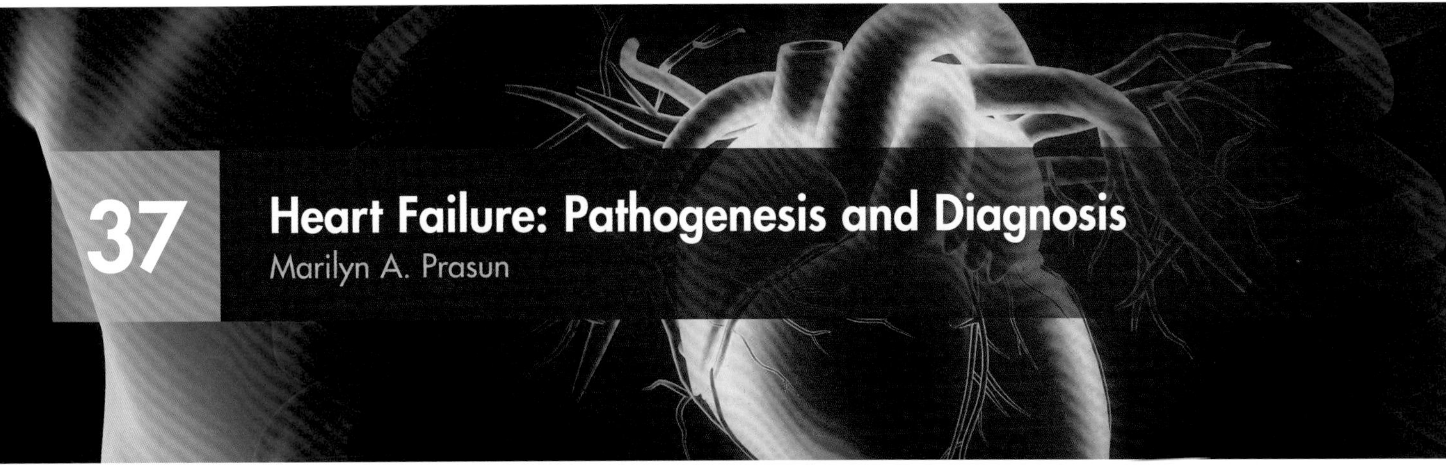

37 Heart Failure: Pathogenesis and Diagnosis

Marilyn A. Prasun

OBJECTIVES

1. Review the pathophysiology of heart failure.
2. Identify current clinical and diagnostic assessment modalities.
3. Discuss treatment strategies for both chronic and acute decompensated heart failure.
4. Examine the transition of care of the patient with heart failure.

KEY QUESTIONS

1. What are the clinical profiles of patients with decompensated heart failure and treatment approaches?
2. What compensatory systems are activated following the initial insult leading to heart failure?
3. Distinguish the clinical differences between heart failure–reduced ejection fraction (HFrEF) and heart failure–preserved ejection fraction (HFpEF)?
4. What diagnostic testing should be included during initial evaluation of the patient with heart failure?
5. List the current recommended pharmacologic and nonpharmacologic treatment of the compensated patient with HFrEF and HFpEF?

HEART FAILURE

Heart failure (HF) is a pathophysiologic state in which an abnormality of cardiac function is responsible for inadequate systemic perfusion. HF is not an event or disease but rather a constellation of signs and symptoms that represent the final pathway of a heterogeneous group of diseases, the end result of most cardiovascular disease states.[1] The extent and severity by which cardiac function is impaired varies greatly. It is the primary reason people over the age of 65 are hospitalized in the United States.[2,3] However, HF hospitalization rates have declined nationally over the past 10 years among the Medicare population, yet rates vary based on race and gender.[3]

The prevalence of the syndrome of HF has increased dramatically throughout the world over the last decade and is projected to continue to increase over the next decade.[4] The increased prevalence of HF is attributable to both the general aging of the worlds' population and advances in the treatment of acute cardiac disease. An estimated 6.2 million adult American people carry the diagnosis, with approximately 1,000,000 new cases diagnosed annually.[4] While the syndrome of HF has been extensively researched, it remains a significant and growing health problem in the United States and worldwide. There is an increasing incidence of HF in the aging population predominantly due to the development of HF risk factors such as, coronary artery disease (CAD), hypertension, diabetes mellitus (DM), and obesity.[5,6] The lifetime risk of developing HF is high (20% to 45%), with highest risk reported in black females (24% to 46%).[4] The American Heart Association (AHA) reports the estimated cost in 2012 for HF was $30.7 billion and projects in 2030 cost to treat HF annually will increase to $69.8 billion.[4]

In the past decade, experimental and clinical studies have demonstrated HF is a multisystem disorder that adversely triggers myocyte changes, alterations in the extracellular matrix and vasculature while signaling neurohormonal activity as an adaptive response. The progression of HF involves succession of these cellular and molecular changes.[7] The quality of life, symptom management, exercise capacity, and perhaps the life expectancy of patients with HF can be altered by the introduction of appropriate medical and nursing interventions.

This chapter reviews major physiologic and pathophysiologic concepts of chronic HF as a basis for understanding its underlying causes as well as its clinical and physical findings. Emphasis also is placed on diagnostic tests as well as medical and nursing interventions in the adult patient with ventricular dysfunction. With this knowledge, the nurse is able to develop and implement a plan of care, to identify patients at risk, and to optimize the management, functional capacity, and outcome of patients living with HF.

Historic Perspective

The understanding of HF has evolved dramatically in the last 100 years. Advances in the understanding of HF, have resulted in significant changes in detection, treatment, and recognition of disease progression. During the 19th century, the altered architecture of the failing heart was implicated as the cause of patient's symptoms. In 1832, James Hope first described *backward failure* as the failure that results as the ventricle fails to pump its volume, causing blood accumulation and subsequent increase in ventricular, atrial, and venous pressures. A primary cause of backward failure was mechanical cardiac obstruction. The term *forward failure*, proposed by MacKenzie in 1913, was applied to a situation in which the primary pathologic process was decreased cardiac output, which ultimately leads to a decrease in vital organ perfusion, and to water and sodium retention.[8] MacKenzie was the first to propose that intrinsic myocardial abnormalities lead to the death of patients with this syndrome.[9] By the mid-1920s, Starling et al. revolutionized the understanding of the syndrome with their animal studies describing the effect of alterations in pressure and flow on myocardial performance. This work formed the basis upon which the syndrome was understood until almost the end of the 20th century. The hemodynamic derangement that was secondary to pressure and flow abnormalities became the accepted paradigm, explaining the therapeutic interventions of the time. If pressure and volume were the two components of myocardial contractility, causing reduced cardiac output, therapeutic interventions were aimed at accurately assessing and altering hemodynamics. While it is now known that cardiac hemodynamics played a role in the syndrome of HF, therapeutic intervention targeted at normalization of hemodynamic derangement did not translate to improved outcomes in patients.

Advances in cellular biochemistry and biophysics in the 1970s to 1980s led to a widening of the lens through which the complexity and progression of HF emerged. Patients with HF were noted to have markedly elevated levels of stress hormones such as norepinephrine (NE). These discoveries led some to hypothesize that while myocardial dysfunction begins the syndrome, progression and subsequent death of the patients may be attributable to dramatic neurohormonal abnormalities. By the early 1990s, studies of medications aimed at altering the neurohormonal milieu within the body solidly supported the neurohormonal/neuroendocrine hypothesis that remains the target of many of the current interventions.[10] However, since the turn of the 20th century, advances in the ability to measure molecular changes in myocytes have led to an ever complex understanding of the collection of complex genetic and molecular disorders that lead to and perpetuate the syndrome.

Etiologies and Definitions

HF is a complex clinical syndrome manifested by shortness of breath, fatigue, and characterized by structural or functional impairment of ventricular filling or ejection of blood and neurohormonal regulation.[1] Any disorder that places the heart under an increased volume or pressure load or that produces primary damage or an increased metabolic demand on the myocardium may result in HF (Table 37-1). Over the last decade, the traditional risk factors for HF were CAD followed by hypertension, DM, obesity, and smoking.[4,6] However, among ethnic minorities in America, a larger proportion of risk for HF was hypertension and left ventricular hypertrophy (LVH).[4] As treatment modalities for both acute and chronic HF improve, the number of patients living with HF grows.

Ventricular dysfunction begins with injury. It is vital for the clinician to identify the underlying and the precipitating causes of HF. Coronary artery disease is frequently the underlying cause of HF in reduced ejection fraction (HFrEF), also known as systolic dysfunction. Hypertension is implicated in both HFrEF and preserved ejection fraction (HFpEF). Patients with systolic dysfunction frequently have aspects of diastolic dysfunction as well.[11] Arrhythmias are common in patients with underlying structural heart disease; and they commonly precipitate an acute decompensation in patients with stable HF. These arrhythmias may take the form of tachyarrhythmias (most commonly atrial fibrillation), marked bradycardia, degrees of heart block, and abnormal intraventricular conduction, such as left bundle-branch block or ventricular arrhythmias. Other precipitating factors include systemic infections, anemia, endocrine abnormalities, and pulmonary emboli placing increased metabolic and hemodynamic demand on the heart. Administration of cardiac depressants or salt-retaining drugs may also precipitate HF; examples may include corticosteroids, nondihydropyridine calcium channel antagonists, and nonsteroidal anti-inflammatory drugs (NSAIDs). Alcohol is a potent myocardial depressant and may be responsible for the development of cardiomyopathy. Nonadherence or inappropriate reduction in evidence-based pharmacologic therapy or dietary excess of sodium are also causes of decompensation in a previously compensated patient.

Stages of HF and Functional Classification

The writing committee of the American College of Cardiology Foundation and the American Heart Association (ACCF/AHA) Task Force decided to emphasize the evolution and progression of HF in their most recent revision of the guidelines.[1] This classification recognizes that HF, like CAD, has established risk factors, that the progression of HF has asymptomatic and symptomatic phases, and that treatments prescribed at each stage can reduce morbidity and mortality. Four stages of HF were identified. Stage A identifies the patient who is at high risk but has no structural heart disease; stage B refers to a patient with structural heart

Table 37-1 • CONDITIONS ASSOCIATED WITH HEART FAILURE

Abnormal Volume Load	Abnormal Pressure Load	Myocardial Abnormalities	Filling Disorders	Increased Metabolic Demand
Aortic valve incompetence	Aortic stenosis	Cardiomyopathy	Mitral stenosis	Anemias
Mitral valve incompetence	Hypertrophic cardiomyopathy	Myocarditis	Tricuspid stenosis	Thyrotoxicosis
Tricuspid valve incompetence	Coarctation of the aorta	Coronary heart disease	Cardiac tamponade	Fever
Left-to-right shunts	Hypertension	Ischemia	Restrictive pericarditis	Beriberi
Secondary hypervolemia	Primary	Infarction	Restrictive cardiomyopathy	Paget disease
	Secondary	Arrhythmias		Arteriovenous fistulas
		Toxic disorders		Pulmonary emboli
		Alcohol		Systemic emboli
		Cocaine		
		Administration of cardiac depressant agents or salt-retaining drugs		

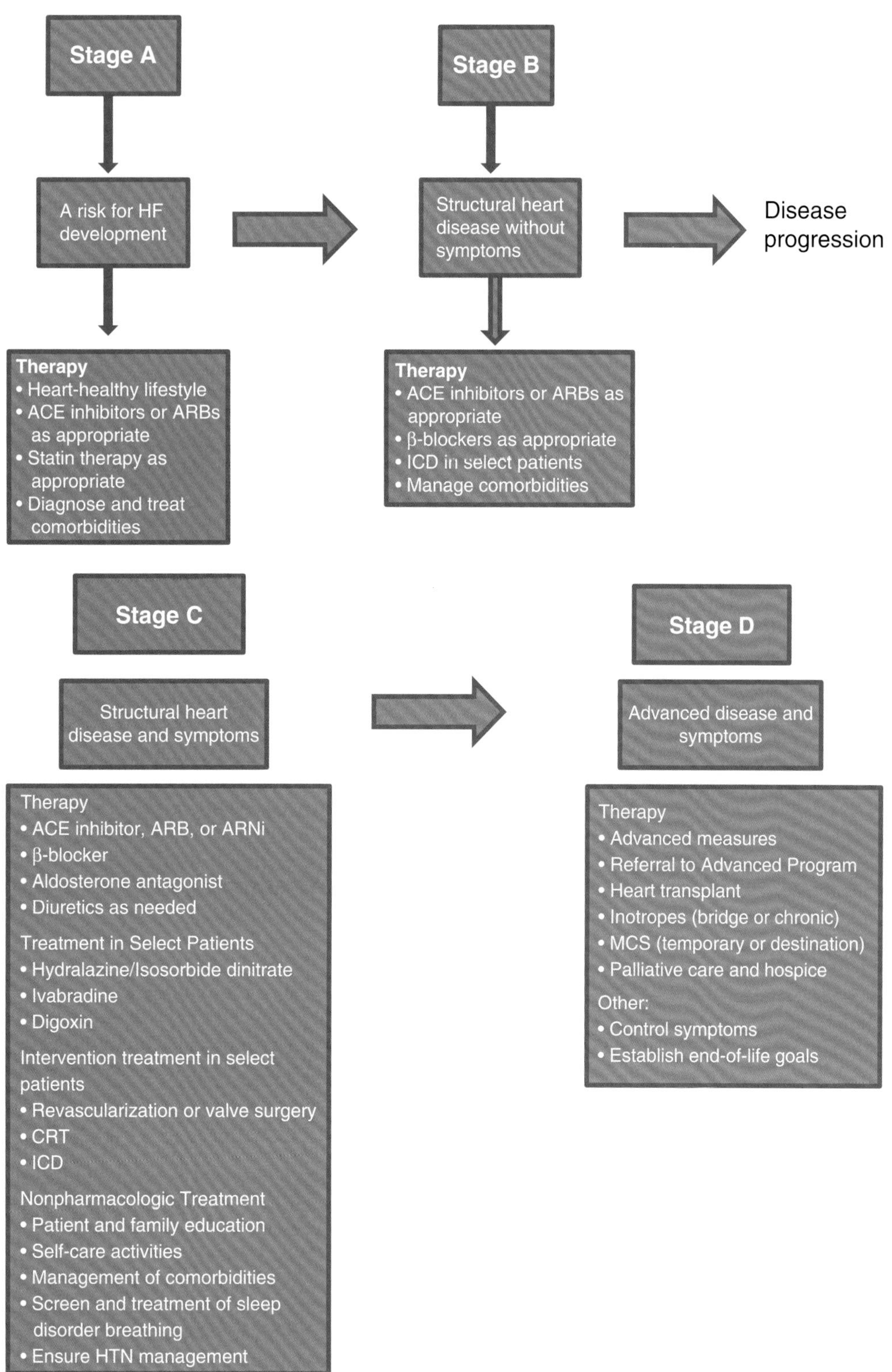

Figure 37-1. Stages in the development of heart failure/recommended therapy by stage. Stages A and B: Early stages of HF and treatment recommendations. Stages C and D: Recommended HF treatment. (Modified from the 2013 ACCF/AHA Guidelines and 2017 ACC/AHA/HFSA Update.)

disease but no symptoms of HF; stage C denotes the patient with structural heart disease and current or previous symptoms of HF; and stage D describes the patient with end-stage disease that requires special interventions (Fig. 37-1). The importance of this staging system arises from the fact that, while treatment options for HF have advanced in the last decade, once myocyte, myocardial, and systemic changes have begun, the only treatment option is altering the trajectory of the syndrome.

As the understanding of the mechanisms underlying both the development and progression of HF has evolved, attention has

Table 37-2 • ESTABLISHED AND HYPOTHESIZED RISK FACTORS FOR HEART FAILURE

Major Risk Factors	Toxic Precipitants	Minor Risk Factors
AsymptomaticLV dysfunction	Chemotherapy (anthracyclines, cyclophosphamide, 5-FU, trastuzumab)	Smoking
Increased LV mass	Cocaine	Dyslipidemia
Age, male gender	NSAIDs	Sleep-disordered breathing
Hypertension, LVH	Doxazosin	Chronic renal disease
Myocardial infarction	Alcohol	Anemia
Diabetes		Sedentary lifestyle
Valvular heart disease		Low socioeconomic status
Obesity		Psychological stress

5-FU, 5-fluorouracil; LV, left ventricle; LVH, left ventricle hypertrophy; NSAIDs, nonsteroidal anti-inflammatory drugs.
Adapted from Schocken DD, Benjamin EJ, Fonarow GC, et al. Prevention of heart failure. A scientific statement from the American Heart Association Councils on Epidemiology And Prevention, Clinical Cardiology, Cardiovascular Nursing, and High Blood Pressure Research; Quality of Care and Outcomes Research Interdisciplinary Working Group; and Functional Genomics and Translational Biology Interdisciplinary Working Group. *Circulation.* 2008;117(19):2544–2565; Table 1.

been placed on identifying the factors that put patients at risk for developing the syndrome (Table 37-2). Although it is not surprising that advancing age, history of CAD, MI, or hypertension are associated with developing HF, a robust association has been seen in patients with both type II DM[6,12] and obesity, and the subsequent syndrome of HF. The worldwide epidemic of type II DM and obesity makes them potentially modifiable targets to reduce the incidence of HF.

The clinical manifestations of acute and chronic failure depend on how rapidly the syndrome of HF develops. Acute HF may be the initial manifestation of heart disease but is more commonly an acute exacerbation of a chronic cardiac condition. The events occur so rapidly that the sympathetic nervous system compensation is ineffective, resulting in the rapid development of pulmonary edema and circulatory collapse (cardiogenic shock). Chronic HF develops over time and is usually the end result of an increasing inability of physiologic mechanisms to compensate.

The New York Heart Association (NYHA) functional classification serves to estimate the severity of symptoms and functional capacity. It is a subjective assessment that can change based on the patient's condition and symptoms. The NYHA classification ranges from I to IV. Class I is no limitation of physical activity and physical activity does not cause HF symptoms; class II is slight limitation of physical activity, comfortable at rest and ordinary physical activity results in HF symptoms; class III is marked limitation of physical activity, comfortable at rest and less than ordinary activity results in HF symptoms; and class IV unable to perform physical activity without symptoms of HF or symptoms of HF at rest.[1,13] Both the ACCF/AHA stages of HF and NYHA functional classifications are used to determine when patients are eligible for various evidence-based HF treatments in clinical practice.[1]

Low and High Cardiac Output Syndromes

In response to high blood pressure (BP) and hypovolemia, low cardiac output syndrome can appear. The word *syndrome* implies that the failure represents a reaction rather than a primary pathologic process. Low cardiac output syndrome is evidenced by impaired peripheral circulation and peripheral vasoconstriction.

Any condition that causes the heart to work harder to supply blood may be categorized as high cardiac output syndrome. Typically, patients with HF present with normal or low cardiac output. A minority of patients present in a high-output state.[14] High cardiac output states require an increased oxygen supply to the peripheral tissues, which can occur only with an increased cardiac output. Reduced systemic vascular resistance (SVR) is characteristic of this condition; it augments peripheral circulation and venous return, which in turn increases stroke volume and cardiac output. High cardiac output states may be caused by increased metabolic requirements, as seen in hyperthyroidism, fever, or may be triggered by conditions such as obesity, arteriovenous fistulas, liver disease, lung disease, and anemia.[14] High-output patients with HF display eccentric left ventricular remodeling, increased B-type natriuretic peptide (BNP) activation, filling pressures, and pulmonary hypertension.[14] While the terms *low output* and *high-output syndromes* are not commonly used in practice, recognizing that processes occur is important.

Pathogenesis and Pathophysiology

While the root of HF is altered myocardial function, a host of compensatory systemic responses lead to the subsequent progressive clinical syndrome (Fig. 37-2). The compensatory response leads to altered myocardial function, ventricular remodeling, changes in hemodynamics, neurohormonal and cytokine activation, and vascular and endothelial dysfunction. Multiple alterations in organ and cellular physiology contribute to HF under various circumstances. Adaptive and maladaptive processes affect the myocardium, kidneys, peripheral vasculature, smooth and skeletal muscle, and multiple reflex control mechanisms.[7,15] Understanding of the mechanism behind both the development and progression of HF over the last decade has continued to evolve (Fig. 37-3).

Changes in myocardial architecture due to injury result in myocardial contractile dysfunction. The changes in architecture come about by alterations in cardiac myocyte biology, gene expression, and in myocardial and ventricular structures.[16] Key features of pathologic cardiac remodeling include cardiac hypertrophy, fibrosis, and cell death (apoptosis).[17] Ventricular hypertrophy is defined by an increase in ventricular mass attributable to increase in the volume of cardiac cells. The increase in ventricular mass is due to an increase in the size of the myocytes, increased number of fibroblasts, and an increase in the extracellular matrix proteins (collagen and fibronectin). Ventricular contractile dysfunction leads to altered systemic perfusion. Alterations in systemic perfusion result in neuroendocrine activation resulting in progressive alterations in myocardial architecture and contractile function. In short, myocardial injury leads to altered systemic perfusion causing neuroendocrine changes that result in further ventricular dysfunction. The remainder of this section examines more closely each of the steps in this process. It is important to recognize that understanding the interplay between each of these steps is a dynamic and rapidly expanding venture.

Myocyte Pathophysiology

The primary goal in preventing and ultimately managing HF is protection and preservation of the myocyte. Myocardial insult and injury occur as decades pass, and the compensatory adaptation often leads to dysfunction. Preventing myocyte

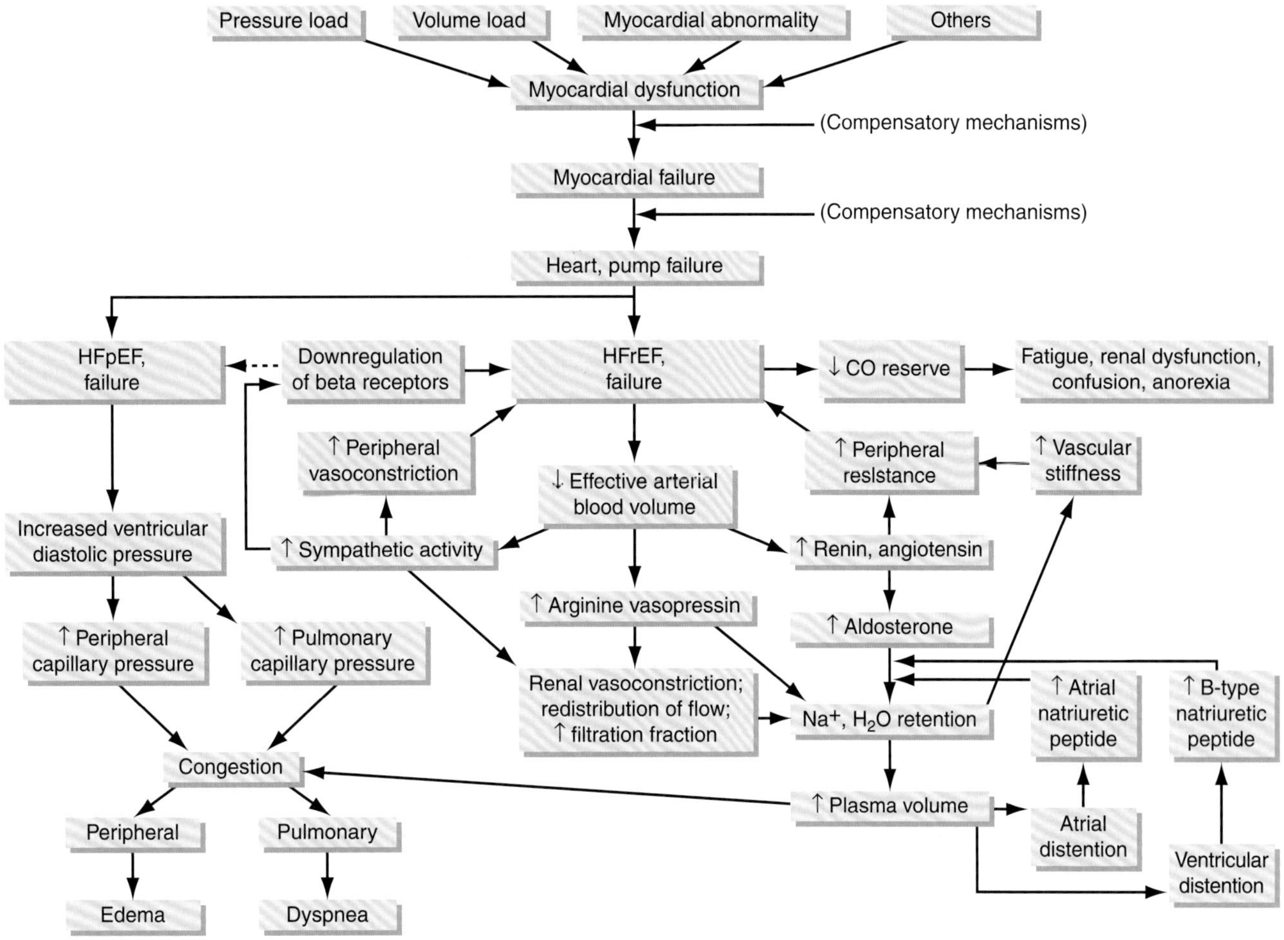

Pressure load
Volume load
Myocardial abnormality
Others
Myocardial dysfunction
(Compensatory mechanisms)
Myocardial failure
(Compensatory mechanisms)
Heart, pump failure
HFpEF, failure
Downregulation of beta receptors
HFrEF, failure
↓ CO reserve
Fatigue, renal dysfunction, confusion, anorexia
↑ Peripheral vasoconstriction
↓ Effective arterial blood volume
↑ Peripheral resistance
↑ Vascular stiffness
Increased ventricular diastolic pressure
↑ Sympathetic activity
↑ Renin, angiotensin
↑ Arginine vasopressin
↑ Aldosterone
↑ Peripheral capillary pressure
↑ Pulmonary capillary pressure
Renal vasoconstriction; redistribution of flow; ↑ filtration fraction
Na^+, H_2O retention
↑ Atrial natriuretic peptide
↑ B-type natriuretic peptide
Congestion
↑ Plasma volume
Atrial distention
Ventricular distention
Peripheral
Pulmonary
Edema
Dyspnea

Figure 37-2. Sequence of events in heart failure. An increased load or myocardial abnormality leads to myocardial failure and eventually heart failure, resulting in increased sympathetic activity, increased activity of the renin–angiotensin–aldosterone system, pulmonary and peripheral congestion and edema, and decreased cardiac output reserve. Both the atrial natriuretic and B-type natriuretic peptides are also released in response to increased plasma volume. (Adapted from Francis GS, Gassler JP, Sonneblick EH. Pathophysiology and diagnosis of heart failure. In: Hurst JW, ed. *The Heart.* 10th ed. New York: McGraw-Hill; 2001.)

hypertrophy, fibrosis, and death becomes the primary goal in altering the trajectory of the syndrome of HF.[17] Understanding the changes that occur within the cardiac myocyte provides insight into the syndrome.

Increased pressure or volume reactivates growth factors present in the embryonic heart but dormant in the adult heart. This fetal gene expression stimulates the hypertrophy of the myocytes and the synthesis and degradation of the extracellular matrix. There is some evidence that extracellular matrix degradation may elicit side-to-side slippage or disarray of myocytes, perhaps caused by dissolution of collagen struts that normally hold cells together. In the myocardium, fibrosis can be divided into interstitial,

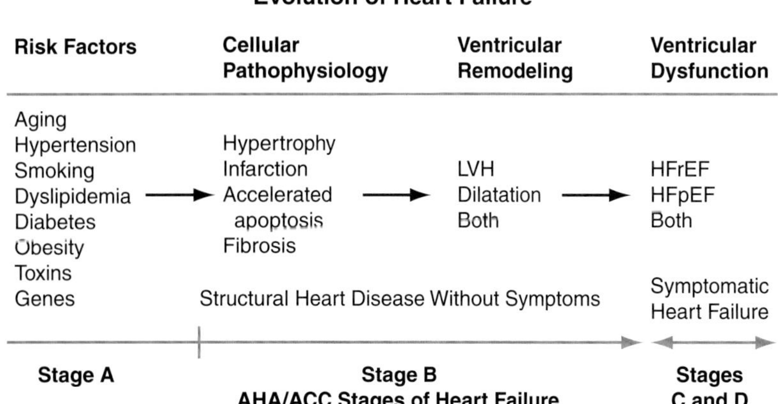

Figure 37-3. The evolution of HF along with AHA/ACC guidelines for the diagnosis and management of HF clinical stages. (Adapted from Schocken DD, Benjamin EJ, Fonarow GC, et al. Prevention of heart failure. A scientific statement from the American Heart Association Councils on Epidemiology and Prevention, Clinical Cardiology, Cardiovascular Nursing, and High Blood Pressure Research; Quality of Care and Outcomes Research Interdisciplinary Working Group; and Functional Genomics and Translational Biology Interdisciplinary Working Group. *Circulation.* 2008;117[19]: 2544–2565.)

replacement, and perivascular. Each is based on cause and anatomical location.[17] Collagen accumulation resulting from fibrosis leads to stiffening of the heart.[18] Myocyte slippage may also be caused by myocyte loss.[19]

Hypertrophied myocytes have alterations in contractile protein synthesis and calcium cycling. Force within the myocyte is a result of the interaction of myosin and actin. Myocyte hypertrophy alters the synthesis of myosin proteins from α-myosin heavy chain toward β-myosin heavy chain. This shift in the myosin subunit alters the kinetics by which it binds to actin, resulting in contraction. Initially, this change produces an energetically favorable state, but chronically this state is unsustainable and failure occurs. Altered expression or alignment of contractile proteins within sarcomeres is important, as increasing mutations in sarcomeric proteins have been linked to inherited cardiomyopathic processes. Alteration in expression and function of the contractile proteins is signaled by mechanical wall stress, angiotensin (AT) II, NE, endothelin (ET), tumor necrosis factor-alpha (TNF-α), inflammatory interleukins, and intracellular calcium signaling. There are changes in the sarcomeric proteins that lead to decreased contraction velocity, reduced stroke volume, and increased ventricular volume.[9,15]

Ventricular contraction and relaxation is a dynamic process controlled by the uptake of calcium by the sarcoplasmic reticulum and the efflux of calcium within the myocyte.[15,19] Myocyte hypertrophy impacts several intracellular proteins involved in calcium cycling. The most consistent change is a significant downregulation of expression and activity of the sarcoplasmic reticulum calcium ATPase (SERCA) pump. While the role of SERCA in calcium handling within the myocyte is complex and remains the topic of study, the net result is a reduction in the availability of peak systolic calcium, and an elevation and prolongation in diastolic calcium, resulting in reduced systolic contraction and delayed diastolic relaxation.

The paracrine function of the heart is markedly altered in HF. Paracrine action is the release of a locally acting endocrine substance, a system in which the target cells are close to the signaling cells. The signal transduction system in the failing myocardium is profoundly altered. The failing myocardium is induced to secrete both atrial and B-type natriuretic peptides (ANP and BNP, respectively). In addition, fibrosis-associated proteins are also released with suppression of tumorigenicity 2 (sST2) and galectin-3 (Gal-3).[20–22]

Actual myocyte loss may also occur by one of two mechanisms: apoptosis or necrosis. Apoptosis is a programmed cell death that is energy dependent, producing cell dropout. Apoptosis is a highly regulated process that causes the cell to shrink, yielding cell fragments that are surrounded by plasma membrane. This process does not invoke an inflammatory or fibrotic response. Apoptosis is stimulated by hypoxia, AT II, TNF-α, myocyte calcium overload, and mitochondrial or cell injury.[23] Two forms of apoptosis appear to affect the course of postinfarction remodeling: ischemic-driven apoptosis at the site of the infarction and load- or receptor-dependent apoptosis at sites remote from the ischemic areas.[24] Necrosis or accidental cell death occurs when the myocyte is deprived of oxygen or energy. Energy starvation of the myocyte results from an increase in energy demand and a reduced capacity for energy production.[15] The inflammatory response that is induced by overload elevates circulating levels of cytokines that in turn release reactive oxygen species and free radicals. Calcium overload increases energy expenditure and slows energy production. All these processes lead to the loss of cellular membrane integrity, causing the cell to swell and eventually burst. This loss of cellular membrane integrity releases proteolytic enzymes that cause cellular disruption. The release of cell contents initiates an inflammatory reaction that leads to scarring and fibrosis. Myocyte necrosis may be localized, as in an MI, or diffuse, from myocarditis or idiopathic cardiomyopathy.[7] The vicious cycle of the overloaded heart is depicted in Figure 37-4.

Ventricular Remodeling

Myocardial remodeling in the failing myocardium involves complex events at the molecular and cellular levels.[25–27] When the heart is presented with an increased workload by either pressure or volume overload, or by myocardial abnormality, a number of physiologic alterations are evoked in an attempt to maintain normal cardiac pumping function. Myocardial contractility (inotropy) and relaxation (lusitropy) are impaired in patients with HF. In addition, systemic hemodynamics, which include both preload and afterload, and ventricular architecture (shape, cavity size, and wall thickness) determine ejection and filling of a failing heart (Fig. 37-5).[7] As diastolic filling increases, ventricular dilatation occurs in response to maladaptive growth response and remodeling of the damaged or chronically overloaded heart. Renal compensatory mechanisms cause sympathetic stimulation, thus increasing the end-diastolic volume or preload. The Frank–Starling response is immediately activated as a consequence of increased diastolic volume. According to the Frank–Starling law, length-dependent changes in contractile performance during diastole increase the force of contraction during systole. The increased preload-augmenting contractility is the major mechanism by which the ventricles maintain an equal output as their stroke volumes vary.[7,15] It may be useful to consider normal and impaired myocardial function within the framework of the Frank–Starling mechanism, as illustrated by analysis of LV function curves (Fig. 37-6). Cardiac output or cardiac index (CI) is used as a measure of ventricular work; LV end-diastolic pressure or pulmonary artery wedge pressure (PAWP) is used as a reflection of preload. The normal relation between ventricular end-diastolic volume and ventricular work is shown in Figure 37-6 by curve 1. Optimal contractility occurs at a diastolic volume of 12 to 18 mm Hg. If the heart is physiologically stressed, as occurs in acute MI, the initial drop in cardiac output stimulates the sympathetic nervous system. An increase in sympathetic tone elevates heart rate (HR) and contractility, illustrated in Figure 37-6 by curve 2. As the cardiac workload increases and myocardial dysfunction persists, HF progresses. HF progression is reflected by further elevation of end-diastolic volume (preload) and ventricular dilatation. This increased preload, in turn, may further contribute to depressed ventricular contractility and the development of congestive symptoms (Fig. 37-6, curve 3).[28]

The normal left ventricle is able to adjust to large changes in aortic impedance (afterload) with small changes in output, in part by calling on the Frank–Starling response and, perhaps, by augmenting the contractile force as an intrinsic property of the normal myocardium. In contrast, the damaged left ventricle loses this compensatory ability and becomes sensitive to even small changes in impedance.[29] Because increased activity of the sympathetic nervous system or the renin–angiotensin–aldosterone system (RAAS) results in vasoconstriction of the small arteries and arterioles, increased impedance of LV filling is imposed, decreasing the stroke volume and cardiac output. Because HF is characterized by heightened activity of these neurohormonal vasoconstrictor systems, a positive feedback loop can be generated in which impaired

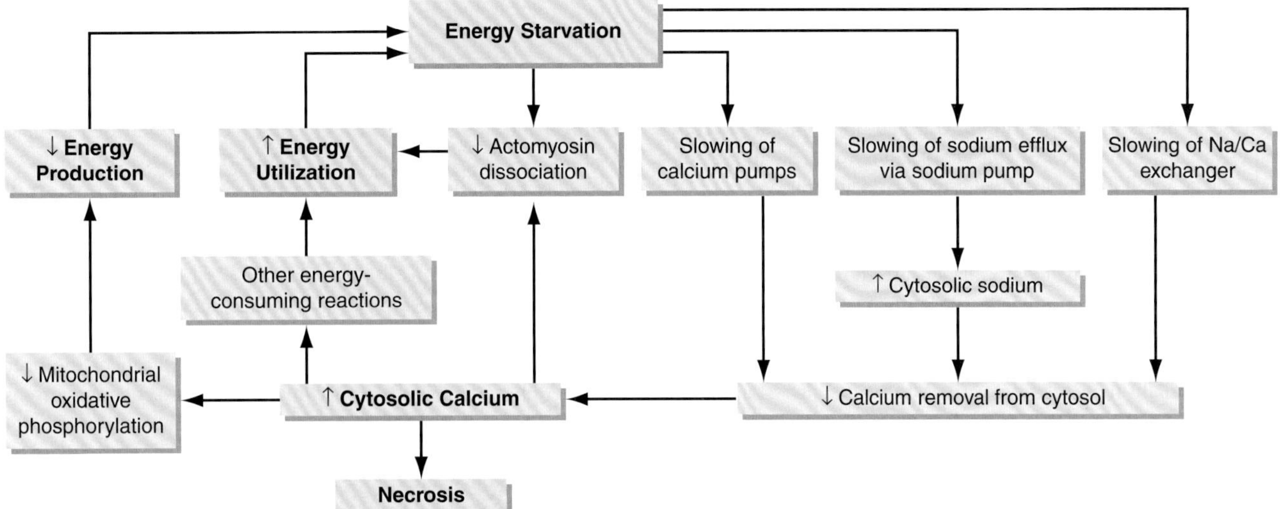

Figure 37-4. Energy starvation contributes to several vicious cycles that cause myocyte necrosis by increasing energy utilization and decreasing energy production. Reduced turnover of the calcium pumps of the sarcoplasmic reticulum and plasma membrane, the Na/Ca exchanger, and the sodium pump impair calcium removal from the cytosol. The resulting increase in cytosolic calcium inhibits actomyosin dissociation, which in addition to impairing relaxation increases energy utilization and so worsens the energy starvation. Aerobic energy production is also inhibited when cytosolic calcium is taken up by the mitochondria, which uncouples oxidative phosphorylation. The resulting increase in cytosolic calcium amplifies these vicious cycles and can lead to necrosis of the energy-starved cells. (From Katz AM, Konstam MA. *Heart Failure: Pathophysiology, Molecular Biology, and Clinical Management.* Philadelphia, PA: Lippincott Williams & Wilkins; 2008; Katz AM. *Physiology of the Heart.* 4th ed. Philadelphia, PA: Lippincott Williams & Wilkins; 2006.)

pump performance increases impedance to LV ejection, further impairing pump performance.

Changes in the composition of the myocardium occur in response to injury or overload and result in structural remodeling, divided into both cellular and noncellular changes. Several of the cellular changes have been discussed in the prior section and include changes within the cardiomyocytes (hypertrophy, apoptosis, and

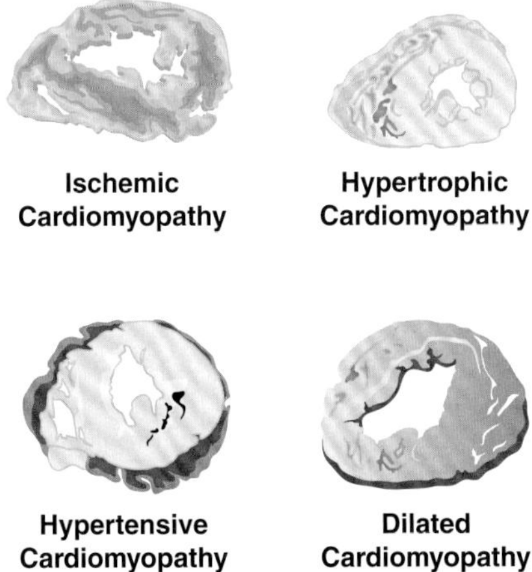

Figure 37-5. Patterns of ventricular hypertrophy and remodeling in various forms of cardiomyopathy. (From Katz AM, Konstam MA. *Heart Failure: Pathophysiology, Molecular Biology, and Clinical Management.* Philadelphia, PA: Lippincott Williams & Wilkins; 2008; Konstam MA. Systolic and diastolic dysfunction in heart failure? Time for a new paradigm. *J Card Fail.* 2003; 9[1]:1–3.)

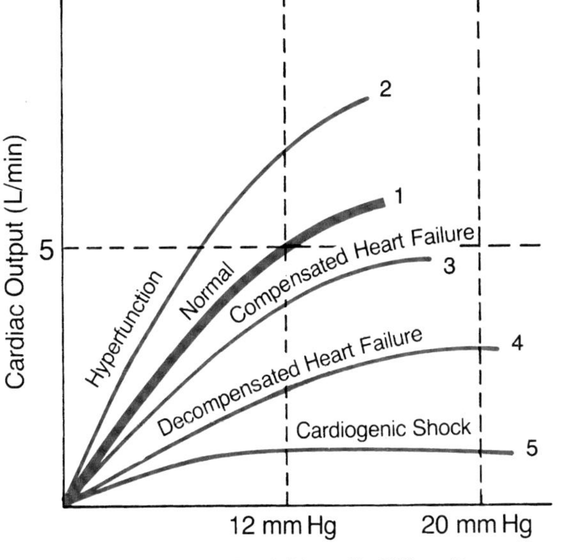

Figure 37-6. Left ventricular function curves. Curve 1: Normal function curve, with a normal cardiac output at optimal filling pressures. Curve 2: Cardiac hyperfunction, with an increased cardiac output at optimal filling pressures. Curve 3: Compensated heart failure, with normal cardiac outputs at higher filling pressures. Curve 4: Decompensated heart failure, with a decrease in cardiac output and elevated filling pressures. Curve 5: Cardiogenic shock, with extremely depressed cardiac output and marked increase in filling pressures. (Adapted from Michaelson CR. *Congestive Heart Failure.* St. Louis, MO: CV Mosby; 1983:61.)

necrosis) but several alterations in other cell types, such as fibroblasts, vascular smooth muscle cells, monocytes and macrophages, also contribute to ventricular remodeling. Noncellular components of the myocardium likewise contribute to remodeling. There is an increase in interstitial deposition of collagen fibers and an increase in perivascular deposition of collagen, leading to thickening of the walls of the small intramyocardial arteries and arterioles.

Throughout the body, there is a fine balance of synthesis and degradation. Fibroblasts within the myocardium produce collagen. Excesses in ventricular collagen are thought to be caused by both an increase in collagen synthesis by the myofibroblasts and an associated reduction in collagenase activity.[7] The balance of synthesis and degradation of myocardial fibrosis is complex. Fibrosis initially may preserve cardiac function; however, under pathologic conditions leads to cardiac functional decline and is a hallmark of pathologic cardiac remodeling.[17] It is intriguing that many of the substances known to be elevated in patients with HF are highly profibrotic and include AT II, ET, NE, aldosterone, and interleukin-6. In contrast, many substances that facilitate degradation seem to be lacking in patients with HF, including bradykinin, prostaglandins, and TNF-α.[15] Thus, myocardial fibrosis, which accounts for a large part of the structural changes seen in patients with HF, may be the ultimate consequence of the loss of regulation that exists between synthesis and degradation.

Neurotransmitters such as NE, secreted at sympathetic nerve junctions within the myocardium, attempt to help the myocardium meet the increasing demands of the body. β-Receptors located within the myocardium serve as the portal to activation. Stimulation of β_1-receptors leads to increased HR, contractility, and speed of relaxation. Myocardial injury leads to neurohormonal activation that prompts a dramatic reduction of both the number and function of β-receptors within the myocardium, resulting in impaired signal transduction and disturbances in myocellular calcium metabolism.

The metabolism of the failing myocardium likewise is altered adversely. In fact, the hyperadrenergic state of HF initiates a metabolic vicious cycle. The principal energy source in a normal myocardium is free fatty acids, but in hypertrophic states, switches to glucose utilization. Myocardial energy generation and utilization may have a profound effect on cellular energy levels. Altered myocardial carbohydrate metabolism and related insulin resistance are currently variables of interest in abnormal myocardial energetics.

Ventricular volume overload and increased diastolic wall stress lead to replication of sarcomeres, elongation of myocytes, and ventricular dilatation or eccentric hypertrophy. Maladaptive growth and changing myocyte phenotype lead to myocyte thickening (seen in diastolic dysfunction and concentric hypertrophy) and myocyte elongation (seen in systolic dysfunction and eccentric hypertrophy).[30] These large, genetically abnormal cells cannot contract as efficiently as normal cells.

Concentric and eccentric hypertrophies impair ventricular filling. Decreased cavity size, as seen in concentric hypertrophy, decreases compliance and thus impedes venous return. Eccentric hypertrophy, which increases end-diastolic volume and pressure, is also accompanied by a decrease in compliance.[17] Mechanisms responsible for diastolic dysfunction include hypertrophy, as described, which causes an increase in passive chamber stiffness (decreased compliance) and decreased active relaxation. Decreased levels of activity of SERCA (sarco/endoplasmic reticulum calcium ATPase) to remove calcium from the cytosol and increased levels of phospholamban (a SERCA inhibitory protein) lead to a net effect of impaired relaxation. This same net effect is seen in myocardial ischemia, abnormal ventricular loading (e.g., hypertrophic or dilated cardiomyopathy), asynchrony, abnormal flux of calcium ions, and hypothyroidism. Of interest, SERCA decreases with age, coincident with impaired diastolic dysfunction.[7,31] Wall stiffness and associated decreased compliance is increased with age and is caused, in part, by diffuse fibrosis. Decreased compliance is also noted in patients with focal scar or aneurysm after MI. Infiltrative cardiomyopathies (e.g., amyloidosis) can also increase wall stiffness. Pericardial constriction or tamponade causes mechanical increased resistance to filling of part or all of the heart.[30] Interactions with LV hypertrophy (LVH), ischemia, and diastolic dysfunction create a vicious cycle in which LVH predisposes to ischemia, the ischemia causes impairment of relaxation in the heart with LVH, and the severity of subendocardial ischemia worsens. Several mechanisms appear to lower subendocardial perfusion pressure. Coronary vascular remodeling occurs with increased medial thickness and perivascular fibrosis. The increased LV mass and inadequate vascular growth result in a loss of coronary vasodilator reserve so that there is a limited ability to increase myocardial perfusion in response to an increased oxygen demand. In addition, increased diastolic pressure exerts a compressive force against the subendocardium and restricts subendocardial perfusion.[30]

Altered Systemic Perfusion Results in Activation of Neurohumoral, Inflammatory, and Metabolic Processes

The major elements of this complex response may be described as activation of the sympathetic nervous system, RAAS, natriuretic peptides, inflammatory systems, and metabolic changes such as insulin resistance. While each of these homeostatic mechanisms represents a beneficial short-term response to impaired cardiac function, they also are associated with detrimental maladaptive long-term consequences (Table 37-3).[32]

The systemic response to a decrease in cardiac output accelerates HR, vasoconstricts arteries and veins, increases the ejection fraction and, by promoting salt and water retention by the kidneys, increases blood volume. Salt and water retention, vasoconstriction, and cardiac stimulation are mediated by signaling molecules that play a regulatory and counterregulatory role in HF (Table 37-4). The various mediators evoke similar and often overlapping responses. When a regulatory signal turns on a process, counterregulatory signals are released to turn off the process.[7,32]

Activation of the Sympathetic Nervous System. The most important stimulus for vasoconstriction in HF is sympathetic activation that releases catecholamines. NE is released from adrenergic (sympathetic) nerve endings within the heart. Plasma levels of NE become elevated and bind to both α-adrenergic and β-adrenergic receptors leading to multiple signaling pathways being activated.[7] NE binds to α_1-adrenergic receptors increasing vascular tone to raise SVR (afterload) and mean systemic filling pressure, thereby augmenting venous return or preload.[7,32]

In HF, stimulation of the sympathetic nervous system represents the most immediately responsive mechanism of compensation. Stimulation of the β-adrenergic receptors in the heart causes an elevation in HR and contractility to raise stroke volume and cardiac output as well as multiple metabolic changes.[7] As plasma levels of NE remain elevated, cardiac NE stores become depleted and other tissue sources are stimulated. Long-term high concentrations of NE have significant adverse effects on myocardial and cardiac myocyte function leading to remodeling.[7] Myocardial remodeling involves hypertrophy, apoptosis of myocytes,

Table 37-3 • NEUROHORMONAL RESPONSE: SHORT- AND LONG-TERM RESPONSES

Mechanism	Short-Term Adaptive	Long-Term Maladaptive
Functional	**Adaptive Response**	**Maladaptive Consequences**
Salt and water retention	↑ Preload, maintain cardiac output	Edema, anasarca, pulmonary congestion
Vasoconstriction	↑ Afterload, maintain blood pressure	↓ Cardiac output, ↑ energy expenditure, cardiac necrosis
Cardiac β-adrenergic drive	↑ Contractility, ↑ relaxation	↑ Cytosolic calcium (arrhythmias, sudden death)
	↑ Heart rate	↑ Cardiac energy demand (cardiac necrosis)
Proinflammatory	**"Anti-Other"**	**"Anti-Self"**
	Antimicrobial, antihelminthic	Cachexia (skeletal catabolism)
	Adaptive hypertrophy	Skeletal muscle myopathy
Proliferative	**Adaptive Hypertrophy**	**Maladaptive Hypertrophy**
Transcriptional activation	Cell thickening (normalize wall stress, maintain cardiac output)	Cell elongation (dilatation, remodeling, increased wall stress)
More sarcomeres	↑ Sarcomere number	Apoptosis
		↑ Cardiac energy demand (cardiac myocyte necrosis)

Adapted from Katz AM, Konstam MA. *Heart Failure: Pathophysiology, Molecular Biology, and Clinical Management.* Philadelphia, PA: Lippincott Williams & Wilkins; 2009.

regression to a cellular phenotype, and changes in the nature of the extracellular matrix.[7,15]

Attenuating the myocardial response to NE is an important counterregulatory change in patients with HF. Chronic sympathetic stimulation inhibits β-receptor synthesis and reduces the ability of the β-receptor to respond to the stimulus of NE. β-Receptor downregulation reduces the amount of receptors available to bind to NE. Mechanisms responsible for β_1-receptor downregulation help protect the failing heart from the adverse effects of sustained sympathetic stimulation.

Activation of the RAAS. The RAAS plays an important role in HF and consists of a cascade of reactions involving angiotensinogen (AGT), renin, and angiotensin-converting enzyme (ACE), which generates AT II as an active by-product, a potent vasoconstrictor (Fig. 37-7).[7,15] AT II as a biologic active product binds to specific receptors. There are four recognized AT receptor sites, but the AT1 receptors, which predominate in adult hearts, exert their regulatory effects in myocytes: vasoconstriction, increased myocardial contractility, cell growth (hypertrophy), and apoptosis (programmed cell death). The AT2 receptor, a "fetal phenotype," promotes counterregulatory effects, including vasodilatation and decrease in growth and proliferation of cells. The AT1 receptor is downregulated in patients with HF.[7,33]

Table 37-4 • REGULATORY AND COUNTERREGULATORY SIGNALING MOLECULES

I. Signaling Molecules Whose Major Role Is Regulatory

Mediators

Catecholamines (peripheral effect)
Renin–angiotensin–aldosterone system (angiotensin II)
Arginine vasopressin or ADH
Endothelin

Responses

Retention of fluid by kidneys
Vasoconstriction
Stimulation of cell growth and proliferation
Increased contractility, relaxation, heart rate

II. Signaling Molecules Whose Major Role Is Counterregulatory

Mediators

Catecholamines (peripheral effect)
Dopamine
Atrial and B-type natriuretic peptide
Nitric oxide
Bradykinin

Effects

Reduced fluid retention by the kidneys
Vasodilatation
Decreased cardiac contractility, relaxation, heart rate
Inhibition of cell growth and proliferation

Adapted from Katz AM, Konstam MA. *Heart Failure: Pathophysiology, Molecular Biology, and Clinical Management.* Philadelphia, PA: Lippincott Williams & Wilkins; 2009.

In addition to the systemic and local RAAS, recent studies have been shown to provide evidence of intracellular RAAS under certain conditions.[34] Alternative mechanisms for synthesis of AT II may be based on the cell type and/or stimulus.[34–36] Cardiac myocytes, renal mesangial and vascular smooth muscle cells when placed under hyperglycemic conditions have been shown to synthesize intracellular AT II.[34–36] The significance of intracellular cardiac RAAS on pathology in the general population is undetermined. However, diabetes is a major factor in the activation of intracellular RAAS which may influence treatment considerations in the future.[7,37]

Aldosterone release by the adrenal gland is also stimulated by AT II as part of RAAS. Aldosterone acts on the distal tubules which results in increased water and sodium reabsorption.[32] Aldosterone has also been found to contribute to myocardial fibrosis, autonomic dysfunction, and arrhythmias. In addition, studies have implicated aldosterone in endothelial dysfunction and prothrombotic effects.[38]

Arginine vasopressin also known as antidiuretic hormone (ADH) is a pituitary hormone that plays a central role in regulation of plasma osmolality and free water clearance. It is released into the circulation in response to hyperosmolarity and AT. It causes vasoconstriction via vasopressin 1 receptors.[8] Endothelin-1 (ET-1) is also a potent vasoconstrictor, which is stimulated by ADH, catecholamines, AT, and growth factors.[39] Two ET receptor sites, ET-A and ET-B, have been identified. The ET-A elicits, in addition to peripheral vasoconstriction, an increase in inotropy, fluid retention, fibrosis, and hypertrophy. The ET-B receptor is less well understood, although it can mediate vasoconstriction and also a vasodilator effect through increased levels of nitric oxide (NO) and prostaglandins. Plasma ET-1 correlates directly with PA pressures and PA resistance and plays a role in pulmonary hypertension seen in patients with HF.[15] Counterregulatory mediators that cause vasodilatation include the natriuretic

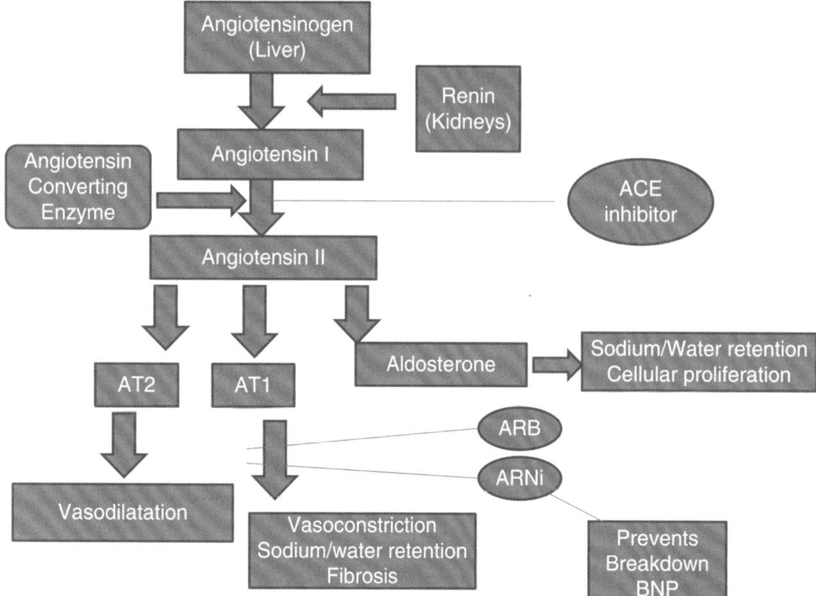

Figure 37-7. The renin–angiotensin–aldosterone system is activated in patients with heart failure. Multiple stimuli may contribute to renal release of renin into the systemic circulation, including increased sympathetic efferent activity, decreased tubular sodium delivery, reduced renal perfusion, and diuretic therapy. Natriuretic peptides (ANP, BNP), and vasopressin (ADH) may inhibit release of renin. Angiotensin I is converted to angiotensin II, which is a potent vasoconstrictor; it promotes sodium reabsorption by increasing aldosterone secretion, and by a direct effect on the tubules, stimulates water intake by acting on the thirst center. (Modified from Paganelli WC, Creager MA, Dzau VJ. Cardiac regulation of renal function. In Cheng TO, ed. *The International Textbook of Cardiology*. New York: Pergamon Press; 1986.)

peptides, NO, bradykinin, dopamine, and some of the prostaglandins, all of which act directly to relax arteriolar smooth muscle. NO, a free-radical gas initially known as endothelial-derived relaxing factor, is synthesized by the vascular endothelium. Inability of the endothelium to respond to vasodilator stimulus of NO may contribute to the exercise intolerance in patients with HF. Bradykinin and related peptides are vasodilators. Bradykinin is a substrate for ACE that is also responsible for the production of AT. In addition, bradykinin also inhibits maladaptive growth.[8,9] Adrenomedullin (AM) is a peptide with vasodilating and natriuretic properties. It also has a positive inotropic effect. Although it is expressed in various organs, the endothelium and smooth muscles are felt to be the main plasma source.[40] Plasma levels of AM are proportionally higher in patients with HF and have been identified as prognostic markers.[40] Dopamine, which is a precursor to NE, is a catecholamine that has central and peripheral effects. At low concentrations, dopamine relaxes smooth muscle; this vasodilatation lowers peripheral resistance and dilates renal blood vessels. Prostaglandin synthesis is stimulated by NE, AT, and ADH. The vasodilators are prostacyclin (PGI_2) and prostaglandin E_2. Because they are short-lived, they act locally to exert their effects, either released from one cell to work on another (paracrine effect) or binding to the same cell that released the prostaglandin (autocrine effect). In patients with HF, these counterregulatory effects are often overwhelmed by the vasoconstrictor response.[15]

Renal compensation is triggered initially by a decrease in kidney perfusion, which decreases glomerular filtration rate (GFR) and activates the RAAS, resulting in an increased SVR and increased sodium and water absorption.[32] Under normal physiologic conditions, these pathways act in concert to maintain volume status, vascular tone, and optimize cardiac output. However, chronic activation of these systems leads to worsening of the syndrome.[7] Mediators of the selective vasoconstrictor response include NE, ADH, AT, and ET.[7] AT II is later converted to AT III which directly stimulates the adrenal glands to produce aldosterone.[7] Aldosterone, a steroid hormone, increases tubular sodium reabsorption along with AT and NE. ADH acts on the collecting ducts to promote water reabsorption. In early HF, catecholamine, ADH, and ET play the major role in stimulating aldosterone secretion.[41] In patients with advanced HF, the most important stimulus for aldosterone release is AT, whose levels are increased with diuretic therapy.[42]

Natriuretic peptides are counterregulatory mediators produced in the body. This family of peptides includes ANP, BNP, and clearance natriuretic peptide (CNP). The heart itself produces ANP and BNP. ANP is stored mainly in the right atria, and an increase in atrial distending pressure, however produced, leads to the release of ANP. BNP, identified initially in the brain, is synthesized in the ventricles and is released in response to increased ventricular pressure and stretch.[43] CNP is produced in blood vessels and in the brain. CNP appears to act primarily as a clearance receptor that regulates levels of the peptides and reduces vascular resistance but has no natriuretic property. Both ANP and BNP promote vasodilatation and sodium excretion.[43] They may also attenuate sympathetic tone, RAAS activity (see Fig. 37-7), ADH, and the growth or hypertrophy of the ventricle.[8,15] All three peptides are elevated in HF.

Heart failure is most accurately depicted as a syndrome of concomitant cardiac and renal dysfunction, each accelerating the progression of the other. Renal dysfunction in patients with HF is common and is an independent risk factor for morbidity and mortality.[44] Studies have demonstrated that an increase in serum creatinine 0.3 mg/dL or more from admission resulted in a significantly higher rate of urgent hospitalization for HF or risk of death.[45] Interestingly, renal dysfunction is equally prevalent in patients with HF with either preserved or reduced ejection fractions.[44] What is not known is whether worsening renal function itself leads to increased morbidity and mortality or if it is a marker of more severe cardiac and renal diseases.

Inflammation. Heart failure is characterized by ongoing inflammation in response to tissue injury. Inflammatory mediators are central to the innate immune system.[7] Cytokines are signaling peptides whose actions include cell growth and cell death through direct toxic effects on the heart and peripheral circulation. The proinflammatory or "stress-activated" cytokines include TNF, interleukin-1 family, interleukin-6 family (e.g., IL-1α, IL-1β, ST2, IL-6, IL-10, IL-18), and chemokines. The cardiac myocytes themselves are capable of synthesizing these proinflammatory cytokines in response to various forms of cardiac injury.[7] The local inflammatory response can appear within minutes and work with specific cytokine inhibitors to regulate the human immune response.[43] More recently, a family of receptors called Toll-like receptors (TLRs) has been identified that has furthered understanding of the innate immune response.[46] The TLRs recognize patterns of host materials that are released during cellular injury and when sustained activation occurs that can lead to LV dysfunction.[47] Local inflammation from the cytokines and other mediators includes deleterious effects of LV remodeling, which include myocyte hypertrophy, alteration in fetal gene expression, contractile defects, fibrosis, and progressive myocyte loss through apoptosis.[7] There may also be promotion of LV remodeling through alterations of the extracellular matrix. Studies have shown that proinflammatory molecules are activated early in HF and continue to increase with worsening symptoms regardless of the etiology.[43,48–50] In addition, there are important signaling interactions between the RAAS, the sympathetic nervous system, and the proinflammatory cytokines that serve to stimulate and further affect cardiac remodeling.[7,51]

Activation of the systemic inflammatory response is found in advanced HF. Cardiac cachexia and skeletal muscle myopathy, which contributes to the fatigue and muscle weakness seen in HF, is a part of the systemic inflammatory response; the elevation of the proinflammatory cytokines correlates with the severity of the syndrome. The knowledge of the role of inflammation has increased significantly yet continues to be studied. Similar to the hemodynamic defense reaction, the inflammatory response may be initially beneficial, but when sustained becomes deleterious.

Metabolic Changes. Calcium transport is critical to normal contractility of the cardiac myocyte and serves in several signaling roles.[52] Alterations in calcium homeostasis contribute as well as result in morphologic changes in the myocyte, which include increased length, sarcomeric disorganization, and changes in the calcium channels.[53] These changes affect the calcium transport and cycling which leads to reduced myocardial contractility and HF.[32]

Diabetes complicates HF but is also a contributor. Insulin resistance alters myocyte metabolism and decreases the myocytes' ability to use lipids and glucose as an energy source. Increased levels of catecholamines and reduced energy stores lead to alterations in fatty acid oxidation, calcium metabolism, and mitochondrial dysfunction resulting in myocardial remodeling and decreased contractility.[54]

Neurohormonal, inflammatory, and metabolic processes interact and collectively contribute to a decline in cardiac function and remodeling. When unchecked, there is further progress of HF leading to increased mortality.

Reduced or Preserved Ejection Fraction

HF is commonly subdivided into two entities. Patients with symptoms of HF and a reduction in left ventricular ejection fraction (LVEF) less than or equal to 40% have been classified as having systolic dysfunction. Patients with symptoms and preserved LVEF are classified as having diastolic dysfunction. However, in many patients with HF abnormalities, systolic and diastolic dysfunctions coexist.[1] While these labels are somewhat useful in describing the pattern of LV dysfunction, they grossly oversimplify the underlying pathophysiology. Instead, HF might best be thought of as a continuous spectrum of closely related clinical entities. The current preferred terms are preserved or reduced LVEF.[1]

Table 37-5 describes the clinical features of HF in patients with reduced and preserved LVEFs. Interestingly, patients with either HFrEF or HFpEF are at risk for rehospitalization and similar inpatient resource utilization.[55] Survival rates of patients with clinical HF symptoms whether LVEF is reduced or preserved vary based on other cofounding variables such as age, gender, ethnicity, evidence-based treatment, and location.[4,55–57]

HF With Reduced Left Ventricular Ejection Fraction. Systolic dysfunction is determined by an impaired pump function with LVEF less than or equal to 40% and an enlarged end-diastolic chamber volume. The left ventricle is dilated, often thin-walled, and may be eccentrically hypertrophied. Dysfunction can be regional, as in MI, or global, as in dilated cardiomyopathy.[8] The principal clinical manifestations of LV systolic dysfunction result from inadequate cardiac output and fluid retention. HFrEF is thought to account for approximately 50% of patients with symptoms of HF.[58] The etiology is commonly secondary to chronic ischemic heart disease attributable to CAD; however, many other risk factors may contribute.[1]

HF With Preserved Left Ventricular Ejection Fraction. HF with preserved ejection fraction implies normal or near-normal

Table 37-5 • COMPARISON OF CLINICAL FEATURES OF HEART FAILURE WITH REDUCED AND PRESERVED EJECTION FRACTIONS

	HF With Reduced LVEF	HF With Preserved LVEF
Sex	More men than women	More women than men
Age (years)	50–60	>60
Etiology	MI or idiopathic DCM	HTN + DM, AF
Clinical progress	Persistent HF	Often episodic HF
↑ LV volumes	+++	0
LV hypertrophy	+/–	+++
Desynchronize	Common	Less common
Mitral inflow pattern	RFP or ARP	ARP
Peak mitral annular systolic velocity	Greatly reduced	Moderately reduced
Peak mitral annular early diastolic velocity	Greatly reduced	Moderately reduced
LA pressure	Elevated	Elevated
LA volume	Elevated	Normal

AF, atrial fibrillation; ARP, abnormal relaxation pattern; DCM, dilated cardiomyopathy; HTN, hypertension; DM, diabetes mellitus; LA, left atrium; RFP, restricted filling pattern; MI, myocardial infarction.
Adapted from Sanderson JE. Heart failure with a normal ejection fraction. *Heart.* 2007;93(2):155--158; Table 1.

ejection fraction in the presence of clinical HF, and is characterized by an increased resistance to filling, with one or both ventricles becoming stiff or noncompliant. The term *diastolic dysfunction* indicates a reduction in early LV relaxation or abnormality in filling, compromising the transfer of blood from the atrium into the ventricle.[7] Further research has led to an increased understanding of the pathophysiology and myocardial remodeling that occurs in HFpEF.[7,58] It is believed HFpEF develops as a result of complex interactions between several pathophysiologic mechanisms which include, yet not limited to, impaired LV relaxation, elevated filling pressures, myocardial stiffness, inflammation, reduced NO bioavailability which trigger LV hypertrophy.[58,59] HFpEF is typically characterized by delayed ventricular relaxation due to distortion of the ventricular chamber and prolongation of the ventricular ejection and elevated LV stiffness at rest and with exercise.[7,60] Ventricle walls are thick, there is an increase in left atrial (LA) size, and reduction in mitral annulus motion is observed. LA volume is often viewed as a morphologic expression of LV diastolic dysfunction. When the mitral valve is open during diastole, the LA is exposed to the loading pressures of the LV. As the LA is chronically exposed to the increased filling pressure of LV, remodeling occurs and results in increased LA size and volume.[7,61,62]

The LV has passive compliance or elastic property that characterizes wall stiffness. Left ventricular diastolic function can be impaired by four types of lusitropic abnormalities: slowed relaxation with decreased rate of pressure fall ($-\Delta P/\Delta t$) during isovolumetric relaxation, delayed filling during early diastole, incomplete relaxation with reduced filling throughout diastole, and decreased compliance or increased stiffness in late diastole. These changes cause abnormal pressure–volume relationships and produce a higher pressure for any given volume. The pressure is transmitted backward to the atria, as noted by elevated pulmonary pressures and decreased cardiac output, leading to dyspnea and fatigue during exercise.[9]

The etiology of HFpEF is most commonly secondary to long-standing systemic hypertension with a prevalence of 60% to 89%.[1,63] In addition, atrial fibrillation, CAD, diabetes, sleep disorders, obesity, pulmonary hypertension, and primary valve disorders are prevalent and can contribute to HFpEF.[1,7,61–63] Changes that occur in the cardiovascular system as a result of aging have a greater impact on diastolic function than on systolic function. Consistency of the association of female gender with HFpEF across numerous subgroups of patients implies that gender itself is an important determinant of LV adaptation, regardless of the underlying pathophysiologic process.[1,4,7] The major consequence of HFpEF relates to elevation of ventricular filling pressures, causing pulmonary and/or systemic congestion.

It has been recognized that patients with HFpEF may have had a reduced or borderline ejection fraction in the past. In the current treatment guidelines (ACCF/AHA), HFpEF categories have been further divided into HFpEF borderline or intermediate with an LVEF 41% to 49% and HFpEF improved with an LVEF greater than 40%.[1] Patients with a borderline ejection fraction are felt to be similar to patients with HFpEF. However, patients who previously had HFrEF may be clinically different from those with HFpEF.[1,64]

During the past 30 years, HFpEF has been increasingly recognized. The different pathophysiologic processes behind HFpEF are not completely understood which has led to limited treatment options and the need for further research.[7] Treatment options for HFpEF will be addressed in the following sections.

Left-Sided Heart Failure

Left-sided HF, associated with elevated pulmonary venous pressure and decreased cardiac output, appears clinically as breathlessness, weakness, fatigue, dizziness, confusion, pulmonary congestion, hypotension, and death.

Weakness or fatigue is precipitated by decreased perfusion to the muscles. Abnormalities of skeletal muscle histology and biochemistry also play a role, along with deficient endothelial function. Patients describe a feeling of heaviness in their arms and legs, and there is a reduction in exercise capacity. Cardiac cachexia is a severe complication of HF and is considered a terminal manifestation. Circulating cytokines are known to be important in tissue catabolism.

Decreased cerebral perfusion caused by low cardiac output leads to changes in mental status, such as restlessness, insomnia, nightmares, or memory loss. Anxiety, agitation, paranoia, and feelings of impending doom may develop as the syndrome progresses.

During the course of HF, pulmonary congestion progresses through three stages: stage 1, early pulmonary congestion; stage 2, interstitial edema; and stage 3, alveolar edema.[65] During the early phase, little measurable increase in interstitial lung fluid is noted. There are few clinical manifestations during this phase.

Interstitial edema usually occurs when the PAWP exceeds 18 mm Hg, leading to a net filtration of fluid into the interstitial space. Clinical manifestations of interstitial edema are varied. Engorged pulmonary vessels, elevated PA pressure, and reduced lung compliance cause increased exertional dyspnea.[42,66] If LV function is severely impaired, orthopnea or a nonproductive cough may be present. Paroxysmal nocturnal dyspnea may also occur because of postural redistribution of blood flow that increases venous return and pulmonary vascular pressure when the patient is in a recumbent position. Congestion of the bronchial mucosa that increases airway resistance and the work of breathing may also contribute to paroxysmal nocturnal dyspnea. Pulmonary crackles are first noted over the lung bases, and as the PAWP increases, they progress toward the apices.

Stage 3 occurs when the PAWP rises to 25 to 28 mm Hg, causing rapid movement of fluid out of the intravascular and interstitial spaces into the alveoli. As the edema progresses, the alveoli no longer remain open because of the large fluid accumulation. At this point, the alveolar–capillary membrane is disrupted, fluid invades the large airways, and the patient describes or exhibits frothy, pink-tinged sputum. Acute pulmonary edema is a catastrophic indicator of HF. These pulmonary congestion stages are broad categories. The correlation between a patient's Pulmonary capillary wedge pressure (PCWP) and clinical symptoms is highly variable and most likely dependent on the duration of illness and individual compensatory mechanisms.

Right-Sided Heart Failure

Right-sided HF, associated with increased systemic venous pressure, gives rise to the clinical signs of jugular venous distention, hepatomegaly, dependent peripheral edema, and ascites.[42] Dependent ascending peripheral edema is a manifestation in which edema begins in the lower legs and ascends to the thighs, genitalia, and abdominal wall. Patients may notice their shoes fitting tightly or marks left on the feet from their shoes or socks. Weight gain is what most patients recognize; consistent self-weighing in the morning helps to detect subtle changes in fluid status. An adult may retain 10 to 15 lb (4 to 7 L) of fluid before edema occurs.

Table 37-6 • CLINICAL INDICATORS AND PHYSICAL FINDINGS OF LEFT AND RIGHT VENTRICULAR FAILURE

Left Ventricular Failure	Right Ventricular Failure
Subjective Findings	
Breathlessness	Lower extremity heaviness
Cough	Abdominal distention
Fatigue and weakness	Gastric distress
Memory loss and confusion	Anorexia, nausea
Diaphoresis	
Palpitations	
Anorexia	
Insomnia	
Objective Findings	
Weight gain	Weight gain
Tachycardia	Neck vein pulsations and distention
Decreased S_1	Increased jugular venous pressure (increased central venous pressure)
S_3 and S_4 gallops	Edema
Crackles (rales)	Hepatomegaly
Pleural effusion	Positive hepatojugular reflux
Diaphoresis	Ascites
Pulsus alternans	
Increased pulmonary artery wedge pressure	
Decreased cardiac index	
Increased systemic vascular resistance	

Congestive hepatomegaly characterized by a large, tender, pulsating liver, and ascites also occurs. Liver engorgement is caused by venous engorgement, whereas ascites results from transudation of fluid from the capillaries into the abdominal cavity. Gastrointestinal symptoms such as nausea and anorexia may be a direct consequence of the increased intra-abdominal pressure.

Another finding related to fluid retention is diuresis at rest. When at rest, the body's metabolic requirements are decreased, and cardiac function improves. This decreases systemic venous pressure, allowing edema fluid to be mobilized and excreted. The recumbent position also increases renal blood flow and GFR, facilitating increased diuresis. Table 37-6 lists the various subjective and objective indicators for LV and right ventricular (RV) failure.

Clinical Assessment and Diagnosis

Patients with HF can present with a wide array of signs and symptoms. The predominant symptoms of HF are breathlessness or dyspnea and fatigue. Orthopnea and paroxysmal nocturnal dyspnea occur in the more advanced stages of HF.

History

The first step of clinical evaluation is to confirm the patient has HF. Although this may seem obvious, patients often present with symptoms that are the result of noncardiac conditions or may have been incorrectly labeled with HF. Conversely, undiagnosed patients may present without signs or symptoms. Therefore, a careful history is important to obtain and identify possible cardiac disorders that contribute to HF and as well to identify patients at increased risk for HF.[1] Cardinal symptoms of HF are dyspnea and fatigue that occur either at rest or with activity. The history should include history of present illness, past medical history, family history, a thorough review of systems, and functional assessment. A risk assessment is also recommended.[1] There are several methods of assessing risk which include biomarkers and a variety of risk models for both HFrEF and HFpEF which serve to assess risk and to guide treatment.[43,67,68] When interviewing the patient, questions regarding the occurrence of symptoms, their severity, factors that exacerbate their symptoms, and progression are critical. Do their symptoms occur at rest and/or with activity? Do they wake up at night with symptoms of shortness of breath (paroxysmal nocturnal dyspnea)? Have they noted weight gain or weight loss? In addition, if family members or significant others are present, they may contribute and provide insight into the patient's state of health. Table 37-7 lists the vital elements in a thorough history, including a history of CAD, hypertension, valvular heart disease, congenital heart defects, or diabetes. Other abnormalities include a history of thyroid, pulmonary, and/or renal disease. A three-generational family history of cardiomyopathy should be explored and include information regarding severity and prognosis.[1] Ascertain if the patient is using possible toxic agents, such as alcohol or cocaine, or has been exposed to radiation or chemotherapy. Does the patient report daytime sleepiness or carry a diagnosis of sleep disorder breathing? Obstructive and central sleep apnea is more prevalent among patients with HF and can contribute to progression through intermittent hypoxia, sympathetic nervous system activation, and endothelial dysfunction consideration of screening the patient for sleep disorders should be considered based on the patient's presentation.[69] Precipitating factors for HF should be assessed, such as—yet not limited to—anemia, infection, nutritional deficiency, or change in medications. Obtaining a description of a patient's exercise capacity and ability to perform activities of daily living is helpful in assessing their degree of limitation. Patients who describe symptoms of presyncope or syncope should be evaluated for arrhythmias, because atrial fibrillation and ventricular arrhythmias are commonly found in this patient population. In patients with decompensation of existing HF, dietary, medication nonadherence, or exacerbating medi-

Table 37-7 • EVALUATION OF THE CAUSE OF HEART FAILURE

Patient History to Include	Family History to Include
Hypertension	Predisposition to atherosclerotic disease
Diabetes	Sudden cardiac death
Dyslipidemia	Myopathy
Valvular heart disease	Conduction system disease
Coronary or peripheral vascular disease	Tachyarrhythmias
Myopathy	Cardiomyopathy (unexplained HF)
Rheumatic fever	Skeletal myopathies
Mediastinal irradiation	
Arrhythmias	
History or symptoms of sleep disorders	
Exposure to cardiotoxic agents	
Current or past heavy alcohol consumption	
Smoking	
Collagen vascular disease	
Anemia	
Thyroid disease	
Pheochromocytoma	
Obesity	

Recent life event and/or stress (Takotsubo).

Adapted from Yancy C, Jessup M, Bozkurt B, et al. 2013 ACCF/AHA guideline for the management of heart failure: A report of the American College of Cardiology Foundation/American Heart Association Task Force on practice guidelines: developed in collaboration with the Heart Rhythm Society: endorsed by the American Association of Cardiovascular and Pulmonary Rehabilitation. *Circulation.* 2013;128:e240–e327.

ations (like NSAIDs) should be investigated. A quality history can take time and requires a good trusting rapport with the patient and family.

Physical Examination

A major goal in assessing the patient with HF is to determine the type and severity of the underlying disease causing HF and the extent of the HF syndrome. Physical examination of the patient with HF focuses on the cardiovascular and pulmonary systems, as well as relevant aspects of the integumentary and gastrointestinal systems. Initial and return appointments should always include weight (gain or loss), body mass index (BMI), BP, HR, and respiratory rate. Orthostatic HR and BP are important for assessing volume status changes.[1]

Cardiovascular Assessment. Determination of the rate, rhythm, and character of the HR is important in patients with HF. The HR is usually elevated in response to a low cardiac out put. Pulsus alternans (alternating pulse) is characterized by an altering strong and weak pulse with a normal rate and interval. Pulsus alternans is associated with altered functioning of the LV causing variance in LV preload. An irregular pulse is usually indicative of an arrhythmia. Increased heart size is common in patients with HF. This cardiac enlargement is detected by precordial palpation, with the apical impulse displaced laterally to the left and downward. In patients with HF, there may be a third heart sound (S_3) that persists when sitting up and is associated with volume overload and impaired diastolic function as determined by the peak filling rate.[70] The S_3 may be one of the early signs of HF yet may be absent in advanced HF.[7,70] A fourth heart sound (S_4) may occur, although it is not in itself a sign of failure but rather a reflection of decreased ventricular compliance associated with ischemic heart disease, outflow obstruction (such as aortic stenosis), high BP, or hypertrophy. When the HR is increased, these two diastolic sounds may merge into a single sound or summation gallop. Murmurs indicate valvular disease. Patients with HF can have a murmur of mitral regurgitation, which radiates to the left axilla. In advanced HF, murmurs of both mitral and tricuspid regurgitation are frequently present. Jugular venous pulses are a means of estimating venous pressure. The A and V waves rise as the mean right atrial (RA) pressure rises. Jugular vein distention above 45 degrees signifies increased CVP and occurs with HF.[70] The abdominojugular test (formerly hepatojugular reflux) is associated with HF and should be performed if jugular vein distention is present.[1,70,71]

Pulmonary Assessment. Persistently elevated PA pressures result in the transudation of fluid from the capillaries into the interstitial spaces and, eventually, into the alveolar spaces. The accumulated fluid may result in pulmonary crackles. Initially, the late inspiratory crackles are heard at the most dependent portions of the lungs; but later, as pulmonary congestion increases, crackles become diffuse and are heard over the entire chest.[70] However, the absence of crackles does not exclude pulmonary edema.[1] Respiratory rate and pattern reflect the severity of the pulmonary compromise, with rapid breathing (tachypnea) or periodic respiratory (Cheyne–Stokes) diaphoresis, tachycardia, and coldness of extremities being noted.[7]

Integumentary Assessment. Patients with HF may or may not present with dependent edema. When present, it is most often detected in the abdomen, feet, ankles, or sacral area. Color and temperature of the skin are also assessed, with major findings being pallor, decreased temperature, cyanosis, and diaphoresis. Cardiac cachexia, with a decrease in tissue mass, may be evident in patients with long-standing HF. Cachexia is defined as a documented, unintentional, nonedematous weight loss of 5 kg or more with a BMI of less than 24 kg/m^2. Although the mechanism of cachexia is not completely understood, it is thought to be related to various cytokines with a poor prognosis.[72]

Gastrointestinal Assessment. Although patients may not report abdominal complaints, a thorough examination is important. Characteristically, HF results in hepatomegaly and congestion may lead to reports of right upper quadrant pain similar to cholecystitis. The liver span is increased and the liver is usually palpable well below the right costal margin. An enlarged spleen may also be palpated in advanced HF. Patients may accumulate abdominal fluid either as ascites or visceral edema. Associated symptoms may include indigestion, nausea, vomiting, and diarrhea.[70]

After establishing the patient's symptoms are the results of HF determination, NYHA functional class and staging are necessary. As noted earlier, NYHA functional class is a subjective measure that can change as symptoms improve or decline. The ACC/AHA staging is progressive and can only move forward. The patient's class and stage serve to help guide evidence-based therapies while recognizing each patient is unique and treatment should always be individualized while incorporating shared decision-making.

Imaging and Laboratory Studies

Transthoracic Doppler echocardiography coupled with Doppler flow studies is one of the most valuable tools and is of particular benefit for specifically assessing ventricular mass, chamber size, valvular changes, pericardial effusion, and ventricular dysfunction.[1] Cardiac chamber dilatation can provide insight into disease progression, valvular regurgitation, and mechanical dyssynchrony. Doppler estimates of pulmonary artery systolic pressure can serve as surrogates for evaluating pulmonary hypertension.[7] In addition, Doppler flow patterns can serve to estimate intracardiac pressure and diastolic staging.[7] HFrEF is defined as an EF less than or equal to 40. Left atrial enlargement with concentric LV hypertrophy and a prolonged time to peak filling are common findings in HFpEF.[7] Reduced myocardial velocities by tissue Doppler imaging (TDI) in the septum and lateral wall are consistent with delayed relaxation.[73] The echocardiogram should quantify numeric estimates of LVEF, ventricular dimension (both left and right), wall thickness, ventricular volumes, chamber geometry, atrial size, valve function, and regional wall motion.[1]

Magnetic resonance (MR) and radionuclide imaging are reliable measurements of EF and have also become important in providing clues to the presence and cause of HF.[1] MR enhancement techniques provide insight into patterns that may indicate the presence of infiltrative diseases such as amyloidosis, or sarcoidosis. Myocardial perfusion studies are also a valuable tool in assessing myocardial ischemia, myocardial infarction, and myocardial viability. The imaging assists in determining infarct size and scar burden among patients post-myocardial infarction. Both MR and radionuclide imaging lose accuracy with high HR.[1]

Cardiac catheterization/coronary arteriography is used in patients with angina or large areas of ischemic or hibernating myocardium. It is recommended for any patient who presents with suspicion of obstructive CAD.[1] A cardiac catheterization provides quantitative evaluation of diastolic dysfunction and shows an increase in PAWP or LV end-diastolic pressure.[1,7] Right heart catheterization is not routinely performed, however assists with complex forms of HF such as restrictive cardiomyopathy, evaluation for cardiac transplant or mechanical circulatory support (MCS) device and can serve to guide therapy.[1,7]

Cardiopulmonary exercise (CPX) testing can provide insight into the functional class of the patient with HF and prognosis. Metabolic exercise testing facilitates evaluation of the source of the patient's reported dyspnea. Increased ventilation (V_2) and carbon dioxide (CO_2) production is a consistent sign of HF.[74] One of the key roles of metabolic stress testing is evaluation of patients with HF for transplant. Current guidelines report relative indications for cardiac transplant are a peak VO_2 at 11 to 14 mL/kg per minute (or 55% predicted) and major limitation of the patient's daily activities, whereas an absolute indication is a peak VO_2 less than 10 mL/kg per minute.[75]

An endomyocardial biopsy is not routinely performed. It can be helpful in diagnosing myocarditis, acute cardiac rejection post-transplant, or an infiltrative process.[1] Although its role is more limited, it can be helpful in guiding treatment.

Genetic testing has evolved in recent years and is more readily available as compared to the past. It is not routinely performed yet can serve to identify at-risk individuals who require close monitoring.

A number of routine laboratory tests useful in the evaluation of HF, including a chest radiograph, should also be included to assess the size of the heart and the pulmonary vascular markings. The electrocardiogram (ECG) is not helpful in assessing the presence or degree of HF, but it demonstrates patterns of ventricular hypertrophy, arrhythmias, conduction abnormalities, and any degree of myocardial ischemia, injury, or infarction.

Laboratory tests include blood chemistries (blood urea nitrogen, serum creatinine, calcium, and electrolytes), glucose, lipid profile, liver function, magnesium level, thyroid-stimulating hormone (TSH), complete blood count, and urinalysis. In addition, BNP or *N*-terminal pro-B-type natriuretic peptide (NT-proBNP) biomarkers of HF should be measured in patients who are at risk to establish a diagnosis. BNP or NT-proBNP is recommended to be obtained prior hospital discharge and in follow-up.[76,77] Other biomarkers of cardiac fibrosis, inflammation, and cardiac injury may provide benefit and in the future may help to guide HF therapy.[77] Measurement of hemoglobin and hematocrit is useful to exclude anemia in patients with HF.[1] Anemia was found to be a common factor in patients with HF and an independent prognostic factor for mortality.[78] Electrolyte imbalances in HF reflect complications of failure as well as the use of diuretics and other drug therapy. Disturbances in sodium, potassium, and magnesium are particularly significant. In patients with severe HF, an increase in total body water dilutes body fluid and is reflected by a decrease in the serum sodium. Diuretics may also contribute to low serum sodium. Hypokalemia, or low serum potassium level, and low serum magnesium may occur as the result of the use of diuretics such as thiazides and loop diuretics, because their mechanism of action leads to excessive excretion of potassium and magnesium. Hyperkalemia, or elevated potassium level, may occur secondary to depressed effective renal blood flow and low GFR. Uric acid levels may also increase as a result of diuretic therapy.

Any impairment of kidney function may be reflected by elevated blood urea nitrogen, creatinine, and a decline in estimated glomerular filtration rate (eGFR) and have been found to be important predictors of outcome.[7,79] Elevated levels of bilirubin, aspartate aminotransferase, and lactate dehydrogenase result from hepatic congestion. Urinalysis may reveal proteinuria, red blood cells, and high specific gravity. TSH in patients with unexplained HF may also be helpful. Elevated serum glucose (diabetes) and lipid abnormalities are risk factors, and these should also be measured.[1]

In patients with decompensation of HF, arterial blood gases usually show a decrease in PaO_2 (partial pressure of oxygen in arterial blood; hypoxemia) and a low $PaCO_2$ (partial pressure of carbon dioxide in arterial blood). In the clinical situation of HF, the alveoli become filled with fluid, causing a decrease in PaO_2, whereas the compensatory attempt to increase the PaO_2 by hyperventilating causes a decrease in the $PaCO_2$, resulting in a mild respiratory alkalosis. Later changes caused by decreased peripheral perfusion result in a buildup of lactic acid, causing metabolic acidosis.

Utilization of biomarkers is currently recommended in the assessment and management of patients with HF.[77] BNP and NT-proBNP are class I recommendations for diagnosis and determining prognosis and a class II recommendation for guiding therapy.[77] Increased stretching of the LV wall as a result of pressure and/or volume stimulates the release of BNP. BNP levels are elevated in HF. When BNP is released into the bloodstream, it is cleaved into an active form (32-amino-acid peptide) BNP and a biologic inert form (76-amino-acid peptide) NT-proBNP.[43] Once bound to the receptor, BNP begins a cascade of events which include natriuresis, diuresis, vasodilatation, inhibition of RAAS, and fibrosis. There are several mechanisms by which BNP is removed and include receptor-mediated (NPR C) enzymatic processes such as neutral endopeptidase, and passively cleared by multiple organs including the kidneys.[7,43,80] BNP is good at differentiating causes of dyspnea. The normal level of BNP is less than 100 pg/mL. NT-proBNP age-stratified approach has been found to improve performance. An NT-proBNP level of less than 300 pg/mL has been found to rule out acute decompensated heart failure (ADHF) (Fig. 37-8).[7]

Other biomarkers to consider in HF include troponin level which is reflective of several mechanisms which include, yet not limited to, inflammation, supply and demand mismatch, cellular

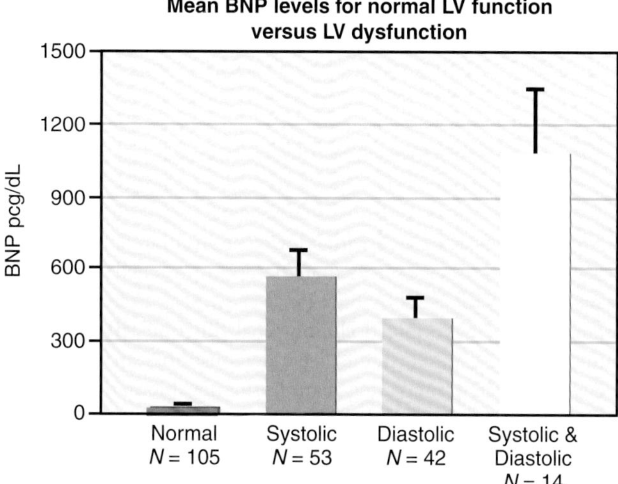

Figure 37-8. BNP values for the different subclasses of LV dysfunction. Normal BNP levels are less than 100 pg/mL. (From Maisel AS, Koon J, Krishnaswamy P, et al. Utility of B-natriuretic peptide as a rapid, point-of-care test for screening patients undergoing echocardiography to determine left ventricular dysfunction. *Am Heart J.* 2001;141[3]:367–374.)

necrosis, and apoptosis. Elevated levels have been associated with increased risk for hospitalization and death.[7] Proinflammatory cytokines are activated following insult. When cytokines are activated for prolonged periods of time as previously noted, they contribute to cardiac remodeling. ST2 was initially reported to be involved in the inflammatory response. The soluble sST2 test tests for risk prediction in both acute and chronic HF and mortality. The sST2 test is a class II recommendation within the updated ACC/AHA/HFSA guidelines.[77] Gal-3 testing is also a class II recommendation.[77] Gal-3 is involved in the initiation of the inflammatory process and is elevated in ADHF. It is predictive of adverse outcomes and is superior among patients with HFpEF as compared to HFrEF.[81] Biomarkers play an important role in diagnosis and management of HF. Continued advances with a potential combination of markers may facilitate greater personalized HF care.

Prognosis

Despite many advances in the treatment of HF in the last decade, it remains a highly lethal syndrome, with a 1-year mortality rate of 29.6% among Medicare beneficiaries and a 50% mortality rate at 5 years.[4,82] Mortality rates were reported to be uneven across states and blacks had a greater 5-year fatality rate than whites.[4,56] Patients with HFrEF frequently die from the syndrome. The mode of death is typically either secondary to progressive LV dysfunction with systemic malperfusion or via a sudden arrhythmic event. Interestingly, patients with HFpEF are more frequently (54.3%) reported to die from noncardiovascular causes.[83] Based on current data, it is estimated 6.2 million adult Americans have HF with projections suggesting the prevalence will increase (46%) by 2030.[4] The incidence of HF is reported to have declined.[83] Among patients hospitalized for HF, 53% were reported to have HFrEF and 47% with HFpEF. Black males had the highest portion of HFrEF admissions (70%) and white females with HFpEF (59%).[4]

While algorithms and computer-based tools have been developed to aid in estimating prognosis and should be utilized in examining risk,[84] it is important to remember that the likelihood of survival can only be determined in populations, not in individuals. A large, population-based study examined the association between application of the AHA/ACC HF staging system and survival. The following 5-year survival rates in patients were determined: stage 0, 99%; stage A, 97%; stage B, 96%; stage C, 75%; and stage D, 20%.[85] Historically, mortality has been linked to NYHA functional class; however, newer algorithms include laboratory measures and quantitative data regarding LV status. Clinical factors associated with a lower survival rate include older age; hyponatremia, decreased hematocrit; widened QRS; and worsening LVEF, NYHA functional class, peak exercise oxygen uptake (VO_2 max), and declining renal function (BUN, creatinine, eGFR).[86] While studies have demonstrated an association between elevated circulating neurohormones, biomarkers (BNP, NT-proBNP, sST2, Gal-3), and outcome, neurohormonal levels are not commonly used in the clinical area to predict survival. Sudden cardiac death remains an ever-present risk. It is estimated that approximately 50% of patients with systolic dysfunction will die of a sudden tachycardic or bradycardic rhythm. Predicting SCD in this population has proven difficult; thus, primary prevention measures, such as implantation of implantable cardioverter defibrillators (ICDs) is indicated in patients with a reduced LVEF less than 0.35%.[1]

Although the ability to evaluate and risk stratify has improved significantly, the ability to predict the outcome for an individual patient can be challenging. Regardless, candid ongoing discussions regarding prognosis are essential and must occur between providers, patients, and families such that expectations can be aligned and shared decision-making can occur as treatment plans are made.

Approach to Treatment

Patients with LV dysfunction often present with exercise intolerance, shortness of breath, and/or fluid retention. Incidental findings of dysfunction also may be found in asymptomatic patients. All patients presenting with HF should undergo a detailed evaluation to: (1) determine the type of cardiac dysfunction, (2) uncover correctable causative factors, (3) determine prognosis, and (4) guide treatment. Recognition of signs and symptoms resulting from an inadequate cardiac output and from systemic and pulmonary congestion is accomplished through a careful history, physical examination, routine laboratory analyses, and diagnostic studies.[1]

There are various principles that guide management of HF. The first and most important step begins with early identification of patients who are known to be at risk for developing the syndrome. The first step is identification and correction of the underlying pathogenic processes, as appropriate, such as aggressive medical management of hypertension, coronary revascularization procedures for CAD, or surgical correction of structural abnormalities.[1] The second step is the removal of the compounding or precipitating causes, such as infection, arrhythmia, and pulmonary emboli. The third step is the treatment and control of HF. Therapy for HF is directed at reducing the workload of the heart and manipulating the various factors that determine cardiac performance, such as contractility, HR, preload, and afterload. One of the greatest advances in managing HF has been the pharmacologic agents that inhibit harmful neurohormonal systems that are activated in support of the failing heart, specifically the RAAS and sympathetic nervous system. Treatment of HF is based on the manner in which the patient clinically presents, which may encompass the extremes from asymptomatic LV failure to acute cardiogenic shock.

The goal of therapy is the support of cardiac function, which may include managing comorbidities (HTN, DM), pharmacologic therapy (initiation and optimization), ICD, and/or, if extremely severe, mechanical assist devices and consideration of transplant. In the case of ischemia caused by CAD, treatment of the underlying process is the management goal. The combination of ischemia and LV dysfunction carries a poor prognosis, and it is this patient group that may benefit from revascularization by percutaneous coronary intervention (PCI) techniques or urgent cardiac surgery.

HFrEF

Coronary heart disease, hypertension, and dilated cardiomyopathy are the most commonly identified causes of LV systolic dysfunction. The writing committee of the ACC/AHA[1] based the therapy guidelines on the four stages of evolution of HF (Fig. 37-1). *Stage A* includes patients who are at high risk for HF yet do not have LV dysfunction. Treatment is aimed at risk factor modification, including management of hypertension, diabetes and lipids, cessation of smoking, and counseling to avoid alcohol and illicit drugs. Patients are encouraged to exercise on a regular basis. Obesity increases the risk of diabetes and hypertension, and steps should be taken to promote strategies to maintain optimal weight. An angiotensin-converting enzyme inhibitor (ACE-I) is indicated in patients with a history of atherosclerotic vascular disease, hypertension, or diabetes. In addition, all patients with a history of atherosclerosis statin therapy should be implemented.

Stage B includes patients who are asymptomatic but who have LV systolic dysfunction and are at significant risk for HF. All of stage A therapies are needed, with the addition of an ACE-I and β-adrenergic blockers unless contraindicated. Valve replacement or repair should be undertaken in patients with hemodynamically significant valvular stenosis or regurgitation. An ICD is considered reasonable in asymptomatic patients with LVEF less than or equal to 0.30% who are 40 days post MI.

Stage C includes patients with LV dysfunction with current or previous symptoms and who need to be treated with all measures used for stages A and B. They should be managed routinely with four types of drugs: a diuretic, a renin–angiotensin blocking agent angiotensin receptor neprilysis inhibitor [ACE-I] or angiotensin receptor blocker [ARB] or ARNi), a β-adrenergic blocker agent, and aldosterone antagonist. For those patients with an intolerance to ACE-Is, an ARB can be used. The new oral combination ARB and neprilysin inhibitor (ARNi) has been recommended for symptomatic patients to be initiated in place of or transition to from an ACE-I or ARB.[77] For those patients with renal insufficiency or angioedema, a hydralazine/nitrate combination can be substituted. The use of an aldosterone antagonist (i.e., spironolactone) for NYHA classes II to IV symptoms should be implemented unless there are contraindications. The addition of digoxin may be beneficial in patients with persistent symptoms to decrease hospitalization if there are no contraindications. In cases where the patient's HR remains above 70 bpm on an optimal dose of β-adrenergic blocker agent and in sinus rhythm ivabradine may be added.[77] Avoid the use of antiarrhythmics, NSAIDs, and most calcium channel blockers. Calcium channel blockers are not recommended for patients with HFrEF and may be harmful. Such risks may not extend to the use of longer-acting calcium channel blockers (e.g., amlodipine). ICD therapy is indicated in patients with an LVEF less than or equal to 0.35% and cardiac resynchronization therapy (CRT) for patients with a left bundle branch block.[1] Nonpharmacologic therapies include a 3-g sodium diet, encouragement of physical activity with referral for cardiac rehabilitation and exercise training, and administration of influenza and pneumococcal vaccines.

Stage D includes patients with refractory end-stage HF. As patients are found to progress, if deemed appropriate, they should be referred early to an advanced heart failure program for evaluation. They should be treated with all measures used for stages A, B, and C. An overview of the specific pharmacologic therapy for systolic dysfunction is described in Table 37-8. It is critical in this group of patients to have meticulous control of fluid retention. Patients who are at the end stage of their disease are at particular risk for hypotension and may be able to tolerate only a small dose of ACE-Is or β-blockers, or they may not be able to tolerate them at all. Despite optimal treatment, some patients do not improve. For these patients, specialized treatment strategies include MCS, continuous inotropic therapy, cardiac transplantation, palliative and/or hospice care.

Circulatory support may include LV assistance devices (LVADs) or extracorporeal devices.[1] For patients who cannot be sustained on medical therapy, LVAD has been a successful bridge to transplantation as well as destination therapy. Low-dose dopamine, dobutamine, or milrinone on an outpatient basis may benefit patients with refractory HF. However, the intermittent or chronic use of these positive inotropic agents remains an area of controversy. All of these agents have been associated with an increase in mortality as a result of markedly higher occurrences of sudden death. Cardiac transplantation plays a role in end-stage patients without contraindications to this procedure and offers excellent long-term outcomes. The goal of therapy for those patients not desiring or eligible for cardiac transplantation is symptom relief. End-of-life considerations deserve attention for this patient population as well, with the focus of hospice care extending to the relief of symptoms.

Table 37-8 • HFrEF PHARMACOLOGIC THERAPIES

Renin–Angiotensin Aldosterone System Inhibition

ACE-I, ARB, or ARNi

Titrate to target dose as tolerated[1,77]

Do not use if creatinine >3.0 mg/dL or potassium >5.0 mEq/L

Begin therapy if systolic blood pressure (SBP) >90 mm Hg without vasodilator therapy or >80 mm Hg and asymptomatic with other vasodilator therapy

Begin therapy if serum sodium >134 mg/dL

Patients who tolerate ACE-I or ARB, replacement by ARNi is recommended[77]

- When transitioning from an ACE-I 36 hours from last dose prior ARNI[77]

Do not hold vasodilator unless SBP <80 mm Hg or signs/symptoms of orthostasis, mental changes, or ↓ urine output

Contraindicated to give ACE-I, ARB, or ARNi concomitantly[77]

Alternative to ACE-I: ARB or hydralazine/nitrate combination

Add aldosterone antagonist

- NYHA classes II–IV
- Creatinine <2.5 mg/dL (men), <2.0 mg/dL (females), or eGFR >30 mL/min per 1.73 m^2
- Serum potassium <5.0 mEq/L[1]

Close laboratory follow-up for renal function and electrolytes is necessary.

IV/oral loop diuretics for volume overload

Maintenance dosing versus aggressive dosing with symptoms

Add thiazide diuretic for synergistic response as needed

Change in loop diuretic may facilitate response (e.g., bumetanide, torsemide)

β-Blocker: Titrate to target dose as tolerated

Use in NYHA classes II and III patients.* May use in NYHA class I patients with history of myocardial infarction or hypertension.†

May use in NYHA class IV patients* who are euvolemic without significant signs/symptoms of volume overload

Do not initiate therapy if history of bronchospasm, heart block, or sick sinus syndrome without permanent pacemaker, hepatic failure, overt congestion, symptomatic hypotension

Digoxin: Dose is based on weight, age, sex, creatinine clearance, and concomitant medication

Given at a low dose of 0.125 mg QD. Maintain serum digoxin level of 0.5–0.9 ng/dL

Ivabradine in NYHA class II–III patients who are in sinus rhythm and receiving evidence-based therapy and maximum tolerated dose of β-blocker with HR >70 bpm.[77]

*Carvedilol (Coreg) is the only β-blocker indicated in mild, moderate, and severe HF and essential hypertension.

†Carvedilol (Coreg) is not indicated in NYHA Class I.

HFpEF

In recent years, the increased frequency of patients with normal or near-normal ejection fraction (HFpEF) or diastolic HF has been reported, which in part may be attributed to the aging population.[4] The aging that occurs in the cardiovascular system has a greater impact on diastolic function than on systolic performance. There is a reduction in the elastic properties of the heart and vascular system that is associated with aging leading to an increase in systolic BP. HF associated with HFpEF is more frequently observed in older women, most with hypertension and LV hypertrophy. In contrast to systolic dysfunction, there were

Table 37-9 • HFpEF GENERAL TREATMENT RECOMMENDATIONS

Blood pressure control based on current recommendations
- ACE inhibitors, ARB, and β-blockers[1,77]

Diuretics to address symptoms of fluid volume overload
- A small change in volume can result in a significant change in cardiac output
- Patients may diurese rapidly leading to hypotension and prerenal azotemia

Coronary revascularization in patients with CAD who are symptomatic or have ischemia[77]
Management of atrial fibrillation based on current guidelines[1,77]
Aldosterone antagonist in select patients
- EF ≥45%, elevated BNP or hospitalization within the year,
- eGFR >30 mL/min, creatinine <2.5 mg/dL, potassium <5.0 mEq/L[77]

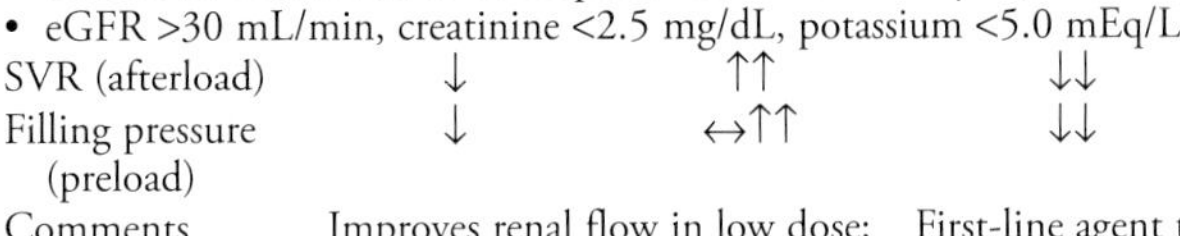

SVR (afterload)	↓	↑↑	↓↓	↑↑↑↑	↓↓↑↑	↑↑↑↑	↓↓↓
Filling pressure (preload)	↓	↔↑↑	↓↓	↔↑↑	↔	↔	↓↓
Comments	Improves renal flow in low dose; first-line drug to restore BP	First-line agent to improve CO, but may be arrhythmogenic	Pure vasoconstrictor compared to dopamine	Increases MVO_2, supports BP	Purest vasoconstrictor	Inotrope of choice in pulmonary hypertension	

few studies on therapy for diastolic dysfunction until recently.[7] The difference in pharmacologic therapy is that the goal of drug therapy in HFpEF is to reduce symptoms by lowering the elevated filling pressures without significantly reducing cardiac output (Table 37-9). The treatment of HFpEF has similarities and dissimilarities to the treatment of HF caused by systolic dysfunction.[1] The first step is the treatment of the underlying cause. Ischemia is relieved through standard medical management and revascularization for CAD. Medical management extends to the use of nitrates, β-adrenergic blockers, and calcium channel blockers. Volume reduction with diuretics is used to control pulmonary congestion and peripheral edema; diuretics should be titrated carefully. Control of systemic hypertension is critically important, with ACE-I assisting in normalizing BP and reducing LV mass in patients with hypertension-induced LVH. Other antihypertensive agents also may be needed. In select patients with HFpEF, the addition of an aldosterone antagonist may be of benefit.[77]

Tachycardia is poorly tolerated, and atrial tachyarrhythmias and even sinus tachycardia have a negative impact on diastolic function. Allowing maximum time for diastolic filling and lowering diastolic filling pressure can be accomplished by rate-slowing agents. Benefits of a slower rate include increased coronary perfusion time, decreased myocardial oxygen requirements, and increased myocardial efficiency. β-Adrenergic blockers and calcium channel blockers (amlodipine or diltiazem) have been used to prevent excessive tachycardia and also have been shown to improve some exercise parameters. Calcium channel blockers have important lusitropic effects that enhance ventricular relaxation, with verapamil usually the drug of choice, particularly in hypertrophic cardiomyopathy. β-Adrenergic blockers also improve LV relaxation by decreasing myocardial oxygen consumption and ischemia.

Atrial fibrillation with rapid ventricular response is poorly tolerated, and electrical or chemical cardioversion can be performed to restore normal sinus rhythm. β-Blockers and/or amiodarone may be required to control and prevent atrial fibrillation. Radiofrequency ablation and atrioventricular (AV) pacing may also be used. Careful assessment and identification of potential factors for triggering or exacerbating atrial fibrillation should be performed. Factors include: electrolyte imbalance, thyroid disease, or medications. Agents with positive inotropic actions are not indicated if systolic function is normal; these agents appear to provide little benefit and have the potential to worsen pathophysiologic processes, such as myocardial ischemia.

Disease Management Programs

Whether in a hospital, clinic, nursing home, or patient's home, the nurse cares for patients across the continuum in all stages and phases of the syndrome of HF. The nurse may be the first person to identify the risk factors for the presence of HF. The best means for reducing the number of patients with HF is by prevention, early identification of HF risk, and implementation of targeted interventions. The importance of early diagnosis is highlighted by evidence that treatment of asymptomatic patients can slow progression and improve clinical outcomes.[87] Screening for high BP, diabetes, dyslipidemia, metabolic syndrome, smoking, atherosclerosis, and breathing and valvular disorders may ensure aggressive treatment and may prevent the subsequent development of HF.

Once a diagnosis of HF has been established, a major goal is determining the type and severity of the underlying disease and the extent of the syndrome. HF remains the number one reason why patients over the age of 65 years require hospitalization.[88] The number of overall HF hospitalizations decreased over a 10-year period between 1998 and 2008 by 31.2% although significant geographic variation was reported.[3] Among Medicare beneficiaries, the risk-adjusted HF hospitalization rate decreased by 29.5% during that same time frame, with black men experiencing the lowest decline.[3] Although the primary symptom on presentation to the hospital for HF is dyspnea, most hospitalizations are related to comorbid conditions and are noncardiac related.[89] Precipitants and modifiable risk for readmission can include failure to manage comorbidities, medication nonadherence, dietary indiscretion, inappropriate medications, and delay in seeking care. Early identification of onset of HF symptoms can prompt therapeutic interventions instituted on an ambulatory basis and prevent rehospitalization. Coordination of care by a nurse-directed multidisciplinary team (including nurses, cardiologists, primary care providers, case managers, dieticians, pharmacists, and cardiac rehabilitation specialists) can provide HF initiatives to guide evidence-based practice, facilitate self-care at home, and coordinate clinical care across the continuum. A growing trend has been to have advanced practice nurses coordinate these programs.[90] However, intense face-to-face follow-up strategies limit the number of patients that can participate, and consideration of a combination of approaches may be optimal.[7] Several multicenter randomized trials have evaluated HF disease management programs with varying results.[7,91,92] Additional approaches to HF management may include home health, telemonitoring, and invasive monitoring.

The goal of HF disease management programs is to reduce symptom burden, improve functional capacity, reduce hospital visits, and reduce rehospitalization. Components of disease management programs include discharge planning, education and counseling, medication optimization, early attention to deterioration, and vigilant follow-up. Nurses are in the optimal position to lead and participate in the various HF disease management strategies to improve patient outcomes. However, appropriate selection and identification of patients most likely to benefit and ensuring nurses who are educated in HF management is critical to success.

Acute Decompensated HF

Acute decompensation of HF leads to more than 1 million hospitalizations annually and are frequently patients 65 years of age or older with comorbid conditions.[4,93] When patients with HF are hospitalized, most are for an exacerbation of chronic HF and are relatively equally divided between HFpEF and HFrEF.[1,94] Other etiologies can lead to hospitalization resulting in a new HF diagnosis and can include, but are not limited to, hypertensive emergencies, anemia, myocardial infarction, and valvular regurgitation. Patients with chronic HFrEF or HFpEF are likely to be using combination therapy, which may include an ACE-I, diuretic, β-blocker, and aldosterone antagonist. There is already activation of the neurohormonal compensatory mechanisms, including increased sympathetic stimulation of the heart, activation of the RAAS, increased vasoconstriction, and fluid retention by the kidneys, increased ventricular preload, LV hypertrophy, and remodeling. When a precipitating event occurs, there is further derangement of these compensatory mechanisms. Factors leading to acute decompensation in chronic HF may include the following: acute myocardial ischemia, poorly treated or untreated hypertension, new-onset atrial fibrillation, concurrent infection (e.g., pneumonia, influenza), medication nonadherence, excess dietary sodium, excessive alcohol intake and or illicit drugs, NSAIDs, and endocrine abnormalities (e.g., poorly controlled diabetes, hyperthyroidism).[1]

Acute decompensated HF is a true medical emergency that warrants an expedient diagnosis and should include identification of factors contributing to decompensation. The severity of decompensation among chronic HF patients may be underappreciated due to their ability to adapt. Comorbidities can also complicate as well as mimic decompensation. Upon arrival, clinical assessment should be undertaken to identify the fluid status and perfusion that will serve to guide therapy.[1,7] When evaluating the status, patients are typically either congested (wet) or not (dry) and have either a reduced cardiac output/peripheral perfusion (cold) or their perfusion is not reduced (warm).[1,95] During the initial assessment, prompt identification, triage, and treatment of emergent situations such as AMI, pulmonary edema, severe hypertension, and/or cardiogenic shock are necessary to prevent further deterioration.

Congestion

When patients present to the hospital with symptoms of congestion, their most frequent complaints are dyspnea, abdominal swelling, and fatigue.[96] Orthopnea and/or dyspnea with minimal exertion indicate increased pulmonary venous pressures (an exception would be severe emphysema).[7] Patients who report dyspnea and fatigue with high levels of exertion may not require hospitalization based on further evaluation. Bendopnea is a term used to describe shortness of breath or "head fullness" during activities requiring bending such as putting on shoes, and is associated with both right- and left-sided filling pressures.[71] Most patients report a combination of symptoms.

Physical assessment can be challenging because patients may or may not have rales and or edema on presentation. Jugular venous pressure is the most visible and reliable index of elevated right-sided filling pressures on physical examination.[71] Hepatomegaly also suggests elevated right-sided pressures. Abdominojugular reflex is often positive with mild elevations in venous volume.[70] When auscultating heart sounds, increased radiation across the precordium of the pulmonary second sound (P2) can reflect increased left-sided filling pressures. Careful assessment of respiratory status can further insight into diagnosis of dyspnea. Note the level of the head of the bed, respiratory rate, depth of respiration, and use of accessory muscles. Congestion usually results in an increased respiratory rate, shallow breaths, and potential use of accessory muscles. Intermittent breathing without frank apnea is common in advanced HF.[7]

Perfusion and Blood Pressure

Hypoperfusion can be missed in a patient who appears orientated with a history of low cardiac output. Careful proper assessment of the patient's BP is key. When the patient has atrial fibrillation or premature beats automated, BP readings will vary. Patients on optimal therapy for chronic HF often have systolic pressures below 100 mm Hg. On the other hand, patients may have low perfusion with higher systolic pressures. A proportional pulse pressure (systolic blood pressure minus diastolic pressure, divided by the diastolic pressure) can provide additional insight.[7]

Warm hands and feet are a good indication of adequate perfusion. However, many patients may be cool due to a number of variables such as anxiety, peripheral vascular disease, or room temperature. Alterations in level of alertness and/or nodding off during evaluation can be a sign of low perfusion. Finally, patients who have a history of hypotension or who have been intolerant of low-dose guideline directed medical therapy (GDMT) potentially have a low baseline perfusion.

Diagnosis

In addition to a thorough history and physical examination, diagnostic evaluation is critical to confirm a diagnosis of acute decompensated HF.[1] Initial laboratory testing should include complete blood count, urinalysis, electrolytes (including calcium and magnesium), renal function, glucose, liver function, TSH, and lipid profile. Cardiac enzymes (troponins I and T) should be considered in the event of suspected AMI or an ischemic event. Troponin levels may be elevated in acute decompensated HF and are prognostic yet should be interpreted in the clinical context.[77] Natriuretic peptide biomarkers (BNP or NT-proBNP) assist in the diagnosis of HF and are recommended to be obtained on presentation and prior hospital discharge.[77,97] Natriuretic peptides are elevated in patients with an HF. In patients with a history of chronic HF, comparing a BNP level obtained when the patient was hemodynamically stable may be helpful when interpreting the results. Other biomarkers of inflammation and myocardial fibrosis such as ST2 and Gal-3 have additive prognostic value.[1]

Patients presenting with acute decompensated HF should undergo a chest x-ray to evaluate congestion, heart size, and other potential sources of dyspnea. A 12-lead ECG provides information regarding rhythm, HR, as well as evidence of ST wave changes suggestive of ischemia or AMI. Transthoracic echocardiography with Doppler flow is an excellent noninvasive tool to obtain information regarding the overall and regional systolic and diastolic function, intravascular volume, valve, and myocardial abnormalities. Echocardiography can rapidly assess for mechanical causes, such as severe mitral regurgitation and papillary muscle rupture, acute ventricular septal defect (VSD), free-wall rupture, and tamponade. The study should report abnormalities, the estimates of the LVEF, ventricular dimensions, wall thickness, ventricular volumes, chamber geometry, and regional wall motion. Echocardiography is easily accessible and therefore is recommended; however, other approaches may be used.

Profile-Guided Therapy

Most patients who present for evaluation with acute decompensated HF can begin treatment based on their clinical profile. For patients who present, warm and dry HF may not be the diagnosis to explain their symptoms. Alternative diagnoses may include, but are not limited to, pneumonia, COPD exacerbation, anemia, and/or hepatic disease.

Warm and Wet

The most common profile of patients presenting to community hospitals (approximately 90%) is warm and wet. The initial goal is to relieve the congestion and reduce the filling pressure below 18 mm Hg. Intravenous loop diuretic therapy is the treatment of choice. Patients on oral diuretic therapy, initial intravenous dose, should equal or exceed their oral daily dose.[1] Intravenous diuretic dosing may be bolus or continuous infusion.[226] In the DOSE trial, the continuous infusion of diuretics was not superior to bolus diuretic therapy.[98,99] If the congestive symptoms fail to improve, increasing the diuretic dose or adding a thiazide diuretic to the treatment plan may be necessary. If initial congestion is not relieved and the patient is tachypnea positive-pressure (BiPAP), ventilation may help to address symptoms and avert urgent intubation.[7] ACE-I and/or β-blocker therapy may be adjusted for those patients who are hypertensive or normotensive with decompensated HF. If the patient's renal function declines, consider temporary reduction in ACE-I, ARB, ARNi, and/or aldosterone antagonist until their renal function improves.[1] Patients on digoxin, should have drug levels measured. Digoxin levels may be abnormally increased during acute decompensation and adjustments of the daily dose may be necessary.

Elevated filling pressures can result from increased intravascular volume, vasoconstriction, severe diastolic dysfunction, or a combination of these.[7] For patients where vasoconstriction is predominant, such as severe hypertension, intravenous vasodilators are recommended. Vasodilators are commonly added to the treatment regimen to facilitate diuresis in patients with pulmonary edema and hypertension such as nitroglycerin (NTG), sodium nitroprusside (SNP), or nesiritide.[100] NTG is commonly used for HF when ischemia is suspected. Regardless of the route of administration, NTG is an effective arterial vasodilator. SNP was the first vasodilator to improve cardiac output in HF and is effective in severe hypertensive crisis.[7] When administering SNP, careful monitoring of the BP is warranted either by automated cuff or invasive monitoring using a pulmonary artery catheter.[7] Nesiritide is a recombinant form of BNP and acts as a systemic vasodilator. Nesiritide is frequently used for pulmonary vasodilatation.[7] The ASCEND-HF trial as previously noted reported no difference in self-reported dyspnea, mortality at 30 days, and renal impairment when compared to placebo.[101] Given the results of ASCEND-HF trial, nesiritide should be considered in select patients with an adequate BP and fluid volume overloaded who are at risk for NTG intolerance and/or SNP toxicity.[101]

Wet and Cold

With prompt diagnosis and treatment, many patients who present to the hospital wet and cold can be stabilized. With low filling pressures, it is not possible to establish effective diuresis. Patients essentially need to warm up and then can dry out. The treatment for hypoperfusion depends on the SVR. If the SVR is high, vasodilators can increase cardiac output and decrease filling pressures. However, this is less common today among patients who have been maintained on GDMT and may represent progression of their disease.[7] Both direct vasodilators and inotropic therapy will increase cardiac output. However, inotropic therapy can increase myocardial demand. For patients who have hypoperfusion without severe vasoconstriction, increased contractility is warranted. A careful review of the patient's current medications and a reduction of their β-blocker therapy should be undertaken. If this has been done, addition of low-dose inotropic therapy is reasonable. Inotropic dosing should be as low as possible to limit the negative effects. Once stabilization and volume reduction has occurred, weaning of the inotropic agent should begin.[7]

Dry and Cold

In the setting of low filling pressures, oral fluid replacement may be considered. Oral fluid replacement, while holding the patient's diuretic, is often better tolerated than intravenous fluids which can lead to congestion. Evaluation of the patient's current medications should be undertaken with adjustments to their diuretic therapy and separation of dosing times of their BP-lowering medications. Further vasodilatation may increase resting cardiac output yet may result in symptomatic orthostatic hypotension.[7] Intravenous inotropic therapy may provide temporary relief.[7] Overall, treatment goals will depend on the clinical situation.

Cardiogenic Shock

Shock is a complex clinical syndrome characterized by impaired cellular metabolism caused by decreased tissue perfusion. Cardiogenic shock is defined by persistent hypotension and tissue perfusion in the presence of adequate intravascular volume and LV filling pressures.[32,102] The inadequacy of tissue perfusion results in cellular hypoxia, the accumulation of cellular metabolic wastes, cellular destruction, and ultimately, organ and system failure. The syndrome begins as an adaptive response to some insult or injury and progresses to multiple organ system failure.

Atherosclerotic heart disease and the complications of ischemia and myocardial infarction (AMI) are the most common causes of cardiogenic shock.[103,104] AMI complicated by cardiogenic shock occurs in about 5% to 15% of the cases, reflecting approximately 40,000 to 50,000 patients in the United States.[105] However, the overall incidence of cardiogenic shock has trended down in recent years and the survival rate has significantly improved with PCI.[106] Acute coronary occlusion first impairs diastolic function, with later diminished systolic function, stroke volume, and BP. This downward spiral leads to progressive myocardial dysfunction and possibly death.[107] Some patients may present in cardiogenic shock on admission, but shock often evolves over several hours. Shock with a delayed onset may result from infarct expansion, reocclusion of a previously patent infarct artery, or decompensation of myocardial function in the infarction zone caused by metabolic abnormalities. Ischemia-related systolic dysfunction also could contribute to the development of cardiogenic shock. One pattern is the "hibernating" myocardium, seen with low tissue perfusion states matched by a decline in compensatory function. The second pattern is the "stunned" myocardium, which is a more prolonged (hours to days) myocardial dysfunction after a relatively brief interruption of myocardial perfusion. These patterns have been reported after PCIs and unstable angina.[108]

Complications of MI include mitral regurgitation, VSD, and free-wall rupture. Significant mitral regurgitation patterns are seen clinically: papillary muscle (usually the posterior papillary muscle) or chordal rupture caused by MI, and mitral regurgitation associated with LV dilatation. Acute VSD abruptly increases pulmonary blood flow and leads to symptoms of biventricular failure within hours to days if not corrected. LV free-wall rupture occurs in less than 0.5% of AMIs but carries a high mortality rate.[109] RV infarction occurs after occlusion of the proximal right coronary artery and is identified in the setting of concomitant inferoposterior LV dysfunction.

Non–MI-related acute valvular problems involve the mitral and aortic valve. Acute mitral regurgitation can be caused by spontaneous chordal rupture, infective endocarditis, inflammatory disorders (e.g., rheumatic fever), or trauma. Acute aortic insufficiency may be caused by infective endocarditis with leaflet destruction (most common), acute aortic dissection, or traumatic injury. Shock may be caused by aortic stenosis with increasing metabolic demands or with concomitant LV failure. Mitral stenosis rarely causes shock without rapid atrial fibrillation.[110] Prosthetic valve dysfunction, especially left-sided, most often causes shock because of valvular insufficiency. Acute prosthetic valvular insufficiency occurs because of dehiscence of the sewing ring, infective endocarditis, or catastrophic mechanical failure.

Amyloidosis, sarcoidosis, and hemochromatosis are examples of infiltrative diseases in their later stages that may be associated with shock. Shock caused by trauma is usually seen secondary to myocardial or aortic rupture, or caused by acute volume loss secondary to hemorrhage.

Compensatory Mechanisms

The following equations illustrate the physiologic relation of the hemodynamic variables. Here CO, cardiac output; SV, stroke volume; HR, heart rate; MAP, mean arterial pressure; and SVR, systemic vascular resistance compose the equations:

$$\text{CO} = \text{SV} \times \text{HR}$$
$$\text{MAP} = \text{CO} \times \text{SVR}$$

In the pathophysiologic state of cardiogenic shock, the decrease in MAP is brought about by an alteration in one of the variables. The reduction in cardiac output results from a decrease in stroke volume:

$$\downarrow \text{CO} = \downarrow \text{SV} \times \text{HR}$$

The deduction in MAP results from the decrease in cardiac output:

$$\downarrow \text{MAP} = \downarrow \text{CO} \times \text{SVR}$$

Compensatory mechanisms consist of reflex reactions to an initial fall in BP. They are activated immediately and increase in intensity in an attempt to restore adequate tissue perfusion.[107] The compensatory mechanisms are directed at the restoration and maintenance of adequate blood volume, cardiac output, and vascular tone. The initial compensatory mechanisms vary with the primary pathophysiologic derangement, but the intermediate and final stages are similar. The initial compensatory mechanisms in cardiogenic shock are an increased HR and increased SVR.

Initial Stage

In cardiogenic shock, the decreased coronary blood flow results in profound local compensatory events. There is an increase in myocardial oxygen extraction and dilatation of the coronary arteries. The myocardial cells shift to anaerobic metabolism and use glycolysis in the production of adenosine triphosphate (ATP).[111] These events occur immediately in response to myocardial ischemia. If compensatory mechanisms are inadequate, myocardial contractility decreases, leading to a decrease in cardiac output and systemic hypoperfusion.

A reduction in arterial BP secondary to decreased blood volume, decreased cardiac output, or increased venous capacitance initiates the body's compensatory mechanisms to maintain adequate tissue perfusion. These mechanisms serve to increase cardiac output and arterial BP through increasing HR, enhancing myocardial contractility, providing selective vasoconstriction, conserving sodium and water, and shifting fluid from the interstitial to the intravascular space.

Specialized nerve endings (mechanoreceptors) in the carotid sinus, aortic arch, heart, and lungs sense the decrease in BP and transmit their impulses to the vasomotor center. The vasomotor center stimulates the sympathetic nervous system, inhibits the parasympathetic nervous system, and initiates the secretion of catecholamines from the adrenal gland. Sympathetic nervous system stimulation unopposed by parasympathetic effects results in increased HR, increased myocardial contractility, and selective vasoconstriction. Reflexes of the sympathetic nervous system are active within 30 seconds of an acute decrease in circulating blood volume and are able to compensate for a 20% loss in blood volume by increasing cardiac output by 20% to 25%.[102] In response to ischemia and sympathetic stimulation, hormones are released from the adrenal medulla, adrenal cortex, anterior and posterior pituitary gland, and kidneys, which further compensate for decreased circulating blood volume. The adrenal medulla releases epinephrine and NE, which enhance vasoconstriction and myocardial contractility, and increase HR. Epinephrine and NE also stimulate glycogenolysis, thus increasing serum glucose. The adrenal cortex releases glucocorticoids, which also increase serum glucose. Decreased renal blood flow results in the release of renin, which initiates a series of reactions in the liver and elsewhere, resulting in the production of AT. AT promotes the release of aldosterone by the adrenal cortex and, in situations of hypovolemia, promotes profound vasoconstriction. Aldosterone enhances renal sodium reabsorption accompanied by increased water reabsorption. ADH is released from the posterior pituitary and further enhances renal water reabsorption. As a result of decreased capillary pressure, Starling capillary forces are altered, and fluid is transferred from the interstitial space to the capillary.

Intermediate Stage

If shock is not recognized and reversed in the initial compensatory stage, it progresses (Fig. 37-9). Compensatory mechanisms are no

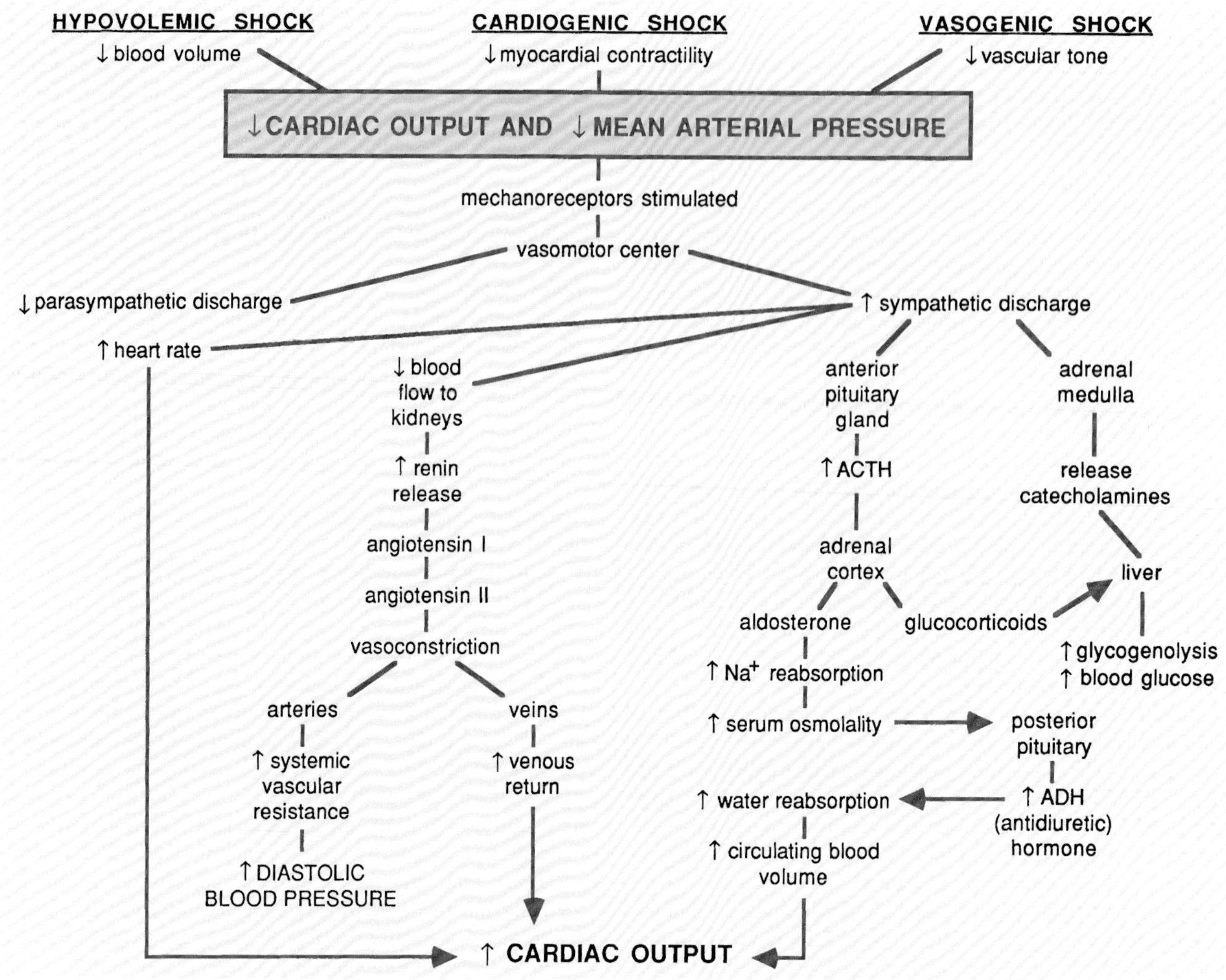

Figure 37-9. Mechanisms to augment cardiac output. (Adapted from Pina IL, Apstein CS, Balady GJ, et al. Exercise and heart failure: a statement from the American Heart Association Committee on exercise, rehabilitation, and prevention. *Circulation.* 2003;107[8]:1210–1225.)

longer able to maintain homeostasis and may become counterproductive. For example, continued profound vasoconstriction in the presence of decreased MAP promotes inadequate tissue perfusion and cellular hypoxia.

Decreased delivery of oxygen and nutrients causes cells to shift to anaerobic metabolic pathways.[107] Increasing amounts of lactic acid are produced and accumulate in the cells because of decreased perfusion. Because anaerobic metabolism is less efficient in meeting the energy requirements of the cells, ATP is depleted. Reduction in the available ATP results in failure of the membrane transport mechanisms, intracellular edema, and rupture of the cell membrane. Progressive tissue ischemia results in increased anaerobic metabolism and the further production of metabolic acidosis.[107]

Impairment of cellular function disrupts all body organs and organ systems. Splanchnic ischemia results in the release of endotoxin from the intestine. The reticuloendothelial (tissue macrophage) system is suppressed by splenic and hepatic ischemia. The continued renal response to ischemia leads to further vasoconstriction, stimulating the release of aldosterone from the adrenal gland and promoting the reabsorption of sodium in the kidney. This response is no longer useful because the increased volume cannot be pumped by the failing heart and results in ventilatory failure. The increased volume begins to pool in tissues secondary to profound venoconstriction and increased capillary permeability.

If the myocardial ischemia is severe and prolonged enough, myocardial cellular injury becomes irreversible.[107] Cytokines are signaling peptides whose actions include cell growth and cell death through direct toxic effects on the heart and peripheral circulation. The proinflammatory or "stress-activated" cytokines include TNF-α and some interleukins (i.e., IL-1β, IL-6, IL-8, IL-12). The cardiac myocytes are capable of synthesizing these proinflammatory cytokines in response to various forms of cardiac injury. The local inflammatory response can appear within minutes of an abnormal stress. Local inflammation of the cytokines and other mediators includes deleterious effects of LV remodeling, which include myocyte hypertrophy, alteration in fetal gene expression, contractile defects, and progressive myocyte loss through apoptosis.[107]

Irreversible Stage

In this stage, the compensatory mechanisms are no longer effective, and hypotension has reached the critical level of adversely affecting the heart and brain. Myocardial hypoperfusion, resulting from hypotension and tachycardia, produces acidosis, which leads to further depression of myocardial function. Decreased cerebral blood flow leads to depressed neuronal function and activity and loss of the central neuronal compensatory mechanisms.[9,32]

The progressive general hypoxia and reduction in cardiac output further deprive body cells of oxygen and nutrients needed for cell growth and result in microcirculatory insufficiency. The microcirculation responds by vasodilatation to secure the necessary nutrients and oxygen for the deprived cells. Microcirculatory vasodilatation, along with systemic vasoconstriction, results in the sequestration of blood in the capillary beds, which further reduces the volume of blood returning to the systemic circulation. With the loss of circulating blood volume and impaired capillary flow, venous return is reduced leading to further decline in cardiac output and arterial pressure.[32]

Diagnosis and Clinical Manifestations

Most patients who present with cardiogenic shock have either a history of cardiovascular disease or risk factors for cardiovascular disease. The diagnosis of shock is made by the history, physical examination, and collection of data from adjunctive diagnostic tests.

Monitoring and Diagnostic Tools

The primary measurements that document the relative adequacy of blood flow include continuous monitoring of arterial BP and monitoring of the ECG with rhythm analysis. The ECG can be diagnostic in the setting of MI. Most patients in shock are tachycardic and may show evidence of supraventricular or ventricular arrhythmias. Low QRS voltage and/or electrical alternans can be seen in cardiac tamponade.[111]

In addition to standard laboratory testing recommended on presentation with decompensated HF, serial cardiac enzymes should be obtained. Serial measurements of arterial blood gases reflect the overall metabolic state of the patient, the adequacy of ventilation, and the adequacy of the circulation in providing for oxygen and metabolic needs. Measurement of mixed venous oxygen content ($S\bar{v}O_2$) by direct blood sampling or by continuous invasive monitoring reflects peripheral oxygen extraction and use. Serial arterial lactate levels can also be measured because the presence of lactic acidosis helps identify critical hypoperfusion.[32]

In seriously ill patients, direct determination of intra-arterial pressure with an arterial line is necessary because systemic arterial pressure determines the perfusion pressure of various organ systems and is predominantly the product of cardiac output and SVR. In HF, a drop in cardiac output is compensated for by an increased SVR in an attempt to maintain the arterial BP in normal range.

Right-sided heart catheterization with a PA quadruple lumen thermodilution catheter can aid in the diagnosis and assessment of the severity of HF. This invasive hemodynamic monitoring can be useful in excluding volume depletion, RV infarction, and mechanical problems (e.g., acute mitral regurgitation). It is also useful for monitoring the response to treatment (including volume, diuretics, inotropic support, vasoactive agents, natriuretic peptide) and manipulation of the variables of cardiac output, preload, and afterload.[107] The hemodynamic variables measured by this catheter are cardiac output by thermodilution; RA pressure; and PA systolic, diastolic, and wedge pressures. The cardiac output is decreased in HF, whereas the RA pressure or central venous pressure is elevated. The PAWP indirectly measures the LV end-diastolic pressure, which is a measure of end-diastolic volume or preload and is elevated in HF.

Derived parameters that may be obtained by the use of the PA catheter include CI and SVR. Body surface area (BSA), measured in square meters, is correlated with the volume of cardiac output (CO) to establish the CI:

$$\text{CI} = \frac{\text{CO}}{\text{BSA}}$$

SVR, measured in dynes per cm^5, reflects the pressure difference of the systemic arteries to the veins.

$$\text{SVR} = \frac{\text{MAP} - \text{RAP}}{\text{CO}} \times 80$$

Besides offering diagnostic information, hemodynamic variables show a strong prognostic value for short-term survival. They showed that clinical signs of hypoperfusion occur with a CI of less than 2.2 L/min per m^2 and clinical signs of pulmonary congestion occur with a PAWP greater than 18 mm Hg. PA catheters are useful in settings MI and cardiogenic shock.[1]

Prognosis

The stages of shock depict a series of pathophysiologic changes that occur if medical and nursing interventions are delayed or inappropriate. The stages do not progress at the same speed in all patients. The length of time tissues are hypoxic is a major factor in determining the occurrence of complications. The initial and intermediate stages of shock are reversible with aggressive management. The irreversible stage is caused by cellular necrosis and multiple organ failure, reducing the chances of recovery.

Approach to Treatment

The main goal of treatment of the metabolic defects produced by shock is the restoration of adequate tissue perfusion.[103]

Initial general management for patients is placement of large-bore venous catheters, and continuous monitoring of BP, pulse oximetry, and ECG. If respiratory failure is imminent with patients with severe hypoxemia, hypercarbia, or metabolic acidosis, then endotracheal intubation may be required with mechanical ventilation. A PA catheter may be placed. Volume expansion may be needed to restore adequate circulation to maintain a PAWP of 14 to 16 mm Hg. Vasopressor support should be used only after preload is adequate to restore the BP. The choice of a particular vasopressor/inotropic agent depends on the clinical circumstance.

Cardiogenic shock can occur in a new onset or in patients with established chronic HF. As previously stated, it is critical to establish the diagnosis, precipitating event, and determine the hemodynamic status: pulmonary congestion without peripheral hypoperfusion versus shock/hypoperfusion. The three major goals of treatment of acute decompensated HF and/or cardiogenic shock are (1) to increase the oxygen supply to the myocardium; (2) to maximize the cardiac output; and (3) to decrease the cardiac workload.

Goal 1: Increase Oxygen Supply to the Myocardium

Increased inspired oxygen concentrations, including the institution of mechanical ventilation with positive end-expiratory pressure, may be required to maintain arterial blood gases within normal limits. Narcotic analgesics are used to control the patient's pain and aid in reducing myocardial oxygen demands.

Aggressive reperfusion of the coronary arteries is recommended to be undertaken by invasive and noninvasive approaches, including percutaneous transluminal coronary angioplasty, atherectomy or stent placement, use of adjunctive antiplatelet therapy, thrombolytic therapy, and coronary artery bypass grafting, which were all associated with lower in-hospital mortality rates than treatment with standard medical therapy.[112,113] Studies suggest that immediate revascularization with PCI, which may include angioplasty, stent placement, and atherectomy, along with adjunctive antiplatelet therapy, improves outcomes in patients with cardiogenic shock.[114,115] Improvement is seen in wall motion in the infarct territory, with increased perfusion of the infarct zone augmenting contraction of remote myocardium, possibly because of recruitment of collateral blood flow. Reperfusion therapy with thrombolytic agents has decreased the occurrence of cardiogenic shock in patients with persistent ST-segment elevation MI.[112] Antithrombotic therapy including antiplatelets and anticoagulation for patients undergoing PCI is well established; however, there is limited evidence in cardiogenic shock. With the lack of specific randomized trials in cardiogenic shock, current recommendations apply for the management of acute coronary syndrome.[103] It is important to recognize the benefits of revascularization even when the risk is high such as post resuscitation. For hospitals without revascularization capability, early thrombolytic therapy along with immediate transfer for PCI or coronary artery bypass grafting may be appropriate.[112]

Goal 2: Maximize Cardiac Output

Because the cardiac output is already compromised, arrhythmias, which occur as a result of ischemia, acid–base alterations, or MI, can cause a further decline in cardiac output. Electrolyte abnormalities should be corrected, because hypokalemia and hypomagnesemia predispose to ventricular arrhythmias. Antiarrhythmic agents, pacing, or cardioversion may be used to maintain a stable heart rhythm. Volume loading is undertaken with caution and in the presence of adequate hemodynamic monitoring. Optimal preload (LV end-diastolic pressure or PAWP) ranges between 14 and 18 mm Hg. However, fluid loading must be abandoned when the increase in filling pressure occurs without increase in cardiac output. Urinary production should be monitored closely for acute renal failure. In this patient population it is essential to maximize nutritional needs as well as glycemic control to avoid hypoglycemia. Patients should also be given venous thromboembolism prophylaxis and stress ulcer prophylaxis.[1]

For patients in cardiogenic shock, simultaneous improvement of both CI and PAWP is important to prevent or reverse multiorgan system dysfunction.[103] These patients are hypoperfused and have pulmonary congestion (cold and wet). For patients with a low BP, NE should be the first choice as a vasopressor.[103] Dopamine is another treatment in patients with systolic pressures less than 80 mm Hg. Tachycardia and increased peripheral resistance are dose dependent with dopamine and can exacerbate myocardial ischemia.[1] Inotropic agents are used to increase systemic and coronary artery perfusion pressure. Dobutamine can be used simultaneously with NE to improve myocardial contractility and increase cardiac output.[103] Dobutamine can precipitate tachyarrhythmias and exacerbate hypotension. Other agents used for positive inotropic effect include phosphodiesterase inhibitors, such as milrinone. Again, current evidence for inotropes and vasodilators in cardiogenic shock is limited and is an area for future study.[116]

Goal 3: Reduce Myocardial Work

The efficacy of vasodilators has been shown in the treatment of cardiogenic shock. The major physiologic effect of vasodilators is a reduction in LV end-diastolic pressure and SVR, with a subsequent increase in stroke volume and improved LV function. Intravenous nitroprusside remains the drug of choice in cardiogenic shock, because it acts rapidly and has a balanced effect, dilating both veins and arterioles, thereby reducing both preload and afterload. NTG can also be used, but it is predominantly a venous vasodilator, and large doses are sometimes required to reduce SVR (afterload). Intravenous NTG may be preferred in patients with acute MI because of its favorable effect on coronary blood flow.[1]

Other Considerations

Right Ventricular Infarction. Interventions include correction of hypovolemia with fluid administration and maintaining RV preload to a mean RA pressure of 15 mm Hg. Inotropic therapy with dobutamine can be used to support cardiac output. AV synchrony is also important, and AV sequential pacing can improve BP and cardiac output. Reperfusion of the occluded coronary artery is also crucial.[117]

Acute Mitral Regurgitation. Management includes afterload reduction, usually with nitroprusside, and IABP as temporizing measures. Inotropic or vasopressor support may also be needed to support BP and cardiac output. Surgical valve repair or replacement is the definitive treatment.[117]

Ventricular Septal Wall Rupture. IABP and supportive pharmacologic agents are necessary. Operative repair is the only option. The timing of the repair remains controversial, although most feel repair should be undertaken within 48 hours of the rupture.[107]

Cardiac Free-Wall Rupture. This condition usually occurs during the first week after MI. This is a catastrophic event. Possible salvage is possible with rapid recognition, pericardiocentesis to relieve acute tamponade, and thoracotomy with repair.[107]

Valvular Heart Disease. Emergency surgery is indicated for aortic dissection that results in acute aortic regurgitation. In cases of severe mitral stenosis, decreasing the HR to improve diastolic filling time improves cardiac output. Mitral valvuloplasty or surgical intervention is indicated.

Extracardiac Obstructive Shock. Pulmonary embolism is best treated with thrombolytic therapy.[118] Cardiac tamponade is treated by pericardiocentesis or pericardial window drain and may require urgent treatment based on the patient's clinical presentation.[119]

Transition of Care

Throughout the hospital course, discharge planning using shared decision-making should be undertaken. Ongoing assessment of symptoms, quality of life, and patient preferences regarding treatment options and end of life should be undertaken. Individual assessment of need for palliative care and incorporation early in hospital management is helpful.[1] Stabilization of symptoms and cardiac function of patients with HF are key goals for hospital discharge. This is done through achieving an optimal fluid state, BP, rhythm and HR control, while managing comorbidities. Patients should be transitioned off intravenous medications and placed on oral medications and monitored to ensure stability. Ambulation on the hospital unit will allow for assessment of symptoms. Assessment of BNP or NT-proBNP is recommended and will provide insight into postdischarge prognosis.[77] Failure to ensure stability prior hospital discharge can contribute to rehospitalization and increased mortality.[7,120] Patients who are unable to achieve stability and treatment options are limited transitioning to palliation and/or hospice may be appropriate.

Reassessment of home medications and precipitating factors leading to the hospitalization should be reviewed, barriers to care addressed, and management discussed. Although there is limited evidence on how to determine a home diuretic dose, patient history, current treatment, and response to diuretics can provide insight. All patients should be placed on GDMT prior discharge unless contraindicated with appropriate laboratory follow-up. Individualized reinforcement of patient and family education is necessary and should occur throughout the hospitalization. HF educational topics were previously discussed, yet should include self-care, plans when symptoms occur, need for adherence, resources, and follow-up.[1]

A successful transition is critical to help to prevent rehospitalization. Patients currently are transitioning not only home but to skilled nursing facilities (SIFs), rehabilitation centers, and hospice. Patients who are transitioning home may be prescribed various supportive services such as, but not limited to, home health, telemonitoring, and/or case management. Nurses are the providers and lead in coordinating and directing many of the transitional care activities.[121] Recognition of factors that impact transition should be considered with inclusion of interdisciplinary team members and resources as needed. Key factors that may influence transition include but are not limited to, heath care provider communication (quality handoffs, complete documentation, and timely access by all providers to necessary information), medication management (coordination and reconciliation of medications, multiple providers, medication cost/access, patient understanding) recognition and management of signs and symptoms (adherence, self-care, recognition of symptoms and awareness of appropriate actions), and 7-day follow-up (access, awareness, transportation).[121] The transitional period is a vulnerable time for patients and caregivers. Ensuring understanding of all instructions and printed information, treatment plan and resources are important. Early outpatient follow-up with phone contact (3 days) and a scheduled appointment (7 days) is recommended.[1]

Summary

Heart failure is chronic condition and requires ongoing diligence in management. Patients, caregivers, health care members, and community medical facilities all share in the responsibility to ensure optimal outcomes while promoting quality of life. It is vital for nursing to participate in understanding the medical aspects as well as psychosocial aspects of this condition.

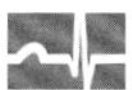

CASE STUDY 1

Patient Profile

Name/Age/Sex: **Mike Jones, 41-year-old black male**

History of Present Illness

Mr. Jones presents to the outpatient clinic today for follow-up. He reports significant fatigue. He denies changes in his level of dyspnea and reports sleeping on his usual 1–2 pillows at night. He indicates he has limited his activity more due to his general fatigue. He denies any changes in his weight and reports adherence to treatment recommendations. He states he has been monitoring his HR and BP over the preceding 2 weeks with his SBP remaining low 90s and HR is consistently in the upper 80s or higher.

Past Medical History

Nonischemic cardiomyopathy
Hypertension
Chronic Kidney Disease (CKD) stage II
Sleep disorder breathing (OSA)
Implantable cardioverter defibrillator (ICD)

Family History

Mother alive, reports HTN and DM
Father alive, reports HTN
Two siblings alive and well; brother reports HTN, sister reports hypothyroidism
Grandparents are deceased, maternal parents report DM, HTN, and CVD; paternal parents' health is unknown

Social History

Works cleaning offices at night for a local cleaning company and details cars during his off time. He denies a prior or current history of smoking, alcohol or illicit drug use. He is engaged and lives with his fiancée and their two children. He walks for exercise when his work schedule allows and attempts to limit sodium in his diet, although he finds it challenging.

Medications/Allergies

No known drug allergies
Lisinopril 5 mg daily
Metoprolol succinate 50 mg daily
Furosemide 20 mg daily as needed
Spironolactone 12.5 mg every other day

Physical Examination

Wt. 198 lb; Ht. 5 ft 10 in; BMI 28.4; HR 90; BP 90/62; orthostatic pressure 92/60; RR 20; oxygen saturation 95%; afebrile
Constitutional: Alert, orientated, well-developed obese gentleman, no acute distress
Neck: No jugular vein distention, no carotid bruit present
Cardiovascular: HR is tachy, rhythm is regular; normal S1, S2, no extra systoles present, no murmur heard, PMI is displaced
Pulmonary: Respirations are easy, no accessory muscles, breath sounds are clear
Abdomen: Soft, obese, nontender, no hepatosplenomegaly
Extremities: Slight pretibial edema, pedal and posterior tibial pulses are present

Testing

Prior cardiac catheterization revealed no obstructive disease
Echocardiogram reveals left ventricular size is mild to moderately enlarged. Left ventricular systolic function is depressed. Left ventricular ejection fraction is 32%. Left ventricular diastolic function is abnormal. Trace mitral regurgitation. Left and right atrial volume is normal
12-Lead ECG reveals sinus tachycardia at a rate of 90 bpm. No acute changes noted

Laboratory Findings

Complete blood count and iron panel normal, sodium 139 mmol/L, potassium 4.2 mmol/L, chloride 103 mmol/L, CO_2 24 mmol/L, BUN 28, Creatinine 1.8 mg/dL, glucose 102 mg/dL,

(continued)

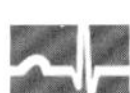 CASE STUDY 1 (*Continued*)

calcium 9.8 mg/dL, anion gap 12, eGFR 60, TSH 3.5 mU/L, BNP 350 pg/dL (unchanged)

Considerations

Treatment Plan

- Addition of ivabradine 5 mg 1 tablet twice daily
- Monitor HR and BP and report results in 1–2 weeks
- Continue other medications as prescribed
- Continue with nightly use of CPAP
- Continue with lifestyle modifications and self-care activities
- Return office visit in 1 month for follow-up with phone contact during the interim

Key Points

The patient was optimized on his current heart failure medications. In the past, uptitration of his ACE-I and attempts at adding daily doses of spironolactone resulted in a decline in his renal function. Further optimization of his β-blocker resulted in hypotension. Although addition of hydralazine and isosorbide is recommended in blacks, once optimized on GDMT, his blood pressure will not support the addition. The patient had self-monitored his HR over the preceding weeks with reported resting HF averaging in the upper 80s. His rhythm was confirmed with a 12-lead ECG as Sinus Tachycardia. Careful assessment of potential factors that could contribute to an elevated HR such as anemia, fluid state, thyroid, further decline in function must all be considered and ruled out.

The addition of a new medication requires shared decision-making with the patient. Consideration of cost, education regarding the medication, purpose, and potential side effects is needed. Ongoing follow-up with the patient is critical to ensure he is tolerating the medication and it is effective.

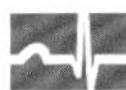 CASE STUDY 2

Patient Profile

Name/Age/Gender: **Shirley Smith, 78-year-old white female**

History of Present Illness

Mrs. Smith is a resident at a local assisted living facility. At 0200, she reported not feeling well indicating it was difficult to breathe lying down. The nursing assistant checked her BP and it was 190/92. She reported shortness of breath but no symptoms of chest pain, back pain, or nausea. She was sent to the ED via EMS for complaints of increased dyspnea and HTN.

Past Medical History

Atrial fibrillation (permanent)
COPD
CKD
Chronic knee pain
HFpEF (LVEF 60%)
Hyperlipidemia
HTN
Morbid obesity
OSA
Pulmonary HTN

Allergies

NKA

Home Medications

Alprazolam 0.25 mg 1 tablet daily PRN for anxiety
Aspirin 81 mg daily
Coumadin 3 mg 1.5 tablets (3 days per week) and 1 tablet (4 days per week)
Norco 5–325 mg 1 tablet Q6H
Ventolin HFA 90 mcg/inhalation Q4H PRN for wheezing
Vit D3 400 units 1.5 tablets daily
Zetia 10 mg daily
Acetaminophen 500 mg 1 tablet BID
Calcium carbonate 1250 mg (500 mg elemental calcium) daily
Furosemide 40 mg 1 tablet BID
Ipratropium-albuterol 0.5–2.5 mg/3-mL inhalation QID
Metoprolol succinate 100 mg daily

Physical Examination

Wt. 225 lb; Ht. 5 ft 2 in; BMI 41.1; HR 100 bpm; BP 200/96; RR 24; oxygen saturation 90%
Constitutional: Alert and oriented, anxious
Neck: JVD to 7 cm
Pulmonary: Respirations are labored, breath sounds are equal, symmetrical chest wall expansion, diminished diffusely particularly in the bases bilaterally
Cardiovascular: Irregular rhythm, no murmur or rub
Abdomen: Soft nontender, obese, normal bowel sounds, (+) hepatojugular reflux
Extremities: Moves all four extremities equally, 2+ LE edema, 2+ pedal and posterior tibial pulses
Skin: Warm, dry, and pink. No rash
Psychiatric: Cooperative, appropriate mood and affect
Clinical profile is Warm and Wet
Treatment goals—Diuresis and Reduction of Blood Pressure

Testing

Chest x-ray: Reveals vascular engorgement and interstitial edema
12-lead ECG: Atrial fibrillation with ventricular response rate 100
Complete blood count within normal limits, sodium 140 mmol/L, potassium 3.8 mmol/L, chloride 102 mmol/L, CO_2 22 mmol/L, BUN 34 mg/dL, Creatinine 1.6 mg/dL, glucose 140 mg/dL, calcium 9.7 mg/dL, anion gap 12, eGFR 40, INR 2.2, troponin I 0.1 ng/mL, BNP 680 pg/mL.

Considerations

Treatment Plan

- IV furosemide 80 mg now
- Admit to telemetry floor
- Blood pressure control
  - Addition of a vasodilator such as IV NTG if patient fails to diurese with diuretic
- Home medications
- Trend troponin
- Cardiology ischemic workup
- Echocardiogram
- Continue warfarin, INR in AM
- Determine precipitating cause

Day 1 Telemetry Unit

- The patient is stable, rhythm remains AF
- BP trending down 164/81; HR 88; RR 22; O_2 Sat 95% on O_2 at 3-L NC

CASE STUDY 2 (*Continued*)

- Good diuretic response was reported (2000-cc output)
- Resumed home medications

Day 2 Hospital Course

- BP continued to improve 136/78; HR 80; RR 20
- Nuclear myocardial perfusion scan:
  - No reversible perfusion defect to indicate ischemia
- Echocardiogram: Mod concentric LVH, LVEF 60%, dilated atria, mild TR
- Hgb 10.4 mg/dL, Hct 32%, potassium 4.0 mmol/L, BUN 37 mg/dL, creatinine 1.6 mg/dL, glucose 100 mg/dL
- The precipitating factor was the patient had an increase in her sodium intake over the prior week (high sodium snacks she had purchased from the vending machine), she was not weighing herself on a regular basis and she had failed to remember to take her metoprolol dose the day of admission
- The dietician met with the patient and contacted the facility to discuss her diet and the importance of low sodium choices
- Individualized education regarding HF, diet, daily weights, monitoring signs and symptoms, and follow-up was discussed
- Ambulated in the hall with assistance without difficulty
- BNP prior discharge 320 pg/dL
- Transition back to the assisted living facility with recommendations for assistance with her medications

Key Points

The patient was followed throughout her hospitalization to ensure resolution of symptoms. If her symptoms had failed to respond to IV diuresis and her pressures remained elevated, consideration of IV vasodilators is warranted. If her respiratory symptoms persist in the setting of declining oxygen saturation, BiPAP may have been beneficial.

The patient responded well to a single dose of IV diuretic and her blood pressure became more controlled. She ruled out for AMI. She received individualized education with recommendations to prevent reoccurrence. She was provided a scale to weigh daily and track her weight. Communication with the assisted living facility was undertaken by the dietician regarding her diet and the importance of avoiding foods high in sodium and low sodium choices. The nurse spoke with the nursing director with recommendations for assistance with her medications to facilitate adherence.

KEY READINGS

Brunwald E. Heart Failure. *JACC: Heart Failure.* 2013;1(1).

Jarvis S, Saman S. Heart failure 1: pathogenesis, presentation and diagnosis. *Nursing Times* [online]. 2017;113(9):49--53.

REFERENCES

1. Yancy C, Jessup M, Bozkurt B, et al. 2013 ACCF/AHA guideline for the management of heart failure: a report of the American College of Cardiology Foundation/American Heart Association Task Force on Practice Guidelines (Writing Committee): developed in collaboration with the American College of Chest Physicians, Heart Rhythm Society and the International Society for Heart and Lung Transplantation: endorsed by the American Association of Cardiovascular and Pulmonary Rehabilitation. *Circulation.* 2013;128(16):e240–e327.
2. Fonarow GC. Epidemiology and risk stratification in acute heart failure. *Am Heart J.* 2008;155(2):200–207.
3. Chen J, Normand ST, Wang Y, et al. National and regional trends in heart failure hospitalization and mortality rates for Medicare beneficiaries, 1998–2008. *JAMA.* 2011;306(15):1669–1678.
4. Benjamin EJ, Muntner P, Alonso A, et al. Heart disease and stroke statistics–2019 update: a report from the American Heart Association. *Circulation.* 2019;139(10):e56–e528.
5. Vigen R, Maddox TM, Allen LA. Aging of the United states population: impact on heart failure. *Curr Heart Fail Rep.* 2012;9(4):369–374.
6. Komanduri S, Jadhao Y, Guduru SS, et al. Prevalence and risk factors of heart failure in the USA: NHANES 2013 – 2014 epidemiological follow-up study. *J Community Hosp Intern Med Perspect.* 2017;7(1):15–20.
7. Mann DL, Felker GM. *Heart Failure: A Companion to Braunwald's Heart Disease.* 3rd ed. Philadelphia, PA: Elsevier; 2016.
8. Zipes DP, Libby P, Bonow RO, et al. *Braunwald's Heart Disease: A Textbook of Cardiovascular Medicine.* 11th ed. Philadelphia, PA: Elsevier; 2018.
9. Katz AM, Konsyam MA. *Heart Failure: Pathophysiology, Molecular Biology, and Clinical Management.* Philadelphia, PA: Lippincott Williams & Williams; 2009.
10. Packer M. The neurohormonal hypothesis: a theory to explain the mechanism of disease progression in heart failure. *J Am Coll Cardiol.* 1992;20(1):248–254.
11. Kane GC, Karon BL, Mahoney DW, et al. Progression of left ventricular diastolic dysfunction and risk of heart failure. *JAMA.* 2011;306(8): 856–863.
12. Dunlay SM, Weston SA, Jacobsen SJ, et al. Risk factors for heart failure: a population-based case-controlled study. *Am J Med.* 2009;122(11): 1023–1028.
13. Athilingam P, D'aoust R, Zambroski C, et al. Predictive validity of NYHA and ACC/AHA classifications of physical and cognitive functioning in heart failure. *Int J Nursing Science.* 2013;3(1):22–32.
14. Reddy YN, Melenovsky V, Redfield MM, et al. High-output heart failure: a 15-year experience. *J Am Coll Cardiol.* 2016;68(5):473–482.
15. Bock G, Goode J. *Heart Failure: Molecules, Mechanisms and Therapeutic Targets.* Chichester, UK: John Wiley & Sons Ltd; 2006.
16. Harvey PA, Leinwand LA. The cell biology of disease: cellular mechanisms of cardiomyopathy. *J Cell Biol.* 2011;194(3):355–365.
17. Piek A, deBoer RA, Sillje HHW. The fibrosis-cell death axis in heart failure. *Heart Fail Rev.* 2016;21(2):199–211.
18. Hein S, Arnon E, Kostin S, et al. Progression from compensated hypertrophy to failure in the pressure-overloaded human heart: structural deterioration and compensatory mechanisms. *Circulation.* 2003; 107(7):984–991.
19. Dorn GW 2nd, Molkentin JD. Manipulating cardiac contractility in heart failure: data from mice and men. *Circulation.* 2004;109(2): 150–158.
20. Ky B, French B, McCloskey K, et al. High-sensitivity ST2 for prediction of adverse outcomes in chronic heart failure. *Circ Heart Fail.* 2011; 4(2):180–187.
21. Gaggin HK, Januzzi JL. Biomarkers and diagnostics in heart failure. *Biochim Biophys Acta.* 2013;1832(12):2442–2450.
22. Edelmann F, Holzendorf V, Wachter R, et al. Galectin-3 in patients with heart failure with preserved ejection fraction: results from the Aldo-DHF trial. *Eur Jo Heart Fail.* 2015;17(2):214–223.
23. Konstantinidis K, Whelan RS, Kitsis RN. Mechanisms of cell death in heart disease. *Arterioscler Thromb Vasc Biol.* 2012;32(7):1552–1562.
24. Abbate A, Biondi-Zoccai GG, Bussani R, et al. Increased myocardial apoptosis in patients with unfavorable left ventricular remodeling and early symptomatic post-infarction heart failure. *J Am Coll Cardiol.* 2003; 41(5):753–760.
25. Sanderson JE. Heart failure with a normal ejection fraction. *Heart.* 2007;93(2):155–158.
26. Dixon JA, Spinale FG. Myocardial remodeling: cellular and extracellular events and targets. *Annu Rev Physiol.* 2011;73:47–68.
27. Abdullah OM, Drakos SG, Diakos NA, et al. Characterization of diffuse fibrosis in failing human heart via diffusion tensor imaging and quantitative histological validation. *NMR Biomedicine.* 2014;27(11):1378–1386.
28. Weil J, Eschenhagen T, Hirt S, et al. Preserved Frank-Starling mechanism in human end stage heart failure. *Cardiovasc Res.* 1998;37(2):541–548.

29. Sokolovsky RE, Zlochiver S, Abboud S. Stroke volume estimation in heart failure patients using bioimpedance: a realistic simulation of the forward problem. *Physiol Meas.* 2008;29(6):S139–S149.
30. Lester SJ, Tajik AJ, Nishimura RA, et al. Unlocking the mysteries of diastolic function: deciphering the Rosetta Stone 10 years later. *J Am Coll Cardiol.* 2008;51(7):679–689.
31. Tang WH, Francis GS. The year in heart failure. *J Am Coll Cardiol.* 2007; 50(24):2344–2351.
32. McCance KL, Huether SE. *Pathophysiology: The Biological Basis for Disease in Adults and Children.* 8th ed. St. Louis, MO: Mosby Elsevier; 2018.
33. Mazhari R, Hare JM. Advances in cell-based therapy for structural heart disease. *Prog Cardiovasc Dis.* 2007;49(6):387–395.
34. Singh VP, Le B, Bhat VB, et al. High glucose induced regulation of intracellular angiotensin II synthesis and nuclear redistribution in cardiac myocytes. *Am J Physiol-Heart Cir Physiol.* 2007;293(2):H939–H948.
35. Kumar R, Yong QC, Thomas CM, et al. Review: intracardiac intracellular angiotensin system in diabetes. *Am J Physiol-Regul Integr Comp Physiol.* 2012;302(5):R510–R517.
36. Singh VP, Baker KM, Kumar R. Activation of the intracellular renin-angiotensin system in cardiac fibroblasts by high glucose: role in extracellular matrix production. *Am J Physiol-Heart Circ Physiol.* 2008;294(4):H16 75–H1684.
37. Kumar R, Singh VP, Baker KM. The intracellular renin-angiotensin system-implications in cardiovascular remodeling. *Curr Opin Nephrol Hypertens.* 2008;17(2):168–173.
38. Pitt B. Aldosterone blockade in patients with chronic heart failure. *Cardiol Clin.* 2008;26(1):15–21.
39. Adiarto S, Heiden S, Vignon-Zellweger N, et al. ET-1 from endothelial cells is required for complete angiotensin II-induced cardiac fibrosis and hypertrophy. *Life Sci.* 2012;91(13–14):651–657.
40. Nishikimi T, Nakagawa Y. Adrenomedullin as a biomarker of heart failure. *Heart Fail Clin.* 2018;14(1):49–55.
41. Takahama H, Kitakaze M. Pathophysiology of cardiorenal syndrome in patients with heart failure: potential therapeutic targets. *Am J Physiol Heart Circ Physiol.* 2017;313(4):H715–H721.
42. Cotter G, Felker GM, Adams KF, et al. The pathophysiology of acute heart failure—is it all about fluid accumulation? *Am Heart J.* 2008; 155(1):9–18.
43. Januzzi J. *Cardiac Biomarkers in Clinical Practice.* Boston, MA: Jones & Bartlett; 2011.
44. Pupalan I, Thomas M, Majoni W, et al. Comorbid heart failure and renal impairment: epidemiology and management. *Cardiorenal Med.* 2012;2(4):281–297.
45. Udani SM, Koyner JL. The effects of heart failure on renal function. *Cardiol Clin.* 2011;28(3):453–465.
46. Ionita MG, Arslan F, de Kleijn DP, et al. Endogenous inflammatory molecules engage Toll-like receptors in cardiovascular disease. *J Innate Immun.* 2010;2(4):307–315.
47. Sakata Y, Dong JW, Vallejo JG, et al. Toll-like receptor 2 modulates left ventricular function following ischemic-reperfusion injury. *Am J Physiol-Heart Circ Physiol.* 2007;292(1):H503–H509.
48. Deswal A, Petersen NJ, Feldman, AM, et al. Cytokines and cytokine receptors in advanced heart failure: an analysis of the cytokine database from the Vesnarinone trial (VEST). *Circulation.* 2001;103(16):2055–2059.
49. Munger MA, Johnson B, Amber IL, et al. Circulating concentrations of proinflammatory cytokines in mild or moderate heart failure secondary to ischemia or idiopathic dilated cardiomyopathy. *Am J Cardiol.* 1996;77(9):723–727.
50. Rauchhaus M, Doehner W, Francis DP, et al. Plasma cytokine parameters and mortality in patients with chronic heart failure. *Circulation.* 2000;102(25):3060–3067.
51. Levick SP, Murray DB, Janicki JS, et al. Sympathetic nervous system modulation of inflammation and remodeling in the hypertensive heart. *Hypertension.* 2010;55(2):270–276.
52. Berridge MJ, Lipp P, Bootman MD. The versatility and universality of calcium signalling. *Nat Rev Mol Cell Biol.* 2000;1(1):11–21.
53. Przemek AG, Ceholski DK, Hajjar RJ. Altered myocardial calcium cycling and energetics in heart failure—a rational approach for disease treatment. *Cell Metab.* 2015;21(2):183–194.
54. Ashrafian H, Frenneaux MP, Opie LH. Metabolic mechanisms in heart failure. *Circulation.* 2007;116(4):434–448.
55. Nichols GA, Reynolds K, Kimes TM, et al. Comparison of risk of re-hospitalization, all-cause mortality and medical care resource utilization in patients with heart failure and preserved versus reduced ejection fraction. *Am J Cardiol.* 2015;116(7):1088–1092.
56. Loehr LR, Rosamond WD, Chang PP, et al. Heart failure incidence and survival (from the Atherosclerosis Risk in Communities study). *Am J Cardiol.* 2008;101(7):1016–1022.
57. Tsao CW, Lyass A, Enserro D, et al. Temporal trends in the incidence of the mortality associated with heart failure with preserved and reduced ejection fraction. *JACC Heart Fail.* 2018;6(8):678–685.
58. Oktay AA, Rich JD, Shah SJ. The emerging epidemic of heart failure with preserved ejection fraction. *Curr Heart Fail Rep.* 2013;10(4):401–410.
59. Paulus WJ, Tschope C. A novel paradigm for heart failure with preserved ejection fraction: comorbidities drive myocardial dysfunction and remodeling through coronary microvascular endothelial inflammation. *J Am Coll Cardiol.* 2013;62(4):263–271.
60. Borlaug BA, Nishimura RA, Sorajja P, et al. Exercise hemodynamics enhance diagnosis of early heart failure with preserved ejection fraction. *Circ Heart Fail.* 2010;3(5):588–595.
61. Nagueh SF, Appleton CP, Gillebert TC, et al. Recommendations for the evaluation of left ventricular diastolic function by echocardiography. *J Am Soc Echocardiogr.* 2009;22(2):107–133.
62. Borlaug BA, Paulus WJ. Heart failure with preserved ejection fraction: pathophysiology, diagnosis and treatment. *Eur Heart J.* 2011;32(6): 670–679.
63. Bhuiyan T, Maurer MS. Heart failure with preserved ejection fraction: persistent diagnosis, therapeutic enigma. *Curr Cardiovasc Risk Rep.* 2011; 5(5):440–449.
64. Punnoose LR, Givertz MM, Lewis EF, et al. Heart failure with recovered ejection fraction: a distinct clinical entity. *J Card Fail.* 2011;17(7): 527–532.
65. Liang KV, Williams AW, Greene EL, et al. Acute decompensated heart failure and the cardiorenal syndrome. *Crit Care Med.* 2008;36(1):S75–S88.
66. Joseph SM, Cedars AM, Ewald GA, et al. Acute decompensated heart failure contemporary medical management. *Tex Heart Inst J.* 2009; 36(6):510–520.
67. Komajda M, Carson PE, Hetzel S, et al. Factors associated with outcome in heart failure with preserved ejection fraction: findings from the Irbesartan in Heart Failure with Preserved Ejection Fraction Study (I-PRESERVE). *Circ Heart Fail.* 2011;1(4):27–35.
68. O'Connor CM, Abraham WT, Albert NM, et al. Predictors of mortality after discharge in patients hospitalized with heart failure: an analysis from the Organized Program to Initiate Lifesaving Treatment in Hospitalized Patients with Heart Failure (OPTIMIZE-HF). *Am Heart J.* 2008;156(4):662–673.
69. Lyons OD, Bradley TD. Heart failure and sleep apnea. *Can J Cardiol.* 2015;31(7):898–908.
70. Jarvis C. *Physical Examination and Health Assessment.* 7th ed. St. Louis, MO: Elsevier; 2016.
71. Drazner MH, Hellkamp AS, Leier CV, et al. Value of clinician assessment of hemodynamics in advanced heart failure: the ESCAPE trial. *Circ Heart Fail.* 2008;1(3):170–177.
72. Dunlay SM, Weston SA, Redfield MM, et al. Tumor necrosis factor-alpha and mortality in heart failure: a community study. *Circulation.* 2008;118(6):625–631.
73. Nagueh SF, Appleton CP, Gillebert TC, et al. Recommendations for the evaluation of left ventricular diastolic dysfunction by echocardiography. *Eur J Echocardiogr.* 2009;10(2):165–193.
74. Chua TP, Ponikowski P, Harrington D, et al. Clinical correlates and prognostic significance of the ventilatory response to exercise in chronic heart failure. *J Am Coll Cardiol.* 1997;29(7):1585–1590.
75. Francis GS, Greenberg BH, Hsu DT, et al. ACCF/AHA/ACP/HFSA/ISHLT 2010 clinical competence statement on management of patients with advanced heart failure and cardiac transplant. *Circulation.* 2010; 122(6):644–672.
76. Januzzi JL, Rehman SU, Mohammed AA, et al. Use of amino-terminal pro-B-type natriuretic peptide to guide outpatient therapy of patients with chronic left ventricular systolic dysfunction. *J Am Coll Cardiol.* 2011;58(18):1881–1891.
77. Yancy CW, Jessup M, Bozkurt B, et al. ACC/AHA/HFSA focused update on the 2013 ACCF/AHA guideline for the management of heart failure: a report of the American College of Cardiology/American Heart Association Task Force on Clinical Practice Guidelines and the Heart Failure Society of America. *Circulation.* 2017;136(6):e138–e161.
78. Migone de Amicis M, Chivite D, Corbella X, et al. Anemia is a mortality prognostic factor in patients initially hospitalized for acute heart failure. *Int Emerg Med.* 2017;12(6):749–756.
79. Fonarow GC, Adams KF, Abraham WT, et al. Risk stratification for in-hospital mortality in acutely decompensated heart failure: classification and regression tree analysis. *JAMA.* 2005;293(5):572–580.

80. Januzzi JL. Natriuretic peptides as biomarkers in heart failure. *J Investig Med.* 2013;61(6):950–955.
81. de Boer RA, Lok DJ, Jaarsma T, et al. Predictive value of plasma Galectin-3 levels in heart failure with reduced and preserved ejection fraction. *Ann Med.* 2011;43(1):60–68.
82. Chen J, Normand S, Wang Y, et al. National and regional trends in heart failure hospitalization and mortality rates for Medicare beneficiaries, 1998–2008. *JAMA.* 2011;306(15):1669–1678.
83. Gerber Y, Weston SA, Redfield MM, et al. A contemporary appraisal of the heart failure epidemic in Olmsted County, Minnesota, 2000 to 2010. *JAMA Intern Med.* 2015;175:996–1004.
84. Mozaffarian D, Anker SD, Anand I, et al. Prediction of mode of death in heart failure: the Seattle Heart Failure Model. *Circulation.* 2007;116(4):392–398.
85. Ammar KA, Jacobsen SJ, Mahoney DW, et al. Prevalence and prognostic significance of heart failure stages: application of the American College of Cardiology/American Heart Association heart failure staging criteria in the community. *Circulation.* 2007;115(12):1563–1570.
86. Patel J, Heywood JT. Mode of death in patients with systolic heart failure. *J Cardiovasc Pharmacol Ther.* 2007;12(2):127–136.
87. Hernandez AF, O'Connor CM. Sparing a little may save a lot: lessons from the Studies of Left Ventricular Dysfunction (SOLVD). *J Am Coll Cardiol.* 2003;42(4):709–711.
88. Hall MJ, Levant S, DeFrances CJ. Hospitalization for congestive heart failure: United States, 2000–2010. *NCHS Data Brief.* 2012;108:1–8.
89. Dunlay SM, Redfeld MM, Weston SA, et al. Hospitalizations after heart failure diagnosis a community perspective. *J Am Coll Cardiol.* 2009;54(18):1695–1702.
90. Lambnisos F, Kalogirou E, Lamnisos F, et al. Effectiveness of heart failure management programmes with nurse-led discharge planning in reducing readmissions: a systematic review and meta-analysis. *Int J Nurs Stud.* 2012;49(5):610–624.
91. Sisk J, Herbert PL, Horowitz CR, et al. Effects on nurse management on the quality of heart failure care in minority communities: a randomized trial. *Ann Intern Med.* 2006;145(4):273–283.
92. DeBusk RF, Miller NH, Parker K, et al. Care management for low risk patients with heart failure: a randomized, control trial. *Ann Intern Med.* 2004;141(8):606–613.
93. Gheorghiade M, Pang PS. Acute heart failure syndromes. *J Am Coll Cardiol.* 2009;53(7):557–573.
94. Yancy CW, Lopatin M, Stevenson LW, et al. Clinical presentation, management and in-hospital outcomes of patients admitted with acute decompensated heart failure with preserved systolic function: a report from the Acute Decompensated Heart Failure National Registry (ADHERE) database. *J Am Coll Cardiol.* 2006;47(1):76–84.
95. Coona J, McGraw M, Murali S. Pharmacotherapy for acute heart failure syndromes. *Am J Health Syst Pharm.* 2011;68(1):21–35.
96. Kato M, Stevenson LW, Palardy M, et al. The worst symptom as defined by patients during heart failure hospitalization: implications for response to therapy. *J Card Fail.* 2012;18(7):524–533.
97. Booth RA, Hill SA, Don-Wauchope A, et al. Performance of BNP and NT-ProBNP for diagnosis of heart failure in primary care patients: a systematic review. *Heart Fail Rev.* 2014;19(4):439–451.
98. Felker GM, Lee K, Bull D, et al. Diuretic strategies in patients with acute decompensated heart failure. *N Engl J Med.* 2011;364(9):797–805.
99. Lala A, McNulty S, Mentz R, et al. Insights from diuretic optimization strategy evaluation in acute decompensated heart failure (DOSE-AHF) and cardiorenal rescue study in acute decompensated heart failure (CARESS-HF). *Circ Heart Fail.* 2015;8(4):741–748.
100. Sanchez CE, Richards DR. Contemporary in-hospital management strategies for acute decompensated heart failure. *Cardiol Rev.* 2011; 19(3):122–129.
101. Publication Committee for the VMAC Investigators. Intravenous nesiritide vs nitroglycerin for treatment of decompensated congestive heart failure: a randomized controlled trial. *JAMA.* 2002;287(12): 1531–1540.
102. Topalian S, Ginsberg F, Parrillo JE. Cardiogenic shock. *Crit Care Med.* 2008;36(1 suppl.):S66–S74.
103. Thiele H, Ohman EM, Desch S, et al. Management of cardiogenic shock. *Eur Heart J.* 2015;36(20):1223–1230.
104. Goldberg RJ, Spencer F, Gore J, et al. Thirty year trends (1975-2005). In the magnitude, management, and hospital death rates associated with cardiogenic shock in patients with acute myocardial infarction: a population-based perspective. *Circulation.* 2009;119(9):1211–1219.
105. Thiele H, Allam B, Chatellier G, et al. Shock in acute myocardial infarction: the Cape Horn for trials? *Eur Heart J.* 2010;31(15):1828–1835.
106. Abdel-Qadir H, Ivanov J, Austin P, et al. Temporal trends in cardiogenic shock treatment and outcomes among Ontario patients with myocardial infarction between 1992 and 2008. *Circ Cardiovasc Qual Outcomes.* 2011;4(4):440–447.
107. Reynolds HR, Hochman JS. Cardiogenic shock: current concepts and improving outcomes. *Circulation.* 2008;117(5):686–697.
108. Minicucci M, Azevedo P, Polegator B, et al. Heart failure after myocardial infarction: clinical implications and treatment. *Clin Cardiol.* 2011;34(7):410–414.
109. Babaev A, Frederick PD, Pasta DJ, et al. Trends in management and outcomes of patients with acute myocardial infarction complicated by cardiogenic shock. *JAMA.* 2005;294(4):448–454.
110. Slater J, Brown RJ, Antonelli TA, et al. Cardiogenic shock due to cardiac free-wall rupture or tamponade after acute myocardial infarction: a report from the SHOCK Trial Registry. Should we emergently revascularize occluded coronaries for cardiogenic shock? *J Am Coll Cardiol.* 2000;36(3 suppl. 1):1117–1122.
111. Oliver C, Marin F, Pineda J, et al. Low QRS voltage in cardiac tamponade: a study of 70 cases. *Int J Cardiol.* 2002;83(1):91–92.
112. Windecker S, Kolh P, Alfonso F, et al. 2014 ESC/EACTS Guidelines on myocardial revascularization: the task force on myocardial revascularization of the European Society of Cardiology (ESC) and the European association for cardio-thoracic surgery (EACTS) developed with the special contribution of the European Association of Percutaneous Cardiovascular Interventions (EAPCI). *Eur Heart J.* 2014;35(37):2541–2619.
113. Steg PG, James SK, Atar D, et al. ESC guidelines for the management of acute myocardial infarction in patients presenting with ST-segment elevation. *Eur Heart J.* 2012;33(20):2569–2619.
114. Hochman JS, Sleeper LA, Webb JG, et al. Early revascularization and long-term survival in cardiogenic shock complicating acute myocardial infarction. *JAMA.* 2006;295(21):2511–2515.
115. Webb JG, Lowe AM, Sanborn TA, et al. Percutaneous coronary intervention for cardiogenic shock in the SHOCK trial. *J Am Coll Cardiol.* 2003;42(8):1380–1386.
116. Unverzagt S, Wachsmuth L, Hirsch K, et al. Inotropic agents and vasodilator strategies for acute myocardial infarction complicated by cardiogenic shock or low cardiac output syndrome (Review). *Cochrane Database System Rev.* 2014;1:1–48.
117. Jeger RV, Harkness SM, Ramanathan K, et al. Emergency revascularization in patients with cardiogenic shock on admission: a report from the SHOCK trial and registry. *Eur Heart J.* 2006;27(6):664–670.
118. Konstantinides S, Torbicki A, Agnelli G, et al. 2014 ESC guidelines on the diagnosis and management of acute pulmonary embolism: Task Force for the diagnosis and management of acute pulmonary embolism of the European Society of Cardiology (ESC). *Eur Heart J.* 2014;35(43):3033–3069.
119. Ristic A, Imazio M, Adler Y, et al. Triage strategy for urgent management of cardiac tamponade: a position statement of the European Society of Cardiology working group on myocardial and pericardial disease. *Eur Heart J.* 2014;35(34):2279–2284.
120. Gupta A, Allen L, Bhatt D, et al. Association of the hospital readmissions reduction program implementation with readmission and mortality outcomes in heart failure. *JAMA.* 2018;3(1):44–53.
121. Albert N, Barnason S, Hernandez A, et al. Transitions of care in heart failure: a scientific statement from the American Heart Association. *Circ Heart Fail.* 2015;8(2):384–409.

38 Heart Failure: Guideline-Directed Medical and Device Therapy

Kelley M. Anderson, Dorothy L. Murphy, Reiko Asano, Karen M. Vuckovic

OBJECTIVES

1. Detail contemporary guideline-directed therapies in individuals with HF. Differentiate HFpEF and HFrEF and the treatment modalities for each. Discern the complexity of comorbidities and heart failure management.
2. Identify the importance of the nurse in the heart failure team to promote management and therapeutic interventions to improve quality of life and symptoms.

KEY QUESTIONS

1. What are the usual recommended therapies for HFpEF and HFrEF?
2. When is cardiac implantable electronic devices, ICD and CRT, indicated?
3. Why is a multidisciplinary team, including the patient, essential for the management of HF?

BACKGROUND

Heart failure (HF) is a pathophysiologic state in which an abnormality of cardiac function results in inadequate systemic perfusion. HF is not an event or disease but rather a constellation of signs and symptoms that represent the final pathway of a heterogeneous group of diseases, the end result of most cardiovascular disease states.[1] The extent and severity by which cardiac function is impaired and symptoms manifest in each individual varies greatly. Established guideline-directed medical therapies (GDMT) provide recommendations for management and treatment options, however, an individualized approach including an understanding of HF type, etiology, symptoms, HF stage, comorbidities, prognosis, ethnicity and patient preferences is required for optimal care. Management of HF involves the patient and caregivers in self-management practices and an interdisciplinary team of healthcare providers. Therapeutic treatments may include management of comorbidities, lifestyle modifications, sodium and fluid restrictions, cardiac rehabilitation, pharmacologic agents, implantable cardiac device therapies, and palliative care. Patients with HF frequently experience symptoms along a spectrum, with periods of exacerbation and stability. The acute or chronic nature of the clinical presentation of symptoms is an important consideration while directing therapeutic management strategies.

As the understanding of this mechanisms underlying both the development and progression of HF have evolved, focus is on identifying the factors that increase the risk for developing the syndrome. While it is not surprising that advancing age, history of ischemic heart disease (IHD), myocardial infarction (MI), or hypertension are associated with developing HF, a robust association has been seen in patients with both type II diabetes mellitus (DM)[2,3] and obesity, and the subsequent syndrome of HF. The worldwide epidemic of type II DM and obesity make them potentially modifiable targets to reduce incidence of HF.

The American College of Cardiology and the American Heart Association (ACC/AHA) Task Force classification stratifies HF into stages based on established risk factors, the progression of HF from asymptomatic to symptomatic phases, and treatments prescribed at each stage known to reduce morbidity and mortality.[1] The four stages of HF include: Stage A, the patient who is at high risk but has no structural heart disease; stage B, the patient with structural heart disease but no symptoms of HF; stage C, the patient with structural heart disease and current or previous symptoms of HF; and stage D, the patient with end-stage disease that requires special interventions. The importance of this staging system arises from the fact that, once myocyte, myocardial, and systemic changes have begun, the primary treatments are altering the trajectory of the syndrome as a cure is seldom an option.

Heart Failure Symptoms and Signs

Symptoms are a key measure to understand HF severity and the basis of the New York Heart Association (NYHA) functional classification system. Improving HF symptoms is a primary goal of GDMTs and fundamentally correlates to health-related quality of life (HRQOL). Symptoms and signs are associated with the type of ventricular dysfunction, that is, whether the dysfunction is left sided, right side, or a combination of both. Left-sided HF, associated with elevated pulmonary venous pressure and decreased cardiac output, appears clinically as breathlessness, weakness, fatigue,

We'd like to thank Laurie A. Soine, PhD, ARNP, ACNP for her contributions to the previous editions.

dizziness, confusion, pulmonary congestion, poor peripheral perfusion, and death. Cardiac cachexia is a severe complication of HF and is considered a terminal manifestation. Decreased cerebral perfusion caused by low cardiac output leads to changes in mental status, such as cognitive impairment, restlessness, insomnia, nightmares, or memory loss. Anxiety, agitation, paranoia, and feelings of impending doom may develop as the syndrome progresses.

Right-sided HF, associated with increased systemic venous pressure, gives rise to the clinical signs of jugular venous distention, hepatomegaly, dependent peripheral edema, and ascites.[4] Weight gain is often recognized by patients; consistent self-weighing in the morning helps to detect subtle changes in fluid status. An adult may retain 10 to 15 lb (4 to 7 L) of fluid before edema occurs. Gastrointestinal symptoms such as nausea and anorexia may be a direct consequence of the increased intra-abdominal pressure.

Another finding related to fluid retention is recumbent diuresis. When at rest, the body's metabolic requirements are decreased, and cardiac function improves. This decreases systemic venous pressure, allowing edema fluid to be mobilized and excreted. Recumbency also increases renal blood flow and glomerular filtration rate (GFR), also increasing diuresis.

APPROACHES TO TREATMENT

Patients with left ventricular (LV) dysfunction often present with exercise intolerance, shortness of breath, and/or fluid retention. Incidental findings of dysfunction may also be found in asymptomatic patients (stage B). All patients presenting with HF, that is LV dysfunction with symptoms, should undergo a detailed evaluation to: (1) determine the type of cardiac dysfunction, (2) uncover correctable causative factors, (3) determine prognosis, (4) identify behaviors that might contribute and accelerate the development of HF, and (5) guide treatment. Recognition of signs and symptoms resulting from an inadequate cardiac output and from systemic and pulmonary congestion is accomplished through a careful history, physical examination, routine laboratory analyses, and diagnostic studies including the evaluation of left ventricular ejection fraction (LVEF).[1]

There are various principles that guide management of HF. The first step is identification and correction of the underlying pathogenic processes, as appropriate, such as hypertension, coronary revascularization procedures for coronary artery disease (CAD), treatment of amyloid, therapies for pulmonary hypertension, or surgical correction of structural abnormalities.[1] The second step is the removal of the compounding or precipitating causes, such as infection, arrhythmia, and pulmonary emboli. In addition, certain medications, including nonsteroidal anti-inflammatory drugs (NSAIDs), may exacerbate HF and their discontinuation should be considered. The third step is the treatment and control of HF. For patients with heart failure with reduced ejection fraction (HFrEF), therapy for HF is directed at reducing the workload of the heart and manipulating the various factors that determine cardiac performance, such as contractility, heart rate, preload, afterload, and LV synchrony. The greatest advance has been in pharmacologic agents that inhibit harmful neurohormonal systems that are activated in support of the failing heart, specifically the renin-angiotensin-aldosterone system (RAAS) and sympathetic nervous system.[1,5,6] Treatment of HF is based on the clinical presentation of the patient, which may encompass the extremes from mildly symptomatic to acute decompensation.

HF ranges clinically from stable chronic HF to acute HF with cardiogenic shock. The goal of therapy is to support pump function, which may include vasodilator therapy, positive inotropic agents, and mechanical devices. In the case of ischemia caused by CAD, treatment of the underlying process is the management goal. The combination of ischemia and LV dysfunction carries a poor prognosis, and it is this patient group that may benefit from revascularization by percutaneous coronary intervention techniques or urgent cardiac surgery.

Heart Failure With Reduced Ejection Fraction (HFrEF)

Coronary heart disease, hypertension, and dilated cardiomyopathy are the most commonly identified causes of LV systolic dysfunction. The 2013 writing committee of the ACC/AHA[1] based the therapy guidelines on the four stages of the evolution of HF (Fig. 38-1). *Stage A* includes patients who are at high risk for HF but do not have LV dysfunction. Treatment is aimed at risk factor modification, including management of hypertension, diabetes and lipids, cessation of smoking, and counseling to avoid alcohol and illicit drugs. Patients are encouraged to exercise on a regular basis. Obesity increases the risk of diabetes and hypertension, and steps should be taken to promote strategies to maintain optimal weight. An angiotensin-converting enzyme inhibitor (ACE-I) is indicated in patients with a history of atherosclerotic vascular disease, hypertension, or diabetes.

Stage B includes patients who are asymptomatic but have structural disease with LV systolic dysfunction and are at significant risk for HF. All of stage A therapies are indicated, with the addition of an ACE-I and β-adrenergic blockers, if appropriate and if there are no contraindications. An overview of the specific pharmacologic therapy for HFrEF is described in Table 38-1. Valve replacement or repair should be undertaken in patients with hemodynamically significant valvular stenosis or regurgitation.

Stage C includes patients with LV dysfunction with current or previous symptoms. In addition to all measures used for stages A and B, stage C patients have a confirmed diagnosis of HF and should be managed routinely with the following types of medications: (1) an ACE-I, angiotensin receptor blocker (ARB) or angiotensin neprilysin receptor inhibitor (ARNI), (2) β-adrenergic blocker agent (β-blocker), (3) diuretic, (4) hydralazine-nitrates for persistently symptomatic African Americans, and (5) mineralocorticoid receptor antagonists (MRA) otherwise known as aldosterone antagonists. For those patients intolerant to ACE-I or an ARNI, an ARB can be used. For those patients with renal insufficiency or angioedema on an ACE-I or ARB, a hydralazine/nitrate combination can be substituted. The use of an MRA or aldosterone antagonist for NYHA classes III and IV symptoms should be considered. Avoid the use of antiarrhythmics, NSAIDs, and most calcium-channel blockers (CCBs). Amlodipine may be considered in the management of hypertension. Nonpharmacologic therapies include a low-sodium diet, encouragement of physical activity, referral for cardiac rehabilitation and exercise training, and administration of influenza and pneumococcal vaccines.

Stage D includes patients with refractory HF who might be eligible for specialized, advanced treatment strategies. Patients should be treated with all measures used for stages A, B, and C. In addition, patients should undergo a thorough evaluation to determine that the diagnosis is correct and that there are no other alternative etiologies or explanations for advanced symptoms.

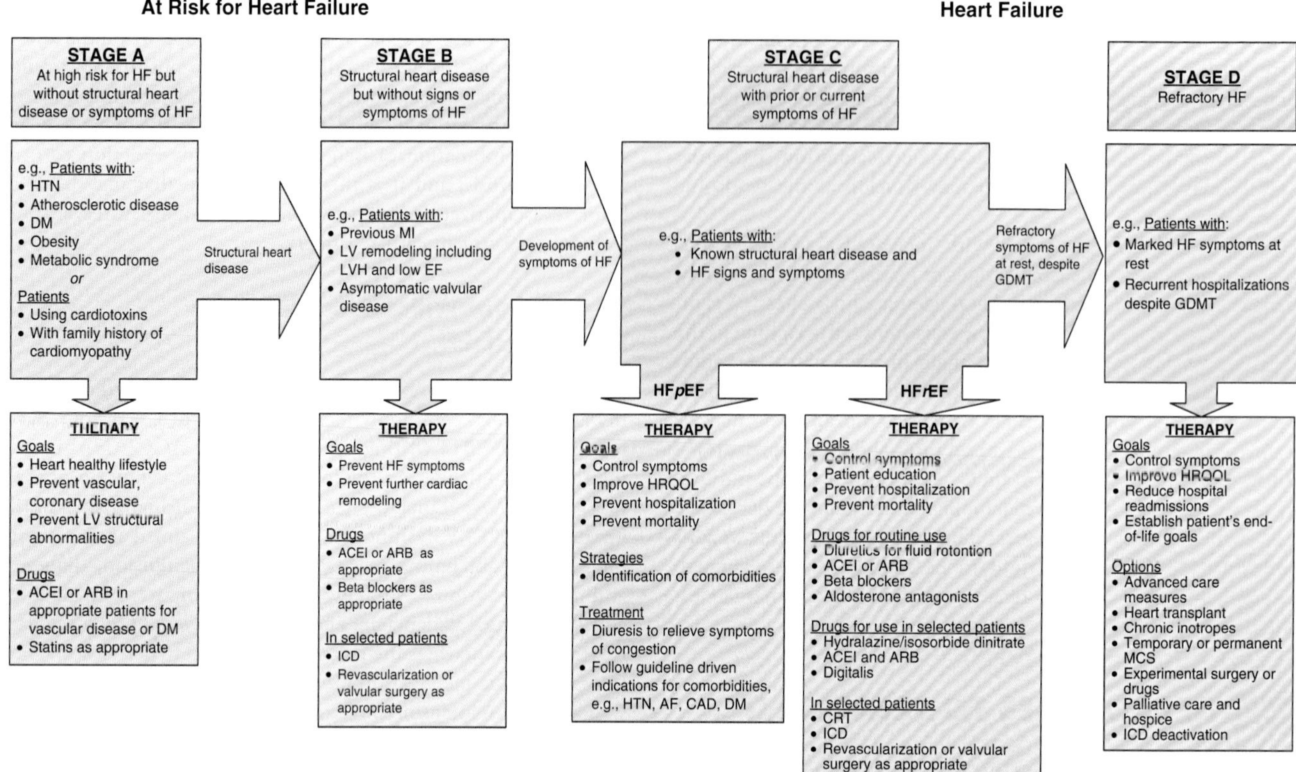

Figure 38-1. Stages in the development of HF and recommended therapy by stage. ACE-I, angiotensin-converting enzyme inhibitor; AF, atrial fibrillation; ARB, angiotensin-receptor blocker; CAD, coronary artery disease; CRT, cardiac resynchronization therapy; DM, diabetes mellitus; EF, ejection fraction; GDMT, guideline-directed medical therapy; HF, heart failure; HFpEF, heart failure with preserved ejection fraction; HFrEF, heart failure with reduced ejection fraction; HRQOL, health-related quality of life; HTN, hypertension; ICD, implantable cardioverter defibrillator; LV, left ventricular; LVH, left ventricular hypertrophy; MCS, mechanical circulatory support; MI, myocardial infarction. (Adapted from Hunt SA, Abraham WT, Chin MH, et al. ACC/AHA 2005 guideline update for the diagnosis and management of chronic heart failure in the adult: a report of the American College of Cardiology/American Heart Association Task Force on Practice Guidelines (Writing Committee to Update the 2001 Guidelines for the Evaluation and Management of Heart Failure): developed in collaboration with the American College of Chest Physicians and the International Society for Heart and Lung Transplantation: endorsed by the Heart Rhythm Society. *Circulation*. 2005;112[12]:e154–e235; Yancy CW, Jessup M, Bozkurt B, et al. 2013 ACCF/AHA guideline for the management of heart failure: a report of the American College of Cardiology Foundation/American Heart Association Task Force on Practice Guidelines. *J Am Coll Cardiol.* 2013;62[16]:e147–e239.)

Stage D patients require meticulous control of fluid retention. Fluid restriction is especially critical in patients with hyponatremia. In addition, fluid and sodium restriction may be helpful for patients who are refractory to diuretics. Patients who are at the end stage of their disease are at particular risk for hypotension and may be able to tolerate only a small dose of ACE-I or β-adrenergic blockers, or they may not be able to tolerate them at all. Despite optimal treatment, some patients do not improve. For these patients, specialized treatment strategies include mechanical circulatory support, continuous inotropic therapy, referral for cardiac transplantation, palliative or hospice care. Circulatory support may include durable and nondurable ventricular assistance devices (VADs).[1] For patients who cannot be sustained on medical therapy, VADs can successfully bridge to transplantation or be used as destination therapy.

Low-dose dopamine, dobutamine, or milrinone may be of benefit in hospitalized patients with severe systolic dysfunction, hypotension, and end-organ hypoperfusion. However, the intermittent or long-term use of these positive inotropic agents has not demonstrated improved outcomes; all of these agents have been associated with an increase in mortality related to arrhythmic events. To minimize adverse effects, it is recommended to use the lowest dose and frequently reassess the ongoing need for inotrope support. Cardiac transplantation plays a role in end-stage patients without contraindications to this procedure and offers excellent long-term outcomes. The goal of therapy for those patients not desiring or eligible for cardiac transplantation is symptom relief, which may include long-term intravenous inotrope support. Relieving symptom, reducing suffering and caregiver support is the focus of palliative care. Palliative care encompasses managing the physical, psychosocial, and spiritual problems associated with chronic illness and palliative care is associated with improved quality of life for the patient with HF and the patient's family. If end-of-life considerations deserve attention for this patient population, patients may transition to hospice care.

Table 38-1 • EVIDENCE-BASED CONSIDERATIONS FOR PHARMACOLOGIC THERAPIES FOR HFrEF

General considerations for ACE-I, ARB, ARNI
Titrate medications to target dose as tolerated
Begin therapy if systolic blood pressure (SBP) >90 mm Hg without vasodilator therapy or >80 mm Hg and asymptomatic with other vasodilator therapy
Do not hold vasodilator unless SBP <80 mm Hg or signs/symptoms of orthostasis, mental changes or ↓ urine output
Renal function should be checked 1–2 weeks after initiation of therapy and dose changes
ACE-I
Do not use if creatinine >3.0 mg/dL or potassium >5.5 mEq/L
Alternative to ACE-I: angiotensin II receptor blocker, angiotensin receptor neprilysin inhibitor, or hydralazine/nitrate combination
ARNI
Do not administer to patients with a history of angioedema
Do not administer within 36 hours switching from or to an ACE-I
Loop diuretics for volume overload (oral or intravenous)
Maintenance dosing vs. aggressive dosing with symptoms
Add thiazide diuretic for synergistic response as needed
Add aldosterone antagonist, spironolactone 25 mg QD (or less) for classes III and IV
β-Adrenergic blockers (bisoprolol, carvedilol, metoprolol succinate)
Patients do not need to be on target dose of ACE-Is before initiation of a β-blocker
Use in NYHA class II and III patients. May use in NYHA class I patients with history of myocardial infarction or hypertension; class IV patients who are euvolemic
May consider in patients with reactive airway disease or asymptomatic bradycardia but use cautiously if symptoms develop
Digoxin
Dose is based on weight, age, sex, creatinine clearance
Use with caution with concomitant medication that cause hyperkalemia
Start at a low dose (0.125 mg QD). Maintain serum digoxin level of 0.8–2.0 ng/dL

Table 38-2 • HFpEF GENERAL TREATMENT

Goal	Treatment
Reduce venous pressure	Decrease central blood volume Salt restriction Diuretics Venodilation ACE-Is/ARB/ARNI Angiotensin II receptor blockers Nitrates Morphine
Maintain atrial contraction, synchrony	Electrical or pharmacologic cardioversion Sequential AV pacing Biventricular pacing
Prevent tachycardia	Digitalis in atrial fibrillation β-adrenergic blockers Calcium-channel blockers
Treat and prevent ischemia	Nitrates, β-Adrenergic blockers, calcium-channel blockers Coronary revascularization (percutaneous coronary intervention or bypass surgery)
Control hypertension and other comorbidities	ACE-Is, other antihypertensive agents Surgical intervention (e.g., aortic valve repair)
Attenuate neurohormonal activation	ACE-Is, β-Adrenergic blockers
Prevent fibrosis and promote regression of fibrosis	ACE-I or angiotensin II receptor blockers Spironolactone Antianginal agents
Improve ventricular relaxation	β-adrenergic blocker Calcium-channel blockers (in hypertropic cardiomyopathy) Systolic unloading agents

Adapted from Gaasch WH, Shick EC. Heart failure with normal left ventricular ejection fraction: a manifestation of diastolic dysfunction. In: Crawford MH, DiMarco JP, eds. *Cardiology*. Section 5. London: Mosby; 2000:6.1–6.8.

Heart Failure With Preserved Ejection Fraction (HFpEF)

The effects of aging, obesity, and inflammation have a significant impact on diastolic dysfunction. Myocardial disorders associated with diastolic dysfunction, include restrictive, infiltrative, and hypertrophic cardiomyopathy. However, several key mechanistic pathways likely contribute to HFpEF (not just diastolic dysfunction) such as atrial dysfunction, ventricular–vascular stiffening, and chronotropic incompetence.[7] In contrast to HFrEF, there are fewer studies on therapy for HFpEF and unsolved issues in basic and clinical research in HFpEF remain. Unfortunately, efficacious therapies for HFrEF have not demonstrated the same benefit in patients with HFpEF. The goals of medication therapy in HFpEF are to reduce symptoms, manage comorbidities, and minimize risk factors (Table 38-2). HFpEF is predominantly a disease of older women, most with hypertension and LV hypertrophy. CAD is common in patients with HFpEF. As in treatment for HFrEF, ischemia is relieved through standard medical management and revascularization for CAD. Medical management extends to the use of nitrates, β-adrenergic blockers, and CCBs. Volume reduction with diuretics is used to control pulmonary congestion and peripheral edema; diuretics should be titrated carefully. Agents with positive inotropic actions are not indicated if systolic function is normal; these agents appear to provide little benefit and have the potential to worsen pathophysiologic processes, such as myocardial ischemia.

Control of systemic hypertension is vital, with ACE-I or ARBS as first-line treatment. Other antihypertensive agents also may be needed; the recommended targets are the same as those used in general hypertensive populations. Comorbidities are common in patients with HFpEF, complicating treatment and creating a diverse patient population. Consequently, the standard approach to treatment that works relatively well for many patients with HFrEF, is not applicable to patients with HFpEF. One of the suggested approaches for HFpEF management has been to use clinical presentation phenotypes to guide treatment and research. This approach is an active area of investigation (Fig. 38-2).[8,9]

PHARMACOLOGIC MANAGEMENT OF HEART FAILURE

Pharmacologic therapies, as outlined in the guidelines, remain the cornerstone of treatment for patients with HFrEF (Table 38-3).[1] Prior to consideration for any advanced or device therapies, patients should be treated to target doses of a combination of agents to inhibit the neuroendocrine activation of the RAAS and sympathetic systems (SNS) while augmenting the activity of natriuretic peptides (NPs) and other vasodilators.[1,5]

For patients with HFpEF, therapeutic decisions are less defined as the clinical trial evidence is much more limited. Testing new

HFpEF Predisposition Phenotypes	Lung Congestion	+Chronotropic Incompetence	+Pulmonary Hypertension (CpcPH)	+Skeletal muscle weakness	+Atrial Fibrillation
Overweight/obesity/ metabolic syndrome/ type 2 DM	• **Diuretics (loop diuretic in DM)** • **Caloric restriction** • Statins • Inorganic nitrite/nitrate • Sacubitril • Spironolactone	+Rate adaptive atrial pacing	+Pulmonary vasodilators (e.g. PDE5I)	**+Exercise training program**	+Cardioversion +Rate Control **+Anticoagulation**
+Arterial hypertension	+ACEI/ARB	+ACEI/ARB +Rate adaptive atrial pacing	+ACEI/ARB +Pulmonary vasodilators (e.g. PDE5I)	+ACEI/ARB **+Exercise training program**	+ACEI/ARB +Cardioversion +Rate Control **+Anticoagulation**
+Renal dysfunction	+Ultrafiltration if needed	+Ultrafiltration if needed +Rate adaptive atrial pacing	+Ultrafiltration if needed +Pulmonary vasodilators (e.g. PDE5I)	+Ultrafiltration if needed **+Exercise training program**	+Ultrafiltration if needed +Cardioversion +Rate Control **+Anticoagulation**
+CAD	+ACEI +Revascularization	+ACEI +Revascularization +Rate adaptive atrial pacing	+ACEI +Revascularization +Pulmonary vasodilators (e.g. PDE5I)	+ACEI +Revascularization **+Exercise training program**	+ACEI +Revascularization +Cardioversion +Rate Control **+Anticoagulation**

HFpEF Clinical Presentation Phenotypes

Figure 38-2. Phenotype-specific HFpEF treatment strategy using a matrix of predisposition phenotypes and clinical presentation phenotypes. A stepwise approach is proposed that begins in the left hand upper corner of the matrix with general treatment recommendations, presumed to be beneficial to the vast majority of HFpEF patients as they address the presentation phenotype of lung congestion and the predisposition phenotype of overweight/obesity present in >80% of HFpEF patients. Subsequently, supplementary (+) recommendations are suggested for additional predisposition-related phenotypic features when moving downward in the matrix and for additional presentation-related phenotypic features when moving rightward in the matrix. Arterial hypertension, renal dysfunction, and coronary artery disease are proposed as additional predisposition phenotypes. Additional clinical presentation phenotypes, in which specific therapeutic interventions could be meaningful, include chronotropic incompetence, pulmonary hypertension (especially combined precapillary and postcapillary pulmonary hypertension [CpcPH]), skeletal muscle weakness, and atrial fibrillation. Only therapeutic measures indicated in bold are currently established. All other therapeutic measures require further testing in specific phenotypes. ACE-I, angiotensin-converting enzyme inhibitor; ARB, angiotensin II receptor blocker; CAD, coronary artery disease; DM, diabetes mellitus; HFpEF, heart failure with preserved ejection fraction; PDE5I, phosphodiesterase 5 inhibitor. (Shah SJ, Kitzman DW, Borlaug BA, et al. Phenotype-specific treatment of heart failure with preserved ejection fraction: a multiorgan roadmap. *Circulation.* 2016;134[1]:73–90.)

therapies against placebo, rather than in addition to known therapies is currently underway.[9]

Inhibitors of the Renin-Angiotensin-Aldosterone System (RAAS)

The consequences of RAAS and SNS activation in the pathogenesis of HF have been established for over 20 years. Attenuating RAAS activation significantly improves HF outcomes, including mortality, and thus remains a core therapy in the management of HF.

Angiotensin-Converting Enzyme Inhibitors (ACE-Is)

The use of ACE-I has been conclusively shown to improve long-term prognosis in HF.[10,11] ACE-I blocks the formation of angiotensin (AT), which reverses vasoconstriction (reducing afterload), and inhibit endocrine, paracrine, and cellular growth effect of AT.[12] ACE-I also diminishes the release of aldosterone (inhibiting sodium retention) and produces venodilation (reducing preload). In addition to blocking AT formation, this medication class increases levels of bradykinin, promotes vasodilatation, and inhibits maladaptive growth of cardiac cells including ventricular remodeling, hypertrophy, fibrosis, and improves endothelial and vascular function. The unique characteristics of this class of neurohormonal inhibitors support the use of ACE-I as first-line drugs in all patients with HFrEF or asymptomatic LV systolic dysfunction.[1,13] Clinical benefits also extend to patients with evidence of atherosclerotic disease. The doses used should be titrated to target levels.

NSAIDs should be avoided in patients in HF, and particularly in those patients using ACE-I therapy.

Angiotensin Receptor Blockers (ARBs)

The ARBs differ in their mechanism of action compared to ACE-I. Rather than inhibiting the production of angiotensin, thereby decreasing the amount of angiotensin available to bind to AT I and AT II receptors; ARBs block the cell surface receptor for AT I.[11] Hemodynamic effects are similar to those of ACE-I with respect to reducing preload and afterload and increasing cardiac output. The potential concern of this class of drug is that the

Table 38-3 • ORAL PHARMACOLOGIC THERAPIES FOR HFrEF STAGE C

Class Medication	Initial Dose (mg)	Mean Dose in Clinical Trials (mg)	Maximum Dose (mg)
Angiotensin-Converting Enzyme Inhibitors (ACE-Is)			
Captopril	6.25 TID	122.7 QD	50 TID
Enalapril	2.5 BID	16.6 QD	10–20 BID
Fosinopril	5–10 QD	N/A	40 QD
Lisinopril	2.5–5 QD	32.5–35.0 QD	20–40 QD
Perindopril	2	N/A	8–16 QD
Quinapril	5 BID	N/A	20 BID
Ramipril	1.25–2.5 QD	N/A	10 QD
Angiotensin Receptor Blockers (ARBs)			
Candesartan	4–8 QD	24 QD	32 QD
Losartan	25–50 QD	129 QD	50–150 QD
Valsartan	20–40 QD	254 QD	160 QD
Angiotensin Receptor-Neprilysin Inhibitor (ARNI)			
Sacubitril/Valsartan	24/26–49/51 BID	375 QD (Target dose 24/26, 49/51 OR 97/103 BID)	97/103 BID
Aldosterone Receptor Antagonists/Mineralocorticoid Receptor Antagonists (MRAs)			
Eplerenone[a]	25 QD	42.6 QD	50 QD
Spironolactone[a]	12.5–25 QD	26 QD	25 QD or BID
β-Adrenergic Blockers			
Bisoprolol	1.25 QD	8.6 QD	10 QD
Carvedilol	3.125 BID	37 QD	50 BID
Carvedilol CR	10 QD	N/A	80 QD
Metoprolol Succinate	6.25–25 QD	159 QD	200 QD
Diuretics (no established target dose)			
Bumetanide (Loop)	0.5–1.0 QD or BID		10 QD
Chlorthalidone (Thiazide)	12.5–25 QD		100 QD
Furosemide[b] (Loop)	20–40 QD		480 QD
Hydrochlorothiazide[c] (Thiazide)	25 QD		200 QD
Metolazone[b],[c] (Thiazide)	2.5 QD		5 QD
Torsemide[b] (Loop)	10–20 QD		200 QD
Isosorbide Dinitrate and Hydralazine			
Fixed-dose combination	20 isosorbide dinitrate/37.5 hydralazine TID	90 isosorbide dinitrate/ ~175 hydralazine	40 isosorbide dinitrate/ 75 hydralazine TID
Isosorbide dinitrate and hydralazine	20–30 isosorbide dinitrate/ 25–50 hydralazine TID or QD	N/A	40 isosorbide dinitrate/ 100 hydralazine TID
I_f Channel Inhibitor			
Ivabradine	5 BID	6.4 BID	7.5 BID
Cardiac Glycoside			
Digoxin	0.125–0.25 QD 0.125 QD or QOD if >70 years of age, impaired renal function or low body mass		Plasma concentration of 0.5–0.9 ng/mL

[a]May increase serum potassium; do not give if serum potassium >4.7 mEq/L.
[b]Watch potassium carefully; may cause hypokalemia.
[c]Give 30 minutes before loop diuretic.

selective blockade of AT I elevates serum AT, and because the AT II receptors are not blocked, this can increase counter regulatory actions of AT II activation.[14]

Combination therapy with ACE-I and ARBs is not recommended.[15,16] ACE-I rather than ARBs continues to be the agent of choice for blockade of the RAAS in HF, and the use of ARBs is usually reserved for patients truly intolerant to ACE-I because of cough.[14,17]

Angiotensin Receptor-Neprilysin Inhibitors (ARNIs)

An ARNI is a combination of an ARB (valsartan) with an inhibitor of neprilysin (sacubitril), which is an enzyme that degrades NPs, bradykinin, adrenomedullin, and other vasoactive peptides. This drug combination blocks the harmful effects of RAAS while increasing levels of potentially beneficial endogenous NPs degraded by neprilysin and was shown to be superior to enalapril in the PARDIGM-HF study.[18] NPs cause vasodilation by promoting smooth muscle relaxation and indirectly by inhibiting RAAS activity and endothelin-1 production (Fig. 38-3).[19,20] Thus, ARNIs have more than one mechanism to attenuate the effects of an upregulated RAAS. As with any ACE-I and ARB, hyperkalemia is a concern. Patients should *not* receive an ARNI concomitantly with an ACE-I or within 36 hours of the last dose of an ACE-I.[5]

Mineral Receptor Antagonists (MRAs)

ACE-I does block the effect of the RAAS, however, after several months of ACE-I treatment, there can be an increase in aldosterone levels. Aldosterone promotes sodium retention (edema), release of cytokines and growth factors, myocardial and vascular

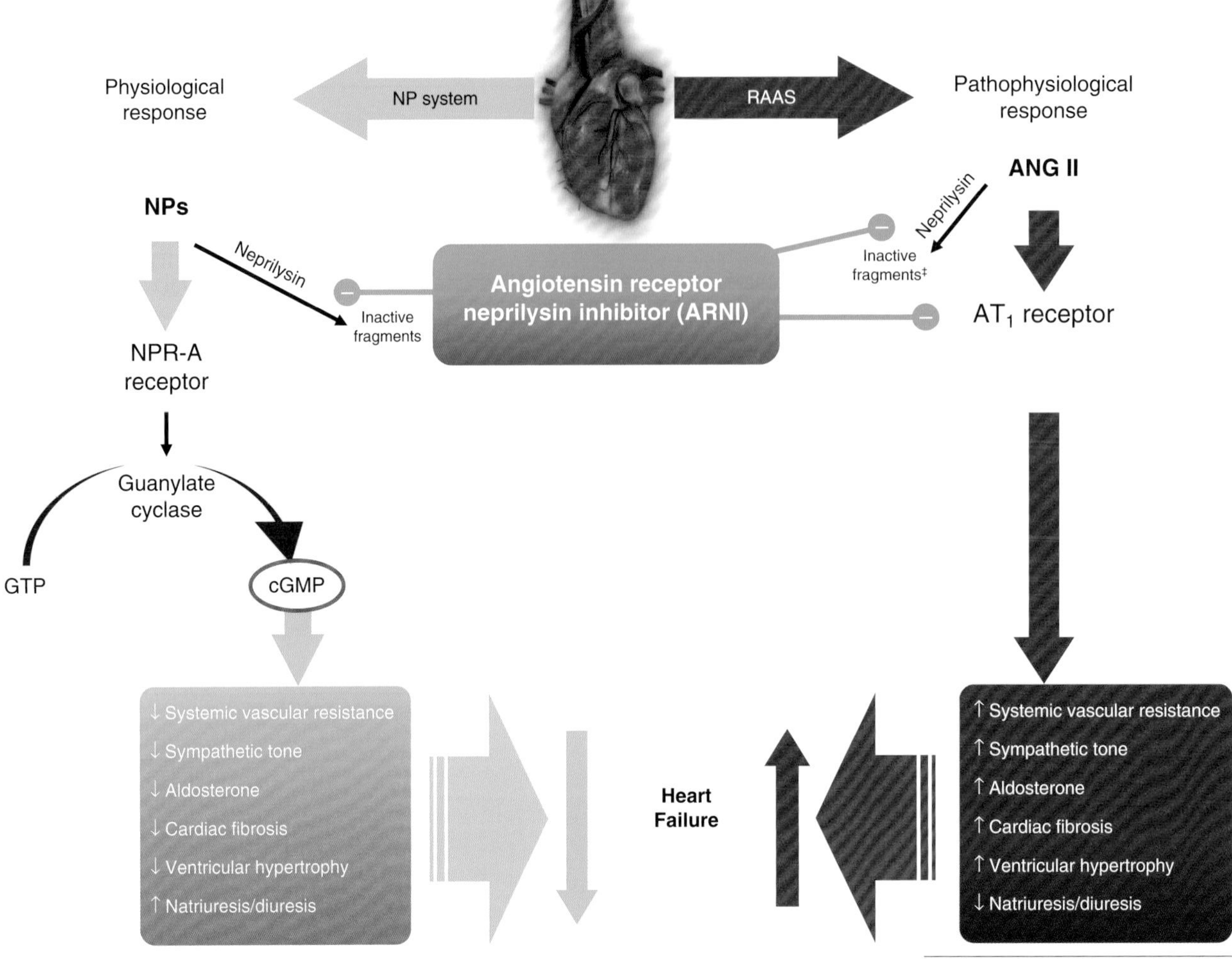

Figure 38-3. Angiotensin receptor neprilysin inhibitors have the potential to modulate two counterregulatory neurohormonal systems in HF: the renin-angiotensin-aldosterone system and natriuretic peptide system. ANG, angiotensin; ARNI, angiotensin receptor neprilysin inhibitor; AT1, angiotensin type 1; cGMP, cyclic guanosine monophosphate; GTP, guanosine-5'-triphosphate; NP, natriuretic peptide (e.g., atrial natriuretic peptide [ANP], B-type natriuretic peptide[BNP], etc.); NPR-A, NP receptor-A; RAAS, renin–angiotensin–aldosterone system; ‡, in vitro evidence. (Langenickel TH, Dole WP. Angiotensin receptor-neprilysin inhibition with LCZ696: a novel approach for the treatment of heart failure. *Drug Discov Today Ther Strateg.* 2012;9[4]:e131–e139.)

fibroses (through autocrine or paracrine effects), baroreceptor dysfunction, and progressive remodeling.[21–23] The addition of a low-dose MRA (spironolactone or eplerenone) to standard therapy for patients with ACC/AHA stage C and/or D (NYHA classes II to IV; LVEF less than or equal to 35%) promotes a therapeutic effect and reduces morbidity and mortality.[1] The benefit of this class of drug is not primarily a diuretic effect; spironolactone lessens myocardial fibrosis, significantly reduces plasma brain natriuretic peptide (BNP) levels, and improves LV remodeling and cardiac sympathetic nerve activity (which may reduce ventricular arrhythmias and SCD).[24] In patients with HFpEF (with EF greater than or equal to 45%), elevated BNP levels or HF admission within 1 year, eGFR greater than 30 mL/min, creatinine less than 2.5 mg/dL, potassium less than 5.0 mEq/L, an MRA may help decrease hospitalizations.[5] Best practice necessitates the monitoring of potassium, renal function, and diuretic dosing while receiving MRA medications in all patients, upon initiation and during follow-up to minimize the risk of hyperkalemia and worsening renal function.

β-Adrenergic Blockers

Cardiac myocytes have three adrenergic receptors (β_1, β_2, and α_1) that are coupled with inotropic and chronotropic responses, cardiac myocyte growth, toxicity, and apoptosis.[25] Although β_1 and β_2 receptors are present in the normal human myocardium, in the failing myocardium β_1 receptors are downregulated and β_2 receptors predominate. Neurohormonal activity in HF can be blunted by administering second- and third-generation β-adrenergic blockers.[26,27] Metoprolol (succinate) and bisoprolol are second-generation selective β_1-adrenergic blockers.[27] Carvedilol is a nonselective β-adrenergic agent, blocking α_1, β_1 and β_2 receptors. At low doses, carvedilol exhibits β_1 selectivity; at higher target doses, it blocks all three adrenergic receptors, allowing for renal and systemic vasodilatation. β-adrenergic blockers protect the failing myocardium from the deleterious effects of the neurohormonal activity associated with HF. β-Adrenergic blockers should be administered to stable patients upon a confirmed diagnosis of HFrEF without delay (ACC/AHA stages C and D).

Table 38-4 • MANAGING SIDE EFFECTS DURING TITRATION OF β-BLOCKERS[a]

Vasodilator effects (dizziness or lightheadedness)
Administer medication with food
Administer β-blocker 2 hours before vasodilator agents or stagger doses of vasodilator medications or other medications affecting blood pressure
Reduce diuretic or vasodilator therapy temporarily
Reduce β-adrenergic blocker dose if symptoms persist after diuretic and vasodilator decreased
Significant bradycardia (heart rate <60–65 bpm with symptoms)
Reduce β-adrenergic blocker dose
Monitor digoxin level and dose, renal function
Stop digoxin or reduce digoxin dose
Clarify concomitant drug use (amiodarone, calcium-channel blockers)
Worsening heart failure (dyspnea, weight gain, edema)
Increase diuretic dose (if QD increase to BID; if BID, consider increasing the dose)
Review and intensify salt restriction
Reduce β-adrenergic blocker dose (if symptoms persist after diuretic increased)

[a]Do not continue titration until symptoms are resolved.

Generally, therapy should be initiated at low doses and uptitrated slowly at 2-week intervals.[1] Patients do need not be taking a high dose of ACE-I prior to the initiation of a β-adrenergic blocker. Table 38-4 describes strategies for management of side effects during titration of β-adrenergic blockers. β-adrenergic blockers have been shown in multiple studies to reduce mortality, morbidity, and improve symptoms.[28–33] However, the positive findings demonstrated in clinical trials is not a class effect, bisoprolol, carvedilol, metropolol succinate are indicated for the treatment of HF. The safety and efficacy of β-adrenergic blockers in asymptomatic LV dysfunction has not been fully studied.

Diuretics

The kidney is the target organ of multiple neurohormonal and hemodynamic changes that occur in HF.[34] Diuretics and dietary salt restriction exert their primary benefit by decreasing extracellular fluid and intravascular blood volume; increasing urinary sodium excretion (natriuresis) and improving signs and symptoms of fluid retention. The elimination of dependent edema reduces tissue pressure, opposes venous pooling, and therefore improves the capacitance of the venous system. Similarly, the decrease in intravascular volume also reduces ventricular preload directly, thereby helping to diminish the filling pressures in the pulmonary and systemic circulations. Loop diuretics have emerged as the preferred agent for patients with HF; thiazide diuretics may be helpful in patients with hypertension. Administration of the MRA spironolactone or eplerenone should be considered (see previous section). Patients may become refractory to a fixed dose of diuretics if they consume large amounts of sodium, take agents that block the effect of diuretics (e.g., NSAIDs) or have renal impairment or perfusion deficits. Diuretic resistance can often be overcome by changing the route or frequency of diuretic administration (intravenous or continuous) or a combination of different diuretic classes with multiple sites of action.[1]

Vasodilator Therapy

The venous and arterial beds are often inappropriately constricted in patients with HF. Venoconstriction tends to displace blood in the thorax causing pulmonary congestion, whereas arteriolar constriction increases the impedance to LV emptying.

Arteriolar dilatation results in a reduction of afterload and may augment cardiac output, whereas venodilation tends to produce a reduction in preload, lowers ventricular filling pressure, and reduces symptoms of pulmonary congestion. Vasodilators may be separated into three categories: venous dilators (preload reducers), arterial dilators (afterload reducers), and mixed venous and arterial dilators (preload and afterload reducers).

Venous Dilators

Nitroglycerin and the closely related isosorbide dinitrate are primarily reducers of preload because they dilate the systemic veins and reduce venous return, ultimately to reduce intracardiac filling pressures. Nitrates are indicated for the treatment of angina in patients with HF.[1]

Arterial Dilators

As a direct arteriolar vasodilator with direct inotropic effects, hydralazine can improve LV function by reducing afterload and myocardial oxygen consumption, augmenting stroke volume, and improving cardiac output.

Combined Venous Arterial Dilators

A combination of hydralazine with isosorbide dinitrate augments the effect of improved preload and afterload, may reduce pathologic remodeling and offers a therapeutic option for patients who cannot tolerate an ACE-I, ARB, or ARNI. The combination of hydralazine with isosorbide dinitrate offers significant benefit for African Americans with HFrEF who remain symptomatic despite guideline-directed therapy.[35] It has been hypothesized that the combination of hydralazine with nitrates enhances nitric oxide (NO) bioavailability; nitrates are NO donors and hydralazine is an antioxidant that reduces NO depletion. The combination of hydralazine with isosorbide dinitrate is available as a fixed dose or administered separately, although adherence may be poor with separate dosing because of the large number of tablets required.

Current Inhibitors or Hyperpolarization-Activated Cyclic Nucleotide–Gated (HCN) Channel Blockers

The hyperpolarization-activated cyclic nucleotide (HCN)–modulated channels are voltage-dependent ion channels (f channels), conducting both Na^+ and K^+ current, that contribute to the pacemaker activity in the sinoatrial (SA) node. Ivabradine is an HCN channel blocker and selective inhibitor of the I_f current within the SA node. Disruption of the I_f current slows firing of the SA node, thereby reducing heart rate. In HF, an elevated heart rate is likely an indicator of sympathetic activation and is associated with worse outcomes. The postulated detrimental effects of an elevated heart rate include increases in myocardial oxygen consumption, increases in shear stress, and decreases in myocardial perfusion.[36] Thus, the benefit of ivabradine is associated with reduced sinus rate. For patients with symptomatic chronic stable HFrEF with an EF less than or equal to 35%, in sinus rhythm with a resting heart rate greater than or equal to 70 beats per minute (bpm), and who are either on a maximum tolerated dose of a β-adrenergic blockers or have a contraindication to β-adrenergic blocker use, treatment with ivabradine may be indicated.[5] Ivabradine reduces the risk of HF-related hospital admission and death from HF in patients with HFrEF.[5] Concurrent treatment should include ACE-I, ARB or ARNI and an MRA.

Cardiac Glycosides

The oral cardiac glycoside, digitalis (most common formulation is digoxin), has important effects in HF, including augmenting contractility (positive inotropy), slowing of the sinus pacemaker and atrioventricular conduction (negative chronotropy and dromotropy), and neurohormonal modulating effects including a sympathoinhibitory effect.[37] Although the hemodynamic, neurohormonal, and electrophysiologic effects of digoxin seem beneficial, data supporting survival are lacking. Evidence from clinical trials indicates digoxin improves symptoms and reduces hospitalizations, especially in symptomatic patients with advanced HFrEF.[38] Digoxin is added to optimal therapy for HFrEF (ACE-I, ARB, or ARNI; β-adrenergic blocker; MRA; and diuretic). The decision to add or withdraw digoxin should be made after careful consideration of the patient's renal function and the risk for digoxin toxicity, as digoxin has a narrow therapeutic window. Dosing is then individualized based upon renal function, ideal body weight, and concomitant medications that may alter serum digoxin levels or serum potassium levels. Prior to initiation and during the use of digoxin, serum electrolytes levels including potassium, magnesium, and calcium should be assessed. In patients with HFrEF, with ideal body weight and creatinine clearance greater than or equal to 30 mL/min, the starting dose is 0.125 mg/day to achieve a serum level between 0.5 and 0.8 ng/mL, higher concentrations are associated with increased mortality.[39,40] In patients with HFrEF with atrial fibrillation and rapid ventricular response, higher doses are not recommended. If amiodarone is added, the dose of digoxin should be reduced as inhibitors of P-glycoprotein efflux transporters can increase serum digoxin levels. Digoxin should be prescribed cautiously, if at all, to patients with cardiac amyloidosis as the medication binds to amyloid fibrils and may increase the risk of digoxin toxicity.

Calcium-Channel Blockers (CCBs)

The potential benefits of CCBs are related to their ability to decrease afterload, slow heart rate and exert an anti-ischemic effect. However, some CCBs have negative inotrope activity and failed to demonstrate any functional or mortality benefit in patient with HF. Amlodipine may be of benefit in patients with HF and diastolic dysfunction because of improvement of diastolic relaxation, control of blood pressure, and prevention of myocardial ischemia. Amlodipine had neutral effects on morbidity and mortality in large clinical trials.

Natriuretic Peptides

NPs, such as nesiritide, are intravenously delivered synthetic compounds that mimic endogenous BNP which promotes diuresis and natriuresis with vasodilatory properties that suppress neurohormonal activation, indirectly improving myocardial performance.[41,42] Nesiritide in the acute setting has been shown to reduce dyspnea, but nesiritide use may worsen renal function and increase mortality and thus it should be used cautiously.[43,44]

Antiarrhythmics

HF is the most arrhythmogenic disorder in cardiovascular disease. Management of arrhythmias in patients with HF is complex and remains far from satisfactory. Many patients with HF experience frequent and complex ventricular tachyarrhythmias, and the imminent risk of sudden cardiac death (SCD) is present for all patients with HF. Experimental and clinical evidence indicates that circulatory neurohormonal and electrolyte deficits of potassium and magnesium interact to provoke malignant ventricular ectopic rhythms. In general, antiarrhythmic therapy in patients with HF is reserved for symptomatic arrhythmias or to control the ventricular response to atrial fibrillation.[1]

Class I and III antiarrhythmics, which are proarrhythmic demonstrated an increased mortality in patients with ventricular arrhythmias in HF.[45] β-Adrenergic blockers can prevent up to 40% to 50% of SCD, which adds to their benefit in managing patients with HF.[30] Amiodarone and dofetilide are the only agents to have neutral effects on mortality and are the preferred agents in HF. Survival of patients with life-threatening arrhythmias is improved with ICD placement as compared with antiarrhythmic pharmacologic therapy.[46,47] Amiodarone is the preferred medication in patients with HF with supraventricular tachycardia not controlled by β-adrenergic blockers or digoxin, or for those patients who are not candidates for ICD placement.[1,48]

Adjunctive Therapy

Omega-3 polyunsaturated acid (PUFA) supplements may be reasonable to use in patients with HFrEF and HFpEF to reduce the risk of cardiovascular events. The therapy has been safe and well tolerated but the optimal dose and formulation of PUFA supplementation remains to be defined.[1]

Other Important Pharmacologic Considerations

Tachycardia

Tachycardia of any etiology, even sinus tachycardia, is poorly tolerated and has a negative impact on diastolic function. This is especially true for patients with HFpEF and atrial fibrillation with a rapid ventricular response. Allowing maximum time for diastolic filling and lowering diastolic filling pressure can be accomplished by rate-slowing agents, such as β-adrenergic blockers or a CCB. Theoretically, benefits of a slower rate include increased coronary perfusion time, decreased myocardial oxygen requirements, and increased myocardial efficiency. β-adrenergic blockers and CCBs (amlodipine or diltiazem) have been used to prevent excessive tachycardia and also have been shown to improve some exercise parameters. CCBs have important lusitropic effects that enhance ventricular relaxation. β-Adrenergic blockers also improve LV relaxation by decreasing myocardial oxygen consumption and ischemia.

Atrial fibrillation with rapid ventricular response is poorly tolerated in patients with HF, and electrical or chemical cardioversion should be considered to restore sinus rhythm. β-adrenergic blockers and/or amiodarone may be required to control and prevent atrial fibrillation. Radiofrequency ablation and atrioventricular pacing may also be used.

Thromboembolism

Patients with chronic HFrEF are at increased risk for thromboembolic formation and events due to the stasis of blood in enlarged hypokinetic atrial and ventricular chambers. Embolization of these thrombi into the systemic circulation can result in transient ischemic attacks and cerebrovascular accidents.[49] However, in large scale clinical trials, the risk of thromboembolism was 1% to 3% per year, even in those with a low EF and echocardiographic evidence of an intracardiac thrombi. Several studies have attempted to determine whether chronic anticoagulation reduces this transient ischemic attack or cerebrovascular accident risk, but their findings are variable.[50,51] Due to an increased risk of major bleeding with anticoagulation, this therapy is recommended only for patients with permanent/persistent/paroxysmal atrial fibrillation and an additional risk factor for embolic stroke, whether they

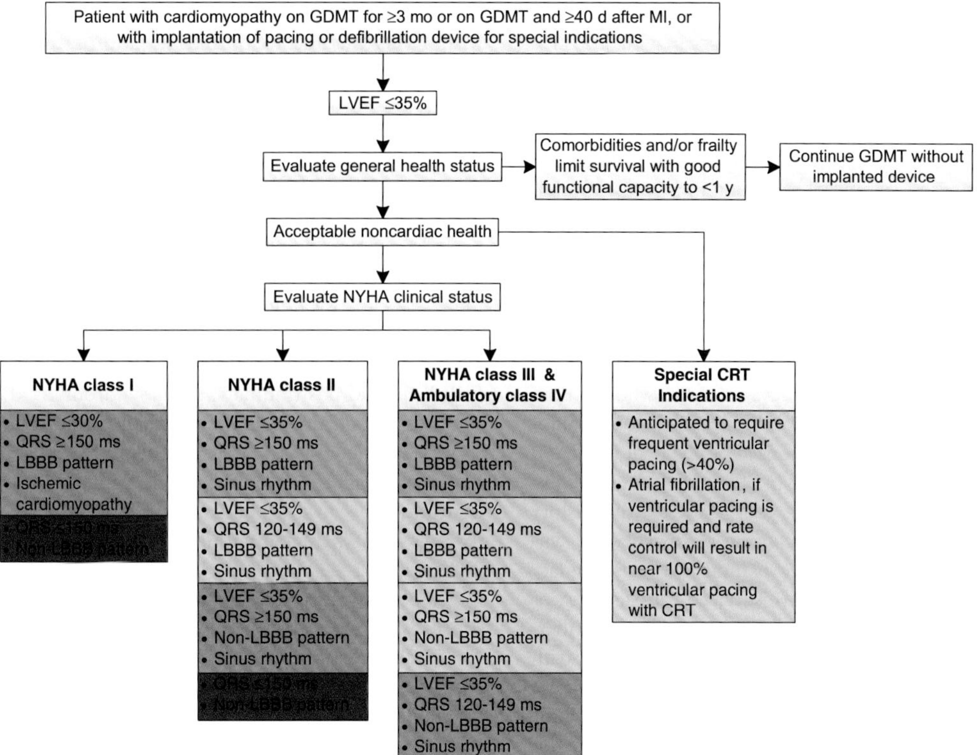

Colors correspond to the class of recommendations in the ACCF/AHA Table 1.

Benefit for NYHA class I and II patients has only been shown in CRT-D trials, and while patients may not experience immediate symptomatic benefit, late remodeling may be avoided along with long-term HF consequences. There are no trials that support CRT-pacing (without ICD) in NYHA class I and II patients. Thus, it is anticipated these patients would receive CRT-D unless clinical reasons or personal wishes make CRT-pacing more appropriate. In patients who are NYHA class III and ambulatory class IV, CRT-D may be chosen but clinical reasons and personal wishes may make CRT-pacing appropriate to improve symptoms and quality of life when an ICD is not expected to produce meaningful benefit in survival.

Figure 38-4. Indications for CRT therapy algorithm. CRT, cardiac resynchronization therapy; CRT-D, cardiac resynchronization therapy defibrillator; GDMT, guideline-directed medical therapy; HF, heart failure; ICD, implantable cardioverter defibrillator; LBBB, left bundle-branch block; LVEF, left ventricular ejection fraction; MI, myocardial infarction; NYHA, New York Heart Association. (Yancy CW, Jessup M, Bozkurt B, et al. 2013 ACCF/AHA guideline for the management of heart failure: a report of the American College of Cardiology Foundation/American Heart Association Task Force on Practice Guidelines. *J Am Coll Cardiol.* 2013;62[16]:e147–e239.)

receive rate of rhythm control.[1] Trials with the newer anticoagulants have comparable efficacy and safety to warfarin. The benefit of low-dose aspirin in patients with HFrEF of a nonischemia etiology is unknown, but patients who are taking aspirin do have an increased risk of HF events.[52]

Pharmacologic Agents to Avoid in HF

Several pharmacologic agents should be avoided in the treatment of HF. Most antiarrhythmic agents, most CCBs (except amlodipine), NSAIDs, and thiazolidinediones should be avoided because these drugs are known to adversely impact clinical outcomes and are potentially harmful. If patients are already taking these agents, attempt to withdraw the medication whenever possible. Nutritional supplementation or hormonal therapy is not recommended for those with HFrEF.[1]

CARDIOVASCULAR IMPLANTABLE ELECTRONIC DEVICES (CIEDs)

In patients with HF, cardiovascular implantable electronic device (CIED) therapy extends to biventricular pacing and implantable cardioverter defibrillators (ICDs), or a combination of these therapies. Implanted cardiac device therapy has become a mainstay of GDMT for patients with HFrEF. Key indications for device therapy are aimed at primary and secondary prevention of SCD and cardiac resynchronization therapy (CRT) aimed at improving health outcomes in patients with reduced LVEF and prolonged QRS duration. The biventricular ICD (BiVICD) combines CRT and ICD technology for those who meet criteria for cardiac resynchronization and ICD therapy. The ACC/AHA recommends CIED based upon disease etiology, HF stage, NYHA class, LVEF, electrocardiographic criteria, and cardiac rhythm (Fig. 38-4).[1] Further, technology is rapidly advancing and becoming more accurate at hemodynamic monitoring to trend heart rate variability, activity, and intrathoracic impedance.

Hemodynamic monitoring provides clinical insight into stability and functional status and detects hypervolemia at subclinical levels. Advances in device technology have ushered in a new era of device therapy for strengthening cardiac contractility in patients with moderate to severe HF with normal QRS.

Device Therapy for Primary Prevention of Sudden Cardiac Death in High-Risk Populations

It is well established that patients with HFrEF have an increased incidence of ventricular tachyarrhythmias, experiencing a nine times higher risk of SCD than the general population.[53] SCD is the primary cause of mortality among patients with HFrEF, with an LVEF less than or equal to 30% the most significant independent risk factor for SCD.[54] The most significant predictor of SCD in patients with HFrEF is a syncopal event with unidentifiable etiology.[53]

The ICD has changed the landscape of cardiovascular care. ICD therapy is associated with a significant reduction in all-cause mortality in patients with ischemic and nonischemic cardiomyopathy.[5,55] ICDs are the treatment of choice for prevention of SCD in patients with LV dysfunction who have documented ventricular tachycardia (VT) or ventricular fibrillation (VF).[1,56] Given the substantial reduction in mortality with ICD therapy, ICD is indicated for the primary prevention of SCD in patients with nonischemic dilated cardiomyopathy or IHD at least 40 days post-MI who have an LVEF of less than or equal to 35% and NYHA class II to III symptoms after at least 3 to 6 months of optimized GDMT, or if after 40 days post-MI, LVEF less than or equal to 30%, NYHA class I and the patient is expected to live for over a year.[1] Patients with history of ventricular tachyarrhythmias, cardiac arrest, or unexplained syncope are at highest risk.[1,55] ICD therapy is indicated for secondary prevention of SCD in patients who have survived cardiac arrest or sustained VT. While there is strong evidence to support ICD therapy, device therapy is considered on an individualized basis with patient's highly involved in shared decision making that considers the patient goals and preferences. Documentation of shared decision making should be included in the medical record. ICD is not recommended in those who do not have a reasonable expectation for meaningful survival greater than 1 year.[1] The benefit of ICD is unclear for patients with a high risk of nonsudden death. Predictors of high risk of nonsudden death include frequent hospitalizations, advanced frailty, or comorbidities such as a systemic malignancy or severe renal dysfunction.[1]

ICD technology has advanced significantly and continues to be highly refined to optimize detection and discrimination of cardiac arrhythmias and deliver specialized treatments. Algorithms are aimed at detecting onset of arrhythmias, ventricular rates, and QRS morphology that discriminates supraventricular tachycardias from VTs. Upon detection of VT or VF, the device responds with an individualized pre-programed pacing, known as antitachycardic pacing (ATP) and/or shock therapy. ATP is a low-voltage pacing function that delivers cycles of pacing to promote the termination of VT. ATP is often successful at terminating sustained monomorphic VT and rarely successful at terminating sustained polymorphic VT. ATP is not uncomfortable and when used as first-line therapy has been shown to reduce shock therapy by 70%.[57] In the event that ATP does not terminate VT with pre-programmed therapy, a high voltage shock is delivered. ICD shock voltage is programmed to maximize clinical benefit balancing defibrillator charge time, delivering adequate electrical output to terminate VT or VF, yet minimize myocardial depression in the long term, and preserve the generator life. Typically, ICD defibrillation is set between 20 and 40 J. In the event that ATP does not terminate a ventricular tachyarrhythmia, ICD shock is delivered and one shock will terminate 80% to 90% of ventricular tachyarrhythmias and two shocks will terminate 98% of ventricular tachyarrhythmias.[58]

Device Limitations and Considerations

While ICD therapy is well supported in primary and secondary prevention of SCD in patients with HFrEF despite optimized therapy, there are considerations for living with a device and device limitations. Common problems encountered in patients with ICDs include inappropriate and/or frequent appropriate shocks, device under-detection of ventricular tachyarrhythmias, psychological distress, and reduced quality of life.

Inappropriate and/or frequent shocks is associated with worsening LV function and mortality. Device technology has advanced and programmable algorithms are able to mitigate device therapy complications and circumvent inappropriate and/or frequent shocks.

ICD implantation has been shown to be associated with a combination of physiologic and psychological sequelae and there is a higher risk of psychological distress with the occurrence of inappropriate and/or frequent shocks. Psychological syndromes include anxiety, depression, social withdrawal, phantom shocks, decreased HRQOL, and posttraumatic stress syndrome.[1,55] Phantom shocks resulting from fear and anxiety have been reported.[55] Inappropriate shocks occur in 10% to 24% of patients. Several large clinical trials have found that inappropriate shock significantly increases the risk of death and is an independent predictor of mortality.[48,59] Mortality rates are 10% higher within the first few days after a first shock, 25% within 1 year and 40% by 2 years.[60] Appropriate shocks also increased mortality when compared with patients without ICD shocks, who receive ATP only.

Misclassification of supraventricular tachycardia accounts for approximately one-third of inappropriate shocks with rapid atrial fibrillation being the primary culprit.[60–62] Ventricular interval regularity stabilizes in rapid atrial fibrillation at rates greater than 170 bpm, making discriminating VT from atrial fibrillation at this rate and interval less reliable.

Interval stability is also unreliable if drugs such as amiodarone cause monomorphic VT to become irregular or induce polymorphic VT to slow into the SVT-VT discrimination zone.[55] Programming technology that allows for faster VT/VF detection rates, longer detection time, and SVT discriminatory settings reduce inappropriate shocks and improves survival.[55] ATP delivery reduces appropriate and inappropriate shocks, syncopal episodes, and improves quality of life.[55] Additionally, antiarrhythmic drugs and catheter ablation can decrease the number of ICD shocks.[55]

Cardiac Resynchronization Therapy

Cardiac remodeling in systolic HF is associated with ventricular conduction delays. Ventricular conduction delays alter cardiac mechanical function causing suboptimal ventricular filling, reduced LV contractility, prolonged mitral regurgitation (MR), and paradoxical septal wall motion.[63] This mechanical distortion is known as ventricular dyssynchrony and occurs in approximately one-third of patients with advanced HF.[1] Ventricular dyssynchrony is associated with reduced exercise function, quality of life, and increases mortality in patients with systolic HF.[53] Ventricular dyssynchrony is defined as a prolonged QRS duration greater than 120 milliseconds (ms) on electrocardiogram (ECG). While ventricular dyssynchrony is identifiable on echocardiogram, there are currently no established imaging criteria of ventricular dyssynchrony to guide device therapy.

CRT or biventricular pacing is the simultaneous pacing of the right and left ventricles with the goal to improve ventricular synchrony. CRT has been shown to improve ventricular contraction, diminish secondary MR, reverse LV remodeling, and sustain LVEF improvement in those with HFrEF and a wide QRS complex.[1] The addition of CRT in patients with HFrEF with QRS prolongation who are on optimized GDMT with sinus rhythm has been shown to significantly decrease mortality and hospitalization, reverse LV remodeling and improve quality of life and exercise capacity.[1] Another clinically important benefit of CRT is that there is an increase in blood pressure that allows for upward titration of neurohormonal antagonist, which can contribute to improved LV function.[1] While CRT has demonstrated improvement in health outcomes in the overall HF population, approximately 25% of patients do not respond to therapy.[53]

CRT is strongly recommended for patients with LVEF of less than or equal to 35% with NYHA class II to IV ambulatory symptoms on GDMT in the setting of sinus rhythm and left bundle branch block with a QRS duration of 150 ms or greater.[1] Further, there is sufficient evidence to support CRT benefit in patients with HFrEF with NYHA class II to IV ambulatory symptoms on GDMT with LVEF less than 35% with an LBBB with QRS duration of 120 to 149 ms.[1] CRT may also be considered for (1) patients with HFrEF on GDMT and NYHA class III to IV ambulatory symptoms on GDMT with a QRS duration 120 to 149 ms without an LBBB pattern, (2) patients with NYHA class II symptoms on GDMT with an LVEF less than or equal to 35% with a non-LBBB pattern QRS duration 150 ms or greater, and (3) patients with an ischemic etiology of HFrEF with NYHA class I symptoms on GDMT with LVEF of less than or equal to 30%, in the presence of an LBBB with QRS duration 150 ms or greater.[1] CRT is not recommended for patients with NYHA class I or II symptoms with a non-LBBB pattern with QRS duration less than 150 ms. Further, CRT is not recommended when a patient's comorbidities or frailty limits survival to less than 1 year (see Fig. 38-4).[1]

Implantable Device-Guided Management

Cardiac implantable electronic device (CIED) technologies continue to alter HF surveillance and disease management. In-person and remote monitoring of implantable devices in HF management for the prognostication of subclinical acute decompensated HF allows for preemptive treatment. Studies evaluating the ability of thoracic impedance, to predict the onset of acute HF have demonstrated mixed findings. The positive predictive value of thoracic impedance to detect worsening HF is 38% to 60% and some studies have shown benefit in impedance-guided therapy.[55,64,65] Not surprisingly, another study found that thoracic impedance monitoring for subclinical acute decompensated HF increases HF-related hospitalizations.[66] Thoracic impedance may detect worsening HF, though can yield false positives in the setting of other etiologies.[67]

Multiparameter telemonitoring has been shown to improve outcomes in patients with HF. The In-TIME trial found that automatic multiparameter telemonitoring may improve clinical outcomes in patients with HF.[66] The In-TIME trial utilized physiologic and technical data to evaluate ventricular and atrial tachyarrhythmias, percentage of biventricular pacing, and patient activity to predict clinical deterioration followed by phone interview to assess the patient's symptoms and a clinic follow up was scheduled. This study found that multiparameter telemonitoring reduced clinical incidence and all-cause mortality, with early identification of tachyarrhythmias and suboptimal device function and patient interviews revealed symptomatic worsening or medication noncompliance, contributing to improved outcomes.[66] Additionally, implantable and wireless remotely monitored pulmonary artery hemodynamic monitoring for elevated pulmonary artery pressure and subsequent preemptive treatment has been shown to reduce hospitalizations by 37%.[68,69]

Cardiac Contractility Modulation

Cardiac contractility modulation (CCM) is a newly FDA-approved therapy for patients with HF aimed at strengthening cardiac muscular contraction. The CCM system includes a pulse generator with an externally rechargeable battery, an atrial lead and two ventricular leads on the right ventricular septum. The CCM device produces nonexcitatory, intermittently delivered, electrical signals during the refractory period, strengthening cardiac contractility. CCM is approved for patients with NYHA class III HF with LVEF 25% to 45% in sinus rhythm and are symptomatic despite optimized medical therapy and not eligible for CRT.[70] CCM has been shown to be safe and significantly improves exercise tolerance, NYHA functional status, and quality of life in patients with HF with LVEF 25% to 45% in sinus rhythm who are not eligible for CRT and symptomatic despite optimized GDMT.[71,72]

Device Deactivation at End of Life

Caregivers and patients experiencing end of life care may have questions about device deactivation. Patients actively dying with an active ICD experience uncomfortable shock, even late in the dying process. Maintaining proactive and open communication with the patient and caregivers about the patient's status and goals for end of life is important. Ethical care encompasses ensuring the patient or decision-making surrogate is fully aware of ICD function and alternatives during the dying process. ICD deactivation requests from patients and caregivers should be honored, providing the patient or decision-making surrogate has been fully informed of the natural dying process and the consequences of device deactivation. Device deactivation should be accompanied by a do not resuscitate order.[55,73]

Cardiovascular External Electronic Devices

The wearable cardioverter defibrillator (WCD) is vest-like apparatus that monitors for cardiac arrhythmias and delivers a shock for ventricular arrhythmias.[74] The WCD is designed for those who are at risk for SCD. The WCD is intended to be worn under the clothing at all times except during bathing or showering. In patients with newly diagnosed cardiomyopathy, approximately 40% of patients on GDMT will experience LV recovery (LVEF greater than 40%) within 6 months and have low risk of mortality.[75] In these patients, WCD as a "bridge to ICD," is considered reasonable (class IIB LOE B-NR), given the safety and effectiveness of the device, however the benefit is uncertain in this population.[76] The Heart Rhythm Society recommends a WCD in patients with a history of SCD or sustained ventricular arrhythmias in whom removal of the ICD is required.[76] WCDs are considered beneficial and safe, successfully treating ventricular arrhythmias is comparable to ICD.[77,78] The rates of inappropriate shock have been found to occur in less than 2% of patients.[74,77,78] Limitations to the WCD is the lack of ATP functionality. Barriers to use include discomfort and interference in lifestyle and activity. Discontinuation due to lifestyle and comfort, may be as high as 25%.[79]

COMPREHENSIVE MANAGEMENT OF HF

Prevention of HF

The nurse may be the primary person to identify the risk factors for or presence of HF. The most effective mechanisms for reducing the incidence of HF is through prevention, early identification of HF risk, and implementation of targeted interventions. The importance of early diagnosis is highlighted by evidence that treatment of asymptomatic patients can slow progression and improve clinical outcomes.[80,81] Screening for hypertension, IHD, diabetes, dyslipidemia, metabolic syndrome, smoking, pulmonary conditions, valvular disorders, and congenital heart disease may ensure aggressive treatment and subsequently prevent or delay the syndrome of HF.

Comorbidities Related to HF Management and Treatment

HF is usually an end-stage condition on the trajectory of other cardiovascular and noncardiovascular diseases, with almost all patients with HF having other illnesses.

Primary etiologies of HF include hypertension and IHD. Other associated conditions that may require concomitant management include tachycardia, dyslipidemia, obesity, diabetes, infectious and noninfectious inflammatory disorders, endocrine abnormalities, toxic substance use disorders, cardiotoxic medications, pregnancy, iron overload, amyloidosis, sarcoidosis, and emotional stress. The management of these etiologies and comorbidities are an essential component in the management of HF, however both healthcare providers and patients have difficulty in managing HF in the context of multiple comorbid conditions.

Hypertension

More than any other modifiable cardiovascular disease risk factor, hypertension is most commonly associated with CVD-related deaths.[82] Systolic and diastolic hypertension are major risk factor for the development of HFpEF and HFrEF, and occurs in approximately 75% of patients with chronic HF.[82] Hypertension is the most common etiology of HFpEF, occurring in 605 to 89% of participants in large studies.[82] HFpEF is most common in older women with hypertension.

Updated guidelines include adjusted parameters for the classification of hypertension, and under the new definitions about 46% of the U.S. adult population has high blood pressure.[82] Current categorizations include normal (less than 120/80 mm Hg), elevated (SBP 120 to 129 mm Hg and DBP less than 80), stage 1 (SBP 130 to 139 mm Hg or DBP 80 to 89 mm Hg), and stage 2 (SBP greater than or equal to 140 mm Hg or DBP greater than or equal to 90 mm Hg).[82]

Multi-modal treatment with lifestyle and antihypertensive therapy is required for most people with hypertension. Overall control of hypertension in adults has been estimated at 55%.[82] In patients at risk for HF, the current guidelines recommend anti hypertensive therapy with a goal BP less than 130/80 mm Hg. The management of hypertension is imperative for the prevention of HF and treatment of HF symptoms and progression. There is robust patient outcome data associated with treatment, effectively reducing the risk of HF by almost 50%.[1] Effective medications include diuretics, ACE-I, ARBs and β-adrenergic blockers. The diagnosis, management, and treatment of hypertension should be provided through recommendations of published guidelines.

Ischemic Heart Disease

There is a known correlation of IHD and the development of HF. After MI the 5-year risk of developing HF is 7% for men and 12% for women 40 to 69 years of age.[1] For patients greater than 70 years, this risk increases to 22% and 25% for men and women, respectively.[1] Many of the interventions and guideline-directed therapies for IHD and HF are synergistic and complementary. The diagnosis, management, and treatment of IHD should be provided through recommendations of published guidelines.

Renal Disease

In the syndrome of HF, the heart and kidneys are interrelated. In all phenotypes of HF, renal disease occurs frequently and is associated with higher morbidity and mortality.[83] Chronic kidney disease, defined as an estimated glomerular filtration rate, eGFR less than 60 mL/min/1.73 m^2 and/or urine albumin:creatinine greater than or equal to 300 mg/g, occurs in approximately 50% of patients with acute and chronic HFrEF and HFpEF.[83] Cardiorenal syndrome is a bidirectional relationship involving the heart and kidneys either acutely or chronically, as both organs have interlinking basic physiologic and pathologic properties. There are five general classifications for cardiorenal syndrome, including: type 1, acute cardiorenal, HF leading to acute kidney disease; type 2, chronic cardiorenal, chronic HF leading to kidney failure; type 3, acute nephrocardiac, acute kidney disease leading to acute HF; type 4, chronic nephrocardiac, chronic kidney disease leading to HF; type 5, secondary, systemic disease resulting in heart and kidney failure.[84] The management of patients with kidney disease and HF is complex and includes the utilization of RAAS, diuretics, and device therapies.

Cognitive Dysfunction

Cognitive dysfunction, including impairments in memory, attention, concentration, learning, psychomotor ability, perceptual skills, problem solving, executive function, and language are common in patients with HF.[85,86] It has been reported that 30% to 50% of patients with HF have diminished cognition.[87,88] Baseline intelligence and NYHA functional class have been shown to predict the degree of impairment.[89] Increased age, presence of comorbidities, and abnormalities of serum sodium, potassium, albumin, and glucose all increased the relative risk of cognitive impairment.[90] Cognitive impairment has been associated with a reduction in self-care[91] and an increased risk for readmissions[92] and mortality.[93]

While the precise mechanisms of impairment remain unclear and multifactorial (Fig. 38-5), primary hypotheses for cognitive impairment in HF include chronic cerebral hypoperfusion and/or hypoxia, and repeated cerebral microembolic events.[94] Small observational studies of patients with HF have shown an association between diminished cerebral blood flow as measured by single-photon emission computed tomography brain imaging and abnormalities noted on neuropsychological testing.[95] Cognitive deficits have been correlated with diminished gray matter volume in patients with HF.[86]

Cognition changes are often barriers to a patient's ability to engage in self-care behaviors and patients with cognitive disorders have less knowledge about HF.[86] Reductions in cognitive abilities are correlated to worse adherence to treatment regimens.[94]

Diabetes Mellitus

There is a positive correlation between HF and DM: Patients with HF are at higher risk of developing DM; those with DM are at higher risk of developing HF.[96] A recent study found the individuals with type 2 DM are two to three times more likely to develop HF.[97] The prevalence of diabetes and HF has rapidly increased in the past three decades[98] and the prognosis for individuals with HF with diabetes is worse than for those without diabetes.[99] Diabetes affects 30 million Americans and is highly associated with factors known to cause HF, such as hypertension and CAD.[100]

The accumulation of lipids in cardiac cells and insulin resistance (IR) cause diabetic cardiomyopathy that leads to HF.[101] In addition, anomalies in glucose metabolism may synergistically act to increase the prevalence of HF. Several genetic disorders,

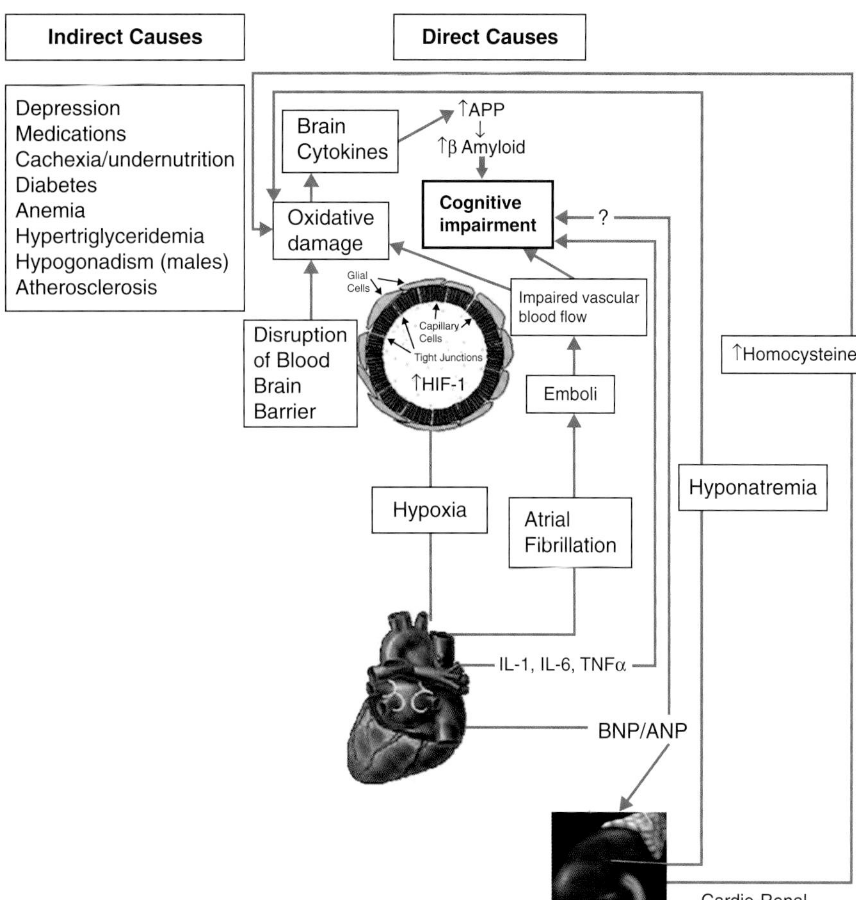

Figure 38-5. The potential factors involved in the pathogenesis of cognitive dysfunction in heart failure. APP, amyloid precursor protein; HIF-1, hypoxia inducible factor-1; IL-1, interleukin 1; IL-6, interleukin-6; TNFα, tumor necrosis factor-α-1; BNP, brain naturetic peptide; ANP, atrial naturetic peptide. (Ampadu J, Morley JE. Heart failure and cognitive dysfunction. *Int J Cardiol.* 2015;178: 12–23.)

such as Alström syndrome and Bardet–Biedl syndrome, are associated with both severe IR and fatal hyperglycemia. Such association prompts us to examine the mechanistic impact of IR on the myocardium. A more common thought is that HF predisposes a person to developing IR or type 2 DM. There are data to suggest that 43% of patients with HF exhibit abnormal glucose metabolism.[102] A recent prospective study suggested that a one standard deviation decrease in insulin sensitivity increased the risk of HF by one-third.[103] Studies have shown that even a 1% increase in hemoglobin A1c increases the risk of HF by 15%.[104] While systemic IR (type 2 DM) is associated with increased mortality in patients with HF,[105] systemic and myocardial IR may be different. Interestingly, cardiac positron emission tomography studies suggest that a failing myocardium has reduced glucose uptake in favor of free fatty acid uptake; in patients with type 2 DM, myocardial glucose uptake is even lower.[106] There is some evidence to support that the use of some SGLT2 inhibitor medications may decrease the incidence of HF and hospitalizations in individuals with DM.[107]

Anemia

Anemia, defined by the World Health Organization as an Hgb less than 12 g/dL in women and less than 13 g/dL in men,[108] is a common problem in patients with HF and reduced LV ejection fraction. Up to 70% of patients with HF have anemia,[109] with anemia more common in HF patient groups with other comorbidities, such as renal dysfunction and advanced age. Moreover, this population experiences poor quality of life and worse prognosis.[109] Anemia occurs secondary to a deficiency in new erythrocyte production relative to the rate of removal of aged erythrocytes. Erythropoietin, primarily produced by the kidneys, is the key component in red blood cell mass. Abnormalities that impact renal perfusion impact the body's response to erythropoietin. In addition, iron deficiency is present in about 30% of anemic patients with HF.[110] Age, female sex, decreased GFR, decreased body mass index, use of ACE-I, increased jugular venous pressure, and lower extremity edema have all been associated with anemia.[111,112]

Chronic anemia is associated with sodium and water retention, reduction of renal blood flow, and neurohormonal activation—all defining characteristics of the HF syndrome. While reduction in hemoglobin in patients with HF has been shown to be an independent predictor of rehospitalization and mortality in many studies,[113–115] it is difficult to determine whether the HF outcome is worsened by the anemia or the anemia is secondary to worsening HF. There are currently no recommendations to treat anemia in patients with HF. The diagnosis and evaluation of potential reversible causes such as nutritional deficiencies should be undertaken, but given the absence of long-term clinical trials, aggressive treatment with transfusions or exogenous erythropoietin is not recommended.[5,116] Patients with iron deficiency, with a ferritin less than 100 ng/mL or 100 to 300 ng/mL with a transferrin saturation less than 20%, may experience an improvement in functional status and quality of life after intravenous iron replacement.[5]

Interestingly, perhaps an alternative hypothesis may be that the anemia associated with HF is an adaptive mechanism.

Hemoglobin is high in oxidative stress and, as such, the reduction in trafficking of such an agent may be a compensatory mechanism. Further work in this area is ongoing and highlights an important point: Observations made in a patient with HF cannot automatically be converted to treatment options without prospective, well-done, randomized clinical trials.[112]

Depression

Patients living with HF have a significant burden of symptoms and are three to four times more likely than the general population to have depression.[117] Moreover, patients with HF and depression have increased hospital readmissions, emergency room visits, morbidity, and mortality.[117] Specifically, one study found that up to 35% of outpatients and 35% to 70% of inpatients had depression.[118] These depressed patients report a significantly higher symptom burden, lower physical and social function, and lower quality of life than nondepressed patients with HF. Depressive symptoms are some of the strongest predictors of decline in health status in patients with HF.[119] Symptoms of depression have been associated with a 56% increased likelihood of hospitalization or death for patients with HF even after controlling for other markers of disease severity.[120] Additionally, depressed patients with HF experience poor prognosis, increased caregiver burden and healthcare utilization.[121] Nonpharmacologic treatments, such as cognitive-behaviorial therapy, has been shown to reduce depressive symptoms. Routine screening for depression in this population of patients with HF is strongly recommended.[121]

Sleep Disturbances

The majority of patients with HF suffer from sleep-disordered breathing.[122] The prevalence of sleep-disordered breathing among individuals with HF is between 50% and 75%.[122] Patients with obstructive sleep apnea have a 2.6 times higher risk of developing HF independent of other risk factors.[122,123] Interestingly, the risk of HF associated with obstructive sleep apnea exceeds that of hypertension, CAD, and stroke. Respiratory events during sleep have long been known to cause hypoxemia, systemic and pulmonary hypertension, sympathetic activation, and reduced stroke volume.[124] Patients with sleep apnea have dynamic ST-segment and T-wave changes on ambulatory ECG monitoring consistent with myocardial ischemia.[125,126] Although the many mechanisms that might link the broad spectrum of sleep disturbances to clinical HF remain uncertain, several hypotheses are plausible. Obstructive sleep apnea is associated with sympathetic hyperactivity[127] that can cause hypoxia—a putative atherogenic factor[128]—and pulmonary hypertension[129]; sympathetic hyperactivity and pulmonary hypertension both lead to and exacerbate the HF syndrome. In patients with HF class II to IV and suspicion of sleep disorder breathing, consider a formal sleep assessment.[5] While there is no current evidence that treating sleep disorders will prevent HF, data are beginning to suggest that treatment of HF with continuous positive airway pressure (CPAP) improves outcomes in patients with documented sleep apnea.[5,130]

Lifestyle Modifications

Current evidence demonstrates the important role of lifestyle interventions as a component of HF prevention.[131] Folsom et al.[131] demonstrated a lower lifetime occurrence of HF in middle-aged adults with greater adherence to the American Heart Association (AHA) Life's Simple 7®. This initiative was a component of the AHA Strategic Planning Task Force to promote optimal cardiovascular health.[132] The 7 cardiovascular metrics include: smoking, body mass index, physical activity, healthy diet, total cholesterol level, blood pressure, fasting plasma glucose—important for the prevention and management of HF.

Smoking Cessation

Cessation of smoking has a dramatic effect on improvement in health status. More than 10% of deaths worldwide due to cardiovascular disease is caused by smoking, which accounts for approximately 1.7 million deaths annually.[133] In the United States alone, smoking contributes to 32% of all deaths due to cardiovascular disease.[134] Patients with HF who continue to smoke have an approximately 30% to 50% higher risk of hospitalization for HF, MI, and death than patients who do not smoke.[135,136] While many patients with HF who have smoked for long periods of time may question the benefit of quitting seemingly late in the course of their lives, there is strong evidence to support that within 2 years of quitting, the increased relative risk of both hospitalization for HF and MI drop similar to those levels in persons who have never smoked.[136] In fact mortality benefits associated with smoking cessation exceed those of many of the standard pharmacologic treatment regimes, such as ACE-I and β-adrenergic blocker therapy in patients with HF. The benefits of smoking cessation accrue rapidly (within 1 year) in patients with HF. Despite this clear benefit, many nurses and healthcare providers are hesitant to address this issue with this patient population.[137] Data suggest that only 9% of smokers hospitalized with HF are counseled to quit smoking.[138] However, there is mounting evidence that smokers who receive assistance from healthcare providers have a 66% greater probability of quitting.[133] Counseling for smoking cessation for current smokers should be encouraged because the risk of developing cardiovascular disease decreases significantly after abstinence even for heavy smokers.[139]

Activity and Exercise

A classic symptom associated with HF is exercise intolerance, characterized by fatigue or shortness of breath. Exploring the pathophysiologic mechanisms underlying these symptoms has been the focus of much study over the last decade.[140] Figure 38-6 depicts the mechanisms in HF for augmenting cardiac output in patients with and without HF.[140] The mechanisms involve both myocardial and peripheral abnormalities, including altered cardiac output in response to exercise, abnormal redistribution of blood flow, reduced mitochondrial volume density, impaired vasodilatory capacity, heightened sympathetic vascular resistance, and impaired sympathetic tone.[141–143]

Exercise limitation leads to worsening of physical function, which leads to poor prognosis and HRQOL.[1] One study found that individuals who needed assistance with ambulation or activities of daily living were considerably more likely to be readmitted to a hospital within 60 days.[144] Exercise programs that are tailored to an individual's physiologic capacity and preferences have been shown to be safe, effective, and to ultimately improve quality of life for individuals with HF, and it is important to incorporate exercise in a comprehensive HF care program.[145] Although exercise is a guideline-recommended treatment that has been shown to improve cardiorespiratory fitness and prognosis as well as quality of life for a wide range of HF populations, specifically for patients with HF with preserved ejection fraction, heart transplants, and LV assisted devices, it is underutilized in practice settings.[145] Exercise may be contraindicated in some patients with HF, Table 38-5 highlights a subset of patients for whom exercise prescriptions should be altered.

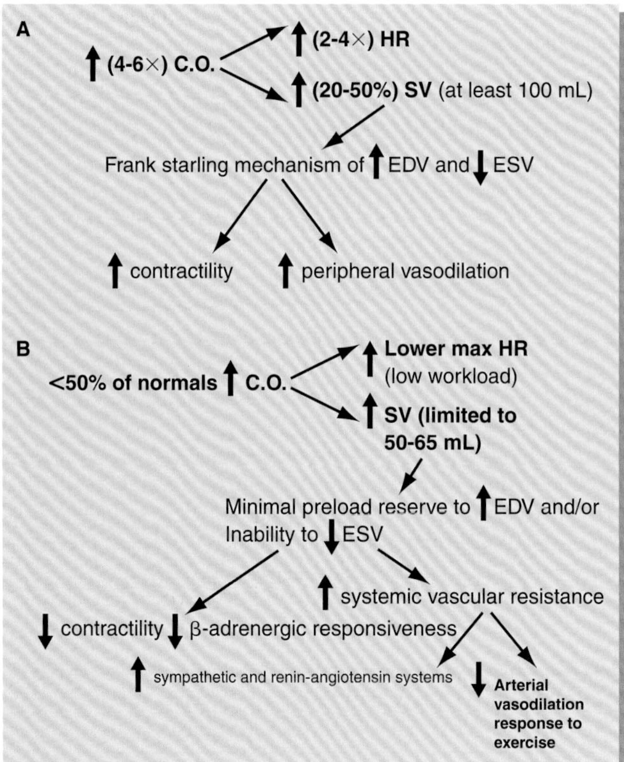

Figure 38-6. Mechanisms to augment cardiac output. A series indicates cardiac output augmentation in a normal heart. B series indicates cardiac output augmentation in HF. (From Pina IL, Apstein CS, Balady GJ, et al. Exercise and heart failure: a statement from the American Heart Association Committee on exercise, rehabilitation, and prevention. *Circulation.* 2003;107[8]: 1210–1225.)

Table 38-5 • RELATIVE AND ABSOLUTE CONTRAINDICATIONS TO EXERCISE TRAINING AMONG PATIENTS WITH STABLE CHRONIC HEART FAILURE

Relative Contraindications	Absolute Contraindications
>4 lb wt gain over previous 1–3 days	Progressive dyspnea at rest over previous 5 days
Continuous or intermittent dobutamine	Ischemia at low levels of exercise
↓ In systolic BP with exercise	Uncontrolled diabetes
NYHA IV	Acute systemic illness or fever
Complex ventricular arrhythmia at rest	Recent embolism
Complex ventricular arrhythmia with exercise	Thrombophlebitis
	Active pericarditis or myocarditis
Supine resting HR >100 beats/min	Severe aortic stenosis
	Myocardial infarction within previous 3 weeks
	New-onset atrial fibrillation with rapid ventricular response

wt, weight; BP, blood pressure; NYHA, New York Heart Association functional class; HR, heart rate.
Adapted from Working Group on Cardiac Rehabilitation & Exercise Physiology and Working Group on Health Failure of the European Society of Cardiology. Recommendations for exercise training in chronic heart failure patients. *Eur Heart J.* 2001;22(2):125–135.

Nutrition—Diet, Sodium, and Fluid

Although a low-sodium diet has been commonly prescribed for patients with HF as a part of self-care management strategy, patients with HF frequently lack a clear understanding of the dietary recommendations.[146] A recent study highlighted a lack of randomized clinical trials to determine the optimal amount of sodium intake and indicated that current recommendations vary widely.[146] Despite the inconsistent guidelines, the consensus is that limiting sodium intake lessens the risk of volume overload. While most clinicians agree that limiting sodium intake is important, the incorporation of this strategy into the lives of patients is more complex.

Lack of knowledge or motivation, poorly perceived benefits or social support, and difficulty in changing eating habits have been identified as factors associated with patient nonadherence to a low-sodium diet.[147] One study found a positive relationship between perceived benefits and long-term adherence to a low-sodium diet.[147] If patients perceive the positive link between low or consistent sodium intake and reduced risk of hospitalization for volume overload, they are more likely to adhere to a reduced sodium diet.[148] Thus, Bennet et al.[148] validated the common sense association that if patients understand the rationale behind the treatment recommendations, adherence is more likely improved. Routine fluid restriction has not been shown to be significantly effective in either short- or long-term volume management[149] in the HF population, regardless of symptoms.[1] Fluid restriction may be indicated for the management of hyponatremia and in patients with advanced HF.[1] End-stage cardiovascular disease patients may experience cardiac cachexia and recommendations for dietary modifications will need adjustments to ensure that the patients have appropriate caloric intake to meet their metabolic needs.

Cardiac Rehabilitation

As the prevalence of HF rapidly increases, it is important to include secondary prevention such as cardiac rehabilitation as a part of HF management.[150] Cardiac rehabilitation is indicated in patients with HF, coronary disease, valvular heart disease, and heart transplantation.[150] Cardiac rehabilitation, which is customized to an individual's needs, is a crucial component of HF treatment.[151] Cardiac rehabilitation programs allow individuals to partner with a multidisciplinary team of healthcare providers—medicine, nursing, exercise physiology, physical and occupational therapy, pharmacology, education, psychology, and sociology—to better manage their disease, lifestyle, and habits.[151] Cardiac rehabilitation programs often include exercise counseling, physical training, heart-healthy living education, and counseling to help reduce stress.[151] The programs are available in healthcare settings (inpatient and outpatient) as well as at home.[151] In general, there are four phases: Phase 1, acute rehabilitation; Phase 2, subacute; Phase 3, intensive outpatient therapy; Phase 4, independent ongoing conditioning.

In 2015, the U.S. Center for Medicare Services (CMS) extended the eligibility to cover cardiac rehabilitation programs for individuals with HFrEF despite the controversy that the program could be harmful for this population.[152] While cardiac rehabilitation has proven to be effective for many patients with cardiovascular diseases, studies have shown some concern when used for patients with HFrEF due to predisposed arrhythmia, fluid overload, and hemodynamic instability.[152] In stable patients with HF, cardiac rehabilitation has demonstrated improvement in functional ability, exercise duration, HRQOL, and mortality.[1]

Management With Diagnostic Studies—Serial Echocardiogram or Biomarkers

Echocardiogram is performed for the initial evaluation of patients presenting with HF symptoms. Routine serial evaluation by echocardiogram is not indicated in the management of patients with HF.[1] Repeat echocardiogram is indicated for significant changes in clinical presentation, recovery from a clinical event, evaluation for electrical device therapy, or after the initiation of therapies that may significantly impact ventricular function.[1]

Measurement of BNP or NT-proBNP is useful for the diagnosis and prognosis of HF, however, current evidence does not support NP-guided therapy due to insufficient data that demonstrate consistent evidence for the improvement in mortality or cardiovascular outcomes in patients with HF.[5] Other biomarkers including troponin, soluble ST2 receptor, galectin-3 are currently not recommended to guide HF therapy or management.[5]

Heart Failure Disease Management

Once a diagnosis of HF has been established, a major goal is determining the type and severity of the underlying disease and the extent of the syndrome. HF remains the primary reason why patients over the age of 65 years require hospitalization.[153] Three-month rehospitalization rates exceed 50%.[154] The primary reason for rehospitalization is volume overload followed by angina and arrhythmias.[155] Common precipitants of readmission include medication nonadherence, dietary indiscretion, inappropriate medications, and delay in seeking care.[156] Identification of the early onset of HF symptoms may prompt therapeutic interventions instituted on an ambulatory basis and prevent rehospitalization. Coordination of care by a nurse-directed multidisciplinary team (including nurses, cardiologists, primary care providers, case managers, dieticians, pharmacists, cardiac rehabilitation specialists, and patients and their caregivers) can provide HF initiatives to guide evidence-based practice, enable self-care at home, and coordinate clinical care across the continuum.[157] A growing trend has been to have advanced practice nurses coordinate these programs.[158]

The goal of HF disease management programs is to reduce symptom burden, improve functional capacity, reduce hospital visits by facilitating guideline-directed therapies and addressing barriers to behavioral change.[1] Components of disease management programs include discharge planning, education and counseling, medication optimization, early attention to deterioration and vigilant follow-up. HF disease management programs have been shown to improve quality of life[154] and patient satisfaction with care.[159] Application of these strategies by nurses has been shown to reduce the likelihood of 90-day readmission by 56%[154,160] and to improve significantly 1-year survival without readmission.[161,162] There is mounting evidence to suggest that HF disease management programs reduce not only readmission but also mortality, therefore these programs are recommended for all HF patients at high risk for reshospitalization.[1,163]

Patient and Family Education

Whether in a hospital, clinic, nursing home, or patient's home, the nurse cares for patients in all stages and phases of the syndrome of HF. The healthcare community is increasingly faced with a growing division between what is known to improve patient outcome and our ability to encourage, engage, apply, and teach these behaviors to the patients and populations we serve. An early study demonstrated that education successfully alters adherence in patients living with chronic diseases.[164] Education and support have been shown to improve self-care behaviors in patients with chronic HF.[165,166] Multidisciplinary education and support interventions have been shown to reduce rehospitalization rates in this patient population.[161,167] Comprehensive discharge planning and postdischarge follow-up of elderly patients with HF has been shown to not only reduce the need for rehospitalization but may even reduce 1-year mortality.[168] However, education alone certainly does not predict patient behavior in the home setting.[169] Patient-related decompensation of chronic HF can be attributed to knowledge deficit and even short one-on-one teaching sessions can significantly reduce rehospitalization and death.[170] Education should focus on understanding of the disease, diet and sodium restrictions, medication administration, physical activity, recognizing signs and symptoms of HF, enhancing social support, and accessing healthcare providers. Table 38-6 presents topics for patient, family, and caregiver education.

Table 38-6 • TOPICS FOR PATIENT, FAMILY, AND CAREGIVER EDUCATION AND COUNSELING

General Counseling
Heart failure definition and the reason for symptoms
Cause or probable cause of heart failure
Expected symptoms
Symptoms of worsening heart failure
What to do if symptoms worsen
Self-monitoring with daily weights
Treatment/care plan
Patient/caregiver responsibilities
Importance of cessation of tobacco use
Role of family members or other caregivers in the treatment/care plan
Availability and value of qualified local support group/online resources
Importance of preventative health, including vaccinations against influenza and pneumococcal disease

Prognosis
Life expectancy
Advance directives
Advice for family members in the event of sudden death

Activity Recommendations
Recreation, leisure, and work activity
Exercise
Sexual activity, sexual difficulties, and coping strategies

Dietary Recommendations
Consistent and restricted sodium intake (2–5 mg/day)
Relationship of excess sodium intake to subsequent symptoms or weight gain
Fluid moderation
Small, frequent meals
Calorie-appropriate diet
Alcohol moderation or restriction if heart failure secondary to alcohol use

Medications
Effects of medications on quality of life and survival
Dosing
Likely side effects and what to do if they occur
Coping mechanisms for complicated medical regimens
Availability of lower-cost medications or financial assistance
Avoiding dangerous interactions with over-the-counter medications, herbal supplements, and home remedies

Educational interventions improve knowledge, medication adherence, symptom monitoring, rehospitalizations, and hospital length of stay.[1] Specialized HF centers have been established to oversee therapeutic options, including complex polypharmacy, device therapy, and investigational agents.[171] Nursing plays a key role in these centers and clinics, coordinating care that impacts the physical, psychological, and social challenges of HF patients. In addition to morbidity and mortality, quality of life is an equally important outcome in patients with HF.[172] Risk factor modification, management of nutrition, biobehavioral therapy, drug management, and exercise training are just some of the interventions shown to benefit patients with HF.[172] Home management of HF may relate to stabilizing the patient's condition after hospital discharge, providing care before cardiac transplantation, or palliative and hospice care for those patients with end-stage HF.[173]

When the patient is admitted to the hospital, the problems associated with HF may have become more advanced and may require supervised administration of medications as well as other measures to reduce edema and improve myocardial performance. The overall plan of care for patients with HF is to reduce cardiac workload, improve cardiac output, prevent complications, and educate the patient regarding follow-up care.

Self-Care

Self-care is defined as a "naturalistic decision-making process involving the choice of behaviors that maintain physiologic stability (self-care maintenance) and the response to symptoms when they occur (self-care management)."[174] Self-care is the process by which persons function on their own behalf to promote health and to prevent and treat disease.[175] Important components of self-care in patients living with HF include recognizing and evaluating symptoms, monitoring and weighing daily, adhering to dietary and activity recommendations, taking medications, smoking cessation and participating in health promotion behaviors.[86,175] There is evidence that supports self-care behaviors improve readmissions, quality of life, and survival.[176]

Self-care in patients with HF has been divided into "maintenance" and "management" processes. Riegel et al.[177] classified the concrete "rule-following" activities of patients with HF as "maintenance" behaviors. However, a patient's independent decision or choice to engage in these activities (restricting dietary sodium intake, home daily weights, and daily exercise) remains complex. Sneed and Paul[178] found that while most patients report consistently adhering to recommended "maintenance" behaviors, only 39% reported engaging in regular exercise while 94% reported consumption of a high-sodium food product within the preceding 24 hours.[177,178] "Management" behaviors, require the integration of multifaceted data, include the perception and/or recognition of symptoms, decisions involved in articulating and reporting changes in status, independent or guided alternatives in treatment plans, and complex evaluation of responses.[177,179] Each of these vital steps is linked to the aforementioned complexity of the phenomena we term behavior. Interventions to promote self-care for individuals with HF include the enhancement of skill development, behavior change, family support, and systems of care of disease management programs and care coordination.[86] In a qualitative systematic review, Harkness et al.[180] describe patients' views of self-care as an adaptation from learning through experiences to maintain their independence and quality of life.

Complexity of Patient Behavior. Patient behavior is a complex phenomenon. Knowledge, motivation,[181] hope,[162] self-efficacy, health beliefs, social support,[182] cognitive capacity,[87] and perceived support[183] are just a few of the variables that have been shown to impact behavior of patients with HF. Each of these variables serves as a filter through which patients perceive and integrate information, and establish resultant behavior. While patients' perceptions of the severity of symptoms of HF have been shown to correlate with the assessments of their healthcare providers,[184] the studies in this area are few. In a small, prospective qualitative study, Riegel and Carlson[179] explored the impact of HF on patients' lives and identified symptoms and misconceptions as major barriers to performing self-care behaviors. Patient education and symptom severity predicted behavior, such as recognizing, reporting, and evaluating symptoms.[185] Reflective listing, negotiating a plan, and bridging the transition to home also lead to a patient's successful adherence to self-care regimens.[175]

Daily Weight. Lack of adherence to a prescribed outpatient regimen, resulting in volume overload and leading to shortness of breath, has been cited as the primary reason patients require rehospitalization.[156,186] In the hospital setting, daily weights provide an assessment of volume status and are a critical tool used by nurses and providers caring for patient with HF. Patient's home monitoring of daily weights has been proposed as an effective way to monitor volume status.[167] There are emerging data to support an association between hospital admission and weight gain beginning 1 week prior to admission.[187] However, little is known about the home self-weighing behavior experience of patients with chronic HF.

Patient-directed home monitoring of daily weights can be an effective tool to detect subtle (2 to 5 lb) changes in volume status, often prior to the development of overt symptoms. Two small studies have shown that while most patients with HF recall being asked to monitor their weights at home, and describe this behavior as "important," only approximately 30% reported engaging in the behavior.[167,188] Daily weights were among the five least frequently performed self-care behaviors.[162]

Most patients with HF are instructed to weigh themselves one time per day. Although the ideal time of this weight has not been studied, it is most likely not as important as the fact that it is performed at a consistent time each day. In general, patients are typically asked to weigh upon rising in the morning, after urinating and prior to dressing or eating. The accuracy or precision of the home device (scale) used for weighing has likewise not been studied. However, the accuracy of the measurement probably is not as important as its reproducibility and the trends of change over time.

Recognizing mild volume overload early, increases the efficacy of treatment interventions, such as augmentation of diuretic dose and heightened sodium restriction. These interventions can interrupt the cycle of progressive sodium and water retention, manifested clinically as shortness of breath, paroxysmal nocturnal dyspnea, and lower extremity edema.

Medication Adherence. Important advances have been made in the pharmacologic treatment of patients with HF, however there remain barriers to medication adherence in patients with HF. Patients who are unable to obtain medications or to take their medications correctly, are unlikely to experience the favorable outcomes observed in clinical trials. Medication nonadherence is highly prevalent in patients with HF.[156,189,190] A positive association between patients' perception of the effects of a medication and subsequent adherence has been demonstrated.[191] Education and support have likewise been shown to significantly increase adherence resulting in improvements in functional outcome and reduced emergency room visits and hospitalization.[192,193]

Social Support

Several investigators have described a relationship between social support and health outcomes in the HF patient population, including hospitalizations and mortality.[1,161,166] Socially isolated, living alone, and unmarried or unpartnered HF patients are at risk for poor self-care, psychosocial distress, and depression.[86] Enhanced social support reduces stress, promotes a healthy lifestyle and improves adherence to treatments and medication regimens, exercise, and dietary adherence.[1,86]

Patient Monitoring—Follow-Up and Remote Technology

Care coordination and transitions of care to facilitate achieving GDMT and prevent rehospitalization is recommended for all patients with chronic HF.[1] These practices include effective communication strategies and medication reconciliation. For the hospitalized patient, early follow-up visits, within 7 to 14 days and telephone follow-up within 3 days of discharge is reasonable.[1] Several clinical studies have demonstrated a decline in hospital readmissions by as much as 50% with aggressive telephone follow-up care. Feldman et al.[157] evaluated the impact of sending e-mail reminders regarding HF-specific clinical recommendations to home health nurses. Patients cared for by nurses receiving the prompts were significantly more likely to recognize their medications, less likely to report salting their food, and more likely to weigh themselves. The Kansas City Cardiomyopathy Questionnaire score and HRQOL were significantly higher in the patients receiving care from a nurse receiving the prompts. Telemanagement of HF undertaken by advanced practice nurses,[194] has been shown to promote consistency of care across healthcare sites.

Telehealth and remote patient monitoring are evolving as components to enhance the care and management of patients with HF. Some of the data on telehealth versus usual care has demonstrated mixed results, with no statistically significant difference in mortality or readmission within 180 days of enrollment in some studies.[195,196] However, Ong et al.[196] reported a significant difference in 180-day QOL scores between groups. Other investigators have reported significantly reduced readmission rate for the monitored group compared to the usual care group.[197,198] In a meta-analysis of 21 randomized control trials that evaluated the effect of remote patient monitoring as an adjunct to usual postdischarge care in reducing HF and all-cause readmissions, the monitoring was associated with a significantly lower number of hospitalizations for HF and for any cause.[199] Similarly, in a systematic review by Inglis et al.[200] of 41 randomized controlled trials evaluating structured telephone support and/or telehealth, significant improvements were noted in HF knowledge and self-care behaviors, and reductions in both mortality and HF-related hospitalizations.

Health-Related Quality of Life

HRQOL or meaningful survival, is decreased in patients with HF.[1] The contributions to HRQOL is multifactorial and associated with gender, ethnicity, age, comorbidities, symptoms, socioeconomic issues, physiologic parameters, and mental health. Rehospitalizations and mortality can be attributed to lack of improvement in HRQOL.[1] Interventions that have demonstrated consistent improvement in HRQOL are CRT therapy, some disease management programs and educational opportunities.[1] Research has been less clear on the impact on HRQOL through self-care practices and exercise.[1]

Palliative Care

Patients with HF, especially late-stage HF, experience multiple symptoms, hospitalizations, and a high mortality rate. Palliative care is a multidisciplinary approach for symptomatic patients with advanced HF to improve HRQOL.[1] The World Health Organization[201] defines palliative care as "...an approach that improves the quality of life of patients and their families facing the problem associated with life-threatening illness, through the prevention and relief of suffering by means of early identification and impeccable assessment and treatment of pain and other problems, physical, psychosocial and spiritual." The integration of palliative care into routine management of end-stage HF continues to develop. Barriers to integration include uncertainty of the disease trajectory, communication issues, silos of care, lack of knowledge, and the complexity of treatment decisions involving device deactivation.[202] In a systematic review, palliative care was associated with decrease in emergency department visits, rehospitalizations, symptom improvement, increased quality of life, and increased documentation of preferences for care.[203]

Shared Decision Making

Patient-centered care is a component of evidence-based practice, as the patient is a part of the healthcare team. This approach ensures that the decisions are guided by the patient's values, goals, values, and preferences.[202] Shared decision making must be provided within the context of health literacy and social determinants of health to ensure ethical and legal mandates to fully inform patients of the risks and benefits of therapies and treatments. In patients with HF there is often a complex balance of healthcare decisions, and these decisions may change over time based on the disease trajectory and expression of the syndrome, necessitating the full involvement of the patient in the decision-making process.

CONCLUSIONS

Summary

HF is a complex syndrome with multiple etiologies, symptoms, and manifestations of the condition in each patient. As an end state to other disorders, HF patients often have concomitant health-related conditions. Ensuring guideline-based care for patients with both HFrEF and HFpEF that are individualized based on the patient's status and goals, contributes to improved patient outcomes in this diverse patient population. Nursing care is an essential component of chronic disease management for the condition of HF.

Future Considerations/Implications

Future considerations include additional research on the optimum therapies for patients with HFpEF. Additional considerations include the utilization of technology to enhance care transitions and chronic care management in the patient with HF.

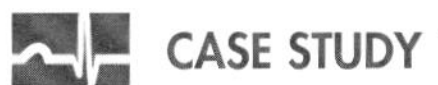

CASE STUDY 1

Patient Profile

Name/Age/Sex: **Max Trout, 52-year-old African American male**

History of Present Illness

Mr. Trout, a 52-year-old African American male with established stage C NYHA class II HF came to the clinic for his 3-month follow-up appointment. He was initially diagnosed with HF approximately 2 years ago. During the 2-year period he has been hospitalized once for acute HF, which was resolved with intravenous diuretics in less than 24 hours. His most recent echocardiogram performed after initiation of target doses of GDMT revealed an LVEF of 30%, unchanged from his initial echocardiogram. He was offered an internal cardioverter defibrillator (ICD) approximately 3 months ago. Although the patient expressed interest during the shared decision-making consult, prior to the procedure he changed his mind and declined ICD therapy at this time. He denies chest pain, edema, paroxysmal nocturnal dyspnea, orthopnea, palpitations, dizziness, and has taken his home medications this AM.

Past Medical History

Type 2 diabetes mellitus, hypertension, and hyperlipidemia

Surgical History

None

Family History

He has a family history of HTN, DM. Father died from complications following triple bypass at the age of 75.

Social History

Denies smoking or the use of illicit drugs or alcohol. He is rather sedentary, although attempts to walk daily. He is self-employed and does not have insurance. Today he reports he can walk 1/2 block before feeling shortness of breath, which he states is his baseline.

Medications

Aspirin 81 mg QD, atorvastatin 40 mg QD, carvedilol 25 mg BID, furosemide 20 mg BID, metformin 500 mg BID, sacubitril-valsartan (97 mg/103 mg) one tablet BID.

Allergies

None

Patient Examination

Vital Signs

BP 148/53; HR 65; Wt. 99 kg; Ht. 177 cm; SaO_2 95% on room air

Physical Examination

General: Awake, alert, and oriented. No distress noted. Appears younger than stated age. No neurologic deficits.

Skin: Intact, warm, dry. No rashes or lesions are noted.

Cardiac: No murmurs, gallops, or rubs are auscultated. S_1 and S_2 are heard and are of normal intensity. He is euvolemic on exam.

Respiratory: Clear to auscultation bilaterally

Abdominal: Abdomen is soft, symmetric, and nontender without distention. No masses, hepatomegaly, or splenomegaly are noted.

Psychiatric: Appropriate mood and affect. Good judgment and insight.

Testing

ECG shows SR with QRS interval measuring 0.11 ms.

Considerations

Key Questions

What is patient's NYHA status?
Is his BP at goal? Does he need any medication changes?

Evidence

Patient is stage C NYHA class II.

Given that the patient is not at goal for BP, has a history of DM, and his EF is relatively unchanged he is started on spironolactone 12.5 mg QD. Recall that starting an MRA requires careful review of potassium levels, renal function, and diuretic dosing. His creatinine has been 1.3 mg/dL, eGFR of 79 mL/min/1.73 m^2 and potassium less than 5.9 mEq/L and so he fits the criteria. The patient is counseled to avoid NSAIDs and to return to the clinic in 3 days and again in a week to recheck renal function and potassium levels. Upon review of his laboratory tests, subsequent monitoring and dosing will be determined by the stability of the patient's renal function, symptoms, and blood pressure readings.

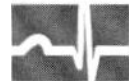

CASE STUDY 2

Patient Profile

Name/Age/Sex: **Ronald Jones, 60-year-old male**

History of Present Illness

Mr. Jones presents with a history of known CAD with a history of drug-eluting stent to the mid LAD 5 years prior, recently experienced an acute anterior MI with thrombectomy and DES to the culprit, totally occluded proximal LAD lesion. The patient was discharged on GDMT including dual antiplatelet therapy. He was fitted for an external cardioverter defibrillator for the primary prevention of sudden cardiac death. He presents for 6-week hospital follow-up. He reports taking all prescribed medications as directed and wears the external cardioverter defibrillator with the exception of when showering. He denies chest pain. He does experience dyspnea with minimal exertional activities. He denies paroxysmal nocturnal dyspnea, orthopnea, palpitations, syncopal or near-syncopal episodes, lower extremity pain, or edema.

Past Medical History

Type 2 diabetes mellitus, hypertension, and hyperlipidemia.

Surgical History

None

Family History

He has a family history of CAD. Father died from MI at age 65.

Social History

Smoking 1 pack per day of cigarettes for 40 years prior to quitting at the age of 59 years old. He denies use of alcohol or recreational substances.
He is active without regular exercise.

Medications

clopidogrel 75 mg PO Q day, metoprolol succinate 25 mg PO Q day, lisinopril 10 mg PO Q day, atorvastatin 80 mg PO Q day, furosemide 40 mg PO Q AM, aspirin 81 mg PO Q day

Allergies

None

(continued)

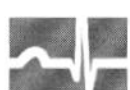 CASE STUDY 2 (*Continued*)

Patient Examination

Vital Signs

BP 100/65; HR 60 bpm; Wt. 79 kg; Ht. 167 cm; SaO_2 97% on room air

Physical Examination

General: Awake, alert and oriented. No distress noted. Appears younger than stated age. No neurologic deficits.

Skin: intact, warm, dry. No rashes or lesions are noted.

Cardiac: No murmurs, gallops, or rubs are auscultated. S_1 and S_2 are heard and are of normal intensity. He is euvolemic on exam

Respiratory: clear to auscultation bilaterally

Abdominal: Abdomen is soft, symmetric, and nontender without distention. No masses, hepatomegaly, or splenomegaly are noted.

Psychiatric: Appropriate mood and affect. Good judgment and insight.

Testing

Echocardiogram post-MI revealed an LVEF of 20%. ECG reveals SR with LBBB with QRS interval 140 ms. Cardioverter defibrillator interrogation reveals no detection of ventricular arrhythmias.

Considerations

Key Questions

Should this patient be considered for a CRT-D?

Evidence

His GDMT and external cardioverter defibrillator, are continued and an echocardiogram for reassessment of LVEF is planned for 6 weeks. The patient follows up 6 weeks later to review the echocardiogram findings. He remains symptomatic with dyspnea with minimal exertional activities. The echocardiogram reveals LVEF 30%. The patient is relieved to hear that his heart function has improved. A discussion about the appropriateness of CRT-D, including indications, benefits, and risks occur. After discussing that CRT-D is recommended after 3 to 6 months of GDMT, the patient requests to continue GDMT and reassess heart function after a few more months of therapy. The patient follows up 3 months later to review his echocardiogram results from 1 week prior. His LVEF is calculated to be 30% to 35%. The patient is referred to a cardiac electrophysiologist and undergoes CRT-D placement. A 3-month post-device placement appointment with echocardiogram reveals that the patient's LVEF improved to 50%. Device interrogation reveals no detection of ventricular arrhythmias or device therapy. The patient reports his dyspnea has improved and he experiences dyspnea only with significant exertional activity.

KEY READINGS

Yancy CW, Jessup M, Bozkurt B, et al. 2013 ACCF/AHA guideline for the management of heart failure: a report of the American College of Cardiology Foundation/American Heart Association Task Force on Practice Guidelines. *J Am Coll Cardiol.* 2013;62(16):e147–e239.

Yancy CW, Jessup M, Bozkurt B, et al. 2017 ACC/AHA/HFSA focused update of the 2013 ACCF/AHA guideline for the management of heart failure: a report of the American College of Cardiology/American Heart Association Task Force on clinical practice guidelines and the Heart Failure Society of America. *J Am Coll Cardiol.* 2017;70(6):776–803.

REFERENCES

1. Yancy CW, Jessup M, Bozkurt B, et al. ACCF/AHA guideline for the management of heart failure: a report of the American College of Cardiology Foundation/American Heart Association Task Force on practice guidelines. *J Am Coll Cardiol.* 2013;62(16):e147–e239.
2. Bell DS. Heart failure: the frequent, forgotten, and often fatal complication of diabetes. *Diabetes Care.* 2003;26(8):2433–2441.
3. Kannel WB, McGee DL. Diabetes and cardiovascular disease. The Framingham study. *JAMA.* 1979;241(19):2035–2038.
4. Cotter G, Felker GM, Adams KF, et al. The pathophysiology of acute heart failure—is it all about fluid accumulation? *Am Heart J.* 2008;155(1):9–18.
5. Yancy CW, Jessup M, Bozkurt B, et al. ACC/AHA/HFSA focused update of the 2013 ACCF/AHA guideline for the management of heart failure. *J Am Coll Cardiol.* 2017;136:e137–e161.
6. Linseman JV, Bristow MR. Drug therapy and heart failure prevention. *Circulation.* 2003;107(9):1234–1236.
7. Borlaug BA. The pathophysiology of heart failure with preserved ejection fraction. *Nat Rev Cardiol.* 2014;11(9):507.
8. Shah SJ, Kitzman DW, Borlaug BA, et al. Phenotype-specific treatment of heart failure with preserved ejection fraction: a multiorgan roadmap. *Circulation.* 2016;134(1):73–90.
9. Pfeffer MA, Shah AM, Borlaug BA. Heart failure with preserved ejection fraction in perspective. *Circ Res.* 2019;124(11):1598–1617.
10. The CONSENSUS Trial Study Group. Effects of enalapril on mortality in severe congestive heart failure. *N Engl J Med.* 1987;316(23):1429–1435.
11. Howard PA, Cheng JWM, Crouch MA, et al. Drug therapy recommendations from the 2005 ACC/AHA guidelines for treatment of chronic heart failure. *Ann Pharmacother.* 2006;40(9):1607–1616.
12. Shibata MC, Tsuyuki RT, Wiebe N. The effects of angiotensin-receptor blockers on mortality and morbidity in heart failure: a systematic review. *Int J Clin Pract.* 2008;62(9):1397–1402.
13. Aronow WS. Epidemiology, pathophysiology, prognosis, and treatment of systolic and diastolic heart failure in elderly patients. *Heart Disease.* 2003;5(4):279–294.
14. Cohn JN, Tognoni G. A randomized trial of the angiotensin-receptor blocker valsartan in chronic heart failure. *N Engl J Med.* 2001;345(23):1667–1675.
15. McMurray JJ, Ostergren J, Swedberg K, et al. Effects of candesartan in patients with chronic heart failure and reduced left-ventricular systolic function taking angiotensin- converting-enzyme inhibitors: the CHARM-added trial. *Lancet.* 2003;362(9386):767–771.
16. Heran BS, Musini VM, Bassett K, et al. Angiotensin receptor blockers for heart failure. *Cochrane Database Syst Rev.* 2012;(4):CD003040.
17. Granger CB, McMurray JJ, Yusuf S, et al. Effects of candesartan in patients with chronic heart failure and reduced left-ventricular systolic function intolerant to angiotensin-converting-enzyme inhibitors: the CHARM-alternative trial. *Lancet.* 2003;362(9386):772–776.
18. McMurray JJ, Packer M, Desai AS, et al. Dual angiotensin receptor and neprilysin inhibition as an alternative to angiotensin-converting enzyme inhibition in patients with chronic systolic heart failure: rationale for and design of the Prospective comparison of ARNI with ACEI to Determine Impact. *Eur J Heart Fail.* 2013;15(9):1062.
19. Langenickel TH, Dole WP. Angiotensin receptor-neprilysin inhibition with LCZ696: a novel approach for the treatment of heart failure. *Drug Discov Today: Ther Strateg.* 2012;9(4):e131–e139.
20. Langenickel TH, Tsubouchi C, Ayalasomayajula S, et al. The effect of LCZ696 (sacubitril/valsartan) on amyloid-β concentrations in cerebrospinal fluid in healthy subjects. *Br J Clin Pharmacol.* 2016;81(5):878–890.
21. Struthers AD. Aldosterone blockade in cardiovascular disease. *Heart.* 2004;90(10):1229–1234.
22. Chai W, Garrelds IM, de Vries R, et al. Nongenomic effects of aldosterone in the human heart: interaction with angiotensin II. *Hypertension.* 2005;46(4):701–706.
23. Khan NU, Movahed A. The role of aldosterone and aldosterone-receptor antagonists in heart failure. *Rev Cardiovasc Med.* 2004;5(2):71–81.

24. Pitt B, Zannad F, Remme WJ, et al. The effect of spironolactone on morbidity and mortality in patients with severe heart failure. Randomized Aldactone Evaluation Study Investigators. *N Engl J Med.* 1999;341(10):709–717.
25. Azuma J, Nonen S. Chronic heart failure: beta-blockers and pharmacogenetics. *Eur J Clin Pharmacol.* 2008;65(1):3–17.
26. Bristow MR, Krause-Steinrauf H, Nuzzo R, et al. Effect of baseline or changes in adrenergic activity on clinical outcomes in the beta-blocker evaluation of survival trial. *Circulation.* 2004;110(11):1437–1442.
27. Gilbert EM, O'Connell JB, Bristow MR. Therapy of idiopathic dilated cardiomyopathy with chronic beta-adrenergic blockade. *Heart Vessels Suppl.* 1991;6:29–39.
28. Tate CW 3rd, Robertson AD, Zolty R, et al. Quality of life and prognosis in heart failure: results of the Beta-Blocker Evaluation of Survival Trial (BEST). *J Card Fail.* 2007;13(9):732–737.
29. Varadarajan P, Joshi N, Appel D, et al. Effect of beta-blocker therapy on survival in patients with severe mitral regurgitation and normal left ventricular ejection fraction. *Am J Cardiol.* 2008;102(5):611–615.
30. Hjalmarson A, Goldstein S, Fagerberg B, et al. Effects of controlled-release metoprolol on total mortality, hospitalizations, and well-being in patients with heart failure: the Metoprolol CR/XL Randomized Intervention Trial in Congestive Heart Failure (MERIT-HF). *JAMA.* 2000;283(10):1295–1302.
31. O'Connor CM, Gattis WA, Zannad F, et al. Beta-blocker therapy in advanced heart failure: clinical characteristics and long-term outcomes. *Eur J Heart Fail.* 1999;1(1):81–88.
32. Houghton T, Freemantle N, Cleland JG. Are beta-blockers effective in patients who develop heart failure soon after myocardial infarction? A meta-regression analysis of randomised trials. *Eur J Heart Fail.* 2000;2(3):333–340.
33. Tatli E, Kurum T. A controlled study of the effects of carvedilol on clinical events, left ventricular function and proinflammatory cytokines levels in patients with dilated cardiomyopathy. *Can J Cardiol.* 2005; 21(4):344–348.
34. Cohn JN. Optimal diuretic therapy for heart failure. *Am J Med.* 2001; 111(7):577.
35. Taylor AL, Ziesche S, Yancy C, et al. Combination of isosorbide dinitrate and hydralazine in blacks with heart failure. *N Engl J Med.* 2004;351(20):2049–2057.
36. Dobre D, Borer JS, Fox K, et al. Heart rate: a prognostic factor and therapeutic target in chronic heart failure. The distinct roles of drugs with heart rate-lowering properties. *Eur J Heart Fail.* 2014;16(1):76–85.
37. Harjola VP, Oikarinen L, Toivonen L, et al. The hemodynamic and pharmacokinetic interactions between chronic use of oral levosimendan and digoxin in patients with NYHA Classes II–III heart failure. *Int J Clin Pharmacol Ther.* 2008;46(8):389–399.
38. Gheorghiade M, van Veldhuisen DJ, Colucci WS. Contemporary use of digoxin in the management of cardiovascular disorders. *Circulation.* 2006;113(21):2556–2564.
39. Ahmed A, Pitt B, Rahimtoola SH, et al. Effects of digoxin at low serum concentrations on mortality and hospitalization in heart failure: a propensity-matched study of the DIG trial. *Int J Cardiol.* 2008;123(2):138–146.
40. Leibundgut G, Pfisterer M, Brunner-La Rocca HP. Drug treatment of chronic heart failure in the elderly. *Drugs and Aging.* 2007;24(12):991–1006.
41. Rutten JHW, Steyerberg EW, Boomsma F, et al. N-terminal pro-brain natriuretic peptide testing in the emergency department: beneficial effects on hospitalization, costs, and outcome. *Am Heart J.* 2008;156(1):71–77.
42. Owan TE, Chen HH, Frantz RP, et al. The effects of nesiritide on renal function and diuretic responsiveness in acutely decompensated heart failure patients with renal dysfunction. *J Card Fail.* 2008;14(4):267–275.
43. Aaronson KD, Sackner-Bernstein J. Risk of death associated with nesiritide in patients with acutely decompensated heart failure. *JAMA.* 2006;296(12):1465–1466.
44. Sackner-Bernstein JD, Skopicki HA, Aaronson KD. Risk of worsening renal function with nesiritide in patients with acutely decompensated heart failure. *Circulation.* 2005;111(12):1487–1491.
45. Echt DS, Liebson PR, Mitchell LB, et al. Mortality and morbidity in patients receiving encainide, flecainide, or placebo. The Cardiac Arrhythmia Suppression Trial. *N Engl J Med.* 1991;324(12):781–788.
46. Chapa DW, Lee HJ, Kao CW, et al. Reducing mortality with device therapy in heart failure patients without ventricular arrhythmias. *Am J Crit Care.* 2008;17(5):443–452; quiz 453.
47. Russo AM, Poole JE, Mark DB, et al. Primary prevention with defibrillator therapy in women: results from the sudden cardiac death in heart failure trial. *J Cardiovasc Electrophysiol.* 2008;19(7):720–724.
48. Bardy GH, Lee KL, Mark DB, et al. Amiodarone or an implantable cardioverter-defibrillator for congestive heart failure. *N Engl J Med.* 2005;352(3):225–237.
49. Fuster V, Gersh BJ, Giuliani ER, et al. The natural history of idiopathic dilated cardiomyopathy. *Am J Cardiol.* 1981; 47(3):525–531.
50. Al-Khadra AS, Salem DN, Rand WM, et al. Warfarin anticoagulation and survival: a cohort analysis from the studies of left ventricular dysfunction. *J Am Coll Cardiol.* 1998;31(4):749–753.
51. Dries DL, Domanski MJ, Waclawiw MA, et al. Effect of antithrombotic therapy on risk of sudden coronary death in patients with congestive heart failure. *Am J Cardiol.* 1997;79(7):909–913.
52. Teerlink JR, Qian M, Bello NA, et al; WARCEF Investigators. Aspirin does not increase heart failure events in heart failure patients: from the WARCEF Trial. *JACC Heart Fail.* 2017;5(8):603–610.
53. Abraham WT. Devices for monitoring and managing heart failure. In: Mann DA, Zipes DP, Libby P, et al., eds. *Braunwald's Heart Disease: A Textbook of Cardiovascular Medicine.* 10th ed. Philadelphia, PA: Elsevier; 2015.
54. Myerburg RJ. Implantable cardioverter-defibrillators after myocardial infarction. *N Engl J Med.* 2008;359(21):2245–2253.
55. Tracy CM, Epstein AE, Darbar D, et al. Focused update incorporating into the ACCF/AHA/HRS 2008 guidelines for device-based therapy for cardiac rhythm abnormalities: a report of the American College of Cardiology Foundation/American Heart Association Task Force on Practice Guidelines and the Heart Rhythm Society. *Circulation.* 2012;127:e283–e353.
56. Mehta PA, Dubrey SW, McIntyre HF, et al. Mode of death in patients with newly diagnosed heart failure in the general population. *Eur J Heart Fail.* 2008;10(11):1108–1116.
57. Wathen M. Implantable cardioverter defibrillator shock reduction using antitachycardia pacing therapies. *Am Heart J.* 2007;153(4):44–52.
58. Swerdlow CD, Wang PJ, Zipes DP. Pacemakers and implantable cardioverter-defibrillators. In: Mann DA, Zipes DP, Libby P, et al., eds. *Braunwald's Heart Disease: A Textbook of Cardiovascular Medicine.* 10th ed. Philadelphia, PA: Elsevier; 2015.
59. Greenberg H, Case RB, Moss AJ, et al. Analysis of mortality events in the Multicenter Automatic Defibrillator Implantation Trial (MADIT-II). *J Am Coll Cardiol.* 2004;43(8):1459–1465.
60. Sweeney ML, Wathen MS, Volosin K, et al. Appropriate and inappropriate ventricular therapies, quality of life and mortality among primary and secondary prevention implantable cardioverter defibrillator patients: results from the Pacing Fast VT Reduces Shock ThErapies (PainFREE Rx II) trial. *Circulation.* 2005;111(2):898–905.
61. Germano JJ, Reynolds M, Essebag V, et al. Frequency and causes of implantable cardioverter-defibrillator therapies: is device therapy proarrythmic? *Am J Cardiol.* 2006;97(8):1255–1261.
62. Van der Heijden AD, Borleffs CJ, Buiten MS, et al. The clinical course of patients with implantable defibrillators: extended experience on clinical outcomes, device replacements, and device-related complications. *Heart Rhythm.* 2015;12(6):1169–1176.
63. Mann DL. Management of patients with heart failure with reduced ejection fraction. In: Mann DA, Zipes DP, Libby P, et al., eds. *Braunwald's Heart Disease: A Textbook of Cardiovascular Medicine.* 10th ed. Philadelphia, PA: Elsevier; 2015.
64. Maines M, Catanzariti D, Cemin C, et al. Usefulness of intrathoracic fluids accumulation monitoring with an implantable biventricular defibrillator in reducing hospitalization in patients with heart failure: a case control study. *J Interv Card Electrophysiol.* 2007;19:201–207.
65. Van Veldhuisen DJ, Braunschweig F, Conraads V, et al. Intrathoracic impedance monitoring, audible patient alerts, and outcome in patients with heart failure. *Circulation.* 2011;124:1719–1726.
66. Hindricks G, Taborsky M, Glikson M, et al. Implant-based multiparameter telemonitoring of patients with heart failure (IN-TIME): a randomized controlled trial. *Lancet North Am Ed.* 2014;384(9943):557–636.
67. Slotwiner D, Varma N, Akar JG, et al. Heart Rhythm Society expert consensus statement on remote interrogation and monitoring for cardiovascular implantable electronic devices. *Heart Rhythm.* 2015;12(7):e70–e95.
68. Abraham WT, Adamson PB, Bourge RC, et al. Wireless pulmonary artery haemodynamic monitoring in chronic heart failure: a randomized controlled trial. *Lancet.* 2011;377:658–666.
69. Bourge RC, Abraham WT, Adamson PB, et al. Randomized controlled trial of an implantable continuous heomodynamic monitor in patients with advanced hear failure: the COMPASS-HF study. *J Am Coll Cardiol.* 2008;51:1073.
70. U.S. Food and Drug Administration. *Optimizer smart system-P180036.* 2019. Available at https://www.fda.gov/medical-devices/recently-approved-devices/optimizer-smart-system-p180036. Accessed April 15, 2019.

71. Abraham WT, Kuck KH, Goldsmith RL, et al. A randomized control trial to evaluate the safety and efficacy of cardiac contractility modulation. *JACC Heart Fail.* 2018;6(10):875–882.
72. Kadish A, Nadamanee K, Volosin K, et al. A randomized controlled trial evaluating the safety and efficacy of cardiac contractility modulation in advanced heart failure. *Am Heart J.* 2011;161:329–337.
73. Goodlin SJ, Bonow RO. Care of patients with end-stage heart disease. In: Mann DA, Zipes DP, Libby P, et al., eds. *Braunwald's Heart Disease: A Textbook of Cardiovascular Medicine.* 10th ed. Philadelphia, PA: Elsevier; 2015.
74. Feldman AM, Klein H, Tchou P, et al. Use of a wearable defibrillator in terminating tachyarrhythmias in patients at high risk for sudden death: results of WEARIT/BIROAD. *Pacing Clin Electrophysiol.* 2004;27(1):4–9.
75. Teeter WA, Thibodeau JT, Krishnasree R, et al. The natural history of new-onset heart failure with a severely depressed left ventricular ejection fraction: implications for timing of implantable cardioverter-defibrillator implantation. *Am Heart J.* 2012;164(3):358–364.
76. Al-Khatib SM, Stevenson WG, Ackerman MJ, et al. 2017 AHA/ACC/HRS guideline for the management of patients with ventricular arrhythmias and the prevention of sudden cardiac death. *Heart Rhythm.* 2017;15(10):e73–e182.
77. Chung MK, Szymkiewicz SJ, Shao MZ, et al. Aggregate national experience with the wearable cardioverter-defibrillator: event rates, compliance, and survival. *J Am Coll Cardiol.* 2010;56(3):194–203.
78. Kutyifa V, Moss AJ, Klein H, et al. Use of the wearable cardioverter defibrillator in high-risk cardiac patients. *Circulation.* 2015;132:1613–1619.
79. Piccini JP, Allen LA, Kudencheck PJ, et al. Wearable cardioverter-defibrillator therapy for prevention of sudden cardiac death. *Circulation.* 2016;133:1715–1727.
80. The SOLVD Investigators. Effect of enalapril on survival in patients with reduced left ventricular ejection fractions and congestive heart failure. *N Engl J Med.* 1991;325(5):293–302.
81. Hernandez AF, O'Connor CM. Sparing a little may save a lot: lessons from the Studies of Left Ventricular Dysfunction (SOLVD). *J Am Coll Cardiol.* 2003;42(4):709–711.
82. Whelton PK, Carey RM, Aronow WS, et al. 2017 ACC/AHA/AAPA/ABC/ACPM/AGS/APhA/ASH/ASPC/NMA/PCNA guideline for the prevention, detection, evaluation, and management of high blood pressure in adults: a report of the American College of Cardiology/American Heart Association Task Force on clinical practice guidelines. *J Am Coll Cardiol.* 2018;71(19):e127–e248.
83. Damman K, Testani JM. The kidney in heart failure: an update. *Eur Heart J.* 2015;36(23):1437–1444.
84. Ronco C, DiLullo L. Cardiorenal syndrome. *Heart Fail Clin.* 2014;10(2):251–280.
85. Dickson VV, Tkacs N, Riegel B. Cognitive influences on self-care decision making in persons with heart failure. *Am Heart J.* 2007;154(3):424–431.
86. Riegel B, Moser DK, Anker SD, et al. State of the science: promoting self-care in persons with heart failure: a scientific statement from the American Heart Association. *Circulation.* 2009;120(12):1141–1163.
87. Bennett SJ, Sauve MJ. Cognitive deficits in patients with heart failure: a review of the literature. *J Cardiovasc Nurs.* 2003;18(3):219–242.
88. Zuccala G, Onder G, Pedone C, et al. Hypotension and cognitive impairment: selective association in patients with heart failure. *Neurology.* 2001;57(11):1986–1992.
89. Vogel R. Oosterman JM, van Harten B, et al. Profile of cognitive impairment in chronic heart failure. *J Am Geriatr Soc.* 2007;55(11):1764–1770.
90. Zuccola T. Correlates of cognitive impairment among patients with heart failure: results of a multicenter survey. *Am J Med.* 2006;118(5):496–502.
91. Davis KK, Himmelfarb CRD, Szanton SL, et al. Predictors of heart failure self-care in patients who screened positive for mild cognitive impairment. *J Cardiovasc Nurs.* 2015;30(2):152–160.
92. Huynh QL, Negishi K, Blizzard L, et al. Mild cognitive impairment predicts death and readmission within 30 days of discharge for heart failure. *Int J Cardiol.* 2016;221:212–217.
93. Murad K, Goff DC, Morgan TM, et al. Burden of comorbidities and functional and cognitive impairments in elderly patients at the initial diagnosis of heart failure and their impact on total mortality: the Cardiovascular Health Study. *JACC Heart Fail.* 2015;3(7):542–550.
94. Ampadu J, Morley JE. Heart failure and cognitive dysfunction. *Int J Cardiol.* 2015;178:12–23.
95. Alves TC, Rays J, Fráguas FR Jr, et al. Localized cerebral blood flow reductions in patients with heart failure: a study using 99mTc-HMPAO SPECT. *J Neuroimaging.* 2005;15(2):150–156.
96. Rosano GMC, Vitale C, Seferovic P. Heart failure in patients with diabetes mellitus. *Cardiac Fail Rev.* 2017;3(1):52.
97. Winell K, Pietila A, Salomaa V. Incidence and prognosis of heart failure in persons with type 2 diabetes compared with individuals without diabetes—a nation-wide study from Finland in 1996–2012. *Ann Med.* 2019;51(2):174–181.
98. Leon BM, Maddox TM. Diabetes and cardiovascular disease: epidemiology, biological mechanisms, treatment recommendations and future research. *World J of Diabetes.* 2015;6(13):1246–1258.
99. Lehrke M, Marx N. Diabetes mellitus and heart failure. *Am J Med.* 2017;130(6S):S40–S50.
100. Centers for Disease Control and Prevention. *National Diabetes Statistics Report, 2017.* Atlanta, GA: Centers for Disease Control and Prevention; 2017.
101. Nakamura M, Sadoshima J. Cardiomyopathy in obesity, insulin resistance or diabetes. *J Physiol.* 2019. doi:10.1113/JP276747.
102. Suskin N, McKelvie RS, Burns RJ, et al. Glucose and insulin abnormalities relate to functional capacity in patients with congestive heart failure. *Eur Heart J.* 2000;21(16):1368–1375.
103. Ingelsson E, Sundstrom J, Arnlov J, et al. Insulin resistance and risk of congestive heart failure. *JAMA.* 2005;294(3):334–341.
104. Stratton IM, Adler AI, Neil HA, et al. Association of glycaemia with macrovascular and microvascular complications of type 2 diabetes (UKPDS 35): prospective observational study. *BMJ.* 2000;321(7258):405–412.
105. Kostis JB, Sanders M. The association of heart failure with insulin resistance and the development of type 2 diabetes. *Am J Hypertens.* 2005;18(5 Pt 1):731–737.
106. Dutka DP, Pitt M, Pagano D, et al. Myocardial glucose transport and utilization in patients with type 2 diabetes mellitus, left ventricular dysfunction, and coronary artery disease. *J Am Coll Cardiol.* 2006;48(11):2225–2231.
107. Diabetes Care. Standards of medical care in diabetes 2019. *Diabetes Care.* 2019;42(suppl 1):S81–S89.
108. World Health Organization (WHO). *Health topics: Anaemia.* (n.d.) Available at https://www.who.int/topics/anaemia/en/
109. Beverborg NG, van Veldhuisen DJ, van der Meer P. Anemia in heart failure: still relevant? *JACC Heart Fail.* 2018;6(3):201–208.
110. Handelman GJ, Levin NW. Iron and anemia in human biology: a review of mechanisms. *Heart Fail Rev.* 2008;13(4):393–404.
111. Dzudie A, Kengne AP, Mbahe S, et al. Chronic heart failure, selected risk factors and co-morbidities among adults treated for hypertension in a cardiac referral hospital in Cameroon. *Eur J Heart Fail.* 2008;10(4):367–372.
112. Westenbrink BD, de Boer RA, Voors AA, et al. Anemia in chronic heart failure: etiology and treatment options. *Curr Opin Cardiol.* 2008;23(2):141–147.
113. Anand IS, Kuskowski MA, Rector TS, et al. Anemia and change in hemoglobin over time related to mortality and morbidity in patients with chronic heart failure: results from Val-HeFT. *Circulation.* 2005; 112(8):1121–1127.
114. Mozaffarian D, Anker SD, Anand I, et al. Prediction of mode of death in heart failure: the seattle heart failure model. *Circulation.* 2007;116(4):392–398.
115. Maggioni AP, Opasich C, Anand I, et al. Anemia in patients with heart failure: prevalence and prognostic role in a controlled trial and in clinical practice. *J Card Fail.* 2005;11(2):91–98.
116. Pfeffer MA, Solomon SD, Singh AK, et al. Uncertainty in the treatment of anemia in chronic kidney disease. *Rev Cardiovasc Med.* 2005;6(suppl 3):S35–S41.
117. Bhatt KN, Kalogeropoulos AP, Dunbar SB, et al. Depression in heart failure: can PHQ-9 help? *Int J Cardiol.* 2016;221:246–250.
118. Newhouse A, Jiang W. Heart failure and depression. *Heart Fail Clin.* 2014;10(2):295–304.
119. Rumsfeld JS, Havranek E, Masoudi FA, et al. Depressive symptoms are the strongest predictors of short-term declines in health status in patients with heart failure. *J Am Coll Cardiol.* 2003;42(10):1811–1817.
120. Sherwood A, Blumenthal JA, Trivedi R, et al. Relationship of depression to death or hospitalization in patients with heart failure. *Arch Intern Med.* 2007;167(4):367–373.
121. Jha MK, Qamar A, Vaduganathan M, et al. Screening and management of depression in patients with cardiovascular disease: JACC State-of-the-Art Review. *J Am Coll Cardiol.* 2019;73(14):1827–1845.
122. Cowie MR, Gallagher AM. Sleep disordered breathing and heart failure: what does the future hold? *JACC Heart Fail.* 2017;5(10):715–723.
123. Shahar E, Whitney CW, Redline S, et al. Sleep-disordered breathing and cardiovascular disease: cross-sectional results of the Sleep Heart Health Study. *Am J Respir Crit Care Med.* 2001;163(1):19–25.
124. Parish JM, Shepard JW Jr. Cardiovascular effects of sleep disorders. *Chest.* 1990;97(5):1220–1226.

125. Hanly P, Sasson Z, Zuberi N, et al. ST-segment depression during sleep in obstructive sleep apnea. *Am J Cardiol.* 1993;71(15):1341–1345.
126. Guilleminault C, Connolly SJ, Winkle RA. Cardiac arrhythmia and conduction disturbances during sleep in 400 patients with sleep apnea syndrome. *Am J Cardiol.* 1983;52(5):490–494.
127. Fletcher EC, Miller J, Schaaf JW, et al. Urinary catecholamines before and after tracheostomy in patients with obstructive sleep apnea and hypertension. *Sleep.* 1987;10(1):35–44.
128. Gainer JL. Hypoxia and atherosclerosis: re-evaluation of an old hypothesis. *Atherosclerosis.* 1987;68(3):263–266.
129. Bradley TD. Right and left ventricular functional impairment and sleep apnea. *Clin Chest Med.* 1992;13(3):459–479.
130. Mansfield DR, Gollogly NC, Kaye DM, et al. Controlled trial of continuous positive airway pressure in obstructive sleep apnea and heart failure. *Am J Respir Crit Care Med.* 2004;169(3):361–366.
131. Folsom AR, Shah AM, Lutsey PL, et al. American Heart Association's Life's Simple 7: avoiding heart failure and preserving cardiac structure and function. *Am J Med.* 2015;128(9):970–976.
132. American Heart Association (AHA). *Life Simple 7.* 2019. Available at https://www.heart.org/en/professional/workplace-health/lifes-simple-7
133. World Health Organization (WHO). *Tobacco free initiative.* 2019. Available at https://www.who.int/tobacco/quitting/summary_data/en/
134. Center for Disease Control and Prevention. *Annual U.S. deaths attributable to smoking 1997–2001.* 2005.
135. Bibbins Domingo K, Lin F, Vittinghoff E, et al. Predictors of heart failure among women with coronary disease. *Circulation.* 2004;110(11): 1424–1430.
136. Suskin N, Sheth T, Negassa A, et al. Relationship of current and past smoking to mortality and morbidity in patients with left ventricular dysfunction. *J Am Coll Cardiol.* 2001;37(6):1677–1682.
137. Goldstein MG, Niaura R, Willey-Lessne C, et al. Physicians counseling smokers. A population-based survey of patients' perceptions of health care provider-delivered smoking cessation interventions. *Arch Intern Med.* 1997;157(12):1313–1319.
138. Nohria A, Chen YT, Morton DJ, et al. Quality of care for patients hospitalized with heart failure at academic medical centers. *Am Heart J.* 1999;137(6):1028–1034.
139. Ahmed AA, Patel K, Nyaku MA, et al. Risk of heart failure and death after prolonged smoking cessation: role of amount and duration of prior smoking. *Circ Heart Fail.* 2015;8(4):694–701.
140. Pina IL, Apstein CS, Balady GJ, et al. Exercise and heart failure: a statement from the American Heart Association Committee on exercise, rehabilitation, and prevention. *Circulation.* 2003;107(8):1210–1225.
141. Drexler H, Coats AJ. Explaining fatigue in congestive heart failure. *Annu Rev Med.* 1996;47:241–256.
142. Kitzman DW. Exercise intolerance. *Prog Cardiovasc Dis.* 2005;47(6): 367–379.
143. Myers J, Froelicher VF. Hemodynamic determinants of exercise capacity in chronic heart failure. *Ann Intern Med.* 1991;115(5):377–386.
144. Anderson KM. Discharge clinical characteristics and 60-day readmission in patients hospitalized with heart failure. *J Cardiovasc Nurs.* 2014;29(3):232–241.
145. Alvarez P, Hannawi B, Guha A. Exercise and heart failure: Advancing knowledge and improving care. *Methodist Debakey Cardiovasc J.* 2016;12(2):110–115.
146. Reilly CM, Anderson KM, Baas L, et al. American Association of Heart Failure Nurses Best Practices paper: literature synthesis and guideline review for dietary sodium restriction. *Heart Lung.* 2015;44(4):289–298.
147. Chung ML, Park L, Frazier SK, et al. Long-term adherence to low-sodium diet in patients with heart failure. *West J Nurs Res.* 2017;39(4): 553–567.
148. Bennett SJ, Lane KA, Welch J, et al. Medication and dietary compliance beliefs in heart failure. *West J Nurs Res.* 2005;27(8):977–993; discussion 994–999.
149. Travers B, O'Loughlin C, Murphy NF, et al. Fluid restriction in the management of decompensated heart failure: no impact on time to clinical stability. *J Card Fail.* 2007;13(2):128–132.
150. Lancellotti P, Ancion A, Pierard L. Cardiac rehabilitation, state of the art 2017. *Rev Med Liege.* 2017;72(11):481–487.
151. American Heart Association (AHA;.. *What is cardiac rehabilitation?* 2016. Available at https://www.heart.org/en/health-topics/cardiac-rehab/what-is-cardiac-rehabilitation. Accessed July 5, 2019.
152. Forman DE, Sanderson BK, Josephson RA, et al. Heart failure as a newly approved diagnosis for cardiac rehabilitation: challenges and opportunities. *J Am Coll Cardiol.* 2015;65(24):2652–2659.
153. Benjamin EJ, Muntner P, Alonso A, et al. Heart disease and stroke statistics-2019 update: a report from the American Heart Association. *Circulation.* 2019;139(10):e56–e528.
154. Rich MW, Beckham V, Wittenberg C, et al. A multidisciplinary intervention to prevent the readmission of elderly patients with congestive heart failure. *N Engl J Med.* 1995;333(18):1190–1195.
155. Bennett SJ, Huster GA, Baker SL, et al. Characterization of the precipitants of hospitalization for heart failure decompensation. *Am J Crit Care.* 1998;7(3):168–174.
156. Vinson JM, Rich MW, Sperry JC, et al. Early readmission of elderly patients with congestive heart failure. *J Am Geriatr Soc.* 1990; 38(12):1290–1295.
157. Feldman PH, Murtaugh CM, Pezzin LE, et al. Just-in-time evidence-based e-mail "reminders" in home health care: impact on patient outcomes. *Health Serv Res.* 2005;40(3):865–885.
158. Ansari M, Shlipak MG, Heidenreich PA, et al. Improving guideline adherence: a randomized trial evaluating strategies to increase [beta]-blocker use in heart failure. *Circulation.* 2003;107(22):2799–2804.
159. Riegel B, Carlson B, Kopp Z, et al. Effect of a standardized nurse case-management telephone intervention on resource use in patients with chronic heart failure. *Arch Intern Med.* 2002;162(6):705–712.
160. Kimmelstiel C, Levine D, Perry K, et al. Randomized, controlled evaluation of short- and long-term benefits of heart failure disease management within a diverse provider network: the SPAN-CHF Trial. *Circulation.* 2004;110(11):1450–1455.
161. Krumholz HM, Amatruda J, Smith GL, et al. Randomized trial of an education and support intervention to prevent readmission of patients with heart failure. *J Am Coll Cardiol.* 2002;39(1):83–89.
162. Stromberg A, Martensson J, Fridlund B, et al. Nurse-led heart failure clinics improve survival and self-care behaviour in patients with heart failure: results from a prospective, randomised trial. *Eur Heart J.* 2003;24(11):1014–1023.
163. Inglis SC, Pearson S, Treen S, et al. Extending the horizon in chronic heart failure: effects of multidisciplinary, home-based intervention relative to usual care. *Circulation.* 2006;114(23):2466–2473.
164. Mazzuca SA. Does patient education in chronic disease have therapeutic value? *J Chronic Dis.* 1982;35(7):521–529.
165. Artinian NT, Magnan M, Sloan M, et al. Self-care behaviors among patients with heart failure. *Heart Lung.* 2002;31(3):161–172.
166. Jaarsma T, Halfens R, Huijer Abu-Saad H, et al. Effects of education and support on self-care and resource utilization in patients with heart failure. *Eur Heart J.* 1999;20(9):673–682.
167. Sulzbach-Hoke LM, Kagan SH, Craig K. Weighing behavior and symptom distress of clinic patients with CHF. *Medsurg Nurs.* 1997;6(5):288–293, 314.
168. Baker DW, Asch SM, Keesey JW, et al. Differences in education, knowledge, self- management activities, and health outcomes for patients with heart failure cared for under the chronic disease model: the improving chronic illness care evaluation. *J Card Fail.* 2005;11(6):405–413.
169. Lee NC, Wasson DR, Anderson MA, et al. A survey of patient education postdischarge. *J Nurs Care Qual.* 1998;13(1):63–70.
170. Koelling TM, Johnson ML, Cody RJ, et al. Discharge education improves clinical outcomes in patients with chronic heart failure. *Circulation.* 2005;111(2):179–185.
171. Fonarow GC. Quality indicators for the management of heart failure in vulnerable elders. *Ann Intern Med.* 2001;135(8 Pt 2):694–702.
172. Grady KL, Dracup K, Kennedy G, et al. Team management of patients with heart failure: a statement for healthcare professionals from the Cardiovascular Nursing Council of the American Heart Association. *Circulation.* 2000;102(19):2443–2456.
173. Bither CJ, Apple S. Home management of the failing heart. Inotropic therapy in the outpatient setting. *Am J Nurs.* 2001;101(12):41–45.
174. Riegel B, Carlson B, Moser DK, et al. Psychometric testing of the self-care of heart failure index. *J Card Fail.* 2004;10(4):350–360.
175. Riegel B, Dickson VV, Hoke L, et al. A motivational counseling approach to improving heart failure self-care: mechanisms of effectiveness. *J Cardiovasc Nurs.* 2006;21(3):232–241.
176. Riegel B, Moser DK. Self-care: an update on the state of the science one decade later. *J Cardiovasc Nurs.* 2018;33(5):404–407.
177. Riegel B, Carlson B, Glaser D. Development and testing of a clinical tool measuring self-management of heart failure. *Heart Lung.* 2002;29(1):4–15.
178. Sneed NV, Paul SC. Readiness for behavioral changes in patients with heart failure. *Am J Crit Care.* 2003;12(5):444–453.
179. Riegel B, Carlson B. Facilitators and barriers to heart failure self-care. *Patient Educ Couns.* 2002;46(4):287–295.

180. Harkness K, Spaling MA, Currie K, et al. A systematic review of patient heart failure self-care strategies. *J Cardiovasc Nurs.* 2015;30(2):121–135.
181. Happ MB, Naylor MD, Roe-Prior P. Factors contributing to rehospitalization of elderly patients with heart failure. *J Cardiovasc Nurs.* 1997;11(4):75–84.
182. Koenig HG. Depression in hospitalized older patients with congestive heart failure. *Gen Hosp Psychiatry.* 1998;20(1):29–43.
183. Yu DS, Lee DT, Woo J. Health-related quality of life in elderly Chinese patients with heart failure. *Res Nurs Health.* 2004;27(5):332–344.
184. Subramanian U, Fihn SD, Weinberger M, et al. A controlled trial of including symptom data in computer-based care suggestions for managing patients with chronic heart failure. *Am J Med.* 2004;116(6):375–384.
185. Chriss PM, Sheposh J, Carlson B, et al. Predictors of successful heart failure self-care maintenance in the first three months after hospitalization. *Heart Lung.* 2004;33(6):345–353.
186. Welsh JD, Heiser RM, Schooler MP, et al. Characteristics and treatment of patients with heart failure in the emergency department. *J Emerg Nurs.* 2002;28(2):126–131.
187. Chaudhry SI, Wang Y, Concato J, et al. Patterns of weight change preceding hospitalization for heart failure. *Circulation.* 2007;116(14):1549–1554.
188. Ni H, Nauman DJ, Hershberger RE. Analysis of trends in hospitalizations for heart failure. *J Card Fail.* 1999;5(2):79–84.
189. Monane M, Bohn RL, Gurwitz JH, et al. Noncompliance with congestive heart failure therapy in the elderly. *Arch Intern Med.* 1994;154(4):433–437.
190. Bagchi AD, Esposito D, Kim M, et al. Utilization of, and adherence to, drug therapy among Medicaid beneficiaries with congestive heart failure. *Clin Ther.* 2007;29(8):1771–1783.
191. Ekman I, Fagerberg B, Lundman B. Health-related quality of life and sense of coherence among elderly patients with severe chronic heart failure in comparison with healthy controls. *Heart Lung.* 2002;31(2):94–101.
192. Goodyer LI, Miskelly F, Milligan P. Does encouraging good compliance improve patients' clinical condition in heart failure? *Br J Clin Pract.* 1995;49(4):173–176.
193. Murray MD, Young J, Hoke S, et al. Pharmacist intervention to improve medication adherence in heart failure: a randomized trial. *Ann Intern Med.* 2007;146(10):714–725.
194. Mueller TM, Vuckovic KM, Knox DA, et al. Telemangement of heart failure: a diuretic treatment algorithm for advanced practice nurses. *Heart Lung.* 2002;31(5):340–347.
195. Chaudhry SI, Mattera JA, Curtis JP, et al. Telemonitoring in patients with heart failure. *N Engl J Med.* 2010;363:2301–2309. Available at http://dx.doi.org/10.1056/NEJMoa1010029
196. Ong MK, Romano PS, Edgington S, et al. Effectiveness of remote patient monitoring after discharge of hospitalized patients with heart failure: the better effectiveness after transition–heart failure (BEAT-HF) randomized clinical trial. *JAMA Intern Med.* 2016;176(3):310–318.
197. Maeng DD, Starr AE, Tomcavage JF, et al. Can telemonitoring reduce hospitalization and cost of care? A health plan's experience in managing patients with heart failure. *Popul Health Manag.* 2014;17(6):340–344.
198. Blum K, Gottlieb S. The effect of a randomized trial of home telemonitoring on medical costs, 30-day readmissions, mortality, and health-related quality of life in a cohort of community-dwelling heart failure patients. *J Card Fail.* 2014;20(7):513–521.
199. Klersy C, Silvestri AD, Gabutti G, et al. Economic impact of remote patient monitoring: an integrated economic model derived from a meta-analysis of randomized controlled trials in heart failure. *Eur J Heart Fail.* 2011;13:450–459.
200. Inglis SC, Clark R A, Dierckx R, et al. Structured telephone support or non-invasive telemonitoring for patients with heart failure. *Cochrane Database Syst Rev.* 2015;(10):CD007228. Available at https://doi.org/10.1002/14651858.CD007228.pub3
201. World Health Organization (WHO). *Definition of Palliative Care.* 2019. Available at https://www.who.int/cancer/palliative/definition/en/. Accessed May 1, 2019.
202. McIlvennan CK, Larry AA. Palliative care in patients with heart failure. *BMJ.* 2016;353:i1010.
203. Diop MS, Rudolph JL, Zimmerman KM, et al. Palliative care interventions for patients with heart failure: a systematic review and meta-analysis. *J Palliat Med.* 2017;20(1):84–92.

39 Therapeutic Intervention for Cardiogenic Shock and End-Stage Heart Failure: Mechanical Circulatory Support and Heart Transplantation

Nicole Dellise, Beth Davidson

OBJECTIVES

1. Describe pathophysiology, etiology, and treatment approach to acute cardiogenic shock.
2. Identify physiologic findings consistent with refractory, end-stage heart failure.
3. Describe treatment options for end-stage heart failure such as durable mechanical circulatory support (MCS), heart transplantation, and palliative/hospice care.

KEY QUESTIONS

1. How do the physiology, etiology, and management of acute cardiogenic shock and refractory end-stage heart failure differ?
2. What are the indications for mechanical circulatory support (MCS), heart transplantation, and palliative/hospice care?
3. What is the role of the cardiac nurse in the evaluation and treatment of cardiogenic shock and end-stage heart failure?

CARDIOGENIC SHOCK

Pathophysiology

Acute heart failure (HF) is a true medical emergency that warrants an expedient diagnosis. If appropriate treatment is not instituted within a short time course, then irreversible decompensation may ensue, leading to a progressive syndrome of shock.[1] At the endpoint on the clinical continuum of left ventricular (LV) failure, cardiogenic shock includes shock caused by ineffective cardiac contractility and myocardial failure. The complexity of acute HF has diverse potential etiologies making a precise definition difficult.

Shock is a complex clinical syndrome characterized by impaired cellular metabolism caused by decreased tissue perfusion. The inadequacy of tissue perfusion results in cellular hypoxia, the accumulation of cellular metabolic wastes, cellular destruction, and ultimately, organ and system failure. The syndrome begins as an adaptive response to some insult or injury and progresses to multiple organ system failure. The pathophysiologic mechanisms of shock include decreased circulating blood volume, decreased cardiac contractility, and increased venous capacitance.[2]

Cardiogenic Shock

Atherosclerotic heart disease and the complications of ischemia and infarction are the most common causes of acute HF.[2] Acute coronary occlusion first impairs diastolic function, with later diminished systolic function, stroke volume, and blood pressure. This downward spiral leads to progressive myocardial dysfunction and possibly death (Fig. 39-1).[1] Shock occurs in approximately 8% of patients with acute LV myocardial infarction (MI), most often of the anterior wall. Angiographic findings of the landmark SHOCK (Should We Emergently Revascularize Occluded Coronaries for Cardiogenic

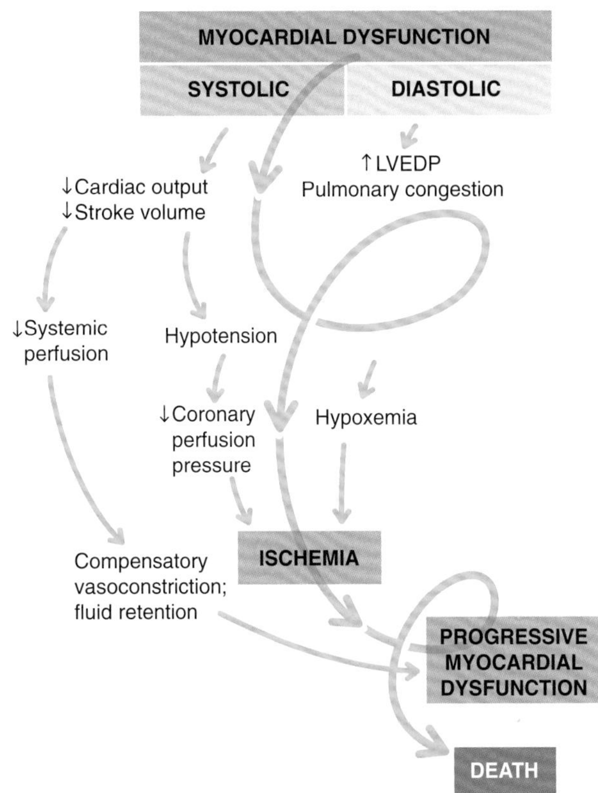

Figure 39-1. The Downward Spiral in Cardiogenic Shock. LVEDP, left ventricular end-diastolic pressure. (From Hollenberg SM. Cardiogenic shock. *Crit Care Clin.* 2001;17[2]:395.)

Shock) trial showed left main coronary artery occlusion in 20% of patients, three-vessel disease in 64%, two-vessel disease in 23%, and single-vessel disease in 13%.[3] Some patients may present in cardiogenic shock on admission, but shock often evolves over several hours. The median delay from onset of MI to development of cardiogenic shock in the SHOCK trial was 5.6 hours.[3] Shock with a delayed onset may result from infarct expansion, reocclusion of a previously patent infarct artery, or decompensation of myocardial function in the infarction zone caused by metabolic abnormalities. Ischemia-related systolic dysfunction also could contribute to the development of cardiogenic shock. One pattern is the "hibernating" myocardium, seen with low tissue perfusion states matched by a decline in compensatory function. The second pattern is the "stunned" myocardium, which is a more prolonged (hours to days) myocardial dysfunction after a relatively brief interruption of myocardial perfusion. These patterns have been reported after percutaneous coronary interventions (PCIs), cardioplegic arrest, and unstable angina.[4,5]

Right ventricular (RV) infarction occurs after occlusion of the proximal right coronary artery and is identified in the setting of concomitant inferoposterior LV dysfunction.

Complications of MI include mitral regurgitation, ventricular septal defect (VSD), and free-wall rupture. Significant mitral regurgitation patterns are seen clinically: papillary muscle (usually the posterior papillary muscle) or chordal rupture caused by MI, and mitral regurgitation associated with LV dilatation. Acute VSD abruptly increases pulmonary blood flow and leads to symptoms of biventricular failure within hours to days if not corrected. LV free-wall rupture occurs in less than 1% of acute MIs but carries a high mortality rate.[6]

Non–MI-related acute valvular problems involve the mitral and aortic valve. Acute mitral regurgitation can be caused by spontaneous chordal rupture, infective endocarditis, inflammatory disorders (e.g., rheumatic fever), or trauma. Acute aortic insufficiency may be caused by infective endocarditis with leaflet destruction (most common), acute aortic dissection, or traumatic injury. Shock may be caused by aortic stenosis with increasing metabolic demands or with concomitant LV failure. Mitral stenosis rarely causes shock without rapid atrial fibrillation.[6] Prosthetic valve dysfunction, especially left sided, most often causes shock because of valvular insufficiency. Acute prosthetic valvular insufficiency occurs because of dehiscence of the sewing ring, infective endocarditis, or catastrophic mechanical failure.

Amyloidosis, sarcoidosis, and hemochromatosis are examples of infiltrative diseases in their later stages that may be associated with shock. Shock caused by trauma is usually seen secondary to myocardial or aortic rupture, or caused by acute volume loss secondary to hemorrhage.

Acute decompensation of chronic HF represents a somewhat different pathophysiologic state, because these patients have a marked reduction in LV systolic function at baseline as compared to those patients with acute HF without prior LV dysfunction.[1] There is already activation of the neurohormonal compensatory mechanisms, including increased sympathetic stimulation of the heart, activation of the renin–angiotensin–aldosterone system (RAAS), increased vasoconstriction, fluid retention by the kidneys, increased ventricular preload, and LV hypertrophy and remodeling. When a precipitating event occurs, there is further derangement of these compensatory mechanisms. Factors leading to acute decompensation in chronic HF may include the following: acute myocardial ischemia, poorly treated or untreated hypertension, new-onset atrial fibrillation, concurrent infections (e.g., pneumonia, influenza), medication noncompliance, excess dietary sodium, cardiac depressant drugs, nonsteroidal anti-inflammatory drugs (NSAIDs), and endocrine abnormalities (e.g., poorly controlled diabetes, hyperthyroidism).[1] Table 39-1 compares clinical and pathophysiologic features of acute and chronic HF.

Extracardiac Obstructive Shock

Pericardial Tamponade. The accumulation of fluid within the pericardial sac increases pressure, causing extracardiac obstruction to filling that results in a decrease in ventricular preload and cardiac output. What determines whether pericardial effusion will cause shock is how rapidly the fluid accumulates. Patients at risk for shock caused by tamponade are those with malignancy (especially lung and breast cancer, lymphoma, leukemia, or melanoma), infection, aortic dissection, or severe pericarditis.

Pulmonary Embolism. When embolic material, such as thrombus, fat, tumor, or air, obstructs 30% or more of the pulmonary vasculature, the RV cannot provide adequate pressure to compensate for the increased resistance to blood flow. RV failure ensues, with increased RV end-diastolic and RA pressures, and finally a decrease in cardiac output and shock.

Compensatory Mechanisms

The following equations illustrate the physiologic relation of the hemodynamic variables. Here CO, cardiac output; SV, stroke volume; HR, heart rate; MAP, mean arterial pressure; and SVR, systemic vascular resistance compose the equations:

$$CO = SV \times HR$$
$$MAP = CO \times SVR$$

Table 39-1 • CLINICAL AND PATHOPHYSIOLOGIC FEATURES OF ACUTE AND CHRONIC HF

Abnormal Volume Load	Abnormal Pressure Load	Myocardial Abnormalities	Filling Disorders	Increased Metabolic Demand
Aortic valve incompetence Mitral valve incompetence Tricuspid valve incompetence Left-to-right shunts Secondary hypervolemia	Aortic stenosis Hypertrophic cardiomyopathy Coarctation of the aorta Hypertension • Primary • Secondary	Cardiomyopathy Myocarditis Coronary heart disease Ischemia Infarction Arrhythmias Toxic disorders • Alcohol • Cocaine Administration of cardiac depressant agents or salt-retaining drugs	Mitral stenosis Tricuspid stenosis Cardiac tamponade Restrictive pericarditis Restrictive cardiomyopathy	Anemias Thyrotoxicosis Fever Beriberi Paget disease Arteriovenous fistulas Pulmonary emboli Systemic emboli

In the pathophysiologic state of cardiogenic shock, the decrease in MAP is brought about by an alteration in one of the variables. The reduction in cardiac output results from a decrease in stroke volume:

$$\downarrow \text{CO} = \downarrow \text{SV} \times \text{HR}$$

The deduction in MAP results from the decrease in cardiac output:

$$\downarrow \text{MAP} = \downarrow \text{CO} \times \text{SVR}$$

Compensatory mechanisms consist of reflex reactions to an initial fall in blood pressure. They are activated immediately and increase in intensity in an attempt to restore adequate tissue perfusion.[1] The compensatory mechanisms are directed at the restoration and maintenance of adequate blood volume, cardiac output, and vascular tone. The initial compensatory mechanisms vary with the primary pathophysiologic derangement, but the intermediate and final stages are similar. The initial compensatory mechanisms in cardiogenic shock are an increased heart rate and increased SVR.

Diagnosis and Clinical Manifestations

The diagnosis of shock is made by the history, physical examination, and collection of data from adjunctive diagnostic tests.

History

Most patients who present with cardiogenic shock have either a history of cardiovascular disease or risk factors for cardiovascular disease. Obtaining a thorough medical and surgical history is vital to plan lifesaving interventions. Much like chronic HF, a history may provide possible causes of the acute decompensation.

Physical Examination

Ongoing assessment of the patient at risk for or in shock, with early detection of subtle changes in the patient's condition, is essential. Subjective and objective data must be correlated with adjunctive clinical measurements, such as the measurement of cardiac output and oxygen consumption. The clinical assessment of the patient provides the basis for medical and nursing interventions.

Cardiovascular Assessment

Low blood pressure is one of the defining characteristics of shock. A MAP of 65 mm Hg is required to maintain adequate myocardial and renal perfusion. Shock is defined clinically as the pathophysiologic state that results from a MAP of less than 65 mm Hg over time. Narrowing of the pulse pressure indicates arteriolar vasoconstriction and a decreasing cardiac output.[7,8] Heart rate usually increases in response to sympathetic stimulation to compensate for decreased stroke volume and to maintain cardiac output. In cardiogenic shock, the pulse is weak and thready.

Distended neck veins may be seen with cardiogenic shock.[9] The presence of an RV heave, jugular venous V waves, and right-sided S_3 or S_4 gallops may suggest pulmonary emboli. Distant heart sounds and an exaggerated pulsus paradoxus (greater than 10 mm Hg) suggest cardiac tamponade. A laterally displaced and sustained LV apical impulse with left-sided S_3 and/or S_4 suggests LV dysfunction.[9]

Pulmonary Assessment

The lungs are fairly resistant to short-term ischemia. Thus, it is unlikely that low blood flow is the sole cause of pulmonary insufficiency associated with shock. Other contributory factors have been implicated, including thromboemboli or fat emboli in the pulmonary tree and the toxic effects of fibrin degradation products that result from intravascular coagulation and serum complement depletion with sequestration of granulocytes in the lung. These factors lead to increased pulmonary capillary permeability. As the ensuing alveolar edema impairs surfactant production, massive atelectasis develops, clinically termed shock lung, systemic inflammatory response syndrome, adult respiratory distress syndrome, or primary pulmonary edema. These conditions are characterized by severe hypoxemia, dyspnea, a marked reduction in lung compliance, and the presence of extensive lung infiltrates.[9]

In cardiogenic shock, failure of the left ventricle leads to acute cardiogenic pulmonary edema. Because of the increase in LV end-diastolic pressure, there is an increase in left atrial (LA) pressure and dilatation. Pressure is increased within the pulmonary capillary bed, forcing plasma or whole blood into the pulmonary interstitial compartment and, finally, into the pulmonary alveoli.

Respiratory rate and depth are initially increased in all forms of shock, and patients may experience dyspnea or air hunger. This increased ventilation represents the body's attempt to eliminate lactic acid resulting from decreased tissue perfusion. Increased respiratory depth also enhances blood return to the right heart. Arterial blood gases initially reveal respiratory alkalosis. As shock progresses, a combined metabolic and respiratory acidosis follows.

Neuroregulatory Assessment

Decreased cerebral blood flow and coagulopathy can lead to a cerebral infarction or cerebral thrombus formation. Alterations in cellular metabolism throughout the body, metabolic acidosis, and the accumulation of toxins further depress cerebral function. Lethargy, stupor, and coma develop as shock progresses. Finally, in the irreversible stage of shock, the vasomotor center in the brain is disrupted, causing failure of the circulatory mechanisms.[9]

Level of consciousness is an indicator of the adequacy of cerebral blood flow. With cerebral ischemia, the patient initially exhibits hypervigilance, restlessness, agitation, and mild confusion. Persistent cerebral hypoxia results in progressive unresponsiveness to verbal stimuli with eventual coma.

Gastrointestinal Assessment

Compensatory vasoconstriction in shock may result in mucosal ischemia, an ileus, and full-thickness gangrene of the bowel. If the bowel wall becomes disrupted, the normal bacterial flora of the intestines enters the abdomen and can then enter the circulation. Gastrointestinal bleeding may also occur. Factors that cause damage to the liver include decreased blood flow, splanchnic vasoconstriction, pooling of blood in the microcirculation, right HF, and bacterial invasion. The subsequent changes include loss of reticuloendothelial (tissue macrophage) system function, increasing the risk of infection; a decreased lactic acid conversion, contributing to metabolic acidosis; altered protein, fat, and carbohydrate metabolism; and altered bilirubin function.[9] Jaundice, increased serum bilirubin levels, and increased serum enzymes are early indicators of liver damage associated with shock. Serum globulin is increased, and serum albumin is decreased.[9]

Renal Assessment

Adequate renal perfusion produces a minimum of 400 mL urine per 24 hours, or 20 mL/h. Impaired renal perfusion in shock results in hourly urine outputs of less than 20 mL/h.[9] The excretion of high volumes of low-solute urine may also represent renal hypoperfusion. Prolonged hypoperfusion may lead to acute tubular necrosis and acute renal failure. Urine output is an indicator of the adequacy of renal perfusion and may decrease early in cardiogenic shock. Oliguria is defined by a urine output of less than 20 mL/h. Urine osmolarity and specific gravity increase, and urine sodium decreases with decreased urine output. An elevated serum creatinine is an early, nonspecific indicator of impaired renal perfusion.

Integumentary Assessment

Skin appearance and temperature provide a clinical measure of peripheral circulation. Progressive peripheral vasoconstriction results in a change from the initial normal skin appearance to cool, moist, pale skin with mottling. In cardiogenic shock, cool, moist skin with barely perceptible peripheral pulses is commonly observed. Capillary refill and peripheral pulses are other indicators of the relative adequacy of cardiac output. Normal capillary refill is almost instantaneous; in cardiogenic shock, capillary refill is often prolonged.

Diagnostic Tools

The primary measurements that document the relative adequacy of blood flow include continuous monitoring of arterial blood pressure and monitoring of the electrocardiogram (ECG) with rhythm analysis. The ECG can be diagnostic in the setting of MI. Most patients in shock are tachycardic and may show evidence of supraventricular or ventricular arrhythmias. Low QRS voltage and/or electrical alternans can be seen in cardiac tamponade.[10]

Transthoracic echocardiography is an excellent tool to obtain noninvasive information regarding the overall and regional systolic and diastolic function, intravascular volume, cardiac hemodynamics, and myocardial abnormalities. Echocardiography can rapidly assess for mechanical causes, such as severe mitral regurgitation and papillary muscle rupture, acute VSD, free-wall rupture, and tamponade. Predictors of short- and long-term mortality from cardiogenic shock relate to the LV ejection fraction (LVEF) and mitral regurgitation on presentation, supporting early use of echocardiography in the course of cardiogenic shock.[8]

Chest radiography may suggest a specific diagnosis. Continuous measurement of urine output and mental status are good indicators of adequate organ perfusion. A complete blood count and serial cardiac enzymes should be obtained. Serial measurements of arterial blood gases reflect the overall metabolic state of the patient, the adequacy of ventilation, and the adequacy of the circulation in providing for oxygen and metabolic needs. Measurement of mixed venous oxygen content ($S\bar{v}O_2$) by direct blood sampling or by continuous invasive monitoring reflects peripheral oxygen extraction and use. Serial arterial lactate levels can also be measured because the presence of lactic acidosis helps identify critical hypoperfusion as marked by anaerobic metabolism.[8]

Measurement of serum BNP is a means to identify those patients with LV dysfunction.[7] Elevation of other substances in the blood that reflect the function of specific organs, such as blood urea nitrogen, creatinine, bilirubin, aspartate aminotransferase, and lactate dehydrogenase, may be useful in the diagnosis of shock.

In seriously ill patients, direct determination of intra-arterial pressure with an arterial line is necessary because systemic arterial pressure determines the perfusion pressure of various organ systems and is predominantly the product of cardiac output and SVR. In HF, a drop in cardiac output is compensated for by an increased SVR in an attempt to maintain the arterial blood pressure in normal range.

Right-sided heart catheterization with a pulmonary artery (PA) quadruple lumen thermodilution catheter can aid in the diagnosis and assessment of the severity of HF.[7,8] This invasive hemodynamic monitoring can be useful in excluding volume depletion, RV infarction, and mechanical problems (e.g., acute mitral regurgitation). It is also useful for monitoring the response to treatment (including volume, diuretics, inotropic support, vasoactive agents, natriuretic peptide) and manipulation of the variables of cardiac output, preload, and afterload.[7] The hemodynamic variables measured by this catheter are cardiac output by thermodilution; RA pressure; and PA systolic, diastolic, and wedge pressures. The cardiac output is decreased in HF, whereas the RA pressure or central venous pressure is elevated. The pulmonary artery wedge pressure (PAWP) indirectly measures the LV end-diastolic pressure, which is a measure of end-diastolic volume or preload and is elevated in HF.

Derived parameters that may be obtained by the use of the PA catheter include cardiac index (CI) and SVR. Body surface area (BSA), measured in square meters, is correlated with the volume of cardiac output (CO) to establish the CI:

$$CI = \frac{CO}{BSA}$$

CI = SVR, measured in dynes/s/cm^5, reflects the pressure difference of the systemic arteries to the veins.

$$SVR = \frac{MAP - RAP}{CO} \times 80$$

Besides offering diagnostic information, hemodynamic variables show a strong prognostic value for short-term survival. In their seminal study, Forrester et al.[11] classified patients with acute MI into four subsets with different mortality rates. The investigators showed that clinical signs of hypoperfusion occur with a CI of less than 2.2 L/min/m^2 and clinical signs of pulmonary congestion occur with a PAWP greater than 18 mm Hg. Subset I shows a patient with normal CI and normal PAWP with no evidence of pulmonary congestion or peripheral hypoperfusion (warm and dry). Subset III shows a patient with a low CI and PAWP, reflecting peripheral hypoperfusion without pulmonary congestion (cool and dry) as seen in patients with hypovolemia. Subset II describes the patient with pulmonary edema with an elevated PAWP but without peripheral hypoperfusion (warm and wet), which may be seen in acute HF or decompensated chronic HF. Subset IV describes the patient with pulmonary edema with hypoperfusion (cold and wet), as seen in cardiogenic shock.[8]

Assessment of tissue metabolism, which is determined by mixed venous oxygen saturation, conventionally required sending a PA blood sample to the laboratory for interpretation. Some PA catheters are designed with a fiberoptic photometric lumen, allowing for continuous monitoring of mixed venous oxygen saturation. Although PA catheters were widely used for over 40 years, their use has decreased in critically ill patients due to data suggestive of increased mortality in certain populations. Current consensus is that PA catheters are useful in cardiogenic shock due to acute MI.[8]

Approach to Treatment

The main goal of treatment of the metabolic defects produced by shock is the restoration of adequate tissue perfusion.[8]

Table 39-2 • VASOPRESSORS AND INOTROPIC AGENTS IN SHOCK

Feature	Dopamine		Dobutamine	Norepinephrine	Epinephrine	Phenylephrine	Milrinone
Dosage (mcg/kg/min)	1–4	4–20	2.5–20	0.05–1	0.05–2	0.5–5	0.375–0.750
Receptor							
α	+	+++	+	++++	++++	++++	0
β_1	+	++	+++	+	++++	0	0
β_2	0	0	++	0	++	0	0
Dopaminergic	+++	++	0	0	0	0	0
Chronotropic (HR)	+	++	++	+	+++	0	+
Inotropic (stroke volume/cardiac output)	+	++/+++	+++	+	+++	0	+++
SVR (afterload)	↓	↑↑	↓↓	↑↑↑↑	↓↓↑↑	↑↑↑↑	↓↓↓
Filling pressure (preload)	↓	↔↑↑	↓↓	↔↑↑	↔	↔	↓↓
Comments	Improves renal flow in low dose; first-line drug to restore BP		First-line agent to improve CO, but may be arrhythmogenic	Pure vasoconstrictor compared to dopamine	Increases MVO_2, supports BP	Purest vasoconstrictor	Inotrope of choice in pulmonary hypertension

Initial general management for patients is placement of large-bore venous catheters, and continuous monitoring of blood pressure, pulse oximetry, and ECG. If respiratory failure is imminent with patients with severe hypoxemia, hypercarbia, or metabolic acidosis, then endotracheal intubation may be required with mechanical ventilation. A PA catheter may be placed. Volume expansion may be needed to restore adequate circulation to maintain a PAWP of 14 to 16 mm Hg. Vasopressor support should be used only after preload is adequate to restore the blood pressure. The choice of a particular vasopressor/inotropic agent depends on the clinical circumstance (Table 39-2).

Acute manifestations of HF can be either in the setting of a new onset or in patients with established chronic HF. It is critical to establish the diagnosis and determine the hemodynamic status: pulmonary congestion without peripheral hypoperfusion versus shock/hypoperfusion (Table 39-3). The three major goals of treatment of acute HF, acute decompensated chronic HF, and cardiogenic shock are (1) to increase the oxygen supply to the myocardium; (2) to maximize the cardiac output; and (3) to decrease the workload of the left ventricle.

Goal 1: Increase Oxygen Supply to the Myocardium. Increased inspired oxygen concentrations, including the institution of mechanical ventilation with positive end-expiratory pressure, may be required to maintain arterial blood gases within normal limits. Narcotic analgesics are used to control the patient's pain and aid in reducing myocardial oxygen demands.

Aggressive reperfusion of the coronary arteries can be undertaken by invasive and noninvasive approaches, including percutaneous transluminal coronary angioplasty, atherectomy or stent placement, use of adjunctive antiplatelet therapy, thrombolytic therapy, and coronary artery bypass grafting, which were all associated with lower in-hospital mortality rates than treatment with standard medical therapy.[12–14] Studies suggest that immediate revascularization with PCI, which may include angioplasty, stent placement, and atherectomy, along with adjunctive antiplatelet therapy, improves outcomes in patients with cardiogenic shock.[14] Improvement is seen in wall motion in the infarct territory, with increased perfusion of the infarct zone augmenting contraction of remote myocardium, possibly because of recruitment of collateral blood flow. Reperfusion therapy with thrombolytic agents has decreased the occurrence of cardiogenic shock in patients with persistent ST-segment elevation MI, but thrombolytic therapy for patients in whom shock has already developed is disappointing and may be attributed to low perfusion pressure.[8] For hospitals without revascularization capability, early thrombolytic therapy along with intra-aortic balloon pumping followed by immediate transfer for PCI or coronary

Table 39-3 • PULMONARY CONGESTION AND HYPOPERFUSION

Clinical Feature	Acute Heart Failure	Decompensated Chronic Heart Failure	Stable Chronic Heart Failure
Symptom severity (shortness of breath and fatigue)	Marked and sudden	Moderate to severe	None to mild or moderate
Pulmonary edema	Common	Frequent	Rare
Peripheral edema	Rare	Frequent	Occasional
Weight gain	None to mild	Very frequent	Occasional
Total-body volume	No change to mild increase	Marked increase	Mild increase
Cardiomegaly	Uncommon	Common	Common
LV systolic function	Hypo-, normo- or hypercontractile	Normal to reduced	Normal to reduced
LV wall stress	Marked increase	Marked increase	Elevated
Activation of sympathetic nervous system	Marked increase	Marked increase	Mild to marked increase
Activation of RAAS	Marked increase	Marked increase	Mild to marked increase
Myocardial ischemia[a]	Common	Occasional	Rare
Hypertensive crisis	Common	Occasional	Rare

[a]For example, acute coronary syndrome, acute mitral regurgitation, aortic stenosis, or ventricular septal defect.
LV, left ventricle; RAAS, renin–angiotensin–aldosterone system.

artery bypass grafting may be appropriate.[8] However, long-term 6-year follow-up data from the SHOCK II trial showed that intra-aortic balloon pump (IABP) support did not improve outcomes in acute MI with cardiogenic shock. Researchers concluded IABP may not offer enough hemodynamic support and it is unknown if stronger temporary mechanical support devices would yield positive outcomes.[13]

Goal 2: Maximize Cardiac Output. Because the cardiac output is already compromised, arrhythmias, which occur as a result of ischemia, acid–base alterations, or MI, can cause a further decline in cardiac output. Electrolyte abnormalities should be corrected, because hypokalemia and hypomagnesemia predispose to ventricular arrhythmias. Antiarrhythmic agents, pacing, or cardioversion may be used to maintain a stable heart rhythm. Volume loading is undertaken with caution and in the presence of adequate hemodynamic monitoring. Optimal preload (LV end-diastolic pressure or PAWP) ranges between 14 and 18 mm Hg. However, fluid loading must be abandoned when the increase in filling pressure occurs without increase in cardiac output.

For patients with adequate intravascular volume, inotropic agents should be initiated. Inotropic agents are used to increase systemic and coronary artery perfusion pressure. Dobutamine can improve myocardial contractility and increase cardiac output and is usually the agent of choice in patients with systolic pressures greater than 80 mm Hg. Dobutamine can precipitate tachyarrhythmias and exacerbate hypotension. Dopamine is preferable in patients with systolic pressures less than 80 mm Hg. Tachycardia and increased peripheral resistance are dose dependent, and can exacerbate myocardial ischemia.[8,9] In some situations, a combination of dopamine and dobutamine can be more effective than one agent alone. When hypotension remains refractory, norepinephrine may be necessary. Other agents used for positive inotropic effect include phosphodiesterase inhibitors, such as milrinone.

Afterload reduction by peripheral vasodilators appears particularly well suited to reducing PAWP and SVR and improving CI. Inotropic agents are also used to increase systemic and coronary artery perfusion pressure. IABP counterpulsation may also be used in certain patients.[8]

Goal 3: Reduce Myocardial Work. The efficacy of vasodilators has been shown in the treatment of cardiogenic shock. The major physiologic effect of vasodilators is a reduction in LV end-diastolic pressure and SVR, with a subsequent increase in stroke volume and improved LV function (Table 39-4).

When to Consider Temporary Mechanical Circulatory Assist Devices

When medications alone do not offer adequate cardiac output and reduction of myocardial workload, temporary mechanical circulatory assist devices should be considered. With early recognition, the often rapid hemodynamic deterioration of patients with acute LV failure can be arrested with circulatory assist devices. The type of device used depends on the degree of myocardial injury, the degree of LV functional impairment, the anticipated length of therapy, as well as other factors (including what is available locally). The purpose of therapy is to stabilize the patient until (1) the left ventricle recovers from acute injury; (2) mechanical problems causing acute failure (e.g., ruptured ventricular septum) can be surgically corrected; (3) heart transplantation can be performed; or (4) a decision is made to place a device as "destination therapy," for patients who are not candidates for transplant. The goal of a circulatory assist device is to stabilize or improve hemodynamics and secondary organ function. The major principles governing all devices are that they (1) decrease or take over LV workload; (2) enhance oxygen supply to the myocardium; and (3) partially or totally support the systemic circulation and thus, other organ perfusion. The extent to which each principle can be achieved depends on the type of device used. An IABP offers only partial support, whereas implantable right ventricular assist devices (RVADs), left ventricular assist devices (LVADs), and biventricular VADs (BiVADs) can assume the total workload of the right, left, or both ventricles, respectively. In addition, there are devices that provide intermediate levels of support (Table 39-5).

Indications and Contraindications

Indications for mechanical assistance include support/off-loading of the heart during high-risk PCI, weaning from cardiopulmonary bypass, as a bridge to recovery (from acute MI or acute myocarditis), as a bridge to transplant, or as a bridge to another device (e.g., a more permanent device). Device selection depends on patient factors such as anticipated duration of need, patient size, as well as local experience and patient preference.

Contraindications to most of these devices include severe aortic or peripheral vascular disease (i.e., dissection, atherosclerosis, or aneurysm), LV or atrial thrombi, coagulopathy, uncontrolled sepsis, significant aortic valve stenosis or regurgitation, recent stroke or neurologic injury, or when invasive or heroic therapy would clearly be futile or inappropriate.

Table 39-4 • VASOACTIVE MEDICATIONS FOR THE TREATMENT OF CARDIOGENIC SHOCK

Drug	Dosing	Advantages	Disadvantages
Nitroglycerin	Sublingual: 0.4 mg (or 1–2 sprays) at 5-minute intervals intravenous: 0.4 μg/kg/min initially; increase as needed	Positive effect on coronary vasculature and in myocardial ischemia infarction	Hypotension; drug tolerance; inadequate afterload reduction in catastrophic disorders (e.g., acute valve insufficiency)
Nitroprusside	Intravenous: 0.1 μg/kg/min initially; increase as needed	Powerful afterload reducer	Hypotension; infusion needs to be watched closely; less favorable effects on coronary vasculature and myocardial ischemia; thiocyanate or cyanide toxicity during high-dose or prolonged infusion; particularly in renal failure
Nesiritide	Intravenous: bolus of 2 μg/kg, followed by 0.01 μg/kg/min infusion; may rebolus 1 μg/kg 1, and increase infusion up to maximum, which is 0.03 μg/kg/min	Useful afterload reducer and diuretic; use in acute decompensated heart failure	Hypotension; has been linked to progressive renal dysfunction; not to be used in patients in cardiogenic shock, moderate renal dysfunction or systolic BP <90 mm Hg

Table 39-5 • COMPARISON OF MCS DEVICES

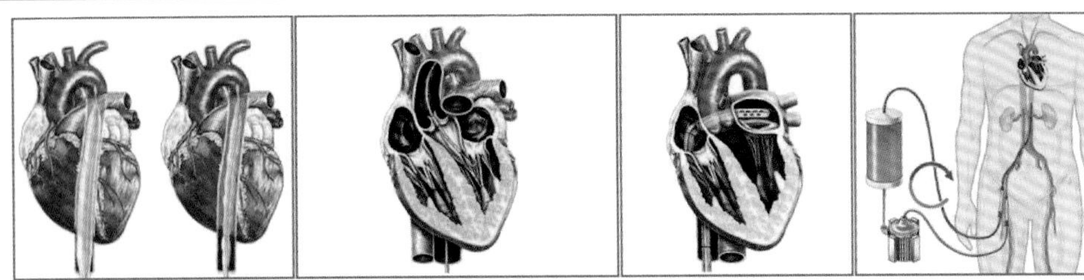

	IABP	Impella	Tandemheart	VA-ECMO
Cardiac Flow	0.3–0.5 L/ min	1–5 L/min (Impella 2.5, Impella CP, Impella 5)	2.5–5 L/min	3–7 L/min
Mechanism	Aorta	LV → AO	LA → AO	RA → AO
Maximum implant days	Weeks	7 days	14 days	Weeks
Sheath size	7–8 Fr	13–14 Fr Impella 5.0–21 Fr	15–17 Fr arterial 21 Fr venous	14–16 Fr arterial 18–21 Fr Venous
Femoral artery size	>4 mm	Impella 2.5 and CP 5–5.5 mm Impella 5–8 mm	8 mm	8 mm
Cardiac synchrony or stable rhythm	Yes	No	No	No
Afterload	↓	↓	↑	↑↑↑
MAP	↑	↑↑	↑↑	↑↑
Cardiac flow	↑	↑↑	↑↑	↑↑
Cardiac power	↑	↑↑	↑↑	↑↑
LVEDP	↓	↓↓	↓↓	↔
PCWP	↓	↓↓	↓↓	↔
LV preload	—	↓↓	↓↓	↓
Coronary perfusion	↑	↑	—	—
Myocardial oxygen demand	↓	↓↓	↔↓	↔

Reprinted with permission from Atkinson TM, Ohman EM, O'Neill WW, et al. A practical approach to mechanical circulatory support in patients undergoing percutaneous coronary intervention: an interventional perspective. *JACC Cardiovasc Interv.* 2016;9(9):871–883.

Types of Temporary Devices

Intra-Aortic Balloon Pump. An IABP is only able to augment cardiac output marginally (500 to 800 mL/min). Thus, with profound ventricular failure, IABP therapy may provide insufficient assistance, and more aggressive therapy may need to be considered. In recent years, a number of other mechanical circulatory assist devices have been developed for short-, intermediate-, and long-term use.

Percutaneous Axial Flow Pump. Axial flow pumps work on the principle of the Archimedes screw. They are composed of a single cannula which is placed retrograde across the aortic valve into the left ventricle. Although they may be placed surgically, a femoral artery approach can be used. The screw turns and draws blood out of the LV and ejects it into the ascending aorta beyond the aortic valve. Figure 39-2 depicts the device. Currently available devices include the Impella 2.5, Impella CP (Cardiac Peripheral), and Impella 5.0 (Abiomed, Inc., Danvers, MA). Because the position of the outflow area must be confirmed to be on the aortic side of the aortic valve, either fluoroscopic or echocardiographic guidance must be utilized. These devices can generate (nonpulsatile) flows of up to 2.5 or 5.0 L/min (depending on the model). Anticoagulation is required. Risks include hemolysis and thrombocytopenia, which are often transient; significant aortic valve disease (stenosis or regurgitation) can contraindicate its use.[15]

Percutaneous Centrifugal Pumps. Another percutaneously placed VAD is the LA to femoral artery VAD (e.g., Tandem-Heart™). A venous catheter is placed in the left atrium via transseptal puncture from the right atrium. An arterial cannula

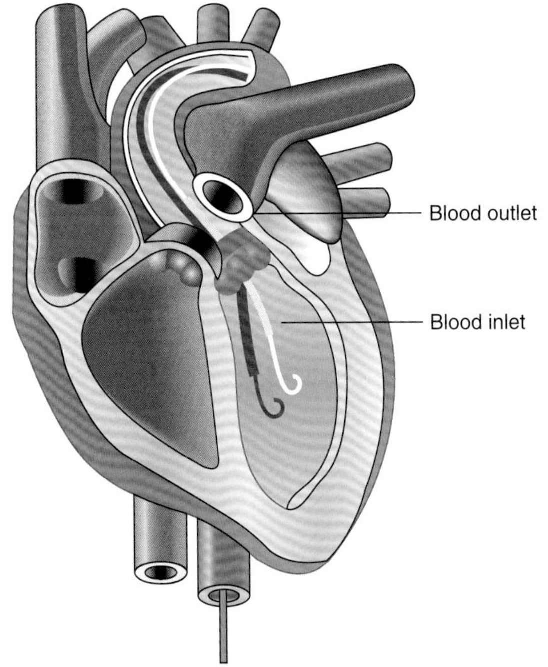

Figure 39-2. Percutaneous Axial Flow Device. The Impella device is placed across the aortic valve, which allows the pump to aspirate blood from the left ventricle and expel it into the ascending aorta. (Courtesy of Abiomed, Inc., Danvers, MA; also from Figure 17, Lee MS, Makkar RR. Percutaneous left ventricular support devices. *Cardiology Clinics.* 2006;24[2]:265–275, vii.)

is inserted in the iliac artery. The pump is a centrifugal model providing continuous flow. The device is used for short-term stabilization, for hemodynamic support during PCIs, or as a bridge to recovery or surgical treatment. It requires anticoagulation (ideal activated clotting time of 250 to 350 seconds). Studies have shown improvement in cardiac output (the pump can move 4 to 5 L/min of blood), CI, and other metabolic parameters. Mortality rates were comparable between IABP and VAD, but there were more complications (e.g., bleeding, acute limb ischemia) with VAD than with IABP.[16]

Cardiopulmonary Assist Devices. Extracorporeal membrane oxygenation (ECMO) devices are designed to remove carbon dioxide from and to add oxygen to venous blood. Blood passes through an artificial membrane lung, bypassing the pulmonary circulation and returning to either the venous or arterial bloodstream. In severe respiratory failure, the venovenous route is used. In severe heart failure, venoarterial bypass is utilized. When used in cardiogenic shock, ECMO is usually paired with either IABP or another mechanical assist device to augment cardiac output. Hemolysis and thromboembolism are significant barriers to extended use.[17]

Nursing Considerations

Cardiogenic shock is an acute, life-threatening, emergent condition leading to hypoperfusion and hypoxia of vital organs. Time to treatment is crucial to avoid irreversible organ damage. Nurses play a critical role in recognizing signs and symptoms of cardiogenic shock and are a vital component to expediting treatment.

Nursing Considerations

- Monitor for signs and symptoms of cardiogenic shock
  - Physical assessment criteria
    - SBP less than 90 mm Hg for greater than or equal to 30 min OR support to maintain SBP greater than or equal to 90 mm Hg AND
    - End-organ hypoperfusion (urine output less than 30 mL/h or cool extremities)
  - Hemodynamic criteria
    - CI less than 2.1 L/min/m^2 and PCWP greater than 15 mm Hg

END-STAGE HEART FAILURE (STAGE D)

Background

The American College of Cardiology (ACC) and American Heart Association (AHA) define end-stage heart failure (HF) or "Stage D" HF as refractory HF symptoms despite maximum medical therapy.[7,18] In 2016, the European Society of Cardiology Heart Failure Association updated the criteria for advanced HF, specifying that these patients remain symptomatic despite optimal guideline–directed medical therapy (Table 39-6).[19] Despite HF being a complex disease process affecting roughly six million Americans over the age of 20, the presence of stage D HF has been largely unknown.[20] It is estimated roughly 5% to 10% of patients living with HF have stage D HF and are more frequently males with dyslipidemia and coronary disease.[20]

This section will review the major physiologic and pathophysiologic concepts of end-stage HF. Additionally, treatment options including mechanical circulatory support (MCS), heart transplant, and palliative care will be explored. With this knowledge, the nurse will be able to identify physical examination findings consistent with end-stage HF, develop nursing care plans that meet needs of this patient population, and understand the nursing role within the cardiac team approach to care for patients with end-stage HF.

Pathophysiology

Chronic hemodynamic stress and neurohormonal activation lead to progressive ventricular remodeling. As the ventricle fails to maintain normal cardiovascular homeostasis, more neurohormones are released, thus causing more remodeling. This cycle continues to the point of life-threatening reduction in blood flow to vital organs (Fig. 39-3), causing refractory heart failure symptoms.

Clinical Manifestations and Approach to Treatment

End-stage heart failure can be recognized by a pattern of clinical characteristics including repeat HF hospitalizations, reduction of

Table 39-6 • HEART FAILURE ASSOCIATION OF THE EUROPEAN SOCIETY OF CARDIOLOGY CRITERIA FOR ADVANCED HEART FAILURE

All the following criteria must be present despite optimal guideline–directed treatment:

1. Severe and persistent symptoms of heart failure (NYHA class III [advanced] or IV).
2. Severe cardiac dysfunction defined by a reduced LVEF less than or equal to 30%, isolated RV failure (e.g. ARVC) or nonoperable severe valve abnormalities or congenital abnormalities or persistently high (or increasing) BNP or NT-proBNP values and data of severe diastolic dysfunction or LV structural abnormalities according to the ESC definition of HFpEF and HFmrEF.[9]
3. Episodes of pulmonary or systemic congestion requiring high-dose intravenous diuretics (or diuretic combinations) or episodes of low output requiring inotropes or vasoactive drugs or malignant arrhythmias causing >1 unplanned visit or hospitalization in the last 12 months.
4. Severe impairment of exercise capacity with inability to exercise or low 6MWTD (<300 m) or pVO_2 (<12—14 mL/kg/min), estimated to be of cardiac origin.

In addition to the above, extracardiac organ dysfunction due to heart failure (e.g. cardiac cachexia, liver, or kidney dysfunction) or type 2 pulmonary hypertension may be present, but are not required criteria.

Criteria 1 and 4 can be met in patients who have cardiac dysfunction (as described in criterion no. 2), but who also have substantial limitation due to other conditions (e.g., severe pulmonary disease, noncardiac cirrhosis, or most commonly by renal disease with mixed etiology). These patients still have limited quality of life and survival due to advanced disease and warrant the same intensity of evaluation as someone in whom the only disease is cardiac, but the therapeutic options for these patients are usually more limited.

ARVC, arrhythmogenic right ventricular cardiomyopathy; BNP, B-type natriuretic peptide; ESC, European Society of Cardiology; HFA, Heart Failure Association; HFmrEF, heart failure with mid-range ejection fraction; HFpEF, heart failure with preserved ejection fraction; LV, left ventricular; LVEF, left ventricular ejection fraction; NT-proBNP, N-terminal pro-B-type natriuretic peptide; NYHA, New York Heart Association; pVO_2, peak exercise oxygen consumption; RV, right ventricular; 6MWTD, 6-minute walk test distance.

Reprinted with permission from Crespo-Leiro MG, Metra M, Lund LH, et al. Advanced heart failure: a position statement of the Heart Failure Association of the European Society of Cardiology. *Eur J Heart Fail.* 2018;20(11):1505–1535.

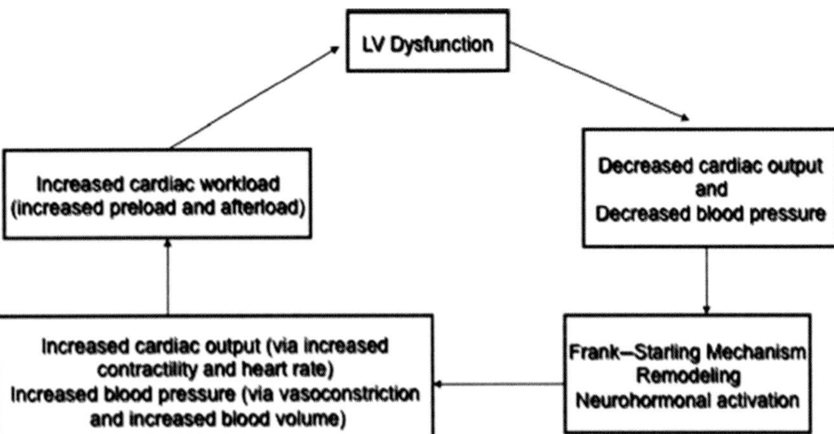

Figure 39-3. The Vicious Cycle of HF. (From Fig. 4. Kemp C, Conte J. The pathophysiology of heart failure. *Cardiovasc Pathol.* 2012;21:365–371.)

guideline-directed medical therapy due to intolerance (i.e., hypotension), increased need for diuretic therapy, end-organ dysfunction, cardiac cachexia, and/or refractory arrhythmias.[18] Diagnostic testing including echocardiogram, biomarkers, exercise testing, cardiopulmonary exercise test, and 6-minute walk test may aid in identification of stage D heart failure.[7] Clinical indicators of end-stage heart failure warranting referral for consideration of advanced heart failure therapy, such as durable mechanical circulatory assist devices and or heart transplantation, can be found in Table 39-7.[20]

Prognosis

Early identification of patients progressing to stage D HF is critical, as prognosis remains poor. In the Randomized Evaluation of Mechanical Assistance for the Treatment of Congestive Heart Failure (REMATCH), patients with stage D HF who were treated medically had a 75% 1-year mortality rate and almost none survived at 2 years.[21] An additional study evaluating patients bridging to end of life on continuous home inotropes had only a 6% survival rate at 1 year.[22] Models such as the Seattle Heart Failure Model and the Heart Failure Survival Score can be helpful in determining prognosis.[7,8]

Table 39-7 • CLINICAL INDICATORS OF ADVANCED HEART FAILURE

- Need for intravenous inotropic therapy for symptomatic relief or to maintain end-organ function
- Peak VO_2 <14 mL/kg/min or <50% of predicted
- Distance on 6 minute walk test <300 m
- ≥2 HF admissions in 12 mo
- >2 unscheduled visits (e.g., ED or clinic) in 12 mo
- Worsening right heart failure and secondary pulmonary hypertension
- Diuretic refractoriness associated with worsening renal function
- Circulatory-renal limitation to RAAS inhibition or β-blocker therapy
- Progressive/persistent NYHA functional class III—IV symptoms
- Increased 1-year mortality (e.g., 20–25%) predicted by HF survival models (e.g., SHFM, HFSS, etc.)
- Progressive renal or hepatic end-organ dysfunction
- Persistent hyponatremia (serum sodium <134 mEq/L)
- Recurrent refractory ventricular tachyarrhythmias; frequent ICD shocks
- Cardiac cachexia
- Inability to perform ADLs

SHFM, Seattle Heart Failure Model; HFSS, Heart Failure Survival Score.
Reprinted with permission from Stewart GC, Givertz MM. Mechanical circulatory support for advanced heart failure: patients and technology in evolution. *Circulation.* 2012;125:1304–1315.

Nursing Considerations

As patients progress to end-stage (stage D) heart failure, medical care becomes increasingly complex. An interdisciplinary approach to patient care is essential to ensure successful outcomes. Early referral to centers offering advanced heart failure therapy, such as LVADs or cardiac transplantation, remains pivotal to allowing patients and medical providers the opportunity to partake in the shared decision process and determine the best treatment option in conjunction with patient goals.

Nursing care for patients with end-stage, D heart failure should focus on recognizing signs and symptoms of disease progression, assessing the patient and caregiver's level of understanding of the disease process, and offering support and education.

MECHANICAL CIRCULATORY SUPPORT DEVICES FOR END-STAGE HEART FAILURE

Background

The first LVAD was placed in 1966.[23] This LVAD was made up of a titanium frame and a polyurethane pump. It was pneumatically powered to assist ventricular function. Within time, first-generation LVADs (Novacor and HeartMate XVE) were created and offered improvements such as improved pumping mechanisms, external power, and external controller. Despite these changes, LVADs remained unfavorable due to limited portability, infection, bleeding, and thrombosis.

MCS devices have drastically improved over the past 20 years. Second-generation LVADs, such as the HeartMate II (Abbott) and Jarvik 2000 (Jarvik), improved patient outcomes. These devices were smaller and used single axial rotatory motor pump to drive circulation.[24–26] Favorable outcomes were demonstrated in the REMATCH trial, showing a 15% increase in survival rate and better quality of life among patients.[22] Third-generation LVADs, such as HeartWare (Medtronic) and HeartMate III (Abbott), are now being used and offer promising advancements.[21] Third-generation LVADs are approved for the use of bridge to transplantation or destination therapy (not eligible for transplantation).[21]

Total artificial heart (TAH) is another form of durable MCS. Different from the LVADs, which only assist workload of the left ventricle, the TAH replaced the native biventricular workload and valves.[26] Regardless of which type of device is used, patients must

Table 39-8 • INDICATIONS AND CONTRAINDICATIONS TO DURABLE MECHANICAL SUPPORT

Indications: Combinations of the Following:
Frequent hospitalizations for heart failure
NYHA class IIIb–IV functional limitations despite maximal therapy
Intolerance of neurohormonal antagonists
Increasing diuretic requirement
Symptomatic despite CRT
Inotropic dependence
End-organ dysfunction attributable to low cardiac output
Contraindications
Absolute
Irreversible hepatic disease
Irreversible renal disease
Irreversible neurologic disease
Medical nonadherence
Severe psychosocial limitations
Relative
Age >80 years for DT
Obesity or malnutrition
Musculoskeletal disease that impairs rehabilitation
Active systemic infection or prolonged intubation
Untreated malignancy
Severe PVD
Active substance abuse
Impaired cognitive function
Unmanaged psychiatric disorder
Lack of social support

Reprinted with permission from Cook JL, Colvin M, Francis GS, et al. Recommendations for the use of mechanical circulatory support: ambulatory and community patient care: a scientific statement from the American Heart Association. *Circulation.* 2017;135:e1145–e1158.

undergo a comprehensive evaluation to determine if they meet eligibility criteria. Indications and contraindications for durable MCS can be found in Table 39-8.[27]

Durable Left Ventricular Assist Devices

HeartMate II

The HeartMate II (Abbott) device is a continuous axial flow device approved for bridge to transplant or destination therapy. Unlike the pulsatile devices, which need a compliance chamber, the HeartMate II is much smaller but also requires somewhat higher levels of anticoagulation. The inflow cannula is placed in the LV apex and the outflow cannula is anastomosed to the ascending aorta. The VAD pump is placed in the abdominal or peritoneal cavity, with a percutaneous lead carrying the electrical cable to an electronic controller and battery packs which are worn on a belt and shoulder holster. Two-year survival rate for this device is 76%. In addition, 81% of patients demonstrate improvement in NYHA class, 6 months after implant.[28]

HeartMate III

The HeartMate III (Abbott) is a third-generation LVAD that replaced the mechanical-bearing axial flow pump design of HeartMate II with a fully magnetically levitated centrifugal flow pump. Early analysis of the Multicenter Study of MagLev Technology in Patients Undergoing Mechanical Circulatory Support Therapy With HeartMate 3 (MOMENTUM 3) trial demonstrated the absence of pump malfunction secondary to thrombus and overall lower stroke rates. Long-term trail data analysis is ongoing.[29] HeartMate III is approved for bridge to transplant and destination therapy. Figure 39-4 illustrates the HeartMate III LVAD.

HeartWare

HeartWare (Medtronic) is a centrifugal, continuous flow durable LVAD approved for bridge to transplant and destination therapy. Designed with an integrated inflow cannula, this device does not require abdominal surgery and formation of a pump pocket during implantation.[30]

Total Artificial Heart

The SynCardia TAH is a pulsatile, durable mechanical circulatory assist device approved for end-stage biventricular HF as a bridge to transplantation.[31] This device consists of two ventricles and four heart valves. Patients are considered for TAH devices if they are ineligible to receive a LVAD due to RV failure but otherwise candidates for bridge to transplantation. Anticoagulation approach to TAH varies by institution but typically includes warfarin and antiplatelet therapy.[27] This device is depicted in Figure 39-5.

Complications

Although great advancements have been made in the field of mechanical circulatory assist devices, complications remain problematic. The majoring of data surrounding adverse events is gathered from the Interagency Registry for Mechanically Assisted Circulatory Support, mostly consisting of LVAD data.[32] Given the fact that TAHs are less commonly implanted, fewer data are available. Display 39-1 outlines common complications.[9]

Careful attention regarding bleeding, the use of blood products, and LVADs in general is important for bridge to transplant patients. Exposure to nonself tissue and blood products causes patients to produce anti-human leukocyte antigen (HLA) antibodies. Because of transfusions at implantation and because the surfaces of the LVADs (and other devices) are thought to activate lymphocytes, patients with LVADs have increased anti-HLA antibody production. These antibodies are associated with transplant rejection and decreased allograft survival and are an area of active research.[33]

Ventricular Recovery and Device Removal

Intriguing research has demonstrated myocardial changes suggestive of "reverse remodeling," that may indicate that support could lead to significant myocardial recovery and explantation without need for transplant. Favorable findings include normalization of LV chamber geometry, regression of myocyte hypertrophy and

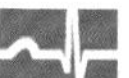 DISPLAY 39-1

Common Complications of Mechanical Circulatory Assist Devices

- Infection (typically from driveline site, pump pocket, or pump)
- Bleeding (secondary to anticoagulation use or acquired von Willebrand disease)
- Stroke (hemorrhagic or thrombotic)
- Pump thrombus (can be devastating, often resulting in surgical replacement of pump, stroke, or death)
- Aortic insufficiency (caused by increased aortic blood flow from continuous flow devices)
- Review hospital adult cardiac life support (ACLS) protocol in LVAD patients, as recommendations for chest compressions may differ from facility to facility.

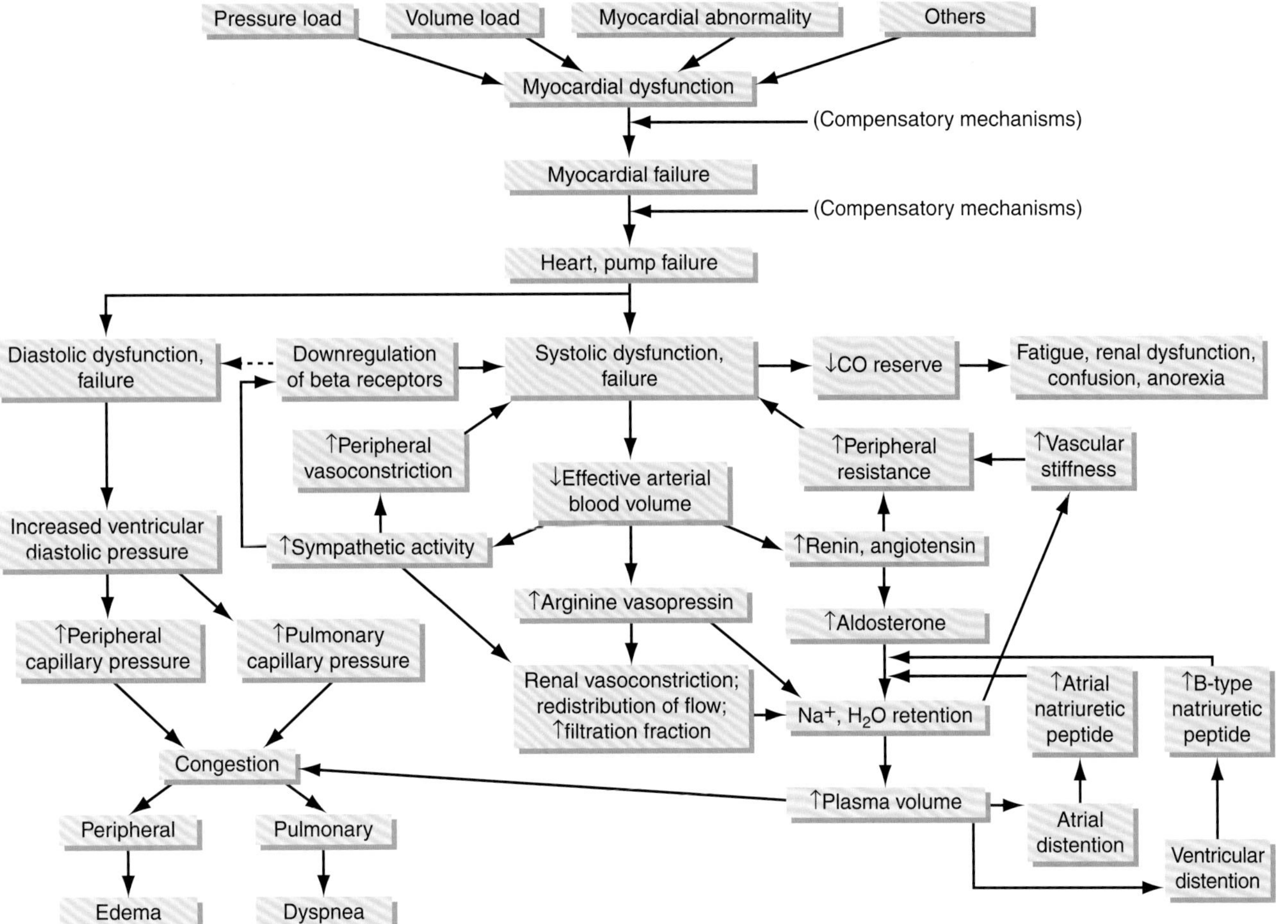

Figure 39-4. Abbott HeartMate. Sequence of events in heart failure. An increased load or myocardial abnormality leads to myocardial failure and eventually heart failure, resulting in increased sympathetic activity, increased activity of the renin–angiotensin–aldosterone system, pulmonary and peripheral congestion and edema, and decreased cardiac output reserve. Both the atrial natriuretic and B-type natriuretic peptides are also released in response to increased plasma volume. (From Francis GS, Gassler JP, Sonneblick EH. Pathophysiology and diagnosis of heart failure. In: Hurst JW, ed. *The Heart*. 10th ed. New York: McGraw-Hill; 2001.)

fibrosis, improvement in myocyte contractile force, restoration of β-adrenergic responsiveness, and altered expression of genes involved in metabolism and apoptosis.[34] In one clinical study, 15 patients with nonischemic cardiomyopathies had aggressive medical therapy (which was composed of an angiotensin-converting enzyme inhibitor (ACE-I), two β-blockers, an aldosterone antagonist, and an angiotensin receptor antagonist) plus LVAD. Of these patients, 11 had sufficient recovery of ventricular function (mean ejection fraction of 0.12 before and 0.64 after) to have the devices explanted.[35] Two of the 11 explanted patients died: one of arrhythmias 24 hours after explant and the other of lung cancer. After a mean 4-year follow-up on the surviving nine patients, the ejection fraction remained normal, and recurrent heart failure was experienced by only one patient (after a period of high alcohol intake).[35]

Nursing Considerations

MCS devices have greatly advanced over the past several years. Despite possible adverse events, they have shown to increase survival rate and improve quality of life for patients with end-stage (stage D) heart failure. Whether used as a bridge to transplant or as destination therapy, durable MCS devices remain a viable treatment option for many. Research in this field is ongoing, and with continuing efforts, technical advancements in the future remain likely.

Nurses caring for patients with durable mechanic circulatory support devices should receive additional training regarding the particular device. General considerations are listed below.

- Patients with LVAD often do not have a pulse due to the lack of pulsatile blood flow.
- Blood pressure should be obtained via Doppler. MAP is typically assessed, with a goal being 60 to 90 mm Hg.
- Heart auscultation will sound like a continuous "hum."
- Driveline exit site should be assessed for signs of bleeding or infection.
- Pump parameters and power source are assessed frequently according to protocol or ordering provider.

CARDIAC TRANSPLANTATION

Background

Despite advances in MCS, heart transplantation remains the surgical gold standard for end-stage heart failure treatment. The first

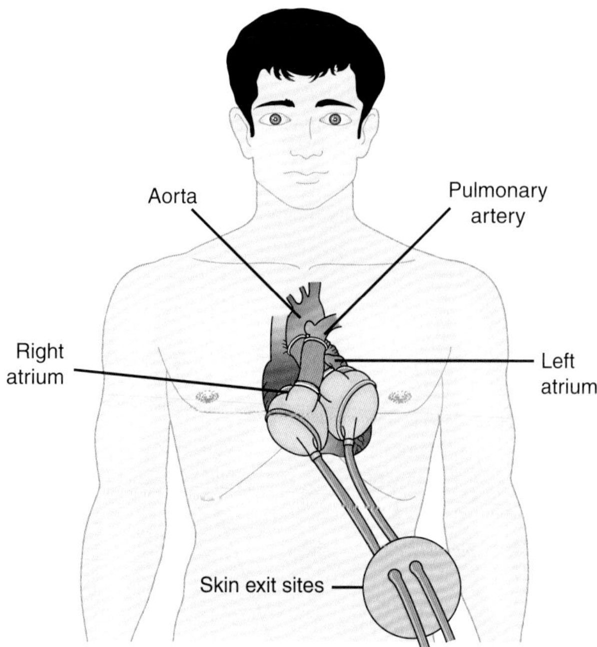

Figure 39-5. Total Artificial Heart. The CardioWest total artificial heart. (From Figure 1, Copeland JG, Smith RG, Arabia FA, et al. Cardiac replacement with a total artificial heart as a bridge to transplantation. *N Engl J Med.* 2004;351, 859–867.)

Table 39-9 • INCLUSION AND EXCLUSION CRITERIA FOR CARDIAC TRANSPLANTATION

Inclusion Criteria	Exclusion Criteria
Symptoms refractory to conventional therapy	Presence of extracardiac end-organ disease
Severe functional limitation—peak VO_2 <14 mL/min/m^2 or <50% predicted	Active substance/tobacco abuse
Severe, limiting cardiac ischemia	Morbid obesity/severe cachexia
Recurrent arrhythmias	Active neoplasm
Reliable social support	Irreversible pulmonary hypertension
Adequate insurance/financial resources	Systemic infection
	Nonadherence
	Psychiatric illness limiting self-care

heart transplant was performed in late 1967 by Dr. Christiaan Barnard in Capetown, South Africa.[36] The development of the endomyocardial biopsy and discovery of cyclosporine made transplantation a viable therapeutic option in the 1970s.[37] Currently, 1-year survival is approximately 85% with a 14-year median survival for those who survive the initial 12 months.[38] The total number of adult and pediatric heart transplants in the United States in 2018 was 3,408.[39] Unfortunately, the need for transplant far exceeds the supply and therefore, transplantation is typically reserved for those with the best chance of survival and improved quality of life.

Evaluation Process

Heart transplantation is considered when patients fail guideline-directed medical therapy and there are no other options that would offer better long-term survival. Although this may vary slightly between transplant centers, the typical inclusion and exclusion criteria encompass both physiologic and psychosocial components. A detailed list can be found in Table 39-9.[40] Patients must undergo an extensive, medical and psychosocial evaluation to determine their candidacy for transplantation. In 2016, the International Society for Heart and Lung Transplantation published an update to the guidelines for the evaluation and listing of heart transplant candidates.[41] Prior to listing for transplant, multiple organ systems (Table 39-10) are evaluated and discussed among a multidisciplinary team. The multidisciplinary team usually consists of heart failure/transplant-trained cardiologists, cardiothoracic surgeons, palliative care specialists, psychiatrist, transplant coordinators, social workers, nurses, and nutrition specialist.

Listing Process

Patients who are deemed acceptable candidates for heart transplantation are listed within the United Network for Organ Sharing (UNOS) database. UNOS is the organization contracted through the Department of Health and Human Services to oversee transplantation in the United States. Candidates are waitlisted by blood type and medical urgency. In 2018, UNOS expanded the adult heart allocation criteria to address the increasing utilization of MCS and ECMO as "bridging" strategies for end-stage heart failure (Table 39-11). Select patients

Table 39-10 • COMMON DIAGNOSTIC TESTS FOR TRANSPLANT EVALUATION

System	Test/Procedure	
Cardiovascular	Electrocardiogram (ECG)	
	Right/left heart catheterization	
	Cardiopulmonary exercise stress test	
	Echocardiogram	
	Carotid/peripheral blood flow studies	
Pulmonary	Chest radiograph	
	Pulmonary function tests (PFTs)	
Renal	Urinalysis	
	24-hour urine collection (creatinine clearance, protein)	
GI	Stool guaiac, ova/parasites	
	Abdominal ultrasound	
	Colonoscopy	
Gender specific	Mammography	
	Papanicolaou smear	
	β-Human chorionic gonadotropin	
	Prostate-specific antigen	
Laboratory	ABO/antibody screen/panel-reactive antibodies	
	HLA typing	
	Blood chemistries	
	Renal/hepatic panels	
	Lipid panel	
	Complete blood count	
	Prothrombin time/partial thromboplastin time/fibrinogen	
	International normalized ratio	
	Glycosylated hemoglobin	
Infectious disease	Tuberculin skin test	Varicella titers
	Human immunodeficiency virus	*Toxoplasma gondii*
	Hepatitis profile	Fungal antibody screen
	Herpes group virus	Lyme titers
	Cytomegalovirus	Epstein–Barr
Psychosocial	Home environment	Emotional stability
	Neurocognitive status	Social support
	Mental illness	Substance use/abuse
	Nonadherence	Insurance/financial resources

Table 39-11 • ADULT HEART ALLOCATION FOR MEDICAL URGENCY STATUS

Status	Criteria
1	VA-ECMO Nondischargeable BiVADs MCS with life-threatening arrhythmias
2	Dischargeable MCS (TAH, RVAD, BiVAD) Nondischargeable LVAD IABP or percutaneous endovascular MCS MCS with malfunction Sustained ventricular tachycardia or ventricular fibrillation
3	Continuous single or multiple IV inotropes + hemodynamic monitoring 30-day exception time (LVADs) MCS with complication
4	Continuous IV inotropes Stable LVAD Congenital heart disease, restrictive cardiomyopathy, retransplant
5	Multiple organ transplant
6	All other candidates

VA-ECMO, venous-arterial extracorporeal membrane oxygenation; MCS, mechanical circulatory support; TAH, total artificial heart; BiVAD, biventricular ventricular assist device; RVAD, right ventricular assist device; LVAD, left ventricular assist device.

may move between status categories based on disease progression and changes in acuity.

Surgical Procedure

There are two surgical procedures for heart transplantation—orthotopic and heterotopic. Orthotopic transplantation is the most common and involves excision of the native heart and replacement with a donor heart. Heterotopic procedures involve a "piggyback" approach, where the donor heart is placed into the recipient right chest cavity with anastomosis of the aorta, superior vena cava, and pulmonary arteries. Heterotopic transplantation has several disadvantages, including increased risk of thromboembolism from the native heart requiring long-term anticoagulation.

Postoperative Considerations

Immunosuppression

For organ transplant recipients, the term immunosuppression refers to the pharmacologic agents that alter the immune system to limit/prevent rejection of the allograft. One of the biggest challenges in transplant medicine remains the "balance" between prevention of rejection while maintaining sufficient immunity to prevent infection. Although immunosuppression protocols can vary greatly by center, the most common regimen includes a combination of triple therapy with a CNI, antiproliferative agent, and corticosteroids (Table 39-12). Therapeutic drug monitoring is critical to maintain appropriate drug levels while preventing both over/underdosing.

Concentrations of calcineurin inhibitors are affected by other medications that are metabolized by the cytochrome P450 3A enzyme (Table 39-13). Appropriate dose titration is essentially if these drugs are used concomitantly. Side-effect management requires diligent surveillance and in general, the degree of immunosuppression can be decreased over time. Most protocols include steroid tapers over the initial 12 months post transplant. Common immunosuppressant adverse effects include Cushing syndrome, hypertension, nephrotoxicity, hyperglycemia, dyslipidemia, tremors, gingival hyperplasia, bone marrow depression, and gastrointestinal distress.

Table 39-12 • COMMON IMMUNOSUPPRESSIVE AGENTS

Immunosuppressant Class	Mechanism of Action
Calcineurin inhibitors (CNIs) • Cyclosporine • Tacrolimus	Suppress T-cell activation
Antiproliferative agents • Azathioprine • Mycophenolate mofetil • Mycophenolate sodium	Inhibit B- and T-cell proliferation
mTOR inhibitors • Sirolimus • Everolimus	Inhibit T-cell proliferation Antineoplastic effects
Corticosteroids • Methylprednisolone • Prednisone	Alter DNA/RNA synthesis inhibit macrophages and T-cells

Complications of Cardiac Transplantation

Although there are a myriad of potential complications post transplant, four of the most common complications can be categorized by timing of occurrence (Display 39-2).

Rejection

Rejection is the process by which the native immune system attempts to destroy the allograft by either cellular or humoral factors. Allograft rejection can occur any time after transplant, but is a major cause of morbidity and mortality within the first year.[42,43] Rejection is classified as hyperacute, acute cellular, acute antibody mediated (AMR), and chronic.

Patients may remain asymptomatic unless rejection is severe. In more extreme cases, signs/symptoms mimic that of acute decompensated heart failure—dyspnea, fatigue, edema, S_3 or S_4 heart sounds, hypotension, and in some instances, LV dysfunction.

Since the introduction of the bioptome, the endomyocardial biopsy is the gold standard by which rejection is diagnosed. Many centers have also adopted the use of gene expression profiling (AlloMap®, CareDx, Brisbane, CA) to replace surveillance biopsies with a simple blood test to determine rejection risk.[40]

Treatment varies depending on time from transplant, severity, and presence/degree of LV dysfunction. In general, the immunosuppressive regimen is "optimized" and may include intravenous

Table 39-13 • DRUGS/HERBALS/FOODS METABOLIZED BY THE CYTOCHROME P450 PATHWAY

Increase CNI Concentrations	Decrease CNI Concentrations
Calcium channel blockers	Antibiotics (nafcillin, rifampin, trimethoprim/sulfamethoxazole)
Macrolide antibiotics (mycins)	Anticonvulsants agents (phenytoin, carbamazepine, phenobarbital)
HMG-CoA reductase inhibitors (statins)	Topiramate
Antifungal agents (azoles)	Octreotide
Protease inhibitors	Herbal supplements (St. John's Wort, *Echinacea*)
Grapefruit	
Red yeast rice	

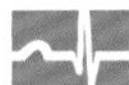 DISPLAY 39-2

Complications of Heart Transplantation

Early Complications	Late Complications
Rejection	Malignancy
Infection	Cardiac allograft vasculopathy (CAV)

or oral steroids, as well as intensification or change in current therapy. In the event of AMR, intravenous immunoglobulin, cyclophosphamide, rituximab and/or plasmapheresis may be warranted.[32,42–44]

Infection

Immunosuppression places the transplant recipient at risk for nosocomial, opportunistic, and community-acquired infections (Table 39-14). Approximately one fourth of patients have one or more major infections in the first two posttransplant months. Bacterial infections occur most frequently in the immediate postoperative period, with the pulmonary system being the most common site.[42] Other viral, bacterial, and fungal infections are also common the first year. Prophylaxis is routinely prescribed when the risk of these infections is highest (Table 39-15). Community-acquired infections are most common after the initial 12 months. Transplant recipients should be monitored closely because standard immunosuppression will inhibit the inflammatory process and decrease clinical signs/symptoms of infection. Infectious disease specialists may be warranted to assist in clinical management and hospitalization is indicated for pulmonary infiltrates, sepsis, and/or persistent fever.[43]

Malignancy

Malignancy remains a significant issue post transplant due to the systemic effects of immunosuppression combined with other carcinogens. With the exception of steroids, all immunosuppressant agents contribute to the risk of malignancy. Transplant recipients have a higher incidence of lymphoproliferative diseases, skin cancers, and Kaposi sarcoma compared to the general population.[43] The overall risk of malignancy in the first 10 years following cardiac transplant is 35%.[43] Skin cancer surveillance and age-appropriate cancer screenings are imperative to minimize the malignancy risk.

Table 39-14 • COMMON INFECTIOUS PATHOGENS

Bacterial	*Pseudomonas aeruginosa*
	Legionella
	Nocardia asteroides
	Listeria monocytogenes
	Salmonella
	Mycobacterium tuberculosis
Viral	Cytomegalovirus (CMV)
	Epstein–Barr virus (EBV)
	Varicella zoster
	Hepatitis B/Hepatitis C
	Influenza
	Enterovirus
	Adenovirus
Fungal	*Candida*
	Aspergillus
	Cryptococcus neoformans
	Pneumocystis jiroveci
	Coccidioides immitis
	Histoplasma capsulatum
	Blastomyces dermatitidis
Parasitic	*Toxoplasmosis*
	Cryptosporidium
	Strongyloides stercoralis

Table 39-15 • PATHOGENS AND PROPHYLACTIC AGENTS

Target Pathogen	Agents
Pneumocystis jiroveci	Sulfamethoxazole/trimethoprim
Nocardia	Dapsone
Toxoplasmosis	Inhaled pentamidine
CMV	Valganciclovir
Herpes simplex I	Acyclovir
Herpes simplex II	Valacyclovir
	Famciclovir
Candida	Nystatin
	Clotrimazole troches
	Fluconazole

Cardiac Allograft Vasculopathy

Cardiac allograft vasculopathy (CAV) can occur anytime post transplant and is a rapid, progressive form of coronary artery disease characterized by concentric diffuse intimal proliferation and luminal stenosis. It is thought to be a form of chronic rejection and remains the most common reason for retransplantation.[43] As many as 50% of heart transplant recipients will develop CAV by 5 years.[40] It is frequently described as a "pruning" of the vessels when visualized by coronary angiogram and single, discrete lesions are less common. Predictors for the development of CAV per the International Society of Heart and Lung Transplantation (ISHLT) registry are older donor age, donor history of hypertension, younger recipient age, greater number of HLA-DR mismatches, and recipient pretransplant diagnosis of ischemic heart disease.[45]

Traditional treatment with percutaneous intervention and bypass surgery is limited due to the diffuse, distal nature of the disease.[40] There is some evidence that rapamycin inhibitors and statin therapy may slow disease progression regardless of lipid levels.[40]

Nursing Implications/Care of the Heart Transplant Recipient

Although MCS utilization is on the rise, heart transplantation remains the gold standard surgical therapy for advanced heart failure. Despite a small increase in the number of transplants in recent years, donor demand still exceeds supply and many patients die while on the UNOS waiting list.[46] The multidisciplinary team can improve clinical outcomes with routine surveillance and attention to the known risks and comorbid conditions.

General nursing care of the heart transplant recipient should focus on screening/prevention of posttransplant complications to improve morbidity and quality of life.

Unique nursing considerations[40] post heart transplantation include:

- Denervation of the transplanted heart
  - Baseline heart rate 90 to 110 bpm
  - Catecholamines to increase/slow heart rate
  - Absence of angina equivalent in setting of myocardial ischemia
  - Atropine ineffective in the treatment of bradycardia
- Aggressive management of cardiovascular risk factors
  - Hyperglycemia
  - Hypertension

Table 39-16 • TOP 10 CONSIDERATIONS FOR DECISION MAKING IN ADVANCED HEART FAILURE

1. Shared decision making is the process through which clinicians and patients share information with each other and work toward decisions about treatment chosen from medically reasonable options that are aligned with the patents' values, goals, and preferences.
2. For patients with advanced heart failure, shared decision making has become both more challenging and more crucial as duration of disease and treatment options have increased.
3. Difficult discussions now will simplify difficult decisions in the future.
4. Ideally, shared decision making is an iterative process that evolves over time as a patient's disease and quality of life change.
5. Attention to the clinical trajectory is required to calibrate expectations and guide timely decisions, but prognostic uncertainly is inevitable and should be included in discussions with patients and caregivers.
6. An annual heart failure review with patients should include discussion of current and potential therapies for both anticipated and unanticipated events.
7. Discussions should include outcomes beyond survival, including major adverse events, symptom burden, functional limitations, loss of independence, quality of life, and obligations for caregivers.
8. As the end of life is anticipated, clinicians should take responsibility for initiating the development of a comprehensive plan for end-of-life care consistent with patient values, preferences, and goals.
9. Assessing and integrating emotional readiness of the patient and family is vital to effective communication.
10. Changes in organizational and reimbursement structures are essential to promote high-quality decision making and delivery of patient-centered health care.

Reprinted with permission from Allen LA, Stevenson LW, Grady KL, et al. Decision making in advanced heart failure: a scientific statement from the American Heart Association. *Circulation*. 2012;125:1928–1952.

- Lipid levels
- Obesity
- Smoking/substance abuse
- Age-appropriate health screenings/cancer surveillance
- Vaccines for infection prevention
- Statin therapy for CAV (regardless of lipid levels)
- Therapeutic drug monitoring to maintain immunosuppressant levels in target range

PALLIATIVE CARE AND HOSPICE

Shared Decision Making

Shared decision making is an individualized process that encompasses the ethical and legal obligation to involve patients in medical decisions.[47] Table 39-16 describes the top 10 considerations for decision making in advanced HF. Conversations between HF providers and patients regarding treatment options should occur early in the disease process. The concept of an "Annual Heart Failure Review" is dedicated time for the HF team to discuss disease trajectory. Additional details regarding the "Annual Heart Failure Review" can be found in Table 39-17.

Palliative Care and Hospice

Palliative care is a treatment option for patients with complex chronic illness whose prognosis is unknown. The aim of palliative care is to improve quality of life and offer additional support to patients and families.[47] Benefits have been proven for those who receive palliative care. A recent randomized controlled trial, the PAL-HF trial, evaluated an interdisciplinary palliative care

Table 39-17 • ANNUAL HEART FAILURE REVIEW

Selected Components That May Be Included in an Annual Heart Failure Review
- Characterization of clinical status
  - Functional ability, symptom burden, mental status, quality of life, and disease trajectory
- Perceptions from caregiver
- Solicitation of patient values, goals, and general care preferences
- Estimation of prognosis
  - Consider incorporating objective modeling data
  - Orient to wide range of uncertainty

Review of Therapies
- Indicated heart failure therapies in appropriate patients (BB, ACE-I/ARB, AA, CRT, ICD)
- Treatment of comorbidities (AF, HTN, DM, CKD, etc.)
- Appropriate preventive care, within the context of symptomatic heart failure
- Planning for future events/advance care planning
- Resuscitation preferences
  - Desire for advanced therapies, major surgery, hospice
  - Standardized documentation of the annual review in the medical record

BB, β-blocker; ACE-I, angiotensin-converting enzyme inhibitor; ARB, angiotensin II receptor blocker; AA, aldosterone antagonist; CRT, cardiac resynchronization therapy; ICD, implantable cardioverter-defibrillator; AF, atrial fibrillation; HTN, hypertension; DM, diabetes mellitus; CKD, chronic kidney disease.
Reprinted with permission from Allen LA, Stevenson LW, Grady KL. Decision making in advanced heart failure: a scientific statement from the American Heart Association. *Circulation*. 2012;125:1928–1952.

intervention for patients with HF and found a benefit in quality of life, anxiety, depression, and spiritual well-being.[48] Palliative care can be integrated into the plan of care concurrent with ongoing HF medical therapy, even before patients reach stage D.

Unlike palliative care, hospice is determinant on expected prognosis and/or life expectancy.[49] In the United States, regulations from the Centers for Medicare & Medicaid Services mandate that two physicians or a physician and a nurse practitioner must attest that patients have less than 6 months to live in order to be eligible for hospice care. Additionally, patients must be willing to halt medical services aimed at curing the terminal illness.[50] Shared decision making becomes of utmost importance when patients near end of life. Figure 39-6 depicts the disease progression through life-prolonging care, palliative care, and hospice.[49]

Deactivating Devices

Deactivation of internal defibrillators (ICDs) should be discussed anytime the patient has a major clinical change.[47] As patients near end of life, this conversation becomes increasingly important to avoid unwanted ICD discharges and discomfort. Additionally, the deactivation of LVADs is also an increasing clinical scenario. Withdrawal of LVAD support most often leads to rapid deterioration and death within minutes. Prior to LVAD deactivation, conversations with the patient (if able) and family regarding prognosis, changes in device benefit, management of symptoms, readiness, and outcomes should be thoroughly discussed.[47]

Nursing Considerations

Nursing care should be aimed at providing physical, social, psychological, and spiritual comfort and support to patients and families.

Physical Assessment:

1. Assess patient's comfort level and provide comfort medications as directed by advanced practice provider or physician.

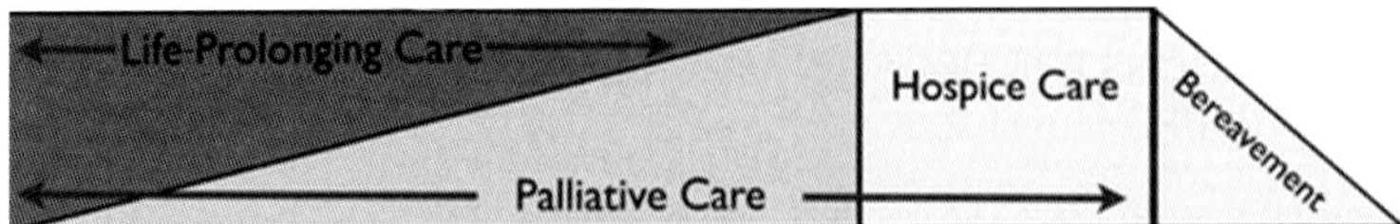

Figure 39-6. Palliative Care Integrative Model. Palliative care is initiated when patients are diagnosed with any serious or advanced chronic illness. As illness progresses, the ratio of palliative care to life-prolonging care gradually increases. Ultimately, life-prolonging care is discontinued according to patient's wishes or when the harm of treatment outweighs its benefit. At this point, the transition to hospice care is made. After death, palliative care services continue and help family members with bereavement. (Used with permission from Alder ED, Goldfinger JZ, Kalman J, et al. Palliative care in the treatment of advanced heart failure. *Circulation.* 2009;120:2597–2606.)

2. Monitor for signs/symptoms of hypoperfusion (see Diagnosis and Clinical Manifestations).

Social Assessment:

1. Encourage family members to express feelings, and convey understanding of their concerns and emotional stress.
2. Provide the family with honest information about the patient's condition.

Psychosocial Assessment:

1. Assess the patient's understanding and acceptance of prognosis.
2. Encourage patient to express feelings.

Spiritual Assessment:

1. Acknowledge the patient's spiritual/religious preference.

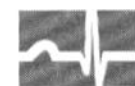 CASE STUDY 1

Patient Profile

Name/Age/Sex: **Nancy Smith, 68-year-old female**

Past Medical History/Problem List

Heart failure with reduced ejection fraction; status post CRT-D; dilated, ischemic cardiomyopathy; coronary artery disease, status post coronary artery bypass grafting greater than 10 years ago; hypertension; diabetes mellitus, type 2; hypothyroidism; depression

Family History

Coronary artery disease

Social History

Married. Mother to three healthy, adult children. Retired grade school teacher. Denies alcohol, tobacco, and illicit drug use

Medications/Allergies

Carvedilol 3.125 mg BID; Entresto 24/26 mg BID; spironolactone 25 QD; furosemide 80 mg BID; levothyroxine 75 mcg QD; metformin 1,000 mg BID; aspirin 81 mg QD; atorvastatin 80 mg QSH

Case Scenario

Ms. Smith presents to clinic for 1 week post hospitalization follow-up visit. She was recently admitted for acute decompensated heart failure exacerbation and required inotropic support for cardiogenic shock. Initial right heart catheterization revealed a RAP 12 mm Hg, PAWP 27 mm Hg, and CI 1.6 L/min/m^2. Lasix drip was initiated, resulting in a total volume removal of 12 L. Inotropic support was slowly weaned and hemodynamics stabilized. Guideline-directed medical therapy was reintroduced at significantly lower doses than previously tolerated. Furosemide was increased from 40 mg BID to 80 mg BID.

Subjective

Ms. Smith reports a 5-lb weight gain since hospital discharge, decreased exercise tolerance, dyspnea with mild exertion, and lower extremity edema. She states, "getting dressed in the morning makes me short of breath." Limits sodium intake to 2 g daily and fluid intake to 2 L daily. Takes all medications as prescribed.

Objective

Vital Signs: BP 92/65 mm Hg; HR 79 bpm; SaO_2 98% on room air; Temp 98.7°F

Physical Examination: Jugular venous distention (JVD) 14 cm. Positive hepatojugular reflux. Positive S_3. 2/6 holosystolic murmur. 1+ bilateral lower extremity pitting edema

Labs: Sodium 131 mEq/mL; potassium 3.8 mEq/mL; BUN 54 mg/dL; creatinine 2.2 mg/dL; proBNP 2,560; uric acid 11.2 mg/dL

Assessment

Ms. Smith has progressed to Stage D, refractory heart failure with NYHA class III symptoms. History is also notable for three hospitalizations within the past 12 months. Most recently, required significant down titration of carvedilol and Entresto (valsartan and sacubitril), as well as escalation of diuretic therapy. Despite medication changes, fluid retention continues to be an issue. Laboratory data is notable for worsening kidney function therefore indicating possible end-organ dysfunction.

Plan

Ms. Smith is currently hemodynamically stable; however, referral for advanced heart therapy is indicated.

Clinical Pearls

- Downtitration of neurohormonal blockade should be recognized as a significant sign of heart failure disease progression.
- Escalation of diuretic therapy, in the context of patient compliance with medication and dietary restrictions, is a sign of heart failure disease progression.
- Multiple heart failure hospitalizations can be a sign of disease progression, but also due to patient noncompliance. Perform a thorough assessment of patient and caregiver knowledge regarding dietary sodium consumption. Conduct a 24-hour food diary recall while interviewing the patient. This can be a pivotal teaching point and allows the nurse to assess patient and caregiver knowledge.

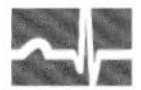

CASE STUDY 2

Patient Profile

Name/Age/Sex: **Clarence Jones, 77-year-old Caucasian male**

Past Medical History/Problem List

Ischemic cardiomyopathy, left ventricular ejection fraction 25%
Deep vein thrombosis and pulmonary embolus, s/p inferior vena cava filter
Peripheral vascular disease
Carotid stenosis and carotid artery stenting
Hypercholesterolemia with statin intolerance
Bilateral hip replacement
Cholecystectomy

Family History

Mother (deceased)—hypertension, coronary artery disease
Father (deceased)—hypertension, coronary artery disease
Sister (deceased)—coronary artery disease/acute myocardial infarction

Social History

Married, two adult children. Residing in assisted-living community, continues to work part-time in community store. No tobacco/substance use

Medications

Torsemide 100 mg twice daily
Amiodarone 200 mg twice daily
Potassium chloride 20 mEq twice daily
Aspirin 81 mg daily
Coumadin 5 mg daily
Midodrine 10 mg three times daily
Milrinone 0.375 mcg/kg/min continuous infusion

Allergies/Intolerances

Penicillin
Levaquin
Phenergan
Statins
Neurohormonal blockade (hypotension)

Case Scenario

Mr. Margolis is a 77-year-old Caucasian male with multiple emergency room visits and hospitalizations for acute decompensated heart failure. Referred to the Advanced HF Clinic for evaluation and underwent placement of an ambulatory pulmonary artery pressure monitor. Unable to tolerate standard guideline-directed medical therapy due to symptomatic hypotension, and filling pressures remain elevated despite escalating diuretic therapy.

During most recent hospitalization, initiated on inotropic therapy and evaluated for destination VAD placement. Ultimately declined as VAD candidate due to advancing age and overall frailty.

Presents to HF Clinic for follow-up and to discuss plan of care.

Subjective

Reports multiple falls in the past 2 weeks, declining exercise tolerance, and poor balance. Mild dyspnea at rest. Frequent episodes of crying, questioning need for antidepressant. Using rolling walker to assist with ambulation.

Objective

Vital Signs: BP 92/58 mm Hg; HR 83 bpm; SaO_2 98% on room air

Physical Examination: Jugular venous distention (JVD) 12 cm. Positive hepatojugular reflux. Positive S_3. 2+ bilateral lower extremity pitting edema

Labs: Sodium 130 mEq/L; potassium 4.1 mEq/L; BUN 55 mg/dL; creatinine 2.0 mg/dL; BNP 1,762

Pulmonary Artery (PA) Sensor: PA diastolic 32 mm Hg

Assessment

Mr. Margolis has NYHA IV Stage D heart failure. Unfortunately, he is not a candidate for advanced therapies. He wishes to avoid additional ER visits and hospitalizations and prefers to remain comfortable at home. After a lengthy shared decision-making discussion with patient, family, and multidisciplinary team including palliative care, he plans to transition to hospice.

Plan

1. Referral to hospice
2. Deactivate ICD to avoid repetitive shocks in the event of ventricular arrhythmias
3. DNR/DNI per living will
4. Initiate antidepressant therapy
5. Flexible diuretic dosing to control congestion

Clinical Pearls

- Multiple ER visits/hospitalizations should be recognized as a sign of disease progression.
- Annual review should include discussion of current and potential therapies for both anticipated and unanticipated events.
- Confirm patient/family goals to guide clinical decision making (shared decision making).
- Acknowledge feelings of anxiety, depression, and fear—active listening and treat accordingly.
- Deactivation of ICD is desirable to avoid unnecessary pain/distress at the end of life.
- Ongoing research is needed to establish best symptom management, caregiver support, advanced care planning, and palliative care/hospice models.

KEY READINGS

Allen LA, Stevenson LW, Grady KL, et al. Decision making in advanced heart failure: a scientific statement from the American Heart Association. *Circulation.* 2012;125(15):1928–1952.

Gelfman LP, Bakitas M, Warner Stevenson L, et al. The state of the science on integrating palliative care in heart failure. *J Palliat Med.* 2017;20(6):592–603.

Yancy CW, Januzzi JL Jr, Allen LA, et al. 2017 ACC expert consensus decision pathway for optimization of heart failure treatment: answers to 10 pivotal issues about heart failure with reduced ejection fraction: a report of the American College of Cardiology Task Force on Expert Consensus Decision Pathways. *J Am Coll Cardiol.* 2018;71(2):201–230.

REFERENCES

1. Reynolds HR, Hochman JS. Cardiogenic shock: current concepts and improving outcomes. *Circulation.* 2008;117(5):686–697.
2. Gheorghaide M, Sopko G, De Luca L, et al. Navigating the crossroads of coronary artery disease and heart failure. *Circulation.* 2006;114(11):1202–1213.
3. Hochman JS, Sleeper LA, Webb JG, et al. Early revascularization in acute myocardial infarction complicated by cardiogenic shock. SHOCK investigators: should we emergently revascularize occluded coronaries for cardiogenic shock. *N Engl J Med.* 1999;341(9):625–634.
4. Bonow RO. The hibernating myocardium: implications for management of congestive heart failure. *Am J Cardiol.* 1995;75(3):17A–25A.
5. Bolli R. Basic and clinical aspects of myocardial stunning. *Prog Cardiovasc Dis.* 1998;40(6):477–516.

6. Babaev A, Frederick PD, Pasta DJ, et al. Trends in management and outcomes of patients with acute myocardial infarction complicated by cardiogenic shock. *JAMA*. 2005;294(4):448–454.
7. Yancy CW, Jessup M, Bozkurt B, et al. 2017 ACC/AHA/HFSA Focused Update of the 2013 ACCF/AHA Guideline for the Management of Heart Failure: a Report of the American College of Cardiology/American Heart Association Task Force on Clinical Practice Guidelines and the Heart Failure Society of America. *Circulation*. 2017;136(6):e137–e161.
8. van Diepen S, Katz JN, Albert NM, et al. Contemporary management of cardiogenic shock: a scientific statement from the American Heart Association. *Circulation*. 2017;136(16):e232–e268.
9. Hiemstra B, Eck RJ, Keus F, et al. Clinical examination for diagnosing circulatory shock. *Curr Opin Crit Care*. 2017;23(4):293–301.
10. Oliver C, Marin F, Pineda J, et al. Low QRS voltage in cardiac tamponade: a study of 70 cases. *Int J Cardiol*. 2002;83(1):91–92.
11. Forrester JS, Diamond G, Chatterjee K, et al. Medical therapy of acute myocardial infarction by application of hemodynamic subsets (second of two parts). *N Engl J Med*. 1976;295:1404–1413.
12. Sanborn TA, Sleeper LA, Bates ER, et al. Impact of thrombolysis, intra-aortic balloon pump counterpulsation, and their combination in cardiogenic shock complicating acute myocardial infarction: a report from the SHOCK Trial Registry. Should we emergently revascularize occluded coronaries for cardiogenic shock? *J Am Coll Cardiol*. 2000;36(3 suppl A):1123–1129.
13. Thiele H, Zeymer U, Thelemann N, et al; IABP-SHOCK II Trial (Intraaortic Balloon Pump in Cardiogenic Shock II) Investigators. Intraaortic balloon pump in cardiogenic shock complicating acute myocardial infarction: long-term 6-year outcome of the randomized IABP-SHOCK II trial. *Circulation*. 2018.
14. Goldberg RJ, Spencer FA, Gore JM, et al. Thirty-year trends (1975 to 2005) in the magnitude of, management of, and hospital death rates associated with cardiogenic shock in patients with acute myocardial infarction. *Circulation*. 2009;119(9):1211–1219.
15. Schrage B, Ibrahim K, Loehn T, et al. Impella support for acute myocardial infarction complicated by cardiogenic shock. *Circulation*. 2019; 139(10):1249–1258.
16. Smith L, Peters A, Mazimba S, et al. Outcomes of patients with cardiogenic shock treated with TandemHeart® percutaneous ventricular assist device: importance of support indication and definitive therapies as determinants of prognosis. *Catheter Cardiovasc Interv*. 2018;92(6):1173–1181.
17. Atkinson TM, Ohman EM, O'Neill WW, et al. A practical approach to mechanical circulatory support in patients undergoing percutaneous coronary intervention: an interventional perspective. *JACC Cardiovasc Interv*. 2016;9(9):871–883.
18. Ponikowski P, Voors AA, Anker SD, et al. 2016 ESC Guidelines for the diagnosis and treatment of acute and chronic heart failure: the Task Force for the diagnosis and treatment of acute and chronic heart failure of the European Society of Cardiology (ESC). Developed with the special contribution of the Heart Failure Association (HFA) of the ESC. *Eur Heart J*. 2016;37(27):2129–2200.
19. Crespo-Leiro MG, Metra M, Lund LH, et al. Advanced heart failure: a position statement of the Heart Failure Association of the European Society of Cardiology. *Eur J Heart Fail*. 2018;20(11):1505–1535.
20. Liu L, Eisen H. Epidemiology of heart failure and the scope of the problem. *Cardiol Clin*. 2014;32:1–8.
21. Stewart GC, Givertz MM. Mechanical circulatory support for advanced heart failure: patients and technology in evolution. *Circulation*. 2012;125: 1304–1315.
22. Rose EA, Gelijns AC, Moskowitz AJ, et al. Long-term use of a left ventricular assist device for end-stage heart failure. *N Engl J Med*. 2001;345:1435–1443.
23. DeBakey ME. Left ventricular bypass pump for cardiac assistance: clinical experience. *Am J Cardiol*. 1971;27:3–11.
24. Birks EJ. Left ventricular assist devices. *Heart*. 2010;96:63–71.
25. Haj-Yahia S, Birks EJ, Rogers P, et al. Midterm experience with the Jarvik 2000 axial flow left ventricular assist device. *J Thorac Cardiovasc Surg*. 2007;134:199–203.
26. Cook JA, Shah KB, Quader MA, et al. The total artificial heart. *J Thorac Dis*. 2015;7:2172–2180.
27. Cook JL, Colvin M, Francis GS, et al. Recommendations for the use of mechanical circulatory support: ambulatory and community patient care: a scientific statement from the American Heart Association. *Circulation*. 2017;135:e1145–e1158.
28. Slaughter MS, Rogers JG, Milano CA, et al. Advanced heart failure treated with continuous-flow left ventricular assist device. *N Engl J Med*. 2009;361(23):2241–2251.
29. Mehra MR, Goldstein DJ, Uriel N, et al. Two-year outcomes with a magnetically levitated cardiac pump in heart failure. *N Engl J Med*. 2018;378(15):1386–1395.
30. Slaughter M, Pagani FD, McGee EC, et al. HeartWare ventricular assist system for bridge to transplant: combined results of the bridge to transplant and continued access protocol trial. *J Heart Lung Transpl*. 2013; 32:675–683.
31. Copeland JG, Smith RG, Arabia FA, et al. Cardiac replacement with a total artificial heart as a bridge to transplantation. *N Engl J Med*. 2004;351(9):859–867.
32. Dumas-Hicks D. Immunosuppression. In: Scheetz L, ed. *Transplantation Nursing Secrets*. Philadelphia, PA: Hanley & Belfus; 2003:67–83.
33. Mancini D, Lietz K. Selection of cardiac transplantation candidates in 2010. *Circulation*. 2010;122:173–183.
34. Kemp C, Conte J. The pathophysiology of heart failure. *Cardiovasc Pathol*. 2012;21:365–371.
35. Birks EJ, Tansley PD, Hardy J, et al. Left ventricular assist device and drug therapy for the reversal of heart failure. *N Engl J Med*. 2006;355(18): 1873–1884.
36. Barnard CN. Human cardiac transplantation: an evaluation of the first two operations performed at the Groote Schuur Hospital, Cape Town. *Am J Cardiol*. 1968;22(4):584–596.
37. Borel JF, Feurer C, Gubler HU, et al. Biological effects of cyclosporin A: a new antilymphocytic agent. *Agents Actions*. 1994;43(3–4):179–186.
38. Yusen RD, Edwards LB, Dipchand AI, et al. The registry of the International Society for Heart and Lung Transplantation: thirty-third adult lung and heart–lung transplant report—2016; focus theme: primary diagnostic indications for transplant. *J Heart Lung Transplant*. 2016;35(10):1170–1184.
39. Organ Procurement and Transplantation Network. Available at https://optn.transplant.hrsa.gov/data/view-data-reports/national-data. Accessed February 21, 2019.
40. Flattery M, Constantino S. Advanced heart failure therapies. In: Paul S, ed. Heart Failure Nursing Certification: Core Curriculum Review. 1st ed. American Association of Heart Failure Nurses; 2012:155–171.
41. Mehra MR, Canter CE, Hannan MM, et al. The 2016 International Society for Heart Lung Transplantation listing criteria for heart transplantation: a 10-year update. *J Heart Lung Transplant*. 2016;35(1):1–23.
42. Lindenfeld J, Miller GG, Shakar SF, et al. Drug therapy in the heart transplant recipient: part I: cardiac rejection and immunosuppressive drugs. *Circulation*. 2004;110:3734–3740.
43. Lindenfeld J, Page RL, Zolty R, et al. Drug therapy in the heart transplant recipient: part III: common medical problems. *Circulation*. 2005; 111:113–117.
44. Cupples S. Heart Transplantation. In: Scheetz L, ed. *Transplantation Nursing Secrets*. Philadelphia, PA: Hanley & Belfus; 2003:85–105.
45. Mehra MR, Crespo-Leiro MG, Dipchand A, et al. International Society for Heart and Lung Transplantation working formulation of a standardized nomenclature for cardiac allograft vasculopathy-2010. *J Heart Lung Transplant*. 2010;29(7):717–727.
46. Organ Procurement and Transplantation Network. *Adult heart allocation*. Available at https://optn.transplant.hrsa.gov/learn/professional-education/adult-heart-allocation. Accessed October 11, 2018.
47. Allen LA, Stevenson LW, Grady KL, et al. Decision making in advanced heart failure a scientific statement from the American Heart Association. *Circulation*. 2012;125;1928–1952.
48. Rogers JG, Chetan BP, Mentz RJ, et al. Palliative care in heart failure: the PAL-HF randomized, controlled trial. *J Am Coll Cardiol*. 2017;70: 331–341.
49. Alder ED, Goldfinger JZ, Kalman J, et al. Palliative care in the treatment of advanced heart failure. *Circulation*. 2009;120:2597–2606.
50. Department of Health and Human Services; Centers for Medicare & Medicaid Services. *Medicare and Medicaid programs: Medicare hospice benefits*. Available at https://www.medicare.gov/Pubs/pdf/02154-Medicare

40 Therapeutic Intervention for Cardiovascular Disease: Future Advances and Approaches

Sarah E. Clarke

OBJECTIVES

1. Illustrate how digital technologies can impact risk factor reduction and timely access to care.
2. Define artificial intelligence and applications within contemporary cardiology.
3. Explain the challenges of clinical decision support systems (CDSSs).
4. Discuss how advanced imaging plays a key role in operator training and case planning.
5. Describe the data contributing to the evolution of minimally invasive surgical and catheter-based technologies.

KEY QUESTIONS

1. How does mobile health impact the healthcare landscape?
2. What safeguards are in place to protect the patient electronic medical record?
3. How does telehealth improve access to care?

INTRODUCTION

In less than 20 years, the face of cardiology has changed dramatically. From 2004 to 2014, there has been a 25.3% decrease in death rates attributable to cardiovascular diseases (CVDs).[1] The management of patients with heart disease has evolved through advancements in drug treatments, interventions, and diagnostic technologies; the American Heart Association's Strategic Initiatives 2020 and Beyond also seeks to address prevention and control risk factors.[2] This has led to technologic advances in digital health, artificial intelligence and its integration in clinical decision support tools, simulation, and advanced imaging and 3D printing.

Due to these technologic advances, a striking evolution has taken place in addressing patient and operator safety, heart team collaboration, and techniques related to minimally invasive device technology. Advances in digital health technology and availability of real time patient-centered data are improving patient safety by ensuring that clinicians have access to a patient's health information in real time at the point of care. Heart team decision making can be facilitated utilizing clinical decision support tools that integrate artificial intelligence and machine learning to provide the best care and outcome possible. The advances in imaging and 3D printing have created the opportunity to simplify procedure complexity and improve patient and operator safety through the use of simulation. Minimally invasive surgical and/or catheter-based cardiac interventions have seen a dramatic increase especially in the management of coronary artery disease, valvular heart disease, and stroke mitigation in patients. The next generation of therapeutic treatments will likely further integrate the above modalities to expand the use of minimally invasive cardiovascular technologies.

DIGITAL HEALTH

Digital health is defined as the social transformation of technologies that collect, share, and analyze patient data and digital information to improve patient health and healthcare delivery.[3] The spectrum of digital health, as defined by the Food and Drug Administration (FDA), includes the use of data from multiple sources that include mobile health (mHealth), health information technology (HIT), wearable devices, telehealth/telemedicine, and personalized medicine.[4] Due to the rapid evolution in this space, the Digital Health Innovation Action Plan seeks to address safety concerns and ensure that all patients receive timely access to quality digital health products. Programs are leveraging ever present internet connectivity to provide real-time data transfer of biophysical measurements and patient-generated data to practitioners for clinical decisions and providing a digital mechanism to facilitate shared decision making.[5] From a research perspective, these technologies have the potential to accelerate, streamline, and optimize clinical research operations and reduce costs. Programs are leveraging omnipresent internet connectivity to provide real-time data transfer of biophysical measurements and patient-generated data to practitioners for clinical decisions and providing a digital mechanism to facilitate shared decision making.[5]

Mobile Health

Mobile health, or mHealth, is defined by the Global Observatory for eHealth of the World Health Organization (WHO's) "medical and public health practice supported by mobile devices, such as mobile phones, patient monitoring devices, personal digital assistants, and other wireless devices."[6] These applications are

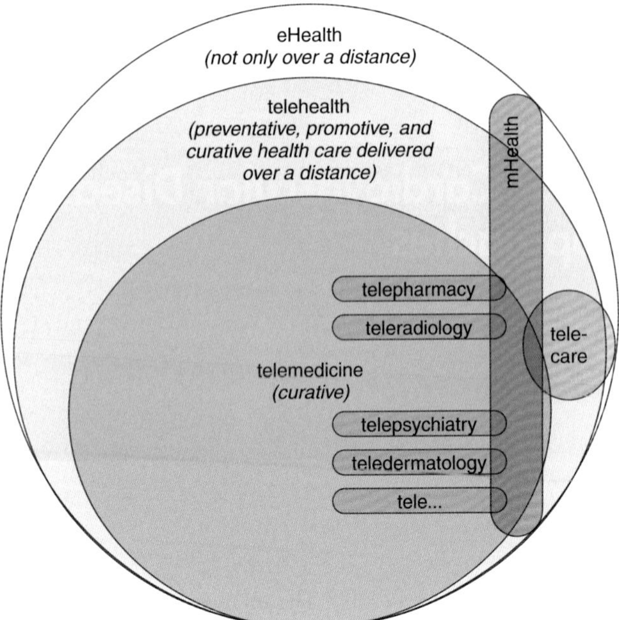

Figure 40-1. Practices Within Telehealth and Relationship to mHealth.

available on mobile devices, such as mobile phones and patient monitoring devices that patients use on a daily basis to support practices that aim to improve general health.[7] In the cardiovascular realm, mHealth aids in cardiovascular prevention such as short-term smoking prevention, weight loss, diabetes management, and cardiac rehabilitation and education.[7] However, the technologic innovations in mobile health create specific challenges in a largely unregulated field that include usability for the patient, system integration and sharing of information with other electronic modalities, data security and privacy, and network access and reliability (Fig. 40-1).[8]

Wearable Devices

Wearable devices are a subset of mHealth that focuses on technology that a patient can wear, such as watches, wristbands, cutaneous patches, and clothing.[10] Advancements in Bluetooth technology and minicomputer chips have accelerated the development of biosensors that transfer the physiologic input into a measurable and interpretable signal.[11] Wearable or implantable technology is expected to play an increasingly significant role in monitoring high-risk patients to prevent hospitalizations or readmissions.[12] Future research and clinical advances with wearable patient monitors will likely replace traditional monitoring devices. Data provided by these monitors may offer a mechanism to monitor a patient's response to interventions such as medication or lifestyle changes, etc. Accessibility of these data for review by designated clinicians is imperative with subsequent documentation of the data and provider response in the patient's electronic medical records.

It is only in the last couple of years that healthcare professionals are realizing that the majority of a patient's health and well-being takes place outside the hospital or clinic setting. Leveraging mHealth technologies for proactive health care can transform disease prevention and management. Atrial fibrillation is of particular interest because it can be difficult to detect and manage.[13] Reliance on episodic office visits and short-term monitoring is no longer necessary as ongoing monitoring with mHealth devices is an opportunity to prevent strokes, manage symptoms, and reduce hospitalizations from atrial fibrillation (Fig. 40-2).[13]

Health Information Technology

The U.S. Department of Health and Human Services defines HIT as the electronic exchange of health information.[14] The desired outcome with the utilization of HIT is to "improve the quality of health care by preventing medical errors, reducing healthcare costs, increasing administrative efficiencies, decreasing paperwork, and expanding access to affordable health care."[14] To move from paper to electronic documentation required government policy to encourage and accelerate the adoption of electronic health records (EHRs).

The Health Information Technology for Clinical and Economic (HITECH) Act in 2009 was designed to incentivize the use of EHRs and address the privacy and security concerns related to electronic transfer of personal health information and strengthen civil and criminal penalties for Health Insurance Portability and Accountability Act (HIPAA) violations.[15] With the advent of EHRs, key challenges that clinicians and patients have faced include seamless EHR interoperability, ease of use for the patient, data integration and proper display of appropriate information that supports clinical decision making, securing and maintaining private data, all the while addressing the cost of care and quality.[16]

Despite these challenges, as of 2017, roughly 96% of hospitals across the United States have adopted a certified EHR (Fig. 40-3).[17] However, due to nonstandardization of EHRs, only 41% of hospitals are able to electronically send, receive, find, and integrate patient information from outside providers.[17] Lastly, just over one third of hospital EHRs have the capability for patients to access their own health information using an application programming interface.[17] Both interoperability and patient access remain a challenge despite the advancements in EHR adoption. As a result, new CMS policy changes have been proposed to facilitate interoperability and expand patient access.[18]

Telemedicine

The Center for Connected Health Policy defines telehealth as a broad collection of methods that deliver medical, health, and education services to consumers.[19] Telemedicine is defined as a subset of telehealth. Telemedicine is the delivery of healthcare to diagnose and monitor through the use of telecommunication tools such as mobile phones, wireless devices, and computers.[5,20] Telemedicine traditionally has had two types of settings: synchronous and asynchronous virtual visits.

Synchronous Virtual Visits

Synchronous visits occur in real time and are live exchanges between clinician and patient, including virtual appointments utilizing smartphones, tablets, or computers with video camera.[21] This format is commonly used in cardiovascular medicine, known as telecardiology, and improves the delivery of specialty care in rural medicine. Patients are able to see specialists without extended travel that may preclude patients from seeking medical attention. The improvements in technology, such as an electronic stethoscope to conduct a physical examination and the ability to electronically review lab results, also permit care for patients in the comfort of their community.[22]

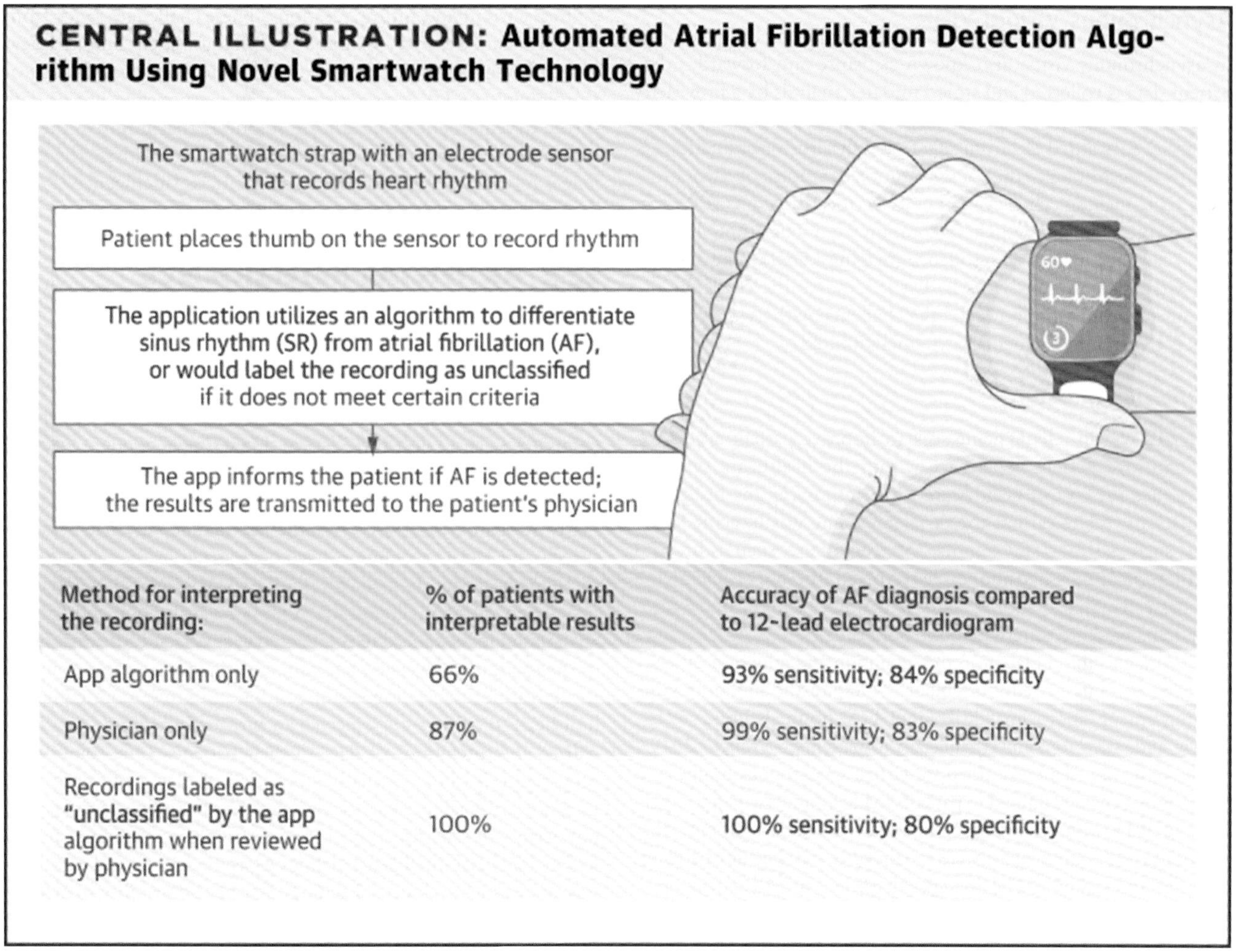

CENTRAL ILLUSTRATION: Automated Atrial Fibrillation Detection Algorithm Using Novel Smartwatch Technology
The smartwatch strap with an electrode sensor that records heart rhythm
Patient places thumb on the sensor to record rhythm
The application utilizes an algorithm to differentiate sinus rhythm (SR) from atrial fibrillation (AF), or would label the recording as unclassified if it does not meet certain criteria
The app informs the patient if AF is detected; the results are transmitted to the patient's physician
60
Method for interpreting the recording:
% of patients with interpretable results
Accuracy of AF diagnosis compared to 12-lead electrocardiogram
App algorithm only
66%
93% sensitivity; 84% specificity
Physician only
87%
99% sensitivity; 83% specificity
Recordings labeled as "unclassified" by the app algorithm when reviewed by physician
100%
100% sensitivity; 80% specificity

Figure 40-2. Automated Atrial Fibrillation Algorithm Using Novel Smartwatch Technology. (Used with permission from Bumgarner JM, Lambert CT, Hussein AA, et al. Smartwatch algorithm for automated detection of atrial fibrillation. *J Am Coll Cardiol.* 2018;71[21]:2381–2388. Elsevier.)

Certified EHR
Basic EHR
71.9%
85.2%*
94%*
96.9%*
96%
83.8%*
75.5%*
59.4%*
44.4%*
27.6%*
9.4%
12.2%
15.6%
2008
2009
2010
2011
2012
2013
2014
2015

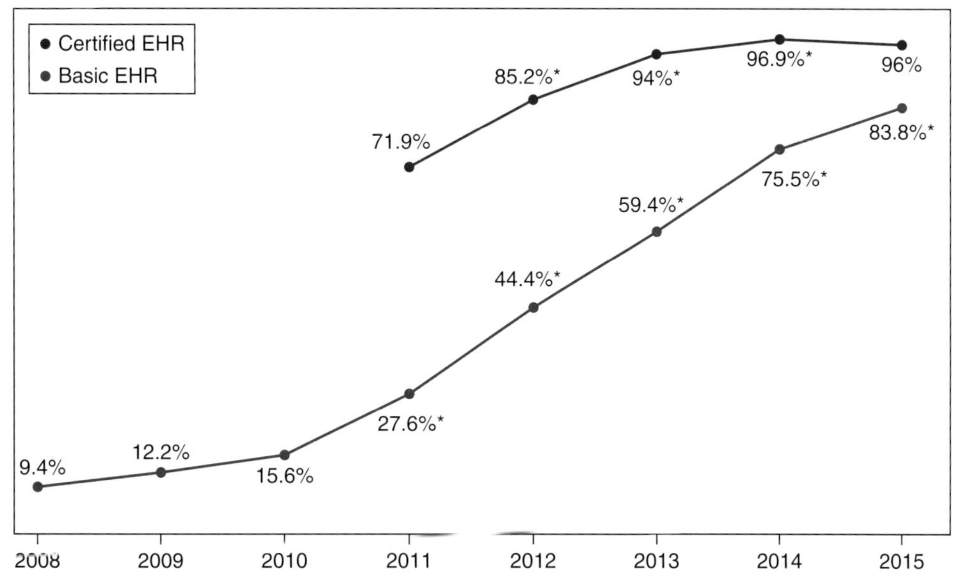

Source: ONC/American Hospital Association (AHA), AHA Annual Survey Information Technology Supplement

Figure 40-3. Percent of non-Federal acute care hospitals with adoption of at least a Basic EHR with notes system and possession of a certified EHR: 2008–2015.

Asynchronous Virtual Visits

In asynchronous visits, also known as "store-and-forward," the patient data is collected and stored for later analysis by a provider. At such time, digital images, clinical information or prerecorded videos are forwarded electronically to a specialist for evaluation.[23] Within telecardiology, the most common examples of asynchronous visits include echocardiograms, electrocardiograms (ECGs), and advanced imaging such as computerized axial tomography (CT) scans and magnetic resonance imaging (MRI). The advantage with asynchronous visits is that it removes the challenge of schedule coordination; however, the challenge with asynchronous visits is that reimbursement is extremely limited.[24]

Telemedicine Goals

The goals within telemedicine seek to improve patient access to care, improve patient experience within the healthcare system, and reduce the cost of health care while improving the health of populations.[20] The earliest use of telemedicine was in acute situations such as stroke and trauma.[5] As technology, such as broadband internet and smartphones, has evolved, the use of telemedicine has expanded to address chronic conditions and extend care to patients who are otherwise homebound.[5]

The major limiting factor in the expansion and adoption of telemedicine pertains to reimbursement.[20] Despite the limitations in reimbursement, approximately 76% of U.S. hospitals utilize technology and video to connect clinicians to patients.[25] Prior to 2019, Medicare reimbursements existed for virtual synchronous health visits but were generally limited to patients living in underserved or rural areas. In 2019, with the passage of the Bipartisan Budget Act of 2018, additional telehealth benefits were expanded to coverage for patients regardless of location.[26] The act states that Medicare Advantage programs may provide telehealth to enrollees. The act is patient focused when it comes to care decisions and allows the patient to determine if they would like to receive treatment remotely or through in-patient visits. The Act also allows eligible Accountable Care Organizations (ACOs) to expand telehealth services.

As mobile technology continues to advance, along with the push toward value-based health care, telemedicine will continue to evolve as healthcare systems seek to expand their network while decreasing cost of episodic care.[5]

Precision Medicine

The FDA defines precision medicine as an innovative approach to address disease prevention and treatment by customizing it to people's genetics, environments, and lifestyles. The goal is to "target the right treatments to the right patients at the right time"[4] and to ensure that the tailored care optimizes treatment for the individual based on the unique personal profile rather than treatment based on the average population.[27] An early example of precision medicine relates to blood transfusions and ensuring the donor and recipient are matched to reduce complications.[28] However, as with all digital health technology, precision medicine presents its own challenges that include: securing and maintaining patient privacy, data extraction from EHRs, and a searchable database that incorporates data from multiple sources (such as public databases and clinical references) to create individualized treatment plans for patients.[29]

Challenges Around Digital Health

With the innumerous ways digital health is rapidly expanding, it is logical that the FDA has created a regulatory task force to address current and future questions. These challenges range from personal data security, wearable technology safety and efficacy, and policy-governing reimbursement.[4] The American College of Cardiology (ACC) is advocating for the responsible use of data in the development of healthcare solutions that improve the clinician delivery of care for patients[30] and seek to address the challenges related to Digital Health and Artificial Intelligence.[31]

ARTIFICIAL INTELLIGENCE

Initially described in 1936 by Alan Turing as "computing machinery and intelligence," the field of artificial intelligence began with the inception of computers in the 1940s.[32] The actual term "Artificial Intelligence (AI)" was not coined until 1956 by American computer scientist John McCarthy. Interestingly enough, artificial intelligence did not create significant public interest until an algorithm-based Deep Blue won a chess match against world champion Garry Kasparov in 1997. Over the last decade, advancements in speech and facial recognition have been made in the gaming and social media arenas. In medicine, the creation of algorithms and deep neural networks has allowed for improved classification and pattern recognition for advanced technology such as CT and MR imaging.[33]

As the source diversity, amount, and character of data available to the cardiovascular care team continue to grow more complex, healthcare providers are expected to provide expeditious, individualized interpretations of data to their patients. One solution to provide this level of personalized precision medicine efficiently is to integrate artificial intelligence with patient phenotypes. Eric Topol, physician and scientist specializing in cardiology, genetics, genomics, and artificial intelligence defines AI as the science and engineering of creating intelligent machines that have the ability to achieve goals like humans via a constellation of technologies.[34] Collaborative partnerships between clinicians and data scientists are imperative for meaningful automation and analysis. Artificial intelligence is an umbrella term that refers to a collection of techniques that mimic human behavior in making decisions. Two subsets of artificial intelligence have evolved: machine learning and deep learning.

Machine Learning

Machine learning is an application of AI using algorithms to supply computers with the ability to automatically learn and improve from prior encounters or datasets, similar to humans, without being explicitly programmed.[32] Machine learning focuses on the development of computer programs that can access data and use it to learn by examining patterns in data. Through this continued examination, machine learning continues to evolve and make more informed decisions. Machine learning can be supervised (human-labeled datasets are processed), unsupervised (pattern identification without human input) or reinforced (algorithms that learn the best way to reach a desired goal).[32,35]

Supervised learning is defined as an algorithm that already has sorted and labeled data. The algorithm learns the general rules that guide the input and output data points. Based on those learnings, the desired outcome for supervised learning is the ability to predict future events on input only.[36] Unsupervised learning is designed to explore unlabeled input data with a desired outcome to infer hidden patterns or structure. When the patterns become apparent, the data points are put together (clustered) and classified.[36] Reinforced learning is where the machine, through trial and error, learns the best way to reach a desired goal that has been programmed.

Deep Learning

Deep learning is a subtype of machine learning that mimics the function of the human brain by utilizing multiple layers of artificial neuronal networks.[9,37] Deep learning models solve complex problems using a data set that can be diverse, unstructured, and interconnected. As the datasets become more elaborate, the data facilitates the ability for the machine to reason and interpret the data with increased accuracy.[9] Artificial intelligence is made up of multiple branches that include predictive systems, expert systems, speech to text, and natural language processing. Each of these branches contributes to the decision capabilities related to artificial intelligence.

Predictive Systems

Predictive systems are defined as "a system that finds relationships between variables in historical datasets and their outcomes."[36] Within the cardiovascular space, there are an extensive number of predictive systems attempting to model the future prevalence and outcomes related to CVD. However, in a review of the vast number of predictive systems, the study concluded that the utility of these predictive models is still unclear due to incomplete data, lack of external validation, and methodologic shortcomings.[38] Based on these findings, the authors recommended external validation of existing predictive models in a comparison study. This may provide information on scalability and the ability to incorporate new data.[38] A population health study investigated the ability of machine learning to quantify risk factors, predict outcomes, and identify biomarkers in an asymptomatic population. By combining machine learning with precision medicine (phenotyping), the authors discovered success in improving prediction accuracy.[39]

Expert Systems

Since the 1970s, expert systems have been artificial intelligence systems that utilize knowledge specific to a field, such as medicine or law, and combine it with a rules engine that dictates how the knowledge is applied.[36] Expert systems seek to improve the accessibility of the information, facilitate the process of decision making, and provide a way to test theories or ideas.[40] In cardiology, examples of expert systems have included smoking cessation,[41] diagnosis of myocardial infarction,[42] and diagnosis of ischemic heart disease (Fig. 40-4).[43]

Speech to Text

In this type of artificial intelligence, audio signals are converted into text and this phenomenon is commonly known as voice or speech recognition.[36] In health care, it is more frequent to see the use of a microphone to dictate directly into the medical health record for clinical documentation. When compared with traditional documentation methods such as scribes, typing, templates, or traditional dictation, the speech-to-text ability provides several advantages that include saving time, the ease of use for physicians, and the ability to record a more accurate depiction of the encounter in the EHR.[44,45]

Natural Language Processing

This type of artificial intelligence utilizes computers to process natural, human language. It includes speech recognition, computer translation, and a feelings analysis.[36] U.S. Department of Veterans Affairs conducted a study to evaluate the automation of Quality Metrics for Heart Failure through the use of natural language processing. They developed a natural language processing system called CHIEF (Congestive Heart Failure Information Extraction Framework) that collected essential data that could be used in a dashboard to identify patients who needed additional medication intervention. The study concluded that CHIEF was highly accurate in identifying patients, real-time completion of data collection, and improved clinical care for inpatient patients at time of discharge which could reduce hospital readmissions.[46]

Big Data

In each of these branches of artificial intelligence, big data is a common factor. Big data refers to extremely large datasets that cannot be searched, interpreted, or analyzed by applying traditional data-processing methods. Big data includes data from multiple sources such as wearable technology, social media, mobile phone applications, environmental and lifestyle-related factors, sociodemographic data, and data from EHRs. Currently, big data utilization is extremely limited due to massive size, heterogeneity, and impermanence of the data (Fig. 40-5).[31] In addition, the rate that data is being generated far exceeds the number of specialists required to analyze it. Despite the limitations, progress is being made in cardiology in research and development, population and precision health, and clinical practice

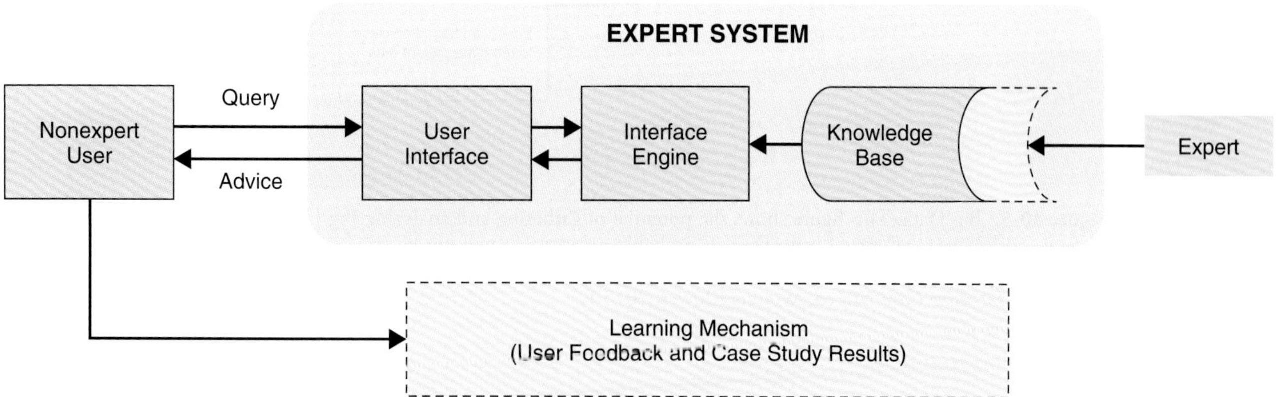

Figure 40-4. Typical Architecture of an Expert System. (Used with permission from Ozden A, Faghri A, Li M, et al. *Procedia Engineering*. 2016;145:752–759. Elsevier.)

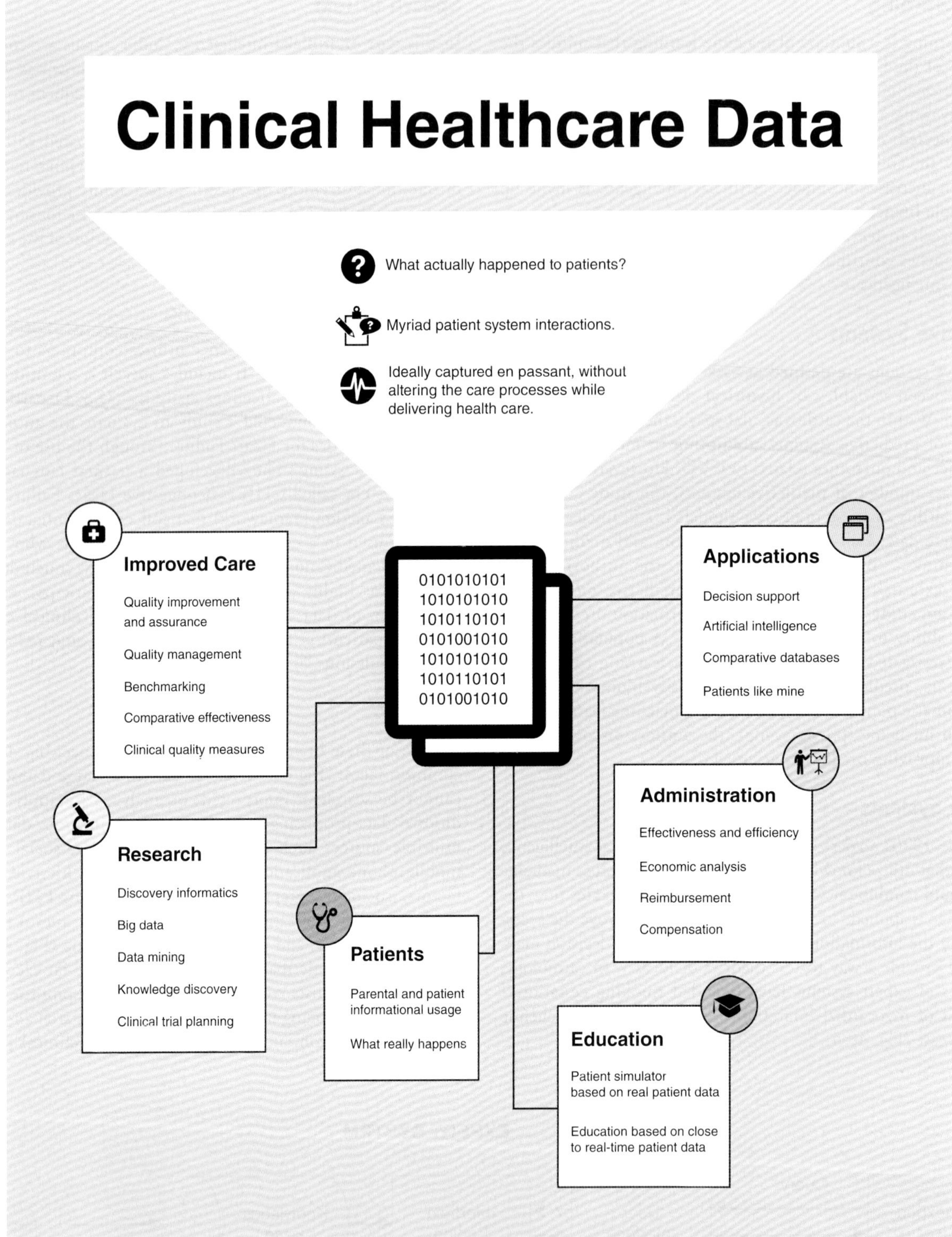

Figure 40-5. Big Data. This figure shows the potential of gathering and analyzing Big Data in multiple critical areas of critical care. There is probably no area that will not be enhanced by the critical application of Big Data analytics. (Used with permission. Shaffner DH, Nichols DG. *Rogers' Textbook of Pediatric Intensive Care*. 5th ed. Wolters Kluwer; 2015.)

and decision support.[47] The use of evidence-based medicine in current practice will definitely be impacted as the applications for machine learning increase.[37]

ARTIFICIAL INTELLIGENCE APPLICATIONS

With the advent of artificial intelligence technologies and applications, the integration of machine learning has played a significant role in the development and evolution of clinical decision support tools, advanced imaging, simulation, and the development of new minimally invasive technologies.[37] From the implementation of expert and predictive systems to the integration of natural language processing, there are multiple artificial intelligence applications that seek to address healthcare challenges such as smoking cessation, undertreatment of specific disease states, and time management for both physicians and patients. With the expansion of artificial intelligence to include virtual and augmented mixed reality technology, the advancements seek to improve the way physician, advanced clinician, and nurse training provides care for patients (see Simulation section).[36] The impact of these collective solutions will continue to evolve as the technology continues to advance (Figs. 40-6 and 40-7).

CLINICAL DECISION SUPPORT SYSTEMS

Introduction

Clinical decision support systems (CDSSs) are computer-based information systems designed to assist clinicians in implementing clinical guidelines and evidence-based practices at the point of care.[48] Accurate use of clinical information is critical to making the proper clinical decision and providing quality care. Pertinent patient data, combined with the clinician's knowledge and expertise is integral to clinical decision making.

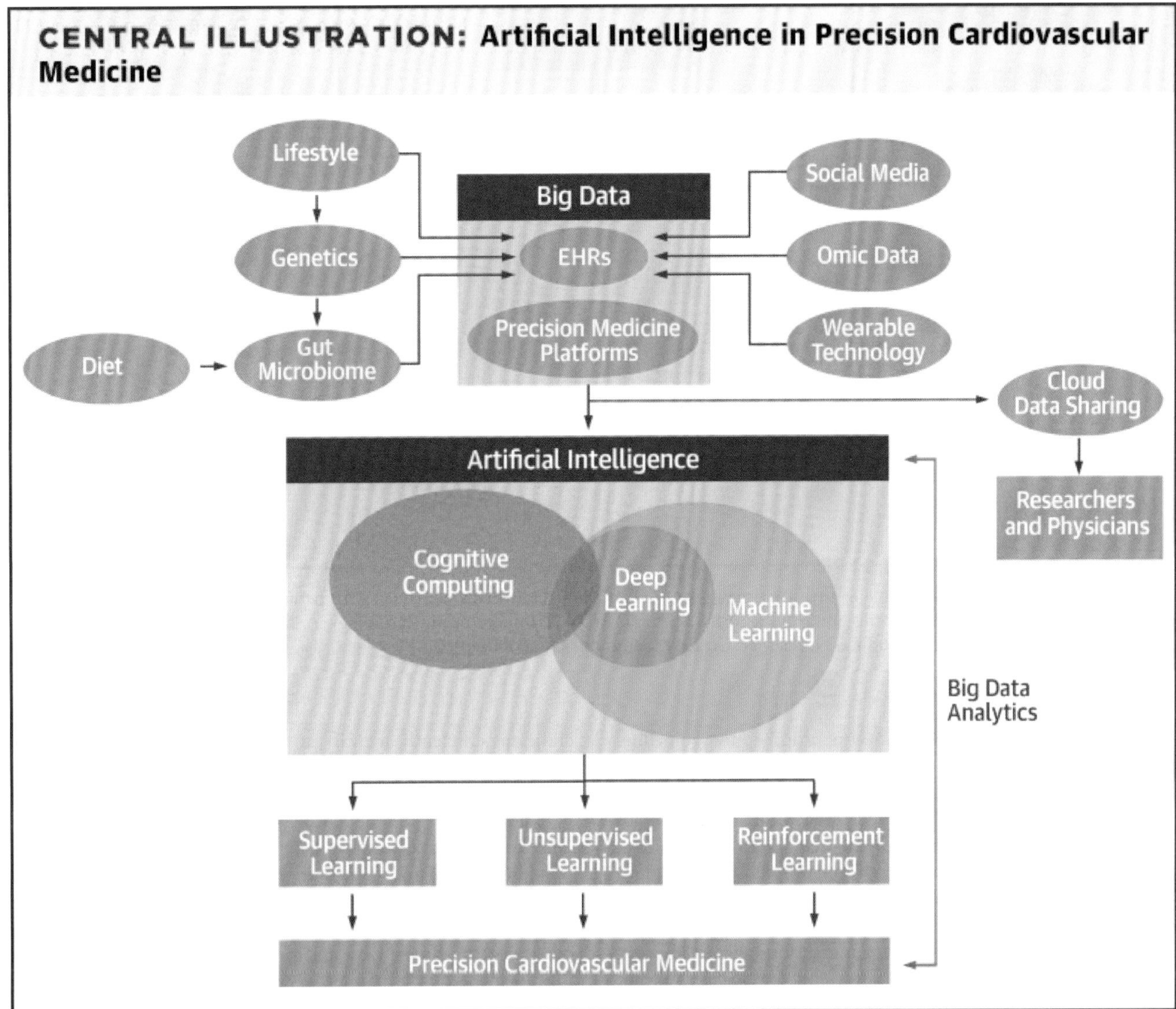

Figure 40-6. Artificial Intelligence in Precision Cardiovascular Medicine. (Used with permission from Krittanawong C, Zhang H, Wang Z, et al. Artificial intelligence in precision cardiovascular medicine. *J Am Coll Cardiol.* 2017;69[21]:2657–2664. Elsevier.)

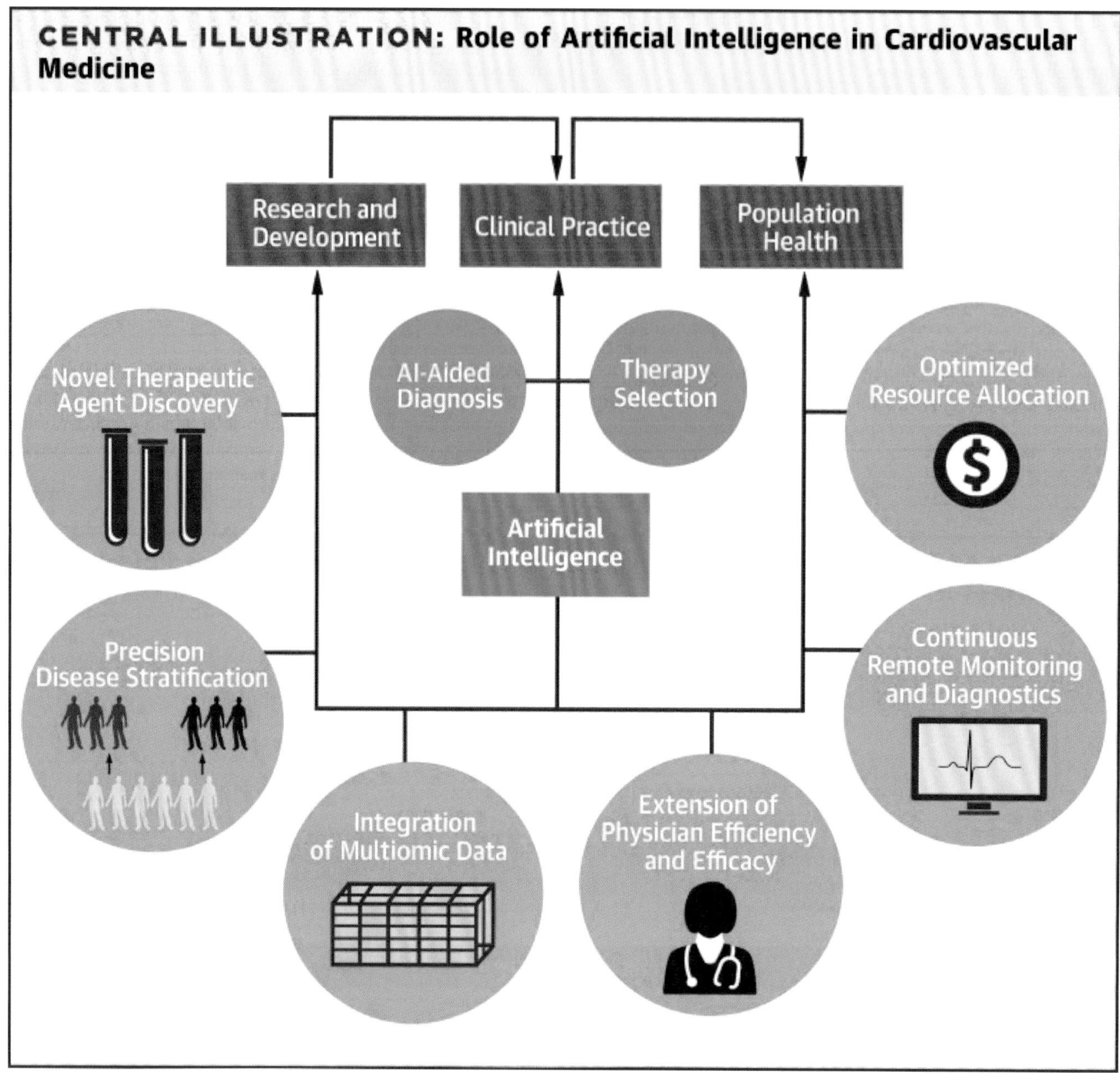

Figure 40-7. Role of Artificial Intelligence in Cardiovascular Medicine. (Used with permission from Johnson KW, Torres Soto J, Glicksberg BS, et al. Artificial intelligence in cardiology. *J Am Coll Cardiol.* 2018;71[23]:2668–2679. Elsevier. Creative Commons CC-BY license.)

Currently, there is a drive to meet appropriate use guidelines for diagnostic tests, imaging, and therapy. In 2014, CMS established a program to increase the rate of *appropriate* advanced diagnostic imaging services provided to Medicare patients. This program, slated to be fully implemented in 2021, mandates that ordering providers consult Appropriate Use Criteria (AUC) through a CDSS.[49] In addition, healthcare reform initiatives include financial incentives for value-based health care. Increasingly, these incentives have been for institutions able to improve patient care by leveraging information technology. Stage 3 meaningful use requirements for EHRs, modified in 2018, call for clinical decision support to improve performance on high-priority health conditions.[50] These directives have launched CDSS to the forefront of healthcare IT. Some of the goals of CDSS are to help clinicians efficiently identify at-risk patients, eliminate inappropriate testing and procedures, interpret clinical data, and inform patient treatment.

There has been much discussion about implementation of CDSSs. There is concern by some who view CDSS technology as "cookbook medicine" aimed at telling practitioners how to treat their patients. Other concerns are the cost of implementation and challenge of keeping the necessary software up to date on the most current clinical data and practice guidelines. Nevertheless, if implemented in a manner in which it is integrated with workflow and accepted by the clinicians and hospital administration, CDSSs have the potential to assist in reducing variations in care, unnecessary tests, and meeting the AUC mandate by CMS, which in turn, reduce healthcare costs.

Disease Prevention

Modifiable risk factors for CVD, such as smoking, hyperlipidemia, hypertension, diabetes, obesity, and physical inactivity can be improved with provider-focused strategies such as guideline education, provider alerts, and audit and feedback techniques. In the literature, the data on CDSS aiding in the prevention of CVD is equivocal. The goal is that CDSS can assist the provider in detecting and managing risk factors by providing customized assessments and treatment recommendations based on individual patient data. There is a paucity of data to support CDSS use for CVD prevention and study results examining changes in CVD risk factors such as systolic and diastolic blood pressure, total and low-density lipoprotein cholesterol, and hemoglobin A1C levels as a result of CDSS implementation are inconsistent.[48,51] More evidence is necessary to determine CDSS's impact on reducing CVD risk.

Patient Identification and Access to Treatment

Guidelines from professional organizations list and define patient criteria for various CVDs. However, a discrepancy exists between the number of patients that meet criteria and those who are referred for definitive treatment.[52,53] Delays in this treatment can result in poor patient outcomes. CDSSs have data to support improved patient identification and access to definitive care by providing clinicians access to published guidelines and treatment algorithms.[54–56] In a systematic review published by Njie et al.,[47] the authors noted increases in the completion of guideline-recommended screening and other preventive care services, diagnostic tests, and treatments.

Patient Assessment

Despite early inconsistent outcomes, the use of CDSS to improve adherence to guideline-based testing has been gaining popularity in the management of hypertension,[51,57,58] diabetes,[59–61] and hyperlipidemia[62,63] management. As outlined above, CMS mandates that ordering professionals must consult with AUC through a clinical decision support mechanism (CDSM) for all Medicare patients receiving applicable advanced imaging care. The American Association of Cardiology (ACC) has designed quality initiatives to assist in bridging the research practice gap. FOCUS is a quality initiative to guide and improve appropriate ordering of cardiovascular imaging and tests.[64]

Patient Treatment

Currently, a heart team approach is recommended in the care of patients with complex coronary disease and valvular heart disease. Patient outcomes can be improved with heart team meetings.[65–69] However, with a limited time for processing large amounts of patient data and in-depth case discussion, the process is potentially error prone. CDSSs have been shown to streamline communication, reduce errors, and improve efficiency,[54,70–72] which may prove valuable in a heart team setting.

Challenges Around Clinical Decision Support Implementation

Usability

CDSSs and dashboards are utilized more consistently and demonstrate improved outcomes when they are easy for clinicians to use. Findings suggest that an effective CDSS must minimize the effort required by clinicians to receive and act on system recommendations.[70] Several commercial platforms exist that incorporate information visualization strategies. However, integrating user-centered design principles is critical for successful implementation.[73] System development is comprehensive and requires clear communication and input from stakeholders such as physicians, nurses, administration, and information technology. Careful attention must be paid to the human–computer interaction to ensure enduring practice changes. CDSS displaying high-density clinically relevant information also helps streamline communications and efficiencies.[71] Subsequently, the CDSS must be easy to use to ensure adoption of the user.

Integration Into Workflow

Previous research shows that clinicians accept computer alerts and recommendations but resist processes that interfere with their daily workflow or challenge their autonomy. CDSSs that do not support users and the work environment can create inefficiencies and prevent goal attainment.[73,74] For clinicians to get the full benefit of CDSSs, these systems must better engage the end user.

Relevance and Context in Decision Making

End-user clinician input was an integral step in the process as their input and use was crucial for wider adoption of CDSS. Accurate and science-based algorithms were vital to clinician trust and utilization.[71,73,75] Availability of the CDSS at the point of care is imperative to provide context and utility.

ADVANCED IMAGING

Through the rapid technology gains in artificial intelligence and algorithm design, advanced imaging has become the gold standard for diagnosis and pre-case procedural planning. An example that demonstrates the accelerated evolution of advanced imaging occurs in transcatheter technology. In the early days of clinical trial with transcatheter aortic valve implant/replacement (TAVI/TAVR), the sizing of the annulus relied solely on transthoracic echocardiogram (TTE) which underestimated the size.[76] In 2010, there was still no defined gold standard in annular measurement sizing.[77]

As the technology evolved, and understanding of the annulus transitioned from a circular structure to elliptical structure, advanced imaging evolved in tandem. Two years later, in 2012, the Society of Cardiovascular Computed Tomography (SCCT) released guidelines to persuade physicians that CT-based imaging provided the best information for preprocedural planning.[78] During this time, 3D transesophageal echocardiogram (TEE) and CT were considered comparable to each other in annular sizing. However, there was concern that 3D TEE still undersized the annulus, anywhere from 9% to 12% when compared to CT.[76] In 6 years, CT moved from being an "optional" imaging platform to being a gold standard for case planning. Most recently, SCCT released an expert consensus document for CT imaging in context with TAVR.[79]

In addition, CT and echocardiogram turn to real-time ultrasound and fluoroscopy fusion technologies to improve the outcomes of these procedures. Within TAVR, TEE and fluoroscopy fusion have created the ability to implant transcatheter valves without the use of contrast dye, which is especially important in renal-compromised patients (Fig. 40-8).[76,80]

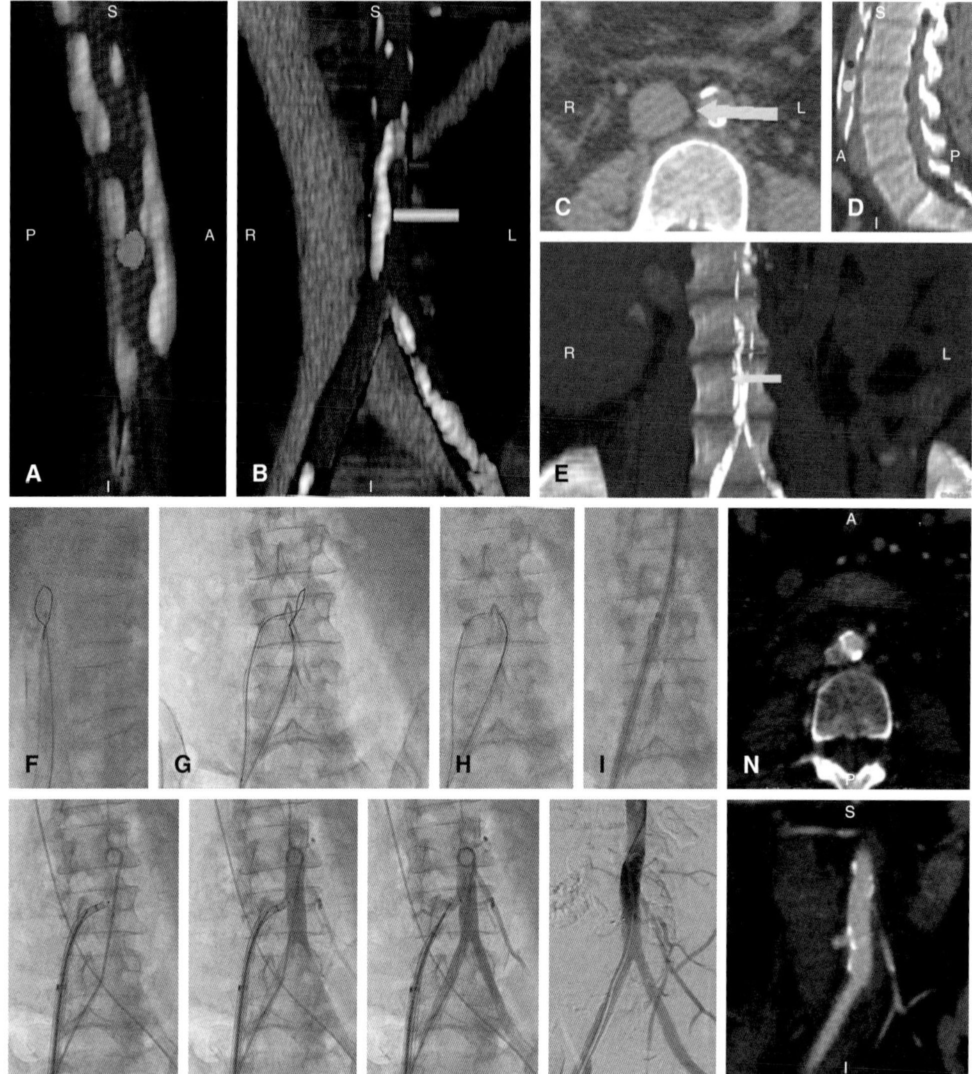

Figure 40-8. Advanced Imaging Used to Plan for Transcaval Approach TAVR. (Used with permission from Greenbaum AB, Babaliaros VS, Chen MY, et al. Transcaval access and closure for transcatheter aortic valve replacement: a prospective investigation. *J Am Coll Cardiol.* 2017;69[5]:511–521. Elsevier.)

As cardiac imaging technologies rapidly expand and evolve, the ACC has created a think tank to address future challenges of cardiac imaging within the constraints of a cost-conscious quality-oriented healthcare system. These challenges include the preservation and enhancement of cardiac imaging within an evolving value-based healthcare system, to identify the role of cardiac imaging in the future, how to ensure continued innovation and research investment, and how to improve patient outcomes while simultaneously maximizing and standardizing imaging data.[81]

3D Printing

Across cardiac imaging, there will be greater use of 3D advanced visualization to create 3D models. 3D printing, also known as additive manufacturing (AM), is a technique of creating a physical structure by arranging numerous thin layers of a material, on top of each other, in a predefined pattern. Initially, a virtual computer-aided design (CAD) model is processed by a 3D printer. Then the printer proceeds to stack each layer of model material on top of the next until the 3D object is created (Farooqi figure). Applications in medicine for 3D printing have gained more visibility in the last 5 years (Fig. 40-9).[82]

Cellular bioprinting techniques have been developed to create cardiovascular tissues. However, 3D printing of the cardiovascular system is costly and difficult, which limits its applicability in disease treatment. Recent advances demonstrate a potential for creating functional cardiovascular tissue on a larger scale. In addition, heart models targeting the myocardium as the minimal functional unit may have the potential to model drug responses, disease states, and potential disease treatments.[83,84]

Advanced visualization in complex cases will see an increase in 3D printed models from medical images. Cardiology, radiology, and other specialties may utilize holographic and true 3D imaging to better understand complex anatomy and for procedural planning. A number of programs in the United States already utilize 3D printing technology to create precision models of the heart and other anatomical structures, to better prepare for procedures.

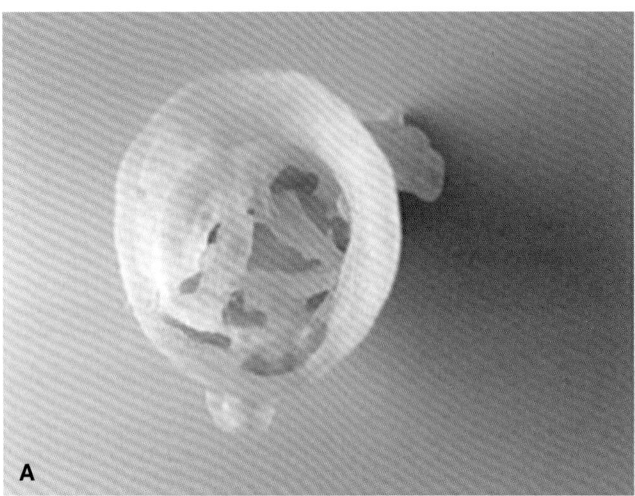
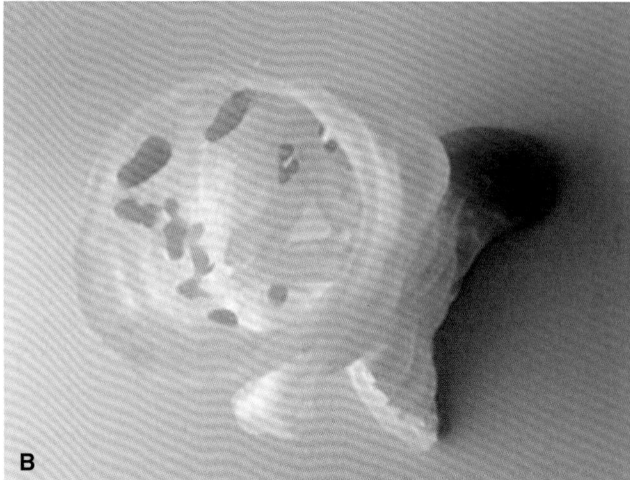

Figure 40-9. (**A, B**) Examples of Prints of the Aortic Valve in a Flexible Transparent Material With Calcifications in Blue Nonflexible Material. (Reprinted from Tuncay V, van Ooijen PMA. 3D printing for heart valve disease: a systematic review. *Eur Radiol Exp*. 2019;3:9. Available at https://doi.org/10.1186/s41747-018-0083-0. Creative Commons Attribution 4.0 International license http://creativecommons.org/licenses/by/4.0.)

SIMULATION TECHNOLOGIES

In the 1960s, early types of simulation technology, such as cardiopulmonary resuscitation mannequins, were integrated into medical training.[85] The mannequins provide a safe environment to teach multiple skills that include practice of CPR, intubation, medication administration, defibrillation, and crisis management.[86]

In the 1980s, computer-aided surgery came into existence due to three key technologies: surgical planning via imaging, live surgical guidance afforded by imaging fusion technology, and surgical robotics.[87] With new advances in artificial technology and advanced algorithms, advanced imaging with 3D planning and fusion technology has allowed for simulation technology that significantly aids in the training of physicians. Simulation technology has advanced such that it has a meaningful impact on patient safety, operator safety, and improving operator technique.

Operator experience is inversely related to procedural risk. Just as airline pilots spend hours in flight simulators for training, medical schools are integrating high-fidelity simulators to decrease procedural risk by novice physician operators.[88] Specifically within interventional cardiology, three studies demonstrated that incorporating simulation training helped improve trainees' technical performance scores compared to their peers who did not have simulation training.[86] This simulation technology not only helps heart surgeons and cardiologists train, but also prepares them for managing challenging clinical scenarios. Within structural heart, advanced imaging has provided the ability to do preprocedure implant planning to predict device and host (patient) interaction[89] and utilize fusion technology for optimal intraprocedural guidance.[90] The entire team can perform patient-specific dry runs and minimize deleterious outcomes related to anatomical complexities.

CONCLUSIONS

Carl Sagan once said, "Imagination will often carry us to worlds that never were. But without it we go nowhere." As we enter the information age of health care, advanced health technologies offer significant opportunities to optimize clinical care delivery, clinical research, and both operator and patient safety. Despite the potential of such technologies, their use in clinical care and research faces major data quality, privacy, and regulatory concerns.

The potential for massive amounts of lifestyle and health data generated by wearables is upon us. Clinicians are utilizing the imaging capabilities offered by CMR, CTA, and PET/CT scans to expedite diagnosis and therapy. Machine learning will generate algorithms that will make these big data useful to impact outcomes and stratify risk and procedural success rate as low, moderate, or high by revealing the degree of disease and specific anatomical considerations.

Techniques and technologies that can improve patient outcomes, reduce cost of care, length of stay, or prevent readmissions must be investigated in today's value-based healthcare environment. New technologies that demonstrate evidence for being able to improve outcomes at lower costs are being fast-tracked. The transition from traditional open surgical procedures to catheter-based interventional procedures warrants a focus on not only improved mortality, but improvements in functional status and quality of life. Durability of catheter-based devices will likely impact the widespread adoption.

KEY READINGS

Bhavnani SP, Parakh K, Atreja A, et al. 2017 roadmap for innovation—ACC health policy statement on healthcare transformation in the era of digital health, big data, and precision health: a report of the American College of Cardiology Task Force on health policy statements and systems of care. *J Am Coll Cardiol*. 2017;70(21):2696–2718.

Doenst T, Diab M, Sponholz C, et al. The opportunities and limitations of minimally invasive cardiac surgery. *Dtsch Arztebl Int*. 2017;114(46):777–784.

Farooqi KM, Mahmood F. Innovations in preoperative planning: insights into another dimension using 3D printing for cardiac disease. *J Cardiothorac Vasc Anesth*. 2018;32(4):1937–1945.

Topol E. *Deep Medicine: How Artificial Intelligence Can Make Healthcare Human Again*. New York, New York: Basic Books; 2019.

REFERENCES

1. Benjamin EJ, Muntner P, Alonso A, et al. Heart Disease and Stroke Statistics-2019 Update: a report from the American Heart Association. *Circulation*. 2019;139(10):e56–e528.
2. Lloyd-Jones DM, Hong Y, Labarthe D, et al. Defining and setting national goals for cardiovascular health promotion and disease reduction: the American Heart Association's strategic Impact Goal through 2020 and beyond. *Circulation*. 2010;121(4):586–613.
3. Sharma A, Harrington RA, McClellan MB, et al. Using digital health technology to better generate evidence and deliver evidence-based care. *J Am Coll Cardiol*. 2018;71(23):2680–2690.
4. Center for Devices and Radiological Health, U.S. Food and Drug Administration. *Precision medicine*. Available at https://www.fda.gov/medical-devices/vitro-diagnostics/precision-medicine. Published August 2, 2019. Accessed July 20, 2019.
5. Dorsey ER, Topol EJ. State of telehealth. *N Engl J Med*. 2016;375(2):154–161.
6. World Health Organization. *MHealth: New Horizons for Health Through Mobile Technologies*. Geneva, Switzerland: World Health Organization; 2011.
7. Chow CK, Ariyarathna N, Islam SMS, et al. mHealth in cardiovascular health care. *Heart Lung Circ*. 2016;25(8):802–807.
8. Gurupur VP, Wan TTH. Challenges in implementing mHealth interventions: a technical perspective. *Mhealth*. 2017;3:32.
9. Seetharam K, Kagiyama N, Sengupta PP. Application of mobile health, telemedicine and artificial intelligence to echocardiography. *Echo Res Pract*. 2019;6(2):R41–R52.
10. Eapen ZJ, Turakhia MP, McConnell MV, et al. Defining a mobile health roadmap for cardiovascular health and disease. *J Am Heart Assoc*. 2016;5(7):e003119.
11. Vasan RS, Benjamin EJ. The future of cardiovascular epidemiology. *Circulation*. 2016;133(25):2626–2633.
12. Amir O, Ben-Gal T, Weinstein JM, et al. Evaluation of remote dielectric sensing (ReDS) technology-guided therapy for decreasing heart failure re-hospitalizations. *Int J Cardiol*. 2017;240:279–284.
13. McConnell MV, Turakhia MP, Harrington RA, et al. Mobile health advances in physical activity, fitness, and atrial fibrillation: moving hearts. *J Am Coll Cardiol*. 2018;71(23):2691–2701.
14. Office for Civil Rights (OCR), HHS.gov. *Health information technology*. Available at https://www.hhs.gov/hipaa/for-professionals/special-topics/health-information-technology/index.html. Published April 19, 2019. Accessed July 18, 2019.
15. Office for Civil Rights (OCR), HHS.gov. *HITECH Act Enforcement Interim Final Rule*. Available at https://www.hhs.gov/hipaa/for-professionals/special-topics/hitech-act-enforcement-interim-final-rule/index.html. Published June 16, 2017. Accessed July 18, 2019.
16. Washington V, DeSalvo K, Mostashari F, et al. The HITECH era and the path forward. *N Engl J Med*. 2017;377(10):904–906.
17. Health IT Dashboard. *Non-federal acute care hospital health IT adoption and use*. Available at https://dashboard.healthit.gov/apps/hospital-health-it-adoption.php. Accessed July 18, 2019.
18. CMS.gov. *CMS advances interoperability & patient access to health data through new proposals*. Available at https://www.cms.gov/newsroom/fact-sheets/cms-advances-interoperability-patient-access-health-data-through-new-proposals. Accessed August 4, 2019.
19. Center for Connected Health Policy. *About telehealth*. Available at https://www.cchpca.org/about/about-telehealth. Accessed August 4, 2019.
20. Tuckson RV, Edmunds M, Hodgkins ML. Telehealth. *N Engl J Med*. 2017;377(16):1585–1592.
21. Mahar JH, Rosencrance JG, Rasmussen PA. Telemedicine: past, present, and future. *Cleve Clin J Med*. 2018;85(12):938–942.
22. Kuehn BM. Telemedicine helps cardiologists extend their reach. *Circulation*. 2016;134(16):1189–1191.
23. Deshpande A, Khoja S, Lorca J, et al. Asynchronous telehealth: a scoping review of analytic studies. *Open Med*. 2009;3(2):e69–e91.
24. mHealthIntelligence. *Telehealth terminology: "store-and-forward" has its fans—and critics*. Available at https://mhealthintelligence.com/news/telehealth-terminology-store-and-forward-has-its-fans-and-critics. Published July 21, 2016. Accessed July 26, 2019.
25. American Hospital Association. *Fact sheet: telehealth*. Available at https://www.aha.org/factsheet/telehealth. Accessed July 20, 2019.
26. CMS.gov. *CMS finalizes policies to bring innovative telehealth benefit to Medicare advantage*. Available at https://www.cms.gov/newsroom/press-releases/cms-finalizes-policies-bring-innovative-telehealth-benefit-medicare-advantage. Accessed July 20, 2019.
27. Leopold JA, Loscalzo J. Emerging role of precision medicine in cardiovascular disease. *Circ Res*. 2018;122(9):1302–1315.
28. Genetics Home Reference. *What is precision medicine?* Available at https://ghr.nlm.nih.gov/primer/precisionmedicine/definition. Accessed August 4, 2019.
29. Haendel MA, Chute CG, Robinson PN. Classification, ontology, and precision medicine. *N Engl J Med*. 2018;379(15):1452–1462.
30. American College of Cardiology. *Digital health*. Available at https://www.acc.org/tools-and-practice-support/advocacy-at-the-acc/acc-health-care-principles/digital-health. Accessed July 26, 2019.
31. Bhavnani SP, Parakh K, Atreja A, et al. 2017 roadmap for innovation—ACC health policy statement on healthcare transformation in the era of digital health, big data, and precision health: a report of the American College of Cardiology Task Force on health policy statements and systems of care. *J Am Coll Cardiol*. 2017;70(21):2696–2718.
32. Warwick K. *Artificial Intelligence: The Basics*. Routledge, United Kingdom; 2013.
33. Pesapane F, Codari M, Sardanelli F. Artificial intelligence in medical imaging: threat or opportunity? Radiologists again at the forefront of innovation in medicine. *Eur Radiol Exp*. 2018;2(1):35.
34. Topol E. *Deep Medicine: How Artificial Intelligence Can Make Healthcare Human Again*. New York, New York: Basic Books; 2019.
35. Vellido A, Martín-Guerrero JD, Lisboa PJG. Making machine learning models interpretable. *ESANN*. 2012. Available at http://citeseerx.ist.psu.edu/viewdoc/download?doi=10.1.1.431.5382&rep=rep1&type=pdf
36. Daugherty PR, James Wilson H. *Human + Machine: Reimagining Work in the Age of AI*. Boston, Massachusetts: Harvard Business Press; 2018.
37. Johnson KW, Torres Soto J, Glicksberg BS, et al. Artificial intelligence in cardiology. *J Am Coll Cardiol*. 2018;71(23):2668–2679.
38. Damen JAAG, Hooft L, Schuit E, et al. Prediction models for cardiovascular disease risk in the general population: systematic review. *BMJ*. 2016;353:i2416.
39. Ambale-Venkatesh B, Yang X, Wu CO, et al. Cardiovascular event prediction by machine learning: the multi-ethnic study of atherosclerosis. *Circ Res*. 2017;121(9):1092–1101.
40. Thomas RF. The benefits of expert systems in health care. practical experiences from CATEG05-ES. In: *AIME 89*. Second European Conference on Artificial Intelligence in Medicine, London, August 29th–31st 1989. Proceedings.
41. Velicer WF, Prochaska JO. An expert system intervention for smoking cessation. *Patient Educ Couns*. 1999;36(2):119–129.
42. Gath SJ, Kulkarni RV. A review: expert system for diagnosis of myocardial infarction. *arXiv [csAI]*. 2014. Available at http://arxiv.org/abs/1401.0245
43. Hossain MS, Haque M, Mustafa R, et al. An expert system to assist the diagnosis of ischemic heart disease. *Int J Integr Care*. 2016;16(6):A31.
44. Goss FR, Blackley SV, Ortega CA, et al. A clinician survey of using speech recognition for clinical documentation in the electronic health record. *Int J Med Inform*. 2019;130:103938.
45. American Medical Association. *8 ways speech-recognition software can work for your practice*. Available at https://www.ama-assn.org/practice-management/sustainability/8-ways-speech-recognition-software-can-work-your-practice. Accessed August 4, 2019.
46. Garvin JH, Kim Y, Gobbel GT, et al. Automating quality measures for heart failure using natural language processing: a descriptive study in the Department of Veterans Affairs. *JMIR Med Inform*. 2018;6(1):e5.
47. Krittanawong C, Zhang H, Wang Z, et al. Artificial intelligence in precision cardiovascular medicine. *J Am Coll Cardiol*. 2017;69(21):2657–2664.
48. Njie GJ, Proia KK, Thota AB, et al. Clinical decision support systems and prevention: a community guide cardiovascular disease systematic review. *Am J Prev Med*. 2015;49(5):784–795.
49. CMS. Appropriate Use Criteria. Available at https://www.cms.gov/medicare/quality-initiatives-patient-assessment-instruments/appropriate-use-criteria-program/index.html. Published February 21, 2019. Accessed July 21, 2019.
50. Clinical Decision Support and Meaningful Use. *HIMSS*. Available at https://www.himss.org/library/clinical-decision-support/meaningful-use. Published December 1, 2015. Accessed July 21, 2019.
51. Anchala R, Pinto MP, Shroufi A, et al. The role of decision support system (DSS) in prevention of cardiovascular disease: a systematic review and meta-analysis. *PLoS One*. 2012;7(10):e47064.
52. Nishimura RA, Otto CM, Bonow RO, et al. 2017 AHA/ACC Focused Update of the 2014 AHA/ACC Guideline for the Management of Patients With Valvular Heart Disease: a report of the American College

of Cardiology/American Heart Association Task Force on Clinical Practice Guidelines. *Circulation.* 2017;135(25):e1159–e1195.

53. Bugiardini R, Ricci B, Cenko E, et al. Delayed care and mortality among women and men with myocardial infarction. *J Am Heart Assoc.* 2017;6(8):e005968.
54. Clarke S, Wilson ML, Terhaar M. Using clinical decision support and dashboard technology to improve heart team efficiency and accuracy in a Transcatheter Aortic Valve Implantation (TAVI) program. *Stud Health Technol Inform.* 2016;225:98–102.
55. Kirby AM, Kruger B, Jain R, et al. Using clinical decision support to improve referral rates in severe symptomatic aortic stenosis: a quality improvement initiative. *Comput Inform Nurs.* 2018;36(11): 525–529.
56. Chatzakis I, Vassilakis K, Lionis C, et al. Electronic health record with computerized decision support tools for the purposes of a pediatric cardiovascular heart disease screening program in Crete. *Comput Methods Programs Biomed.* 2018;159:159–166.
57. Hetlevik I, Holmen J, Krüger O. Implementing clinical guidelines in the treatment of hypertension in general practice. Evaluation of patient outcome related to implementation of a computer-based clinical decision support system. *Scand J Prim Health Care.* 1999;17(1):35–40.
58. Hicks LS, Sequist TD, Ayanian JZ, et al. Impact of computerized decision support on blood pressure management and control: a randomized controlled trial. *J Gen Intern Med.* 2008;23(4):429–441.
59. Conway N, Adamson KA, Cunningham SG, et al. Decision support for diabetes in Scotland: implementation and evaluation of a clinical decision support system. *J Diabetes Sci Technol.* 2018;12(2): 381–388.
60. Schnipper JL, Linder JA, Palchuk MB, et al. Effects of documentation-based decision support on chronic disease management. *Am J Manag Care.* 2010;16(12 Suppl HIT):SP72–SP81.
61. Hetlevik I, Holmen J, Krüger O, et al. Implementing clinical guidelines in the treatment of diabetes mellitus in general practice. Evaluation of effort, process, and patient outcome related to implementation of a computer-based decision support system. *Int J Technol Assess Health Care.* 2000;16(1):210–227.
62. Scheitel MR, Kessler ME, Shellum JL, et al. Effect of a novel clinical decision support tool on the efficiency and accuracy of treatment recommendations for cholesterol management. *Appl Clin Inform.* 2017;8(1):124–136.
63. Chang TS, Buchipudi A, Fonarow GC, et al. Physicians voluntarily using an EHR-based CDS tool improved patients' guideline-related statin prescription rates: a retrospective cohort study. *Appl Clin Inform.* 2019;10(3):421–445.
64. American College of Cardiology. *AUC mandate information.* Available at https://www.acc.org/tools-and-practice-support/quality-programs/imaging-in-focus/auc-mandate-information. Accessed July 21, 2019.
65. Dubois C, Coosemans M, Rega F, et al. Prospective evaluation of clinical outcomes in all-comer high-risk patients with aortic valve stenosis undergoing medical treatment, transcatheter or surgical aortic valve implantation following heart team assessment. *Interact Cardiovasc Thorac Surg.* 2013;17(3):492–500.
66. Chelliah R, Showkathali R, Brickham B, et al. Multi-disciplinary clinic: next step in "heart team" approach for TAVI. *Heart.* 2014;100(Suppl 3): A58–A59.
67. Boureau AS, Trochu JN, Colliard C, et al. Determinants in treatment decision-making in older patients with symptomatic severe aortic stenosis. *Maturitas.* 2015;82(1):128–133.
68. Dworakowski R, MacCarthy PA, Monaghan M, et al. Transcatheter aortic valve implantation for severe aortic stenosis—a new paradigm for multidisciplinary intervention: a prospective cohort study. *Am Heart J.* 2010;160(2):237–243.
69. Hong SJ, Hong MK, Ko YG, et al. Multidisciplinary team approach for identifying potential candidate for transcatheter aortic valve implantation. *Yonsei Med J.* 2014;55(5):1246–1252.
70. Ahern DK, Stinson LJ, Uebelacker LA, et al. E-health blood pressure control program. *J Med Pract Manage.* 2012;28(2):91–100.
71. Koopman RJ, Kochendorfer KM, Moore JL, et al. A diabetes dashboard and physician efficiency and accuracy in accessing data needed for high-quality diabetes care. *Ann Fam Med.* 2011;9(5):398–405.
72. Waitman LR, Phillips IE, McCoy AB, et al. Adopting real-time surveillance dashboards as a component of an enterprisewide medication safety strategy. *Jt Comm J Qual Patient Saf.* 2011;37(7):326–332.
73. Dolan JG, Veazie PJ, Russ AJ. Development and initial evaluation of a treatment decision dashboard. *BMC Med Inform Decis Mak.* 2013;13:51.
74. McMenamin J, Nicholson R, Leech K. Patient Dashboard: the use of a colour-coded computerised clinical reminder in Whanganui regional general practices. *J Prim Health Care.* 2011;3(4):307–310.
75. Batley NJ, Osman HO, Kazzi AA, et al. Implementation of an emergency department computer system: design features that users value. *J Emerg Med.* 2011;41(6):693–700.
76. Bleakley C, Monaghan MJ. The pivotal role of imaging in TAVR procedures. *Curr Cardiol Rep.* 2018;20(2):9.
77. Serruys PW, Piazza N, Cribier A, et al. *Transcatheter Aortic Valve Implantation: Tips and Tricks to Avoid Failure.* New York, New York: CRC Press; 2009.
78. tctMD/the heart beat. *New CT guidelines for TAVR emphasize standardization, 4-D acquisition, and postprocedural imaging.* Available at https:// www.tctmd.com/news/new-ct-guidelines-tavr-emphasize-standardization-4-d-acquisition-and-postprocedural-imaging. Accessed July 28, 2019.
79. Blanke P, Weir-McCall JR, Achenbach S, et al. Computed tomography imaging in the context of transcatheter aortic valve implantation (TAVI)/ transcatheter aortic valve replacement (TAVR): an expert consensus document of the Society of Cardiovascular Computed Tomography. *J Cardiovasc Comput Tomogr.* 2019;13(1):1–20.
80. Balzer J, Zeus T, Hellhammer K, et al. Initial clinical experience using the EchoNavigator(®)-system during structural heart disease interventions. *World J Cardiol.* 2015;7(9):562–570.
81. Douglas PS, Cerqueira MD, Berman DS, et al. The future of cardiac imaging: report of a think tank convened by the American College of Cardiology. *JACC Cardiovasc Imaging.* 2016;9(10):1211–1223.
82. Farooqi KM, Mahmood F. Innovations in preoperative planning: insights into another dimension using 3D printing for cardiac disease. *J Cardiothorac Vasc Anesth.* 2018;32(4):1937–1945.
83. Cui H, Miao S, Esworthy T, et al. 3D bioprinting for cardiovascular regeneration and pharmacology. *Adv Drug Deliv Rev.* 2018;132: 252–269.
84. Kurokawa YK, George SC. Tissue engineering the cardiac microenvironment: multicellular microphysiological systems for drug screening. *Adv Drug Deliv Rev.* 2016;96:225–233.
85. Cooper JB, Taqueti VR. A brief history of the development of mannequin simulators for clinical education and training. *Postgrad Med J.* 2008;84(997):563–570.
86. Joshi A, Wragg A. Simulator training in interventional cardiology. *Interv Cardiol.* 2016;11(1):70–73.
87. Joskowicz L. Computer-aided surgery meets predictive, preventive, and personalized medicine. *EPMA J.* 2017;8(1):1–4.
88. Westerdahl DE. The necessity of high-fidelity simulation in cardiology training programs. *J Am Coll Cardiol.* 2016;67(11):1375–1378.
89. FEOPS. *The predictive value of FEops' simulation technology.* Available at https://www.feops.com/technology. Accessed August 3, 2019.
90. Biaggi P, Fernandez-Golfín C, Hahn R, et al. Hybrid imaging during transcatheter structural heart interventions. *Curr Cardiovasc Imaging Rep.* 2015;8(9):33.

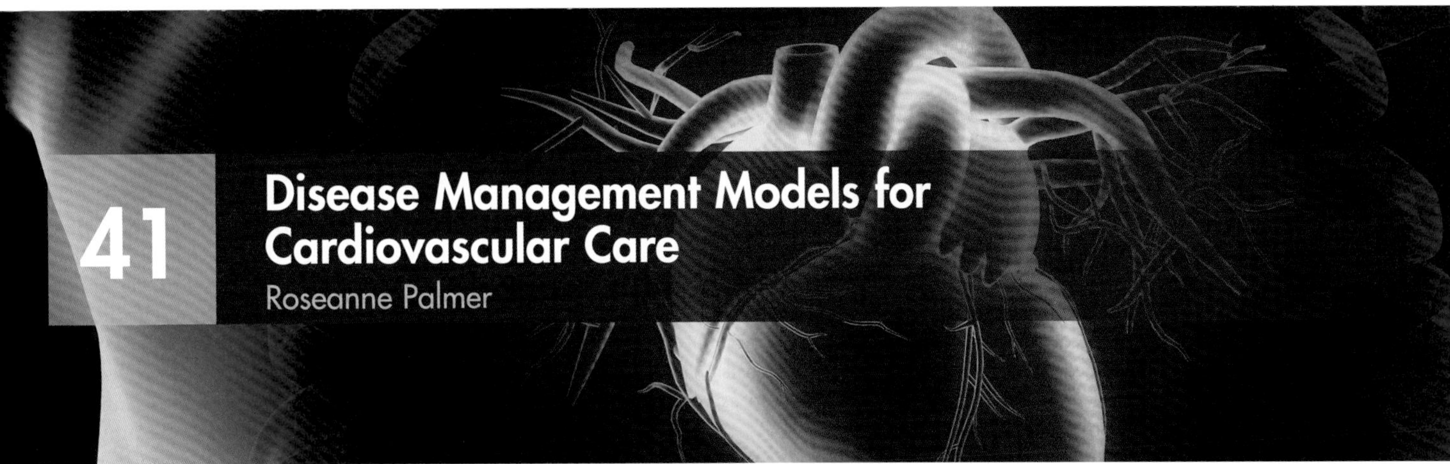

41 Disease Management Models for Cardiovascular Care

Roseanne Palmer

OBJECTIVES

1. Highlight the impact of cardiovascular disease management programs on patient outcomes.
2. Describe the essential role of cardiovascular nursing as part of multispecialty care team.

KEY QUESTIONS

1. What are the major contributors to avoidable hospitalizations?
2. How do disease models affect patient care?
3. What are the major complexities of caring for patients with multiple comorbid conditions?

BACKGROUND

Since the mid-1990s, disease management programs (DMPs) have served as an important method of caring for patients with chronic illness. The goal of these programs is to improve patient outcomes, increase quality of life, and decrease healthcare utilization and cost. Disease management has been adopted on the basis of results of numerous randomized controlled trials showing that patients with cardiovascular conditions such as heart failure (HF), coronary heart disease, diabetes, and hypertension are better supported through methods involving a team approach, coordinated delivery of care, systematic education, and documentation of outcomes directed at improving program delivery. The trend toward caring for patients through DMPs has spread rapidly and not only involves researchers, but also numerous healthcare organizations, the government, and for-profit organizations. These organizations are attempting to improve chronic disease care and reduce costly emergency department visits and hospitalizations. Data from managed care organizations indicate that at least 88% of such organizations have implemented at least one DMP.[1] The aim of this chapter is to review disease management models for cardiovascular care and how they can affect the care provided by the cardiovascular team.

CHRONIC CONDITIONS AND AGING

In a healthcare system faced with an overburden of chronic illnesses, disease management is a concept likely to enable Americans to live differently in the future. Improving health status is necessary in any society whose population is growing older with a healthcare system that is focused on managing the acute aspects of illness. By 2030 all baby boomers will be 65 years of age.[1] Moreover, life expectancy has increased 44% between 1900 and 1950, 13% between 1950 and 2000, and is projected to increase by 9% between 2000 and 2050. In 1997, the average life expectancy was 79 years for women and 74 years for men. As of 2016, life expectancy was 81.1 years for women and 76.1 years for men.[2]

In 2014, 60% of Americans had at least one chronic condition and 42% had multiple chronic conditions.[3] This figure is expected to increase by 1% per year through the year 2030, where the number will increase by 46 million Americans.[4] It is forecasted that women will experience the major burden of chronic diseases. Many of these conditions are related to the vascular system including hypertension, which is the leading chronic condition in those younger and older than 65 years. Currently, heart disease is the leading cause of death in both men and women, responsible for approximately 1 in 4 deaths.[5] Other chronic conditions prevalent in those older than 65 years include pulmonary disease, diabetes mellitus, arthritis, and chronic mental health disorders. Treatment is complicated by the coexistence of multiple medical conditions and the social and psychological sequelae that accompany them.[4] Cardiovascular disease (CVD) is the leading cause of morbidity and mortality in the United States as well as in other parts of the world. CVD is burdensome to the individual living with chronic illness, their families, and to the healthcare system.

Current DMPs focus primarily on guideline-directed care of a single-disease entity. Approximately one in four Americans is living with a major comorbid condition (MCC) according to data from the U.S. Department of Health and Human Services (HHS).[6] HHS has proposed a paradigm shift from single-disease management strategies to a framework that addresses the complexities of living with multiple disease processes.[6] The HHS has designed a strategic map with an overarching vision of optimizing health outcomes and quality of life for people living with MCCs. Notably, recommendations for changes in payment systems driving away from fee-for-service models that disincentivize collaboration to a system of coordination-of-care is a top priority. The identification of quality metrics that better align with collaborative models of care and ultimately improved patient outcomes are highlighted as part of this work. Also, there is emphasis on identifying regional, socioeconomic, age, gender, sexual orientation, and other potential disparities in access and quality of care that may exist within the subset of persons with MCC.

COST OF CHRONIC DISEASE

It is estimated that three quarters of all healthcare expenditures go to caring for individuals with chronic conditions. National health expenditures grew 3.9%, to $3.5 trillion in 2017, or $10,739 per person, and accounted for 17.9% of gross domestic product (GDP).[7] Numerous healthcare plans, including Medicaid and Medicare have implemented DMP to improve high-cost care. Whether DMP will succeed in significantly lowering the costs associated with managing chronic disease remains to be seen as the evidence of cost-effectiveness remains limited.[8]

In addition to the physical and psychosocial burdens to the person living with MCC, there are substantial financial implications involving the individual and health systems. It is estimated that three quarters of all healthcare expenditures go to providing care for individuals with chronic conditions. With healthcare expenditures exceeding $1.7 trillion annually, regulatory agencies have a heightened interest in containing costs through guideline-directed medical therapies (GDMTs). Initiatives implemented under the Affordable Care Act have shown promising results. However, despite the gains made in 2015, the United States continues to experience a 30-day all-cause hospital readmissions at a rate of 17.8% for Medicare patients.[9]

The resources to manage those with an acute illness are quite different from those with a chronic condition. Physicians, nurses, and other care team members, often in intensive, hospital-based care requiring the use of expensive technology, provide acute care services. In contrast, effective chronic care requires a comprehensive approach that combines social, educational, vocational, and medical services provided in a variety of settings that increasingly focus on the home as the setting of care. The scope of chronic care is broad, encompassing social, community, and personal services as well as medical and rehabilitative care. Much of chronic care requires education and support of patients and family members to maximize self-management.

In the late 1990s, Wagner et al.[10] identified five important elements associated with improved outcomes for those with chronic conditions such as hypertension and diabetes. Successful programs tended to be those that (1) incorporated guidelines and protocols in practice; (2) used a multidisciplinary team (MDT) with careful allocation of tasks and ongoing patient contact; (3) provided counseling, education, information feedback, and other support to patients; (4) offered access to necessary clinical expertise such as referral to specialists, collaborative care models, and computer-decision support; and (5) used supportive information systems that offer reminders for preventive care and follow-up as well as feedback to providers on patient compliance and service use. Various disease management models have been developed to meet the needs of those with chronic conditions, incorporating many of these elements associated with chronic care delivery.

CONTROLLING READMISSIONS

The financial impact of preventable admissions is well documented in the literature. Guarav, Heidenreich, and Fonarrow[8] described the significant bearing heart failure (HF) has on healthcare economics. One in five Americans is at risk to developing HF at a cost of more than $1 million annually for hospitalizations and $39.2 billion annually for indirect costs. Guarav et al. quantified associated costs of systolic HF and concurred guideline-directed care is cost efficient and can substantially reduce overall healthcare expenditures.[8] Likewise, a position paper by the Austrian Society of Cardiology cites HF as having a poor prognosis and is the most common discharge diagnosis with a greater than 50% readmission rate within 6 month of discharge.[11] Through a systematic review of more than 40 trials, they determined that models of care that include multi-professional follow-ups with patients via clinic, phone contact and home care, as well as strategies for self-care and facilitated access during times of decompensation, significantly reduced all-cause readmission and mortality rates as well as associated costs. This is especially true for DMP-targeted patients who are at high risk for decompensating. The most effective programs are those that help patients understand the various components of their disease and how to respond to changes in symptoms.

The Austrian Society of Cardiology also notes that coordination of care is paramount given the HF patient comorbidities and propensity to be managed by multiple providers.[11] Ruppar et al. take this concept one step further by suggesting DMP incorporate interventions aimed at assurance of medication compliance due to the significant correlation between lack of medication adherence, loss of function, and increased morbidity and mortality.[12] Similarly, Cutler and Everett[13] identified medication adherence to be a major contributor of avoidable hospitalizations resulting in over $100 billion additional expenditures each year citing lack of care coordination as a major causative factor.

Yancy et al. agree that optimizing adherence is achieved through models of care that incorporate a team-based approach.[14] Teams comprised of at least two providers working collaboratively, with the patient and their families, to develop treatment strategies that align with the individual patient's preferences and goals have consistently demonstrated superiority. This is in respect to morbidity and mortality and, perhaps most importantly, quality of life. The Expert Consensus Document for Optimizing Heart Failure Treatment gives voice to the significant complexity that exists in caring for patients with CVD.[14] This is due to the need for multiple care providers across numerous care settings such as acute care, rehabilitation services, electrophysiologists, cardiovascular interventionalists, cardiovascular surgeons, and ambulatory care providers to name a few. Understanding that 50% of the cardiovascular population have four or more MCC and 25% of patients have six or more, it is clear that MCC in combination with the ensuing need for numerous care providers increases the proclivity for miscommunications, polypharmacy complications, inefficiencies, and reduced health optimization. The consensus document highlights the codirectional relationship that occurs with MCC noting that the presence of one condition increases the risk of developing additional conditions. Subsequent prognoses become exponentially worse and increasingly more difficult to manage. Symptom recognition can become challenging in the setting of MCC and practitioners must be vigilant in responding to subtle changes. Referral, collaboration, and inclusion of clinical experts as part of the care team are key components of clinical optimization through comprehensive DMP.

Common conditions that coexist in the cardiology population include coronary artery disease, rhythm disturbances, valvular heart disease, hypertension, dyslipidemia, diabetes, anemia, sleep disorders, peripheral vascular disease, cerebrovascular disease, lung, renal, and thyroid diseases. Living with any combination of these conditions often requires life-altering treatment decisions.

Attention to ongoing reassessment of their goals and preferences is paramount. To that end, guidance from our professional societies provides evidence-based consensus for the management of HF that is intended to inform practice, improve quality of care, and align with patients' preferences and values.[15]

Management of hypertension is now recognized as having a significant role in HF outcomes. Randomized clinical trials demonstrate blood pressure control to be a significant contributor in the reduction of HF incidence and overall cardiovascular death, therefore GDMT are now considered to be a Class 1 recommendation for treating hypertension in patients with HF.[14] Similarly, concomitant sleep disorders are also understood to be common in patients with HF. A noteworthy finding relative to sleep apnea in patients with HF is the association of CPAP therapy with the reduction of incidence in progression to permanent atrial fibrillation.[16]

As an adjunct to GDMT, Ory et al. proposed placing emphasis on building self-management skills for patients.[17] They reviewed more than one thousand participants of community-based chronic disease self-management programs (CDSMPs), performing evaluations at baseline, at 6 months, and 12-month intervals. Significant reduction in emergency department presentations at 12 months and reduction in hospital admissions from baseline to 6 months were noted. The findings highlight the substantial relationship between quality of life and overall reduction in health expenditure for patients who have definitive strategies for self-management. Furthermore, it exemplifies opportunities to align with the Institute for Healthcare Improvement (IHI) Triple Aim framework that embodies improving the patient experience, population health, and cost containment.[18]

SYSTEM BURDEN

DMP should be designed to reduce symptom burden. Programs that engage patients and give control over aspects of their disease through self-management skills have proven to be successful. Enhancing the ability to understand their disease trajectory, associated symptom burdens, and providing the requisite skills for early recognition of symptoms and risk reduction have a positive influence in overall secondary outcomes. For example, in a randomized clinical trial that followed patients with atrial fibrillation over the course of 15 months, Abed et al. concluded that initiatives directed at risk factor management and weight reduction had an overall positive influence in reduction of symptom burden and cardiac remodeling.[19]

In setting the stage for CDSMP, there is movement toward home-based and community-based programs. Stewart et al. analyzed three randomized trials totaling more than 1000 patients with chronic heart disease in order to understand the impact of nurse-led home-based interventions (HBI).[20] The studied population included patients hospitalized with heart disease without HF, atrial fibrillation without HF, and patients with HF alone. They followed the patients over a 5-year period and studied days alive and days out of the hospital. The authors noted a significant difference in achieving days alive and fewer hospital days for the patients who were participating in an HBI model as opposed to the patients who received standard medical management.[19] The HBI patients received a home visit by a cardiac nurse within 1 to 2 weeks following discharge from the hospital as well as follow-up visits with their MDT based on their specific clinical needs. The success of these interventions led the researchers to conclude that nurse-led HBI postdischarge should not be limited to HF diagnosis but rather be considered standard of care for patients hospitalized with any form of chronic heart disease. The data was compelling in that there were approximately 600 fewer hospital days per 100 patients for those managed in HBI program across all heart disease entities.[19]

Stewart et al. noted that although there is substantial evidence to support DMP and cardiac rehabilitation programs for people with HF, much more research is needed in the area prevention and management of people with other forms of heart disease.[21] The AHA's 2017 report on heart disease and stroke further validates this philosophy.[22] As authors Benjamin et al. noted, the data suggests the prevalence of atrial fibrillation and its adverse consequences is increasing.[23] Utilizing a meta-analysis of more than 12,000 people showing clinically significant reduction in stroke and all-cause cardiovascular mortality, the AHA envisions an approach to cardiovascular health that incorporates twofold strategies in which we improve health for those with existing disease and maintain health for those currently without disease.[24]

Congruent with thought leaders from other regulatory bodies, the AHA proposes that this can best be accomplished through combined approaches that focus on policies rewarding health systems who optimize patient health and develop broader population health programs in schools, workplace, and communities.[23] Aligned with this thinking, the National Council on Aging (NCOA) warns that 80% of the adult population has at least one chronic disease and without self-management education, many will struggle to maintain health.[24] Partnering with the U.S. Administration for Community Living, NCOA aims to implement community programs with workshops that incorporate attention to emotional and psychosocial issues of chronic disease, pain management, medication management, healthy meal planning, improving physical strength, flexibility and endurance, and also strategies for effective communication with providers and loved ones. In addition, findings from Pozehl, McGuire, and Norman identifies gaps in current research within subsets of DMP.[25] Their review focused on cardiac rehabilitation (CR) guidelines, which revealed recommendations specifically related to the HF population are very limited.

Despite the existence of explicit guidelines outlining the core components of CR programs which include risk factor and nutritional counseling, patient assessment, psychosocial interventions, and exercise and training, Pozehl et al. found that guidance related to HF management and other cardiac subsets was a high-level view and lacked specificity.[25] To further widen the gap in optimizing outcomes, the authors reported a significant underutilization of CR of the eligible patients with myocardial infarction actually participating and less than 20% in those with HF. Thomas et al. suggested that improvements in this arena could avert more than 25,000 untimely deaths and 180,000 preventable hospitalizations each year.[26] They proposed institution of quality measures aimed at addressing access and participation in CR programs. As such, a phenomenal opportunity exists for cardiovascular nursing to take the lead in moving best practice forward.

DISEASE MANAGEMENT: DEFINITION AND MODELS

Disease management is a term that has been used for more than a decade to encompass the way in which care is delivered to individuals, but more specifically to groups of patients. Many associate the term with managed care and a way to control healthcare services.[14] Although numerous definitions for this term exist, Ellrodt et al.[16] defined disease management as an approach to patient care that emphasizes coordinated comprehensive care along a continuum of disease and across healthcare delivery systems.

The most comprehensive definition for disease management has been developed by the Disease Management Association of America (DMAA), a nonprofit trade association.[27] The DMAA states that disease management is a system of coordinated healthcare interventions and communications for populations with conditions in which patient self-care efforts are significant. Disease management components include the following: (1) population identification processes; (2) evidence-based practice guidelines; (3) collaborative practice models, which include nurses, physicians, and other support service providers; (4) patient self-management education; (5) process and outcomes measurement, evaluation, and management; and (6) routine reporting and feedback. This organization suggests that full-service disease management involves all six components.

Case management was a term used early in the course to describe the role of caring for patients with chronic illness with a primary focus of management of patients at high risk for expensive outcomes. Case managers often would undertake a broad assessment of the medical, functional, social, and emotional needs of individuals by developing written plans of care and incorporating community resources to support patients. Education about symptom management, compliance with medications, diet and medical follow-up, and ways of accessing the emergency department are often part of the care provided by case managers.

Another model of disease management offers programs that are specific to patient-focused diagnoses such as HF or diabetes. Often undertaken by nurses, these DMPs follow guidelines for a particular disease, utilize standardized education related to the disease, and often use technology to monitor a patient's condition. Follow-up is often long term as well noting that conditions like HF and diabetes are not amenable to care and that patients are likely to lapse into old behaviors. Three likely contributors are noted to cause a decline in adherence: lapses in attention, excessive daytime sleepiness, and dosing frequency. These factors represent three of the five World Health Organization dimensions as predictors of nonadherence.[28]

DMPs have been identified as essential components in the care of patients with chronic illness for over two decades. The primary aim of DMP is to improve patient outcomes, increase quality of life, and decrease preventable healthcare utilization and cost through guideline-driven practice. Evidence from numerous randomized controlled trials over the years continues to demonstrate that patients living with cardiovascular conditions such as HF, coronary artery disease, atrial fibrillation, and hypertension have superior outcomes when they are engaged in programs that include MDTs, coordinated delivery of care, focused education to both patients and providers, and attention to quality indicators. DMP has become the standard of care for patients with certain chronic diseases such as HF, and to a large extent, that is due to regulatory requirements and transparencies in reporting quality data.

Evolving evidence-based disease management guidance will likely enable Americans to live differently in the future by moving away from practices that provide focused, resource-intensive care during acute events to more systematic strategies that give rise to maintaining health over time. Conditions that were previously considered fatal have instead come to be thought of as chronic illnesses. McMurray postulated as treatments become more complex, patient care becomes increasingly segmented as it is delivered by multiple specialists.[29]

Clinical trials have demonstrated the positive influence of nurse-led home-based HF programs on health outcomes measured by days alive and days out of the hospital among other quality indicators. McCabe et al. noted that DMP aimed at managing comorbid CVD improved patient outcomes and reduced costly recidivism rates.[30]

Models of Disease Management in Cardiovascular Care by Nurses

Since the early 1970s, unique models for delivering care to individuals with chronic conditions by nurses have evolved. Much of this early work in disease management occurred in hypertension control in the United States and Europe.[31,32] Most often, attempts were made to deliver high-quality care in various settings that were convenient to the population being studied. In one of the first DMPs,[32] patients with hypertension, diabetes, or cardiac disease chose to be followed by specially trained nurses in decentralized clinics close to their homes or in a hospital-based outpatient clinic for chronic disease that was staffed by internists. After 2 years, hypertension control rates were superior in those patients cared for by specially trained nurses, and they had 50% fewer hospital admission days. The authors of this study attributed the success of the nurse-run clinics to greater follow-up and time devoted to helping patients manage their chronic conditions.

Studies suggest that the convenience of helping individuals manage their health in settings conducive to work and home offered an optimal opportunity for disease management to be brought to the patient. Since the 1970s, disease management by nurses has been applied not only to hypertension,[31–40] but also to other aspects of cardiovascular management, including dyslipidemia,[41–44] tobacco dependence,[45–49] diabetes,[50–54] coronary artery disease,[55–68] and HF.[21,68–84] Much of the early work before the term disease management was coined occurred in managing patients after myocardial infarction using a multidisciplinary approach to managing risk factors, adherence to diet, exercise, medications, and medical regimens to improve functioning and quality of life through the provision of individual and group education, counseling, and behavioral interventions, which included the patient and family as part of rehabilitation.[85]

Disease Management in Low-Income Populations

Recent work has shown the benefit of disease management in low-income and minority populations who may be at greatest risk of CVD. Much of the disease and disability burden from CVDs are in people under the age of 70 years in low- and middle-income countries.[86] Research has shown that disadvantaged groups are at greater risk for CVD. Rates of smoking, heavy drinking, obesity, and diabetes are more prevalent among the poor.[86] There are two types of prevention that can be associated with disease management, primordial and primary. Primordial prevention has a goal of stopping development of risk factors before they occur. Policy change is an example of primordial prevention. Primary prevention focuses on risk factor reduction by targeting persons at risk for disease development, or those already diagnosed. An example of a primary prevention program is a smoking cessation program.[86]

The World Health Organization (WHO) substantiates this concern regarding health disparity.[4] It is noted that of the more than 17 million deaths from CVD occur globally each year, the highest risk burden remains in low-income areas. The WHO guidance urges reduction in preventable incidence of heart attack and stroke through consideration of comprehensive cardiovascular risk assessment as part of basic health care rather than independent treatment decisions addressing singular risk factors.[4] According to WHO, lone entities such as hypertension, diabetes, or obesity should be considered as entry points for comprehensive, integrated cardiovascular DMP.[4] It is also noted that sustainable healthcare financing must ensure access to basic care.

Future Research by Nurses

Ongoing innovative nursing research is needed to continue to advance the successes of DMP. Research is needed to determine the most cost-effective models, how to support long-term adherence including the frequency of interactions to ensure maintenance of health behavior changes, and if improved outcomes in reduction in rehospitalizations are achieved through DMP. Nurses who have conducted successful trials are also well positioned to disseminate and study the translation of these models into clinical practice settings.

COMPONENTS OF DISEASE MANAGEMENT SYSTEMS

Identifying a Patient Population

Effective disease management involves a process of identifying at-risk populations, coordinating systems of care delivery, obtaining outcomes, and managing outcomes most appropriately to improve care. Most often, DMPs are developed for chronic conditions that are costly, such as coronary artery disease, diabetes, HF, renal failure, and chronic obstructive pulmonary disease. Populations are moderate- to high-risk individuals. They may be identified through hospital discharge records as high users of care,[63] through health plan databases when the aim is to reduce costs associated with certain conditions,[50] or through a team of individuals such as nurses and physicians aiming to improve the quality of care through a quality-improvement process to meet national guidelines.[58]

Coordinating Delivery Systems for Disease Management

There is variation in the design of DMP evidenced by differences in the frequency of interactions with patients, the use of face-to-face visits versus telephone follow-up, the intervals between follow-up evaluations, and the ability to use monitoring devices. There can also be wide variability in the number of program resources and the level of clinic expertise on the MDT. However, research provides guidance to create appropriate structure and frequency of patient interactions. Components include understanding the unique needs of the patient population as a whole, as well as individuals, and tailoring interventions accordingly; engaging the patient to determine which mode of contact will best meet their needs; understanding the typical timeframe in which untoward outcomes, problematic behaviors, and lack of adherence occur.

Although disease management models have operated in a variety of settings including clinics, hospitals, and work sites, investigators have also used telephones and the Internet to deliver care and structure interactions with the patient to optimize care within the home setting.[57,87,88] There is much diversity related to structured interventions among these programs, most have incorporated patient education, multidisciplinary or physician–nurse teams, and specialized follow-up. Furthermore, the development of algorithms and protocols for delivering structured care has been crucial to the success of disease management systems.

Disease management involves a process of care delivery. Because the process of care delivery is different from the typical structure within an office visit or hospital that is well known to most healthcare professionals; many different models for care delivery in disease management exist today. Although populations differ, interventions have varied, such as a single face-to-face visit with telephone follow-up to comprehensive management teams comprising multiple team members.[89,90] This is because of the system's approach to care uses multiple interventions, specifying primary and secondary goals is key to developing intervention activities. Goals for a DMP are often to improve patient and caregiver knowledge of the disease, enhance self-management through skill building, increase medication and treatment adherence, and improve health-related outcomes.[91,92]

Irrespective of whether clinical interventions are in-person or electronic interactions, by design, interactions occur more frequently in the early phases of the patient's participation in DMP and become less frequent as patients and family members become competent with self-management behaviors and pharmacotherapies. It is important to remain adaptable as symptoms fluctuate. Being aware of the patients' multiple conditions and how they challenge care delivery in terms of coordination of care and communication is critical.

Education as a Part of Disease Management

Education and collaboration are key components of DMP. Most often, education focuses on lifestyle changes including diet, exercise, and smoking cessation. Education provides necessary understanding of the disease as well as methods to self-monitor symptoms, such as, lower extremity edema, weight gain, increasing dyspnea, blood glucose monitoring, and blood pressure trending. The format for education differs from one program to another. Some have used face-to-face individualized education,[50,57] whereas others have used a group approach followed by individualized education.[67,68] A review of programs offering structured educational interventions for CVD[93] found that more than two thirds of successful programs, many directed by nurses, were focused on behavioral approaches directed at skill building. Rather than providing information, these programs succeeded by offering a range of health behavior skills, such as contracting, goal setting, self-monitoring, feedback, and problem solving.[94] Many used theories of stages of change,[95] social learning (most specifically, self-efficacy),[96,97] and relapse prevention training[92,93] to plan successful educational interventions. In addition, offering educational materials in multiple formats (e.g., print, audio, video) has also been shown to increase adherence to long-term behavioral changes. Adult learners differ in their preferred ways of gaining knowledge and skills and these multimedia approaches giving them an opportunity for reinforcement of information.[94]

Whether delivered individually or in a group format, successful nurse-directed programs focused on specific skill building rather than simply providing generalized information. Additionally, programs that incorporate feedback and strategies to prevent relapse glean the best outcomes.

Communication With Physicians and Other Personnel

The frequency of interactions with other personnel in the disease management team is important to overall care. One of the failures of the current system in the United States in managing those with chronic conditions has been the frequency of visits to multiple physician providers and the lack of communication among them. In the setting of DMP, nurses generally assume the role of coordinating care between multiple providers. The evolution of the electronic health records has in some cases narrowed the communication gap, however, complete integration of these systems within and outside most healthcare networks has yet to be fully realized. As such, the development of systematic approaches to clear and timely communication to facilitate coordinated care among all providers is an essential component of every DMP. An essential role of the nurse as a member of the DMP team is to ensure coordination of care and communication as to optimize best possible outcomes.[98] The frequency of interactions with healthcare professionals across multiple settings within the disease management team is important to overall care but can also result in confusion and missteps without a clear communication strategy. One of the failures of the current system in the United States in managing people with MCC has been the frequency of visits to multiple providers and the lack of effective communication.[6,13,98] Communication with the patient and family is imperative to screen for signs of social isolation, depression, economic burden, and functional decline. These symptoms can subtly emerge as a result of living with MCC. Vigilant monitoring can provide a timeframe to provide support and intervention.

The frequency of phone-based interactions and the format for receiving information about the care being delivered to patients as part of disease management should be addressed as part of the development of algorithms and protocols. Interactions with physicians most often relate changes in symptoms and medications and need to be addressed by the team. Physician champions who can facilitate problem solving and offer expertise to nurses in the absence of primary care or specialty physicians facilitate success with program implementation.

Anticipating the needs of patients and family members, nurses also play a role in coordinating the care delivered by other healthcare professionals, such as social workers, pharmacists, dieticians, and psychologists. These disciplines offer specialized expertise in defined fields often required for managing long-term chronic conditions.

Measuring Clinical and Resource Utilization Outcomes

Irrespective of a research or clinical initiative in disease management, collecting outcome data is crucial to evaluating programmatic value and sustainability. Metrics to be evaluated are dependent on the DMP, however with the trend toward reporting transparency, it is wise to have a clear vision of essential quality measures. These may include patient outcomes such as mortality rates and readmission rates, resource utilization, quality-of-life elements, patient and provider satisfaction, and program costs and profitability. Program costs and profitability may ultimately substantiate the need for the program or additional resources. Health insurance companies and payers are obviously interested in outcomes associated with a reduction in emergency department visits, hospitalizations, length of hospital stay, and costs of care. Depending on the organization, the information may be readily available through facility reporting structures. Otherwise developing tools to efficiently track important data elements will be necessary.

Quality-of-life indicators are perhaps the most valuable data element for DMP. Although this can be subjective and difficult to assess, measurement tools exist to evaluate components including markers for symptoms, functional status, health perceptions, and overall well-being. Regulatory agencies are beginning to consider quality-of-life tools as part of mandated standard practice in certain disease domains. The first FDA health status approved tool, the Kansas City Cardiomyopathy Questionnaire (KCCQ),[21] is an accepted tool that measures multiple domains of quality of life in HF patients including the impact of dyspnea and fatigue on patient's sense of well-being.

Measuring functional status of patients, which may be significantly impacted as a result of DMPs, should also be considered in developing outcome measures for disease management. As with quality-of-life measurements, there are evidence-based tools that can be easily incorporated into the routine assessment of patients. In addition to their significance as quality data points, they can be utilized as trend markers for patient progress or identifying decompensation over time.

Measures of patient satisfaction are an important marketing tool for DMPs. Most large organizations are committed to measuring patient satisfaction as part of quality assurance, however these are not DMP specific. This may be an opportunity for future nursing research. Individualized measures that have significance to the DMP team provide opportunities to better understand areas for process improvement, celebration of success, or potentially the need for program or resource restructuring. This type of evaluation is helpful in determining whether nonclinical tasks can be allocated to other personnel allowing nurses to work at the top of their license.

Training and Role Qualifications

Nurses who coordinate DMP require sound clinical expertise and the ability to manage multiple competing demands in the midst of a rapidly moving target. As noted, exceptional assessment skills and clinical judgment, innate leadership characteristics, and interpersonal skills are essential for success. Specific credentials may vary by institution, state, or local regulatory agencies. Core competencies in chronic disease management may be mastered through a curriculum that includes knowledge of the disease process, medical management of risk factors, treatment protocols, lifestyle, and psychosocial interventions; however, as in most nursing roles, much of the requisite knowledge is obtained in real time, on the job training. Professional nursing societies frequently offer regional training, national training, and web-based continuing education (CEU) specific to cardiovascular medicine. Literature provides a wealth of evidence-based information, helpful guidelines, protocols, and tools to support the role of the nurse on the Heart Team.

Opportunities

Discussions have ensued regarding how best to encourage the adoption and implementation of DMP globally and across all socioeconomic, cultural, age, and gender barriers. Nurses are well positioned to take on this challenge through ongoing research and practice. In addition, seeking to understand how concomitant chronic illnesses are interrelated and how they impact care will be an important role for nursing. Quality of life will be a fundamental goal as we move to develop future GDMT. Nurses have established themselves as essential members of the DMP through their astute awareness of an evolving clinical picture, patient advocacy, as well as the number of remarkable gains they have made over time in improving patient outcomes. As new and evolving challenges continue to confront and stress our health systems, nursing research will become increasingly more important and will likely be in the forefront of positive change. It is also important for DMP to better understand how the use of telemonitoring affects patient outcome. Technology is expanding in such a way that at every turn there is a new device ready for market. How do we ensure, for example, that wearable devices are providing accurate information as they may be used to adjust medications or treatment regimes? And, if they are indeed deemed reliable, what opportunities exist to secure funding to ensure equitable access.

In considering self-management programs, there are unexplored opportunities to consider, such as, community-based facilitated peer groups in which participants discuss topics. Examples of topics are adopting exercise programs; use of technique such as guided relaxation or anger management; fatigue and sleep management; use of medications and community resources; managing the emotions of fear, depression, or social isolation; and, training in how to communicate with healthcare professionals, in particular techniques to begin shared decision-making conversations for healthcare decisions. In addressing quality-of-life issues, one component that begs further exploration is the patients' feeling of uncertainty the midst of a confusing healthcare journey. Impersonal, confounding and confusing information and communication are generally reported to be the impetus for feeling loss of control. While perhaps difficult to study, engagement in self-management programs will likely help to increase patients and their support persons' sense of control as does engaging in nurse-led DMP.

Finally, as regulatory agencies continue to direct practice through mandatory requirements that are attached to reimbursement, nurses have the opportunity, or perhaps the obligation, to put their voice on the decision-making table on behalf of patient advocacy and program viability.

TRAINING AND JOB QUALIFICATIONS FOR DISEASE MANAGEMENT

The Emergence of Nursing Roles and Disease Management

Since the early 1970s, nurses have been instrumental in developing and implementing models of care aimed at improving outcomes for individuals with chronic conditions. Case Management was the early, innovative, nursing model with a primary focus of managing patients at high risk for expensive therapies and costly readmissions. Nurses in case management roles were responsible for clinical, functional, and psychosocial assessment of individuals, developing plans of care, securing durable medical equipment, and incorporating community resources to support transition to home or next level of care. Education related to symptom management, medications, diet, follow-up evaluations, and access to emergency care were elements of the nursing scope of practice. Additionally, nurse responsibility included care coordination with physician, home health nurses, and social service providers. Current DMPs are commonly managed by nurses. Nurses utilize evidence-based research as guiding principles for practice standards and protocol development. Long-term follow-up and monitoring of patient progress and health status through the use of technology, such as telehealth and wearable devices, are frequently incorporated into the nursing role.

Much of the early work in disease management in the United States and Europe focused on hypertension control. In one of the first disease management studies,[32] patients with hypertension were randomized to monitoring by specially trained nurses in decentralized clinics within their communities, or by a physician in a hospital-based outpatient clinic. At the end of the 2-year study, hypertension control was superior in those patients cared for in the nurse management arm. Fifty percent fewer hospital admission days were noted in the nurse management group. Success was attributed to the nurse-run clinics, greater follow-up, and targeted time devoted to helping patients manage their chronic conditions. These early studies lay the groundwork to understand how we can optimize the individuals' potential for success. Offering care and treatment access that is convenient to their home and place of work increase likelihood of successful outcomes. Similar results were noted in research focused on minority, multiethnic, and low-income population. By adding bilingual case manager to programs, the managers were able to more effectively counsel patients in the intervention group about sodium intake, fluid retention, medication adherence, and self-reported symptoms, and served as a liaison between patients and physicians.[99] As with prior studies, patients who were managed by the nurse-led group had fewer hospitalizations, functional improvement, and quality-of-life based on the Minnesota Living with Heart Failure Questionnaire.[100] Current research continues to demonstrate the added value of nurse-led home-based DMP in improved quality of life, cost-containment, and reduction in readmission rates and all-cause mortality.[101] MDTs have emerged to address the complex care of patients with comorbid conditions and their treatment options. The MDT plays a pivotal role in the delivery of healthcare service and disease. As an example, the MDT to determine options for treatment to include evaluates patients with aortic stenosis who are under consideration for transcatheter aortic valve replacement (TAVR): medical management, surgical intervention, or transcatheter intervention. Options are discussed with patients to determine the best course of treatment. The patient is considered a part of the treatment team and a shared decision-making process is utilized to elicit patient preferences and goals of treatment. The efficacy and success of the MDT will likely drive similar team-based models via national consensus determinations for CVD management.

UNRESOLVED ISSUES FOR DISEASE MANAGEMENT

Although disease management has not yet reached widespread application in clinical practice, it holds promise as a new way of delivering care to those at high risk for and those with established CVD. The success of nurse utilization to coordinate DMPs has most often resulted in more frequent medication changes, an increase in the use of combination drug regimens, less expensive medications, and an increase in short-term adherence. These results are in large part because of the use of defined protocols and increased patient contact time for education and behavioral

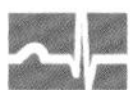 DISPLAY 41-1

Important Lessons for Program Implementation in Disease Management

Physician leadership/support is key to program viability
Ongoing marketing is essential
Program modifications save time and resources
Protocols require annual updates and alignment with national guidelines
Defining caseload requirements and reevaluating is necessary for quality control

counseling. In addition, a greater achievement of goals such as a reduction in blood pressure, cholesterol, and glucose control has been realized. A by-product of comprehensive care in patients has produced a reduction in utilization for all causes (emergency department visits and hospitalizations), something not expected by many in the field.[102] As noted in Display 41-1, organizations implementing DMPs for more than 10 years suggest several important lessons for those developing new programs. In addition, Stewart and Horowitz[82] have highlighted a number of factors that appear to be important in the overall development of those DMPs that successfully reduced rehospitalization rates and costs for HF. These are highlighted in Display 41-2.

Many challenges continue to confront those involved in disease management, offering future opportunities for research and for those conducting clinical programs. DMPs have typically focused on what is often called a "single-disease state" or "carve out." These specialty programs for high-cost patient populations treat only a single chronic condition such as diabetes or HF. However, many individuals have predisposing risk factors and comorbid conditions that determine their functional status and prognosis. For example, more than half of all rehospitalizations for HF are caused by coexisting conditions that impact the disease, such as hypertension and coronary artery disease, or unrelated conditions, such as chronic obstructive pulmonary disease.[87] Moreover, the overlap of cardiovascular risk factors (dyslipidemia, obesity, hypertension, alcohol use, and smoking) is significant. Thus, the need for managing multiple risk factors concurrently is noteworthy and requires continued research. As adherence to guidelines by physicians and systems becomes more common place, allowing achievement of better patient outcomes, a more central role for nurses in disease management is likely to reside with an elderly and aging population that is burdened by multiple diseases and associated conditions. Naylor et al. have started to address many of the factors associated with the older adults,[103] early findings suggested promise for the future.

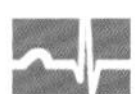 DISPLAY 41-2

Key Features of Successful Programs of Care in CHF

- A commitment to individualized health care
- A multidisciplinary approach to managing the patient
- A major role for a specialist nurse to assess patient needs and provide for ongoing management within a supportive multidisciplinary environment
- At least one home visit for a comprehensive assessment of the patients' circumstances
- The promotion of self-care behaviors
- Increased levels of monitoring in "high-risk" patients
- The application of optimal, evidence-based pharmacologic treatment with flexible protocols for changes in patient status and titration to maximal tolerated doses

Adapted with permission from Stewart S, Horowitz J. Specialist nurse management programmes: economic benefits in the management of heart failure. *Pharmacoeconomics*. 2003;21(4):225–240.

A second challenge relates to intervention components and the duration of follow-up. Although disease management models focus on multiple interventions, there is large variation in the frequency of contact, the context for what is provided to patients, and whether patients are followed up for 1 month, 1 year, or indefinitely. It is likely that those who demonstrate high accountability through good patient outcomes at a reasonable cost and that also offset the high costs of acute exacerbations will likely prevail.

Does home telemonitoring for chronic disease improve patient outcomes? The use of electronic blood pressure monitors, blood glucose meters, and voice recognition technology offers data that can be concealed during infrequent office visits. A *Cochrane Review* evaluated the use of home telemonitoring on improvement of patient outcomes.[104] Their review suggests that irrespective of nationality, socioeconomic status, or age, patients are relatively adherent with telemonitoring programs and technologies. Studies in patients with cardiologic problems showed significant benefit on clinical outcomes from the use of such devices. However, research is still needed on the cost-effectiveness of the use of these technologies, the impact on service utilization, and the acceptance by healthcare professionals such as case managers.

Although disease management models have been effectively implemented in research and clinical practice, it is likely that such programs will be delivered only to subgroups of patients in the future, because of cost. Peer support models for self-management of chronic conditions have also been tested.[105,106] These offer significant promise as an alternative modality supporting self-management of symptoms in individuals with chronic conditions. The Chronic Disease Management Program is a community-based, peer-led program designed to help those individuals with chronic conditions such as CVD, arthritis, pulmonary disease, and stroke.[107] This program, which is offered to 10 to 15 participants over 7 weeks in 2.5-hour group sessions and led by a trained peer leader, focuses on improving self-management skills based on self-efficacy theory, drawing on peers for support. Weekly sessions focus on action planning and feedback, modeling of behaviors and problem solving by participants for one another, group problem solving, and individual decision making. Supported by a program guide entitled "*Living a Healthy Life with Chronic Conditions*," weekly content includes the following: adopting exercise programs; use of cognitive symptom management techniques, such as guided relaxation and distraction; fatigue and sleep management; use of medications and community resources; managing the emotions of fear, anger, and depression; training in communication with healthcare professionals and others; health-related problem solving; and decision making.

A final important challenge facing disease management relates to the transitional aspects of care and the healthcare delivery system. Acute care that has been linked to the hospital must truly be linked to the delivery of chronic care. A problem confronting some patients has been the perceived loss of control over the healthcare system.[108] Nelson found that impersonal service, healthcare system navigation, and, for many, feeling discounted by the medical care system are problems many older adult patients face today. Conversely, those patients participating in nurse case management frequently cited feeling cared for and receiving support. Structured appropriately, disease management models must help to support a successful transition from home to hospital and other settings. Ensuring a smooth transition with the disease manager operating in partnership with the patient at the center is likely to reduce the sense of loss of control for patients and families. More opportunities will arise to improve care as communication technologies improve and our capability to monitor patients in the home environment is extended.

In summary, disease management models offer the promise of better care for millions of individuals with multiple risk factors and known CVDs. Although much has been studied, the challenge of implementation of those models showing improved outcomes must continue, and further research is needed about best methods for dissemination. Much of this challenge rests in the hands of nurses who participate in research in disease management and those who are in newly defined disease management roles.

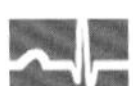

CASE STUDY 1

Patient Profile

Name/Age/Sex: **Stanley Frank, 85-year-old male**

History of Present Illness

Mr. Frank presents to his PCP for his regular checkup. He is retired and lives with his wife, his adult children live out of state. He is very active and enjoys travel, hiking, tennis, and volunteerism. He verbalizes that he is feeling well with no complaints. On physical examination, his PCP auscultates a change in his longstanding murmur and orders an echocardiogram and a follow-up appointment. He returns in 3 months at which time the echocardiogram is reviewed and reveals moderate to severe aortic stenosis. Because Mr. Frank continues to be asymptomatic, they agree that he will return in 1 year with a possible repeat echocardiogram. He returns to his PCP in generally good health but does note some intermittent fatigue with strenuous activity, a stress echo is ordered. There was no evidence of ischemia, however the examination was stopped early due to complaint of fatigue and shortness of breath. Mr. Frank's subsequent clinic visits were on behalf of his wife who sustained significant orthopedic trauma in an auto accident. She became quite debilitated and much of his time was devoted to her care; as a result he essentially became lost to follow up. He presumed his increasing fatigue and activity intolerance to be due to the exhausting work of being a primary care provider to his wife. When he returned to his PCP 3 years later, he had unintended weight loss, lower extremity edema, and NYHA Class III–IV dyspnea at rest. He was noted to be anemic and his echocardiogram now showed significant cardiomyopathy and critical aortic stenosis. He was referred for a Structural Heart evaluation and subsequently scheduled urgently for a transcatheter aortic valve replacement (TAVR). In the days just prior to his procedure, his wife was admitted with pneumonia, which caused him to delay his TAVR by several weeks. Fortunately, visiting nurse services were now in place to assist with the care of Mrs. Frank following her discharge home.

Past Medical History

Hypertension, AAA repair, PPM s/p Complete heart block, radiation therapy for prostate cancer.

Surgical History

AAA repair, prostate biopsy

Family History

Mother—breast cancer, Father—hypertension

Social History

Denies alcohol, tobacco, or illicit drug use

Medications

Lisinopril 10 mg po q daily, Acetaminophen PRN

Allergies

NKDA

Patient Examination

Vital Signs

BP 120/72; Resp 16 breaths per minute; Temp 37°C; HR 70 beats per minute; Ht. 171 cm; Wt. 75 kg

Physical Examination

General: Awake, alert, and oriented. No distress noted.

Skin: Warm, well perfused, intact

Cardiac: Systolic murmur at LUSB, harsh, III/VI.

Respiratory: Lung sounds are clear in all lobes bilaterally without rales, rhonchi, or wheezes.

Abdominal: Abdomen is soft, symmetric, and nontender without distention. No masses, hepatomegaly, or splenomegaly are noted.

Psychiatric: Appropriate mood and affect. Good judgment and insight. No visual or auditory hallucinations. No suicidal or homicidal ideation.

Testing

Echocardiogram: AVA 0.8 cm^2, Mean gradient 42 mm Hg, Vmax 3.9 m/s

ECG-paced rhythm

Considerations

Key Questions

- What is the management for severe asymptomatic aortic stenosis?
- What it the evaluation model for patients with aortic stenosis?

Evidence

- According to the 2014 AHA/ACC Guideline for the Management of Patients With Valvular Heart Disease: Executive Summary patients with severe asymptomatic aortic stenosis should be monitored every 6 to 12 months for development of symptoms or worsening valvular disease. It should be noted that asymptomatic AS continues to be studied and this recommendation may change in the future.
- According to the 2019 AATS/ACC/ASE/SCAI/STS Expert Consensus Systems of Care Document: A Proposal to Optimize Care for Patients With Valvular Heart Disease patients should undergo a thorough evaluation within a Structural Valve program. The program should have an MDT in place.

KEY READINGS

Ellrodt G, Cook DJ, Lee J, et al. Evidence-based disease management. *JAMA*. 1997;278:1687–1692.

Hisashige A. The effectiveness and efficiency of disease management programs for patients with chronic diseases. *Glob J Health Sci.* 2012;5(2):27–48.

REFERENCES

1. Hisashige A. The effectiveness and efficiency of disease management programs for patients with chronic diseases. *Glob J Health Sci.* 2012;5(2):27–48.
2. Centers for Disease Control and Prevention. Life expectancy at birth. Available at https://www.cdc.gov/nchs/data/hus/2017/fig20.pdf. Accessed March 24, 2019.
3. Buttorff C, Teague R, Melissa B. *Multiple Chronic Conditions in the United States*. Santa Monica, California: RAND Corporation, TL-221-PFCD; 2017. Available at https://www.rand.org/pubs/tools/TL221.html. Accessed March 24, 2019.
4. World Health Organization (WHO). *Global status report on noncommunicable diseases 2014*. Geneva: WHO; 2014. Available at http://apps.who.int/iris/bitstream/handle/10665/148114/9789241564854_eng.pdf;jsessionid=1216 55C04CA213DE3D85434786714CAF?sequence=1. Accessed October 10, 2019.
5. Centers for Disease Control and Prevention. *Heart facts*. Available at https://www.cdc.gov/heartdisease/facts.htm. Updated December 2, 2019, Accessed December 16, 2019.
6. U.S. Department of Health and Human Services. *Multiple Chronic Conditions-A strategic Framework: Optimum Health and Quality of Life for Individuals with Multiple Chronic Conditions.* Washington, DC: National Center for Health Statistics; 2006. Deaths. Preliminary data for 2005. Available at www.nlm.nih.gov/medlineplus/healthstatistics.html. Accessed October 10, 2019.
7. Centers for Medicare and Medicaid Services. *NHE fact sheet*. Available at https://www.cms.gov/research-statistics-data-and-systems/statistics-trends-and-reports/nationalhealthexpenddata/nhe-fact-sheet.html. Accessed October 10, 2019.
8. Guarav B, Heidenreich PA, Fonarow GC. Incremental cost-effectiveness of guideline-directed medical therapies for heart failure. *J Am Coll Cardiol.* 2013;61(13):1440–1446.
9. Kolte D, Khera S, Sardar R, et al. Thirty day readmissions after transcatheter aortic valve replacement in the United States: insights from the National Readmission Database. *Circ Cardiovasc Interv.* 2017;10(1):e004472. Available at http://circinterventions.ahajournals.org/content/10/1/e004472.long. Accessed October 10, 2019.
10. Wagner EH, Austin B, Von Korff M. Organizing care for patients with chronic illness. *Milbank Quarterly.* 1996;74(4):511–542.
11. Moerti D, Altenberger J, Bauer N, et al. Disease management programs in chronic heart failure: position statement of the Heart Failure Working Group and the Working Group of the Cardiological Assistance and Care Personnel of the Austrian Society of Cardiology. *Wien Klin Wochenschr.* 2017;129(23):869–878.
12. Ruppar TM, Cooper PS, Mehr DR, et al. Medication adherence interventions improve heart failure mortality and readmission rates: Systematic review and meta-analysis of controlled trials. *J Am Heart Assoc.* 2016;5(6):e002606. Available at https://www.ncbi.nlm.nih.gov/pmc/articles/PMC4937243/. Accessed October 10, 2019.
13. Cutler DM, Everett W. Thinking outside the pillbox—Medication adherence as a priority for health care reform. *N Engl J Med.* 2010;362(17):1553–1555.
14. Yancy CW, Januzzi JL, Allen LA, et al. 2017 ACC Expert Consensus Decision Pathway for optimization of heart failure treatment: Answers to 10 pivotal issues about heart failure with reduced ejection fraction: a report of the American College of Cardiology Task Force on Expert Consensus Decision Pathways. *JACC.* 2018;72(2):201–230.
15. Ellrodt G, Cook DJ, Lee J, et al. Evidence-based disease management. *JAMA.* 1997;278:1687–1692.
16. Yancy CW, Jessup M, Bozkurt B, et al. 2017 ACC/AHA/HFSA Focused Update of the 2013 ACCF/AHA Guideline for the Management of Heart Failure: A Report of the American College of Cardiology/American Heart Association Task Force on Clinical Practice Guidelines and the Heart Failure Society of America. *Circulation.* 2017;136(6):e137–e161. doi:10.1161/CIR.0000000000000509
17. Ory MG, Ahn S, Jiang L, et al. Success of a national study of the chronic disease self-management program: meeting the Triple Aim of health care reform. *Medical Care.* 2013;51(11):992–998.
18. IHI Triple Aim Initiative. Institute for Healthcare Improvement. Available at http://www.ihi.org/Engage/Initiatives/TripleAim/Pages/default.aspx. Accessed October 10, 2019.
19. Abed HS, Wittert GA, Leong DP et al. Effect of weight reduction and cardiometabolic risk factor management on symptom burden and severity in patients with atrial fibrillation. *JAMA.* 2013;301(19):2050–2060.
20. Stewart S, Willey JF, Ball J, et al. Impact of nurse led multidisciplinary home-based intervention on event-free survival across the spectrum of chronic heart disease composite analysis of health outcomes in 1226 patients from 3 randomized trials. *Circulation.* 2016;133:1867–1877.
21. Stewart S, Horowitz J, Pearson S. Effects of a home-based intervention among patients with congestive heart failure discharged from acute hospital care. *Arch Intern Med.* 1998;158:1067–1072.
22. Benjamin EJ, Muntner P, Alonso A, et al. Heart disease and stroke statistics—2019 update: a report from the American Heart Association. *Circulation.* 2019;139(10):e56–e528.
23. Benjamin EJ, Blaha MJ, Chiuve SE, et al. Heart Disease and stroke statistics—2017 update: a report from the American Heart Association. *Circulation.* 2017;135(10).e146 e603. Available at Downloads/CIR.0000000000000485.full.pdf. Accessed October 10, 2019.
24. National Council on Aging, Chronic Disease Self Management Programs. Available at https://www.ncoa.org/healthy-aging/chronic-disease/chronic-disease-self-management-programs/. Downloaded July 7, 2018.
25. Pozehl B, McGuire R, Norman J. Team-based care for cardiac rehabilitation and exercise training in heart failure. *Heart Fail Clin.* 2015;11(3):431–449. Available at https://www.sciencedirect.com/science/article/pii/S1551713615000215?via%3Dihub. Accessed October 10, 2019.
26. Thomas RJ, Balady G, Banka G, et al. 2018 ACC/AHA clinical performance and quality measures for cardiac rehabilitation: a report of the American College of Cardiology/American Heart Association Task Force on Performance Measures. *Circ Cardiovasc Qual Outcomes.* 2018;11(4):e000037. Available at http://circoutcomes.ahajournals.org/content/11/4/e000037.full. Accessed October 10, 2019.
27. Disease Management Association of America. *The definition of disease management.* 2008. Available at http://www.dmaa.org/definition.html. Accessed June 13, 2008.
28. Riegel B, Lee CS, Ratcliffe SJ, et al. Predictors of objectively measured medication non-adherence in adults with heart failure. *Circ Heart Fail.* 2012;5:430–436.
29. McMurray JV. Disease management programs in cardiology. *Circulation.* 2016;133:1836–1837.
30. McCabe PJ, DeVon HA. Home-based management of patients with atrial fibrillation. *Lancet.* 2015;385:752–753. Available at https://www.thelancet.com/journals/lancet/article/PIIS0140-6736(14)62013-4/fulltext. Accessed October 10, 2019.
31. Alderman MH, Shoenbaum EF. Detection and treatment of hypertension at the work site. *N Engl J Med.* 1975;293:65–68.
32. Runyan KW Jr. The Memphis chronic disease program. Comparison in outcome and the nurse's extended role. *JAMA.* 1975;231:264–267.
33. Denver EA, Barnard M, Woolfson RG, et al. Management of uncontrolled hypertension in a nurse-led clinic compared with conventional care for patients with Type 2 diabetes. *Diabetes Care.* 2003;26:2256–2260.
34. Gabbay RA, Lendel I, Saleem TM, et al. Nurse case management improves blood pressure, emotional stress and diabetes complication screening. *Diabetes Res Clin Pract.* 2006;71:28–35.
35. Hill MN, Bone LJ, Hilton SC, et al. A clinical trial to improve high blood pressure care in young urban black men: recruitment, follow-up, and outcomes. *Am J Hypertens.* 1999;12:548–554.
36. Logan AG, Milne BJ, Achber C, et al. Work-site treatment of hypertension by specially trained nurses. A controlled trial. *Lancet.* 1979;2:1175–1178.
37. Perry HM, Schnapner JW, Meyer G, et al. Clinical program for screening and treatment of hypertension in veterans. *J Natl Med Assoc.* 1982;74:433–444.
38. Pheley AM, Terry P, Peitz L, et al. Evaluation of a nurse-based hypertension management program: screening, management, and outcomes. *J Cardiovasc Nurs.* 1995;9:54–61.
39. Reichgott MJ, Pearson S, Hill MN. The nurse practitioner's role in complex patient management: hypertension. *J Natl Med Assoc.* 1983;75:1197–1204.
40. Tobe SW, Pylypchuk G, Wentworth J, et al. Effect of nurse-directed hypertension treatment among First Nations people with existing hypertension and diabetes mellitus: The Diabetes Risk Evaluation and Microalbuminuria (DREAM) randomized controlled trial. *CMAJ.* 2006;174:1267–1271.
41. Allen J, Blumenthal RS, Margolis S, et al. Nurse case management of hypercholesterolemia in patients with coronary heart disease: results of a randomized clinical trial. *Am Heart J.* 2002;144:678–686.

42. Becker DM, Rqueno JV, Yook RM, et al. Nurse mediated cholesterol management compared with enhanced primary care in siblings of individuals with premature coronary disease. *Arch Intern Med.* 1998;158:1533–1539.
43. Blair TP, Bryant J, Bocuzzi S. Treatment of hypercholesterolemia by a clinical nurse using a stepped-care protocol in a non-volunteer population. *Arch Intern Med.* 1988;148:1046–1048.
44. Shaffer J, Wexler LF. Reducing low-density lipoprotein cholesterol levels in an ambulatory care system. *Arch Intern Med.* 1995;155:2330–2335.
45. Hollis JF, Lichtenstein E, Vogt TM, et al. Nurse-assisted counseling for smokers in primary care. *Ann Intern Med.* 1993;118:521–525.
46. Martin K, Froelicher E, Miller HN. Women's Initiative for Nonsmoking (WINS) II: The intervention. *Heart Lung.* 2000;29:438–445.
47. Miller NH, Smith PM, DeBusk RF, et al. Smoking cessation in hospitalized patients. Results of a randomized trial. *Arch Intern Med.* 1997;157:409–415.
48. Rigotti NA, McKool KM, Shiffman S. Predictors of smoking cessation after coronary artery bypass graft surgery: results of a randomized trial with 5-year follow-up. *Ann Intern Med.* 1994;120:287–293.
49. Taylor CB, Miller NH, Killen JD, et al. Smoking cessation after acute myocardial infarction: effects of a nurse-managed intervention. *Ann Intern Med.* 1990;13:118–123.
50. Aubert RE, Herman WH, Waters J, et al. Nurse case management to improve glycemic control in diabetic patients in a health maintenance organization. A randomized, controlled trial. *Ann Intern Med.* 1998;129:605–612.
51. Peters AL, Davidson MB, Ossorio RC. Management of patients with diabetes by nurses with support of specialists. *HMO Pract.* 1995;9:8–13.
52. Piette JD, Weinberger M, Kraemer FB, et al. Impact of automated calls with nurse follow-up on diabetes treatment outcomes in a Department of Veterans Affairs Health Care System: a randomized controlled trial. *Diabetes Care.* 2001;24:202–208.
53. Taylor CB, Houston Miller N, Reilly KR, et al. Evaluation of a nurse-care management system to improve outcomes in patients with complicated diabetes. *Diabetes Care.* 2003;26:1058–1053.
54. Weinberger M, Kirkman MS, Samsa GP, et al. A nurse-coordinated intervention for primary care patients with non-insulin-dependent diabetes mellitus: impact on glycemic control and health-related quality of life. *J Gen Intern Med.* 1995;10:59–66.
55. Campbell NC, Ritchie LD, Thain J, et al. Secondary prevention in coronary heart disease: a randomized trial of nurse led clinics in primary care. *Heart.* 1998;80(5):447–452.
56. Cupples ME, McKnight A. Randomized controlled trial of health promotion in general practice for patients at high cardiovascular risk. *BMJ.* 1994;309(6960):993–996.
57. DeBusk RF, Miller NH, Superko HR, et al. A case management system for coronary risk factor modification following acute myocardial infarction. *Ann Intern Med.* 1994;120:721–729.
58. Fonarow GC, Gawlinksi A, Moughrabi S, et al. Improved treatment of coronary heart disease by implementation of a Cardiac Hospitalization Atherosclerosis Management Program (CHAMP). *Am J Cardiol.* 2001;87:819–822.
59. Fonarow G, Gawlinski A, Watson K. In-hospital initiation of cardiovascular protective therapies to improve treatment rates and clinical outcomes: The University of California–Los Angeles, Cardiovascular Hospitalization Atherosclerosis Management Program. *Crit Pathw Cardiol.* 2003;2:61–70.
60. Gordon NF, English CD, Contractor AS, et al. Effectiveness of three models for comprehensive cardiovascular disease risk reduction. *Am J Cardiol.* 2002;89:1263–1268.
61. Haskell WL, Alderman EL, Fair JM, et al. Effects of intensive multiple risk factor reduction on coronary atherosclerosis and clinical cardiac events in men and women with coronary artery disease. The Stanford Coronary Risk Intervention Project (SCRIP). *Circulation.* 1994;89:975–990.
62. Murchie P, Campbell N, Ritchie LD, et al. Secondary prevention clinics for coronary heart disease: four year follow up of a randomized controlled trial in primary care. *BMJ.* 2003;326:84.
63. Naylor M, Brooten D, Campbell R, et al. Comprehensive discharge planning and home follow-up of hospitalized elders. *JAMA.* 1999;281(7):613–620.
64. O'Malley PG, Feurstein IM, Taylor AJ. Impact of electron beam tomography, with or without case management, on motivation, behavioral change, and cardiovascular risk profile. *JAMA.* 2003;289(17):2215–2223.
65. Pozen MW, Stechmiller J, Harris W, et al. A nurse rehabilitator's impact on patients with myocardial infarction. *Med Care.* 1977;15: 830–837.
66. Sivarajan ES, Bruce RA, Almes MJ, et al. In-hospital exercise after myocardial infarction does not improve treadmill performance. *N Engl J Med.* 1981;305:357–362.
67. Sivarajan ES, Bruce RA, Lindskog BD, et al. Treadmill test responses to an early exercise program after myocardial infarction: a randomized study. *Circulation.* 1982;65:1420–1428.
68. Sivarajan ES, Newton KM, Almes MJ, et al. Limited effects of outpatient teaching and counseling after myocardial infarction: a controlled study. *Heart Lung.* 1983;12:65–73.
69. Benatar DB, Ghitelman M, Avitall J. Outcomes of chronic heart failure. *Arch Intern Med.* 2003;163:347–351.
70. Blue LL, McMurray E, Davie JJ, et al. Randomized controlled trial of specialist nurse intervention in heart failure. *BMJ.* 2001;323:715–718.
71. Cline CMJ, Israelsson B, Willenheimer RB, et al. Cost effective management programme for heart failure reduces hospitalization. *Heart.* 1998;80:442–446.
72. Ekman I, Andersson B, Ehnforst M, et al. Feasibility of a nurse-monitored, outpatient-care programme for elderly patients with moderate-to-severe, chronic heart failure. *Eur Heart J.* 1998;19:1254–1260.
73. Fonarow G, Stevenson LW, Walden JA, et al. Impact of a comprehensive heart failure management program on hospital readmission and functional status of patients with advanced heart failure. *J Am Coll Cardiol.* 1997;30:725–732.
74. Jaarsma T, Halfens R, Huijer Abu-Saad H, et al. Effects of education and support on self-care and resource utilization in patients with heart failure. *Eur Heart J.* 1999;20:673–682.
75. Jaarsma T, van der Wal MH, Lesman-Leegle I, et al. Effect of moderate or intensive disease management program on outcomes in patients with heart failure. *Arch Intern Med.* 2008;168:316–324.
76. Kasper E, Gerstenblith G, Hefter G, et al. A randomized trial of the efficacy of multidisciplinary care in heart failure outpatients at high risk of hospital readmission. *J Am Coll Cardiol.* 2002;39(3):471–480.
77. Kornowski R, Zeeli D, Averbuch M, et al. Intensive home-care surveillance prevents hospitalization and improves morbidity rates among elderly patients with severe congestive heart failure. *Am Heart J.* 1995;129: 762–766.
78. Laramee AS, Levinsky SK, Sargent J, et al. Case management in a heterogeneous congestive heart failure population. *Arch Intern Med.* 2003;163:809–817.
79. Reigel BC, Kopp Z, LePetri B, et al. Effect of a standardized nurse case-management telephone intervention on resource use in patients with chronic heart failure. *Arch Intern Med.* 2002;162:705–712.
80. Rich MW, Beckham V, Wittenberg C, et al. A multidisciplinary intervention to prevent the readmission of elderly patients with congestive heart failure. *N Engl J Med.* 1995;333(18):1190–1195.
81. Stewart S, Marley JE, Horowitz JD. Effects of a multidisciplinary, home-based intervention on planned readmissions and survival among patients with chronic congestive heart failure: a randomized controlled study. *Lancet.* 1999;354:1077–1083.
82. Stewart S, Horowitz J. Specialist nurse management programmes. *Pharmacoeconomics.* 2003;21(4):225–240.
83. Weinberger M, Oddone E, Henderson WG. Does increased access to primary care reduce hospital readmissions? *N Engl J Med.* 1996;334(22):1441–1447.
84. West J, Miller NH, Parker KM, et al. A comprehensive management system for heart failure improves clinical outcomes and reduces medical resource utilization. *Am J Cardiol.* 1997;79(1):58–63.
85. Sivarajan ES, Newton KM. Symposium on cardiac rehabilitation: exercise, education and counseling for patients with coronary artery disease. *Clin Sports Med.* 1984;2:349–369.
86. Yeates K, Lohfeld L, Sleeth J, et al. A global perspective on cardiovascular disease in vulnerable populations. *Can J Cardiol.* 2015;31(9):1081–1093.
87. DeBusk RF, Miller NH, Parker KM, et al. Care management for low-risk patients with heart failure. *Ann Intern Med.* 2004;141:606–613.
88. Chaudhry SI, Phillips CO, Stewart SS, et al. Telemonitoring for patients with chronic heart failure: a systematic review. *J Cardiovasc Fail.* 2007;13:56–62.
89. Rich MW. Heart failure disease management programs: efficacy and limitations. *Am J Med.* 2001;110(5):410–412.
90. Stewart S, Vanderbrock AJ, Pearson S, et al. Prolonged beneficial effects of a home-based intervention on unplanned readmissions and morality among patients with congestive heart failure. *Arch Intern Med.* 1999;159:257–261.
91. Ott CR, Sivarajan ES, Newton KM, et al. A randomized study of early cardiac rehabilitation: the sickness impact profile as an assessment tool. *Heart Lung.* 1983;12(2):162–170.

92. Sivarajan FE, Kozuki Y. Application of theory to smoking cessation intervention. Women's Initiative for Non-smoking IV. *Int J Nurs Studies*. 2002;39:1–15.
93. Mullen PD, Mains DA, Velez R. A meta-analysis of controlled trials of cardiac patient education. *Patient Educ Couns*. 1992;19:143–162.
94. Miller NH, Taylor CB. Education, communication and methods of intervention. In: Giles E, Moore S, eds. *Lifestyle Management for Patients with Coronary Heart Disease*. Champaign, IL: Human Kinetics; 1995:21–30.
95. Prochaska JO, DiClemente CC. Stages and process of self-change of smoking: toward an integrative model of change. *J Consult Clin Psychol*. 1983;51:390–395.
96. Bandura A. *Self-Efficacy: The Exercise of Control*. New York: W. H. Freeman; 1997.
97. Bandura A. *Social Learning Theory*. Englewood Cliffs, NJ: Prentice-Hall; 1977.
98. Free C, Phillips G, Galli L, et al. The effectiveness of mobile-health technology-based health behaviour change or disease management interventions for health care consumers: a systematic review. *PLoS Med*. 2013;10(1):e1001362. Available at http://journals.plos.org/plosmedicine/article?id=10.1371/journal.pmed.1001362. Accessed October 10, 2019.
99. Sisk JE, Hebert PL, Horowitz CR, et al. Effects of nurse management on the quality of heart failure care in minority communities. *Ann Intern Med*. 2006;145:273–283.
100. Rector TS, Kubo SH, Cohn JN. Validity of the Minnesota living with heart failure questionnaire as a measure of therapeutic response to enalapril or placebo. *Am J Cardiol*. 1993;71:1106–1107.
101. Fergenbaum J, Bermingham S, Krahn M, et al. Care in the home for the management of chronic heart failure: systematic review and cost-effectiveness analysis. *J Cardiovasc Nurs*. 2015:30(4 Suppl 1):S44–S51. Available at https://insights.ovid.com/pubmed?pmid=25658188. Accessed October 10, 2019.
102. Ades P, Kottke T, Miller HN, et al. Task force #3–getting results: who, where, and how? 33rd Bethesda Conference? *J Am Coll Cardiol*. 2002;40(4):615–630.
103. Naylor MD, Brooten DA, Campbell RL, et al. Transitional care of older adults hospitalized with heart failure: a randomized, controlled trial. *J Am Geriatr Soc*. 2004;52:675–684.
104. Pare G, Jaana M, Sicotte C. Systematic review of home telemonitoring for chronic diseases: the evidence base. *J Am Med Inform Assoc*. 2007;14:269–277.
105. Lorig K, Ritter P, Stewart A, et al. Chronic disease self-management program. 2-year health status and health care utilization outcomes. *Med Care*. 2001;39(11):1217–1223.
106. Lorig K, Sobel DS, Stewart AL, et al. Evidence suggesting that a chronic disease self-management program can improve health status while reducing hospitalization: a randomized trial. *Med Care*. 1999;37(1):5–14.
107. Wootton R. Twenty years of telemedicine in chronic disease management—an evidence synthesis. *J Telemed Telecare*. 2012;18(4):211–220. Available at http://journals.sagepub.com/doi/full/10.1258/jtt.2012.120219. Accessed October 10, 2019.
108. Nelson J, Arnold-Powers P. Community case management for frail, elderly clients: the nurse case managers role. *J Nurs Administr*. 2001;31(9):444–450.

42 Global and Population Health

Christina R. Paganelli

OBJECTIVES

1. Describe the global epidemiology of cardiovascular disease.
2. List population-level primary and secondary prevention interventions for reducing cardiovascular disease risk factors.
3. Describe the challenges of implementing population-level secondary prevention measures.

KEY QUESTIONS

1. How can nursing research impact CVD morbidity and mortality in those populations facing the greatest burden?
2. In what ways are nurses as policy makers positioned to mitigate CVD morbidity and mortality?
3. As front-line healthcare professionals, how can nurses reduce CVD risk at the population level?

BACKGROUND

Historical State and Context

In recent decades there has been an epidemiologic transition globally. This transition is characterized by a shift in primary causes of morbidity and mortality from communicable and infectious diseases and nutritional deficiencies to noncommunicable diseases (NCDs).[1] This transition is a result of global industrialization, urbanization, changes in lifestyle, medical innovation, and improvements in understanding diseases.[2] By 2030, the global burden of mortality attributable to NCDs will be five times that of communicable disease.[3] In 2016, 71% of global mortality was attributable to NCDs and 44% of NCD mortality attributable to cardiovascular disease (CVD).[4]

Yusuf and colleagues integrated CVD into this epidemiologic transition and the result was a five-stage model that highlights the changing epidemiology of CVD morbidity and mortality[5–7]:

- Stage 1 is characterized by circulatory diseases secondary to infections such as rheumatic heart disease.
- Stage 2 is characterized by a lower infectious disease burden and improved nutritional status, but an increased risk of hypertension.
- Stage 3 is marked by an increase in high-risk behaviors including smoking, drinking, and decreased physical activity.
- Stage 4 represents an increase in efforts to prevent, diagnose, and treat CVD resulting in morbidity at more advanced ages.
- Stage 5 is characterized by health regression and social upheaval in which there is a renewed increase in CVD morbidity and mortality as a result of infection as well as an increase in high-risk behaviors such as drinking. The result is an increase in CVD in younger populations.

These stages are not mutually exclusive and there may be populations within a single country experiencing different stages of this transition. For example, in rural areas of a country such as India, where the population is still cultivating much of its own food, many people still participate in significant physical activity as a result of their occupation and there is limited water and sanitation infrastructure; thus, this transition may still be in the early stages. Yet, in urban areas of India where there is significant industrialization, more pollution, fewer green spaces, less physical activity and more consumption of processed foods, the transition is more advanced.

Epidemiology and Demographics

In 2016, CVD accounted for 32% of global mortality.[8] Between 2000 and 2016 CVD mortality increased by 21%.[9] However, due to population-level risk-reduction measures, namely tobacco reduction interventions and advances in care, age-specific mortality has declined and counterbalances the absolute increases in deaths as a result of population growth and aging.[10] Accounting for over half of all CVD mortality, ischemic heart disease is the largest contributor to CVD mortality.[4] In 2016, stroke was attributed to 31% of all CVD mortality (Fig. 42-1).[4] Combined, ischemic heart disease and stroke were responsible for over 25% of all deaths (all-cause) worldwide.

The morbidity and mortality of CVD does not impact every population equally. Where a person lives influences their risk for CVD mortality as much as being obese or hypertensive.[10] Using the country income classifications established by the World Bank, it is evident that in many respects those living in low- and middle-income countries (LMICs), compared to high-income countries (HICs), suffer the most from CVD despite having the lowest burden (Fig. 42-2).[11] LMICs contribute to 80% of all CVD mortality; populations in LMICs have the highest risk of experiencing a

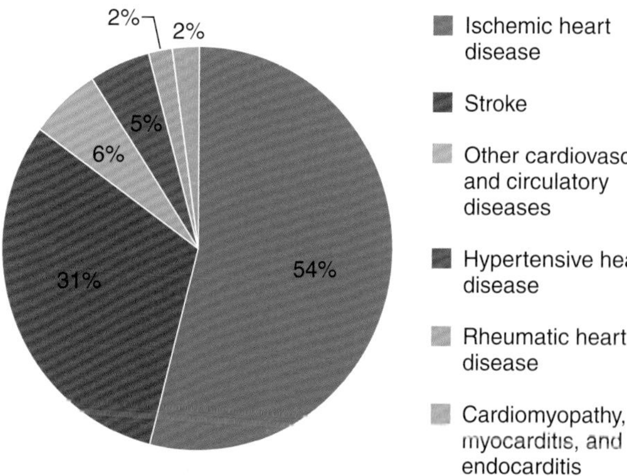

Figure 42-1. Global CVD mortality by cause 2016. (From World Health Organization. *Global health estimates 2016: Deaths by Cause, Age, Sex, by Country and by Region, 2000–2016.* Geneva: 2018.)

cardiovascular event and the highest case fatality rate despite having the lowest absolute numbers of CVD.[12,13] In fact, deaths due to CVD have decreased significantly in HICs. This is largely due to decreases in smoking, and increases in the availability of medical and surgical treatment.[10,14] Using Disability-Adjusted Life Years (DALYs) as the standardized measure of disease morbidity, populations living in LMICs experience 75% of the global morbidity attributable to CVD.[8] Ischemic heart disease and stroke are the top two causes of deaths globally irrespective of the country income level with the exception of low-income countries where they are the third and fifth most frequent causes, respectively.[4]

Current State and Context

Increased globalization and urbanization, particularly in LMICs, are the biggest drivers related to increases in CVD morbidity and mortality.[10,11,15,16] Described as a "public health emergency in slow motion," a global response has been mounting over the last decade.[7] In 2011, the World Health Organization (WHO) convened a United Nations (UN) High Level Meeting on the prevention and control of NCDs at the UN General Assembly. At this time the WHO set a global target for the reduction of "premature deaths from NCDs by 25% by 2025."[17,18] All 194 WHO Member States endorsed this target at the World Health Assembly in 2012. In 2013, the WHO released a Global Action Plan for the Prevention and Control of NCDs, which sets targets for risk factors associated with CVD[17]:

- **Target 1:** A 25% relative reduction in the risk of premature mortality from CVD, cancer, diabetes, or chronic diseases
- **Target 2:** At least a 10% reduction in the harmful use of alcohol, as appropriate, within the national context

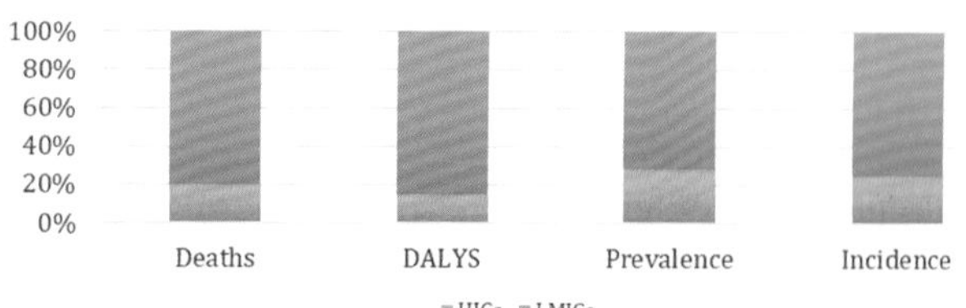

Figure 42-2. CVD morbidity and mortality stratified by World Bank Country Income. *Global Burden of Disease Collaborative Network. Global Burden of Disease Study 2016 (GBD 2016) Results.* Seattle, United States; 2018. Available at http://ghdx.healthdata.org/gbd-results-tool. Accessed September 7, 2018.

- **Target 3:** A 10% relative reduction in prevalence of insufficient physical activity
- **Target 4:** A 30% relative reduction in the mean population intake of salt/sodium
- **Target 5:** A 30% reduction in the prevalence of current tobacco use
- **Target 6:** A 25% relative reduction in the prevalence of raised blood pressure
- **Target 7:** Halt the rise in obesity and diabetes
- **Target 8:** At least 50% of eligible people receive drug therapy and counseling to prevent heart attacks and strokes
- **Target 9:** An 80% availability of the affordable basic technologies and medicines, to treat NCDs in both public and private settings

As suggested by the above targets, the largest contributing lifestyle risk factors for CVD are tobacco use, poor diet, physical inactivity, excessive alcohol and obesity. These risk factors are directly associated with precursors to CVD including hypertension, elevated blood sugar and cholesterol, and type 2 diabetes.[7] In 2011, the WHO released a report outlining "best-buy" interventions, those that have been demonstrated to be cost-effective and feasible to implement in LMICs.[19] Since 2016 the WHO has released several population-level initiatives aimed at reducing CVD risk (Table 42-1).

PRIMARY PREVENTION OF CVD AT THE POPULATION LEVEL

Population-level risk factors for developing CVD do not differ largely from individual-level risk factors contributing to CVD morbidity and mortality. Individual risk factors such as smoking, physical inactivity, dyslipidemia, obesity, hypertension, alcohol consumption, and type 2 diabetes all contribute to the global burden of CVD. In addition to these health and lifestyle risk factors, there are social, environmental, and economic risk factors that contribute to global CVD morbidity and mortality. Collectively these risk factors can be placed under the umbrella of "social determinants of health." The WHO defines social determinants of health as "the circumstance in which people are born, grow, live, work and age and the health systems put in place to deal with illness."[20] Social determinants of health are impactful and influence lifestyle and behavioral risk factors at the population level, particularly in the context of prevention and management of CVD morbidity and mortality in LMICs.

Significant data exist identifying effective primary prevention interventions, and those that reduce the risk of CVD morbidity and mortality prior to the onset of disease, at both the population and individual levels. Population-level interventions are effective because even a small risk reduction in a large number of people will reduce the overall CVD risk and burden significantly. Successful efforts to address the burden are likely to require a mix of population and individual-based interventions.[21] While still being debated, there is growing consensus that population-wide approaches to prevention of CVD are more effective and cost-efficient than implementing strategies to reduce individual risk, and there is evidence to suggest that a focus on individual-level interventions at the expense of population-level interventions will only widen inequality gaps.[7] As will be evident through this chapter, most population-level primary prevention interventions require multidisciplinary stakeholder and community buy-in from both the public and private sectors.

Table 42-1 • WHO GLOBAL INITIATIVES TO PREVENT AND REDUCE CVD

Global Hearts (WHO and CDC): Launched in 2016, a joint initiative between the WHO and CDC includes three technical packages aimed at scaling up prevention and control of CVD.	
MPOWER *Tobacco control*	Monitor use and prevention policies Protect people from exposure to tobacco smoke Offer interventions and support smoking cessation Warn of the dangers of tobacco Enforce regulation of marketing, advertising, and promotion of tobacco products Raise taxes
SHAKE *Salt reduction*	Surveillance of salt use Harness and promote industry reforms to reduce salt Adopt labeling and marketing standards and regulation Knowledge Educate and empower individuals to reduce salt intake Environment Supporting settings that promote healthy eating
HEARTS *Management of CVD in primary care*	Healthy lifestyle promotion including counseling on tobacco cessation, diet, physical activity and self-care Evidence-based treatment protocols Access to essential medicines and technologies Risk-based management including total CV risk assessment, treatment, and referral Team-based care and task sharing to improve patient care Systems for monitoring patient registries and evaluation of programs
REPLACE **Launched in 2018, this WHO initiative offers a guide for governments to reduce intake of industrially produced trans fats by 2023.**	
	REview dietary sources of industrially-produced trans fat and the landscape for policy change Promote the replacement of industrially-produced trans fats with healthier fats and oils Legislate and enact regulatory actions to eliminate the use of industrially-produced trans fats Assess and monitor trans fat consumption and content in the food supply Create awareness of negative health impacts among policy-makers, food producers, and suppliers and the public Enforce compliance with policies and regulations
SAFER **Launched in 2018, this WHO alcohol initiative outlines strategies to help governments reduce the harmful use of alcohol.**	
	Strengthen restrictions on alcohol availability Advance and enforce drunk driving counter measures Facilitate access to screening, interventions, and treatment Enforce bans and restrictions on advertising and promotion Raise prices through excise taxes
BreatheLife2030 **Launched in 2016, this collaboration between the WHO, Climate and Air Coalition, United Nations Environment, and the World Bank aims to mobilize communities to reduce the health impacts of air pollution.**	

Tobacco

It is well established that tobacco use and secondhand smoke significantly increase CVD morbidity and mortality. In 2016, global burden of disease (GBD) data estimated that tobacco is attributable to 21% of all CVD morbidity (DALYs) and more than 15% of all CVD mortality.[8,22,23] While smoking prevalence has declined globally, this decline has almost exclusively been limited to HICs. For example, in the United States smoking prevalence has decreased by more than 30% in the last two decades.[24,25] In contrast, smoking rates, especially in adolescents in LMICs, continue to increase and 80% of the world's 1 billion smokers live in LMICs.[26]

Population-level interventions including limiting smoking in public places and workplaces, taxation, advertising bans, packaging regulations, and cessation programs are deployed to reduce the prevalence and incidence of smoking and are included in the WHO "best buys interventions."[19] In 1995, the WHO established the Framework Convention on Tobacco Control (FCTC), which was subsequently adopted by the World Health Assembly in 2003 and took effect in 2005. Created to standardize and promote tobacco control policy, the FCTC set the goal of reducing smoking prevalence 30% by the year 2025. In 2008, the FCTC created the MPOWER Package to assist in country-level implementation of tobacco control policies. The MPOWER package, later integrated into the larger WHO Global Hearts Initiative, consists of seven interventions including monitoring tobacco use, protecting people from tobacco smoke, offering cessation support, warning about the dangers of tobacco, enforcing bans on advertising and raising taxes on tobacco products.[27] Since its initiation, 190 countries have signed onto the WHO FCTC.[28] Thus far, taxation has been shown to be the most effective intervention to reduce tobacco-attributable CVDs.[10] Unfortunately, while the implementation of WHO FCTC recommendations and MPOWER interventions have strengthened since 2007, only about 45% of suggested policies have been implemented in LMICs and smoking remains affordable in these countries.[10,23] Further, global tobacco companies are a powerful lobby and have shown themselves to be effective in evading advertising restrictions and influencing government officials to delay or halt the introduction of tobacco control policy, leaving the opportunity for more improvements in tobacco control.[26]

Obesity/Diet

In 2016, the WHO estimated that worldwide there were 1.9 billion overweight adults, of which, 650 million (13%) were considered obese.[29] In 2016, GBD data indicated that 16% of CVD deaths and 20% of CVD DALYs were attributable to obesity.[8]

Over recent decades there has been a change in the global food supply and the foods that people consume. These changes have been associated with rising incidences of obesity, type 2 diabetes, and CVD. There have been five specific changes in diet that have contributed to increases in obesity and CVD: (1) increases in refined carbohydrates, (2) increase intake in vegetable oils, (3) increased consumption of meat and animal protein, (4) increases in consumption of packaged and processed foods, and (5) increases in added sugars.[30,31] These changes are compounded by the fact that the consumption of fruits and vegetables, widely believed to serve as a protective factor against CVD, remains below the recommended daily intake, especially in LMICs.[31] Similar to strategies to reduce and discourage tobacco use, public policy is also being used at local and national levels to support reduced consumption of foods that contribute to CVD including, sodium, sugar-sweetened beverages, trans fats, and alcohol.

Sodium

The 2012 guidelines from the WHO suggest adults consume less than 2000 mg of sodium or 5 g of salt daily.[32] The GBD suggest that global daily sodium intake is close to 10 g/day and that 12% of CVD mortality is attributable to diets high in sodium.[8] Reducing sodium intake reduces morbidity and mortality at the individual level, and there have been studies suggesting that population-level interventions to reduce sodium consumption have been successful.[33] Interventions such as those encompassed in the WHO's REPLACE initiative have largely consisted of establishing sodium content targets for foods, mass media and consumer education, labeling requirements and, taxation on high-salt foods have been shown to be the most effective population-level measures to reduce sodium consumption.[34]

Sugar-Sweetened Beverages

Another shift in global dietary habits is the increased consumption of sugar-sweetened beverages. The consumption of sugar-sweetened beverages including fruit juice and soda has increased since 1997 from 9.4 to 11.2 gallons per capita annually.[30] The excess calories and added sugar in sugar-sweetened beverages are associated with several risk factors for CVD including obesity and diabetes.[35,36] While individual-level interventions aimed at changing lifestyle have been difficult to implement and evaluate, there is increasing evidence that taxes on sugar-sweetened beverages are effective in reducing their consumption in both LMICs and HICs.[36] A study in Mexico found that 70% of added sugars came from sugar-sweetened beverages, representing nearly 10% of their total energy intake.[37] In an effort to reduce sugar consumption in 2014 the Mexican government implemented a tax on all nonalcoholic sugar-sweetened beverages. The result after 2 years was a 7.3% reduction in sales of sugar-sweetened beverages.[35] The results of these taxes can be twofold: they can not only reduce consumption, but also pressure the soft drink industry to reduce the amount of added sugar in their beverages. This is exactly what is happening in the United Kingdom where companies like Fanta are reducing the amount of added sugar to below the threshold of sugar levels subject to taxation.[38] While it is understood that a reduction in sales is not equivalent to a reduction in CVD risk, similar to tobacco taxes, the greatest reductions in sales occurred in households of lower socioeconomic status which are often the populations that bear the greatest burden of CVD and have the highest proportion of their energy coming from added sugars.[35,38] While there is increasing evidence that excise taxes are beneficial, there is widespread agreement that public education campaigns to raise awareness and support behavior change are also a critical component to be successful.

Trans Fat

Trans fat can be both naturally or artificially occurring but are largely artificial and prevalent in industrially produced food. Increasing the risk of coronary artery disease, the WHO estimates that consumption of artificially produced trans fat results in more than 500,000 CVD deaths and more than 5 million DALYs annually.[39] In recent decades both national and local governments have taken steps to reduce the consumption of trans fat. Interventions have ranged from establishing labeling and packaging requirements, to limiting the amount of trans fat in food, and even going as far as completely banning trans fat. The movement to reduce and ultimately eliminate the addition of trans fat to food has been in effect in HIC for some time. In 2003, Denmark was the first country to implement a policy eliminating artificial trans fat in foods.[40] While many countries including Brazil, Canada, Chile, India, and South Africa followed suit by introducing package labeling requirements and imposing limitations on artificial trans fat, data suggest that banning the addition of trans fat will have the greatest population-level impact.[40,41]

Many LMICs have been slow to implement such policies. In 2018, the WHO reported that 20 HICs have instituted mandatory bans or limits on trans fat while only 3 LMICs have instituted such bans.[40] Recently the WHO released a call for all countries to eliminate artificial trans fat worldwide by 2023 and introduced the REPLACE initiative, which offers governments a guide to reduce the intake of industrially produced trans fats.[39] Similar to policy interventions to reduce consumption of tobacco and sugar-sweetened beverages, banning trans fat seems to most significantly impact those in the lowest socioeconomic groups, further substantiating the importance of trans fat regulation in LMICs.[41]

Alcohol

While there is broad consensus that heavy alcohol consumption increases risk for CVD morbidity and mortality especially coronary artery disease and myocardial infarction, over the past decades there has been increasing evidence that moderate alcohol consumption could serve as a protective factor against CVD. In 2004, the INTERHEART study, a large international case-control study identified a protective effect against myocardial infarction with moderate alcohol consumption.[42] Since then there have been several studies supporting the finding that moderate consumption of alcohol can reduce risk of CVD. In 2011, a systematic review and meta-analysis by Ronksley et al. found that moderate alcohol consumption reduces risk of all causes of CVD mortality and morbidity.[43] However, a large study in 2018 has confirmed more recent research that alcohol provides no significant protective factor against CVD.[44] Researchers in the 2018 study identify methodologic flaws in previous studies supporting moderate alcohol consumption and their findings state that there is "no safe quantity" that can be consumed.[44] While alcohol consumption is highest in HIC, data suggest that consumption in LMICs is increasing.[45] Through the SAFER initiative, the WHO has recommended several strategies for reducing the harmful use of alcohol including enacting and enforcing bans on alcohol advertising, restricting access to alcohol, restricting marketing of alcoholic beverages, and increasing alcohol taxes as policy measures to reduce risk-taking behaviors.[46] The implications of the most recent research on recommendations for population-level risk-reduction measures related to alcohol remains to be seen.

Air Pollution

For nearly 20 years there has been convincing evidence that indicates that environmental exposure to air pollution has significant negative impacts on CVD morbidity and mortality.[47,48] In 2016, it was estimated that over 20% of DALYs lost to CVD and 18% of CVD deaths were attributable to air pollution.[8] Household air pollution is largely a result of indoor cook stoves while outdoor air pollution is caused by traffic and industry emissions that increase fine particulate matter.[49] Franklin et al. describe the mechanism by which exposure to fine particulate matter increasing CVD risk as result of a "spillover of proinflammatory or oxidative stress mediators generated in the lungs into the systemic circulation; the incitement of autonomic nervous system imbalance, characterized by sympathetic predominance; and, the penetration of certain particles or components directly into the cardiovascular tissues."[47] Although the health impacts of exposure are dose dependent, both short- and long-term exposure have shown to impact CVD morbidity and mortality. Short-term impacts associated with exposure to fine particulate matter include increased risk of hypertension, myocardial infarction, stroke, and acute heart failure.[50–52] In addition to the short-term effects, long-term effects of exposure to fine particulate matter include an increased risk of ischemic heart disease and an 11% higher risk in CVD mortality.[50] LMICs experience an increased risk of CVD morbidity and mortality due to increasing levels of fine particulate matter resulting from rapid and increasing industrialization and the use of indoor cook stoves in LMICs.[53]

Population-level interventions to reduce exposure to indoor and outdoor air pollution include establishing efficient transit options, regulation of land use to promote walking and biking, incentivizing the use of clean fuels and establish emission controls. There are limited data identifying specific interventions that result in improved CVD outcomes. One study in Australia found that reducing fine particulate matter using a combination of coordinated interventions including community education, public incentives, and law enforcement did result in a decrease in overall CVD mortality.[54] There has been some public criticism that the international health community has not meaningfully addressed air pollution and NCDs, including scrutiny of the absence of recommendations for specific interventions and lack of international targets aimed at reducing NCD and CVD risk attributable to air pollution as part of larger NCD action packages. While exposure to air pollution is not unique among CVD risk factors in that population interventions require a coordinated response at the local, national, and international levels, unlike the other risk factors, reducing risk exposure to air pollution demands a highly coordinated effort across many facets of government and the private sector to ultimately reduce CVD mortality and morbidity. BreatheLife2030 is a collaboration between health and climate experts that supports communities to mobilize their communities to reduce the harmful health impacts of air pollution.[55]

Physical Inactivity

Since the 1990s, deaths attributable to physical inactivity have increased 15% in HICs and increased 25% in LMICs.[10] In 2016, GBD data indicated that physical inactivity was attributable to 22 million DALYs and over 7% of CVD deaths.[8] The WHO estimates that currently one in four adults and 3 in 4 adolescents do not meet the global recommendations for physical activity.[56] Currently the WHO recommends adults engage in at least 150 minutes of moderate intensity and 75 minutes of vigorous activity weekly. Populations that typically experience higher levels of physical inactivity include women and older adults.[57] Physical activity also varies across socioeconomic groups and urban versus rural settings. In general, in LMICs the higher the socioeconomic level the less active the population, except in urban areas, where a lower socioeconomic class is correlated with higher levels of physical activity and higher socioeconomic classes with lower levels of physical activity.[58] In HICs occupational physical activity has decreased due to advances in technology and decreased physical labor, but at the same time, leisure physical activity has increased in part, due to coordinated efforts by urban planners, employers, and healthcare organizations to increase physical activity.[10,57] Similar to HICs, occupational physical activity has also decreased in LMICs, however, in contrast to HICs, leisure physical activity has not increased in LMICs.[10] Rapid urbanization has been cited as a cause for the lack of physical activity increases in LMICs.[59]

Many countries have established national action plans to increase physical activity, however, LMICs have been slower than HICs to adopt such plans and policies.[60] Cross-sectoral intervention has been particularly challenging to implement in LMICs and there remains room for research identifying effective interventions.[60] That said, there have been some successful community-wide interventions identified in LMICs. For example, several studies in Latin America demonstrated the effectiveness of utilizing public settings such as parks to provide physical activity classes and closing streets to automobiles to support pedestrian and bicycle traffic as strategies to increase physical activity.[59,61] The WHO set a target to reduce physical inactivity by 10% by 2025 and created a global action plan that demands coordinated multi-sectoral participation to implement.[56]

SECONDARY AND TERTIARY PREVENTION OF CVD FROM A POPULATION PERSPECTIVE

Once a person has been diagnosed with CVD, management of the disease becomes imperative to reduce the risk of significant morbidity, disability, and mortality. There is significant disability attributed to CVD globally. The absolute number of DALYs attributable to CVD increased by 20% globally from 2000 to 2016 and by 36% in LMICs versus 10% in HICs.[9] Years of life lost to disability (YLD) due to CVD increased by 47% between 2000 and 2016 globally and by 56% in LMICs and 21% in HICs.[9]

Effective management of conditions such as hypertension and diabetes in order to reduce the risk of recurrence and incidence of additional cardiovascular events and subsequently the risk of further disability and mortality is known as secondary prevention. Largely pharmacologic, secondary preventions have been found to be crucial and cost-effective in the management and prevention of CVD morbidity and mortality.[62] Reducing the risk of long-term disability or impairment from CVD is known as tertiary prevention.[63] In this section we will look at challenges and opportunities for secondary and tertiary prevention globally.

Medication Availability and Adherence

Pharmacologic interventions are potentially the most effective strategy for secondary prevention. For example, the use of β-blockers, statins, and angiotensin-converting enzyme inhibitors

(ACE-Is) and anti-platelet drugs such aspirin have been shown to significantly reduce the risk of major cardiovascular events by up to 25% each and by up to 75% when used together.[64] The WHO has released a list of essential medicines every 2 years since 1975. This comprehensive list includes generic and cost-effective medications that are the foundation of pharmacotherapy secondary prevention and that should be available worldwide.

Yet there exists a discrepancy between the use of these medications in HICs versus LMICs. In India, it is reported that only 8% of individuals with CVD are receiving statins compared with 80% in HICs, and that the use of inexpensive antiplatelets such as aspirin varied sevenfold between low-income countries and HICs.[2,10,65] One study found that aspirin was not available in 20% to 30% of rural communities in LMICs.[66] In LMICs, only 31% of patients with hypertension were aware of their hypertension and fewer than 30% of those were being treated. In contrast, in HICs 49% of patients were aware of their hypertension and nearly 50% were being treated.[10,67] It is estimated that globally fewer than one in five patients with hypertension are receiving secondary prevention, although the percentage of those being treated is increasing in HICs.[10] The WHO study on Prevention of Recurrences of Myocardial Infarction and StrokE (WHO-PREMISE) study found that in some LMICs, fewer than 40% of acute MI patients received ACE-I and only 20% received statins, compared with HICs where 40% of patients received ACE-Is and almost 70% received statins.[16] A study by Yusuf et al. found that a country's economic status accounted for more than 60% of a patient's use of medication in secondary prevention.[65]

Access to pharmacotherapy as secondary prevention in LMICs can be influenced by a number of factors including availability, affordability, accessibility, acceptability, and the quality of medicines. Wirtz et al. provides a thorough review of how these five dimensions impact access to secondary prevention.[68]

- *Affordability* reflects a patient's ability to pay for a medication. Wirtz et al. report that in LMICs a 1-month supply of one generic CVD medication can cost, on average, 2 days of a government wage.[68] This leaves many with low-wage jobs and the unemployed unable to afford secondary prevention.
- *Availability* refers to the supply of medicine versus the demand. Many factors can influence the availability of medications including supply change management and staff capacity and performance. In 2011, Cameron et al. found that the availability of medications to treat chronic diseases in LMICs was 38% in public institutions and 64% in private institutions.[69] In 2016, Wirtz et al. found availability of CVD medications in LMICs to be 26% in public institutions and 57% in private institutions.[68,69]
- *Accessibility* describes a patient's ability to be prescribed medications and ability to obtain the medication. This can be influenced by a number of factors including the distance to the clinic or dispensary as well as the ability to be seen by a provider as well as duration of consultation time. In LMICs, absenteeism of workers in public institutions can be as high as 35% to 68%, resulting in longer wait times or reduced clinic hours.[68]
- *Acceptability* of a medication refers to adherence of the medication by patients as well as how the medication is prescribed by healthcare professionals. Acceptability can be influenced by the complexity of the medication regimen, medication side effects, a patient's attitude and beliefs about the medication and their illness, and healthcare professionals' perception of a patient's ability to afford and manage the medication.[70,71] The use of a fixed-dose combination of medications or "polypill" has been shown to simplify treatment regimens and increase acceptability and has been identified by the WHO as a best buy in the prevention and treatment of CVD.[46] The use of polypills has been shown to work in other disease areas including the use of combination antiretroviral in the treatment of human immunodeficiency virus and antibiotics to cure tuberculosis.[7,68]
- *Quality* of the medication refers to whether the ingredients meet the national standards for purity and concentration, and thereby influences patient access to the medication. This is a problem across HICs as well as LMICs. One study found that 2 out of 10 CVD drugs purchased at retail outlets were substandard in their quality or concentration of ingredients.[68]

Whether it is because the dispensary is out of medication, the patient can't afford the medication, or the regimen is too complicated, a number of potential barriers exist for patients seeking secondary prevention, especially in LMICs. Addressing these barriers include establishing national medicine policies to ensure supply and decrease cost; health workforce development to ensure patients can be seen and prescribed medication; and building public–private partnerships with the pharmaceutical industry to drive down cost and increase availability of generic medications. The overall goal is to increase secondary prevention measures and ultimately significantly reduce CVD morbidity and mortality.

mHealth

Mobile phones are virtually ubiquitous globally. In 2017, it was estimated that there were over 6 billion mobile phone users worldwide and 60% or 3.6 million of mobile phone users were living in LMICs.[72] Broadly described as "mHealth," mobile phones have the potential to improve lifestyle and management of CVD worldwide. In 2015, the American Heart Association released a statement suggesting that mHealth has the potential to significantly impact health communication, provide support for behavior change, and improve medication adherence.[73] mHealth presents a unique opportunity to efficiently and affordably provide patient support for healthy behaviors and medication adherence in a way that is convenient for the patient.

While there needs to be more research to evaluate the effectiveness of using mHealth, initial studies have shown them to be effective in both HICs and LMICs.[72,74,75] A U.S.-based study found that participation in a text messaging program resulted in improved glycemic control and cost savings for patients with diabetes.[76] mHealth has already demonstrated utility in infectious disease in LMICs. Two large randomized trials in Kenya showed that using short message systems, or text messages significantly improved antiretroviral medication adherence in people living with HIV.[72] In Mexico mHealth was used with patients with poorly controlled hypertension to provide weekly support calls customized to the patient. The result was a reduction in systolic blood pressure and improvements in lifestyle risk factors.[72] Further evidence on the effectiveness of mHealth in the prevention and management of CVD is needed, particularly in LMICs, yet early results and evidence of the use of mHealth in management of NCDs and CVD are promising.

Cardiac Rehabilitation

The goal of tertiary prevention is to reduce the risk of long-term disability. By slowing, stabilizing, and promoting regression of

CVD, cardiac rehabilitation has been identified as a cost-effective method for reducing CVD morbidity and mortality.[64,77] The WHO defines cardiac rehabilitation as the "sum of activities required to influence favorably the underlying cause of the disease, as well as to provide the best possible physical, mental and social conditions, so that the patients may, by their own efforts, preserve or resume when lost, as normal a place as possible in the community."[78] Turk-Adawi, Sarrafzadegan, and Grace found that the exercises, education, and risk reduction included in cardiac rehabilitation improve functional capacity, decrease hospital readmission, and reduce mortality by up to 25% in HIC.[77]

Worldwide, fewer than 40% of countries have cardiac rehabilitation and there is great disparity in its availability across country income levels.[77] Turk et al. found that cardiac rehabilitation is available in 68% of HICs, 21% to 28% of middle-income countries and only 8% of low-income countries, with a density of one program per 6 million people in low-income countries.[77] When available, there are several factors that can influence utilization of cardiac rehabilitation. In both HICs and LMICs, barriers to utilization include lack of physician referrals as a result of inadequate knowledge about cardiac rehabilitation and a perception about patients' ability or inability to participate.[77] A 2017 systematic review by Ragupathi et al. identified the absence of physical referral as the biggest barrier to cardiac rehabilitation in LMICs where cardiac rehabilitation is available.[79]

Strategies for increasing the provision and utilization of cardiac rehabilitation include redistribution/dedication of resources and systematic integration of cardiac rehabilitation into care that includes patient referral that is independent of physician bias and leveraging health technology to provide expanded patient support. For example, there has been demonstrated success integrating mHealth and cardiac rehab services. In HICs, integration of a cardiac rehab program and mHealth showed positive results in health behavior change and compliance, physical activity, and clinical outcomes.[80] While such strategies need further evaluation in the context of LMICs, there is opportunity to tailor and adapt existing approaches for delivering cardiac rehabilitation to benefit more patients, especially in LMICs.

CVD IN SPECIAL POPULATIONS

HIV

Currently UNAIDS estimates that there are nearly 37 million people living HIV (PLHIV).[84] As treatment for HIV has evolved and as HIV is increasingly being managed as a chronic illness, the epidemiology of HIV and the associated comorbidities have also changed. Recent studies suggest that PLHIV who initiate antiretroviral therapy (ART) early in the disease progression, experience a life expectancy similar of that to their HIV-negative peers, and this holds true in both HICs and LMICs.[85] PLHIV currently taking antiretroviral medications can expect to live longer and thus are at more risk for developing chronic conditions such as CVD.

There is convincing evidence that PLHIV are at an increased risk for developing cardiac problems.[86] The reasons for this increased risk are not entirely clear but are likely a result of prolonged exposure to the virus, ongoing immunologic dysfunction, and adverse effects associated with ART.[87] HIV infection is associated with hyperlipidemia, and increased blood pressure/hypertension is the most prevalent CVD risk factor in PLHIV.[86] For PLHIV taking ART, in particular protease inhibitors, further increases LDL and HDL and their risk for cardiometabolic and glycemic risk factors including lipids and glucose abnormalities also increases.[88,89] PLHIV have an increased risk for cardiovascular events as well. Data from HICs suggest that PLHIV taking ART have almost a twofold increased risk of heart failure over HIV-negative matched controls.[87] Currently the majority of data on PLHIV and CVD is derived from HICs. The fact that populations living in LMICs experience the highest incidence of both HIV and CVD morbidity and mortality, additional research in LMICs is needed to effectively implement prevention and management interventions in this unique population.[4]

STRUCTURAL HEART DISEASE

Congenital Heart Disease

The incidence of congenital heart disease (CHD) is estimated to be between 8 and 12 per 1000 live-births.[11,90,91] Of those born with CHD, between 5 and 6 per 1000 births is considered complex and requires surgical intervention.[92] Data on CHD incidence, mortality, and morbidity in LMICs are limited. There are several factors that suggest that the CHD burden in LMICs is significant. That fact that LMICs typically have higher fertility rates and lower rates of voluntary termination of pregnancy suggests that the absolute number of CHD births annually may be higher in LMICs than in HICs.[92] It is estimated that 94% of all congenital anomalies occur in LMICs and in 2016 the WHO estimated that more than 30% of all congenital anomalies were cardiac in nature, further suggesting that the majority of CHD incidence occurs in LMICs.[9,93] However, because there is limited prenatal screening and postnatal diagnosis in LMICs, and even less so in low-income countries, exact rates of incidence and mortality are not known.

While additional research is needed to fully understand the impact of CHD in LMICs, methods that consider the CHD burden in terms beyond strict incidence rates may be useful. Hoffman suggests that because the burden of caring and supporting those with CHD falls on individuals who are typically the wage earners in a household, a more useful method for studying the burden of CHD is looking at the incidence of CHD per the number of wage earners.[90] This allows the burden of CHD to be considered in the context of the age distribution across a specific population. For example, in countries with younger populations as is the case in many LMICs where a smaller proportion of the population is considered to be a wage earner, the burden of CHD per wage earner is greater than in populations with a more even age distribution.

It is estimated that only 25% of the world's population has access to cardiac surgery.[90] Given that roughly 50% of infants born with CHD require surgical intervention and the variance in availability of surgical treatment between HICs and LMICs it is not surprising that the outcomes for children born with CHD differ significantly between LMICs and HICs.[92] The discrepancy in outcomes between LMICs and HICs is further highlighted by the ratio of cardiac surgeons to population. In North America, the ratio is estimated to be 1 cardiac surgeon per 3.5 million population while the estimated ratio in Africa is 1 cardiac surgeon per 38 million population.[90] The result of this 10-fold difference is that most children with minor CHD in LMICs may never be diagnosed and the defect may resolve without intervention, meanwhile children with complex CHD in LMICs experience more dire outcomes due to the absence of surgical intervention.

Due to drastically improved survival rates for children born with CHD in HICs, the prevalence of those living with CHD has increased. It is estimated that over 85% of children born with CHD in HICs survive into adult years.[94] Improved survival rates are largely attributed to improvements in diagnostic methods, medical management, surgical interventions, and postoperative care.[95] The current prevalence for CHD in HICs is estimated to be 6.12 per 1000 people and the number of adults with CHD now outnumbers the number of children.[94] Currently the life expectancy for those with moderate defects is 77 years (± 10 years) and 70 years (± 13 years) for those with complex defects.[91]

There are unique population-level considerations with this epidemiologic shift. There is now a need for specialized care for adults living with CHD and this sector of cardiology is the fastest growing sector within the specialty of cardiology.[95] Adults with CHD are predisposed to a variety of both cardiovascular and other comorbidities. The specific nature and complexity of their CHD influences their degree of risk but in general, adults with CHD face an increased risk for cardiovascular comorbidities including arrhythmias, sudden cardiac death, heart failure, coronary artery disease, endocarditis, and pulmonary hypertension.[91,94,95] Non-cardiovascular comorbidities include lung, renal, and hepatic diseases.[91] Adults with CHD also face increased risk of persistent neurocognitive deficits associated with childhood CHD. These deficits have the potential to impact the education, employment, and relationships of adults with CHD.

From a population perspective, options for CHD prevention are limited. Only 20% of CHD cases have identifiable causes.[92] Population-level prevention measures include rubella vaccination and folic acid and vitamin B_{12} supplementation for all women of childbearing age as well as providing primary and prenatal care to support women in managing pre-existing metabolic disorders such as diabetes.[92]

There are limited data to support the positive predictive value of prenatal, neonatal, and school-age screening of CHD.[92] Prenatal and neonatal screenings are time consuming and resource intensive, making them impractical in many LMICs. Further, screenings are most useful in detecting complex CHD. This may be useful in situations where surgical intervention is available; however, few people in LMICs have the necessary resources to travel for care if it is not already readily available. School-age screening can be conducted with minimal resources and can be integrated into other health screenings, but without more specialized follow-up care such screenings are unlikely to alter outcomes.[92] Primary and secondary prevention of CVD at the population level requires a longer-term investment of resources including improved disease surveillance to better understand the CHD burden and support prioritization of surgical and palliative interventions, strengthening surgical capacity including enhancing health facility infrastructure and workforce development for skilled nursing, specialized physicians and anesthesia and others.

Rheumatic Heart Disease

While rheumatic heart disease (RHD) is no longer a significant health threat in HICs, it continues to contribute to cardiac morbidity and mortality in LMICs, with higher prevalence in South Asia, Africa, and the Pacific Islands.[96] In 2016, GBD data indicated that RHD was attributed to approximately 314,000 deaths, 57% of which occurred in LMICs and that of the global incidence of RHD, 80% occurred in LMICs.[8] RHD was responsible for 9.8 million DALYs globally, of which 7 million were in LMICs.[8] In fact, RHD was the single largest contributor to CVD morbidity and mortality for children, adolescents, and young adults living in LMICs.[97]

There is currently some debate as to the accuracy of prevalence statistics. This is in large part because definitive diagnosis of RHD requires microbiology and/or echocardiography, which are not widely available in LMICs. One study has indicated that screening of school children for RHD found a 10-fold higher prevalence than initially estimated.[92] In addition, recurrent acute rheumatic fever, which is caused by untreated group A streptococcal pharyngitis, can result in asymptomatic and clinically undetectable infection. A study in Uganda found that of 309 newly diagnosis cases of RHD, none had a confirmed history of acute rheumatic fever.[97] It is estimated that 50% to 75% of all cases of acute rheumatic fever have no history of systematic pharyngitis.[92] The fact that acute rheumatic fever can be asymptomatic and often goes undetected further complicates estimation of RHD prevalence. Individual risk factors associated with RHD are those most associated with poverty and include poor sanitation, undernutrition, and living in rural or overcrowded locations.[92,96,97] Poor access to primary healthcare, insufficient access to medicines, and limited availability of cardiac surgery contribute to RHD morbidity and mortality at the population level.[92,96,97]

The WHO and World Heart Federation have called for a 25% reduction in premature mortality due to RHD by 2025. However, there are few studies documenting the effectiveness of primary and secondary interventions at the population level. A dated study in the U.S. military indicated that prophylactic treatment with antibiotics (penicillin) can reduce RHD incidence by 80%.[92] This study did not demonstrate a reduction in mortality and has not been replicated in populations where RHD is endemic.[92] Short of vaccine development, primary prevention including testing and treatment of streptococcal pharyngitis as part of routine child health coupled with campaigns aimed at community education are the most promising interventions for reducing RHD-attributable morbidity and mortality. Other primary prevention measures include minimizing exposure to risk factors such as reducing overcrowding, strengthening primary care services, and improving sanitation. Secondary prevention using regular penicillin prophylaxis in those with known RHD is effective but the possibility of surgical intervention is very low in most endemic areas. Reducing RHD morbidity and mortality through surgical interventions may be impractical in endemic areas.

CONCLUSIONS

Summary

NCDs and specifically, CVD represent a significant and growing burden globally. Increasingly there has been a global focus on primary prevention of CVD lifestyle and behavioral risk factors including reducing tobacco use, increasing physical activity, limiting trans fat, sodium, and sugar-sweetened beverages. Some risk factors that are not exclusively behavioral in nature, such as exposure to air pollution, require more international and intersectoral efforts to mitigate.

Despite these efforts, CVD morbidity and mortality remains a significant burden on vulnerable populations and the greatest burden is borne in populations with the fewest resources. There is a substantial evidence base demonstrating the effectiveness and feasibility of interventions that reduce CVD risk and it is imperative that such knowledge is applied to stem CVD morbidity and mortality in LMICs.

Future Considerations and Implications

Nurses play a critical role in the primary and secondary prevention of CVD morbidity and mortality globally and are uniquely positioned to impact CVD morbidity and mortality in a variety of ways. As researchers, nurses have the capability to study the feasibility and validate the effectiveness of evidence-based interventions to prevent and manage CVD. As policy makers, nurses have the capacity to implement and regulate public policy that reduces population exposure to risk factors. Also, because nurses are often the front-line healthcare professionals who have the most contact with individual patients, nurses are positioned to play a pivotal role in promoting healthy behaviors and supporting patients to engage in primary and secondary prevention activities. As stated earlier, even small reductions in individual CVD risk can culminate in significant reductions in population CVD risk.

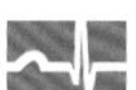 CASE STUDY

Nurse-led Initiatives in the Management of Hypertension

Patient Profile

Nurses and the role they play in primary care are fundamental in the successful management of CVD. Few LMICs offer specialized cardiovascular care and primary care facilities and the nurses that work in them serve as the first line in the treatment and prevention of CVD. This case study demonstrates the opportunities and potential that exists for nurses to affect CVD.

In 2014, researchers at the Icahn and Duke Schools of Medicine, in collaboration with Centro Nacional de Investigaciones in Madrid and Moi University and the Academic Model Providing Access to Healthcare in Kenya, embarked on a research study to evaluate the effectiveness of task-shifting in two rural divisions in western Kenya. "Task-shifting" refers to the delegation of certain tasks from higher-level healthcare professionals (e.g., physicians) to less specialized professionals (e.g., nurses). At the time of the study's initiation, GBD data indicated that nearly 30,000 deaths and 722,000 DALYs were attributable to CVD in Kenya.[8] The estimated physician to patient ratio in 2014 was 0.204 per 1000 people and 0.48 nurses per 1000 people.[81] This is well below the WHO threshold of a minimum of 2.3 physicians and nurses per 1000 population.[82]

The primary outcome for evaluating the efficacy of this model were changes in systolic blood pressure. The intervention consisted of community wide in-home measurement of blood pressures and those participants with elevated blood pressure (systolic greater than 140 or diastolic greater than 90) were referred to a nurse run dispensary for further evaluation. Once at the dispensary repeat blood pressures were taken and those with a second elevated pressure were enrolled into the program. High-risk individuals including those who were symptomatic or had other high-risk factors were referred to more specialized care at the health center. For those enrolled in the program nurse management for hypertension included lifestyle counseling and prescription of medications that included clear algorithms for escalating pharmacotherapy and referrals to specialized care.

While this study is ongoing, initial results are positive and significant with an average decrease of 22.1 mm Hg from baseline systolic blood pressures.[83] This pilot program has demonstrated the initial feasibility of a hypertension management by nurses but will require that the barriers identified are addressed prior to larger-scale implementation.

KEY READINGS

Bansilal S, Castellano JM, Fuster V. Global burden of CVD: focus on secondary prevention of cardiovascular disease. *Int J Cardiol.* 2015;201:S1–S7.

Dougherty S, Beaton A, Nascimento BR, et al. Prevention and control of rheumatic heart disease: overcoming core challenges in resource-poor environments. *Ann Pediatr Cardiol.* 2018;11(1):68–78.

Joseph P, Leong D, Mckee M, et al. Reducing the global burden of cardiovascular disease part 1 the epidemiology and risk factors. *Circ Res.* 2017;121(6):677–694.

Leong DP, Joseph PG, McKee M, et al. Reducing the global burden of cardiovascular disease, part 2: prevention and treatment of cardiovascular disease. *Circ Res.* 2017;121(6):695–710.

REFERENCES

1. Omran A. The epidemiologic transition: a theory of the epidemiology of population change. *Milbank Mem Fund Q.* 1971;49(1):509–538.
2. Bowry ADK, Lewey J, Dugani SB, et al. The burden of cardiovascular disease in low- and middle-income countries: epidemiology and management. *Can J Cardiol.* 2015;31:1151–1159.
3. Lozano R, Naghavi M, Lim SS, et al. Global and regional mortality from 235 causes of death for 20 age groups in 1990 and 2010: a systematic analysis for the global burden of disease study 2010. *Lancet.* 2012;380: 2095–2128.
4. World Health Organization. *Global health estimates 2016: Deaths by Cause, Age, Sex, by Country and by Region, 2000–2016.* Geneva: 2018.
5. Yusuf S, Reddy S, Ôunpuu S, et al. *Global burden of cardiovascular diseases part I: general considerations, the epidemiologic transition, risk factors, and impact of urbanization.* 2001. Available at http://www.circulationaha.org. Accessed August 29, 2018.
6. Okwuosa IS, Lewsey SC, Adesiyun T, et al. Worldwide disparities in cardiovascular disease: challenges and solutions. *Int J Cardiol.* 2016;202: 433–440.
7. Yeates K, Lohfeld L, Sleeth J, et al. A global perspective on cardiovascular disease in vulnerable populations. *Can J Cardiol.* 2015;31(9): 1081–1093.
8. *Global Burden of Disease Collaborative Network. Global Burden of Disease Study 2016 (GBD 2016) Results.* Seattle, United States; 2018. Available at http://ghdx.healthdata.org/gbd-results-tool. Accessed September 7, 2018.
9. World Health Organization. *WHO Global Disease Burden and mortality estimates; 2016.* 2016. Available at http://www.who.int/healthinfo/global_burden_disease/estimates/en/
10. Prabhakaran D, Anand S, Watkins D, et al. Cardiovascular, respiratory, and related disorders: key messages from disease control priorities, 3rd edition. *Lancet.* 2018;391(10126):1224–1236.
11. Mcaloon CJ, Boylan LM, Hamborg T, et al. The changing face of cardiovascular disease 2000–2012: an analysis of the world health organisation global health estimates data. *Int J Cardiol.* 2016;224:256–264.
12. Deaton C, Froelicher E, Wu L, et al. The global burden of cardiovascular disease. *Eur J Cardiovasc Nurs.* 2011;10(2 suppl):S5–S13.

13. Yusuf S, Rangarajan S, Teo K, et al. Cardiovascular risk and events in 17 low-, middle-, and high-income countries. *N Engl J Med.* 2014;371(9): 818–827.
14. Roth GA, Forouzanfar MH, Moran AE, et al. Demographic and epidemiologic drivers of global cardiovascular mortality. *N Engl J Med.* 2015;372(14):1333–1341.
15. Feigin VL, Norrving B, Mensah GA. Primary prevention of cardiovascular disease through population-wide motivational strategies: insights from using smartphones in stroke prevention. *BMJ Global Health.* 2017;2(2):e000306.
16. Bansilal S, Castellano JM, Fuster V. Global burden of CVD: focus on secondary prevention of cardiovascular disease. *Int J Cardiol.* 2015;201:S1–S7.
17. World Health Organization. 2013–2020 Global action plan for the prevention and control of noncommunicable diseases. Geneva; 2013. Available at http://www.unaids.org/sites/default/files/media_asset/UNAIDS_FactSheet_en.pdf. Accessed August 1, 2018.
18. United Nations General Assembly. High-level meeting on prevention and control of noncommunicable diseases. In: *WHO UN High-Level Meeting on Prevention and Control of Noncommunicable Diseases UN General Assembly.* New York. 2018.
19. World Health Organization. From burden to best buys: reducing the economic impact of non-communicable diseases in low-and middle-income countries. 2011. Available at www.who.int. Accessed September 11, 2018.
20. World Health Organization. *Social determinants of health.* 2018. Available at http://www.who.int/social_determinants/en/
21. Gaziano T, Abrahams-Gessel S, Surka S, et al. Cardiovascular disease screening by community health workers can be cost-effective in low-resource countries. *Health Aff.* 2015;34(9):1538–1545.
22. Laslett LJ, Alagona P, Clark BA, et al. The worldwide environment of cardiovascular disease: prevalence, diagnosis, therapy, and policy issues. A report from the American College of Cardiology. *J Am Coll Cardiol.* 2012; 60:S1–S49.
23. Wang L, Mamudu HM, Collins C, et al. High prevalence of tobacco use and exposure to secondhand tobacco smoke among adolescents in low- and middle-income countries. *Ann Transl Med.* 2017;5(1):795–805.
24. Centers for Disease Control. *Cigarette smoking among adults United States 1998. MMWR. morbidity and mortality weekly report.* 1998. Available at https://www.cdc.gov/mmwr/preview/mmwrhtml/mm4939a1.htm
25. Centers for Disease Control and Prevention. *Current cigarette smoking among adults in the United States. Smoking and tobacco use fast facts and fact sheets.* 2016. Available at https://www.cdc.gov/tobacco/data_statistics/fact_sheets/adult_data/cig_smoking/index.htm
26. Anderson CL, Becher H, Winkler V, et al. Tobacco control progress in low and middle income countries in comparison to high income countries. *Int J Environ Res Public Health.* 2016;13(10):E1039.
27. Burroughs Pena MS, Bloomfield GS. Cardiovascular disease research and the development agenda in low- and middle-income countries HHS public access. *Global Heart.* 2015;10(1):71–73.
28. World Health Organization. *Framework convention on tobacco control.* 2018. Available at http://www.who.int/fctc/signatories_parties/en/. Accessed August 27, 2018.
29. World Health Organization. *Obesity and overweight. Fact sheet.* 2018. Available at http://www.who.int/news-room/fact-sheets/detail/obesity-and-overweight. Accessed August 30, 2018.
30. Basu S. The transitional dynamics of caloric ecosystems: changes in the food supply around the world. *Critical Public Health.* 2015;25(3):248–264.
31. Anand SS, Hawkes C, De Souza RJ, et al. Food consumption and its impact on cardiovascular disease: importance of solutions focused on the globalized food system a report from the workshop convened by the World heart federation. *J Am Coll Cardiol.* 2015;66(14):1590–1614.
32. World Health Organization. *Guidelines: sodium intake for adults and children.* Geneva; 2012. Available at http://apps.who.int/iris/bitstream/handle/10665/77985/9789241504836_eng.pdf;jsessionid=3CF529587B648BD567C7B083FAD04897?sequence=1
33. Hope SF, Webster J, Trieu K, et al. A systematic review of economic evaluations of population-based sodium reduction interventions. *PLoS One.* 2017;12(3):e0173600.
34. Hyseni L, Elliot-Green A, Lloyd-Williams F, et al. Systematic review of dietary salt reduction policies: evidence for an effectiveness hierarchy? *PLoS One.* 2017;12(5):e0177535.
35. Cochero A, Rivera-Dommarco J, Popkin BM, et al. In Mexico, evidence of sustained consumer response two years after implementing a sugar-sweetened beverage tax. *Health Aff.* 2017;36(3):564–571.
36. Basu S, Madsen K. Effectiveness and equity of sugar-sweetened beverage taxation. *PLoS Med.* 2017;14(6):e1002327.
37. Aburto TC, Pedraza LS, Sánchez-Pimienta TG, et al. Results from the national health and nutrition survey. *J Nutr.* 2012;146(9):1881S–1887S.
38. Hashem K, Rosborough J. Why tax sugar sweetened beverages? *J Pediatr Gastroenterol Nutr.* 2017;65(4):358–359.
39. World Health Organization. *WHO plan to eliminate industrially-produced trans-fatty acids from global food supply.* 2018. Available at http://www.who.int/news-room/detail/14-05-2018-who-plan-to-eliminate-industrially-produced-trans-fatty-acids-from-global-food-supply. Accessed August 31, 2018.
40. World Health Organization. *Policies to eliminate industrially-produced trans fat consumption.* 2018. Available at http://www.who.int/docs/default-source/documents/replace-transfats/replace-act-information-sheet.pdf. Accessed August 31, 2018.
41. Downs SM, Bloem MZ, Zheng M, et al. *The impact of policies to reduce trans fat consumption: a systematic review of the evidence.* 2017. Available at August 31, 2018, from http://www.ovid.com/site/catalog/databases/901. Accessed August 31, 2018.
42. Yusuf S, Hawken S, Ôunpuu S, et al. Effect of potentially modifiable risk factors associated with myocardial infarction in 52 countries (the INTERHEART Study) case control study. *Lancet.* 2004;364:937–952.
43. Ronksley PE, Brien SE, Turner BJ. Association of alcohol consumption with selected cardiovascular disease outcomes: a systematic review and meta-analysis. *Br Med J.* 2011;342:d671.
44. GBD 2016 Alcohol Collaborators. Articles Alcohol use and burden for 195 countries and territories, 1990–2016: a systematic analysis for the Global Burden of Disease Study 2016. *Lancet.* 2018;392(10152): 1015–1035.
45. Esser MB, Jernigan DH. Policy approaches for regulating alcohol marketing in a global context: a public health perspective. *Annu Rev Public Health.* 2018;39:385–401.
46. World Health Organization. Chapter 4-Reducing risks and preventing disease: population-wide interventions. In: *Global Status Report on NCDs.* 2010. 47–60. Available at http://www.who.int/nmh/publications/ncd_report_chapter4.pdf. Accessed August 31, 2018.
47. Franklin BA, Brook R, Arden Pope C. Air pollution and cardiovascular disease. *Curr Probl Cardiol.* 2015;40(5):207–238.
48. Brook RD, Rajagopalan S, Arden, C, et al. AHA scientific statement particulate matter air pollution and cardiovascular disease an update to the scientific statement from the American heart association. *Circulation.* 2010;121(21):2331–2378.
49. Chowdhury R, Lawrence R, van Daalen K, et al. Reducing NCDs globally: the under-recognised role of environmental risk factors. *Lancet.* 2018; 392(10143):212.
50. Bourdrel T, Bind MA, Béjot Y, et al. Effets cardiovasculaires de la pollution de l'air. *Arch Cardiovasc Dis.* 2017;110(11):634–642.
51. Franchini M, Mannucci PM. Air pollution and cardiovascular disease. *Thromb Res.* 2012;129(3):230–234.
52. Forastiere F, Agabiti N. Assessing the link between air pollution and heart failure. *Lancet.* 2013;382(9897):1008–1010.
53. Lee KK, Miller MR, Shah A. Special review air pollution and stroke. *J Stroke.* 2018;20(1):2–11.
54. Martinelli N, Olivieri O, Girelli D. Air particulate matter and cardiovascular disease: a narrative review. *Eur J Intern Med.* 2013;24(4):295–302.
55. World Health Organization. *Breathe life – a global campaign for clean air.* 2018. Available at http://breathelife2030.org/. Accessed March 8, 2019.
56. World Health Organization. *Global Action Plan on Physical Activity 2018–20130.* Geneva; 2018. Available at http://apps.who.int/iris/bitstream/handle/10665/272722/9789241514187-eng.pdf. Accessed September 1, 2018.
57. Hallal PC, Andersen LB, Bull FC, et al. Physical Activity 1 Global physical activity levels: surveillance progress, pitfalls, and prospects. *Lancet.* 2012;380:247–257.
58. Allen L, Williams J, Townsend N, et al. Socioeconomic status and non-communicable disease behavioural risk factors in low-income and lower-middle-income countries: a systematic review. *Lancet Global Health.* 2017;5(3):e277–e289.
59. Sallis JF, Bull F, Guthold R, et al. Physical activity 2016: progress and challenges progress in physical activity over the olympic quadrennium. *Lancet.* 2016;388(10051):1325–1336.
60. Koyanagi A, Stubbs B, Vancampfort D. Correlates of low physical activity across 46 low- and middle-income countries: a cross-sectional analysis of community-based data. *Prev Med.* 2018;106:107–113.
61. Pratt M, Perez LG, Goenka S, et al. Can population levels of physical activity be increased? Global evidence and experience. *Prog Cardiovasc Dis.* 2014;57:356–367.

62. Banerjee A, Khandelwal S, Nambiar L, et al. Health system barriers and facilitators to medication adherence for the secondary prevention of cardiovascular disease: a systematic review. *Open Heart*. 2016;3(2):e000438.
63. Aminde LN, Fongwen Takah N, Zapata-Diomedi B, et al. Primary and secondary prevention interventions for cardiovascular disease in low-income and middle-income countries: a systematic review of economic evaluations. *Cost Eff Resour Alloc*. 2018;16:22.
64. Mendis S, Fukino K, Cameron A, et al. The availability and affordability of selected essential. *Bull World Health Organ*. 2007;85(4):279–288.
65. Yusuf S, Islam S, Chow CK, et al. Use of secondary prevention drugs for cardiovascular disease in the community in high-income, middle-income, and low-income countries (the PURE Study): a prospective epidemiological survey. *Lancet*. 2011;378(9798):1231–1243.
66. Leong DP, Joseph PG, McKee M, et al. Reducing the global burden of cardiovascular disease, part 2: prevention and treatment of cardiovascular disease. *Circ Res*. 2017;121(6):695–710.
67. Chow CK, Teo KK, Rangarajan S, et al. Prevalence, awareness, treatment, and control of hypertension in rural and urban communities in high-, middle-, and low-income countries. *JAMA*. 2013;310(9):959–968.
68. Wirtz VJ, Kaplan WA, Kwan GF, et al. Access to medications for cardiovascular diseases in low- and middle-income countries HHS public access. *Circulation*. 2016;133(21):2076–2085.
69. Cameron A, Roubos I, Ewen M, et al. Differences in the availability of medicines for chronic and acute conditions in the public and private sectors of developing countries. *Bull World Health Organ*. 2011;89(6):412–421.
70. Khatib R, Schwalm JD, Yusuf S, et al. Patient and healthcare provider barriers to hypertension awareness, treatment and follow up: a systematic review and meta-analysis of qualitative and quantitative studies. *PLoS One*. 2014;9(1):e84238.
71. Bigdeli M, Jacobs B, Tomson G, et al. Access to medicines from a health system perspective. *Health Policy Plan*. 2013;28:692–704.
72. Piette JD, List J, Rana GK, et al. . Mobile health devices as tools for worldwide cardiovascular risk reduction and disease management. *Circulation*. 2015;132(21):2012–2027.
73. Burke L, Ma J, Azar KM, et al. Current science on consumer use of mobile health for cardiovascular disease prevention: a scientific statement from the American Heart Association. *Circulation*. 2015;132:1157–1213.
74. Redfern J, Thiagalingam A, Jan S, et al. Development of a set of mobile phone text messages designed for prevention of recurrent cardiovascular events. *Eur J Prev Cardiol*. 2014;21(4):492–499.
75. Chow CK, Islam SMS, Farmer A, et al. Text2PreventCVD: protocol for a systematic review and individual participant data meta-analysis of text message-based interventions for the prevention of cardiovascular diseases. *BMJ Open*. 2016;6(10):1–8.
76. Nundy S, Dick JJ, Nocon RS, et al. Mobile phone diabetes project led to improved glycemic control and net savings for Chicago plan participants. *Health Aff*. 2014;33(2):265–272.
77. Turk-Adawi K, Sarrafzadegan N, Grace S. Global availability of cardiac rehabilitation. *Nat Rev Cardiol*. 2014;11(10):586–596.
78. World Health Organization. *Prevention of Cardiovascular Disease Guidelines for Assessment and Management of Cardiovascular Risk*. Geneva; 2007. Available at www.inis.ie. Accessed September 3, 2018.
79. Ragupathi L, Stribling J, Yakunina Y, et al. Availability, use, and barriers to cardiac rehabilitation in LMIC. *Global Heart*. 2017;12(4):323–334.
80. Munro J, Angus N, Leslie SJ. Patient focused internet-based approaches to cardiovascular rehabilitation—a systematic review. *J Telemed Telecare*. 2013;19(6):347–353.
81. World Health Organization. *Density of physicians and nurses (per 1,000 population)*. Global health observatory data. 2018. Available at http://www.who.int/gho/health_workforce/physicians_density/en/
82. World Health Organization. *Achieving the health-related MDGs. It takes a workforce!*. 2018. Available at http://www.who.int/hrh/workforce_mdgs/en/
83. Kumar A, Kamano J, Too K, et al. Effect of nurse-based management of hypertension in rural western Kenya. *J Am Coll Cardiol*.2016;67(13): 1944.
84. UNAIDS. *2017 Global HIV Statistics*. UNAIDS. 2018. Available at http://www.unaids.org/sites/default/files/media_asset/UNAIDS_FactSheet_en.pdf
85. Maartens G, Meintjes G. Improved life expectancy of people living with HIV: who is left behind? *Lancet HIV*. 2017;4:e324–e326.
86. Patel P, Rose CE, Collins PY, et al. Noncommunicable diseases among HIV-infected persons in low-income and middle-income countries. *AIDS*. 2018;32(suppl 1):S5–S20.
87. Bloomfield GS, Khazanie P, Morris A, et al. HIV and non-communicable cardiovascular and pulmonary diseases in low- and middle-income countries in the ART Era: what we know and best directions for future research. *J Acquir Immune Defic Syndr*. 2014;67(1):40–53.
88. Ali MK, Magee MJ, Dave JA, et al. HIV and metabolic, body, and bone disorders: what we know from low-and middle-income countries, *J Acquir Immune Defic Syndr*. 2014;67:S27–S39.
89. Barr AL, Young EH, Smeeth L, et al. The need for an integrated approach for chronic disease research and care in Africa. *Global Health Epidemiol Genom*. 2016;1:e19.
90. Hoffman JI. The global burden of congenital heart disease. *Cardiovasc J Afr*. 2013;24(4):141–145.
91. Steiner JM, Kovacs AH. Adults with congenital heart disease – Facing morbidities and uncertain early mortality. *Prog Pediatr Cardiol*. 2018;48: 75–81.
92. Prabhakaran D, Anand S, Gaziano T, et al. Structural heart disease. In: *Disease Control Priorities Network Cardiovascular, Respiratory and Related Disorders*. 3rd ed. Washington, DC: World Bank; 2017:191–208.
93. Sitkin NA, Ozgediz D, Donkor P, et al. Congenital anomalies in low- and middle-income countries: the unborn child of global surgery. *World J Surg*. 2015;39(1):36–40.
94. Webb G, Mulder BJ, Aboulhosn J, et al. The care of adults with congenital heart disease across the globe: current assessment and future perspective: a position statement from the International Society for Adult Congenital Heart Disease (ISACHD). *Int J Cardiol*. 2015;195:326–333.
95. Ávila P, Ee Mercier LA, Dore A, et al. Adult congenital heart disease: a growing epidemic. *Can J Cardiol*. 2014;30:410–419.
96. Watkins DA, Johnson CO, Colquhoun SM, et al. Global, regional, and national burden of rheumatic heart disease, 1990–2015. *N Engl J Med*. 2017; 377(8):713–722.
97. Curry C, Zuhlke L, Mocumbi A, et al. Acquired heart disease in low-income and middle-income countries. *Arch Dis Child*. 2018;10:73–77.

43 Quality in Cardiovascular Care

Katie N. Jaschke

OBJECTIVES

1. Identify definitions of quality in health care.
2. Explore the history and practice of quality care.
3. Determine how quality care affects patient outcomes.

KEY QUESTIONS

1. Why does a goal need to have measurable criteria?
2. How are clinical practice guidelines (CPGs) developed?

BACKGROUND

The Institute of Medicine (IOM) has defined quality of health care as "the degree to which health services for individuals and populations increase the likelihood of desired health outcomes and are consistent with current professional knowledge."[1]

When quality care is discussed it would be remiss not to mention medical errors are now the third leading cause of death in the United States.[2] Because of the importance of patient outcomes, one of the top priorities for healthcare organizations is to achieve high-quality care with low complications independent of patient acuity. The IOM landmark paper, Crossing the Quality Chasm, highlights the development of a strategy to improve quality in health care.[3] Six domains were developed with core needs for health care to be safe, effective, patient-centered, timely, efficient, and equitable. When discussing healthcare improvements, quality is centric to all of these elements.

HISTORY OF QUALITY DETERMINANTS

Avedis Donabedian was a professor of medical care organization at the University of Michigan. He was a nonpracticing physician who focused his studies on quality of care.[4] In 1966, Dr. Avedis Donabedian, physician and founder of the study of quality in health care and medical outcomes research published "Evaluating the Quality of Medical Care." As part of his work, he concluded quality is a diverse concept that neither a unifying construct nor a single measure could be developed to define a singular quality concept.[5] Donabedian postulated that good structure should promote good processes and therefore promote good outcomes. He also specified that there are two kinds of outcomes: technical and interpersonal. Technical outcomes involve the physical and functional aspects of care. This includes absence of complications, disease reduction, reduction in disability, and lowering mortality. Interpersonal outcomes include patient satisfaction on care and quality of life as perceived by the patient.[6]

As part of his work, he proposed using structure, outcomes, and process as a way to evaluate quality of care. Structure includes settings of care, qualification of providers, and the administrative systems where the care takes place.[4] Determination of outcome quality evaluates the patient recovery, restoration of function, as well as mortality. Finally, processes are the components of care delivered (Fig. 43-1).

Florence Nightingale

In nursing it is noted the concept of quality began with Florence Nightingale. Nightingale was among the first to develop a theoretical approach to quality improvement (QI). Her work addressed nursing interventions and health quality by identifying and working to eliminate factors that hindered patient care.[7] The concept of evidence-based QI was evident when she demonstrated that basic sanitation and hygiene standards led to decreased mortality when caring for soldiers wounded in the Crimean War.[8] She used medical statistics to reveal the nature of infection in hospitals and on the battlefield. Nightingale assembled data and evidence to establish guidelines for healthcare reform.[9] Nightingale supervised the modernization of nursing, was a government advisor on

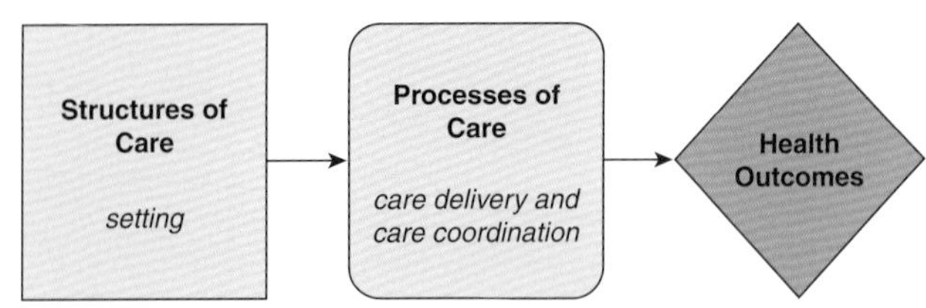

Figure 43-1. Donabedian quality. (Used with permission from Frontera WR, DeLisa JA, Gans BM, et al. *DeLisa's Physical Medicine and Rehabilitation: Principles and Practice*. 6th ed. Philadelphia, PA: Wolters Kluwer; 2019.)

Army health reform, organized sanitary improvements in Britain and India, and influenced hospital design. Gathering evidence to support the need for such reforms, Nightingale utilized observation, record keeping, and statistical analysis to validate her work in each of these developments.[9]

DEFINING QUALITY IN HEALTH CARE

There are five perspectives from which quality can be viewed: patient/client, medicine, nursing, purchaser, and provider.[10] Each of these perspectives will have varied viewpoints dependent on the user. Many think of outcomes as the determination of quality, however outcomes are only one aspect of quality care. Patients can experience good outcomes despite inferior care while others may experience undesirable outcomes in spite of receiving the best possible care. The World Health Organization (WHO) of quality of care is "the extent to which the health care services provided to individuals and patient populations improve the desired health outcomes. In order to achieve this, health care must be safe, effective, timely, efficient, equitable, and people-centered."[11] The IOM (2019) defines healthcare quality as "the degree to which health services for individuals and populations increase the likelihood of desired health outcomes and are consistent with current professional knowledge"[12] The second portion of the IOM definition states that high-quality care is up to date, a task that for anyone who has been to a national cardiology conference knows, it a challenging feat to say the least. *The Journal of the American College of Cardiology (JACC)* publishes a journal with new science weekly. *JACC* also publishes seven subspecialized journals adding to the near 50 ranked cardiovascular journals.[13,14] In addition to publications, hundreds of studies are presented as abstracts year round at conferences. It is easy to see the complexity of defining quality care.

MEASURING QUALITY

Defining and measuring quality in health care is quite challenging and is often an everlasting cycle. Quality measures are tools that help to quantify healthcare processes, outcomes, patient perceptions, and organizational structure. These measures are associated with the ability to provide high-quality health care and relate the goals to care. A quality measurement tool must be objective, based on scientific evidence, and not affect or distort the results.[15] Figure 43-2 demonstrates the steps in auditing quality control. The first, and likely most important step, is identifying a measurable goal. The criterion, or standard, specified is the mark against which success is measured. The tool must contain various elements. The tool should be reliable. A reliable tool results in the same reading regardless of who does the measuring or where and when the measurement is performed. Second, the tool should be valid and measure what it is intended to measure. Finally, the tool should be standardized. A standard tool defines the data elements, how data is collected, and a method for data analysis. A standard tool should be performed in the same way regardless of who is performing or applying the tool.[15]

For example, the agreed upon standard may be that a surgical site is checked every 15 minutes for 1 hour, then every 30 minutes

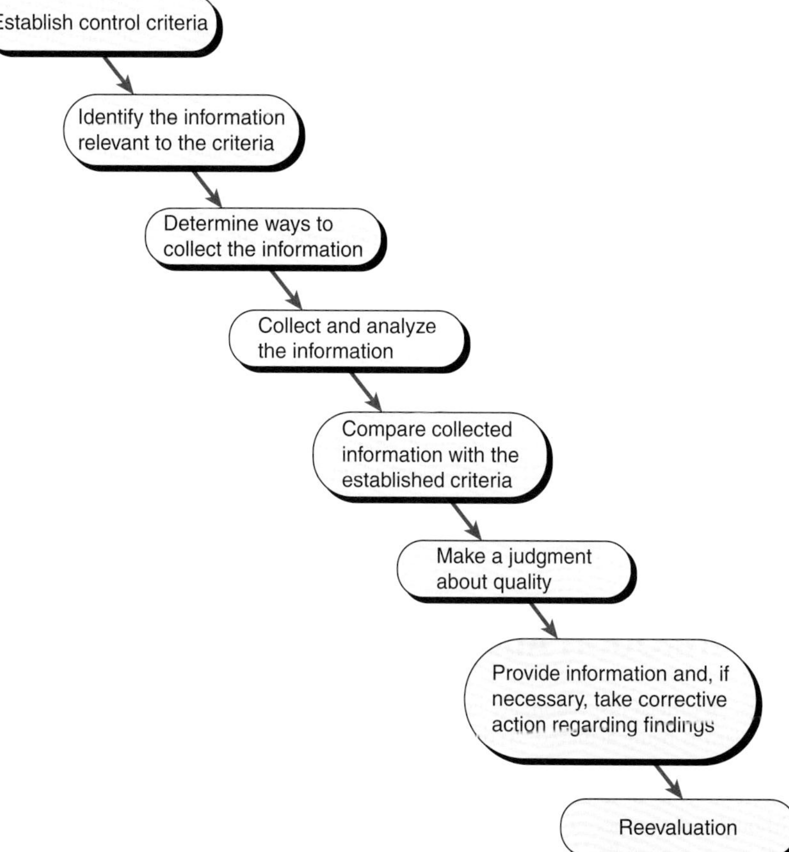

Figure 43-2. Steps in auditing quality control. (Used with permission from Marquis BL, Huston CJ. *Leadership and Management Tools for the New Nurse*. Philadelphia, PA: Wolters Kluwer; 2012.)

for an hour, followed by hourly for a total 4 hours. All the nurses who work on this unit should be well educated on this standard and how evaluation will occur. In this case the nurse performance will be evaluated to note if the standard is achieved. Another way to establish standards is to use *benchmarking*, which is the process of measuring products, practices, and services against the best-performing organizations.[16] Benchmarking allows a hospital to compare themselves to similar health care systems and use top-rated institutions as a role model for achievement. Often, the wheel does not need to be reinvented and adopting processes from high-performing organizations can help drive QI.

The next steps involved are to identify what information will need to be collected, how to gather that information, and how to synthesize the data. In the example of patient management following a coronary angiogram, frequency and number of access site assessments, as well as pulse checks would be the information that could be collected. The best way to accumulate this data would likely to be abstract patients' charts or create a query via the EMR that would pull the data and provide a report. Once the data is collected, it can be analyzed.

The analysis should then be compared to the standard. If the unit fell short of their quality goal, the manager may need to investigate contributing factors and create an action plan for correction. The standard itself may need to be reevaluated to ensure that it is appropriate and attainable. The last step in the process is to reevaluate and start the process again from the top. The same standard can be reevaluated after corrective action or if the standard is met with confidence, the unit may choose to focus on a new goal.[16]

DEVELOPING STANDARDS

A standard is a prespecified level of quality developed by an organization or profession that serves as a guide for practice. Standards must be objective, measurable, and achievable.[16] A policy and procedural document will usually reference the hospital standards for nursing care. Standards are created, adopted, and revised through consensus-based processes managed by standards developing organizations (SDOs). The SDOs are composed of members that use the standards, typically organizations such as hospitals, laboratories, and pharmacies.[17]

Efforts have been made to create more universal standards, rather than location-specific policies. The American Nurses Association (ANA) publishes standards for nursing practice.[18] As well, the Agency for Healthcare Research and Quality (AHRQ) developed diagnosis-related standardized clinical practice guidelines (CPGs) to provide best practice recommendations based on extensive literature review.[19] The National Guideline Clearinghouse was developed in 1998 to provide an evidence-based database of CPGs.[16]

QUALITY CONTROL THROUGH AUDITS

Audits, an official inspection, are useful tools to measure whether a standard is being achieved. Audits can be conducted retrospectively, concurrently, or prospectively to the services provided. Different types of audits are utilized in the healthcare setting. Although other types of audits exist, we will focus on outcome audits, process audits, and structure audits. Outcomes are the result or consequence of care. For example, familiar outcomes that are often audited in the healthcare setting are mortality, length of stay, and complications. Nursing-sensitive indicators, outcomes impacted by quality nursing care, may include ventilator-associated pneumonia, catheter-associated urinary tract infections (CAUTI), falls, and skin break down. It is important to recognize that many factors contribute to outcomes. Audits can help identify behaviors or processes that can be altered to improve these outcomes. Process audits look at the process of care with the assumption that it directly impacts the quality of care. A structure audit examines the resources in the environment in which care is being provided, such as, staffing ratios, call lights within reach, and number of code carts on the unit. The structure of the environment is often separate from the healthcare worker, the patient, and the relationship between them.[16]

To incorporate all three types of audits, picture an inpatient unit whose outcome report card demonstrates increasing CAUTI rates (outcome audit). A process audit could be conducted to investigate how often Foley care and patient baths were documented in the chart. A structural audit might look at staffing ratios to see if there was a difference in quarters where the unit had lower CAUTI rates. Another example of a structural audit would be to look at whether the unit was stocked with adequate supplies to provide Foley care per hospital protocol or if the unit recently changed products to provide Foley care.

EVOLUTION OF QUALITY IN HEALTH CARE

Quality in health care is the responsibly of everyone within the organization. From an individual perspective, participation in quality control promotes professionalism by providing feedback on outcomes. This allows nurse to identify areas of opportunity, strategically plan to make improvements, and implement a developed action plan. This often requires a team effort that fosters a collaborative and a healthy work environment. In today's healthcare climate, most organizations have quality departments and dedicated staff whose sole responsibility is to improve patient outcomes and experience. While quality personnel may not have much direct contact with patients, they often work closely with nurse- and physician-led quality councils or committees who provide direct patient care.[16]

THE NEED FOR SURVEILLANCE

Surveillance is an essential component of quality efforts. According to the Centers for Disease Control and Prevention (CDC), surveillance is defined as "the ongoing, systematic collection, analysis, interpretation, and dissemination of data regarding a health-related event for use in public health action to reduce morbidity and mortality and to improve health."[19] Surveillance is the continuous, systematic collection, analysis, and interpretation of data.[20] The data is utilized in planning, implementation, and evaluation of health practices.[21] Surveillance can serve multiple purposes. It can serve as an early warning for impending issues. As data is reviewed findings can help guide practice. Secondly, impacts of interventions can be determined and measured toward specific goals. Finally, surveillance can help to monitor and clarify the epidemiology of health problems to guide priorities.[21] The evolution of quality control in health care was accelerated by external stimuli. Prior to the implementation of surveillance programs, healthcare organizations had little motivation to control costs or demonstrate evidence of high quality. The rising cost of health care caught the attention of the federal government who began to push for increased regulation and accountability.

The Joint Commission

The stated mission of The Joint Commission is: "To continuously improve health care for the public, in collaboration with other stakeholders, by evaluating health care organizations and inspiring them to excel in providing safe and effective care of the highest quality and value."[22] Founded in 1951, *The Joint Commission* (JC) is an independent, nonprofit organization whose vision is that "all people always experience the safest, high quality, best-value health care across all settings."[22] Through on-site surveys and quarterly reporting, the JC evaluates and provides accreditation to more than 21,000 organizations. From the JC website, an individual can search by organization, service, or location to identify accredited organizations and/ or certified programs. An accredited hospital may also have program-specific certifications or advanced certifications. The JC has several cardiology-specific certifications, such as, Comprehensive Cardiac Center, as well as, disease specific certifications (acute coronary syndrome, cardiac valve repair and replacement, hypertension, etc.). Their easy to search website allows patients and their loved ones to identify and choose centers who have a proven record of quality in care.[16,22]

Centers for Medicare & Medicaid Services

In 1965, legislation signed by President Lyndon B. Johnson laid the foundation for what would become *The Centers for Medicare & Medicaid Services* (CMS), increasing access to health care, especially among elderly and low-income Americans.[23] CMS implements quality initiatives to assure quality health care for Medicare Beneficiaries through accountability and public disclosure. CMS uses quality measures in its various quality initiatives that include QI, pay for reporting, and public reporting.

CMS develops quality measures to be utilized in QI, public reporting, and pay-for-reporting programs. CMS has been largely responsible for the establishment of value-based programs aimed to shift health care from a fee or service model to incentivizing providers based on the quality and value of care.[23]

The original value-based programs put in place by CMS include End-Stage Renal Disease Quality Incentive Program (ESRD QIP), Hospital Value-Based Purchasing (VBP) Program, Hospital Readmission Reduction Program (HRRP), Value Modifier (VM) Program, and Hospital Acquired Conditions (HAC) Reduction Program. The ESRD-QIP reduced payments to dialysis facilities who did not meet specified performance standards. Likewise, the HRRP and HAC reduction programs penalize hospitals with *excessive* readmission rates or hospital-acquired conditions. The VM Program adjusts payment per claim to physicians based on their performance. In 2018, this expanded to include advanced practice providers. The Hospital VBP Program withholds 2% of Medicare payments from participating hospitals to fund incentivized payments based on performance. A large criticism of this program has been including patient experience/ satisfaction as a marker for quality. The existence of these programs magnifies the plea from the government for more accountable healthcare practices.[16,24]

CMS continues to monitor quality of healthcare organizations and conditions. "Meaningful Measures" framework is a CMS initiative designed to identify the highest priorities for quality measurement and improvement. It involves assessing core issues that are critical to providing high-quality care and improving individual outcomes. The Meaningful Measure Areas serve as the connectors between CMS strategic goals and individual measures/ initiatives that demonstrate how high-quality outcomes for our beneficiaries are being achieved. Examples of Meaningful Measure Areas include *Healthcare-Associated Infections* and *Prevention and Treatment of Opioid and Substance Use Disorders* (Fig. 43-3).[24]

Prospective Payment System

A prospective payment system (PPS) is a method of reimbursement in which Medicare payment is made based on a predetermined, fixed amount. The payment amount for a particular service is derived based on the classification system of that service (e.g., diagnosis-related groups for inpatient hospital services). CMS uses separate PPSs for reimbursement to acute inpatient hospitals, home health agencies, hospice, hospital outpatient, inpatient psychiatric facilities, inpatient rehabilitation facilities, long-term care hospitals, and skilled nursing facilities.[25] Reimbursement based on DRGs, rather than the actual cost accrued, forced hospitals to monitor quality and compelled them to contain costs. The advantage of reimbursement based on a PPS is that it actively refutes the fee-for-service system that could lead to unnecessary tests and services. However, the critique has been that patients may be discharged too early or not receive needed tests or services leading to inferior quality of care.[16]

Professional Standards Review Organizations

In 1972, amendments to the Social Security act included Professional Standards Review Organizations (PSROs) whose role in health care would be to determine "necessity, appropriateness, and quality of medical care."[26] PSROs report to and advise CMS on potential misuse or abuse of resource utilization or poor quality of care. The purpose of PSRO review is to determine (1) the medical necessity of services provided; (2) the services furnished or proposed to be furnished on an inpatient basis could have been effectively furnished on an outpatient basis or more economically in an inpatient healthcare facility of a different type.[27] Instituting PSROs was one of the first efforts by the government to hold healthcare organizations accountable for providing high-quality, high-value care.[16,28]

QUALITY REGISTRIES

Prospective registries began as components of randomized clinical trials. Ongoing surveillance of patient outcomes provides a better understanding of whether trial data can be applied to a larger population and allows for subgroup analysis. The American College of Cardiology (ACC) developed the National Cardiovascular Data Registry (NCDR) in 1987 "to define clinical characteristics and outcomes of patients undergoing cardiac catheterization and coronary interventions"; currently, the NCDR boasts more than 1500 participating U.S. hospitals with over 12 million patient records.[29] The Society of Thoracic Surgery (STS) registry is the largest, most successful registry; founded in 1989, it now houses over 5.8 million surgical cases. Since the 1980s, the number of registries continues to surge with new registries being added every few months. Figure 43-4 presents a few of the available

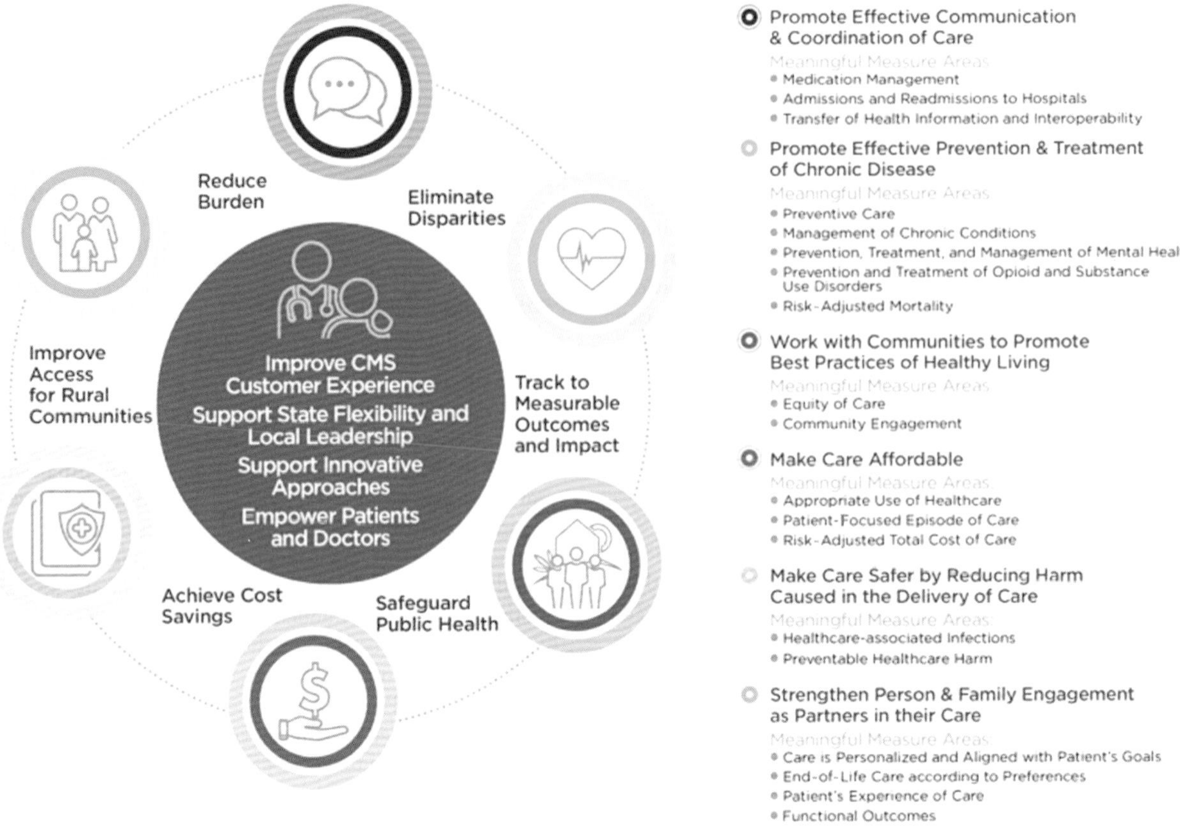

Figure 43-3. Meaningful measures.

cardiovascular registries sponsored by the ACC and European Society of Cardiology (ESC).

It is important to understand the limitations of registry data. It is currently not feasible to rely on the EMR for data collection due to the substantial amount of data (often >80 individual data points) and variability in definitions among different registries. Institutions often must employ nurses, at their own expense, to manually abstract data. For example, the NCDR PCI registry defines acute kidney injury (AKI) as any one of the following: (1) Increase in serum creatinine of >0.3 mg/dL from baseline. (2) Increase in serum creatinine of >50% from baseline. (3) New requirement for dialysis (NCDR).[30] In contrast to NCDR which bases its definition on serum creatinine and new dialysis, the STS registry also takes into account GFR, urine output, and duration of kidney function loss. While AKI is a yes/no choice in the NCDR PCI registry, the STS registry categorizes patients into various levels of kidney dysfunction postoperatively (risk, injury, failure, loss, and end-stage kidney disease). For example, a patient in the STS registry would be coded as renal injury if he/she experienced an increase in serum creatinine level × 3.0, or decrease in GFR by 50%, or urine output <0.5 mL/ kg/h for 12 hours.[31]

NCDR	ESC
IMPACT	ELECTRa
TVT	Euro-Endo
ACTION-GTWG	ROPAC
LAAO	TCVT

Figure 43-4. Examples of current registries. (Created by Katie N. Jaschke, used with permission.)

The quality of the data is dependent on the accuracy of data collection, as well as, the institutions' access to the patients' information outside of the institution. It is unrealistic to assume that registry data can be 100% precise. Organizations can run reports on mortality, readmission, and complications within their own health system; however, collecting this data becomes complex and challenging if a patient presents to or follows up at an outside facility. "Linking the Social Security database for 30-day mortality with the STS registry showed good concordance for in-hospital death, but 30-day death was only 60% sensitive."[29] It is easy to see how this would impact quality measurement, reporting, and improvement initiatives. Despite the limitations, the value of registry data is indisputable. These massive data banks have become essential to the development of practice guidelines, monitoring postmarket safety for new devices, and ensuring compliance with appropriate use criteria. Participating organizations receive their performance data and can benchmark themselves against similar institutions, providing valuable insight into the construction of quality initiatives.

ROLE OF THE CARDIOVASCULAR NURSE IN QUALITY

For nurses whose professional roles have expanded beyond direct patient care to include influencing policy, a review of healthcare quality can improve professional and transprofessional communications by increasing understanding, clarifying its definition, and

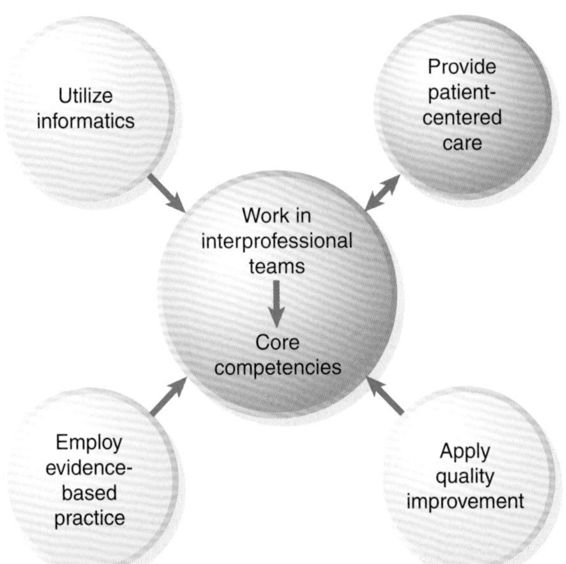

Figure 43-5. Interprofessional teamwork and Institute of Medicine core competencies. (Used with permission from Hinkle JL, Cheever KH. *Brunner & Suddarth's Textbook of Medical-Surgical Nursing*. Philadelphia, PA: Wolters Kluwer; 2017.)

contributing to a shared meaning among stakeholders.[32] "Nurses have an obligation to reasonably ensure that the care they provide is evidence-based and that work processes are consumer-centric."[33] Accountability for applying QI and utilization of evidence-based care are among core competencies (Fig. 43-5) for all healthcare professionals as described by the Institute of Medicine.[34] The nurse should give consideration to the complex relationships between clinical research, registry data, practice guidelines, health systems policy, and QI (Fig. 43-6). Taking into account potential conflicts of interest and limitations in study design and registry data, guidelines are recommended based on the best available evidence. Nevertheless, many guidelines are based on expert opinion. While it is not the individual nurses' responsibility be familiar with all guidelines and graded recommendations, it is imperative that a nurse know where to find reliable information to provide to patients. *UpToDate* is an example of a clinical decision resource to that is associated with improved patient outcomes and hospital performance. CPGs are graded based on evidence and quality of data (Fig. 43-7).

Nurses are at the forefront of patient care and in an optimal position to question practice. Why do we do it this way? Is there a better way? What does the evidence say? Research, evidence-based practice, and QI projects are three ways nurses can become involved in answering clinical questions. The lines between these three methodologies can become blurry. Research involves a systematic, rigorous study protocol, either qualitative or quantitative, to test a hypothesis. Research strives to develop new or add to existing knowledge and protocols must be reviewed by an Institutional Review Board (IRB) to protect human subjects. Evidence-based practice starts with a clinical question. Existing literature, patient preferences, and expert opinion are gathered and examined. The goal is to translate best evidence into clinical practice. QI is somewhere in between and ideally suited for nurses. QI does not have to follow a rigorous IRB approved study protocol and does not require an extensive literature review. However, many QI projects are submitted to the IRB to ensure they are truly QI and do not meet criteria for research. If the IRB deems a project within the scope of QI, the project protocol can be altered or changed throughout the duration of the project. The goal of QI is to improve a process or a patient outcome; results typically are for internal use and not generalizable outside the institution (Fig. 43-8).

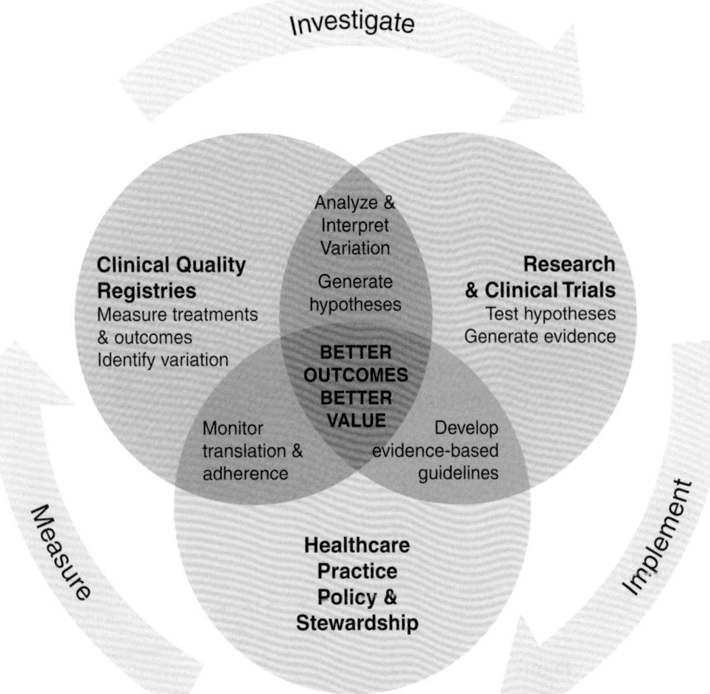

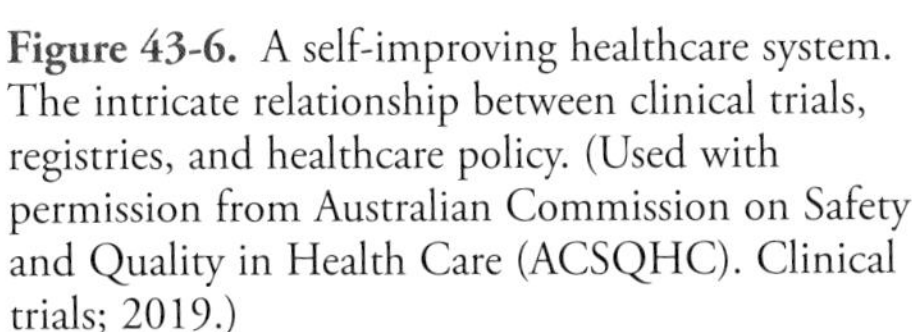
Figure 43-6. A self-improving healthcare system. The intricate relationship between clinical trials, registries, and healthcare policy. (Used with permission from Australian Commission on Safety and Quality in Health Care (ACSQHC). Clinical trials; 2019.)

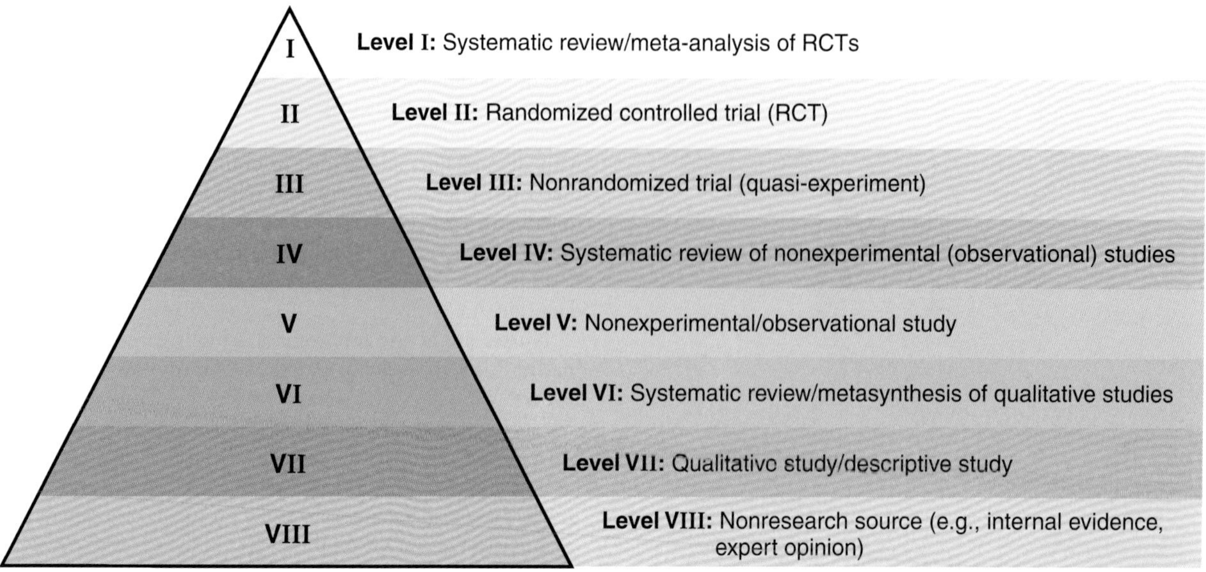

Figure 43-7. Grading of the level of evidence. (Used with permission from Polit D, Beck C. *Nursing Research*. 11th ed. Philadelphia, PA: Wolters Kluwer; 2020.)

QUALITY IMPROVEMENT MODELS

Contemporary health care in America has seen a transition from *quality assurance* (QA) to *quality improvement* (QI). The difference is in the titles; QA focuses on maintaining a desired level of existing quality. QI promotes ongoing improvement with the mindset that processes can always be better.

Total Quality Management

Total quality management (TQM), also known as *continuous quality improvement (CQI)*, is a QI model developed by Dr. W. Edward Deming based on his 14 quality management principles. Deming felt that good quality means a predictable degree of uniformity and dependability with a quality standard suited to the customer.[35] It emphasizes the value of quality over profit understanding that high quality will attract a larger consumer base, thus potentially increasing profit. No matter how high the quality of service may be currently, the TQM philosophy asserts that it can always be better. A vital component to achieving continuous improvement is the empowerment of the employees as their unique knowledge of their role and how it plays into system processes is critically important to identifying issues and addressing them proactively, rather than reactively. There is not a centralized QI department; the data collection is conducted by the actual employees allowing for constant feedback between the employees, customers, and administration. Engaging the employees in turn provides them with a sense of teamwork and value leading to higher productivity and job satisfaction.

Six Sigma

By the late 1980s, TQM had evolved into Six Sigma, the most widely adopted process improvement toolset today. Originating at the Motorola Corporation, Six Sigma accelerated in popularity after the corporation won the Malcolm Baldrige National Quality Award in 1988 and was later successfully implemented at General Electric. Six Sigma strives to minimize defects and process variability to maximize quality and profitability.[36] Improving on the successes of TQM, Six Sigma builds its foundation on a team approach requiring management participation and defines a sequence of steps to follow. Two main project methodologies of Six Sigma are DMAIC and DMADV. DMAIC (Define, Measure, Analyze, Improve, Control) aims to modify and control a current process versus DMADV (Define, Measure, Analyze, Design, Verify) in which a process is completely redesigned.

Lean. Lean thinking, based on Toyota's production system, is a methodology with an emphasis on waste elimination. Lean principles were introduced in the 1991 book *The Machine that Changed the World*. With lean management, every step in a process is analyzed with the goal to disregard any step that does not add value. Lean is a set of operating philosophies and methods that help create a maximum value for patients with an emphasis on reducing waste and waits. The focus of lean methodology is

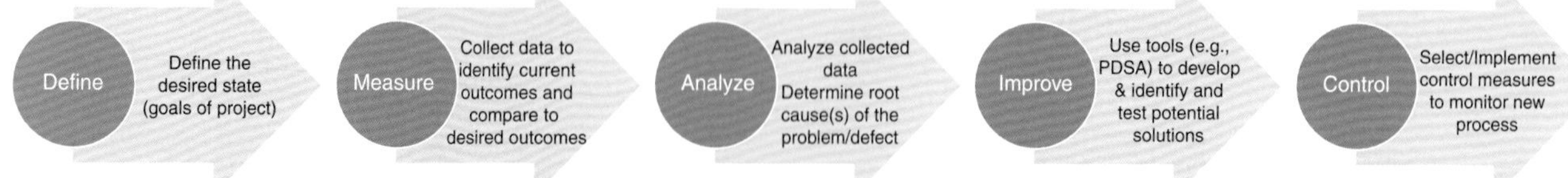

Figure 43-8. Six Sigma DMAIC (define, measure, analyze, improve, and control) quality improvement approach. (Used with permission from Rundio A. *Nurse Management & Executive Practice*. Philadelphia, PA: Wolters Kluwer; 2018.)

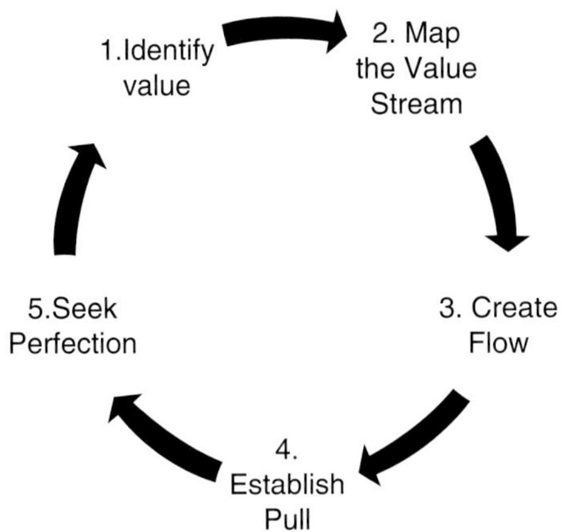

Figure 43-9. Lean thinking. (Used with permission from Mayhall CG. *Hospital Epidemiology and Infection Control.* 4th ed. Philadelphia, PA: Wolters Kluwer; 2011.)

of the customer's needs, employee involvement and continuous improvement.[37] Lean aims to change the organization thinking and values, which leads to organizational transformations of behaviors and culture. The focus is on efficient resource utilization and questions value add (Fig. 43-9).

CONCLUSION

Healthcare professionals, healthcare systems, healthcare organizations, are all in a state of evolution. They share the struggles of development in a world that is changing at incredible speed. Nearly everyone involved in the practice of Medicine is highly trained and committed to providing the highest quality of care. Because of all the changes in health care, the ways in which quality is perceived, pursued, and ensured continues to develop. Many of what has driven the changes in health care has been the need for insuring quality across the entire healthcare system.

KEY READING

The influencer change framework. The Influencer Change Model is a systematic approach to changing behavior, based on the book *Influencer: The Power to Change Anything* (Patterson, Grenny, Maxfield, McMillan, & Switzler, 2008).

REFERENCES

1. Institute of Medicine. *IOM definition of quality.* 2019. Available at http://iom.nationalacademies.org/Global/News%20Announcements/Crossing-the-Quality-Chasm-TheIOM-Health-Care-Quality-Initiative
2. Mackary M, Daniel M. Medical error—the third leading cause of death in the US. *BMJ.* 2016; 353:i2139.
3. Committee on Quality Health Care in America, Institute of Medicine. *Crossing the Quality Chasm: a New Health System for the 21st Century.* Washington, DC: National Academy Press; 2001.
4. Ayanian J, Markel H. Donabedians lasting framework for healthcare quality. *N Engl J Med.* 2016;375:205–207.
5. Donabedian A. Evaluating the quality of medical care. 1966. *Milbank Q.* 2005;83(4):691–729.
6. Ameh S, Gómez-Olivé FX, Kahn K, et al. Relationships between structure, process and outcome to assess quality of integrated chronic disease management in a rural South African setting: applying a structural equation model. *BMC Health Serv Res.* 2017;17(1):229.
7. Nightingale, Florence. *Notes On Nursing: What It Is, and What It Is Not.* New York: Appleton-Century; 1946.
8. Kudzma EC. Florence Nightingale and healthcare reform. *Nurs Sci Q.* 2006;19(1):61–64.
9. Aravind M, Chung KC. Evidence-based medicine and hospital reform: tracing origins back to Florence Nightingale. *Plast Reconstr Surg.* 2010;125(1):403–409.
10. Attree M. Towards a conceptual model of quality care. *Int J Nurs Stud.* 1996;33(1):13–28.
11. World Health Organization. *What is quality care and why is it important website.* Available at https://www.who.int/maternal_child_adolescent/topics/quality-of-care/definition/en/. Updated December 1, 2019. Accessed December 28, 2019.
12. World Health Organization. *Quality of care.* Available at https://www.who.int/management/quality/assurance/QualityCare_B.Def.pdf. Accessed December 28, 2019.
13. Journal of the American College of Cardiology. *JACC Journals.* 2019. Available at http://www.onlinejacc.org/content/74/24
14. Scimago Lab. *Scimago institutions rankings.* 2019. Available at https://www.scimagojr.com/journalrank.php?category=2705
15. *AHRQ Understanding Quality Measurement.* Content last reviewed October 2018. Agency for Healthcare Research and Quality, Rockville, MD. Available at https://www.ahrq.gov/professionals/quality-patient-safety/quality-resources/tools/chtoolbx/understand/index.html
16. Marquis BL, Huston CJ. *Leadership and Management Tools for the New Nurse: A Case Study Approach.* Philadelphia, PA: Wolters Kluwer/Lippincott Williams & Wilkins; 2012.
17. Agency for Healthcare Research and Quality (AHRQ) Quality Indicators Overview. Available at https://www.qualityindicators.ahrq.gov/FAQs_Support/FAQ_QI_Overview.aspx. Accessed December 28, 2019.
18. Sawyer LM, Berkowitz B, Haber JE, et al. Expanding American Nurses Association nursing quality indicators to community-based practices. *Outcomes Manag.* 2002;6(2):53–61.
19. AHRQ Guideline Clearinghouse. Available at https://www.ahrq.gov/gam/index.html. Accessed December 28, 2019.
20. German RR, Lee LM, Horan JM, et al; Guidelines Working Group Centers for Disease Control and Prevention (CDC). Updated guidelines for evaluating public health surveillance systems: recommendations from the guidelines working group. *MMWR Recomm Rep.* 2001;50(RR-13):1–35; quiz CE1–7.
21. World Health Organization. *Who Global Surveillance and Monitoring System.* Available at https://www.who.int/medicines/regulation/ssffc/surveillance/en/.
22. The Joint Commission. *History of the Joint Commission.* 2019. Available at https://www.jointcommission.org/about_us/history.aspx
23. Centers for Medicare & Medicaid Services. *History.* 2019. Available at https://www.cms.gov/About-CMS/Agency-information/History/
24. CMS Meaningful Measures Hub. Available at https://www.cms.gov/Medicare/Quality-Initiatives-Patient-Assessment-Instruments/QualityInitiativesGenInfo/MMF/General-info-Sub-Page. Updated September 10, 2019. Accessed December 28, 2019.
25. CMS Prospective Payment Systems. Available at https://www.cms.gov/Medicare/Medicare-Fee-for-Service-Payment/ProspMedicareFeeSvcPmtGen/index. Updated November 29, 2019. Accessed December 28, 2019.
26. Ellis GL. PSRO: current status of the professional standards review organization program. *Am J Occup Ther.* 1976;30(6):370–375.
27. Social Security Administration. *HI 00208.080 Role of Professional Standards Review Organizations (PSRO's).* Available at https://secure.ssa.gov/apps10/poms.nsf/lnx/0600208080. Updated September 23, 2003. Accessed December 28, 2019.
28. Centers for Medicare & Medicaid Services. *Prospective payment systems.* 2019. Available at https://www.cms.gov/Medicare/Medicare-Fee-for-Service-Payment/ProspMedicareFeeSvcPmtGen/index.html
29. Faxon DP, Burgess A. Cardiovascular registries: too much of a good thing? *Circ Cardiovasc Interv.* 2016;9(4):e003866.
30. National Cardiovascular Data Registry [NCDR]. *CathPCI: Acute kidney injury (risk-adjusted) specifications and testing overview [PDF file].* n.d. Available at https://www.ncdr.com/WebNCDR/docs/default-source/ncdr-general-documents/cathpci_kidney-injury-overview_comment-period.pdf?sfvrsn=2
31. Jacobs J, Shahian D, D'Agostina R, et al. The Society of Thoracic Surgery National Database 2018 annual report. *Ann Thorac Surg.* 2018;106(6):1603–1611.
32. Allen-Duck A, Robinson J, Stewart M. Healthcare quality: a concept analysis. *Nurs Forum.* 2017;52(4):377–386.
33. Huber D. *Leadership & nursing care management.* 6th ed. St. Louis, MO: Elsevier; 2018.
34. Bormann L. *Institute of Medicine core competencies for health professionals: Foundation for care coordination in practice [PDF file].* 2016. Available at

https://www.wku.edu/nursing/documents/organizations/institute_of_medicine_core_competencies.pdf

35. Institute for Healthcare Improvement (IHI) Think Improvement, Not Inspection. Available at http://www.ihi.org/resources/Pages/ImprovementStories/ThinkImprovementNotInspection.aspx. Accessed December 28, 2019.
36. Almorsy L, Khalifa M. Lean six sigma in health care: improving utilization and redirecting waste. *Stud Health Technol Inform.* 2016;226:194–197.
37. Lawal AK, Rotter T, Kinsman L, et al. Lean management in health care: definition, concepts, methodology and effects reported (systematic review protocol). *Syst Rev.* 2014;3:103.

44 Advanced Practice Nursing and Cardiovascular Care

Kimberly A. Guibone

OBJECTIVES

1. Discuss the history of the role of the Advanced Practice Nurse.
2. Highlight the function of the Advanced Practice Nurse in the Cardiology practice.

KEY QUESTIONS

1. How were the first Advanced Practice Nurses utilized?
2. Why is the role of the Advanced Practice Nurse important to the field of Cardiology?

Advanced practice nursing encompasses the registered nurse role with expanded training including, but not limited to, expert knowledge of disease processes, diagnoses and intervention, and care for individuals or populations attained through theoretical and evidence-based education at the graduate level.[1] The formal title emerged in the mid-1960s, though what is now defined as advanced practice nursing can be traced back to the 1800s and earlier.[2] Today, advancements in health management and the increasing need for access to health care, including consultation and multidisciplinary care, have led to a global call for optimization of advanced practice nursing in many areas, including cardiovascular care.

HISTORY

Historical depictions of nurses practicing at an expanded role exist as solutions by pioneering nurses to meet the needs of the poorest of populations, and those in distant and remote areas void of medical services. Development of the Henry Street Settlement in 1893 by Lillian Wald is one of the earliest examples. Lillian Wald was a graduate nurse from the New York Training School in Manhattan. Rapid industrialization of the time and worker immigration had led to pockets of impoverished communities unable to obtain medical assistance due to the inability to provide payment. Lillian Wald recognized the critical need and as the founder of what is now public health nursing developed a program for nurses going out into the grossly underserved community providing supplies, assessing needs, and dispensing medications and remedies based on their nursing experience. By 1890, she had a recorded staff of 12 nurses who made 26,600 home visits.[3]

In parallel timeline, nurse-led anesthesia presented with the discovery of chloroform rapidly expanding the abilities for surgical intervention paired with the exponential increase in its use brought on by wartime-wounded soldiers. In Minnesota, to standardize procedure, surgeon Dr. W.W. Mayo hired a nurse to administer anesthesia. Through foresight of the nurse, Alice Magaw, outcomes were tracked and later published demonstrating the effectiveness of chloroform and secondarily that such chloroform was administered by nurse anesthetists. The Mayo Clinic introduced the first program to formally train nurse anesthetists which became highly successful and broadly recognized. However, with the early 1900's rapid development of anesthesiology as a specialty, the medical profession began to take notice and questioned as to whether or not nurses were practicing medicine without a license. The New York State Medical Society initiated the argument that such violated state law. The Ohio State Medical Board went on to mandate that anesthesia could only be administered by physicians. The culmination resulted in a 1917 Kentucky lawsuit (Frank v. South) of which the appellate court ruled that anesthesia provided by nurse anesthetist Margaret Hatfield was allowable only if under the supervision of a licensed physician.[4] This was a foreshadowing of ongoing interprofessional and legal conflict of the advanced practice nurse (APN) and scope of practice.

In 1925, nursing pioneer, Mary Breckinridge, developed the Frontier Nursing Service (FNS). At the time, the area of Appalachian community of Leslie County, Kentucky was broad, sparsely populated, inaccessible, and deeply impoverished with one of the highest maternal and infant mortality rates in the country. Coming from a heritage of public servants, Mary Breckinridge became a district nursing volunteer in France at the end of World War I and gained experience working alongside European midwives. Upon her return, she attended graduate courses in public health and nursing. Aware of the severity of need of the Appalachian people, she returned to Europe to become a certified midwife. She then founded the FNS in Kentucky, setting up eight decentralized clinics over rugged territory and serving three counties accomplishing a marked decrease in overall mortality. FNS nurses traveled by horseback, treating a spectrum of maladies.

Treatments included administration of ether, medications, and emergency care based on their assessment and diagnosis. Later, in response to Margaret Hatfield and Frank v. South, Mary Breckinridge established a Medical Advisory Committee to create a guideline manual for legal protection of FNS practice autonomy given the physical absence of a physician in the vicinity.[3]

These foundations created by early leaders demonstrated the impact and outcomes of advanced practice nursing. As the practice grew, the expanded nursing role that was openly accepted and unchallenged to meet the needs of the poor and remote populations became questioned in the more affluent areas of which there were a greater number of physicians and a population that could pay for service. This demarcation of practice would underscore the importance of role development and scope of practice.

The early 20th century launched a period of territorial definition of practice for medical doctors. Medical doctors led the way in establishing licensure guidelines and their legislative adoption in each state. In doing so, the practice of medicine was codified using broad definitions of care and claiming exclusive performance of diagnosis, cure, prescription of medicines, and any therapy that "severs or penetrates the tissues of human beings."[1] This would later include the practice authority to impact policy and delegate care that could take place only under medical supervision.[5] The rapid growth of hospitals after World War II brought nursing care out of the community and into the hospital setting reinforcing the medical model and deterring the nursing autonomy that had long been practiced.[1]

The American Nurses Association (ANA) was founded in 1896 as a unifying organization to advance and protect the profession of nursing. Efforts were aimed at defining practice, broadening academic curriculums, and seeking input to legislature. In 1955, the ANA developed a model of nursing that would later be adopted by many states. Inadvertently, the proactive intent to elucidate nursing practice and meet the purposes of licensing legislation unwittingly enforced boundaries consistent to that of the medical model which would later serve as barriers to advanced practice nursing.[3]

"The practice of professional nursing means the performance for compensation of any act in the observation, care and counsel of the ill ... or in the maintenance of health or prevention of illness ... or the administration of medications and treatments *as prescribed by a licensed physician... The foregoing shall not be deemed to include acts of diagnosis or prescription of therapeutic or corrective measures*" (ANA, 1955, p. 1474).

Much of the development of advanced practice nursing for the rest of the 20th century would focus efforts on regaining this scope.

In 1965, Loretta Ford, along with pediatrician Henry Silver, proposed and created the first nurse practitioner (NP) program at the University of Colorado. As a longtime public health nurse, she had seen the gravity of need for pediatric care in the community. Recognizing the crisis, a specialized graduate nurse program was developed to educate pediatric nurses to provide broader care in rural clinics. The novelty was that of collaboration between physician and NP as colleagues rather than the APN functioning as a physician substitute or physician extender.[3]

The 1970s was a period of growth and development for the Clinical Nurse Specialist (CNS). The concept originated in the psychiatric nursing arena where it was recognized that specialization was advantageous in caring for specific patient group subtypes, specifically the mentally ill to match and implement newer therapies of intervention and management. Hildegard Peplau who promoted the therapeutic value of the nurse–patient relationship spearheaded much of this work. Her many works included creating the foundation for her vision of the psychiatric nurse with specialization to go out into the homes and the community treating patients with the same roles, goals, and functions as that of the physician.[6] Following suit, specialization training programs in several areas began to form independently and in 1975, the ANA formally identified the CNS role as that of an expert practitioner and change agent requiring graduate-level education and certification.[1] The CNS grew in popularity and later transcended to a role less directly involved in direct patient care and more instrumental in education, improving nursing practice and contributing to evidence-based bodies of knowledge and role development. The role was initially highly valued by institutions as its impact was demonstrated in improved outcomes and patient care systems. However, the rapid rise of the CNS implementation was followed by a plunge as economic changes in the 1990s led to hospital financial strain and federal Medicare reimbursement restructuring that did not include the CNS as a reimbursable role.[1]

Furthermore, the 1980s experienced a marked shift in physician practice. An increasing number of trained physicians led to expanding practice outreach into the community and the prediction of a physician glut led to scrutiny of the APN role and value within the territory of medicine. In 1986, the Senate Committee on Appropriations requested a review by the Office of Technology Assessment (OTA) to examine the evidence on the quality and costs of the care NPs, certified nurse midwives (CNMs), and physician assistants (PAs) provided. More specifically, the questions asked included what contributions NPs, CNMs, and PAs added to meeting the nation's healthcare needs and questioned the impact on healthcare costs related to their role. Extensive review of evidence supported that, within defined areas of competence, NPs, PAs, and CNMs provided care whose quality was equivalent to that of care provided by physicians and was cost-effective from a societal perspective (OTA-HCS-37, 1986).

Argument persisted regarding broad variations in training, education, and scope. Baseline regulation of practice required graduation from a specialty program and certification. Additional legal jurisdiction and parameters were imposed on a state-by-state basis, as nurse practice acts, varying in content and definitions of practice regardless of training or education. For all states, certification by a national professional body was required for licensure to meet the state's responsibility to protect its public. Concerns were raised, as there was variation in certification programs and an uneven enforcement of criteria to enter these programs. After a 1995 Boards of Nursing Delegation Assembly, the National Council of State Boards of Nursing (NCSBN) was tasked to collaborate with the various specialties to produce psychometrically sound, legally defensible NP examinations providing a standard for regulatory purposes.[7]

CONSENSUS MODEL FOR APRN REGULATION

Over the next several years, the NCSBN working with the APRN Advisory Panel defined standards to meet accreditation for certification programs. In 2002, the NCSBN published the Criteria for Evaluating APRN Certification Programs, which included requirements of education concentrated in the specialty, 500 supervised clinical hours, and clinical expertise directly related to the role and specialty. In 2003, the APRN Advisory Panel initiated a draft vision paper to address among items, the regulatory concerns given the proliferation of APRN subspecialty areas and needed direction for a future APRN regulatory model.[8]

Soon to follow in 2004, combined efforts were put forth by the American Association of Colleges of Nursing (AACN) and the National Organization of Nurse Practitioner Faculties (NONPF) in a proposal to the Alliance for Nursing Accreditation to also draft a vision paper to standardize the regulatory credentialing of APNs. An invitation was sent to multiple organizations to participate in a focused conference to address all educational, regulatory, and practice aspects of the APN. Streamlining of input produced a subgroup, the APN Work Group, retitled the APRN Consensus Work Group, which was tasked with developing a statement of recommendations.[9]

In 2006, the parallel efforts of the APRN Advisory Panel and the APRN Consensus Work Group were identified and the two groups joined forces with representatives of each forming the APRN Joint Dialogue Group. Over the next 2 years, the group worked together to systematically produce a widely vetted Consensus Model for APRN Regulation published in July 2008.[8]

The aim of the document was to address the lack of a uniform model of regulation of APRNs across states. With the expansion in numbers of APRNs and their value to the healthcare system, the variations in recognition of role by state-to-state licensing bodies were viewed as a barrier to scope of practice and patient access to care. The document was a proposal to define APRN practice, define the APRN regulatory model, identify titles to be used, define specialty, describe the emergence of new roles and population foci, and present strategies for implementation.[8] The model addressed lack of common definitions of APRN roles, lack of standardization of APRN educational programs, proliferation of APRN specialties and subspecialties, and lack of common legal recognition of APRNs across states. Goals were to ensure public safety, facilitate mobility of APRNs, advocate appropriate scope of practice, and increase access to health care. The regulatory model necessitated the components of licensure, accreditation, certification, and education (LACE) throughout. Target full implementation date was set for 2015.

The definition of the APRN was specified in language pertaining to characteristics, accountability, and responsibility (Table 44-1). Changes included titling as APRN that would be legally protected and required to be included in legal representation of roles such as that of legal signature.[8]

The regulatory model of the APRN recognized licensure at two levels: that of role and that of population foci. The four designated APRN roles were certified registered nurse anesthetist (CRNA), CNM, CNS, and certified nurse practitioner (CNP). The population foci referred to the four roles and their education, training, and licensure specific to one of the population foci. The population foci included family/individual across the life span, adult gerontology, neonatal, pediatrics, women's health/gender related, and psychiatric mental health. Competencies were required to be met at the level of role and foci for certification and licensure (Fig. 44-1).[8]

Table 44-1 • DEFINITION OF ADVANCED PRACTICE REGISTERED NURSE (APRN)

1. One who has completed an accredited graduate-level education program preparing him/her for one of the four recognized APRN roles.
2. One who has passed a national certification examination that measures APRN, role- and population-focused competencies, and who maintains continued competence as evidenced by recertification in the role and population through the national certification program.
3. One who has acquired advanced clinical knowledge and skills preparing him/her to provide direct care to patients, as well as a component of indirect care: however, the defining factor for all APRNs is that a significant component of the education and practice focuses on direct care of individuals.
4. One whose practice builds on the competencies of registered nurses (RNs) by demonstrating a greater depth and breadth of knowledge, a greater synthesis of data, increased complexity of skills and interventions, and a greater role autonomy.
5. One who is educationally prepared to assume responsibility and accountability for health promotion and/or maintenance as well as the assessment, diagnosis, and management of patient problems, which includes the use and prescription of pharmacologic and nonpharmacologic interventions.
6. One who has clinical expertise of sufficient depth and breadth to reflect the intended license.
7. One who has obtained a license to practice as an APRN in one of the four APRN roles: certified registered nurse anesthetist (CRNA), certified nurse midwife (CNM), clinical nurse specialist (CNS), or certified nurse practitioner (CNP).

APRN Consensus Work Group & the National Council of State Boards of Nursing APRN Advisory Committee. *APRN Joint Dialogue Group Report*. 2008. Available at https://www.oplc.nh.gov/nursing/documents/aprn-consensus-model.pdf

INSTITUTE OF MEDICINE: THE FUTURE OF NURSING REPORT

The ACA was a revolutionary restructuring of the U.S. healthcare system, comparable to the introduction of Medicare and Medicaid in 1965. The enactment predicted facilitation of access to health care to approximately 32 million Americans. Much of the ACA design to accommodate these numbers and to improve the quality of health care was based on the recognition and utilization of nursing as the largest most impactful group within the healthcare force numbering at greater than three million.[10]

In anticipation of needed restructuring to allow for improvements in the scope and practice of nursing, the Robert Wood Johnson Foundation partnered with the Institute of Medicine (IOM) to formally address and make recommendations to transform the nursing profession. The experts were tasked to provide action plans addressing the nursing shortage, the congested nursing education system, and nursing retention at the local, state, and federal levels. Identified barriers included the broad continuum of care from birth to death, prevention to disease state, and coordination of such in an increasing variety of settings that nursing provided. Newly identified was the need for diversity in both the patient population and the nursing profession to provide culturally competent care.[11]

Evidence-based review and expert consensus collaboration established a 2-year Initiative on the Future of Nursing with key messages identified as a framework for the subsequent recommendations. The key messages included nurses practicing to their full extent, improvement in educational attainment and advancement for nursing, ability to partnership with other professionals in addressing healthcare redesign, and structured workforce planning with formalized review (Table 44-2).[11]

Operationalizing the key messages necessitated a mandate of significant change across the nursing profession. The historic, political, and conflicting regulatory structure had already limited practice to the extent of full licensure and education in many locations and arenas. For the APRN, broad discrepancies ranged from

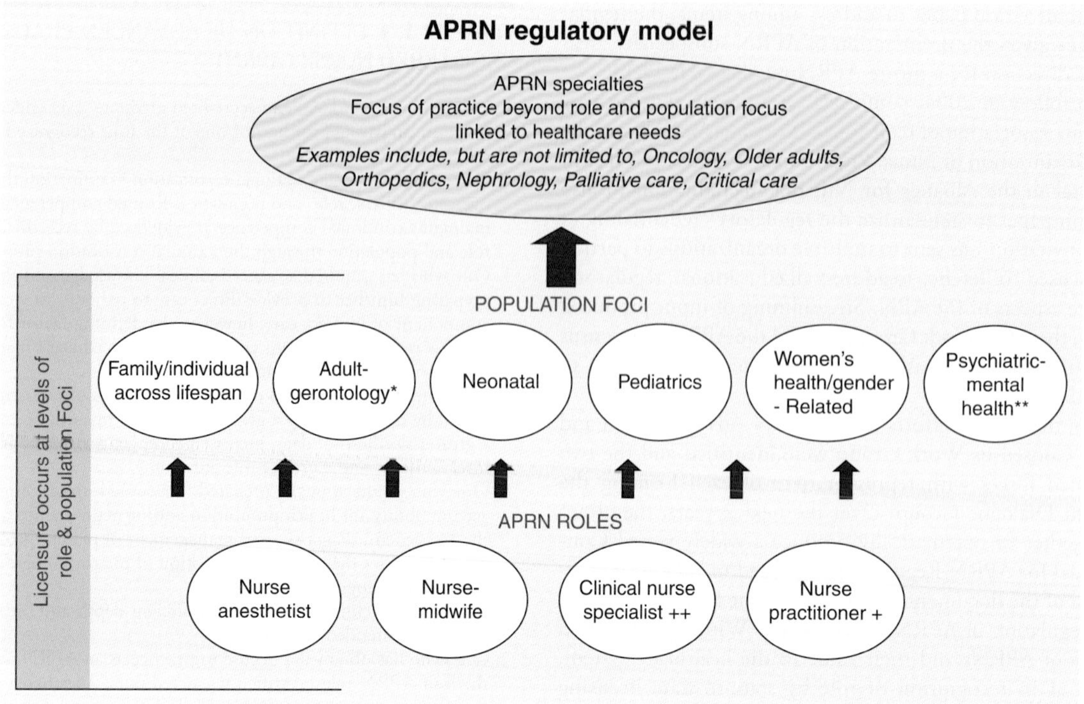

Figure 44-1. APRN regulatory model.
+The certified nurse practitioner (CNP) is prepared with the acute care CNP competencies and/or the primary care CNP competencies. At this point in time, the acute care and primary care CNP delineation applies only to the pediatric and adult-gerontology CNP population foci. Scope of practice of the primary care or acute care CNP is not setting specific but is based on patient care needs. Programs may prepare individuals across both the primary care and acute care CNP competencies. If programs prepare graduates across both sets of roles, the graduate must be prepared with the consensus-based competencies for both roles and must successfully obtain certification in both the acute and the primary care CNP roles. CNP certification in the acute care or primary care roles must match the educational preparation for CNPs in these roles.
*The population focus, adult gerontology, encompasses the young adult to the older adult, including the frail elderly. APRNs educated and certified in the adult-gerontology population are educated and certified across both areas of practice and will be titled Adult-Gerontology CNP or CNS. All APRNs in any of the four roles providing care to the adult population (e.g., family or gender specific) must be prepared to meet the growing needs of the older adult population. Therefore, the education program should include didactic and clinical education experiences necessary to prepare APRNs with these enhanced skills and knowledge.
**The population focus, psychiatric/mental health, encompasses education and practice across the life span.
++The clinical nurse specialist is educated and assessed through national certification processes across the continuum from wellness through acute care.

allowing full practice to restricting prescriptive authority or ability to see patients without physician supervision based on state-specific nurse practice acts, many of which were compounded by vague interpretation. Despite uniform licensure, the APRN role was greatly dependent on state of practice rather than extent of education or training.[4]

Table 44-2 • INITIATIVE ON THE FUTURE OF NURSING: KEY MESSAGES

1. Nurses should practice to the full extent of their education and training.
2. Nurses should achieve higher levels of education and training through an improved education system that promotes seamless academic progression.
3. Nurses should be full partners with physicians and other professionals, in redesigning health care in the United States.
4. Effective workforce planning and policy making require better data collection and an improved information infrastructure.

IOM (Institute of Medicine). *The Future of Nursing: Leading Change, Advancing Health.* Washington, DC: The National Academies Press; 2011.

Proposed solutions to bridging the gap included the federal government leveraging optimization of the APRN role by disseminating best practice and incentivizing policies to promote full evidenced-based practice to all providers nationwide. Such would press the Centers for Medicare and Medicaid Services to meet responsibility of access to care for its beneficiaries (IOM, 2011, p. 5). In addition, identification of the high level of nursing education and training required to match the needs of the broadening areas of practice, increase in complexity of patients, and rapid technologic advancements suggested a requirement of a minimum baccalaureate level of education. Necessary funding and mechanisms of support strategies would need to be incorporated to defray the strain on current educational resources. Shortages in primary care, research, and faculty also promulgated streamlining advancement to APRN, PhD, and doctoral programs (DNP). Revised capacity and curriculum are required to reduce the nursing shortage and facilitate advanced practice to provide quality care to patients.[11]

The nursing role should include that of leadership, which should be incorporated into education and training. Nursing leaders should be full partners with physicians, administrators, and health policy decision makers to truly collaborate in redesigning and addressing ongoing changes in healthcare delivery.[11] The Doctor of Nursing Practice (DNP) is an advanced nursing degree at the doctorate level to include training in organizational and systems leadership, information systems technology, healthcare policy, and interprofessional collaboration.[1] The IOM calls for future state of all APRNs to be educated at the doctoral level to provide safe patient care along with leadership and innovation to continually improve practice, systems, and policy.[12]

Transformation of change in the practice environment, optimization of roles, and influx of access to health care will need statistical and scientific systems of measure to evaluate implementation and effect on outcomes. Additionally, examining the practice model interrelationship with reimbursement, policy, and technologic advancements will require aggressive and ongoing data collection. In recognition of this, the ACA mandated formation of the National Health Care Workforce Analysis with a responsibility to monitor training and education to meet the growing healthcare force and to address barriers between the local, state, and federal levels. The ACA also granted the National Center for Workforce Analysis to fund workforce data collection and studies.[11]

APRN PRACTICE IN CARDIOVASCULAR CARE

Cardiovascular disease (CVD) is the leading cause of death in the United States, with one death occurring every 37 seconds.[13] Nearly half of all Americans (121.5 million adults) have CVD. Projections suggest upward of 30 million Americans that will be diagnosed by 2035 at the cost of $1.1 trillion in care.[14] Increasing patient numbers, growing elderly population, technologic advancements, and improved access to health care all contribute to the demand for cardiovascular care providers. The APRN is widely suited to address the spectrum of disease management, preventative care, research, public health, and systems management.

Education and training for the cardiovascular APRN includes successful completion of an accredited graduate-level program, certification, and licensure. Most commonly, expertise is achieved through experience, job training, and self-directed learning. Currently, there is no APRN cardiology subspecialty certification; however, newer academic programs are now offering focus courses. Need for improved transition to practice as outlined in the IOM report prompted the ANCC in 2014 to develop an accreditation for residency and fellowship transition-to-practice program to set the global standard titled the Practice Transition Accreditation Program (PTAP). Institutions can apply for accreditation of a voluntary APRN fellowship program that meets criteria as outlined in the application. These would include practice-based learning, preceptorship, and specified institutional support. To date, there are only a few APRN fellowship programs specific to cardiovascular care.[15] These programs generally are 12-month advanced fellowship training programs providing preceptorship in both inpatient and outpatient cardiovascular care and professional and leadership development.

The APRN role differs from that of the expert cardiovascular nurse. The expert cardiovascular nurse acquires a mastery of cardiovascular care of a specific cardiovascular population achieved through advanced experiential and clinical training often over many years. The APRN also encompasses advanced knowledge in care of the cardiovascular patient. However, in addition to advanced knowledge of cardiovascular care, the APRN is also proficient in the competencies that define the APRN scope of practice, including acquisition of new practice and skills which may be congruent to aspects of physician practice, autonomy, prescriptive authority, responsibility for health maintenance, disease prevention, diagnosis, and treatment. This includes guidance and coaching, consultation, evidence-based practice, leadership, collaboration, and ethical decision making.[1]

Under the umbrella of cardiovascular care, the APRN impacts patient outcomes through roles in the inpatient acute setting, outpatient clinical setting, clinical efficiency and process improvement, research, and leadership in administration, service line management, and national policy. In 2015, the American College of Cardiology (ACC), a long-standing credentialing medical association with a focus on education and advancements in cardiovascular care, published a policy statement on cardiovascular team-based care. The aim of the paper was to formally state the necessity of advanced practice providers to meet the need of a growing population of complex patients in a climate of healthcare reform, cost containment, and desire to improve outcomes. The concept of team-based care was introduced as a model to provide multidisciplinary collaborative care promoting higher quality and better outcomes along with greater patient and provider satisfaction. The following are examples of advanced practice nursing in cardiovascular care.

HEART FAILURE APRN

Heart failure (HF) affects approximately 6.5 million people in the United States and carries a high morbidity and mortality rate at significant economic cost.[13] Projections show that the prevalence of HF will increase 46% from 2012 to 2030, estimating greater than 8 million adults affected by HF.[16] The condition is generally chronic in nature requiring ongoing care and management and intermittent hospitalizations. The mechanism of congestive heart failure is related to the heart's inability to pump sufficient blood to the organs and tissues resulting in impaired function. Inadequate forward flow is evidenced in pedal edema, pulmonary edema, liver congestion, renal insufficiency, decreased activity tolerance, and shortness of breath. Prognosis is poor at 40% to 50% mortality at 5 years.[16] Contributing factors are coronary artery disease, diabetes, hypertension, obesity, valvular heart disease, high salt diet, smoking, sedentary lifestyle, and excessive alcohol intake. Goals of care are directed at lifestyle modifications, guideline-directed medical therapy (GDMT), and patient and provider monitoring to facilitate evidence-based practices.

In 2010, the American Heart Association (AHA) developed the 2020 Impact Goals to reduce the incidence of CVD addressing the need for weight management, optimized diet, exercise, and smoking cessation with a goal to reduce the incidence of CVD by 20% in 2020 (Lloyd-Jones et al., 2010). National guidelines promote a team model of interdisciplinary care. Recommendations address individual-focused approaches, healthcare systems approaches, and broader population-targeted interventions.[16] The holistic and patient relationship characteristic of APRN practice provides a model conducive to managing this challenging population.

Heart failure clinics include or are often led by APRNs highly trained and experienced in HF management who also work closely with HF specialty–trained cardiologists. The HF APRN is responsible for ongoing monitoring of the heart failure patient, medication titration, optimization of GDMT, patient and family education, triage for acute exacerbations, and transition from hospital to home. Data has shown that HF clinics with two or more advanced practice providers are likely to have greater patient compliance with guideline-recommended care, better delivery of individualized HF education, and counseling that leads to decision making and a provider–patient relationship of trust.[17] Moreover, outpatient HF APRN–led visits when grouped with nutritionist, medication, and mental health counseling have been shown to increase HF self-care skills, compliance with GDMT, patient empowerment, and a reduction in the readmission rate by one third.[18]

In the inpatient acute care setting APRNs have been shown to correlate with reduced readmission rates in the heart failure and myocardial infarction (MI) patient population. Comparison of a medical team with an APRN with that of a medical team without an APRN showed significantly fewer postdischarge presentations to the emergency department (ED) and patient readmissions.[19] The inpatient HF APRN responsibilities may include daily rounding, patient management, and complex care transition. In a comparison of physician discharge instructions to that of the APRN discharge, the APRN placed greater emphasis on symptom identification, and was more likely to confirm a scheduled visit for follow-up.[20] As member of the multidisciplinary HF team, the APRN is an active participant in formulating treatment plans and reviewing strategies to improve practice and processes.

The APRN CNS has also been shown to impart a critical role in reducing heart failure readmissions through program development and education. Various programs describe the impact of the CNS in developing handoff tools, mechanisms for follow-up, patient education, and systems improvement. The APRN CNS may oversee content and training to all members of the care team, including mechanisms for review or reeducation in response to staff turnover and new clinical information. Such interventions are measurable in outcomes and effect on improved staff competency, patient adherence, and reduced readmission rates.[21]

CARDIAC TRANSPLANT/ VENTRICULAR ASSIST DEVICE APRN

Advanced heart failure can lead to reduced left ventricular function, unresponsiveness to medications, organ compromise, need for continuous inotropic support, and significantly reduced quality of life. Options are then directed toward evaluation for cardiac transplant, left ventricular assist devices (LVADs) to bridge to cardiac transplant while waiting for a donor organ or as a destination therapy, or palliative care. Detailed guidelines and requirements exist for transplant and LVAD therapies both clinically and institutionally.

An LVAD is a surgically implanted continuous-flow pump that directs blood from the left ventricle to the ascending aorta. This compensates for the impaired left ventricular function by increasing cardiac output. To power the LVAD, a lead ("driveline") exits the abdomen to connect to a power source, usually a battery. The LVAD can be a temporary "bridge" while waiting for donor organ availability. For patients that do not meet criteria for transplant due to conditions such as advanced age, malignancy, severe kidney disease, or morbid obesity, the LVAD can be implanted as a destination therapy to improve the quantity and quality of life.[22] Significant ongoing care and monitoring is required. Potential complications include right-sided heart failure, stroke, arrhythmia, respiratory failure, device-related infection, bleeding, and pump thrombosis. Only approximately 30% of patients are free of any adverse event at 1 year.[23]

Care for the LVAD patient requires an extensive multidisciplinary team. The VAD coordinator may be an APRN who works closely with the patient and team throughout the process of patient selection, candidacy, coordination of care, and transition to home care. Criteria for inclusion include the availability of a caregiver to be with the patient around the clock for 3 to 6 months. The education and training of patient and caregiver is extensive as is the training of all staff members involved in patient care. Most LVAD clinical APRNs are certified in critical care.

Continual outpatient care is required. The APRN closely follows these patients with clinic visits and follow-up. Particular attention is given to monitoring the driveline for infection. Ongoing psychological support and reinforcement of education are critical parts of the standard of care in these complex patients. The APRN may be the liaison for recurrent hospitalizations to provide clinical information and direct care, as well as participate in providing 24-hour on-call coverage for patient and first-responder calls.[24]

DISEASE APRN

The increase in cardiovascular care needs with an aging and growing population combined with improved access to care with the Affordable Care Act predicts a foreseeable shortage in primary care and chronic cardiovascular care providers. APRN training and scope of practice translates as a viable solution as providers for CVD treatment and preventative care. The effectiveness of outpatient CVD care and delivery between physicians and advanced practice providers has been shown to be comparable in outcomes,[25] without an increased cost in healthcare resources utilization.[26]

Coronary and post-MI patients are at risk for hospital readmission. Guidelines elucidate the importance of primary and secondary prevention for coronary disease.[18] Patients are generally seen 1 to 2 weeks post discharge in clinic as medication and therapy adherence has been shown to be more likely with early follow-up.[27] Many of these patients are seen by an APRN in a cardiology clinic for evaluation, medication reconciliation, and reinforcement of lifestyle modification education. Contrary to assumption that highly complex patients are deferred to physician care, these patients are more likely to be followed by the APRN using a team-based care model as they often require more frequent visits, closer monitoring, and medication titrations.[27]

Innovative care practices have been introduced to improve patient care and reduce cost for care of the chest pain patient. An example is the role of the APRN in the ED. For patients presenting with chest pain, once acute coronary syndrome (ACS) is ruled out, risk stratification for stable coronary disease is determined by an experienced cardiology APRN using a diagnostic algorithm and protocol. The identified patients suggestive of stable coronary disease rather than musculoskeletal pain are referred to an APRN-led chest pain clinic to be seen within 72 hours for cardiac stress testing and additional evaluation.[28]

Development of a non–ED-based cardiac direct access clinic has also been shown to reduce ED visits and hospital admissions. As an urgent care for cardiology patients, most commonly chest pain, arrhythmia, or congestive heart failure, patients are referred for same-day evaluation and observation. A physician sees patients initially and the associated observational cardiac care unit is managed by APRNs.[29]

For all patients recovering from a cardiac event, cardiac rehabilitation is indicated as secondary prevention and has been shown to significantly reduce readmissions, recurrence, and death.[30] Cardiac rehabilitation is a multidisciplinary structured guided program incorporating physical activity, nutritional education, support groups, and strategies to return to work and implement long-term lifestyle modification. Of the post-MI patients who participate in a cardiac rehabilitation program, 75% to 85% have demonstrated improvement.[30] The program takes place in an outpatient setting and includes medical supervision, counseling, and cardiac testing over a period of 36 sessions. Despite the success of cardiac rehabilitation, only 30% of affected patients are referred.[30] Reasons include need for referral education and access to care. Since inception, only physicians were allowed to oversee a cardiac rehabilitation center, greatly limiting the number of centers due to physician availability, cost, and location especially in remote or rural areas with fewer physicians. Recognizing the need to improve access and acknowledging the scope of practice of APRNs, multisocietal efforts were put forth to change legislature. In 2018, the Improving Access to Cardiac and Pulmonary Rehabilitation Act was passed allowing advanced practice providers to supervise cardiac rehabilitation services under Medicare beginning in 2024.

ARRHYTHMIA/ ELECTROPHYSIOLOGY APRN

Arrhythmia management is a rapidly growing specialty area. Interventions include pharmacology, lifestyle modification, and interventional therapies and devices. Many of the heart rhythm disorders require invasive testing and knowledge of underlying pathophysiology of conduction disease and treatment modalities.

The APRN in the arrhythmia or electrophysiology clinic would be responsible for advanced interpretation of electrocardiograms (ECGs), monitoring patients, and titrating medications for heart rate or rhythm control. Atrial fibrillation is one of the most common arrhythmias affecting nearly six million folks in the United States. The majority of these patients are on anticoagulation therapy needing regulation and monitoring for complications as well as underlying causes and available therapies. Many have multiple cardiovascular issues and need to be seen regularly. Other outpatient roles include pacemaker device interrogation, or autonomic testing centers overseeing autonomic testing such as tilt-table evaluation.

APRNs in the acute care setting manage the care of electrophysiology patients as part of a team, or by performing history and physicals for consultation. They may also work directly in the procedure lab, assisting with pacemaker implantation, catheter access for invasive studies, and other clinical procedures. Often, they also see the patients in clinic as part of their postprocedure follow-up.

Innovative APRN roles include that of injectable loop recorder implantation in the ambulatory setting. A loop recorder is subcutaneous implantable device used for continuous heart rhythm monitoring often used to assess for arrhythmias as the etiology for syncope or palpitations. The advanced practice provider–led practice has been shown to correlate with a low infection rate and a high rate of success.[31] Another example is that of an independently run outpatient cardioversion program. After specialized training and credentialing, under guideline-directed protocol, the APRN along with an anesthesiologist performs elective cardioversions in selected patients. Management includes preprocedural, periprocedural, and postprocedural care. Outcomes of the autonomously performed procedure show 95% success rate, low rate of complications, and high patient satisfaction.[32]

STRUCTURAL HEART APRN

Structural heart disease is a recent and rapidly growing specialty referring to treatment of noncoronary cardiac diseases such as heart valves and other structures of the heart via catheter-based interventions. As an alternative to conventional surgery, less invasive transcatheter therapies can be used for valve replacements, valve repairs, atrial septal defect closures, patent foramen ovale closures, left atrial appendage closures, and paravalvular leak closures. Devices and technique development are ongoing and the field includes an awareness of research and current evidence.[33]

The advent of transcatheter aortic valve replacement (TAVR) introduced a change in practice of evaluation and care for the structural heart disease patient. The role of Valve Coordinator was established, evolved to be that of most often an APRN with advanced clinical expertise and significant cardiovascular experience. The role includes patient screening and workup, procedural care, and coordination of care throughout. Advent of care for the structural heart patient necessitated formation of the Heart Team, a multidisciplinary team approach to decision making, patient selection, and preprocedure planning often including cardiac surgeons, interventional cardiologists, imaging experts, nursing staff, and various specialties as appropriate. The Valve Coordinator is the mainstay of any structural heart program. Responsibilities span direct clinical care, program development, research, and outreach.[34]

APRNs may also be involved in inpatient postprocedural care of the structural patient. Innovative centers may also have APRNs directly involved in the technical procedure. Many of the valve diseases have the sequelae of congestive heart failure for which structural heart disease care and heart failure care overlap requiring collaborative practice.

CRITICAL CARE APRN

Integration of APRNs into critical care units was introduced in the 1980s and has continued to increase. The APRN's ability to diagnose, treat, and manage acutely ill patients is an adjunct to comprehensive care. Coronary care units treat critically ill patients in cardiogenic shock secondary to a variety of etiologies and competency includes working knowledge of invasive monitoring, pacemaker management, heart pump devices, vasoactive medications, and emergency response. The APRN may manage patients in collaboration with an intensivist, or may be combined with physician staff to make up a team with overlapping responsibilities.[35]

The responsibilities may include participating in daily rounds, formulating and implementing plans of care, procedures such as invasive lines, admitting patients, and coordinating care. The APRN is also trained to focus on the holistic needs of the patient, family, and involved staff. This may include multidisciplinary discussions on goals of care and end-of-life care. In many intensive care units, the APRN is the consistent provider often involved in training residents, overseeing care standards, and serving as a resource.

Cardiothoracic surgery intensive care units care for postcardiac surgery patients. Much like the coronary care units, the APRNs function in around-the-clock coverage in managing the care of cardiac surgery patients to facilitate recovery and transfer to floor as well as manage surgical and cardiac complications. In addition to invasive line placement, the APRN may also remove and place chest tubes, remove pacing wires, remove intra-aortic balloon pumps, and manage mechanical support therapies.[36]

The critical care APRN role often requires extensive orientation and site training, and more recently institutions are trending toward developing designated training fellowship programs.[35]

EDUCATION/RESEARCH APRN

The APRN practice includes ongoing continual education for self, staff, patients, and healthcare systems. APRNs may participate in formalized research trials, conduct original research, and apply evidence-based improvements in cardiovascular care at all levels. This is particularly central in the APRN CNS role. The APRN CNS is integral in improving quality measurements, identifying and developing best practice standards, and increasing staff education.

The APRN CNS often leads protocol development and safe implementation of new therapies. One such example is development of postcardiac arrest–induced hypothermia protocol in the coronary care unit. Studies have shown that induced hypothermia post cardiac arrest may reduce edema associated with ischemic brain injury, thereby increasing the chances of meaningful recovery.[37] In this case, the APRN CNS abreast of new evidenced-based therapies conducted an extensive literature review on the subject, recruited critical care staff members to engage, and distributed data-driven information to physician teams, pharmacy, and the medical director. The APRN CNS led development of an evidenced-based site-specific protocol, vetted it through necessary departmental, clinical, and administrative approval, and spearheaded extensive education to all parties involved. Successful implementation was evidenced in outcomes tracking and utilization of therapy.[38]

The APRN CNS also oversees ongoing quality improvement and staff development. Specific to heart failure, much of outcome success is dependent on patient lifestyle modification and adherence to medical therapy achieved through patient education. This teaching is often introduced and reinforced in the inpatient setting. To review staff preparedness, a CNS-driven study was performed looking at nursing knowledge of heart failure education across several sites within a hospital system. Data suggested gaps in knowledge and provided guidance in a needs assessment to design and implement educational strategies to improve nursing knowledge, standardize education within the system, and improve patient outcomes.[39]

Quality improvement, application of research to practice, promoting best practice, and reducing cost are focal points for the APRN. In addition is the responsibility to contribute to evidence-based care and encourage publications, disseminate quality improvement projects, and attend and participate in conferences and national meetings.

LEADERSHIP

The term "Advanced" practice is inclusive of associated leadership characteristics and attributes. Improving patient outcomes, contributing to and applying evidence-based care, and affecting health systems and healthcare reform are within the scope of definition. Ongoing development of the role recognized the need for additional formalized education and training in the areas of leadership, organizational management, and policy. In 2004, the AACN released a position paper on the DNP as an additional tier to advanced practice nursing recognizing that many existing APRN programs already carried a credit load comparable to doctorate level training in other health specialties and the need to consolidate titling and formalize curricula. The DNP tract diverges to both clinical and research-focused options. Both incorporate scientific underpinnings for practice, systems thinking, information technology, healthcare policy, population health, and prevention.[40]

Ongoing healthcare changes, challenges, and complexities require leadership competencies. Leadership can be exercised at many levels. Clinically, the APRN ensures that quality care is achieved and maintained. This may be in the form of direct patient advocacy, active lifelong learning to stay abreast of the newest information, identifying areas for potential improvement, and spearheading change through protocol development, staff education, and group leadership. Patient care teams are often led by APRNs and require coordination of care and adept communication skills to facilitate multidisciplinary collaboration and interplay. Improving practice, the APRN leader may share clinical information through presenting talks or written documents and publications.[41]

Broader leadership at the systems level requires APRN knowledge of organizational function and the ability to identify gaps and influence change through the engagement of others. This may be a formal title as that of lead APRN, director, or administrator or less formal as that of participating in a task force, hospitalwide committees, or entrepreneurial ventures. Systems leadership also includes promotion of the role and further development of nursing practice and profession.[42]

Professionally, the APRN models, mentors, and educates other healthcare professionals on the role and function. Collaboration with multidisciplinary colleagues allows for mentorship and facilitation of empowerment to advanced practice. Active membership and participation in professional organizations encourages leadership in the profession and may parlay into healthcare policy and role advocacy. Local, state, and national committees and organizations are opportunities for advancing leadership development.[42]

FUTURE

Convergence of multifactorial changes in healthcare policy and patient complexity has promulgated the value and necessity of APRN practice. APRNs now exceed 270,000 in number with an additional 30% growth anticipated by 2028, far greater than that of many other professions. The majority of APRNs practice in primary care settings. The aging population's focus on preventative care and improved access to care has exponentially increased the demand for providers. Additionally, specific to cardiovascular care, demographics show that nearly half of the current cardiologists are older than 55 years, very few are women, and significant disparities exist in racial and ethnic backgrounds. Numbers of physicians going into the field of cardiology are decreasing as cost of training and changes in reimbursement deter candidates. Professional cardiology organizations have acknowledged the value of advanced practice providers in meeting cardiovascular care needs.[43]

Regulatory challenges persist in aligning APRN skill set with practice autonomy. State occupational licensing laws continue to determine whether the APRN requires full physician supervision, physician supervision for prescribing only, or no physician supervision. More autonomous APRN practice has been shown to increase the number of routine checkups and other measures of healthcare quality and reduce overall cost.[44] Currently, less than 25 states allow full practice authority and federal regulations still exist that are barriers to care. More importantly, increasing practice authority has demonstrated patterns of APRN growth not competitive to physicians, but rather complementary by broadening care to rural and underserved areas of physician scarcity.[44] The APRN needs to actively participate in advocacy efforts at institutional, state, or federal policy levels.

Maintaining quality program and certification standards is paramount for professional integrity and legitimacy. The increase in demand and growth of APRNs has led to downstream impact on availability of faculty and resources for training. As more APRNs are graduating into practice, fewer are seeking faculty positions and those in current positions are advancing in age. The AACN and federal funding efforts are being put forth to improve faculty development and retention through incentives such as educational loan repayment programs in exchange for an agreement to teaching 4 years at an accredited nursing program.[45] Critical review has suggested that clinical content of APRN programs may be more generalist in content. Transition of the newly graduated APRN into acute care specialties may identify a gap between education and practice. In response, institutions are developing and implementing postgraduate residency programs to facilitate standardized onboarding and role success. These are generally structured 12-month programs rotating through various specialties.[45]

The APRN role is unique in advancing nursing practice through development of intellectual capacity for advanced decision making, complex patient care, and foray into healthcare policy and forward improvements in quality of care. As a profession, it is important to include mechanisms to assure continued standards, continued growth, and succession planning. Professional development through mentoring, precepting, and teaching is implicit. Leading and participating in research, professional organization membership, and publication are necessary for profession protection and evolution. The APRN is burgeoning as a cardinal role in addressing the current issues in health care.

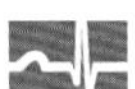 CASE STUDY

Heart Failure

Patient Profile

52-year-old Caucasian male with history of hypertension, type 2 diabetes, chronic kidney disease (CKD), obesity, coronary artery disease (CAD) with prior surgical coronary artery bypass grafting (CABG), mixed pulmonary parenchymal disease, and heart failure with preserved ejection fraction (HFpEF) who presents to the Nurse Practitioner Heart Failure Clinic for follow-up of his cardiac issues.

His dyspnea is determined to be multifactorial, including mild obstructive lung disease, diastolic dysfunction, and obesity. His ejection fraction is preserved at 52%. Invasive cardiopulmonary exercise testing showed marked increases of his pulmonary capillary wedge pressure and pulmonary artery pressures during exercise with a significantly reduced oxygen consumption. Today he reports persistent shortness of breath and fatigue. He has intermittent mild 3/10 chest discomfort. He takes 100 mg of torsemide daily and increases the dose to 200 mg when he experiences abdominal bloating or pedal edema. Baseline weight is 220 lb.

History significant for:
Hypertension
Type 2 diabetes
Dyslipidemia
CAD s/p CABG, chronic chest pain secondary to microvascular disease
HFpEF
Paroxysmal atrial fibrillation
History of remote myocarditis
Mild obstructive lung disease
Obesity
Hypothyroidism
CKD

Social History

He is a businessman now working only part time due to decreased activity tolerance. He is divorced, lives alone with a son living nearby. He is independent with activities of daily living and lives in an apartment with elevator access. He is a never smoker and former moderate alcohol intake, none for the last 3 years.

Family History

No family history of early myocardial infarction, arrhythmia, cardiomyopathies, or sudden cardiac death.

Allergies

No known allergies

Medications

Atorvastatin 40 mg daily
Carvedilol 50 mg twice a day
Diltiazem HCl 420 mg extended release daily
Lisinopril 10 mg daily
Ranolazine 500 mg twice a day
Empagliflozin 10 mg daily
Glipizide 10 mg twice a day
Levothyroxine 150 mg daily
Metformin 1000 mg daily
Spironolactone 2 mg daily
Torsemide 100 mg daily

Physical Examination

The patient is a well-groomed, well-appearing male in no acute distress and resting comfortably in a chair.
Ambulating independently. He is awake, alert, and fully oriented and conversant. He is responding appropriately to questions. There are no focal neurologic abnormalities. He has appropriate mood and affect.

Vital Signs

B/P 146/84; HR 78; O_2 Sat 98%; Wt. 224.2 and stable
Pt did not take any of his home medications prior to this clinic visit.
The head is normocephalic and atraumatic. Normal facial expressions and contours without asymmetries, involuntary movements, edema, masses, or lesions. Alignment of eyes is good and equal. The sclerae are anicteric.

(continued)

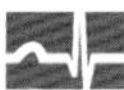 CASE STUDY (*Continued*)

Heart Failure

The neck is supple. The trachea is midline with good tone.
Respirations are symmetric with good expansion, unlabored, and regular. Lung sounds are clear to auscultation with good air movement.
JVP is at 8 cm H_2O. Regular heart rate and rhythm with normal S1, physiologically split S2. No murmurs, rubs, or gallops.
The abdomen is rotund, nontender, and nondistended with active bowel sounds.
The extremities are warm, dry, and well perfused. No edema to upper or lower extremities.
No varicosities, redness, or stasis pigmentation to lower extremities.

Laboratory Data

Hemoglobin 14.5 g/dL
Hematocrit 43.1%
Blood urea nitrogen 30 mg/dL
Creatinine 2.0 mg/dL
Alanine aminotransferase (ALT) 31 IU/L
Asparate aminotransferase (AST) 21 IU/L
NTproBNP 296 pg/mL

Review of Recent Management

Frequent clinic visits and follow-up calls with titration of diuretics.
Two referrals to outpatient infusion APRN clinic for intravenous diuretics.
Extensive and ongoing education regarding diet, medications, disease, and lifestyle modifications.
Consideration for implantable heart failure–monitoring system declined by insurance carrier.
Optimizing medical therapy adding ACE-I, uptitrated diltiazem for continued chest discomfort.

Assessment

53-year-old male with history of hypertension, T2DM, chronic kidney disease, obesity, coronary artery disease (CAD) post CABG, mixed pulmonary parenchymal disease, and heart failure with preserved ejection fraction appearing euvolemic on examination today. NYHA Heart Failure Classification III.

Plan: No plan for medication changes as patient is currently on stable doses of guideline-directed medical therapy (GDMT). Reinforced heart failure teaching and parameters to contact office. Confirmed understanding of self-monitoring and adjustment of diuretic dosing. Discussed at length a weight loss program as an intervention to reduce hypertension, left ventricular dysfunction, CAD, and restrictive pulmonary dysfunction. Plan is to refer patient to a structured medical weight loss program. He is agreeable. He will also be referred to an academic medical center for consideration for clinical trial options. Follow-up calls will continue to monitor patient and return to clinic. Social work consulted to assist with reimbursement approval for implantable hemodynamic monitoring.

Summary/APRN Role

Heart failure is a chronic and progressive disease with intermittent periods of decompensation requiring hospitalization. Management is a combination of preventing disease progression, self-care teaching, and close monitoring. APRN-led teams have been shown to improve patient quality of life and reduce hospital readmissions (Black et al., 2017).

APRN Competencies

Advanced-level knowledge and understanding of pathophysiology of heart failure and comorbid conditions.
Prescriptive authority facilitating frequent titration of medications using evidence-based guideline-directed medical therapy.
Complex decision making directing need for intravenous diuretic therapy in the setting of concomitant renal dysfunction.
Understanding of appropriate testing and interpretation to treat and diagnose, including laboratory values, chest x-ray, electrocardiogram (ECG), echocardiogram, cardiac exercise testing, etc.
Patient education and staff education to implement nonpharmacologic lifestyle modification interventions, including low sodium diet, fluid restriction, exercise activity, and self-monitoring parameters.
Advanced physical assessment skills specific to cardiac disease and holistic measures, including screening for depression, anxiety, and level of social support.
Healthcare systems knowledge of reimbursement and access.
Participation in research and continued learning.
Utilization of evidence-based risk-scoring tools to predict trajectory of disease, tailoring of therapies, and incorporation of patient shared decision making.
Leadership in coordinating multidisciplinary team-based care.

KEY READINGS

Black S, Frazier S, Haydo M. A nurse practitioner directed, interdisciplinary model for heart failure transitional care. *J Cardiovasc Nurs.* 2017;32(5):424–425.

Bowers M. Managing patients with heart failure. *J Nurse Pract.* 2013;9(10)634–641.

Yancy CW, Jessup M, Bozkurt B, et al. 2017 ACC/AHA/HFSA Focused Update of the 2013 ACCF/AHA Guideline for the management of heart failure: a report of the American College of Cardiology/American Heart Association Task Force on Clinical Practice Guidelines and the Heart Failure Society of America. *J Am Coll Cardiol.* 2017;70(6):776–803.

REFERENCES

1. Hamric AB. A definition of advanced practice nursing. In: Hamric AB, Hanson CM, Tracy MF, et al., eds. *Advanced Practice Nursing: An Integrative Approach.* 5th ed. St. Louis, MO: Saunders; 2014.
2. Gray M, Ratliff C, Mawyer R. A brief history of advanced practice nursing and its implications for WOC advanced nursing practice. *J Wound Ostomy Continence Nurs.* 2000;27(1):48–54.
3. Keeling AW. *Historical perspectives on an expanded role for nursing. OJIN.* 2015;20(2):Manuscript 2.
4. Cockerham AZ, Keeling AW. Historical and developmental aspects of advanced practice nursing. In: Hamric AB, Hanson CM, Tracy MF, et al., eds. *Advanced Practice Nursing an Integrative Approach.* 5th ed. St. Louis, MI: Elsevier Saunders; 2014.
5. Safriet BJ. Closing the gap between can and may in healthcare providers' scope of practice: a primer for policymakers. *Faculty Scholarship Series.* 2002;442:301–334.
6. Haber J, Hildegard E. Peplau: the psychiatric nursing legacy of a legend. *J Am Psychiatr Nurses Assoc.* 2004;6(2):56–62.
7. National Council of State Boards of Nursing (NCSBN). *History of APRN.* Available at https://www.ncsbn.org/737.htm. 2020
8. APRN Consensus Work Group & the National Council of State Boards of Nursing APRN Advisory Committee. *Consensus model for APRN regulation: Licensure, accreditation, certification & education [Press release].*

Available at https://www.ncsbn.org/Consensus_Model_for_APRN_Regulation_July_2008.pdf. Accessed July 7, 2008.
9. Hanson C, Hamric A. Reflections on the continuing evolution of advanced practice nursing. *Nurs Outlook.* 2003;51(5):203–211.
10. The Patient Protection and Affordable Care Act, Public Law 111–148 Authenticated U.S. Government Information §§ 1001–10909. 2010.
11. Institute of Medicine. *The Future of Nursing: Leading Change, Advancing Health.* Washington, DC: National Academy of Sciences; 2011.
12. Vincent D, Reed PG. Affordable Care Act: overview and implications for advancing nursing. *Nurs Sci Q.* 2014;27(3):254–259.
13. Centers for Disease Control and Prevention (CDC). Available at https://www.cdc.gov/heartdisease/facts.htm#:~:text=Heart%20disease%20is%20the%20leading,1%20in%20every%204%20deaths. Accessed March 1, 2020.
14. Benjamin EJ, Muntner P, Alonso A, et al; American Heart Association Council on Epidemiology and Prevention Statistics Committee and Stroke Statistics Subcommittee. Heart disease and stroke statistics—2019 update: a report from the American Heart Association. *Circulation.* 2019;139(10):e56–e528.
15. Windey M, Cosme C. American Nurses Credentialing Center Practice Transition Accreditation Program Update. *J Nurses Prof Dev.* 2017;33(4):205–206.
16. Mozaffarian D, Benjamin EJ, Go AS, et al. Heart disease and stroke statistics—2016 update: a report from the American Heart Association. *Circulation.* 2016;133:e38–e360.
17. Albert NM, Fonarow GC, Yancy CW, et al. Outpatient cardiology practices with advanced practice nurses and physician assistants provide similar delivery of recommended therapies (findings from IMPROVE HF). *Am J Cardiol.* 2010;105(12):1773–1779.
18. Smith SC, Benjamin EJ, Bonow RO, et al. AHA/ACCF secondary prevention and risk reduction therapy for patients with coronary and other atherosclerotic vascular disease: 2011 update: a guideline from the American Heart Association and American College of Cardiology Foundation. *Circulation.* 2011;124:2458–2473.
19. David D, Britting L, Dalton J. Cardiac acute care nurse practitioner and 30-day readmission. *J Cardiovasc Nurs.* 2015;30(3):248–255.
20. David D, Howard E, Dalton J, et al. Self-care in heart failure hospital discharge instructions—differences between nurse practitioner and physician providers. *J Nurse Pract.* 2018;14(1):18–25.
21. Wood RL, Migliore LA, Nasshan SJ, et al. Confronting challenges in reducing heart failure 30-day readmissions: lessons learned with implications for evidence-based practice. *Worldviews Evid Based Nurs.* 2019;16(1):43–50.
22. Martonik H. Caring for patients with a left ventricular assist device. *Am Nurse Today.* 2017;12(5):20–25. Available at AmericanNurseToday.com
23. Pinney SP, Anyanwu AC, Lala A, et al. Left ventricular assist devices for lifelong support. *J Am Coll Cardiol.* 2017;69(23):2845–2861.
24. Casida J, Johnson C, Schroeder SE. Missing link: clarity and impact of nurse practitioners' roles on outcomes of ventricular assist device programs in the United States. *AACN Adv Crit Care.* Summer 2019;30(2):181–184.
25. Virani SS, Akeroyd JM, Ramsey DJ, et al. Comparative effectiveness of outpatient cardiovascular disease and diabetes care delivery between advanced practice providers and physician providers in primary care: Implications for care under the Affordable Care Act. *Am Heart J.* 2016;181:74–82.
26. Virani SS, Akeroyd JM, Ramsey DJ, et al. Health care resource utilization for outpatient cardiovascular disease and diabetes care delivery among advance practice providers and physician providers in primary care. *Popul Health Manag.* 2018;21:209–216.
27. Rymer JA, Chen AY, Thomas L, et al. Advanced practice provider versus physician-only outpatient follow-up after acute myocardial infarction. *J Am Heart Assoc.* 2018;7(17):e008481.
28. Ingram SJ, McKee G, Quirke MB, et al. Discharge of non-acute coronary syndrome chest pain patients from emergency care to an advanced nurse practitioner-led chest pain clinic. *J Cardiovasc Nurs.* 2017;32(2):E1–E8.
29. Cajiao K, Estrada-Roman A, McCarthy K, et al. The impact of a non-emergency department based cardiac direct access unit on hospital. *J Am Coll Cardiol.* 2019;73:(9 Suppl 1):231.
30. Thomas RJ, Balady G, Banka G, et al. 2018 ACC/AHA clinical performance and quality measures for cardiac rehabilitation. *J Am Coll Cardiol.* 2018;71(16):1814–1837.
31. Kipp R, Kopp D, Teelin T, et al. Injectable loop recorder implantation in an ambulatory setting by advanced practice providers: analysis of outcomes. *Pacing Clin Electrophysiol.* 2017;40(9):982–985.
32. Strzelcsyk TA, Kaplan RM, Medler M, et al. Outcomes associated with electrical cardioversion for atrial fibrillation when performed autonomously by an advanced practice provider. *JACC Clin Electrophysiol.* 2017;3(12):1447–1452.
33. Steinberg DH, Staubach S, Franke J, et al. Defining structural heart disease in the adult patient: current scope, inherent challenges and future directions. *Eur Heart J Suppl.* 2010;12(Suppl_E):E2–E9.
34. Perpetua EM, Clarke SE, Guibone KA, et al. Surveying the landscape of structural heart disease coordinator: an exploratory study of the coordinator role. *Structural Heart.* 2019;3(3):201–210.
35. Dykstra AC, Marini J. Integration of nurse practitioners into the critical care team. *ICU Management Practice.* 2017;4:238–240.
36. Jensen L, Scherr K. Impact of the nurse practitioner role in cardiothoracic surgery. *Dynamics.* 2004 Fall;15(3):14–19.
37. Holzer M, Bernard SA, Hachim-Idrissi S, et al. Hypothermia for neuroprotection after cardiac arrest: systematic review and individual patient data meta-analysis. *Crit Care Med.* 2005;33:414–418.
38. Kosik TM. Induced hypothermia for patients with cardiac arrest. *Crit Care Nurse.* 2007;27(5):36–42.
39. Mahramus TL, Penoyer DA, Sole ML, et al. Clinical nurse specialist assessment of nurses' knowledge of heart failure. *Clin Nurse Spec.* 2013;27(4):198–204.
40. American Association of Colleges of Nursing. *AACN position statement on the practice document in nursing.* Available at http://www.aacn.nche.edu/publications/position/DNPpositionstatement.pdf. 2004. Accessed March 1, 2020.
41. Tracy MF, Hanson CM. Leadership. In: Hamric AB, Hanson CM, Tracy MF, et al., eds. *Advanced Practice Nursing: An Integrative Approach.* 5th ed. St. Louis, MO: Elsevier; 2014:266–298.
42. Lamb A, Misener RM, Lukosius DB, et al. Describing the leadership capabilities of advanced practice nurses using a qualitative descriptive study. *Nurs Open.* 2018;500:400–413.
43. Narang A, Sinha SS, Rajagopalan B, et al. The supply and demand of the cardiovascular workforce striking the right balance. *J Am Coll Cardiol.* 2016;68(15):1680–1689.
44. McMichael BJ. Beyond physicians: the effect of licensing and liability laws on the supply of nurse practitioners and physician assistants. *J Empir Leg Stud.* 2018;15(4):732–771.
45. Harris C. Bridging the gap between acute care nurse practitioners education and practice: the need for postgraduate residency programs. *J Nurse Practitioners.* 2014;10(5):331–336. Available at www.npjournal.org

45 Leadership and Team-Based Care

Elizabeth M. Perpetua

OBJECTIVES

1. Envision the future of nursing and reflect upon the leadership development necessary to bring this vision to fruition.
2. Describe the competencies, skill sets, and outcomes of effective leadership in cardiac nursing.
3. Define team-based care and describe cardiac nursing's role in the future of team-based care.
4. Describe the competencies, skill sets, and outcomes of effective team-based care in cardiac nursing.
5. Introduce professional development considerations for cardiac nursing leadership and team-based care.

KEY QUESTIONS

1. What is leadership? Can anyone be a leader?
2. How do leadership and management differ?
3. What are the characteristics and skill sets of an effective leader or team?
4. How does an effective leader or an effective team impact performance and outcomes?
5. What is the role of professional development in leadership and team-based care?

A VISION FOR NURSING LEADERSHIP

The Institute of Medicine landmark paper, *Future of Nursing: Leading Change, Advancing Health*, powerfully articulated a transformative vision of our profession.[1] Four key tenets were outlined:

1. **Transform Practice:** Nurses should practice to the full extent of their education and training.
2. **Transform Education:** Nurses should achieve higher levels of education and training through an improved education system that promotes seamless academic progression.
3. **Transform Planning and Policy:** Effective workforce planning and policy making require better data collection and improved information infrastructure.
4. **Transform Leadership:** Nurses should be full partners with physicians and other health professionals in redesigning health care.[1]

Now more than ever, each and every nurse is called upon to lead. Leadership does not require a formal title or role; rather, the operating definition of leader is someone who inspires positive, transformative change in people, teams, or organizations. The change proposed here is the shared vision described in these critical messages in *Future of Nursing*. As cardiovascular disease has the highest morbidity and mortality of any disease worldwide, the opportunities for cardiac nurses to engage in leadership abound. Let each nurse do what we can from right where we are in our current roles: nursing students, front-line nurses, nurse managers, nurse researchers, advanced practice nurses, chief nursing officers.

The purpose of this chapter is to (1) define leadership and team-based care; (2) describe competencies, skill sets, and outcomes of effective leadership and team-based care; and (3) introduce professional development considerations for leadership and team-based care. Important aims of this chapter are to cultivate the spirit and skills of leadership and to empower nurses to use their voices to share their knowledge and experience. To that end, incorporated throughout this chapter are **reflective journaling** exercises. This journaling is informed by reflective practice, which is the intentional self-assessment, analysis, and synthesis of strengths and opportunities for professional leadership development and improvement.[2] An introductory journaling practice incorporating elements of mindfulness, emotional intelligence, and logic modeling is described in Display 45-1 with foundational exercises in Displays 45-2 to 45-5. Openness and curiosity are key whilst reading this chapter and engaging in these reflective journal exercises. This process requires courage and vulnerability and this introspection may be experienced as exhilarating, uncomfortable, or even indulgent or trite, at first. This practice aims to reinforce that the most important voice to listen to is your own. While much knowledge can be sought in texts such as this, reflective practice answers the most important questions within ourselves. After all, it is said that we do not learn from experience, but from reflecting on our experience.[3] May this text and your work empower and further your development as a leader.

DISPLAY 45-1

Introduction to Reflective Journaling

1. Designate time and space for reflective practice.
   a. Give yourself time to work through the exercise (5 min for a question, 15–30 min for an exercise)
   b. Give yourself a space to work on the exercise: a journal to record your work (audio, video, handwritten, electronic) and a comfortable, inviting place to engage in reflective practice
2. Commit to recall the prompted scenario(s) systematically with curiosity, neutrality, and the intention to seek authenticity.
3. Recall and collect the following as data points of the scenario(s) systematically and as these data arise.
   a. Why, who, what, where, when
   b. Thoughts, wants, emotions
   c. Body experience (e.g., sympathetic nervous system responses) and the sequence or relationship with specific data points (e.g., pulse racing and palms racing with anxiety; sensation of heart and chest expanding with gratitude)
   d. Orientation to self and others
   e. How, how much and how well
4. Complete the reflection process and record it in your journal.
5. Review the recorded reflection, adding any new data and annotating insights or themes.
6. Record specifically any opportunities for improvement and connect the rationale to core values and/or desired goals or outcomes and associated anticipated emotions.
7. Rewrite a brief summary of the scenario with the new process and insights.
8. Visualize the scenario systematically per step #3, emphasizing the heightened, positive desired emotions.
9. Integrate the scenario systematically, emphasizing the heightened, positive desired emotions paired with values and goals and their experience in the body.
10. Designate time and space for self-care after reflective practice—hydration, nutrition, exercise, deep breathing, leisure activity, rest.

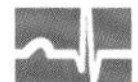
DISPLAY 45-2

Reflective Journal Exercise: Who is a Leader?

Take 5 min and write down the names of inspiring leaders. Consider their qualities, their accomplishments.
Do not read on until you have done so.

After your list and reflection is complete, then consider the following questions:
- Is your name on this list?
- Are any of the names you wrote down nurses?
- Are nurses considered leaders? Why or why not?
- What beliefs, insights, or biases were revealed by this exercise? What did you learn?

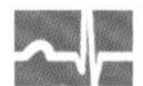
DISPLAY 45-3

Reflective Journal Exercise: Leadership Self-Awareness—You are a Leader

Reflect now upon a time you were extraordinarily inspired by a leader.
Recall as many details as you can using the reflective practice instructions introduced in Display 45-1.

Now consider this insight: You recognize in others the qualities you have in yourself. In other words, you and this leader that inspires you are alike.
- We are often inspired by qualities that we possess but have yet to develop or may not yet fully recognize or own in ourselves.
- What are the stories and characteristics of this leader that ignite and empower you?
- What thoughts, emotions, stories, or goals arise during this exercise? What old stories or new insights arise, and which of these serve you and your goals?

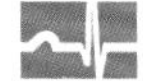
DISPLAY 45-4

Reflective Journal Exercise: Leadership Awareness—We are ALL Leaders

The simple definition provided for leadership in this chapter suggests that *anyone* can lead. Recall an individual who inspired meaningful change in your organization or in your career. What was this leader's vision or goal?

Consider the motivations, values, words, actions that influenced you to work toward this leader's vision or goal. Recall your relationship with this leader, your interactions with one another. What path and processes were created or facilitated?
- Why was this experience particularly meaningful to you? What potential in you manifested? Recall the details—what did this look and feel like to you? How did this impact you and your life? Perhaps there is a signature or footprint in your communication, decisions, and behaviors directly shaped by this individual or time in your life.
- Notice the thoughts and feelings that arise during this reflection, and without judgment or attachment to a "correct" answer, recall the role or position this person had: Was this a manager, supervisor, or individual with overt authority, a title? How did this leader and experience influence your perspective, attitudes, behaviors?
- How did interprofessional dynamics or relationships obstruct or catalyze leadership success for this leader? For you?
- Was the vision or goal realized? Sustained? If so, why? If not, why not? What did you learn about your own perceptions and relationships as a result? What might you consider or do differently in the future?

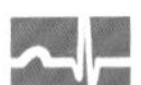 DISPLAY 45-5

Reflective Journal Exercise: Define and Evaluate Leadership

How do you define and evaluate leadership?
What is your personal definition of leadership?

- Provide 1–2 specific examples of your accomplishments as a leader.
- Provide 1–2 specific scenarios that exemplify your leadership style.
- Provide as much detail as you can. What compelled you to select these particular scenarios?
- How do you evaluate leadership style and performance?
- Have you used any assessment tools in the past? If so, what did these assessments reveal?

DEFINING LEADERSHIP

Leadership, a core standard of the cardiac nurse, is defined across disciplines and in this chapter as the ability to develop and influence people and processes toward a shared vision or goal.[2,4,5] Nurses believe we know effective leadership when we see it: lives are saved and health care teams and organizations are transformed because of it.[6–8] Numerous benefits have been associated with effective leadership: improved nursing recruitment engagement, retention, role satisfaction; patient experience and outcomes; cost savings and increased value.[9–12] Therein lies the opportunity for cardiac nurses who strive to understand, meet, and model this core standard.

Overcoming the Nursing Paradoxes

Paradox of Numbers

Nurses are the largest profession in health care and provide up to 95% of the direct patient care in hospitals. Opinion leaders however perceive nurses as minimally influential to healthcare reform, access to health care, healthcare decision making, or revenue generation.[13] If there are more nurses providing more care than any other health profession, then why is nursing's perceived impact so disproportionate to its presence and contribution?[14]

Paradox of Trust

For 18 years in a row, nursing has ranked highest among all professions for honesty and ethics. In 2019, 85% of 1021 respondents ranked nurses as very high/highly honest and ethical, with engineers (66%) and medical doctors (65%) ranked as second and third, respectively.[15] With trust one may expect much needed support, resources, even activism however nursing advocates—the public, colleagues, leadership and even nurses themselves—are challenged to describe what nurses know or do.

Navigating the Polarity Trap

The incongruence of nursing's role and perceived impact has been attributed to many factors: a demographic historically stigmatized and oppressed, predominantly comprised of a membership that identifies as women[16]; the healthcare hierarchy in which disempowerment, blame, and bullying is normalized and prevalent toward and among nurses[17]; and the elimination of billing for hospital nursing services[18] which systematically decoupled revenue from the work nurses perform. Nursing may be subsequently described in dichotomous polarities—taskmasters instead of evidence-based critical thinkers; doing and implementing as opposed to directing and leading; or direct costs on a budget unassociated with revenue generation or contribution to quality patient outcomes.[13] To overcome the polarity trap nurses must make their voices heard and be prepared to go beyond the comfortable diatribe of "just doing the job" or "the art and science of caring."[1,13,14] Nurses must be (1) positioned to lead from a platform of our knowledge, competencies, and skills and (2) armed with evidence that substantiates the impact of our profession.

Providing Multigenerational Mentorship

Transforming nursing leadership means attention must be paid to the multigenerational dynamics of mentoring nurse leaders.[19] In practice this profession has four generations of nurses, for whom traits, values, historical influences, and motivations for remaining in practice vary dramatically (Fig. 45-1). As the veteran and baby boomer generation retires, millennials are increasingly likely to exit the workforce due to a lack of job satisfaction.[20] Emerging nurse leaders also report idealistic and possibly unrealistic expectations of their leaders, anticipating high-level advocacy while recognizing the competing demands of frontline staff and administrative responsibilities. A landmark editorial sought to dispel myths and misperceptions between millennials and mentors with the aim of inspiring and improving intergenerational mentorship (Table 45-1).[21] Highly engaged nurse leaders, both established and emerging, are important to sustaining and advancing the profession of nursing.

LEADERSHIP COMPETENCIES

Going from silence to voice involves knowledge of the leadership competencies in one's specialty and role. This section provides an overview of these competencies and curates resources for further reading.

Preventative Cardiology Nurses Association, a prime example of professional leadership, drafted leadership competencies in 2006. To follow, the American College of Cardiology convened several professional organizations to create the Scope and Standards of Cardiovascular Nursing. The competencies for leadership, differentiated for the scope of registered nurses (RNs) and advanced practice registered nurses (APRNs), are listed in Table 45-2. These competencies of the cardiovascular nurse are generally aligned with the three leadership domains (personal, group, and organizational levels) and the related competency clusters identified by the American Nurses Association (Table 45-3). For example, the nurse competent leading the organization in change management will effectively manage others' resistance to organizational change and is straightforward about the consequences of an expected decision or action. A review of the full document is outside of the scope of this chapter however highly recommended.

Leadership competencies are specific to the level of education or licensure (scope), position, or role, and typically endorsed by a professional society or certification.[22,23] Additional APRN competencies are notable for the expanded clinical scope of diagnosis

Generational cohort	Birth years	Traits/characteristics	Core values	History influence	Percentage of RN workforce
Veteran	1925–1945	Traditionalist Silent generation 'Do the right thing' Conservative Independent	Self-sacrifice Values rules Conformity Dedicated/Loyal	WWII Great Depression	2
Baby Boomer	1946–1964	'Live to work' Workaholics Team players Favours job security Well educated	Commitment Optimistic Personal growth Involvement	Civil Rights Vietnam War Equal rights Birth control pills	40
Generation X	1965–1980	'Work to Live' Latch–Key Kids Independent Informal Innovative	Work-life balance Diversity Global thinkers Self-reliance	Watergate Challenger shuttle explosion AIDS	40
Millennial	1981–2000	Ability to multi-task technology savvy Crave instant & continuous feedback Confident Wants to be a part of something/sense of belonging	Values meaningful work Civic minded Social responsibility Teamwork Confidence Sociability	Internet Advancement of technology Terrorist attack of 9/11 Death of Princess Diana Columbine shooting	15

Note: Adapted from Farrell & Hurt, 2014; Murphy, 2011; Stanley, 2010; Strauss & Howe, 1991; Smith-Trudeau, 2016; Sullivan-Havens et al., 2013.

Figure 45-1. The multigenerational nursing workforce. (Used with permission from Hisel M. Measuring work engagement in a multigenerational nursing workforce. *J Nurs Manag*. 2020;28(2):294–305.)

and therapy prescription, and the related clinical, health policy, and health system change.[24,25]

LEADERSHIP VERSUS MANAGEMENT

The tenet that anyone can lead stands in contrast to the stereotype that leaders must be charismatic extroverts whose titles confer authority. In fact, leaders may manage and managers may lead, but not all leaders manage nor all managers lead. A manager may be described as focused on navigating and maintaining the *how* (i.e., transactions and implementation) whereas the leader may be described as focused on the *why* (i.e., the purpose, mission, vision, values, goals). Leadership and management are not mutually exclusive but interdependent. To illustrate this, the American Organization of Nurse Executives model (Fig. 45-2) blends nursing leadership and management and identifies competencies for nurse managers at the personal, group, and organization levels.[22] Reflective practice exercises (e.g., Display 45-6) may provide further insight of the distinction between management and leadership.

How might cardiac nurses' leadership capabilities be perceived or evaluated by peers, supervisors, and other disciplines? Research is limited. Evaluation of leadership competencies has found that the following activities may be indicative of leadership competency but must be weighed on a case-by-case basis[26]:

- Health system leadership through policy work and development, change management or change agent roles, committees

Table 45-1 • CONSIDERATIONS FOR MENTORING MILLENNIALS

Millennial			Mentor	
Myth	**Reality**	**Perspective**	**Avoid**	**Embrace**
Impatient	Efficient	Accustomed to rapid information and distillation	Inertia	Innovation
Entitled	Motivated	Do not view social distinctions in the hierarchy in the same way as previous generations	Hierarchy	Autonomy
Lazy	Balanced	Motivated by purpose, organizational mission, and skill over "time in rank" or traditional advancement metrics	Busywork	Purpose
Narcissistic	Empowered	Desire early advancement based on vision and deliverables	Subordinate	Leadership
Social	Collaborative	Have a greater sense of global consciousness	Uniformity	Diversity
Needy	Engaged	Used to instant responses due to social media and technology	Isolation	Community

Adapted from Waljee JF, Chopra V, Saint S. Mentoring millennials. *JAMA*. 2018;319(15):1547–1548.

Table 45-2 • LEADERSHIP, SCOPE AND STANDARDS FOR CARDIOVASCULAR NURSES

Standard: The cardiovascular registered nurse demonstrates leadership in the practice setting and the profession

Oversees the nursing care given by others while retaining accountability for the quality of care given to the patient

Supports the vision, associated goals, and plan to implement and measure progress of an individual patient or progress within the context of the healthcare organization

Demonstrates commitment to continuous lifelong learning and education for self and others

Mentors colleagues for the advancement of nursing practice, the profession and quality health care

Treats colleagues with respect, trust, and dignity

Develops communication and conflict resolution skills

Participates in professional organizations

Communicates effectively with patients and colleagues

Seeks ways to advance nursing autonomy and accountability

Participates in efforts to impact healthcare policy

Standard: Additional advanced practice registered nurse competencies

Seeks ways to advance nursing autonomy and accountability

Participates in efforts to impact healthcare policy

Leads decision-making groups and organizations to improve the professional practice environment and patient outcomes

Provides direction to enhance the effectiveness of the interprofessional team

Promotes advanced practice nursing and role development by interpreting its role for patients, families, and others

Models expert practice to interprofessional team members and patients

Mentors colleagues in the acquisition of clinical knowledge, skills, abilities and judgment

Adapted from American Nurses Association. Cardiovascular nursing: Scope and standards of practice (2nd ed). 2015, American Nurses Association: Silver Spring, MD.

Table 45-3 • AMERICAN NURSES' ASSOCIATION LEADERSHIP INSTITUTE COMPETENCIES

Leading Yourself	Leading Others	Leading the Organization
Adaptability Openness to influence, flexibility	**Communication** Communicating effectively	**Business acumen** Seeks broad business knowledge
Image Executive image	**Conflict** Confronting problem employees	**Change** Change management
Initiative Builds relationship	**Employee development** Development and empowerment	**Decision making** Decisiveness
Learning capacity Knowledge of job, business	**Relationships** Building collaborative relationships	**Influence** Strategic perspective
Self-awareness		**Problem solving** Getting information, making sense of it, problem identification
		System thinking Acts systemically
		Vision and strategy Strategic planning
		Project management Organizes

Adapted from American Nurses Association. ANA Leadership Institute Competency Model. 2018, July; https://www.nursingworld.org/-4a0a2e/globalassets/docs/ce/177626-ana-leadership-booklet-new-final.pdf.

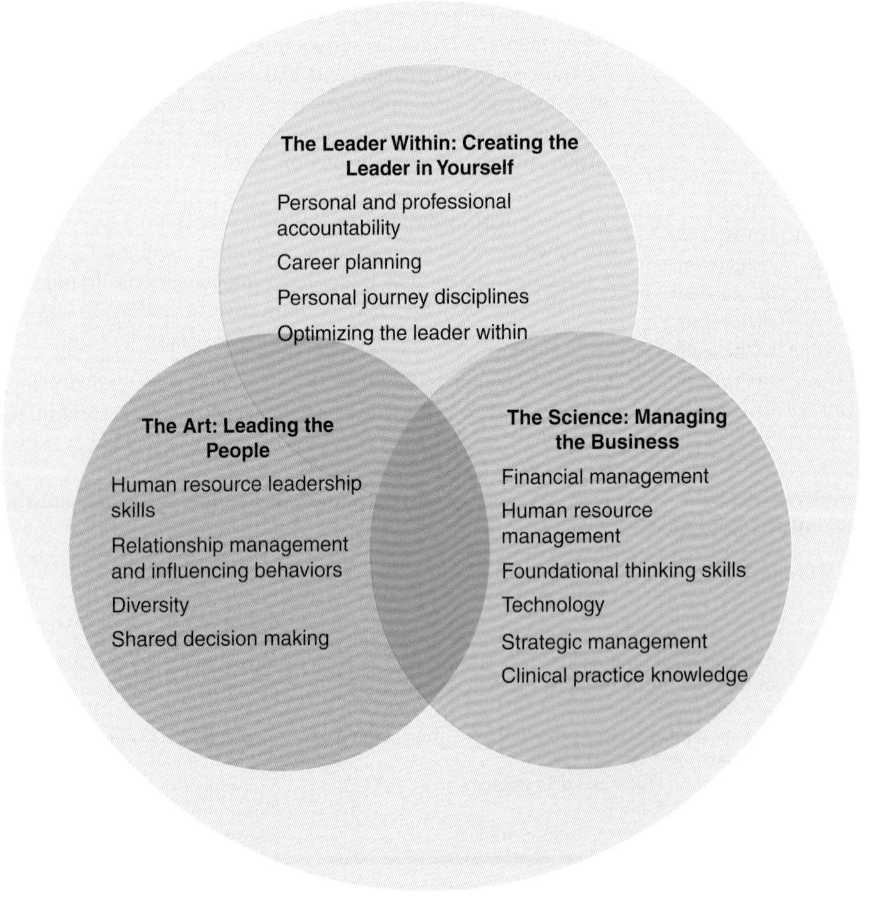

Figure 45-2. American Organization of Nurse Executives nurse manager competencies. (Adapted from American Organization of Nurse Executives. Chicago, IL: AONE; 2015. http://www.aone.org/resources/nurse-leader-competencies.shtml.)

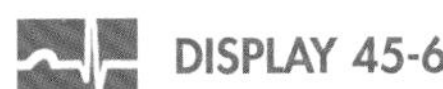

DISPLAY 45-6

Reflective Journaling Exercise: Leadership and Management

Name a current **manager** in your organization. Using a specific scenario as the context for this exercise, would you describe this manager as a leader? Why or why not?

Name a current **leader** in your organization. Using a specific scenario as the context for this exercise, would you describe this leader as a manager? Why or why not?

and advisory board work, development or evaluation of initiatives, practice inquiry

- Clinical collaboration and scholarship including research and publication, presentations, professional recognition, grant writing, consulting activities
- Role model or mentorship activities including teaching, formal mentoring including for any of the above[26]

LEADERSHIP IN TEAM-BASED CARE

Cardiac nurses are agents of change. Out of necessity, this specialty has brought to bear some of the most advanced, complex life-saving therapies from bench to bedside in a very short amount of time. Translation of research to practice may take on average up to 18 years; cardiology has never had the luxury of time. Our specialty's mantras is "time is muscle." Our metrics are door-to-balloon times of 90 minutes. From the coronary care unit to coronary artery stenting, and now with transcatheter valve therapies or advanced heart failure therapies, cardiac nurses have been instrumental in translation and implementation of these innovations. With deep and broad end-user knowledge and relationship with nearly all team members and service lines involved in the care of the patients, the cardiac nurse is often a maven, connector, and salesperson who ensures patient safety and quality of nursing care are matched to the pioneering technology or protocols. The ever-growing complexity of health care and specialization (Fig. 45-3) has resulted in many leadership opportunities for the cardiac nurse in team-based care. The paradigm shift to interdisciplinary team care (Table 45-4) continues to drive these roles to the forefront.

Table 45-4 • PARADIGM SHIFTS DRIVING TEAM-BASED CARE

Prior Paradigm	Paradigm Shift
Physician-centric	Patient-centered
Acute, inpatient care	Prevention
Department or therapy-based	Disease or condition-based
Single episodes or encounters of care	Continuum of care
Fragmentation	Coordination, triage, and access to care
Centralization within silos	Collaboration and specialization
Standardized but not individualized	Protocolized and personalized
Paternal, hierarchical	Transparency, shared decision-making
Volumes	Quality and value
Quantity of life	Quality of life

In addition to conventional nurse manager or director positions, novel roles have emerged in care coordination, research, program development, and strategy. The titles for these positions may vary at the hospital or health system level however cardiac nurses and advanced practice providers roles increasingly function as critical members of the Heart Team.[27] These roles are described in the literature for heart failure[28]; advanced heart failure including ventricular assist device or mechanical circulatory system teams and transplant[29]; electrophysiology particularly for atrial fibrillation, device management, and neuro-electrophysiology[30]; congenital heart disease[31]; valvular and structural heart disease[32,33]; and chest pain units.[34] Professional society guidelines have specific recommendations for advanced practice providers in team-based care.[35] Cardiac nurses are also named as key team members in the regulatory requirements (i.e., Centers for Medicare and Medicaid Services [CMS]) of patients receiving certain therapies such as transcatheter aortic valve replacement and transcatheter mitral valve repair or edge-to-edge repair.[36,37] As a member of the care team, the cardiac nurse can have an important role in advocacy and policy change (Display 45-7).

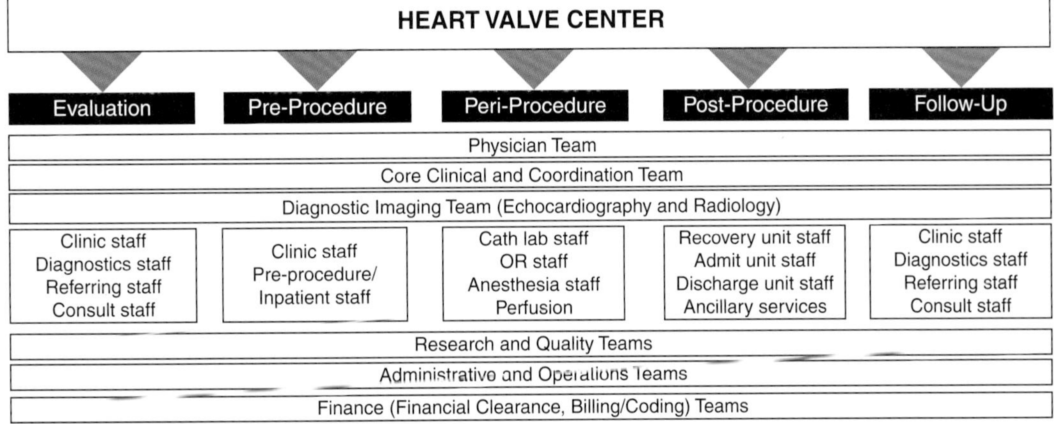

Figure 45-3. The Heart Valve Center: A Team of Teams. This figure provides an example of the multidisciplinary, team-based care required across the continuum for patients with valvular heart disease. (Used with permission from Perpetua EM. 2019. Program Development and Optimization of Health Services [C/o Empath Health Services]).

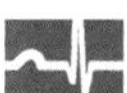 DISPLAY 45-7

Nursing Advocacy and Team Based-Care

In the U.S., Centers for Medicare Services (CMS) may issue a national coverage determination (NCD) for certain medical treatments. An NCD is a form of utilization management and guideline implementation; the document specifies eligibility criteria for hospital provision of services and for CMS payment of services. In cardiology for example there is an NCD for pacemakers, cardiac rehabilitation, and transcatheter aortic valve replacement (TAVR). New evidence from clinical trials, guidelines from professional societies, and changes in "state of the art" practice may prompt Medicare Evidence Development and Coverage Advisory Committee (MEDCAC) review for revision of an outmoded NCD. A MEDCAC panel convenes up to 100 experts across all stakeholders and the public in a formal meeting per the Federal Register. MEDCAC then judges the strength of evidence and makes recommendations to CMS.

In July 2018, a MEDCAC panel convened in Bethesda, MD at the Department of Health and Human Services to review the TAVR NCD. Specifically minimum procedure volume thresholds and their relationship to quality and access to care were discussed. This chapter's author had the opportunity to present during the formal proceedings.

Excerpted from the CMS Medicare Evidence Development Advisory Committee Panel Transcript for Transcatheter Aortic Valve Replacement

July 25, 2018

Dr. Bach: Thank you very much. We have Liz Perpetua, so name, affiliation, disclosures, and 1 min. Thank you.

Ms. Perpetua: Good day. I'm Liz Perpetua. I'm a nurse practitioner and consultant from Seattle, Washington. I have been caring for TAVR patients and coordinating their journey in TAVR for the last 10 yr in community hospitals and academic medical centers alike. My disclosures include consulting fees from Edwards and Abbott for valve disease patient education, and consulting directly with hospitals for structural heart program launch and optimization.

I'd like to speak today to the role of the clinician coordinator in the TAVR program. We often spend the most time with the patient and serve as a "boots-on-the-ground" translator and enforcer of the NCD. We establish and adhere to clinical pathways that ensure NCD compliance, safety, and quality.

So what do minimum volume requirements really mean to patients? Do they really allow for the right care for the right patient in the right place at the right time? Data today have shown us that gains in outcomes are minimal with increased volume requirements and that living better, not longer, is what patients want. They want choice with shared decision-making and care locally. For some, safe care may mean partnership with small and large programs in the spirit of patient-centered systems of care.

It's the patient that absorbs the consequences of failure to meet volume requirements to the NCD. Patients may refuse therapy because of costs and hardship, or they can't incur these things for treatment or travel to another place. Due to delays in care, lack of access to beds, we see clinical decline and death. This is happening now and stands only to get worse with further restriction and an increase in minimal volume requirements. There are also significant implications for patients and programs if the NCD creates two standards of care—one for TAVR and none for SAVR—for a single disease state.

Direct measures of quality are what matter, and assurance of parity, not serendipity in access to quality programs. It's my hope, and the hope of nurses, that the NCD will measure and provide what matters: direct measures of quality and access to patients for a therapy that is already underutilized and sorely needed.

Let the NCD enable, not prohibit, patient-centered care in which the goal is the right care in the right place at the right time, based on direct measures of quality and shared decision making with the patient at the center. Thank you very much.

End of excerpt

LEADERSHIP STYLES

Understanding leadership styles and their characteristics can be useful to the developing cardiac nurse leader.[38] Some styles are more closely coupled with healthcare hierarchy and service.[39] Lewin, one of the earliest theorists, characterized leadership by control over others: *autocratic (authoritative); democratic (participative)*; and *laissez faire (delegative)*.[40] The autocratic style was historically used in the rank and file particularly when trainees (medical interns, new graduates nurses) were involved. This style relies upon increased control over followers and demographic, clinical, and managerial characteristics such as educational degree, years of experience, clinical proficiency, or the number of subordinates, which do not necessarily correlate with leadership effectiveness.[41] The autocratic, transactional, managerial style has made way for participatory and transformational leadership styles.

Leadership theories prominent in health care and particularly in nursing include Greenleaf[42] servant leadership; transformational leadership as coined by Bass[43]; and Kouzes and Posner[39] exemplary leadership theory. Characteristics of servant leaders are well matched to nursing: listening, empathy, healing, awareness, persuasion, conceptualization, foresight, stewardship, commitment to the growth of people, and community building.[42] Transformational leadership qualities appear to be similarly aligned with servant leadership and the nursing profession: emphasizing inherent motivation and positive development of people; appealing to high ideals, promoting cooperation and harmony, using persuasive appeals, providing individual coaching and mentoring, raising awareness of and fostering high moral and ethical standards, using authentic, consistent means (i.e., "walking the talk"), and encouraging others to focus on the common good.[43] Kouzes and Pozner[39] describe also the four strategies of the exemplary, transformational leader: model the way; inspire a shared vision; challenge the process; enable others to act; encourage the heart. The modus operandi of the servant leader is to serve the people before one's self through direct service whereas the transformational leader serves the organization through results. Collectively, the servant leader, transformational leader, and exemplary leader influence through authenticity and service toward a greater good at the level of the individual, community, or organization.

Table 45-5 • TWELVE COMPETENCIES OF EMOTIONAL INTELLIGENCE

Self-Awareness	Self-Management	Social Awareness	Relationship Management
Emotional self-awareness	Emotional self-control Adaptability Achievement orientation Positive outlook	Empathy Organizational awareness	Influence Coach and mentor Conflict management Teamwork Inspirational leadership

Adapted from Goleman D, Boyatzis A. Emotional intelligence has 12 elements. Which do you need to work on? *Harv Bus Rev.* 2017. https://hbr.org/2017/02/emotional-intelligence-has-12-elements-which-do-you-need-to-work-on

SKILL SETS FOR LEADERSHIP AND TEAM-BASED CARE

There are many theory-based, educational, and certification programs in health care and nursing leadership. Selected resources applicable to nursing and health care are listed here and are strongly recommended for further reading. Expanded review follows for some of these theories and frameworks.

- Emotional Intelligence (Goleman)[5,44]
- Dare to Lead (Brown)[4]
- Managing Change (Kotter)[45]
- Dysfunctions of a Team (Lencioni)[46]
- Principles for Effective Teams (Institute of Medicine)[47]
- Team Strategies to Enhance Performance and Patient Safety (Team STEPPS, Agency for Healthcare Quality and Research)[48]

Emotional Intelligence

At the core of leadership are skill sets that produce results. Goleman et al.[5,44] revealed that it is emotional intelligence—*self-awareness, self-regulation, or the managing of one's self,*[49] *social awareness,* and *relationship management*—and 12 competencies that made the most positive impact on a leader's results (Table 45-5).[50] Six leadership styles (Table 45-6) and their characteristics emerged from their research. Autocratic styles, classified as commanding or pacesetting, was found to negatively impact organizations. The democratic or delegative styles, characterized as democratic, affiliative, coaching, and visionary, were found to positively impact organizations. In health care and especially at more senior levels with physicians, commanding or pacesetting styles may be used more frequently than anticipated.[51] Women have been found to have a greater preference for more effective, relational styles such as coaching, affiliative, and visionary leadership.[51] Of note, all styles may be utilized by an individual leader, depending on the needs and situation. Emotional intelligence is now widely adopted as critical for effective leadership development and recognized as the skill set that gets results.[51]

Dare to Lead

Current research increasingly supports leadership as a constellation of teachable, measurable competencies and skill sets with emotional intelligence at the forefront. Brown, recognized for research in vulnerability and daring leadership,[4] proposed four skill sets in the Dare to Lead certification training:

- Living values: Leadership requires self-awareness and self-regulation, for which core values serve to anchor the leader.
- Braving trust: Leadership requires psychological safety, or a "safe container," which is promoted by clear roles and shared goals, as well as congruence with values and actions.
- Rumble with vulnerability: Leadership requires the ability to communicate effectively, resolve conflict and manage change.
- Learning to rise: Leadership requires resilience and the ability to self-regulate, lean into values, rumble with vulnerability and brave trust in order to try again despite failure or imperfection.

Theory and skills from social work, technology innovation, health care and business include many common themes for effective leadership and teams. The five operating tenets that repeatedly arise are

Table 45-6 • LEADERSHIP STYLES

Leadership Styles	Modus Operandi	Style in a Phrase	Emotional Intelligence Traits	When to Use the Style	Overall Impact
Visionary	Mobilize people toward vision	"Come with me"	Self-confidence, empathy, change catalyst	To bring a clear direction or when changes require a new vision	Most strongly positive
Coaching	Develops people for the future	"Try this"	Developing others, empathy, self-awareness	To help an employee improve performance or develop long-term strengths	Positive
Affiliative	Creates harmony and builds emotional bonds	"People come first"	Empathy, building relationships, communication	To heal rifts in a team or to motivate people during stressful circumstances	Positive
Democratic	Cultivates consensus through participation	"What do you think?"	Collaboration, team leadership, communication	To build buy-in or consensus, or to get input from valuable employees	Positive
Pacesetting	Sets high standards for performance	"Do as I do, now"	Conscientiousness, drive to achieve, initiative	To get quick results from a highly motivated and competent team	Negative
Commanding	Demands immediate compliance	"Do what I tell you"	Drive to achieve, initiative, self-control	In a crisis, to kick start a turnaround or with problem employees	Negative

Adapted from Goleman D. Leadership that gets results. *Harv Bus Rev.* 2000;78(2):78–90.

Principle	Definition	Impact on Clinician Well-Being
Shared Goals	The team establishes shared goals that can be clearly articulated, understood, and supported by all members [a]	
Clear Roles	Clear expectations for each team member's functions, responsibilities, and accountabilities to optimize team efficiency and effectiveness [a]	Role clarity has been associated with improved clinician well-being [b] A fully staffed team that is not over patient capacity is associated with decreased burnout [c]
Mutual Trust (psychological safety)	Team members trust one another and feel safe enough within the team to admit a mistake, ask a question, offer new data, or try a new skill without fear of embarrassment or punishment [a]	A strong team climate promotes clinician well-being and member retention [d,e]
Effective Communication	The team prioritizes and continuously refines its communications skills and has consistent channels for efficient, bidirectional communication [a]	Effective communication is associated with decreased clinician burnout [f] Participatory decision making is associated with lower burnout scores [g]
Measurable Processes and Outcomes	Reliable and ongoing assessment of team structure, function, and performance that is provided as actionable feedback to all team members to improve performance [a]	Emotional exhaustion is associated with low personal accomplishment, so reiteration of accomplishments could decrease burnout [h]

Figure 45-4. Principles of effective team-based care: definitions and impact on clinician well-being. Notes: [a] Mitchell P, Wynia R, Golden B, et al; Institute of Medicine. *Core Principles and Values of Effective Team-Based Health Care*. Discussion Paper. Washington, DC; 2012; [b] So TTC, West MA, Dawson JF. Team-based working and employee well-being: A crosscultural comparison of United Kingdom and Hong Kong health services. *Eur J Work Organ Psychol.* 2011;20(3):305–325; [c] Brunetto Y, Wharton RF, Shacklock K. Supervisor-nurse relationships, teamwork, role ambiguity and wellbeing: Public versus private sector nurses. *Asia Pac J Hum Resour.* 2011;49(2):143–164; [d] Cheng C, Bartram T, Karimi L, et al. The role of team climate in the management of emotional labour: Implications for nurse retention. *J Adv Nurs.* 2013;69(12):2812–2825; [e] Estryn-Béhar M, Van der Heijden BI, Oginska H, et al; NEXT Study Group. The impact of social work environment, teamwork characteristics, burnout, and personal factors upon intent to leave among European nurses. *Med Care.* 2007;45:939–950; [f] Bodenheimer T, Willard-Grace R. Teamlets in primary care: Enhancing the patient and clinician experience. *J Am Board Fam Med.* 2016;29(1):135–138; [g] Helfrich CD, Dolan ED, Simonetti J, et al. Elements of team-based care in a patient-centered medical home are associated with lower burnout among VA primary care employees. *J Gen Intern Med.* 2014;29(Suppl 2):S659–S666; [h] Catt S, Fallowfield L, Jenkins V, et al. The informational roles and psychological health of members of 10 oncology multidisciplinary teams in the UK. *Br J Cancer.* 2005;93(10):1092–1097. (Used with permission from Smith CD, Balatbat C, Corbridge S, et al. Implementing optimal team-based care to reduce clinician burnout. In: *NAM Perspectives*. Washington, DC: Discussion Paper, National Academy of Medicine; 2018. doi: 10.31478/201809c.)

Table 45-7 • SYNTHESIZING PRINCIPLES AND SKILL SETS IN LEADERSHIP AND TEAM-BASED CARE

	Lencioni	**Institute of Medicine**	**Google**	**Brown**
Principle and Skill Set	**5 Dysfunctions of a Team**	**5 Principles of Effective Teams**	**5 Dynamics of Productive Teams**	**4 Skillsets of Daring Leadership**
Trust	Absence of trust	Mutual trust	Psychological safety	Braving trust
Communication	Fear of conflict	Effective communication	Clarity	Rumbling with vulnerability
Roles and Structure	Fear of commitment	Clear roles	Structure	Living into our values
Goals and Accountability	Avoidance of accountability	Shared goals	Meaning and dependability	
Process, Results, and Outcomes	Inattention to results	Measurable processes and outcomes	Impact	Learning to rise

shared goals, clear roles, mutual trust, effective communication, and measurable processes and outcomes. These tenets are echoed by the Institute of Medicine's Principles of Effective Team-Based Care,[12] depicted in Figure 45-4. While a full review is outside of the scope of this chapter, it is strongly encouraged that cardiac nurses seeking leadership knowledge and skills familiarize themselves with these resources and their availability in their organization.

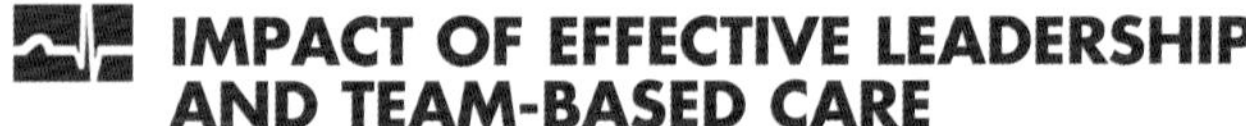

IMPACT OF EFFECTIVE LEADERSHIP AND TEAM-BASED CARE

Effective leadership and team-based care has been shown to deeply and broadly improve processes and outcomes. An important systematic review included 21 studies of which 57% identified a

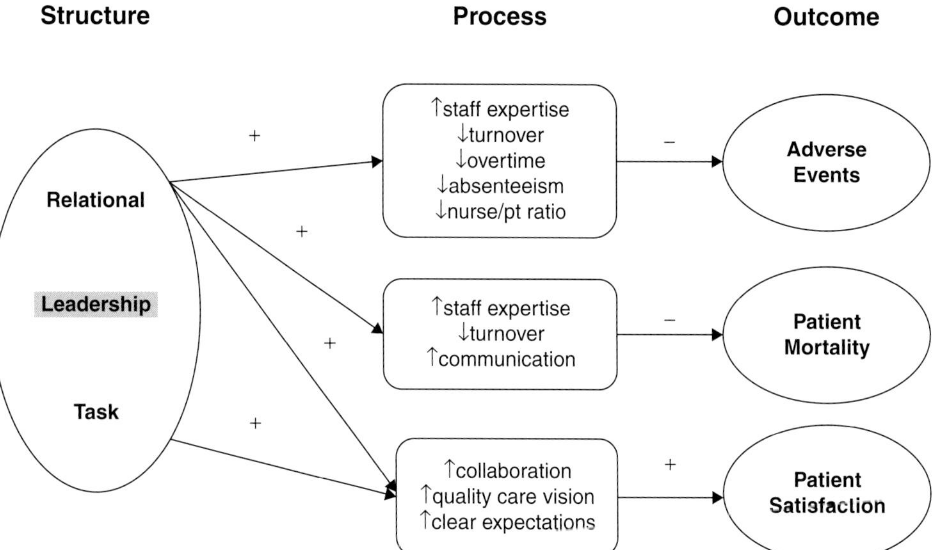

Figure 45-5. Impact of nursing leadership on processes and outcomes. (Used with permission from Wong CA, Cummings GG, Ducharme L. The relationship between nursing leadership and patient outcomes: a systematic review update. *J Nurs Manag.* 2013;21:709–724; creative common license 4.0.)

statistically significant improvement in patient satisfaction and improvement in at least one of the specified patient outcomes.[8] In another systematic review specific to nursing leadership, Wong et al. found that a relational-based leadership style was highly associated with positive impacts on processes including increased staff expertise and lower turnover, overtime, absenteeism, as well as a lower nurse to patient ratio which was in turn associated with a lower rate of adverse events. Similarly, increased staff expertise also resulted in decreased turnover and increased communication which decreased patient mortality. The relational leader involved in work resulted in increased collaboration, increased clarity in expectations, vision, and quality of care, and overall increased patient satisfaction. These impacts are depicted in Figure 45-5. The principles and skill sets of effective leadership and team-based care are summarized in Table 45-7.

CALL TO ACTION

Leadership knowledge and skills are not born; these are teachable and to be acquired, practiced. Opportunities abound. A leadership plan using SMART goals (specific, measurable, actionable, realistic and time based, ideally tied to core values) is a critical tool for intentionally developing and practicing leadership skills.

Self-awareness is first; there are many psychometric assessments available including the Myers Briggs Trait Inventory; Big 5 OCEAN evaluation; VIA strengths assessment; Gallup Strength Finders assessment; Hogan assessment; emotional intelligence evaluations; growth or fixed mindset testing; and conflict competence assessments. An employer may provide some of these assessments at reduced or nominal costs or offer continuing education funds; many courses offer continuing education credits that may be applied to license or certification renewals.

Next is intentional investment in one's self. There are certainly formal avenues such as educational and certification programs, as well as professional development in societies or other organizations. Consider pursue mentorship or coaching. Participate on committees. Join practice councils or launch journal clubs. Find someone who is doing what you want to be doing; ask questions, make connections. Every moment and conversation is an opportunity to show up as a leader. Pursue creative and novel paths for public speaking, scholarly writing or peer review, teaching and inservicing, participating in research, policy, digital innovation, or entrepreneurship. Do this within the field of nursing, specialty of cardiac nursing, and in multidisciplinary arenas that include physicians, administrators, and other agents of influence and change. Emotional intelligence, social intelligence, and relationship management are underpinnings for all interactions and goals on a leadership plan.

Professional development as a cardiac nurse, and as a leader, is personal. What is meaningful to you? What are your core values and what does living these values look and feel like to you? Are you listening to your own voice? How will you use your voice in service of what is important to you? What is your capacity to do this, given the quality of your health and your relationships? Leadership begins by leading one's self, and, for many nurses who have put service *before* self, bridging the gap between self-care *and* service of others. Let us care for ourselves and for others, use our voices, and listen as we wish to be heard. The call to action for nurse leaders begins with acknowledging ourselves and each other as individuals—our similarities, differences, and unique contributions. We are stronger together, rising the tide by empowering one another and our profession as a whole.

KEY READINGS

Brown B. *Dare to Lead: Brave Work, Tough Conversations, Whole Hearts.* New York, NY: Random House; 2018. (Please note that there is an online workbook available in PDF that includes core values exercises and more.)

Buresh B, Gordon S. *From Silence to Voice: What Nurses Know and Must Communicate to the Public.* 3rd ed. Ithaca, NY: Cornell University Press; 2013.

Goleman D. Leadership that gets results. *Harvard Business Review.* 2000;78(2):78–90.

Institute of Medicine. *Future of Nursing: Leading Change, Advancing Health.* Washington, DC: National Academies Press; 2011.

REFERENCES

1. Institute of Medicine. *Future of Nursing: Leading Change, Advancing Health*. Washington, DC: National Academies Press; 2011.
2. American Nurses Association. ANA Leadership Institute Competency Model. 2018, July. https://www.nursingworld.org/~4a0a2e/globalassets/docs/ce/177626-ana-leadership-booklet-new-final.pdf.
3. Dwyer CA. The Future of Assessment: Shaping Teaching and Learning. 2008. New York: Lawrence Erlbaum Associates.
4. Brown B. *Dare to Lead: Brave Work, Tough Conversations, Whole Hearts*. New York, NY: Random House; 2018.
5. Goleman D. Leadership that gets results. *Harv Bus Rev*. 2000;78(2):78–90.
6. Hughes V. Standout nurse leaders…What's in the research? *Nurs Manag*. 2017;48(9):16–24.
7. Wong CA, Cummings GG, Ducharme L. The relationship between nursing leadership and patient outcomes: a systematic review update. *J Nurs Manag*. 2013;21(5):709–724.
8. Will KK, Johnson ML, Lamb G. Team-based care and patient satisfaction in the hospital setting: a systematic review. *J Patient Cent Res Rev*. 2019;6(2):158–171.
9. Aiken LH, Clarke SP, Sloane DM, et al. Hospital nurse staffing and patient mortality, nurse burnout, and job dissatisfaction. *JAMA*. 2002;288(16):1987–1993.
10. Aiken LH, Sloane DM, Bruyneel L, et al. Nurse staffing and education and hospital mortality in nine European countries: a retrospective observational study. *Lancet*. 2014;383(9931):1824–1830.
11. Allen JK, Dennison Himmelfarb CR, Szanton SL, et al. Cost-effectiveness of nurse practitioner/community health worker care to reduce cardiovascular health disparities. *J Cardiovasc Nurs*. 2014;29(4):308–314.
12. Mitchell P, Wynia R, Golden B, et al; Institute of Medicine. *Core principles and values of effective team-based health care*. Washington, DC: National Academies Press; 2012.
13. Robert Wood Johnson Foundation. Nursing leadership from bedside to boardroom: Opinion leaders' perceptions. 2010.
14. Buresh B, Gordon S. *From Silence to Voice. What Nurses Know and Must Communicate to the Public*. 3rd ed. Cornell University Press; 2013.
15. Reinhart R. Gallup survey: nurses continue to rate highest in honesty, ethics. 2019. https://news.gallup.com/poll/274673/nurses-continue-rate-highest-honesty-ethics.aspx. June 8, 2020.
16. Roberts SJ. Oppressed group behavior: implications for nursing. *ANS Adv Nurs Sci*. 1983;5(4):21–30.
17. Stein LI. The doctor-nurse game. *Arch Gen Psychiatry*. 1967;16(6):699–703.
18. Welton JM, Harris K. Hospital billing and reimbursement: charging for inpatient nursing care. *J Nurs Adm*. 2007;37(4):164–166.
19. Lanuza DM, Davidson PM, Dunbar SB, et al. Preparing nurses for leadership roles in cardiovascular disease prevention. *Eur J Cardiovasc Nurs*. 2011;10(2_suppl):S51–S57.
20. Hisel ME. Measuring work engagement in a multigenerational nursing workforce. *J Nurs Manag*. 2020;28(2):294–305.
21. Waljee JF, Chopra V, Saint S. Mentoring millennials. *JAMA*. 2018;319(15):1547–1548.
22. American Organization of Nurse Executives. *AONE Nurse Manager Competencies*. Chicago, IL: AONE; 2015. http://www.aone.org/resources/nurse-leader-competencies.shtml.
23. Khoury CM, Blizzard R, Wright Moore L, et al. Nursing leadership from bedside to boardroom: a Gallup national survey of opinion leaders. *J Nurs Adm*. 2011;41(7–8):299–305.
24. Heinen M, van Oostveen C, Peters J, et al. An integrative review of leadership competencies and attributes in advanced nursing practice. *J Adv Nurs*. 2019;75(11):2378–2392.
25. Lamb A, Martin-Misener R, Bryant-Lukosius D, et al. Describing the leadership capabilities of advanced practice nurses using a qualitative descriptive study. *Nurs Open*. 2018;5(3):400–413.
26. Watson C. Assessing leadership in nurse practitioner candidates. *Aust J Adv Nurs*. 2008;26(1):67–76.
27. Coylewright M, Mack MJ, Holmes JDR, et al. A call for an evidence-based approach to the heart team for patients with severe aortic stenosis. *J Am Coll Cardiol*. 2015;65(14):1472–1480.
28. Crespo-Leiro MG, Metra M, Lund LH, et al. Advanced heart failure: a position statement of the Heart Failure Association of the European Society of Cardiology. *Eur J Heart Fail*. 2018;20(11):1505–1535.
29. Creaser JW, Rourke D, Vandenbogaart E, et al. Outcomes of biventricular mechanical support patients discharged to home to await heart transplantation. *J Cardiovasc Nurs*. 2015;30(4):E13–E20.
30. Alkhouli M, Graff-Radford J, Holmes DR. The heart-brain team—towards optimal team-based coordinated care. *JAMA Cardiol*. 2018;3(3):187–188.
31. Sillman C, Morin J, Thomet C, et al. Adult congenital heart disease nurse coordination: essential skills and role in optimizing team-based care a position statement from the International Society for Adult Congenital Heart Disease (ISACHD). *Int J Cardiol*. 2017;229:125–131.
32. Perpetua EM, Clarke SE, Guibone KA, et al. Surveying the landscape of structural heart disease coordination: an exploratory study of the coordinator role. *Structural Heart*. 2019;3(3):201–210.
33. Otto CM, Kumbhani DJ, Alexander KP, et al. 2017 ACC expert consensus decision pathway for transcatheter aortic valve replacement in the management of adults with aortic stenosis. A Report of the American College of Cardiology Task Force on Clinical Expert Consensus Documents. *J Am Coll Cardiol*. 2017;69(10):1313–1346.
34. Zhu Z, Islam S, Bergmann SR. Effectiveness and outcomes of a nurse practitioner-run chest pain evaluation unit. *J Am Assoc Nurs Pract*. 2016;28(11):591–595.
35. Brush JE, Handberg EM, Biga C, et al. 2015 ACC health policy statement on cardiovascular team-based care and the role of advanced practice providers. *J Am Coll Cardiol*. 2015;65(19):2118–2136.
36. Centers for Medicare and Medicaid Services. National Coverage Determination for Transcatheter Aortic Valve Replacement. 2019. https://www.cms.gov/medicare-coverage-database/details/nca-decision-memo.aspx?NCAId = 293. Accessed March 31, 2017.
37. Centers for Medicare and Medicaid Services. National coverage determination decision memo for percutaneous left atrial appendage closure therapy. 2015.
38. Marshall E, Broome M. *Transformational Leadership in Nursing*. 2nd ed. New York, NY: Springer; 2016.
39. Kouzes J, Pozner B. *The Leadership Challenge: How to Make Extraordinary Things Happen in Organizations*. San Francisco, CA: Jossey-Bass; 2012.
40. Lewin K. *Resolving Social Conflicts; Selected Papers on Group Dynamics*. Oxford, England: Harper; 1948.
41. Fujino Y, Tanaka M, Yonemitsu Y, et al. The relationship between characteristics of nursing performance and years of experience in nurses with high emotional intelligence. *Int J Nurs Pract*. 2015;21(6):876–881.
42. Greenleaf RK. *Servant Leadership: A Journey Into the Nature of Legitimate Power and Greatness*. New York: Paulist Press; 1977.
43. Bass B. From transactional to transformational leadership: learning to share the vision. *Org Dyn*. 1990;18(3):19–31.
44. Goleman D. What makes a leader. *Harv Bus Rev*. 1998;76(6):93–102.
45. Kotter JP. What leaders really do. *Harv Bus Rev*. 1990;68(3):103–111.
46. Lencioni PM, Okabayashi K. *The Five Dysfunctions of a Team. 123Library*. 1st ed. San Francisco, CA: Jossey-Bass; 2012.
47. Edmondson AC, Lei Z. Psychological safety: the history, renaissance, and future of an interpersonal construct. *Ann Rev Org Psychol Org Behav*. 2014;1(1):23–43.
48. Quality AfH. Team STEPPS 2.0 Fundamentals. 2019. https://www.ahrq.gov/teamstepps/instructor/fundamentals/index.html. June 8, 2020.
49. Drucker PF. Managing oneself. *Harv Bus Rev*. 1999;77:64.
50. Goleman D, Boyatzis A. Emotional intelligence has 12 elements. Which do you need to work on? *Harv Bus Rev*. 2017. https://hbr.org/2017/02/emotional-intelligence-has-12-elements-which-do-you-need-to-work-on
51. Saxena A, Desanghere L, Stobart K, et al. Goleman's leadership styles at different hierarchical levels in medical education. *BMC Med Educ*. 2017;17(1):169.

INDEX

Note: Page numbers followed by *f* indicate figures, *t* tables, *d* display.

B

C

D

E

I

T

U

V

W

X

Y

Z

CCS1020